OPTUM360°®

EXPERT

Current Procedural Coding Expert

CPT® codes with Medicare essentials for enhanced accuracy

2022

optum360coding.com

Notice

The *2022 Current Procedural Coding Expert* is designed to be an accurate and authoritative source of information about the CPT® coding system. Every effort has been made to verify the accuracy of the listings, and all information is believed reliable at the time of publication. Absolute accuracy cannot be guaranteed, however. This publication is made available with the understanding that the publisher is not engaged in rendering legal or other services that require a professional license.

American Medical Association Notice

Fee schedules, relative value units, conversion factors and/or related components are not assigned by the AMA, are not part of CPT, and the AMA is not recommending their use. The AMA does not directly or indirectly practice medicine or dispense medical services. The AMA assumes no liability for data contained or not contained herein.

CPT is a registered trademark of the American Medical Association.

Our Commitment to Accuracy

Optum360 is committed to producing accurate and reliable materials.

To report corrections, please email accuracy@optum.com. You can also reach customer service by calling 1.800.464.3649, option 1.

Copyright

Made in the USA

ISBN 978-1-62254-744-9

Acknowledgments

Gregory A. Kemp, MA, *Product Manager*
Stacy Perry, *Manager, Desktop Publishing*
Elizabeth Leibold, RHIT, *Subject Matter Expert*
Anita Schmidt, BS, RHIA, AHIMA-approved ICD-10-CM/PCS Trainer, *Subject Matter Expert*
LaJuana Green, RHIA, CCS, *Subject Matter Expert*
Tracy Betzler, *Senior Desktop Publishing Specialist*
Hope M. Dunn, *Senior Desktop Publishing Specialist*
Katie Russell, *Desktop Publishing Specialist*
Kate Holden, *Editor*

About the Contributors

Elizabeth Leibold, RHIT

Ms. Leibold has more than 25 years of experience in the health care profession. She has served in a variety of roles, ranging from patient registration to billing and collections, and has an extensive background in both physician and hospital outpatient coding and compliance. She has worked for large health care systems and health information management services companies, and has wide-ranging experience in facility and professional component coding, along with CPT expertise in interventional procedures, infusion services, emergency department, observation, and ambulatory surgery coding. Her areas of expertise include chart-to-claim coding audits and providing staff education to both tenured and new coding staff. She is an active member of the American Health Information Management Association (AHIMA) and West Tennessee Health Information Management Association (WTHIMA).

Anita Schmidt, BS, RHIA, AHIMA-approved ICD-10-CM/PCS Trainer

Ms. Schmidt has expertise in ICD-10-CM/PCS, DRG, and CPT with more than 15 years' experience in coding in multiple settings, including inpatient, observation, and same-day surgery. Her experience includes analysis of medical record documentation, assignment of ICD-10-CM and PCS codes, and DRG validation. She has conducted training for ICD-10-CM/PCS and electronic health record. She has also collaborated with clinical documentation specialists to identify documentation needs and potential areas for physician education. Most recently she has been developing content for resource and educational products related to ICD-10-CM, ICD-10-PCS, DRG, and CPT. Ms. Schmidt is an AHIMA-approved ICD-10-CM/PCS trainer and is an active member of the American Health Information Management Association (AHIMA) and the Minnesota Health Information Management Association.

LaJuana Green, RHIA, CCS

Ms. Green is a Registered Health Information Administrator with over 35 years of experience in multiple areas of information management. She has proven expertise in the analysis of medical record documentation, assignment of ICD-10-CM and PCS codes, DRG validation, and CPT code assignment in ambulatory surgery units and the hospital outpatient setting. Her experience includes serving as a director of a health information management department, clinical technical editing, new technology research and writing, medical record management, utilization review activities, quality assurance, tumor registry, medical library services, and chargemaster maintenance. Ms. Green is an active member of the American Health Information Management Association (AHIMA).

Contents

Introduction

Welcome to Optum360's *Current Procedural Coding Expert*, an exciting Medicare coding and reimbursement tool and definitive procedure coding source that combines the work of the Centers for Medicare and Medicaid Services (CMS), American Medical Association (AMA), and Optum360 experts with the technical components you need for proper reimbursement and coding accuracy. Handy snap in tabs are included to indicate those sections used most often for easy reference.

This approach to CPT® Medicare coding utilizes innovative and intuitive ways of communicating the information you need to code claims accurately and efficiently. *Includes* and *Excludes* notes, similar to those found in the ICD-10-CM manual, help determine what services are related to the codes you are reporting. Icons help you crosswalk the code you are reporting to laboratory and radiology procedures necessary for proper reimbursement. CMS-mandated icons and relative value units (RVUs) help you determine which codes are most appropriate for the service you are reporting. Add to that additional information identifying age and sex edits, ambulatory surgery center (ASC) and ambulatory payment classification (APC) indicators, and Medicare coverage and payment rule citations, and *Current Procedural Coding Expert* provides the best in Medicare procedure reporting.

Current Procedural Coding Expert includes the information needed to submit claims to federal contractors and most commercial payers, and is correct at the time of printing. However, CMS, federal contractors, and commercial payers may change payment rules at any time throughout the year. *Current Procedural Coding Expert* includes effective codes that will not be published in the AMA's Current Procedural Terminology (CPT) book until the following year. Commercial payers will announce changes through monthly news or information posted on their websites. CMS will post changes in policy on its website at http://www.cms.gov/transmittals. National and local coverage determinations (NCDs and LCDs) provide universal and individual contractor guidelines for specific services. The existence of a procedure code does not imply coverage under any given insurance plan.

Current Procedural Coding Expert is based on the AMA's Current Procedural Terminology coding system, which is copyrighted and owned by the physician organization. The CPT codes are the nation's official, Health Information Portability and Accountability Act (HIPAA) compliant code set for procedures and services provided by physicians, ambulatory surgery centers (ASCs), and hospital outpatient services, as well as laboratories, imaging centers, physical therapy clinics, urgent care centers, and others.

Getting Started with *Current Procedural Coding Expert*

Current Procedural Coding Expert is an exciting tool combining the most current material at the time of our publication from the AMA's CPT 2022, CMS's online manual system, the Correct Coding initiative, CMS fee schedules, official Medicare guidelines for reimbursement and coverage, the Integrated Outpatient Code Editor (I/OCE), and Optum360's own coding expertise.

These coding rules and guidelines are incorporated into more specific section notes and code notes. Section notes are listed under a range of codes and apply to all codes in that range. Code notes are found under individual codes and apply to the single code.

Material is presented in a logical fashion for those billing Medicare, Medicaid, and many private payers. The format, based on customer comments, better addresses what customers tell us they need in a comprehensive Medicare procedure coding guide.

Designed to be easy to use and full of information, this product is an excellent companion to your AMA CPT manual, and other Optum360 and Medicare resources.

In anticipation of severe acute respiratory syndrome coronavirus 2 (SARS-CoV-2) (COVID-19) vaccines receiving Emergency Use Authorization (EUA) and/or FDA approval, and in order to expedite the availability of codes for coding and reimbursement, the AMA released a set of codes (0001A–0104A, 91300–91310) to be utilized upon receipt of EUA or FDA approval. In *Current Procedural Coding Expert*, these codes have been designated as placeholders and **PLACEHOLDER ONLY** appears next to the code. When the AMA releases an official code descriptor, Optum360 will update the corresponding electronic files and will provide updates to customers to allow them to update their *Current Procedural Coding Expert* book.

For mid-year code updates, official errata changes, correction notices, and any other changes pertinent to the information in *Current Procedural Coding Expert*, see our product update page at https://www.optum360coding.com/ProductUpdates/. The password for 2022 is PROCEDURE2022.

Note: The AMA releases code changes quarterly as well as errata or corrections to CPT codes and guidelines and posts them on their website. Some of these changes may not appear in the AMA's CPT book until the following year. *Current Procedural Coding Expert* incorporates the most recent errata or release notes found on the AMA's website at our publication time, including new, revised and deleted codes. *Current Procedural Coding Expert* identifies these new or revised codes from the AMA website errata or release notes with an icon similar to the AMA's current new ● and revised ▲ icons. For purposes of this publication, new CPT codes and revisions that won't be in the AMA book until the next edition are indicated with a ● and a ▲ icon. CPT codes that are new or revised during 2021 but do not appear in the AMA's CPT code book until 2023 are identified in appendix B as "Web Release New, Revised, and Deleted Codes." For the next year's edition of *Current Procedural Coding Expert*, these codes will appear with standard black new or revised icons, as appropriate, to correspond with those changes as indicated in the AMA's CPT book.

General Conventions

Many of the sources of information in this book can be determined by color.

- All CPT codes and descriptions and the Evaluation and Management guidelines from the American Medical Association are in **black text**.
- Includes, Excludes, and other notes appear in **blue text**. The resources used for this information are a variety of Medicare policy manuals, the *National Correct Coding Initiative Policy Manual* (NCCI), AMA resources and guidelines, and specialty association resources and our Optum360 clinical experts.

Resequencing of CPT Codes

The American Medical Association (AMA) employs a numbering methodology of resequencing, which is the practice of displaying codes outside of their numerical order according to the description relationship. According to the AMA, there are instances in which a new code is needed within an existing grouping of codes, but an unused code number is not available. In these situations, the AMA will resequence the codes. In other words, it will assign a code that is not in numeric sequence with the related codes.

An example of resequencing from *Current Procedural Coding Expert* follows:

	21555	**Excision, tumor, soft tissue of neck or anterior thorax, subcutaneous; less than 3 cm**
#	21552	**3 cm or greater**
	21556	**Excision, tumor, soft tissue of neck or anterior thorax, subfascial (eg, intramuscular); less than 5 cm**
#	21554	**5 cm or greater**

In *Current Procedural Coding Expert* the resequenced codes are listed twice. They appear in their resequenced position as shown above as well as in their original numeric position with a note indicating that the code is out of numerical sequence and where it can be found. (See example below.)

21554 **Resequenced code. See code following 21556.**

This differs from the AMA CPT book, in which the coder is directed to a code range that contains the resequenced code and description, rather than to a specific location.

Resequenced codes will appear in brackets in the headers, section notes, and code ranges. For example:

27327-27339 [27337, 27339] Excision Soft Tissue Tumors Femur/Knee. Codes [27337, 27339] are included in section 27327-27339 in their resequenced positions.

Code also toxoid/vaccine (90476-90749 [90619, 90620, 90621, 90625, 90630, 90644, 90672, 90673, 90674, 90750, 90756])

This shows codes 90619, 90620, 90621, 90625, 90630, 90644, 90672, 90673, 90674, 90750, and 90756 are resequenced in this range of codes.

Code Ranges for Medicare Billing

Appendix E identifies all resequenced CPT codes. Optum360 will display the resequenced coding as assigned by the AMA in its CPT products so that the user may understand the code description relationships.

Each particular group of CPT codes in *Current Procedural Coding Expert* is organized in a more intuitive fashion for Medicare billing, being grouped by the Medicare rules and regulations as found in the official CMS online manuals that govern payment of these particular procedures and services, as in this example:

99221-99233 Inpatient Hospital Visits: Initial and Subsequent

CMS: 100-4,11,40.1.3 Independent Attending Physician Services; 100-4,12,30.6.10 Consultation Services; 100-4,12,30.6.15.1 Prolonged Services With Direct Face-to-Face Patient Contact; 100-4,12,30.6.4 Services Furnished Incident to Physician's Service; 100-4,12,30.6.9 Hospital Visit and Critical Care on Same Day

Icons

● **New Codes**
Codes that have been added since the last edition of the AMA CPT book was printed.

▲ **Revised Codes**
Codes that have been revised since the last edition of the AMA CPT book was printed.

● **New Web Release**
Codes that are new for the current year but will not be in the AMA CPT book until 2023.

▲ **Revised Web Release**
Codes that have been revised for the current year, but will not be in the AMA CPT book until 2023.

Resequenced Codes
Codes that are out of numeric order but apply to the appropriate category.

★ **Telemedicine Services**
Codes that may be reported for telemedicine services. Modifier 95 must be appended to code.

❍ **Reinstated Code**
Codes that have been reinstated since the last edition of the book was printed.

Pink Color Bar—Not Covered by Medicare
Services and procedures identified by this color bar are never covered benefits under Medicare. Services and procedures that are not covered may be billed directly to the patient at the time of the service.

Gray Color Bar—Unlisted Procedure
Unlisted CPT codes report procedures that have not been assigned a specific code number. An unlisted code delays payment due to the extra time necessary for review.

Green Color Bar—Resequenced Codes
Resequenced codes are codes that are out of numeric sequence—they are indicated with a green color bar. They are listed twice, in their resequenced position as well as in their original numeric position with a note that the code is out of numerical sequence and where the resequenced code and description can be found.

INCLUDES **Includes notes**
Includes notes identify procedures and services that would be bundled in the procedure code. These are derived from AMA, CMS, NCCI, and Optum360 coding guidelines. This is not meant to be an all-inclusive list.

EXCLUDES **Excludes notes**
Excludes notes may lead the user to other codes. They may identify services that are not bundled and may be separately reported, OR may lead the user to another more appropriate code. These are derived from AMA, CMS, NCCI, and Optum360 coding guidelines. This is not meant to be an all-inclusive list.

Code Also This note identifies an additional code that should be reported with the service and may relate to another CPT code or an appropriate HCPCS code(s) that should be reported along with the CPT code when appropriate.

Code First Found under add-on codes, this note identifies codes for primary procedures that should be reported first, with the add-on code reported as a secondary code.

Laboratory/Pathology Crosswalk
This icon denotes CPT codes in the laboratory and pathology section of CPT that may be reported separately with the primary CPT code.

Radiology Crosswalk
This icon denotes codes in the radiology section that may be used with the primary CPT code being reported.

TC **Technical Component Only**
Codes with this icon represent only the technical component (staff and equipment costs) of a procedure or service. Do not use either modifier 26 (professional component) or TC (technical component) with these codes.

26 **Professional Component**
Only codes with this icon represent the physician's work or professional component of a procedure or service. Do not use either modifier 26 (professional component) or TC (technical component) with these codes.

50 **Bilateral Procedure**
This icon identifies codes that can be reported bilaterally when the same surgeon provides the service for the same patient on the same date. Medicare allows payment for both procedures at 150 percent of the usual amount for one procedure. The modifier does not apply to bilateral procedures inclusive to one code.

80 **Assist-at-Surgery Allowed**
Services noted by this icon are allowed an assistant at surgery with a Medicare payment equal to 16 percent of the allowed amount for the global surgery for that procedure. No documentation is required.

80 **Assist-at-Surgery Allowed with Documentation**
Services noted by this icon are allowed an assistant at surgery with a Medicare payment equal to 16 percent of the allowed amount for the global surgery for that procedure. Documentation is required.

+ **Add-on Codes**
This icon identifies procedures reported in addition to the primary procedure. The icon "+" denotes add-on codes. An add-on code is neither a stand-alone code nor subject to multiple procedure rules since it describes work in addition to the primary procedure.

According to Medicare guidelines, add-on codes may be identified in the following ways:

- The code is found on Change Request (CR) 7501 or successive CRs as a Type I, Type II, or Type III add-on code.
- The add-on code most often has a global period of "ZZZ" in the Medicare Physician Fee Schedule Database.
- The code is found in the CPT book with the icon "+" appended. Add-on code descriptors typically include the phrases "each additional" or "(List separately in addition to primary procedure)."

(50) **Optum Modifier 50 Exempt**
Codes identified by this icon indicate that the procedure should not be reported with modifier 50 (Bilateral procedures).

⊘ **Modifier 51 Exempt**
Codes identified by this icon indicate that the procedure should not be reported with modifier 51 (Multiple procedures).

(51) **Optum Modifier 51 Exempt**
Codes identified by this Optum360 icon indicate that the procedure should not be reported with modifier 51 (Multiple procedures). Any code with this icon is backed by official AMA guidelines but was not identified by the AMA with their modifier 51 exempt icon.

Correct Coding Initiative (CCI)
Current Procedural Coding Expert identifies those codes with corresponding CCI edits. The CCI edits define correct coding practices that serve as the basis of the national Medicare policy for paying claims. The code noted is the major service/procedure. The code may represent a column 1 code within the column 1/column 2 correct coding edits table or a code pair that is mutually exclusive of each other.

CLIA Waived Test
This symbol is used to distinguish those laboratory tests that can be performed using test systems that are waived from regulatory oversight established by the Clinical Laboratory Improvement Amendments of 1988 (CLIA). The applicable CPT code for a CLIA waived test may be reported by providers who perform the testing but do not hold a CLIA license.

(63) **Modifier 63 Exempt**
This icon identifies procedures performed on infants that weigh less than 4 kg. Due to the complexity of performing procedures on infants less than 4 kg, modifier 63 may be added to the surgery codes to inform the payers of the special circumstances involved.

A2–Z3 **ASC Payment Indicators**
This icon identifies ASC status payment indicators. They indicate how the ASC payment rate was derived and/or how the procedure, item, or service is treated under the revised ASC payment system. For more information about these indicators and how they affect billing, consult Optum360's *Revenue Cycle Pro.*

A2 Surgical procedure on ASC list in 2007; payment based on OPPS relative payment weight.

B5 Alternative code may be available; no payment made.

D5 Deleted/discontinued code; no payment made.

F4 Corneal tissue acquisition; hepatitis B vaccine; paid at reasonable cost.

G2 Non-office-based surgical procedure added in CY 2008 or later; payment based on OPPS relative payment weight.

H2 Brachytherapy source paid separately when provided integral to a surgical procedure on ASC list; payment based on OPPS rate.

J7 OPPS pass-through device paid separately when provided integral to a surgical procedure on ASC list; payment contractor-priced.

J8 Device-intensive procedure; paid at adjusted rate.

K2 Drugs and biologicals paid separately when provided integral to a surgical procedure on ASC list; payment based on OPPS rate.

K7 Unclassified drugs and biologicals; payment contractor-priced.

L1 Influenza vaccine; pneumococcal vaccine. Packaged item/service; no separate payment made.

L6 New technology intraocular lens (NTIOL); special payment.

N1 Packaged service/item; no separate payment made.

P2 Office-based surgical procedure added to ASC list in CY 2008 or later with MPFS nonfacility practice expense (PE) RVUs; payment based on OPPS relative payment weight.

P3 Office-based surgical procedure added to ASC list in CY 2008 or later with MPFS nonfacility PE RVUs; payment based on MPFS nonfacility PE RVUs.

R2 Office-based surgical procedure added to ASC list in CY 2008 or later without MPFS nonfacility PE RVUs; payment based on OPPS relative payment weight.

Z2 Radiology or diagnostic service paid separately when provided integral to a surgical procedure on ASC list; payment based on OPPS relative payment weight.

Z3 Radiology or diagnostic service paid separately when provided integral to a surgical procedure on ASC list; payment based on MPFS nonfacility PE RVUs.

A **Age Edit**
This icon denotes codes intended for use with a specific age group, such as neonate, newborn, pediatric, and adult. This edit is based on age specifications in the CPT code descriptors, the product/service represented by the code *may* have age restrictions, and/or updates from the Integrated Outpatient Code Editor (I/OCE). Carefully review the code description to ensure the code you report most appropriately reflects the patient's age.

M **Maternity**
This icon identifies procedures that by definition should be used only for maternity patients generally between 9 and 64 years of age based on CMS I/OCE designations.

♀ **Female Only**
This icon identifies procedures designated by CMS for females only based on CMS I/OCE designations.

♂ **Male Only**
This icon identifies procedures designated by CMS for males only based on CMS I/OCE designations.

Facility RVU
This icon precedes the facility RVU from CMS's 2018 physician fee schedule (PFS). It can be found under the code description.

New codes include no RVU information.

Nonfacility RVU
This icon precedes the nonfacility RVU from CMS's 2018 PFS. It can be found under the code description.

New codes include no RVU information.

FUD: Global days are sometimes referred to as "follow-up days" or FUDs. The global period is the time following surgery during which routine care by the physician is considered postoperative and included in the surgical fee. Office visits or

Introduction

other routine care related to the original surgery cannot be separately reported if provided during the global period. The statuses are:

000	No follow-up care included in this procedure
010	Normal postoperative care is included in this procedure for ten days
090	Normal postoperative care is included in the procedure for 90 days
MMM	Maternity codes; usual global period does not apply
XXX	The global concept does not apply to the code
YYY	The carrier is to determine whether the global concept applies and establishes postoperative period, if appropriate, at time of pricing
ZZZ	The code is related to another service and is always included in the global period of the other service

CMS: This notation indicates that there is a specific CMS guideline pertaining to this code in the CMS Online Manual System which includes the internet-only manual (IOM) *National Coverage Determinations Manual* (NCD). These CMS sources present the rules for submitting these services to the federal government or its contractors and a link to the IOMs is included in appendix G of this book.

AMA: This indicates discussion of the code in the American Medical Association's *CPT Assistant* newsletter. Use the citation to find the correct issue. This includes citations for the current year and the preceding six years. In the event no citations can be found during this time period, the most recent citations that can be found are used.

Drug Not Approved by FDA
The AMA CPT Editorial Panel is publishing new vaccine product codes prior to Food and Drug Administration approval. This symbol indicates which of these codes are pending FDA approval at press time.

A–Y **OPPS Status Indicators (OPSI)**
Status indicators identify how individual CPT codes are paid or not paid under the latest available hospital outpatient prospective payment system (OPPS). The same status indicator is assigned to all the codes within an ambulatory payment classification (APC). Consult your payer or other resource to learn which CPT codes fall within various APCs.

A Services furnished to a hospital outpatient that are paid under a fee schedule or payment system other than OPPS. For example:
- Ambulance services
- Separately payable clinical diagnostic laboratory services
- Separately payable non-implantable prosthetics and orthotics
- Physical, occupational, and speech therapy
- Diagnostic mammography
- Screening mammography

B Codes that are not recognized by OPPS when submitted on an outpatient hospital Part B bill type (12x and 13x)

C Inpatient procedures

D Discontinued codes

E1 Items, codes, and services:
- Not covered by any Medicare outpatient benefit category
- Statutorily excluded by Medicare
- Not reasonable and necessary

E2 Items, codes, and services for which pricing information and claims data are not available

F Corneal tissue acquisition; certain CRNA services and hepatitis B vaccines

G Pass-through drugs and biologicals

H Pass-through device categories

J1 Hospital Part B services paid through a comprehensive APC

J2 Hospital Part B services that may be paid through a comprehensive APC

K Nonpass-through drugs and nonimplantable biologicals, including therapeutic radiopharmaceuticals

L Influenza vaccine; pneumococcal pneumonia vaccine

M Items and services not billable to the MAC

N Items and services packaged into APC rates

P Partial hospitalization

Q1 STV-packaged codes

Q2 T-packaged codes

Q3 Codes that may be paid through a composite APC

Q4 Conditionally packaged laboratory tests

R Blood and blood products

S Procedure or service, not discounted when multiple

T Procedure or service, multiple procedure reduction applies

U Brachytherapy sources

V Clinic or emergency department visit

Y Nonimplantable durable medical equipment

Appendixes

Appendix A: Modifiers—This appendix identifies modifiers. A modifier is a two-position alpha or numeric code that is appended to a CPT or HCPCS code to clarify the services being reported. Modifiers provide a means by which a service can be altered without changing the procedure code. They add more information, such as anatomical site, to the code. In addition, they help eliminate the appearance of duplicate billing and unbundling. Modifiers are used to increase the accuracy in reimbursement and coding consistency, ease editing, and capture payment data.

Appendix B: New, Revised, and Deleted Codes—This is a list of new, revised, and deleted CPT codes for the current year. This appendix also includes a list of web release new, revised, and deleted codes, which indicate official code changes in *Current Procedural Coding Expert* that will not be in the CPT code book until the following year.

Appendix C: Evaluation and Management Extended Guidelines—This appendix presents an overview of evaluation and management (E/M) services that augment the official AMA CPT E/M services. It includes tables that distinguish documentation components of each E/M code and the federal documentation guidelines (1995 and 1997) currently in use by the Centers for Medicare and Medicaid Services (CMS).

Appendix D: Crosswalk of Deleted Codes—This appendix is a cross-reference from a deleted CPT code to an active code when one is available. The deleted code cross-reference will also appear under the deleted code description in the tabular section of the book.

Appendix E: Resequenced Codes—This appendix contains a list of codes that are not in numeric order in the book. AMA resequenced some of the code numbers to relocate codes in the same category but not in numeric sequence. In addition to the list of codes, this appendix provides the page number where the resequenced code may be found.

Appendix F: Add-on, Optum Modifier 50 Exempt, Modifier 51 Exempt, Optum Modifier 51 Exempt, Modifier 63 Exempt, and Modifier 95 Telemedicine Services—This list includes add-on codes that cannot be reported alone, codes that are exempt from modifiers 50 and 51, codes that should not be reported with modifier 63, and codes identified by the ★

icon to which modifier 95 may be appended when the service is provided as a synchronous telemedicine service.

Appendix G: Medicare Internet-only Manual (IOMs)—Previously, this appendix contained a verbatim printout of the Medicare Internet-only Manual references pertaining to specific codes. This appendix now contains a link to the IOMs on the Centers for Medicare and Medicaid Services website. The IOM references applicable to specific codes can still be found at the code level. For example:

93784-93790 Ambulatory Blood Pressure Monitoring

CMS: 100-3,20.19 Ambulatory Blood Pressure Monitoring (20.19); 100-4,32,10.1 Ambulatory Blood Pressure Monitoring Billing Requirements

Appendix H: Quality Payment Program (QPP)—Previously, this appendix contained lists of the numerators and denominators applicable to the Medicare PQRS. However, with the implementation of the Quality Payment Program (QPP) mandated by passage of the Medicare Access and Chip Reauthorization Act (MACRA) of 2015, the PQRS system will be obsolete. This appendix now contains information pertinent to that legislation as well as a brief overview of the proposed changes for the following year, as is available by the date of this publication.

Appendix I: Medically Unlikely Edits—This appendix contains the published medically unlikely edits (MUEs). These edits establish maximum daily allowable units of service. The edits will be applied to the services provided to the same patient, for the same CPT code, on the same date of service when billed by the same provider. Included are the physician and facility edits.

Appendix J: Inpatient-Only Procedures—This appendix identifies services with the status indicator "C." Medicare will not pay an OPPS hospital or ASC when these procedures are performed on a Medicare patient as an outpatient. Physicians should refer to this list when scheduling Medicare patients for surgical procedures. CMS updates this list quarterly.

Appendix K: Place of Service and Type of Service—This appendix contains lists of place-of-service codes that should be used on professional claims and type-of-service codes used by the Medicare Common Working File.

Appendix L: Multianalyte Assays with Algorithmic Analyses —This appendix lists the administrative codes for multianalyte assays with algorithmic analyses. The AMA updates this list three times a year.

Appendix M: Glossary—This appendix contains general terms and definitions that may be helpful for coding and reimbursement.

Appendix N: Listing of Sensory, Motor, and Mixed Nerves—This appendix lists a summary of each sensory, motor, and mixed nerve with its appropriate nerve conduction study code.

Appendix O: Vascular Families—Appendix O contains a table of vascular families starting with the aorta. Additional information can be found in the interventional radiology illustrations located behind the index.

Appendix P: Interventional Radiology Illustrations—This appendix contains illustrations specific to interventional radiology procedures.

Appendix Q: Severe Acute Respiratory Syndrome Coronavirus 2 (SARS-CoV-2) (coronavirus disease [COVID-19]) Vaccine and Administration Codes—This appendix contains a table providing a link between each individual SARS-CoV-2 (COVID-19) vaccine code and its corresponding vaccine administration code, along with other pertinent information related to each vaccine.

Appendix R: Digital Medicine Services—This appendix contains a table providing definitions of terms in digital medicine services and classifies CPT codes related to those services.

Note: All data current as of November 1, 2021.

Anatomical Illustrations

Body Planes and Movements

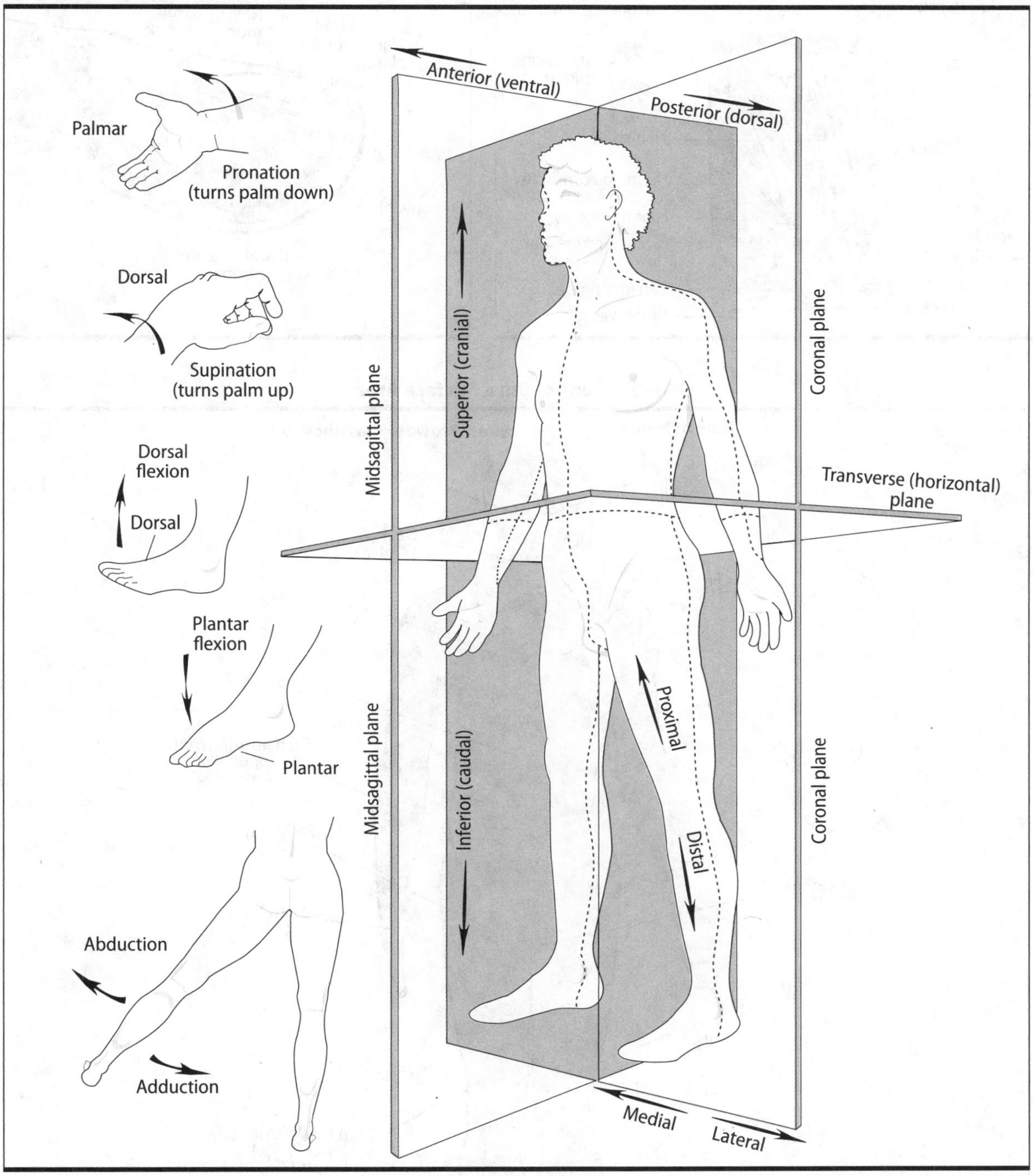

Integumentary System

Skin and Subcutaneous Tissue

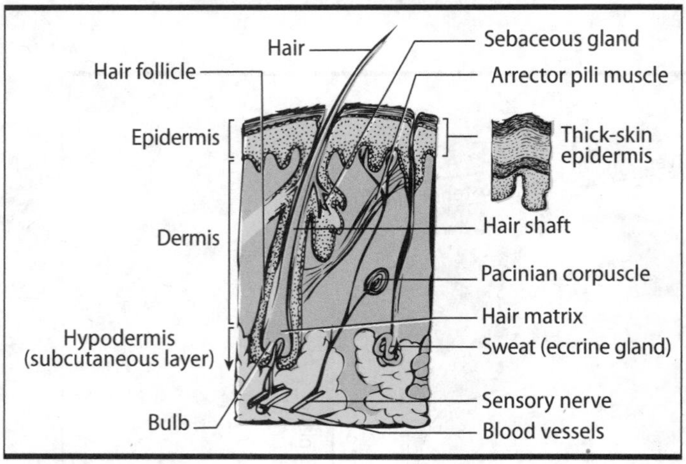

Nail Anatomy

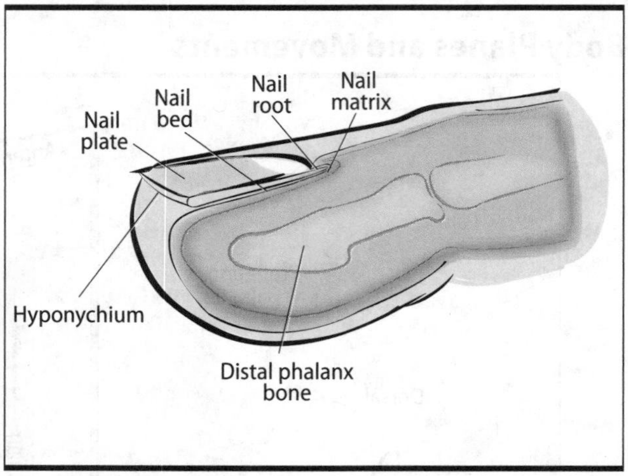

Assessment of Burn Surface Area

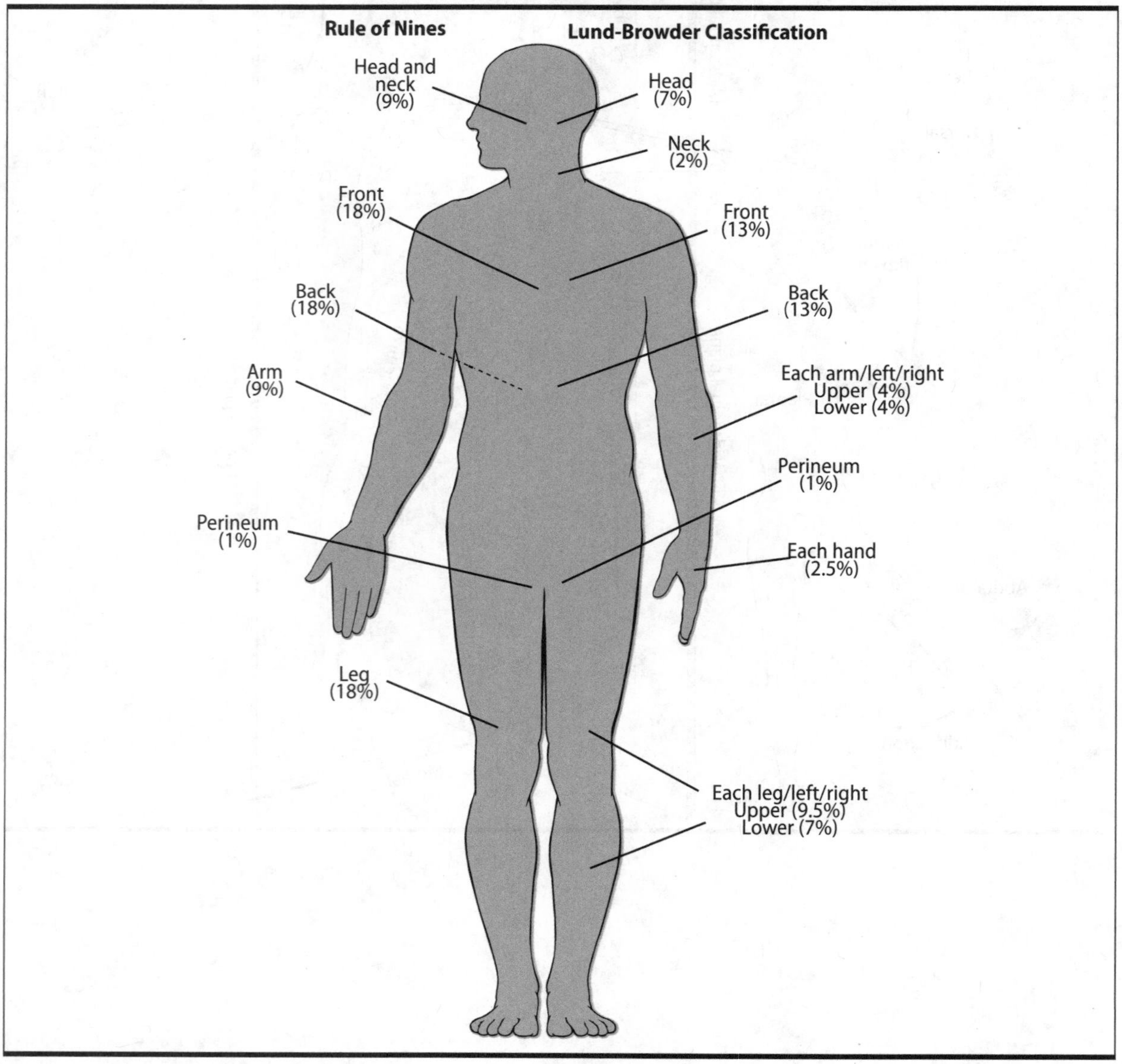

Musculoskeletal System

Bones and Joints

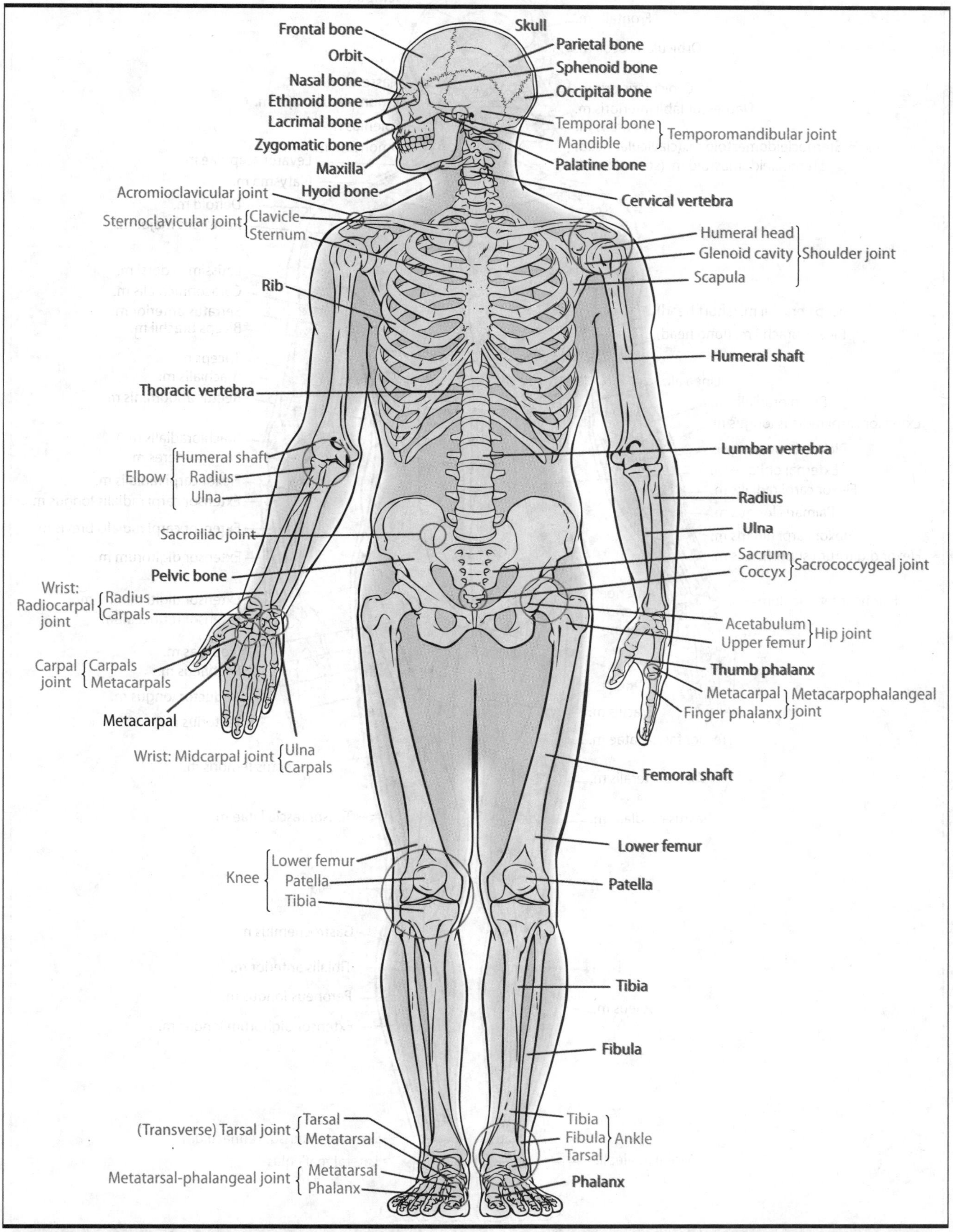

Muscles

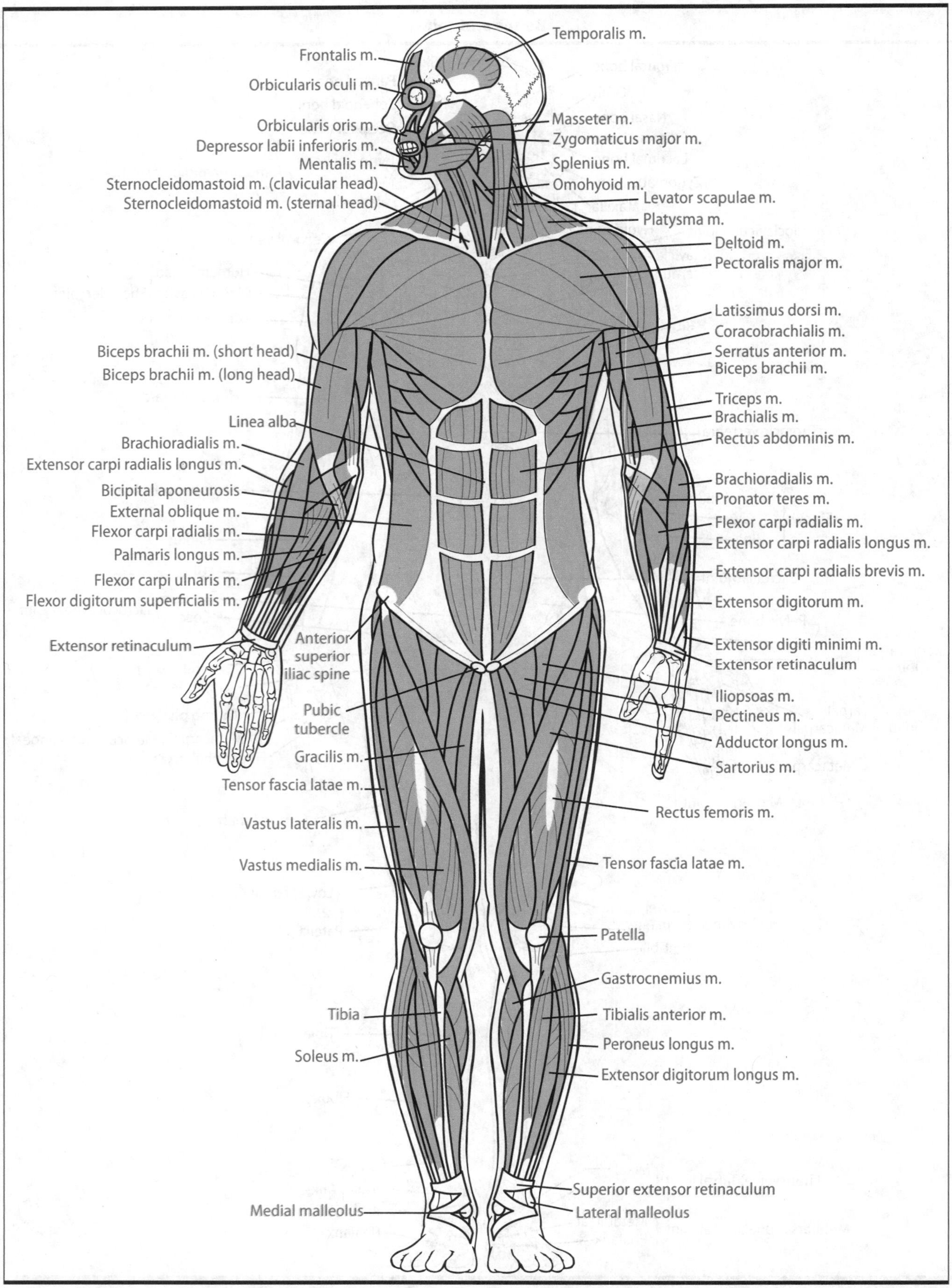
Temporalis m.
Frontalis m.
Orbicularis oculi m.
Orbicularis oris m.
Depressor labii inferioris m.
Mentalis m.
Sternocleidomastoid m. (clavicular head)
Sternocleidomastoid m. (sternal head)
Masseter m.
Zygomaticus major m.
Splenius m.
Omohyoid m.
Levator scapulae m.
Platysma m.
Deltoid m.
Pectoralis major m.
Latissimus dorsi m.
Coracobrachialis m.
Serratus anterior m.
Biceps brachii m.
Biceps brachii m. (short head)
Biceps brachii m. (long head)
Triceps m.
Brachialis m.
Linea alba
Rectus abdominis m.
Brachioradialis m.
Extensor carpi radialis longus m.
Bicipital aponeurosis
External oblique m.
Flexor carpi radialis m.
Palmaris longus m.
Flexor carpi ulnaris m.
Flexor digitorum superficialis m.
Brachioradialis m.
Pronator teres m.
Flexor carpi radialis m.
Extensor carpi radialis longus m.
Extensor carpi radialis brevis m.
Extensor digitorum m.
Extensor retinaculum
Anterior superior iliac spine
Extensor digiti minimi m.
Extensor retinaculum
Pubic tubercle
Iliopsoas m.
Pectineus m.
Adductor longus m.
Sartorius m.
Gracilis m.
Tensor fascia latae m.
Vastus lateralis m.
Rectus femoris m.
Vastus medialis m.
Tensor fascia latae m.
Patella
Gastrocnemius m.
Tibia
Tibialis anterior m.
Peroneus longus m.
Soleus m.
Extensor digitorum longus m.
Superior extensor retinaculum
Medial malleolus
Lateral malleolus

Head and Facial Bones

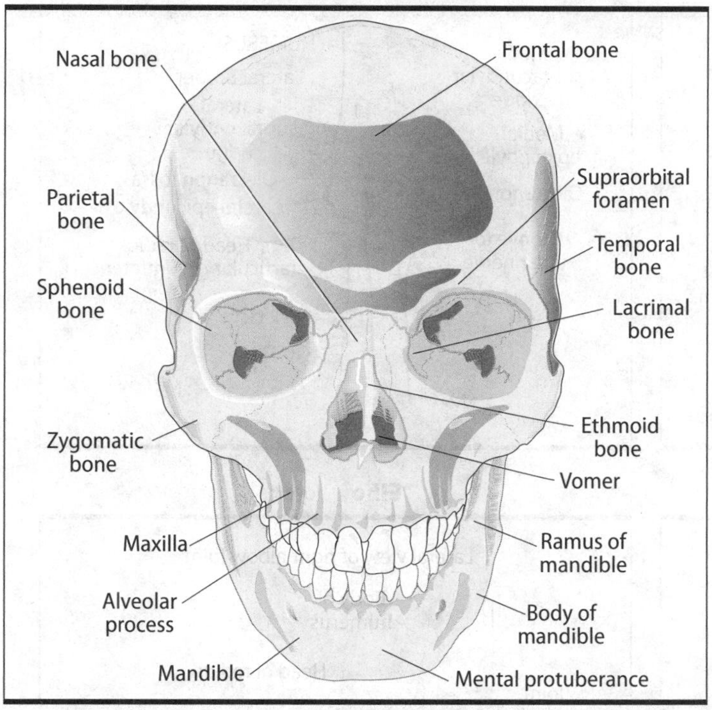
Nasal bone
Frontal bone
Supraorbital foramen
Parietal bone
Temporal bone
Sphenoid bone
Lacrimal bone
Ethmoid bone
Zygomatic bone
Vomer
Maxilla
Ramus of mandible
Alveolar process
Body of mandible
Mandible
Mental protuberance

Nose

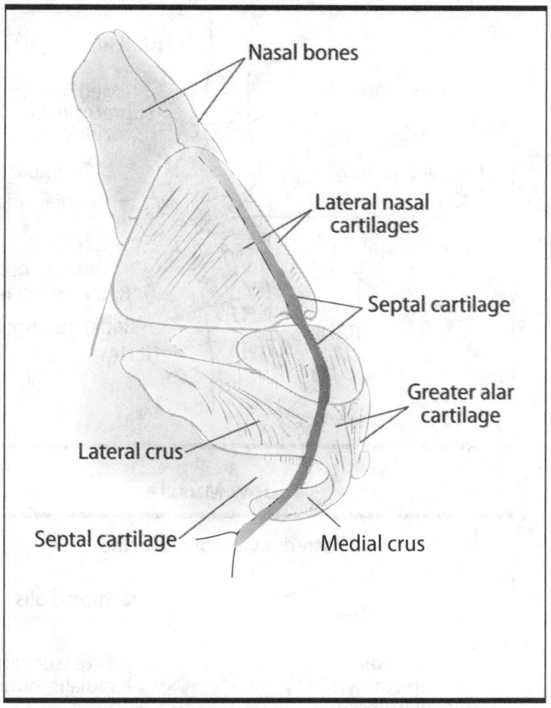
Nasal bones
Lateral nasal cartilages
Septal cartilage
Greater alar cartilage
Lateral crus
Septal cartilage
Medial crus

Shoulder (Anterior View)

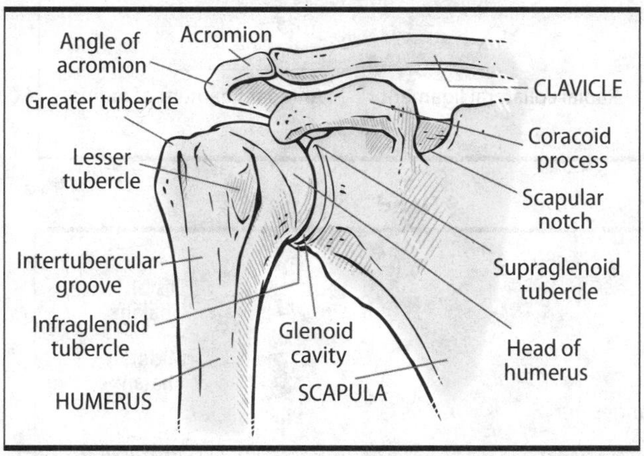
Angle of acromion
Acromion
CLAVICLE
Greater tubercle
Coracoid process
Lesser tubercle
Scapular notch
Intertubercular groove
Supraglenoid tubercle
Infraglenoid tubercle
Glenoid cavity
Head of humerus
HUMERUS
SCAPULA

Shoulder (Posterior View)

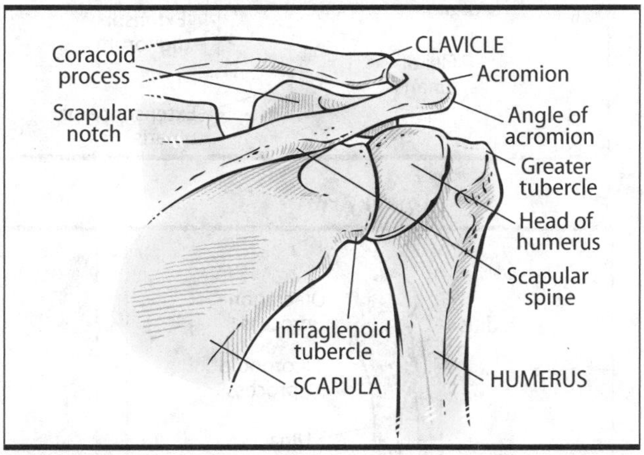
Coracoid process
CLAVICLE
Acromion
Scapular notch
Angle of acromion
Greater tubercle
Head of humerus
Scapular spine
Infraglenoid tubercle
SCAPULA
HUMERUS

Shoulder Muscles

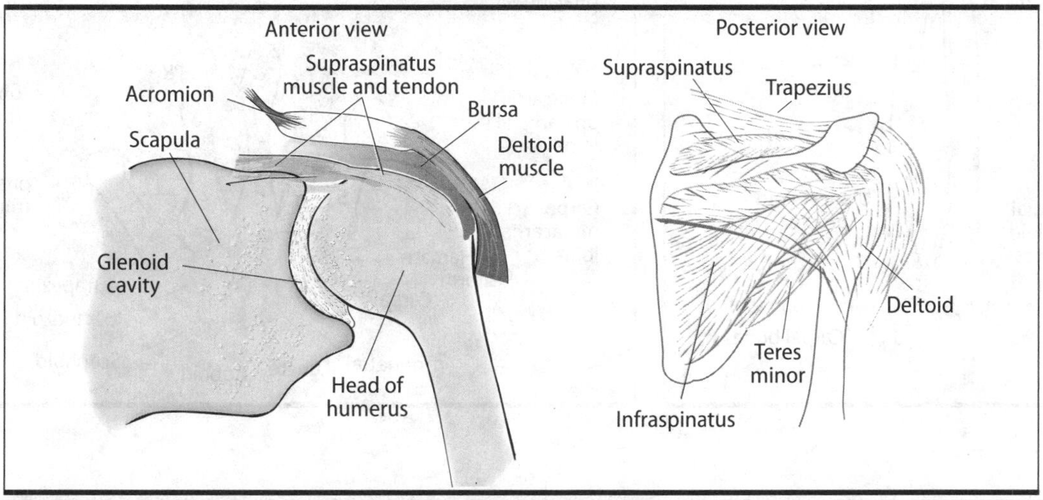
Anterior view
Supraspinatus muscle and tendon
Acromion
Bursa
Scapula
Deltoid muscle
Glenoid cavity
Head of humerus
Posterior view
Supraspinatus
Trapezius
Deltoid
Teres minor
Infraspinatus

Elbow (Anterior View)

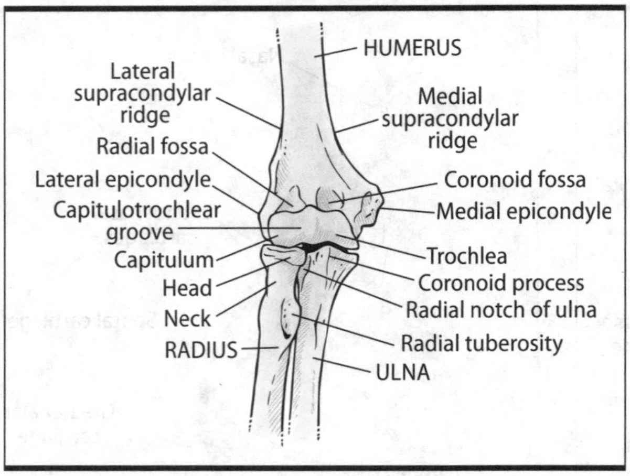

Elbow (Posterior View)

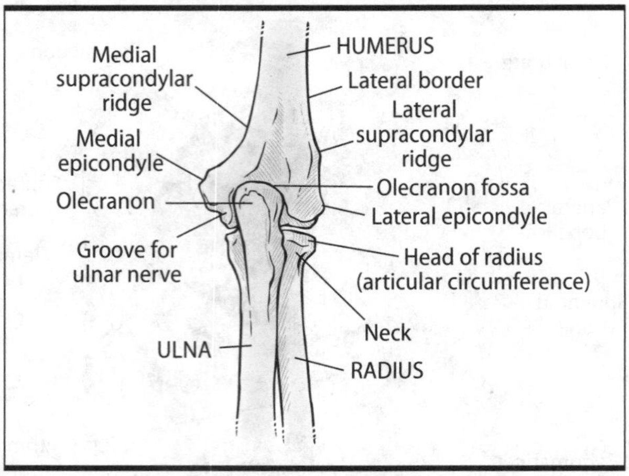

Elbow Muscles

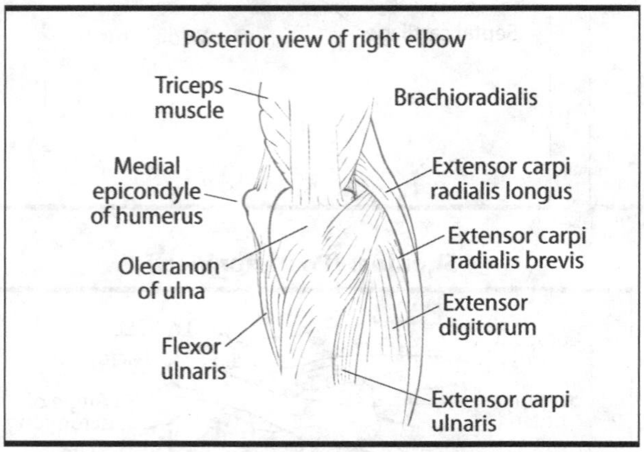

Elbow Joint

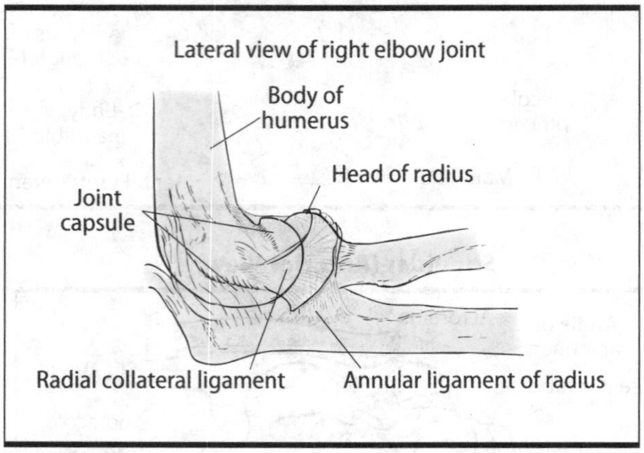

Lower Arm

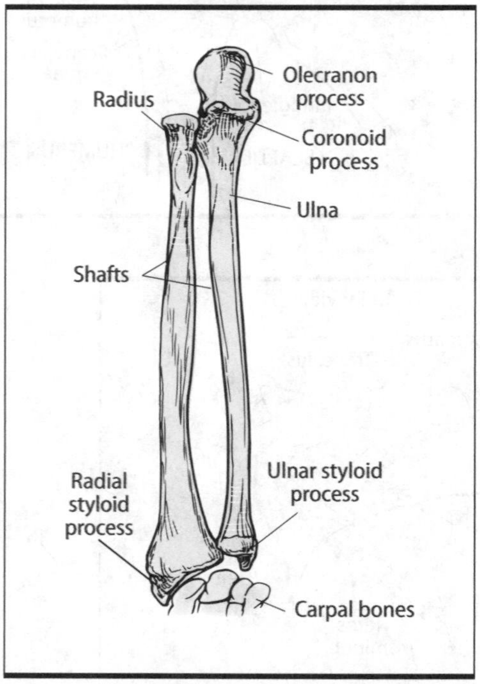

Hand

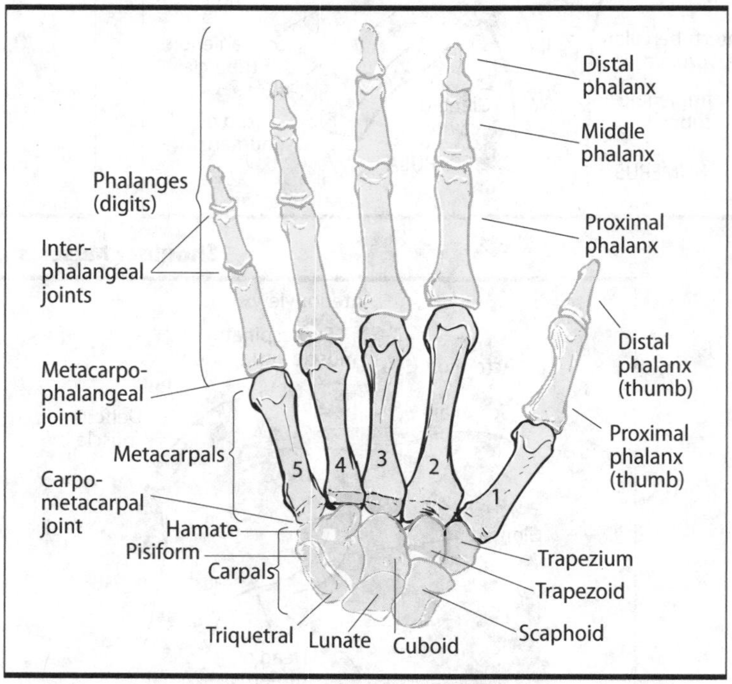

Hip (Anterior View)

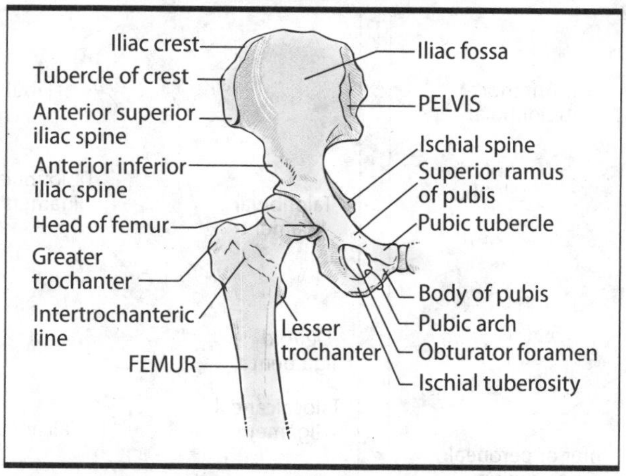
Iliac crest
Tubercle of crest
Anterior superior iliac spine
Anterior inferior iliac spine
Head of femur
Greater trochanter
Intertrochanteric line
FEMUR
Lesser trochanter
Iliac fossa
PELVIS
Ischial spine
Superior ramus of pubis
Pubic tubercle
Body of pubis
Pubic arch
Obturator foramen
Ischial tuberosity

Hip (Posterior View)

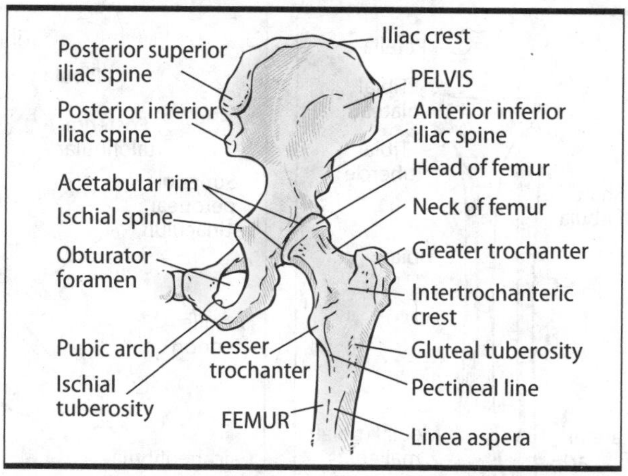
Posterior superior iliac spine
Posterior inferior iliac spine
Acetabular rim
Ischial spine
Obturator foramen
Pubic arch
Ischial tuberosity
Lesser trochanter
FEMUR
Iliac crest
PELVIS
Anterior inferior iliac spine
Head of femur
Neck of femur
Greater trochanter
Intertrochanteric crest
Gluteal tuberosity
Pectineal line
Linea aspera

Knee (Anterior View)

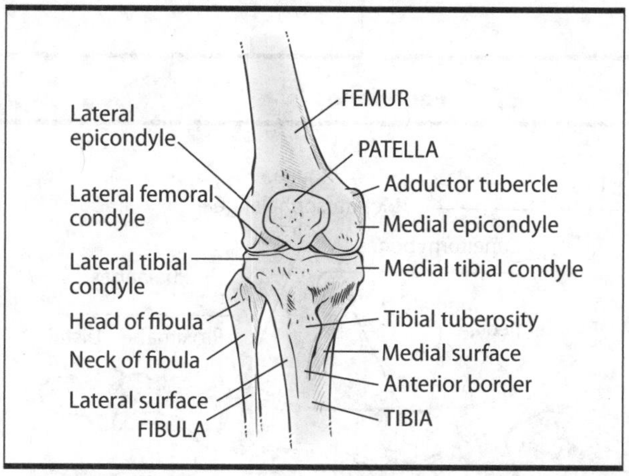
Lateral epicondyle
Lateral femoral condyle
Lateral tibial condyle
Head of fibula
Neck of fibula
Lateral surface
FIBULA
FEMUR
PATELLA
Adductor tubercle
Medial epicondyle
Medial tibial condyle
Tibial tuberosity
Medial surface
Anterior border
TIBIA

Knee (Posterior View)

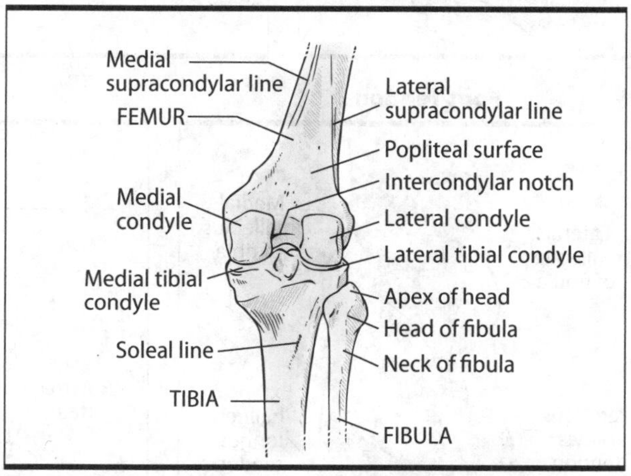
Medial supracondylar line
FEMUR
Medial condyle
Medial tibial condyle
Soleal line
TIBIA
Lateral supracondylar line
Popliteal surface
Intercondylar notch
Lateral condyle
Lateral tibial condyle
Apex of head
Head of fibula
Neck of fibula
FIBULA

Knee Joint (Anterior View)

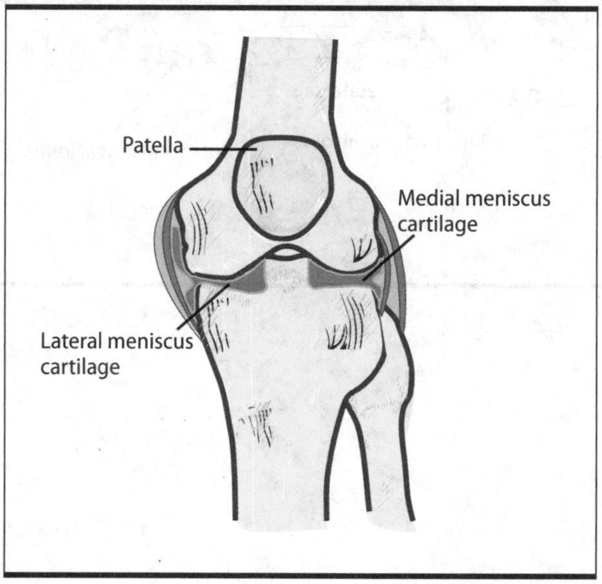
Patella
Medial meniscus cartilage
Lateral meniscus cartilage

Knee Joint (Lateral View)

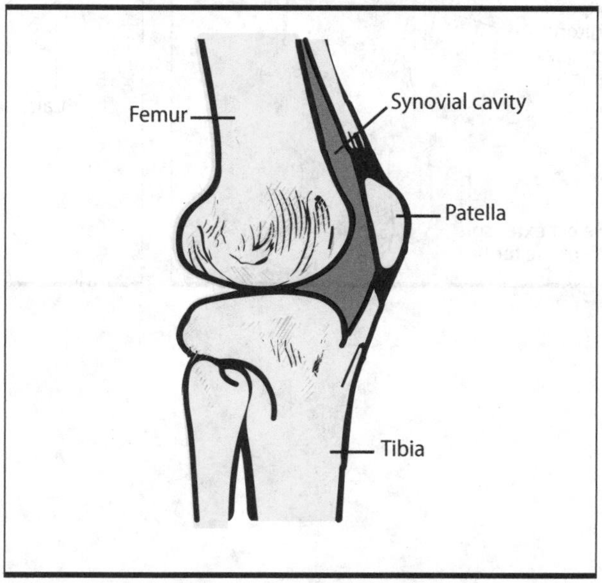
Femur
Synovial cavity
Patella
Tibia

Lower Leg

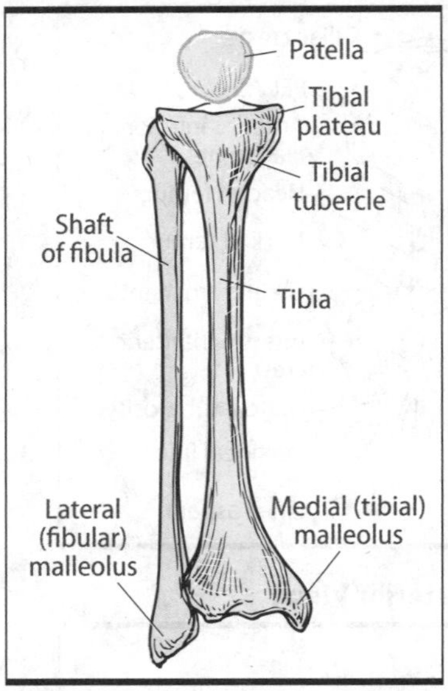
Patella
Tibial plateau
Tibial tubercle
Shaft of fibula
Tibia
Lateral (fibular) malleolus
Medial (tibial) malleolus

Ankle Ligament (Lateral View)

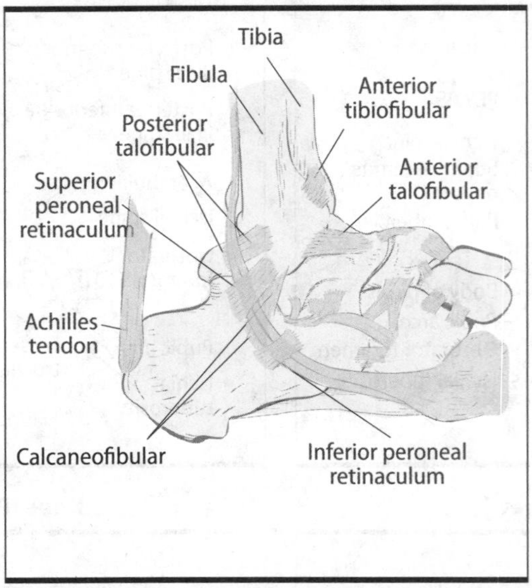
Tibia
Fibula
Anterior tibiofibular
Posterior talofibular
Anterior talofibular
Superior peroneal retinaculum
Achilles tendon
Calcaneofibular
Inferior peroneal retinaculum

Ankle Ligament (Posterior View)

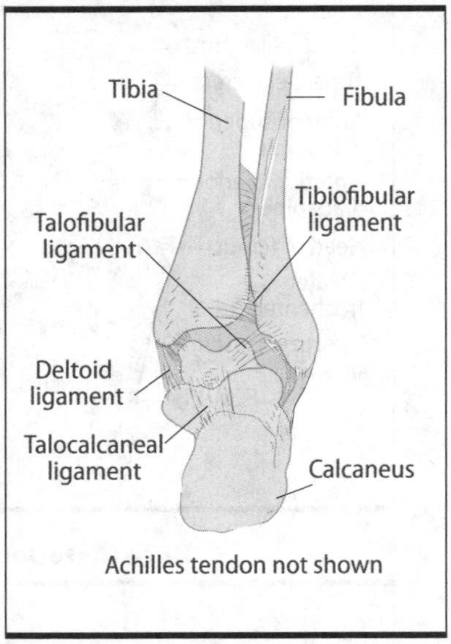
Tibia
Fibula
Tibiofibular ligament
Talofibular ligament
Deltoid ligament
Talocalcaneal ligament
Calcaneus
Achilles tendon not shown

Foot Tendons

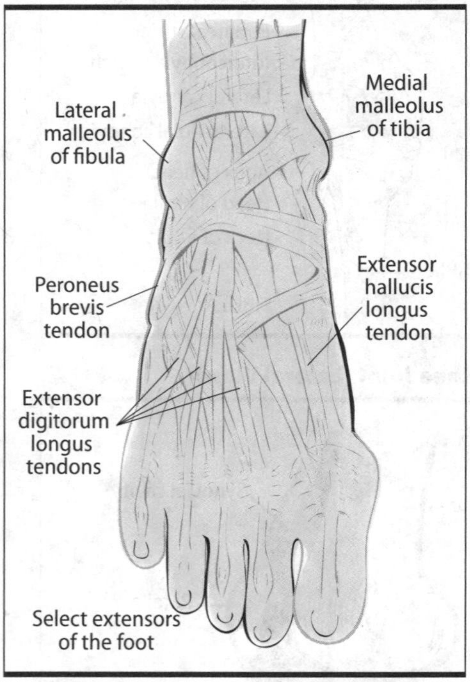
Lateral malleolus of fibula
Medial malleolus of tibia
Peroneus brevis tendon
Extensor hallucis longus tendon
Extensor digitorum longus tendons
Select extensors of the foot

Foot Bones

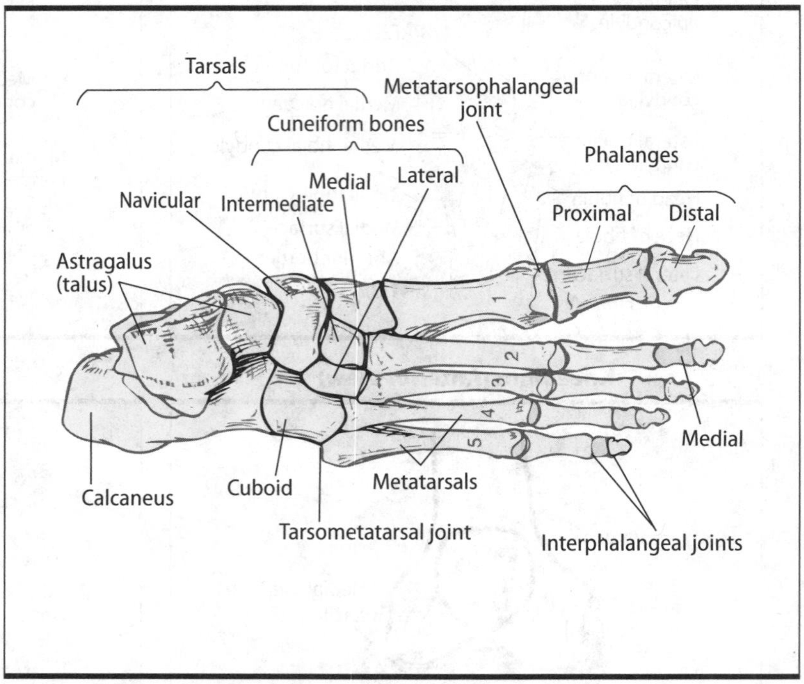
Tarsals
Metatarsophalangeal joint
Cuneiform bones
Phalanges
Medial
Lateral
Navicular
Intermediate
Proximal
Distal
Astragalus (talus)
1
2
3
4
5
Medial
Calcaneus
Cuboid
Metatarsals
Tarsometatarsal joint
Interphalangeal joints

Respiratory System

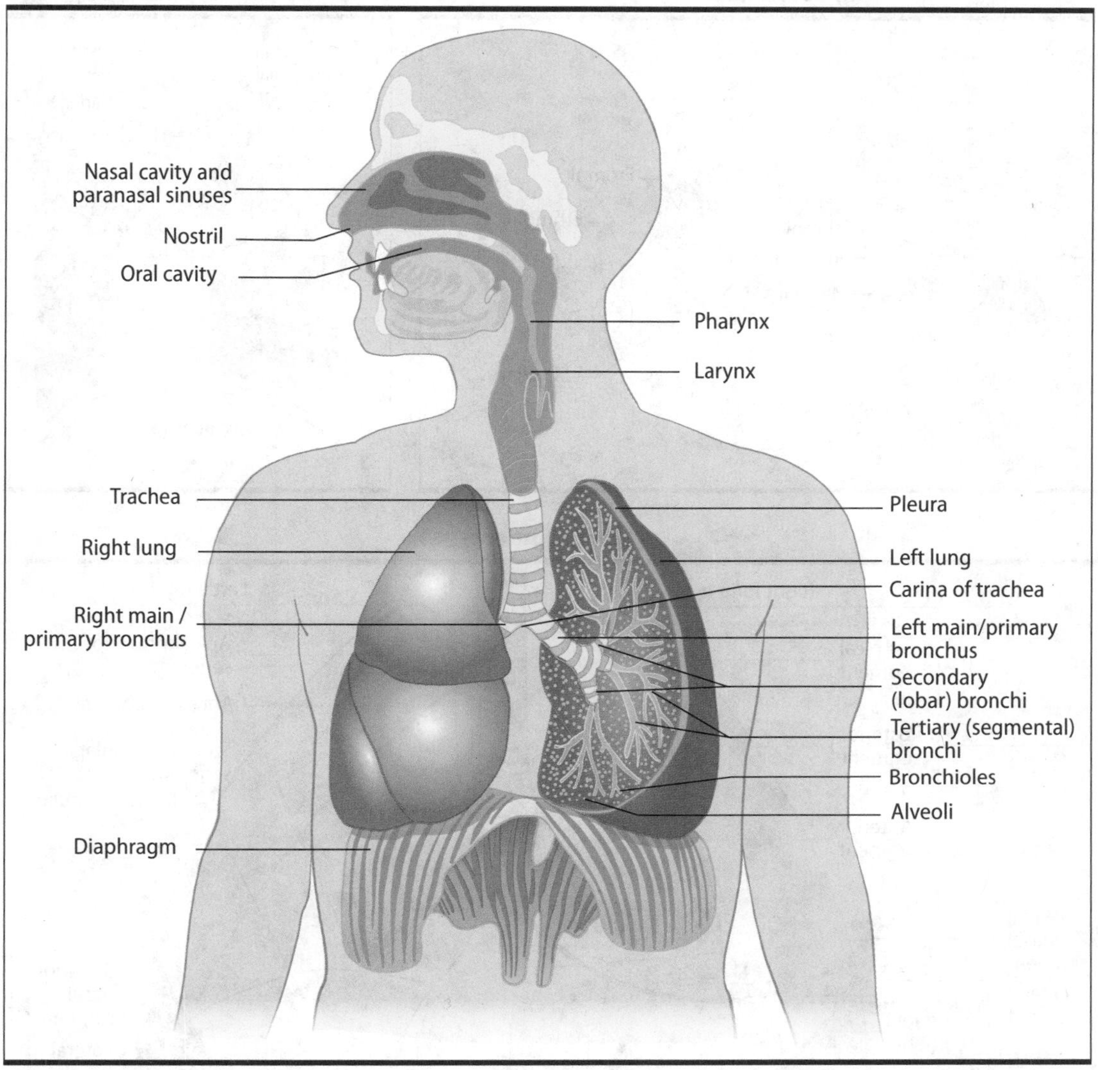
Nasal cavity and paranasal sinuses
Nostril
Oral cavity
Pharynx
Larynx
Trachea
Right lung
Right main / primary bronchus
Diaphragm
Pleura
Left lung
Carina of trachea
Left main/primary bronchus
Secondary (lobar) bronchi
Tertiary (segmental) bronchi
Bronchioles
Alveoli

Upper Respiratory System

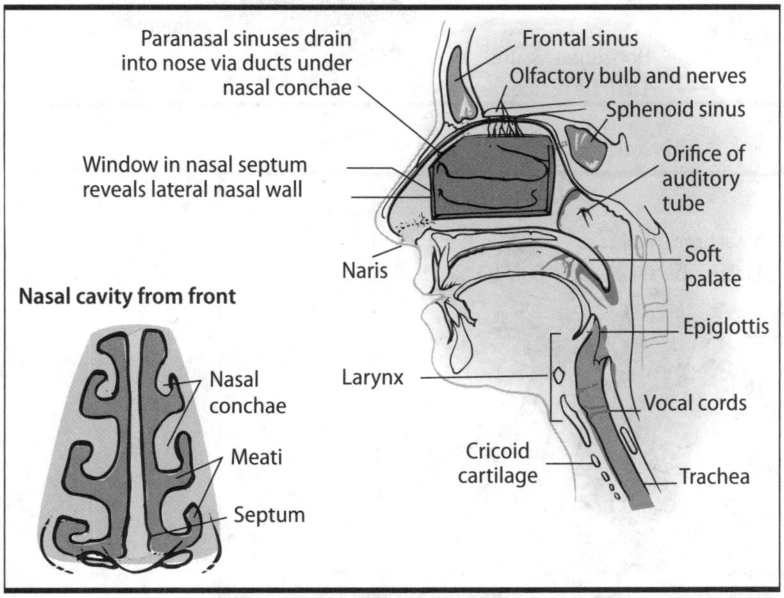
Paranasal sinuses drain into nose via ducts under nasal conchae
Window in nasal septum reveals lateral nasal wall
Naris
Nasal cavity from front
Nasal conchae
Meati
Septum
Larynx
Cricoid cartilage
Frontal sinus
Olfactory bulb and nerves
Sphenoid sinus
Orifice of auditory tube
Soft palate
Epiglottis
Vocal cords
Trachea

Nasal Turbinates

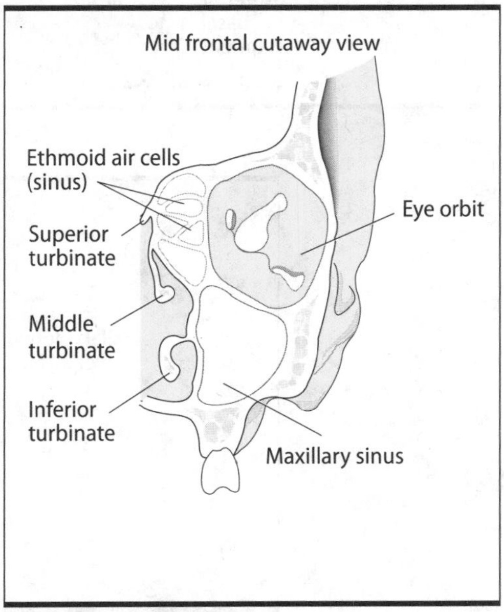
Mid frontal cutaway view
Ethmoid air cells (sinus)
Superior turbinate
Middle turbinate
Inferior turbinate
Eye orbit
Maxillary sinus

Paranasal Sinuses

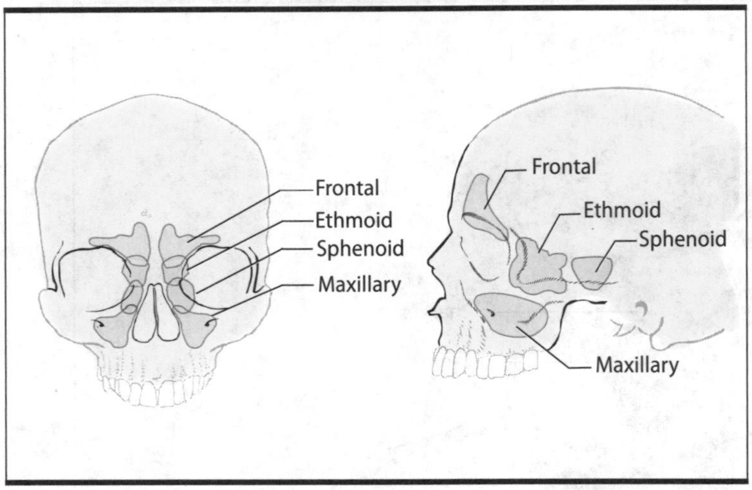
Frontal
Ethmoid
Sphenoid
Maxillary
Frontal
Ethmoid
Sphenoid
Maxillary

Lower Respiratory System

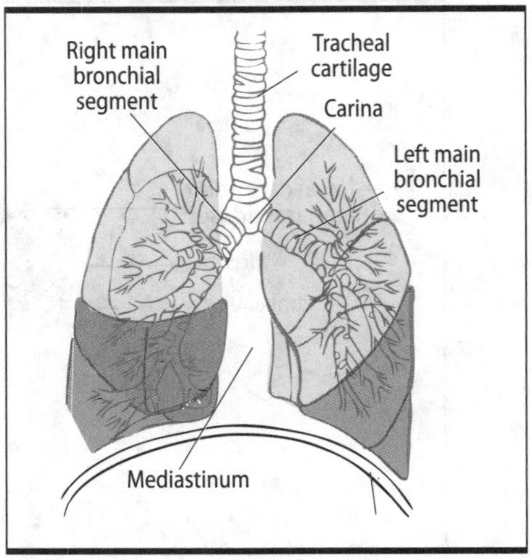
Right main bronchial segment
Tracheal cartilage
Carina
Left main bronchial segment
Mediastinum

Lung Segments

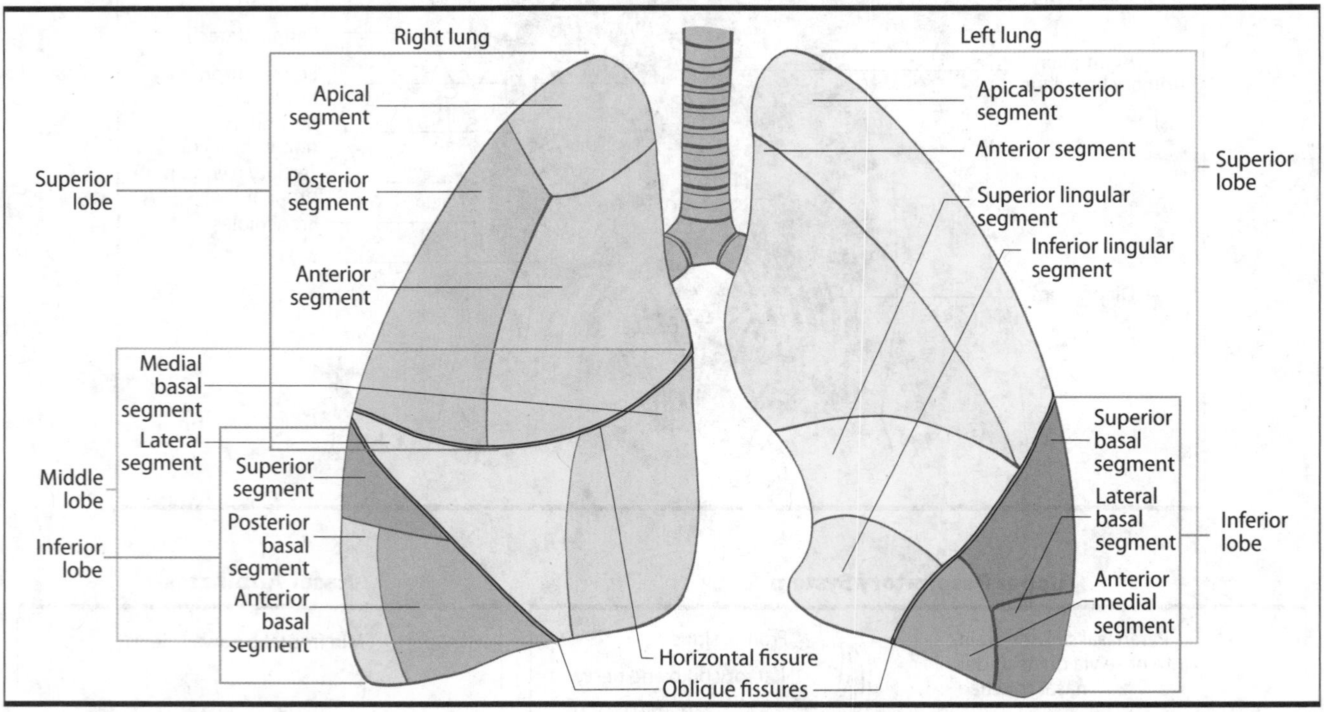
Right lung
Left lung
Apical segment
Superior lobe
Posterior segment
Anterior segment
Medial basal segment
Lateral segment
Middle lobe
Superior segment
Inferior lobe
Posterior basal segment
Anterior basal segment
Apical-posterior segment
Anterior segment
Superior lobe
Superior lingular segment
Inferior lingular segment
Superior basal segment
Lateral basal segment
Inferior lobe
Anterior medial segment
Horizontal fissure
Oblique fissures

Alveoli

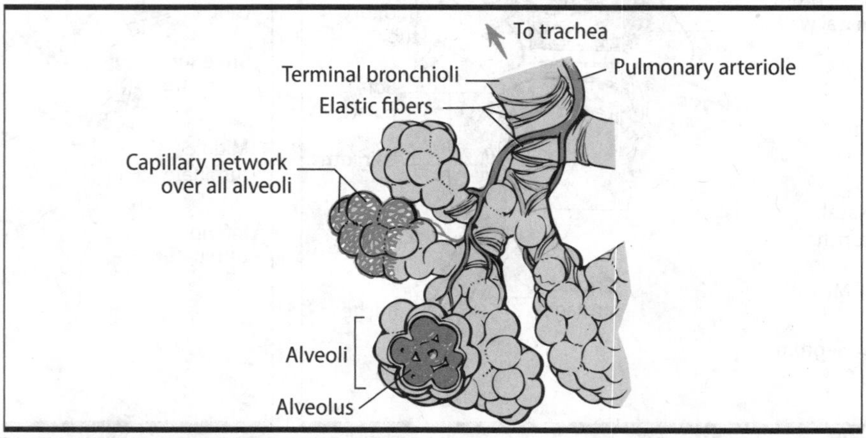
To trachea
Terminal bronchioli
Pulmonary arteriole
Elastic fibers
Capillary network over all alveoli
Alveoli
Alveolus

Arterial System

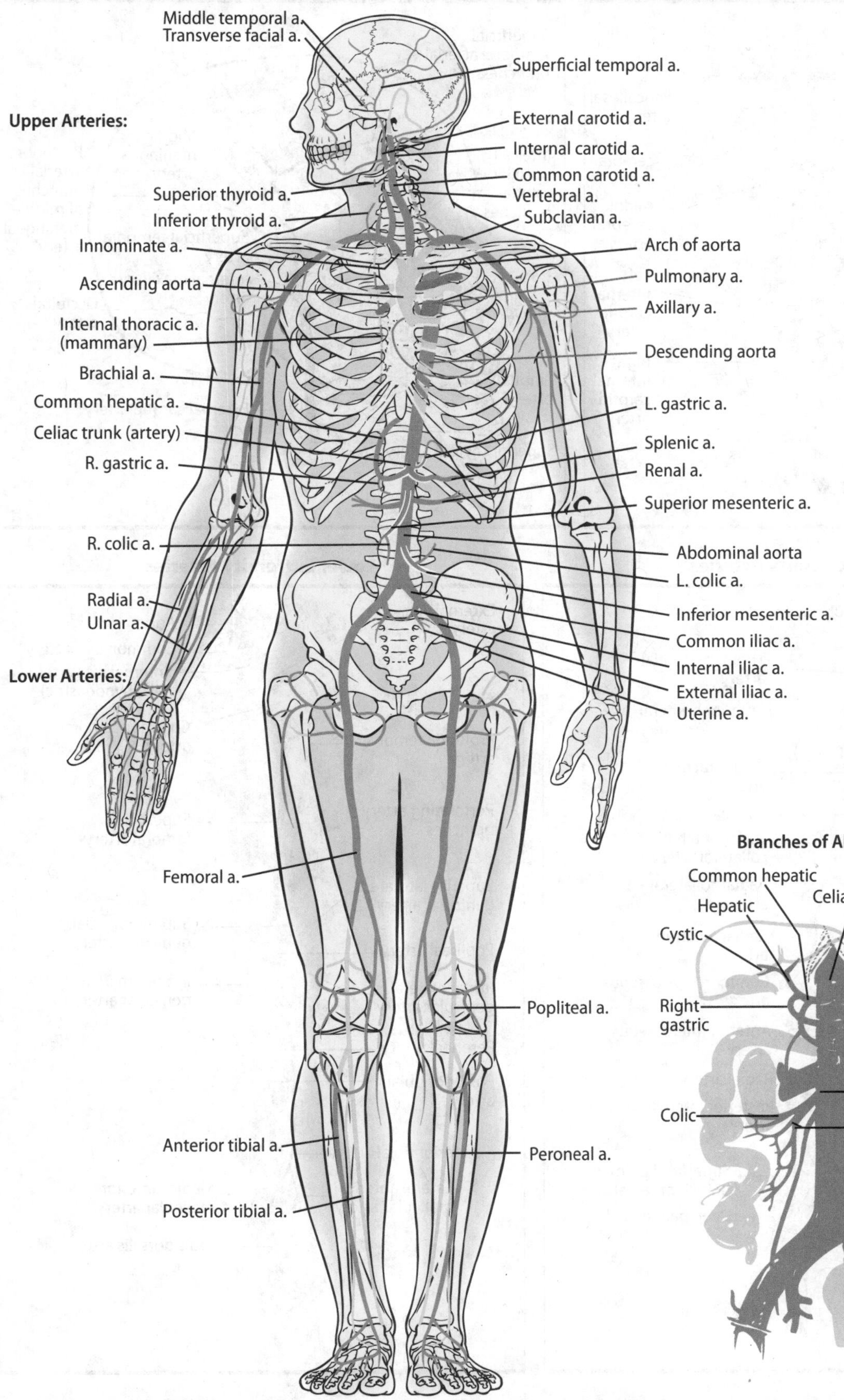
Middle temporal a.
Transverse facial a.
Superficial temporal a.
Upper Arteries:
External carotid a.
Internal carotid a.
Common carotid a.
Superior thyroid a.
Vertebral a.
Inferior thyroid a.
Subclavian a.
Innominate a.
Arch of aorta
Ascending aorta
Pulmonary a.
Axillary a.
Internal thoracic a. (mammary)
Descending aorta
Brachial a.
Common hepatic a.
L. gastric a.
Celiac trunk (artery)
Splenic a.
R. gastric a.
Renal a.
Superior mesenteric a.
R. colic a.
Abdominal aorta
L. colic a.
Radial a.
Inferior mesenteric a.
Ulnar a.
Common iliac a.
Internal iliac a.
Lower Arteries:
External iliac a.
Uterine a.
Femoral a.
Popliteal a.
Anterior tibial a.
Peroneal a.
Posterior tibial a.

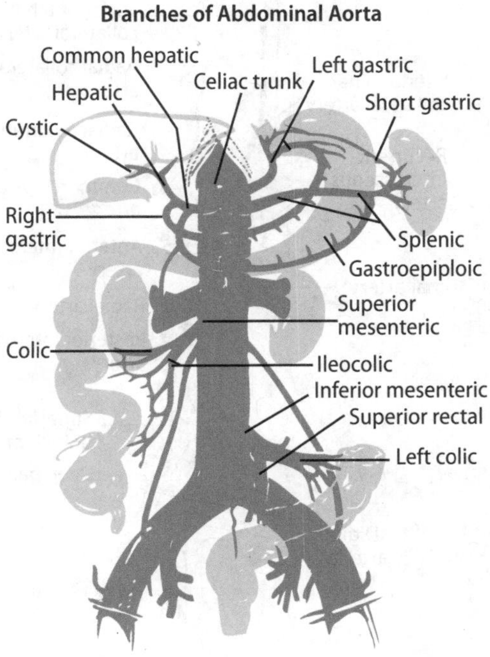
Branches of Abdominal Aorta
Common hepatic
Left gastric
Celiac trunk
Hepatic
Short gastric
Cystic
Right gastric
Splenic
Gastroepiploic
Superior mesenteric
Colic
Ileocolic
Inferior mesenteric
Superior rectal
Left colic

Internal Carotid and Arteries and Branches

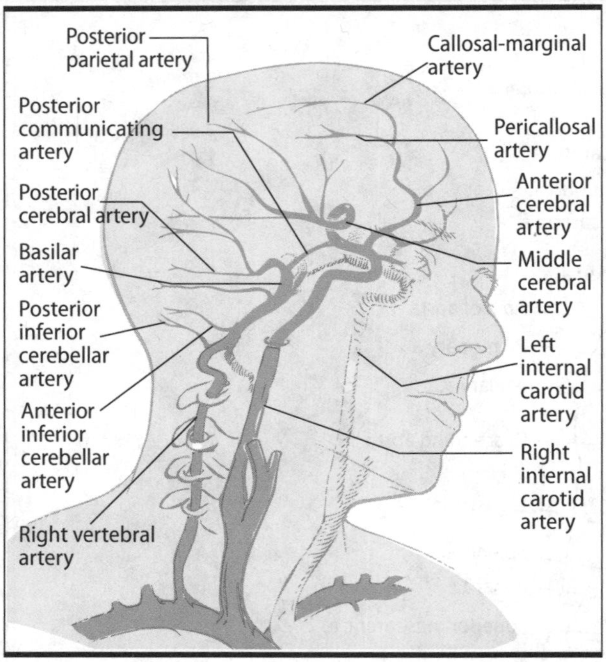
Posterior parietal artery
Callosal-marginal artery
Posterior communicating artery
Pericallosal artery
Posterior cerebral artery
Anterior cerebral artery
Basilar artery
Middle cerebral artery
Posterior inferior cerebellar artery
Left internal carotid artery
Anterior inferior cerebellar artery
Right internal carotid artery
Right vertebral artery

External Carotid Arteries and Branches

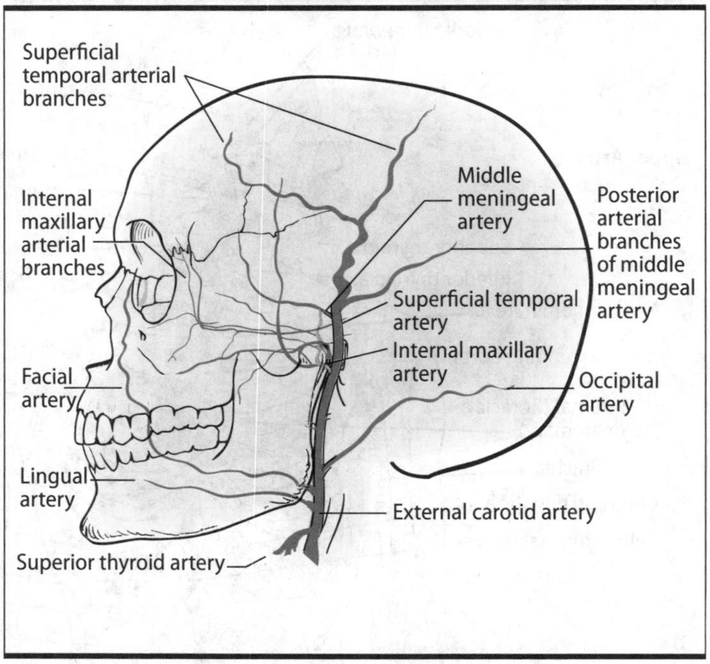
Superficial temporal arterial branches
Middle meningeal artery
Posterior arterial branches of middle meningeal artery
Internal maxillary arterial branches
Superficial temporal artery
Internal maxillary artery
Facial artery
Occipital artery
Lingual artery
External carotid artery
Superior thyroid artery

Upper Extremity Arteries

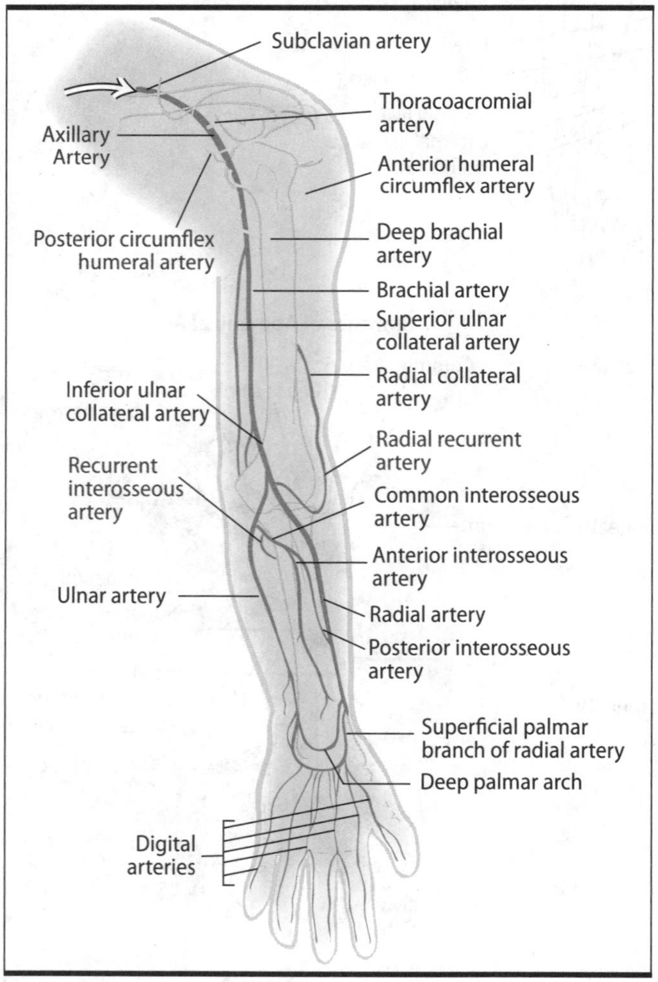
Subclavian artery
Thoracoacromial artery
Axillary Artery
Anterior humeral circumflex artery
Posterior circumflex humeral artery
Deep brachial artery
Brachial artery
Superior ulnar collateral artery
Radial collateral artery
Inferior ulnar collateral artery
Radial recurrent artery
Recurrent interosseous artery
Common interosseous artery
Anterior interosseous artery
Ulnar artery
Radial artery
Posterior interosseous artery
Superficial palmar branch of radial artery
Deep palmar arch
Digital arteries

Lower Extremity Arteries

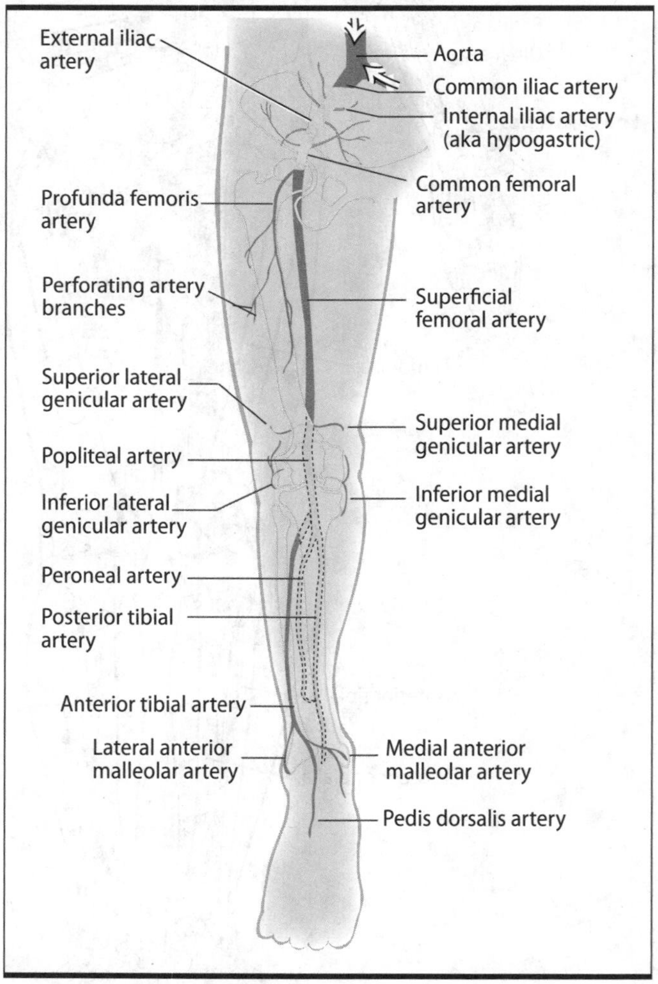
External iliac artery
Aorta
Common iliac artery
Internal iliac artery (aka hypogastric)
Common femoral artery
Profunda femoris artery
Perforating artery branches
Superficial femoral artery
Superior lateral genicular artery
Superior medial genicular artery
Popliteal artery
Inferior lateral genicular artery
Inferior medial genicular artery
Peroneal artery
Posterior tibial artery
Anterior tibial artery
Lateral anterior malleolar artery
Medial anterior malleolar artery
Pedis dorsalis artery

Venous System

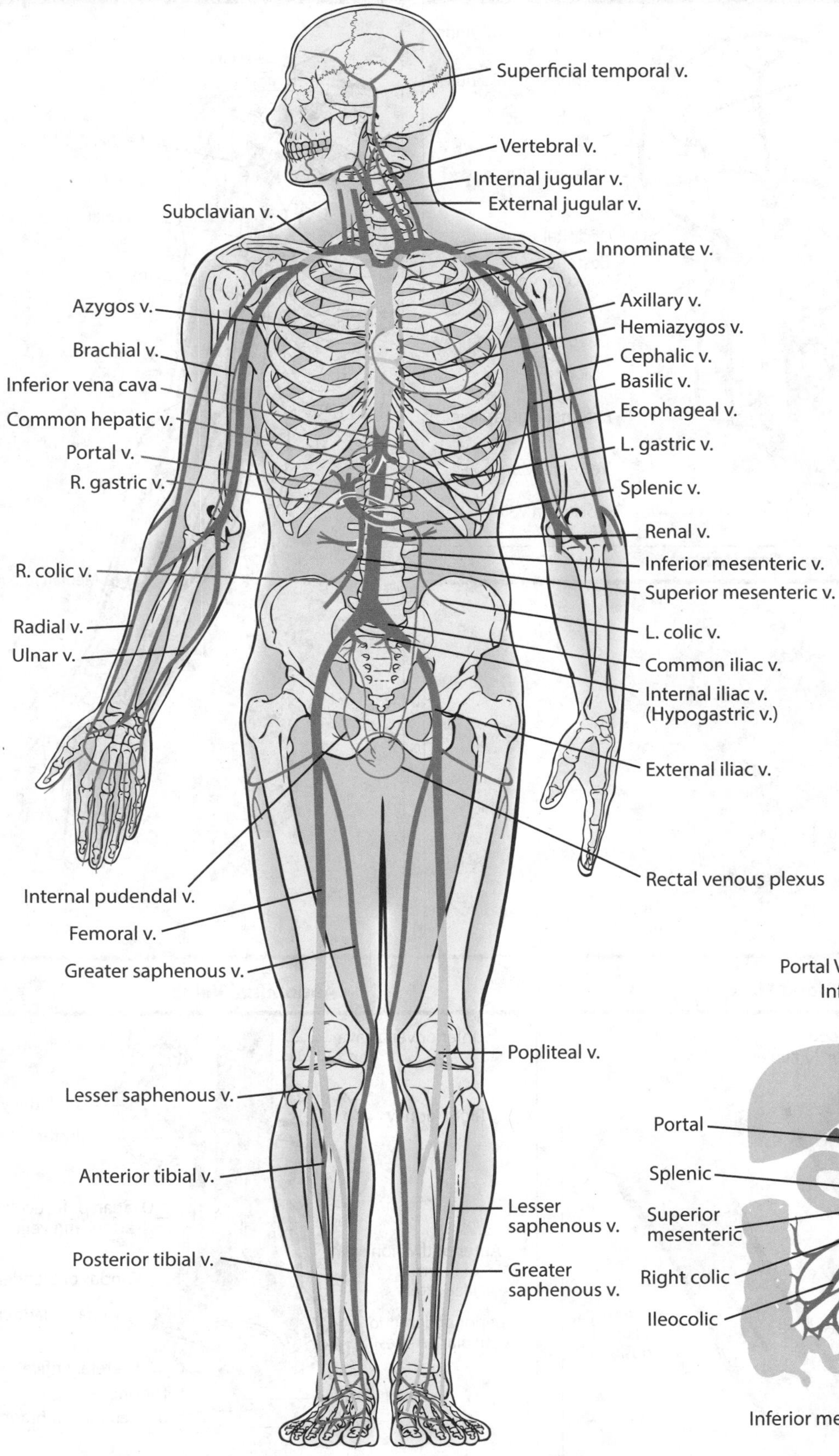
Superficial temporal v.
Vertebral v.
Internal jugular v.
External jugular v.
Subclavian v.
Innominate v.
Azygos v.
Axillary v.
Hemiazygos v.
Brachial v.
Cephalic v.
Inferior vena cava
Basilic v.
Esophageal v.
Common hepatic v.
Portal v.
L. gastric v.
R. gastric v.
Splenic v.
Renal v.
Inferior mesenteric v.
R. colic v.
Superior mesenteric v.
Radial v.
L. colic v.
Ulnar v.
Common iliac v.
Internal iliac v.
(Hypogastric v.)
External iliac v.
Rectal venous plexus
Internal pudendal v.
Femoral v.
Greater saphenous v.
Popliteal v.
Lesser saphenous v.
Anterior tibial v.
Lesser saphenous v.
Posterior tibial v.
Greater saphenous v.

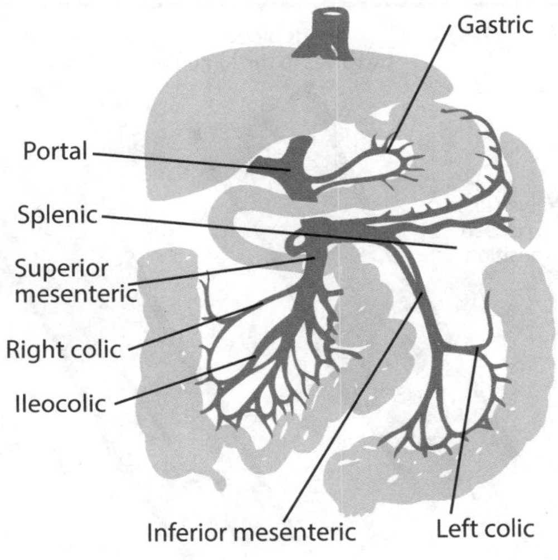
Portal Venous Circulation
Inferior vena cava
Gastric
Portal
Splenic
Superior mesenteric
Right colic
Ileocolic
Inferior mesenteric
Left colic

Head and Neck Veins

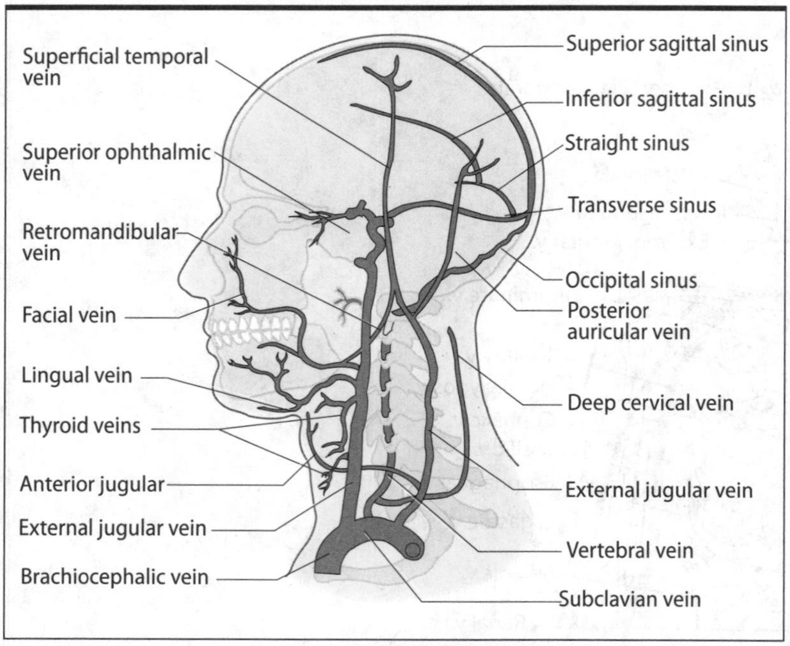
Superficial temporal vein
Superior sagittal sinus
Inferior sagittal sinus
Superior ophthalmic vein
Straight sinus
Transverse sinus
Retromandibular vein
Occipital sinus
Posterior auricular vein
Facial vein
Lingual vein
Deep cervical vein
Thyroid veins
Anterior jugular
External jugular vein
External jugular vein
Vertebral vein
Brachiocephalic vein
Subclavian vein

Upper Extremity Veins

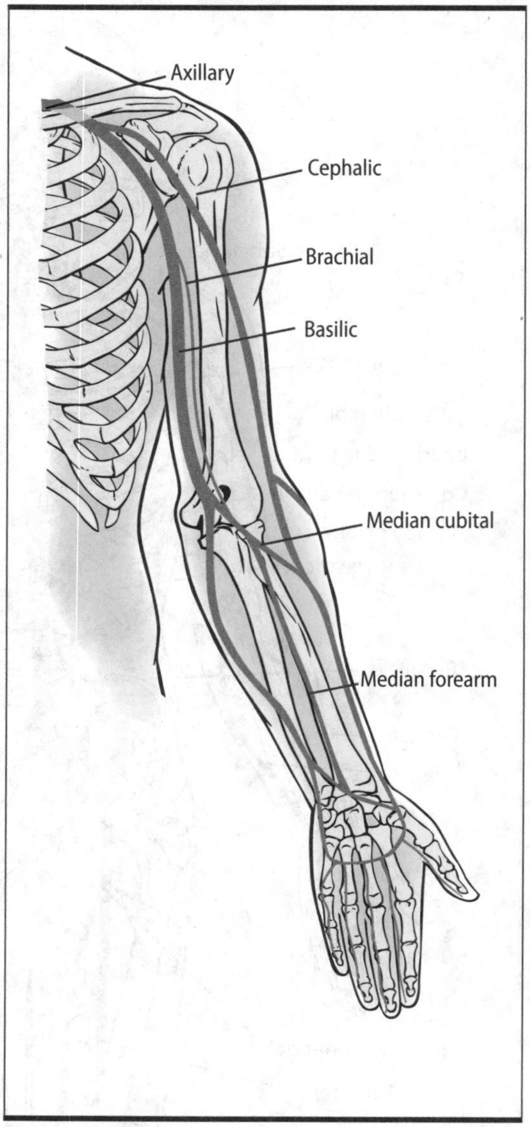
Axillary
Cephalic
Brachial
Basilic
Median cubital
Median forearm

Venae Comitantes

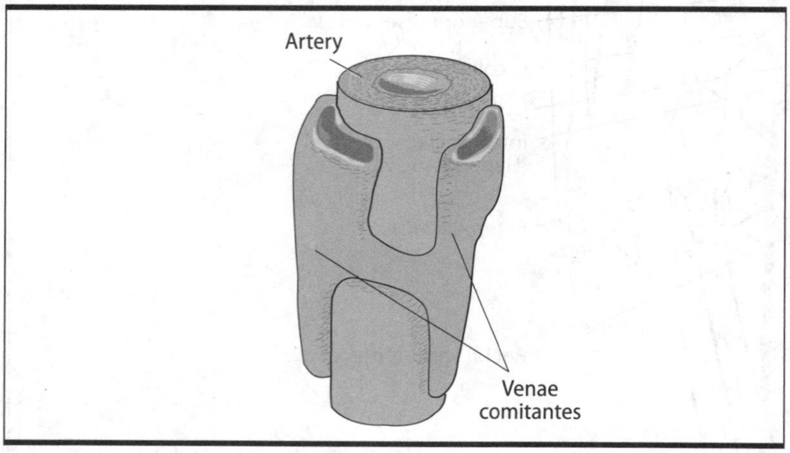
Artery
Venae comitantes

Venous Blood Flow

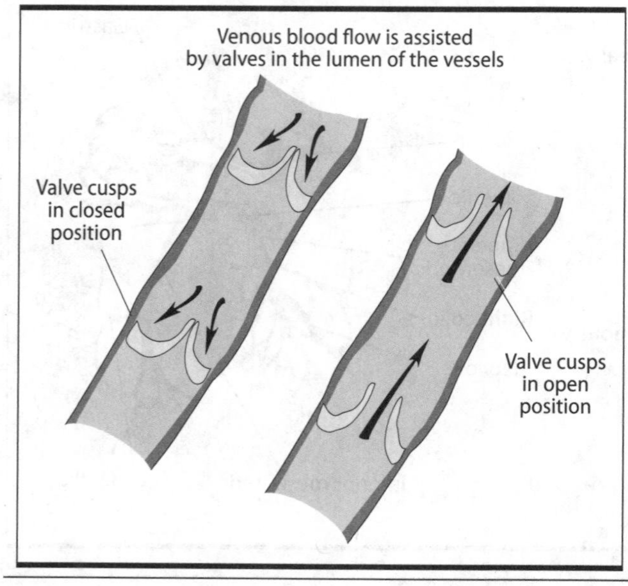
Venous blood flow is assisted by valves in the lumen of the vessels
Valve cusps in closed position
Valve cusps in open position

Abdominal Veins

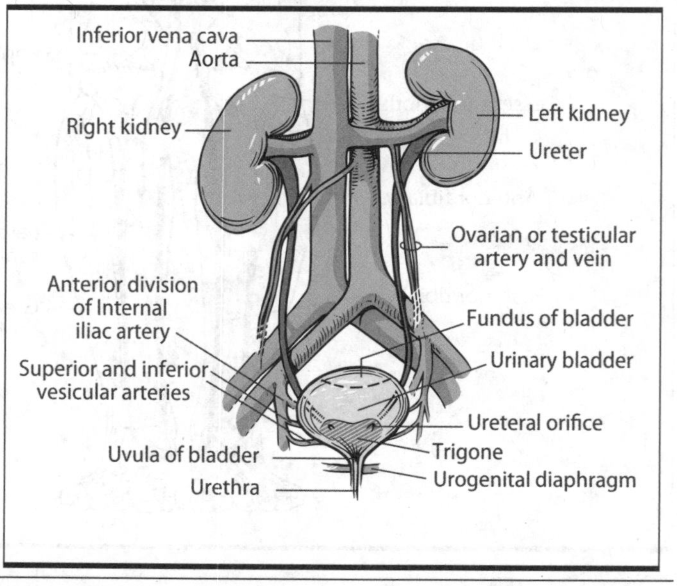
Inferior vena cava
Aorta
Right kidney
Left kidney
Ureter
Ovarian or testicular artery and vein
Anterior division of Internal iliac artery
Fundus of bladder
Superior and inferior vesicular arteries
Urinary bladder
Ureteral orifice
Uvula of bladder
Trigone
Urethra
Urogenital diaphragm

Cardiovascular System

Coronary Veins

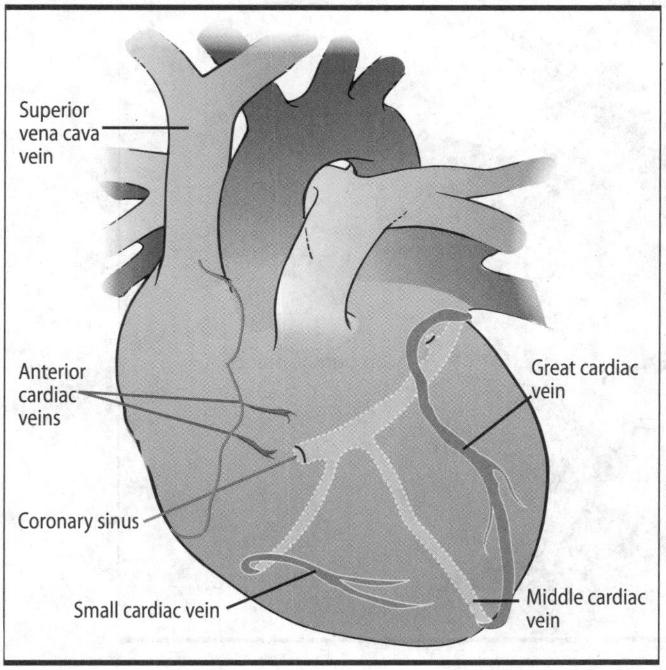

Anatomy of the Heart

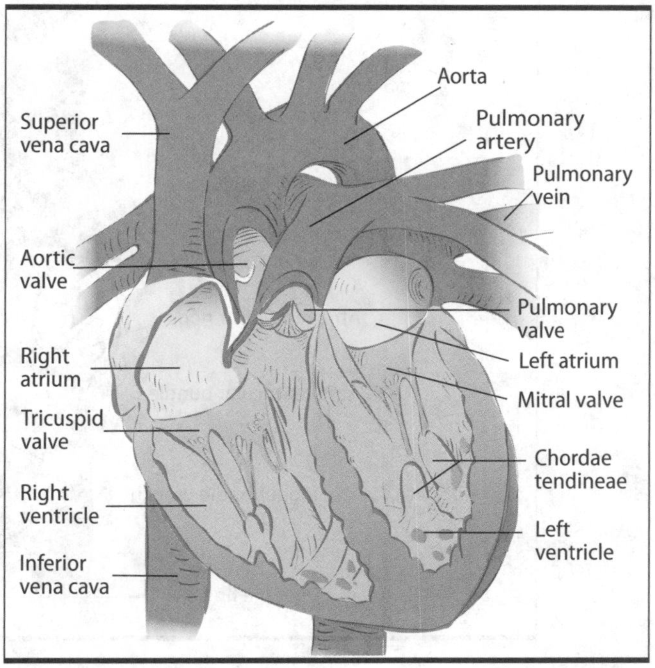

Heart Cross Section

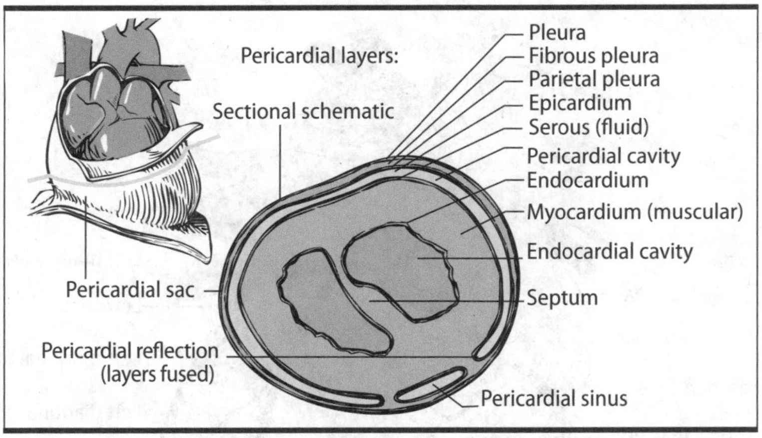

Heart Valves

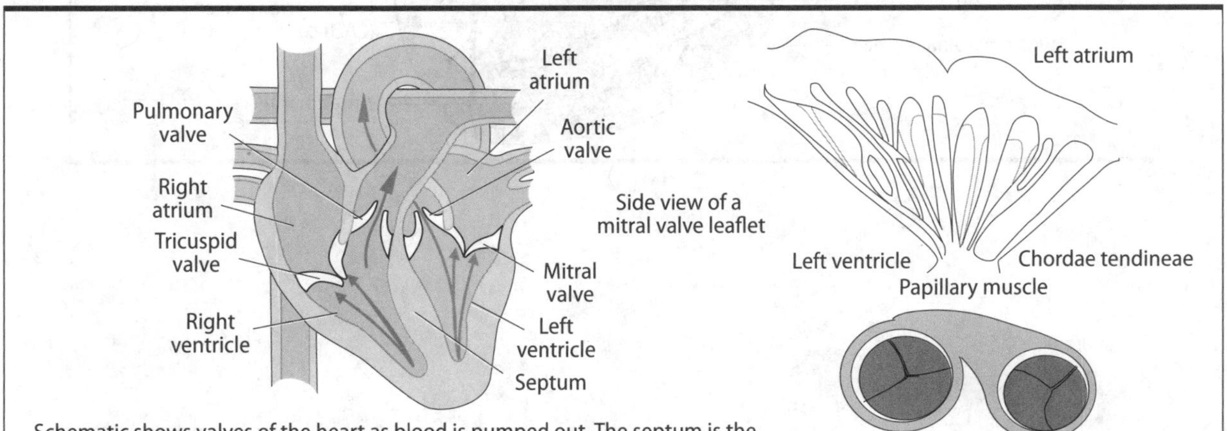

Schematic shows valves of the heart as blood is pumped out. The septum is the wall dividing the left and right ventricles. The papillary muscles and chordae tendineae (above right) function to open and close the atrioventricular valves

Overhead view of aortic (left) and pulmonary valves while closed

Heart Conduction System

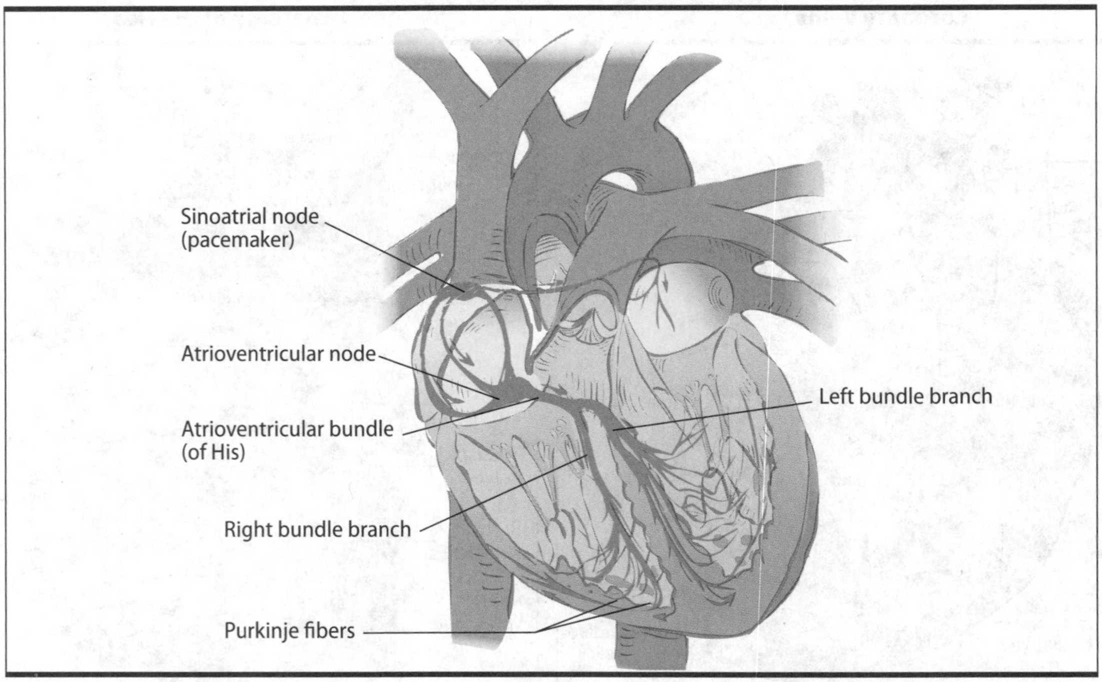
Sinoatrial node
(pacemaker)
Atrioventricular node
Atrioventricular bundle
(of His)
Right bundle branch
Purkinje fibers
Left bundle branch

Coronary Arteries

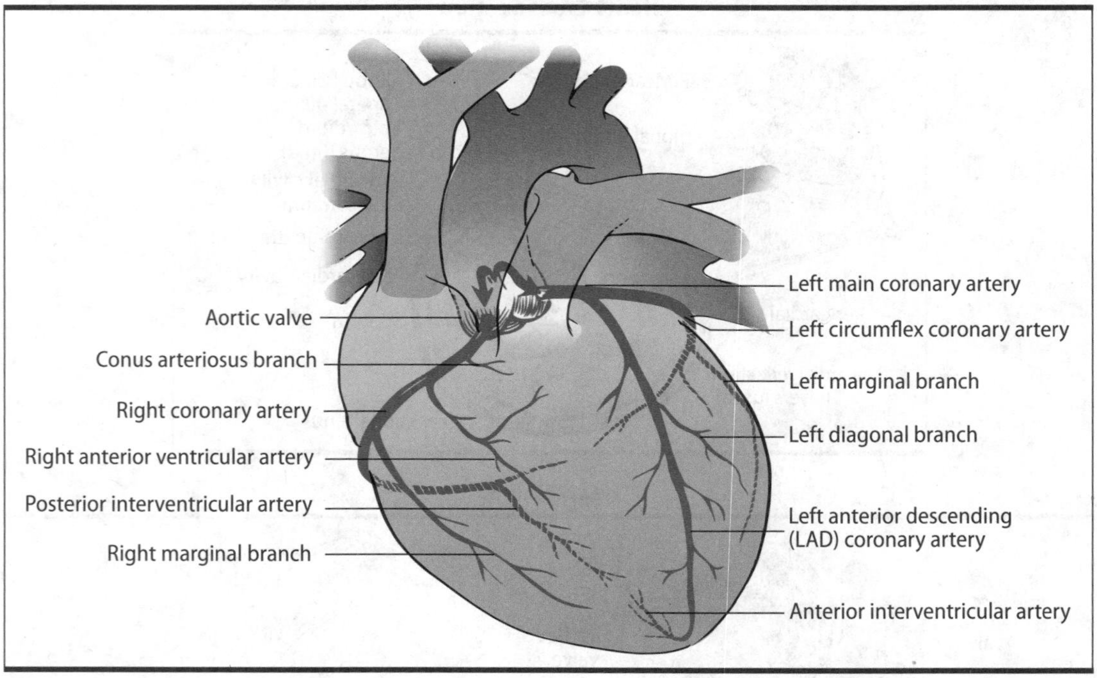
Aortic valve
Conus arteriosus branch
Right coronary artery
Right anterior ventricular artery
Posterior interventricular artery
Right marginal branch
Left main coronary artery
Left circumflex coronary artery
Left marginal branch
Left diagonal branch
Left anterior descending
(LAD) coronary artery
Anterior interventricular artery

Lymphatic System

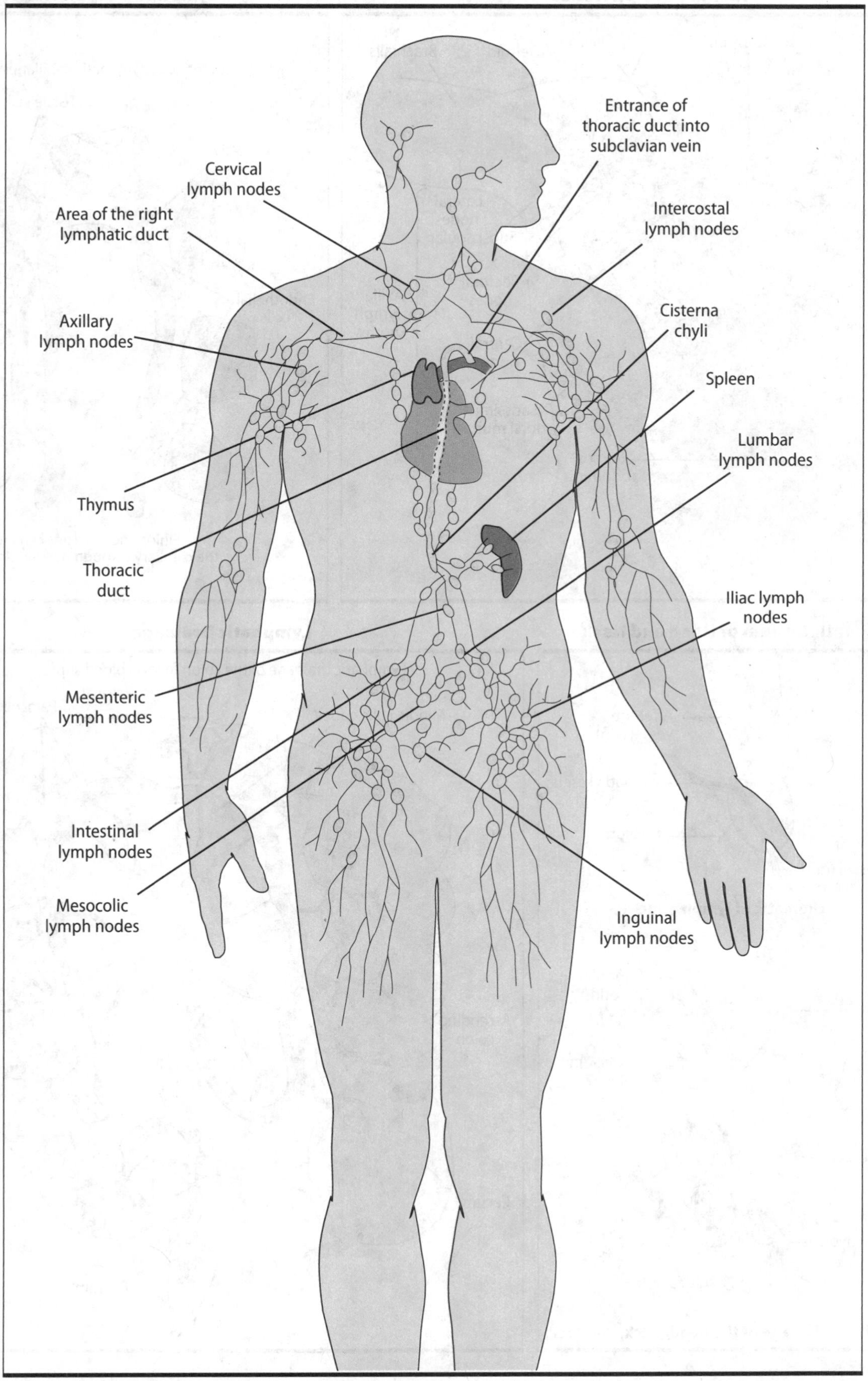

Axillary Lymph Nodes

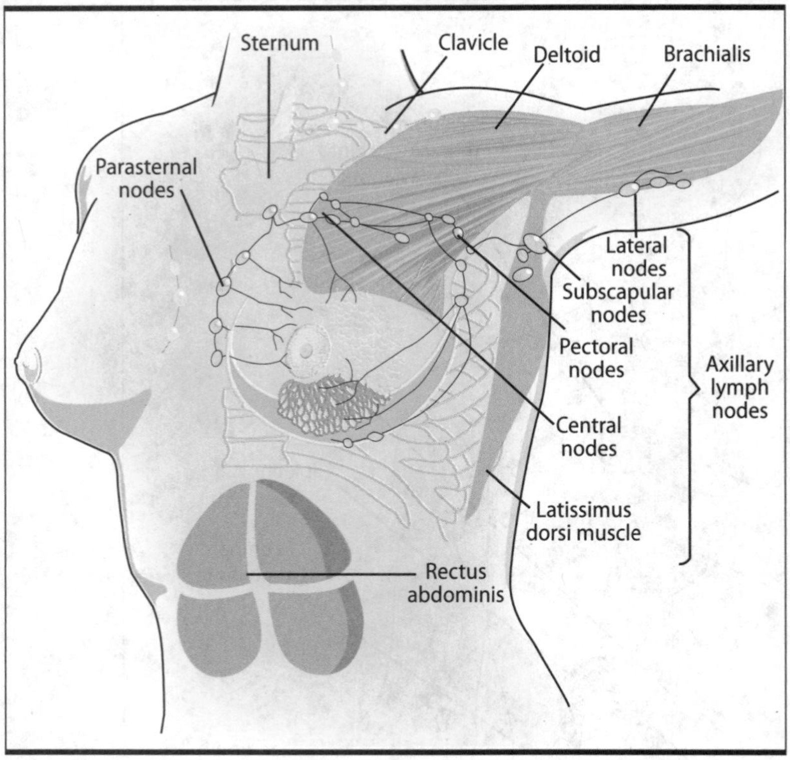

Lymphatic Capillaries

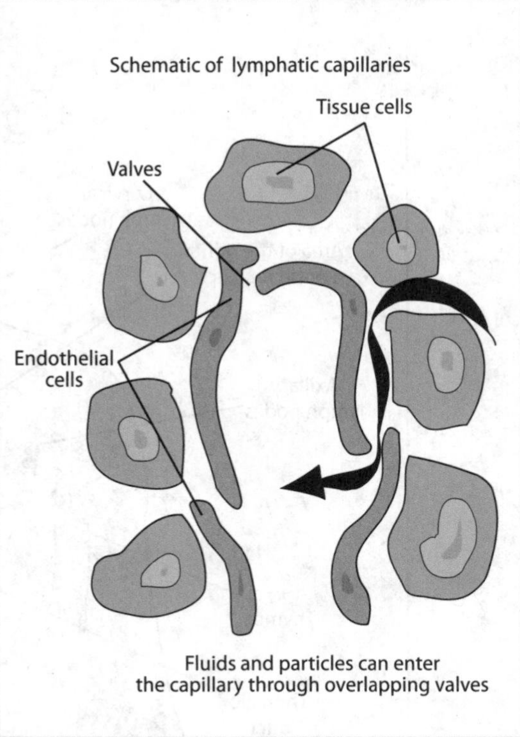

Lymphatic System of Head and Neck

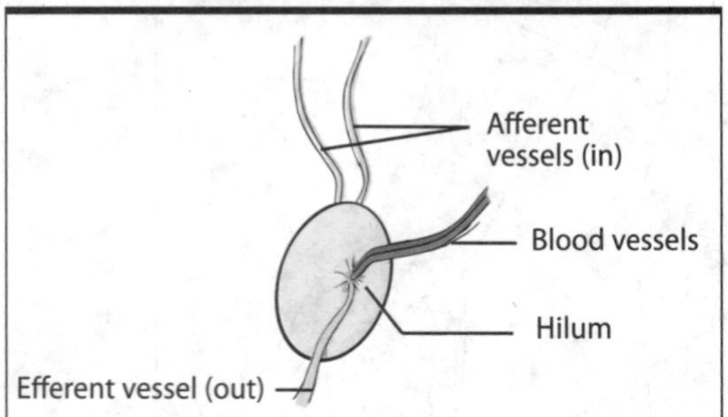

Schematic of lymph node

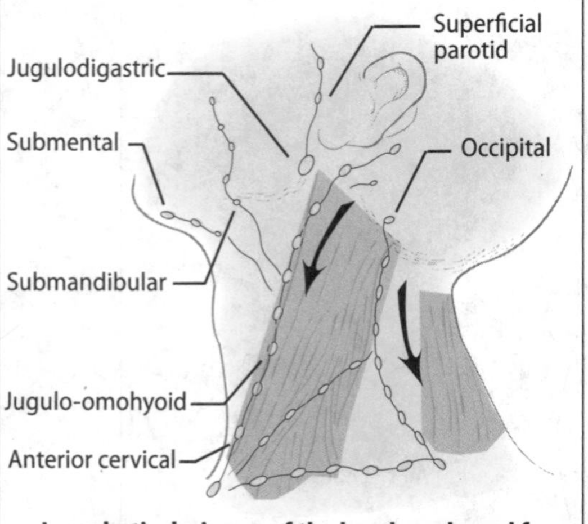

Lymphatic drainage of the head, neck, and face

Lymphatic Drainage

Lymphatic drainage of the colon follows blood supply

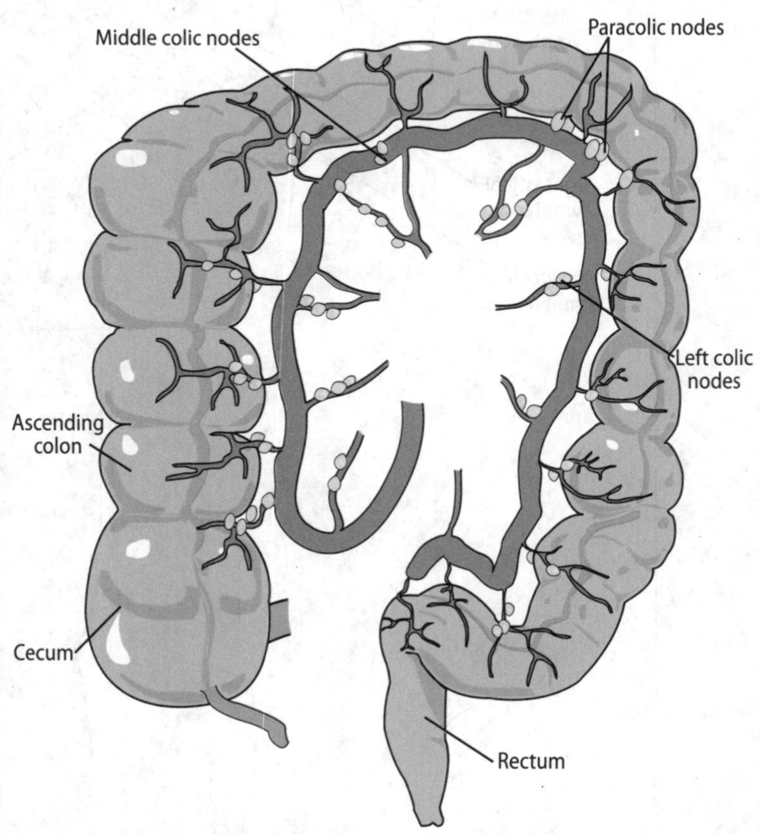

Spleen Internal Structures

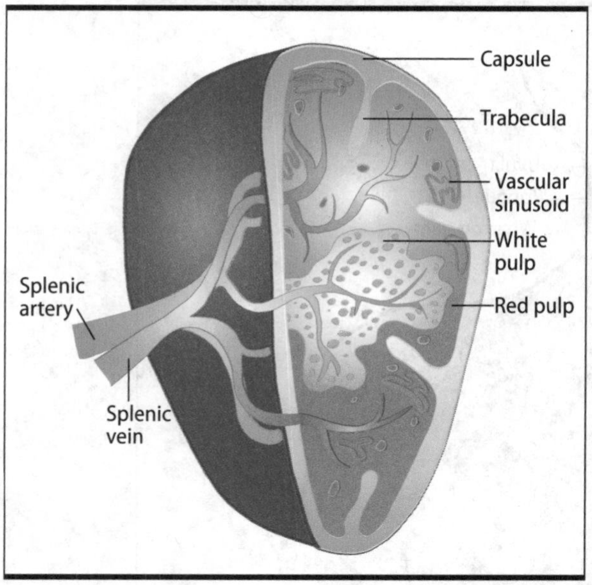

Spleen External Structures

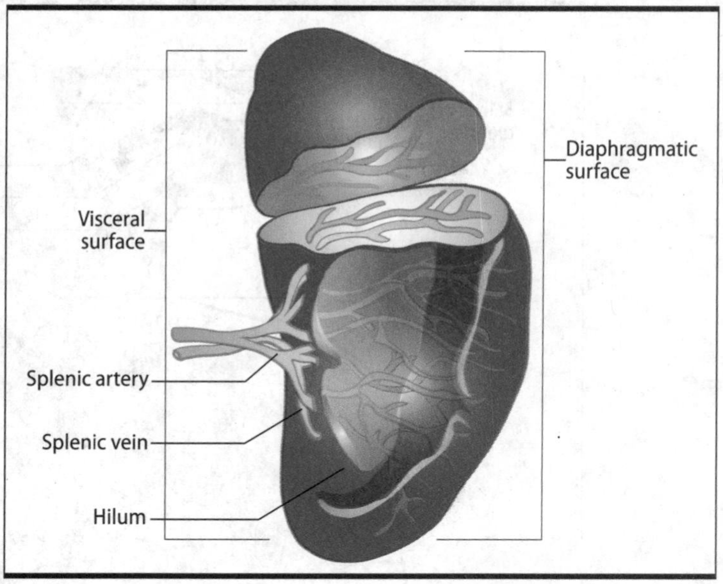

Anatomical Illustrations—Lymphatic System

Digestive System

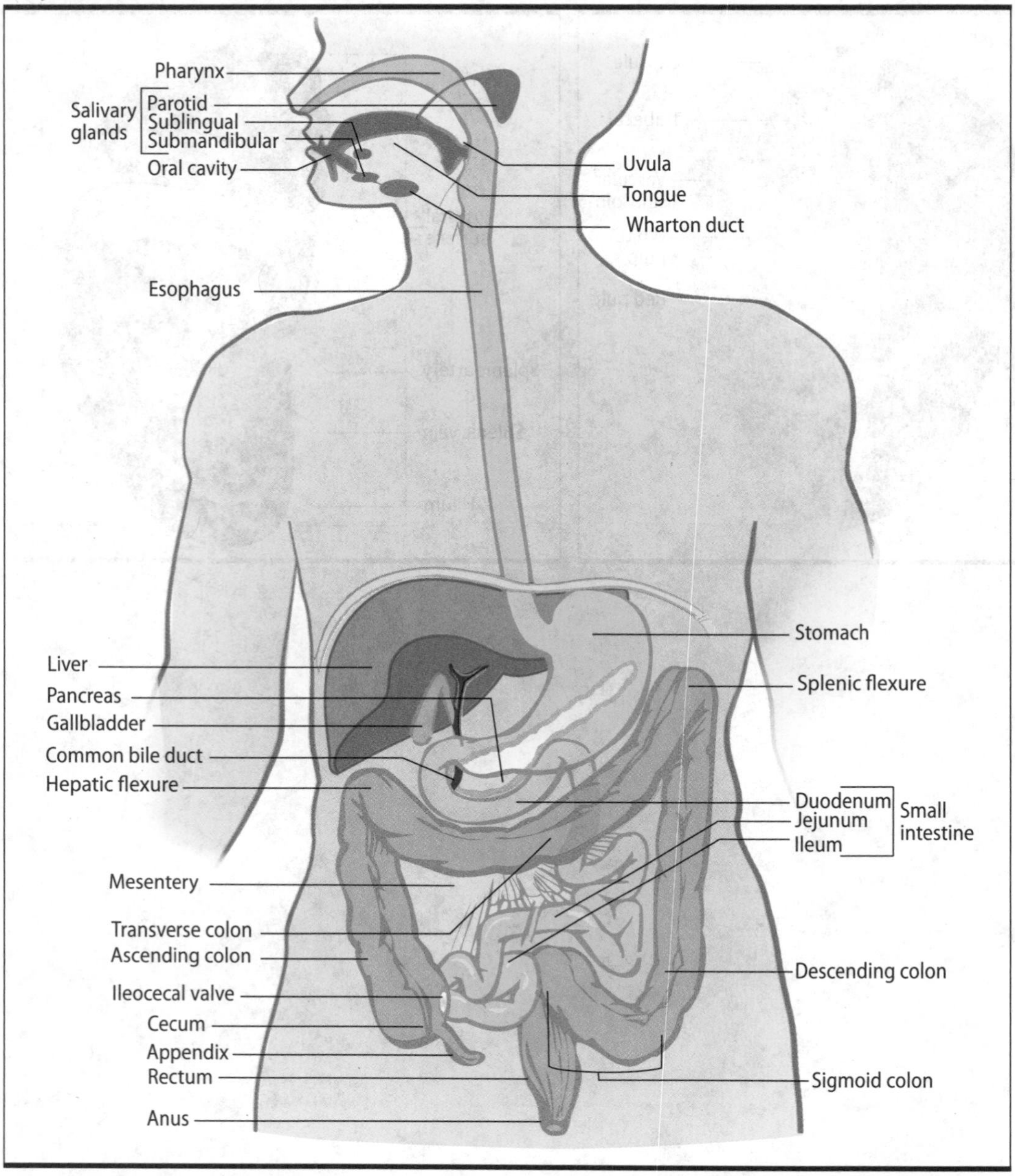
Pharynx
Salivary glands
Parotid
Sublingual
Submandibular
Oral cavity
Uvula
Tongue
Wharton duct
Esophagus
Stomach
Liver
Splenic flexure
Pancreas
Gallbladder
Common bile duct
Hepatic flexure
Duodenum
Jejunum
Ileum
Small intestine
Mesentery
Transverse colon
Ascending colon
Descending colon
Ileocecal valve
Cecum
Appendix
Rectum
Sigmoid colon
Anus

Gallbladder

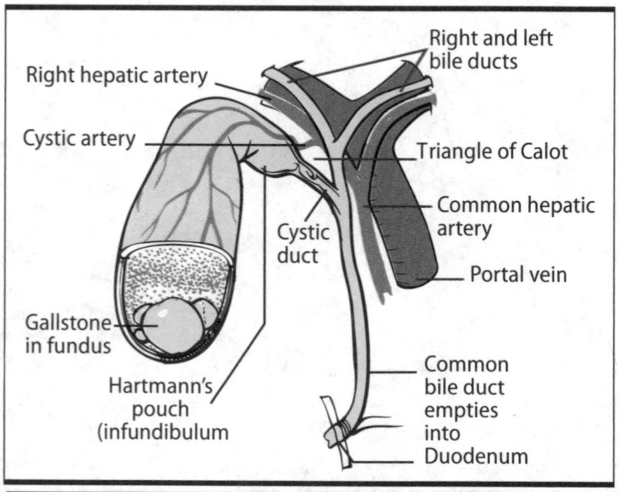
Right and left bile ducts
Right hepatic artery
Cystic artery
Triangle of Calot
Common hepatic artery
Cystic duct
Portal vein
Gallstone in fundus
Hartmann's pouch (infundibulum
Common bile duct empties into Duodenum

Stomach

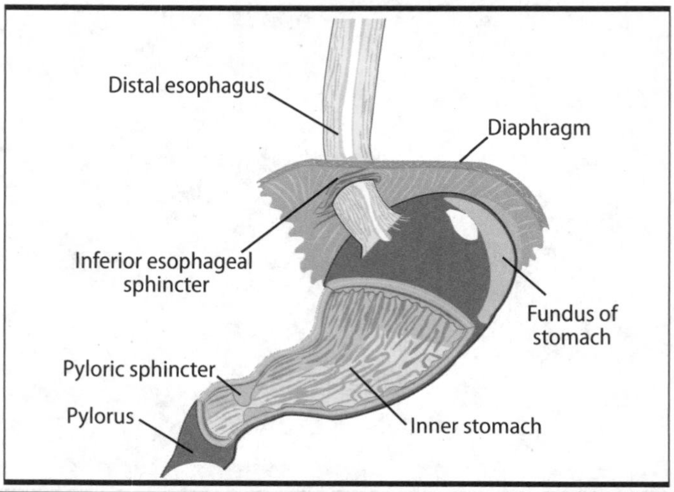
Distal esophagus
Diaphragm
Inferior esophageal sphincter
Fundus of stomach
Pyloric sphincter
Pylorus
Inner stomach

Mouth (Upper)

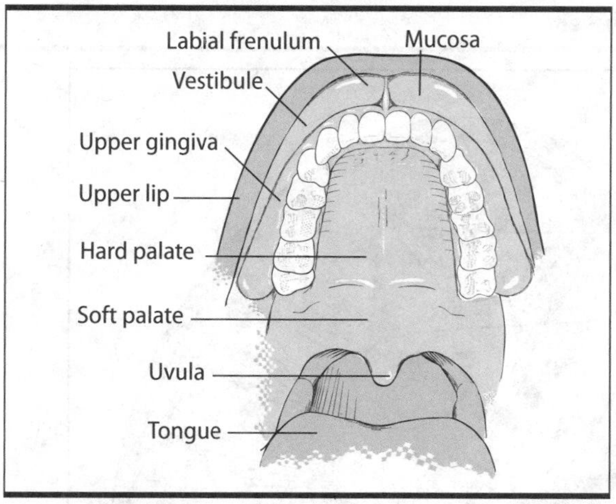

Mouth (Lower)

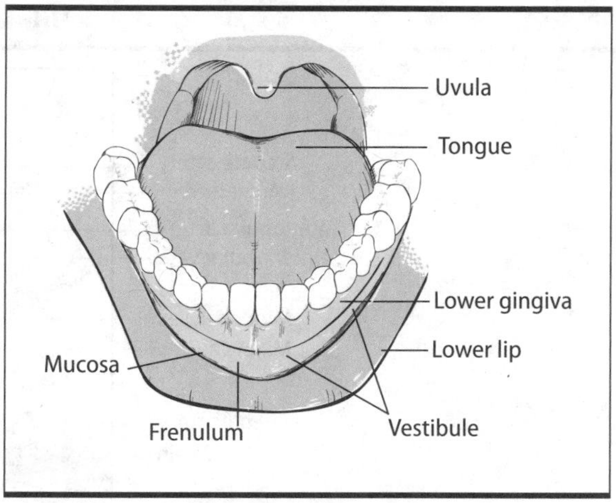

Pancreas

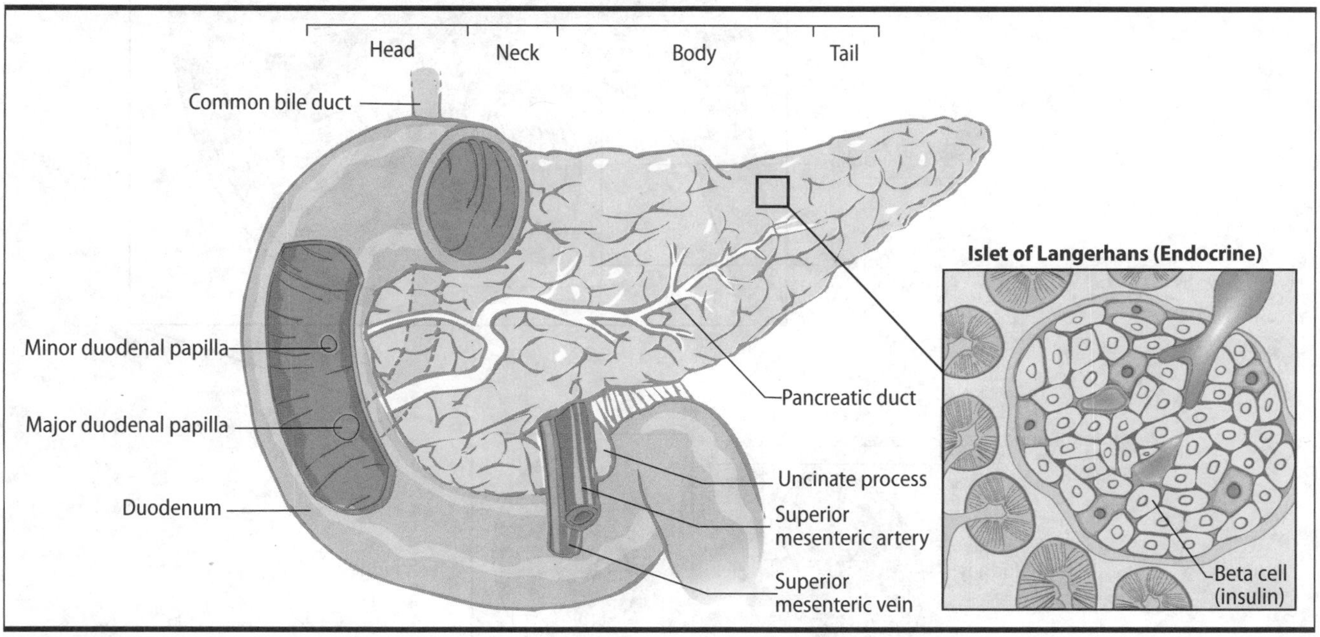

Liver

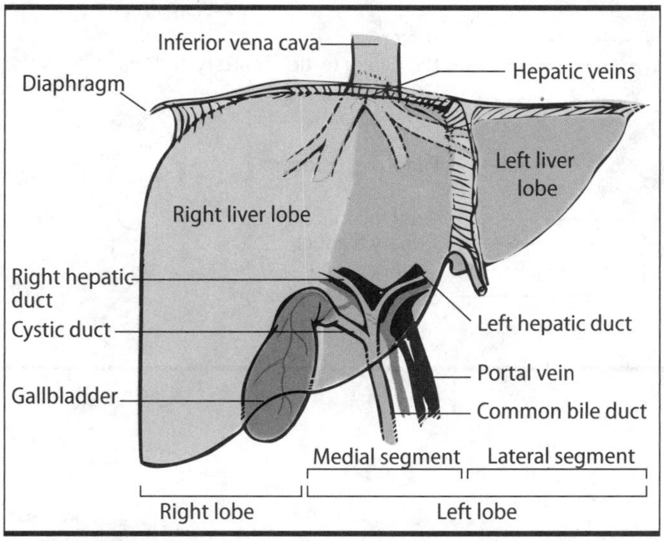

Anus

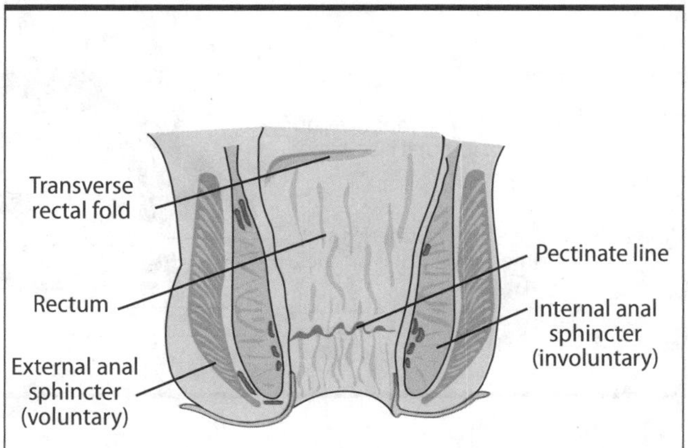

Detail cutaway of lower rectum and anus

Genitourinary System

Urinary System

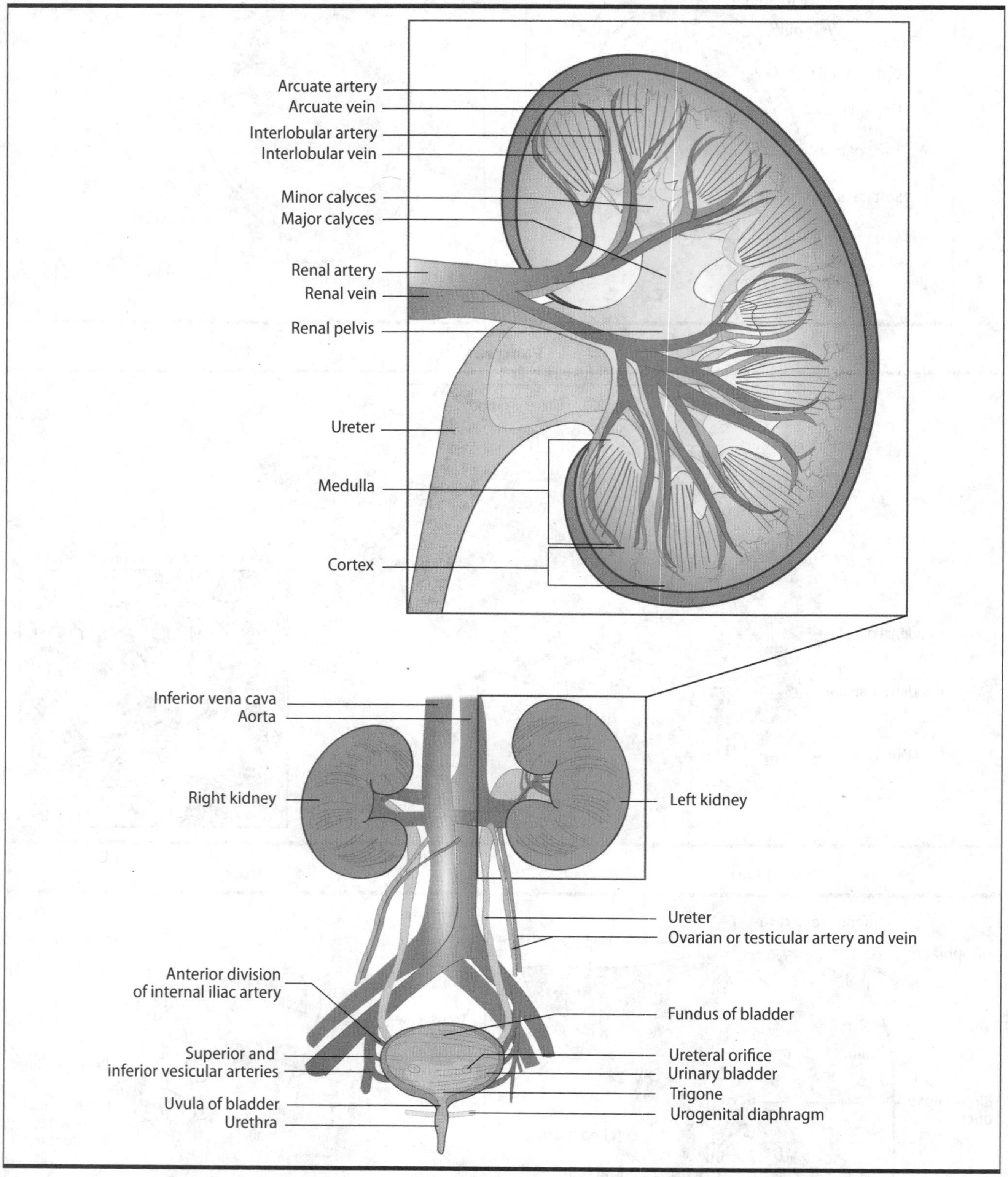
Arcuate artery
Arcuate vein
Interlobular artery
Interlobular vein
Minor calyces
Major calyces
Renal artery
Renal vein
Renal pelvis
Ureter
Medulla
Cortex
Inferior vena cava
Aorta
Right kidney
Left kidney
Ureter
Ovarian or testicular artery and vein
Anterior division
of internal iliac artery
Fundus of bladder
Superior and
inferior vesicular arteries
Ureteral orifice
Urinary bladder
Trigone
Uvula of bladder
Urethra
Urogenital diaphragm

Nephron

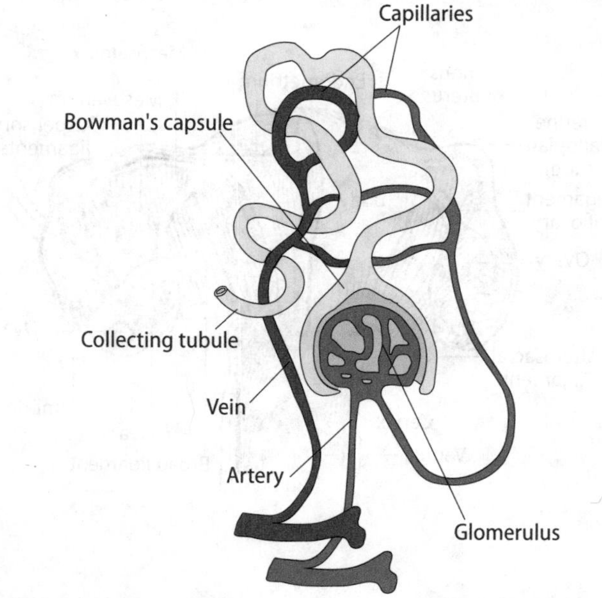

Schematic of nephron, the tiny filtering mechanism of the kidney

Male Genitourinary

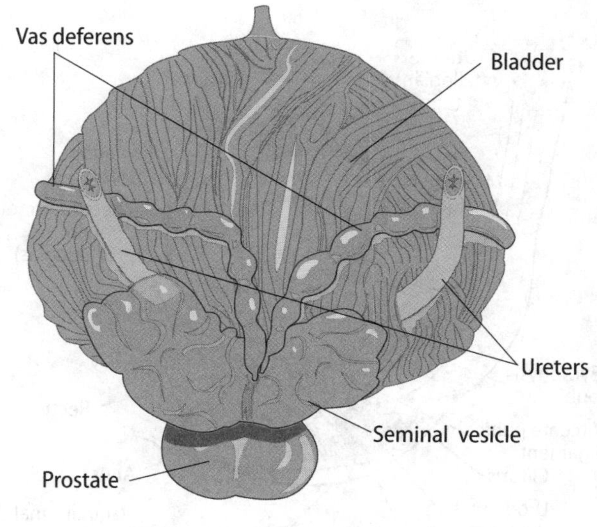

Posterior view of male bladder and prostate

Testis and Associate Structures

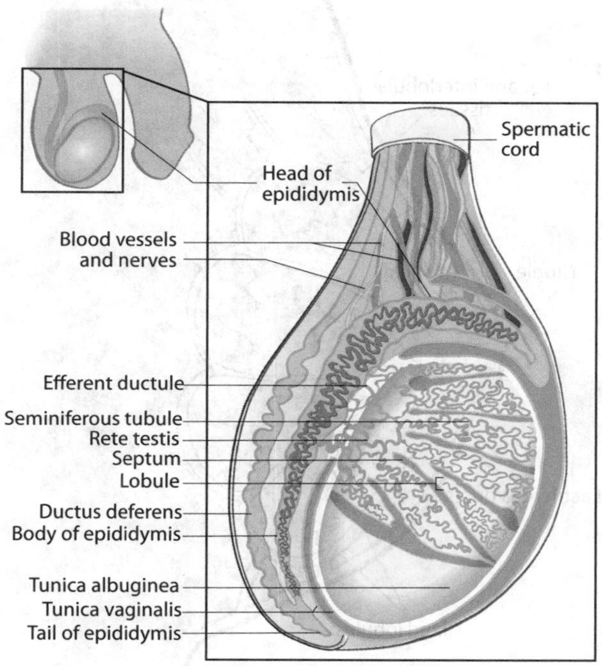

Male Genitourinary System

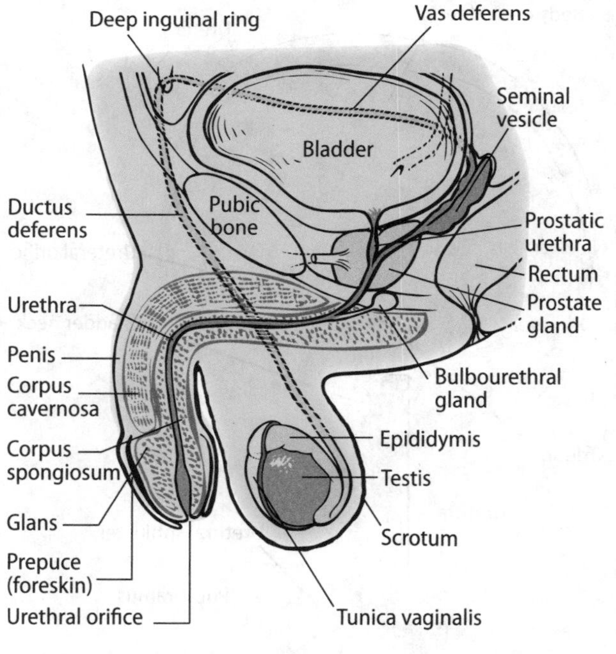

Female Genitourinary

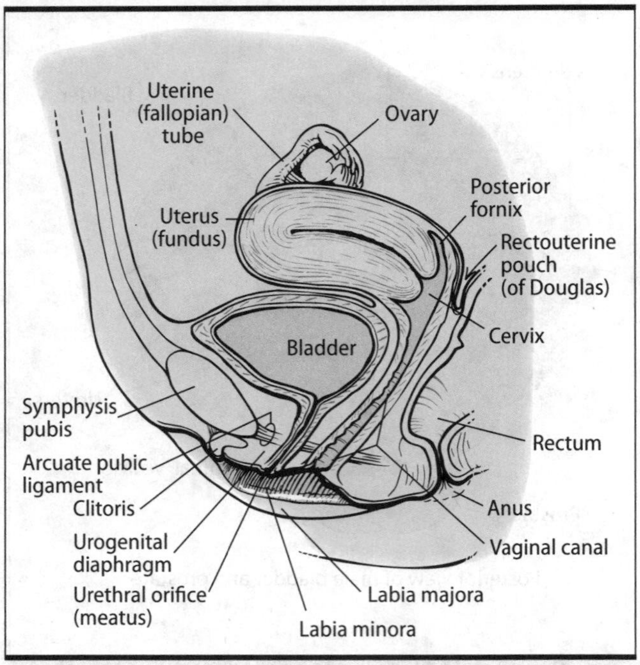

Female Reproductive System

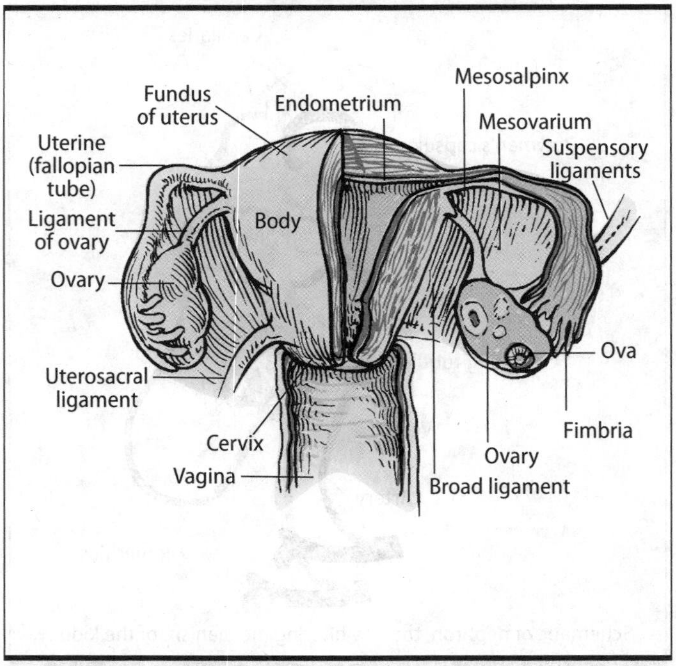

Female Bladder

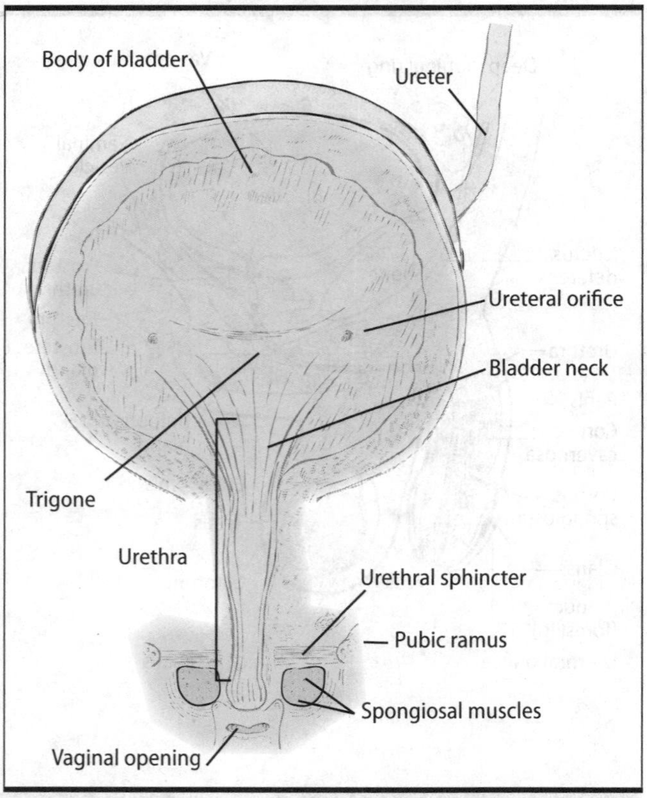

Female Breast

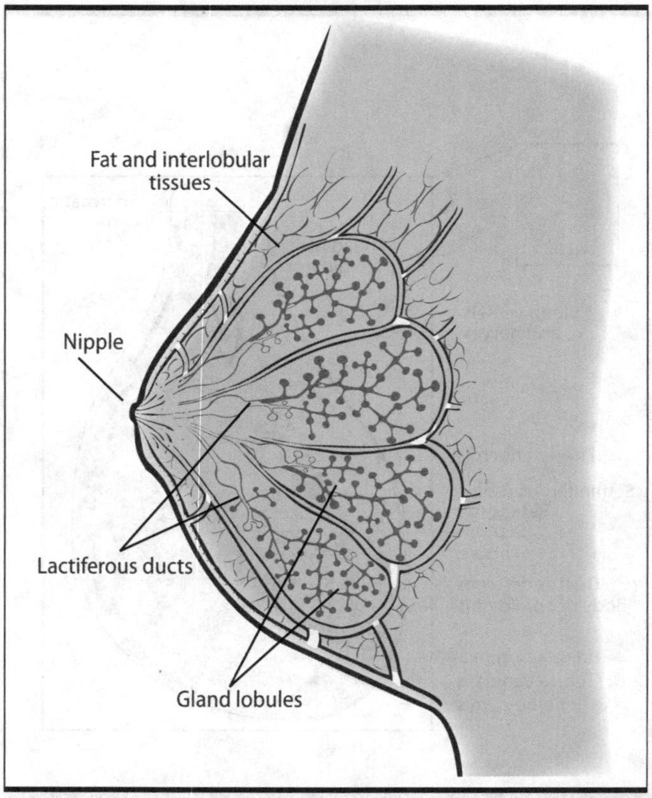

Endocrine System

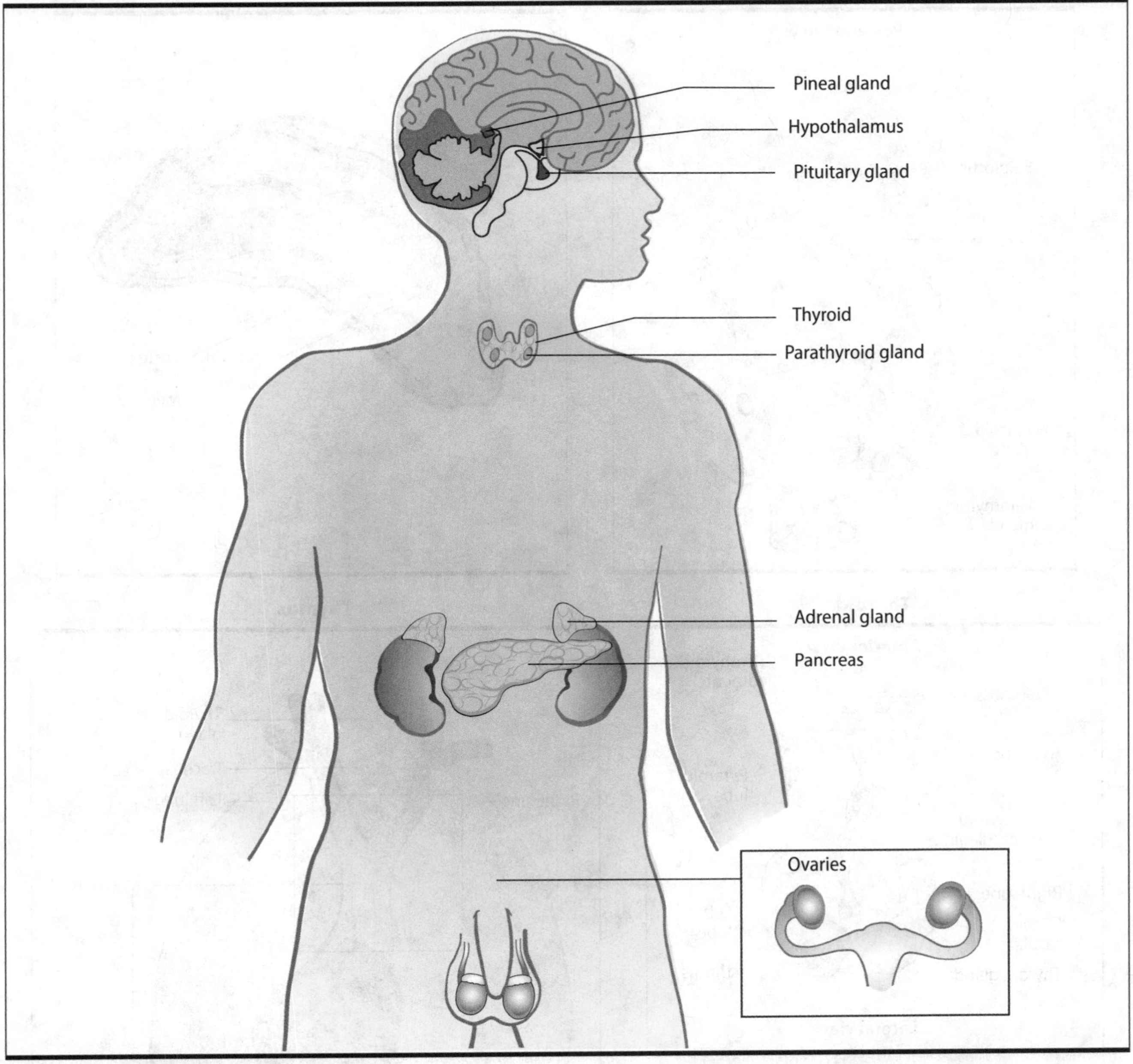

Structure of an Ovary

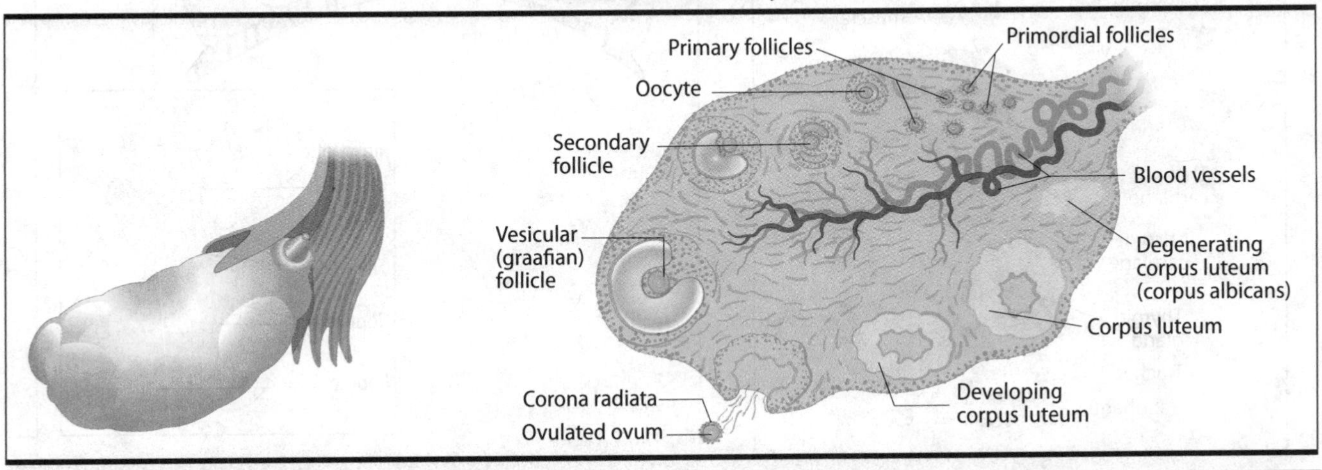

Thyroid and Parathyroid Glands

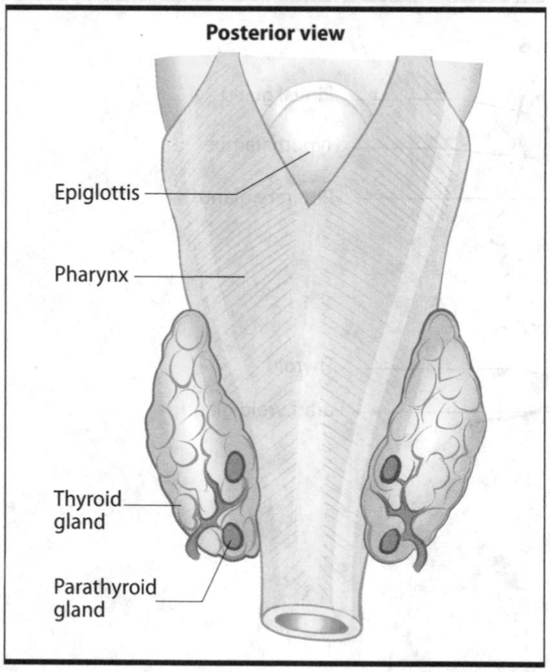

Adrenal Gland

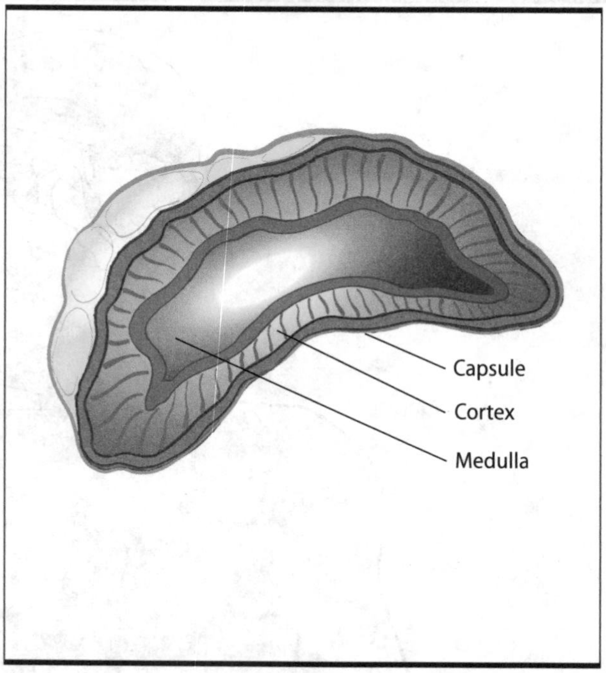

Thyroid

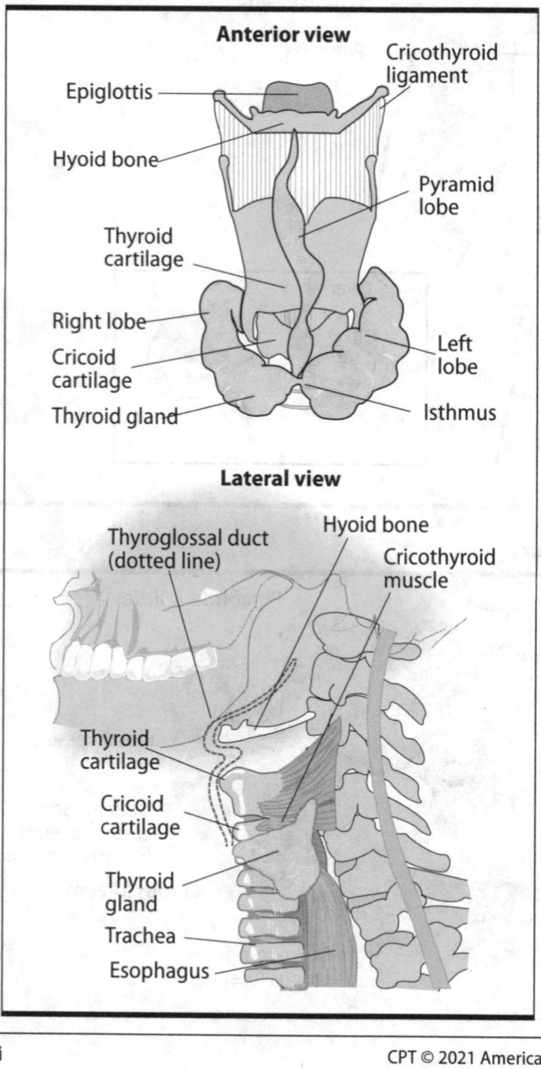

Thymus

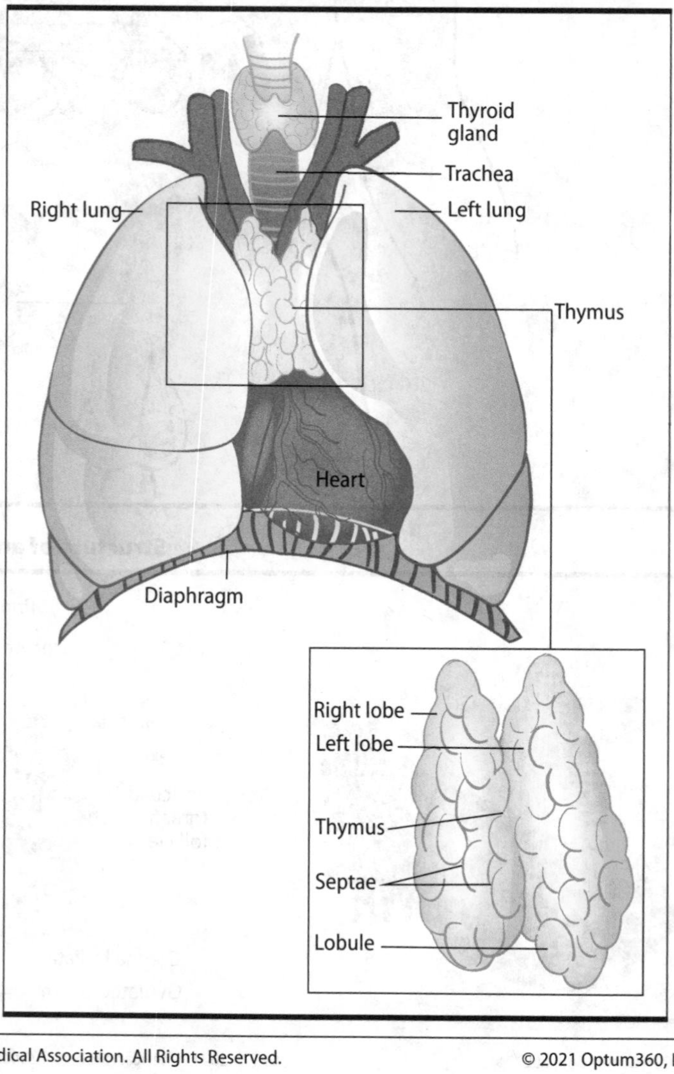

Nervous System

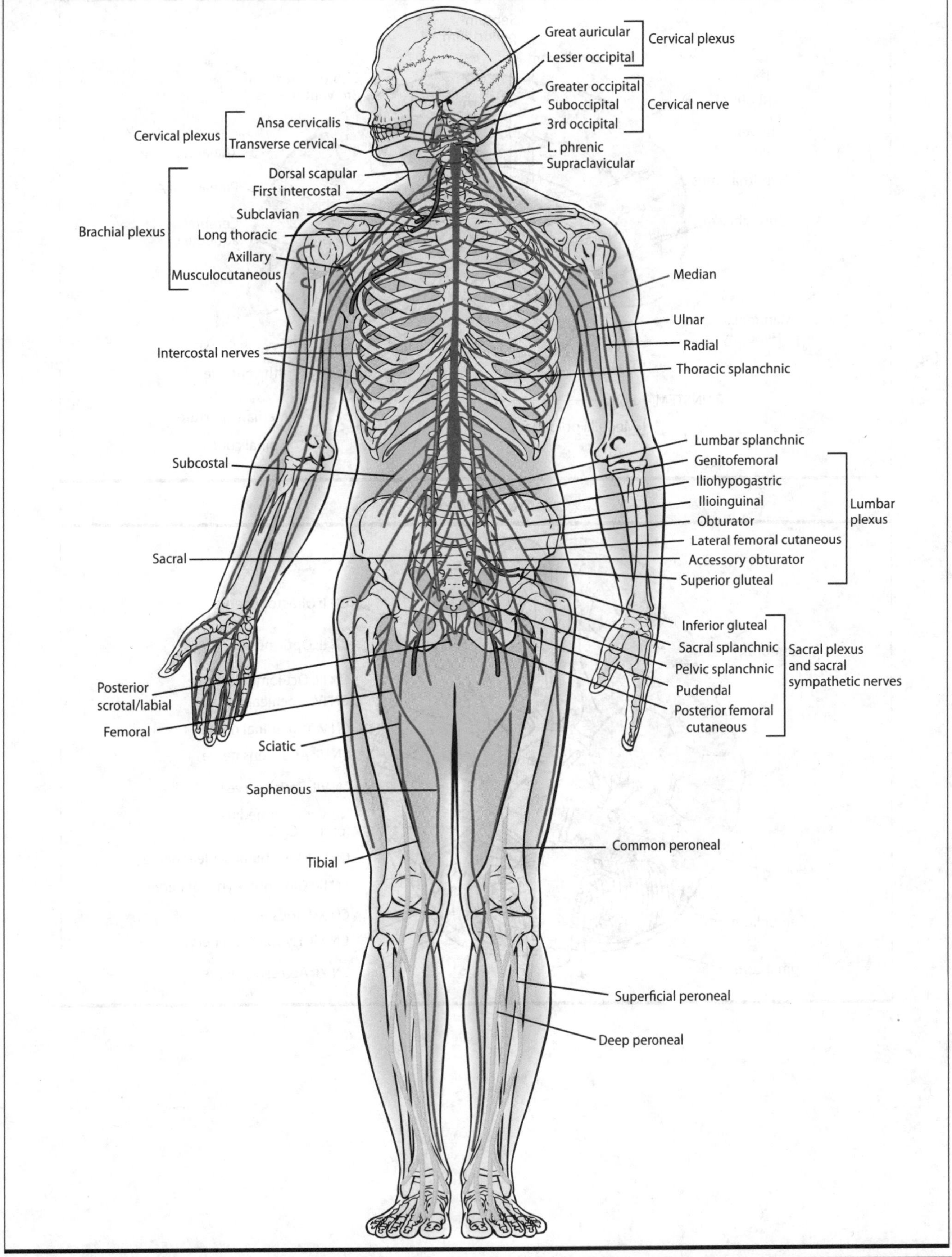

Brain

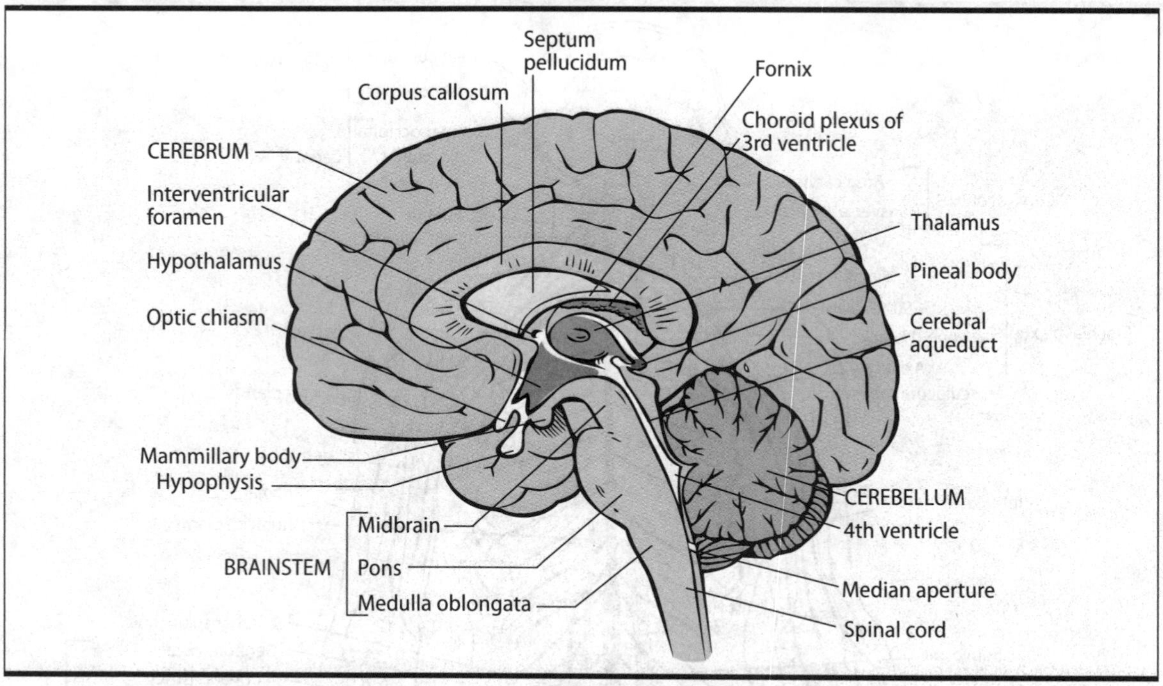
Septum pellucidum
Fornix
Corpus callosum
Choroid plexus of 3rd ventricle
CEREBRUM
Interventricular foramen
Thalamus
Hypothalamus
Pineal body
Optic chiasm
Cerebral aqueduct
Mammillary body
Hypophysis
CEREBELLUM
Midbrain
4th ventricle
BRAINSTEM
Pons
Median aperture
Medulla oblongata
Spinal cord

Cranial Nerves

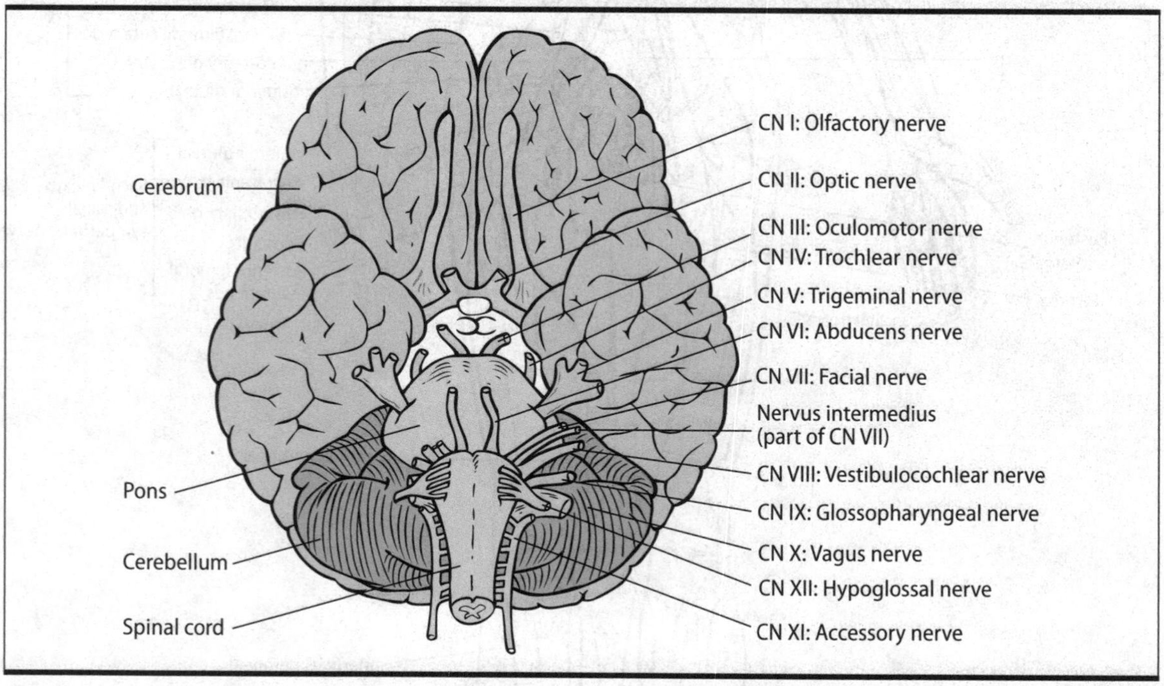
CN I: Olfactory nerve
Cerebrum
CN II: Optic nerve
CN III: Oculomotor nerve
CN IV: Trochlear nerve
CN V: Trigeminal nerve
CN VI: Abducens nerve
CN VII: Facial nerve
Nervus intermedius (part of CN VII)
Pons
CN VIII: Vestibulocochlear nerve
CN IX: Glossopharyngeal nerve
CN X: Vagus nerve
Cerebellum
CN XII: Hypoglossal nerve
Spinal cord
CN XI: Accessory nerve

Spinal Cord and Spinal Nerves

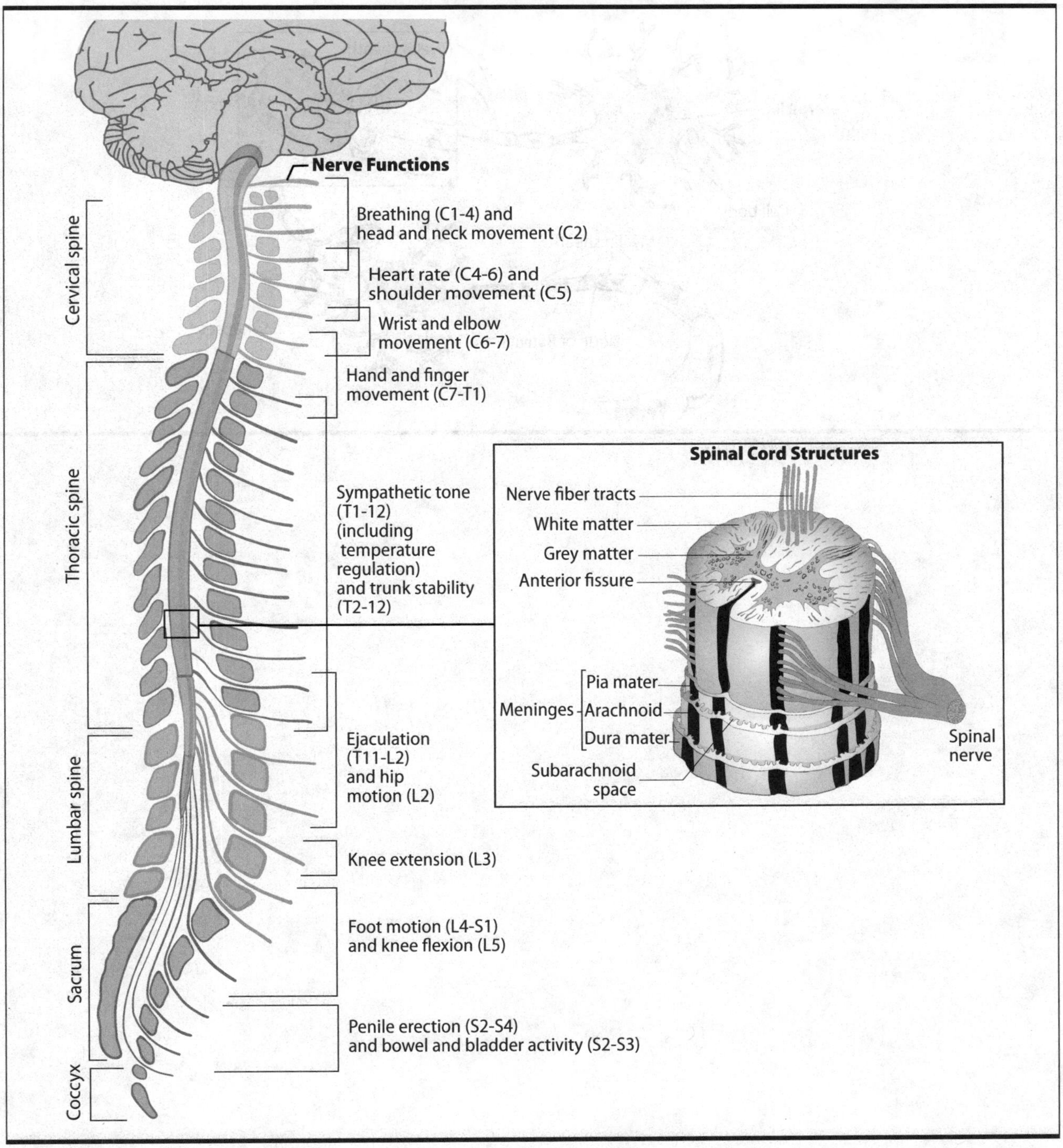
Nerve Functions
Cervical spine
Thoracic spine
Lumbar spine
Sacrum
Coccyx
Breathing (C1-4) and head and neck movement (C2)
Heart rate (C4-6) and shoulder movement (C5)
Wrist and elbow movement (C6-7)
Hand and finger movement (C7-T1)
Sympathetic tone (T1-12) (including temperature regulation) and trunk stability (T2-12)
Ejaculation (T11-L2) and hip motion (L2)
Knee extension (L3)
Foot motion (L4-S1) and knee flexion (L5)
Penile erection (S2-S4) and bowel and bladder activity (S2-S3)
Spinal Cord Structures
Nerve fiber tracts
White matter
Grey matter
Anterior fissure
Meninges
Pia mater
Arachnoid
Dura mater
Subarachnoid space
Spinal nerve

Nerve Cell

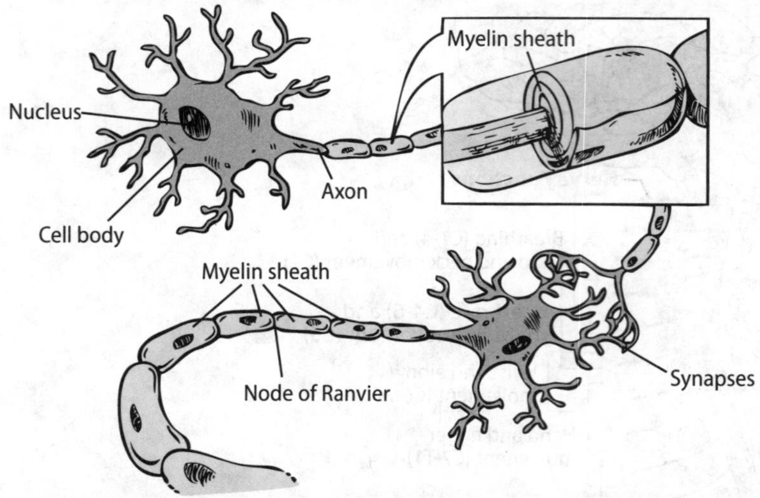
Myelin sheath
Nucleus
Axon
Cell body
Myelin sheath
Synapses
Node of Ranvier

Eye

Eye Structure

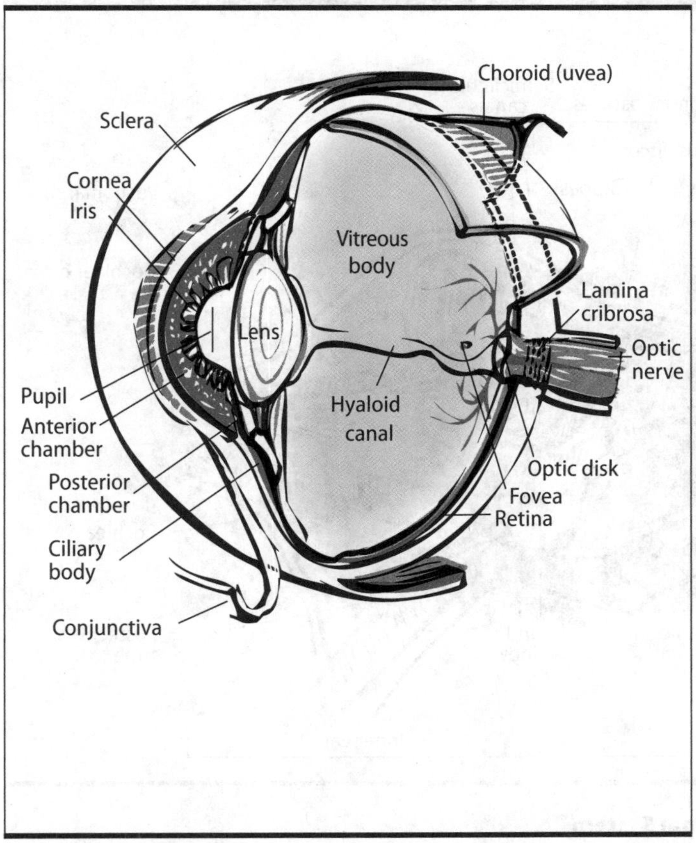

Posterior Pole of Globe/Flow of Aqueous Humor

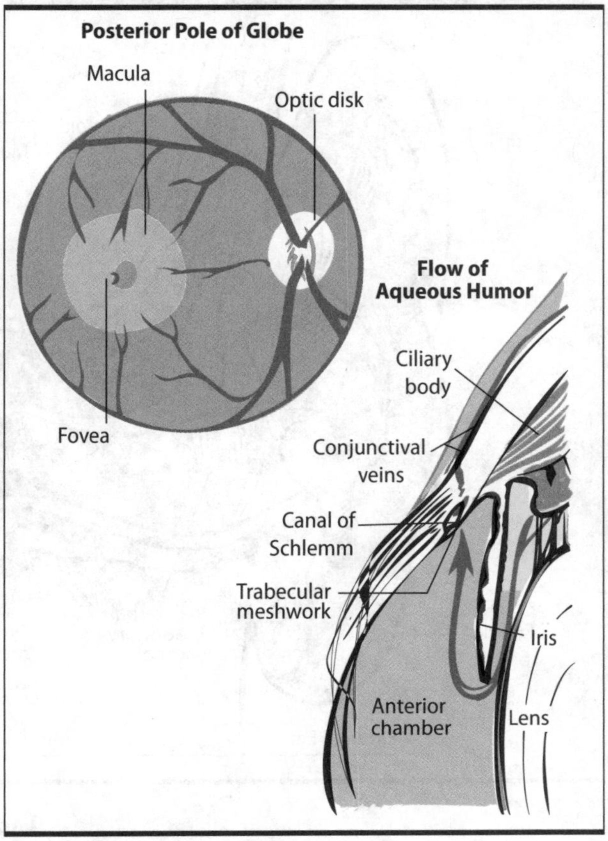

Eye Musculature

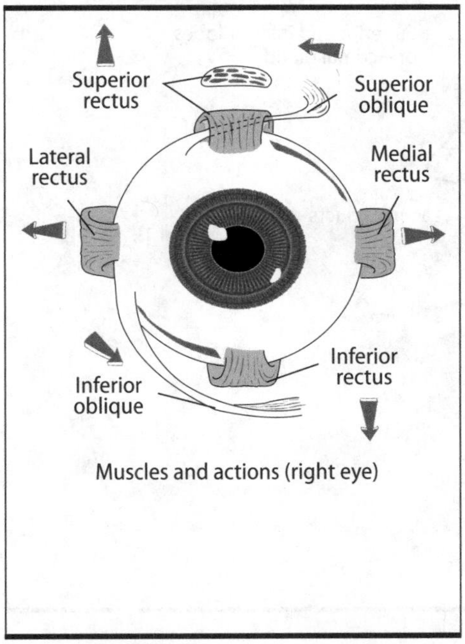

Eyelid Structures

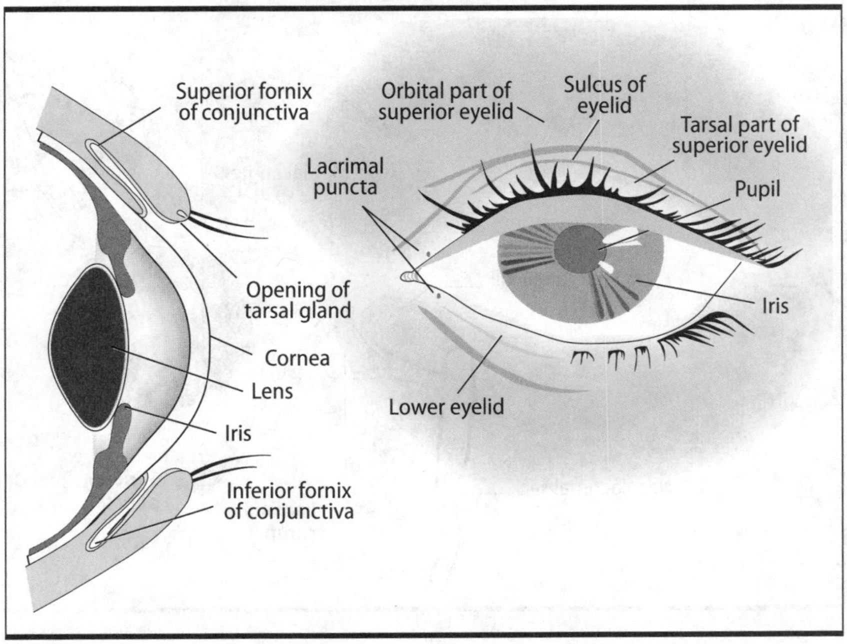

Anatomical Illustrations—Eye

Ear and Lacrimal System

Ear Anatomy

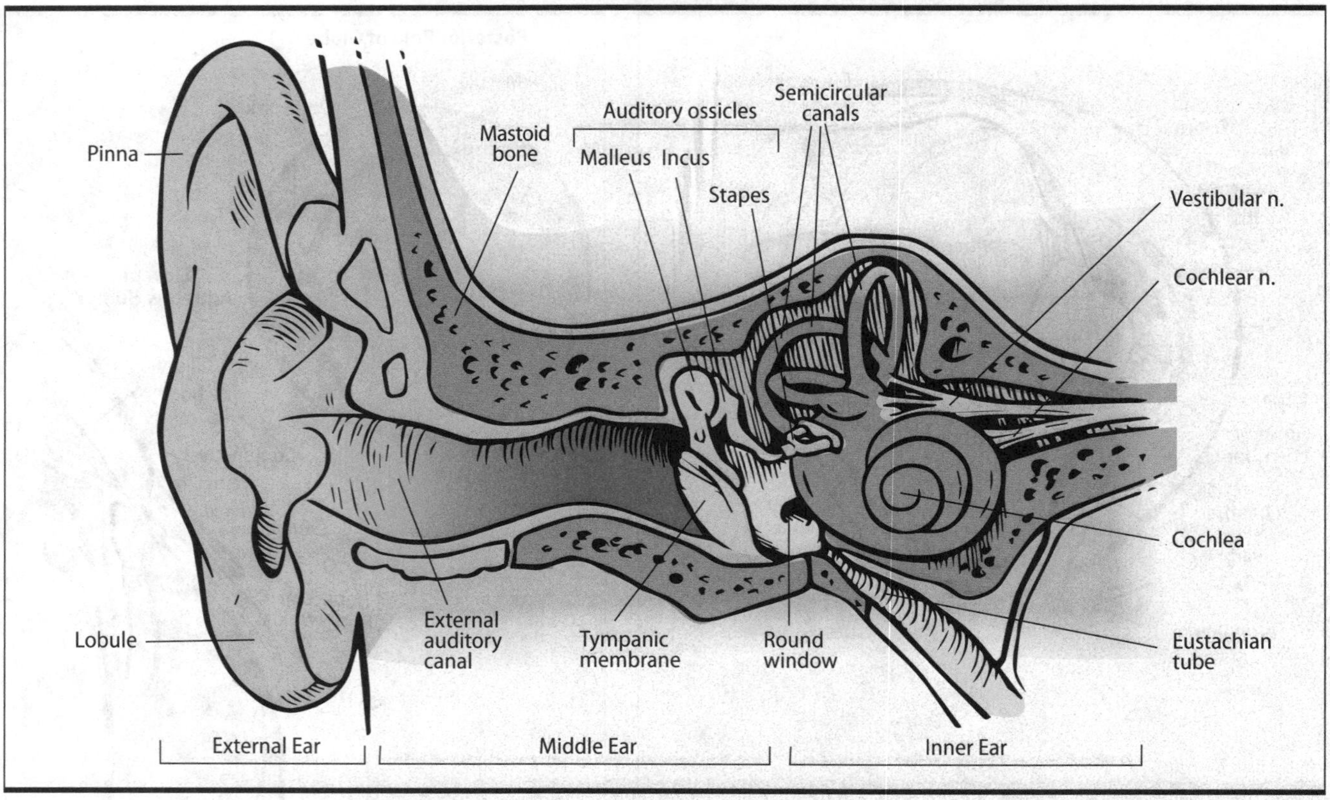

Lacrimal System

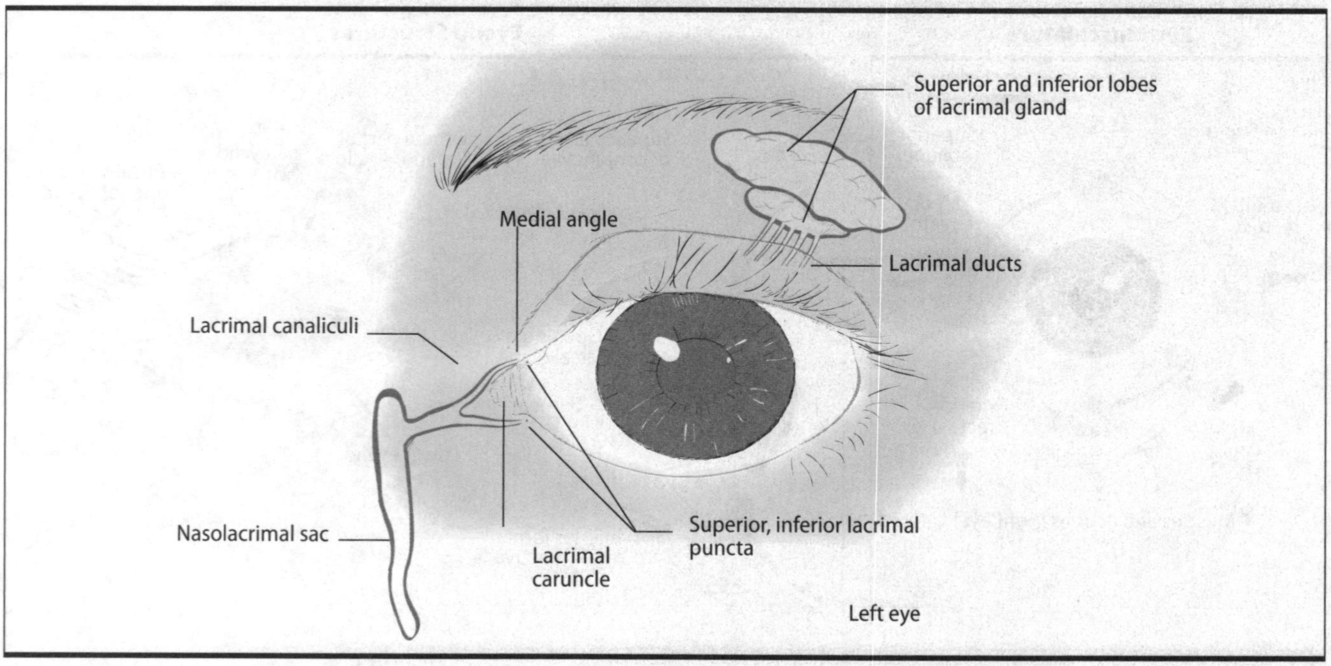

0-Numeric

A

 [Resequenced]

 [Resequenced]

 [Resequenced]

 [Resequenced]

[Resequenced]

B

 [Resequenced]

 [Resequenced]

[Resequenced]

 [Resequenced]

 [Resequenced]

 [Resequenced]

 [Resequenced]

D

 [Resequenced]

E

 [Resequenced]

[Resequenced]

[Resequenced]

 [Resequenced]

F

H

 [Resequenced]

I

 [Resequenced]

 [Resequenced]

J

K

[Resequenced]

 [Resequenced]

[Resequenced]

[Resequenced]

[Resequenced]

N

 [Resequenced]

 [Resequenced]

[Resequenced]

 [Resequenced]

 [Resequenced]

 [Resequenced]

 [Resequenced]

Q

[Resequenced]

 [Resequenced]

S

 [Resequenced]

[Resequenced]

[Resequenced]

[Resequenced]

 [Resequenced]

 [Resequenced]

U

[Resequenced]

[Resequenced]

V

 [Resequenced]

00100-00126 Anesthesia for Cleft Lip, Ear, ECT, Eyelid, and Salivary Gland Procedures

CMS: 100-04,12,140.1 Qualified Nonphysician Anesthetists; 100-04,12,140.3 Payment for Qualified Nonphysician Anesthetists; 100-04,12,140.3.3 Billing Modifiers; 100-04,12,140.3.4 General Billing Instructions; 100-04,12,140.4.1 An Anesthesiologist and Qualified Nonphysician Anesthetist Work Together; 100-04,12,140.4.2 Anesthetist and Anesthesiologist in a Single Procedure; 100-04,12,140.4.3 Payment for Medical /Surgical Services by CRNAs; 100-04,12,140.4.4 Conversion Factors for Anesthesia Services; 100-04,12,140.5 Payment for Anesthesia Services Furnished by a Teaching CRNA; 100-04,4,250.3.2 Anesthesia in a Hospital Outpatient Setting

00100 **Anesthesia for procedures on salivary glands, including biopsy**
0.00 0.00 **FUD** XXX N
AMA: 2019,Oct,10; 2018,Jan,8; 2017,Dec,8; 2017,Jan,8; 2016,Jan,13

00102 **Anesthesia for procedures involving plastic repair of cleft lip**
0.00 0.00 **FUD** XXX N
AMA: 2019,Oct,10; 2018,Jan,8; 2017,Dec,8; 2017,Jan,8; 2016,Jan,13

00103 **Anesthesia for reconstructive procedures of eyelid (eg, blepharoplasty, ptosis surgery)**
0.00 0.00 **FUD** XXX N
AMA: 2019,Oct,10; 2018,Jan,8; 2017,Dec,8; 2017,Jan,8; 2016,Jan,13

00104 **Anesthesia for electroconvulsive therapy**
0.00 0.00 **FUD** XXX N
AMA: 2019,Oct,10; 2018,Jan,8; 2017,Dec,8; 2017,Jan,8; 2016,Jan,13

00120 **Anesthesia for procedures on external, middle, and inner ear including biopsy; not otherwise specified**
0.00 0.00 **FUD** XXX N
AMA: 2019,Oct,10; 2018,Jan,8; 2017,Dec,8; 2017,Jan,8; 2016,Jan,13

00124 **otoscopy**
0.00 0.00 **FUD** XXX N
AMA: 2019,Oct,10; 2018,Jan,8; 2017,Dec,8; 2017,Jan,8; 2016,Jan,13

00126 **tympanotomy**
0.00 0.00 **FUD** XXX N
AMA: 2019,Oct,10; 2018,Jan,8; 2017,Dec,8; 2017,Jan,8; 2016,Jan,13

00140-00148 Anesthesia for Eye Procedures

CMS: 100-04,12,140.1 Qualified Nonphysician Anesthetists; 100-04,12,140.3 Payment for Qualified Nonphysician Anesthetists; 100-04,12,140.3.3 Billing Modifiers; 100-04,12,140.3.4 General Billing Instructions; 100-04,12,140.4.1 An Anesthesiologist and Qualified Nonphysician Anesthetist Work Together; 100-04,12,140.4.2 Anesthetist and Anesthesiologist in a Single Procedure; 100-04,12,140.4.3 Payment for Medical /Surgical Services by CRNAs; 100-04,12,140.4.4 Conversion Factors for Anesthesia Services; 100-04,12,140.5 Payment for Anesthesia Services Furnished by a Teaching CRNA; 100-04,4,250.3.2 Anesthesia in a Hospital Outpatient Setting

00140 **Anesthesia for procedures on eye; not otherwise specified**
0.00 0.00 **FUD** XXX N
AMA: 2019,Oct,10; 2018,Jan,8; 2017,Dec,8; 2017,Jan,8; 2016,Jan,13

00142 **lens surgery**
0.00 0.00 **FUD** XXX N
AMA: 2019,Oct,10; 2018,Jan,8; 2017,Dec,8; 2017,Jan,8; 2016,Jan,13

00144 **corneal transplant**
0.00 0.00 **FUD** XXX N
AMA: 2019,Oct,10; 2018,Jan,8; 2017,Dec,8; 2017,Jan,8; 2016,Jan,13

00145 **vitreoretinal surgery**
0.00 0.00 **FUD** XXX N
AMA: 2019,Oct,10; 2018,Jan,8; 2017,Dec,8; 2017,Jan,8; 2016,Jan,13

00147 **iridectomy**
0.00 0.00 **FUD** XXX N
AMA: 2019,Oct,10; 2018,Jan,8; 2017,Dec,8; 2017,Jan,8; 2016,Jan,13

00148 **ophthalmoscopy**
0.00 0.00 **FUD** XXX N
AMA: 2019,Oct,10; 2018,Jan,8; 2017,Dec,8; 2017,Jan,8; 2016,Jan,13

00160-00326 Anesthesia for Face and Head Procedures

CMS: 100-04,12,140.1 Qualified Nonphysician Anesthetists; 100-04,12,140.3 Payment for Qualified Nonphysician Anesthetists; 100-04,12,140.3.3 Billing Modifiers; 100-04,12,140.3.4 General Billing Instructions; 100-04,12,140.4.1 An Anesthesiologist and Qualified Nonphysician Anesthetist Work Together; 100-04,12,140.4.2 Anesthetist and Anesthesiologist in a Single Procedure; 100-04,12,140.4.4 Conversion Factors for Anesthesia Services; 100-04,12,140.5 Payment for Anesthesia Services Furnished by a Teaching CRNA; 100-04,4,250.3.2 Anesthesia in a Hospital Outpatient Setting

00160 **Anesthesia for procedures on nose and accessory sinuses; not otherwise specified**
0.00 0.00 **FUD** XXX N
AMA: 2019,Oct,10; 2018,Jan,8; 2017,Dec,8; 2017,Jan,8; 2016,Jan,13

00162 **radical surgery**
0.00 0.00 **FUD** XXX N
AMA: 2019,Oct,10; 2018,Jan,8; 2017,Dec,8; 2017,Jan,8; 2016,Jan,13

00164 **biopsy, soft tissue**
0.00 0.00 **FUD** XXX N
AMA: 2019,Oct,10; 2018,Jan,8; 2017,Dec,8; 2017,Jan,8; 2016,Jan,13

00170 **Anesthesia for intraoral procedures, including biopsy; not otherwise specified**
0.00 0.00 **FUD** XXX N
AMA: 2019,Oct,10; 2018,Jan,8; 2017,Dec,8; 2017,Jan,8; 2016,Jan,13

00172 **repair of cleft palate**
0.00 0.00 **FUD** XXX N
AMA: 2019,Oct,10; 2018,Jan,8; 2017,Dec,8; 2017,Jan,8; 2016,Jan,13

00174 **excision of retropharyngeal tumor**
0.00 0.00 **FUD** XXX N
AMA: 2019,Oct,10; 2018,Jan,8; 2017,Dec,8; 2017,Jan,8; 2016,Jan,13

00176 **radical surgery**
0.00 0.00 **FUD** XXX C
AMA: 2019,Oct,10; 2018,Jan,8; 2017,Dec,8; 2017,Jan,8; 2016,Jan,13

00190 **Anesthesia for procedures on facial bones or skull; not otherwise specified**
0.00 0.00 **FUD** XXX N
AMA: 2019,Oct,10; 2018,Jan,8; 2017,Dec,8; 2017,Jan,8; 2016,Jan,13

00192 **radical surgery (including prognathism)**
0.00 0.00 **FUD** XXX C
AMA: 2019,Oct,10; 2018,Jan,8; 2017,Dec,8; 2017,Jan,8; 2016,Jan,13

00210 **Anesthesia for intracranial procedures; not otherwise specified**
0.00 0.00 **FUD** XXX N
AMA: 2019,Oct,10; 2018,Jan,8; 2017,Dec,8; 2017,Jan,8; 2016,Jan,13

00211 **craniotomy or craniectomy for evacuation of hematoma**
0.00 0.00 **FUD** XXX C
AMA: 2019,Oct,10; 2018,Jan,8; 2017,Dec,8; 2017,Jan,8; 2016,Jan,13

00212 **subdural taps**
0.00 0.00 **FUD** XXX N
AMA: 2019,Oct,10; 2018,Jan,8; 2017,Dec,8; 2017,Jan,8; 2016,Jan,13

00214 **burr holes, including ventriculography**
0.00 0.00 **FUD** XXX C
AMA: 2019,Oct,10; 2018,Jan,8; 2017,Dec,8; 2017,Jan,8; 2016,Jan,13

00215 **cranioplasty or elevation of depressed skull fracture, extradural (simple or compound)**
0.00 0.00 FUD XXX C
AMA: 2019,Oct,10; 2018,Jan,8; 2017,Dec,8; 2017,Jan,8; 2016,Jan,13

00216 **vascular procedures**
0.00 0.00 FUD XXX N
AMA: 2019,Oct,10; 2018,Jan,8; 2017,Dec,8; 2017,Jan,8; 2016,Jan,13

00218 **procedures in sitting position**
0.00 0.00 FUD XXX N
AMA: 2019,Oct,10; 2018,Jan,8; 2017,Dec,8; 2017,Jan,8; 2016,Jan,13

00220 **cerebrospinal fluid shunting procedures**
0.00 0.00 FUD XXX N
AMA: 2019,Oct,10; 2018,Jan,8; 2017,Dec,8; 2017,Jan,8; 2016,Jan,13

00222 **electrocoagulation of intracranial nerve**
0.00 0.00 FUD XXX N
AMA: 2019,Oct,10; 2018,Jan,8; 2017,Dec,8; 2017,Jan,8; 2016,Jan,13

00300 **Anesthesia for all procedures on the integumentary system, muscles and nerves of head, neck, and posterior trunk, not otherwise specified**
0.00 0.00 FUD XXX N
AMA: 2019,Oct,10; 2018,Jan,8; 2017,Dec,8; 2017,Jan,8; 2016,Jan,13

00320 **Anesthesia for all procedures on esophagus, thyroid, larynx, trachea and lymphatic system of neck; not otherwise specified, age 1 year or older**
0.00 0.00 FUD XXX N
AMA: 2019,Oct,10; 2018,Jan,8; 2017,Dec,8; 2017,Jan,8; 2016,Jan,13

00322 **needle biopsy of thyroid**
EXCLUDES *Cervical spine and spinal cord procedures (00600, 00604, 00670)*
0.00 0.00 FUD XXX N
AMA: 2019,Oct,10; 2018,Jan,8; 2017,Dec,8; 2017,Jan,8; 2016,Jan,13

00326 **Anesthesia for all procedures on the larynx and trachea in children younger than 1 year of age** A
INCLUDES Anesthesia for patient of extreme age, younger than 1 year and older than 70 (99100)
0.00 0.00 FUD XXX N
AMA: 2019,Oct,10; 2018,Jan,8; 2017,Dec,8; 2017,Jan,8; 2016,Jan,13

00350-00352 Anesthesia for Neck Vessel Procedures

CMS: 100-04,12,140.1 Qualified Nonphysician Anesthetists; 100-04,12,140.3 Payment for Qualified Nonphysician Anesthetists; 100-04,12,140.3.3 Billing Modifiers; 100-04,12,140.3.4 General Billing Instructions; 100-04,12,140.4.1 An Anesthesiologist and Qualified Nonphysician Anesthetist Work Together; 100-04,12,140.4.2 Anesthetist and Anesthesiologist in a Single Procedure; 100-04,12,140.4.3 Payment for Medical /Surgical Services by CRNAs; 100-04,12,140.4.4 Conversion Factors for Anesthesia Services; 100-04,12,140.5 Payment for Anesthesia Services Furnished by a Teaching CRNA; 100-04,4,250.3.2 Anesthesia in a Hospital Outpatient Setting

EXCLUDES *Arteriography (01916)*

00350 **Anesthesia for procedures on major vessels of neck; not otherwise specified**
0.00 0.00 FUD XXX N
AMA: 2019,Oct,10; 2018,Jan,8; 2017,Dec,8; 2017,Jan,8; 2016,Jan,13

00352 **simple ligation**
0.00 0.00 FUD XXX N
AMA: 2019,Oct,10; 2018,Jan,8; 2017,Dec,8; 2017,Jan,8; 2016,Jan,13

00400-00529 Anesthesia for Chest/Pectoral Girdle Procedures

CMS: 100-04,12,140.1 Qualified Nonphysician Anesthetists; 100-04,12,140.3 Payment for Qualified Nonphysician Anesthetists; 100-04,12,140.3.3 Billing Modifiers; 100-04,12,140.3.4 General Billing Instructions; 100-04,12,140.4.1 An Anesthesiologist and Qualified Nonphysician Anesthetist Work Together; 100-04,12,140.4.2 Anesthetist and Anesthesiologist in a Single Procedure; 100-04,12,140.4.3 Payment for Medical /Surgical Services by CRNAs; 100-04,12,140.4.4 Conversion Factors for Anesthesia Services; 100-04,12,140.5 Payment for Anesthesia Services Furnished by a Teaching CRNA; 100-04,4,250.3.2 Anesthesia in a Hospital Outpatient Setting

00400 **Anesthesia for procedures on the integumentary system on the extremities, anterior trunk and perineum; not otherwise specified**
0.00 0.00 FUD XXX N
AMA: 2019,Oct,10; 2018,Jan,8; 2017,Dec,8; 2017,Jan,8; 2016,Jan,13

00402 **reconstructive procedures on breast (eg, reduction or augmentation mammoplasty, muscle flaps)**
0.00 0.00 FUD XXX N
AMA: 2019,Oct,10; 2018,Jan,8; 2017,Dec,8; 2017,Jan,8; 2016,Jan,13

00404 **radical or modified radical procedures on breast**
0.00 0.00 FUD XXX N
AMA: 2019,Oct,10; 2018,Jan,8; 2017,Dec,8; 2017,Jan,8; 2016,Jan,13

00406 **radical or modified radical procedures on breast with internal mammary node dissection**
0.00 0.00 FUD XXX N
AMA: 2019,Oct,10; 2018,Jan,8; 2017,Dec,8; 2017,Jan,8; 2016,Jan,13

00410 **electrical conversion of arrhythmias**
0.00 0.00 FUD XXX N
AMA: 2019,Oct,10; 2018,Jan,8; 2017,Dec,8; 2017,Jan,8; 2016,Jan,13

00450 **Anesthesia for procedures on clavicle and scapula; not otherwise specified**
0.00 0.00 FUD XXX N
AMA: 2019,Oct,10; 2018,Jan,8; 2017,Dec,8; 2017,Jan,8; 2016,Jan,13

00454 **biopsy of clavicle**
0.00 0.00 FUD XXX N
AMA: 2019,Oct,10; 2018,Jan,8; 2017,Dec,8; 2017,Jan,8; 2016,Jan,13

00470 **Anesthesia for partial rib resection; not otherwise specified**
0.00 0.00 FUD XXX N
AMA: 2019,Oct,10; 2018,Jan,8; 2017,Dec,8; 2017,Jan,8; 2016,Jan,13

00472 **thoracoplasty (any type)**
0.00 0.00 FUD XXX N
AMA: 2019,Oct,10; 2018,Jan,8; 2017,Dec,8; 2017,Jan,8; 2016,Jan,13

00474 **radical procedures (eg, pectus excavatum)**
0.00 0.00 FUD XXX C
AMA: 2019,Oct,10; 2018,Jan,8; 2017,Dec,8; 2017,Jan,8; 2016,Jan,13

00500 **Anesthesia for all procedures on esophagus**
0.00 0.00 FUD XXX N
AMA: 2019,Oct,10; 2018,Jan,8; 2017,Dec,8; 2017,Jan,8; 2016,Jan,13

00520 **Anesthesia for closed chest procedures; (including bronchoscopy) not otherwise specified**
0.00 0.00 FUD XXX N
AMA: 2019,Oct,10; 2018,Jan,8; 2017,Dec,8; 2017,Jan,8; 2016,Jan,13

00522 **needle biopsy of pleura**
0.00 0.00 FUD XXX N
AMA: 2019,Oct,10; 2018,Jan,8; 2017,Dec,8; 2017,Jan,8; 2016,Jan,13

26/TC PC/TC Only A2-Z3 ASC Payment 50 Bilateral ♂ Male Only ♀ Female Only Facility RVU Non-Facility RVU CCI CLIA
FUD Follow-up Days CMS: IOM AMA: CPT Asst A-Y OPPSI 80/80 Surg Assist Allowed / w/Doc Lab Crosswalk Radiology Crosswalk
2

00524 **pneumocentesis**
0.00 0.00 FUD XXX C
AMA: 2019,Oct,10; 2018,Jan,8; 2017,Dec,8; 2017,Jan,8; 2016,Jan,13

00528 **mediastinoscopy and diagnostic thoracoscopy not utilizing 1 lung ventilation**
EXCLUDES *Tracheobronchial reconstruction (00539)*
0.00 0.00 FUD XXX N
AMA: 2019,Oct,10; 2018,Jan,8; 2017,Dec,8; 2017,Jan,8; 2016,Jan,13

00529 **mediastinoscopy and diagnostic thoracoscopy utilizing 1 lung ventilation**
0.00 0.00 FUD XXX N
AMA: 2019,Oct,10; 2018,Jan,8; 2017,Dec,8; 2017,Jan,8; 2016,Jan,13

00530 Anesthesia for Cardiac Pacemaker Procedure

CMS: 100-03,10.6 Anesthesia in Cardiac Pacemaker Surgery; 100-04,12,140.1 Qualified Nonphysician Anesthetists; 100-04,12,140.3 Payment for Qualified Nonphysician Anesthetists; 100-04,12,140.3.3 Billing Modifiers; 100-04,12,140.3.4 General Billing Instructions; 100-04,12,140.4.1 An Anesthesiologist and Qualified Nonphysician Anesthetist Work Together; 100-04,12,140.4.2 Anesthetist and Anesthesiologist in a Single Procedure; 100-04,12,140.4.3 Payment for Medical /Surgical Services by CRNAs; 100-04,12,140.4.4 Conversion Factors for Anesthesia Services; 100-04,12,140.5 Payment for Anesthesia Services Furnished by a Teaching CRNA; 100-04,4,250.3.2 Anesthesia in a Hospital Outpatient Setting

00530 **Anesthesia for permanent transvenous pacemaker insertion**
0.00 0.00 FUD XXX N
AMA: 2019,Oct,10; 2018,Jan,8; 2017,Dec,8; 2017,Jan,8; 2016,Jan,13

00532-00550 Anesthesia for Heart and Lung Procedures

CMS: 100-04,12,140.1 Qualified Nonphysician Anesthetists; 100-04,12,140.3 Payment for Qualified Nonphysician Anesthetists; 100-04,12,140.3.3 Billing Modifiers; 100-04,12,140.3.4 General Billing Instructions; 100-04,12,140.4.1 An Anesthesiologist and Qualified Nonphysician Anesthetist Work Together; 100-04,12,140.4.2 Anesthetist and Anesthesiologist in a Single Procedure; 100-04,12,140.4.3 Payment for Medical /Surgical Services by CRNAs; 100-04,12,140.4.4 Conversion Factors for Anesthesia Services; 100-04,12,140.5 Payment for Anesthesia Services Furnished by a Teaching CRNA; 100-04,4,250.3.2 Anesthesia in a Hospital Outpatient Setting

00532 **Anesthesia for access to central venous circulation**
0.00 0.00 FUD XXX N
AMA: 2019,Oct,10; 2018,Jan,8; 2017,Dec,8; 2017,Jan,8; 2016,Jan,13

00534 **Anesthesia for transvenous insertion or replacement of pacing cardioverter-defibrillator**
EXCLUDES *Transthoracic approach (00560)*
0.00 0.00 FUD XXX N
AMA: 2019,Oct,10; 2018,Jan,8; 2017,Dec,8; 2017,Jan,8; 2016,Jan,13

00537 **Anesthesia for cardiac electrophysiologic procedures including radiofrequency ablation**
0.00 0.00 FUD XXX N
AMA: 2019,Oct,10; 2018,Jan,8; 2017,Dec,8; 2017,Jan,8; 2016,Jan,13

00539 **Anesthesia for tracheobronchial reconstruction**
0.00 0.00 FUD XXX N
AMA: 2019,Oct,10; 2018,Jan,8; 2017,Dec,8; 2017,Jan,8; 2016,Jan,13

00540 **Anesthesia for thoracotomy procedures involving lungs, pleura, diaphragm, and mediastinum (including surgical thoracoscopy); not otherwise specified**
EXCLUDES *Thoracic spine and spinal cord procedures via anterior transthoracic approach (00625-00626)*
0.00 0.00 FUD XXX C
AMA: 2019,Oct,10; 2018,Jan,8; 2017,Dec,8; 2017,Jan,8; 2016,Jan,13

00541 **utilizing 1 lung ventilation**
EXCLUDES *Thoracic spine and spinal cord procedures via anterior transthoracic approach (00625-00626)*
0.00 0.00 FUD XXX N
AMA: 2019,Oct,10; 2018,Jan,8; 2017,Dec,8; 2017,Jan,8; 2016,Jan,13

00542 **decortication**
0.00 0.00 FUD XXX C
AMA: 2019,Oct,10; 2018,Jan,8; 2017,Dec,8; 2017,Jan,8; 2016,Jan,13

00546 **pulmonary resection with thoracoplasty**
0.00 0.00 FUD XXX C
AMA: 2019,Oct,10; 2018,Jan,8; 2017,Dec,8; 2017,Jan,8; 2016,Jan,13

00548 **intrathoracic procedures on the trachea and bronchi**
0.00 0.00 FUD XXX N
AMA: 2019,Oct,10; 2018,Jan,8; 2017,Dec,8; 2017,Jan,8; 2016,Jan,13

00550 **Anesthesia for sternal debridement**
0.00 0.00 FUD XXX N
AMA: 2019,Oct,10; 2018,Jan,8; 2017,Dec,8; 2017,Jan,8; 2016,Jan,13

00560-00580 Anesthesia for Open Heart Procedures

CMS: 100-04,12,140.1 Qualified Nonphysician Anesthetists; 100-04,12,140.3 Payment for Qualified Nonphysician Anesthetists; 100-04,12,140.3.3 Billing Modifiers; 100-04,12,140.3.4 General Billing Instructions; 100-04,12,140.4.1 An Anesthesiologist and Qualified Nonphysician Anesthetist Work Together; 100-04,12,140.4.2 Anesthetist and Anesthesiologist in a Single Procedure; 100-04,12,140.4.3 Payment for Medical /Surgical Services by CRNAs; 100-04,12,140.4.4 Conversion Factors for Anesthesia Services; 100-04,12,140.5 Payment for Anesthesia Services Furnished by a Teaching CRNA; 100-04,4,250.3.2 Anesthesia in a Hospital Outpatient Setting

00560 **Anesthesia for procedures on heart, pericardial sac, and great vessels of chest; without pump oxygenator**
0.00 0.00 FUD XXX C
AMA: 2019,Oct,10; 2018,Jan,8; 2017,Dec,8; 2017,Jan,8; 2016,Jan,13

00561 **with pump oxygenator, younger than 1 year of age** A
INCLUDES Anesthesia complicated by utilization of controlled hypotension (99135)
Anesthesia complicated by utilization of total body hypothermia (99116)
Anesthesia for patient of extreme age, younger than 1 year and older than 70 (99100)
0.00 0.00 FUD XXX C
AMA: 2019,Oct,10; 2018,Jan,8; 2017,Dec,8; 2017,Jan,8; 2016,Jan,13

00562 **with pump oxygenator, age 1 year or older, for all noncoronary bypass procedures (eg, valve procedures) or for re-operation for coronary bypass more than 1 month after original operation** A
0.00 0.00 FUD XXX C
AMA: 2019,Oct,10; 2018,Jan,8; 2017,Dec,8; 2017,Jan,8; 2016,Jan,13

00563 **with pump oxygenator with hypothermic circulatory arrest**
0.00 0.00 FUD XXX N
AMA: 2019,Oct,10; 2018,Jan,8; 2017,Dec,8; 2017,Jan,8; 2016,Jan,13

00566 **Anesthesia for direct coronary artery bypass grafting; without pump oxygenator**
0.00 0.00 FUD XXX N
AMA: 2019,Oct,10; 2018,Jan,8; 2017,Dec,8; 2017,Jan,8; 2016,Jan,13

00567 **with pump oxygenator**
0.00 0.00 FUD XXX C
AMA: 2019,Oct,10; 2018,Jan,8; 2017,Dec,8; 2017,Jan,8; 2016,Jan,13

00580 **Anesthesia for heart transplant or heart/lung transplant**
0.00 0.00 FUD XXX C
AMA: 2019,Oct,10; 2018,Jan,8; 2017,Dec,8; 2017,Jan,8; 2016,Jan,13

00600-00670 Anesthesia for Spinal Procedures

CMS: 100-04,12,140.1 Qualified Nonphysician Anesthetists; 100-04,12,140.3 Payment for Qualified Nonphysician Anesthetists; 100-04,12,140.3.3 Billing Modifiers; 100-04,12,140.3.4 General Billing Instructions; 100-04,12,140.4.1 An Anesthesiologist and Qualified Nonphysician Anesthetist Work Together; 100-04,12,140.4.2 Anesthetist and Anesthesiologist in a Single Procedure; 100-04,12,140.4.3 Payment for Medical /Surgical Services by CRNAs; 100-04,12,140.4.4 Conversion Factors for Anesthesia Services; 100-04,12,140.5 Payment for Anesthesia Services Furnished by a Teaching CRNA; 100-04,4,250.3.2 Anesthesia in a Hospital Outpatient Setting

00600 **Anesthesia for procedures on cervical spine and cord; not otherwise specified**

EXCLUDES *Percutaneous image-guided spine and spinal cord anesthesia services (01937-01942)*

0.00 0.00 **FUD** XXX N

AMA: 2019,Oct,10; 2018,Jan,8; 2017,Dec,8; 2017,Jan,8; 2016,Jan,13

00604 **procedures with patient in the sitting position**

0.00 0.00 **FUD** XXX C

AMA: 2019,Oct,10; 2018,Jan,8; 2017,Dec,8; 2017,Jan,8; 2016,Jan,13

00620 **Anesthesia for procedures on thoracic spine and cord, not otherwise specified**

0.00 0.00 **FUD** XXX N

AMA: 2019,Oct,10; 2018,Jan,8; 2017,Dec,8; 2017,Jan,8; 2016,Jan,13

00625 **Anesthesia for procedures on the thoracic spine and cord, via an anterior transthoracic approach; not utilizing 1 lung ventilation**

EXCLUDES *Anesthesia services for thoracotomy procedures other than spine (00540-00541)*

0.00 0.00 **FUD** XXX N

AMA: 2019,Oct,10; 2018,Jan,8; 2017,Dec,8; 2017,Jan,8; 2016,Jan,13

00626 **utilizing 1 lung ventilation**

EXCLUDES *Anesthesia services for thoracotomy procedures other than spine (00540-00541)*

0.00 0.00 **FUD** XXX N

AMA: 2019,Oct,10; 2018,Jan,8; 2017,Dec,8; 2017,Jan,8; 2016,Jan,13

00630 **Anesthesia for procedures in lumbar region; not otherwise specified**

0.00 0.00 **FUD** XXX N

AMA: 2019,Oct,10; 2018,Jan,8; 2017,Dec,8; 2017,Jan,8; 2016,Jan,13

00632 **lumbar sympathectomy**

0.00 0.00 **FUD** XXX C

AMA: 2019,Oct,10; 2018,Jan,8; 2017,Dec,8; 2017,Jan,8; 2016,Jan,13

00635 **diagnostic or therapeutic lumbar puncture**

0.00 0.00 **FUD** XXX N

AMA: 2019,Oct,10; 2018,Jan,8; 2017,Dec,8; 2017,Jan,8; 2016,Jan,13

00640 **Anesthesia for manipulation of the spine or for closed procedures on the cervical, thoracic or lumbar spine**

0.00 0.00 **FUD** XXX N

AMA: 2019,Oct,10; 2018,Jan,8; 2017,Dec,8; 2017,Jan,8; 2016,Jan,13

00670 **Anesthesia for extensive spine and spinal cord procedures (eg, spinal instrumentation or vascular procedures)**

0.00 0.00 **FUD** XXX C

AMA: 2019,Oct,10; 2018,Jan,8; 2017,Dec,8; 2017,Jan,8; 2016,Jan,13

00700-00882 Anesthesia for Abdominal Procedures

CMS: 100-04,12,140.1 Qualified Nonphysician Anesthetists; 100-04,12,140.3 Payment for Qualified Nonphysician Anesthetists; 100-04,12,140.3.3 Billing Modifiers; 100-04,12,140.3.4 General Billing Instructions; 100-04,12,140.4.1 An Anesthesiologist and Qualified Nonphysician Anesthetist Work Together; 100-04,12,140.4.2 Anesthetist and Anesthesiologist in a Single Procedure; 100-04,12,140.4.3 Payment for Medical /Surgical Services by CRNAs; 100-04,12,140.4.4 Conversion Factors for Anesthesia Services; 100-04,12,140.5 Payment for Anesthesia Services Furnished by a Teaching CRNA; 100-04,4,250.3.2 Anesthesia in a Hospital Outpatient Setting

00700 **Anesthesia for procedures on upper anterior abdominal wall; not otherwise specified**

0.00 0.00 **FUD** XXX N

AMA: 2019,Oct,10; 2018,Jan,8; 2017,Dec,8; 2017,Jan,8; 2016,Jan,13

00702 **percutaneous liver biopsy**

0.00 0.00 **FUD** XXX N

AMA: 2019,Oct,10; 2018,Jan,8; 2017,Dec,8; 2017,Jan,8; 2016,Jan,13

00730 **Anesthesia for procedures on upper posterior abdominal wall**

0.00 0.00 **FUD** XXX N

AMA: 2019,Oct,10; 2018,Jan,8; 2017,Dec,8; 2017,Jan,8; 2016,Jan,13

00731 **Anesthesia for upper gastrointestinal endoscopic procedures, endoscope introduced proximal to duodenum; not otherwise specified**

EXCLUDES *Combination upper and lower endoscopic gastrointestinal procedures (00813)*

0.00 0.00 **FUD** XXX N

AMA: 2019,Oct,10; 2018,Jan,8; 2017,Dec,8

00732 **endoscopic retrograde cholangiopancreatography (ERCP)**

EXCLUDES *Combination upper and lower endoscopic gastrointestinal procedures (00813)*

0.00 0.00 **FUD** XXX N

AMA: 2019,Oct,10; 2018,Jan,8; 2017,Dec,8

00750 **Anesthesia for hernia repairs in upper abdomen; not otherwise specified**

0.00 0.00 **FUD** XXX N

AMA: 2019,Oct,10; 2018,Jan,8; 2017,Dec,8; 2017,Jan,8; 2016,Jan,13

00752 **lumbar and ventral (incisional) hernias and/or wound dehiscence**

0.00 0.00 **FUD** XXX N

AMA: 2019,Oct,10; 2018,Jan,8; 2017,Dec,8; 2017,Jan,8; 2016,Jan,13

00754 **omphalocele**

0.00 0.00 **FUD** XXX N

AMA: 2019,Oct,10; 2018,Jan,8; 2017,Dec,8; 2017,Jan,8; 2016,Jan,13

00756 **transabdominal repair of diaphragmatic hernia**

0.00 0.00 **FUD** XXX N

AMA: 2019,Oct,10; 2018,Jan,8; 2017,Dec,8; 2017,Jan,8; 2016,Jan,13

00770 **Anesthesia for all procedures on major abdominal blood vessels**

0.00 0.00 **FUD** XXX N

AMA: 2019,Oct,10; 2018,Jan,8; 2017,Dec,8; 2017,Jan,8; 2016,Jan,13

00790 **Anesthesia for intraperitoneal procedures in upper abdomen including laparoscopy; not otherwise specified**

0.00 0.00 **FUD** XXX N

AMA: 2019,Oct,10; 2018,Jan,8; 2017,Dec,8; 2017,Jan,8; 2016,Jan,13

00792 **partial hepatectomy or management of liver hemorrhage (excluding liver biopsy)**

0.00 0.00 **FUD** XXX C

AMA: 2019,Oct,10; 2018,Jan,8; 2017,Dec,8; 2017,Jan,8; 2016,Jan,13

00794 **pancreatectomy, partial or total (eg, Whipple procedure)**
0.00 0.00 FUD XXX C
AMA: 2019,Oct,10; 2018,Jan,8; 2017,Dec,8; 2017,Jan,8; 2016,Jan,13

00796 **liver transplant (recipient)**
EXCLUDES *Physiological support during liver harvest (01990)*
0.00 0.00 FUD XXX C
AMA: 2019,Oct,10; 2018,Jan,8; 2017,Dec,8; 2017,Jan,8; 2016,Jan,13

00797 **gastric restrictive procedure for morbid obesity**
0.00 0.00 FUD XXX N
AMA: 2019,Oct,10; 2018,Jan,8; 2017,Dec,8; 2017,Jan,8; 2016,Jan,13

00800 **Anesthesia for procedures on lower anterior abdominal wall; not otherwise specified**
0.00 0.00 FUD XXX N
AMA: 2019,Oct,10; 2018,Jan,8; 2017,Dec,8; 2017,Jan,8; 2016,Jan,13

00802 **panniculectomy**
0.00 0.00 FUD XXX C
AMA: 2019,Oct,10; 2018,Jan,8; 2017,Dec,8; 2017,Jan,8; 2016,Jan,13

00811 **Anesthesia for lower intestinal endoscopic procedures, endoscope introduced distal to duodenum; not otherwise specified**
0.00 0.00 FUD XXX N
AMA: 2019,Oct,10; 2018,Jan,8; 2017,Dec,8

00812 **screening colonoscopy**
INCLUDES Anesthesia services for all screening colonoscopy irrespective of findings
0.00 0.00 FUD XXX N
AMA: 2019,Oct,10; 2018,Jan,8; 2017,Dec,8

00813 **Anesthesia for combined upper and lower gastrointestinal endoscopic procedures, endoscope introduced both proximal to and distal to the duodenum**
0.00 0.00 FUD XXX N
AMA: 2019,Oct,10; 2018,Jan,8; 2017,Dec,8

00820 **Anesthesia for procedures on lower posterior abdominal wall**
0.00 0.00 FUD XXX N
AMA: 2019,Oct,10; 2018,Jan,8; 2017,Dec,8; 2017,Jan,8; 2016,Jan,13

00830 **Anesthesia for hernia repairs in lower abdomen; not otherwise specified**
EXCLUDES *Anesthesia for hernia repairs on infants one year old or less (00834, 00836)*
0.00 0.00 FUD XXX N
AMA: 2019,Oct,10; 2018,Jan,8; 2017,Dec,8; 2017,Jan,8; 2016,Jan,13

00832 **ventral and incisional hernias**
EXCLUDES *Anesthesia for hernia repairs on infants one year old or less (00834, 00836)*
0.00 0.00 FUD XXX N
AMA: 2019,Oct,10; 2018,Jan,8; 2017,Dec,8; 2017,Jan,8; 2016,Jan,13

00834 **Anesthesia for hernia repairs in the lower abdomen not otherwise specified, younger than 1 year of age** A
INCLUDES Anesthesia for patient of extreme age, younger than 1 year and older than 70 (99100)
0.00 0.00 FUD XXX N
AMA: 2019,Oct,10; 2018,Jan,8; 2017,Dec,8; 2017,Jan,8; 2016,Jan,13

00836 **Anesthesia for hernia repairs in the lower abdomen not otherwise specified, infants younger than 37 weeks gestational age at birth and younger than 50 weeks gestational age at time of surgery** A
INCLUDES Anesthesia for patient of extreme age, younger than 1 year and older than 70 (99100)
0.00 0.00 FUD XXX N
AMA: 2019,Oct,10; 2018,Jan,8; 2017,Dec,8; 2017,Jan,8; 2016,Jan,13

00840 **Anesthesia for intraperitoneal procedures in lower abdomen including laparoscopy; not otherwise specified**
0.00 0.00 FUD XXX N
AMA: 2019,Oct,10; 2018,Jan,8; 2017,Dec,8; 2017,Jan,8; 2016,Jan,13

00842 **amniocentesis** M ♀
0.00 0.00 FUD XXX N
AMA: 2019,Oct,10; 2018,Jan,8; 2017,Dec,8; 2017,Jan,8; 2016,Jan,13

00844 **abdominoperineal resection**
0.00 0.00 FUD XXX C
AMA: 2019,Oct,10; 2018,Jan,8; 2017,Dec,8; 2017,Jan,8; 2016,Jan,13

00846 **radical hysterectomy** ♀
0.00 0.00 FUD XXX C
AMA: 2019,Oct,10; 2018,Jan,8; 2017,Dec,8; 2017,Jan,8; 2016,Jan,13

00848 **pelvic exenteration**
0.00 0.00 FUD XXX C
AMA: 2019,Oct,10; 2018,Jan,8; 2017,Dec,8; 2017,Jan,8; 2016,Jan,13

00851 **tubal ligation/transection** ♀
0.00 0.00 FUD XXX N
AMA: 2019,Oct,10; 2018,Jan,8; 2017,Dec,8; 2017,Jan,8; 2016,Jan,13

00860 **Anesthesia for extraperitoneal procedures in lower abdomen, including urinary tract; not otherwise specified**
0.00 0.00 FUD XXX N
AMA: 2019,Oct,10; 2018,Jan,8; 2017,Dec,8; 2017,Jan,8; 2016,Jan,13

00862 **renal procedures, including upper one-third of ureter, or donor nephrectomy**
0.00 0.00 FUD XXX N
AMA: 2019,Oct,10; 2018,Jan,8; 2017,Dec,8; 2017,Jan,8; 2016,Jan,13

00864 **total cystectomy**
0.00 0.00 FUD XXX C
AMA: 2019,Oct,10; 2018,Jan,8; 2017,Dec,8; 2017,Jan,8; 2016,Jan,13

00865 **radical prostatectomy (suprapubic, retropubic)** ♂
0.00 0.00 FUD XXX C
AMA: 2019,Oct,10; 2018,Jan,8; 2017,Dec,8; 2017,Jan,8; 2016,Jan,13

00866 **adrenalectomy**
0.00 0.00 FUD XXX C
AMA: 2019,Oct,10; 2018,Jan,8; 2017,Dec,8; 2017,Jan,8; 2016,Jan,13

00868 **renal transplant (recipient)**
EXCLUDES *Anesthesia for donor nephrectomy (00862)*
Physiological support during kidney harvest (01990)
0.00 0.00 FUD XXX C
AMA: 2019,Oct,10; 2018,Jan,8; 2017,Dec,8; 2017,Jan,8; 2016,Jan,13

00870 **cystolithotomy**
0.00 0.00 FUD XXX N
AMA: 2019,Oct,10; 2018,Jan,8; 2017,Dec,8; 2017,Jan,8; 2016,Jan,13

Anesthesia

00794 — 00870

● New Code ▲ Revised Code ○ Reinstated ● New Web Release ▲ Revised Web Release + Add-on Unlisted Not Covered # Resequenced
⑤⓪ Optum Mod 50 Exempt ⊘ AMA Mod 51 Exempt ⑤ Optum Mod 51 Exempt ⑥③ Mod 63 Exempt ✓ Non-FDA Drug ★ Telemedicine M Maternity A Age Edit

00872 **Anesthesia for lithotripsy, extracorporeal shock wave; with water bath**
0.00 0.00 FUD XXX N
AMA: 2019,Oct,10; 2018,Jan,8; 2017,Dec,8; 2017,Jan,8; 2016,Jan,13

00873 **without water bath**
0.00 0.00 FUD XXX N
AMA: 2019,Oct,10; 2018,Jan,8; 2017,Dec,8; 2017,Jan,8; 2016,Jan,13

00880 **Anesthesia for procedures on major lower abdominal vessels; not otherwise specified**
0.00 0.00 FUD XXX N
AMA: 2019,Oct,10; 2018,Jan,8; 2017,Dec,8; 2017,Jan,8; 2016,Jan,13

00882 **inferior vena cava ligation**
0.00 0.00 FUD XXX C
AMA: 2019,Oct,10; 2018,Jan,8; 2017,Dec,8; 2017,Jan,8; 2016,Jan,13

00902-00952 Anesthesia for Genitourinary Procedures

CMS: 100-04,12,140.1 Qualified Nonphysician Anesthetists; 100-04,12,140.3 Payment for Qualified Nonphysician Anesthetists; 100-04,12,140.3.3 Billing Modifiers; 100-04,12,140.3.4 General Billing Instructions; 100-04,12,140.4.1 An Anesthesiologist and Qualified Nonphysician Anesthetist Work Together; 100-04,12,140.4.2 Anesthetist and Anesthesiologist in a Single Procedure; 100-04,12,140.4.3 Payment for Medical /Surgical Services by CRNAs; 100-04,12,140.4.4 Conversion Factors for Anesthesia Services; 100-04,12,140.5 Payment for Anesthesia Services Furnished by a Teaching CRNA; 100-04,4,250.3.2 Anesthesia in a Hospital Outpatient Setting

EXCLUDES *Procedures on perineal skin, muscles, and nerves (00300, 00400)*

00902 **Anesthesia for; anorectal procedure**
0.00 0.00 FUD XXX N
AMA: 2019,Oct,10; 2018,Jan,8; 2017,Dec,8; 2017,Jan,8; 2016,Jan,13

00904 **radical perineal procedure**
0.00 0.00 FUD XXX C
AMA: 2019,Oct,10; 2018,Jan,8; 2017,Dec,8; 2017,Jan,8; 2016,Jan,13

00906 **vulvectomy** ♀
0.00 0.00 FUD XXX N
AMA: 2019,Oct,10; 2018,Jan,8; 2017,Dec,8; 2017,Jan,8; 2016,Jan,13

00908 **perineal prostatectomy** ♂
0.00 0.00 FUD XXX C
AMA: 2019,Oct,10; 2018,Jan,8; 2017,Dec,8; 2017,Jan,8; 2016,Jan,13

00910 **Anesthesia for transurethral procedures (including urethrocystoscopy); not otherwise specified**
0.00 0.00 FUD XXX N
AMA: 2019,Oct,10; 2018,Jan,8; 2017,Dec,8; 2017,Jan,8; 2016,Jan,13

00912 **transurethral resection of bladder tumor(s)**
0.00 0.00 FUD XXX N
AMA: 2019,Oct,10; 2018,Jan,8; 2017,Dec,8; 2017,Jan,8; 2016,Jan,13

00914 **transurethral resection of prostate** ♂
0.00 0.00 FUD XXX N
AMA: 2019,Oct,10; 2018,Jan,8; 2017,Dec,8; 2017,Jan,8; 2016,Jan,13

00916 **post-transurethral resection bleeding**
0.00 0.00 FUD XXX N
AMA: 2019,Oct,10; 2018,Jan,8; 2017,Dec,8; 2017,Jan,8; 2016,Jan,13

00918 **with fragmentation, manipulation and/or removal of ureteral calculus**
0.00 0.00 FUD XXX N
AMA: 2019,Oct,10; 2018,Jan,8; 2017,Dec,8; 2017,Jan,8; 2016,Jan,13

00920 **Anesthesia for procedures on male genitalia (including open urethral procedures); not otherwise specified** ♂
0.00 0.00 FUD XXX N
AMA: 2019,Oct,10; 2018,Jan,8; 2017,Dec,8; 2017,Jan,8; 2016,Jan,13

00921 **vasectomy, unilateral or bilateral** ♂
0.00 0.00 FUD XXX N
AMA: 2019,Oct,10; 2018,Jan,8; 2017,Dec,8; 2017,Jan,8; 2016,Jan,13

00922 **seminal vesicles** ♂
0.00 0.00 FUD XXX N
AMA: 2019,Oct,10; 2018,Jan,8; 2017,Dec,8; 2017,Jan,8; 2016,Jan,13

00924 **undescended testis, unilateral or bilateral** ♂
0.00 0.00 FUD XXX N
AMA: 2019,Oct,10; 2018,Jan,8; 2017,Dec,8; 2017,Jan,8; 2016,Jan,13

00926 **radical orchiectomy, inguinal** ♂
0.00 0.00 FUD XXX N
AMA: 2019,Oct,10; 2018,Jan,8; 2017,Dec,8; 2017,Jan,8; 2016,Jan,13

00928 **radical orchiectomy, abdominal** ♂
0.00 0.00 FUD XXX N
AMA: 2019,Oct,10; 2018,Jan,8; 2017,Dec,8; 2017,Jan,8; 2016,Jan,13

00930 **orchiopexy, unilateral or bilateral** ♂
0.00 0.00 FUD XXX N
AMA: 2019,Oct,10; 2018,Jan,8; 2017,Dec,8; 2017,Jan,8; 2016,Jan,13

00932 **complete amputation of penis** ♂
0.00 0.00 FUD XXX C
AMA: 2019,Oct,10; 2018,Jan,8; 2017,Dec,8; 2017,Jan,8; 2016,Jan,13

00934 **radical amputation of penis with bilateral inguinal lymphadenectomy** ♂
0.00 0.00 FUD XXX C
AMA: 2019,Oct,10; 2018,Jan,8; 2017,Dec,8; 2017,Jan,8; 2016,Jan,13

00936 **radical amputation of penis with bilateral inguinal and iliac lymphadenectomy** ♂
0.00 0.00 FUD XXX C
AMA: 2019,Oct,10; 2018,Jan,8; 2017,Dec,8; 2017,Jan,8; 2016,Jan,13

00938 **insertion of penile prosthesis (perineal approach)** ♂
0.00 0.00 FUD XXX N
AMA: 2019,Oct,10; 2018,Jan,8; 2017,Dec,8; 2017,Jan,8; 2016,Jan,13

00940 **Anesthesia for vaginal procedures (including biopsy of labia, vagina, cervix or endometrium); not otherwise specified** ♀
0.00 0.00 FUD XXX N
AMA: 2019,Oct,10; 2018,Jan,8; 2017,Dec,8; 2017,Jan,8; 2016,Jan,13

00942 **colpotomy, vaginectomy, colporrhaphy, and open urethral procedures** ♀
0.00 0.00 FUD XXX N
AMA: 2019,Oct,10; 2018,Jan,8; 2017,Dec,8; 2017,Jan,8; 2016,Jan,13

00944 **vaginal hysterectomy** ♀
0.00 0.00 FUD XXX C
AMA: 2019,Oct,10; 2018,Jan,8; 2017,Dec,8; 2017,Jan,8; 2016,Jan,13

00948 **cervical cerclage** ♀
0.00 0.00 FUD XXX N
AMA: 2019,Oct,10; 2018,Jan,8; 2017,Dec,8; 2017,Jan,8; 2016,Jan,13

00950 **culdoscopy** ♀ N
0.00 0.00 FUD XXX
AMA: 2019,Oct,10; 2018,Jan,8; 2017,Dec,8; 2017,Jan,8; 2016,Jan,13

00952 **hysteroscopy and/or hysterosalpingography** ♀ N
0.00 0.00 FUD XXX
AMA: 2019,Oct,10; 2018,Jan,8; 2017,Dec,8; 2017,Jan,8; 2016,Jan,13

01112-01522 Anesthesia for Lower Extremity Procedures

CMS: 100-04,12,140.1 Qualified Nonphysician Anesthetists; 100-04,12,140.3 Payment for Qualified Nonphysician Anesthetists; 100-04,12,140.3.3 Billing Modifiers; 100-04,12,140.3.4 General Billing Instructions; 100-04,12,140.4.1 An Anesthesiologist and Qualified Nonphysician Anesthetist Work Together; 100-04,12,140.4.2 Anesthetist and Anesthesiologist in a Single Procedure; 100-04,12,140.4.3 Payment for Medical /Surgical Services by CRNAs; 100-04,12,140.4.4 Conversion Factors for Anesthesia Services; 100-04,12,140.5 Payment for Anesthesia Services Furnished by a Teaching CRNA; 100-04,4,250.3.2 Anesthesia in a Hospital Outpatient Setting

01112 **Anesthesia for bone marrow aspiration and/or biopsy, anterior or posterior iliac crest** N
0.00 0.00 FUD XXX
AMA: 2019,Oct,10; 2018,Jan,8; 2017,Dec,8; 2017,Jan,8; 2016,Jan,13

01120 **Anesthesia for procedures on bony pelvis** N
0.00 0.00 FUD XXX
AMA: 2019,Oct,10; 2018,Jan,8; 2017,Dec,8; 2017,Jan,8; 2016,Jan,13

01130 **Anesthesia for body cast application or revision** N
0.00 0.00 FUD XXX
AMA: 2019,Oct,10; 2018,Jan,8; 2017,Dec,8; 2017,Jan,8; 2016,Jan,13

01140 **Anesthesia for interpelviabdominal (hindquarter) amputation** C
0.00 0.00 FUD XXX
AMA: 2019,Oct,10; 2018,Jan,8; 2017,Dec,8; 2017,Jan,8; 2016,Jan,13

01150 **Anesthesia for radical procedures for tumor of pelvis, except hindquarter amputation** C
0.00 0.00 FUD XXX
AMA: 2019,Oct,10; 2018,Jan,8; 2017,Dec,8; 2017,Jan,8; 2016,Jan,13

01160 **Anesthesia for closed procedures involving symphysis pubis or sacroiliac joint** N
0.00 0.00 FUD XXX
AMA: 2019,Oct,10; 2018,Jan,8; 2017,Dec,8; 2017,Jan,8; 2016,Jan,13

01170 **Anesthesia for open procedures involving symphysis pubis or sacroiliac joint** N
0.00 0.00 FUD XXX
AMA: 2019,Oct,10; 2018,Jan,8; 2017,Dec,8; 2017,Jan,8; 2016,Jan,13

01173 **Anesthesia for open repair of fracture disruption of pelvis or column fracture involving acetabulum** N
0.00 0.00 FUD XXX
AMA: 2019,Oct,10; 2018,Jan,8; 2017,Dec,8; 2017,Jan,8; 2016,Jan,13

01200 **Anesthesia for all closed procedures involving hip joint** N
0.00 0.00 FUD XXX
AMA: 2019,Oct,10; 2018,Jan,8; 2017,Dec,8; 2017,Jan,8; 2016,Jan,13

01202 **Anesthesia for arthroscopic procedures of hip joint** N
0.00 0.00 FUD XXX
AMA: 2019,Oct,10; 2018,Jan,8; 2017,Dec,8; 2017,Jan,8; 2016,Jan,13

01210 **Anesthesia for open procedures involving hip joint; not otherwise specified** N
0.00 0.00 FUD XXX
AMA: 2019,Oct,10; 2018,Jan,8; 2017,Dec,8; 2017,Jan,8; 2016,Jan,13

01212 **hip disarticulation** C
0.00 0.00 FUD XXX
AMA: 2019,Oct,10; 2018,Jan,8; 2017,Dec,8; 2017,Jan,8; 2016,Jan,13

01214 **total hip arthroplasty** C
0.00 0.00 FUD XXX
AMA: 2019,Oct,10; 2018,Jan,8; 2017,Dec,8; 2017,Jan,8; 2016,Jan,13

01215 **revision of total hip arthroplasty** N
0.00 0.00 FUD XXX
AMA: 2019,Oct,10; 2018,Jan,8; 2017,Dec,8; 2017,Jan,8; 2016,Jan,13

01220 **Anesthesia for all closed procedures involving upper two-thirds of femur** N
0.00 0.00 FUD XXX
AMA: 2019,Oct,10; 2018,Jan,8; 2017,Dec,8; 2017,Jan,8; 2016,Jan,13

01230 **Anesthesia for open procedures involving upper two-thirds of femur; not otherwise specified** N
0.00 0.00 FUD XXX
AMA: 2019,Oct,10; 2018,Jan,8; 2017,Dec,8; 2017,Jan,8; 2016,Jan,13

01232 **amputation** C
0.00 0.00 FUD XXX
AMA: 2019,Oct,10; 2018,Jan,8; 2017,Dec,8; 2017,Jan,8; 2016,Jan,13

01234 **radical resection** C
0.00 0.00 FUD XXX
AMA: 2019,Oct,10; 2018,Jan,8; 2017,Dec,8; 2017,Jan,8; 2016,Jan,13

01250 **Anesthesia for all procedures on nerves, muscles, tendons, fascia, and bursae of upper leg** N
0.00 0.00 FUD XXX
AMA: 2019,Oct,10; 2018,Jan,8; 2017,Dec,8; 2017,Jan,8; 2016,Jan,13

01260 **Anesthesia for all procedures involving veins of upper leg, including exploration** N
0.00 0.00 FUD XXX
AMA: 2019,Oct,10; 2018,Jan,8; 2017,Dec,8; 2017,Jan,8; 2016,Jan,13

01270 **Anesthesia for procedures involving arteries of upper leg, including bypass graft; not otherwise specified** N
0.00 0.00 FUD XXX
AMA: 2019,Oct,10; 2018,Jan,8; 2017,Dec,8; 2017,Jan,8; 2016,Jan,13

01272 **femoral artery ligation** C
0.00 0.00 FUD XXX
AMA: 2019,Oct,10; 2018,Jan,8; 2017,Dec,8; 2017,Jan,8; 2016,Jan,13

01274 **femoral artery embolectomy** C
0.00 0.00 FUD XXX
AMA: 2019,Oct,10; 2018,Jan,8; 2017,Dec,8; 2017,Jan,8; 2016,Jan,13

01320 **Anesthesia for all procedures on nerves, muscles, tendons, fascia, and bursae of knee and/or popliteal area** N
0.00 0.00 FUD XXX
AMA: 2019,Oct,10; 2018,Jan,8; 2017,Dec,8; 2017,Jan,8; 2016,Jan,13

01340 **Anesthesia for all closed procedures on lower one-third of femur** N
0.00 0.00 FUD XXX
AMA: 2019,Oct,10; 2018,Jan,8; 2017,Dec,8; 2017,Jan,8; 2016,Jan,13

01360 **Anesthesia for all open procedures on lower one-third of femur** N
0.00 0.00 FUD XXX
AMA: 2019,Oct,10; 2018,Jan,8; 2017,Dec,8; 2017,Jan,8; 2016,Jan,13

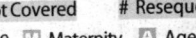

Anesthesia

01380—01522

01380 Anesthesia for all closed procedures on knee joint
0.00 0.00 FUD XXX N
AMA: 2019,Oct,10; 2018,Jan,8; 2017,Dec,8; 2017,Jan,8; 2016,Jan,13

01382 Anesthesia for diagnostic arthroscopic procedures of knee joint
0.00 0.00 FUD XXX N
AMA: 2019,Oct,10; 2018,Jan,8; 2017,Dec,8; 2017,Jan,8; 2016,Jan,13

01390 Anesthesia for all closed procedures on upper ends of tibia, fibula, and/or patella
0.00 0.00 FUD XXX N
AMA: 2019,Oct,10; 2018,Jan,8; 2017,Dec,8; 2017,Jan,8; 2016,Jan,13

01392 Anesthesia for all open procedures on upper ends of tibia, fibula, and/or patella
0.00 0.00 FUD XXX N
AMA: 2019,Oct,10; 2018,Jan,8; 2017,Dec,8; 2017,Jan,8; 2016,Jan,13

01400 Anesthesia for open or surgical arthroscopic procedures on knee joint; not otherwise specified
0.00 0.00 FUD XXX N
AMA: 2019,Oct,10; 2018,Jan,8; 2017,Dec,8; 2017,Jan,8; 2016,Jan,13

01402 total knee arthroplasty
0.00 0.00 FUD XXX C
AMA: 2019,Oct,10; 2018,Jan,8; 2017,Dec,8; 2017,Jan,8; 2016,Jan,13

01404 disarticulation at knee
0.00 0.00 FUD XXX C
AMA: 2019,Oct,10; 2018,Jan,8; 2017,Dec,8; 2017,Jan,8; 2016,Jan,13

01420 Anesthesia for all cast applications, removal, or repair involving knee joint
0.00 0.00 FUD XXX N
AMA: 2019,Oct,10; 2018,Jan,8; 2017,Dec,8; 2017,Jan,8; 2016,Jan,13

01430 Anesthesia for procedures on veins of knee and popliteal area; not otherwise specified
0.00 0.00 FUD XXX N
AMA: 2019,Oct,10; 2018,Jan,8; 2017,Dec,8; 2017,Jan,8; 2016,Jan,13

01432 arteriovenous fistula
0.00 0.00 FUD XXX N
AMA: 2019,Oct,10; 2018,Jan,8; 2017,Dec,8; 2017,Jan,8; 2016,Jan,13

01440 Anesthesia for procedures on arteries of knee and popliteal area; not otherwise specified
0.00 0.00 FUD XXX N
AMA: 2019,Oct,10; 2018,Jan,8; 2017,Dec,8; 2017,Jan,8; 2016,Jan,13

01442 popliteal thromboendarterectomy, with or without patch graft
0.00 0.00 FUD XXX C
AMA: 2019,Oct,10; 2018,Jan,8; 2017,Dec,8; 2017,Jan,8; 2016,Jan,13

01444 popliteal excision and graft or repair for occlusion or aneurysm
0.00 0.00 FUD XXX C
AMA: 2019,Oct,10; 2018,Jan,8; 2017,Dec,8; 2017,Jan,8; 2016,Jan,13

01462 Anesthesia for all closed procedures on lower leg, ankle, and foot
0.00 0.00 FUD XXX N
AMA: 2019,Oct,10; 2018,Jan,8; 2017,Dec,8; 2017,Jan,8; 2016,Jan,13

01464 Anesthesia for arthroscopic procedures of ankle and/or foot
0.00 0.00 FUD XXX N
AMA: 2019,Oct,10; 2018,Jan,8; 2017,Dec,8; 2017,Jan,8; 2016,Jan,13

01470 Anesthesia for procedures on nerves, muscles, tendons, and fascia of lower leg, ankle, and foot; not otherwise specified
0.00 0.00 FUD XXX N
AMA: 2019,Oct,10; 2018,Jan,8; 2017,Dec,8; 2017,Jan,8; 2016,Jan,13

01472 repair of ruptured Achilles tendon, with or without graft
0.00 0.00 FUD XXX N
AMA: 2019,Oct,10; 2018,Jan,8; 2017,Dec,8; 2017,Jan,8; 2016,Jan,13

01474 gastrocnemius recession (eg, Strayer procedure)
0.00 0.00 FUD XXX N
AMA: 2019,Oct,10; 2018,Jan,8; 2017,Dec,8; 2017,Jan,8; 2016,Jan,13

01480 Anesthesia for open procedures on bones of lower leg, ankle, and foot; not otherwise specified
0.00 0.00 FUD XXX N
AMA: 2019,Oct,10; 2018,Jan,8; 2017,Dec,8; 2017,Jan,8; 2016,Jan,13

01482 radical resection (including below knee amputation)
0.00 0.00 FUD XXX N
AMA: 2019,Oct,10; 2018,Jan,8; 2017,Dec,8; 2017,Jan,8; 2016,Jan,13

01484 osteotomy or osteoplasty of tibia and/or fibula
0.00 0.00 FUD XXX N
AMA: 2019,Oct,10; 2018,Jan,8; 2017,Dec,8; 2017,Jan,8; 2016,Jan,13

01486 total ankle replacement
0.00 0.00 FUD XXX C
AMA: 2019,Oct,10; 2018,Jan,8; 2017,Dec,8; 2017,Jan,8; 2016,Jan,13

01490 Anesthesia for lower leg cast application, removal, or repair
0.00 0.00 FUD XXX N
AMA: 2019,Oct,10; 2018,Jan,8; 2017,Dec,8; 2017,Jan,8; 2016,Jan,13

01500 Anesthesia for procedures on arteries of lower leg, including bypass graft; not otherwise specified
0.00 0.00 FUD XXX N
AMA: 2019,Oct,10; 2018,Jan,8; 2017,Dec,8; 2017,Jan,8; 2016,Jan,13

01502 embolectomy, direct or with catheter
0.00 0.00 FUD XXX C
AMA: 2019,Oct,10; 2018,Jan,8; 2017,Dec,8; 2017,Jan,8; 2016,Jan,13

01520 Anesthesia for procedures on veins of lower leg; not otherwise specified
0.00 0.00 FUD XXX N
AMA: 2019,Oct,10; 2018,Jan,8; 2017,Dec,8; 2017,Jan,8; 2016,Jan,13

01522 venous thrombectomy, direct or with catheter
0.00 0.00 FUD XXX N
AMA: 2019,Oct,10; 2018,Jan,8; 2017,Dec,8; 2017,Jan,8; 2016,Jan,13

01610-01680 Anesthesia for Shoulder Procedures

CMS: 100-04,12,140.1 Qualified Nonphysician Anesthetists; 100-04,12,140.3 Payment for Qualified Nonphysician Anesthetists; 100-04,12,140.3.3 Billing Modifiers; 100-04,12,140.3.4 General Billing Instructions; 100-04,12,140.4.1 An Anesthesiologist and Qualified Nonphysician Anesthetist Work Together; 100-04,12,140.4.2 Anesthetist and Anesthesiologist in a Single Procedure; 100-04,12,140.4.3 Payment for Medical /Surgical Services by CRNAs; 100-04,12,140.4.4 Conversion Factors for Anesthesia Services; 100-04,12,140.5 Payment for Anesthesia Services Furnished by a Teaching CRNA; 100-04,4,250.3.2 Anesthesia in a Hospital Outpatient Setting

INCLUDES Acromioclavicular joint
Humeral head and neck
Shoulder joint
Sternoclavicular joint

01610 **Anesthesia for all procedures on nerves, muscles, tendons, fascia, and bursae of shoulder and axilla**
0.00 0.00 **FUD** XXX N
AMA: 2019,Oct,10; 2018,Jan,8; 2017,Dec,8; 2017,Jan,8; 2016,Jan,13

01620 **Anesthesia for all closed procedures on humeral head and neck, sternoclavicular joint, acromioclavicular joint, and shoulder joint**
0.00 0.00 **FUD** XXX N
AMA: 2019,Oct,10; 2018,Jan,8; 2017,Dec,8; 2017,Jan,8; 2016,Jan,13

01622 **Anesthesia for diagnostic arthroscopic procedures of shoulder joint**
0.00 0.00 **FUD** XXX N
AMA: 2019,Oct,10; 2018,Jan,8; 2017,Dec,8; 2017,Jan,8; 2016,Jan,13

01630 **Anesthesia for open or surgical arthroscopic procedures on humeral head and neck, sternoclavicular joint, acromioclavicular joint, and shoulder joint; not otherwise specified**
0.00 0.00 **FUD** XXX N
AMA: 2019,Oct,10; 2018,Jan,8; 2017,Dec,8; 2017,Jan,8; 2016,Jan,13

01634 **shoulder disarticulation**
0.00 0.00 **FUD** XXX C
AMA: 2019,Oct,10; 2018,Jan,8; 2017,Dec,8; 2017,Jan,8; 2016,Jan,13

01636 **interthoracoscapular (forequarter) amputation**
0.00 0.00 **FUD** XXX C
AMA: 2019,Oct,10; 2018,Jan,8; 2017,Dec,8; 2017,Jan,8; 2016,Jan,13

01638 **total shoulder replacement**
0.00 0.00 **FUD** XXX C
AMA: 2019,Oct,10; 2018,Jan,8; 2017,Dec,8; 2017,Jan,8; 2016,Jan,13

01650 **Anesthesia for procedures on arteries of shoulder and axilla; not otherwise specified**
0.00 0.00 **FUD** XXX N
AMA: 2019,Oct,10; 2018,Jan,8; 2017,Dec,8; 2017,Jan,8; 2016,Jan,13

01652 **axillary-brachial aneurysm**
0.00 0.00 **FUD** XXX C
AMA: 2019,Oct,10; 2018,Jan,8; 2017,Dec,8; 2017,Jan,8; 2016,Jan,13

01654 **bypass graft**
0.00 0.00 **FUD** XXX C
AMA: 2019,Oct,10; 2018,Jan,8; 2017,Dec,8; 2017,Jan,8; 2016,Jan,13

01656 **axillary-femoral bypass graft**
0.00 0.00 **FUD** XXX C
AMA: 2019,Oct,10; 2018,Jan,8; 2017,Dec,8; 2017,Jan,8; 2016,Jan,13

01670 **Anesthesia for all procedures on veins of shoulder and axilla**
0.00 0.00 **FUD** XXX N
AMA: 2019,Oct,10; 2018,Jan,8; 2017,Dec,8; 2017,Jan,8; 2016,Jan,13

01680 **Anesthesia for shoulder cast application, removal or repair, not otherwise specified**
0.00 0.00 **FUD** XXX N
AMA: 2019,Oct,10; 2018,Jan,8; 2017,Dec,8; 2017,Jan,8; 2016,Jan,13

01710-01860 Anesthesia for Upper Extremity Procedures

CMS: 100-04,12,140.1 Qualified Nonphysician Anesthetists; 100-04,12,140.3 Payment for Qualified Nonphysician Anesthetists; 100-04,12,140.3.3 Billing Modifiers; 100-04,12,140.3.4 General Billing Instructions; 100-04,12,140.4.1 An Anesthesiologist and Qualified Nonphysician Anesthetist Work Together; 100-04,12,140.4.2 Anesthetist and Anesthesiologist in a Single Procedure; 100-04,12,140.4.3 Payment for Medical /Surgical Services by CRNAs; 100-04,12,140.4.4 Conversion Factors for Anesthesia Services; 100-04,12,140.5 Payment for Anesthesia Services Furnished by a Teaching CRNA; 100-04,4,250.3.2 Anesthesia in a Hospital Outpatient Setting

01710 **Anesthesia for procedures on nerves, muscles, tendons, fascia, and bursae of upper arm and elbow; not otherwise specified**
0.00 0.00 **FUD** XXX N
AMA: 2019,Oct,10; 2018,Jan,8; 2017,Dec,8; 2017,Jan,8; 2016,Jan,13

01712 **tenotomy, elbow to shoulder, open**
0.00 0.00 **FUD** XXX N
AMA: 2019,Oct,10; 2018,Jan,8; 2017,Dec,8; 2017,Jan,8; 2016,Jan,13

01714 **tenoplasty, elbow to shoulder**
0.00 0.00 **FUD** XXX N
AMA: 2019,Oct,10; 2018,Jan,8; 2017,Dec,8; 2017,Jan,8; 2016,Jan,13

01716 **tenodesis, rupture of long tendon of biceps**
0.00 0.00 **FUD** XXX N
AMA: 2019,Oct,10; 2018,Jan,8; 2017,Dec,8; 2017,Jan,8; 2016,Jan,13

01730 **Anesthesia for all closed procedures on humerus and elbow**
0.00 0.00 **FUD** XXX N
AMA: 2019,Oct,10; 2018,Jan,8; 2017,Dec,8; 2017,Jan,8; 2016,Jan,13

01732 **Anesthesia for diagnostic arthroscopic procedures of elbow joint**
0.00 0.00 **FUD** XXX N
AMA: 2019,Oct,10; 2018,Jan,8; 2017,Dec,8; 2017,Jan,8; 2016,Jan,13

01740 **Anesthesia for open or surgical arthroscopic procedures of the elbow; not otherwise specified**
0.00 0.00 **FUD** XXX N
AMA: 2019,Oct,10; 2018,Jan,8; 2017,Dec,8; 2017,Jan,8; 2016,Jan,13

01742 **osteotomy of humerus**
0.00 0.00 **FUD** XXX N
AMA: 2019,Oct,10; 2018,Jan,8; 2017,Dec,8; 2017,Jan,8; 2016,Jan,13

01744 **repair of nonunion or malunion of humerus**
0.00 0.00 **FUD** XXX N
AMA: 2019,Oct,10; 2018,Jan,8; 2017,Dec,8; 2017,Jan,8; 2016,Jan,13

01756 **radical procedures**
0.00 0.00 **FUD** XXX C
AMA: 2019,Oct,10; 2018,Jan,8; 2017,Dec,8; 2017,Jan,8; 2016,Jan,13

01758 **excision of cyst or tumor of humerus**
0.00 0.00 **FUD** XXX N
AMA: 2019,Oct,10; 2018,Jan,8; 2017,Dec,8; 2017,Jan,8; 2016,Jan,13

01760 **total elbow replacement**
0.00 0.00 **FUD** XXX N
AMA: 2019,Oct,10; 2018,Jan,8; 2017,Dec,8; 2017,Jan,8; 2016,Jan,13

01770 **Anesthesia for procedures on arteries of upper arm and elbow; not otherwise specified**
0.00 0.00 **FUD** XXX
AMA: 2019,Oct,10; 2018,Jan,8; 2017,Dec,8; 2017,Jan,8; 2016,Jan,13

01772 **embolectomy**
0.00 0.00 **FUD** XXX
AMA: 2019,Oct,10; 2018,Jan,8; 2017,Dec,8; 2017,Jan,8; 2016,Jan,13

01780 **Anesthesia for procedures on veins of upper arm and elbow; not otherwise specified**
0.00 0.00 **FUD** XXX
AMA: 2019,Oct,10; 2018,Jan,8; 2017,Dec,8; 2017,Jan,8; 2016,Jan,13

01782 **phleborrhaphy**
0.00 0.00 **FUD** XXX
AMA: 2019,Oct,10; 2018,Jan,8; 2017,Dec,8; 2017,Jan,8; 2016,Jan,13

01810 **Anesthesia for all procedures on nerves, muscles, tendons, fascia, and bursae of forearm, wrist, and hand**
0.00 0.00 **FUD** XXX
AMA: 2019,Oct,10; 2018,Jan,8; 2017,Dec,8; 2017,Jan,8; 2016,Jan,13

01820 **Anesthesia for all closed procedures on radius, ulna, wrist, or hand bones**
0.00 0.00 **FUD** XXX
AMA: 2019,Oct,10; 2018,Jan,8; 2017,Dec,8; 2017,Jan,8; 2016,Jan,13

01829 **Anesthesia for diagnostic arthroscopic procedures on the wrist**
0.00 0.00 **FUD** XXX
AMA: 2019,Oct,10; 2018,Jan,8; 2017,Dec,8; 2017,Jan,8; 2016,Jan,13

01830 **Anesthesia for open or surgical arthroscopic/endoscopic procedures on distal radius, distal ulna, wrist, or hand joints; not otherwise specified**
0.00 0.00 **FUD** XXX
AMA: 2019,Oct,10; 2018,Jan,8; 2017,Dec,8; 2017,Jan,8; 2016,Jan,13

01832 **total wrist replacement**
0.00 0.00 **FUD** XXX
AMA: 2019,Oct,10; 2018,Jan,8; 2017,Dec,8; 2017,Jan,8; 2016,Jan,13

01840 **Anesthesia for procedures on arteries of forearm, wrist, and hand; not otherwise specified**
0.00 0.00 **FUD** XXX
AMA: 2019,Oct,10; 2018,Jan,8; 2017,Dec,8; 2017,Jan,8; 2016,Jan,13

01842 **embolectomy**
0.00 0.00 **FUD** XXX
AMA: 2019,Oct,10; 2018,Jan,8; 2017,Dec,8; 2017,Jan,8; 2016,Jan,13

01844 **Anesthesia for vascular shunt, or shunt revision, any type (eg, dialysis)**
0.00 0.00 **FUD** XXX
AMA: 2019,Oct,10; 2018,Jan,8; 2017,Dec,8; 2017,Jan,8; 2016,Jan,13

01850 **Anesthesia for procedures on veins of forearm, wrist, and hand; not otherwise specified**
0.00 0.00 **FUD** XXX
AMA: 2019,Oct,10; 2018,Jan,8; 2017,Dec,8; 2017,Jan,8; 2016,Jan,13

01852 **phleborrhaphy**
0.00 0.00 **FUD** XXX
AMA: 2019,Oct,10; 2018,Jan,8; 2017,Dec,8; 2017,Jan,8; 2016,Jan,13

01860 **Anesthesia for forearm, wrist, or hand cast application, removal, or repair**
0.00 0.00 **FUD** XXX
AMA: 2019,Oct,10; 2018,Jan,8; 2017,Dec,8; 2017,Jan,8; 2016,Jan,13

01916-01942 Anesthesia for Interventional Radiology Procedures

01916 **Anesthesia for diagnostic arteriography/venography**
EXCLUDES *Anesthesia for therapeutic interventional radiological procedures involving arterial system (01924-01926)*
Anesthesia for therapeutic interventional radiological procedures involving venous/lymphatic system (01930-01933)
0.00 0.00 **FUD** XXX
AMA: 2019,Oct,10; 2018,Jan,8; 2017,Dec,8; 2017,Jan,8; 2016,Jan,13

01920 **Anesthesia for cardiac catheterization including coronary angiography and ventriculography (not to include Swan-Ganz catheter)**
0.00 0.00 **FUD** XXX
AMA: 2019,Oct,10; 2018,Jan,8; 2017,Dec,8; 2017,Jan,8; 2016,Jan,13

01922 **Anesthesia for non-invasive imaging or radiation therapy**
0.00 0.00 **FUD** XXX
AMA: 2019,Oct,10; 2018,Jan,8; 2017,Dec,8; 2017,Jan,8; 2016,Jan,13

01924 **Anesthesia for therapeutic interventional radiological procedures involving the arterial system; not otherwise specified**
0.00 0.00 **FUD** XXX
AMA: 2019,Oct,10; 2018,Jan,8; 2017,Dec,8; 2017,Jan,8; 2016,Jan,13

01925 **carotid or coronary**
0.00 0.00 **FUD** XXX
AMA: 2019,Oct,10; 2018,Jan,8; 2017,Dec,8; 2017,Jan,8; 2016,Jan,13

01926 **intracranial, intracardiac, or aortic**
0.00 0.00 **FUD** XXX
AMA: 2019,Oct,10; 2018,Jan,8; 2017,Dec,8; 2017,Jan,8; 2016,Jan,13

01930 **Anesthesia for therapeutic interventional radiological procedures involving the venous/lymphatic system (not to include access to the central circulation); not otherwise specified**
0.00 0.00 **FUD** XXX
AMA: 2019,Oct,10; 2018,Jan,8; 2017,Dec,8; 2017,Jan,8; 2016,Jan,13

01931 **intrahepatic or portal circulation (eg, transvenous intrahepatic portosystemic shunt[s] [TIPS])**
0.00 0.00 **FUD** XXX
AMA: 2019,Oct,10; 2018,Jan,8; 2017,Dec,8; 2017,Jan,8; 2016,Jan,13

01932 **intrathoracic or jugular**
0.00 0.00 **FUD** XXX
AMA: 2019,Oct,10; 2018,Jan,8; 2017,Dec,8; 2017,Jan,8; 2016,Jan,13

01933 **intracranial**
0.00 0.00 **FUD** XXX
AMA: 2019,Oct,10; 2018,Jan,8; 2017,Dec,8; 2017,Jan,8; 2016,Jan,13

~~**01935** **Anesthesia for percutaneous image guided procedures on the spine and spinal cord; diagnostic**~~
To report, see (01937-01942)

~~**01936** **therapeutic**~~
To report, see (01937-01942)

● **01937** **Anesthesia for percutaneous image-guided injection, drainage or aspiration procedures on the spine or spinal cord; cervical or thoracic**

EXCLUDES *Anesthesia for percutaneous image-guided destruction (01939)*

● **01938** **lumbar or sacral**

EXCLUDES *Anesthesia for percutaneous image-guided destruction (01940)*

● **01939** **Anesthesia for percutaneous image-guided destruction procedures by neurolytic agent on the spine or spinal cord; cervical or thoracic**

EXCLUDES *Anesthesia for percutaneous injection, drainage or aspiration (01937)*

● **01940** **lumbar or sacral**

EXCLUDES *Anesthesia for percutaneous injection, drainage or aspiration (01938)*

● **01941** **Anesthesia for percutaneous image-guided neuromodulation or intravertebral procedures (eg, kyphoplasty, vertebroplasty) on the spine or spinal cord; cervical or thoracic**

● **01942** **lumbar or sacral**

01951-01953 Anesthesia for Burn Procedures

CMS: 100-04,12,140.1 Qualified Nonphysician Anesthetists; 100-04,12,140.3 Payment for Qualified Nonphysician Anesthetists; 100-04,12,140.3.3 Billing Modifiers; 100-04,12,140.3.4 General Billing Instructions; 100-04,12,140.4.1 An Anesthesiologist and Qualified Nonphysician Anesthetist Work Together; 100-04,12,140.4.2 Anesthetist and Anesthesiologist in a Single Procedure; 100-04,12,140.4.3 Payment for Medical /Surgical Services by CRNAs; 100-04,12,140.4.4 Conversion Factors for Anesthesia Services; 100-04,12,140.5 Payment for Anesthesia Services Furnished by a Teaching CRNA; 100-04,4,250.3.2 Anesthesia in a Hospital Outpatient Setting

01951 **Anesthesia for second- and third-degree burn excision or debridement with or without skin grafting, any site, for total body surface area (TBSA) treated during anesthesia and surgery; less than 4% total body surface area** N

0.00 0.00 **FUD** XXX

AMA: 2019,Oct,10; 2018,Jan,8; 2017,Dec,8; 2017,Jan,8; 2016,Jan,13

01952 **between 4% and 9% of total body surface area** N

0.00 0.00 **FUD** XXX

AMA: 2019,Oct,10; 2018,Jan,8; 2017,Dec,8; 2017,Jan,8; 2016,Jan,13

\+ **01953** **each additional 9% total body surface area or part thereof (List separately in addition to code for primary procedure)**

Code first (01952)

0.00 0.00 **FUD** XXX N

AMA: 2019,Oct,10; 2018,Jan,8; 2017,Dec,8; 2017,Jan,8; 2016,Jan,13

01958-01969 Anesthesia for Obstetric Procedures

CMS: 100-04,12,140.1 Qualified Nonphysician Anesthetists; 100-04,12,140.3 Payment for Qualified Nonphysician Anesthetists; 100-04,12,140.3.3 Billing Modifiers; 100-04,12,140.3.4 General Billing Instructions; 100-04,12,140.4.1 An Anesthesiologist and Qualified Nonphysician Anesthetist Work Together; 100-04,12,140.4.2 Anesthetist and Anesthesiologist in a Single Procedure; 100-04,12,140.4.3 Payment for Medical /Surgical Services by CRNAs; 100-04,12,140.4.4 Conversion Factors for Anesthesia Services; 100-04,12,140.5 Payment for Anesthesia Services Furnished by a Teaching CRNA; 100-04,4,250.3.2 Anesthesia in a Hospital Outpatient Setting

01958 **Anesthesia for external cephalic version procedure** M

0.00 0.00 **FUD** XXX N

AMA: 2019,Oct,10; 2018,Jan,8; 2017,Dec,8; 2017,Jan,8; 2016,Jan,13

01960 **Anesthesia for vaginal delivery only** M ♀

0.00 0.00 **FUD** XXX N

AMA: 2019,Oct,10; 2018,Jan,8; 2017,Dec,8; 2017,Jan,8; 2016,Jan,13

01961 **Anesthesia for cesarean delivery only** M ♀

0.00 0.00 **FUD** XXX N

AMA: 2019,Oct,10; 2018,Jan,8; 2017,Dec,8; 2017,Jan,8; 2016,Jan,13

01962 **Anesthesia for urgent hysterectomy following delivery** M ♀

0.00 0.00 **FUD** XXX N

AMA: 2019,Oct,10; 2018,Jan,8; 2017,Dec,8; 2017,Jan,8; 2016,Jan,13

01963 **Anesthesia for cesarean hysterectomy without any labor analgesia/anesthesia care** M ♀

0.00 0.00 **FUD** XXX N

AMA: 2019,Oct,10; 2018,Jan,8; 2017,Dec,8; 2017,Jan,8; 2016,Jan,13

01965 **Anesthesia for incomplete or missed abortion procedures** M ♀

0.00 0.00 **FUD** XXX N

AMA: 2019,Oct,10; 2018,Jan,8; 2017,Dec,8; 2017,Jan,8; 2016,Jan,13

01966 **Anesthesia for induced abortion procedures** M ♀

0.00 0.00 **FUD** XXX N

AMA: 2019,Oct,10; 2018,Jan,8; 2017,Dec,8; 2017,Jan,8; 2016,Jan,13

01967 **Neuraxial labor analgesia/anesthesia for planned vaginal delivery (this includes any repeat subarachnoid needle placement and drug injection and/or any necessary replacement of an epidural catheter during labor)** M ♀

0.00 0.00 **FUD** XXX N

AMA: 2019,Oct,10; 2018,Jan,8; 2017,Dec,8; 2017,Jan,8; 2016,Jan,13

\+ **01968** **Anesthesia for cesarean delivery following neuraxial labor analgesia/anesthesia (List separately in addition to code for primary procedure performed)** M ♀

Code first (01967)

0.00 0.00 **FUD** XXX N

AMA: 2019,Oct,10; 2018,Jan,8; 2017,Dec,8; 2017,Jan,8; 2016,Jan,13

\+ **01969** **Anesthesia for cesarean hysterectomy following neuraxial labor analgesia/anesthesia (List separately in addition to code for primary procedure performed)** M ♀

Code first (01967)

0.00 0.00 **FUD** XXX N

AMA: 2019,Oct,10; 2018,Jan,8; 2017,Dec,8; 2017,Jan,8; 2016,Jan,13

01990-01999 Anesthesia Miscellaneous

CMS: 100-04,12,140.1 Qualified Nonphysician Anesthetists; 100-04,12,140.3 Payment for Qualified Nonphysician Anesthetists; 100-04,12,140.3.3 Billing Modifiers; 100-04,12,140.3.4 General Billing Instructions; 100-04,12,140.4.1 An Anesthesiologist and Qualified Nonphysician Anesthetist Work Together; 100-04,12,140.4.2 Anesthetist and Anesthesiologist in a Single Procedure; 100-04,12,140.4.3 Payment for Medical /Surgical Services by CRNAs; 100-04,12,140.4.4 Conversion Factors for Anesthesia Services; 100-04,12,140.5 Payment for Anesthesia Services Furnished by a Teaching CRNA; 100-04,4,250.3.2 Anesthesia in a Hospital Outpatient Setting

01990 **Physiological support for harvesting of organ(s) from brain-dead patient**

0.00 0.00 **FUD** XXX C

AMA: 2019,Oct,10; 2018,Jan,8; 2017,Dec,8; 2017,Jan,8; 2016,Jan,13

01991 **Anesthesia for diagnostic or therapeutic nerve blocks and injections (when block or injection is performed by a different physician or other qualified health care professional); other than the prone position**

EXCLUDES *Bier block for pain management (64999)*
Moderate Sedation (99151-99153, 99155-99157)
Pain management via intra-arterial or IV therapy (96373-96374)
Regional or local anesthesia arms or legs for surgical procedure

0.00 0.00 **FUD** XXX N

AMA: 2019,Oct,10; 2018,Jan,8; 2017,Dec,8; 2017,Jan,8; 2016,Jan,13

01992 **prone position**

EXCLUDES *Bier block for pain management (64999)*
Moderate sedation (99151-99153, 99155-99157)
Pain management via intra-arterial or IV therapy (96373-96374)
Regional or local anesthesia arms or legs for surgical procedure

0.00 0.00 **FUD** XXX N

AMA: 2019,Oct,10; 2018,Jan,8; 2017,Dec,8; 2017,Jan,8; 2016,Jan,13

01996 **Daily hospital management of epidural or subarachnoid continuous drug administration**

INCLUDES Continuous epidural or subarachnoid drug services performed after insertion epidural or subarachnoid catheter

0.00 0.00 **FUD** XXX N

AMA: 2019,Oct,10; 2018,Jan,8; 2017,Dec,8; 2017,Sep,6; 2017,Jan,8; 2016,Jan,13

01999 **Unlisted anesthesia procedure(s)**

0.00 0.00 **FUD** XXX N

AMA: 2019,Oct,10; 2018,Jan,8; 2017,Dec,8; 2017,Jan,8; 2016,Jan,13

10004-10012 [10004, 10005, 10006, 10007, 10008, 10009, 10010, 10011, 10012] Fine Needle Aspiration

EXCLUDES *Core needle biopsy, lung or mediastinum (32408)*
Percutaneous localization clip placement during breast biopsy (19081-19086)
Percutaneous needle biopsy:
Abdominal or retroperitoneal mass (49180)
Epididymis (54800)
Kidney (50200)
Liver (47000-47001)
Lymph node (38505)
Muscle (20206)
Nucleus pulposus, paravertebral tissue, intervertebral disc (62267)
Pancreas (48102)
Pleura (32400)
Prostate (55700, 55706)
Salivary gland (42400)
Spinal cord (62269)
Testis (54500)
Thyroid (60100)
Soft tissue percutaneous fluid drainage by catheter using image guidance (10030)
Thyroid cyst (60300)

Code also multiple biopsies on same service date:
FNA biopsies using same imaging guidance: report imaging add-on code for second and successive procedures
FNA biopsies separate lesions, different imaging guidance: append modifier 59 to codes for additional imaging modality used
FNA and core needle biopsy same lesion, same imaging guidance, procedure includes imaging guidance for core needle procedure
FNA and core needle biopsies separate lesions, same or different imaging guidance, append modifier 59 to code for core needle biopsy and imaging guidance

10004 **Resequenced code. See code following 10021.**
10005 **Resequenced code. See code following 10021.**
10006 **Resequenced code. See code following 10021.**
10007 **Resequenced code. See code following 10021.**
10008 **Resequenced code. See code following 10021.**
10009 **Resequenced code. See code following 10021.**
10010 **Resequenced code. See code following 10021.**
10011 **Resequenced code. See code following 10021.**
10012 **Resequenced code. See code following 10021.**

10021 Fine needle aspiration biopsy, without imaging guidance; first lesion
(88172-88173, [88177])
1.60 2.80 FUD XXX T P3 80
AMA: 2019,May,10; 2019,Apr,4; 2019,Feb,8; 2018,Jan,8; 2017,Jan,8; 2016,Jan,13

+ # 10004 each additional lesion (List separately in addition to code for primary procedure)
EXCLUDES *Fine needle biopsy using other imaging methods for same lesion ([10005, 10006, 10007, 10008, 10009, 10010, 10011, 10012])*
Imaging guidance (76942)
Code first (10021)
(88172-88173, [88177])
1.25 1.48 FUD ZZZ N1 80
AMA: 2019,Apr,4; 2019,Feb,8

 # 10005 Fine needle aspiration biopsy, including ultrasound guidance; first lesion
INCLUDES Imaging guidance (76942)
(88172-88173, [88177])
2.10 3.59 FUD XXX G2 80
AMA: 2019,May,10; 2019,Feb,8; 2019,Apr,4

+ # 10006 each additional lesion (List separately in addition to code for primary procedure)
INCLUDES Imaging guidance (76942)
Code first ([10005])
(88172-88173, [88177])
1.42 1.70 FUD ZZZ N1 80
AMA: 2019,Apr,4; 2019,Feb,8

 # 10007 Fine needle aspiration biopsy, including fluoroscopic guidance; first lesion
INCLUDES Imaging guidance (77002)
(88172-88173, [88177])
2.70 8.09 FUD XXX P3 80
AMA: 2019,Apr,4; 2019,Feb,8

+ # 10008 each additional lesion (List separately in addition to code for primary procedure)
INCLUDES Imaging guidance (77002)
Code first ([10007])
(88172-88173, [88177])
1.76 4.79 FUD ZZZ N1 80
AMA: 2019,Apr,4; 2019,Feb,8

 # 10009 Fine needle aspiration biopsy, including CT guidance; first lesion
INCLUDES Imaging guidance (77012)
(88172-88173, [88177])
3.28 13.3 FUD XXX G2 80
AMA: 2019,Apr,4; 2019,Feb,8

+ # 10010 each additional lesion (List separately in addition to code for primary procedure)
INCLUDES Imaging guidance (77012)
Code first ([10009])
(88172-88173, [88177])
2.38 8.02 FUD ZZZ N1 80
AMA: 2019,Apr,4; 2019,Feb,8

 # 10011 Fine needle aspiration biopsy, including MR guidance; first lesion
INCLUDES Imaging guidance (77021)
(88172-88173, [88177])
0.00 0.00 FUD XXX R2 80
AMA: 2019,Apr,4; 2019,Feb,8

+ # 10012 each additional lesion (List separately in addition to code for primary procedure)
INCLUDES Imaging guidance (77021)
Code first ([10011])
(88172-88173, [88177])
0.00 0.00 FUD ZZZ N1 80
AMA: 2019,Apr,4; 2019,Feb,8

10030-10180 Treatment of Lesions: Skin and Subcutaneous Tissues

EXCLUDES *Excision benign lesion (11400-11471)*

10030 Image-guided fluid collection drainage by catheter (eg, abscess, hematoma, seroma, lymphocele, cyst), soft tissue (eg, extremity, abdominal wall, neck), percutaneous
INCLUDES Radiologic guidance (75989, 76942, 77002-77003, 77012, 77021)
EXCLUDES *Percutaneous drainage with imaging guidance:*
Peritoneal or retroperitoneal collections (49406)
Visceral collections (49405)
Transvaginal or transrectal drainage with imaging guidance peritoneal or retroperitoneal collections (49407)
Code also every instance of fluid collection drained using a separate catheter (10030)
3.98 17.5 FUD 000 T G2 80
AMA: 2019,Apr,4; 2018,Jan,8; 2017,Aug,9; 2017,Jan,8; 2016,Jan,13

10035 Placement of soft tissue localization device(s) (eg, clip, metallic pellet, wire/needle, radioactive seeds), percutaneous, including imaging guidance; first lesion

INCLUDES Radiologic guidance (76942, 77002, 77012, 77021)

EXCLUDES *Sites with more specific code descriptor, such as breast*
Reporting code more than one time per site, regardless number markers used

Code also each additional target on same or opposite side (10036)

2.46 12.8 **FUD** 000 T N1 80 50

AMA: 2018,Jan,8; 2017,Jan,8; 2016,Jun,3

\+ **10036 each additional lesion (List separately in addition to code for primary procedure)**

INCLUDES Radiologic guidance (76942, 77002, 77012, 77021)

EXCLUDES *Sites with more specific code descriptor, such as breast*
Reporting code more than one time per site, regardless number markers used

Code first (10035)

1.25 11.7 **FUD** ZZZ N N1 80

AMA: 2018,Jan,8; 2017,Jan,8; 2016,Jun,3

10040 Acne surgery (eg, marsupialization, opening or removal of multiple milia, comedones, cysts, pustules)

1.53 3.11 **FUD** 010 Q1 N1

AMA: 2018,Jan,8; 2017,Jan,8; 2016,Jan,13

10060 Incision and drainage of abscess (eg, carbuncle, suppurative hidradenitis, cutaneous or subcutaneous abscess, cyst, furuncle, or paronychia); simple or single

2.87 3.44 **FUD** 010 T P3

AMA: 2018,Jan,8; 2017,Jan,8; 2016,Jan,13

10061 complicated or multiple

5.16 5.87 **FUD** 010 T P3

AMA: 2018,Jan,8; 2017,Jan,8; 2016,Jan,13

10080 Incision and drainage of pilonidal cyst; simple

2.95 5.99 **FUD** 010 T P3

AMA: 2018,Jan,8; 2017,Jan,8; 2016,Jan,13

10081 complicated

EXCLUDES *Excision pilonidal cyst (11770-11772)*

4.93 8.67 **FUD** 010 T P3

AMA: 2018,Jan,8; 2017,Jan,8; 2016,Jan,13

10120 Incision and removal of foreign body, subcutaneous tissues; simple

2.94 4.31 **FUD** 010 T P3

AMA: 2018,Jan,8; 2017,Jan,8; 2016,Jan,13

10121 complicated

EXCLUDES *Debridement associated with fracture or dislocation (11010-11012)*
Exploration penetrating wound (20100-20103)

5.33 7.76 **FUD** 010 J A2

AMA: 2018,Jan,8; 2017,Jan,8; 2016,Jan,13

10140 Incision and drainage of hematoma, seroma or fluid collection

(76942, 77002, 77012, 77021)

3.40 4.77 **FUD** 010 J P3

AMA: 2018,Jan,8; 2017,Jan,8; 2016,Jan,13

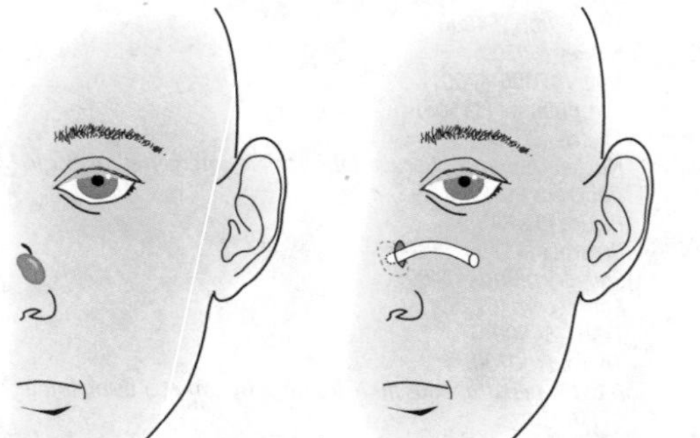
Hematoma may be decompressed with a hemostat
Drain may be placed to allow further drainage

10160 Puncture aspiration of abscess, hematoma, bulla, or cyst

(76942, 77002, 77012, 77021)

2.71 3.71 **FUD** 010 T P3

AMA: 2018,Jan,8; 2017,Aug,9; 2017,Jan,8; 2016,Jan,13

10180 Incision and drainage, complex, postoperative wound infection

EXCLUDES *Wound dehiscence (12020-12021, 13160)*

5.10 7.12 **FUD** 010 J A2

AMA: 2018,Jan,8; 2017,Jan,8; 2016,Jan,13

11000-11012 Removal of Foreign Substances and Infected/Devitalized Tissue

EXCLUDES *Debridement:*
Burns (16000-16030)
Deeper tissue (11042-11047 [11045, 11046])
Nails (11720-11721)
Nonelective debridement/active care management (97597-97598)
Wounds (11042-11047 [11045, 11046])
Dermabrasions (15780-15783)
Pressure ulcer excision (15920-15999)

11000 Debridement of extensive eczematous or infected skin; up to 10% of body surface

EXCLUDES *Necrotizing soft tissue infection:*
Abdominal wall (11005-11006)
External genitalia and perineum (11004, 11006)

0.82 1.61 **FUD** 000 T P3

AMA: 2018,Feb,10; 2018,Jan,8; 2017,Jan,8; 2016,Jan,13

\+ **11001 each additional 10% of the body surface, or part thereof (List separately in addition to code for primary procedure)**

EXCLUDES *Necrotizing soft tissue infection:*
Abdominal wall (11005-11006)
External genitalia and perineum (11004, 11006)

Code first (11000)

0.41 0.62 **FUD** ZZZ N N1

AMA: 2018,Feb,10; 2018,Jan,8; 2017,Jan,8; 2016,Jan,13

11004 Debridement of skin, subcutaneous tissue, muscle and fascia for necrotizing soft tissue infection; external genitalia and perineum

Code also skin grafts or flaps, when performed (14000-14350, 15040-15770 [15769], 15771-15776)

16.6 16.6 **FUD** 000 C

AMA: 2019,Nov,14; 2018,Feb,10; 2018,Jan,8; 2017,Jan,8; 2016,Jan,13

11005 **abdominal wall, with or without fascial closure**

Code also skin grafts or flaps, when performed (14000-14350, 15040-15770 [15769], 15771-15776)

22.6 22.6 **FUD** 000 C 80

AMA: 2019,Nov,14; 2018,Feb,10; 2018,Jan,8; 2017,Jan,8; 2016,Jan,13

11006 **external genitalia, perineum and abdominal wall, with or without fascial closure**

EXCLUDES *Orchiectomy (54520)*

Testicular transplant (54680)

Code also skin grafts or flaps, when performed (14000-14350, 15040-15770 [15769], 15771-15776)

20.4 20.4 **FUD** 000 C

AMA: 2019,Nov,14; 2018,Jan,8; 2017,Jan,8; 2016,Jan,13

\+ **11008** **Removal of prosthetic material or mesh, abdominal wall for infection (eg, for chronic or recurrent mesh infection or necrotizing soft tissue infection) (List separately in addition to code for primary procedure)**

EXCLUDES *Debridement (11000-11001, 11010-11044 [11045, 11046])*

Insertion mesh (49568)

Code also skin grafts or flaps, when performed (14000-14350, 15040-15770 [15769], 15771-15776)

Code first (10180, 11004-11006)

7.99 7.99 **FUD** ZZZ C 80

AMA: 2019,Jan,14; 2018,Jan,8; 2017,Jan,8; 2016,Jan,13

11010 **Debridement including removal of foreign material at the site of an open fracture and/or an open dislocation (eg, excisional debridement); skin and subcutaneous tissues**

7.96 13.5 **FUD** 010 T A2

AMA: 2018,Jan,8; 2017,Jan,8; 2016,Jan,13

11011 **skin, subcutaneous tissue, muscle fascia, and muscle**

8.68 15.4 **FUD** 000 T A2

AMA: 2018,Jan,8; 2017,Jan,8; 2016,Jan,13

11012 **skin, subcutaneous tissue, muscle fascia, muscle, and bone**

12.0 19.3 **FUD** 000 J A2

AMA: 2018,Jan,8; 2017,Jan,8; 2016,Jan,13

11042-11047 [11045, 11046] Removal of Infected/Devitalized Tissue

INCLUDES Debridement reported by size and depth

Debridement reported for multiple wounds by adding total surface area wounds with same depth

Injuries, wounds, chronic ulcers, infections

EXCLUDES *Debridement:*

Burn (16020-16030)

Eczematous or infected skin (11000-11001)

Nails (11720-11721)

Necrotizing soft tissue infection external genitalia, perineum, or abdominal wall (11004-11006)

Non-elective debridement/active care management same wound (97597-97602)

Dermabrasions (15780-15783)

Excision pressure ulcers (15920-15999)

Code also each additional single wound with different depths

Code also modifier 59 for additional wound debridement

Code also multiple wound groups with different depths

11042 **Debridement, subcutaneous tissue (includes epidermis and dermis, if performed); first 20 sq cm or less**

1.75 3.57 **FUD** 000 T A2

AMA: 2018,Jan,8; 2017,Jan,8; 2016,Oct,3; 2016,Aug,9; 2016,Feb,13; 2016,Jan,13

\+ # **11045** **each additional 20 sq cm, or part thereof (List separately in addition to code for primary procedure)**

Code first (11042)

0.77 1.19 **FUD** ZZZ N N1 80

AMA: 2018,Jan,8; 2017,Jan,8; 2016,Oct,3; 2016,Aug,9; 2016,Jan,13

11043 **Debridement, muscle and/or fascia (includes epidermis, dermis, and subcutaneous tissue, if performed); first 20 sq cm or less**

4.47 6.64 **FUD** 000 T A2

AMA: 2020,Apr,8; 2018,Jan,8; 2017,Jan,8; 2016,Oct,3; 2016,Aug,9; 2016,Jan,13

\+ # **11046** **each additional 20 sq cm, or part thereof (List separately in addition to code for primary procedure)**

Code first (11043)

1.62 2.12 **FUD** ZZZ N N1 80

AMA: 2018,Jan,8; 2017,Jan,8; 2016,Oct,3; 2016,Aug,9; 2016,Jan,13

11044 **Debridement, bone (includes epidermis, dermis, subcutaneous tissue, muscle and/or fascia, if performed); first 20 sq cm or less**

6.58 8.93 **FUD** 000 J A2

AMA: 2018,Jan,8; 2017,Jan,8; 2016,Oct,3; 2016,Aug,9; 2016,Jan,13

11045 **Resequenced code. See code following 11042.**

11046 **Resequenced code. See code following 11043.**

\+ **11047** **each additional 20 sq cm, or part thereof (List separately in addition to code for primary procedure)**

Code first (11044)

2.86 3.53 **FUD** ZZZ N N1 80

AMA: 2018,Jan,8; 2017,Jan,8; 2016,Oct,3; 2016,Aug,9; 2016,Jan,13

11055-11057 Excision Benign Hypertrophic Skin Lesions

CMS: 100-04,32,80.8 CSF Edits: Routine Foot Care

EXCLUDES *Destruction benign lesions other than cutaneous vascular proliferative lesions or skin tags (17110-17111)*

11055 **Paring or cutting of benign hyperkeratotic lesion (eg, corn or callus); single lesion**

0.46 1.78 **FUD** 000 Q1 N1

AMA: 2018,Jan,8; 2017,Jan,8; 2016,Jan,13

11056 **2 to 4 lesions**

0.65 1.90 **FUD** 000 Q1 N1

AMA: 2018,Jan,8; 2017,Jan,8; 2016,Jan,13

11057 **more than 4 lesions**

0.85 2.31 **FUD** 000 T P3

AMA: 2018,Jan,8; 2017,Jan,8; 2016,Jan,13

11102-11107 Surgical Biopsy Skin and Mucous Membranes

INCLUDES Attaining tissue for pathologic exam

EXCLUDES *Biopsies performed during related procedures*

Biopsy:

Anterior 2/3 tongue (41100)

Conjunctiva (68100)

Ear (69100)

Eyelid ([67810])

Floor of mouth (41108)

Intranasal (30100)

Lip (40490)

Nail (11755)

Penis (54100)

Perineum/vulva (56605-56606)

Vestibule of mouth (40808)

11102 **Tangential biopsy of skin (eg, shave, scoop, saucerize, curette); single lesion**

1.12 2.84 **FUD** 000 P3

AMA: 2020,May,13; 2019,Dec,9; 2019,Jan,9

\+ **11103** **each separate/additional lesion (List separately in addition to code for primary procedure)**

Code first different biopsy techniques used for additional separate lesions, when performed (11102, 11104, 11106)

0.66 1.51 **FUD** ZZZ N1

AMA: 2020,May,13; 2019,Dec,9; 2019,Jan,9

11104 **Punch biopsy of skin (including simple closure, when performed); single lesion**

1.40 3.57 **FUD** 000 P3

AMA: 2019,Dec,9; 2019,Jan,9

● New Code ▲ Revised Code ○ Reinstated ● New Web Release ▲ Revised Web Release + Add-on Unlisted Not Covered # Resequenced

⑩ Optum Mod 50 Exempt ⊘ AMA Mod 51 Exempt ⑤ Optum Mod 51 Exempt ⑥ Mod 63 Exempt ✗ Non-FDA Drug ★ Telemedicine M Maternity A Age Edit

\+ **11105** **each separate/additional lesion (List separately in addition to code for primary procedure)**
Code first different biopsy techniques used for additional separate lesions, when performed (11104, 11106)
0.76 | 1.72 | FUD ZZZ | N1
AMA: 2019,Dec,9; 2019,Jan,9

11106 **Incisional biopsy of skin (eg, wedge) (including simple closure, when performed); single lesion**
1.74 | 4.26 | FUD 000 | P3
AMA: 2019,Dec,9; 2019,Jan,9

\+ **11107** **each separate/additional lesion (List separately in addition to code for primary procedure)**
Code first (11106)
0.93 | 2.04 | FUD ZZZ | N1
AMA: 2019,Dec,9; 2019,Jan,9

11200-11201 Skin Tag Removal - All Techniques

INCLUDES
- Chemical destruction
- Electrocauterization
- Electrosurgical destruction
- Ligature strangulation
- Removal with or without local anesthesia
- Sharp excision or scissoring

11200 **Removal of skin tags, multiple fibrocutaneous tags, any area; up to and including 15 lesions**
2.10 | 2.52 | FUD 010 | Q1 N1
AMA: 2018,Jan,8; 2017,Jan,8; 2016,Jan,13

\+ **11201** **each additional 10 lesions, or part thereof (List separately in addition to code for primary procedure)**
Code first (11200)
0.48 | 0.54 | FUD ZZZ | N N1
AMA: 2018,Jan,8; 2017,Jan,8; 2016,Jan,13

11300-11313 Skin Lesion Removal: Shaving

INCLUDES
- Local anesthesia
- Partial thickness excision by horizontal slicing
- Wound cauterization

11300 **Shaving of epidermal or dermal lesion, single lesion, trunk, arms or legs; lesion diameter 0.5 cm or less**
0.99 | 2.84 | FUD 000 | Q1 N1 80
AMA: 2019,Jan,9; 2018,Feb,10; 2018,Jan,8; 2017,Dec,14; 2017,Jan,8; 2016,Jan,13

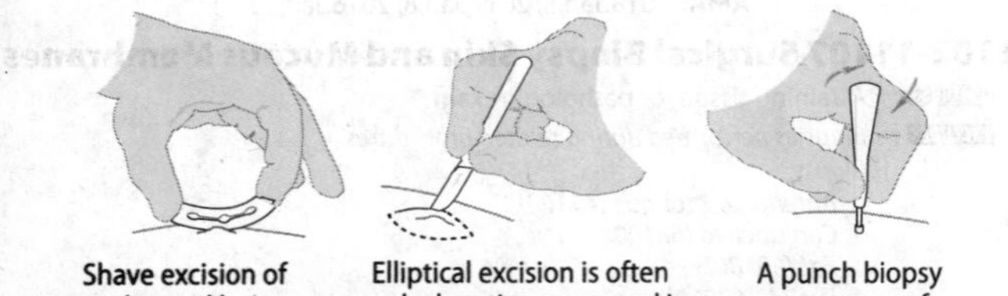

Shave excision of an elevated lesion; technique also used to biopsy

Elliptical excision is often used when tissue removal is larger than 4 mm or when deep pathology is suspected

A punch biopsy cuts a core of tissue as the tool is twisted downward

11301 **lesion diameter 0.6 to 1.0 cm**
1.50 | 3.45 | FUD 000 | Q1 N1 80
AMA: 2019,Jan,9; 2018,Feb,10; 2018,Jan,8; 2017,Dec,14; 2017,Jan,8; 2016,Jan,13

11302 **lesion diameter 1.1 to 2.0 cm**
1.76 | 3.99 | FUD 000 | Q1 N1 80
AMA: 2019,Jan,9; 2018,Feb,10; 2018,Jan,8; 2017,Dec,14; 2017,Jan,8; 2016,Jan,13

11303 **lesion diameter over 2.0 cm**
2.07 | 4.39 | FUD 000 | Q1 N1 80
AMA: 2019,Jan,9; 2018,Feb,10; 2018,Jan,8; 2017,Dec,14; 2017,Jan,8; 2016,Jan,13

11305 **Shaving of epidermal or dermal lesion, single lesion, scalp, neck, hands, feet, genitalia; lesion diameter 0.5 cm or less**
1.12 | 2.90 | FUD 000 | Q1 N1 80
AMA: 2019,Jan,9; 2018,Feb,10; 2018,Jan,8; 2017,Dec,14; 2017,Jan,8; 2016,Jan,13

11306 **lesion diameter 0.6 to 1.0 cm**
1.45 | 3.50 | FUD 000 | Q1 N1 80
AMA: 2019,Jan,9; 2018,Feb,10; 2018,Jan,8; 2017,Dec,14; 2017,Jan,8; 2016,Jan,13

11307 **lesion diameter 1.1 to 2.0 cm**
1.87 | 4.09 | FUD 000 | T P2 80
AMA: 2019,Jan,9; 2018,Feb,10; 2018,Jan,8; 2017,Dec,14; 2017,Jan,8; 2016,Jan,13

11308 **lesion diameter over 2.0 cm**
2.11 | 4.37 | FUD 000 | Q1 N1 80
AMA: 2019,Jan,9; 2018,Feb,10; 2018,Jan,8; 2017,Dec,14; 2017,Jan,8; 2016,Jan,13

11310 **Shaving of epidermal or dermal lesion, single lesion, face, ears, eyelids, nose, lips, mucous membrane; lesion diameter 0.5 cm or less**
1.34 | 3.29 | FUD 000 | T P3 80
AMA: 2019,Jan,9; 2018,Feb,10; 2018,Jan,8; 2017,Dec,14; 2017,Jan,8; 2016,Jan,13

11311 **lesion diameter 0.6 to 1.0 cm**
1.88 | 3.86 | FUD 000 | T P2 80
AMA: 2019,Jan,9; 2018,Feb,10; 2018,Jan,8; 2017,Dec,14; 2017,Jan,8; 2016,Jan,13

11312 **lesion diameter 1.1 to 2.0 cm**
2.17 | 4.51 | FUD 000 | T P3 80
AMA: 2019,Jan,9; 2018,Feb,10; 2018,Jan,8; 2017,Dec,14; 2017,Jan,8; 2016,Jan,13

11313 **lesion diameter over 2.0 cm**
2.82 | 5.27 | FUD 000 | T P3 80
AMA: 2019,Jan,9; 2018,Feb,10; 2018,Jan,8; 2017,Dec,14; 2017,Jan,8; 2016,Jan,13

11400-11446 Skin Lesion Removal: Benign

INCLUDES
- Biopsy on same lesion
- Cicatricial lesion excision
- Full thickness removal including margins
- Lesion measurement before excision at largest diameter plus margin
- Local anesthesia
- Simple, nonlayered closure

EXCLUDES
- *Adjacent tissue transfer: report only adjacent tissue transfer (14000-14302)*
- *Biopsy eyelid ([67810])*
- *Destruction:*
  - *Benign lesions, any method (17110-17111)*
  - *Cutaneous vascular proliferative lesions (17106-17108)*
  - *Destruction of eyelid lesion (67850)*
  - *Malignant lesions (17260-17286)*
  - *Premalignant lesions (17000, 17003-17004)*
- *Escharotomy (16035-16036)*
- *Excision and reconstruction eyelid (67961-67975)*
- *Excision chalazion (67800-67808)*
- *Eyelid procedures involving more than skin (67800 and subsequent codes)*
- *Laser fenestration for scars (0479T-0480T)*
- *Shave removal (11300-11313)*

Code also:
- Complex closure (13100-13153)
- Each separate lesion
- Intermediate closure (12031-12057)
- Modifier 22 when excision complicated or unusual
- Reconstruction (15002-15261, 15570-15770)

11400 **Excision, benign lesion including margins, except skin tag (unless listed elsewhere), trunk, arms or legs; excised diameter 0.5 cm or less**
2.33 | 3.57 | FUD 010 | T P3
AMA: 2019,Nov,3; 2018,Sep,7; 2018,Feb,10; 2018,Jan,8; 2017,Jan,8; 2016,Apr,3; 2016,Jan,13

11401 **excised diameter 0.6 to 1.0 cm**
2.96 | 4.35 | FUD 010 | T P3
AMA: 2019,Nov,3; 2018,Sep,7; 2018,Feb,10; 2018,Jan,8; 2017,Jan,8; 2016,Apr,3; 2016,Jan,13

11402 **excised diameter 1.1 to 2.0 cm**
3.29 | 4.78 | FUD 010 | T P3
AMA: 2019,Nov,3; 2018,Sep,7; 2018,Feb,10; 2018,Jan,8; 2017,Jan,8; 2016,Apr,3; 2016,Jan,13

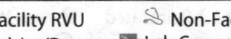

26/TC PC/TC Only | A2-Z3 ASC Payment | 50 Bilateral | ♂ Male Only | ♀ Female Only | Facility RVU | Non-Facility RVU | CCI | CLIA
FUD Follow-up Days | CMS: IOM | AMA: CPT Asst | A-Y OPPSI | 80/80 Surg Assist Allowed / w/Doc | Lab Crosswalk | Radiology Crosswalk

11403 **excised diameter 2.1 to 3.0 cm**
4.23 5.58 **FUD** 010 T P3
AMA: 2019,Nov,3; 2018,Sep,7; 2018,Feb,10; 2018,Jan,8; 2017,Jan,8; 2016,Apr,3; 2016,Jan,13

11404 **excised diameter 3.1 to 4.0 cm**
4.66 6.34 **FUD** 010 J A2
AMA: 2019,Nov,3; 2018,Sep,7; 2018,Feb,10; 2018,Jan,8; 2017,Jan,8; 2016,Apr,3; 2016,Jan,13

11406 **excised diameter over 4.0 cm**
7.09 9.07 **FUD** 010 J A2
AMA: 2019,Nov,3; 2018,Sep,7; 2018,Feb,10; 2018,Jan,8; 2017,Jan,8; 2016,Apr,3; 2016,Jan,13

11420 **Excision, benign lesion including margins, except skin tag (unless listed elsewhere), scalp, neck, hands, feet, genitalia; excised diameter 0.5 cm or less**
2.34 3.60 **FUD** 010 J P3
AMA: 2019,Nov,3; 2018,Sep,7; 2018,Feb,10; 2018,Jan,8; 2017,Jan,8; 2016,Apr,3; 2016,Jan,13

11421 **excised diameter 0.6 to 1.0 cm**
3.15 4.49 **FUD** 010 T P3
AMA: 2019,Nov,3; 2018,Sep,7; 2018,Feb,10; 2018,Jan,8; 2017,Jan,8; 2016,Apr,3; 2016,Jan,13

11422 **excised diameter 1.1 to 2.0 cm**
3.88 5.11 **FUD** 010 J P3
AMA: 2019,Nov,3; 2018,Sep,7; 2018,Feb,10; 2018,Jan,8; 2017,Jan,8; 2016,Apr,3; 2016,Jan,13

11423 **excised diameter 2.1 to 3.0 cm**
4.45 5.81 **FUD** 010 J P3
AMA: 2019,Nov,3; 2018,Sep,7; 2018,Feb,10; 2018,Jan,8; 2017,Jan,8; 2016,Apr,3; 2016,Jan,13

11424 **excised diameter 3.1 to 4.0 cm**
5.11 6.71 **FUD** 010 J A2
AMA: 2019,Nov,3; 2018,Sep,7; 2018,Feb,10; 2018,Jan,8; 2017,Jan,8; 2016,Apr,3; 2016,Jan,13

11426 **excised diameter over 4.0 cm**
7.89 9.63 **FUD** 010 J A2
AMA: 2019,Nov,3; 2018,Sep,7; 2018,Feb,10; 2018,Jan,8; 2017,Jan,8; 2016,Apr,3; 2016,Jan,13

11440 **Excision, other benign lesion including margins, except skin tag (unless listed elsewhere), face, ears, eyelids, nose, lips, mucous membrane; excised diameter 0.5 cm or less**
2.96 3.91 **FUD** 010 T P3
AMA: 2019,Nov,3; 2019,Jan,14; 2018,Sep,7; 2018,Feb,10; 2018,Jan,8; 2017,Jan,8; 2016,Apr,3; 2016,Jan,13

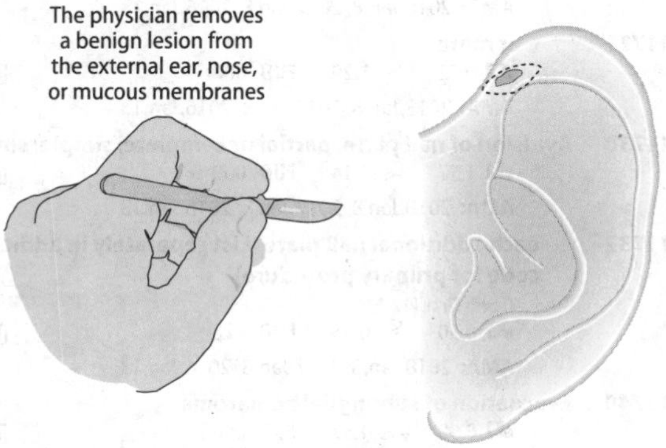

The physician removes a benign lesion from the external ear, nose, or mucous membranes

11441 **excised diameter 0.6 to 1.0 cm**
3.73 4.88 **FUD** 010 T P3
AMA: 2019,Nov,3; 2019,Jan,14; 2018,Sep,7; 2018,Feb,10; 2018,Jan,8; 2017,Jan,8; 2016,Apr,3; 2016,Jan,13

11442 **excised diameter 1.1 to 2.0 cm**
4.14 5.43 **FUD** 010 T P3
AMA: 2019,Nov,3; 2019,Jan,14; 2018,Sep,7; 2018,Feb,10; 2018,Jan,8; 2017,Jan,8; 2016,Apr,3; 2016,Jan,13

11443 **excised diameter 2.1 to 3.0 cm**
5.08 6.45 **FUD** 010 J P3
AMA: 2019,Nov,3; 2019,Jan,14; 2018,Sep,7; 2018,Feb,10; 2018,Jan,8; 2017,Jan,8; 2016,Apr,3; 2016,Jan,13

11444 **excised diameter 3.1 to 4.0 cm**
6.49 8.09 **FUD** 010 J A2
AMA: 2019,Nov,3; 2019,Jan,14; 2018,Sep,7; 2018,Feb,10; 2018,Jan,8; 2017,Jan,8; 2016,Apr,3; 2016,Jan,13

11446 **excised diameter over 4.0 cm**
9.33 11.1 **FUD** 010 J A2
AMA: 2019,Nov,3; 2019,Jan,14; 2018,Sep,7; 2018,Feb,10; 2018,Jan,8; 2017,Jan,8; 2016,Apr,3; 2016,Jan,13

11450-11471 Treatment of Hidradenitis: Excision and Repair

Code also closure by skin graft or flap (14000-14350, 15040-15770 [15769], 15771-15776)

11450 **Excision of skin and subcutaneous tissue for hidradenitis, axillary; with simple or intermediate repair**
7.36 11.6 **FUD** 090 J A2 50
AMA: 2019,Nov,3; 2018,Sep,7; 2018,Feb,10; 2018,Jan,8; 2017,Jan,8; 2016,Aug,9; 2016,Jan,13

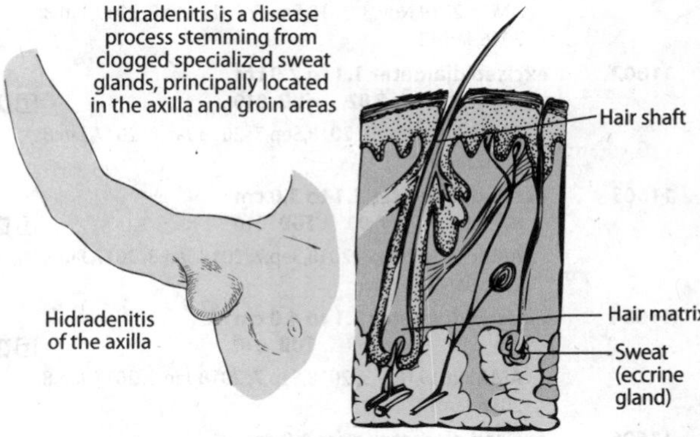

11451 **with complex repair**
9.41 14.5 **FUD** 090 J A2 80 50
AMA: 2019,Nov,3; 2018,Sep,7; 2018,Feb,10; 2018,Jan,8; 2017,Jan,8; 2016,Aug,9; 2016,Jan,13

11462 **Excision of skin and subcutaneous tissue for hidradenitis, inguinal; with simple or intermediate repair**
7.01 11.3 **FUD** 090 J A2 80 50
AMA: 2019,Nov,3; 2018,Sep,7; 2018,Feb,10; 2018,Jan,8; 2017,Jan,8; 2016,Aug,9; 2016,Jan,13

11463 **with complex repair**
9.42 14.3 **FUD** 090 J A2 80 50
AMA: 2019,Nov,3; 2018,Sep,7; 2018,Feb,10; 2018,Jan,8; 2017,Jan,8; 2016,Aug,9; 2016,Jan,13

11470 **Excision of skin and subcutaneous tissue for hidradenitis, perianal, perineal, or umbilical; with simple or intermediate repair**
8.08 12.0 **FUD** 090 J A2
AMA: 2019,Nov,3; 2018,Sep,7; 2018,Feb,10; 2018,Jan,8; 2017,Jan,8; 2016,Aug,9; 2016,Jan,13

11471 **with complex repair**
10.0 15.0 **FUD** 090 J A2 80
AMA: 2019,Nov,3; 2018,Sep,7; 2018,Feb,10; 2018,Jan,8; 2017,Jan,8; 2016,Aug,9; 2016,Jan,13

11600-11646 Skin Lesion Removal: Malignant

INCLUDES Biopsy on same lesion
Excision additional margin at same operative session
Full thickness removal including margins
Lesion measurement before excision at largest diameter plus margin
Local anesthesia
Simple, nonlayered closure

EXCLUDES *Adjacent tissue transfer. Report only adjacent tissue transfer (14000-14302)*
Destruction (17260-17286)
Excision additional margin at subsequent operative session (11600-11646)

Code also:
Complex closure (13100-13153)
Each separate lesion
Intermediate closure (12031-12057)
Modifier 22 when excision complicated or unusual
Reconstruction (15002-15261, 15570-15770)

11600 **Excision, malignant lesion including margins, trunk, arms, or legs; excised diameter 0.5 cm or less**
3.46 5.61 FUD 010 T P3
AMA: 2019,Nov,3; 2018,Sep,7; 2018,Jan,8; 2017,Jan,8; 2016,Jan,13

11601 **excised diameter 0.6 to 1.0 cm**
4.29 6.52 FUD 010 T P3
AMA: 2019,Nov,3; 2018,Sep,7; 2018,Jan,8; 2017,Jan,8; 2016,Jan,13

11602 **excised diameter 1.1 to 2.0 cm**
4.63 7.02 FUD 010 T P3
AMA: 2019,Nov,3; 2018,Sep,7; 2018,Jan,8; 2017,Jan,8; 2016,Jan,13

11603 **excised diameter 2.1 to 3.0 cm**
5.54 8.00 FUD 010 T P3
AMA: 2019,Nov,3; 2018,Sep,7; 2018,Jan,8; 2017,Jan,8; 2016,Jan,13

11604 **excised diameter 3.1 to 4.0 cm**
6.12 8.93 FUD 010 T A2
AMA: 2019,Nov,3; 2018,Sep,7; 2018,Jan,8; 2017,Jan,8; 2016,Jan,13

11606 **excised diameter over 4.0 cm**
9.24 12.8 FUD 010 J A2
AMA: 2019,Nov,3; 2018,Sep,7; 2018,Jan,8; 2017,Jan,8; 2016,Jan,13

11620 **Excision, malignant lesion including margins, scalp, neck, hands, feet, genitalia; excised diameter 0.5 cm or less**
3.50 5.64 FUD 010 J P3
AMA: 2019,Nov,3; 2018,Sep,7; 2018,Jan,8; 2017,Jan,8; 2016,Jan,13

11621 **excised diameter 0.6 to 1.0 cm**
4.27 6.55 FUD 010 T P3
AMA: 2019,Nov,3; 2018,Sep,7; 2018,Jan,8; 2017,Jan,8; 2016,Jan,13

11622 **excised diameter 1.1 to 2.0 cm**
4.93 7.30 FUD 010 T P3
AMA: 2019,Nov,3; 2018,Sep,7; 2018,Jan,8; 2017,Jan,8; 2016,Jan,13

11623 **excised diameter 2.1 to 3.0 cm**
6.03 8.52 FUD 010 J P3
AMA: 2019,Nov,3; 2018,Sep,7; 2018,Jan,8; 2017,Jan,8; 2016,Jan,13

11624 **excised diameter 3.1 to 4.0 cm**
6.85 9.65 FUD 010 J A2
AMA: 2019,Nov,3; 2018,Sep,7; 2018,Jan,8; 2017,Jan,8; 2016,Jan,13

11626 **excised diameter over 4.0 cm**
8.44 11.6 FUD 010 J A2
AMA: 2019,Nov,3; 2018,Sep,7; 2018,Jan,8; 2017,Jan,8; 2016,Jan,13

11640 **Excision, malignant lesion including margins, face, ears, eyelids, nose, lips; excised diameter 0.5 cm or less**
EXCLUDES *Eyelid excision involving more than skin (67800-67808, 67840-67850, 67961-67966)*
3.59 5.77 FUD 010 T P3
AMA: 2019,Nov,3; 2018,Sep,7; 2018,Jan,8; 2017,Jan,8; 2016,Jan,13

11641 **excised diameter 0.6 to 1.0 cm**
EXCLUDES *Eyelid excision involving more than skin (67800-67808, 67840-67850, 67961-67966)*
4.45 6.78 FUD 010 T P3
AMA: 2019,Nov,3; 2018,Sep,7; 2018,Jan,8; 2017,Jan,8; 2016,Jan,13

11642 **excised diameter 1.1 to 2.0 cm**
EXCLUDES *Eyelid excision involving more than skin (67800-67808, 67840-67850, 67961-67966)*
5.30 7.73 FUD 010 T P3
AMA: 2019,Nov,3; 2018,Sep,7; 2018,Jan,8; 2017,Jan,8; 2016,Jan,13

11643 **excised diameter 2.1 to 3.0 cm**
EXCLUDES *Eyelid excision involving more than skin (67800-67808, 67840-67850, 67961-67966)*
6.55 9.06 FUD 010 J P3
AMA: 2019,Nov,3; 2018,Sep,7; 2018,Jan,8; 2017,Jan,8; 2016,Jan,13

11644 **excised diameter 3.1 to 4.0 cm**
EXCLUDES *Eyelid excision involving more than skin (67800-67808, 67840-67850, 67961-67966)*
8.14 11.1 FUD 010 J A2
AMA: 2019,Nov,3; 2018,Sep,7; 2018,Jan,8; 2017,Jan,8; 2016,Jan,13

11646 **excised diameter over 4.0 cm**
EXCLUDES *Eyelid excision involving more than skin (67800-67808, 67840-67850, 67961-67966)*
11.2 14.5 FUD 010 J A2
AMA: 2019,Nov,3; 2018,Sep,7; 2018,Jan,8; 2017,Jan,8; 2016,Jan,13

11719-11765 Nails and Supporting Structures

CMS: 100-02,15,290 Foot Care
EXCLUDES *Drainage paronychia or onychia (10060-10061)*

11719 **Trimming of nondystrophic nails, any number**
0.22 0.41 FUD 000 Q1 N1
AMA: 2018,Jan,8; 2017,Jan,8; 2016,Jan,13

11720 **Debridement of nail(s) by any method(s); 1 to 5**
0.42 0.93 FUD 000 Q1 N1
AMA: 2018,Jan,8; 2017,Jan,8; 2016,Jan,13

11721 **6 or more**
0.72 1.29 FUD 000 Q1 N1
AMA: 2018,Jan,8; 2017,Jan,8; 2016,Jan,13

11730 **Avulsion of nail plate, partial or complete, simple; single**
1.57 3.14 FUD 000 Q1 N1
AMA: 2018,Jan,8; 2017,Jan,8; 2016,Jan,13

\+ **11732** **each additional nail plate (List separately in addition to code for primary procedure)**
Code first (11730)
0.50 0.95 FUD ZZZ N N1
AMA: 2018,Jan,8; 2017,Jan,8; 2016,Jan,13

11740 **Evacuation of subungual hematoma**
0.90 1.52 FUD 000 Q1 N1
AMA: 2018,Jan,8; 2017,Jan,8; 2016,Jan,13

11750 **Excision of nail and nail matrix, partial or complete (eg, ingrown or deformed nail), for permanent removal;**
EXCLUDES *Pinch graft (15050)*
2.92 4.41 FUD 010 T P3
AMA: 2018,Jan,8; 2017,Jan,8; 2016,Jan,13

11755 Biopsy of nail unit (eg, plate, bed, matrix, hyponychium, proximal and lateral nail folds) (separate procedure)
🚑 1.79 ⚕ 3.47 **FUD** 000 [T] [P3] [80] 📖
AMA: 2019,Jan,9; 2018,Jan,8; 2017,Jan,8; 2016,Jan,13

11760 Repair of nail bed
🚑 3.27 ⚕ 5.46 **FUD** 010 [T] [P3] 📖
AMA: 2018,Jan,8; 2017,Jan,8; 2016,Jan,13

11762 Reconstruction of nail bed with graft
🚑 5.33 ⚕ 8.15 **FUD** 010 [T] [P3] 📖
AMA: 2018,Jan,8; 2017,Jan,8; 2016,Jan,13

11765 Wedge excision of skin of nail fold (eg, for ingrown toenail)
[INCLUDES] Cotting's operation
🚑 2.64 ⚕ 4.80 **FUD** 010 [Q1] [N1] 📖
AMA: 2018,Jan,8; 2017,Jan,8; 2016,Jan,13

11770-11772 Treatment Pilonidal Cyst: Excision
[EXCLUDES] Incision of pilonidal cyst (10080-10081)

11770 Excision of pilonidal cyst or sinus; simple
🚑 5.34 ⚕ 8.92 **FUD** 010 [J] [A2] 📖

11771 extensive
🚑 12.7 ⚕ 17.2 **FUD** 090 [J] [A2] 📖

11772 complicated
🚑 16.6 ⚕ 20.9 **FUD** 090 [J] [A2] 📖
AMA: 2018,Jan,8; 2017,Jan,8; 2016,Jan,13

11900-11901 Treatment of Lesions: Injection
[EXCLUDES] Injection local anesthesia performed preoperatively
Injection veins (36470-36471)
Intralesional chemotherapy (96405-96406)

11900 Injection, intralesional; up to and including 7 lesions
🚑 0.90 ⚕ 1.54 **FUD** 000 [Q1] [N1] 📖
AMA: 2018,Jan,8; 2017,Jan,8; 2016,Jan,13

11901 more than 7 lesions
🚑 1.36 ⚕ 1.97 **FUD** 000 [Q1] [N1] 📖
AMA: 2018,Jan,8; 2017,Jan,8; 2016,Jan,13

11920-11971 Tattoos, Tissue Expanders, and Dermal Fillers
CMS: 100-02,16,10 Exclusions from Coverage; 100-02,16,120 Cosmetic Procedures; 100-02,16,180 Services Related to Noncovered Procedures

11920 Tattooing, intradermal introduction of insoluble opaque pigments to correct color defects of skin, including micropigmentation; 6.0 sq cm or less
🚑 3.23 ⚕ 5.33 **FUD** 000 [T] [P3] [80] 📖
AMA: 2018,Jan,8; 2017,Jan,8; 2016,Aug,9

11921 6.1 to 20.0 sq cm
🚑 3.81 ⚕ 6.08 **FUD** 000 [T] [P3] [80] 📖
AMA: 2018,Jan,8; 2017,Jan,8; 2016,Aug,9

+ 11922 each additional 20.0 sq cm, or part thereof (List separately in addition to code for primary procedure)
Code first (11921)
🚑 0.86 ⚕ 1.71 **FUD** ZZZ [N] [N1] [80] 📖

11950 Subcutaneous injection of filling material (eg, collagen); 1 cc or less
🚑 1.51 ⚕ 2.26 **FUD** 000 [T] [P3] [80] 📖
AMA: 2019,Aug,10; 2018,Jan,8; 2017,Jan,8; 2016,Jan,13

11951 1.1 to 5.0 cc
🚑 1.98 ⚕ 2.80 **FUD** 000 [T] [P3] [80] 📖
AMA: 2019,Aug,10; 2018,Jan,8; 2017,Jan,8; 2016,Jan,13

11952 5.1 to 10.0 cc
🚑 3.03 ⚕ 4.13 **FUD** 000 [T] [P3] [80] 📖
AMA: 2019,Aug,10; 2018,Jan,8; 2017,Jan,8; 2016,Jan,13

11954 over 10.0 cc
🚑 3.21 ⚕ 4.41 **FUD** 000 [T] [P3] [80] 📖
AMA: 2019,Aug,10; 2018,Jan,8; 2017,Jan,8; 2016,Jan,13

11960 Insertion of tissue expander(s) for other than breast, including subsequent expansion
[EXCLUDES] Breast reconstruction with tissue expander(s) (19357)
Decompression, nerve (64722-64726)
Endoscopic release transverse carpal ligament (29848)
Neuroplasty (64702-64721)
Removal tissue expander without implant insertion (11971)
Secondary closure, surgical wound or dehiscence (13160)
🚑 28.1 ⚕ 28.1 **FUD** 090 [T] [A2] 📖
AMA: 1991,Win,1

11970 Replacement of tissue expander with permanent implant
🚑 17.6 ⚕ 17.6 **FUD** 090 [J] [J8] [50] 📖
AMA: 2018,Jan,8; 2017,Jan,8; 2016,Jan,13

11971 Removal of tissue expander without insertion of implant
[EXCLUDES] Insertion/replacement tissue expander (11960, 11970)
🚑 9.31 ⚕ 13.7 **FUD** 090 [Q2] [A2] [80] [50] 📖
AMA: 2018,Jan,8; 2017,Jan,8; 2016,Jan,13

11976-11983 Drug Implantation

11976 Removal, implantable contraceptive capsules ♀
🚑 2.73 ⚕ 4.15 **FUD** 000 [Q2] [P3] [80] 📖
AMA: 1992,Win,1; 1991,Win,1

11980 Subcutaneous hormone pellet implantation (implantation of estradiol and/or testosterone pellets beneath the skin)
🚑 1.61 ⚕ 2.69 **FUD** 000 [Q1] [N1] 📖
AMA: 2018,Jan,8; 2017,Jan,8; 2016,Jan,13

▲ 11981 Insertion, drug-delivery implant (ie, bioresorbable, biodegradable, non-biodegradable)
[EXCLUDES] Removal bioresorbable/biodegradable drug-delivery implant (17999)
Insertion deep drug-delivery device:
Intra-articular (20704)
Intramedullary (20702)
Subfascial (20700)
🚑 1.86 ⚕ 2.96 **FUD** 000 [Q1] [N1] [80] 📖
AMA: 2018,Jan,8; 2017,Jan,8; 2016,Jan,13

11982 Removal, non-biodegradable drug delivery implant
[EXCLUDES] Removal deep drug-delivery device:
Intra-articular (20705)
Intramedullary (20703)
Subfascial (20701)
🚑 2.87 ⚕ 4.49 **FUD** XXX [Q1] [N1] [80] 📖

11983 Removal with reinsertion, non-biodegradable drug delivery implant
🚑 3.01 ⚕ 4.15 **FUD** 000 [Q1] [N1] [80] 📖

12001-12021 Suturing of Superficial Wounds

INCLUDES Administration local or topical anesthesia
Hemostasis
Repair that involves:
Routine debridement and decontamination
Simple one layer closure
Superficial tissues
Sutures, staples, tissue adhesives
Total length several repairs in same code category
Simple:
Exploration nerves, blood vessels, tendons
Vessel ligation, in wound

EXCLUDES *Complex repair nerves, blood vessels, tendons (see appropriate anatomical section)*
Debridement requiring:
Comprehensive cleaning
Removal significant tissue
Removal soft tissue and/or bone, no fracture/dislocation, performed separately (11042-11047 [11045, 11046])
Removal soft tissue and/or bone with open fracture/dislocation (11010-11012)
Deep tissue repair (12031-13153)
Major exploration (20100-20103)
Repair/closure limited to:
Adhesive strips only, see appropriate E/M service
Chemical cauterization, see appropriate E/M service
Electrocauterization, see appropriate E/M service
Secondary closure/dehiscence (13160)
Repair nerves, blood vessels, tendons (See appropriate anatomical section. These repairs include simple and intermediate closure. Report complex closure with modifier 59.)

Code also modifier 59 added to less complicated procedure code when reporting more than one wound repair classification

12001 **Simple repair of superficial wounds of scalp, neck, axillae, external genitalia, trunk and/or extremities (including hands and feet); 2.5 cm or less**
1.27 | 2.53 | FUD 000 | Q1 N1
AMA: 2018,Sep,7; 2018,Jan,8; 2017,Dec,14; 2017,Jan,8; 2016,Jan,13

12002 **2.6 cm to 7.5 cm**
1.67 | 3.08 | FUD 000 | Q1 N1
AMA: 2018,Sep,7; 2018,Jan,8; 2017,Jan,8; 2016,Jan,13

12004 **7.6 cm to 12.5 cm**
2.15 | 3.69 | FUD 000 | Q1 N1
AMA: 2018,Sep,7; 2018,Jan,8; 2017,Jan,8; 2016,Jan,13

12005 **12.6 cm to 20.0 cm**
2.71 | 4.69 | FUD 000 | Q1 A2
AMA: 2018,Sep,7; 2018,Jan,8; 2017,Jan,8; 2016,Jan,13

12006 **20.1 cm to 30.0 cm**
3.33 | 5.54 | FUD 000 | Q2 A2
AMA: 2018,Sep,7; 2018,Jan,8; 2017,Jan,8; 2016,Jan,13

12007 **over 30.0 cm**
4.15 | 6.37 | FUD 000 | T A2
AMA: 2018,Sep,7; 2018,Jan,8; 2017,Jan,8; 2016,Jan,13

12011 **Simple repair of superficial wounds of face, ears, eyelids, nose, lips and/or mucous membranes; 2.5 cm or less**
1.57 | 3.09 | FUD 000 | Q1 N1
AMA: 2018,Sep,7; 2018,Jan,8; 2017,Jan,8; 2016,Nov,7; 2016,Jan,13

12013 **2.6 cm to 5.0 cm**
1.72 | 3.29 | FUD 000 | Q1 N1
AMA: 2018,Sep,7; 2018,Jan,8; 2017,Jan,8; 2016,Jan,13

12014 **5.1 cm to 7.5 cm**
2.14 | 3.88 | FUD 000 | Q1 N1
AMA: 2018,Sep,7; 2018,Jan,8; 2017,Jan,8; 2016,Jan,13

12015 **7.6 cm to 12.5 cm**
2.78 | 4.84 | FUD 000 | Q1 G2
AMA: 2018,Sep,7; 2018,Jan,8; 2017,Jan,8; 2016,Jan,13

12016 **12.6 cm to 20.0 cm**
3.77 | 6.16 | FUD 000 | Q1 A2
AMA: 2018,Sep,7; 2018,Jan,8; 2017,Jan,8; 2016,Jan,13

12017 **20.1 cm to 30.0 cm**
4.48 | 4.48 | FUD 000 | Q1 A2 80
AMA: 2018,Sep,7; 2018,Jan,8; 2017,Jan,8; 2016,Jan,13

12018 **over 30.0 cm**
5.08 | 5.08 | FUD 000 | Q1 A2 80
AMA: 2018,Sep,7; 2018,Jan,8; 2017,Jan,8; 2016,Jan,13

12020 **Treatment of superficial wound dehiscence; simple closure**
EXCLUDES *Secondary closure major/complex wound or dehiscence (13160)*
5.43 | 8.41 | FUD 010 | T A2
AMA: 2019,Nov,3; 2018,Jan,8; 2017,Jan,8; 2016,Jan,13

12021 **with packing**
EXCLUDES *Secondary closure major/complex wound or dehiscence (13160)*
4.01 | 4.90 | FUD 010 | T A2
AMA: 2019,Nov,3; 2018,Jan,8; 2017,Jan,8; 2016,Jan,13

12031-12057 Suturing of Intermediate Wounds

INCLUDES Administration local anesthesia
Repair that involves:
Closure contaminated single layer wound
Layered closure (e.g., subcutaneous tissue, superficial fascia)
Limited undermining
Removal foreign material (e.g., gravel, glass)
Routine debridement and decontamination
Simple:
Exploration nerves, blood vessels, tendons in wound
Vessel ligation, in wound
Total length several repairs in same code category

EXCLUDES *Debridement requiring:*
Removal soft tissue and/or bone, no fracture/dislocation, performed separately (11042-11047 [11045, 11046])
Removal soft tissue/bone due to open fracture/dislocation (11010-11012)
Major exploration (20100-20103)
Repair nerves, blood vessels, tendons (See appropriate anatomical section. These repairs include simple and intermediate closure. Report complex closure with modifier 59.)
Secondary closure major/complex wound or dehiscence (13160)
Wound repair involving more than layered closure

Code also modifier 59 added to less complicated procedure code when reporting more than one wound repair classification

12031 **Repair, intermediate, wounds of scalp, axillae, trunk and/or extremities (excluding hands and feet); 2.5 cm or less**
4.36 | 7.17 | FUD 010 | T P2
AMA: 2019,Nov,3; 2018,Sep,7; 2018,Jan,8; 2017,Jan,8; 2016,Jan,13

12032 **2.6 cm to 7.5 cm**
5.58 | 8.65 | FUD 010 | T P2
AMA: 2019,Nov,3; 2018,Sep,7; 2018,Jan,8; 2017,Jan,8; 2016,Jan,13

12034 **7.6 cm to 12.5 cm**
5.99 | 8.92 | FUD 010 | T A2
AMA: 2019,Nov,3; 2018,Sep,7; 2018,Jan,8; 2017,Jan,8; 2016,Jan,13

12035 **12.6 cm to 20.0 cm**
6.94 | 11.0 | FUD 010 | T A2
AMA: 2019,Nov,3; 2018,Sep,7; 2018,Jan,8; 2017,Jan,8; 2016,Jan,13

12036 **20.1 cm to 30.0 cm**
8.05 | 12.1 | FUD 010 | T A2
AMA: 2019,Nov,3; 2018,Sep,7; 2018,Jan,8; 2017,Jan,8; 2016,Jan,13

12037 **over 30.0 cm**
9.53 | 14.0 | FUD 010 | T A2 80
AMA: 2019,Nov,3; 2018,Sep,7; 2018,Jan,8; 2017,Jan,8; 2016,Jan,13

12041 **Repair, intermediate, wounds of neck, hands, feet and/or external genitalia; 2.5 cm or less**
4.22 | 7.19 | FUD 010 | Q2 P2
AMA: 2019,Nov,3; 2018,Sep,7; 2018,Jan,8; 2017,Jan,8; 2016,Jan,13

12042 **2.6 cm to 7.5 cm**
5.64 8.54 **FUD** 010 T P2
AMA: 2019,Nov,3; 2018,Sep,7; 2018,Jan,8; 2017,Jan,8; 2016,Jan,13

12044 **7.6 cm to 12.5 cm**
6.16 10.6 **FUD** 010 T A2
AMA: 2019,Nov,3; 2018,Sep,7; 2018,Jan,8; 2017,Jan,8; 2016,Jan,13

12045 **12.6 cm to 20.0 cm**
7.71 11.4 **FUD** 010 T A2
AMA: 2019,Nov,3; 2018,Sep,7; 2018,Jan,8; 2017,Jan,8; 2016,Jan,13

12046 **20.1 cm to 30.0 cm**
9.01 13.8 **FUD** 010 T A2 80
AMA: 2019,Nov,3; 2018,Sep,7; 2018,Jan,8; 2017,Jan,8; 2016,Jan,13

12047 **over 30.0 cm**
10.1 15.4 **FUD** 010 T A2 80
AMA: 2019,Nov,3; 2018,Sep,7; 2018,Jan,8; 2017,Jan,8; 2016,Jan,13

12051 **Repair, intermediate, wounds of face, ears, eyelids, nose, lips and/or mucous membranes; 2.5 cm or less**
4.85 7.73 **FUD** 010 T P2
AMA: 2019,Nov,3; 2018,Sep,7; 2018,Jan,8; 2017,Jan,8; 2016,Jan,13

12052 **2.6 cm to 5.0 cm**
5.85 8.55 **FUD** 010 T P2
AMA: 2019,Nov,3; 2018,Sep,7; 2018,Jan,8; 2017,Jan,8; 2016,Jan,13

12053 **5.1 cm to 7.5 cm**
6.20 10.1 **FUD** 010 T P2
AMA: 2019,Nov,3; 2018,Sep,7; 2018,Jan,8; 2017,Jan,8; 2016,Jan,13

12054 **7.6 cm to 12.5 cm**
6.35 10.7 **FUD** 010 Q2 A2
AMA: 2019,Nov,3; 2018,Sep,7; 2018,Jan,8; 2017,Jan,8; 2016,Jan,13

12055 **12.6 cm to 20.0 cm**
8.66 13.9 **FUD** 010 T A2
AMA: 2019,Nov,3; 2018,Sep,7; 2018,Jan,8; 2017,Jan,8; 2016,Jan,13

12056 **20.1 cm to 30.0 cm**
11.0 16.0 **FUD** 010 Q2 A2 80
AMA: 2019,Nov,3; 2018,Sep,7; 2018,Jan,8; 2017,Jan,8; 2016,Jan,13

12057 **over 30.0 cm**
12.3 17.0 **FUD** 010 T A2 80
AMA: 2019,Nov,3; 2018,Sep,7; 2018,Jan,8; 2017,Jan,8; 2016,Jan,13

13100-13160 Suturing of Complicated Wounds

INCLUDES Creation limited defect for repair
Debridement complicated wounds/avulsions
Repair with layered closure that involves at least one of the following:
- Debridement wound edges
- Exposure underlying structures, such as bone, cartilage, tendon, or named neovascular structure
- Extensive undermining
- Free margin involvement helical or nostril rim or vermillion border
- Retention suture placement

Simple:
- Exploration nerves, vessels, tendons in wound
- Vessel ligation in wound

Total length several repairs in same code category

EXCLUDES *Excision:*
- *Benign lesions (11400-11446)*
- *Extensive debridement open fracture/dislocation (11010-11012)*
- *Extensive debridement penetrating or blunt trauma not associated with open fracture/dislocation (11042-11047 [11045, 11046])*
- *Malignant lesions (11600-11646)*
- *Surgical preparation wound bed (15002-15005)*

Extensive exploration (20100-20103)
Repair nerves, blood vessel, tendons (See appropriate anatomical section. These repairs include simple and intermediate closure. Report complex closure with modifier 59.)

Code also modifier 59 added to less complicated procedure code when reporting more than one wound repair classification

13100 **Repair, complex, trunk; 1.1 cm to 2.5 cm**
EXCLUDES *Complex repair 1.0 cm or less (12001, 12031)*
5.81 9.72 **FUD** 010 T A2
AMA: 2019,Nov,14; 2019,Nov,3; 2018,Sep,7; 2018,Jan,8; 2017,Apr,9; 2017,Jan,8; 2016,Jan,13

13101 **2.6 cm to 7.5 cm**
7.14 11.4 **FUD** 010 T A2
AMA: 2019,Dec,14; 2019,Nov,3; 2018,Sep,7; 2018,Jan,8; 2017,Apr,9; 2017,Jan,8; 2016,Jan,13

+ **13102** **each additional 5 cm or less (List separately in addition to code for primary procedure)**
Code first (13101)
2.14 3.46 **FUD** ZZZ N N1
AMA: 2019,Nov,14; 2019,Nov,3; 2018,Sep,7; 2018,Jan,8; 2017,Apr,9; 2017,Jan,8; 2016,Jan,13

13120 **Repair, complex, scalp, arms, and/or legs; 1.1 cm to 2.5 cm**
EXCLUDES *Complex repair 1.0 cm or less (12001, 12031)*
6.68 10.1 **FUD** 010 T A2
AMA: 2019,Nov,3; 2018,Sep,7; 2018,Jan,8; 2017,Jan,8; 2016,Jan,13

13121 **2.6 cm to 7.5 cm**
7.67 12.2 **FUD** 010 T A2
AMA: 2019,Nov,3; 2018,Sep,7; 2018,Jan,8; 2017,Jan,8; 2016,Jan,13

+ **13122** **each additional 5 cm or less (List separately in addition to code for primary procedure)**
Code first (13121)
2.42 3.74 **FUD** ZZZ N N1
AMA: 2019,Nov,3; 2018,Sep,7; 2018,Jan,8; 2017,Jan,8; 2016,Jan,13

13131 **Repair, complex, forehead, cheeks, chin, mouth, neck, axillae, genitalia, hands and/or feet; 1.1 cm to 2.5 cm**
EXCLUDES *Complex repair 1.0 cm or less (12001, 12011, 12031, 12041, 12051)*
7.04 11.1 **FUD** 010 T A2
AMA: 2019,Nov,3; 2018,Sep,7; 2018,Jan,8; 2017,Apr,9; 2017,Jan,8; 2016,Jan,13

13132 **2.6 cm to 7.5 cm**
8.81 13.5 **FUD** 010 T A2
AMA: 2019,Nov,3; 2018,Sep,7; 2018,Jan,8; 2017,Apr,9; 2017,Jan,8; 2016,Jan,13

+ 13133 each additional 5 cm or less (List separately in addition to code for primary procedure)

Code first (13132)

Facility RVU 3.77 Non-Facility RVU 5.06 FUD ZZZ N N1 CCI

AMA: 2019,Nov,3; 2018,Sep,7; 2018,Jan,8; 2017,Apr,9; 2017,Jan,8; 2016,Jan,13

13151 Repair, complex, eyelids, nose, ears and/or lips; 1.1 cm to 2.5 cm

EXCLUDES *Complex repair 1.0 cm or less (12011, 12051)*

Facility RVU 8.25 Non-Facility RVU 12.1 FUD 010 T A2 CCI

AMA: 2019,Nov,3; 2018,Sep,7; 2018,Jan,8; 2017,Jan,8; 2016,Jan,13

13152 2.6 cm to 7.5 cm

Facility RVU 9.74 Non-Facility RVU 14.3 FUD 010 T A2 CCI

AMA: 2019,Nov,3; 2018,Sep,7; 2018,Jan,8; 2017,Jan,8; 2016,Jan,13

+ 13153 each additional 5 cm or less (List separately in addition to code for primary procedure)

Code first (13152)

Facility RVU 4.02 Non-Facility RVU 5.45 FUD ZZZ N N1 CCI

AMA: 2019,Nov,3; 2018,Sep,7; 2018,Jan,8; 2017,Jan,8; 2016,Jan,13

13160 Secondary closure of surgical wound or dehiscence, extensive or complicated

EXCLUDES *Insertion tissue expander, other than breast (11960)*
Packing or simple secondary wound closure (12020-12021)

Facility RVU 22.9 Non-Facility RVU 22.9 FUD 090 T A2 CCI

AMA: 2019,Nov,3; 2018,Jan,8; 2017,Jan,8; 2016,Jan,13

14000-14350 Reposition Contiguous Tissue

INCLUDES Excision (with or without lesion) with repair by adjacent tissue transfer or tissue rearrangement
Size includes primary (due to excision) and secondary (due to flap design)
Z-plasty, W-plasty, VY-plasty, rotation flap, advancement flap, double pedicle flap, random island flap

EXCLUDES *Closure wounds by undermining surrounding tissue without additional incisions (13100-13160)*
Full thickness closure:
Eyelid (67930-67935, 67961-67975)
Lip (40650-40654)

Code also skin graft necessary to repair secondary defect (15040-15731)

14000 Adjacent tissue transfer or rearrangement, trunk; defect 10 sq cm or less

INCLUDES Burrow's operation

EXCLUDES *Excision lesion with repair by adjacent tissue transfer or tissue rearrangement (11400-11446, 11600-11646)*

Facility RVU 14.3 Non-Facility RVU 17.8 FUD 090 T A2 CCI

AMA: 2018,Jan,8; 2017,Oct,9; 2017,Jan,8; 2016,Jan,13

Example of common Z-plasty. Lesion is removed with oval-shaped incision

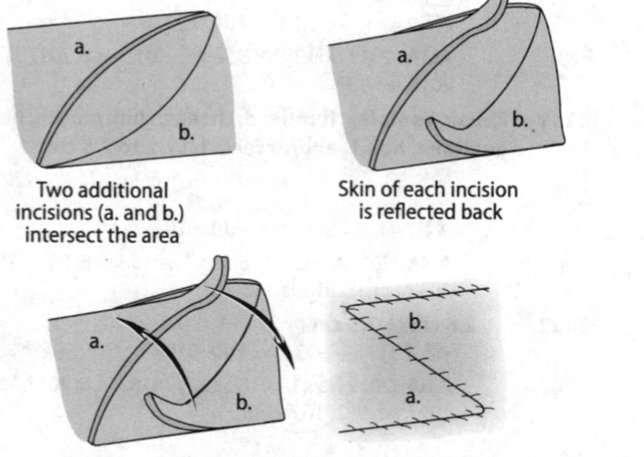

Two additional incisions (a. and b.) intersect the area

Skin of each incision is reflected back

The flaps are then transposed and the repair is closed

An adjacent flap, or other rearrangement flap, is performed to repair a defect

14001 defect 10.1 sq cm to 30.0 sq cm

EXCLUDES *Excision lesion with repair by adjacent tissue transfer or tissue rearrangement (11400-11446, 11600-11646)*

Facility RVU 18.7 Non-Facility RVU 22.8 FUD 090 T A2 CCI

AMA: 2018,Jan,8; 2017,Oct,9; 2017,Jan,8; 2016,Jan,13

14020 Adjacent tissue transfer or rearrangement, scalp, arms and/or legs; defect 10 sq cm or less

EXCLUDES *Excision lesion with repair by adjacent tissue transfer or tissue rearrangement (11400-11446, 11600-11646)*

Facility RVU 16.0 Non-Facility RVU 19.8 FUD 090 T A2 CCI

AMA: 2018,Jan,8; 2017,Jan,8; 2016,Jan,13

14021 defect 10.1 sq cm to 30.0 sq cm

EXCLUDES *Excision lesion with repair by adjacent tissue transfer or tissue rearrangement (11400-11446, 11600-11646)*

Facility RVU 20.5 Non-Facility RVU 24.7 FUD 090 T A2 CCI

AMA: 2018,Jan,8; 2017,Jan,8; 2016,Jan,13

14040 Adjacent tissue transfer or rearrangement, forehead, cheeks, chin, mouth, neck, axillae, genitalia, hands and/or feet; defect 10 sq cm or less

INCLUDES Krimer's palatoplasty

EXCLUDES *Excision lesion with repair by adjacent tissue transfer or tissue rearrangement (11400-11446, 11600-11646)*

Facility RVU 18.1 Non-Facility RVU 21.7 FUD 090 T A2 CCI

AMA: 2018,Jan,8; 2017,Nov,6; 2017,Jan,8; 2016,Jan,13

14041 defect 10.1 sq cm to 30.0 sq cm

EXCLUDES *Excision lesion with repair by adjacent tissue transfer or tissue rearrangement (11400-11446, 11600-11646)*

Facility RVU 22.3 Non-Facility RVU 26.7 FUD 090 T A2 CCI

AMA: 2018,Jan,8; 2017,Nov,6; 2017,Jan,8; 2016,Jan,13

14060 Adjacent tissue transfer or rearrangement, eyelids, nose, ears and/or lips; defect 10 sq cm or less

INCLUDES Denonvillier's operation

EXCLUDES *Excision lesion with repair by adjacent tissue transfer or tissue rearrangement (11400-11446, 11600-11646)*
Eyelid, full thickness (67961-67966)

Facility RVU 19.0 Non-Facility RVU 21.9 FUD 090 T A2 CCI

AMA: 2018,Jan,8; 2017,Nov,6; 2017,Jan,8; 2016,Jan,13

14061 defect 10.1 sq cm to 30.0 sq cm

EXCLUDES *Excision lesion with repair by adjacent tissue transfer or tissue rearrangement (11400-11446, 11600-11646)*
Eyelid, full thickness (67961 and subsequent codes)

Facility RVU 23.4 Non-Facility RVU 28.3 FUD 090 T A2 CCI

AMA: 2018,Jan,8; 2017,Nov,6; 2017,Jan,8; 2016,Jan,13

14301 Adjacent tissue transfer or rearrangement, any area; defect 30.1 sq cm to 60.0 sq cm

EXCLUDES *Excision lesion with repair by adjacent tissue transfer or tissue rearrangement (11400-11446, 11600-11646)*

Facility RVU 25.0 Non-Facility RVU 30.8 FUD 090 T G2 80 CCI

AMA: 2018,Jan,8; 2017,Nov,6; 2017,Apr,9; 2017,Jan,8; 2016,Jan,13

+ 14302 each additional 30.0 sq cm, or part thereof (List separately in addition to code for primary procedure)

EXCLUDES *Excision lesion with repair by adjacent tissue transfer or tissue rearrangement (11400-11446, 11600-11646)*

Code first (14301)

Facility RVU 6.31 Non-Facility RVU 6.31 FUD ZZZ N N1 80 CCI

AMA: 2018,Jan,8; 2017,Nov,6; 2017,Jan,8; 2016,Jan,13

14350 Filleted finger or toe flap, including preparation of recipient site

Facility RVU 19.6 Non-Facility RVU 19.6 FUD 090 T A2 80 CCI

AMA: 2018,Jan,8; 2017,Jan,8; 2016,Jan,13

15002-15005 Development of Base for Tissue Grafting

INCLUDES Add together surface area multiple wounds in same anatomical locations as indicated in code descriptor groups, such as face and scalp. Do not add together multiple wounds at different anatomical site groups such as trunk and face
Ankle or wrist when code description describes leg or arm
Cleaning and preparing viable wound surface for grafting or negative pressure wound therapy used to heal wound primarily
Code selection based on defect size and location
Percentage applies to children younger than age 10
Removal nonviable tissue in nonchronic wounds for primary healing
Square centimeters applies to children and adults age 10 or older

EXCLUDES *Chronic wound management on wounds left to heal by secondary intention (11042-11047 [11045, 11046], 97597-97598)*
Necrotizing soft tissue infections for specific anatomical locations (11004-11008)

15002 Surgical preparation or creation of recipient site by excision of open wounds, burn eschar, or scar (including subcutaneous tissues), or incisional release of scar contracture, trunk, arms, legs; first 100 sq cm or 1% of body area of infants and children

EXCLUDES *Linear scar revision (13100-13153)*
6.45 10.0 **FUD** 000 T A2 80
AMA: 2019,Nov,3; 2018,Jan,8; 2017,Jan,8; 2016,Jan,13

\+ **15003 each additional 100 sq cm, or part thereof, or each additional 1% of body area of infants and children (List separately in addition to code for primary procedure)**

Code first (15002)
1.32 2.11 **FUD** ZZZ N N1 80
AMA: 2019,Nov,3; 2018,Jan,8; 2017,Jan,8; 2016,Jan,13

15004 Surgical preparation or creation of recipient site by excision of open wounds, burn eschar, or scar (including subcutaneous tissues), or incisional release of scar contracture, face, scalp, eyelids, mouth, neck, ears, orbits, genitalia, hands, feet and/or multiple digits; first 100 sq cm or 1% of body area of infants and children

7.65 11.4 **FUD** 000 T A2 80
AMA: 2019,Nov,3; 2018,Jan,8; 2017,Jan,8; 2016,Jan,13

\+ **15005 each additional 100 sq cm, or part thereof, or each additional 1% of body area of infants and children (List separately in addition to code for primary procedure)**

Code first (15004)
2.66 3.50 **FUD** ZZZ N N1 80
AMA: 2019,Nov,3; 2018,Jan,8; 2017,Jan,8; 2016,Jan,13

15040 Obtain Autograft

INCLUDES Ankle or wrist when code description describes leg or arm
Percentage applies to children younger than age 10
Square centimeters applies to children and adults age 10 or older

15040 Harvest of skin for tissue cultured skin autograft, 100 sq cm or less

3.60 7.47 **FUD** 000 T A2
AMA: 2018,Jan,8; 2017,Jan,8; 2016,Jan,13

15050 Pinch Graft

INCLUDES Autologous skin graft harvest and application
Current graft removal
Fixation and anchoring skin graft
Simple cleaning

EXCLUDES *Removal devitalized tissue from wound(s), non-selective debridement, without anesthesia (97602)*

Code also graft or flap necessary to repair donor site

15050 Pinch graft, single or multiple, to cover small ulcer, tip of digit, or other minimal open area (except on face), up to defect size 2 cm diameter

13.0 16.7 **FUD** 090 T A2
AMA: 2018,Jan,8; 2017,Jan,8; 2016,Jun,8; 2016,Jan,13

15100-15261 Skin Grafts and Replacements

INCLUDES Add together surface area multiple wounds in same anatomical locations as indicated in code descriptor groups, such as face and scalp. Do not add together multiple wounds at different anatomical site groups such as trunk and face
Ankle or wrist when code description describes leg or arm
Autologous skin graft harvest and application
Code selection based on recipient site location and graft size and type
Current graft removal
Fixation and anchoring skin graft
Percentage applies to children younger than age 10
Simple cleaning
Simple tissue debridement
Square centimeters applies to children and adults age 10 or older

EXCLUDES *Debridement without immediate primary closure, when wound grossly contaminated and extensive cleaning needed, or when necrotic or contaminated tissue removed (11042-11047 [11045, 11046], 97597-97598)*
Removal devitalized tissue from wound(s), non-selective debridement, without anesthesia (97602)

Code also:
Graft or flap necessary to repair donor site
Primary procedure requiring skin graft for definitive closure

15100 Split-thickness autograft, trunk, arms, legs; first 100 sq cm or less, or 1% of body area of infants and children (except 15050)

20.5 24.5 **FUD** 090 T A2
AMA: 2018,Jan,8; 2017,Jan,8; 2016,Jun,8; 2016,Jan,13

\+ **15101 each additional 100 sq cm, or each additional 1% of body area of infants and children, or part thereof (List separately in addition to code for primary procedure)**

Code first (15100)
3.24 5.40 **FUD** ZZZ N N1
AMA: 2018,Jan,8; 2017,Jan,8; 2016,Jun,8; 2016,Jan,13

15110 Epidermal autograft, trunk, arms, legs; first 100 sq cm or less, or 1% of body area of infants and children

19.9 23.1 **FUD** 090 T A2
AMA: 2018,Jan,8; 2017,Jan,8; 2016,Jan,13

\+ **15111 each additional 100 sq cm, or each additional 1% of body area of infants and children, or part thereof (List separately in addition to code for primary procedure)**

Code first (15110)
3.02 3.33 **FUD** ZZZ N N1
AMA: 2018,Jan,8; 2017,Jan,8; 2016,Jan,13

15115 Epidermal autograft, face, scalp, eyelids, mouth, neck, ears, orbits, genitalia, hands, feet, and/or multiple digits; first 100 sq cm or less, or 1% of body area of infants and children

19.6 22.8 **FUD** 090 T A2
AMA: 2018,Jan,8; 2017,Jan,8; 2016,Jan,13

\+ **15116 each additional 100 sq cm, or each additional 1% of body area of infants and children, or part thereof (List separately in addition to code for primary procedure)**

Code first (15115)
4.39 4.81 **FUD** ZZZ N N1
AMA: 2018,Jan,8; 2017,Jan,8; 2016,Jan,13

15120 Split-thickness autograft, face, scalp, eyelids, mouth, neck, ears, orbits, genitalia, hands, feet, and/or multiple digits; first 100 sq cm or less, or 1% of body area of infants and children (except 15050)

EXCLUDES *Other eyelid repair (67961-67975)*
19.9 24.3 **FUD** 090 T A2
AMA: 2018,Jan,8; 2017,Jan,8; 2016,Jun,8; 2016,Jan,13

\+ **15121 each additional 100 sq cm, or each additional 1% of body area of infants and children, or part thereof (List separately in addition to code for primary procedure)**

EXCLUDES *Other eyelid repair (67961-67975)*
Code first (15120)
3.90 6.05 **FUD** ZZZ N N1
AMA: 2018,Jan,8; 2017,Jan,8; 2016,Jun,8; 2016,Jan,13

15130 **Dermal autograft, trunk, arms, legs; first 100 sq cm or less, or 1% of body area of infants and children**
17.1 20.6 FUD 090
AMA: 2018,Jan,8; 2017,Jan,8; 2016,Jan,13

+ **15131** **each additional 100 sq cm, or each additional 1% of body area of infants and children, or part thereof (List separately in addition to code for primary procedure)**
Code first (15130)
2.65 2.86 FUD ZZZ
AMA: 2018,Jan,8; 2017,Jan,8; 2016,Jan,13

15135 **Dermal autograft, face, scalp, eyelids, mouth, neck, ears, orbits, genitalia, hands, feet, and/or multiple digits; first 100 sq cm or less, or 1% of body area of infants and children**
21.7 25.0 FUD 090
AMA: 2018,Jan,8; 2017,Jan,8; 2016,Jan,13

+ **15136** **each additional 100 sq cm, or each additional 1% of body area of infants and children, or part thereof (List separately in addition to code for primary procedure)**
Code first (15135)
2.65 2.83 FUD ZZZ
AMA: 2018,Jan,8; 2017,Jan,8; 2016,Jan,13

15150 **Tissue cultured skin autograft, trunk, arms, legs; first 25 sq cm or less**
18.4 20.3 FUD 090
AMA: 2018,Jan,8; 2017,Jan,8; 2016,Jan,13

+ **15151** **additional 1 sq cm to 75 sq cm (List separately in addition to code for primary procedure)**
EXCLUDES *Grafts over 75 sq cm (15152)*
Reporting code more than one time per session
Code first (15150)
3.19 3.45 FUD ZZZ
AMA: 2018,Jan,8; 2017,Jan,8; 2016,Jan,13

+ **15152** **each additional 100 sq cm, or each additional 1% of body area of infants and children, or part thereof (List separately in addition to code for primary procedure)**
Code first (15151)
4.22 4.47 FUD ZZZ
AMA: 2018,Jan,8; 2017,Jan,8; 2016,Jan,13

15155 **Tissue cultured skin autograft, face, scalp, eyelids, mouth, neck, ears, orbits, genitalia, hands, feet, and/or multiple digits; first 25 sq cm or less**
21.1 23.0 FUD 090
AMA: 2018,Jan,8; 2017,Jan,8; 2016,Jan,13

+ **15156** **additional 1 sq cm to 75 sq cm (List separately in addition to code for primary procedure)**
EXCLUDES *Grafts over 75 sq cm (15157)*
Reporting code more than one time per session
Code first (15155)
4.39 4.64 FUD ZZZ
AMA: 2018,Jan,8; 2017,Jan,8; 2016,Jan,13

+ **15157** **each additional 100 sq cm, or each additional 1% of body area of infants and children, or part thereof (List separately in addition to code for primary procedure)**
Code first (15156)
4.82 5.19 FUD ZZZ
AMA: 2018,Jan,8; 2017,Jan,8; 2016,Jan,13

15200 **Full thickness graft, free, including direct closure of donor site, trunk; 20 sq cm or less**
19.2 23.9 FUD 090
AMA: 2018,Jan,8; 2017,Jan,8; 2016,Jun,8; 2016,Jan,13

+ **15201** **each additional 20 sq cm, or part thereof (List separately in addition to code for primary procedure)**
Code first (15200)
2.26 4.20 FUD ZZZ
AMA: 2018,Jan,8; 2017,Jan,8; 2016,Jun,8; 2016,Jan,13

15220 **Full thickness graft, free, including direct closure of donor site, scalp, arms, and/or legs; 20 sq cm or less**
17.4 21.9 FUD 090
AMA: 2018,Jan,8; 2017,Jan,8; 2016,Jun,8; 2016,Jan,13

+ **15221** **each additional 20 sq cm, or part thereof (List separately in addition to code for primary procedure)**
Code first (15220)
2.03 3.86 FUD ZZZ
AMA: 2018,Jan,8; 2017,Jan,8; 2016,Jun,8; 2016,Jan,13

15240 **Full thickness graft, free, including direct closure of donor site, forehead, cheeks, chin, mouth, neck, axillae, genitalia, hands, and/or feet; 20 sq cm or less**
EXCLUDES *Fingertip graft (15050)*
Syndactyly repair fingers (26560-26562)
23.0 26.6 FUD 090
AMA: 2018,Jan,8; 2017,Jan,8; 2016,Jun,8; 2016,Jan,13

+ **15241** **each additional 20 sq cm, or part thereof (List separately in addition to code for primary procedure)**
Code first (15240)
3.18 5.22 FUD ZZZ
AMA: 2018,Jan,8; 2017,Jan,8; 2016,Jun,8; 2016,Jan,13

15260 **Full thickness graft, free, including direct closure of donor site, nose, ears, eyelids, and/or lips; 20 sq cm or less**
EXCLUDES *Other eyelid repair (67961-67975)*
24.1 28.5 FUD 090
AMA: 2018,Jan,8; 2017,Jan,8; 2016,Jun,8; 2016,Jan,13

+ **15261** **each additional 20 sq cm, or part thereof (List separately in addition to code for primary procedure)**
EXCLUDES *Other eyelid repair (67961-67975)*
Code first (15260)
3.96 5.99 FUD ZZZ
AMA: 2018,Jan,8; 2017,Jan,8; 2016,Jun,8; 2016,Jan,13

15271-15278 Skin Substitute Graft Application

INCLUDES Add together surface area multiple wounds in same anatomical locations as indicated in code descriptor groups, such as face and scalp. Do not add together multiple wounds at different anatomical site groups such as trunk and face
Ankle or wrist when code description describes leg or arm
Code selection based on defect site location and size
Fixation and anchoring skin graft
Graft types include:
Biological material used for tissue engineering (e.g., scaffold) for growing skin
Nonautologous human skin such as:
Acellular
Allograft
Cellular
Dermal
Epidermal
Homograft
Nonhuman grafts
Percentage applies to children younger than age 10
Removing current graft
Simple cleaning
Simple tissue debridement
Square centimeters applies to children and adults age 10 or older

EXCLUDES *Application nongraft dressing*
Injected skin substitutes
Removal devitalized tissue from wound(s), non-selective debridement, without anesthesia (97602)
Skin application procedures, low cost (C5271-C5278)

Code also:
Biologic implant for soft tissue reinforcement (15777)
Primary procedure requiring skin graft for definitive closure
Supply high-cost skin substitute product (C1849, C9363, Q4101, Q4103-Q4110, Q4116, Q4121-Q4123, Q4126-Q4128, Q4132-Q4133, Q4137-Q4138, Q4140-Q4141, Q4143, Q4146-Q4148, Q4150-Q4161, Q4163-Q4164, Q4167, Q4169, Q4173, Q4175, Q4176, Q4178-Q4184, Q4186-Q4188, Q4190, Q4193-Q4198, Q4200-Q4201, Q4203, Q4205, Q4208-Q4209, Q4211, Q4219, Q4222, Q4226, Q4227, Q4232, Q4234, Q4237-Q4239, Q4249)

15271 **Application of skin substitute graft to trunk, arms, legs, total wound surface area up to 100 sq cm; first 25 sq cm or less wound surface area**

EXCLUDES *Total wound area greater than or equal to 100 sq cm (15273-15274)*
2.45 4.29 **FUD** 000 T G2
AMA: 2018,Jan,8; 2017,Oct,9; 2017,Jan,8; 2016,Jan,13

\+ **15272** **each additional 25 sq cm wound surface area, or part thereof (List separately in addition to code for primary procedure)**

EXCLUDES *Total wound area greater than or equal to 100 sq cm (15273-15274)*
Code first (15271)
0.51 0.75 **FUD** ZZZ N N1
AMA: 2018,Jan,8; 2017,Jan,8; 2016,Jan,13

15273 **Application of skin substitute graft to trunk, arms, legs, total wound surface area greater than or equal to 100 sq cm; first 100 sq cm wound surface area, or 1% of body area of infants and children**

EXCLUDES *Total wound surface area up to 100 cm (15271-15272)*
5.84 8.73 **FUD** 000 T G2
AMA: 2018,Jan,8; 2017,Jan,8; 2016,Jan,13

\+ **15274** **each additional 100 sq cm wound surface area, or part thereof, or each additional 1% of body area of infants and children, or part thereof (List separately in addition to code for primary procedure)**

EXCLUDES *Total wound surface area up to 100 cm (15271-15272)*
Code first (15273)
1.32 2.26 **FUD** ZZZ N N1
AMA: 2018,Jan,8; 2017,Jan,8; 2016,Jan,13

15275 **Application of skin substitute graft to face, scalp, eyelids, mouth, neck, ears, orbits, genitalia, hands, feet, and/or multiple digits, total wound surface area up to 100 sq cm; first 25 sq cm or less wound surface area**

EXCLUDES *Total wound area greater than or equal to 100 sq cm (15277-15278)*
2.75 4.48 **FUD** 000 T G2
AMA: 2018,Jan,8; 2017,Jan,8; 2016,Jan,13

\+ **15276** **each additional 25 sq cm wound surface area, or part thereof (List separately in addition to code for primary procedure)**

EXCLUDES *Total wound area greater than or equal to 100 sq cm (15277-15278)*
Code first (15275)
0.75 0.98 **FUD** ZZZ N N1
AMA: 2018,Jan,8; 2017,Jan,8; 2016,Jan,13

15277 **Application of skin substitute graft to face, scalp, eyelids, mouth, neck, ears, orbits, genitalia, hands, feet, and/or multiple digits, total wound surface area greater than or equal to 100 sq cm; first 100 sq cm wound surface area, or 1% of body area of infants and children**

EXCLUDES *Total surface area up to 100 sq cm (15275-15276)*
6.60 9.55 **FUD** 000 T G2
AMA: 2018,Jan,8; 2017,Jan,8; 2016,Jan,13

\+ **15278** **each additional 100 sq cm wound surface area, or part thereof, or each additional 1% of body area of infants and children, or part thereof (List separately in addition to code for primary procedure)**

EXCLUDES *Total surface area up to 100 sq cm (15275-15276)*
Code first (15277)
1.66 2.54 **FUD** ZZZ N N1
AMA: 2018,Jan,8; 2017,Jan,8; 2016,Jan,13

15570-15731 Wound Reconstruction: Skin Flaps

INCLUDES Ankle or wrist when code description describes leg or arm
Code selection based on recipient site when flap attached in transfer or to final site and based on donor site when tube created for transfer later or when flap delayed prior to transfer
Fixation and anchoring skin graft
Simple tissue debridement
Tube formation for later transfer

EXCLUDES *Contiguous tissue transfer flaps (14040-14041, 14060-14061, 14301-14302)*
Debridement without immediate primary closure (11042-11047 [11045, 11046], 97597-97598)
Excision:
Benign lesion (11400-11471)
Burn eschar or scar (15002-15005)
Malignant lesion (11600-11646)
Microvascular repair (15756-15758)
Primary procedure--see appropriate anatomical site

Code also:
Application extensive immobilization apparatus
Repair donor site with skin grafts or flaps

15570 Formation of direct or tubed pedicle, with or without transfer; trunk
INCLUDES Flaps without vascular pedicle
21.1 26.2 **FUD** 090 T A2
AMA: 2018,Jan,8; 2017,Jan,8; 2016,Jan,13

Pedicle flap

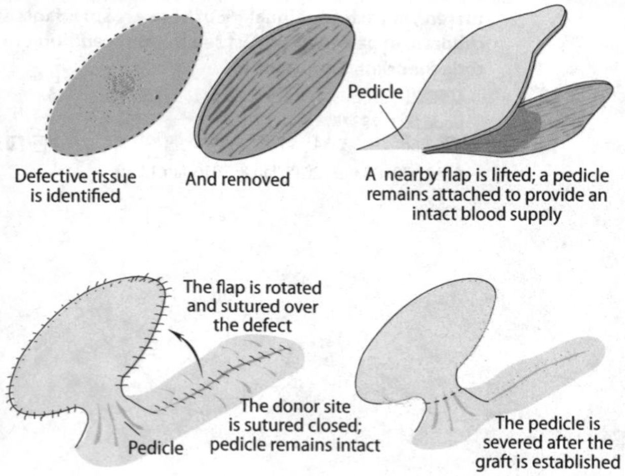
Pedicle
Defective tissue is identified
And removed
A nearby flap is lifted; a pedicle remains attached to provide an intact blood supply
The flap is rotated and sutured over the defect
Pedicle
The donor site is sutured closed; pedicle remains intact
The pedicle is severed after the graft is established

15572 scalp, arms, or legs
INCLUDES Flaps without vascular pedicle
21.2 25.3 **FUD** 090 T A2
AMA: 2018,Jan,8; 2017,Jan,8; 2016,Jan,13

15574 forehead, cheeks, chin, mouth, neck, axillae, genitalia, hands or feet
INCLUDES Flaps without vascular pedicle
21.6 25.7 **FUD** 090 T A2
AMA: 2018,Jan,8; 2017,Jan,8; 2016,Jan,13

15576 eyelids, nose, ears, lips, or intraoral
INCLUDES Flaps without vascular pedicle
19.1 22.9 **FUD** 090 T A2
AMA: 2018,Jan,8; 2017,Jan,8; 2016,Jan,13

15600 Delay of flap or sectioning of flap (division and inset); at trunk
5.96 9.47 **FUD** 090 T A2 80
AMA: 2019,Jun,14; 2018,Jan,8; 2017,Jan,8; 2016,Jan,13

15610 at scalp, arms, or legs
6.89 10.2 **FUD** 090 T A2 80
AMA: 2018,Jan,8; 2017,Jan,8; 2016,Jan,13

15620 at forehead, cheeks, chin, neck, axillae, genitalia, hands, or feet
9.26 12.6 **FUD** 090 T A2
AMA: 2018,Jan,8; 2017,Jan,8; 2016,Jan,13

15630 at eyelids, nose, ears, or lips
9.77 13.0 **FUD** 090 T A2
AMA: 2018,Jan,8; 2017,Jan,8; 2016,Jan,13

15650 Transfer, intermediate, of any pedicle flap (eg, abdomen to wrist, Walking tube), any location
EXCLUDES *Defatting, revision, or rearranging transferred pedicle flap or skin graft (13100-14302)*
Eyelids, ears, lips, and nose - refer to anatomical area
10.9 14.5 **FUD** 090 T A2 80
AMA: 2018,Jan,8; 2017,Jan,8; 2016,Jan,13

15730 Midface flap (ie, zygomaticofacial flap) with preservation of vascular pedicle(s)
26.3 42.9 **FUD** 090 T G2
AMA: 2018,Apr,10; 2018,Jan,8; 2017,Nov,6

15731 Forehead flap with preservation of vascular pedicle (eg, axial pattern flap, paramedian forehead flap)
EXCLUDES *Muscle, myocutaneous, or fasciocutaneous flap head or neck (15733)*
28.6 32.0 **FUD** 090 T A2 80
AMA: 2018,Jan,8; 2017,Nov,6; 2017,Jan,8; 2016,Jan,13

15733-15738 Wound Reconstruction: Muscle Flaps

INCLUDES Code based on donor site
EXCLUDES *Contiguous tissue transfer flaps (14040-14041, 14060-14061, 14301-14302)*
Microvascular repair (15756-15758)

Code also:
Application extensive immobilization apparatus
Repair donor site with skin grafts or flaps

15733 Muscle, myocutaneous, or fasciocutaneous flap; head and neck with named vascular pedicle (ie, buccinators, genioglossus, temporalis, masseter, sternocleidomastoid, levator scapulae)
INCLUDES Repair extracranial defect by anterior pericranial flap on vascular pedicle (15731)
29.9 29.9 **FUD** 090 T A2
AMA: 2018,Apr,10; 2018,Jan,8; 2017,Nov,6

15734 trunk
43.6 43.6 **FUD** 090 T A2 80
AMA: 2018,Aug,10; 2018,Jan,8; 2017,Nov,6; 2017,Jan,8; 2016,Jan,13

15736 upper extremity
35.3 35.3 **FUD** 090 T A2
AMA: 2018,Jan,8; 2017,Nov,6; 2017,Jan,8; 2016,Jan,13

15738 lower extremity
37.4 37.4 **FUD** 090 T A2 80
AMA: 2018,Jan,8; 2017,Nov,6; 2017,Jan,8; 2016,Jan,13

15740-15758 Wound Reconstruction: Other

INCLUDES Fixation and anchoring skin graft
Routine dressing
Simple tissue debridement

EXCLUDES *Adjacent tissue transfer (14000-14302)*
Excision:
Benign lesion (11400-11471)
Burn eschar or scar (15002-15005)
Malignant lesion (11600-11646)
Flaps without vascular pedicle addition (15570-15576)
Primary procedure--see appropriate anatomical section
Skin graft for repair donor site (15050-15278)

Code also repair donor site with skin grafts or flaps (14000-14350, 15050-15278)

15740 Flap; island pedicle requiring identification and dissection of an anatomically named axial vessel
EXCLUDES *V-Y subcutaneous flaps, random island flaps, and other flaps from adjacent areas (14000-14302)*
24.2 28.8 **FUD** 090 T A2
AMA: 2018,Jan,8; 2017,Dec,14; 2017,Jan,8; 2016,Jan,13

15750 **neurovascular pedicle**

EXCLUDES *V-Y subcutaneous flaps, random island flaps, and other flaps from adjacent areas (14000-14302)*

26.4 26.4 FUD 090 T A2 80

AMA: 2018,Jan,8; 2017,Dec,14

15756 **Free muscle or myocutaneous flap with microvascular anastomosis**

INCLUDES Operating microscope (69990)

66.0 66.0 FUD 090 C 80

AMA: 2019,Dec,5; 2018,Jan,8; 2017,Jan,8; 2016,Feb,12; 2016,Jan,13

15757 **Free skin flap with microvascular anastomosis**

INCLUDES Operating microscope (69990)

65.5 65.5 FUD 090 C 80

AMA: 2019,Dec,5; 2018,Jan,8; 2017,Jan,8; 2016,Apr,8; 2016,Feb,12; 2016,Jan,13

15758 **Free fascial flap with microvascular anastomosis**

INCLUDES Operating microscope (69990)

66.0 66.0 FUD 090 C 80

AMA: 2019,Dec,5; 2018,Jan,8; 2017,Jan,8; 2016,Feb,12; 2016,Jan,13

15760-15774 [15769] Other Grafts

EXCLUDES *Adjacent tissue transfer (14000-14302)*
Excision:
Benign lesion (11400-11471)
Burn eschar or scar (15002-15005)
Malignant lesion (11600-11646)
Flaps without vascular pedicle addition (15570-15576)
Microvascular repair (15756-15758)
Primary procedure (see appropriate anatomical site)
Repair donor site with skin grafts or flaps (14000-14350, 15050-15278)

15760 **Graft; composite (eg, full thickness of external ear or nasal ala), including primary closure, donor area**

INCLUDES Fixation and anchoring skin graft
Routine dressing
Simple tissue debridement

20.0 24.1 FUD 090 T A2

AMA: 2018,Jan,8; 2017,Jan,8; 2016,Jan,13

15769 **Resequenced code. See code following 15770.**

15770 **derma-fat-fascia**

INCLUDES Fixation and anchoring skin graft
Routine dressing
Simple tissue debridement

19.0 19.0 FUD 090 T A2 80

AMA: 2019,Oct,5; 2018,Jan,8; 2017,Jan,8; 2016,Jan,13

\# **15769** **Grafting of autologous soft tissue, other, harvested by direct excision (eg, fat, dermis, fascia)**

INCLUDES Excisional graft harvest and recipient site placement

EXCLUDES *Autologous grafts specific tissue types, such as skin, bone, nerve, tendon, fascia lata, or vessels*
Autologous white blood cell concentrate injection (0481T)
Harvesting adipose tissue for adipose-derived regenerative cell therapy (0489T-0490T)
Platelet-rich plasma injection (0232T)
Suction assisted lipectomy (15876-15879)

13.8 13.8 FUD 090 G2

15771 **Grafting of autologous fat harvested by liposuction technique to trunk, breasts, scalp, arms, and/or legs; 50 cc or less injectate**

INCLUDES Add together injectate volume harvested from each anatomical area indicated in code description, such as face and neck, to report total volume. Do not add together injectate harvested from different anatomical site groups, such as trunk and face
Code based on recipient site

EXCLUDES *Autologous white blood cell concentrate injection (0481T)*
Liposuction not for grafting purposes (15876-15879)
Obtaining tissue for adipose-derived regenerative cell therapy (0489T-0490T)
Platelet-rich plasma injection (0232T)
Subcutaneous injection filling material, at same anatomical site (11950-11954)
Reporting code more than one time per session

13.7 16.5 FUD 090 G2

AMA: 2020,Apr,10

\+ **15772** **each additional 50 cc injectate, or part thereof (List separately in addition to code for primary procedure)**

Code first (15771)

4.07 5.22 FUD ZZZ

AMA: 2020,Apr,10

15773 **Grafting of autologous fat harvested by liposuction technique to face, eyelids, mouth, neck, ears, orbits, genitalia, hands, and/or feet; 25 cc or less injectate**

INCLUDES Add together injectate volume harvested from each anatomical area indicated in code description, such as face and neck, to report total volume. Do not add together injectate harvested from different anatomical site groups, such as trunk and face
Code based on recipient site

EXCLUDES *Autologous white blood cell concentrate injection (0481T)*
Liposuction not for grafting purposes (15876-15879)
Obtaining tissue for adipose-derived regenerative cell therapy (0489T-0490T)
Platelet-rich plasma injection (0232T)
Reporting code more than one time per session
Subcutaneous injection filling material, at same anatomical site (11950-11954)

13.9 16.7 FUD 090 G2

\+ **15774** **each additional 25 cc injectate, or part thereof (List separately in addition to code for primary procedure)**

Code first (15773)

3.91 5.06 FUD ZZZ

15775-15839 Plastic, Reconstructive, and Aesthetic Surgery

CMS: 100-02,16,10 Exclusions from Coverage; 100-02,16,120 Cosmetic Procedures; 100-02,16,180 Services Related to Noncovered Procedures

15775 **Punch graft for hair transplant; 1 to 15 punch grafts**

EXCLUDES *Strip transplant (15220)*

6.42 8.74 **FUD** 000 T A2 80

AMA: 2018,Jan,8; 2017,Jan,8; 2016,Jan,13

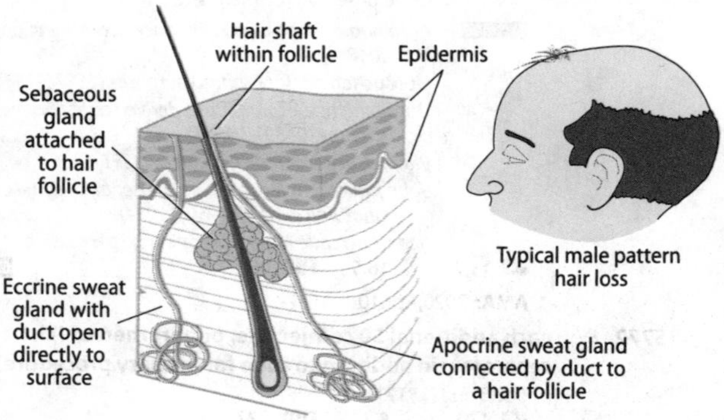

15776 **more than 15 punch grafts**

EXCLUDES *Strip transplant (15220)*

10.2 14.5 **FUD** 000 T A2 80

AMA: 2018,Jan,8; 2017,Jan,8; 2016,Jan,13

\+ **15777** **Implantation of biologic implant (eg, acellular dermal matrix) for soft tissue reinforcement (ie, breast, trunk) (List separately in addition to code for primary procedure)**

EXCLUDES *Application high cost skin substitute to external wound (15271-15278)*
Application low cost skin substitute to external wound (C5271-C5278)
Mesh implantation for:
Open repair ventral or incisional hernia (49560-49566) and (49568)
Repair devitalized soft tissue infection (11004-11006) and (49568)
Repair pelvic floor (57267)
Repair anorectal fistula with plug (46707)
Reporting modifier 50 for bilateral breast procedure. Report once for each side when performed bilaterally
Soft tissue reinforcement with biologic implants other than in the breast or trunk (17999)

Code also:
Supply biologic implant
Synthetic or nonbiological implant to reinforce abdominal wall (0437T)

Code first primary procedure

6.25 6.25 **FUD** ZZZ N N1

AMA: 2019,Nov,14; 2019,Jan,14; 2018,Jan,8; 2017,Jan,8; 2016,Jan,13

15780 **Dermabrasion; total face (eg, for acne scarring, fine wrinkling, rhytids, general keratosis)**

19.3 25.2 **FUD** 090 J P3 80

AMA: 2018,Jan,8; 2017,Jan,8; 2016,Jan,13

15781 **segmental, face**

12.3 15.6 **FUD** 090 T P2

AMA: 1997,Nov,1

15782 **regional, other than face**

11.2 15.3 **FUD** 090 J P3 80

AMA: 1997,Nov,1

15783 **superficial, any site (eg, tattoo removal)**

10.6 13.6 **FUD** 090 T P2 80

AMA: 2018,Jan,8; 2017,Jan,8; 2016,Jan,13

15786 **Abrasion; single lesion (eg, keratosis, scar)**

3.85 6.87 **FUD** 010 Q1 N1

AMA: 1997,Nov,1

\+ **15787** **each additional 4 lesions or less (List separately in addition to code for primary procedure)**

Code first (15786)

0.50 1.27 **FUD** ZZZ N N1

AMA: 1997,Nov,1

15788 **Chemical peel, facial; epidermal**

6.55 12.2 **FUD** 090 Q1 N1

AMA: 1997,Nov,1; 1993,Win,1

15789 **dermal**

11.6 15.3 **FUD** 090 T P2

AMA: 1997,Nov,1; 1993,Win,1

15792 **Chemical peel, nonfacial; epidermal**

6.61 10.9 **FUD** 090 Q1 N1 80

AMA: 1997,Nov,1; 1993,Win,1

15793 **dermal**

10.0 13.6 **FUD** 090 Q1 N1 80

AMA: 1997,Nov,1; 1993,Win,1

15819 **Cervicoplasty**

22.7 22.7 **FUD** 090 T G2 80

AMA: 1997,Nov,1

15820 **Blepharoplasty, lower eyelid;**

14.5 16.2 **FUD** 090 T A2 80 50

AMA: 2018,Jan,8; 2017,Jan,8; 2016,Jan,13

15821 **with extensive herniated fat pad**

15.5 17.4 **FUD** 090 T A2 80 50

AMA: 2018,Jan,8; 2017,Jan,8; 2016,Jan,13

15822 **Blepharoplasty, upper eyelid;**

11.2 12.9 **FUD** 090 T A2 50

AMA: 2018,Jan,8; 2017,Jan,8; 2016,Jan,13

15823 **with excessive skin weighting down lid**

15.5 17.4 **FUD** 090 T A2 50

AMA: 2018,Jan,8; 2017,Jan,8; 2016,Jan,13

15824 **Rhytidectomy; forehead**

EXCLUDES *Repair brow ptosis (67900)*

0.00 0.00 **FUD** 000 T A2 80 50

AMA: 2018,Jan,8; 2017,Apr,9

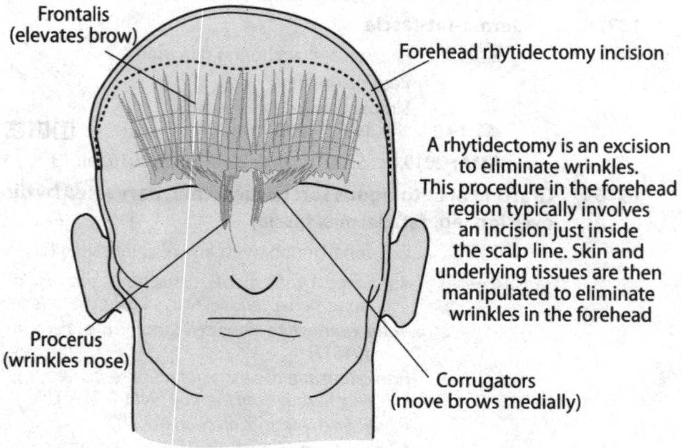

15825 **neck with platysmal tightening (platysmal flap, P-flap)**

0.00 0.00 **FUD** 000 T A2 80 50

AMA: 2018,Jan,8; 2017,Apr,9

15826 **glabellar frown lines**

0.00 0.00 **FUD** 000 T A2 80 50

AMA: 1997,Nov,1

15828 **cheek, chin, and neck**

0.00 0.00 **FUD** 000 T A2 80 50

AMA: 1997,Nov,1

15829 **superficial musculoaponeurotic system (SMAS) flap**

0.00 0.00 **FUD** 000 T A2 80 50

AMA: 1997,Nov,1

15830 **Excision, excessive skin and subcutaneous tissue (includes lipectomy); abdomen, infraumbilical panniculectomy**

EXCLUDES *For same wound:*
Adjacent tissue transfer, trunk (14000-14001, 14302)
Complex wound repair, trunk (13100-13102)
Intermediate wound repair, trunk (12031-12032, 12034-12037)
Other abdominoplasty (17999)

Code also, when performed (15847)
33.9 33.9 FUD 090 J A2 80

15832 **thigh**
26.5 26.5 FUD 090 J A2 80 50
AMA: 1997,Nov,1

15833 **leg**
25.2 25.2 FUD 090 J A2 80 50
AMA: 1997,Nov,1

15834 **hip**
25.7 25.7 FUD 090 J A2 80 50
AMA: 1997,Nov,1

15835 **buttock**
26.9 26.9 FUD 090 J A2 80
AMA: 1997,Nov,1

15836 **arm**
22.6 22.6 FUD 090 J A2 80 50
AMA: 1997,Nov,1

15837 **forearm or hand**
20.6 24.7 FUD 090 J G2 80
AMA: 1997,Nov,1

15838 **submental fat pad**
18.5 18.5 FUD 090 J G2 80
AMA: 1998,Feb,1; 1997,Nov,1

15839 **other area**
21.2 25.4 FUD 090 J A2 80
AMA: 1997,Nov,1

15840-15845 Reanimation of the Paralyzed Face

INCLUDES Routine dressing and supplies

EXCLUDES *Intravenous fluorescein evaluation blood flow in graft or flap (15860)*
Nerve:
Decompression (69720, 69725, 69955)
Pedicle transfer (64905, 64907)
Suture (64831-64876, 69740, 69745)

Code also repair donor site with skin grafts or flaps

15840 **Graft for facial nerve paralysis; free fascia graft (including obtaining fascia)**
28.9 28.9 FUD 090 T A2
AMA: 1997,Nov,1

15841 **free muscle graft (including obtaining graft)**
51.2 51.2 FUD 090 T A2 80
AMA: 1997,Nov,1

15842 **free muscle flap by microsurgical technique**
INCLUDES Operating microscope (69990)
78.5 78.5 FUD 090 T G2 80
AMA: 2016,Feb,12

15845 **regional muscle transfer**
28.8 28.8 FUD 090 T A2 80
AMA: 1998,Feb,1; 1997,Nov,1

15847 Removal of Excess Abdominal Tissue Add-on

CMS: 100-02,16,10 Exclusions from Coverage; 100-02,16,120 Cosmetic Procedures; 100-02,16,180 Services Related to Noncovered Procedures

\+ **15847** **Excision, excessive skin and subcutaneous tissue (includes lipectomy), abdomen (eg, abdominoplasty) (includes umbilical transposition and fascial plication) (List separately in addition to code for primary procedure)**

EXCLUDES *Abdominal wall hernia repair (49491-49587)*
Other abdominoplasty (17999)

Code first (15830)
0.00 0.00 FUD YYY N N1 80

15850-15852 Suture Removal/Dressing Change: Anesthesia Required

15850 **Removal of sutures under anesthesia (other than local), same surgeon**
1.14 2.57 FUD XXX T G2
AMA: 2018,Jan,8; 2017,Jan,8; 2016,Jan,13

15851 **Removal of sutures under anesthesia (other than local), other surgeon**
1.31 2.85 FUD 000 T P3
AMA: 2018,Jan,8; 2017,Jan,8; 2016,Jan,13

15852 **Dressing change (for other than burns) under anesthesia (other than local)**
EXCLUDES *Dressing change for burns (16020-16030)*
1.34 1.34 FUD 000 Q1 N1
AMA: 1997,Nov,1

15860 Injection for Vascular Flow Determination

15860 **Intravenous injection of agent (eg, fluorescein) to test vascular flow in flap or graft**
3.13 3.13 FUD 000 Q1 N1 80
AMA: 2002,May,7; 1997,Nov,1

15876-15879 Liposuction

CMS: 100-02,16,10 Exclusions from Coverage; 100-02,16,120 Cosmetic Procedures; 100-02,16,180 Services Related to Noncovered Procedures

EXCLUDES *Liposuction for autologous fat grafting (15771-15774)*
Obtaining tissue for adipose-derived regenerative cell therapy (0489T-0490T)

15876 **Suction assisted lipectomy; head and neck**
0.00 0.00 FUD 000 T A2 80
AMA: 2019,Oct,5; 2019,Aug,10; 2018,Sep,12

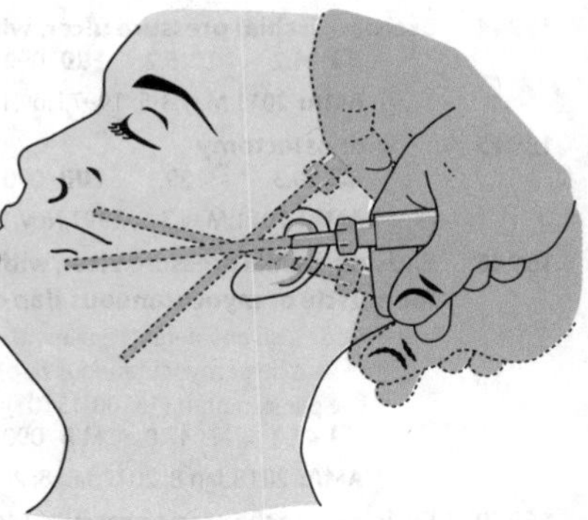

Cannula typically inserted through incision in front of ear

15877 **trunk**
0.00 0.00 FUD 000 T A2 80
AMA: 2019,Oct,5; 2019,Aug,10; 2018,Sep,12; 2018,Jan,8; 2017,Jan,8; 2016,Jan,13

15878 **upper extremity**
0.00 0.00 FUD 000 T A2 80 50
AMA: 2019,Oct,5; 2019,Aug,10; 2018,Sep,12

15879 **lower extremity**
0.00 0.00 FUD 000 T A2 80 50
AMA: 2019,Oct,5; 2019,Aug,10; 2018,Sep,12

15920-15999 Treatment of Decubitus Ulcers

Code also free skin graft to repair ulcer or donor site

15920 **Excision, coccygeal pressure ulcer, with coccygectomy; with primary suture**
17.8 17.8 FUD 090 J A2 80
AMA: 2011,May,3-5; 1997,Nov,1

15922 **with flap closure**
22.8 22.8 FUD 090 T A2 80
AMA: 2011,May,3-5; 1997,Nov,1

15931 Excision, sacral pressure ulcer, with primary suture;
20.1 20.1 FUD 090 J A2
AMA: 2011,May,3-5; 1997,Nov,1

15933 with ostectomy
24.5 24.5 FUD 090 J A2 80
AMA: 2011,May,3-5; 1997,Nov,1

15934 Excision, sacral pressure ulcer, with skin flap closure;
27.3 27.3 FUD 090 T A2
AMA: 2011,May,3-5; 1997,Nov,1

15935 with ostectomy
31.6 31.6 FUD 090 T A2 80
AMA: 2011,May,3-5; 1997,Nov,1

15936 Excision, sacral pressure ulcer, in preparation for muscle or myocutaneous flap or skin graft closure;
Code also any defect repair with:
Muscle or myocutaneous flap (15734, 15738)
Split skin graft (15100-15101)
26.0 26.0 FUD 090 T A2
AMA: 2011,May,3-5; 1998,Nov,1

15937 with ostectomy
Code also any defect repair with:
Muscle or myocutaneous flap (15734, 15738)
Split skin graft (15100-15101)
29.8 29.8 FUD 090 T A2
AMA: 2011,May,3-5; 1998,Nov,1

15940 Excision, ischial pressure ulcer, with primary suture;
20.1 20.1 FUD 090 J A2
AMA: 2011,May,3-5; 1997,Nov,1

15941 with ostectomy (ischiectomy)
26.4 26.4 FUD 090 J A2 80
AMA: 2011,May,3-5; 1997,Nov,1

15944 Excision, ischial pressure ulcer, with skin flap closure;
26.2 26.2 FUD 090 T A2 80
AMA: 2011,May,3-5; 1997,Nov,1

15945 with ostectomy
29.3 29.3 FUD 090 T A2 80
AMA: 2011,May,3-5; 1997,Nov,1

15946 Excision, ischial pressure ulcer, with ostectomy, in preparation for muscle or myocutaneous flap or skin graft closure
Code also any defect repair with:
Muscle or myocutaneous flap (15734, 15738)
Split skin graft (15100-15101)
47.0 47.0 FUD 090 T A2
AMA: 2018,Jan,8; 2017,Jan,8; 2016,Jan,13

15950 Excision, trochanteric pressure ulcer, with primary suture;
17.6 17.6 FUD 090 J A2
AMA: 2011,May,3-5; 1997,Nov,1

15951 with ostectomy
25.3 25.3 FUD 090 J A2 80
AMA: 2011,May,3-5; 1997,Nov,1

15952 Excision, trochanteric pressure ulcer, with skin flap closure;
26.3 26.3 FUD 090 T A2 80
AMA: 2011,May,3-5; 1997,Nov,1

15953 with ostectomy
28.9 28.9 FUD 090 T A2
AMA: 2011,May,3-5; 1997,Nov,1

15956 Excision, trochanteric pressure ulcer, in preparation for muscle or myocutaneous flap or skin graft closure;
Code also any defect repair with:
Muscle or myocutaneous flap (15734, 15738)
Split skin graft (15100-15101)
33.3 33.3 FUD 090 T A2
AMA: 2011,May,3-5; 1998,Nov,1

15958 with ostectomy
Code also any defect repair with:
Muscle or myocutaneous flap (15734-15738)
Split skin graft (15100-15101)
34.0 34.0 FUD 090 T A2
AMA: 2011,May,3-5; 1998,Nov,1

15999 Unlisted procedure, excision pressure ulcer
0.00 0.00 FUD YYY T 80
AMA: 2011,May,3-5; 1997,Nov,1

16000-16036 Burn Care

INCLUDES Local care burn surface only
EXCLUDES *Application skin grafts and flaps including all services described in: (15100-15777)*
E/M services
Laser fenestration for scars (0479T-0480T)

16000 Initial treatment, first degree burn, when no more than local treatment is required
1.33 2.09 FUD 000 Q1 N1
AMA: 2018,Jan,8; 2017,Jan,8; 2016,Jan,13

16020 Dressings and/or debridement of partial-thickness burns, initial or subsequent; small (less than 5% total body surface area)
INCLUDES Wound coverage other than skin graft
1.56 2.35 FUD 000 Q1 N1
AMA: 2018,Jan,8; 2017,Jan,8; 2016,Jan,13

16025 medium (eg, whole face or whole extremity, or 5% to 10% total body surface area)
INCLUDES Wound coverage other than skin graft
3.16 4.26 FUD 000 T A2
AMA: 2018,Jan,8; 2017,Jan,8; 2016,Jan,13

16030 large (eg, more than 1 extremity, or greater than 10% total body surface area)
INCLUDES Wound coverage other than skin graft
3.82 5.40 FUD 000 T A2
AMA: 2018,Jan,8; 2017,Jan,8; 2016,Jan,13

16035 Escharotomy; initial incision
EXCLUDES *Debridement scraping of burn (16020-16030)*
5.71 5.71 FUD 000 T G2
AMA: 2018,Jan,8; 2017,Jan,8; 2016,Jan,13

+ 16036 each additional incision (List separately in addition to code for primary procedure)
EXCLUDES *Debridement or scraping burn (16020-16030)*
Code first (16035)
2.37 2.37 FUD ZZZ C
AMA: 2018,Jan,8; 2017,Jan,8; 2016,Jan,13

17000-17004 Destruction Any Method: Premalignant Lesion

CMS: 100-03,140.5 Laser Procedures

EXCLUDES *Cryotherapy acne (17340)*
Destruction, skin:
Benign lesions other than cutaneous vascular proliferative lesions (17110-17111)
Cutaneous vascular proliferative lesions (17106-17108)
Malignant lesions (17260-17286)
Destruction lesion:
Anus (46900-46917, 46924)
Conjunctiva (68135)
Eyelid (67850)
Penis (54050-54057, 54065)
Vagina (57061, 57065)
Vestibule of mouth (40820)
Vulva (56501, 56515)
Destruction or excision skin tags (11200-11201)
Escharotomy (16035-16036)
Excision benign lesion (11400-11446)
Laser fenestration for scars (0479T-0480T)
Localized chemotherapy treatment see appropriate office visit service code
Paring or excision benign hyperkeratotic lesion (11055-11057)
Shaving skin lesions (11300-11313)
Treatment inflammatory skin disease via laser (96920-96922)

17000 **Destruction (eg, laser surgery, electrosurgery, cryosurgery, chemosurgery, surgical curettement), premalignant lesions (eg, actinic keratoses); first lesion**
1.53 1.85 **FUD** 010 Q1 N1
AMA: 2018,Jan,8; 2017,Dec,14; 2017,Jan,8; 2016,Apr,3; 2016,Jan,13

+ **17003** **second through 14 lesions, each (List separately in addition to code for first lesion)**
Code first (17000)
0.06 0.17 **FUD** ZZZ N N1
AMA: 2018,Jan,8; 2017,Dec,14; 2017,Jan,8; 2016,Apr,3; 2016,Jan,13

17004 **Destruction (eg, laser surgery, electrosurgery, cryosurgery, chemosurgery, surgical curettement), premalignant lesions (eg, actinic keratoses), 15 or more lesions**
EXCLUDES *Reporting code for destruction less than 15 lesions (17000-17003)*
2.85 4.31 **FUD** 010 T P3
AMA: 2018,Jan,8; 2017,Dec,14; 2017,Jan,8; 2016,Apr,3; 2016,Jan,13

17106-17250 Destruction Any Method: Vascular Proliferative Lesion

CMS: 100-02,16,10 Exclusions from Coverage; 100-02,16,120 Cosmetic Procedures

EXCLUDES *Cryotherapy acne (17340)*
Destruction, skin:
Malignant lesions (17260-17286)
Premalignant lesions (17000-17004)
Destruction lesion:
Anus (46900-46917, 46924)
Conjunctiva (68135)
Eyelid (67850)
Penis (54050-54057, 54065)
Vagina (57061, 57065)
Vestibule of mouth (40820)
Vulva (56501, 56515)
Destruction or excision skin tags (11200-11201)
Escharotomy (16035-16036)
Excision benign lesion (11400-11446)
Laser fenestration for scars (0479T-0480T)
Localized chemotherapy treatment see appropriate office visit service code
Paring or excision benign hyperkeratotic lesion (11055-11057)
Shaving skin lesions (11300-11313)
Treatment inflammatory skin disease via laser (96920-96922)

17106 **Destruction of cutaneous vascular proliferative lesions (eg, laser technique); less than 10 sq cm**
7.84 9.72 **FUD** 090 T P2
AMA: 2019,Sep,10; 2018,Jan,8; 2017,Dec,14; 2017,Jan,8; 2016,Apr,3; 2016,Jan,13

17107 **10.0 to 50.0 sq cm**
10.1 12.7 **FUD** 090 T P2
AMA: 2018,Jan,8; 2017,Dec,14; 2017,Jan,8; 2016,Apr,3; 2016,Jan,13

17108 **over 50.0 sq cm**
15.0 18.1 **FUD** 090 T P3 80
AMA: 2018,Jan,8; 2017,Dec,14; 2017,Jan,8; 2016,Apr,3; 2016,Jan,13

17110 **Destruction (eg, laser surgery, electrosurgery, cryosurgery, chemosurgery, surgical curettement), of benign lesions other than skin tags or cutaneous vascular proliferative lesions; up to 14 lesions**
1.91 3.17 **FUD** 010 Q1 N1
AMA: 2020,Apr,10; 2018,Jan,8; 2017,Dec,14; 2017,Jan,8; 2016,Apr,3; 2016,Jan,13

17111 **15 or more lesions**
EXCLUDES *Destruction neurofibromas, 50-100 lesions (0419T-0420T)*
2.34 3.72 **FUD** 010 Q1 N1
AMA: 2018,Jan,8; 2017,Dec,14; 2017,Jan,8; 2016,Apr,3; 2016,Jan,13

17250 **Chemical cauterization of granulation tissue (ie, proud flesh)**
EXCLUDES *Chemical cauterization when applied for wound hemostasis*
Excision/removal codes for same lesion
Wound care management (97597-97598, 97602)
1.05 2.31 **FUD** 000 Q1 N1
AMA: 2018,Jan,8; 2017,Dec,14; 2017,Jan,8; 2016,Apr,3; 2016,Jan,13

17260-17286 Destruction, Any Method: Malignant Lesion

CMS: 100-03,140.5 Laser Procedures

EXCLUDES *Cryotherapy acne (17340)*
Destruction, skin:
Benign lesions other than cutaneous vascular proliferative lesions (17110-17111)
Cutaneous vascular proliferative lesions (17106-17108)
Premalignant lesions (17000-17004)
Destruction lesion:
Anus (46900-46917, 46924)
Conjunctiva (68135)
Eyelid (67850)
Penis (54050-54057, 54065)
Vestibule of mouth (40820)
Vulva (56501-56515)
Destruction or excision skin tags (11200-11201)
Escharotomy (16035-16036)
Excision benign lesion (11400-11446)
Laser fenestration for scars (0479T-0480T)
Localized chemotherapy treatment see appropriate office visit service code
Paring or excision benign hyperkeratotic lesion (11055-11057)
Shaving skin lesion (11300-11313)
Treatment inflammatory skin disease via laser (96920-96922)

17260 **Destruction, malignant lesion (eg, laser surgery, electrosurgery, cryosurgery, chemosurgery, surgical curettement), trunk, arms or legs; lesion diameter 0.5 cm or less**
2.03 2.71 **FUD** 010 Q1 N1
AMA: 2018,Jan,8; 2017,Dec,14; 2017,Jan,8; 2016,Jan,13

17261 **lesion diameter 0.6 to 1.0 cm**
2.58 4.11 **FUD** 010 Q1 N1
AMA: 2018,Jan,8; 2017,Dec,14; 2017,Jan,8; 2016,Jan,13

17262 **lesion diameter 1.1 to 2.0 cm**
3.30 5.01 **FUD** 010 Q1 N1
AMA: 2018,Jan,8; 2017,Dec,14; 2017,Jan,8; 2016,Jan,13

17263 **lesion diameter 2.1 to 3.0 cm**
3.55 5.45 **FUD** 010 Q1 N1
AMA: 2018,Jan,8; 2017,Dec,14; 2017,Jan,8; 2016,Jan,13

17264 **lesion diameter 3.1 to 4.0 cm**
3.79 5.84 **FUD** 010 T P3
AMA: 2018,Jan,8; 2017,Dec,14; 2017,Jan,8; 2016,Jan,13

17266 **lesion diameter over 4.0 cm**
4.47 6.66 **FUD** 010 T P3
AMA: 2018,Jan,8; 2017,Dec,14; 2017,Jan,8; 2016,Jan,13

17270 **Destruction, malignant lesion (eg, laser surgery, electrosurgery, cryosurgery, chemosurgery, surgical curettement), scalp, neck, hands, feet, genitalia; lesion diameter 0.5 cm or less**
2.74 4.22 **FUD** 010 T P2
AMA: 2018,Jan,8; 2017,Dec,14; 2017,Jan,8; 2016,Jan,13

17271 **lesion diameter 0.6 to 1.0 cm**
3.14 4.67 **FUD** 010 T P2
AMA: 2018,Jan,8; 2017,Dec,14; 2017,Jan,8; 2016,Jan,13

17272 **lesion diameter 1.1 to 2.0 cm**
3.63 5.33 **FUD** 010 Q1 N1
AMA: 2018,Jan,8; 2017,Dec,14; 2017,Jan,8; 2016,Jan,13

17273 **lesion diameter 2.1 to 3.0 cm**
4.11 5.94 **FUD** 010 T P3
AMA: 2018,Jan,8; 2017,Dec,14; 2017,Jan,8; 2016,Jan,13

17274 **lesion diameter 3.1 to 4.0 cm**
5.04 7.01 **FUD** 010 T P3
AMA: 2018,Jan,8; 2017,Dec,14; 2017,Jan,8; 2016,Jan,13

17276 **lesion diameter over 4.0 cm**
5.86 8.07 **FUD** 010 T P3
AMA: 2018,Jan,8; 2017,Dec,14; 2017,Jan,8; 2016,Jan,13

17280 **Destruction, malignant lesion (eg, laser surgery, electrosurgery, cryosurgery, chemosurgery, surgical curettement), face, ears, eyelids, nose, lips, mucous membrane; lesion diameter 0.5 cm or less**
2.48 3.94 **FUD** 010 Q1 N1
AMA: 2018,Jan,8; 2017,Dec,14; 2017,Jan,8; 2016,Jan,13

17281 **lesion diameter 0.6 to 1.0 cm**
3.54 5.09 **FUD** 010 T P3
AMA: 2018,Jan,8; 2017,Dec,14; 2017,Jan,8; 2016,Jan,13

17282 **lesion diameter 1.1 to 2.0 cm**
3.97 5.82 **FUD** 010 T P3
AMA: 2018,Jan,8; 2017,Dec,14; 2017,Jan,8; 2016,Jan,13

17283 **lesion diameter 2.1 to 3.0 cm**
4.97 6.94 **FUD** 010 T P3
AMA: 2018,Jan,8; 2017,Dec,14; 2017,Jan,8; 2016,Jan,13

17284 **lesion diameter 3.1 to 4.0 cm**
5.80 7.90 **FUD** 010 T P3
AMA: 2018,Jan,8; 2017,Dec,14; 2017,Jan,8; 2016,Jan,13

17286 **lesion diameter over 4.0 cm**
7.86 10.1 **FUD** 010 T P3
AMA: 2018,Jan,8; 2017,Dec,14; 2017,Jan,8; 2016,Jan,13

17311-17315 Mohs Surgery

INCLUDES Surgical/pathology services performed by same physician or other qualified health care provider:
- Evaluation skin margins by surgeon
- Pathology exam on Mohs surgery specimen (by Mohs surgeon) (88302-88309)
- Routine frozen section stain (88314)
- Tumor removal, mapping, preparation, and examination lesion

EXCLUDES *Frozen section if no prior diagnosis determination has been performed (88331)*

Code also:
- Any special histochemical stain on frozen section, nonroutine and append modifier 59 (88311-88314, 88342)
- Biopsy when no prior diagnosis determination has been performed, biopsy indeterminate, or performed more than 90 days preoperatively and append modifier 59 (11102, 11104, 11106)
- Complex repair (13100-13160)
- Flaps or grafts (14000-14350, 15050-15770)
- Intermediate repair (12031-12057)
- Simple repair (12001-12021)

17311 **Mohs micrographic technique, including removal of all gross tumor, surgical excision of tissue specimens, mapping, color coding of specimens, microscopic examination of specimens by the surgeon, and histopathologic preparation including routine stain(s) (eg, hematoxylin and eosin, toluidine blue), head, neck, hands, feet, genitalia, or any location with surgery directly involving muscle, cartilage, bone, tendon, major nerves, or vessels; first stage, up to 5 tissue blocks**
10.4 18.8 **FUD** 000 T P2
AMA: 2018,Jan,8; 2017,Jan,8; 2016,Jan,13

\+ **17312** **each additional stage after the first stage, up to 5 tissue blocks (List separately in addition to code for primary procedure)**
Code first (17311)
5.55 11.3 **FUD** ZZZ N N1
AMA: 2018,Jan,8; 2017,Jan,8; 2016,Jan,13

17313 **Mohs micrographic technique, including removal of all gross tumor, surgical excision of tissue specimens, mapping, color coding of specimens, microscopic examination of specimens by the surgeon, and histopathologic preparation including routine stain(s) (eg, hematoxylin and eosin, toluidine blue), of the trunk, arms, or legs; first stage, up to 5 tissue blocks**
9.34 17.6 **FUD** 000 T P2
AMA: 2018,Jan,8; 2017,Jan,8; 2016,Jan,13

\+ **17314** **each additional stage after the first stage, up to 5 tissue blocks (List separately in addition to code for primary procedure)**
Code first (17313)
5.14 10.8 **FUD** ZZZ N N1
AMA: 2018,Jan,8; 2017,Jan,8; 2016,Jan,13

\+ **17315** **Mohs micrographic technique, including removal of all gross tumor, surgical excision of tissue specimens, mapping, color coding of specimens, microscopic examination of specimens by the surgeon, and histopathologic preparation including routine stain(s) (eg, hematoxylin and eosin, toluidine blue), each additional block after the first 5 tissue blocks, any stage (List separately in addition to code for primary procedure)**
Code first (17311-17314)
1.47 2.22 **FUD** ZZZ N N1
AMA: 2018,Jan,8; 2017,Jan,8; 2016,Jan,13

17340-17999 Treatment for Active Acne and Permanent Hair Removal

CMS: 100-02,16,10 Exclusions from Coverage; 100-02,16,120 Cosmetic Procedures

17340 **Cryotherapy (CO2 slush, liquid N2) for acne**
1.40 1.49 **FUD** 010 Q1 N1
AMA: 2018,Jan,8; 2017,Jan,8; 2016,Jan,13

17360 **Chemical exfoliation for acne (eg, acne paste, acid)**
2.77 3.61 **FUD** 010 Q1 N1
AMA: 2018,Jan,8; 2017,Jan,8; 2016,Jan,13

17380 **Electrolysis epilation, each 30 minutes**

EXCLUDES *Actinotherapy (96900)*

0.00 0.00 FUD 000 T R2 80

AMA: 2018,Jan,8; 2017,Jan,8; 2016,Jan,13

17999 **Unlisted procedure, skin, mucous membrane and subcutaneous tissue**

0.00 0.00 FUD YYY Q1 80

AMA: 2019,Sep,10; 2019,Mar,10; 2019,Jan,14; 2018,Jan,8; 2017,Dec,13; 2017,Jan,8; 2016,May,13; 2016,Jan,13

19000-19030 Treatment of Breast Abscess and Cyst with Injection, Aspiration, Incision

19000 **Puncture aspiration of cyst of breast;**

(76942, 77021)

1.26 3.12 FUD 000 T P3

AMA: 2018,Jan,8; 2017,Jan,8; 2016,Jan,13

\+ 19001 **each additional cyst (List separately in addition to code for primary procedure)**

Code first (19000)

(76942, 77021)

0.62 0.77 FUD ZZZ N N1

AMA: 2018,Jan,8; 2017,Jan,8; 2016,Jan,13

19020 **Mastotomy with exploration or drainage of abscess, deep**

8.93 13.5 FUD 090 J A2 50

AMA: 2018,Jan,8; 2017,Jan,8; 2016,Jan,13

19030 **Injection procedure only for mammary ductogram or galactogram**

(77053-77054)

2.23 4.74 FUD 000 N N1 50

AMA: 2018,Jan,8; 2017,Jan,8; 2016,Jan,13

19081-19086 Breast Biopsy with Imaging Guidance

CMS: 100-03,220.13 Percutaneous Image-guided Breast Biopsy; 100-04,12,40.7 Bilateral Procedures; 100-04,13,80.1 Physician Presence; 100-04,13,80.2 S&I Multiple Procedure Reduction

INCLUDES Breast biopsy with placement localization devices
Fluoroscopic guidance for needle placement (77002)
Magnetic resonance guidance for needle placement (77021)
Radiological examination, surgical specimen (76098)
Ultrasonic guidance for needle placement (76942)

EXCLUDES *Biopsy breast without imaging guidance (19100-19101)*
Lesion removal without concentration on surgical margins (19110-19126)
Open biopsy after placement localization device (19101)
Partial mastectomy (19301-19302)
Placement localization devices only (19281-19288)
Total mastectomy (19303-19307)

Code also additional biopsies performed with different imaging modalities

19081 **Biopsy, breast, with placement of breast localization device(s) (eg, clip, metallic pellet), when performed, and imaging of the biopsy specimen, when performed, percutaneous; first lesion, including stereotactic guidance**

4.82 17.3 FUD 000 J G2 80 50

AMA: 2019,Apr,4; 2018,Jan,8; 2017,Jan,8; 2016,Jun,3; 2016,Jan,13

\+ 19082 **each additional lesion, including stereotactic guidance (List separately in addition to code for primary procedure)**

Code first (19081)

2.42 13.9 FUD ZZZ N N1 80

AMA: 2019,Apr,4; 2018,Jan,8; 2017,Jan,8; 2016,Jun,3; 2016,Jan,13

19083 **Biopsy, breast, with placement of breast localization device(s) (eg, clip, metallic pellet), when performed, and imaging of the biopsy specimen, when performed, percutaneous; first lesion, including ultrasound guidance**

4.56 17.1 FUD 000 J G2 80 50

AMA: 2019,Apr,4; 2018,Jan,8; 2017,Jan,8; 2016,Jun,3; 2016,Jan,13

\+ 19084 **each additional lesion, including ultrasound guidance (List separately in addition to code for primary procedure)**

Code first (19083)

2.25 13.6 FUD ZZZ N N1 80

AMA: 2019,Apr,4; 2018,Jan,8; 2017,Jan,8; 2016,Jun,3; 2016,Jan,13

19085 **Biopsy, breast, with placement of breast localization device(s) (eg, clip, metallic pellet), when performed, and imaging of the biopsy specimen, when performed, percutaneous; first lesion, including magnetic resonance guidance**

5.28 26.1 FUD 000 J G2 80 50

AMA: 2019,Apr,4; 2018,Jan,8; 2017,Jan,8; 2016,Jun,3; 2016,Jan,13

\+ 19086 **each additional lesion, including magnetic resonance guidance (List separately in addition to code for primary procedure)**

Code first (19085)

2.65 21.9 FUD ZZZ N N1 80

AMA: 2019,Apr,4; 2018,Jan,8; 2017,Jan,8; 2016,Jun,3; 2016,Jan,13

19100-19101 Breast Biopsy Without Imaging Guidance

EXCLUDES *Biopsy breast with imaging guidance (19081-19086)*
Lesion removal without concentration on surgical margins (19110-19126)
Partial mastectomy (19301-19302)
Total mastectomy (19303-19307)

19100 **Biopsy of breast; percutaneous, needle core, not using imaging guidance (separate procedure)**

EXCLUDES *Fine needle aspiration:*
With imaging guidance ([10005, 10006, 10007, 10008, 10009, 10010, 10011, 10012])
Without imaging guidance (10021, [10004])

2.03 4.32 FUD 000 J A2 50

AMA: 2018,Jan,8; 2017,Jan,8; 2016,Jan,13

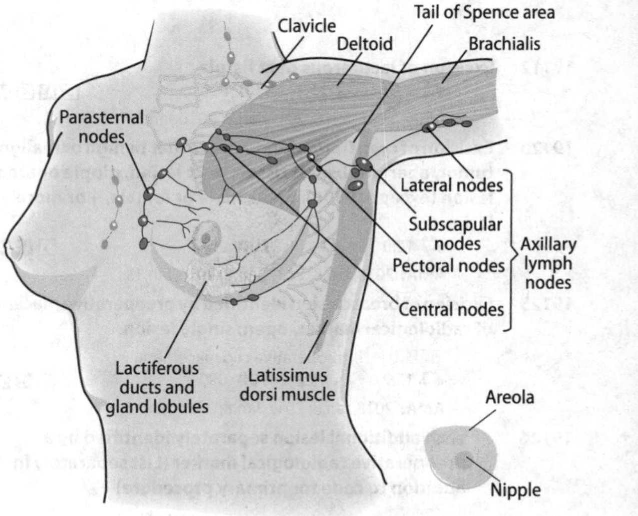

19101 **open, incisional**

Code also placement localization device with imaging guidance (19281-19288)

6.45 9.62 FUD 010 J A2 50

AMA: 2018,Jan,8; 2017,Jan,8; 2016,Jan,13

19105 Treatment of Fibroadenoma: Cryoablation

CMS: 100-04,13,80.1 Physician Presence; 100-04,13,80.2 S&I Multiple Procedure Reduction

INCLUDES Adjacent lesions treated with one cryoprobe
Ultrasound guidance (76940, 76942)

EXCLUDES *Cryoablation malignant breast tumors (0581T)*

19105 **Ablation, cryosurgical, of fibroadenoma, including ultrasound guidance, each fibroadenoma**
6.14 · 77.6 · **FUD** 000 · J J8 50
AMA: 2007,Mar,7-8

19110-19126 Excisional Procedures: Breast

INCLUDES Open removal breast mass without concentration on surgical margins

Code also placement localization device with imaging guidance (19281-19288)

19110 **Nipple exploration, with or without excision of a solitary lactiferous duct or a papilloma lactiferous duct**
9.94 · 13.9 · **FUD** 090 · J A2 50
AMA: 2018,Jan,8; 2017,Jan,8; 2016,Jan,13

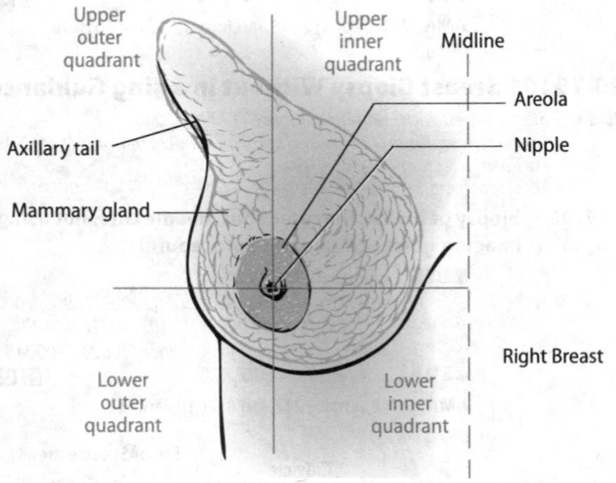

19112 **Excision of lactiferous duct fistula**
9.12 · 13.2 · **FUD** 090 · J A2 80 50
AMA: 2018,Jan,8; 2017,Jan,8; 2016,Jan,13

19120 **Excision of cyst, fibroadenoma, or other benign or malignant tumor, aberrant breast tissue, duct lesion, nipple or areolar lesion (except 19300), open, male or female, 1 or more lesions**
12.0 · 14.5 · **FUD** 090 · J A2 50
AMA: 2018,Jan,8; 2017,Jan,8; 2016,Jan,13

19125 **Excision of breast lesion identified by preoperative placement of radiological marker, open; single lesion**
INCLUDES Intraoperative clip placement
13.2 · 15.8 · **FUD** 090 · J A2 50
AMA: 2018,Jan,8; 2017,Jan,8; 2016,Jan,13

+ **19126** **each additional lesion separately identified by a preoperative radiological marker (List separately in addition to code for primary procedure)**
INCLUDES Intraoperative clip placement
Code first (19125)
4.68 · 4.68 · **FUD** ZZZ · N N1
AMA: 2018,Jan,8; 2017,Jan,8; 2016,Jan,13

19281-19288 Placement of Localization Markers

INCLUDES Placement localization devices only

EXCLUDES *Biopsy breast without imaging guidance (19100-19101)*
When performed on same lesion:
Fluoroscopic guidance for needle placement (77002)
Localization device placement with biopsy breast (19081-19086)
Magnetic resonance guidance for needle placement (77021)
Ultrasonic guidance for needle placement (76942)

Code also:
Open excision of breast lesion when performed after localization device placement (19110-19126)
Open incisional breast biopsy when performed after localization device placement (19101)
Radiography surgical specimen (76098)

19281 **Placement of breast localization device(s) (eg, clip, metallic pellet, wire/needle, radioactive seeds), percutaneous; first lesion, including mammographic guidance**
2.91 · 6.90 · **FUD** 000 · Q1 N1 80 50
AMA: 2018,Jan,8; 2017,Jan,8; 2016,Jun,3; 2016,Jan,13

+ **19282** **each additional lesion, including mammographic guidance (List separately in addition to code for primary procedure)**
Code first (19281)
1.46 · 4.92 · **FUD** ZZZ · N N1 80
AMA: 2018,Jan,8; 2017,Jan,8; 2016,Jun,3; 2016,Jan,13

19283 **Placement of breast localization device(s) (eg, clip, metallic pellet, wire/needle, radioactive seeds), percutaneous; first lesion, including stereotactic guidance**
2.93 · 7.74 · **FUD** 000 · Q1 N1 80 50
AMA: 2018,Jan,8; 2017,Jan,8; 2016,Jun,3; 2016,May,13; 2016,Jan,13

+ **19284** **each additional lesion, including stereotactic guidance (List separately in addition to code for primary procedure)**
Code first (19283)
1.49 · 5.90 · **FUD** ZZZ · N N1 80
AMA: 2018,Jan,8; 2017,Jan,8; 2016,Jun,3; 2016,May,13; 2016,Jan,13

19285 **Placement of breast localization device(s) (eg, clip, metallic pellet, wire/needle, radioactive seeds), percutaneous; first lesion, including ultrasound guidance**
2.49 · 12.9 · **FUD** 000 · Q1 N1 80 50
AMA: 2018,Jan,8; 2017,Jan,8; 2016,Jun,3; 2016,May,13; 2016,Jan,13

+ **19286** **each additional lesion, including ultrasound guidance (List separately in addition to code for primary procedure)**
Code first (19285)
1.25 · 11.9 · **FUD** ZZZ · N N1 80
AMA: 2018,Jan,8; 2017,Jan,8; 2016,Jun,3; 2016,May,13; 2016,Jan,13

19287 **Placement of breast localization device(s) (eg clip, metallic pellet, wire/needle, radioactive seeds), percutaneous; first lesion, including magnetic resonance guidance**
3.72 · 22.1 · **FUD** 000 · Q1 N1 80 50
AMA: 2018,Jan,8; 2017,Jan,8; 2016,Jun,3; 2016,May,13; 2016,Jan,13

+ **19288** **each additional lesion, including magnetic resonance guidance (List separately in addition to code for primary procedure)**
Code first (19287)
1.87 · 19.7 · **FUD** ZZZ · N N1 80
AMA: 2018,Jan,8; 2017,Jan,8; 2016,Jun,3; 2016,May,13; 2016,Jan,13

19294-19298 Radioelement Application

+ **19294** **Preparation of tumor cavity, with placement of a radiation therapy applicator for intraoperative radiation therapy (IORT) concurrent with partial mastectomy (List separately in addition to code for primary procedure)**
  Code first (19301-19302)
  4.71 4.71 FUD ZZZ N N1 80
  AMA: 2020,May,9

19296 **Placement of radiotherapy afterloading expandable catheter (single or multichannel) into the breast for interstitial radioelement application following partial mastectomy, includes imaging guidance; on date separate from partial mastectomy**
  6.11 114. FUD 000 J J8 80 50
  AMA: 2020,May,9; 2018,Jan,8; 2017,Jan,8; 2016,Jan,13

+ **19297** **concurrent with partial mastectomy (List separately in addition to code for primary procedure)**
  Code first (19301-19302)
  2.75 2.75 FUD ZZZ N N1 80
  AMA: 2020,May,9; 2019,Apr,10; 2018,Jan,8; 2017,Jan,8; 2016,Jan,13

19298 **Placement of radiotherapy after loading brachytherapy catheters (multiple tube and button type) into the breast for interstitial radioelement application following (at the time of or subsequent to) partial mastectomy, includes imaging guidance**
  9.22 28.4 FUD 000 J G2 80 50
  AMA: 2020,May,9; 2018,Jan,8; 2017,Jan,8; 2016,Jan,13

19300-19307 Mastectomies: Partial, Simple, Radical

CMS: 100-04,12,40.7 Bilateral Procedures
INCLUDES Intraoperative clip placement
EXCLUDES *Insertion prosthesis (19340, 19342)*

19300 **Mastectomy for gynecomastia** ♂
  EXCLUDES *Removal breast tissue for:*
  Other than gynecomastia (19318)
  Treatment or prevention breast cancer (19301-19307)
  12.1 15.8 FUD 090 J A2 50
  AMA: 2020,May,9; 2018,Jan,8; 2017,Jan,8; 2016,Jan,13

19301 **Mastectomy, partial (eg, lumpectomy, tylectomy, quadrantectomy, segmentectomy);**
  EXCLUDES *Insertion radiotherapy afterloading balloon during separate encounter (19296)*
  Code also:
  3D volumetric specimen imaging, when performed (0694T)
  Insertion radiotherapy afterloading balloon catheter, when performed at same time (19297)
  Insertion radiotherapy afterloading brachytherapy catheter, when performed at same time (19298)
  Intraoperative radiofrequency spectroscopy margin assessment and report (0546T)
  Tumor cavity preparation with intraoperative radiation therapy applicator, when performed (19294)
  19.0 19.0 FUD 090 J A2 80 50
  AMA: 2020,May,9; 2018,Jan,8; 2017,Oct,9; 2017,Jan,8; 2016,Jan,13

19302 **with axillary lymphadenectomy**
  EXCLUDES *Insertion radiotherapy afterloading balloon during separate encounter (19296)*
  Code also:
  3D volumetric specimen imaging, when performed (0694T)
  Insertion radiotherapy afterloading balloon catheter, when performed at same time (19297)
  Insertion radiotherapy afterloading brachytherapy catheter, when performed at same time (19298)
  Intraoperative radiofrequency spectroscopy margin assessment and report (0546T)
  Tumor cavity preparation with intraoperative radiation therapy applicator, when performed (19294)
  25.9 25.9 FUD 090 J A2 80 50
  AMA: 2020,Nov,12; 2020,May,9; 2019,Feb,8; 2018,Jan,8; 2017,Jan,8; 2016,Jan,13

19303 **Mastectomy, simple, complete**
  EXCLUDES *Excision pectoral muscles and axillary or internal mammary lymph nodes*
  Removal breast tissue for:
  Gynecomastia (19300)
  Other than gynecomastia (19318)
  27.8 27.8 FUD 090 J A2 80 50
  AMA: 2020,May,9; 2019,Dec,4; 2018,Jan,8; 2017,Jan,8; 2016,Jan,13

19305 **Mastectomy, radical, including pectoral muscles, axillary lymph nodes**
  33.0 33.0 FUD 090 C 80 50
  AMA: 2020,May,9; 2018,Jan,8; 2017,Jan,8; 2016,Jan,13

19306 **Mastectomy, radical, including pectoral muscles, axillary and internal mammary lymph nodes (Urban type operation)**
  34.6 34.6 FUD 090 C 80 50
  AMA: 2020,May,9; 2018,Jan,8; 2017,Jan,8; 2016,Jan,13

19307 **Mastectomy, modified radical, including axillary lymph nodes, with or without pectoralis minor muscle, but excluding pectoralis major muscle**
  34.6 34.6 FUD 090 J G2 80 50
  AMA: 2020,May,9; 2019,Feb,8; 2018,Jan,8; 2017,Jan,8; 2016,Jan,13

19316-19499 Plastic, Reconstructive, and Aesthetic Breast Procedures

CMS: 100-03,140.2 Breast Reconstruction Following Mastectomy; 100-04,12,40.7 Bilateral Procedures
Code also biologic implant for tissue reinforcement (15777)

19316 **Mastopexy**
  22.3 22.3 FUD 090 J A2 80 50
  AMA: 2018,Jan,8; 2017,Jan,8; 2016,Jan,13

19318 **Breast reduction**
  INCLUDES Aries-Pitanguy mammaplasty
  Biesenberger mammaplasty
  31.5 31.5 FUD 090 J A2 80 50
  AMA: 2020,May,9; 2018,Jan,8; 2017,Jan,8; 2016,Jan,13

19325 **Breast augmentation with implant**
  EXCLUDES *Flap or graft (15100-15650)*
  Code also fat grafting, when performed (15771-15772)
  18.6 18.6 FUD 090 J G2 80 50
  AMA: 2018,Jan,8; 2017,Jan,8; 2016,Jan,13

19328 **Removal of intact breast implant**
  EXCLUDES *Removal tissue expander (11970-11971)*
  Revision peri-implant capsule, breast (19370)
  14.4 14.4 FUD 090 Q2 A2 50
  AMA: 2018,Jan,8; 2017,Jan,8; 2016,Jan,13

19330 **Removal of ruptured breast implant, including implant contents (eg, saline, silicone gel)**
  EXCLUDES *Insertion new breast implant during same operative session (19342)*
  Removal ruptured tissue expander (11970-11971)
  18.1 18.1 FUD 090 Q2 A2 50
  AMA: 2018,Jan,8; 2017,Jan,8; 2016,Jan,13

19340 Insertion of breast implant on same day of mastectomy (ie, immediate)

EXCLUDES *Preparation moulage for custom breast implant (19396)*
Supply prosthetic implant (99070, C1789, L8600)

28.6 28.6 FUD 090 J A2 50

AMA: 2020,May,9; 2018,Jan,8; 2017,Jan,8; 2016,Jan,13

19342 Insertion or replacement of breast implant on separate day from mastectomy

EXCLUDES *Preparation moulage for custom breast implant (19396)*
Removal intact breast implant (19328)
Removal tissue expander with insertion breast implant (11970)
Supply prosthetic implant (99070, C1789, L8600)

26.7 26.7 FUD 090 J A2 80 50

AMA: 2020,May,9; 2018,Jan,8; 2017,Jan,8; 2016,Jan,13

19350 Nipple/areola reconstruction

INCLUDES Adjacent tissue transfer, trunk (14000-14001)
Full-thickness graft, trunk (15200-15201)
Split-thickness autograft, trunk, arms, legs (15100)
Tattooing to correct skin color defects (11920-11922)

19.4 23.8 FUD 090 J A2 50

AMA: 2018,Jan,8; 2017,Jan,8; 2016,Aug,9; 2016,Jan,13

19355 Correction of inverted nipples

17.7 21.5 FUD 090 J A2 80 50

AMA: 2018,Jan,8; 2017,Jan,8; 2016,Jan,13

19357 Tissue expander placement in breast reconstruction, including subsequent expansion(s)

43.1 43.1 FUD 090 J J8 80 50

AMA: 2018,Jan,8; 2017,Jan,8; 2016,Jan,13

19361 Breast reconstruction; with latissimus dorsi flap

INCLUDES Closure donor site
Harvesting skin graft
Inset shaping flap into breast

EXCLUDES *Implant prosthesis with latissimus dorsi implant:*
performed different day than mastectomy (19342)
performed same day as mastectomy (19340)
Insertion tissue expander with latissimus dorsi flap (19357)

45.4 45.4 FUD 090 C 80 50

AMA: 2019,Nov,14; 2018,Jan,8; 2017,Jan,8; 2016,Jan,13

19364 with free flap (eg, fTRAM, DIEP, SIEA, GAP flap)

INCLUDES Closure donor site
Harvesting skin graft
Inset shaping flap into breast
Microvascular repair
Operating microscope (69990)

79.7 79.7 FUD 090 C 80 50

AMA: 2020,Dec,11; 2019,Nov,14; 2018,Jan,8; 2017,Jan,8; 2016,Feb,12; 2016,Jan,13

19367 with single-pedicled transverse rectus abdominis myocutaneous (TRAM) flap

INCLUDES Closure donor site
Harvesting skin graft
Inset shaping flap into breast

51.5 51.5 FUD 090 C 80 50

AMA: 2019,Nov,14; 2018,Jan,8; 2017,Jan,8; 2016,Jan,13

19368 with single-pedicled transverse rectus abdominis myocutaneous (TRAM) flap, requiring separate microvascular anastomosis (supercharging)

INCLUDES Closure donor site
Harvesting skin graft
Inset shaping flap into breast
Operating microscope (69990)

63.2 63.2 FUD 090 C 80 50

AMA: 2019,Nov,14; 2018,Jan,8; 2017,Jan,8; 2016,Feb,12; 2016,Jan,13

19369 with bipedicled transverse rectus abdominis myocutaneous (TRAM) flap

INCLUDES Closure donor site
Harvesting skin graft
Inset shaping flap into breast

59.0 59.0 FUD 090 C 80 50

AMA: 2019,Nov,14; 2018,Jan,8; 2017,Jan,8; 2016,Jan,13

19370 Revision of peri-implant capsule, breast, including capsulotomy, capsulorrhaphy, and/or partial capsulectomy

EXCLUDES *Removal and replacement with new implant (19342)*
Removal intact breast implant (19328)

19.9 19.9 FUD 090 J A2 50

AMA: 2018,Jan,8; 2017,Jan,8; 2016,Jan,13

19371 Peri-implant capsulectomy, breast, complete, including removal of all intracapsular contents

EXCLUDES *Removal and replacement with new implant (19342)*
Removal intact breast implant (19328)
Removal ruptured breast implant (19330)
Revision peri-implant capsule on same breast (19370)

22.5 22.5 FUD 090 J A2 50

AMA: 2018,Jan,8; 2017,Jan,8; 2016,Jan,13

19380 Revision of reconstructed breast (eg, significant removal of tissue, re-advancement and/or re-inset of flaps in autologous reconstruction or significant capsular revision combined with soft tissue excision in implant-based reconstruction)

INCLUDES Removal portion or reshaping flap
Revision flap position on chest wall
Revision scar(s)
When performed on same breast:
- Breast reduction (19318)
- Mastopexy (19316)
- Repair complex, trunk (13100-13102)
- Repair intermediate, trunk (12031-12037)
- Revision peri-implant capsule, breast (19370)
- Suction assisted lipectomy; trunk (15877)

EXCLUDES *Autologuous fat graft (15771-15772)*
Implant replacement (19342)

22.4 22.4 FUD 090 J A2 50

AMA: 2019,Nov,14; 2018,Jan,8; 2017,Dec,13; 2017,Jan,8; 2016,Jan,13

19396 Preparation of moulage for custom breast implant

4.17 8.23 FUD 000 J G2 80 50

AMA: 2018,Jan,8; 2017,Jan,8; 2016,Jan,13

19499 Unlisted procedure, breast

0.00 0.00 FUD YYY J 80 50

AMA: 2019,Aug,10; 2019,Apr,10; 2018,Jan,8; 2017,Jan,8; 2016,Dec,16; 2016,Jan,13

20100-20103 Exploratory Surgery of Traumatic Wound

INCLUDES Debridement
Expanded dissection wound for exploration
Extraction foreign material
Open examination
Tying or coagulation small vessels

EXCLUDES *Cutaneous/subcutaneous incision and drainage procedures (10060-10061)*
Laparotomy (49000-49010)
Repair major vessels:
Abdomen (35221, 35251, 35281)
Chest (35211, 35216, 35241, 35246, 35271, 35276)
Extremity (35206-35207, 35226, 35236, 35256, 35266, 35286)
Neck (35201, 35231, 35261)
Thoracotomy (32100-32160)

20100 Exploration of penetrating wound (separate procedure); neck
17.4 17.4 FUD 010 T G2 80 50
AMA: 2018,Jan,8; 2017,Jan,8; 2016,Jan,13

20101 chest
6.10 13.7 FUD 010 T G2
AMA: 2018,Jan,8; 2017,Jan,8; 2016,Jan,13

20102 abdomen/flank/back
7.43 14.7 FUD 010 T G2
AMA: 2020,Jan,6; 2018,Jan,8; 2017,Jan,8; 2016,Jan,13

20103 extremity
9.99 16.6 FUD 010 T G2 80
AMA: 2018,Jan,8; 2017,Jan,8; 2016,Jan,13

20150 Epiphyseal Bar Resection

20150 Excision of epiphyseal bar, with or without autogenous soft tissue graft obtained through same fascial incision
29.0 29.0 FUD 090 J G2 80 50
AMA: 1996,Nov,1

20200-20206 Muscle Biopsy

EXCLUDES *Removal of muscle tumor (see appropriate anatomic section)*

20200 Biopsy, muscle; superficial
2.73 5.95 FUD 000 J A2
AMA: 2020,NovBULL,1

20205 deep
4.48 8.35 FUD 000 J A2

20206 Biopsy, muscle, percutaneous needle
EXCLUDES *Fine needle aspiration (10021, [10004, 10005, 10006, 10007, 10008, 10009, 10010, 10011, 10012])*
(76942, 77002, 77012, 77021)
(88172-88173)
1.67 6.76 FUD 000 J A2
AMA: 2019,Apr,4

20220-20225 Percutaneous Bone Biopsy

EXCLUDES *Bone marrow aspiration(s) or biopsy(ies) (38220-38222)*

20220 Biopsy, bone, trocar, or needle; superficial (eg, ilium, sternum, spinous process, ribs)
(77002, 77012, 77021)
2.06 4.79 FUD 000 J A2
AMA: 2018,Jan,8; 2017,Jan,8; 2016,Jan,13

20225 deep (eg, vertebral body, femur)
EXCLUDES *When performed at same level:*
Percutaneous sacral augmentation (sacroplasty) (0200T-0201T)
Percutaneous vertebroplasty (22510-22515)
(77002, 77012, 77021)
3.07 14.7 FUD 000 J A2
AMA: 2018,Jan,8; 2017,Jan,8; 2016,Jan,13

20240-20251 Open Bone Biopsy

EXCLUDES *Sequestrectomy or incision and drainage of bone abscess of:*
Calcaneus (28120)
Carpal bone (25145)
Clavicle (23170)
Humeral head (23174)
Humerus (24134)
Olecranon process (24138)
Radius (24136, 25145)
Scapula (23172)
Skull (61501)
Talus (28120)
Ulna (24138, 24145)

20240 Biopsy, bone, open; superficial (eg, sternum, spinous process, rib, patella, olecranon process, calcaneus, tarsal, metatarsal, carpal, metacarpal, phalanx)
4.21 4.21 FUD 000 J A2
AMA: 2018,Jan,8; 2017,Jan,8; 2016,Jan,13

20245 deep (eg, humeral shaft, ischium, femoral shaft)
10.1 10.1 FUD 000 J A2
AMA: 2018,Jan,8; 2017,Jan,8; 2016,Jan,13

20250 Biopsy, vertebral body, open; thoracic
11.3 11.3 FUD 010 J A2
AMA: 2018,Jan,8; 2017,Jan,8; 2016,Jan,13

20251 lumbar or cervical
12.4 12.4 FUD 010 J A2 80
AMA: 2018,Jan,8; 2017,Jan,8; 2016,Jan,13

20500-20501 Injection Fistula/Sinus Tract

EXCLUDES *Arthrography injection of:*
Ankle (27648)
Elbow (24220)
Hip (27093, 27095)
Sacroiliac joint (27096)
Shoulder (23350)
Temporomandibular joint (TMJ) (21116)
Wrist (25246)
Autologous adipose-derived regenerative cells injection (0489T-0490T)

20500 Injection of sinus tract; therapeutic (separate procedure)
(76080)
2.49 3.25 FUD 010 T P3

20501 diagnostic (sinogram)
EXCLUDES *Contrast injection or injections for radiological evaluation existing gastrostomy, duodenostomy, jejunostomy, gastro-jejunostomy, or cecostomy (or other colonic) tube from percutaneous approach (49465)*
(76080)
1.09 3.62 FUD 000 N N1

20520-20525 Foreign Body Removal

20520 Removal of foreign body in muscle or tendon sheath; simple
4.22 6.03 FUD 010 J P3

20525 deep or complicated
7.11 13.6 FUD 010 J A2

20526-20561 [20560, 20561] Therapeutic Injections: Tendons, Trigger Points

20526 Injection, therapeutic (eg, local anesthetic, corticosteroid), carpal tunnel
1.66 2.20 FUD 000 T P3 50
AMA: 2018,Jan,8; 2017,Jan,8; 2016,Jan,13

20527 Injection, enzyme (eg, collagenase), palmar fascial cord (ie, Dupuytren's contracture)
EXCLUDES *Post injection palmar fascial cord manipulation (26341)*
1.90 2.43 FUD 000 T P3 50
AMA: 2018,Jan,8; 2017,Jan,8; 2016,Jan,13

20550 **Injection(s); single tendon sheath, or ligament, aponeurosis (eg, plantar "fascia")**

EXCLUDES *Autologous WBC injection (0481T)*
Morton's neuroma (64455, 64632)
Platelet rich plasma injection (0232T)

(76942, 77002, 77021)

1.13 1.51 FUD 000 T P3 50

AMA: 2018,Jan,8; 2017,Jan,8; 2016,Jan,13

20551 **single tendon origin/insertion**

EXCLUDES *Autologous WBC injection (0481T)*
Platelet rich plasma injection (0232T)

(76942, 77002, 77021)

1.15 1.53 FUD 000 T P3

AMA: 2018,Jan,8; 2017,Dec,13; 2017,Jan,8; 2016,Jan,13

20552 **Injection(s); single or multiple trigger point(s), 1 or 2 muscle(s)**

EXCLUDES *Autologous WBC injection (0481T)*
Needle insertion(s) without injection(s) for same muscle(s) ([20560, 20561])
Platelet rich plasma injection (0232T)

(76942, 77002, 77021)

1.11 1.59 FUD 000 T P3

AMA: 2020,Feb,9; 2018,Jan,8; 2017,Dec,13; 2017,Jun,10; 2017,Jan,8; 2016,Jan,13

20553 **single or multiple trigger point(s), 3 or more muscles**

EXCLUDES *Needle insertion(s) without injection(s) for same muscle(s) ([20560, 20561])*

(76942, 77002, 77021)

1.25 1.82 FUD 000 T P3

AMA: 2020,Feb,9; 2018,Dec,8; 2018,Dec,8; 2018,Jan,8; 2017,Jun,10; 2017,Jan,8; 2016,Jan,13

\# **20560** **Needle insertion(s) without injection(s); 1 or 2 muscle(s)**

INCLUDES Dry needling and trigger-point acupuncture

0.47 0.74 FUD XXX

AMA: 2020,Feb,9

\# **20561** **3 or more muscles**

INCLUDES Dry needling and trigger-point acupuncture

0.71 1.10 FUD XXX

AMA: 2020,Feb,9

20555-20561 [20560, 20561] Placement of Catheters/Needles for Brachytherapy

Code also interstitial radioelement application (77770-77772, 77778)

20555 **Placement of needles or catheters into muscle and/or soft tissue for subsequent interstitial radioelement application (at the time of or subsequent to the procedure)**

EXCLUDES *Interstitial radioelement:*
Devices placed into breast (19296-19298)
Placement needle, catheters, or devices into muscle or soft tissue head and neck (41019)
Placement needles or catheters into pelvic organs or genitalia (55920)
Placement needles or catheters into prostate (55875)

(76942, 77002, 77012, 77021)

9.48 9.48 FUD 000 J A2 80

AMA: 2018,Jan,8; 2017,Jan,8; 2016,Jan,13

20560 **Resequenced code. See code following 20553.**

20561 **Resequenced code. See code before 20555.**

20600-20611 Aspiration and/or Injection of Joint

CMS: 100-03,150.7 Prolotherapy, Joint Sclerotherapy, and Ligamentous Injections with Sclerosing Agents

20600 **Arthrocentesis, aspiration and/or injection, small joint or bursa (eg, fingers, toes); without ultrasound guidance**

EXCLUDES *Autologous adipose-derived regenerative cells injection (0489T-0490T)*
Platelet rich plasma (PRP) injections (0232T)
Ultrasound guidance (76942)

(77002, 77012, 77021)

1.04 1.44 FUD 000 T P3 50

AMA: 2018,Sep,12; 2018,Jan,8; 2017,Aug,9; 2017,Jan,8; 2016,Jan,13

20604 **with ultrasound guidance, with permanent recording and reporting**

INCLUDES Ultrasound guidance (76942)

EXCLUDES *Autologous adipose-derived regenerative cells injection (0489T-0490T)*
Platelet rich plasma (PRP) injections (0232T)

(77002, 77012, 77021)

1.32 2.17 FUD 000 T P3 50

AMA: 2018,Sep,12; 2018,Jan,8; 2017,Jan,8; 2016,Jan,13

20605 **Arthrocentesis, aspiration and/or injection, intermediate joint or bursa (eg, temporomandibular, acromioclavicular, wrist, elbow or ankle, olecranon bursa); without ultrasound guidance**

EXCLUDES *Ultrasound guidance (76942)*

(77002, 77012, 77021)

1.08 1.49 FUD 000 T P3 50

AMA: 2018,Jan,8; 2017,Aug,9; 2017,Jan,8; 2016,Jan,13

20606 **with ultrasound guidance, with permanent recording and reporting**

INCLUDES Ultrasound guidance (76942)

EXCLUDES *Platelet rich plasma (PRP) injections (0232T)*

(77002, 77012, 77021)

1.53 2.28 FUD 000 T P3 50

AMA: 2018,Jan,8; 2017,Jan,8; 2016,Jan,13

20610 **Arthrocentesis, aspiration and/or injection, major joint or bursa (eg, shoulder, hip, knee, subacromial bursa); without ultrasound guidance**

EXCLUDES *Injection contrast for knee arthrography (27369)*
Platelet rich plasma (PRP) injections (0232T)
Ultrasound guidance (76942)

(77002, 77012, 77021)

1.32 1.77 FUD 000 T P3 50

AMA: 2019,Aug,7; 2018,Jan,8; 2017,Apr,9; 2017,Jan,8; 2016,Jan,13

20611 **with ultrasound guidance, with permanent recording and reporting**

INCLUDES Ultrasound guidance (76942)

EXCLUDES *Injection contrast for knee arthrography (27369)*
Platelet rich plasma (PRP) injections (0232T)

(77002, 77012, 77021)

1.76 2.58 FUD 000 T P3 50

AMA: 2019,Aug,7; 2018,Jan,8; 2017,Jan,8; 2016,Jan,13

20612-20615 Aspiration and/or Injection of Cyst

20612 **Aspiration and/or injection of ganglion cyst(s) any location**

Code also modifier 59 for multiple ganglion aspirations or injections

1.19 1.76 FUD 000 T P3

20615 **Aspiration and injection for treatment of bone cyst**

EXCLUDES *Bone marrow lesions bone-substitute material injection (0707T)*

4.60 7.10 FUD 010 T P3

20650-20697 Procedures Related to Bony Fixation

20650 **Insertion of wire or pin with application of skeletal traction, including removal (separate procedure)**

4.54 6.08 FUD 010 J A2

26/TC PC/TC Only A2-Z3 ASC Payment 50 Bilateral ♂ Male Only ♀ Female Only Facility RVU Non-Facility RVU CCI CLIA
FUD Follow-up Days CMS: IOM AMA: CPT Asst A-Y OPPSI 80/80 Surg Assist Allowed / w/Doc Lab Crosswalk Radiology Crosswalk

20660 Application of cranial tongs, caliper, or stereotactic frame, including removal (separate procedure)

7.00 7.00 FUD 000 Q2 G2

AMA: 2018,Jan,8; 2017,Jan,8; 2016,Jan,13

20661 Application of halo, including removal; cranial

14.4 14.4 FUD 090 C

AMA: 2018,Jan,8; 2017,Jan,8; 2016,Jan,13

20662 pelvic

14.8 14.8 FUD 090 J R2 80

20663 femoral

13.6 13.6 FUD 090 J R2 80 50

20664 Application of halo, including removal, cranial, 6 or more pins placed, for thin skull osteology (eg, pediatric patients, hydrocephalus, osteogenesis imperfecta)

25.0 25.0 FUD 090 C

AMA: 2018,Jan,8; 2017,Jan,8; 2016,Jan,13

20665 Removal of tongs or halo applied by another individual

2.68 3.19 FUD 010 Q1 G2 80

AMA: 2018,Jan,8; 2017,Jan,8; 2016,Jan,13

20670 Removal of implant; superficial (eg, buried wire, pin or rod) (separate procedure)

4.18 10.5 FUD 010 Q2 A2

AMA: 2018,Jan,3; 2018,Jan,8; 2017,Jan,8; 2016,Jan,13

20680 deep (eg, buried wire, pin, screw, metal band, nail, rod or plate)

EXCLUDES *Removal and reinsertion sinus tarsi implant ([0511T])*
Removal sinus tarsi implant ([0510T])

12.1 17.6 FUD 090 Q2 A2 80

AMA: 2018,Jan,3; 2018,Jan,8; 2017,Jan,8; 2016,Nov,9; 2016,Jan,13

20690 Application of a uniplane (pins or wires in 1 plane), unilateral, external fixation system

Code also:
For replacement traction device during or after global period
Traction device supplies

17.2 17.2 FUD 090 J J8

AMA: 2018,Jan,3; 2018,Jan,8; 2017,Jan,8; 2016,Jan,13

20692 Application of a multiplane (pins or wires in more than 1 plane), unilateral, external fixation system (eg, Ilizarov, Monticelli type)

Code also:
For replacement traction device during or after global period
Traction device supplies

32.2 32.2 FUD 090 J J8 80

AMA: 2019,May,10; 2018,Jan,8; 2018,Jan,3; 2017,Jan,8; 2016,Jan,13

20693 Adjustment or revision of external fixation system requiring anesthesia (eg, new pin[s] or wire[s] and/or new ring[s] or bar[s])

12.7 12.7 FUD 090 J A2

AMA: 2018,Jan,3; 2018,Jan,8; 2017,Jan,8; 2016,Jan,13

20694 Removal, under anesthesia, of external fixation system

9.72 12.2 FUD 090 Q2 A2

AMA: 2018,Jan,3; 2018,Jan,8; 2017,Jan,8; 2016,Jan,13

20696 Application of multiplane (pins or wires in more than 1 plane), unilateral, external fixation with stereotactic computer-assisted adjustment (eg, spatial frame), including imaging; initial and subsequent alignment(s), assessment(s), and computation(s) of adjustment schedule(s)

EXCLUDES *Application multiplane external fixation system (20692)*
Osteotomy with insertion intramedullary lengthening device, humerus (0594T)
Removal and replacement each strut (20697)

34.4 34.4 FUD 090 J J8 80

AMA: 2018,Jan,3; 2018,Jan,8; 2017,Jan,8; 2016,Jan,13

20697 exchange (ie, removal and replacement) of strut, each

EXCLUDES *Application multiplane external fixation system (20692)*
Exchange strut for multiplane external fixation system (20697)

58.9 58.9 FUD 000 ⊘ J P2 80 TC

AMA: 2018,Jan,3; 2018,Jan,8; 2017,Jan,8; 2016,Jan,13

20700-20705 Drug Delivery Device

+ **20700 Manual preparation and insertion of drug-delivery device(s), deep (eg, subfascial) (List separately in addition to code for primary procedure)**

INCLUDES Combining therapeutic agents, including antibiotics, with carrier substance during operative episode
Forming resulting mixture into drug delivery devices (beads, nails, spacers)
Insertion therapeutic device/agent once per anatomic location

EXCLUDES *Insertion drug delivery implant, non-biodegradable (11981)*
Insertion prefabricated drug device

Code first (11010-11012, 11043, [11046], 11044, 11047, 20240-20251, 21010, 21025-21026, 21501-21510, 21627-21630, 22010-22015, 23030-23044, 23170-23184, 23334-23335, 23930-24000, 24134-24140, 24147, 24160, 25031-25040, 25145-25151, 26070, 26230-26236, 26990-26992, 27030, 27070-27071, 27090, 27301-27303, 27310, 27360, 27603-27604, 27610, 27640-27641, 28001-28003, 28020, 28120-28122)

2.44 2.44 FUD ZZZ 80

+ **20701 Removal of drug-delivery device(s), deep (eg, subfascial) (List separately in addition to code for primary procedure)**

INCLUDES Removal therapeutic device/agent once per anatomic location from subfascial tissues

EXCLUDES *Removal drug delivery device, performed alone (20680)*
Removal drug delivery implant, non-biodegradable (11982)

Code first (11010-11012, 11043, [11046], 11044, 11047, 20240-20251, 21010, 21025-21026, 21501-21510, 21627-21630, 22010-22015, 23030-23044, 23170-23184, 23334-23335, 23930-24000, 24134-24140, 24147, 24160, 25031-25040, 25145-25151, 26070, 26230-26236, 26990-26992, 27030, 27070-27071, 27090, 27301-27303, 27310, 27360, 27603-27604, 27610, 27640-27641, 28001-28003, 28020, 28120-28122)

1.82 1.82 FUD ZZZ 80

+ **20702 Manual preparation and insertion of drug-delivery device(s), intramedullary (List separately in addition to code for primary procedure)**

INCLUDES Combining therapeutic agents, including antibiotics, with carrier substance during operative episode
Forming resulting mixture into drug delivery devices (beads, nails, spacers)
Insertion therapeutic device/agent once per anatomic location into intramedullary spaces

EXCLUDES *Insertion drug delivery implant, non-biodegradable (11981)*
Insertion prefabricated drug device

Code first (20680-20692, 20694, 20802-20805, 20838, 21510, 23035, 23170, 23180, 23184, 23515, 23615, 23935, 24134, 24138-24140, 24147, 24430, 24516, 25035, 25145-25151, 25400, 25515, 25525-25526, 25545, 25574-25575, 27245, 27259, 27360, 27470, 27506, 27640, 27720)

4.06 4.06 FUD ZZZ 80

+ **20703 Removal of drug-delivery device(s), intramedullary (List separately in addition to code for primary procedure)**

INCLUDES Removal therapeutic device/agent once per anatomic location from intramedullary spaces

EXCLUDES *Removal drug delivery device, performed alone (20680)*
Removal drug delivery implant, non-biodegradable (11982)

Code first (20690-20692, 20694, 20802-20805, 20838, 21510, 23035, 23170, 23180, 23184, 23515, 23615, 23935, 24134, 24138-24140; 24147, 24430, 24516, 25035, 25145-25151, 25400, 25515, 25525-25526, 25545, 25574-25575, 27245, 27259, 27360, 27470, 27506, 27640, 27720)

2.91 2.91 FUD ZZZ 80

+ **20704 Manual preparation and insertion of drug-delivery device(s), intra-articular (List separately in addition to code for primary procedure)**

INCLUDES Combining therapeutic agents, including antibiotics, with carrier substance during operative episode
Forming resulting mixture into drug delivery devices (beads, nails, spacers)
Insertion therapeutic device/agent once per anatomic location into intra-articular spaces

EXCLUDES *Insertion drug delivery implant, non-biodegradable (11981)*
Insertion prefabricated drug device
Removal hip prosthesis (27091)
Removal knee prosthesis (27488)

Code first (22864-22865, 23040-23044, 23334, 24000, 24160, 25040, 25250-25251, 26070-26080, 26990, 27030, 27090, 27301, 27310, 27603, 27610, 28020)

4.23 4.23 **FUD** ZZZ 80

+ **20705 Removal of drug-delivery device(s), intra-articular (List separately in addition to code for primary procedure)**

INCLUDES Removal therapeutic device/agent once per anatomic location from intra-articular space(s)

EXCLUDES *Open treatment femoral neck fracture/internal fixation or prosthetic replacement (27236)*
Partial knee replacement (27446)
Partial or total hip replacement (27125-27130)
Patella arthroplasty with prosthesis (27438)
Removal drug delivery device, performed alone (20680)
Removal drug delivery implant, non-biodegradable (11982)
Removal hip prosthesis (27091)
Removal knee prosthesis (27488)
Removal shoulder prosthesis (23335)
Revision hip arthroplasty (27134-27138)
Revision knee arthroplasty (27486-27487)

Code first (22864-22865, 23040-23044, 23334, 24000, 24160, 25040, 25250-25251, 26070-26080, 26990, 27030, 27090, 27301, 27310, 27603, 27610, 28020)

3.48 3.48 **FUD** ZZZ 80

20802-20838 Reimplantation Procedures

EXCLUDES *Repair incomplete amputation (see individual repair codes for bone(s), ligament(s), tendon(s), nerve(s), or blood vessel(s) and append modifier 52)*

20802 Replantation, arm (includes surgical neck of humerus through elbow joint), complete amputation

79.5 79.5 **FUD** 090 C 80 50

AMA: 1997,Apr,4

20805 Replantation, forearm (includes radius and ulna to radial carpal joint), complete amputation

94.7 94.7 **FUD** 090 C 80 50

AMA: 1997,Apr,4

20808 Replantation, hand (includes hand through metacarpophalangeal joints), complete amputation

114. 114. **FUD** 090 C 80 50

AMA: 1997,Apr,4

20816 Replantation, digit, excluding thumb (includes metacarpophalangeal joint to insertion of flexor sublimis tendon), complete amputation

59.5 59.5 **FUD** 090 C 80

AMA: 2018,Jan,8; 2017,Jan,8; 2016,Jan,13

20822 Replantation, digit, excluding thumb (includes distal tip to sublimis tendon insertion), complete amputation

51.2 51.2 **FUD** 090 J G2 80

AMA: 1997,Apr,4

20824 Replantation, thumb (includes carpometacarpal joint to MP joint), complete amputation

59.7 59.7 **FUD** 090 C 80 50

AMA: 1997,Apr,4

20827 Replantation, thumb (includes distal tip to MP joint), complete amputation

52.6 52.6 **FUD** 090 C 80 50

AMA: 1997,Apr,4

20838 Replantation, foot, complete amputation

80.6 80.6 **FUD** 090 C 80 50

AMA: 1997,Apr,4

20900-20924 Bone and Tissue Autografts

EXCLUDES *Acquisition autogenous bone, bone marrow, cartilage, tendon, fascia lata or other grafts through distinct incision unless included in code description*
Autologous fat graft obtained by liposuction (15771-15774)
Bone graft procedures on spine (20930-20938)
Other autologous soft tissue grafts (fat, dermis, fascia) harvested by direct excision ([15769])

20900 Bone graft, any donor area; minor or small (eg, dowel or button)

5.33 11.6 **FUD** 000 J A2 80

AMA: 2020,May,13; 2018,Jul,14; 2018,Jan,8; 2017,Jan,8; 2016,Jan,13

20902 major or large

8.20 8.20 **FUD** 000 J A2 80

AMA: 2020,May,13; 2018,Jul,14; 2018,Jan,8; 2017,Jan,8; 2016,Jan,13

20910 Cartilage graft; costochondral

EXCLUDES *Graft with ear cartilage (21235)*

13.5 13.5 **FUD** 090 T A2 80

AMA: 2020,May,13; 2018,Jul,14; 2018,Jan,8; 2017,Jan,8; 2016,Jan,13

20912 nasal septum

EXCLUDES *Graft with ear cartilage (21235)*

13.6 13.6 **FUD** 090 T A2 80

AMA: 2020,May,13; 2018,Jul,14

20920 Fascia lata graft; by stripper

11.5 11.5 **FUD** 090 T A2

AMA: 2020,May,13; 2018,Jul,14; 2018,Jan,8; 2017,Jan,8; 2016,Jan,13

20922 by incision and area exposure, complex or sheet

13.9 17.0 **FUD** 090 T A2 80

AMA: 2020,May,13; 2018,Jul,14; 2018,Jan,8; 2017,Jan,8; 2016,Jan,13

20924 Tendon graft, from a distance (eg, palmaris, toe extensor, plantaris)

14.6 14.6 **FUD** 090 J A2 80

AMA: 2020,May,13; 2018,Jul,14

20930-20939 Bone Allograft and Autograft of Spine

EXCLUDES *Acquisition autogenous bone, bone marrow, cartilage, tendon, fascia lata, or other grafts through distinct incision unless included in code description*
Autologous fat graft obtained by liposuction (15771-15774)
Other autologous soft tissue grafts (fat, dermis, fascia) harvested by direct excision ([15769])

+ **20930 Allograft, morselized, or placement of osteopromotive material, for spine surgery only (List separately in addition to code for primary procedure)**

Code first (22319, 22532-22533, 22548-22558, 22590-22612, 22630, 22633-22634, 22800-22812)

0.00 0.00 **FUD** XXX N N1

AMA: 2020,May,13; 2019,May,7; 2018,Jul,14; 2018,Jan,8; 2017,Mar,7; 2017,Jan,8; 2016,Jan,13

+ **20931 Allograft, structural, for spine surgery only (List separately in addition to code for primary procedure)**

Code first (22319, 22532-22533, 22548-22558, 22590-22612, 22630, 22633-22634, 22800-22812)

3.22 3.22 **FUD** ZZZ N N1

AMA: 2020,May,13; 2019,May,7; 2018,Jul,14; 2018,Jan,8; 2017,Mar,7; 2017,Jan,8; 2016,Jan,13

\+ **20932** **Allograft, includes templating, cutting, placement and internal fixation, when performed; osteoarticular, including articular surface and contiguous bone (List separately in addition to code for primary procedure)**

EXCLUDES *Allograft, intercalary (20933-20934)*
Injection contrast for ankle arthrography (27648)
Osteotomy, femur (27448)
Radical resection tumor:
Clavicle (23200)
Fibula (27646)
Ischial tuberosity/greater trochanter femur (27078)
Radial head or neck (24152)
Talus or calcaneus (27647)
Removal hip prosthesis (27090-27091)

Code also insertion joint prosthesis
Code first (23210, 23220, 24150, 25170, 27075-27077, 27365, 27645, 27704)
20.6 20.6 FUD ZZZ N1 80
AMA: 2020,May,13; 2019,May,7

\+ **20933** **hemicortical intercalary, partial (ie, hemicylindrical) (List separately in addition to code for primary procedure)**

EXCLUDES *Allograft, intercalary, complete (20934)*
Allograft, osteoarticular (20932)
Arthroplasty procedures, hip (27130, 27132, 27134, 27138)
Bone graft (20955-20957, 20962)
Excision cyst with allograft (23146, 23156, 24116, 24126, 25126, 25136, 27356, 27638, 28103, 28107)
Injection contrast for ankle arthrography (27648)
Open treatment femoral fractures (27236, 27244)
Osteotomy, femur (27448)
Radical resection tumor:
Clavicle (23200)
Fibula (27646)
Ischial tuberosity/greater trochanter femur (27078)
Radial head or neck (24152)
Talus or calcaneus (27647)
Removal hip prosthesis (27090-27091)

Code also insertion joint prosthesis
Code first (23210, 23220, 24150, 25170, 27075-27077, 27365, 27645, 27704)
18.9 18.9 FUD ZZZ N1 80
AMA: 2020,May,13; 2019,May,7

\+ **20934** **intercalary, complete (ie, cylindrical) (List separately in addition to code for primary procedure)**

EXCLUDES *Allograft, intercalary, partial (20933)*
Allograft, osteoarticular (20932)
Excision cyst with allograft (23146, 23156)
Injection contrast for ankle arthrography (27648)
Osteotomy, femur (27448)
Radical resection tumor:
Clavicle (23200)
Fibula (27646)
Ischial tuberosity/greater trochanter femur (27078)
Radial head or neck (24152)
Talus or calcaneus (27647)
Removal hip prosthesis (27090-27091)

Code also insertion joint prosthesis
Code first (23210, 23220, 24150, 25170, 27075-27077, 27365, 27645, 27704)
20.6 20.6 FUD ZZZ N1 80
AMA: 2020,May,13; 2019,May,7

\+ **20936** **Autograft for spine surgery only (includes harvesting the graft); local (eg, ribs, spinous process, or laminar fragments) obtained from same incision (List separately in addition to code for primary procedure)**

Code first (22319, 22532-22533, 22548-22558, 22590-22612, 22630, 22633-22634, 22800-22812)
0.00 0.00 FUD XXX N N1
AMA: 2020,May,13; 2018,Jul,14; 2018,Jan,8; 2017,Mar,7; 2017,Jan,8; 2016,Jan,13

\+ **20937** **morselized (through separate skin or fascial incision) (List separately in addition to code for primary procedure)**

Code first (22319, 22532-22533, 22548-22558, 22590-22612, 22630, 22633-22634, 22800-22812)
4.85 4.85 FUD ZZZ N N1 80
AMA: 2020,May,13; 2018,Jul,14; 2018,Jan,8; 2017,Mar,7; 2017,Jan,8; 2016,Jan,13

\+ **20938** **structural, bicortical or tricortical (through separate skin or fascial incision) (List separately in addition to code for primary procedure)**

EXCLUDES *Bone marrow for bone grafting in spinal surgery (20939)*

Code first (22319, 22532-22533, 22548-22558, 22590-22612, 22630, 22633-22634, 22800-22812)
5.34 5.34 FUD ZZZ N N1 80
AMA: 2020,May,13; 2018,Jul,14; 2018,Jan,8; 2017,Mar,7; 2017,Jan,8; 2016,Jan,13

\+ **20939** **Bone marrow aspiration for bone grafting, spine surgery only, through separate skin or fascial incision (List separately in addition to code for primary procedure)**

EXCLUDES *Bone marrow aspiration for other than bone grafting in spinal surgery (20999)*
Diagnostic bone marrow aspiration (38220, 38222)
Platelet rich plasma injection (0232T)
Reporting with modifier 50. Report once for each side when performed bilaterally

Code first (22319, 22532-22534, 22548, 22551-22552, 22554, 22556, 22558, 22590, 22595, 22600, 22610, 22612, 22630, 22633-22634, 22800, 22802, 22804, 22808, 22810, 22812)
2.03 2.03 FUD ZZZ N N1 80
AMA: 2018,May,3

20950 Measurement of Intracompartmental Pressure

20950 **Monitoring of interstitial fluid pressure (includes insertion of device, eg, wick catheter technique, needle manometer technique) in detection of muscle compartment syndrome**
2.56 7.43 FUD 000 T G2 80
AMA: 2018,Jan,8; 2017,Jan,8; 2016,Jan,13

20955-20973 Bone and Osteocutaneous Grafts

INCLUDES Operating microscope (69990)

20955 **Bone graft with microvascular anastomosis; fibula**
70.9 70.9 FUD 090 C 80
AMA: 2019,Dec,5; 2019,May,7; 2018,Jan,8; 2017,Jan,8; 2016,Feb,12; 2016,Jan,13

20956 **iliac crest**
76.5 76.5 FUD 090 C 80
AMA: 2019,Dec,5; 2019,May,7; 2018,Jan,8; 2017,Jan,8; 2016,Feb,12; 2016,Jan,13

20957 **metatarsal**
79.6 79.6 FUD 090 C 80
AMA: 2019,Dec,5; 2019,May,7; 2018,Jan,8; 2017,Jan,8; 2016,Feb,12; 2016,Jan,13

20962 **other than fibula, iliac crest, or metatarsal**
76.9 76.9 FUD 090 C 80
AMA: 2019,Dec,5; 2019,May,7; 2016,Feb,12

20969 **Free osteocutaneous flap with microvascular anastomosis; other than iliac crest, metatarsal, or great toe**
78.6 78.6 FUD 090 C 80
AMA: 2019,Dec,5; 2019,Oct,10; 2018,Jan,8; 2017,Jan,8; 2016,Feb,12; 2016,Jan,13

20970 **iliac crest**
82.6 82.6 FUD 090 C 80
AMA: 2019,Dec,5; 2018,Jan,8; 2017,Jan,8; 2016,Feb,12; 2016,Jan,13

20972 **metatarsal**
82.4 82.4 FUD 090 J G2 80
AMA: 2019,Dec,5; 2018,Jan,8; 2017,Jan,8; 2016,Feb,12; 2016,Jan,13

20973 **great toe with web space**

EXCLUDES *Great toe wrap-around with bone graft (26551)*

87.0 87.0 FUD 090 J R2 80 50

AMA: 2019,Dec,5; 2018,Jan,8; 2017,Jan,8; 2016,Feb,12; 2016,Jan,13

20974-20979 Osteogenic Stimulation

CMS: 100-03,150.2 Osteogenic Stimulation

20974 **Electrical stimulation to aid bone healing; noninvasive (nonoperative)**

1.45 2.26 FUD 000 A

AMA: 2018,Jan,8; 2017,Jan,8; 2016,Jan,13

20975 **invasive (operative)**

5.18 5.18 FUD 000 N N1 80

AMA: 2002,Apr,13; 2000,Nov,8

20979 **Low intensity ultrasound stimulation to aid bone healing, noninvasive (nonoperative)**

0.93 1.53 FUD 000 Q1 N1

AMA: 2018,Jan,8; 2017,Jan,8; 2016,Jan,13

20982-20999 General Musculoskeletal Procedures

20982 **Ablation therapy for reduction or eradication of 1 or more bone tumors (eg, metastasis) including adjacent soft tissue when involved by tumor extension, percutaneous, including imaging guidance when performed; radiofrequency**

EXCLUDES *Radiologic guidance (76940, 77002, 77013, 77022)*

10.5 110. FUD 000 J G2 50

AMA: 2018,Jan,8; 2017,Jan,8; 2016,Jan,13

20983 **cryoablation**

EXCLUDES *Radiologic guidance (76940, 77002, 77013, 77022)*

10.3 170. FUD 000 J G2 50

AMA: 2018,Jan,8; 2017,Jan,8; 2016,Jan,13

\+ **20985** **Computer-assisted surgical navigational procedure for musculoskeletal procedures, image-less (List separately in addition to code for primary procedure)**

EXCLUDES *Image guidance derived from intraoperative and preoperative obtained images (0054T-0055T)*
Stereotactic computer-assisted navigational procedure; cranial or intradural (61781-61783)

Code first primary procedure

4.24 4.24 FUD ZZZ N N1 80

AMA: 2018,Jan,8; 2017,Jan,8; 2016,Jan,13

20999 **Unlisted procedure, musculoskeletal system, general**

0.00 0.00 FUD YYY T 80

AMA: 2018,May,3; 2018,Jan,8; 2017,Jan,8; 2016,Jan,13

21010 Temporomandibular Joint Arthrotomy

21010 **Arthrotomy, temporomandibular joint**

EXCLUDES *Cutaneous/subcutaneous abscess and hematoma drainage (10060-10061)*
Excision foreign body from dentoalveolar site (41805-41806)

22.0 22.0 FUD 090 J A2 80 50

AMA: 2002,Apr,13

21011-21016 Excision Soft Tissue Tumors Face and Scalp

INCLUDES Any necessary elevation tissue planes or dissection
Measurement tumor and necessary margin at greatest diameter prior to excision
Simple and intermediate repairs
Excision types:
Fascial or subfascial soft tissue tumors: simple and marginal resection tumors found either in or below deep fascia, not including bone or excision substantial amount normal tissue; primarily benign and intramuscular tumors
Radical resection soft tissue tumor: wide resection tumor involving substantial margins normal tissue and may include tissue removal from one or more layers; most often malignant or aggressive benign
Subcutaneous: simple and marginal resection tumors in subcutaneous tissue above deep fascia; most often benign

EXCLUDES *Complex repair*
Excision benign cutaneous lesions (eg, sebaceous cyst) (11420-11426)
Radical resection cutaneous tumors (eg, melanoma) (11620-11646)
Significant vessel exploration or neuroplasty

21011 **Excision, tumor, soft tissue of face or scalp, subcutaneous; less than 2 cm**

7.38 10.3 FUD 090 J P3 80

AMA: 2018,Sep,7; 2018,Jan,8; 2017,Jan,8; 2016,Jan,13

21012 **2 cm or greater**

9.72 9.72 FUD 090 J R2 80

AMA: 2018,Sep,7; 2018,Jan,8; 2017,Jan,8; 2016,Jan,13

21013 **Excision, tumor, soft tissue of face and scalp, subfascial (eg, subgaleal, intramuscular); less than 2 cm**

11.5 15.1 FUD 090 J P3 80

AMA: 2018,Sep,7; 2018,Jan,8; 2017,Jan,8; 2016,Jan,13

21014 **2 cm or greater**

15.0 15.0 FUD 090 J R2 80

AMA: 2018,Sep,7; 2018,Jan,8; 2017,Jan,8; 2016,Jan,13

21015 **Radical resection of tumor (eg, sarcoma), soft tissue of face or scalp; less than 2 cm**

EXCLUDES *Removal of cranial tumor for osteomyelitis (61501)*

20.3 20.3 FUD 090 J G2

AMA: 2018,Sep,7; 2018,Jan,8; 2017,Jan,8; 2016,Jan,13

21016 **2 cm or greater**

29.0 29.0 FUD 090 J G2 80

AMA: 2018,Sep,7; 2018,Jan,8; 2017,Jan,8; 2016,Jan,13

21025-21070 Procedures of Cranial and Facial Bones

INCLUDES Any necessary elevation tissue planes or dissection
Measurement tumor and necessary margins prior to excision
Radical resection bone tumor involves resection tumor (may include entire bone) and wide margins normal tissue primarily for malignant or aggressive benign tumors
Simple and intermediate repairs

EXCLUDES *Complex repair*
Excision soft tissue tumors, face and scalp (21011-21016)
Radical resection cutaneous tumors (e.g., melanoma) (11620-11646)
Significant vessel exploration, neuroplasty, reconstruction, or complex bone repair

21025 **Excision of bone (eg, for osteomyelitis or bone abscess); mandible**

19.9 23.6 FUD 090 J A2

AMA: 2018,Sep,7; 2018,Jan,8; 2017,Jan,8; 2016,Jan,13

21026 **facial bone(s)**

12.9 16.0 FUD 090 J A2

AMA: 2018,Sep,7

21029 **Removal by contouring of benign tumor of facial bone (eg, fibrous dysplasia)**
17.9 | 21.8 | FUD 090 | J A2 80
AMA: 2018,Sep,7

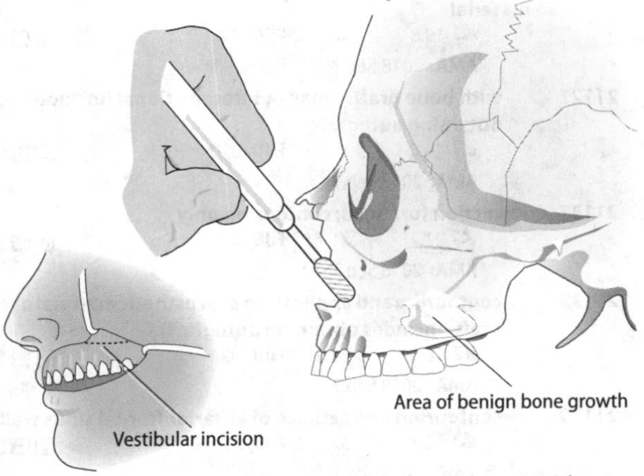

Burrs, files, and osteotomes used to remove bone

21030 **Excision of benign tumor or cyst of maxilla or zygoma by enucleation and curettage**
11.1 | 14.0 | FUD 090 | J P3 50
AMA: 2018,Sep,7; 2018,Jan,8; 2017,Jan,8; 2016,Jan,13

21031 **Excision of torus mandibularis**
8.03 | 11.1 | FUD 090 | J P3 50
AMA: 2018,Sep,7

21032 **Excision of maxillary torus palatinus**
8.21 | 11.3 | FUD 090 | J P3
AMA: 2018,Sep,7

21034 **Excision of malignant tumor of maxilla or zygoma**
33.0 | 37.5 | FUD 090 | J A2 80
AMA: 2018,Sep,7; 2018,Jan,8; 2017,Jan,8; 2016,Jan,13

21040 **Excision of benign tumor or cyst of mandible, by enucleation and/or curettage**
INCLUDES Removal benign tumor or cyst without osteotomy
EXCLUDES *Removal benign tumor or cyst with osteotomy (21046-21047)*
11.1 | 14.1 | FUD 090 | J A2
AMA: 2018,Sep,7; 2018,Jan,8; 2017,Jan,8; 2016,Jan,13

21044 **Excision of malignant tumor of mandible;**
25.0 | 25.0 | FUD 090 | J A2 80
AMA: 2018,Sep,7

21045 **radical resection**
Code also bone graft procedure (21215)
34.6 | 34.6 | FUD 090 | C 80
AMA: 2018,Sep,7

21046 **Excision of benign tumor or cyst of mandible; requiring intra-oral osteotomy (eg, locally aggressive or destructive lesion[s])**
30.0 | 30.0 | FUD 090 | J A2 80
AMA: 2018,Sep,7; 2018,Jan,8; 2017,Jan,8; 2016,Jan,13

21047 **requiring extra-oral osteotomy and partial mandibulectomy (eg, locally aggressive or destructive lesion[s])**
36.7 | 36.7 | FUD 090 | J A2 80
AMA: 2018,Sep,7; 2018,Jan,8; 2017,Jan,8; 2016,Jan,13

21048 **Excision of benign tumor or cyst of maxilla; requiring intra-oral osteotomy (eg, locally aggressive or destructive lesion[s])**
30.5 | 30.5 | FUD 090 | J R2 80
AMA: 2018,Sep,7; 2018,Jan,8; 2017,Jan,8; 2016,Jan,13

21049 **requiring extra-oral osteotomy and partial maxillectomy (eg, locally aggressive or destructive lesion[s])**
34.7 | 34.7 | FUD 090 | J G2 80
AMA: 2018,Sep,7; 2018,Jan,8; 2017,Jan,8; 2016,Jan,13

21050 **Condylectomy, temporomandibular joint (separate procedure)**
25.2 | 25.2 | FUD 090 | J A2 80 50
AMA: 2018,Sep,7

21060 **Meniscectomy, partial or complete, temporomandibular joint (separate procedure)**
22.9 | 22.9 | FUD 090 | J A2 80 50
AMA: 2018,Sep,7

21070 **Coronoidectomy (separate procedure)**
18.3 | 18.3 | FUD 090 | J A2 80 50
AMA: 2018,Sep,7

21073 Temporomandibular Joint Manipulation with Anesthesia

21073 **Manipulation of temporomandibular joint(s) (TMJ), therapeutic, requiring an anesthesia service (ie, general or monitored anesthesia care)**
EXCLUDES *Closed treatment TMJ dislocation (21480, 21485)*
Manipulation TMJ without general or MAC anesthesia (97140, 98925-98929, 98943)
7.19 | 10.9 | FUD 090 | T P3 80 50
AMA: 2018,Sep,7; 2018,Jan,8; 2018,Jan,3; 2017,Jan,8; 2016,Jan,13

21076-21089 Medical Impressions for Fabrication Maxillofacial Prosthesis

INCLUDES Design, preparation, and professional services rendered by physician or other qualified health care professional
EXCLUDES *Application or removal caliper or tongs (20660, 20665)*
Professional services rendered for outside laboratory designed and prepared prosthesis

21076 **Impression and custom preparation; surgical obturator prosthesis**
23.1 | 27.6 | FUD 010 | T P3 80
AMA: 2018,Sep,7; 2018,Jan,8; 2017,Jan,8; 2016,Jan,13

21077 **orbital prosthesis**
53.4 | 64.0 | FUD 090 | J P3 80 50
AMA: 2018,Sep,7; 2018,Jan,8; 2017,Jan,8; 2016,Jan,13

21079 **interim obturator prosthesis**
38.8 | 46.6 | FUD 090 | J P3
AMA: 2018,Sep,7; 2018,Jan,8; 2017,Jan,8; 2016,Jan,13

21080 **definitive obturator prosthesis**
40.4 | 49.8 | FUD 090 | J P3
AMA: 2018,Sep,7; 2018,Jan,8; 2017,Jan,8; 2016,Jan,13

21081 **mandibular resection prosthesis**
37.0 | 45.7 | FUD 090 | J P3 80
AMA: 2018,Sep,7; 2018,Jan,8; 2017,Jan,8; 2016,Jan,13

21082 **palatal augmentation prosthesis**
34.0 | 42.4 | FUD 090 | J P3 80
AMA: 2018,Sep,7; 2018,Jan,8; 2017,Jan,8; 2016,Jan,13

21083 **palatal lift prosthesis**
31.6 | 40.4 | FUD 090 | J P3 80
AMA: 2018,Sep,7; 2018,Jan,8; 2017,Jan,8; 2016,Jan,13

21084 **speech aid prosthesis**
36.5 | 46.2 | FUD 090 | J P3 80
AMA: 2018,Sep,7; 2018,Jan,8; 2017,Jan,8; 2016,Jan,13

21085 **oral surgical splint**
15.7 | 21.0 | FUD 010 | T P2 80
AMA: 2018,Sep,7; 2018,Jan,8; 2017,Sep,14; 2017,Jan,8; 2016,Jan,13

21086 **auricular prosthesis**
39.4 | 47.6 | FUD 090 | J P3 80 50
AMA: 2018,Sep,7; 2018,Jan,8; 2017,Jan,8; 2016,Jan,13

21087 **nasal prosthesis**
42.7 | 51.1 | FUD 090 | J P3 80
AMA: 2018,Sep,7; 2018,Jan,8; 2017,Jan,8; 2016,Jan,13

21088 **facial prosthesis**
0.00 | 0.00 | FUD 090 | J R2 80
AMA: 2018,Sep,7; 2018,Jan,8; 2017,Jan,8; 2016,Jan,13

21089 **Unlisted maxillofacial prosthetic procedure**
0.00 | 0.00 | FUD YYY | T
AMA: 2018,Sep,7; 2018,Jan,8; 2017,Jan,8; 2016,Jan,13

21100-21110 Application Fixation Device

21100 **Application of halo type appliance for maxillofacial fixation, includes removal (separate procedure)**
10.6 | 18.9 | FUD 090 | J A2 80
AMA: 2018,Sep,7

21110 **Application of interdental fixation device for conditions other than fracture or dislocation, includes removal**
EXCLUDES *Interdental fixation device removal by different provider (20670-20680)*
19.5 | 23.3 | FUD 090 | Q2 P2
AMA: 2018,Sep,7; 2018,Jan,8; 2017,Jan,8; 2016,Jan,13

21116 Injection for TMJ Arthrogram

CMS: 100-02,15,150.1 Treatment of Temporomandibular Joint (TMJ) Syndrome; 100-04,13,80.1 Physician Presence; 100-04,13,80.2 S&I Multiple Procedure Reduction

21116 **Injection procedure for temporomandibular joint arthrography**
(70332)
1.34 | 5.62 | FUD 000 | N N1 50
AMA: 2018,Sep,7; 2018,Jan,8; 2017,Jan,8; 2016,May,13; 2016,Jan,13

21120-21299 Repair/Reconstruction Craniofacial Bones

EXCLUDES *Cranioplasty (21179-21180, 62120, 62140-62147)*

21120 **Genioplasty; augmentation (autograft, allograft, prosthetic material)**
15.0 | 19.2 | FUD 090 | J G2
AMA: 2018,Sep,7

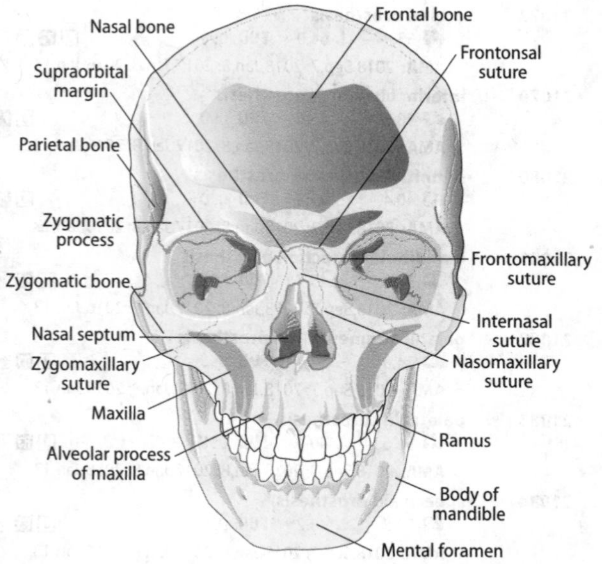

21121 **sliding osteotomy, single piece**
17.8 | 20.9 | FUD 090 | J A2 80
AMA: 2018,Sep,7

21122 **sliding osteotomies, 2 or more osteotomies (eg, wedge excision or bone wedge reversal for asymmetrical chin)**
22.1 | 22.1 | FUD 090 | J A2 80
AMA: 2018,Sep,7

21123 **sliding, augmentation with interpositional bone grafts (includes obtaining autografts)**
26.1 | 26.1 | FUD 090 | J A2 80
AMA: 2018,Sep,7

21125 **Augmentation, mandibular body or angle; prosthetic material**
19.8 | 80.8 | FUD 090 | J A2 80
AMA: 2018,Sep,7

21127 **with bone graft, onlay or interpositional (includes obtaining autograft)**
24.6 | 112. | FUD 090 | J A2 80
AMA: 2018,Sep,7

21137 **Reduction forehead; contouring only**
21.7 | 21.7 | FUD 090 | J G2 80
AMA: 2018,Sep,7

21138 **contouring and application of prosthetic material or bone graft (includes obtaining autograft)**
26.5 | 26.5 | FUD 090 | J G2 80
AMA: 2018,Sep,7

21139 **contouring and setback of anterior frontal sinus wall**
32.1 | 32.1 | FUD 090 | J G2 80
AMA: 2018,Sep,7

21141 **Reconstruction midface, LeFort I; single piece, segment movement in any direction (eg, for Long Face Syndrome), without bone graft**
39.4 | 39.4 | FUD 090 | C 80
AMA: 2018,Sep,7

21142 **2 pieces, segment movement in any direction, without bone graft**
40.5 | 40.5 | FUD 090 | C 80
AMA: 2018,Sep,7

21143 **3 or more pieces, segment movement in any direction, without bone graft**
41.0 | 41.0 | FUD 090 | C 80
AMA: 2018,Sep,7

21145 **single piece, segment movement in any direction, requiring bone grafts (includes obtaining autografts)**
46.2 | 46.2 | FUD 090 | C 80
AMA: 2018,Sep,7

21146 **2 pieces, segment movement in any direction, requiring bone grafts (includes obtaining autografts) (eg, ungrafted unilateral alveolar cleft)**
48.2 | 48.2 | FUD 090 | C 80
AMA: 2018,Sep,7

21147 **3 or more pieces, segment movement in any direction, requiring bone grafts (includes obtaining autografts) (eg, ungrafted bilateral alveolar cleft or multiple osteotomies)**
50.8 | 50.8 | FUD 090 | C 80
AMA: 2018,Sep,7

21150 **Reconstruction midface, LeFort II; anterior intrusion (eg, Treacher-Collins Syndrome)**
47.3 | 47.3 | FUD 090 | J G2 80
AMA: 2018,Sep,7

21151 **any direction, requiring bone grafts (includes obtaining autografts)**
52.0 | 52.0 | FUD 090 | C 80
AMA: 2018,Sep,7

21154 **Reconstruction midface, LeFort III (extracranial), any type, requiring bone grafts (includes obtaining autografts); without LeFort I**
56.4 | 56.4 | FUD 090 | C 80
AMA: 2018,Sep,7

21155 **with LeFort I**
62.2 | 62.2 | FUD 090 | C 80
AMA: 2018,Sep,7

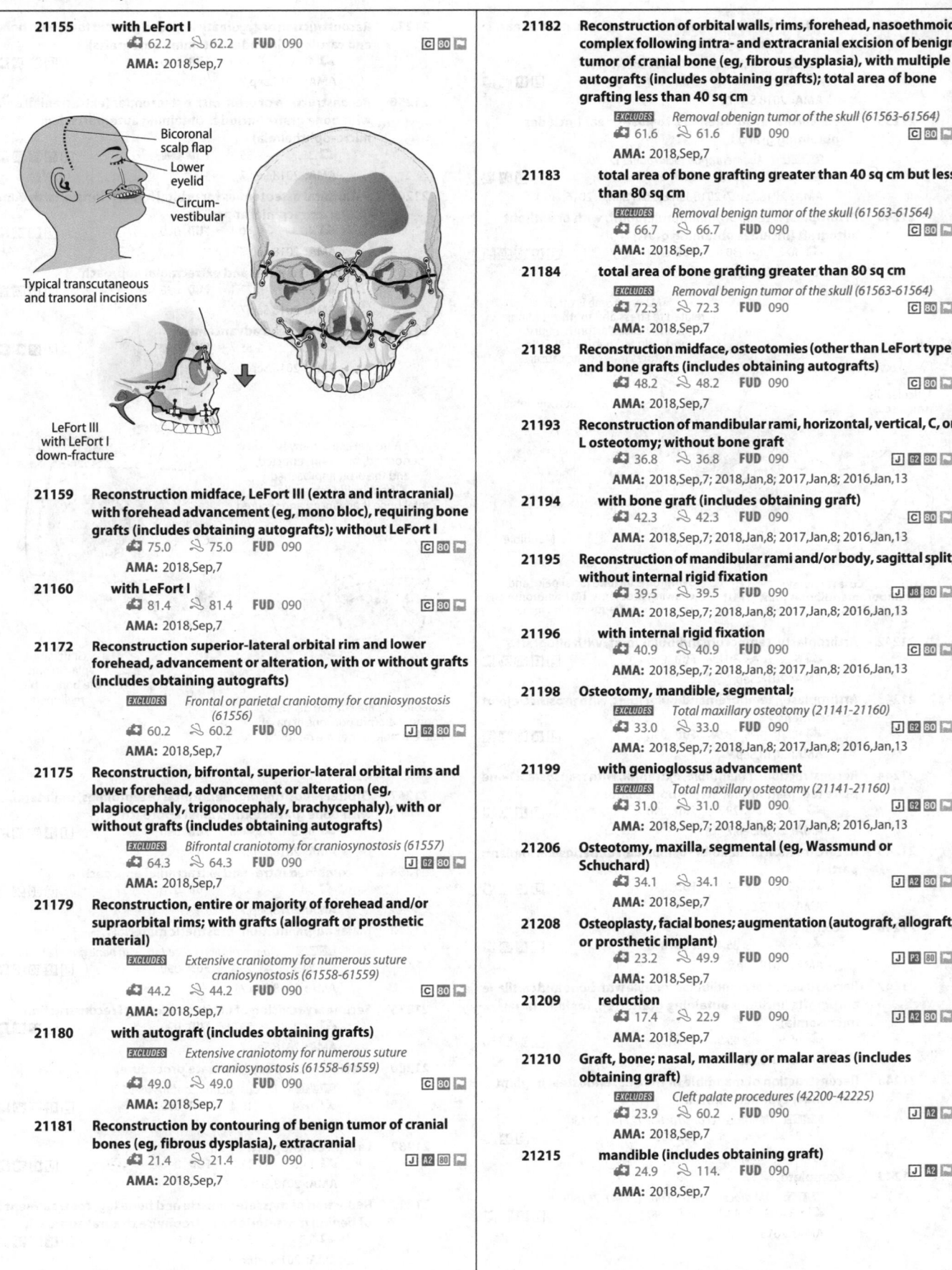

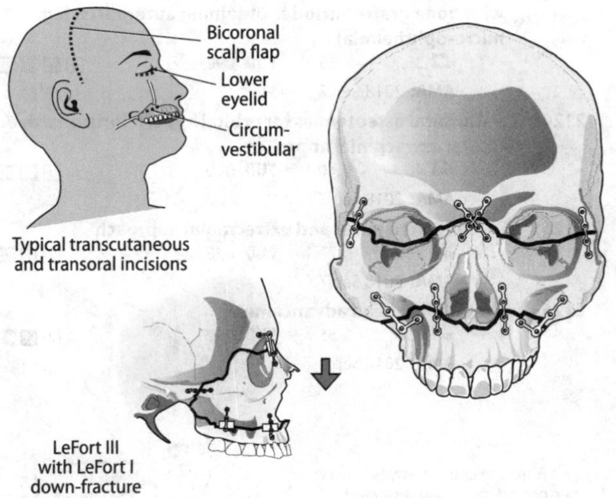

21159 **Reconstruction midface, LeFort III (extra and intracranial) with forehead advancement (eg, mono bloc), requiring bone grafts (includes obtaining autografts); without LeFort I**
75.0 | 75.0 | FUD 090 | C 80
AMA: 2018,Sep,7

21160 **with LeFort I**
81.4 | 81.4 | FUD 090 | C 80
AMA: 2018,Sep,7

21172 **Reconstruction superior-lateral orbital rim and lower forehead, advancement or alteration, with or without grafts (includes obtaining autografts)**
EXCLUDES *Frontal or parietal craniotomy for craniosynostosis (61556)*
60.2 | 60.2 | FUD 090 | J G2 80
AMA: 2018,Sep,7

21175 **Reconstruction, bifrontal, superior-lateral orbital rims and lower forehead, advancement or alteration (eg, plagiocephaly, trigonocephaly, brachycephaly), with or without grafts (includes obtaining autografts)**
EXCLUDES *Bifrontal craniotomy for craniosynostosis (61557)*
64.3 | 64.3 | FUD 090 | J G2 80
AMA: 2018,Sep,7

21179 **Reconstruction, entire or majority of forehead and/or supraorbital rims; with grafts (allograft or prosthetic material)**
EXCLUDES *Extensive craniotomy for numerous suture craniosynostosis (61558-61559)*
44.2 | 44.2 | FUD 090 | C 80
AMA: 2018,Sep,7

21180 **with autograft (includes obtaining grafts)**
EXCLUDES *Extensive craniotomy for numerous suture craniosynostosis (61558-61559)*
49.0 | 49.0 | FUD 090 | C 80
AMA: 2018,Sep,7

21181 **Reconstruction by contouring of benign tumor of cranial bones (eg, fibrous dysplasia), extracranial**
21.4 | 21.4 | FUD 090 | J A2 80
AMA: 2018,Sep,7

21182 **Reconstruction of orbital walls, rims, forehead, nasoethmoid complex following intra- and extracranial excision of benign tumor of cranial bone (eg, fibrous dysplasia), with multiple autografts (includes obtaining grafts); total area of bone grafting less than 40 sq cm**
EXCLUDES *Removal obenign tumor of the skull (61563-61564)*
61.6 | 61.6 | FUD 090 | C 80
AMA: 2018,Sep,7

21183 **total area of bone grafting greater than 40 sq cm but less than 80 sq cm**
EXCLUDES *Removal benign tumor of the skull (61563-61564)*
66.7 | 66.7 | FUD 090 | C 80
AMA: 2018,Sep,7

21184 **total area of bone grafting greater than 80 sq cm**
EXCLUDES *Removal benign tumor of the skull (61563-61564)*
72.3 | 72.3 | FUD 090 | C 80
AMA: 2018,Sep,7

21188 **Reconstruction midface, osteotomies (other than LeFort type) and bone grafts (includes obtaining autografts)**
48.2 | 48.2 | FUD 090 | C 80
AMA: 2018,Sep,7

21193 **Reconstruction of mandibular rami, horizontal, vertical, C, or L osteotomy; without bone graft**
36.8 | 36.8 | FUD 090 | J G2 80
AMA: 2018,Sep,7; 2018,Jan,8; 2017,Jan,8; 2016,Jan,13

21194 **with bone graft (includes obtaining graft)**
42.3 | 42.3 | FUD 090 | C 80
AMA: 2018,Sep,7; 2018,Jan,8; 2017,Jan,8; 2016,Jan,13

21195 **Reconstruction of mandibular rami and/or body, sagittal split; without internal rigid fixation**
39.5 | 39.5 | FUD 090 | J J8 80
AMA: 2018,Sep,7; 2018,Jan,8; 2017,Jan,8; 2016,Jan,13

21196 **with internal rigid fixation**
40.9 | 40.9 | FUD 090 | C 80
AMA: 2018,Sep,7; 2018,Jan,8; 2017,Jan,8; 2016,Jan,13

21198 **Osteotomy, mandible, segmental;**
EXCLUDES *Total maxillary osteotomy (21141-21160)*
33.0 | 33.0 | FUD 090 | J G2 80
AMA: 2018,Sep,7; 2018,Jan,8; 2017,Jan,8; 2016,Jan,13

21199 **with genioglossus advancement**
EXCLUDES *Total maxillary osteotomy (21141-21160)*
31.0 | 31.0 | FUD 090 | J G2 80
AMA: 2018,Sep,7; 2018,Jan,8; 2017,Jan,8; 2016,Jan,13

21206 **Osteotomy, maxilla, segmental (eg, Wassmund or Schuchard)**
34.1 | 34.1 | FUD 090 | J A2 80
AMA: 2018,Sep,7

21208 **Osteoplasty, facial bones; augmentation (autograft, allograft, or prosthetic implant)**
23.2 | 49.9 | FUD 090 | J P3 80
AMA: 2018,Sep,7

21209 **reduction**
17.4 | 22.9 | FUD 090 | J A2 80
AMA: 2018,Sep,7

21210 **Graft, bone; nasal, maxillary or malar areas (includes obtaining graft)**
EXCLUDES *Cleft palate procedures (42200-42225)*
23.9 | 60.2 | FUD 090 | J A2
AMA: 2018,Sep,7

21215 **mandible (includes obtaining graft)**
24.9 | 114. | FUD 090 | J A2
AMA: 2018,Sep,7

21230 Graft; rib cartilage, autogenous, to face, chin, nose or ear (includes obtaining graft)

EXCLUDES *Augmentation facial bones (21208)*

21.3 21.3 FUD 090 J A2 80

AMA: 2018,Sep,7

21235 ear cartilage, autogenous, to nose or ear (includes obtaining graft)

EXCLUDES *Augmentation facial bones (21208)*

16.2 20.7 FUD 090 J A2

AMA: 2018,Sep,7; 2018,Jan,8; 2017,Jan,8; 2016,Jan,13

21240 Arthroplasty, temporomandibular joint, with or without autograft (includes obtaining graft)

30.8 30.8 FUD 090 J A2 80 50

AMA: 2018,Sep,7

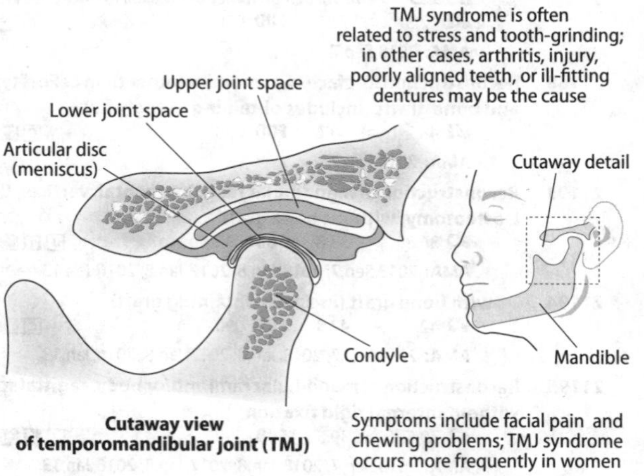
TMJ syndrome is often related to stress and tooth-grinding; in other cases, arthritis, injury, poorly aligned teeth, or ill-fitting dentures may be the cause
Upper joint space
Lower joint space
Articular disc (meniscus)
Cutaway detail
Condyle
Mandible
Cutaway view of temporomandibular joint (TMJ)
Symptoms include facial pain and chewing problems; TMJ syndrome occurs more frequently in women

21242 Arthroplasty, temporomandibular joint, with allograft

30.0 30.0 FUD 090 J A2 80 50

AMA: 2018,Sep,7

21243 Arthroplasty, temporomandibular joint, with prosthetic joint replacement

48.9 48.9 FUD 090 J J8 80 50

AMA: 2018,Sep,7

21244 Reconstruction of mandible, extraoral, with transosteal bone plate (eg, mandibular staple bone plate)

29.3 29.3 FUD 090 J J8 80

AMA: 2018,Sep,7

21245 Reconstruction of mandible or maxilla, subperiosteal implant; partial

26.8 34.5 FUD 090 J A2 80

AMA: 2018,Sep,7

21246 complete

25.4 25.4 FUD 090 J A2 80

AMA: 2018,Sep,7

21247 Reconstruction of mandibular condyle with bone and cartilage autografts (includes obtaining grafts) (eg, for hemifacial microsomia)

45.9 45.9 FUD 090 C 80 50

AMA: 2018,Sep,7

21248 Reconstruction of mandible or maxilla, endosteal implant (eg, blade, cylinder); partial

EXCLUDES *Midface reconstruction (21141-21160)*

25.3 31.1 FUD 090 J A2

AMA: 2018,Sep,7

21249 complete

EXCLUDES *Midface reconstruction (21141-21160)*

33.4 40.1 FUD 090 J A2 80

AMA: 2018,Sep,7

21255 Reconstruction of zygomatic arch and glenoid fossa with bone and cartilage (includes obtaining autografts)

40.6 40.6 FUD 090 C 80 50

AMA: 2018,Sep,7

21256 Reconstruction of orbit with osteotomies (extracranial) and with bone grafts (includes obtaining autografts) (eg, micro-ophthalmia)

35.7 35.7 FUD 090 J G2 80 50

AMA: 2018,Sep,7

21260 Periorbital osteotomies for orbital hypertelorism, with bone grafts; extracranial approach

40.1 40.1 FUD 090 J G2 80

AMA: 2018,Sep,7

21261 combined intra- and extracranial approach

71.1 71.1 FUD 090 J G2 80

AMA: 2018,Sep,7

21263 with forehead advancement

65.7 65.7 FUD 090 J G2 80

AMA: 2018,Sep,7

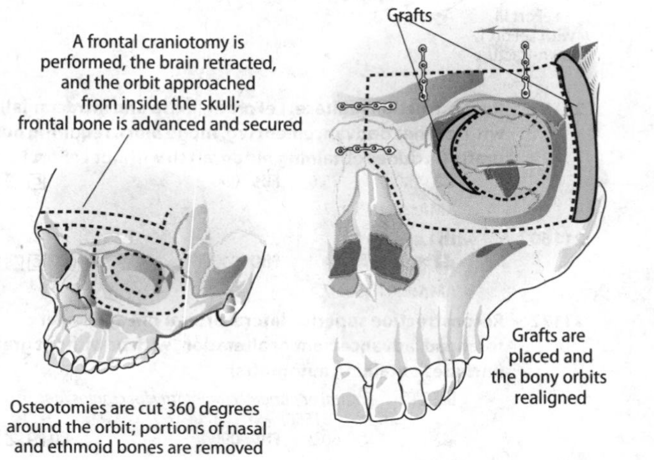
Grafts
A frontal craniotomy is performed, the brain retracted, and the orbit approached from inside the skull; frontal bone is advanced and secured
Grafts are placed and the bony orbits realigned
Osteotomies are cut 360 degrees around the orbit; portions of nasal and ethmoid bones are removed

21267 Orbital repositioning, periorbital osteotomies, unilateral, with bone grafts; extracranial approach

46.8 46.8 FUD 090 J J8 80 50

AMA: 2018,Sep,7

21268 combined intra- and extracranial approach

58.8 58.8 FUD 090 C 80 50

AMA: 2018,Sep,7

21270 Malar augmentation, prosthetic material

EXCLUDES *Augmentation procedure with bone graft (21210)*

21.7 29.1 FUD 090 J A2 80 50

AMA: 2018,Sep,7

21275 Secondary revision of orbitocraniofacial reconstruction

24.1 24.1 FUD 090 J G2 80

AMA: 2018,Sep,7

21280 Medial canthopexy (separate procedure)

EXCLUDES *Reconstruction canthus (67950)*

16.4 16.4 FUD 090 J A2 80 50

AMA: 2018,Sep,7

21282 Lateral canthopexy

11.0 11.0 FUD 090 J A2 50

AMA: 2018,Sep,7

21295 Reduction of masseter muscle and bone (eg, for treatment of benign masseteric hypertrophy); extraoral approach

5.39 5.39 FUD 090 T A2 80 50

AMA: 2018,Sep,7

26/TC PC/TC Only A2-Z3 ASC Payment 50 Bilateral ♂ Male Only ♀ Female Only Facility RVU Non-Facility RVU CCI CLIA
FUD Follow-up Days CMS: IOM AMA: CPT Asst A-Y OPPSI 80/80 Surg Assist Allowed / w/Doc Lab Crosswalk Radiology Crosswalk

21296 **intraoral approach**
11.6 11.6 FUD 090 J A2 80 50
AMA: 2018,Sep,7

21299 **Unlisted craniofacial and maxillofacial procedure**
0.00 0.00 FUD YYY T 80
AMA: 2018,Sep,7

21310-21499 Care of Fractures/Dislocations of the Cranial and Facial Bones

EXCLUDES *Closed treatment skull fracture, report with appropriate E/M service*
Open treatment skull fracture (62000-62010)

21310 ~~**Closed treatment of nasal bone fracture without manipulation**~~

▲ **21315** **Closed treatment of nasal bone fracture with manipulation; without stabilization**
EXCLUDES *Closed treatment without manipulation or stabilization, report appropriate E/M service*
4.31 7.80 FUD 010 T A2
AMA: 2019,Nov,12; 2019,Sep,3; 2018,Sep,7; 2018,Jan,3

▲ **21320** **with stabilization**
EXCLUDES *Closed treatment without maniputaion or stabilization, report appropriate E/M service*
3.83 7.23 FUD 010 J A2
AMA: 2019,Sep,3; 2018,Sep,7

21325 **Open treatment of nasal fracture; uncomplicated**
12.4 12.4 FUD 090 J A2 80
AMA: 2018,Sep,7

21330 **complicated, with internal and/or external skeletal fixation**
16.0 16.0 FUD 090 J A2 80
AMA: 2018,Sep,7

21335 **with concomitant open treatment of fractured septum**
20.3 20.3 FUD 090 J A2
AMA: 2018,Sep,7

21336 **Open treatment of nasal septal fracture, with or without stabilization**
18.2 18.2 FUD 090 J A2 80
AMA: 2018,Sep,7

21337 **Closed treatment of nasal septal fracture, with or without stabilization**
8.41 11.7 FUD 090 J A2 80
AMA: 2019,Sep,3; 2018,Sep,7

21338 **Open treatment of nasoethmoid fracture; without external fixation**
18.8 18.8 FUD 090 J J8 80
AMA: 2018,Sep,7

21339 **with external fixation**
21.3 21.3 FUD 090 J A2 80
AMA: 2018,Sep,7

21340 **Percutaneous treatment of nasoethmoid complex fracture, with splint, wire or headcap fixation, including repair of canthal ligaments and/or the nasolacrimal apparatus**
21.3 21.3 FUD 090 J A2 80
AMA: 2018,Sep,7

21343 **Open treatment of depressed frontal sinus fracture**
30.7 30.7 FUD 090 C 80
AMA: 2018,Sep,7

21344 **Open treatment of complicated (eg, comminuted or involving posterior wall) frontal sinus fracture, via coronal or multiple approaches**
39.7 39.7 FUD 090 C 80
AMA: 2018,Sep,7

21345 **Closed treatment of nasomaxillary complex fracture (LeFort II type), with interdental wire fixation or fixation of denture or splint**
17.9 22.2 FUD 090 T A2 80
AMA: 2018,Sep,7

21346 **Open treatment of nasomaxillary complex fracture (LeFort II type); with wiring and/or local fixation**
27.4 27.4 FUD 090 J G2
AMA: 2018,Sep,7

21347 **requiring multiple open approaches**
29.0 29.0 FUD 090 C 80
AMA: 2018,Sep,7

21348 **with bone grafting (includes obtaining graft)**
31.0 31.0 FUD 090 C 80
AMA: 2018,Sep,7

21355 **Percutaneous treatment of fracture of malar area, including zygomatic arch and malar tripod, with manipulation**
9.18 12.2 FUD 010 J A2 80 50
AMA: 2018,Sep,7

21356 **Open treatment of depressed zygomatic arch fracture (eg, Gillies approach)**
10.7 14.2 FUD 010 J A2 80 50
AMA: 2018,Sep,7

21360 **Open treatment of depressed malar fracture, including zygomatic arch and malar tripod**
14.6 14.6 FUD 090 J G2 80 50
AMA: 2018,Sep,7

21365 **Open treatment of complicated (eg, comminuted or involving cranial nerve foramina) fracture(s) of malar area, including zygomatic arch and malar tripod; with internal fixation and multiple surgical approaches**
31.6 31.6 FUD 090 J G2 80 50
AMA: 2018,Sep,7

21366 **with bone grafting (includes obtaining graft)**
36.5 36.5 FUD 090 C 80 50
AMA: 2018,Sep,7

21385 **Open treatment of orbital floor blowout fracture; transantral approach (Caldwell-Luc type operation)**
21.5 21.5 FUD 090 J G2 80 50
AMA: 2018,Sep,7

21386 **periorbital approach**
18.7 18.7 FUD 090 J G2 80 50
AMA: 2018,Sep,7

21387 **combined approach**
22.5 22.5 FUD 090 J G2 80 50
AMA: 2018,Sep,7

21390 **periorbital approach, with alloplastic or other implant**
22.9 22.9 FUD 090 J G2 80 50
AMA: 2020,Dec,11; 2018,Sep,7

21395 **periorbital approach with bone graft (includes obtaining graft)**
29.0 29.0 FUD 090 J G2 80 50
AMA: 2018,Sep,7

21400 **Closed treatment of fracture of orbit, except blowout; without manipulation**
4.59 5.77 FUD 090 T A2 80 50
AMA: 2018,Sep,7

21401 **with manipulation**
9.23 14.7 FUD 090 T A2 80 50
AMA: 2018,Sep,7

21406 **Open treatment of fracture of orbit, except blowout; without implant**
16.5 16.5 FUD 090 J G2 80 50
AMA: 2020,Dec,11; 2018,Sep,7

21407 **with implant**
18.4 18.4 FUD 090 J G2 80 50
AMA: 2020,Dec,11; 2018,Sep,7

21408 **with bone grafting (includes obtaining graft)**
26.1 26.1 FUD 090 J G2 80 50
AMA: 2018,Sep,7

Musculoskeletal System
21296 — 21408

● New Code ▲ Revised Code ○ Reinstated ● New Web Release ▲ Revised Web Release + Add-on Unlisted Not Covered # Resequenced
⑤⓪ Optum Mod 50 Exempt ⊘ AMA Mod 51 Exempt ⑤① Optum Mod 51 Exempt ⑥③ Mod 63 Exempt ✗ Non-FDA Drug ★ Telemedicine M Maternity A Age Edit

21421 Closed treatment of palatal or maxillary fracture (LeFort I type), with interdental wire fixation or fixation of denture or splint
16.1 19.1 FUD 090 J A2 80
AMA: 2018,Sep,7

21422 Open treatment of palatal or maxillary fracture (LeFort I type);
18.4 18.4 FUD 090 C 80
AMA: 2018,Sep,7

21423 complicated (comminuted or involving cranial nerve foramina), multiple approaches
22.0 22.0 FUD 090 C 80
AMA: 2018,Sep,7

21431 Closed treatment of craniofacial separation (LeFort III type) using interdental wire fixation of denture or splint
19.9 19.9 FUD 090 C 80
AMA: 2018,Sep,7

21432 Open treatment of craniofacial separation (LeFort III type); with wiring and/or internal fixation
20.7 20.7 FUD 090 C 80
AMA: 2018,Sep,7

21433 complicated (eg, comminuted or involving cranial nerve foramina), multiple surgical approaches
50.5 50.5 FUD 090 C 80
AMA: 2018,Sep,7

21435 complicated, utilizing internal and/or external fixation techniques (eg, head cap, halo device, and/or intermaxillary fixation)
EXCLUDES *Removal internal or external fixation (20670)*
40.7 40.7 FUD 090 C 80
AMA: 2018,Sep,7

21436 complicated, multiple surgical approaches, internal fixation, with bone grafting (includes obtaining graft)
59.2 59.2 FUD 090 C 80
AMA: 2018,Sep,7

21440 Closed treatment of mandibular or maxillary alveolar ridge fracture (separate procedure)
14.0 17.3 FUD 090 J P3 80
AMA: 2018,Sep,7

21445 Open treatment of mandibular or maxillary alveolar ridge fracture (separate procedure)
17.9 22.2 FUD 090 J A2 80
AMA: 2018,Sep,7

21450 Closed treatment of mandibular fracture; without manipulation
13.4 16.4 FUD 090 T J8 80
AMA: 2018,Sep,7

21451 with manipulation
18.0 21.5 FUD 090 T A2 80
AMA: 2018,Sep,7

21452 Percutaneous treatment of mandibular fracture, with external fixation
12.0 20.1 FUD 090 J J8 80
AMA: 2018,Sep,7

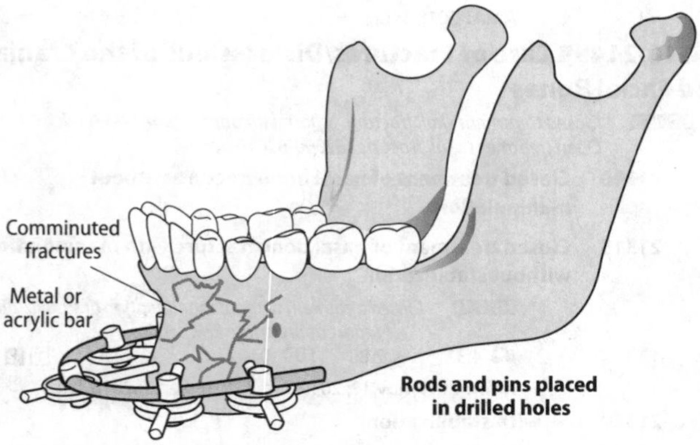

21453 Closed treatment of mandibular fracture with interdental fixation
23.6 27.6 FUD 090 J A2 80
AMA: 2018,Sep,7; 2018,Jan,8; 2017,Jan,8; 2016,Jan,13

21454 Open treatment of mandibular fracture with external fixation
15.6 15.6 FUD 090 J J8 80
AMA: 2018,Sep,7

21461 Open treatment of mandibular fracture; without interdental fixation
28.8 57.4 FUD 090 J J8
AMA: 2018,Sep,7

21462 with interdental fixation
31.9 61.4 FUD 090 J J8 80
AMA: 2018,Sep,7

21465 Open treatment of mandibular condylar fracture
24.1 24.1 FUD 090 J J8 80 50
AMA: 2018,Sep,7

21470 Open treatment of complicated mandibular fracture by multiple surgical approaches including internal fixation, interdental fixation, and/or wiring of dentures or splints
34.5 34.5 FUD 090 J J8 80
AMA: 2018,Sep,7; 2018,Jan,8; 2017,Jan,8; 2016,Jan,13

21480 Closed treatment of temporomandibular dislocation; initial or subsequent
0.91 3.07 FUD 000 T A2 50
AMA: 2018,Sep,7

21485 complicated (eg, recurrent requiring intermaxillary fixation or splinting), initial or subsequent
20.6 25.2 FUD 090 T A2 80 50
AMA: 2018,Sep,7

21490 Open treatment of temporomandibular dislocation
EXCLUDES *Closed treatment larynx fracture, report with appropriate E/M service*
Interdental wiring (21497)
23.7 23.7 FUD 090 J A2 80 50
AMA: 2018,Sep,7

21497 Interdental wiring, for condition other than fracture
16.4 19.6 FUD 090 T A2 80
AMA: 2018,Sep,7; 2018,Jan,8; 2017,Jan,8; 2016,Jan,13

21499 Unlisted musculoskeletal procedure, head
EXCLUDES *Unlisted procedures craniofacial or maxillofacial areas (21299)*
0.00 0.00 FUD YYY T 80
AMA: 2018,Sep,7

21501-21510 Surgical Incision for Drainage: Chest and Soft Tissues of Neck

EXCLUDES *Biopsy flank or back (21920-21925)*
Simple incision and drainage abscess or hematoma (10060, 10140)
Tumor removal flank or back (21930-21936)

21501 **Incision and drainage, deep abscess or hematoma, soft tissues of neck or thorax;**
EXCLUDES *Deep incision and drainage posterior spine (22010-22015)*
9.37 13.4 **FUD** 090 J A2
AMA: 2018,Sep,7; 2018,Jan,8; 2017,Jan,8; 2016,Jan,13

21502 **with partial rib ostectomy**
14.5 14.5 **FUD** 090 J A2 80
AMA: 2018,Sep,7

21510 **Incision, deep, with opening of bone cortex (eg, for osteomyelitis or bone abscess), thorax**
12.9 12.9 **FUD** 090 C 80
AMA: 2018,Sep,7

21550 Soft Tissue Biopsy of Chest or Neck

EXCLUDES *Biopsy bone (20220-20251)*
Soft tissue needle biopsy (20206)

21550 **Biopsy, soft tissue of neck or thorax**
4.47 7.50 **FUD** 010 J G2
AMA: 2018,Sep,7

21552-21558 [21552, 21554] Excision Soft Tissue Tumors Chest and Neck

INCLUDES Any necessary elevation tissue planes or dissection
Measurement tumor and necessary margin at greatest diameter prior to excision
Resection without removal significant normal tissue
Simple and intermediate repairs
Excision types:
Fascial or subfascial soft tissue tumors: simple and marginal resection tumors found either in or below deep fascia, not involving bone or excision substantial amount normal tissue; primarily benign and intramuscular tumors
Radical resection soft tissue tumor: wide resection tumor, involving substantial margins normal tissue and may involve tissue removal from one or more layers; most often malignant or aggressive benign
Subcutaneous: simple and marginal resection tumors in subcutaneous tissue above deep fascia; most often benign

EXCLUDES *Complex repair*
Excision benign cutaneous lesions (eg, sebaceous cyst) (11400-11426)
Radical resection cutaneous tumors (eg, melanoma) (11600-11626)
Significant vessel exploration or neuroplasty

21552 **Resequenced code. See code following 21555.**

21554 **Resequenced code. See code following 21556.**

21555 **Excision, tumor, soft tissue of neck or anterior thorax, subcutaneous; less than 3 cm**
8.79 12.2 **FUD** 090 J G2
AMA: 2018,Sep,7; 2018,Jan,8; 2017,Jan,8; 2016,Jan,13

21552 **3 cm or greater**
12.8 12.8 **FUD** 090 J G2 80
AMA: 2018,Sep,7

21556 **Excision, tumor, soft tissue of neck or anterior thorax, subfascial (eg, intramuscular); less than 5 cm**
15.2 15.2 **FUD** 090 J G2
AMA: 2018,Sep,7

21554 **5 cm or greater**
21.0 21.0 **FUD** 090 J G2 80
AMA: 2018,Sep,7

21557 **Radical resection of tumor (eg, sarcoma), soft tissue of neck or anterior thorax; less than 5 cm**
27.4 27.4 **FUD** 090 J G2 80
AMA: 2020,Apr,10; 2018,Sep,7; 2018,Jan,8; 2017,Jan,8; 2016,Jan,13

21558 **5 cm or greater**
38.7 38.7 **FUD** 090 J G2 80
AMA: 2020,Apr,10; 2018,Sep,7

21600-21632 Bony Resection Chest and Neck

21600 **Excision of rib, partial**
EXCLUDES *Extensive debridement (11044, 11047)*
Radical resection, chest wall/rib cage for tumor (21601)
15.9 15.9 **FUD** 090 J A2 80
AMA: 2018,Sep,7; 2018,Jan,8; 2017,Jan,8; 2016,Jan,13

21601 **Excision of chest wall tumor including rib(s)**
EXCLUDES *Exploratory thoracotomy (32100)*
Resection apical lung tumor (32503-32504)
Thoracentesis (32554-32555)
Tube thoracostomy (32551)
34.1 34.1 **FUD** 090 G2 80
AMA: 2019,Dec,4

21602 **Excision of chest wall tumor involving rib(s), with plastic reconstruction; without mediastinal lymphadenectomy**
EXCLUDES *Exploratory thoracotomy (32100)*
Resection apical lung tumor (32503-32504)
Thoracentesis (32554-32555)
Tube thoracostomy (32551)
45.8 45.8 **FUD** 090 80
AMA: 2019,Dec,4

21603 **with mediastinal lymphadenectomy**
EXCLUDES *Exploratory thoracotomy (32100)*
Resection apical lung tumor (32503-32504)
Thoracentesis (32554-32555)
Tube thoracostomy (32551)
50.7 50.7 **FUD** 090 80
AMA: 2019,Dec,4

21610 **Costotransversectomy (separate procedure)**
34.5 34.5 **FUD** 090 J A2 80
AMA: 2018,Sep,7

21615 **Excision first and/or cervical rib;**
17.8 17.8 **FUD** 090 C 80 50
AMA: 2018,Sep,7; 2018,Jan,8; 2017,Jan,8; 2016,Jan,13

21616 **with sympathectomy**
20.7 20.7 **FUD** 090 C 80 50
AMA: 2018,Sep,7

21620 **Ostectomy of sternum, partial**
14.5 14.5 **FUD** 090 C 80
AMA: 2018,Sep,7

21627 **Sternal debridement**
EXCLUDES *Debridement with sternotomy closure (21750)*
15.4 15.4 **FUD** 090 C 80
AMA: 2018,Sep,7; 2018,Jan,8; 2017,Jan,8; 2016,Jan,13

21630 **Radical resection of sternum;**
35.1 35.1 **FUD** 090 C 80
AMA: 2018,Sep,7

21632 **with mediastinal lymphadenectomy**
34.9 34.9 **FUD** 090 C 80
AMA: 2018,Sep,7

21685-21750 Repair/Reconstruction Chest and Soft Tissues Neck

EXCLUDES *Repair simple wounds (12001-12007)*

21685 **Hyoid myotomy and suspension**
28.2 28.2 **FUD** 090 J G2 80
AMA: 2018,Sep,7; 2018,Jan,8; 2017,Jan,8; 2016,Jan,13

21700 **Division of scalenus anticus; without resection of cervical rib**
10.3 10.3 **FUD** 090 J A2 80 50
AMA: 2018,Sep,7

21705 **with resection of cervical rib**
15.5 15.5 **FUD** 090 C 80 50
AMA: 2018,Sep,7; 2018,Jan,8; 2017,Jan,8; 2016,Jan,13

21720 Division of sternocleidomastoid for torticollis, open operation; without cast application

EXCLUDES *Transection spinal accessory and cervical nerves (63191, 64722)*

15.0 15.0 FUD 090 J A2 80

AMA: 2018,Sep,7

21725 with cast application

EXCLUDES *Transection spinal accessory and cervical nerves (63191, 64722)*

15.5 15.5 FUD 090 T A2 80

AMA: 2018,Sep,7

21740 Reconstructive repair of pectus excavatum or carinatum; open

29.7 29.7 FUD 090 C 80

AMA: 2018,Sep,7

21742 minimally invasive approach (Nuss procedure), without thoracoscopy

0.00 0.00 FUD 090 J G2 80

AMA: 2018,Sep,7

21743 minimally invasive approach (Nuss procedure), with thoracoscopy

0.00 0.00 FUD 090 J G2 80

AMA: 2019,Nov,14; 2018,Sep,7

21750 Closure of median sternotomy separation with or without debridement (separate procedure)

19.7 19.7 FUD 090 C 80

AMA: 2018,Sep,7; 2018,Jan,8; 2017,Jan,8; 2016,Jan,13

21811-21825 Fracture Care: Ribs and Sternum

EXCLUDES *Closed treatment uncomplicated rib fractures, report appropriate E/M services*

21811 Open treatment of rib fracture(s) with internal fixation, includes thoracoscopic visualization when performed, unilateral; 1-3 ribs

17.2 17.2 FUD 000 J 80 50

AMA: 2018,Sep,7; 2018,Jan,8; 2017,Jan,8; 2016,Jan,13

21812 4-6 ribs

21.0 21.0 FUD 000 J 80 50

AMA: 2018,Sep,7; 2018,Jan,8; 2017,Jan,8; 2016,Jan,13

21813 7 or more ribs

28.7 28.7 FUD 000 J 80 50

AMA: 2018,Sep,7; 2018,Jan,8; 2017,Jan,8; 2016,Jan,13

21820 Closed treatment of sternum fracture

4.10 4.08 FUD 090 T A2

AMA: 2018,Sep,7

21825 Open treatment of sternum fracture with or without skeletal fixation

EXCLUDES *Treatment sternoclavicular dislocation (23520-23532)*

15.6 15.6 FUD 090 C 80

AMA: 2018,Sep,7

21899 Unlisted Procedures of Chest or Neck

CMS: 100-04,4,180.3 Unlisted Service or Procedure

21899 Unlisted procedure, neck or thorax

0.00 0.00 FUD YYY T 80

AMA: 2018,Sep,7; 2018,Jan,8; 2017,Jan,8; 2016,Jan,13

21920-21925 Biopsy Soft Tissue of Back and Flank

EXCLUDES *Soft tissue needle biopsy (20206)*

21920 Biopsy, soft tissue of back or flank; superficial

4.55 7.30 FUD 010 J P3

AMA: 2018,Sep,7

21925 deep

10.4 13.4 FUD 090 J A2

AMA: 2018,Sep,7

21930-21936 Excision Soft Tissue Tumors Back or Flank

INCLUDES Any necessary elevation tissue planes or dissection
Measurement tumor and necessary margin at greatest diameter prior to excision
Simple and intermediate repairs
Excision types:
Fascial or subfascial soft tissue tumors: simple and marginal resection tumors found either in or below deep fascia, not involving bone or excision substantial amount normal tissue; most often benign and intramuscular tumors
Radical resection soft tissue tumor: wide resection of tumor, involving substantial margins normal tissue and may include tissue removal from one or more layers; most often malignant or aggressive benign
Subcutaneous: simple and marginal resection tumors in subcutaneous tissue above deep fascia; most often benign

EXCLUDES *Complex repair*
Excision benign cutaneous lesions (eg, sebaceous cyst) (11400-11406)
Radical resection cutaneous tumors (eg, melanoma) (11600-11606)
Significant vessel exploration or neuroplasty

21930 Excision, tumor, soft tissue of back or flank, subcutaneous; less than 3 cm

10.4 13.8 FUD 090 J G2

AMA: 2018,Sep,7; 2018,Jan,8; 2017,Jan,8; 2016,Jan,13

21931 3 cm or greater

13.6 13.6 FUD 090 J G2 80

AMA: 2018,Sep,7

21932 Excision, tumor, soft tissue of back or flank, subfascial (eg, intramuscular); less than 5 cm

19.0 19.0 FUD 090 J G2 80

AMA: 2018,Sep,7

21933 5 cm or greater

21.3 21.3 FUD 090 J G2 80

AMA: 2018,Sep,7

21935 Radical resection of tumor (eg, sarcoma), soft tissue of back or flank; less than 5 cm

29.7 29.7 FUD 090 J G2

AMA: 2018,Sep,7

21936 5 cm or greater

40.9 40.9 FUD 090 J G2 80

AMA: 2018,Sep,7

22010-22015 Incision for Drainage of Deep Spinal Abscess

EXCLUDES *Incision and drainage hematoma (10060, 10140)*
Injection:
Chemonucleolysis (62292)
Discography (62290-62291)
Facet joint (64490-64495, [64633, 64634, 64635, 64636])
Myelography (62284)
Needle/trocar biopsy (20220-20225)

22010 Incision and drainage, open, of deep abscess (subfascial), posterior spine; cervical, thoracic, or cervicothoracic

27.7 27.7 FUD 090 C 80

AMA: 2018,Sep,7

22015 lumbar, sacral, or lumbosacral

EXCLUDES *Incision and drainage, complex, postoperative wound infection (10180)*
Incision and drainage, open, deep abscess (subfascial), posterior spine; cervical, thoracic, or cervicothoracic (22010)
Removal posterior nonsegmental instrumentation (eg, Harrington rod) (22850)
Removal posterior segmental instrumentation (22852)

27.2 27.2 FUD 090 C

AMA: 2018,Sep,7

22100-22103 Partial Resection Vertebral Component

EXCLUDES *Back or flank biopsy (21920-21925)*
Bone biopsy (20220-20251)
Bone grafting procedures (20930-20938)
Harvest bone graft (20931, 20938)
Injection:
Chemonucleolysis (62292)
Discography (62290-62291)
Facet joint (64490-64495, [64633, 64634, 64635, 64636])
Myelography (62284)
Osteotomy (22210-22226)
Reconstruction after vertebral body resection (22585, 63082, 63086, 63088, 63091)
Removal tumor flank or back (21930)
Soft tissue needle biopsy (20206)
Spinal reconstruction with bone graft or vertebral body prosthesis:
Cervical (20931, 20938, 22554, 63081)
Lumbar (20931, 20938, 22558, 63087, 63090)
Thoracic (20931, 20938, 22556, 63085, 63087)
Vertebral corpectomy (63081-63091)

22100 Partial excision of posterior vertebral component (eg, spinous process, lamina or facet) for intrinsic bony lesion, single vertebral segment; cervical
24.8 24.8 **FUD** 090 J 62 80
AMA: 2018,Sep,7; 2018,Jan,8; 2017,Mar,7; 2017,Jan,8; 2016,Jan,13

22101 thoracic
25.1 25.1 **FUD** 090 J 62 80
AMA: 2018,Sep,7; 2018,Jan,8; 2017,Mar,7; 2017,Jan,8; 2016,Jan,13

22102 lumbar
Code also posterior spinous process distraction device insertion, when applicable (22867-22870)
23.4 23.4 **FUD** 090 J 62 80
AMA: 2018,Sep,7; 2018,Jan,8; 2017,Mar,7; 2017,Jan,8; 2016,Jan,13

+ **22103 each additional segment (List separately in addition to code for primary procedure)**
Code first (22100-22102)
4.09 4.09 **FUD** ZZZ N N1 80
AMA: 2018,Sep,7

22110-22116 Partial Resection Vertebral Component without Decompression

EXCLUDES *Back or flank biopsy (21920-21925)*
Bone biopsy (20220-20251)
Bone grafting procedures (20930-20938)
Harvest bone graft (20931, 20938)
Injection:
Chemonucleolysis (62292)
Discography (62290-62291)
Facet joint (64490-64495, [64633, 64634, 64635, 64636])
Myelography (62284)
Osteotomy (22210-22226)
Reconstruction after vertebral body resection (22585, 63082, 63086, 63088, 63091)
Removal tumor flank or back (21930)
Soft tissue needle biopsy (20206)
Spinal reconstruction with bone graft or vertebral body prosthesis:
Cervical (20931, 20938, 22554, 22853-22854 [22859], 63081)
Lumbar (20931, 20938, 22558, 22853-22854 [22859], 63087, 63090)
Thoracic (20931, 20938, 22556, 22853-22854 [22859], 63085, 63087)
Vertebral corpectomy (63081-63091)

22110 Partial excision of vertebral body, for intrinsic bony lesion, without decompression of spinal cord or nerve root(s), single vertebral segment; cervical
30.1 30.1 **FUD** 090 C 80
AMA: 2018,Sep,7; 2018,Jan,8; 2017,Mar,7; 2017,Jan,8; 2016,Jan,13

22112 thoracic
32.7 32.7 **FUD** 090 C 80
AMA: 2018,Sep,7; 2018,Jan,8; 2017,Mar,7; 2017,Jan,8; 2016,Jan,13

22114 lumbar
32.4 32.4 **FUD** 090 C 80
AMA: 2018,Sep,7; 2018,Jan,8; 2017,Mar,7; 2017,Jan,8; 2016,Jan,13

+ **22116 each additional vertebral segment (List separately in addition to code for primary procedure)**
Code first (22110-22114)
4.12 4.12 **FUD** ZZZ C 80
AMA: 2018,Sep,7

22206-22216 Spinal Osteotomy: Posterior/Posterolateral Approach

EXCLUDES *Decompression spinal cord and/or nerve roots (63001-63308)*
Injection:
Chemonucleolysis (62292)
Discography (62290-62292)
Facet joint (64490-64495, [64633, 64634, 64635, 64636])
Myelography (62284)
Vertebral corpectomy (63081-63091)

Code also:
Arthrodesis (22590-22632)
Bone grafting procedures (20930-20938)
Spinal instrumentation (22840-22855 [22859])

22206 Osteotomy of spine, posterior or posterolateral approach, 3 columns, 1 vertebral segment (eg, pedicle/vertebral body subtraction); thoracic
EXCLUDES *Osteotomy spine, posterior or posterolateral approach, lumbar (22207)*
Procedures performed at same level (22210-22226, 22830, 63001-63048, 63055-63066, 63075-63091, 63101-63103)
71.3 71.3 **FUD** 090 C 80
AMA: 2018,Sep,7; 2018,Jan,8; 2017,Mar,7; 2017,Jan,8; 2016,Jan,13

22207 lumbar
EXCLUDES *Osteotomy spine, posterior or posterolateral approach, thoracic (22206)*
Procedures performed at same level (22210-22226, 22830, 63001-63048, 63055-63066, 63075-63091, 63101-63103)
69.8 69.8 **FUD** 090 C 80
AMA: 2018,Sep,7; 2018,Jan,8; 2017,Mar,7; 2017,Jan,8; 2016,Jan,13

+ **22208 each additional vertebral segment (List separately in addition to code for primary procedure)**
EXCLUDES *Procedures performed at same level (22210-22226, 22830, 63001-63048, 63055-63066, 63075-63091, 63101-63103)*
Code first (22206, 22207)
17.1 17.1 **FUD** ZZZ C 80
AMA: 2018,Sep,7; 2018,Jan,8; 2017,Jan,8; 2016,Jan,13

22210 **Osteotomy of spine, posterior or posterolateral approach, 1 vertebral segment; cervical**
51.7 51.7 **FUD** 090 C 80
AMA: 2018,Sep,7; 2018,Jan,8; 2017,Mar,7; 2017,Jan,8; 2016,Jan,13

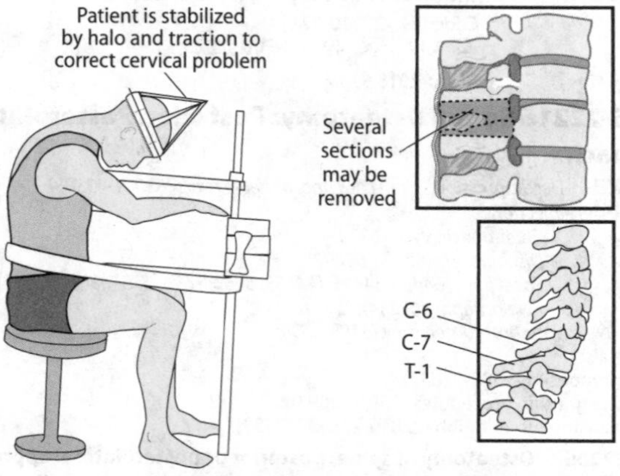
Patient is stabilized by halo and traction to correct cervical problem
Several sections may be removed
C-6
C-7
T-1

Physician removes spinous processes, lamina

22212 **thoracic**
43.2 43.2 **FUD** 090 C 80
AMA: 2018,Sep,7; 2018,Jan,8; 2017,Mar,7; 2017,Jan,8; 2016,Jan,13

22214 **lumbar**
43.4 43.4 **FUD** 090 C 80
AMA: 2018,Sep,7; 2018,Jan,8; 2017,Mar,7; 2017,Jan,8; 2016,Jan,13

\+ **22216** **each additional vertebral segment (List separately in addition to primary procedure)**
Code first (22210-22214)
10.5 10.5 **FUD** ZZZ C 80
AMA: 2018,Sep,7; 2018,Jan,8; 2017,Jan,8; 2016,Jan,13

22220-22226 Spinal Osteotomy: Anterior Approach

EXCLUDES *Decompression spinal cord and/or nerve roots (63001-63308)*
Injection:
Chemonucleolysis (62292)
Discography (62290-62291)
Facet joint (64490-64495, [64633, 64634, 64635, 64636])
Myelography (62284)
Needle/trocar biopsy (20220-20225)
Verterbral corpectomy (63081-63091)

Code also:
Arthrodesis (22590-22632)
Bone grafting procedures (20930-20938)
Spinal instrumentation (22840-22855 [22859])

22220 **Osteotomy of spine, including discectomy, anterior approach, single vertebral segment; cervical**
47.0 47.0 **FUD** 090 C 80
AMA: 2018,Sep,7; 2018,Jan,8; 2017,Mar,7; 2017,Jan,8; 2016,Jan,13

22222 **thoracic**
51.1 51.1 **FUD** 090 C 80
AMA: 2018,Sep,7; 2018,Jan,8; 2017,Mar,7; 2017,Jan,8; 2016,Jan,13

22224 **lumbar**
46.1 46.1 **FUD** 090 C 80
AMA: 2018,Sep,7; 2018,Jan,8; 2017,Mar,7; 2017,Jan,8; 2016,Jan,13

\+ **22226** **each additional vertebral segment (List separately in addition to code for primary procedure)**
Code first (22220-22224)
10.5 10.5 **FUD** ZZZ C 80
AMA: 2018,Sep,7

22310-22315 Closed Treatment Vertebral Fractures

EXCLUDES *Injection:*
Chemonucleolysis (62292)
Discography (62290-62291)
Facet joint (64490-64495, [64633, 64634, 64635, 64636])
Myelography (62284)
Percutaneous vertebroplasty at same level (22510-22515)
Vertebral fracture care by arthrodesis (22590-22632)

Code also:
Arthrodesis (22590-22632)
Bone grafting procedures (20930-20938)
Spinal instrumentation (22840-22855 [22859])

22310 **Closed treatment of vertebral body fracture(s), without manipulation, requiring and including casting or bracing**
8.38 8.70 **FUD** 090 T A2
AMA: 2018,Sep,7; 2018,Jan,8; 2017,Mar,7; 2017,Jan,8; 2016,Jan,13

22315 **Closed treatment of vertebral fracture(s) and/or dislocation(s) requiring casting or bracing, with and including casting and/or bracing by manipulation or traction**
EXCLUDES *Spinal manipulation (97140)*
22.2 25.3 **FUD** 090 J A2
AMA: 2018,Sep,7; 2018,Jan,8; 2017,Mar,7; 2017,Jan,8; 2016,Jan,13

22318-22319 Open Treatment Odontoid Fracture: Anterior Approach

EXCLUDES *Injection:*
Chemonucleolysis (62292)
Discography (62290-62291)
Facet joint (64490-64495, [64633, 64634, 64635, 64636])
Myelography (62284)
Needle/trocar biopsy (20220-20225)

Code also:
Arthrodesis for fracture care (22590-22632)
Bone grafting procedures (20930-20938)
Spinal instrumentation (22840-22855 [22859])

22318 **Open treatment and/or reduction of odontoid fracture(s) and or dislocation(s) (including os odontoideum), anterior approach, including placement of internal fixation; without grafting**
47.6 47.6 **FUD** 090 C 80
AMA: 2018,Sep,7; 2018,Jan,8; 2017,Mar,7; 2017,Jan,8; 2016,Jan,13

22319 **with grafting**
53.6 53.6 **FUD** 090 C 80
AMA: 2018,Sep,7; 2018,May,3; 2018,Jan,8; 2017,Mar,7; 2017,Jan,8; 2016,Jan,13

22325-22328 Open Treatment Vertebral Fractures: Posterior Approach

EXCLUDES *Injection:*
Chemonucleolysis (62292)
Discography (62290-62291)
Facet joint (64490-64495, [64633, 64634, 64635, 64636])
Myelography (62284)
Needle/trocar biopsy (20220-20225)
Spine decompression (63001-63091)
Vertebral corpectomy (63081-63091)

Code also:
Arthrodesis (22590-22632)
Bone grafting procedures (20930-20938)
Spinal instrumentation (22840-22855 [22859])

22325 **Open treatment and/or reduction of vertebral fracture(s) and/or dislocation(s), posterior approach, 1 fractured vertebra or dislocated segment; lumbar**
EXCLUDES *Percutaneous vertebral augmentation performed at same level (22514-22515)*
Percutaneous vertebroplasty performed at same level (22511-22512)
41.9 41.9 **FUD** 090 C 80
AMA: 2018,Sep,7; 2018,Jan,8; 2017,Aug,9; 2017,Mar,7; 2017,Jan,8; 2016,Jan,13

22326 **cervical**

EXCLUDES *Percutaneous vertebroplasty performed at same level (22510, 22512)*

43.4 43.4 FUD 090 C 80

AMA: 2018,Sep,7; 2018,Jan,8; 2017,Mar,7; 2017,Jan,8; 2016,Jan,13

22327 **thoracic**

EXCLUDES *Percutaneous vertebral augmentation performed at same level (22515)*

Percutaneous vertebroplasty performed at same level (22510, 22512-22513)

43.7 43.7 FUD 090 C 80

AMA: 2018,Sep,7; 2018,Jan,8; 2017,Mar,7; 2017,Jan,8; 2016,Jan,13

\+ **22328** **each additional fractured vertebra or dislocated segment (List separately in addition to code for primary procedure)**

Code first (22325-22327)

8.25 8.25 FUD ZZZ C 80

AMA: 2018,Sep,7

22505 Spinal Manipulation with Anesthesia

EXCLUDES *Manipulation not requiring anesthesia (97140)*

22505 **Manipulation of spine requiring anesthesia, any region**

3.76 3.76 FUD 010 J A2

AMA: 2018,Sep,7; 2018,Jan,8; 2017,Jan,8; 2016,Jan,13

22510-22515 Percutaneous Vertebroplasty/Kyphoplasty

INCLUDES Radiological guidance

When performed at same level:

Bone biopsy (20225)

Closed treatment vertebral fractures (22310, 22315)

Open treatment/reduction vertebral fractures (22325, 22327)

EXCLUDES *Sacroplasty/augmentation (0200T-0201T)*

Thermal destruction lumbar or sacral intraosseous basivertebral nerve ([64628, 64629])

22510 **Percutaneous vertebroplasty (bone biopsy included when performed), 1 vertebral body, unilateral or bilateral injection, inclusive of all imaging guidance; cervicothoracic**

12.5 47.9 FUD 010 J G2

AMA: 2018,Sep,7; 2018,Jan,8; 2017,Jan,8; 2016,Jan,13

22511 **lumbosacral**

11.7 47.3 FUD 010 J G2

AMA: 2018,Sep,7; 2018,Jan,8; 2017,Jan,8; 2016,Jan,13

\+ **22512** **each additional cervicothoracic or lumbosacral vertebral body (List separately in addition to code for primary procedure)**

Code first (22510-22511)

5.96 24.4 FUD ZZZ N N1

AMA: 2018,Sep,7; 2018,Jan,8; 2017,Jan,8; 2016,Jan,13

22513 **Percutaneous vertebral augmentation, including cavity creation (fracture reduction and bone biopsy included when performed) using mechanical device (eg, kyphoplasty), 1 vertebral body, unilateral or bilateral cannulation, inclusive of all imaging guidance; thoracic**

15.0 203. FUD 010 J G2

AMA: 2018,Sep,7; 2018,Jan,8; 2017,Jan,8; 2016,Jan,13

22514 **lumbar**

14.0 202. FUD 010 J G2

AMA: 2018,Sep,7; 2018,Jan,8; 2017,Jan,8; 2016,Jan,13

\+ **22515** **each additional thoracic or lumbar vertebral body (List separately in addition to code for primary procedure)**

Code first (22513-22514)

6.39 105. FUD ZZZ N N1

AMA: 2018,Sep,7; 2018,Jan,8; 2017,Jan,8; 2016,Jan,13

22526-22527 Percutaneous Annuloplasty

CMS: 100-04,32,220.1 Thermal Intradiscal Procedures (TIPS)

INCLUDES Fluoroscopic guidance (77002, 77003)

EXCLUDES *Injection:*

Chemonucleolysis (62292)

Discography (62290-62291)

Facet joint (64490-64495, [64633, 64634, 64635, 64636])

Myelography (62284)

Needle/trocar biopsy (20220-20225)

Procedure performed by other methods (22899)

22526 **Percutaneous intradiscal electrothermal annuloplasty, unilateral or bilateral including fluoroscopic guidance; single level**

9.76 65.0 FUD 010 E

AMA: 2018,Sep,7; 2018,Jan,8; 2017,Jan,8; 2016,Jan,13

\+ **22527** **1 or more additional levels (List separately in addition to code for primary procedure)**

Code first (22526)

4.44 53.1 FUD ZZZ E

AMA: 2018,Sep,7; 2018,Jan,8; 2017,Jan,8; 2016,Jan,13

22532-22534 Spinal Fusion: Lateral Extracavitary Approach

EXCLUDES *Corpectomy (63101-63103)*

Exploration spinal fusion (22830)

Fracture care (22310-22328)

Injection:

Chemonucleolysis (62292)

Discography (62290-62291)

Facet joint (64490-64495, [64633, 64634, 64635, 64636])

Myelography (62284)

Laminectomy (63001-63017)

Needle/trocar biopsy (20220-20225)

Osteotomy (22206-22226)

Code also:

Bone grafting procedures (20930-20938)

Spinal instrumentation (22840-22855 [22859])

22532 **Arthrodesis, lateral extracavitary technique, including minimal discectomy to prepare interspace (other than for decompression); thoracic**

52.1 52.1 FUD 090 C 80

AMA: 2020,May,13; 2018,Sep,7; 2018,May,3; 2018,Jan,8; 2017,Mar,7; 2017,Feb,9; 2017,Jan,8; 2016,Jan,13

22533 **lumbar**

48.0 48.0 FUD 090 C 80

AMA: 2020,May,13; 2018,Sep,7; 2018,May,3; 2018,Jan,8; 2017,Mar,7; 2017,Feb,9; 2017,Jan,8; 2016,Jan,13

\+ **22534** **thoracic or lumbar, each additional vertebral segment (List separately in addition to code for primary procedure)**

Code first (22532-22533)

10.5 10.5 FUD ZZZ C 80

AMA: 2020,May,13; 2018,Sep,7; 2018,May,3; 2017,Feb,9

Musculoskeletal System

22326 — 22534

22548-22634 Spinal Fusion: Anterior and Posterior Approach

EXCLUDES *Corpectomy (63081-63091)*
Exploration spinal fusion (22830)
Fracture care (22310-22328)
Injection:
Chemonucleolysis (62292)
Discography (62290-62291)
Facet joint (64490-64495, [64633, 64634, 64635, 64636])
Myelography (62284)
Laminectomy (63001-63017)
Needle/trocar biopsy (20220-20225)
Osteotomy (22206-22226)

Code also:
Bone grafting procedures (20930-20938)
Spinal instrumentation (22840-22855 [22859])

22548 Arthrodesis, anterior transoral or extraoral technique, clivus-C1-C2 (atlas-axis), with or without excision of odontoid process

EXCLUDES *Laminectomy or laminotomy with disc removal (63020-63042)*

56.4 56.4 **FUD** 090 C 80

AMA: 2020,May,13; 2018,Sep,7; 2018,May,3; 2018,Jan,8; 2017,Mar,7; 2017,Jan,8; 2016,Jan,13

22551 Arthrodesis, anterior interbody, including disc space preparation, discectomy, osteophytectomy and decompression of spinal cord and/or nerve roots; cervical below C2

INCLUDES Operating microscope (69990)

49.3 49.3 **FUD** 090 J J8 80

AMA: 2020,May,13; 2018,Sep,7; 2018,Aug,10; 2018,May,3; 2018,Jan,8; 2017,Mar,7; 2017,Jan,8; 2016,May,13; 2016,Feb,12; 2016,Jan,13

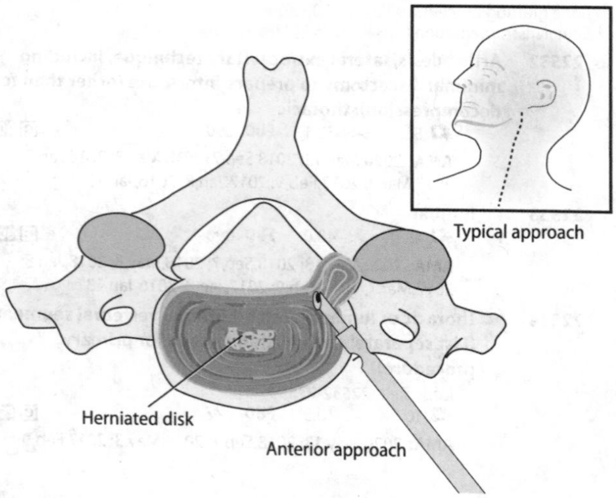

+ **22552 cervical below C2, each additional interspace (List separately in addition to code for separate procedure)**

INCLUDES Operating microscope (69990)

Code first (22551)

11.5 11.5 **FUD** ZZZ N N1 80

AMA: 2020,May,13; 2018,Sep,7; 2018,Aug,10; 2018,May,3; 2018,Jan,8; 2017,Mar,7; 2017,Jan,8; 2016,Feb,12; 2016,Jan,13

22554 Arthrodesis, anterior interbody technique, including minimal discectomy to prepare interspace (other than for decompression); cervical below C2

EXCLUDES *Anterior discectomy and interbody fusion during same operative session (regardless if performed by multiple surgeons) (22551)*
Discectomy, anterior, with decompression spinal cord and/or nerve root(s), cervical (even by separate individual) (63075-63076)

36.3 36.3 **FUD** 090 J J8 80

AMA: 2020,May,13; 2018,Sep,7; 2018,May,3; 2018,Jan,8; 2017,Mar,7; 2017,Jan,8; 2016,Jan,13

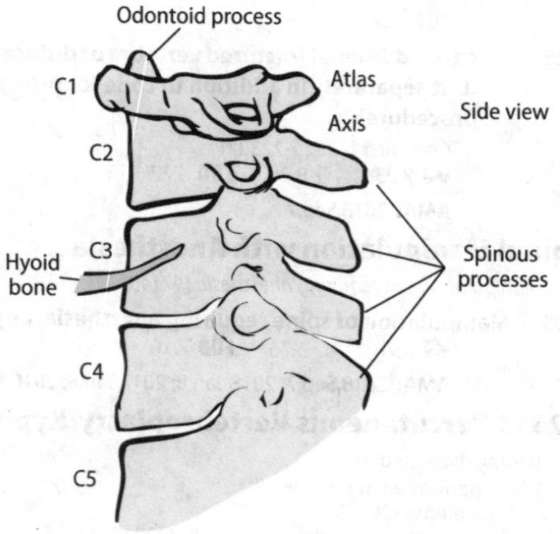

22556 thoracic

48.1 48.1 **FUD** 090 C 80

AMA: 2020,May,13; 2018,Sep,7; 2018,May,3; 2018,Jan,8; 2017,Mar,7; 2017,Jan,8; 2016,Jan,13

22558 lumbar

EXCLUDES *Arthrodesis using pre-sacral interbody technique (22586)*

44.3 44.3 **FUD** 090 C 80

AMA: 2020,May,13; 2018,Sep,7; 2018,May,3; 2018,Jan,8; 2017,Mar,7; 2017,Feb,9; 2017,Jan,8; 2016,Jan,13

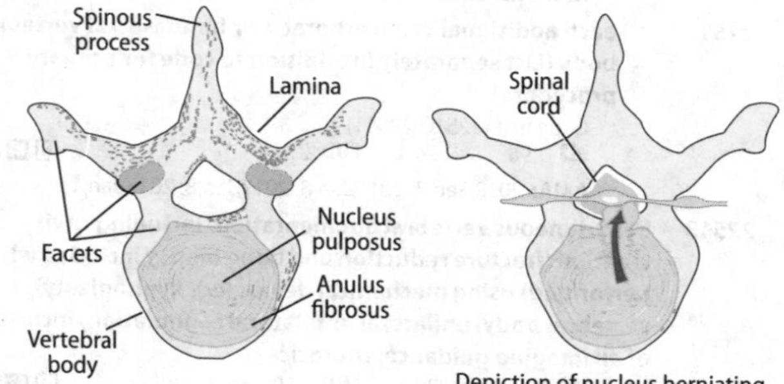

Thoracic vertebra (superior views)

Depiction of nucleus herniating through anulus and pressuring spinal nerve

+ **22585 each additional interspace (List separately in addition to code for primary procedure)**

EXCLUDES *Anterior discectomy and interbody fusion during same operative session (regardless if performed by multiple surgeons) (22552)*
Discectomy, anterior, with decompression spinal cord and/or nerve root(s), cervical (even by separate individual) (63075)

Code first (22554-22558)

9.51 9.51 **FUD** ZZZ N N1 80

AMA: 2020,May,13; 2018,Sep,7; 2018,Jan,8; 2017,Jan,8; 2016,Jan,13

22586 **Arthrodesis, pre-sacral interbody technique, including disc space preparation, discectomy, with posterior instrumentation, with image guidance, includes bone graft when performed, L5-S1 interspace**

INCLUDES Radiologic guidance (77002-77003, 77011-77012)

EXCLUDES *Allograft and autograft spinal bone (20930-20938)*
Pelvic fixation, other than sacrum (22848)
Posterior non-segmental instrumentation (22840)

59.6 59.6 **FUD** 090 C 80

AMA: 2020,May,13; 2018,Sep,7

22590 **Arthrodesis, posterior technique, craniocervical (occiput-C2)**

EXCLUDES *Posterior intrafacet implant insertion (0219T-0222T)*

45.6 45.6 **FUD** 090 C 80

AMA: 2020,May,13; 2018,Sep,7; 2018,May,3; 2018,Jan,8; 2017,Mar,7; 2017,Jan,8; 2016,Jan,13

Skull and cervical vertebrae; posterior view

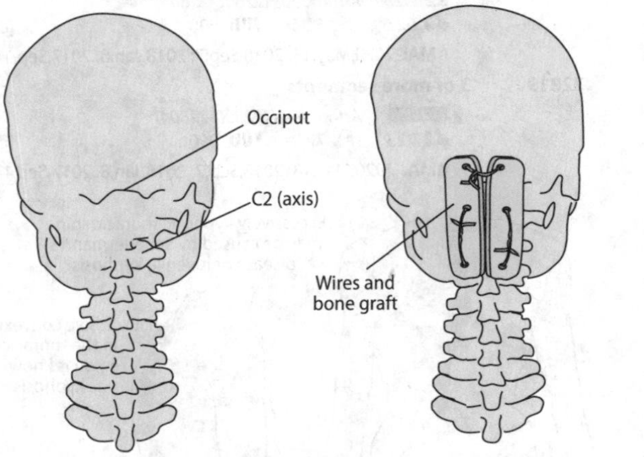

The physician fuses skull to C2 (axis) to stabilize cervical vertebrae; anchor holes are drilled in the occiput of the skull

22595 **Arthrodesis, posterior technique, atlas-axis (C1-C2)**

EXCLUDES *Posterior intrafacet implant insertion (0219T-0222T)*

43.5 43.5 **FUD** 090 C 80

AMA: 2020,May,13; 2018,Sep,7; 2018,May,3; 2018,Jan,8; 2017,Mar,7; 2017,Jan,8; 2016,Jan,13

▲ **22600** **Arthrodesis, posterior or posterolateral technique, single interspace; cervical below C2 segment**

EXCLUDES *Posterior intrafacet implant insertion (0219T-0222T)*

37.4 37.4 **FUD** 090 C 80

AMA: 2020,May,13; 2018,Sep,7; 2018,May,3; 2018,Jan,8; 2017,Mar,7; 2017,Jan,8; 2016,Jan,13

▲ **22610** **thoracic (with lateral transverse technique, when performed)**

EXCLUDES *Posterior intrafacet implant insertion (0219T-0222T)*

36.7 36.7 **FUD** 090 C 80

AMA: 2020,May,13; 2018,Sep,7; 2018,May,3; 2018,Jan,8; 2017,Mar,7; 2017,Jan,8; 2016,Jan,13

▲ **22612** **lumbar (with lateral transverse technique, when performed)**

EXCLUDES *Arthrodesis at same interspace using:*
Posterior interbody technique in combination with posterior/posterolateral technique (22633)
Posterior interbody technique only (22630)
Posterior intrafacet implant insertion (0219T-0222T)

46.0 46.0 **FUD** 090 J J8 80

AMA: 2020,May,13; 2018,Sep,7; 2018,May,3; 2018,Jan,8; 2017,Mar,7; 2017,Feb,9; 2017,Jan,8; 2016,Jan,13

▲ + **22614** **each additional interspace (List separately in addition to code for primary procedure)**

EXCLUDES *Additional interspace athrodesis using:*
Posterior interbody technique in combination with posterior/posterolateral technique (22634)
Posterior interbody technique only (22632)
Posterior intrafacet implant insertion (0219T-0222T)

Code first initial interspace arthrodesis using posterior/posterolateral technique (22600, 22610, 22612)

Code first initial interspace athrodesis using posterior interbody technique in combination with posterior/posterolateral technique (22633)

Code first initial interspace athrodesis using posterior interbody technique (22630)

11.4 11.4 **FUD** ZZZ N N1 80

AMA: 2020,May,13; 2018,Sep,7; 2018,Jan,8; 2017,Feb,9; 2017,Jan,8; 2016,Jan,13

22630 **Arthrodesis, posterior interbody technique, including laminectomy and/or discectomy to prepare interspace (other than for decompression), single interspace; lumbar**

EXCLUDES *Athrodesis at same interspace using:*
Posterior/posterolateral technique in combination with posterior interbody technique (22633)
Posterior/posterolateral technique only (22612)

Code also decompression nerves or spinal components on same vertebral segment or interspace, when performed ([63052])

45.5 45.5 **FUD** 090 C 80

AMA: 2020,May,13; 2018,Sep,7; 2018,May,3; 2018,Jan,8; 2017,Mar,7; 2017,Feb,9; 2017,Jan,8; 2016,Jan,13

+ **22632** **each additional interspace (List separately in addition to code for primary procedure)**

EXCLUDES *Additional interspace athrodesis using:*
Posterior/posterolateral technique in combination with posterior interbody technique (22634)
Posterior/posterolateral technique only (22614)

Code also decompression nerves or spinal components on same vertebral segment or interspace, when performed ([63053])

Code first initial interspace athrodesis using posterior interbody technique (22630)

Code first initial interspace athrodesis using posterior/posterolateral technique (22612)

Code first initial interspace athrodesis using posterior/posterolateral technique in combination with posterior interbody technique (22633)

9.36 9.36 **FUD** ZZZ C 80

AMA: 2020,May,13; 2018,Sep,7; 2018,Jan,8; 2017,Feb,9; 2017,Jan,8; 2016,Jan,13

▲ **22633 Arthrodesis, combined posterior or posterolateral technique with posterior interbody technique including laminectomy and/or discectomy sufficient to prepare interspace (other than for decompression), single interspace; lumbar**

EXCLUDES *Athrodesis at same interspace using:*
Posterior/posterolateral technique only (22612)
Posterior interbody technique only (22630)

Code also decompression nerves or spinal components on same vertebral segment or interspace, when performed ([63052])

53.8 53.8 FUD 090 C 80

AMA: 2020,May,13; 2018,Sep,7; 2018,Jul,14; 2018,May,9; 2018,May,3; 2018,Jan,8; 2017,Mar,7; 2017,Feb,9; 2017,Jan,8; 2016,Oct,11; 2016,Jan,13

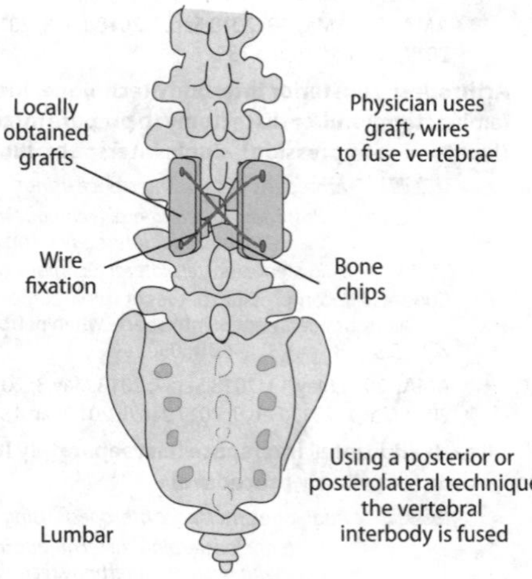
Locally obtained grafts
Physician uses graft, wires to fuse vertebrae
Wire fixation
Bone chips
Using a posterior or posterolateral technique the vertebral interbody is fused
Lumbar

▲ + **22634 each additional interspace and segment (List separately in addition to code for primary procedure)**

EXCLUDES *Additional interspace athrodesis using:*
Posterior/posterolateral technique only (22614)
Posterior interbody technique only (22632)

Code also decompression nerves or spinal components on same vertebral segment or interspace, when performed ([63053])

Code first (22633)

14.4 14.4 FUD ZZZ C 80

AMA: 2020,May,13; 2018,Sep,7; 2018,Jul,14; 2018,May,3; 2018,Jan,8; 2017,Mar,7; 2017,Feb,9; 2017,Jan,8; 2016,Jan,13

22800-22819 Procedures to Correct Anomalous Spinal Vertebrae

CMS: 100-03,150.2 Osteogenic Stimulation

EXCLUDES *Facet injection (64490-64495, [64633, 64634, 64635, 64636])*
Vertebral body tethering (0656T-0657T)

Code also:
Bone grafting procedures (20930-20938)
Modifier 62 when two surgeons perform distinct arthrodesis portion
Spinal instrumentation (22840-22855 [22859])

22800 Arthrodesis, posterior, for spinal deformity, with or without cast; up to 6 vertebral segments

39.3 39.3 FUD 090 C 80

AMA: 2020,May,13; 2018,Sep,7; 2018,May,3; 2018,Jan,8; 2017,Sep,14; 2017,Mar,7; 2017,Feb,9; 2017,Jan,8; 2016,Jan,13

22802 7 to 12 vertebral segments

61.0 61.0 FUD 090 C 80

AMA: 2020,May,13; 2018,Sep,7; 2018,Jul,14; 2018,May,3; 2018,Jan,8; 2017,Sep,14; 2017,Mar,7; 2017,Feb,9; 2017,Jan,8; 2016,Jan,13

22804 13 or more vertebral segments

70.3 70.3 FUD 090 C 80

AMA: 2020,May,13; 2018,Sep,7; 2018,May,3; 2018,Jan,8; 2017,Sep,14; 2017,Mar,7; 2017,Feb,9; 2017,Jan,8; 2016,Jan,13

22808 Arthrodesis, anterior, for spinal deformity, with or without cast; 2 to 3 vertebral segments

INCLUDES Smith-Robinson arthrodesis

53.1 53.1 FUD 090 C 80

AMA: 2020,May,13; 2018,Sep,7; 2018,May,3; 2018,Jan,8; 2017,Sep,14; 2017,Mar,7; 2017,Jan,8; 2016,Jan,13

22810 4 to 7 vertebral segments

60.2 60.2 FUD 090 C 80

AMA: 2020,May,13; 2018,Sep,7; 2018,May,3; 2018,Jan,8; 2017,Sep,14; 2017,Mar,7; 2017,Jan,8; 2016,Jan,13

22812 8 or more vertebral segments

63.9 63.9 FUD 090 C 80

AMA: 2020,May,13; 2018,Sep,7; 2018,May,3; 2018,Jan,8; 2017,Sep,14; 2017,Mar,7; 2017,Jan,8; 2016,Jan,13

22818 Kyphectomy, circumferential exposure of spine and resection of vertebral segment(s) (including body and posterior elements); single or 2 segments

EXCLUDES *Arthrodesis (22800-22804)*

62.6 62.6 FUD 090 C 80

AMA: 2020,May,13; 2018,Sep,7; 2018,Jan,8; 2017,Sep,14

22819 3 or more segments

EXCLUDES *Arthrodesis (22800-22804)*

72.2 72.2 FUD 090 C 80

AMA: 2020,May,13; 2018,Sep,7; 2018,Jan,8; 2017,Sep,14

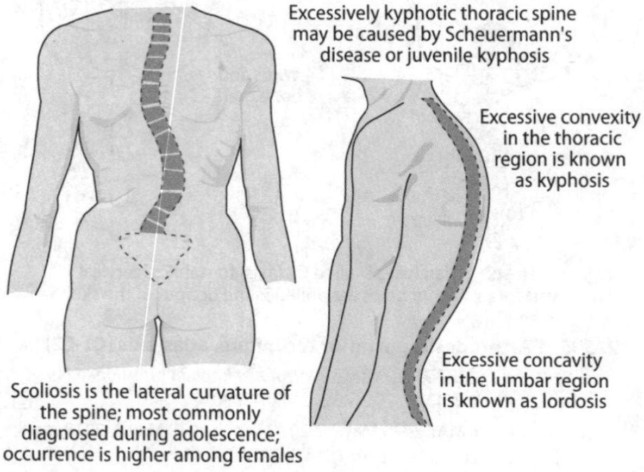
Excessively kyphotic thoracic spine may be caused by Scheuermann's disease or juvenile kyphosis
Excessive convexity in the thoracic region is known as kyphosis
Excessive concavity in the lumbar region is known as lordosis
Scoliosis is the lateral curvature of the spine; most commonly diagnosed during adolescence; occurrence is higher among females

22830 Surgical Exploration Previous Spinal Fusion

CMS: 100-03,150.2 Osteogenic Stimulation

EXCLUDES *Arthrodesis (22532-22819)*
Bone grafting procedures (20930-20938)
Instrumentation removal (22850, 22852, 22855)
Spinal decompression (63001-63103)

Code also spinal instrumentation (22840-22855 [22859])

22830 Exploration of spinal fusion

23.6 23.6 FUD 090 C 80

AMA: 2018,Sep,7; 2018,Jan,8; 2017,Jan,8; 2016,Jan,13

22840-22848 Posterior, Anterior, Pelvic Spinal Instrumentation

INCLUDES Removal or revision previously placed spinal instrumentation during same session as insertion new instrumentation at levels including all or part of previously instrumented segments (22849, 22850, 22852, 22855)

EXCLUDES *Arthrodesis (22532-22534, 22548-22812)*
Bone grafting procedures (20930-20938)
Exploration spinal fusion (22830)
Fracture treatment (22325-22328)
Reporting more than one instrumentation code per incision

\+ **22840** **Posterior non-segmental instrumentation (eg, Harrington rod technique, pedicle fixation across 1 interspace, atlantoaxial transarticular screw fixation, sublaminar wiring at C1, facet screw fixation) (List separately in addition to code for primary procedure)**

Code first (22100-22102, 22110-22114, 22206-22207, 22210-22214, 22220-22224, 22310-22327, 22532-22533, 22548-22558, 22590-22612, 22630, 22633-22634, 22800-22812, 63001-63030, 63040-63042, 63045-63047, 63050-63056, 63064, 63075, 63077, 63081, 63085, 63087, 63090, 63101-63102, 63170-63290, 63300-63307)

22.2 22.2 **FUD** ZZZ N N1 80

AMA: 2020,May,13; 2018,Sep,7; 2018,Jan,8; 2017,Jun,10; 2017,Feb,9; 2017,Jan,8; 2016,Jan,13

\+ **22841** **Internal spinal fixation by wiring of spinous processes (List separately in addition to code for primary procedure)**

Code first (22100-22102, 22110-22114, 22206-22207, 22210-22214, 22220-22224, 22310-22327, 22532-22533, 22548-22558, 22590-22612, 22630, 22633-22634, 22800-22812, 63001-63030, 63040-63042, 63045-63047, 63050-63056, 63064, 63075, 63077, 63081, 63085, 63087, 63090, 63101-63102, 63170-63290, 63300-63307)

0.00 0.00 **FUD** XXX C

AMA: 2020,May,13; 2018,Sep,7; 2018,Jan,8; 2017,Feb,9; 2017,Jan,8; 2016,Jan,13

\+ **22842** **Posterior segmental instrumentation (eg, pedicle fixation, dual rods with multiple hooks and sublaminar wires); 3 to 6 vertebral segments (List separately in addition to code for primary procedure)**

Code first (22100-22102, 22110-22114, 22206-22207, 22210-22214, 22220-22224, 22310-22327, 22532-22533, 22548-22558, 22590-22612, 22630, 22633-22634, 22800-22812, 63001-63030, 63040-63042, 63045-63047, 63050-63056, 63064, 63075, 63077, 63081, 63085, 63087, 63090, 63101-63102, 63170-63290, 63300-63307)

22.1 22.1 **FUD** ZZZ N N1 80

AMA: 2020,May,13; 2018,Sep,7; 2018,Jan,8; 2017,Feb,9; 2017,Jan,8; 2016,Jan,13

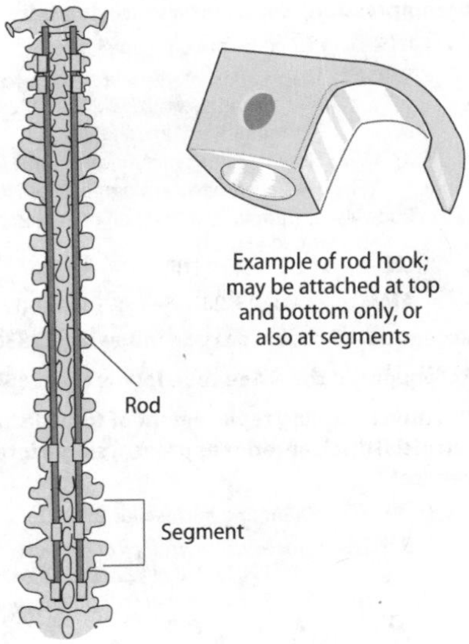

\+ **22843** **7 to 12 vertebral segments (List separately in addition to code for primary procedure)**

Code first (22100-22102, 22110-22114, 22206-22207, 22210-22214, 22220-22224, 22310-22327, 22532-22533, 22548-22558, 22590-22612, 22630, 22633-22634, 22800-22812, 63001-63030, 63040-63042, 63045-63047, 63050-63056, 63064, 63075, 63077, 63081, 63085, 63087, 63090, 63101-63102, 63170-63290, 63300-63307)

23.8 23.8 **FUD** ZZZ C 80

AMA: 2020,May,13; 2018,Sep,7; 2018,Jul,14; 2018,Jan,8; 2017,Jan,8; 2016,Jan,13

\+ **22844** **13 or more vertebral segments (List separately in addition to code for primary procedure)**

Code first (22100-22102, 22110-22114, 22206-22207, 22210-22214, 22220-22224, 22310-22327, 22532-22533, 22548-22558, 22590-22612, 22630, 22633-22634, 22800-22812, 63001-63030, 63040-63042, 63045-63047, 63050-63056, 63064, 63075, 63077, 63081, 63085, 63087, 63090, 63101-63102, 63170-63290, 63300-63307)

28.6 28.6 **FUD** ZZZ C 80

AMA: 2020,May,13; 2018,Sep,7; 2018,Jan,8; 2017,Jan,8; 2016,Jan,13

\+ **22845** **Anterior instrumentation; 2 to 3 vertebral segments (List separately in addition to code for primary procedure)**

INCLUDES Dwyer instrumentation technique

EXCLUDES *Vertebral body tethering (0656T)*

Code first (22100-22102, 22110-22114, 22206-22207, 22210-22214, 22220-22224, 22310-22327, 22532-22533, 22548-22558, 22590-22612, 22630, 22633-22634, 22800-22812, 63001-63030, 63040-63042, 63045-63047, 63050-63056, 63064, 63075, 63077, 63081, 63085, 63087, 63090, 63101-63102, 63170-63290, 63300-63307)

21.1 21.1 **FUD** ZZZ N N1 80

AMA: 2020,May,13; 2018,Sep,7; 2018,Jan,8; 2017,Mar,7; 2017,Jan,8; 2016,May,13; 2016,Jan,13

\+ **22846** **4 to 7 vertebral segments (List separately in addition to code for primary procedure)**

INCLUDES Dwyer instrumentation technique

EXCLUDES *Vertebral body tethering (0656T)*

Code first (22100-22102, 22110-22114, 22206-22207, 22210-22214, 22220-22224, 22310-22327, 22532-22533, 22548-22558, 22590-22612, 22630, 22633-22634, 22800-22812, 63001-63030, 63040-63042, 63045-63047, 63050-63056, 63064, 63075, 63077, 63081, 63085, 63087, 63090, 63101-63102, 63170-63290, 63300-63307)

22.0 22.0 **FUD** ZZZ C 80

AMA: 2020,May,13; 2018,Sep,7; 2018,Jan,8; 2017,Jan,8; 2016,May,13; 2016,Jan,13

\+ **22847** **8 or more vertebral segments (List separately in addition to code for primary procedure)**

INCLUDES Dwyer instrumentation technique

EXCLUDES *Vertebral body tethering (0657T)*

Code first (22100-22102, 22110-22114, 22206-22207, 22210-22214, 22220-22224, 22310-22327, 22532-22533, 22548-22558, 22590-22612, 22630, 22633-22634, 22800-22812, 63001-63030, 63040-63042, 63045-63047, 63050-63056, 63064, 63075, 63077, 63081, 63085, 63087, 63090, 63101-63102, 63170-63290, 63300-63307)

23.4 23.4 **FUD** ZZZ C 80

AMA: 2020,May,13; 2018,Sep,7; 2018,Jan,8; 2017,Jan,8; 2016,May,13; 2016,Jan,13

\+ **22848** **Pelvic fixation (attachment of caudal end of instrumentation to pelvic bony structures) other than sacrum (List separately in addition to code for primary procedure)**

Code first (22100-22102, 22110-22114, 22206-22207, 22210-22214, 22220-22224, 22310-22327, 22532-22533, 22548-22558, 22590-22612, 22630, 22633-22634, 22800-22812, 63001-63030, 63040-63042, 63045-63047, 63050-63056, 63064, 63075, 63077, 63081, 63085, 63087, 63090, 63101-63102, 63170-63290, 63300-63307)

10.4 10.4 **FUD** ZZZ C 80

AMA: 2020,May,13; 2018,Sep,7; 2018,Jan,8; 2017,Jan,8; 2016,Jan,13

22849-22855 [22859] Miscellaneous Spinal Instrumentation

EXCLUDES *Arthrodesis (22532-22534, 22548-22812)*
Bone grafting procedures (20930-20938)
Exploration spinal fusion (22830)
Facet injection (64490-64495, [64633, 64634, 64635, 64636])
Fracture treatment (22325-22328)

22849 Reinsertion of spinal fixation device

INCLUDES Removal of instrumentation at the same level (22850, 22852, 22855)

37.7 37.7 FUD 090 C 80

AMA: 2020,May,13; 2018,Sep,7; 2018,Jan,8; 2017,Jun,10; 2017,Jan,8; 2016,May,13; 2016,Jan,13

22850 Removal of posterior nonsegmental instrumentation (eg, Harrington rod)

21.0 21.0 FUD 090 C 80

AMA: 2020,May,13; 2018,Sep,7; 2018,Jan,8; 2017,Jun,10; 2017,Jan,8; 2016,May,13; 2016,Jan,13

22852 Removal of posterior segmental instrumentation

20.2 20.2 FUD 090 C 80

AMA: 2020,May,13; 2018,Sep,7; 2018,Jan,8; 2017,Jun,10; 2017,Jan,8; 2016,Jan,13

+ **22853 Insertion of interbody biomechanical device(s) (eg, synthetic cage, mesh) with integral anterior instrumentation for device anchoring (eg, screws, flanges), when performed, to intervertebral disc space in conjunction with interbody arthrodesis, each interspace (List separately in addition to code for primary procedure)**

Code also:
Intervertebral bone device/graft application (20930-20931, 20936-20938)
Subsequent disc spaces undergoing device insertion when disc spaces are not connected (22853-22854, [22859])

Code first (22100-22102, 22110-22114, 22206-22207, 22210-22214, 22220-22224, 22310-22327, 22532-22533, 22548-22558, 22590-22612, 22630, 22633-22634, 22800-22812, 63001-63030, 63040, 63042, 63045-63047, 63050-63056, 63064, 63075, 63077, 63081, 63085, 63087, 63090, 63101-63102, 63170-63290, 63300-63307)

7.52 7.52 FUD ZZZ N N1 80

AMA: 2020,May,13; 2018,Sep,7; 2018,Jul,14; 2018,Jan,8; 2017,Aug,9; 2017,Mar,7

+ **22854 Insertion of intervertebral biomechanical device(s) (eg, synthetic cage, mesh) with integral anterior instrumentation for device anchoring (eg, screws, flanges), when performed, to vertebral corpectomy(ies) (vertebral body resection, partial or complete) defect, in conjunction with interbody arthrodesis, each contiguous defect (List separately in addition to code for primary procedure)**

Code also:
Intervertebral bone device/graft application (20930-20931, 20936-20938)
Subsequent disc spaces undergoing device insertion when disc spaces are not connected (22853-22854, [22859])

Code first (22100-22102, 22110-22114, 22206-22207, 22210-22214, 22220-22224, 22310-22327, 22532-22533, 22548-22558, 22590-22612, 22630, 22633-22634, 22800-22812, 63001-63030, 63040, 63042, 63045-63047, 63050-63056, 63064, 63075, 63077, 63081, 63085, 63087, 63090, 63101-63102, 63170-63290, 63300-63307)

9.74 9.74 FUD ZZZ N N1 80

AMA: 2020,May,13; 2018,Sep,7; 2018,Jan,8; 2017,Mar,7

+ # **22859 Insertion of intervertebral biomechanical device(s) (eg, synthetic cage, mesh, methylmethacrylate) to intervertebral disc space or vertebral body defect without interbody arthrodesis, each contiguous defect (List separately in addition to code for primary procedure)**

Code also:
Intervertebral bone device/graft application (20930-20931, 20936-20938)
Subsequent disc spaces undergoing device insertion when disc spaces are not connected (22853-22854, [22859])

Code first (22100-22102, 22110-22114, 22206-22207, 22210-22214, 22220-22224, 22310-22327, 22532-22533, 22548-22558, 22590-22612, 22630, 22633-22634, 22800-22812, 63001-63030, 63040-63042, 63045-63047, 63050-63056, 63064, 63075, 63077, 63081, 63085, 63087, 63090, 63101-63102, 63170-63290, 63300-63307)

9.74 9.74 FUD ZZZ N N1 80

AMA: 2020,May,13; 2018,Sep,7; 2018,Jan,8; 2017,Mar,7

22855 Removal of anterior instrumentation

32.1 32.1 FUD 090 C 80

AMA: 2020,May,13; 2018,Sep,7; 2018,Jan,8; 2017,Jun,10; 2017,Jan,8; 2016,Jan,13

22856-22865 [22858, 22859] Artificial Disc Replacement

EXCLUDES *Fluoroscopy*
Spinal decompression (63001-63048)

22856 Total disc arthroplasty (artificial disc), anterior approach, including discectomy with end plate preparation (includes osteophytectomy for nerve root or spinal cord decompression and microdissection); single interspace, cervical

INCLUDES Operating microscope (69990)

EXCLUDES *Application intervertebral biomechanical device(s) at same level (22853-22854, [22859])*
Arthrodesis at same level (22554)
Discectomy at same level (63075)
Insertion instrumentation at same level (22845)

Code also arthroplasty more than one interspace, when performed ([22858])

47.3 47.3 FUD 090 J J8 80

AMA: 2020,May,13; 2018,Sep,7; 2018,Jan,8; 2017,Jan,8; 2016,Feb,12; 2016,Jan,13

+ # **22858 second level, cervical (List separately in addition to code for primary procedure)**

Code first (22856)

14.8 14.8 FUD ZZZ N N1 80

AMA: 2020,May,13; 2018,Sep,7; 2018,Jan,8; 2017,Jan,8; 2016,Feb,12; 2016,Jan,13

22857 Total disc arthroplasty (artificial disc), anterior approach, including discectomy to prepare interspace (other than for decompression), single interspace, lumbar

INCLUDES Operating microscope (69990)

EXCLUDES *Application intervertebral biomechanical device(s) at same level (22853-22854, [22859])*
Arthrodesis at same level (22558)
Insertion instrumentation at same level (22845)
Retroperitoneal exploration (49010)

Code also arthroplasty more than one interspace, when performed (0163T)

51.4 51.4 FUD 090 C 80

AMA: 2020,May,13; 2018,Sep,7; 2016,Feb,12

22858 **Resequenced code. See code following 22856.**

22859 **Resequenced code. See code following 22854.**

22861 Revision including replacement of total disc arthroplasty (artificial disc), anterior approach, single interspace; cervical

INCLUDES Operating microscope (69990)

EXCLUDES *Procedures performed at same level (22845, 22853-22854, [22859], 22864, 63075)*
Revision additional cervical arthroplasty (0098T)

66.9 66.9 FUD 090 C 80

AMA: 2020,May,13; 2018,Sep,7; 2016,Feb,12

22862 **lumbar**

EXCLUDES *Arthroplasty revision more than one interspace (0165T)*
Procedures performed at same level (22558, 22845, 22853-22854, [22859], 22865, 49010)

66.8 66.8 FUD 090 C 80

AMA: 2020,May,13; 2018,Sep,7; 2018,Jan,8; 2017,Jan,8; 2016,Jan,13

22864 **Removal of total disc arthroplasty (artificial disc), anterior approach, single interspace; cervical**

INCLUDES Operating microscope (69990)

EXCLUDES *Cervical total disc arthroplasty with additional interspace removal (0095T)*
Revision total disc arthroplasty (22861)

59.7 59.7 FUD 090 C 80

AMA: 2020,May,13; 2018,Sep,7

22865 **lumbar**

EXCLUDES *Arthroplasty more than one level (0164T)*
Exploration, retroperitoneal area with or without biopsy(s) (49010)

65.1 65.1 FUD 090 C 80

AMA: 2020,May,13; 2018,Sep,7; 2018,Jan,8; 2017,Jan,8; 2016,Jan,13

22867-22899 Spinal Distraction/Stabilization Device

22867 **Insertion of interlaminar/interspinous process stabilization/distraction device, without fusion, including image guidance when performed, with open decompression, lumbar; single level**

EXCLUDES *Interlaminar/interspinous stabilization/distraction device insertion (22869, 22870)*
Procedures at same level (22532-22534, 22558, 22612, 22614, 22630, 22632-22634, 22800, 22802, 22804, 22840-22842, 22869-22870, 63005, 63012, 63017, 63030, 63035, 63042, 63044, 63047-63048, 77003)

28.2 28.2 FUD 090 J J8 80

AMA: 2020,May,13; 2018,Sep,7; 2018,Jan,8; 2017,Feb,9

+ **22868** **second level (List separately in addition to code for primary procedure)**

EXCLUDES *Interlaminar/interspinous stabilization/distraction device insertion (22869-22870)*
Procedures at same level (22532-22534, 22558, 22612, 22614, 22630, 22632-22634, 22800, 22802, 22804, 22840-22842, 22869-22870, 63005, 63012, 63017, 63030, 63035, 63042, 63044, 63047-63048, 77003)

Code first (22867)

7.08 7.08 FUD ZZZ N N1 80

AMA: 2020,May,13; 2018,Sep,7; 2018,Jan,8; 2017,Feb,9

22869 **Insertion of interlaminar/interspinous process stabilization/distraction device, without open decompression or fusion, including image guidance when performed, lumbar; single level**

EXCLUDES *Procedures at the same level (22532-22534, 22558, 22612, 22614, 22630, 22632-22634, 22800, 22802, 22804, 22840-22842, 63005, 63012, 63017, 63030, 63035, 63042, 63044, 63047-63048, 77003)*

12.8 12.8 FUD 090 J J8 80

AMA: 2020,May,13; 2018,Sep,7; 2018,Jan,8; 2017,Feb,9

+ **22870** **second level (List separately in addition to code for primary procedure)**

EXCLUDES *Procedures at the same level (22532-22534, 22558, 22612, 22614, 22630, 22632-22634, 22800, 22802, 22804, 22840-22842, 63005, 63012, 63017, 63030, 63035, 63042, 63044, 63047-63048, 77003)*

Code first (22869)

3.62 3.62 FUD ZZZ N N1 80

AMA: 2020,May,13; 2018,Sep,7; 2018,Jan,8; 2017,Feb,9

22899 **Unlisted procedure, spine**

0.00 0.00 FUD YYY T 80

AMA: 2020,Jun,14; 2018,Sep,7; 2018,May,10; 2018,Jan,8; 2017,Feb,9; 2017,Jan,8; 2016,Jan,13

22900-22999 Musculoskeletal Procedures of Abdomen

INCLUDES Any necessary elevation tissue planes or dissection
Measurement tumor and necessary margin at greatest diameter prior to excision
Simple and intermediate repairs
Excision types:
Fascial or subfascial soft tissue tumors: simple and marginal resection tumors found either in or below deep fascia, not involving bone or excision substantial amount normal tissue; primarily benign and intramuscular tumors
Radical resection soft tissue tumor: wide resection tumor involving substantial margins normal tissue and may include tissue removal from one or more layers; most often malignant or aggressive benign
Subcutaneous: simple and marginal resection tumors in subcutaneous tissue above deep fascia; most often benign

EXCLUDES *Complex repair*
Excision benign cutaneous lesions (eg, sebaceous cyst) (11400-11406)
Radical resection cutaneous tumors (eg, melanoma) (11600-11606)
Significant vessel exploration or neuroplasty

22900 **Excision, tumor, soft tissue of abdominal wall, subfascial (eg, intramuscular); less than 5 cm**

16.3 16.3 FUD 090 J G2 80

AMA: 2018,Sep,7

22901 **5 cm or greater**

19.3 19.3 FUD 090 J G2 80

AMA: 2018,Sep,7

22902 **Excision, tumor, soft tissue of abdominal wall, subcutaneous; less than 3 cm**

9.57 13.1 FUD 090 J G2 80

AMA: 2018,Sep,7

22903 **3 cm or greater**

12.6 12.6 FUD 090 J G2 80

AMA: 2018,Sep,7

22904 **Radical resection of tumor (eg, sarcoma), soft tissue of abdominal wall; less than 5 cm**

30.5 30.5 FUD 090 J G2 80

AMA: 2018,Sep,7

22905 **5 cm or greater**

38.5 38.5 FUD 090 J G2 80

AMA: 2018,Sep,7

22999 **Unlisted procedure, abdomen, musculoskeletal system**

0.00 0.00 FUD YYY T 80

AMA: 2018,Sep,7

23000-23044 Surgical Incision Shoulder: Drainage, Foreign Body Removal, Contracture Release

23000 **Removal of subdeltoid calcareous deposits, open**

EXCLUDES *Arthroscopic removal calcium deposits bursa (29999)*

10.5 16.4 FUD 090 J A2 80 50

AMA: 2018,Sep,7

23020 **Capsular contracture release (eg, Sever type procedure)**

EXCLUDES *Simple incision and drainage (10040-10160)*

19.9 19.9 FUD 090 J A2 80 50

AMA: 2018,Sep,7

23030 **Incision and drainage, shoulder area; deep abscess or hematoma**

7.20 12.4 FUD 010 J A2

AMA: 2018,Sep,7

23031 **infected bursa**
6.01 11.5 **FUD** 010 J A2 50
AMA: 2018,Sep,7

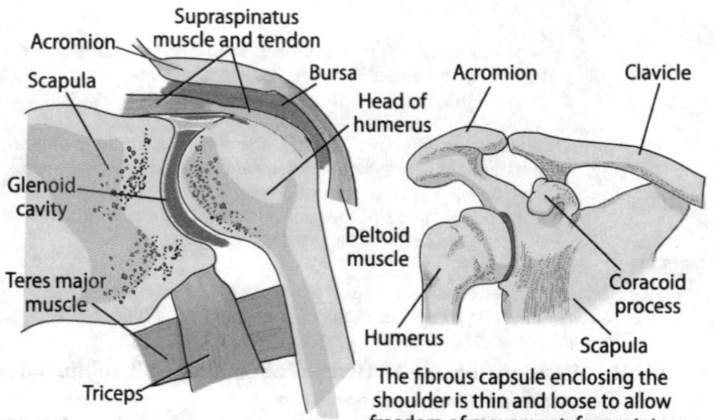

Section of left shoulder

The fibrous capsule enclosing the shoulder is thin and loose to allow freedom of movement; four rotator cuff muscles (supraspinatous, infraspinatous, teres minor, and scapularis) work together to hold the head of the humerus in the glenoid cavity

23035 **Incision, bone cortex (eg, osteomyelitis or bone abscess), shoulder area**
19.6 19.6 **FUD** 090 J A2 80 50
AMA: 2018,Sep,7

23040 **Arthrotomy, glenohumeral joint, including exploration, drainage, or removal of foreign body**
20.7 20.7 **FUD** 090 J A2 80 50
AMA: 2018,Sep,7

23044 **Arthrotomy, acromioclavicular, sternoclavicular joint, including exploration, drainage, or removal of foreign body**
16.3 16.3 **FUD** 090 J A2 50
AMA: 2018,Sep,7

23065-23066 Shoulder Biopsy

EXCLUDES *Soft tissue needle biopsy (20206)*

23065 **Biopsy, soft tissue of shoulder area; superficial**
4.81 6.34 **FUD** 010 J P3 50
AMA: 2018,Sep,7

23066 **deep**
10.4 16.2 **FUD** 090 J A2 50
AMA: 2018,Sep,7

23071-23078 [23071, 23073] Excision Soft Tissue Tumors of Shoulder

INCLUDES Any necessary elevation tissue planes or dissection
Measurement tumor and necessary margin at greatest diameter prior to excision
Simple and intermediate repairs
Excision types:
Fascial or subfascial soft tissue tumors: simple and marginal resection tumors found either in or below deep fascia, not involving bone or excision substantial amount normal tissue; primarily benign and intramuscular tumors
Radical resection soft tissue tumor: wide resection tumor, involving substantial margins normal tissue and may involve tissue removal from one or more layers; most often malignant or aggressive benign
Subcutaneous: simple and marginal resection tumors in subcutaneous tissue above deep fascia; most often benign

EXCLUDES *Complex repair*
Excision benign cutaneous lesions (eg, sebaceous cyst) (11400-11406)
Radical resection cutaneous tumors (eg, melanoma) (11600-11606)
Significant vessel exploration or neuroplasty

23071 **Resequenced code. See code following 23075.**

23073 **Resequenced code. See code following 23076.**

23075 **Excision, tumor, soft tissue of shoulder area, subcutaneous; less than 3 cm**
9.44 14.3 **FUD** 090 J G2 50
AMA: 2018,Sep,7; 2018,Jan,8; 2017,Jan,8; 2016,Jan,13

\# **23071** **3 cm or greater**
12.1 12.1 **FUD** 090 J G2 80 50
AMA: 2018,Sep,7

23076 **Excision, tumor, soft tissue of shoulder area, subfascial (eg, intramuscular); less than 5 cm**
15.6 15.6 **FUD** 090 J G2 50
AMA: 2018,Sep,7; 2018,Jan,8; 2017,Jan,8; 2016,Jan,13

\# **23073** **5 cm or greater**
20.1 20.1 **FUD** 090 J G2 80 50
AMA: 2018,Sep,7

23077 **Radical resection of tumor (eg, sarcoma), soft tissue of shoulder area; less than 5 cm**
32.7 32.7 **FUD** 090 J R2 80 50
AMA: 2018,Sep,7

23078 **5 cm or greater**
41.4 41.4 **FUD** 090 J G2 80 50
AMA: 2018,Sep,7

23100-23195 Bone and Joint Procedures of Shoulder

INCLUDES Acromioclavicular joint
Clavicle
Head and neck of humerus
Scapula
Shoulder joint
Sternoclavicular joint

23100 **Arthrotomy, glenohumeral joint, including biopsy**
14.5 14.5 **FUD** 090 J A2 80 50
AMA: 2018,Sep,7

23101 **Arthrotomy, acromioclavicular joint or sternoclavicular joint, including biopsy and/or excision of torn cartilage**
13.1 13.1 **FUD** 090 J A2 50
AMA: 2018,Sep,7

23105 **Arthrotomy; glenohumeral joint, with synovectomy, with or without biopsy**
18.3 18.3 **FUD** 090 J A2 80 50
AMA: 2018,Sep,7

23106 **sternoclavicular joint, with synovectomy, with or without biopsy**
14.3 14.3 **FUD** 090 J A2 50
AMA: 2018,Sep,7

23107 **Arthrotomy, glenohumeral joint, with joint exploration, with or without removal of loose or foreign body**
19.0 19.0 **FUD** 090 J A2 80 50
AMA: 2018,Sep,7

23120 **Claviculectomy; partial**
INCLUDES Mumford operation
EXCLUDES *Arthroscopic claviculectomy (29824)*
16.8 16.8 **FUD** 090 J A2 80 50
AMA: 2018,Sep,7; 2018,Jan,8; 2017,Jan,8; 2016,Jan,13

23125 **total**
20.4 20.4 **FUD** 090 J A2 80 50
AMA: 2018,Sep,7

23130 **Acromioplasty or acromionectomy, partial, with or without coracoacromial ligament release**
17.6 17.6 **FUD** 090 J A2 50
AMA: 2018,Sep,7; 2018,Jan,8; 2017,Jan,8; 2016,Jan,13

23140 **Excision or curettage of bone cyst or benign tumor of clavicle or scapula;**
15.9 15.9 **FUD** 090 J A2 50
AMA: 2018,Sep,7

23145 **with autograft (includes obtaining graft)**
20.0 20.0 **FUD** 090 J A2 80 50
AMA: 2018,Sep,7

23146 **with allograft**
17.9 17.9 **FUD** 090 J A2 80 50
AMA: 2019,May,7; 2018,Sep,7

23150 **Excision or curettage of bone cyst or benign tumor of proximal humerus;**
19.2 19.2 **FUD** 090 J A2 80 50
AMA: 2018,Sep,7

23155 **with autograft (includes obtaining graft)**
22.7 22.7 **FUD** 090 J A2 80 50
AMA: 2018,Sep,7

23156 **with allograft**
19.4 19.4 **FUD** 090 J A2 80 50
AMA: 2019,May,7; 2018,Sep,7

23170 **Sequestrectomy (eg, for osteomyelitis or bone abscess), clavicle**
16.2 16.2 **FUD** 090 J A2 50
AMA: 2018,Sep,7

23172 **Sequestrectomy (eg, for osteomyelitis or bone abscess), scapula**
16.3 16.3 **FUD** 090 J A2 80 50
AMA: 2018,Sep,7

23174 **Sequestrectomy (eg, for osteomyelitis or bone abscess), humeral head to surgical neck**
21.9 21.9 **FUD** 090 J A2 80 50
AMA: 2018,Sep,7

23180 **Partial excision (craterization, saucerization, or diaphysectomy) bone (eg, osteomyelitis), clavicle**
19.1 19.1 **FUD** 090 J A2 50
AMA: 2018,Sep,7

23182 **Partial excision (craterization, saucerization, or diaphysectomy) bone (eg, osteomyelitis), scapula**
19.0 19.0 **FUD** 090 J A2 80 50
AMA: 2018,Sep,7

23184 **Partial excision (craterization, saucerization, or diaphysectomy) bone (eg, osteomyelitis), proximal humerus**
21.1 21.1 **FUD** 090 J A2 80 50
AMA: 2018,Sep,7

23190 **Ostectomy of scapula, partial (eg, superior medial angle)**
16.5 16.5 **FUD** 090 J A2 80 50
AMA: 2018,Sep,7

23195 **Resection, humeral head**
EXCLUDES *Arthroplasty with replacement with implant (23470)*
21.5 21.5 **FUD** 090 J A2 80 50
AMA: 2018,Sep,7

23200-23220 Radical Resection of Bone Tumors of Shoulder

INCLUDES Any necessary elevation tissue planes or dissection
Excision adjacent soft tissue during bone tumor resection (23071-23078 [23071, 23073])
Measurement tumor and necessary margin at greatest diameter prior to excision
Radical resection cutaneous tumors (e.g., melanoma)
Resection tumor (may include entire bone) and wide margins normal tissues primarily for malignant or aggressive benign tumors
Simple and intermediate repairs

EXCLUDES *Complex repair*
Significant vessel exploration, neuroplasty, reconstruction, or complex bone repair

23200 **Radical resection of tumor; clavicle**
43.6 43.6 **FUD** 090 C 80 50
AMA: 2019,May,7; 2018,Sep,7

23210 **scapula**
51.2 51.2 **FUD** 090 C 80 50
AMA: 2019,May,7; 2018,Sep,7

23220 **Radical resection of tumor, proximal humerus**
56.3 56.3 **FUD** 090 C 80 50
AMA: 2019,May,7; 2018,Sep,7

23330-23335 Removal Implant/Foreign Body from Shoulder

EXCLUDES *Bursal arthrocentesis or needling (20610)*
K-wire or pin insertion (20650)
K-wire or pin removal (20670, 20680)

23330 **Removal of foreign body, shoulder; subcutaneous**
4.76 8.00 **FUD** 010 T A2 80 50
AMA: 2018,Sep,7; 2018,Jan,8; 2017,Jan,8; 2016,Jan,13

23333 **deep (subfascial or intramuscular)**
13.2 13.2 **FUD** 090 J G2 80 50
AMA: 2018,Sep,7; 2018,Jan,8; 2017,Jan,8; 2016,Jan,13

23334 **Removal of prosthesis, includes debridement and synovectomy when performed; humeral or glenoid component**
EXCLUDES *Foreign body removal (23330, 23333)*
Prosthesis removal and replacement in same shoulder (eg, glenoid and/or humeral components) (23473-23474)
30.8 30.8 **FUD** 090 J G2 50
AMA: 2018,Sep,7; 2018,Jan,8; 2017,Jan,8; 2016,Jan,13

23335 **humeral and glenoid components (eg, total shoulder)**
EXCLUDES *Foreign body removal (23330, 23333)*
Prosthesis removal and replacement in same shoulder (eg, glenoid and/or humeral components) (23473-23474)
36.7 36.7 **FUD** 090 C 50
AMA: 2018,Sep,7; 2018,Jan,8; 2017,Jan,8; 2016,Jan,13

23350 Injection for Shoulder Arthrogram

23350 **Injection procedure for shoulder arthrography or enhanced CT/MRI shoulder arthrography**
EXCLUDES *Shoulder biopsy (29805-29826)*
(73040, 73201-73202, 73222-73223, 77002)
1.47 3.97 **FUD** 000 N N1 50
AMA: 2018,Sep,7; 2018,Jan,8; 2017,Jan,8; 2016,May,13; 2016,Jan,13

23395-23491 Repair/Reconstruction of Shoulder

23395 **Muscle transfer, any type, shoulder or upper arm; single**
37.0 37.0 **FUD** 090 J A2 80
AMA: 2018,Sep,7

23397 **multiple**
32.9 32.9 **FUD** 090 J A2 80
AMA: 2018,Sep,7

23400 **Scapulopexy (eg, Sprengels deformity or for paralysis)**
28.0 28.0 **FUD** 090 J A2 80 50
AMA: 2018,Sep,7

23405 **Tenotomy, shoulder area; single tendon**
17.8 17.8 **FUD** 090 J A2 80
AMA: 2018,Sep,7

23406 **multiple tendons through same incision**
22.2 22.2 **FUD** 090 J A2 80
AMA: 2018,Sep,7

23410 **Repair of ruptured musculotendinous cuff (eg, rotator cuff) open; acute**
EXCLUDES *Arthroscopic repair (29827)*
23.6 23.6 **FUD** 090 J A2 80 50
AMA: 2018,Sep,7; 2018,Jan,8; 2017,Jan,8; 2016,Jan,13

23412 **chronic**
EXCLUDES *Arthroscopic repair (29827)*
24.5 24.5 **FUD** 090 J A2 80 50
AMA: 2018,Sep,7; 2018,Jan,8; 2017,Jan,8; 2016,Jan,13

23415 **Coracoacromial ligament release, with or without acromioplasty**
EXCLUDES *Arthroscopic repair (29826)*
20.1 20.1 **FUD** 090 J A2 50
AMA: 2018,Sep,7; 2018,Jan,8; 2017,Jan,8; 2016,Jan,13

23420 Reconstruction of complete shoulder (rotator) cuff avulsion, chronic (includes acromioplasty)
28.0 28.0 FUD 090 J A2 80 50
AMA: 2018,Sep,7; 2018,Jan,8; 2017,Jan,8; 2016,Jan,13

23430 Tenodesis of long tendon of biceps
EXCLUDES *Arthroscopic biceps tenodesis (29828)*
21.4 21.4 FUD 090 J A2 80 50
AMA: 2018,Sep,7

23440 Resection or transplantation of long tendon of biceps
21.7 21.7 FUD 090 J A2 80 50
AMA: 2018,Sep,7

23450 Capsulorrhaphy, anterior; Putti-Platt procedure or Magnuson type operation
EXCLUDES *Arthroscopic thermal capsulorrhaphy (29999)*
27.3 27.3 FUD 090 J J8 80 50
AMA: 2018,Sep,7

23455 with labral repair (eg, Bankart procedure)
EXCLUDES *Arthroscopic repair (29806)*
28.7 28.7 FUD 090 J J8 80 50
AMA: 2018,Sep,7

23460 Capsulorrhaphy, anterior, any type; with bone block
INCLUDES Bristow procedure
31.5 31.5 FUD 090 J A2 80 50
AMA: 2018,Sep,7

23462 with coracoid process transfer
EXCLUDES *Open thermal capsulorrhaphy (23929)*
30.9 30.9 FUD 090 J A2 80 50
AMA: 2018,Sep,7

23465 Capsulorrhaphy, glenohumeral joint, posterior, with or without bone block
EXCLUDES *Sternoclavicular and acromioclavicular joint repair (23530, 23550)*
32.3 32.3 FUD 090 J G2 80 50
AMA: 2018,Sep,7

23466 Capsulorrhaphy, glenohumeral joint, any type multi-directional instability
32.0 32.0 FUD 090 J A2 80 50
AMA: 2018,Sep,7

23470 Arthroplasty, glenohumeral joint; hemiarthroplasty
34.7 34.7 FUD 090 J J8 80 50
AMA: 2018,Sep,7; 2018,Jan,8; 2017,Jan,8; 2016,Jan,13

23472 total shoulder (glenoid and proximal humeral replacement (eg, total shoulder))
EXCLUDES *Proximal humerus osteotomy (24400)*
Removal total shoulder components (23334-23335)
41.9 41.9 FUD 090 C 80 50
AMA: 2018,Sep,7; 2018,Jan,8; 2017,Jan,8; 2016,Jan,13

23473 Revision of total shoulder arthroplasty, including allograft when performed; humeral or glenoid component
EXCLUDES *Removal prosthesis only (glenoid and/or humeral component) same shoulder/same operative sessions (23334-23335)*
46.7 46.7 FUD 090 J J8 80 50
AMA: 2018,Sep,7; 2018,Jan,8; 2017,Jan,8; 2016,Jan,13

23474 humeral and glenoid component
EXCLUDES *Removal prosthesis only (glenoid and/or humeral component) same shoulder/same operative sessions (23334-23335)*
50.5 50.5 FUD 090 C 80 50
AMA: 2018,Sep,7; 2018,Jan,8; 2017,Jan,8; 2016,Jan,13

23480 Osteotomy, clavicle, with or without internal fixation;
23.7 23.7 FUD 090 J A2 50
AMA: 2018,Sep,7

23485 with bone graft for nonunion or malunion (includes obtaining graft and/or necessary fixation)
27.6 27.6 FUD 090 J J8 80 50
AMA: 2018,Sep,7

23490 Prophylactic treatment (nailing, pinning, plating or wiring) with or without methylmethacrylate; clavicle
24.6 24.6 FUD 090 J A2 80 50
AMA: 2018,Sep,7

23491 proximal humerus
29.3 29.3 FUD 090 J J8 80 50
AMA: 2018,Sep,7

23500-23680 Treatment of Shoulder Fracture/Dislocation

23500 Closed treatment of clavicular fracture; without manipulation
6.37 6.24 FUD 090 T A2 50
AMA: 2018,Sep,7

23505 with manipulation
9.61 10.2 FUD 090 J A2 50
AMA: 2018,Sep,7

23515 Open treatment of clavicular fracture, includes internal fixation, when performed
20.7 20.7 FUD 090 J J8 80 50
AMA: 2018,Sep,7; 2018,Jan,8; 2017,Jan,8; 2016,Jan,13

23520 Closed treatment of sternoclavicular dislocation; without manipulation
6.73 6.72 FUD 090 J A2 80 50
AMA: 2018,Sep,7

23525 with manipulation
10.2 11.1 FUD 090 T A2 80 50
AMA: 2018,Sep,7

23530 Open treatment of sternoclavicular dislocation, acute or chronic;
16.5 16.5 FUD 090 J A2 80 50
AMA: 2018,Sep,7

23532 with fascial graft (includes obtaining graft)
17.7 17.7 FUD 090 J J8 80 50
AMA: 2018,Sep,7

23540 Closed treatment of acromioclavicular dislocation; without manipulation
6.64 6.67 FUD 090 T A2 50
AMA: 2018,Sep,7

23545 with manipulation
8.93 9.91 FUD 090 T A2 80 50
AMA: 2018,Sep,7

23550 Open treatment of acromioclavicular dislocation, acute or chronic;
16.3 16.3 FUD 090 J A2 80 50
AMA: 2018,Sep,7

23552 with fascial graft (includes obtaining graft)
18.8 18.8 FUD 090 J J8 80 50
AMA: 2019,Nov,14; 2018,Sep,7

23570 Closed treatment of scapular fracture; without manipulation
6.89 6.69 FUD 090 T A2 50
AMA: 2018,Sep,7

23575 with manipulation, with or without skeletal traction (with or without shoulder joint involvement)
10.8 11.6 FUD 090 J A2 80 50
AMA: 2018,Sep,7

23585 Open treatment of scapular fracture (body, glenoid or acromion) includes internal fixation, when performed
28.2 28.2 FUD 090 J A2 80 50
AMA: 2018,Sep,7; 2018,Jan,8; 2017,Jan,8; 2016,Jan,13

23600 Closed treatment of proximal humeral (surgical or anatomical neck) fracture; without manipulation
8.92 9.45 FUD 090 T P2 50
AMA: 2018,Sep,7

23605 with manipulation, with or without skeletal traction
12.2 13.4 FUD 090 J A2 50
AMA: 2018,Sep,7

23615 Open treatment of proximal humeral (surgical or anatomical neck) fracture, includes internal fixation, when performed, includes repair of tuberosity(s), when performed;
25.5 25.5 FUD 090 J J8 80 50
AMA: 2018,Sep,7; 2018,Jan,8; 2017,Jan,8; 2016,Jan,13

23616 with proximal humeral prosthetic replacement
35.7 35.7 FUD 090 J J8 80 50
AMA: 2018,Sep,7

23620 Closed treatment of greater humeral tuberosity fracture; without manipulation
7.32 7.65 FUD 090 T P2 50
AMA: 2018,Sep,7

23625 with manipulation
10.1 10.9 FUD 090 J A2 50
AMA: 2018,Sep,7

23630 Open treatment of greater humeral tuberosity fracture, includes internal fixation, when performed
22.4 22.4 FUD 090 J A2 80 50
AMA: 2018,Sep,7

23650 Closed treatment of shoulder dislocation, with manipulation; without anesthesia
8.36 9.18 FUD 090 T A2 50
AMA: 2018,Sep,7

23655 requiring anesthesia
11.5 11.5 FUD 090 J A2 50
AMA: 2018,Sep,7

23660 Open treatment of acute shoulder dislocation
EXCLUDES *Chronic dislocation repair (23450-23466)*
16.8 16.8 FUD 090 J A2 80 50
AMA: 2018,Sep,7; 2018,Jan,8; 2017,Jan,8; 2016,Jan,13

23665 Closed treatment of shoulder dislocation, with fracture of greater humeral tuberosity, with manipulation
11.4 12.3 FUD 090 J A2 50
AMA: 2019,Feb,10; 2018,Sep,7

23670 Open treatment of shoulder dislocation, with fracture of greater humeral tuberosity, includes internal fixation, when performed
25.2 25.2 FUD 090 J A2 80 50
AMA: 2018,Sep,7

23675 Closed treatment of shoulder dislocation, with surgical or anatomical neck fracture, with manipulation
14.4 15.9 FUD 090 J A2 50
AMA: 2018,Sep,7

23680 Open treatment of shoulder dislocation, with surgical or anatomical neck fracture, includes internal fixation, when performed
26.7 26.7 FUD 090 J J8 80 50
AMA: 2018,Sep,7

23700-23929 Other/Unlisted Shoulder Procedures

23700 Manipulation under anesthesia, shoulder joint, including application of fixation apparatus (dislocation excluded)
5.63 5.63 FUD 010 J A2 50
AMA: 2018,Sep,7; 2018,Jan,8; 2017,Jan,8; 2016,Jan,13

23800 Arthrodesis, glenohumeral joint;
29.6 29.6 FUD 090 J G2 80 50
AMA: 2020,May,13; 2018,Sep,7

23802 with autogenous graft (includes obtaining graft)
37.0 37.0 FUD 090 J G2 80 50
AMA: 2020,May,13; 2018,Sep,7

23900 Interthoracoscapular amputation (forequarter)
40.0 40.0 FUD 090 C 80
AMA: 2018,Sep,7

23920 Disarticulation of shoulder;
32.4 32.4 FUD 090 C 80 50
AMA: 2018,Sep,7

23921 secondary closure or scar revision
13.5 13.5 FUD 090 T A2 50
AMA: 2018,Sep,7

23929 Unlisted procedure, shoulder
0.00 0.00 FUD YYY T 80
AMA: 2018,Sep,7

23930-24006 Surgical Incision Elbow/Upper Arm

EXCLUDES *Simple incision and drainage procedures (10040-10160)*

23930 Incision and drainage, upper arm or elbow area; deep abscess or hematoma
6.12 10.2 FUD 010 J A2 50
AMA: 2018,Sep,7

23931 bursa
4.48 8.19 FUD 010 J A2 50
AMA: 2018,Sep,7

23935 Incision, deep, with opening of bone cortex (eg, for osteomyelitis or bone abscess), humerus or elbow
14.7 14.7 FUD 090 J A2 80 50
AMA: 2018,Sep,7

24000 Arthrotomy, elbow, including exploration, drainage, or removal of foreign body
13.7 13.7 FUD 090 J A2 80 50
AMA: 2018,Sep,7

24006 Arthrotomy of the elbow, with capsular excision for capsular release (separate procedure)
20.5 20.5 FUD 090 J A2 80 50
AMA: 2018,Sep,7

24065-24066 Biopsy of Elbow/Upper Arm

EXCLUDES *Soft tissue needle biopsy (20206)*

24065 Biopsy, soft tissue of upper arm or elbow area; superficial
4.71 7.41 FUD 010 J P3 50
AMA: 2018,Sep,7

24066 deep (subfascial or intramuscular)
12.0 18.0 FUD 090 J A2 50
AMA: 2018,Sep,7

24071-24079 [24071, 24073] Excision Soft Tissue Tumors Elbow/Upper Arm

INCLUDES Any necessary elevation tissue planes or dissection
Measurement tumor and necessary margin at greatest diameter prior to excision
Excision types:
Fascial or subfascial soft tissue tumors: simple and marginal resection tumors found either in or below deep fascia, not involving bone or excision substantial amount normal tissue; primarily benign and intramuscular tumors
Radical resection soft tissue tumor: wide resection tumor involving substantial margins normal tissue and may involve tissue removal from one or more layers; most often malignant or aggressive benign
Subcutaneous: simple and marginal resection tumors found in subcutaneous tissue above deep fascia; most often benign

EXCLUDES *Complex repair*
Excision benign cutaneous lesion (eg, sebaceous cyst) (11400-11406)
Radical resection cutaneous tumors (eg, melanoma) (11600-11606)
Significant vessel exploration or neuroplasty

24071 Resequenced code. See code following 24075.

24073 Resequenced code. See code following 24076.

24075 Excision, tumor, soft tissue of upper arm or elbow area, subcutaneous; less than 3 cm
9.47 14.8 FUD 090 J G2 50
AMA: 2018,Sep,7

24071 3 cm or greater
11.7 11.7 FUD 090 J G2 80 50
AMA: 2018,Sep,7

24076 Excision, tumor, soft tissue of upper arm or elbow area, subfascial (eg, intramuscular); less than 5 cm
15.6 15.6 FUD 090 J G2 50
AMA: 2018,Sep,7

\# **24073 5 cm or greater**
19.9 19.9 FUD 090 J G2 80 50
AMA: 2018,Sep,7

24077 Radical resection of tumor (eg, sarcoma), soft tissue of upper arm or elbow area; less than 5 cm
29.9 29.9 FUD 090 J G2 50
AMA: 2018,Sep,7

24079 5 cm or greater
38.3 38.3 FUD 090 J G2 80 50
AMA: 2018,Sep,7

24100-24149 Bone/Joint Procedures Upper Arm/Elbow

24100 Arthrotomy, elbow; with synovial biopsy only
12.0 12.0 FUD 090 J A2 80 50
AMA: 2018,Sep,7

24101 with joint exploration, with or without biopsy, with or without removal of loose or foreign body
14.4 14.4 FUD 090 J A2 80 50
AMA: 2018,Sep,7

24102 with synovectomy
17.7 17.7 FUD 090 J A2 80 50
AMA: 2018,Sep,7

24105 Excision, olecranon bursa
10.1 10.1 FUD 090 J A2 50
AMA: 2018,Sep,7

24110 Excision or curettage of bone cyst or benign tumor, humerus;
16.8 16.8 FUD 090 J A2 50
AMA: 2018,Sep,7

24115 with autograft (includes obtaining graft)
21.2 21.2 FUD 090 J A2 80 50
AMA: 2018,Sep,7

24116 with allograft
24.8 24.8 FUD 090 J A2 80 50
AMA: 2019,May,7; 2018,Sep,7

24120 Excision or curettage of bone cyst or benign tumor of head or neck of radius or olecranon process;
15.3 15.3 FUD 090 J A2 80 50
AMA: 2018,Sep,7

24125 with autograft (includes obtaining graft)
17.9 17.9 FUD 090 J A2 80 50
AMA: 2018,Sep,7

24126 with allograft
18.7 18.7 FUD 090 J J8 80 50
AMA: 2019,May,7; 2018,Sep,7

24130 Excision, radial head
EXCLUDES *Radial head arthroplasty with implant (24366)*
14.6 14.6 FUD 090 J A2 50
AMA: 2018,Sep,7

24134 Sequestrectomy (eg, for osteomyelitis or bone abscess), shaft or distal humerus
21.4 21.4 FUD 090 J A2 80 50
AMA: 2018,Sep,7

24136 Sequestrectomy (eg, for osteomyelitis or bone abscess), radial head or neck
18.2 18.2 FUD 090 J A2 50
AMA: 2018,Sep,7

24138 Sequestrectomy (eg, for osteomyelitis or bone abscess), olecranon process
19.6 19.6 FUD 090 J A2 80 50
AMA: 2018,Sep,7

24140 Partial excision (craterization, saucerization, or diaphysectomy) bone (eg, osteomyelitis), humerus
20.2 20.2 FUD 090 J A2 80 50
AMA: 2018,Sep,7

24145 Partial excision (craterization, saucerization, or diaphysectomy) bone (eg, osteomyelitis), radial head or neck
17.1 17.1 FUD 090 J A2 50
AMA: 2018,Sep,7

24147 Partial excision (craterization, saucerization, or diaphysectomy) bone (eg, osteomyelitis), olecranon process
17.9 17.9 FUD 090 J A2 50
AMA: 2018,Sep,7

24149 Radical resection of capsule, soft tissue, and heterotopic bone, elbow, with contracture release (separate procedure)
EXCLUDES *Capsular and soft tissue release (24006)*
33.8 33.8 FUD 090 J G2 80 50
AMA: 2018,Sep,7

24150-24152 Radical Resection Bone Tumor Upper Arm

INCLUDES Any necessary elevation tissue planes or dissection
Excision adjacent soft tissue during bone tumor resection (24071-24079 [24071, 24073])
Measurement tumor and necessary margin at greatest diameter prior to excision
Resection tumor (may include entire bone) and wide margins normal tissue primarily for malignant or aggressive benign tumors
Simple and intermediate repairs

EXCLUDES *Complex repair*
Significant vessel exploration, neuroplasty, reconstruction, or complex bone repair

24150 Radical resection of tumor, shaft or distal humerus
44.8 44.8 FUD 090 J G2 80 50
AMA: 2019,May,7; 2018,Sep,7

24152 Radical resection of tumor, radial head or neck
38.9 38.9 FUD 090 J G2 80 50
AMA: 2019,May,7; 2018,Sep,7

24155 Elbow Arthrectomy

24155 Resection of elbow joint (arthrectomy)
24.6 24.6 FUD 090 J A2 80 50
AMA: 2018,Sep,7

24160-24201 Removal Implant/Foreign Body from Elbow/Upper Arm

EXCLUDES *Bursal or joint arthrocentesis or needling (20605)*
K-wire or pin insertion (20650)
K-wire or pin removal (20670, 20680)

24160 Removal of prosthesis, includes debridement and synovectomy when performed; humeral and ulnar components
INCLUDES Prosthesis removal and replacement in same elbow (eg, humeral and/or ulnar component(s)) (24370-24371)
EXCLUDES *Foreign body removal (24200-24201)*
Hardware removal other than prosthesis (20680)
36.3 36.3 FUD 090 Q2 A2 50
AMA: 2018,Sep,7; 2018,Jan,8; 2017,Jan,8; 2016,Jan,13

24164 radial head
EXCLUDES *Foreign body removal (24200-24201)*
Hardware removal other than prosthesis (20680)
20.8 20.8 FUD 090 Q2 A2 50
AMA: 2018,Sep,7; 2018,Jan,8; 2017,Jan,8; 2016,Jan,13

24200 Removal of foreign body, upper arm or elbow area; subcutaneous
4.05 6.20 FUD 010 J P3 80 50
AMA: 2018,Sep,7; 2018,Jan,8; 2017,Jan,8; 2016,Jan,13

24201 deep (subfascial or intramuscular)
10.4 15.8 FUD 090 J A2 50
AMA: 2018,Sep,7; 2018,Jan,8; 2017,Jan,8; 2016,Jan,13

24220 Injection for Elbow Arthrogram

24220 Injection procedure for elbow arthrography

EXCLUDES *Injection tennis elbow (20550)*

(73085)

1.95 4.71 FUD 000 N N1 80 50

AMA: 2018,Sep,7; 2018,Jan,8; 2017,Jan,8; 2016,May,13; 2016,Jan,13

24300-24498 Repair/Reconstruction of Elbow/Upper Arm

24300 Manipulation, elbow, under anesthesia

EXCLUDES *External fixation (20690, 20692)*

12.0 12.0 FUD 090 J G2 50

AMA: 2018,Sep,7

24301 Muscle or tendon transfer, any type, upper arm or elbow, single (excluding 24320-24331)

21.6 21.6 FUD 090 J A2 80

AMA: 2018,Sep,7

24305 Tendon lengthening, upper arm or elbow, each tendon

16.7 16.7 FUD 090 J A2 80

AMA: 2018,Sep,7

24310 Tenotomy, open, elbow to shoulder, each tendon

13.4 13.4 FUD 090 J A2 80

AMA: 2018,Sep,7

24320 Tenoplasty, with muscle transfer, with or without free graft, elbow to shoulder, single (Seddon-Brookes type procedure)

22.5 22.5 FUD 090 J A2 80

AMA: 2018,Sep,7

24330 Flexor-plasty, elbow (eg, Steindler type advancement);

20.7 20.7 FUD 090 J A2 80 50

AMA: 2018,Sep,7

24331 with extensor advancement

22.7 22.7 FUD 090 J A2 80 50

AMA: 2018,Sep,7

24332 Tenolysis, triceps

17.6 17.6 FUD 090 J G2 50

AMA: 2018,Sep,7

24340 Tenodesis of biceps tendon at elbow (separate procedure)

17.7 17.7 FUD 090 J A2 80 50

AMA: 2018,Sep,7

24341 Repair, tendon or muscle, upper arm or elbow, each tendon or muscle, primary or secondary (excludes rotator cuff)

21.4 21.4 FUD 090 J A2 80 50

AMA: 2018,Sep,7

24342 Reinsertion of ruptured biceps or triceps tendon, distal, with or without tendon graft

22.3 22.3 FUD 090 J A2 80 50

AMA: 2018,Sep,7; 2018,Jan,8; 2017,Apr,9

24343 Repair lateral collateral ligament, elbow, with local tissue

20.4 20.4 FUD 090 J G2 80 50

AMA: 2018,Sep,7

24344 Reconstruction lateral collateral ligament, elbow, with tendon graft (includes harvesting of graft)

31.5 31.5 FUD 090 J J8 80 50

AMA: 2018,Sep,7

24345 Repair medial collateral ligament, elbow, with local tissue

20.2 20.2 FUD 090 J A2 80 50

AMA: 2018,Sep,7

24346 Reconstruction medial collateral ligament, elbow, with tendon graft (includes harvesting of graft)

31.7 31.7 FUD 090 J G2 80 50

AMA: 2018,Sep,7

24357 Tenotomy, elbow, lateral or medial (eg, epicondylitis, tennis elbow, golfer's elbow); percutaneous

EXCLUDES *Arthroscopy, elbow, surgical; debridement (29837-29838)*

11.9 11.9 FUD 090 J G2 80 50

AMA: 2018,Sep,7; 2018,Jan,8; 2017,Jan,8; 2016,Jan,13

24358 debridement, soft tissue and/or bone, open

EXCLUDES *Arthroscopy, elbow, surgical; debridement (29837-29838)*

15.1 15.1 FUD 090 J G2 80 50

AMA: 2018,Sep,7; 2018,Jan,8; 2017,Jan,8; 2016,Jan,13

24359 debridement, soft tissue and/or bone, open with tendon repair or reattachment

EXCLUDES *Arthroscopy, elbow, surgical; debridement (29837-29838)*

19.0 19.0 FUD 090 J G2 80 50

AMA: 2018,Sep,7; 2018,Jan,8; 2017,Jan,8; 2016,Jan,13

24360 Arthroplasty, elbow; with membrane (eg, fascial)

26.0 26.0 FUD 090 J J8 80 50

AMA: 2018,Sep,7

24361 with distal humeral prosthetic replacement

29.1 29.1 FUD 090 J J8 80 50

AMA: 2018,Sep,7

24362 with implant and fascia lata ligament reconstruction

30.6 30.6 FUD 090 J J8 80 50

AMA: 2018,Sep,7

24363 with distal humerus and proximal ulnar prosthetic replacement (eg, total elbow)

EXCLUDES *Total elbow implant revision (24370-24371)*

41.9 41.9 FUD 090 J J8 80 50

AMA: 2018,Sep,7; 2018,Jan,8; 2017,Jan,8; 2016,Jan,13

24365 Arthroplasty, radial head;

18.4 18.4 FUD 090 J J8 80 50

AMA: 2018,Sep,7

24366 with implant

19.6 19.6 FUD 090 J J8 80 50

AMA: 2018,Sep,7

24370 Revision of total elbow arthroplasty, including allograft when performed; humeral or ulnar component

EXCLUDES *Prosthesis removal without replacement in same elbow (eg, humeral and/or ulnar component/s) (24160)*

44.7 44.7 FUD 090 J J8 80 50

AMA: 2018,Sep,7; 2018,Jan,8; 2017,Jan,8; 2016,Jan,13

24371 humeral and ulnar component

EXCLUDES *Prosthesis removal without replacement in same elbow (eg, humeral and/or ulnar component/s) (24160)*

51.3 51.3 FUD 090 J J8 80 50

AMA: 2018,Sep,7; 2018,Jan,8; 2017,Jan,8; 2016,Jan,13

24400 Osteotomy, humerus, with or without internal fixation

EXCLUDES *Osteotomy with insertion intramedullary lengthening device, humerus (0594T)*

23.7 23.7 FUD 090 J A2 80 50

AMA: 2018,Sep,7; 2018,Jan,8; 2017,Jan,8; 2016,Jan,13

24410 Multiple osteotomies with realignment on intramedullary rod, humeral shaft (Sofield type procedure)

EXCLUDES *Osteotomy with insertion intramedullary lengthening device, humerus (0594T)*

30.5 30.5 FUD 090 J G2 80 50

AMA: 2018,Sep,7

24420 Osteoplasty, humerus (eg, shortening or lengthening) (excluding 64876)

EXCLUDES *Osteotomy with insertion intramedullary lengthening device, humerus (0594T)*

29.5 29.5 FUD 090 J A2 80 50

AMA: 2018,Sep,7

Musculoskeletal System

24220 — 24420

24430 **Repair of nonunion or malunion, humerus; without graft (eg, compression technique)**

EXCLUDES *Repair proximal radius and/or ulna (25400-25420)*

30.4 30.4 FUD 090 J J8 80 50

AMA: 2018,Sep,7

24435 **with iliac or other autograft (includes obtaining graft)**

EXCLUDES *Repair proximal radius and/or ulna (25400-25420)*

31.0 31.0 FUD 090 J J8 80 50

AMA: 2018,Sep,7

24470 **Hemiepiphyseal arrest (eg, cubitus varus or valgus, distal humerus)**

19.3 19.3 FUD 090 J A2 80 50

AMA: 2018,Sep,7

24495 **Decompression fasciotomy, forearm, with brachial artery exploration**

21.3 21.3 FUD 090 J A2 80 50

AMA: 2018,Sep,7

24498 **Prophylactic treatment (nailing, pinning, plating or wiring), with or without methylmethacrylate, humeral shaft**

24.9 24.9 FUD 090 J J8 80 50

AMA: 2018,Sep,7

24500-24685 Treatment of Fracture/Dislocation of Elbow/Upper Arm

INCLUDES Treatment for either closed or open fractures or dislocations

24500 **Closed treatment of humeral shaft fracture; without manipulation**

9.35 10.2 FUD 090 T A2 50

AMA: 2018,Sep,7

24505 **with manipulation, with or without skeletal traction**

12.9 14.3 FUD 090 J A2 50

AMA: 2018,Sep,7

24515 **Open treatment of humeral shaft fracture with plate/screws, with or without cerclage**

25.3 25.3 FUD 090 J J8 80 50

AMA: 2018,Sep,7

24516 **Treatment of humeral shaft fracture, with insertion of intramedullary implant, with or without cerclage and/or locking screws**

EXCLUDES *Osteotomy with insertion intramedullary lengthening device, humerus (0594T)*

24.7 24.7 FUD 090 J J8 80 50

AMA: 2018,Sep,7; 2018,Jan,8; 2018,Jan,3; 2017,Jan,8; 2016,Jan,13

24530 **Closed treatment of supracondylar or transcondylar humeral fracture, with or without intercondylar extension; without manipulation**

9.96 10.9 FUD 090 T A2 50

AMA: 2018,Sep,7

24535 **with manipulation, with or without skin or skeletal traction**

16.3 17.6 FUD 090 J A2 50

AMA: 2018,Sep,7

24538 **Percutaneous skeletal fixation of supracondylar or transcondylar humeral fracture, with or without intercondylar extension**

21.5 21.5 FUD 090 J A2 50

AMA: 2018,Sep,7; 2018,Jan,8; 2017,Jan,8; 2016,Jan,13

24545 **Open treatment of humeral supracondylar or transcondylar fracture, includes internal fixation, when performed; without intercondylar extension**

26.7 26.7 FUD 090 J J8 80 50

AMA: 2018,Sep,7

24546 **with intercondylar extension**

29.9 29.9 FUD 090 J J8 80 50

AMA: 2018,Sep,7

24560 **Closed treatment of humeral epicondylar fracture, medial or lateral; without manipulation**

8.41 9.43 FUD 090 T A2 50

AMA: 2018,Sep,7

24565 **with manipulation**

14.1 15.3 FUD 090 J A2 50

AMA: 2018,Sep,7

24566 **Percutaneous skeletal fixation of humeral epicondylar fracture, medial or lateral, with manipulation**

20.6 20.6 FUD 090 J A2 50

AMA: 2018,Sep,7

24575 **Open treatment of humeral epicondylar fracture, medial or lateral, includes internal fixation, when performed**

21.0 21.0 FUD 090 J J8 80 50

AMA: 2018,Sep,7

24576 **Closed treatment of humeral condylar fracture, medial or lateral; without manipulation**

8.75 9.80 FUD 090 T A2 50

AMA: 2018,Sep,7

24577 **with manipulation**

14.4 15.8 FUD 090 J A2 50

AMA: 2018,Sep,7

24579 **Open treatment of humeral condylar fracture, medial or lateral, includes internal fixation, when performed**

EXCLUDES *Closed treatment without manipulation (24530, 24560, 24576, 24650, 24670)*

Repair with manipulation (24535, 24565, 24577, 24675)

24.0 24.0 FUD 090 J J8 80 50

AMA: 2018,Sep,7

24582 **Percutaneous skeletal fixation of humeral condylar fracture, medial or lateral, with manipulation**

23.3 23.3 FUD 090 J A2 50

AMA: 2018,Sep,7

24586 **Open treatment of periarticular fracture and/or dislocation of the elbow (fracture distal humerus and proximal ulna and/or proximal radius);**

31.2 31.2 FUD 090 J G2 80 50

AMA: 2018,Sep,7

24587 **with implant arthroplasty**

EXCLUDES *Distal humerus arthroplasty with implant (24361)*

31.4 31.4 FUD 090 J J8 80 50

AMA: 2018,Sep,7

24600 **Treatment of closed elbow dislocation; without anesthesia**

9.71 10.6 FUD 090 T A2 50

AMA: 2018,Sep,7

24605 **requiring anesthesia**

13.5 13.5 FUD 090 J A2 50

AMA: 2018,Sep,7

24615 **Open treatment of acute or chronic elbow dislocation**

20.6 20.6 FUD 090 J A2 80 50

AMA: 2018,Sep,7

24620 **Closed treatment of Monteggia type of fracture dislocation at elbow (fracture proximal end of ulna with dislocation of radial head), with manipulation**

15.8 15.8 FUD 090 J A2 80 50

AMA: 2018,Sep,7

24635 **Open treatment of Monteggia type of fracture dislocation at elbow (fracture proximal end of ulna with dislocation of radial head), includes internal fixation, when performed**

19.3 19.3 FUD 090 J J8 80 50

AMA: 2018,Sep,7

24640 **Closed treatment of radial head subluxation in child, nursemaid elbow, with manipulation** A

2.26 2.89 FUD 010 T P3 80 50

AMA: 2018,Sep,7

24650 **Closed treatment of radial head or neck fracture; without manipulation**
6.96 7.51 **FUD** 090 T P2 50
AMA: 2018,Sep,7

24655 **with manipulation**
11.4 12.6 **FUD** 090 J A2 50
AMA: 2018,Sep,7

24665 **Open treatment of radial head or neck fracture, includes internal fixation or radial head excision, when performed;**
18.8 18.8 **FUD** 090 J A2 80 50
AMA: 2018,Sep,7

24666 **with radial head prosthetic replacement**
21.1 21.1 **FUD** 090 J J8 80 50
AMA: 2018,Sep,7

24670 **Closed treatment of ulnar fracture, proximal end (eg, olecranon or coronoid process[es]); without manipulation**
7.53 8.28 **FUD** 090 T A2 50
AMA: 2018,Sep,7

24675 **with manipulation**
11.9 13.1 **FUD** 090 J A2 50
AMA: 2018,Sep,7

24685 **Open treatment of ulnar fracture, proximal end (eg, olecranon or coronoid process[es]), includes internal fixation, when performed**
EXCLUDES *Arthrotomy, elbow (24100-24102)*
18.8 18.8 **FUD** 090 J J8 80 50
AMA: 2018,Sep,7; 2018,Jan,3

24800-24999 Other/Unlisted Elbow/Upper Arm Procedures

24800 **Arthrodesis, elbow joint; local**
23.9 23.9 **FUD** 090 J A2 80 50
AMA: 2020,May,13; 2018,Sep,7

24802 **with autogenous graft (includes obtaining graft)**
28.9 28.9 **FUD** 090 J G2 80 50
AMA: 2020,May,13; 2018,Sep,7

24900 **Amputation, arm through humerus; with primary closure**
21.3 21.3 **FUD** 090 C 80 50
AMA: 2018,Sep,7

24920 **open, circular (guillotine)**
21.1 21.1 **FUD** 090 C 80 50
AMA: 2018,Sep,7

24925 **secondary closure or scar revision**
16.3 16.3 **FUD** 090 J A2 80 50
AMA: 2018,Sep,7

24930 **re-amputation**
22.3 22.3 **FUD** 090 C 80 50
AMA: 2018,Sep,7

24931 **with implant**
26.9 26.9 **FUD** 090 C 80 50
AMA: 2020,NovBULL,2; 2018,Sep,7

24935 **Stump elongation, upper extremity**
33.6 33.6 **FUD** 090 J G2 80 50
AMA: 2018,Sep,7

24940 **Cineplasty, upper extremity, complete procedure**
0.00 0.00 **FUD** 090 C 80 50
AMA: 2018,Sep,7

24999 **Unlisted procedure, humerus or elbow**
0.00 0.00 **FUD** YYY T 80 50
AMA: 2018,Sep,7

25000-25001 Incision Tendon Sheath of Wrist

25000 **Incision, extensor tendon sheath, wrist (eg, deQuervains disease)**
EXCLUDES *Carpal tunnel release (64721)*
9.70 9.70 **FUD** 090 J A2 50
AMA: 2018,Sep,7

25001 **Incision, flexor tendon sheath, wrist (eg, flexor carpi radialis)**
9.88 9.88 **FUD** 090 J G2 50
AMA: 2018,Sep,7

25020-25025 Decompression Fasciotomy Forearm/Wrist

25020 **Decompression fasciotomy, forearm and/or wrist, flexor OR extensor compartment; without debridement of nonviable muscle and/or nerve**
EXCLUDES *Brachial artery exploration (24495)*
Superficial incision and drainage (10060-10160)
16.4 16.4 **FUD** 090 J A2 50
AMA: 2018,Sep,7

25023 **with debridement of nonviable muscle and/or nerve**
EXCLUDES *Debridement (11000-11044 [11045, 11046])*
Decompression fasciotomy with exploration brachial artery exploration (24495)
Superficial incision and drainage (10060-10160)
34.4 34.4 **FUD** 090 J A2 80 50
AMA: 2018,Sep,7

25024 **Decompression fasciotomy, forearm and/or wrist, flexor AND extensor compartment; without debridement of nonviable muscle and/or nerve**
22.5 22.5 **FUD** 090 J A2 50
AMA: 2018,Sep,7

25025 **with debridement of nonviable muscle and/or nerve**
34.8 34.8 **FUD** 090 J A2 80 50
AMA: 2018,Sep,7

25028-25040 Incision for Drainage/Foreign Body Removal

25028 **Incision and drainage, forearm and/or wrist; deep abscess or hematoma**
17.0 17.0 **FUD** 090 J A2 50
AMA: 2018,Sep,7

25031 **bursa**
10.0 10.0 **FUD** 090 J A2 80 50
AMA: 2018,Sep,7

25035 **Incision, deep, bone cortex, forearm and/or wrist (eg, osteomyelitis or bone abscess)**
16.8 16.8 **FUD** 090 J A2 80 50
AMA: 2018,Sep,7

25040 **Arthrotomy, radiocarpal or midcarpal joint, with exploration, drainage, or removal of foreign body**
16.1 16.1 **FUD** 090 J A2 80 50
AMA: 2018,Sep,7

25065-25066 Biopsy Forearm/Wrist

EXCLUDES *Soft tissue needle biopsy (20206)*

25065 **Biopsy, soft tissue of forearm and/or wrist; superficial**
4.59 7.37 **FUD** 010 J P3 50
AMA: 2018,Sep,7

25066 **deep (subfascial or intramuscular)**
10.3 10.3 **FUD** 090 J A2 50
AMA: 2018,Sep,7

25071-25078 [25071, 25073] Excision Soft Tissue Tumors Forearm/Wrist

INCLUDES Any necessary elevation tissue planes or dissection
Measurement tumor and necessary margin at greatest diameter prior to excision
Simple and intermediate repairs
Excision types:
Fascial or subfascial soft tissue tumors: simple and marginal resection tumors found either in or below deep fascia, not involving bone or excision substantial amount normal tissue; primarily benign and intramuscular tumors
Radical resection soft tissue tumor: wide resection tumor involving substantial margins normal tissue and may include tissue removal from one or more layers; most often malignant or aggressive benign
Subcutaneous: simple and marginal resection tumors in subcutaneous tissue above deep fascia; most often benign

EXCLUDES *Complex repair*
Excision benign cutaneous lesions (eg, sebaceous cyst) (11400-11406)
Radical resection cutaneous tumors (eg, melanoma) (11600-11606)
Significant vessel exploration or neuroplasty

25071 **Resequenced code. See code following 25075.**

25073 **Resequenced code. See code following 25076.**

25075 **Excision, tumor, soft tissue of forearm and/or wrist area, subcutaneous; less than 3 cm**
9.09 14.5 FUD 090 J G2 50
AMA: 2018,Sep,7

\# 25071 **3 cm or greater**
12.2 12.2 FUD 090 J G2 80 50
AMA: 2018,Sep,7

25076 **Excision, tumor, soft tissue of forearm and/or wrist area, subfascial (eg, intramuscular); less than 3 cm**
14.9 14.9 FUD 090 J G2 50
AMA: 2018,Sep,7

\# 25073 **3 cm or greater**
15.4 15.4 FUD 090 J G2 80 50
AMA: 2018,Sep,7

25077 **Radical resection of tumor (eg, sarcoma), soft tissue of forearm and/or wrist area; less than 3 cm**
25.6 25.6 FUD 090 J G2 50
AMA: 2018,Sep,7

25078 **3 cm or greater**
33.6 33.6 FUD 090 J G2 80 50
AMA: 2018,Sep,7

25085-25240 Procedures of Bones/Joints Lower Arm/Wrist

25085 **Capsulotomy, wrist (eg, contracture)**
12.9 12.9 FUD 090 J A2 80 50
AMA: 2018,Sep,7

25100 **Arthrotomy, wrist joint; with biopsy**
10.0 10.0 FUD 090 J A2 80 50
AMA: 2018,Sep,7

25101 **with joint exploration, with or without biopsy, with or without removal of loose or foreign body**
11.6 11.6 FUD 090 J A2 80 50
AMA: 2018,Sep,7

25105 **with synovectomy**
13.9 13.9 FUD 090 J A2 80 50
AMA: 2018,Sep,7

25107 **Arthrotomy, distal radioulnar joint including repair of triangular cartilage, complex**
17.7 17.7 FUD 090 J A2 80 50
AMA: 2018,Sep,7

25109 **Excision of tendon, forearm and/or wrist, flexor or extensor, each**
15.4 15.4 FUD 090 J G2 50
AMA: 2018,Sep,7

25110 **Excision, lesion of tendon sheath, forearm and/or wrist**
9.84 9.84 FUD 090 J A2 50
AMA: 2018,Sep,7

25111 **Excision of ganglion, wrist (dorsal or volar); primary**
EXCLUDES *Excision ganglion hand or finger (26160)*
9.24 9.24 FUD 090 J A2 50
AMA: 2018,Sep,7

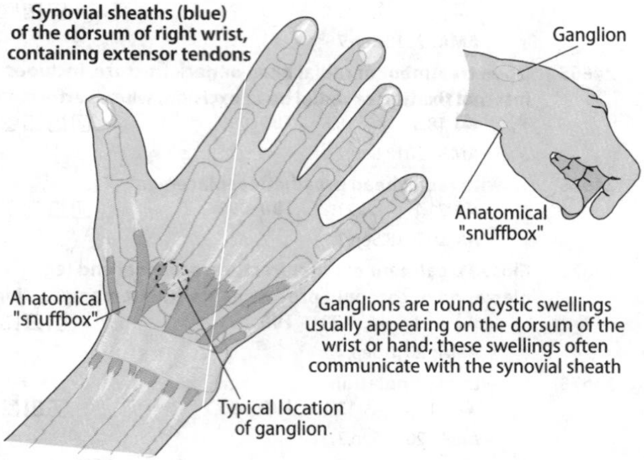

25112 **recurrent**
EXCLUDES *Excision ganglion hand or finger (26160)*
11.1 11.1 FUD 090 J A2 50
AMA: 2018,Sep,7

25115 **Radical excision of bursa, synovia of wrist, or forearm tendon sheaths (eg, tenosynovitis, fungus, Tbc, or other granulomas, rheumatoid arthritis); flexors**
EXCLUDES *Finger synovectomy (26145)*
21.8 21.8 FUD 090 J A2 50
AMA: 2018,Sep,7; 2018,Jan,8; 2017,Jan,8; 2016,Jan,13

25116 **extensors, with or without transposition of dorsal retinaculum**
EXCLUDES *Finger synovectomy (26145)*
17.3 17.3 FUD 090 J A2 80 50
AMA: 2018,Sep,7

25118 **Synovectomy, extensor tendon sheath, wrist, single compartment;**
EXCLUDES *Finger synovectomy (26145)*
10.9 10.9 FUD 090 J A2 50
AMA: 2018,Sep,7; 2018,Jan,8; 2017,Jan,8; 2016,Jan,13

25119 **with resection of distal ulna**
EXCLUDES *Finger synovectomy (26145)*
14.2 14.2 FUD 090 J A2 80 50
AMA: 2018,Sep,7

25120 **Excision or curettage of bone cyst or benign tumor of radius or ulna (excluding head or neck of radius and olecranon process);**
EXCLUDES *Removal bone cyst or tumor radial head, neck, or olecranon process (24120-24126)*
14.4 14.4 FUD 090 J A2 80 50
AMA: 2018,Sep,7

25125 **with autograft (includes obtaining graft)**
16.9 16.9 FUD 090 J A2 80 50
AMA: 2018,Sep,7

25126 **with allograft**
17.2 17.2 FUD 090 J A2 80 50
AMA: 2019,May,7; 2018,Sep,7

25130 **Excision or curettage of bone cyst or benign tumor of carpal bones;**
12.9 12.9 FUD 090 J A2 80 50
AMA: 2018,Sep,7

25135 **with autograft (includes obtaining graft)**
16.0 16.0 FUD 090 J A2 80 50
AMA: 2018,Sep,7

25136 **with allograft**
14.2 14.2 FUD 090 J A2 80 50
AMA: 2019,May,7; 2018,Sep,7

25145 **Sequestrectomy (eg, for osteomyelitis or bone abscess), forearm and/or wrist**
14.9 14.9 FUD 090 J A2 80 50
AMA: 2018,Sep,7

25150 **Partial excision (craterization, saucerization, or diaphysectomy) of bone (eg, for osteomyelitis); ulna**
16.2 16.2 FUD 090 J A2 50
AMA: 2018,Sep,7

25151 **radius**
EXCLUDES *Partial removal radial head, neck, or olecranon process (24145, 24147)*
16.8 16.8 FUD 090 J A2 80 50
AMA: 2018,Sep,7

25170 **Radical resection of tumor, radius or ulna**
INCLUDES Any necessary elevation tissue planes or dissection
Excision adjacent soft tissue during bone tumor resection (25071-25078 [25071, 25073])
Measurement tumor and necessary margin at greatest diameter prior to excision
Resection tumor (may include entire bone) and wide margins normal tissues primarily for malignant or aggressive benign tumors
Resection without removal significant normal tissue
Simple and intermediate repairs
EXCLUDES *Complex repair*
Radical resection cutaneous tumors (e.g., melanoma) (11600-11646)
Significant vessel exploration, neuroplasty, reconstruction, or complex bone repair
42.5 42.5 FUD 090 J G2 80 50
AMA: 2019,May,7; 2018,Sep,7

25210 **Carpectomy; 1 bone**
EXCLUDES *Carpectomy with insertion implant (25441-25445)*
14.0 14.0 FUD 090 J A2 80
AMA: 2018,Sep,7

25215 **all bones of proximal row**
17.8 17.8 FUD 090 J A2 80 50
AMA: 2019,Dec,14; 2019,Feb,10; 2018,Sep,7

25230 **Radial styloidectomy (separate procedure)**
12.4 12.4 FUD 090 J A2 50
AMA: 2018,Sep,7

25240 **Excision distal ulna partial or complete (eg, Darrach type or matched resection)**
EXCLUDES *Acquisition fascia for interposition (20920, 20922)*
Implant replacement (25442)
12.3 12.3 FUD 090 J A2 80 50
AMA: 2018,Sep,7

25246 Injection for Wrist Arthrogram

25246 **Injection procedure for wrist arthrography**
EXCLUDES *Excision superficial foreign body (20520)*
(73115)
2.14 5.25 FUD 000 N N1 50
AMA: 2018,Sep,7; 2018,Jan,8; 2017,Jan,8; 2016,Jan,13

25248-25251 Removal Foreign Body of Wrist

EXCLUDES *Excision superficial foreign body (20520)*
K-wire, pin, or rod insertion (20650)
K-wire, pin, or rod removal (20670, 20680)

25248 **Exploration with removal of deep foreign body, forearm or wrist**
11.8 11.8 FUD 090 J A2 50
AMA: 2018,Sep,7

25250 **Removal of wrist prosthesis; (separate procedure)**
15.2 15.2 FUD 090 Q2 A2 80 50
AMA: 2018,Sep,7

25251 **complicated, including total wrist**
20.7 20.7 FUD 090 Q2 A2 80 50
AMA: 2018,Sep,7

25259 Manipulation of Wrist with Anesthesia

25259 **Manipulation, wrist, under anesthesia**
EXCLUDES *Application external fixation (20690, 20692)*
12.1 12.1 FUD 090 J G2 50
AMA: 2018,Sep,7; 2018,Jan,8; 2017,Jan,8; 2016,Jan,13

25260-25492 Repair/Reconstruction of Forearm/Wrist

25260 **Repair, tendon or muscle, flexor, forearm and/or wrist; primary, single, each tendon or muscle**
18.1 18.1 FUD 090 J A2
AMA: 2018,Sep,7

25263 **secondary, single, each tendon or muscle**
18.1 18.1 FUD 090 J A2 80
AMA: 2018,Sep,7

25265 **secondary, with free graft (includes obtaining graft), each tendon or muscle**
21.4 21.4 FUD 090 J A2 80
AMA: 2018,Sep,7

25270 **Repair, tendon or muscle, extensor, forearm and/or wrist; primary, single, each tendon or muscle**
14.1 14.1 FUD 090 J A2 80
AMA: 2018,Sep,7

25272 **secondary, single, each tendon or muscle**
15.9 15.9 FUD 090 J A2 80
AMA: 2018,Sep,7

25274 **secondary, with free graft (includes obtaining graft), each tendon or muscle**
19.1 19.1 FUD 090 J A2 80
AMA: 2018,Sep,7

25275 **Repair, tendon sheath, extensor, forearm and/or wrist, with free graft (includes obtaining graft) (eg, for extensor carpi ulnaris subluxation)**
19.3 19.3 FUD 090 J A2 80 50
AMA: 2018,Sep,7

25280 **Lengthening or shortening of flexor or extensor tendon, forearm and/or wrist, single, each tendon**
16.3 16.3 FUD 090 J A2 80
AMA: 2018,Sep,7

25290 **Tenotomy, open, flexor or extensor tendon, forearm and/or wrist, single, each tendon**
12.5 12.5 FUD 090 J A2
AMA: 2018,Sep,7

25295 **Tenolysis, flexor or extensor tendon, forearm and/or wrist, single, each tendon**
15.1 15.1 FUD 090 J A2
AMA: 2018,Sep,7; 2018,Jan,8; 2017,Jan,8; 2016,Jan,13

25300 **Tenodesis at wrist; flexors of fingers**
19.7 19.7 FUD 090 J A2 80 50
AMA: 2018,Sep,7

25301 **extensors of fingers**
18.5 18.5 FUD 090 J A2 80 50
AMA: 2018,Sep,7

25310 **Tendon transplantation or transfer, flexor or extensor, forearm and/or wrist, single; each tendon**
17.8 17.8 FUD 090 J A2 80
AMA: 2018,Sep,7; 2018,Jan,8; 2017,Jan,8; 2016,Jan,13

25312 **with tendon graft(s) (includes obtaining graft), each tendon**
20.7 20.7 FUD 090 J A2 80
AMA: 2018,Sep,7

25315 **Flexor origin slide (eg, for cerebral palsy, Volkmann contracture), forearm and/or wrist;**
22.2 22.2 **FUD** 090 J A2 80 50
AMA: 2018,Sep,7

25316 **with tendon(s) transfer**
26.4 26.4 **FUD** 090 J A2 80 50
AMA: 2018,Sep,7

25320 **Capsulorrhaphy or reconstruction, wrist, open (eg, capsulodesis, ligament repair, tendon transfer or graft) (includes synovectomy, capsulotomy and open reduction) for carpal instability**
28.3 28.3 **FUD** 090 J A2 80 50
AMA: 2018,Sep,7

25332 **Arthroplasty, wrist, with or without interposition, with or without external or internal fixation**
EXCLUDES *Acquiring fascia for interposition (20920, 20922)*
Arthroplasty with prosthesis (25441-25446)
24.3 24.3 **FUD** 090 J A2 80 50
AMA: 2019,Feb,10; 2018,Sep,7; 2018,Jan,8; 2017,Jan,8; 2016,Jan,13

25335 **Centralization of wrist on ulna (eg, radial club hand)**
27.2 27.2 **FUD** 090 J A2 80 50
AMA: 2018,Sep,7; 2018,May,10

25337 **Reconstruction for stabilization of unstable distal ulna or distal radioulnar joint, secondary by soft tissue stabilization (eg, tendon transfer, tendon graft or weave, or tenodesis) with or without open reduction of distal radioulnar joint**
EXCLUDES *Acquiring fascia lata graft (20920, 20922)*
25.5 25.5 **FUD** 090 J A2 50
AMA: 2018,Sep,7

25350 **Osteotomy, radius; distal third**
19.4 19.4 **FUD** 090 J J8 80 50
AMA: 2018,Sep,7

25355 **middle or proximal third**
22.0 22.0 **FUD** 090 J A2 80 50
AMA: 2018,Sep,7

25360 **Osteotomy; ulna**
18.8 18.8 **FUD** 090 J A2 80 50
AMA: 2018,Sep,7

25365 **radius AND ulna**
26.4 26.4 **FUD** 090 J A2 80 50
AMA: 2018,Sep,7

25370 **Multiple osteotomies, with realignment on intramedullary rod (Sofield type procedure); radius OR ulna**
29.0 29.0 **FUD** 090 J A2 80 50
AMA: 2018,Sep,7

25375 **radius AND ulna**
27.5 27.5 **FUD** 090 J A2 80 50
AMA: 2018,Sep,7

25390 **Osteoplasty, radius OR ulna; shortening**
22.1 22.1 **FUD** 090 J J8 80 50
AMA: 2018,Sep,7

25391 **lengthening with autograft**
28.7 28.7 **FUD** 090 J J8 80 50
AMA: 2018,Sep,7

25392 **Osteoplasty, radius AND ulna; shortening (excluding 64876)**
29.3 29.3 **FUD** 090 J A2 80 50
AMA: 2018,Sep,7

25393 **lengthening with autograft**
32.6 32.6 **FUD** 090 J A2 80 50
AMA: 2018,Sep,7

25394 **Osteoplasty, carpal bone, shortening**
22.6 22.6 **FUD** 090 J G2 80 50
AMA: 2018,Sep,7

25400 **Repair of nonunion or malunion, radius OR ulna; without graft (eg, compression technique)**
23.1 23.1 **FUD** 090 J J8 80 50
AMA: 2018,Sep,7

25405 **with autograft (includes obtaining graft)**
29.9 29.9 **FUD** 090 J J8 80 50
AMA: 2018,Sep,7

25415 **Repair of nonunion or malunion, radius AND ulna; without graft (eg, compression technique)**
27.9 27.9 **FUD** 090 J J8 80 50
AMA: 2018,Sep,7

25420 **with autograft (includes obtaining graft)**
33.7 33.7 **FUD** 090 J J8 80 50
AMA: 2018,Sep,7

25425 **Repair of defect with autograft; radius OR ulna**
27.8 27.8 **FUD** 090 J A2 80 50
AMA: 2018,Sep,7

25426 **radius AND ulna**
32.4 32.4 **FUD** 090 J J8 80 50
AMA: 2018,Sep,7

25430 **Insertion of vascular pedicle into carpal bone (eg, Hori procedure)**
21.0 21.0 **FUD** 090 J G2 50
AMA: 2018,Sep,7

25431 **Repair of nonunion of carpal bone (excluding carpal scaphoid (navicular)) (includes obtaining graft and necessary fixation), each bone**
22.7 22.7 **FUD** 090 J G2 80 50
AMA: 2018,Sep,7

25440 **Repair of nonunion, scaphoid carpal (navicular) bone, with or without radial styloidectomy (includes obtaining graft and necessary fixation)**
22.1 22.1 **FUD** 090 J A2 80 50
AMA: 2018,Sep,7

25441 **Arthroplasty with prosthetic replacement; distal radius**
27.0 27.0 **FUD** 090 J J8 80 50
AMA: 2018,Sep,7; 2018,Jan,8; 2017,Aug,9; 2017,Jan,8; 2016,Jan,13

25442 **distal ulna**
23.2 23.2 **FUD** 090 J J8 80 50
AMA: 2018,Sep,7; 2018,Jan,8; 2017,Aug,9; 2017,Jan,8; 2016,Jan,13

25443 **scaphoid carpal (navicular)**
22.6 22.6 **FUD** 090 J J8 80 50
AMA: 2018,Sep,7; 2018,Jan,8; 2017,Jan,8; 2016,Jan,13

25444 **lunate**
23.7 23.7 **FUD** 090 J J8 80 50
AMA: 2018,Sep,7; 2018,Jan,8; 2017,Jan,8; 2016,Jan,13

25445 **trapezium**
20.8 20.8 **FUD** 090 J J8 50
AMA: 2018,Sep,7; 2018,Jan,8; 2017,Jan,8; 2016,Jan,13

25446 **distal radius and partial or entire carpus (total wrist)**
33.8 33.8 **FUD** 090 J J8 80 50
AMA: 2018,Sep,7; 2018,Jan,8; 2017,Jan,8; 2016,Jan,13

25447 **Arthroplasty, interposition, intercarpal or carpometacarpal joints**
EXCLUDES *Wrist arthroplasty (25332)*
23.8 23.8 **FUD** 090 J A2 80 50
AMA: 2018,Sep,7; 2018,Jan,8; 2017,Jan,8; 2016,Jan,13

25449 **Revision of arthroplasty, including removal of implant, wrist joint**
29.8 29.8 **FUD** 090 J A2 80 50
AMA: 2018,Sep,7

26/TC PC/TC Only · A2-Z3 ASC Payment · 50 Bilateral · ♂ Male Only · ♀ Female Only · Facility RVU · Non-Facility RVU · CCI · CLIA
FUD Follow-up Days · **CMS:** IOM · **AMA:** CPT Asst · A-Y OPPSI · 80/80 Surg Assist Allowed / w/Doc · Lab Crosswalk · Radiology Crosswalk

25450 **Epiphyseal arrest by epiphysiodesis or stapling; distal radius OR ulna**
17.7 17.7 FUD 090 J A2 50
AMA: 2018,Sep,7

25455 **distal radius AND ulna**
20.9 20.9 FUD 090 J A2 50
AMA: 2018,Sep,7

25490 **Prophylactic treatment (nailing, pinning, plating or wiring) with or without methylmethacrylate; radius**
20.7 20.7 FUD 090 J A2 80 50
AMA: 2018,Sep,7

25491 **ulna**
21.3 21.3 FUD 090 J A2 80 50
AMA: 2018,Sep,7

25492 **radius AND ulna**
26.1 26.1 FUD 090 J A2 80 50
AMA: 2018,Sep,7

25500-25695 Treatment of Fracture/Dislocation of Forearm/Wrist

Code also external fixation, when performed (20690, 20692)

25500 **Closed treatment of radial shaft fracture; without manipulation**
7.25 7.98 FUD 090 T P2 50
AMA: 2018,Sep,7

25505 **with manipulation**
13.2 14.4 FUD 090 J A2 50
AMA: 2018,Sep,7

25515 **Open treatment of radial shaft fracture, includes internal fixation, when performed**
19.2 19.2 FUD 090 J J8 80 50
AMA: 2018,Sep,7

25520 **Closed treatment of radial shaft fracture and closed treatment of dislocation of distal radioulnar joint (Galeazzi fracture/dislocation)**
15.5 16.4 FUD 090 J A2 50
AMA: 2018,Sep,7

25525 **Open treatment of radial shaft fracture, includes internal fixation, when performed, and closed treatment of distal radioulnar joint dislocation (Galeazzi fracture/ dislocation), includes percutaneous skeletal fixation, when performed**
22.6 22.6 FUD 090 J J8 80 50
AMA: 2018,Sep,7

25526 **Open treatment of radial shaft fracture, includes internal fixation, when performed, and open treatment of distal radioulnar joint dislocation (Galeazzi fracture/ dislocation), includes internal fixation, when performed, includes repair of triangular fibrocartilage complex**
27.5 27.5 FUD 090 J A2 80 50
AMA: 2018,Sep,7

25530 **Closed treatment of ulnar shaft fracture; without manipulation**
6.88 7.52 FUD 090 T P2 50
AMA: 2018,Sep,7

25535 **with manipulation**
13.0 14.0 FUD 090 T A2 50
AMA: 2018,Sep,7

25545 **Open treatment of ulnar shaft fracture, includes internal fixation, when performed**
17.9 17.9 FUD 090 J J8 80 50
AMA: 2018,Sep,7; 2018,Jan,8; 2017,Jan,8; 2016,Jan,13

25560 **Closed treatment of radial and ulnar shaft fractures; without manipulation**
7.31 8.15 FUD 090 T P2 50
AMA: 2018,Sep,7

25565 **with manipulation**
13.2 14.7 FUD 090 J A2 50
AMA: 2018,Sep,7

25574 **Open treatment of radial AND ulnar shaft fractures, with internal fixation, when performed; of radius OR ulna**
19.4 19.4 FUD 090 J J8 80 50
AMA: 2018,Sep,7; 2018,Jan,8; 2017,Jan,8; 2016,Jan,13

25575 **of radius AND ulna**
25.9 25.9 FUD 090 J J8 80 50
AMA: 2018,Sep,7

25600 **Closed treatment of distal radial fracture (eg, Colles or Smith type) or epiphyseal separation, includes closed treatment of fracture of ulnar styloid, when performed; without manipulation**
INCLUDES Closed treatment ulnar styloid fracture (25650)
9.06 9.51 FUD 090 T P2 50
AMA: 2018,Sep,7; 2018,Jan,8; 2017,Jan,8; 2016,Jan,13

25605 **with manipulation**
INCLUDES Closed treatment ulnar styloid fracture (25650)
14.7 15.5 FUD 090 J A2 50
AMA: 2018,Sep,7; 2018,Jan,8; 2017,Jan,8; 2016,Jan,13

25606 **Percutaneous skeletal fixation of distal radial fracture or epiphyseal separation**
EXCLUDES *Closed treatment ulnar styloid fracture (25650)*
Open repair ulnar styloid fracture (25652)
Percutaneous repair ulnar styloid fracture (25651)
19.1 19.1 FUD 090 J A2 50
AMA: 2018,Sep,7

25607 **Open treatment of distal radial extra-articular fracture or epiphyseal separation, with internal fixation**
EXCLUDES *Closed treatment ulnar styloid fracture (25650)*
Open repair ulnar styloid fracture (25652)
Percutaneous repair ulnar styloid fracture (25651)
21.1 21.1 FUD 090 J J8 80 50
AMA: 2018,Sep,7; 2018,Jan,8; 2017,Jan,8; 2016,Jan,13

25608 **Open treatment of distal radial intra-articular fracture or epiphyseal separation; with internal fixation of 2 fragments**
EXCLUDES *Closed treatment ulnar styloid fracture (25650)*
Open repair ulnar styloid fracture (25652)
Open treatment distal radial intra-articular fracture or epiphyseal separation; with internal fixation of 3 or more fragments (25609)
Percutaneous repair ulnar styloid fracture (25651)
23.7 23.7 FUD 090 J J8 80 50
AMA: 2018,Sep,7; 2018,Jan,8; 2017,Jan,8; 2016,Jan,13

25609 **with internal fixation of 3 or more fragments**
EXCLUDES *Closed treatment ulnar styloid fracture (25650)*
Open repair ulnar styloid fracture (25652)
Percutaneous repair ulnar styloid fracture (25651)
30.2 30.2 FUD 090 J J8 80 50
AMA: 2018,Sep,7; 2018,Jan,8; 2017,Jan,8; 2016,Jan,13

25622 **Closed treatment of carpal scaphoid (navicular) fracture; without manipulation**
8.07 8.76 FUD 090 T P2 50
AMA: 2018,Sep,7

25624 **with manipulation**
12.6 13.8 FUD 090 J A2 80 50
AMA: 2018,Sep,7

25628 **Open treatment of carpal scaphoid (navicular) fracture, includes internal fixation, when performed**
20.7 20.7 FUD 090 J A2 80 50
AMA: 2018,Sep,7

25630 **Closed treatment of carpal bone fracture (excluding carpal scaphoid [navicular]); without manipulation, each bone**
8.13 8.77 FUD 090 T P2 50
AMA: 2018,Sep,7

25635 **with manipulation, each bone**
11.9 13.1 **FUD** 090 J A2 80 50
AMA: 2018,Sep,7

25645 **Open treatment of carpal bone fracture (other than carpal scaphoid [navicular]), each bone**
16.4 16.4 **FUD** 090 J A2 80 50
AMA: 2018,Sep,7

25650 **Closed treatment of ulnar styloid fracture**
EXCLUDES *Closed treatment distal radial fracture (25600, 25605)*
Open treatment distal radial extra-articular fracture or epiphyseal separation, with internal fixation (25607-25609)
8.70 9.35 **FUD** 090 T P2 50
AMA: 2018,Sep,7; 2018,Jan,8; 2017,Jan,8; 2016,Jan,13

25651 **Percutaneous skeletal fixation of ulnar styloid fracture**
14.0 14.0 **FUD** 090 J G2 80 50
AMA: 2018,Sep,7

25652 **Open treatment of ulnar styloid fracture**
17.9 17.9 **FUD** 090 J J8 50
AMA: 2018,Sep,7; 2018,Jan,8; 2017,Jan,8; 2016,Jan,13

25660 **Closed treatment of radiocarpal or intercarpal dislocation, 1 or more bones, with manipulation**
11.9 11.9 **FUD** 090 T A2 80 50
AMA: 2018,Sep,7

25670 **Open treatment of radiocarpal or intercarpal dislocation, 1 or more bones**
17.5 17.5 **FUD** 090 J J8 80 50
AMA: 2018,Sep,7

25671 **Percutaneous skeletal fixation of distal radioulnar dislocation**
15.3 15.3 **FUD** 090 J A2 50
AMA: 2018,Sep,7

25675 **Closed treatment of distal radioulnar dislocation with manipulation**
11.3 12.5 **FUD** 090 T A2 80 50
AMA: 2018,Sep,7

25676 **Open treatment of distal radioulnar dislocation, acute or chronic**
18.2 18.2 **FUD** 090 J A2 80 50
AMA: 2018,Sep,7

25680 **Closed treatment of trans-scaphoperilunar type of fracture dislocation, with manipulation**
15.0 15.0 **FUD** 090 T A2 80 50
AMA: 2018,Sep,7

25685 **Open treatment of trans-scaphoperilunar type of fracture dislocation**
21.2 21.2 **FUD** 090 J A2 80 50
AMA: 2018,Sep,7

25690 **Closed treatment of lunate dislocation, with manipulation**
13.9 13.9 **FUD** 090 J A2 80 50
AMA: 2018,Sep,7

25695 **Open treatment of lunate dislocation**
18.2 18.2 **FUD** 090 J A2 80 50
AMA: 2018,Sep,7

25800-25830 Wrist Fusion

25800 **Arthrodesis, wrist; complete, without bone graft (includes radiocarpal and/or intercarpal and/or carpometacarpal joints)**
21.1 21.1 **FUD** 090 J J8 80 50
AMA: 2020,May,13; 2018,Sep,7

25805 **with sliding graft**
24.4 24.4 **FUD** 090 J J8 80 50
AMA: 2020,May,13; 2018,Sep,7

25810 **with iliac or other autograft (includes obtaining graft)**
24.9 24.9 **FUD** 090 J J8 80 50
AMA: 2020,May,13; 2018,Sep,7

25820 **Arthrodesis, wrist; limited, without bone graft (eg, intercarpal or radiocarpal)**
18.1 18.1 **FUD** 090 J J8 80 50
AMA: 2020,May,13; 2018,Sep,7

25825 **with autograft (includes obtaining graft)**
21.9 21.9 **FUD** 090 J J8 80 50
AMA: 2020,May,13; 2018,Sep,7; 2018,Jan,8; 2017,Jan,8; 2016,Jan,13

25830 **Arthrodesis, distal radioulnar joint with segmental resection of ulna, with or without bone graft (eg, Sauve-Kapandji procedure)**
28.1 28.1 **FUD** 090 J A2 80 50
AMA: 2020,May,13; 2018,Sep,7

25900-25999 Amputation Through Forearm/Wrist

25900 **Amputation, forearm, through radius and ulna;**
20.5 20.5 **FUD** 090 C 80 50
AMA: 2018,Sep,7

25905 **open, circular (guillotine)**
20.2 20.2 **FUD** 090 C 80 50
AMA: 2018,Sep,7

25907 **secondary closure or scar revision**
17.6 17.6 **FUD** 090 J A2 80 50
AMA: 2018,Sep,7

25909 **re-amputation**
19.7 19.7 **FUD** 090 J G2 80 50
AMA: 2018,Sep,7

25915 **Krukenberg procedure**
33.7 33.7 **FUD** 090 C 80 50
AMA: 2018,Sep,7

25920 **Disarticulation through wrist;**
20.5 20.5 **FUD** 090 C 80 50
AMA: 2018,Sep,7

25922 **secondary closure or scar revision**
17.7 17.7 **FUD** 090 J A2 80 50
AMA: 2018,Sep,7

25924 **re-amputation**
20.0 20.0 **FUD** 090 C 80 50
AMA: 2018,Sep,7

25927 **Transmetacarpal amputation;**
24.0 24.0 **FUD** 090 C 80 50
AMA: 2018,Sep,7

25929 **secondary closure or scar revision**
17.2 17.2 **FUD** 090 T A2 80 50
AMA: 2018,Sep,7

25931 **re-amputation**
22.1 22.1 **FUD** 090 J G2 50
AMA: 2018,Sep,7

25999 **Unlisted procedure, forearm or wrist**
0.00 0.00 **FUD** YYY T 80 50
AMA: 2019,Feb,10; 2018,Sep,7

26010-26037 Incision Hand/Fingers

26010 **Drainage of finger abscess; simple**
3.97 8.62 FUD 010 T P2
AMA: 2018,Sep,7

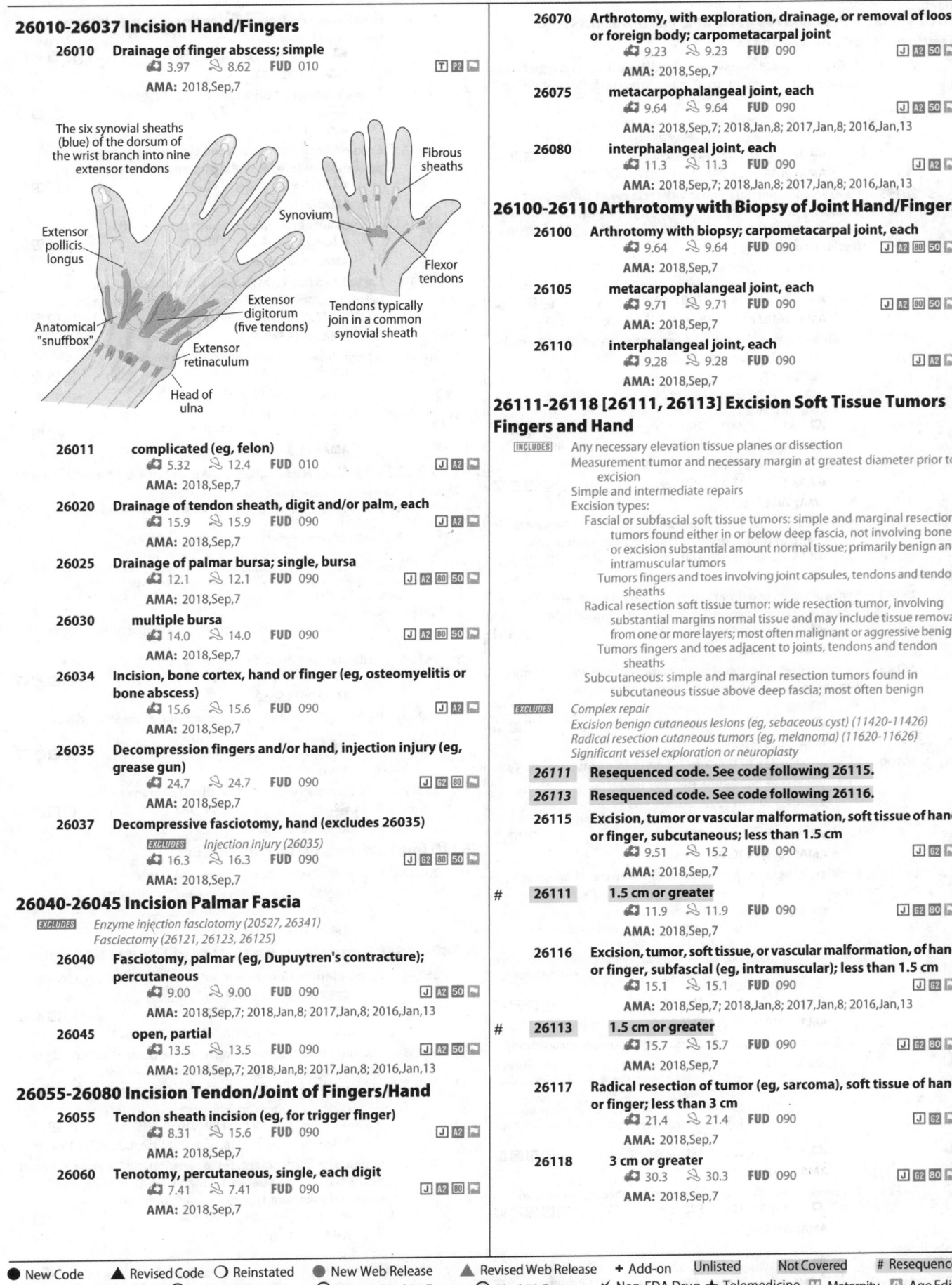

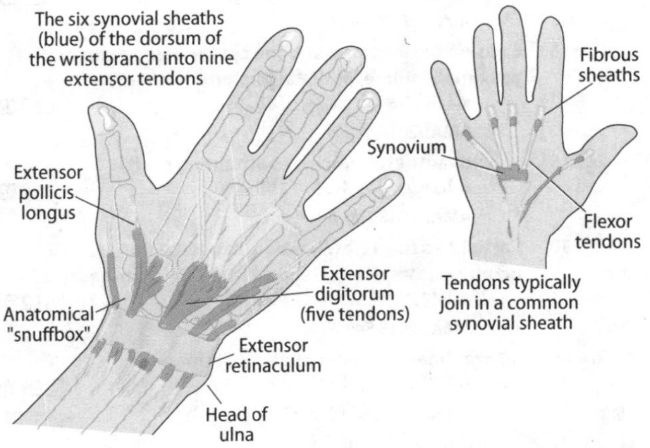

26011 **complicated (eg, felon)**
5.32 12.4 FUD 010 J A2
AMA: 2018,Sep,7

26020 **Drainage of tendon sheath, digit and/or palm, each**
15.9 15.9 FUD 090 J A2
AMA: 2018,Sep,7

26025 **Drainage of palmar bursa; single, bursa**
12.1 12.1 FUD 090 J A2 80 50
AMA: 2018,Sep,7

26030 **multiple bursa**
14.0 14.0 FUD 090 J A2 80 50
AMA: 2018,Sep,7

26034 **Incision, bone cortex, hand or finger (eg, osteomyelitis or bone abscess)**
15.6 15.6 FUD 090 J A2
AMA: 2018,Sep,7

26035 **Decompression fingers and/or hand, injection injury (eg, grease gun)**
24.7 24.7 FUD 090 J G2 80
AMA: 2018,Sep,7

26037 **Decompressive fasciotomy, hand (excludes 26035)**
EXCLUDES *Injection injury (26035)*
16.3 16.3 FUD 090 J G2 80 50
AMA: 2018,Sep,7

26040-26045 Incision Palmar Fascia

EXCLUDES *Enzyme injection fasciotomy (20527, 26341)*
Fasciectomy (26121, 26123, 26125)

26040 **Fasciotomy, palmar (eg, Dupuytren's contracture); percutaneous**
9.00 9.00 FUD 090 J A2 50
AMA: 2018,Sep,7; 2018,Jan,8; 2017,Jan,8; 2016,Jan,13

26045 **open, partial**
13.5 13.5 FUD 090 J A2 50
AMA: 2018,Sep,7; 2018,Jan,8; 2017,Jan,8; 2016,Jan,13

26055-26080 Incision Tendon/Joint of Fingers/Hand

26055 **Tendon sheath incision (eg, for trigger finger)**
8.31 15.6 FUD 090 J A2
AMA: 2018,Sep,7

26060 **Tenotomy, percutaneous, single, each digit**
7.41 7.41 FUD 090 J A2 80
AMA: 2018,Sep,7

26070 **Arthrotomy, with exploration, drainage, or removal of loose or foreign body; carpometacarpal joint**
9.23 9.23 FUD 090 J A2 50
AMA: 2018,Sep,7

26075 **metacarpophalangeal joint, each**
9.64 9.64 FUD 090 J A2 50
AMA: 2018,Sep,7; 2018,Jan,8; 2017,Jan,8; 2016,Jan,13

26080 **interphalangeal joint, each**
11.3 11.3 FUD 090 J A2
AMA: 2018,Sep,7; 2018,Jan,8; 2017,Jan,8; 2016,Jan,13

26100-26110 Arthrotomy with Biopsy of Joint Hand/Fingers

26100 **Arthrotomy with biopsy; carpometacarpal joint, each**
9.64 9.64 FUD 090 J A2 80 50
AMA: 2018,Sep,7

26105 **metacarpophalangeal joint, each**
9.71 9.71 FUD 090 J A2 80 50
AMA: 2018,Sep,7

26110 **interphalangeal joint, each**
9.28 9.28 FUD 090 J A2
AMA: 2018,Sep,7

26111-26118 [26111, 26113] Excision Soft Tissue Tumors Fingers and Hand

INCLUDES Any necessary elevation tissue planes or dissection
Measurement tumor and necessary margin at greatest diameter prior to excision
Simple and intermediate repairs
Excision types:
Fascial or subfascial soft tissue tumors: simple and marginal resection tumors found either in or below deep fascia, not involving bone or excision substantial amount normal tissue; primarily benign and intramuscular tumors
Tumors fingers and toes involving joint capsules, tendons and tendon sheaths
Radical resection soft tissue tumor: wide resection tumor, involving substantial margins normal tissue and may include tissue removal from one or more layers; most often malignant or aggressive benign
Tumors fingers and toes adjacent to joints, tendons and tendon sheaths
Subcutaneous: simple and marginal resection tumors found in subcutaneous tissue above deep fascia; most often benign

EXCLUDES *Complex repair*
Excision benign cutaneous lesions (eg, sebaceous cyst) (11420-11426)
Radical resection cutaneous tumors (eg, melanoma) (11620-11626)
Significant vessel exploration or neuroplasty

26111 **Resequenced code. See code following 26115.**

26113 **Resequenced code. See code following 26116.**

26115 **Excision, tumor or vascular malformation, soft tissue of hand or finger, subcutaneous; less than 1.5 cm**
9.51 15.2 FUD 090 J G2
AMA: 2018,Sep,7

\# **26111** **1.5 cm or greater**
11.9 11.9 FUD 090 J G2 80
AMA: 2018,Sep,7

26116 **Excision, tumor, soft tissue, or vascular malformation, of hand or finger, subfascial (eg, intramuscular); less than 1.5 cm**
15.1 15.1 FUD 090 J G2
AMA: 2018,Sep,7; 2018,Jan,8; 2017,Jan,8; 2016,Jan,13

\# **26113** **1.5 cm or greater**
15.7 15.7 FUD 090 J G2 80
AMA: 2018,Sep,7

26117 **Radical resection of tumor (eg, sarcoma), soft tissue of hand or finger; less than 3 cm**
21.4 21.4 FUD 090 J G2
AMA: 2018,Sep,7

26118 **3 cm or greater**
30.3 30.3 FUD 090 J G2 80
AMA: 2018,Sep,7

26121-26236 Procedures of Bones, Fascia, Joints and Tendons Hands and Fingers

26121 **Fasciectomy, palm only, with or without Z-plasty, other local tissue rearrangement, or skin grafting (includes obtaining graft)**
EXCLUDES *Enzyme injection fasciotomy (20527, 26341)*
Fasciotomy (26040, 26045)
17.2 17.2 **FUD** 090 J A2 50
AMA: 2018,Sep,7; 2018,Jan,8; 2017,Jan,8; 2016,Jan,13

26123 **Fasciectomy, partial palmar with release of single digit including proximal interphalangeal joint, with or without Z-plasty, other local tissue rearrangement, or skin grafting (includes obtaining graft);**
EXCLUDES *Enzyme injection fasciotomy (20527, 26341)*
Fasciotomy (26040, 26045)
24.0 24.0 **FUD** 090 J A2 50
AMA: 2018,Sep,7; 2018,Jan,8; 2017,Jan,8; 2016,Jan,13

\+ **26125** **each additional digit (List separately in addition to code for primary procedure)**
EXCLUDES *Enzyme injection fasciotomy (20527, 26341)*
Fasciotomy (26040, 26045)
Code first (26123)
7.89 7.89 **FUD** ZZZ N N1
AMA: 2018,Sep,7; 2018,Jan,8; 2017,Jan,8; 2016,Jan,13

26130 **Synovectomy, carpometacarpal joint**
13.4 13.4 **FUD** 090 J A2 50
AMA: 2018,Sep,7

26135 **Synovectomy, metacarpophalangeal joint including intrinsic release and extensor hood reconstruction, each digit**
15.9 15.9 **FUD** 090 J A2 80
AMA: 2018,Sep,7

26140 **Synovectomy, proximal interphalangeal joint, including extensor reconstruction, each interphalangeal joint**
14.5 14.5 **FUD** 090 J A2
AMA: 2018,Sep,7

26145 **Synovectomy, tendon sheath, radical (tenosynovectomy), flexor tendon, palm and/or finger, each tendon**
EXCLUDES *Wrist synovectomy (25115-25116)*
14.7 14.7 **FUD** 090 J A2
AMA: 2018,Sep,7

26160 **Excision of lesion of tendon sheath or joint capsule (eg, cyst, mucous cyst, or ganglion), hand or finger**
EXCLUDES *Trigger finger (26055)*
Wrist ganglion removal (25111-25112)
9.04 16.3 **FUD** 090 J A2
AMA: 2019,Jul,10; 2018,Sep,7

26170 **Excision of tendon, palm, flexor or extensor, single, each tendon**
EXCLUDES *Excision extensor tendon, with implantation synthetic rod for delayed tendon graft, hand or finger, each rod (26415)*
Excision flexor tendon, with implantation synthetic rod for delayed tendon graft, hand or finger, each rod (26390)
11.6 11.6 **FUD** 090 J A2 80
AMA: 2018,Sep,7; 2018,Jan,8; 2017,Jan,8; 2016,Jan,13

26180 **Excision of tendon, finger, flexor or extensor, each tendon**
EXCLUDES *Excision extensor tendon, with implantation synthetic rod for delayed tendon graft, hand or finger, each rod (26415)*
Excision flexor tendon, with implantation synthetic rod for delayed tendon graft, hand or finger, each rod (26390)
12.7 12.7 **FUD** 090 J A2 80
AMA: 2018,Sep,7

26185 **Sesamoidectomy, thumb or finger (separate procedure)**
15.8 15.8 **FUD** 090 J A2 80 50
AMA: 2018,Sep,7

26200 **Excision or curettage of bone cyst or benign tumor of metacarpal;**
13.0 13.0 **FUD** 090 J A2 80
AMA: 2018,Sep,7

26205 **with autograft (includes obtaining graft)**
17.3 17.3 **FUD** 090 J A2
AMA: 2018,Sep,7

26210 **Excision or curettage of bone cyst or benign tumor of proximal, middle, or distal phalanx of finger;**
12.7 12.7 **FUD** 090 J A2
AMA: 2018,Sep,7

26215 **with autograft (includes obtaining graft)**
16.2 16.2 **FUD** 090 J A2
AMA: 2018,Sep,7

26230 **Partial excision (craterization, saucerization, or diaphysectomy) bone (eg, osteomyelitis); metacarpal**
14.4 14.4 **FUD** 090 J A2 80
AMA: 2018,Sep,7

26235 **proximal or middle phalanx of finger**
14.1 14.1 **FUD** 090 J A2 80
AMA: 2019,Jul,10; 2018,Sep,7

26236 **distal phalanx of finger**
12.6 12.6 **FUD** 090 J A2
AMA: 2019,Jul,10; 2018,Sep,7

26250-26262 Radical Resection Bone Tumor of Hand/Finger

INCLUDES Any necessary elevation tissue planes or dissection
Excision adjacent soft tissue during bone tumor resection (26111-26118 [26111, 26113])
Measurement tumor and necessary margin at greatest diameter prior to excision
Resection tumor (may include entire bone) and wide margins normal tissue primarily for malignant or aggressive benign tumors
Simple and intermediate repairs

EXCLUDES *Complex repair*
Significant vessel exploration, neuroplasty, reconstruction, or complex bone repair

26250 **Radical resection of tumor, metacarpal**
30.8 30.8 **FUD** 090 J A2 80
AMA: 2018,Sep,7

26260 **Radical resection of tumor, proximal or middle phalanx of finger**
23.0 23.0 **FUD** 090 J A2 80
AMA: 2018,Sep,7

26262 **Radical resection of tumor, distal phalanx of finger**
18.1 18.1 **FUD** 090 J A2 80
AMA: 2018,Sep,7

26320 Implant Removal Hand/Finger

26320 **Removal of implant from finger or hand**
EXCLUDES *Excision foreign body (20520, 20525)*
9.98 9.98 **FUD** 090 Q2 A2
AMA: 2018,Sep,7

26340-26548 Repair/Reconstruction of Fingers and Hand

26340 **Manipulation, finger joint, under anesthesia, each joint**
EXCLUDES *Application external fixation (20690, 20692)*
9.67 9.67 **FUD** 090 J G2 50
AMA: 2018,Sep,7; 2018,Jan,8; 2017,Jan,8; 2016,Jan,13

26341 **Manipulation, palmar fascial cord (ie, Dupuytren's cord), post enzyme injection (eg, collagenase), single cord**
EXCLUDES *Enzyme injection fasciotomy (20527)*
Code also custom orthotic fabrication and/or fitting
2.17 2.90 **FUD** 010 T P3 50
AMA: 2018,Sep,7; 2018,Jan,8; 2017,Jan,8; 2016,Jan,13

26350 **Repair or advancement, flexor tendon, not in zone 2 digital flexor tendon sheath (eg, no man's land); primary or secondary without free graft, each tendon**
20.8 20.8 **FUD** 090 J A2
AMA: 2018,Sep,7

26352 **secondary with free graft (includes obtaining graft), each tendon**
23.3 23.3 FUD 090 J A2 80
AMA: 2018,Sep,7

26356 **Repair or advancement, flexor tendon, in zone 2 digital flexor tendon sheath (eg, no man's land); primary, without free graft, each tendon**
22.8 22.8 FUD 090 J A2
AMA: 2018,Sep,7; 2018,Jan,8; 2017,Dec,14; 2017,Jan,8; 2016,Jan,13

26357 **secondary, without free graft, each tendon**
25.6 25.6 FUD 090 J A2 80
AMA: 2018,Sep,7

26358 **secondary, with free graft (includes obtaining graft), each tendon**
28.3 28.3 FUD 090 J A2 80
AMA: 2018,Sep,7

26370 **Repair or advancement of profundus tendon, with intact superficialis tendon; primary, each tendon**
21.9 21.9 FUD 090 J A2 80
AMA: 2018,Sep,7; 2018,Jan,8; 2017,Jan,8; 2016,Jan,13

26372 **secondary with free graft (includes obtaining graft), each tendon**
25.7 25.7 FUD 090 J A2 80
AMA: 2018,Sep,7

26373 **secondary without free graft, each tendon**
24.7 24.7 FUD 090 J A2 80
AMA: 2018,Sep,7

26390 **Excision flexor tendon, with implantation of synthetic rod for delayed tendon graft, hand or finger, each rod**
23.6 23.6 FUD 090 J J8 80
AMA: 2018,Sep,7

26392 **Removal of synthetic rod and insertion of flexor tendon graft, hand or finger (includes obtaining graft), each rod**
27.5 27.5 FUD 090 J A2 80
AMA: 2018,Sep,7

26410 **Repair, extensor tendon, hand, primary or secondary; without free graft, each tendon**
16.5 16.5 FUD 090 J A2
AMA: 2018,Sep,7

26412 **with free graft (includes obtaining graft), each tendon**
19.7 19.7 FUD 090 J A2 80
AMA: 2018,Sep,7

26415 **Excision of extensor tendon, with implantation of synthetic rod for delayed tendon graft, hand or finger, each rod**
23.7 23.7 FUD 090 J A2 80
AMA: 2018,Sep,7

26416 **Removal of synthetic rod and insertion of extensor tendon graft (includes obtaining graft), hand or finger, each rod**
25.7 25.7 FUD 090 J A2
AMA: 2018,Sep,7; 2018,Jan,8; 2017,Jan,8; 2016,Jan,13

26418 **Repair, extensor tendon, finger, primary or secondary; without free graft, each tendon**
16.2 16.2 FUD 090 J A2
AMA: 2018,Sep,7; 2018,Jan,8; 2017,Jan,8; 2016,Jan,13

26420 **with free graft (includes obtaining graft) each tendon**
20.6 20.6 FUD 090 J A2 80
AMA: 2018,Sep,7

26426 **Repair of extensor tendon, central slip, secondary (eg, boutonniere deformity); using local tissue(s), including lateral band(s), each finger**
14.4 14.4 FUD 090 J A2
AMA: 2018,Sep,7

26428 **with free graft (includes obtaining graft), each finger**
21.3 21.3 FUD 090 J A2 80
AMA: 2018,Sep,7

26432 **Closed treatment of distal extensor tendon insertion, with or without percutaneous pinning (eg, mallet finger)**
14.7 14.7 FUD 090 J A2
AMA: 2018,Sep,7

26433 **Repair of extensor tendon, distal insertion, primary or secondary; without graft (eg, mallet finger)**
EXCLUDES *Trigger finger (26055)*
15.6 15.6 FUD 090 J A2
AMA: 2018,Sep,7

26434 **with free graft (includes obtaining graft)**
EXCLUDES *Trigger finger (26055)*
18.2 18.2 FUD 090 J A2 80
AMA: 2018,Sep,7

26437 **Realignment of extensor tendon, hand, each tendon**
17.5 17.5 FUD 090 J A2
AMA: 2018,Sep,7

26440 **Tenolysis, flexor tendon; palm OR finger, each tendon**
17.4 17.4 FUD 090 J A2
AMA: 2018,Sep,7; 2018,Jan,8; 2017,Jan,8; 2016,Jan,13

26442 **palm AND finger, each tendon**
27.1 27.1 FUD 090 J A2
AMA: 2018,Sep,7

26445 **Tenolysis, extensor tendon, hand OR finger, each tendon**
16.1 16.1 FUD 090 J A2
AMA: 2018,Sep,7; 2018,Jan,8; 2017,Jan,8; 2016,Jan,13

26449 **Tenolysis, complex, extensor tendon, finger, including forearm, each tendon**
19.9 19.9 FUD 090 J A2 80
AMA: 2018,Sep,7

26450 **Tenotomy, flexor, palm, open, each tendon**
11.4 11.4 FUD 090 J A2 80
AMA: 2018,Sep,7

26455 **Tenotomy, flexor, finger, open, each tendon**
12.1 12.1 FUD 090 J A2 80
AMA: 2018,Sep,7

26460 **Tenotomy, extensor, hand or finger, open, each tendon**
11.1 11.1 FUD 090 J A2
AMA: 2018,Sep,7

26471 **Tenodesis; of proximal interphalangeal joint, each joint**
18.0 18.0 FUD 090 J A2 80
AMA: 2018,Sep,7

26474 **of distal joint, each joint**
17.7 17.7 FUD 090 J A2 80
AMA: 2018,Sep,7

26476 **Lengthening of tendon, extensor, hand or finger, each tendon**
16.7 16.7 FUD 090 J A2
AMA: 2018,Sep,7

26477 **Shortening of tendon, extensor, hand or finger, each tendon**
16.3 16.3 FUD 090 J A2
AMA: 2018,Sep,7

26478 **Lengthening of tendon, flexor, hand or finger, each tendon**
18.2 18.2 FUD 090 J A2 80
AMA: 2018,Sep,7; 2018,Jan,8; 2017,Jan,8; 2016,Jan,13

26479 **Shortening of tendon, flexor, hand or finger, each tendon**
17.6 17.6 FUD 090 J A2 80
AMA: 2018,Sep,7

26480 **Transfer or transplant of tendon, carpometacarpal area or dorsum of hand; without free graft, each tendon**
21.1 21.1 FUD 090 J A2 80
AMA: 2018,Sep,7; 2018,Jan,8; 2017,Jan,8; 2016,Jan,13

26483 **with free tendon graft (includes obtaining graft), each tendon**
Facility RVU 24.4 Non-Facility RVU 24.4 **FUD** 090 J A2 80
AMA: 2018,Sep,7

26485 **Transfer or transplant of tendon, palmar; without free tendon graft, each tendon**
Facility RVU 22.7 Non-Facility RVU 22.7 **FUD** 090 J A2 80
AMA: 2018,Sep,7

26489 **with free tendon graft (includes obtaining graft), each tendon**
Facility RVU 27.1 Non-Facility RVU 27.1 **FUD** 090 J A2 80
AMA: 2018,Sep,7

26490 **Opponensplasty; superficialis tendon transfer type, each tendon**
EXCLUDES *Thumb fusion (26820)*
Facility RVU 22.5 Non-Facility RVU 22.5 **FUD** 090 J A2 80
AMA: 2018,Sep,7

26492 **tendon transfer with graft (includes obtaining graft), each tendon**
EXCLUDES *Thumb fusion (26820)*
Facility RVU 25.0 Non-Facility RVU 25.0 **FUD** 090 J A2 80
AMA: 2018,Sep,7

26494 **hypothenar muscle transfer**
EXCLUDES *Thumb fusion (26820)*
Facility RVU 23.3 Non-Facility RVU 23.3 **FUD** 090 J A2 80
AMA: 2018,Sep,7

26496 **other methods**
EXCLUDES *Thumb fusion (26820)*
Facility RVU 24.9 Non-Facility RVU 24.9 **FUD** 090 J A2 80
AMA: 2018,Sep,7

26497 **Transfer of tendon to restore intrinsic function; ring and small finger**
Facility RVU 25.2 Non-Facility RVU 25.2 **FUD** 090 J A2 80
AMA: 2018,Sep,7

26498 **all 4 fingers**
Facility RVU 33.2 Non-Facility RVU 33.2 **FUD** 090 J A2 80
AMA: 2018,Sep,7

26499 **Correction claw finger, other methods**
Facility RVU 24.2 Non-Facility RVU 24.2 **FUD** 090 J A2 80
AMA: 2018,Sep,7

26500 **Reconstruction of tendon pulley, each tendon; with local tissues (separate procedure)**
Facility RVU 18.2 Non-Facility RVU 18.2 **FUD** 090 J A2 80
AMA: 2018,Sep,7

26502 **with tendon or fascial graft (includes obtaining graft) (separate procedure)**
Facility RVU 20.8 Non-Facility RVU 20.8 **FUD** 090 J A2 80
AMA: 2018,Sep,7

26508 **Release of thenar muscle(s) (eg, thumb contracture)**
Facility RVU 18.6 Non-Facility RVU 18.6 **FUD** 090 J A2 80 50
AMA: 2018,Sep,7

26510 **Cross intrinsic transfer, each tendon**
Facility RVU 16.7 Non-Facility RVU 16.7 **FUD** 090 J A2 80
AMA: 2018,Sep,7

26516 **Capsulodesis, metacarpophalangeal joint; single digit**
Facility RVU 20.5 Non-Facility RVU 20.5 **FUD** 090 J A2 80 50
AMA: 2018,Sep,7

26517 **2 digits**
Facility RVU 24.1 Non-Facility RVU 24.1 **FUD** 090 J A2 80 50
AMA: 2018,Sep,7

26518 **3 or 4 digits**
Facility RVU 24.4 Non-Facility RVU 24.4 **FUD** 090 J A2 80 50
AMA: 2018,Sep,7

26520 **Capsulectomy or capsulotomy; metacarpophalangeal joint, each joint**
EXCLUDES *Carpometacarpal joint arthroplasty (25447)*
Facility RVU 18.2 Non-Facility RVU 18.2 **FUD** 090 J A2
AMA: 2018,Sep,7

26525 **interphalangeal joint, each joint**
EXCLUDES *Carpometacarpal joint arthroplasty (25447)*
Facility RVU 18.9 Non-Facility RVU 18.9 **FUD** 090 J A2
AMA: 2018,Sep,7; 2018,Jan,8; 2017,Jan,8; 2016,Jan,13

26530 **Arthroplasty, metacarpophalangeal joint; each joint**
EXCLUDES *Carpometacarpal joint arthroplasty (25447)*
Facility RVU 15.4 Non-Facility RVU 15.4 **FUD** 090 J J8 80
AMA: 2018,Sep,7

26531 **with prosthetic implant, each joint**
EXCLUDES *Carpometacarpal joint arthroplasty (25447)*
Facility RVU 18.0 Non-Facility RVU 18.0 **FUD** 090 J J8 80
AMA: 2018,Sep,7; 2018,Jan,8; 2017,Jan,8; 2016,Jan,13

26535 **Arthroplasty, interphalangeal joint; each joint**
EXCLUDES *Carpometacarpal joint arthroplasty (25447)*
Facility RVU 12.4 Non-Facility RVU 12.4 **FUD** 090 J A2
AMA: 2018,Sep,7

26536 **with prosthetic implant, each joint**
EXCLUDES *Carpometacarpal joint arthroplasty (25447)*
Facility RVU 20.8 Non-Facility RVU 20.8 **FUD** 090 J J8 80
AMA: 2018,Sep,7

26540 **Repair of collateral ligament, metacarpophalangeal or interphalangeal joint**
Facility RVU 19.3 Non-Facility RVU 19.3 **FUD** 090 J A2 80
AMA: 2018,Sep,7

26541 **Reconstruction, collateral ligament, metacarpophalangeal joint, single; with tendon or fascial graft (includes obtaining graft)**
Facility RVU 22.5 Non-Facility RVU 22.5 **FUD** 090 J A2 80
AMA: 2018,Sep,7; 2018,Jan,8; 2017,Jan,8; 2016,Jan,13

26542 **with local tissue (eg, adductor advancement)**
Facility RVU 19.9 Non-Facility RVU 19.9 **FUD** 090 J A2 80
AMA: 2018,Sep,7; 2018,Jan,8; 2017,Jan,8; 2016,Jan,13

26545 **Reconstruction, collateral ligament, interphalangeal joint, single, including graft, each joint**
Facility RVU 19.9 Non-Facility RVU 19.9 **FUD** 090 J A2 80
AMA: 2018,Sep,7

26546 **Repair non-union, metacarpal or phalanx (includes obtaining bone graft with or without external or internal fixation)**
Facility RVU 28.9 Non-Facility RVU 28.9 **FUD** 090 J A2 80 50
AMA: 2018,Sep,7

26548 **Repair and reconstruction, finger, volar plate, interphalangeal joint**
Facility RVU 22.2 Non-Facility RVU 22.2 **FUD** 090 J A2 80
AMA: 2018,Sep,7

26550-26556 Reconstruction Procedures with Finger and Toe Transplants

26550 **Pollicization of a digit**
Facility RVU 46.8 Non-Facility RVU 46.8 **FUD** 090 J A2 80 50
AMA: 2018,Sep,7

26551 **Transfer, toe-to-hand with microvascular anastomosis; great toe wrap-around with bone graft**
INCLUDES Operating microscope (69990)
EXCLUDES *Big toe with web space (20973)*
Facility RVU 95.1 Non-Facility RVU 95.1 **FUD** 090 C 80 50
AMA: 2018,Sep,7; 2018,Jan,8; 2017,Jan,8; 2016,Feb,12; 2016,Jan,13

26553 **other than great toe, single**
INCLUDES Operating microscope (69990)
94.5 94.5 FUD 090 C 80 50
AMA: 2018,Sep,7; 2018,Jan,8; 2017,Jan,8; 2016,Feb,12; 2016,Jan,13

26554 **other than great toe, double**
INCLUDES Operating microscope (69990)
109. 109. FUD 090 C 80 50
AMA: 2018,Sep,7; 2018,Jan,8; 2017,Jan,8; 2016,Feb,12; 2016,Jan,13

26555 **Transfer, finger to another position without microvascular anastomosis**
39.6 39.6 FUD 090 J A2 80
AMA: 2018,Sep,7

26556 **Transfer, free toe joint, with microvascular anastomosis**
INCLUDES Operating microscope (69990)
EXCLUDES *Big toe to hand transfer (20973)*
98.2 98.2 FUD 090 C 80
AMA: 2018,Sep,7; 2018,Jan,8; 2017,Jan,8; 2016,Feb,12; 2016,Jan,13

26560-26596 Repair of Other Deformities of the Fingers/Hand

26560 **Repair of syndactyly (web finger) each web space; with skin flaps**
16.5 16.5 FUD 090 J A2 80
AMA: 2018,Sep,7

26561 **with skin flaps and grafts**
27.5 27.5 FUD 090 J A2 80
AMA: 2018,Sep,7

26562 **complex (eg, involving bone, nails)**
38.8 38.8 FUD 090 J A2 80
AMA: 2018,Sep,7

26565 **Osteotomy; metacarpal, each**
19.0 19.0 FUD 090 J A2 80
AMA: 2018,Sep,7

26567 **phalanx of finger, each**
19.9 19.9 FUD 090 J A2 80
AMA: 2018,Sep,7; 2018,Jan,8; 2017,Jan,8; 2016,Jan,13

26568 **Osteoplasty, lengthening, metacarpal or phalanx**
26.1 26.1 FUD 090 J A2 80
AMA: 2018,Sep,7

26580 **Repair cleft hand**
INCLUDES Barsky's procedure
43.7 43.7 FUD 090 J A2 80 50
AMA: 2018,Sep,7

26587 **Reconstruction of polydactylous digit, soft tissue and bone**
EXCLUDES *Soft tissue removal only (11200)*
30.0 30.0 FUD 090 J A2 80
AMA: 2018,Sep,7; 2018,Jan,8; 2017,Jan,8; 2016,Jan,13

26590 **Repair macrodactylia, each digit**
40.7 40.7 FUD 090 J A2 80
AMA: 2018,Sep,7; 2018,Jan,8; 2017,Jan,8; 2016,Jan,13

26591 **Repair, intrinsic muscles of hand, each muscle**
13.0 13.0 FUD 090 J A2 80
AMA: 2018,Sep,7; 2018,Jan,8; 2017,Jan,8; 2016,Jan,13

26593 **Release, intrinsic muscles of hand, each muscle**
17.6 17.6 FUD 090 J A2
AMA: 2018,Sep,7

26596 **Excision of constricting ring of finger, with multiple Z-plasties**
EXCLUDES *Graft repair or scar contracture release (11042, 14040-14041, 15120, 15240)*
21.6 21.6 FUD 090 J A2 80
AMA: 2018,Sep,7

26600-26785 Treatment of Fracture/Dislocation of Fingers and Hand

INCLUDES Closed, percutaneous, and open treatment fractures or dislocations

26600 **Closed treatment of metacarpal fracture, single; without manipulation, each bone**
7.94 8.39 FUD 090 T P2
AMA: 2018,Sep,7

26605 **with manipulation, each bone**
8.45 9.33 FUD 090 T A2
AMA: 2018,Sep,7

26607 **Closed treatment of metacarpal fracture, with manipulation, with external fixation, each bone**
13.9 13.9 FUD 090 J A2 80
AMA: 2018,Sep,7

26608 **Percutaneous skeletal fixation of metacarpal fracture, each bone**
13.8 13.8 FUD 090 J A2 80
AMA: 2018,Sep,7

26615 **Open treatment of metacarpal fracture, single, includes internal fixation, when performed, each bone**
16.5 16.5 FUD 090 J A2
AMA: 2018,Sep,7

26641 **Closed treatment of carpometacarpal dislocation, thumb, with manipulation**
9.97 11.0 FUD 090 T P2 80 50
AMA: 2018,Sep,7

26645 **Closed treatment of carpometacarpal fracture dislocation, thumb (Bennett fracture), with manipulation**
11.3 12.3 FUD 090 J A2 80 50
AMA: 2018,Sep,7

26650 **Percutaneous skeletal fixation of carpometacarpal fracture dislocation, thumb (Bennett fracture), with manipulation**
13.7 13.7 FUD 090 J A2 50
AMA: 2018,Sep,7

26665 **Open treatment of carpometacarpal fracture dislocation, thumb (Bennett fracture), includes internal fixation, when performed**
18.0 18.0 FUD 090 J A2 50
AMA: 2018,Sep,7

26670 **Closed treatment of carpometacarpal dislocation, other than thumb, with manipulation, each joint; without anesthesia**
8.87 9.86 FUD 090 T P2 80
AMA: 2018,Sep,7

26675 **requiring anesthesia**
12.0 13.1 FUD 090 J A2 80
AMA: 2018,Sep,7

26676 **Percutaneous skeletal fixation of carpometacarpal dislocation, other than thumb, with manipulation, each joint**
14.5 14.5 FUD 090 J A2
AMA: 2018,Sep,7

26685 **Open treatment of carpometacarpal dislocation, other than thumb; includes internal fixation, when performed, each joint**
16.5 16.5 FUD 090 J A2
AMA: 2018,Sep,7

26686 **complex, multiple, or delayed reduction**
18.0 18.0 FUD 090 J A2 80
AMA: 2018,Sep,7

26700 **Closed treatment of metacarpophalangeal dislocation, single, with manipulation; without anesthesia**
8.86 9.55 FUD 090 T P2
AMA: 2018,Sep,7

26705 **requiring anesthesia**
10.9 11.9 FUD 090 J A2 80
AMA: 2018,Sep,7

26706 **Percutaneous skeletal fixation of metacarpophalangeal dislocation, single, with manipulation**
12.6 12.6 FUD 090 J A2
AMA: 2018,Sep,7

26715 **Open treatment of metacarpophalangeal dislocation, single, includes internal fixation, when performed**
16.4 16.4 FUD 090 J A2 80
AMA: 2018,Sep,7

26720 **Closed treatment of phalangeal shaft fracture, proximal or middle phalanx, finger or thumb; without manipulation, each**
5.26 5.62 FUD 090 T P2
AMA: 2018,Sep,7

26725 **with manipulation, with or without skin or skeletal traction, each**
8.73 9.75 FUD 090 T P2
AMA: 2018,Sep,7

26727 **Percutaneous skeletal fixation of unstable phalangeal shaft fracture, proximal or middle phalanx, finger or thumb, with manipulation, each**
13.5 13.5 FUD 090 J A2
AMA: 2018,Sep,7

26735 **Open treatment of phalangeal shaft fracture, proximal or middle phalanx, finger or thumb, includes internal fixation, when performed, each**
17.1 17.1 FUD 090 J A2
AMA: 2018,Sep,7

26740 **Closed treatment of articular fracture, involving metacarpophalangeal or interphalangeal joint; without manipulation, each**
6.25 6.60 FUD 090 T P2
AMA: 2018,Sep,7

26742 **with manipulation, each**
9.64 10.6 FUD 090 J A2
AMA: 2018,Sep,7

26746 **Open treatment of articular fracture, involving metacarpophalangeal or interphalangeal joint, includes internal fixation, when performed, each**
21.3 21.3 FUD 090 J A2
AMA: 2018,Sep,7

26750 **Closed treatment of distal phalangeal fracture, finger or thumb; without manipulation, each**
5.35 5.32 FUD 090 T P2
AMA: 2018,Sep,7

26755 **with manipulation, each**
7.77 8.99 FUD 090 T G2
AMA: 2018,Sep,7

26756 **Percutaneous skeletal fixation of distal phalangeal fracture, finger or thumb, each**
12.1 12.1 FUD 090 J A2 80
AMA: 2018,Sep,7

26765 **Open treatment of distal phalangeal fracture, finger or thumb, includes internal fixation, when performed, each**
14.3 14.3 FUD 090 J A2
AMA: 2018,Sep,7

26770 **Closed treatment of interphalangeal joint dislocation, single, with manipulation; without anesthesia**
7.41 8.08 FUD 090 T G2
AMA: 2018,Sep,7

26775 **requiring anesthesia**
9.96 11.0 FUD 090 T P2
AMA: 2018,Sep,7

26776 **Percutaneous skeletal fixation of interphalangeal joint dislocation, single, with manipulation**
12.8 12.8 FUD 090 J A2
AMA: 2018,Sep,7

26785 **Open treatment of interphalangeal joint dislocation, includes internal fixation, when performed, single**
15.7 15.7 FUD 090 J A2
AMA: 2018,Sep,7

26820-26863 Fusion of Joint(s) of Fingers or Hand

26820 **Fusion in opposition, thumb, with autogenous graft (includes obtaining graft)**
22.2 22.2 FUD 090 J J8 80 50
AMA: 2020,May,13; 2018,Sep,7

26841 **Arthrodesis, carpometacarpal joint, thumb, with or without internal fixation;**
21.2 21.2 FUD 090 J A2 80 50
AMA: 2020,May,13; 2018,Sep,7

26842 **with autograft (includes obtaining graft)**
22.8 22.8 FUD 090 J A2 80 50
AMA: 2020,May,13; 2018,Sep,7

26843 **Arthrodesis, carpometacarpal joint, digit, other than thumb, each;**
21.6 21.6 FUD 090 J J8 80
AMA: 2020,May,13; 2018,Sep,7; 2018,Jan,8; 2017,Jan,8; 2016,Jan,13

26844 **with autograft (includes obtaining graft)**
23.9 23.9 FUD 090 J J8 80
AMA: 2020,May,13; 2018,Sep,7

26850 **Arthrodesis, metacarpophalangeal joint, with or without internal fixation;**
20.2 20.2 FUD 090 J A2 80
AMA: 2020,May,13; 2018,Sep,7

26852 **with autograft (includes obtaining graft)**
23.2 23.2 FUD 090 J A2 80
AMA: 2020,May,13; 2018,Sep,7

26860 **Arthrodesis, interphalangeal joint, with or without internal fixation;**
15.9 15.9 FUD 090 J A2
AMA: 2020,May,13; 2018,Sep,7; 2018,Jan,8; 2017,Jan,8; 2016,Jan,13

\+ **26861** **each additional interphalangeal joint (List separately in addition to code for primary procedure)**
Code first (26860)
2.98 2.98 FUD ZZZ N N1
AMA: 2020,May,13; 2018,Sep,7; 2018,Jan,8; 2017,Jan,8; 2016,Jan,13

26862 **with autograft (includes obtaining graft)**
21.1 21.1 FUD 090 J A2 80
AMA: 2020,May,13; 2018,Sep,7

\+ **26863** **with autograft (includes obtaining graft), each additional joint (List separately in addition to code for primary procedure)**
Code first (26862)
6.62 6.62 FUD ZZZ N N1 80
AMA: 2020,May,13; 2018,Sep,7

26910-26989 Amputations and Unlisted Procedures Finger/Hand

26910 **Amputation, metacarpal, with finger or thumb (ray amputation), single, with or without interosseous transfer**
EXCLUDES *Repositioning (26550, 26555)*
Transmetacarpal amputation hand (25927)
21.1 21.1 FUD 090 J A2
AMA: 2018,Sep,7

26951 **Amputation, finger or thumb, primary or secondary, any joint or phalanx, single, including neurectomies; with direct closure**
EXCLUDES *Repair necessitating flaps or grafts (15050-15758)*
Transmetacarpal amputation hand (25927)
19.1 19.1 FUD 090 J A2
AMA: 2018,Sep,7

26952 **with local advancement flaps (V-Y, hood)**
EXCLUDES *Repair necessitating flaps or grafts (15050-15758)*
Transmetacarpal amputation hand (25927)
18.9 18.9 FUD 090 J A2
AMA: 2018,Sep,7

26989 **Unlisted procedure, hands or fingers**
0.00 0.00 FUD YYY T
AMA: 2018,Sep,7

26990-26992 Incision for Drainage of Pelvis or Hip

EXCLUDES *Simple incision and drainage procedures (10040-10160)*

26990 **Incision and drainage, pelvis or hip joint area; deep abscess or hematoma**
18.8 18.8 FUD 090 J A2
AMA: 2018,Sep,7

26991 **infected bursa**
15.1 20.4 FUD 090 J A2 80
AMA: 2018,Sep,7

26992 **Incision, bone cortex, pelvis and/or hip joint (eg, osteomyelitis or bone abscess)**
28.5 28.5 FUD 090 C 80
AMA: 2018,Sep,7; 2018,Jan,8; 2017,Jan,8; 2016,Jan,13

27000-27006 Tenotomy Procedures of Hip

27000 **Tenotomy, adductor of hip, percutaneous (separate procedure)**
11.6 11.6 FUD 090 J A2 50
AMA: 2018,Sep,7

27001 **Tenotomy, adductor of hip, open**
15.6 15.6 FUD 090 J A2 80 50
AMA: 2018,Sep,7

27003 **Tenotomy, adductor, subcutaneous, open, with obturator neurectomy**
17.0 17.0 FUD 090 J A2 80 50
AMA: 2018,Sep,7

27005 **Tenotomy, hip flexor(s), open (separate procedure)**
20.8 20.8 FUD 090 C 80 50
AMA: 2018,Sep,7

27006 **Tenotomy, abductors and/or extensor(s) of hip, open (separate procedure)**
20.7 20.7 FUD 090 J G2 80 50
AMA: 2018,Sep,7

27025-27036 Surgical Incision of Hip

27025 **Fasciotomy, hip or thigh, any type**
26.5 26.5 FUD 090 C 80 50
AMA: 2018,Sep,7

27027 **Decompression fasciotomy(ies), pelvic (buttock) compartment(s) (eg, gluteus medius-minimus, gluteus maximus, iliopsoas, and/or tensor fascia lata muscle), unilateral**
25.8 25.8 FUD 090 J G2 80 50
AMA: 2018,Sep,7

27030 **Arthrotomy, hip, with drainage (eg, infection)**
27.0 27.0 FUD 090 C 80 50
AMA: 2018,Sep,7

27033 **Arthrotomy, hip, including exploration or removal of loose or foreign body**
28.1 28.1 FUD 090 J A2 80 50
AMA: 2018,Sep,7; 2018,Jan,8; 2017,Jan,8; 2016,Jan,13

27035 **Denervation, hip joint, intrapelvic or extrapelvic intra-articular branches of sciatic, femoral, or obturator nerves**
EXCLUDES *Transection obturator nerve (64763, 64766)*
32.8 32.8 FUD 090 J A2 80 50
AMA: 2018,Sep,7; 2018,Jan,8; 2017,Jan,8; 2016,Jan,13

27036 **Capsulectomy or capsulotomy, hip, with or without excision of heterotopic bone, with release of hip flexor muscles (ie, gluteus medius, gluteus minimus, tensor fascia latae, rectus femoris, sartorius, iliopsoas)**
29.1 29.1 FUD 090 C 80 50
AMA: 2018,Sep,7

27040-27041 Biopsy of Hip/Pelvis

EXCLUDES *Soft tissue needle biopsy (20206)*

27040 **Biopsy, soft tissue of pelvis and hip area; superficial**
5.70 9.83 FUD 010 J A2 50
AMA: 2018,Sep,7

27041 **deep, subfascial or intramuscular**
20.1 20.1 FUD 090 J A2 50
AMA: 2018,Sep,7

27043-27059 [27043, 27045, 27059] Excision Soft Tissue Tumors Hip/ Pelvis

INCLUDES Any necessary elevation tissue planes or dissection
Measurement tumor and necessary margin at greatest diameter prior to excision
Simple and intermediate repairs
Excision types:
Fascial or subfascial soft tissue tumors: simple and marginal resection tumors found either in or below deep fascia, not involving bone or excision substantial amount normal tissue; primarily benign and intramuscular tumors
Radical resection soft tissue tumor: wide resection tumor involving substantial margins normal tissue and may involve tissue removal from one or more layers; mostly malignant or aggressive benign,
Subcutaneous: simple and marginal resection tumors found in subcutaneous tissue above deep fascia; most often benign

EXCLUDES *Complex repair*
Excision benign cutaneous lesions (eg, sebaceous cyst) (11400-11406)
Radical resection cutaneous tumors (eg, melanoma) (11600-11606)
Significant vessel exploration, neuroplasty, reconstruction, or complex bone repair

27043 **Resequenced code. See code following 27047.**

27045 **Resequenced code. See code following 27048.**

27047 **Excision, tumor, soft tissue of pelvis and hip area, subcutaneous; less than 3 cm**
10.4 13.6 FUD 090 J G2 50
AMA: 2018,Sep,7

\# **27043** **3 cm or greater**
13.5 13.5 FUD 090 J G2 50
AMA: 2018,Sep,7

27048 **Excision, tumor, soft tissue of pelvis and hip area, subfascial (eg, intramuscular); less than 5 cm**
17.6 17.6 FUD 090 J G2 80 50
AMA: 2018,Sep,7

\# **27045** **5 cm or greater**
21.3 21.3 FUD 090 J G2 80 50
AMA: 2018,Sep,7

27049 **Radical resection of tumor (eg, sarcoma), soft tissue of pelvis and hip area; less than 5 cm**
38.6 38.6 FUD 090 J G2 80 50
AMA: 2018,Sep,7

\# **27059** **5 cm or greater**
52.6 52.6 FUD 090 J G2 80 50
AMA: 2018,Sep,7

27050-27071 [27059] Procedures of Bones and Joints of Hip and Pelvis

27050 **Arthrotomy, with biopsy; sacroiliac joint**
11.5 11.5 FUD 090 J A2 80
AMA: 2018,Sep,7

27052 **hip joint**
16.6 16.6 FUD 090 J A2 80 50
AMA: 2018,Sep,7

27054 **Arthrotomy with synovectomy, hip joint**
19.8 19.8 FUD 090 C 80 50
AMA: 2018,Sep,7

27057 **Decompression fasciotomy(ies), pelvic (buttock) compartment(s) (eg, gluteus medius-minimus, gluteus maximus, iliopsoas, and/or tensor fascia lata muscle) with debridement of nonviable muscle, unilateral**
29.2 29.2 FUD 090 J G2 80 50
AMA: 2018,Sep,7

27059 **Resequenced code. See code following 27049.**

27060 **Excision; ischial bursa**
13.4 13.4 FUD 090 J A2 50
AMA: 2018,Sep,7

27062 **trochanteric bursa or calcification**
EXCLUDES *Arthrocentesis (20610)*
13.0 13.0 FUD 090 J A2 50
AMA: 2018,Sep,7

27065 **Excision of bone cyst or benign tumor, wing of ilium, symphysis pubis, or greater trochanter of femur; superficial, includes autograft, when performed**
15.0 15.0 FUD 090 J A2 80 50
AMA: 2018,Sep,7

27066 **deep (subfascial), includes autograft, when performed**
23.1 23.1 FUD 090 J A2 80 50
AMA: 2018,Sep,7

27067 **with autograft requiring separate incision**
29.8 29.8 FUD 090 J A2 80 50
AMA: 2018,Sep,7

27070 **Partial excision, wing of ilium, symphysis pubis, or greater trochanter of femur, (craterization, saucerization) (eg, osteomyelitis or bone abscess); superficial**
25.3 25.3 FUD 090 C 80 50
AMA: 2018,Sep,7

27071 **deep (subfascial or intramuscular)**
27.2 27.2 FUD 090 C 80 50
AMA: 2018,Sep,7

27075-27078 Radical Resection Bone Tumor of Hip/Pelvis

INCLUDES Any necessary elevation tissue planes or dissection
Excision adjacent soft tissue during bone tumor resection (27043-27049 [27043, 27045, 27059])
Measurement tumor and necessary margin at greatest diameter prior to excision
Resection tumor (may include entire bone) and wide margins normal tissue primarily for malignant or aggressive benign tumors
Simple and intermediate repairs

EXCLUDES *Complex repair*
Significant vessel exploration, neuroplasty, reconstruction, or complex bone repair

27075 **Radical resection of tumor; wing of ilium, 1 pubic or ischial ramus or symphysis pubis**
60.5 60.5 FUD 090 C 80
AMA: 2019,May,7; 2018,Sep,7

27076 **ilium, including acetabulum, both pubic rami, or ischium and acetabulum**
73.3 73.3 FUD 090 C 80
AMA: 2019,May,7; 2018,Sep,7

27077 **innominate bone, total**
81.8 81.8 FUD 090 C 80
AMA: 2019,May,7; 2018,Sep,7

27078 **ischial tuberosity and greater trochanter of femur**
59.6 59.6 FUD 090 C 80 50
AMA: 2019,May,7; 2018,Sep,7

27080 Excision of Coccyx

EXCLUDES *Surgical excision decubitus ulcers (15920, 15922, 15931-15958)*

27080 **Coccygectomy, primary**
14.7 14.7 FUD 090 J A2 80
AMA: 2018,Sep,7

27086-27091 Removal Foreign Body or Hip Prosthesis

27086 **Removal of foreign body, pelvis or hip; subcutaneous tissue**
4.82 8.78 FUD 010 J A2 80 50
AMA: 2018,Sep,7; 2018,Jan,8; 2017,Jan,8; 2016,Jan,13

27087 **deep (subfascial or intramuscular)**
17.7 17.7 FUD 090 J A2 80 50
AMA: 2018,Sep,7

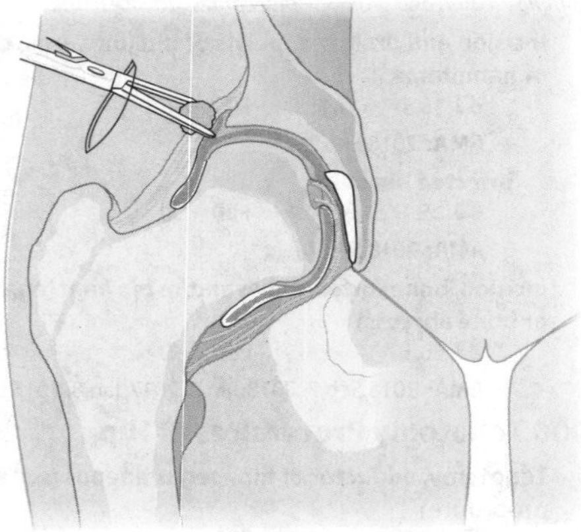

A foreign body is removed from the pelvis or hip

27090 **Removal of hip prosthesis; (separate procedure)**
24.0 24.0 FUD 090 C 80 50
AMA: 2019,May,7; 2018,Sep,7

27091 **complicated, including total hip prosthesis, methylmethacrylate with or without insertion of spacer**
46.0 46.0 FUD 090 C 80 50
AMA: 2019,May,7; 2018,Sep,7; 2018,Jan,8; 2017,Jan,8; 2016,Jan,13

27093-27096 Injection for Arthrogram Hip/Sacroiliac Joint

27093 **Injection procedure for hip arthrography; without anesthesia**
(73525)
2.01 5.72 FUD 000 N N1 50
AMA: 2018,Sep,7; 2018,Jan,8; 2017,Jan,8; 2016,Jan,13

27095 **with anesthesia**
(73525)
2.43 8.36 FUD 000 N N1 50
AMA: 2018,Sep,7; 2018,Jan,8; 2017,Jan,8; 2016,Jan,13; 2016,Jan,11

27096 **Injection procedure for sacroiliac joint, anesthetic/steroid, with image guidance (fluoroscopy or CT) including arthrography when performed**
INCLUDES Confirmation intra-articular needle placement with CT or fluoroscopy
Fluoroscopic guidance (77002-77003)
EXCLUDES *Procedure performed without fluoroscopy or CT guidance (20552)*
2.39 4.61 FUD 000 B 50
AMA: 2018,Sep,7; 2018,Jan,8; 2017,Jan,8; 2016,Jan,13

27097-27187 Revision/Reconstruction Hip and Pelvis

INCLUDES Closed, open and percutaneous treatment fractures and dislocations

27097 **Release or recession, hamstring, proximal**
19.7 19.7 FUD 090 J A2 80 50
AMA: 2018,Sep,7

27098 **Transfer, adductor to ischium**
20.0 20.0 FUD 090 J A2 80 50
AMA: 2018,Sep,7

27100 Transfer external oblique muscle to greater trochanter including fascial or tendon extension (graft)

INCLUDES Eggers procedure

23.6 23.6 FUD 090 J A2 80 50

AMA: 2018,Sep,7

27105 Transfer paraspinal muscle to hip (includes fascial or tendon extension graft)

25.0 25.0 FUD 090 J A2 80 50

AMA: 2018,Sep,7

27110 Transfer iliopsoas; to greater trochanter of femur

28.0 28.0 FUD 090 J J8 80 50

AMA: 2018,Sep,7

27111 to femoral neck

26.0 26.0 FUD 090 J A2 80 50

AMA: 2018,Sep,7

27120 Acetabuloplasty; (eg, Whitman, Colonna, Haygroves, or cup type)

37.5 37.5 FUD 090 C 80 50

AMA: 2018,Sep,7

27122 resection, femoral head (eg, Girdlestone procedure)

31.7 31.7 FUD 090 C 80 50

AMA: 2018,Sep,7

27125 Hemiarthroplasty, hip, partial (eg, femoral stem prosthesis, bipolar arthroplasty)

EXCLUDES *Hip replacement following hip fracture (27236)*

32.7 32.7 FUD 090 C 80 50

AMA: 2018,Sep,7; 2018,Jan,8; 2017,Jan,8; 2016,Jan,13

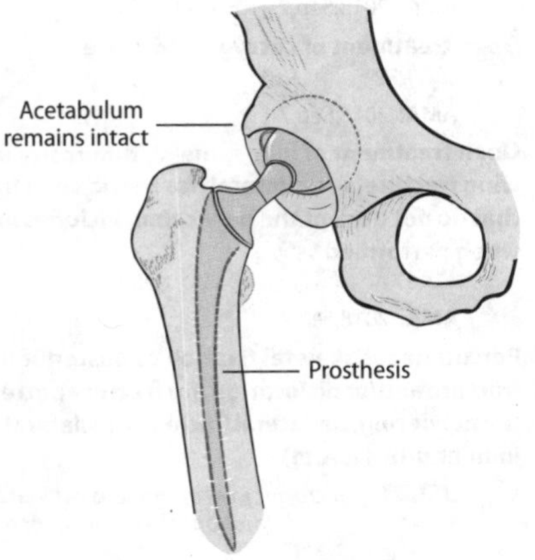

27130 Arthroplasty, acetabular and proximal femoral prosthetic replacement (total hip arthroplasty), with or without autograft or allograft

39.2 39.2 FUD 090 C J8 80 50

AMA: 2019,May,7; 2018,Sep,7; 2018,Jan,8; 2017,Jan,8; 2016,Jan,13

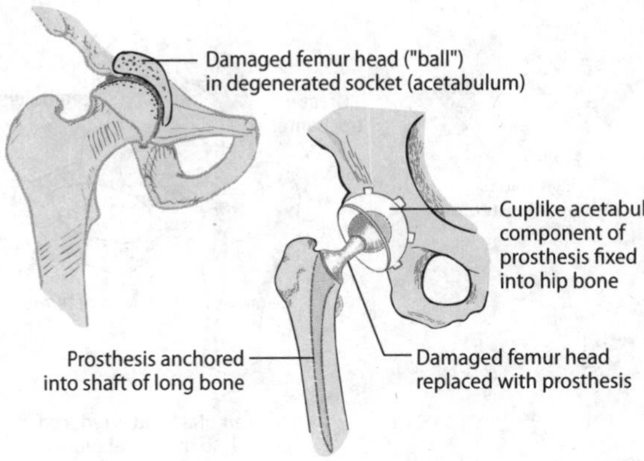

27132 Conversion of previous hip surgery to total hip arthroplasty, with or without autograft or allograft

48.3 48.3 FUD 090 C 80 50

AMA: 2019,May,7; 2018,Sep,7; 2018,Jan,8; 2017,Sep,14; 2017,Jan,8; 2016,Jan,13

27134 Revision of total hip arthroplasty; both components, with or without autograft or allograft

55.3 55.3 FUD 090 C 80 50

AMA: 2019,May,7; 2018,Sep,7; 2018,Jan,8; 2017,Jan,8; 2016,Jan,13

27137 acetabular component only, with or without autograft or allograft

42.5 42.5 FUD 090 C 80 50

AMA: 2018,Sep,7; 2018,Jan,8; 2017,Jan,8; 2016,Jan,13

27138 femoral component only, with or without allograft

44.1 44.1 FUD 090 C 80 50

AMA: 2019,May,7; 2018,Sep,7; 2018,Jan,8; 2017,Jan,8; 2016,Jan,13

27140 Osteotomy and transfer of greater trochanter of femur (separate procedure)

25.8 25.8 FUD 090 C 80 50

AMA: 2018,Sep,7

27146 Osteotomy, iliac, acetabular or innominate bone;

INCLUDES Salter osteotomy

36.9 36.9 FUD 090 C 80 50

AMA: 2018,Sep,7; 2018,Jan,8; 2017,Jan,8; 2016,Jan,13

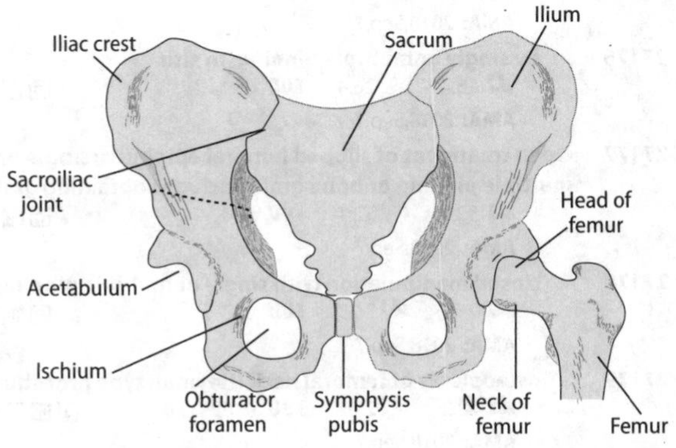

27147 **with open reduction of hip**
INCLUDES Pemberton osteotomy
41.9 41.9 FUD 090 C 80 50
AMA: 2018,Sep,7

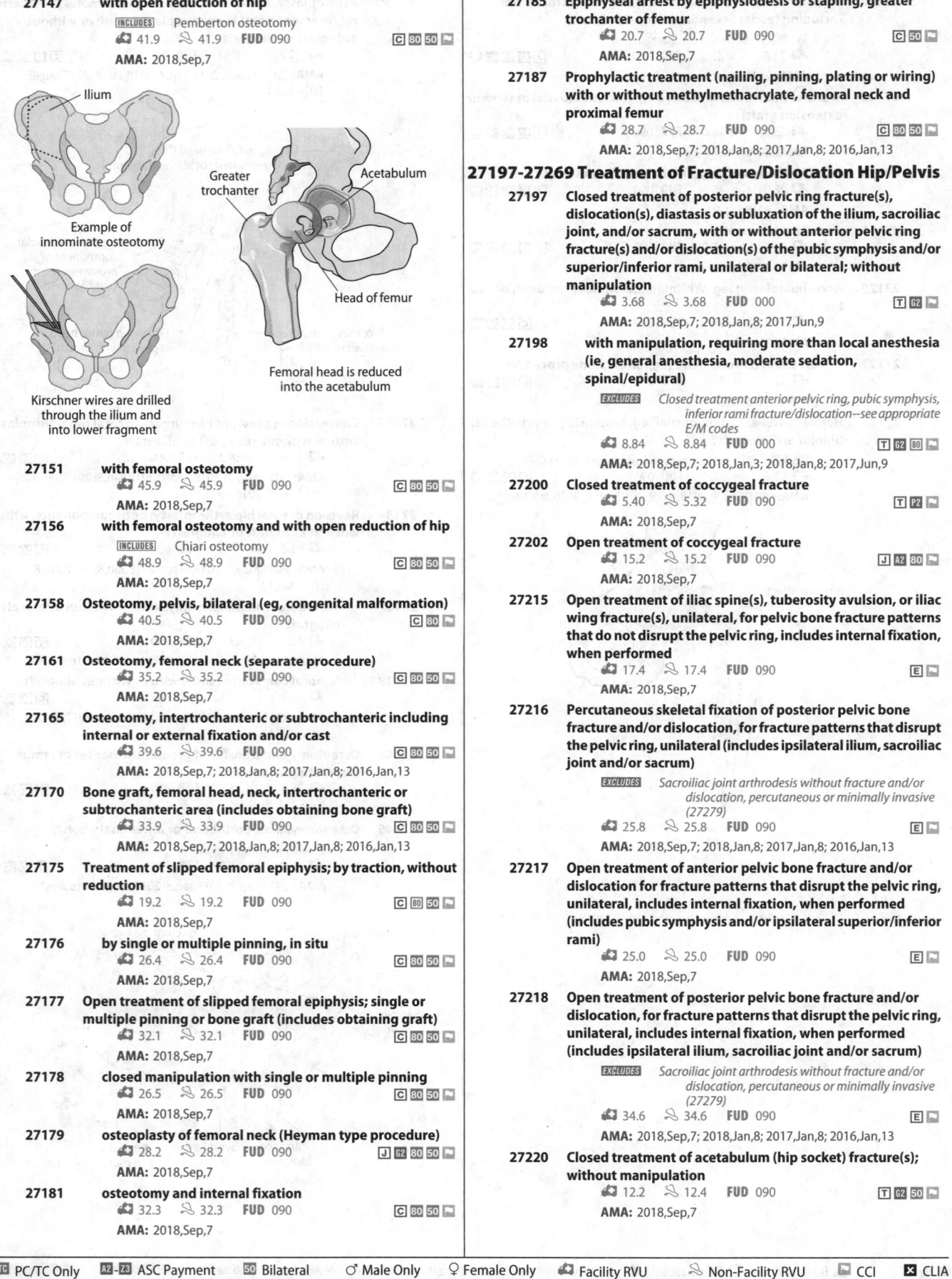

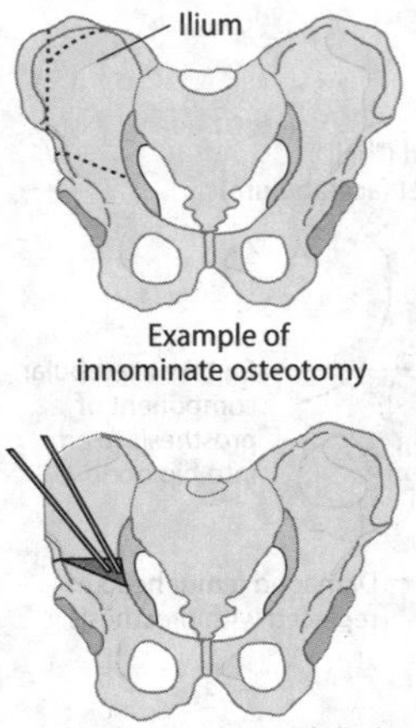

Example of innominate osteotomy
Kirschner wires are drilled through the ilium and into lower fragment

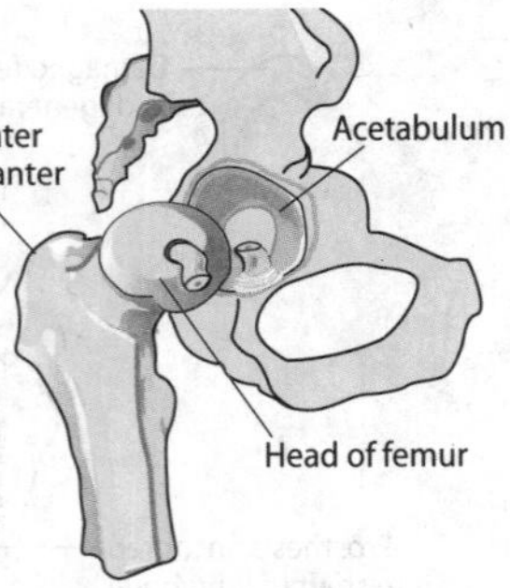

Femoral head is reduced into the acetabulum

27151 **with femoral osteotomy**
45.9 45.9 FUD 090 C 80 50
AMA: 2018,Sep,7

27156 **with femoral osteotomy and with open reduction of hip**
INCLUDES Chiari osteotomy
48.9 48.9 FUD 090 C 80 50
AMA: 2018,Sep,7

27158 **Osteotomy, pelvis, bilateral (eg, congenital malformation)**
40.5 40.5 FUD 090 C 80
AMA: 2018,Sep,7

27161 **Osteotomy, femoral neck (separate procedure)**
35.2 35.2 FUD 090 C 80 50
AMA: 2018,Sep,7

27165 **Osteotomy, intertrochanteric or subtrochanteric including internal or external fixation and/or cast**
39.6 39.6 FUD 090 C 80 50
AMA: 2018,Sep,7; 2018,Jan,8; 2017,Jan,8; 2016,Jan,13

27170 **Bone graft, femoral head, neck, intertrochanteric or subtrochanteric area (includes obtaining bone graft)**
33.9 33.9 FUD 090 C 80 50
AMA: 2018,Sep,7; 2018,Jan,8; 2017,Jan,8; 2016,Jan,13

27175 **Treatment of slipped femoral epiphysis; by traction, without reduction**
19.2 19.2 FUD 090 C 80 50
AMA: 2018,Sep,7

27176 **by single or multiple pinning, in situ**
26.4 26.4 FUD 090 C 80 50
AMA: 2018,Sep,7

27177 **Open treatment of slipped femoral epiphysis; single or multiple pinning or bone graft (includes obtaining graft)**
32.1 32.1 FUD 090 C 80 50
AMA: 2018,Sep,7

27178 **closed manipulation with single or multiple pinning**
26.5 26.5 FUD 090 C 80 50
AMA: 2018,Sep,7

27179 **osteoplasty of femoral neck (Heyman type procedure)**
28.2 28.2 FUD 090 J G2 80 50
AMA: 2018,Sep,7

27181 **osteotomy and internal fixation**
32.3 32.3 FUD 090 C 80 50
AMA: 2018,Sep,7

27185 **Epiphyseal arrest by epiphysiodesis or stapling, greater trochanter of femur**
20.7 20.7 FUD 090 C 50
AMA: 2018,Sep,7

27187 **Prophylactic treatment (nailing, pinning, plating or wiring) with or without methylmethacrylate, femoral neck and proximal femur**
28.7 28.7 FUD 090 C 80 50
AMA: 2018,Sep,7; 2018,Jan,8; 2017,Jan,8; 2016,Jan,13

27197-27269 Treatment of Fracture/Dislocation Hip/Pelvis

27197 **Closed treatment of posterior pelvic ring fracture(s), dislocation(s), diastasis or subluxation of the ilium, sacroiliac joint, and/or sacrum, with or without anterior pelvic ring fracture(s) and/or dislocation(s) of the pubic symphysis and/or superior/inferior rami, unilateral or bilateral; without manipulation**
3.68 3.68 FUD 000 T G2
AMA: 2018,Sep,7; 2018,Jan,8; 2017,Jun,9

27198 **with manipulation, requiring more than local anesthesia (ie, general anesthesia, moderate sedation, spinal/epidural)**
EXCLUDES *Closed treatment anterior pelvic ring, pubic symphysis, inferior rami fracture/dislocation--see appropriate E/M codes*
8.84 8.84 FUD 000 T G2 80
AMA: 2018,Sep,7; 2018,Jan,3; 2018,Jan,8; 2017,Jun,9

27200 **Closed treatment of coccygeal fracture**
5.40 5.32 FUD 090 T P2
AMA: 2018,Sep,7

27202 **Open treatment of coccygeal fracture**
15.2 15.2 FUD 090 J A2 80
AMA: 2018,Sep,7

27215 **Open treatment of iliac spine(s), tuberosity avulsion, or iliac wing fracture(s), unilateral, for pelvic bone fracture patterns that do not disrupt the pelvic ring, includes internal fixation, when performed**
17.4 17.4 FUD 090 E
AMA: 2018,Sep,7

27216 **Percutaneous skeletal fixation of posterior pelvic bone fracture and/or dislocation, for fracture patterns that disrupt the pelvic ring, unilateral (includes ipsilateral ilium, sacroiliac joint and/or sacrum)**
EXCLUDES *Sacroiliac joint arthrodesis without fracture and/or dislocation, percutaneous or minimally invasive (27279)*
25.8 25.8 FUD 090 E
AMA: 2018,Sep,7; 2018,Jan,8; 2017,Jan,8; 2016,Jan,13

27217 **Open treatment of anterior pelvic bone fracture and/or dislocation for fracture patterns that disrupt the pelvic ring, unilateral, includes internal fixation, when performed (includes pubic symphysis and/or ipsilateral superior/inferior rami)**
25.0 25.0 FUD 090 E
AMA: 2018,Sep,7

27218 **Open treatment of posterior pelvic bone fracture and/or dislocation, for fracture patterns that disrupt the pelvic ring, unilateral, includes internal fixation, when performed (includes ipsilateral ilium, sacroiliac joint and/or sacrum)**
EXCLUDES *Sacroiliac joint arthrodesis without fracture and/or dislocation, percutaneous or minimally invasive (27279)*
34.6 34.6 FUD 090 E
AMA: 2018,Sep,7; 2018,Jan,8; 2017,Jan,8; 2016,Jan,13

27220 **Closed treatment of acetabulum (hip socket) fracture(s); without manipulation**
12.2 12.4 FUD 090 T G2 50
AMA: 2018,Sep,7

27222 **with manipulation, with or without skeletal traction**
28.1 28.1 **FUD** 090 C 50
AMA: 2018,Sep,7

27226 **Open treatment of posterior or anterior acetabular wall fracture, with internal fixation**
30.4 30.4 **FUD** 090 C 80 50
AMA: 2018,Sep,7

27227 **Open treatment of acetabular fracture(s) involving anterior or posterior (one) column, or a fracture running transversely across the acetabulum, with internal fixation**
47.9 47.9 **FUD** 090 C 80 50
AMA: 2018,Sep,7

27228 **Open treatment of acetabular fracture(s) involving anterior and posterior (two) columns, includes T-fracture and both column fracture with complete articular detachment, or single column or transverse fracture with associated acetabular wall fracture, with internal fixation**
54.3 54.3 **FUD** 090 C 80 50
AMA: 2018,Sep,7

27230 **Closed treatment of femoral fracture, proximal end, neck; without manipulation**
13.6 13.8 **FUD** 090 T A2 50
AMA: 2018,Sep,7

27232 **with manipulation, with or without skeletal traction**
21.6 21.6 **FUD** 090 C 50
AMA: 2018,Sep,7

27235 **Percutaneous skeletal fixation of femoral fracture, proximal end, neck**
26.2 26.2 **FUD** 090 J G2 50
AMA: 2018,Sep,7; 2018,Jan,8; 2017,Jan,8; 2016,Jan,13

27236 **Open treatment of femoral fracture, proximal end, neck, internal fixation or prosthetic replacement**
34.4 34.4 **FUD** 090 C 80 50
AMA: 2019,May,7; 2018,Sep,7; 2018,Jan,8; 2017,Jan,8; 2016,Nov,9; 2016,Jan,13

27238 **Closed treatment of intertrochanteric, peritrochanteric, or subtrochanteric femoral fracture; without manipulation**
13.3 13.3 **FUD** 090 J A2 50
AMA: 2018,Sep,7; 2018,Jan,8; 2017,Jan,8; 2016,Jan,13

27240 **with manipulation, with or without skin or skeletal traction**
27.5 27.5 **FUD** 090 C 50
AMA: 2018,Sep,7; 2018,Jan,8; 2017,Jan,8; 2016,Jan,13

27244 **Treatment of intertrochanteric, peritrochanteric, or subtrochanteric femoral fracture; with plate/screw type implant, with or without cerclage**
35.5 35.5 **FUD** 090 C 80 50
AMA: 2019,May,7; 2018,Sep,7; 2018,Jan,8; 2017,Jan,8; 2016,Jan,13

27245 **with intramedullary implant, with or without interlocking screws and/or cerclage**
35.5 35.5 **FUD** 090 C 80 50
AMA: 2018,Sep,7; 2018,Jan,8; 2017,Jan,8; 2016,Jan,13

27246 **Closed treatment of greater trochanteric fracture, without manipulation**
11.1 11.1 **FUD** 090 T A2 50
AMA: 2018,Sep,7

27248 **Open treatment of greater trochanteric fracture, includes internal fixation, when performed**
21.5 21.5 **FUD** 090 C 80 50
AMA: 2018,Sep,7

27250 **Closed treatment of hip dislocation, traumatic; without anesthesia**
5.33 5.33 **FUD** 000 T A2 50
AMA: 2018,Sep,7

27252 **requiring anesthesia**
21.8 21.8 **FUD** 090 J A2 50
AMA: 2018,Sep,7

27253 **Open treatment of hip dislocation, traumatic, without internal fixation**
27.2 27.2 **FUD** 090 C 80 50
AMA: 2018,Sep,7

27254 **Open treatment of hip dislocation, traumatic, with acetabular wall and femoral head fracture, with or without internal or external fixation**
EXCLUDES *Acetabular fracture treatment (27226-27227)*
36.4 36.4 **FUD** 090 C 80 50
AMA: 2018,Sep,7

27256 **Treatment of spontaneous hip dislocation (developmental, including congenital or pathological), by abduction, splint or traction; without anesthesia, without manipulation**
6.78 8.73 **FUD** 010 T G2 80 50
AMA: 2018,Sep,7

27257 **with manipulation, requiring anesthesia**
10.4 10.4 **FUD** 010 J A2 80 50
AMA: 2018,Sep,7

27258 **Open treatment of spontaneous hip dislocation (developmental, including congenital or pathological), replacement of femoral head in acetabulum (including tenotomy, etc);**
INCLUDES Lorenz's operation
32.1 32.1 **FUD** 090 C 80 50
AMA: 2018,Sep,7

27259 **with femoral shaft shortening**
44.7 44.7 **FUD** 090 C 80 50
AMA: 2018,Sep,7

27265 **Closed treatment of post hip arthroplasty dislocation; without anesthesia**
11.5 11.5 **FUD** 090 T A2 50
AMA: 2018,Sep,7

27266 **requiring regional or general anesthesia**
16.8 16.8 **FUD** 090 J A2 50
AMA: 2018,Sep,7

27267 **Closed treatment of femoral fracture, proximal end, head; without manipulation**
12.5 12.5 **FUD** 090 J G2 80 50
AMA: 2018,Sep,7; 2018,Jan,8; 2017,Jan,8; 2016,Jan,13

27268 **with manipulation**
15.6 15.6 **FUD** 090 C 80 50
AMA: 2018,Sep,7; 2018,Jan,8; 2017,Jan,8; 2016,Jan,13

27269 **Open treatment of femoral fracture, proximal end, head, includes internal fixation, when performed**
EXCLUDES *Arthrotomy, hip (27033)*
Open treatment hip dislocation, traumatic, without internal fixation (27253)
35.8 35.8 **FUD** 090 C 80 50
AMA: 2018,Sep,7; 2018,Jan,8; 2017,Jan,8; 2016,Jan,13

27275 Hip Manipulation with Anesthesia

27275 **Manipulation, hip joint, requiring general anesthesia**
5.26 5.26 **FUD** 010 J A2
AMA: 2018,Sep,7; 2018,Jan,8; 2017,Jan,8; 2016,May,13; 2016,Jan,11; 2016,Jan,13

27279-27286 Arthrodesis of Hip and Pelvis

27279 **Arthrodesis, sacroiliac joint, percutaneous or minimally invasive (indirect visualization), with image guidance, includes obtaining bone graft when performed, and placement of transfixing device**
25.3 25.3 **FUD** 090 J J8 80 50
AMA: 2020,May,13; 2018,Sep,7

27280 **Arthrodesis, open, sacroiliac joint, including obtaining bone graft, including instrumentation, when performed**

EXCLUDES *Sacroiliac joint arthrodesis without fracture and/or dislocation, percutaneous or minimally invasive (27279)*

39.2 39.2 FUD 090 C 80 50

AMA: 2020,May,13; 2018,Sep,7; 2018,Jan,8; 2017,Jan,8; 2016,Jan,13

27282 **Arthrodesis, symphysis pubis (including obtaining graft)**

24.7 24.7 FUD 090 C 80

AMA: 2020,May,13; 2018,Sep,7

27284 **Arthrodesis, hip joint (including obtaining graft);**

46.6 46.6 FUD 090 C 80 50

AMA: 2020,May,13; 2018,Sep,7

27286 **with subtrochanteric osteotomy**

47.6 47.6 FUD 090 C 80 50

AMA: 2020,May,13; 2018,Sep,7; 2018,Jan,8; 2017,Jan,8; 2016,Jan,13

27290-27299 Amputations and Unlisted Procedures of Hip and Pelvis

27290 **Interpelviabdominal amputation (hindquarter amputation)**

46.9 46.9 FUD 090 C 80

AMA: 2018,Sep,7; 2018,Jan,8; 2017,Jan,8; 2016,Jan,13

27295 **Disarticulation of hip**

36.4 36.4 FUD 090 C 80 50

AMA: 2018,Sep,7; 2018,Jan,8; 2017,Jan,8; 2016,Jan,13

27299 **Unlisted procedure, pelvis or hip joint**

0.00 0.00 FUD YYY T 80 50

AMA: 2018,Sep,7; 2018,Jan,8; 2017,Jan,8; 2016,Jun,8; 2016,Jan,13

27301-27310 Incisional Procedures Femur or Knee

EXCLUDES *Superficial incision and drainage (10040-10160)*

27301 **Incision and drainage, deep abscess, bursa, or hematoma, thigh or knee region**

14.5 19.4 FUD 090 J A2 50

AMA: 2018,Sep,7; 2018,Jan,8; 2017,Jan,8; 2016,Jan,13

27303 **Incision, deep, with opening of bone cortex, femur or knee (eg, osteomyelitis or bone abscess)**

18.5 18.5 FUD 090 C 80 50

AMA: 2018,Sep,7

27305 **Fasciotomy, iliotibial (tenotomy), open**

EXCLUDES *Ober-Yount (gluteal-iliotibial) fasciotomy (27025)*

13.8 13.8 FUD 090 J A2 80 50

AMA: 2018,Sep,7

27306 **Tenotomy, percutaneous, adductor or hamstring; single tendon (separate procedure)**

9.87 9.87 FUD 090 J A2 80 50

AMA: 2018,Sep,7; 2018,Jan,8; 2017,Aug,9

27307 **multiple tendons**

13.8 13.8 FUD 090 J A2 80 50

AMA: 2018,Sep,7; 2018,Jan,8; 2017,Aug,9

27310 **Arthrotomy, knee, with exploration, drainage, or removal of foreign body (eg, infection)**

21.1 21.1 FUD 090 J A2 80 50

AMA: 2018,Sep,7; 2018,Jan,8; 2017,Jan,8; 2016,Jan,13

27323-27324 Biopsy Femur or Knee

EXCLUDES *Soft tissue needle biopsy (20206)*

27323 **Biopsy, soft tissue of thigh or knee area; superficial**

5.08 7.91 FUD 010 J A2 50

AMA: 2018,Sep,7; 2018,Jan,8; 2017,Jan,8; 2016,Jan,13

27324 **deep (subfascial or intramuscular)**

11.6 11.6 FUD 090 J A2 50

AMA: 2018,Sep,7; 2018,Jan,8; 2017,Jan,8; 2016,Jan,13

27325-27326 Neurectomy

27325 **Neurectomy, hamstring muscle**

16.1 16.1 FUD 090 J A2 80 50

AMA: 2018,Sep,7

27326 **Neurectomy, popliteal (gastrocnemius)**

14.9 14.9 FUD 090 J A2 80 50

AMA: 2018,Sep,7

27327-27339 [27329, 27337, 27339] Excision Soft Tissue Tumors Femur/ Knee

INCLUDES Any necessary elevation tissue planes or dissection
Measurement tumor and necessary margin at greatest diameter prior to excision
Simple and intermediate repairs
Excision types:
Fascial or subfascial soft tissue tumors: simple and marginal resection tumors found either in or below deep fascia, not including bone or excision substantial amount normal tissue; primarily benign and intramuscular tumors
Radical resection soft tissue tumor: wide resection tumor involving substantial margins normal tissue and may involve tissue removal from one or more layers; most often malignant or aggressive benign
Subcutaneous: simple and marginal resection tumors in subcutaneous tissue above deep fascia; most often benign

EXCLUDES *Complex repair*
Excision benign cutaneous lesions (eg, sebaceous cyst) (11400-11406)
Radical resection cutaneous tumors (eg, melanoma) (11600-11606)
Significant vessel exploration or neuroplasty

27327 **Excision, tumor, soft tissue of thigh or knee area, subcutaneous; less than 3 cm**

9.00 13.5 FUD 090 J G2 50

AMA: 2018,Sep,7

\# **27337** **3 cm or greater**

12.1 12.1 FUD 090 J G2 80 50

AMA: 2018,Sep,7

27328 **Excision, tumor, soft tissue of thigh or knee area, subfascial (eg, intramuscular); less than 5 cm**

18.0 18.0 FUD 090 J G2 50

AMA: 2018,Sep,7; 2018,Jan,8; 2017,Jan,8; 2016,Nov,9

27329 **Resequenced code. See code following 27360.**

\# **27339** **5 cm or greater**

21.7 21.7 FUD 090 J G2 80 50

AMA: 2018,Sep,7

27330-27360 [27337, 27339] Resection Procedures Thigh/Knee

27330 **Arthrotomy, knee; with synovial biopsy only**

11.8 11.8 FUD 090 J A2 50

AMA: 2018,Sep,7; 2018,Jan,8; 2017,Jan,8; 2016,Jan,13

27331 **including joint exploration, biopsy, or removal of loose or foreign bodies**

13.6 13.6 FUD 090 J A2 80 50

AMA: 2018,Sep,7; 2018,Jan,8; 2017,Jan,8; 2016,Jan,13

27332 **Arthrotomy, with excision of semilunar cartilage (meniscectomy) knee; medial OR lateral**
18.5 18.5 FUD 090 J A2 80 50
AMA: 2018,Sep,7

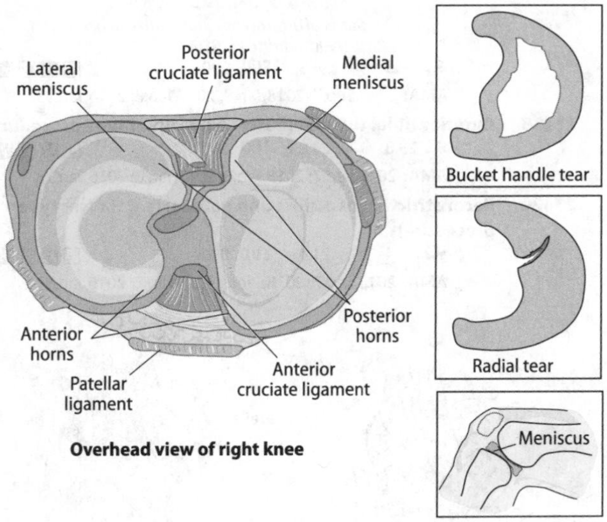

Overhead view of right knee

27333 **medial AND lateral**
16.9 16.9 FUD 090 J A2 80 50
AMA: 2018,Sep,7; 2018,Jan,8; 2017,Jan,8; 2016,Jan,13

27334 **Arthrotomy, with synovectomy, knee; anterior OR posterior**
19.7 19.7 FUD 090 J A2 80 50
AMA: 2018,Sep,7

27335 **anterior AND posterior including popliteal area**
22.0 22.0 FUD 090 J A2 80 50
AMA: 2018,Sep,7

27337 **Resequenced code. See code following 27327.**

27339 **Resequenced code. See code before 27330.**

27340 **Excision, prepatellar bursa**
10.6 10.6 FUD 090 J A2 50
AMA: 2018,Sep,7

27345 **Excision of synovial cyst of popliteal space (eg, Baker's cyst)**
13.9 13.9 FUD 090 J A2 80 50
AMA: 2018,Sep,7

27347 **Excision of lesion of meniscus or capsule (eg, cyst, ganglion), knee**
15.1 15.1 FUD 090 J A2 80 50
AMA: 2018,Sep,7

27350 **Patellectomy or hemipatellectomy**
18.8 18.8 FUD 090 J A2 80 50
AMA: 2018,Sep,7

27355 **Excision or curettage of bone cyst or benign tumor of femur;**
17.4 17.4 FUD 090 J A2 80 50
AMA: 2018,Sep,7

27356 **with allograft**
21.3 21.3 FUD 090 J G2 80 50
AMA: 2019,May,7; 2018,Sep,7

27357 **with autograft (includes obtaining graft)**
23.5 23.5 FUD 090 J A2 80 50
AMA: 2018,Sep,7; 2018,Jan,8; 2017,Jan,8; 2016,Jan,13

\+ **27358** **with internal fixation (List in addition to code for primary procedure)**
Code first (27355-27357)
8.03 8.03 FUD ZZZ N N1 80
AMA: 2018,Sep,7

27360 **Partial excision (craterization, saucerization, or diaphysectomy) bone, femur, proximal tibia and/or fibula (eg, osteomyelitis or bone abscess)**
24.7 24.7 FUD 090 J A2 80 50
AMA: 2018,Sep,7

27329-27365 [27329] Radical Resection Tumor Knee/Thigh

INCLUDES
Any necessary elevation tissue planes or dissection
Excision adjacent soft tissue during bone tumor resection
Measurement tumor and necessary margin at greatest diameter prior to excision
Radical resection bone tumor: resection tumor (may include entire bone) and wide margins normal tissue primarily for malignant or aggressive benign tumors
Radical resection soft tissue tumor: wide resection tumor involving substantial margins normal tissue that may include tissue removal from one or more layers; most often malignant or aggressive benign
Simple and intermediate repairs

EXCLUDES
Complex repair
Radical resection cutaneous tumors (eg, melanoma) (11600-11606)
Significant vessel exploration, neuroplasty, reconstruction, or complex bone repair

\# **27329** **Radical resection of tumor (eg, sarcoma), soft tissue of thigh or knee area; less than 5 cm**
30.1 30.1 FUD 090 J G2 80 50
AMA: 2018,Sep,7

27364 **5 cm or greater**
45.2 45.2 FUD 090 J G2 80 50
AMA: 2018,Sep,7

27365 **Radical resection of tumor, femur or knee**
EXCLUDES *Soft tissue tumor excision thigh or knee area (27329, 27364)*
59.6 59.6 FUD 090 C 80 50
AMA: 2019,May,7; 2018,Sep,7

27369 Injection for Arthrogram of Knee

EXCLUDES
Arthrocentesis, aspiration and/or injection, knee (20610-20611)
Arthroscopy, knee (29871)

27369 **Injection procedure for contrast knee arthrography or contrast enhanced CT/MRI knee arthrography**
Code also fluoroscopic guidance, when performed for CT/MRI arthrography (73701-73702, 73722-73723, 77002)
(73580, 73701-73702, 73722-73723)
1.17 4.06 FUD 000 N1 50
AMA: 2019,Aug,7

27372 Foreign Body Removal Femur or Knee

EXCLUDES
Arthroscopic procedures (29870-29887)
Removal knee prosthesis (27488)

27372 **Removal of foreign body, deep, thigh region or knee area**
11.4 17.0 FUD 090 J A2 80 50
AMA: 2018,Sep,7

27380-27499 Repair/Reconstruction of Femur or Knee

27380 **Suture of infrapatellar tendon; primary**
17.5 17.5 FUD 090 J A2 80 50
AMA: 2018,Sep,7

27381 **secondary reconstruction, including fascial or tendon graft**
23.0 23.0 FUD 090 J J8 80 50
AMA: 2018,Sep,7

27385 **Suture of quadriceps or hamstring muscle rupture; primary**
16.9 16.9 FUD 090 J A2 80 50
AMA: 2018,Sep,7; 2018,Jan,8; 2017,Aug,9

27386 **secondary reconstruction, including fascial or tendon graft**
24.3 24.3 FUD 090 J A2 80 50
AMA: 2020,Apr,10; 2018,Sep,7

27390 **Tenotomy, open, hamstring, knee to hip; single tendon**
12.9 12.9 FUD 090 J A2 80 50
AMA: 2018,Sep,7

27391 **multiple tendons, 1 leg**
16.2 16.2 FUD 090 J A2 80
AMA: 2018,Sep,7

27392 **multiple tendons, bilateral**
20.5 20.5 FUD 090 J A2 80
AMA: 2018,Sep,7

27393 **Lengthening of hamstring tendon; single tendon**
14.6 14.6 FUD 090 J A2 80 50
AMA: 2018,Sep,7

27394 **multiple tendons, 1 leg**
18.8 18.8 FUD 090 J A2 80
AMA: 2018,Sep,7

27395 **multiple tendons, bilateral**
25.4 25.4 FUD 090 J A2 80
AMA: 2018,Sep,7

27396 **Transplant or transfer (with muscle redirection or rerouting), thigh (eg, extensor to flexor); single tendon**
17.6 17.6 FUD 090 J A2 80 50
AMA: 2018,Sep,7

27397 **multiple tendons**
26.4 26.4 FUD 090 J G2 80 50
AMA: 2018,Sep,7

27400 **Transfer, tendon or muscle, hamstrings to femur (eg, Egger's type procedure)**
20.0 20.0 FUD 090 J A2 80 50
AMA: 2018,Sep,7

27403 **Arthrotomy with meniscus repair, knee**
EXCLUDES *Arthroscopic treatment (29882)*
18.5 18.5 FUD 090 J A2 80 50
AMA: 2019,May,10; 2018,Sep,7

27405 **Repair, primary, torn ligament and/or capsule, knee; collateral**
19.5 19.5 FUD 090 J A2 80 50
AMA: 2018,Sep,7; 2018,Jan,8; 2017,Jan,8; 2016,Jan,13

27407 **cruciate**
EXCLUDES *Reconstruction (27427)*
22.9 22.9 FUD 090 J A2 80 50
AMA: 2018,Sep,7

27409 **collateral and cruciate ligaments**
EXCLUDES *Reconstruction (27427-27429)*
27.9 27.9 FUD 090 J A2 80 50
AMA: 2018,Sep,7

27412 **Autologous chondrocyte implantation, knee**
EXCLUDES *Arthrotomy, knee (27331)*
Autologous fat graft obtained by liposuction (15771-15774)
Manipulation knee joint under general anesthesia (27570)
Obtaining chondrocytes (29870)
Other autologous soft tissue grafts (fat, dermis, fascia) harvested by direct excision ([15769])
47.8 47.8 FUD 090 J G2 80 50
AMA: 2018,Sep,7

27415 **Osteochondral allograft, knee, open**
EXCLUDES *Arthroscopic procedure (29867)*
Osteochondral autograft knee (27416)
39.6 39.6 FUD 090 J J8 80 50
AMA: 2019,Apr,10; 2018,Sep,7; 2018,Jan,8; 2017,Jan,8; 2016,Jan,13

27416 **Osteochondral autograft(s), knee, open (eg, mosaicplasty) (includes harvesting of autograft[s])**
EXCLUDES *Procedures in same compartment (29874, 29877, 29879, 29885-29887)*
Procedures performed at same surgical session (27415, 29870-29871, 29875, 29884)
Surgical arthroscopy knee with osteochondral autograft(s) (29866)
28.3 28.3 FUD 090 J G2 80 50
AMA: 2018,Sep,7; 2018,Jan,8; 2017,Jan,8; 2016,Jan,13

27418 **Anterior tibial tubercleplasty (eg, Maquet type procedure)**
23.8 23.8 FUD 090 J A2 80 50
AMA: 2018,Sep,7; 2018,Jan,8; 2017,Jan,8; 2016,Jan,13

27420 **Reconstruction of dislocating patella; (eg, Hauser type procedure)**
21.4 21.4 FUD 090 J A2 80 50
AMA: 2018,Sep,7; 2018,Jan,8; 2017,Jan,8; 2016,Jan,13

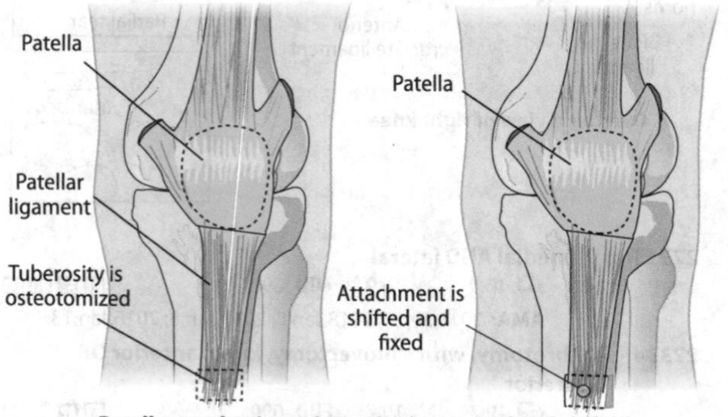

Patellar tendon insertion point is resected and shifted

27422 **with extensor realignment and/or muscle advancement or release (eg, Campbell, Goldwaite type procedure)**
21.4 21.4 FUD 090 J A2 80 50
AMA: 2018,Sep,7; 2018,Jan,8; 2017,Jan,8; 2016,Jan,13

27424 **with patellectomy**
21.5 21.5 FUD 090 J A2 80 50
AMA: 2018,Sep,7

27425 **Lateral retinacular release, open**
EXCLUDES *Arthroscopic release (29873)*
12.9 12.9 FUD 090 J A2 50
AMA: 2018,Sep,7; 2018,Jan,8; 2017,Jan,8; 2016,Jan,13

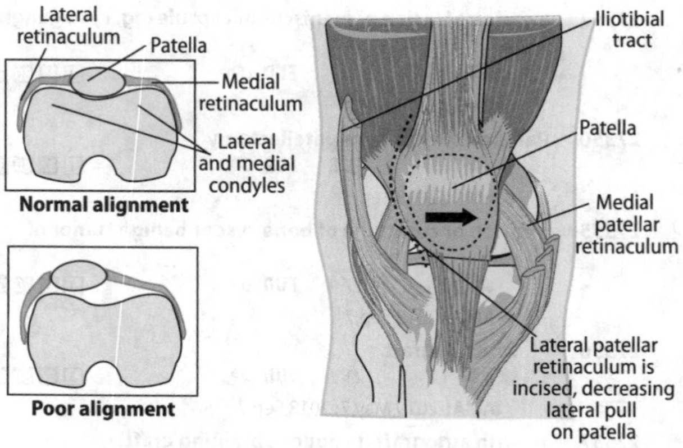

27427 **Ligamentous reconstruction (augmentation), knee; extra-articular**
EXCLUDES *Primary repair ligament(s) (27405, 27407, 27409)*
20.5 20.5 FUD 090 J J8 80 50
AMA: 2018,Sep,7; 2018,Jan,8; 2017,Jan,8; 2016,Jan,13

27428 **intra-articular (open)**
EXCLUDES *Primary repair ligament(s) (27405, 27407, 27409)*
32.2 32.2 FUD 090
AMA: 2018,Sep,7; 2018,Jan,8; 2017,Jan,8; 2016,Jan,13

27429 **intra-articular (open) and extra-articular**
EXCLUDES *Primary repair ligament(s) (27405, 27407, 27409)*
36.2 36.2 FUD 090
AMA: 2018,Sep,7; 2018,Jan,8; 2017,Jan,8; 2016,Jan,13

27430 **Quadricepsplasty (eg, Bennett or Thompson type)**
21.2 21.2 FUD 090
AMA: 2018,Sep,7

27435 **Capsulotomy, posterior capsular release, knee**
23.2 23.2 FUD 090
AMA: 2018,Sep,7

27437 **Arthroplasty, patella; without prosthesis**
19.0 19.0 FUD 090
AMA: 2018,Sep,7

27438 **with prosthesis**
24.3 24.3 FUD 090
AMA: 2018,Sep,7

27440 **Arthroplasty, knee, tibial plateau;**
23.0 23.0 FUD 090
AMA: 2018,Sep,7

27441 **with debridement and partial synovectomy**
23.8 23.8 FUD 090
AMA: 2018,Sep,7

27442 **Arthroplasty, femoral condyles or tibial plateau(s), knee;**
25.2 25.2 FUD 090
AMA: 2018,Sep,7; 2018,Jan,8; 2017,Jan,8; 2016,Jun,8

27443 **with debridement and partial synovectomy**
23.4 23.4 FUD 090
AMA: 2018,Sep,7

27445 **Arthroplasty, knee, hinge prosthesis (eg, Walldius type)**
EXCLUDES *Removal knee prosthesis (27488)*
Revision knee arthroplasty (27487)
36.1 36.1 FUD 090
AMA: 2018,Sep,7

27446 **Arthroplasty, knee, condyle and plateau; medial OR lateral compartment**
EXCLUDES *Removal knee prosthesis (27488)*
Revision knee arthroplasty (27487)
33.4 33.4 FUD 090
AMA: 2018,Sep,7; 2018,Jan,8; 2017,Dec,13

27447 **medial AND lateral compartments with or without patella resurfacing (total knee arthroplasty)**
EXCLUDES *Removal knee prosthesis (27488)*
Revision knee arthroplasty (27487)
39.1 39.1 FUD 090
AMA: 2018,Sep,7; 2018,Jan,8; 2017,Jan,8; 2016,Jan,13

27448 **Osteotomy, femur, shaft or supracondylar; without fixation**
23.7 23.7 FUD 090
AMA: 2019,May,7; 2018,Sep,7

27450 **with fixation**
29.3 29.3 FUD 090
AMA: 2018,Sep,7

27454 **Osteotomy, multiple, with realignment on intramedullary rod, femoral shaft (eg, Sofield type procedure)**
37.4 37.4 FUD 090
AMA: 2018,Sep,7

27455 **Osteotomy, proximal tibia, including fibular excision or osteotomy (includes correction of genu varus [bowleg] or genu valgus [knock-knee]); before epiphyseal closure**
27.5 27.5 FUD 090
AMA: 2018,Sep,7

27457 **after epiphyseal closure**
27.8 27.8 FUD 090
AMA: 2018,Sep,7

27465 **Osteoplasty, femur; shortening (excluding 64876)**
36.1 36.1 FUD 090
AMA: 2018,Sep,7

27466 **lengthening**
34.0 34.0 FUD 090
AMA: 2018,Sep,7

27468 **combined, lengthening and shortening with femoral segment transfer**
38.8 38.8 FUD 090
AMA: 2018,Sep,7

27470 **Repair, nonunion or malunion, femur, distal to head and neck; without graft (eg, compression technique)**
33.9 33.9 FUD 090
AMA: 2018,Sep,7

27472 **with iliac or other autogenous bone graft (includes obtaining graft)**
36.4 36.4 FUD 090
AMA: 2018,Sep,7

27475 **Arrest, epiphyseal, any method (eg, epiphysiodesis); distal femur**
19.1 19.1 FUD 090
AMA: 2018,Sep,7

27477 **tibia and fibula, proximal**
21.1 21.1 FUD 090
AMA: 2018,Sep,7

27479 **combined distal femur, proximal tibia and fibula**
26.5 26.5 FUD 090
AMA: 2018,Sep,7

27485 **Arrest, hemiepiphyseal, distal femur or proximal tibia or fibula (eg, genu varus or valgus)**
19.3 19.3 FUD 090
AMA: 2018,Sep,7

27486 **Revision of total knee arthroplasty, with or without allograft; 1 component**
40.5 40.5 FUD 090
AMA: 2018,Sep,7; 2018,Apr,10; 2018,Jan,8; 2017,Jan,8; 2016,Jan,13

27487 **femoral and entire tibial component**
50.7 50.7 FUD 090
AMA: 2018,Sep,7; 2018,Jan,8; 2017,Jan,8; 2016,Jan,13

27488 **Removal of prosthesis, including total knee prosthesis, methylmethacrylate with or without insertion of spacer, knee**
34.6 34.6 FUD 090
AMA: 2018,Sep,7; 2018,Jan,8; 2017,Jan,8; 2016,Jan,13

27495 **Prophylactic treatment (nailing, pinning, plating, or wiring) with or without methylmethacrylate, femur**
32.5 32.5 FUD 090
AMA: 2018,Sep,7

27496 **Decompression fasciotomy, thigh and/or knee, 1 compartment (flexor or extensor or adductor);**
15.7 15.7 FUD 090
AMA: 2018,Sep,7

27497 **with debridement of nonviable muscle and/or nerve**
16.7 16.7 FUD 090
AMA: 2018,Sep,7

27498 **Decompression fasciotomy, thigh and/or knee, multiple compartments;**
18.8 18.8 FUD 090
AMA: 2018,Sep,7

27499 **with debridement of nonviable muscle and/or nerve**
20.2 20.2 FUD 090
AMA: 2018,Sep,7

27500-27566 Treatment of Fracture/Dislocation of Femur/Knee

INCLUDES   Closed, percutaneous, and open treatment fractures and dislocations

27500   **Closed treatment of femoral shaft fracture, without manipulation**
🔹 13.8   ⚖ 15.0   **FUD** 090   T A2 50 ▭
AMA: 2018,Sep,7

27501   **Closed treatment of supracondylar or transcondylar femoral fracture with or without intercondylar extension, without manipulation**
🔹 14.3   ⚖ 14.5   **FUD** 090   T A2 80 50 ▭
AMA: 2018,Sep,7

27502   **Closed treatment of femoral shaft fracture, with manipulation, with or without skin or skeletal traction**
🔹 21.9   ⚖ 21.9   **FUD** 090   J A2 50 ▭
AMA: 2018,Sep,7; 2018,Jan,8; 2017,Jan,8; 2016,Jan,13

27503   **Closed treatment of supracondylar or transcondylar femoral fracture with or without intercondylar extension, with manipulation, with or without skin or skeletal traction**
🔹 23.1   ⚖ 23.1   **FUD** 090   J A2 80 50 ▭
AMA: 2018,Sep,7

27506   **Open treatment of femoral shaft fracture, with or without external fixation, with insertion of intramedullary implant, with or without cerclage and/or locking screws**
🔹 38.6   ⚖ 38.6   **FUD** 090   C 80 50 ▭
AMA: 2018,Sep,7; 2018,Jan,8; 2017,Jan,8; 2016,Jan,13

27507   **Open treatment of femoral shaft fracture with plate/screws, with or without cerclage**
🔹 28.0   ⚖ 28.0   **FUD** 090   C 80 50 ▭
AMA: 2018,Sep,7

27508   **Closed treatment of femoral fracture, distal end, medial or lateral condyle, without manipulation**
🔹 14.3   ⚖ 15.0   **FUD** 090   T A2 50 ▭
AMA: 2018,Sep,7

27509   **Percutaneous skeletal fixation of femoral fracture, distal end, medial or lateral condyle, or supracondylar or transcondylar, with or without intercondylar extension, or distal femoral epiphyseal separation**
🔹 18.6   ⚖ 18.6   **FUD** 090   J J8 80 50 ▭
AMA: 2018,Dec,10; 2018,Dec,10; 2018,Sep,7

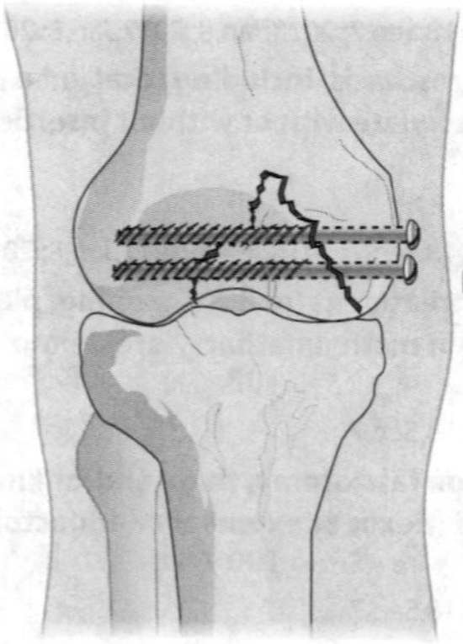

Pins are placed percutaneously

27510   **Closed treatment of femoral fracture, distal end, medial or lateral condyle, with manipulation**
🔹 19.6   ⚖ 19.6   **FUD** 090   J A2 50 ▭
AMA: 2018,Sep,7

27511   **Open treatment of femoral supracondylar or transcondylar fracture without intercondylar extension, includes internal fixation, when performed**
🔹 28.8   ⚖ 28.8   **FUD** 090   C 80 50 ▭
AMA: 2018,Sep,7

27513   **Open treatment of femoral supracondylar or transcondylar fracture with intercondylar extension, includes internal fixation, when performed**
🔹 35.9   ⚖ 35.9   **FUD** 090   C 80 50 ▭
AMA: 2018,Sep,7

27514   **Open treatment of femoral fracture, distal end, medial or lateral condyle, includes internal fixation, when performed**
🔹 27.9   ⚖ 27.9   **FUD** 090   C 80 50 ▭
AMA: 2018,Sep,7

27516   **Closed treatment of distal femoral epiphyseal separation; without manipulation**
🔹 13.8   ⚖ 14.7   **FUD** 090   T A2 50 ▭
AMA: 2018,Sep,7

27517   **with manipulation, with or without skin or skeletal traction**
🔹 19.6   ⚖ 19.6   **FUD** 090   J A2 80 50 ▭
AMA: 2018,Sep,7

27519   **Open treatment of distal femoral epiphyseal separation, includes internal fixation, when performed**
🔹 25.8   ⚖ 25.8   **FUD** 090   C 80 50 ▭
AMA: 2018,Sep,7

27520   **Closed treatment of patellar fracture, without manipulation**
🔹 8.46   ⚖ 9.21   **FUD** 090   T A2 50 ▭
AMA: 2018,Sep,7

27524   **Open treatment of patellar fracture, with internal fixation and/or partial or complete patellectomy and soft tissue repair**
🔹 21.6   ⚖ 21.6   **FUD** 090   J 62 80 50 ▭
AMA: 2018,Sep,7

27530   **Closed treatment of tibial fracture, proximal (plateau); without manipulation**
EXCLUDES   Arthroscopic repair (29855-29856)
🔹 8.05   ⚖ 8.63   **FUD** 090   T A2 50 ▭
AMA: 2018,Sep,7

27532   **with or without manipulation, with skeletal traction**
EXCLUDES   Arthroscopic repair (29855-29856)
🔹 16.5   ⚖ 17.7   **FUD** 090   J A2 50 ▭
AMA: 2018,Sep,7

27535   **Open treatment of tibial fracture, proximal (plateau); unicondylar, includes internal fixation, when performed**
EXCLUDES   Arthroscopic repair (29855-29856)
🔹 25.9   ⚖ 25.9   **FUD** 090   C 80 50 ▭
AMA: 2018,Sep,7

27536   **bicondylar, with or without internal fixation**
EXCLUDES   Arthroscopic repair (29855-29856)
🔹 34.2   ⚖ 34.2   **FUD** 090   C 80 50 ▭
AMA: 2018,Sep,7

27538   **Closed treatment of intercondylar spine(s) and/or tuberosity fracture(s) of knee, with or without manipulation**
EXCLUDES   Arthroscopic repair (29850-29851)
🔹 12.7   ⚖ 13.6   **FUD** 090   T A2 80 50 ▭
AMA: 2018,Sep,7

27540   **Open treatment of intercondylar spine(s) and/or tuberosity fracture(s) of the knee, includes internal fixation, when performed**
🔹 23.4   ⚖ 23.4   **FUD** 090   C 80 50 ▭
AMA: 2018,Sep,7

27550 **Closed treatment of knee dislocation; without anesthesia**
13.8 14.9 **FUD** 090 T A2 80 50
AMA: 2018,Sep,7

27552 **requiring anesthesia**
18.1 18.1 **FUD** 090 J A2 80 50
AMA: 2018,Sep,7

27556 **Open treatment of knee dislocation, includes internal fixation, when performed; without primary ligamentous repair or augmentation/reconstruction**
25.3 25.3 **FUD** 090 C 80 50
AMA: 2018,Sep,7

27557 **with primary ligamentous repair**
30.2 30.2 **FUD** 090 C 80 50
AMA: 2018,Sep,7

27558 **with primary ligamentous repair, with augmentation/reconstruction**
34.5 34.5 **FUD** 090 C 80 50
AMA: 2018,Sep,7

27560 **Closed treatment of patellar dislocation; without anesthesia**
EXCLUDES *Recurrent dislocation (27420-27424)*
9.66 10.5 **FUD** 090 T A2 50
AMA: 2018,Sep,7

27562 **requiring anesthesia**
EXCLUDES *Recurrent dislocation (27420-27424)*
13.9 13.9 **FUD** 090 T A2 80 50
AMA: 2018,Sep,7

27566 **Open treatment of patellar dislocation, with or without partial or total patellectomy**
EXCLUDES *Recurrent dislocation (27420-27424)*
25.8 25.8 **FUD** 090 J A2 80 50
AMA: 2018,Sep,7

27570 Knee Manipulation with Anesthesia

27570 **Manipulation of knee joint under general anesthesia (includes application of traction or other fixation devices)**
4.34 4.34 **FUD** 010 J A2 50
AMA: 2018,Sep,7; 2018,Jan,8; 2017,Jan,8; 2016,Jan,13

27580 Knee Arthrodesis

27580 **Arthrodesis, knee, any technique**
42.1 42.1 **FUD** 090 C 80 50
AMA: 2020,May,13; 2018,Sep,7

27590-27599 Amputations and Unlisted Procedures at Femur or Knee

27590 **Amputation, thigh, through femur, any level;**
23.0 23.0 **FUD** 090 C 80 50
AMA: 2018,Sep,7; 2018,Jan,8; 2017,Dec,13

27591 **immediate fitting technique including first cast**
27.9 27.9 **FUD** 090 C 80 50
AMA: 2018,Sep,7

27592 **open, circular (guillotine)**
19.5 19.5 **FUD** 090 C 80 50
AMA: 2018,Sep,7

27594 **secondary closure or scar revision**
14.6 14.6 **FUD** 090 J A2 50
AMA: 2018,Sep,7

27596 **re-amputation**
20.6 20.6 **FUD** 090 C 50
AMA: 2018,Sep,7

27598 **Disarticulation at knee**
INCLUDES Batch-Spittler-McFaddin operation
Callander knee disarticulation
Gritti amputation
20.6 20.6 **FUD** 090 C 80 50
AMA: 2018,Sep,7

27599 **Unlisted procedure, femur or knee**
0.00 0.00 **FUD** YYY T 80 50
AMA: 2019,Apr,10; 2018,Dec,10; 2018,Dec,10; 2018,Sep,7; 2018,Apr,10; 2018,Jan,8; 2017,Aug,9; 2017,Mar,10; 2017,Jan,8; 2016,Nov,9; 2016,Jun,8; 2016,Jan,13

27600-27602 Decompression Fasciotomy of Leg

EXCLUDES *Fasciotomy with debridement (27892-27894)*
Simple incision and drainage (10140-10160)

27600 **Decompression fasciotomy, leg; anterior and/or lateral compartments only**
11.7 11.7 **FUD** 090 J A2 50
AMA: 2018,Sep,7

27601 **posterior compartment(s) only**
12.8 12.8 **FUD** 090 J A2 50
AMA: 2018,Sep,7

27602 **anterior and/or lateral, and posterior compartment(s)**
13.9 13.9 **FUD** 090 J A2 80 50
AMA: 2018,Sep,7

27603-27612 Incisional Procedures Lower Leg and Ankle

27603 **Incision and drainage, leg or ankle; deep abscess or hematoma**
11.2 15.3 **FUD** 090 J A2 50
AMA: 2018,Sep,7

27604 **infected bursa**
9.61 13.6 **FUD** 090 J A2 80 50
AMA: 2018,Sep,7

27605 **Tenotomy, percutaneous, Achilles tendon (separate procedure); local anesthesia**
5.34 9.83 **FUD** 010 J A2 80 50
AMA: 2018,Sep,14; 2018,Sep,7

27606 **general anesthesia**
7.99 7.99 **FUD** 010 J A2 50
AMA: 2018,Sep,7; 2018,Sep,14

27607 **Incision (eg, osteomyelitis or bone abscess), leg or ankle**
17.5 17.5 **FUD** 090 J A2 50
AMA: 2018,Sep,7

27610 **Arthrotomy, ankle, including exploration, drainage, or removal of foreign body**
18.7 18.7 **FUD** 090 J A2 50
AMA: 2018,Sep,7

27612 **Arthrotomy, posterior capsular release, ankle, with or without Achilles tendon lengthening**
EXCLUDES *Lengthening or shortening tendon (27685)*
16.0 16.0 **FUD** 090 J A2 80 50
AMA: 2018,Sep,7

27613-27614 Biopsy Lower Leg and Ankle

EXCLUDES *Needle biopsy (20206)*

27613 **Biopsy, soft tissue of leg or ankle area; superficial**
4.60 7.22 **FUD** 010 J P3 50
AMA: 2018,Sep,7

27614 **deep (subfascial or intramuscular)**
11.7 16.6 **FUD** 090 J A2 50
AMA: 2018,Sep,7

27615-27634 [27632, 27634] Excision Soft Tissue Tumors Lower Leg/Ankle

INCLUDES Any necessary elevation tissue planes or dissection
Measurement tumor and necessary margin at greatest diameter prior to excision
Resection without removal significant normal tissue
Simple and intermediate repairs
Excision types:
- Fascial or subfascial soft tissue tumors: simple and marginal resection most often benign and intramuscular tumors found either in or below deep fascia, not involving bone
- Resection tumor (may include entire bone) and wide margins normal tissue primarily for malignant or aggressive benign tumors
- Subcutaneous: simple and marginal resection most often benign tumors found in subcutaneous tissue above deep fascia

EXCLUDES *Complex repair*
Excision benign cutaneous lesions (eg, sebaceous cyst) (11400-11406)
Radical resection cutaneous tumors (eg, melanoma) (11600-11606)
Significant vessel exploration or neuroplasty

27615 **Radical resection of tumor (eg, sarcoma), soft tissue of leg or ankle area; less than 5 cm**
29.6 29.6 **FUD** 090 J G2 80 50
AMA: 2018,Sep,7

27616 **5 cm or greater**
36.6 36.6 **FUD** 090 J G2 80 50
AMA: 2018,Sep,7

27618 **Excision, tumor, soft tissue of leg or ankle area, subcutaneous; less than 3 cm**
8.83 13.2 **FUD** 090 J G2 50
AMA: 2018,Sep,7; 2018,Jan,8; 2017,Jan,8; 2016,Jan,13

\# **27632** **3 cm or greater**
11.9 11.9 **FUD** 090 J G2 80 50
AMA: 2018,Sep,7

27619 **Excision, tumor, soft tissue of leg or ankle area, subfascial (eg, intramuscular); less than 5 cm**
13.3 13.3 **FUD** 090 J G2 50
AMA: 2018,Sep,7

\# **27634** **5 cm or greater**
19.7 19.7 **FUD** 090 J G2 80 50
AMA: 2018,Sep,7

27620-27641 [27632, 27634] Bone and Joint Procedures Ankle/Leg

27620 **Arthrotomy, ankle, with joint exploration, with or without biopsy, with or without removal of loose or foreign body**
12.9 12.9 **FUD** 090 J A2 80 50
AMA: 2018,Sep,7

27625 **Arthrotomy, with synovectomy, ankle;**
16.4 16.4 **FUD** 090 J A2 80 50
AMA: 2018,Sep,7

27626 **including tenosynovectomy**
17.4 17.4 **FUD** 090 J A2 80 50
AMA: 2018,Sep,7

27630 **Excision of lesion of tendon sheath or capsule (eg, cyst or ganglion), leg and/or ankle**
10.4 15.9 **FUD** 090 J A2 50
AMA: 2018,Sep,7

27632 **Resequenced code. See code following 27618.**

27634 **Resequenced code. See code following 27619.**

27635 **Excision or curettage of bone cyst or benign tumor, tibia or fibula;**
16.7 16.7 **FUD** 090 J A2 50
AMA: 2018,Sep,7; 2018,Jan,8; 2017,Jan,8; 2016,Jan,13

27637 **with autograft (includes obtaining graft)**
21.5 21.5 **FUD** 090 J A2 80 50
AMA: 2018,Sep,7

27638 **with allograft**
22.0 22.0 **FUD** 090 J A2 80 50
AMA: 2019,May,7; 2018,Sep,7

27640 **Partial excision (craterization, saucerization, or diaphysectomy), bone (eg, osteomyelitis); tibia**
EXCLUDES *Excision exostosis (27635)*
23.9 23.9 **FUD** 090 J A2 50
AMA: 2018,Sep,7; 2018,Jan,8; 2017,Jan,8; 2016,Jan,13

27641 **fibula**
EXCLUDES *Excision exostosis (27635)*
19.0 19.0 **FUD** 090 J A2 50
AMA: 2018,Sep,7

27645-27647 Radical Resection Bone Tumor Ankle/Leg

INCLUDES Any necessary elevation tissue planes or dissection
Excision adjacent soft tissue during bone tumor resection (27615-27619 [27632, 27634])
Measurement tumor and necessary margin at greatest diameter prior to excision
Resection tumor (may include entire bone) and wide margins normal tissue primarily for malignant or aggressive benign tumors
Simple and intermediate repairs

EXCLUDES *Complex repair*
Significant vessel exploration, neuroplasty, reconstruction, or complex bone repair

27645 **Radical resection of tumor; tibia**
51.2 51.2 **FUD** 090 C 80 50
AMA: 2019,May,7; 2018,Sep,7

27646 **fibula**
44.6 44.6 **FUD** 090 C 80 50
AMA: 2019,May,7; 2018,Sep,7

27647 **talus or calcaneus**
29.3 29.3 **FUD** 090 J A2 80 50
AMA: 2019,May,7; 2018,Sep,7

27648 Injection for Ankle Arthrogram

EXCLUDES *Arthroscopy (29894-29898)*

27648 **Injection procedure for ankle arthrography**
(73615)
1.52 5.22 **FUD** 000 N N1 80 50
AMA: 2019,May,7; 2018,Sep,7; 2018,Jan,8; 2017,Jan,8; 2016,Jan,13

27650-27745 Repair/Reconstruction Lower Leg/Ankle

27650 **Repair, primary, open or percutaneous, ruptured Achilles tendon;**
18.9 18.9 **FUD** 090 J A2 80 50
AMA: 2020,Jun,14; 2018,Sep,7; 2018,Jan,8; 2017,Jan,8; 2016,Jan,13

27652 **with graft (includes obtaining graft)**
19.1 19.1 **FUD** 090 J J8 50
AMA: 2018,Sep,7; 2018,Jan,8; 2017,Jan,8; 2016,Jan,13

27654 **Repair, secondary, Achilles tendon, with or without graft**
20.4 20.4 **FUD** 090 J A2 80 50
AMA: 2020,Jun,14; 2020,Apr,8; 2018,Sep,7; 2018,Jan,8; 2017,Jan,8; 2016,Dec,16; 2016,Jan,13

27656 **Repair, fascial defect of leg**
11.4 18.2 **FUD** 090 J A2 80 50
AMA: 2018,Sep,7

27658 **Repair, flexor tendon, leg; primary, without graft, each tendon**
10.6 10.6 **FUD** 090 J A2 80
AMA: 2018,Sep,7

27659 **secondary, with or without graft, each tendon**
13.5 13.5 **FUD** 090 J A2 80
AMA: 2018,Sep,7; 2018,Jan,8; 2017,Jan,8; 2016,Jan,13

27664 **Repair, extensor tendon, leg; primary, without graft, each tendon**
10.3 10.3 **FUD** 090 J A2 80
AMA: 2018,Sep,7; 2018,Jan,8; 2017,Jan,8; 2016,Jan,13

27665 **secondary, with or without graft, each tendon**
11.9 11.9 FUD 090 J A2 80
AMA: 2018,Sep,7

27675 **Repair, dislocating peroneal tendons; without fibular osteotomy**
14.1 14.1 FUD 090 J A2 80 50
AMA: 2018,Sep,7

27676 **with fibular osteotomy**
17.2 17.2 FUD 090 J A2 80 50
AMA: 2018,Sep,7

27680 **Tenolysis, flexor or extensor tendon, leg and/or ankle; single, each tendon**
12.2 12.2 FUD 090 J A2
AMA: 2018,Sep,7; 2018,Jan,8; 2017,Jan,8; 2016,Jan,13

27681 **multiple tendons (through separate incision[s])**
15.7 15.7 FUD 090 J A2 50
AMA: 2018,Sep,7

27685 **Lengthening or shortening of tendon, leg or ankle; single tendon (separate procedure)**
13.3 19.0 FUD 090 J A2 80 50
AMA: 2018,Sep,7; 2018,Sep,14; 2018,Jan,8; 2017,Jan,8; 2016,Jan,13

27686 **multiple tendons (through same incision), each**
15.6 15.6 FUD 090 J A2 50
AMA: 2018,Sep,7; 2018,Jan,8; 2017,Jan,8; 2016,Jan,13

27687 **Gastrocnemius recession (eg, Strayer procedure)**
13.0 13.0 FUD 090 J A2 80 50
AMA: 2018,Sep,7

27690 **Transfer or transplant of single tendon (with muscle redirection or rerouting); superficial (eg, anterior tibial extensors into midfoot)**
INCLUDES Toe extensors considered single tendon with transplant into midfoot
18.4 18.4 FUD 090 J A2 80 50
AMA: 2018,Sep,7

27691 **deep (eg, anterior tibial or posterior tibial through interosseous space, flexor digitorum longus, flexor hallucis longus, or peroneal tendon to midfoot or hindfoot)**
INCLUDES Barr procedure
Toe extensors considered single tendon with transplant into midfoot
21.4 21.4 FUD 090 J A2 80 50
AMA: 2018,Sep,7

+ **27692** **each additional tendon (List separately in addition to code for primary procedure)**
INCLUDES Toe extensors considered single tendon with transplant into midfoot
Code first (27690-27691)
3.01 3.01 FUD ZZZ N N1 80
AMA: 2018,Sep,7

27695 **Repair, primary, disrupted ligament, ankle; collateral**
13.6 13.6 FUD 090 J A2 50
AMA: 2018,Nov,11; 2018,Sep,7; 2018,Jan,8; 2017,Jan,8; 2016,Jan,13

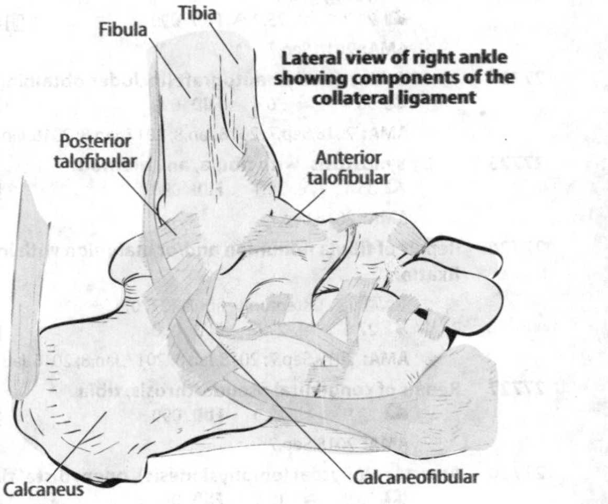

27696 **both collateral ligaments**
16.0 16.0 FUD 090 J A2 50
AMA: 2018,Nov,11; 2018,Sep,7; 2018,Jan,8; 2017,Jan,8; 2016,Jan,13

27698 **Repair, secondary, disrupted ligament, ankle, collateral (eg, Watson-Jones procedure)**
18.3 18.3 FUD 090 J A2 80 50
AMA: 2018,Sep,7; 2018,Jan,8; 2017,Jan,8; 2016,Jan,13

27700 **Arthroplasty, ankle;**
17.6 17.6 FUD 090 J J8 80 50
AMA: 2018,Sep,7

27702 **with implant (total ankle)**
27.7 27.7 FUD 090 C 80 50
AMA: 2018,Sep,7

27703 **revision, total ankle**
32.2 32.2 FUD 090 C 80 50
AMA: 2018,Sep,7

27704 **Removal of ankle implant**
16.5 16.5 FUD 090 Q2 A2 50
AMA: 2019,May,7; 2018,Sep,7

27705 **Osteotomy; tibia**
EXCLUDES *Genu varus or genu valgus repair (27455-27457)*
21.8 21.8 FUD 090 J J8 80 50
AMA: 2018,Sep,7

27707 **fibula**
EXCLUDES *Genu varus or genu valgus repair (27455-27457)*
11.4 11.4 FUD 090 J A2 50
AMA: 2018,Sep,7

27709 **tibia and fibula**
EXCLUDES *Genu varus or genu valgus repair (27455-27457)*
33.6 33.6 FUD 090 J J8 80 50
AMA: 2018,Sep,7

27712 **multiple, with realignment on intramedullary rod (eg, Sofield type procedure)**
EXCLUDES *Genu varus or genu valgus repair (27455-27457)*
31.8 31.8 FUD 090 C 80 50
AMA: 2018,Sep,7

27715 **Osteoplasty, tibia and fibula, lengthening or shortening**
INCLUDES Anderson tibial lengthening
30.9 30.9 FUD 090 C 80 50
AMA: 2018,Sep,7

27720 Repair of nonunion or malunion, tibia; without graft, (eg, compression technique)
25.1 25.1 FUD 090 J J8 80 50
AMA: 2018,Sep,7

27722 with sliding graft
25.7 25.7 FUD 090 J J8 80 50
AMA: 2018,Sep,7

27724 with iliac or other autograft (includes obtaining graft)
36.4 36.4 FUD 090 C 80 50
AMA: 2018,Sep,7; 2018,Jan,8; 2017,Jan,8; 2016,Jan,13

27725 by synostosis, with fibula, any method
35.1 35.1 FUD 090 C 80 50
AMA: 2018,Sep,7

27726 Repair of fibula nonunion and/or malunion with internal fixation
INCLUDES Osteotomy; fibula (27707)
27.6 27.6 FUD 090 J J8 50
AMA: 2018,Sep,7; 2018,Jan,8; 2017,Jan,8; 2016,Jan,13

27727 Repair of congenital pseudarthrosis, tibia
29.9 29.9 FUD 090 C 80 50
AMA: 2018,Sep,7

27730 Arrest, epiphyseal (epiphysiodesis), open; distal tibia
16.9 16.9 FUD 090 J A2 50
AMA: 2018,Sep,7

27732 distal fibula
12.9 12.9 FUD 090 J A2 50
AMA: 2018,Sep,7

27734 distal tibia and fibula
18.9 18.9 FUD 090 J A2 50
AMA: 2018,Sep,7

27740 Arrest, epiphyseal (epiphysiodesis), any method, combined, proximal and distal tibia and fibula;
EXCLUDES *Epiphyseal arrest proximal tibia and fibula (27477)*
20.4 20.4 FUD 090 J G2 80 50
AMA: 2018,Sep,7

27742 and distal femur
EXCLUDES *Epiphyseal arrest proximal tibia and fibula (27477)*
22.4 22.4 FUD 090 J A2 80 50
AMA: 2018,Sep,7

27745 Prophylactic treatment (nailing, pinning, plating or wiring) with or without methylmethacrylate, tibia
21.7 21.7 FUD 090 J J8 80 50
AMA: 2018,Sep,7

27750-27848 Treatment of Fracture/Dislocation Lower Leg/Ankle

INCLUDES Treatment open or closed fracture or dislocation

27750 Closed treatment of tibial shaft fracture (with or without fibular fracture); without manipulation
9.18 9.91 FUD 090 T A2 50
AMA: 2018,Sep,7; 2018,Jan,8; 2017,Jan,8; 2016,Jan,13

27752 with manipulation, with or without skeletal traction
14.1 15.4 FUD 090 J A2 50
AMA: 2018,Sep,7; 2018,Jan,8; 2018,Jan,3; 2017,Jan,8; 2016,Jan,13

27756 Percutaneous skeletal fixation of tibial shaft fracture (with or without fibular fracture) (eg, pins or screws)
16.6 16.6 FUD 090 J A2 80 50
AMA: 2018,Sep,7; 2018,Jan,8; 2017,Jan,8; 2016,Jan,13

27758 Open treatment of tibial shaft fracture (with or without fibular fracture), with plate/screws, with or without cerclage
25.8 25.8 FUD 090 J J8 80 50
AMA: 2018,Sep,7; 2018,Jan,8; 2017,Jan,8; 2016,Jan,13

27759 Treatment of tibial shaft fracture (with or without fibular fracture) by intramedullary implant, with or without interlocking screws and/or cerclage
28.8 28.8 FUD 090 J J8 80 50
AMA: 2018,Sep,7; 2018,Jan,8; 2017,Jan,8; 2016,Jan,13

27760 Closed treatment of medial malleolus fracture; without manipulation
8.81 9.56 FUD 090 T A2 50
AMA: 2018,Sep,7

27762 with manipulation, with or without skin or skeletal traction
12.4 13.7 FUD 090 J A2 50
AMA: 2018,Sep,7

27766 Open treatment of medial malleolus fracture, includes internal fixation, when performed
17.4 17.4 FUD 090 J A2 50
AMA: 2018,Sep,7

27767 Closed treatment of posterior malleolus fracture; without manipulation
EXCLUDES *Treatment bimalleolar ankle fracture (27808-27814)*
Treatment trimalleolar ankle fracture (27816-27823)
8.20 8.24 FUD 090 T P2 50
AMA: 2018,Sep,7

27768 with manipulation
EXCLUDES *Treatment bimalleolar ankle fracture (27808-27814)*
Treatment trimalleolar ankle fracture (27816-27823)
12.7 12.7 FUD 090 J G2 50
AMA: 2018,Sep,7

27769 Open treatment of posterior malleolus fracture, includes internal fixation, when performed
EXCLUDES *Treatment bimalleolar ankle fracture (27808-27814)*
Treatment trimalleolar ankle fracture (27816-27823)
21.0 21.0 FUD 090 J G2 50
AMA: 2018,Sep,7

27780 Closed treatment of proximal fibula or shaft fracture; without manipulation
8.08 8.80 FUD 090 T A2 50
AMA: 2018,Sep,7; 2018,Jan,8; 2017,Jan,8; 2016,Jan,13

27781 with manipulation
11.3 12.3 FUD 090 J A2 50
AMA: 2018,Sep,7

27784 Open treatment of proximal fibula or shaft fracture, includes internal fixation, when performed
20.5 20.5 FUD 090 J A2 50
AMA: 2018,Sep,7; 2018,Jan,8; 2017,Jan,8; 2016,Jan,13

27786 Closed treatment of distal fibular fracture (lateral malleolus); without manipulation
8.25 9.01 FUD 090 T A2 50
AMA: 2018,Sep,7

27788 with manipulation
11.1 12.2 FUD 090 T A2 50
AMA: 2018,Sep,7

27792 Open treatment of distal fibular fracture (lateral malleolus), includes internal fixation, when performed
EXCLUDES *Repair tibia and fibula shaft fracture (27750-27759)*
18.6 18.6 FUD 090 J J8 50
AMA: 2018,Sep,7; 2018,Jan,8; 2017,Jan,8; 2016,Jan,13

27808 Closed treatment of bimalleolar ankle fracture (eg, lateral and medial malleoli, or lateral and posterior malleoli or medial and posterior malleoli); without manipulation
8.70 9.57 FUD 090 T A2 50
AMA: 2018,Sep,7

27810 with manipulation
12.1 13.3 FUD 090 J A2 50
AMA: 2018,Sep,7

27814 **Open treatment of bimalleolar ankle fracture (eg, lateral and medial malleoli, or lateral and posterior malleoli, or medial and posterior malleoli), includes internal fixation, when performed**
22.1 22.1 FUD 090 J J8 80 50
AMA: 2018,Sep,7; 2018,Jan,8; 2017,Jan,8; 2016,Feb,13

27816 **Closed treatment of trimalleolar ankle fracture; without manipulation**
8.28 9.27 FUD 090 T A2 50
AMA: 2018,Sep,7

27818 **with manipulation**
12.4 13.9 FUD 090 J A2 50
AMA: 2018,Sep,7

27822 **Open treatment of trimalleolar ankle fracture, includes internal fixation, when performed, medial and/or lateral malleolus; without fixation of posterior lip**
24.9 24.9 FUD 090 J J8 80 50
AMA: 2018,Sep,7

27823 **with fixation of posterior lip**
28.0 28.0 FUD 090 J J8 80 50
AMA: 2018,Sep,7

27824 **Closed treatment of fracture of weight bearing articular portion of distal tibia (eg, pilon or tibial plafond), with or without anesthesia; without manipulation**
8.71 9.02 FUD 090 T A2 50
AMA: 2018,Sep,7

27825 **with skeletal traction and/or requiring manipulation**
14.2 15.7 FUD 090 J A2 80 50
AMA: 2018,Sep,7

27826 **Open treatment of fracture of weight bearing articular surface/portion of distal tibia (eg, pilon or tibial plafond), with internal fixation, when performed; of fibula only**
24.2 24.2 FUD 090 J J8 80 50
AMA: 2018,Sep,7

27827 **of tibia only**
32.0 32.0 FUD 090 J J8 80 50
AMA: 2018,Sep,7

27828 **of both tibia and fibula**
38.1 38.1 FUD 090 J J8 80 50
AMA: 2018,Sep,7; 2018,Jan,8; 2017,Jan,8; 2016,Jan,13

27829 **Open treatment of distal tibiofibular joint (syndesmosis) disruption, includes internal fixation, when performed**
20.0 20.0 FUD 090 J J8 80 50
AMA: 2018,Sep,7; 2018,Jan,8; 2017,Jan,8; 2016,Feb,13; 2016,Jan,13

27830 **Closed treatment of proximal tibiofibular joint dislocation; without anesthesia**
10.2 11.1 FUD 090 T A2 80 50
AMA: 2018,Sep,7

27831 **requiring anesthesia**
11.6 11.6 FUD 090 J A2 80 50
AMA: 2018,Sep,7

27832 **Open treatment of proximal tibiofibular joint dislocation, includes internal fixation, when performed, or with excision of proximal fibula**
21.8 21.8 FUD 090 J J8 80 50
AMA: 2018,Sep,7

27840 **Closed treatment of ankle dislocation; without anesthesia**
10.7 10.7 FUD 090 T A2 50
AMA: 2018,Sep,7

27842 **requiring anesthesia, with or without percutaneous skeletal fixation**
14.2 14.2 FUD 090 J A2 50
AMA: 2018,Sep,7

27846 **Open treatment of ankle dislocation, with or without percutaneous skeletal fixation; without repair or internal fixation**
EXCLUDES *Arthroscopy (29894-29898)*
20.6 20.6 FUD 090 J A2 80 50
AMA: 2018,Sep,7

27848 **with repair or internal or external fixation**
EXCLUDES *Arthroscopy (29894-29898)*
23.0 23.0 FUD 090 J J8 80 50
AMA: 2018,Sep,7

27860 Ankle Manipulation with Anesthesia

27860 **Manipulation of ankle under general anesthesia (includes application of traction or other fixation apparatus)**
4.91 4.91 FUD 010 J A2 80 50
AMA: 2018,Sep,7

27870-27871 Arthrodesis Lower Leg/Ankle

27870 **Arthrodesis, ankle, open**
EXCLUDES *Arthroscopic arthrodesis ankle (29899)*
29.5 29.5 FUD 090 J J8 80 50
AMA: 2020,May,13; 2018,Sep,7

27871 **Arthrodesis, tibiofibular joint, proximal or distal**
19.8 19.8 FUD 090 J J8 80 50
AMA: 2020,May,13; 2018,Sep,7

27880-27889 Amputations of Lower Leg/Ankle

27880 **Amputation, leg, through tibia and fibula;**
INCLUDES Burgess amputation
26.3 26.3 FUD 090 C 80 50
AMA: 2018,Sep,7

27881 **with immediate fitting technique including application of first cast**
24.8 24.8 FUD 090 C 80 50
AMA: 2018,Sep,7

27882 **open, circular (guillotine)**
17.2 17.2 FUD 090 C 80 50
AMA: 2018,Sep,7

27884 **secondary closure or scar revision**
16.5 16.5 FUD 090 J A2 50
AMA: 2018,Sep,7

27886 **re-amputation**
18.9 18.9 FUD 090 C 50
AMA: 2018,Sep,7

27888 **Amputation, ankle, through malleoli of tibia and fibula (eg, Syme, Pirogoff type procedures), with plastic closure and resection of nerves**
18.9 18.9 FUD 090 C 80 50
AMA: 2018,Sep,7

27889 **Ankle disarticulation**
18.6 18.6 FUD 090 J A2 50
AMA: 2018,Sep,7

27892-27899 Decompression Fasciotomy Lower Leg

EXCLUDES *Decompression fasciotomy without debridement (27600-27602)*

27892 **Decompression fasciotomy, leg; anterior and/or lateral compartments only, with debridement of nonviable muscle and/or nerve**
15.8 15.8 FUD 090 J A2 80 50
AMA: 2018,Sep,7

27893 **posterior compartment(s) only, with debridement of nonviable muscle and/or nerve**
17.5 17.5 FUD 090 J A2 80 50
AMA: 2018,Sep,7

27894 **anterior and/or lateral, and posterior compartment(s), with debridement of nonviable muscle and/or nerve**
24.3 24.3 FUD 090 J A2 80 50
AMA: 2018,Sep,7

Musculoskeletal System

27814 — 27894

27899 **Unlisted procedure, leg or ankle**
0.00 0.00 FUD YYY
AMA: 2020,Apr,8; 2018,Sep,7; 2018,Jan,8; 2017,Jan,8; 2016,Dec,16; 2016,Jan,13

28001-28008 Surgical Incision Foot/Toe

EXCLUDES *Simple incision and drainage (10060-10160)*

28001 **Incision and drainage, bursa, foot**
4.90 8.03 FUD 010
AMA: 2018,Sep,7

28002 **Incision and drainage below fascia, with or without tendon sheath involvement, foot; single bursal space**
9.20 12.7 FUD 010
AMA: 2018,Sep,7

28003 **multiple areas**
16.0 20.1 FUD 090
AMA: 2018,Sep,7

28005 **Incision, bone cortex (eg, osteomyelitis or bone abscess), foot**
16.6 16.6 FUD 090
AMA: 2018,Sep,7

28008 **Fasciotomy, foot and/or toe**
EXCLUDES *Plantar fascia division (28250)*
Plantar fasciectomy (28060, 28062)
8.46 12.5 FUD 090
AMA: 2018,Sep,7

28010-28011 Tenotomy/Toe

EXCLUDES *Open tenotomy (28230-28234)*
Simple incision and drainage (10140-10160)

28010 **Tenotomy, percutaneous, toe; single tendon**
5.99 6.69 FUD 090
AMA: 2018,Sep,7

28011 **multiple tendons**
8.10 9.09 FUD 090
AMA: 2018,Sep,7

28020-28024 Arthrotomy Foot/Toe

EXCLUDES *Simple incision and drainage (10140-10160)*

28020 **Arthrotomy, including exploration, drainage, or removal of loose or foreign body; intertarsal or tarsometatarsal joint**
10.4 15.5 FUD 090
AMA: 2018,Sep,7

28022 **metatarsophalangeal joint**
9.36 14.0 FUD 090
AMA: 2018,Sep,7

28024 **interphalangeal joint**
8.67 13.1 FUD 090
AMA: 2018,Sep,7

28035 Tarsal Tunnel Release

EXCLUDES *Other nerve decompression (64722)*
Other neuroplasty (64704)

28035 **Release, tarsal tunnel (posterior tibial nerve decompression)**
10.2 15.2 FUD 090
AMA: 2018,Sep,7

28039-28047 [28039, 28041] Excision Soft Tissue Tumors Foot/Toe

INCLUDES Any necessary elevation tissue planes or dissection
Measurement tumor and necessary margin at greatest diameter prior to excision
Simple and intermediate repairs
Excision types:
- Fascial or subfascial soft tissue tumors: simple and marginal resection tumors found either in or below deep fascia, not involving bone or excision substantial amount normal tissue; primarily benign and intramuscular tumors
  - Tumors fingers and toes involving joint capsules, tendons and tendon sheaths
- Radical resection soft tissue tumor: wide resection tumor, involving substantial margins normal tissue and may involve tissue removal from one or more layers; most often malignant or aggressive benign
  - Tumors fingers and toes adjacent to joints, tendons and tendon sheaths
- Subcutaneous: simple and marginal resection tumors in subcutaneous tissue above deep fascia; most often benign

EXCLUDES *Complex repair*
Excision benign cutaneous lesions (eg, sebaceous cyst) (11420-11426)
Radical resection cutaneous tumors (eg, melanoma) (11620-11626)
Significant vessel exploration, neuroplasty, or reconstruction

28039 **Resequenced code. See code following 28043.**

28041 **Resequenced code. See code following 28045.**

28043 **Excision, tumor, soft tissue of foot or toe, subcutaneous; less than 1.5 cm**
7.52 11.3 FUD 090
AMA: 2018,Sep,7

\# **28039** **1.5 cm or greater**
9.94 14.3 FUD 090
AMA: 2018,Sep,7

28045 **Excision, tumor, soft tissue of foot or toe, subfascial (eg, intramuscular); less than 1.5 cm**
9.97 14.0 FUD 090
AMA: 2018,Sep,7

\# **28041** **1.5 cm or greater**
13.0 13.0 FUD 090
AMA: 2018,Sep,7

28046 **Radical resection of tumor (eg, sarcoma), soft tissue of foot or toe; less than 3 cm**
20.6 20.6 FUD 090
AMA: 2018,Sep,7

28047 **3 cm or greater**
30.1 30.1 FUD 090
AMA: 2018,Sep,7

28050-28160 Resection Procedures Foot/Toes

28050 **Arthrotomy with biopsy; intertarsal or tarsometatarsal joint**
8.03 12.1 FUD 090
AMA: 2002,Apr,13; 1998,Nov,1

28052 **metatarsophalangeal joint**
8.15 12.8 FUD 090
AMA: 2002,Apr,13

28054 **interphalangeal joint**
6.77 10.8 FUD 090
AMA: 2002,Apr,13

28055 **Neurectomy, intrinsic musculature of foot**
11.0 11.0 FUD 090

28060 **Fasciectomy, plantar fascia; partial (separate procedure)**
EXCLUDES *Plantar fasciotomy (28008, 28250)*
10.3 15.0 FUD 090
AMA: 2018,Jan,8; 2017,Jan,8; 2016,Jan,13

28062 **radical (separate procedure)**
EXCLUDES *Plantar fasciotomy (28008, 28250)*
11.7 16.7 FUD 090
AMA: 2002,Apr,13

28070 Synovectomy; intertarsal or tarsometatarsal joint, each
10.1 15.2 FUD 090 J A2
AMA: 2002,Apr,13

28072 metatarsophalangeal joint, each
9.26 14.1 FUD 090 J A2
AMA: 2002,Apr,13

28080 Excision, interdigital (Morton) neuroma, single, each
10.6 15.1 FUD 090 J A2 80
AMA: 2018,Jan,8; 2017,Jan,8; 2016,Jan,13

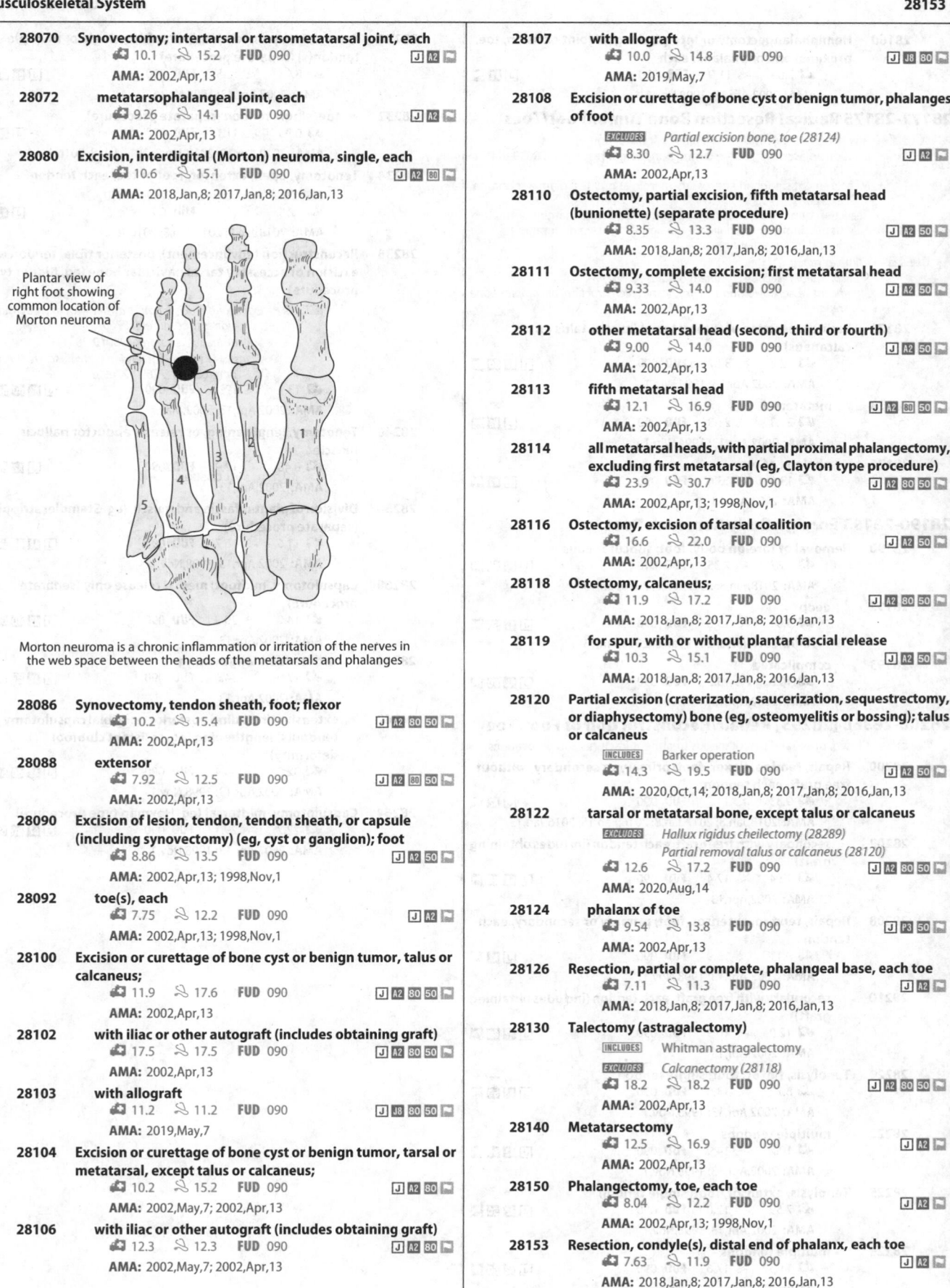

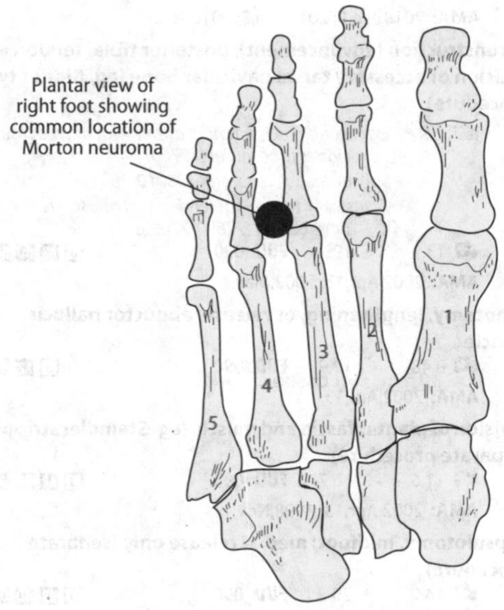

Morton neuroma is a chronic inflammation or irritation of the nerves in the web space between the heads of the metatarsals and phalanges

28086 Synovectomy, tendon sheath, foot; flexor
10.2 15.4 FUD 090 J A2 80 50
AMA: 2002,Apr,13

28088 extensor
7.92 12.5 FUD 090 J A2 80 50
AMA: 2002,Apr,13

28090 Excision of lesion, tendon, tendon sheath, or capsule (including synovectomy) (eg, cyst or ganglion); foot
8.86 13.5 FUD 090 J A2 50
AMA: 2002,Apr,13; 1998,Nov,1

28092 toe(s), each
7.75 12.2 FUD 090 J A2
AMA: 2002,Apr,13; 1998,Nov,1

28100 Excision or curettage of bone cyst or benign tumor, talus or calcaneus;
11.9 17.6 FUD 090 J A2 80 50
AMA: 2002,Apr,13

28102 with iliac or other autograft (includes obtaining graft)
17.5 17.5 FUD 090 J A2 80 50
AMA: 2002,Apr,13

28103 with allograft
11.2 11.2 FUD 090 J J8 80 50
AMA: 2019,May,7

28104 Excision or curettage of bone cyst or benign tumor, tarsal or metatarsal, except talus or calcaneus;
10.2 15.2 FUD 090 J A2 80
AMA: 2002,May,7; 2002,Apr,13

28106 with iliac or other autograft (includes obtaining graft)
12.3 12.3 FUD 090 J A2 80
AMA: 2002,May,7; 2002,Apr,13

28107 with allograft
10.0 14.8 FUD 090 J J8 80
AMA: 2019,May,7

28108 Excision or curettage of bone cyst or benign tumor, phalanges of foot
EXCLUDES *Partial excision bone, toe (28124)*
8.30 12.7 FUD 090 J A2
AMA: 2002,Apr,13

28110 Ostectomy, partial excision, fifth metatarsal head (bunionette) (separate procedure)
8.35 13.3 FUD 090 J A2 50
AMA: 2018,Jan,8; 2017,Jan,8; 2016,Jan,13

28111 Ostectomy, complete excision; first metatarsal head
9.33 14.0 FUD 090 J A2 50
AMA: 2002,Apr,13

28112 other metatarsal head (second, third or fourth)
9.00 14.0 FUD 090 J A2 50
AMA: 2002,Apr,13

28113 fifth metatarsal head
12.1 16.9 FUD 090 J A2 80 50
AMA: 2002,Apr,13

28114 all metatarsal heads, with partial proximal phalangectomy, excluding first metatarsal (eg, Clayton type procedure)
23.9 30.7 FUD 090 J A2 80 50
AMA: 2002,Apr,13; 1998,Nov,1

28116 Ostectomy, excision of tarsal coalition
16.6 22.0 FUD 090 J A2 50
AMA: 2002,Apr,13

28118 Ostectomy, calcaneus;
11.9 17.2 FUD 090 J A2 80 50
AMA: 2018,Jan,8; 2017,Jan,8; 2016,Jan,13

28119 for spur, with or without plantar fascial release
10.3 15.1 FUD 090 J A2 50
AMA: 2018,Jan,8; 2017,Jan,8; 2016,Jan,13

28120 Partial excision (craterization, saucerization, sequestrectomy, or diaphysectomy) bone (eg, osteomyelitis or bossing); talus or calcaneus
INCLUDES Barker operation
14.3 19.5 FUD 090 J A2 50
AMA: 2020,Oct,14; 2018,Jan,8; 2017,Jan,8; 2016,Jan,13

28122 tarsal or metatarsal bone, except talus or calcaneus
EXCLUDES *Hallux rigidus cheilectomy (28289)*
Partial removal talus or calcaneus (28120)
12.6 17.2 FUD 090 J A2 80 50
AMA: 2020,Aug,14

28124 phalanx of toe
9.54 13.8 FUD 090 J P3 50
AMA: 2002,Apr,13

28126 Resection, partial or complete, phalangeal base, each toe
7.11 11.3 FUD 090 J A2
AMA: 2018,Jan,8; 2017,Jan,8; 2016,Jan,13

28130 Talectomy (astragalectomy)
INCLUDES Whitman astragalectomy
EXCLUDES *Calcanectomy (28118)*
18.2 18.2 FUD 090 J A2 80 50
AMA: 2002,Apr,13

28140 Metatarsectomy
12.5 16.9 FUD 090 J A2
AMA: 2002,Apr,13

28150 Phalangectomy, toe, each toe
8.04 12.2 FUD 090 J A2
AMA: 2002,Apr,13; 1998,Nov,1

28153 Resection, condyle(s), distal end of phalanx, each toe
7.63 11.9 FUD 090 J A2
AMA: 2018,Jan,8; 2017,Jan,8; 2016,Jan,13

28160 **Hemiphalangectomy or interphalangeal joint excision, toe, proximal end of phalanx, each**
7.69 | 11.9 | FUD 090 | J A2
AMA: 2002,Apr,13; 1998,Nov,1

28171-28175 Radical Resection Bone Tumor Foot/Toes

INCLUDES Any necessary elevation tissue planes or dissection
Excision adjacent soft tissue during bone tumor resection (28039-28047 [28039, 28041])
Measurement tumor and necessary margin at greatest diameter prior to excision
Resection tumor (may include entire bone) and wide margins normal tissue primarily for malignant or aggressive benign tumors
Simple and intermediate repairs

EXCLUDES *Complex repair*
Radical tumor resection calcaneus or talus (27647)
Significant vessel exploration, neuroplasty, reconstruction, or complex bone repair

28171 **Radical resection of tumor; tarsal (except talus or calcaneus)**
32.2 | 32.2 | FUD 090 | J A2 80
AMA: 2002,Apr,13; 1994,Win,1

28173 **metatarsal**
21.3 | 21.3 | FUD 090 | J A2
AMA: 2002,Apr,13; 1994,Win,1

28175 **phalanx of toe**
13.6 | 13.6 | FUD 090 | J A2
AMA: 2002,Apr,13

28190-28193 Foreign Body Removal: Foot

28190 **Removal of foreign body, foot; subcutaneous**
3.85 | 7.35 | FUD 010 | T P3 50
AMA: 2018,Jan,8; 2017,Jan,8; 2016,Jan,13

28192 **deep**
9.01 | 13.5 | FUD 090 | J A2 50
AMA: 2018,Jan,8; 2017,Jan,8; 2016,Jan,13

28193 **complicated**
10.6 | 15.2 | FUD 090 | J A2 50
AMA: 2002,Apr,13

28200-28360 [28295] Repair/Reconstruction of Foot/Toe

INCLUDES Closed, open, and percutaneous treatment fractures and dislocations

28200 **Repair, tendon, flexor, foot; primary or secondary, without free graft, each tendon**
9.33 | 14.2 | FUD 090 | J A2
AMA: 2018,Jan,8; 2017,Jan,8; 2016,Feb,15; 2016,Jan,13

28202 **secondary with free graft, each tendon (includes obtaining graft)**
12.4 | 17.4 | FUD 090 | J A2 80
AMA: 2002,Apr,13

28208 **Repair, tendon, extensor, foot; primary or secondary, each tendon**
9.11 | 13.9 | FUD 090 | J A2
AMA: 2002,Apr,13; 1998,Nov,1

28210 **secondary with free graft, each tendon (includes obtaining graft)**
12.0 | 16.9 | FUD 090 | J A2 80
AMA: 2002,Apr,13

28220 **Tenolysis, flexor, foot; single tendon**
8.72 | 13.0 | FUD 090 | J P3 50
AMA: 2002,Apr,13; 1998,Nov,1

28222 **multiple tendons**
10.2 | 14.9 | FUD 090 | J A2 50
AMA: 2002,Apr,13; 1998,Nov,1

28225 **Tenolysis, extensor, foot; single tendon**
7.59 | 12.0 | FUD 090 | J A2 50
AMA: 2002,Apr,13; 1998,Nov,1

28226 **multiple tendons**
11.3 | 17.6 | FUD 090 | J A2 50
AMA: 2002,Apr,13; 1998,Nov,1

28230 **Tenotomy, open, tendon flexor; foot, single or multiple tendon(s) (separate procedure)**
8.16 | 12.5 | FUD 090 | J P3 50
AMA: 2002,Apr,13; 1998,Nov,1

28232 **toe, single tendon (separate procedure)**
6.95 | 11.1 | FUD 090 | J P3
AMA: 2020,Apr,10; 2018,Jan,8; 2017,Jan,8; 2016,Jan,13

28234 **Tenotomy, open, extensor, foot or toe, each tendon**
EXCLUDES *Tendon transfer (27690-27691)*
7.59 | 11.8 | FUD 090 | J A2
AMA: 2018,Jan,8; 2017,Jan,8; 2016,Jan,13

28238 **Reconstruction (advancement), posterior tibial tendon with excision of accessory tarsal navicular bone (eg, Kidner type procedure)**
EXCLUDES *Extensor hallucis longus transfer with big toe fusion (Jones procedure) (28760)*
Subcutaneous tenotomy (28010-28011)
Transfer or transplant tendon with muscle redirection or rerouting (27690-27692)
13.9 | 19.2 | FUD 090 | J A2 80 50
AMA: 2002,Apr,13; 2002,May,7

28240 **Tenotomy, lengthening, or release, abductor hallucis muscle**
8.46 | 12.9 | FUD 090 | J A2 50
AMA: 2002,Apr,13

28250 **Division of plantar fascia and muscle (eg, Steindler stripping) (separate procedure)**
11.6 | 16.7 | FUD 090 | J A2 80 50
AMA: 2002,Apr,13; 1998,Nov,1

28260 **Capsulotomy, midfoot; medial release only (separate procedure)**
14.9 | 20.2 | FUD 090 | J A2 80 50
AMA: 2002,Apr,13

28261 **with tendon lengthening**
27.0 | 34.6 | FUD 090 | J A2 80 50
AMA: 2002,Apr,13

28262 **extensive, including posterior talotibial capsulotomy and tendon(s) lengthening (eg, resistant clubfoot deformity)**
32.5 | 40.4 | FUD 090 | J A2 80 50
AMA: 2002,Apr,13; 1998,Nov,1

28264 **Capsulotomy, midtarsal (eg, Heyman type procedure)**
22.2 | 29.1 | FUD 090 | J A2 80 50
AMA: 2002,Apr,13; 1998,Nov,1

28270 **Capsulotomy; metatarsophalangeal joint, with or without tenorrhaphy, each joint (separate procedure)**
9.64 14.2 FUD 090 J A2 50
AMA: 2018,Jan,8; 2017,Jan,8; 2016,Jan,13

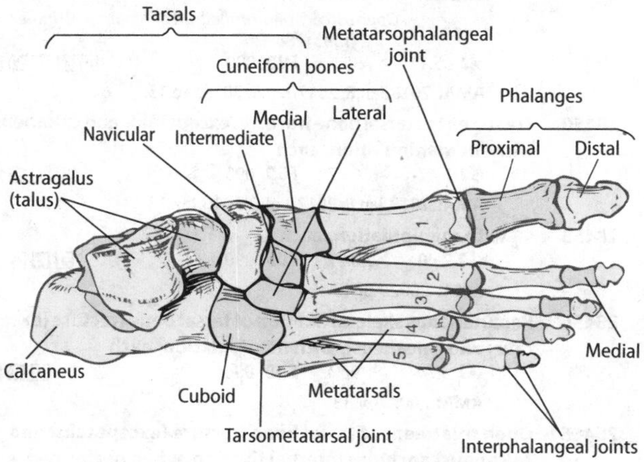

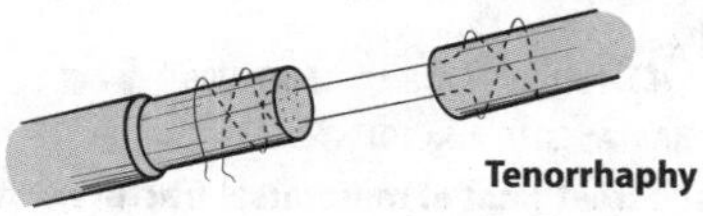

28272 **interphalangeal joint, each joint (separate procedure)**
7.25 11.2 FUD 090 J P3 50
AMA: 2018,Jan,8; 2017,Jan,8; 2016,Jan,13

28280 **Syndactylization, toes (eg, webbing or Kelikian type procedure)**
10.0 14.8 FUD 090 J A2 80 50
AMA: 2002,Apr,13; 1998,Nov,1

28285 **Correction, hammertoe (eg, interphalangeal fusion, partial or total phalangectomy)**
10.9 15.5 FUD 090 J A2 50
AMA: 2018,Jan,8; 2017,Jan,8; 2016,Jun,8; 2016,Jan,13

28286 **Correction, cock-up fifth toe, with plastic skin closure (eg, Ruiz-Mora type procedure)**
8.56 12.8 FUD 090 J A2 50
AMA: 2002,Apr,13; 1998,Nov,1

28288 **Ostectomy, partial, exostectomy or condylectomy, metatarsal head, each metatarsal head**
12.4 17.5 FUD 090 J A2
AMA: 2002,Apr,13; 1998,Nov,1

28289 **Hallux rigidus correction with cheilectomy, debridement and capsular release of the first metatarsophalangeal joint; without implant**
13.2 20.5 FUD 090 J A2 80 50
AMA: 2020,Aug,14; 2020,Jul,13; 2018,Jan,8; 2017,Jan,8; 2016,Dec,3; 2016,Jan,13

28291 **with implant**
14.1 21.0 FUD 090 J J8 80 50
AMA: 2020,Aug,14; 2018,Jan,8; 2017,Nov,10; 2017,Jan,8; 2016,Dec,3

28292 **Correction, hallux valgus (bunionectomy), with sesamoidectomy, when performed; with resection of proximal phalanx base, when performed, any method**
13.9 21.3 FUD 090 J A2 80 50
AMA: 2018,Jan,8; 2017,Jan,8; 2016,Dec,3; 2016,Jan,13

28295 **Resequenced code. See code following 28296.**

28296 **with distal metatarsal osteotomy, any method**
14.8 26.1 FUD 090 J A2 80 50
AMA: 2020,Jul,13; 2018,Sep,14; 2018,Jan,8; 2017,Jan,8; 2016,Dec,3; 2016,Jan,13

\# **28295** **with proximal metatarsal osteotomy, any method**
16.1 28.5 FUD 090 J G2 80 50
AMA: 2018,Jan,8; 2017,Jan,8; 2016,Dec,3

28297 **with first metatarsal and medial cuneiform joint arthrodesis, any method**
17.4 30.2 FUD 090 J J8 80 50
AMA: 2018,Jan,8; 2017,Jan,8; 2016,Dec,3; 2016,Jan,13

28298 **with proximal phalanx osteotomy, any method**
INCLUDES Akin procedure
14.3 24.3 FUD 090 J J8 80 50
AMA: 2018,Jan,8; 2017,Jan,8; 2016,Dec,3; 2016,Jan,13

28299 **with double osteotomy, any method**
16.8 29.1 FUD 090 J A2 80 50
AMA: 2018,Jan,8; 2017,Jan,8; 2016,Dec,3; 2016,Apr,8; 2016,Jan,13

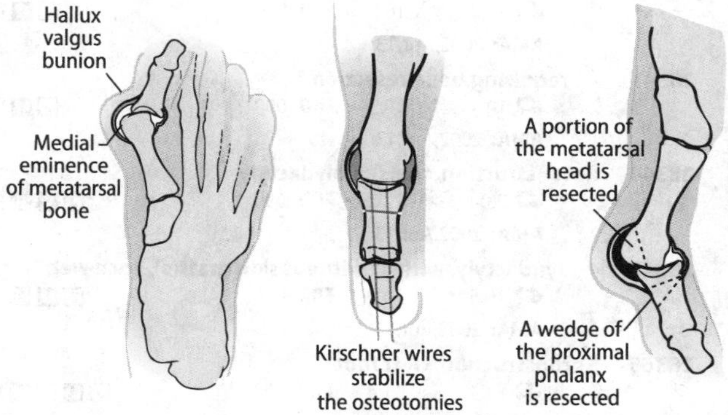

28300 **Osteotomy; calcaneus (eg, Dwyer or Chambers type procedure), with or without internal fixation**
18.7 18.7 FUD 090 J J8 80 50
AMA: 2002,Apr,13; 1998,Nov,1

28302 **talus**
20.6 20.6 FUD 090 J A2 80 50
AMA: 2002,Apr,13

28304 **Osteotomy, tarsal bones, other than calcaneus or talus;**
17.3 23.6 FUD 090 J A2 80 50
AMA: 2002,Apr,13; 1998,Nov,1

28305 **with autograft (includes obtaining graft) (eg, Fowler type)**
19.3 19.3 FUD 090 J J8 80 50
AMA: 2002,Apr,13; 1998,Nov,1

28306 **Osteotomy, with or without lengthening, shortening or angular correction, metatarsal; first metatarsal**
11.6 17.6 FUD 090 J A2 80 50
AMA: 2018,Jan,8; 2017,Jan,8; 2016,Jan,13

28307 **first metatarsal with autograft (other than first toe)**
11.9 17.9 FUD 090 J A2 80 50
AMA: 2002,Apr,13; 1998,Nov,1

28308 **other than first metatarsal, each**
10.9 16.4 FUD 090 J A2 80 50
AMA: 2002,Apr,13; 1998,Nov,1

28309 **multiple (eg, Swanson type cavus foot procedure)**
25.5 25.5 FUD 090 J J8 80 50
AMA: 2018,Jan,8; 2017,Jan,8; 2016,Jan,13

28310 **Osteotomy, shortening, angular or rotational correction; proximal phalanx, first toe (separate procedure)**
10.3 15.7 FUD 090 J A2 50
AMA: 2018,Jan,8; 2017,Jan,8; 2016,Jan,13

28312 **other phalanges, any toe**
9.12 14.4 FUD 090 J A2
AMA: 2002,Apr,13

28313 **Reconstruction, angular deformity of toe, soft tissue procedures only (eg, overlapping second toe, fifth toe, curly toes)**
10.2 15.1 FUD 090 J A2
AMA: 2002,Apr,13; 1998,Nov,1

28315 **Sesamoidectomy, first toe (separate procedure)**
9.37 13.9 FUD 090 J A2 50
AMA: 2002,Apr,13

28320 **Repair, nonunion or malunion; tarsal bones**
17.5 17.5 FUD 090 J J8 80 50
AMA: 2002,Apr,13; 1998,Nov,1

28322 **metatarsal, with or without bone graft (includes obtaining graft)**
16.5 22.5 FUD 090 J J8 80
AMA: 2002,Apr,13

28340 **Reconstruction, toe, macrodactyly; soft tissue resection**
11.8 16.5 FUD 090 J A2
AMA: 2002,Apr,13

28341 **requiring bone resection**
14.1 19.3 FUD 090 J A2
AMA: 2002,Apr,13

28344 **Reconstruction, toe(s); polydactyly**
8.04 12.2 FUD 090 J A2 50
AMA: 2002,Apr,13

28345 **syndactyly, with or without skin graft(s), each web**
10.5 14.9 FUD 090 J A2 80
AMA: 2002,Apr,13

28360 **Reconstruction, cleft foot**
31.4 31.4 FUD 090 J G2 80 50
AMA: 2002,Apr,13

28400-28675 Treatment of Fracture/Dislocation of Foot/Toe

28400 **Closed treatment of calcaneal fracture; without manipulation**
6.55 7.09 FUD 090 T A2 50
AMA: 2002,Apr,13

28405 **with manipulation**
INCLUDES Bohler reduction
10.0 11.1 FUD 090 T A2 80 50
AMA: 2002,Apr,13

28406 **Percutaneous skeletal fixation of calcaneal fracture, with manipulation**
15.1 15.1 FUD 090 J A2 80 50
AMA: 2002,Apr,13

28415 **Open treatment of calcaneal fracture, includes internal fixation, when performed;**
32.2 32.2 FUD 090 J J8 80 50
AMA: 2002,Apr,13

28420 **with primary iliac or other autogenous bone graft (includes obtaining graft)**
37.1 37.1 FUD 090 J J8 80 50
AMA: 2002,Apr,13

28430 **Closed treatment of talus fracture; without manipulation**
6.03 6.85 FUD 090 T P2 50
AMA: 2002,Apr,13

28435 **with manipulation**
9.31 10.4 FUD 090 J A2 80 50
AMA: 2002,Apr,13

28436 **Percutaneous skeletal fixation of talus fracture, with manipulation**
12.9 12.9 FUD 090 J G2 50
AMA: 2002,Apr,13

28445 **Open treatment of talus fracture, includes internal fixation, when performed**
30.2 30.2 FUD 090 J J8 80 50
AMA: 2002,Apr,13

28446 **Open osteochondral autograft, talus (includes obtaining graft[s])**
INCLUDES Osteotomy; fibula (27707)
Osteotomy; tibia (27705)
EXCLUDES *Arthroscopically aided osteochondral talus graft (29892)*
Open osteochondral allograft or repairs with industrial grafts (28899)
35.1 35.1 FUD 090 J G2 80 50
AMA: 2018,Jan,8; 2017,Jan,8; 2016,Jan,13

28450 **Treatment of tarsal bone fracture (except talus and calcaneus); without manipulation, each**
5.47 6.07 FUD 090 T P2
AMA: 2018,Jan,8; 2017,Jan,8; 2016,Jan,13

28455 **with manipulation, each**
7.40 8.27 FUD 090 J P3 80
AMA: 2002,Apr,13

28456 **Percutaneous skeletal fixation of tarsal bone fracture (except talus and calcaneus), with manipulation, each**
9.74 9.74 FUD 090 J A2
AMA: 2002,Apr,13

28465 **Open treatment of tarsal bone fracture (except talus and calcaneus), includes internal fixation, when performed, each**
18.1 18.1 FUD 090 J J8
AMA: 2019,Aug,10

28470 **Closed treatment of metatarsal fracture; without manipulation, each**
5.85 6.26 FUD 090 T P2
AMA: 2002,Apr,13

28475 **with manipulation, each**
6.52 7.37 FUD 090 T P2
AMA: 2002,Apr,13

28476 **Percutaneous skeletal fixation of metatarsal fracture, with manipulation, each**
10.5 10.5 FUD 090 J A2 80
AMA: 2002,Apr,13

28485 **Open treatment of metatarsal fracture, includes internal fixation, when performed, each**
15.8 15.8 FUD 090 J J8
AMA: 2019,Aug,10

28490 **Closed treatment of fracture great toe, phalanx or phalanges; without manipulation**
3.57 4.12 FUD 090 T P3 50
AMA: 2002,Apr,13

28495 **with manipulation**
4.25 5.10 FUD 090 T P2 50
AMA: 2002,Apr,13

28496 **Percutaneous skeletal fixation of fracture great toe, phalanx or phalanges, with manipulation**
6.93 12.9 FUD 090 J A2 50
AMA: 2002,Apr,13

28505 **Open treatment of fracture, great toe, phalanx or phalanges, includes internal fixation, when performed**
14.3 19.1 FUD 090 J A2 50
AMA: 2002,Apr,13

28510 **Closed treatment of fracture, phalanx or phalanges, other than great toe; without manipulation, each**
3.41 3.47 FUD 090 T P3
AMA: 2002,Apr,13

28515 **with manipulation, each**
4.08 4.67 FUD 090 T P2
AMA: 2002,Apr,13

28525 **Open treatment of fracture, phalanx or phalanges, other than great toe, includes internal fixation, when performed, each**
11.6 16.5 FUD 090 J A2 80
AMA: 2002,Apr,13

28530 **Closed treatment of sesamoid fracture**
2.88 3.30 FUD 090 T P3 80 50
AMA: 2002,Apr,13

28531 **Open treatment of sesamoid fracture, with or without internal fixation**
5.22 9.73 FUD 090 J A2 50
AMA: 2002,Apr,13

28540 **Closed treatment of tarsal bone dislocation, other than talotarsal; without anesthesia**
5.01 5.57 FUD 090 T P2 80 50
AMA: 2002,Apr,13

28545 **requiring anesthesia**
7.62 8.67 FUD 090 J G2 80 50
AMA: 2002,Apr,13

28546 **Percutaneous skeletal fixation of tarsal bone dislocation, other than talotarsal, with manipulation**
9.85 16.7 FUD 090 J A2 80 50
AMA: 2002,Apr,13

28555 **Open treatment of tarsal bone dislocation, includes internal fixation, when performed**
18.7 24.6 FUD 090 J J8 80 50
AMA: 2002,Apr,13

28570 **Closed treatment of talotarsal joint dislocation; without anesthesia**
5.52 6.57 FUD 090 T P2 80 50
AMA: 2002,Apr,13

28575 **requiring anesthesia**
9.57 10.6 FUD 090 J A2 80 50
AMA: 2002,Apr,13

28576 **Percutaneous skeletal fixation of talotarsal joint dislocation, with manipulation**
11.1 11.1 FUD 090 J A2 80 50
AMA: 2002,Apr,13

28585 **Open treatment of talotarsal joint dislocation, includes internal fixation, when performed**
19.6 25.0 FUD 090 J J8 80 50
AMA: 2018,Jan,8; 2017,Jan,8; 2016,Jan,13

28600 **Closed treatment of tarsometatarsal joint dislocation; without anesthesia**
5.35 6.26 FUD 090 T P2 80
AMA: 2002,Apr,13

28605 **requiring anesthesia**
8.57 9.58 FUD 090 T A2 80
AMA: 2002,Apr,13

28606 **Percutaneous skeletal fixation of tarsometatarsal joint dislocation, with manipulation**
11.1 11.1 FUD 090 J A2
AMA: 2002,Apr,13

28615 **Open treatment of tarsometatarsal joint dislocation, includes internal fixation, when performed**
23.4 23.4 FUD 090 J J8 80
AMA: 2002,Apr,13

28630 **Closed treatment of metatarsophalangeal joint dislocation; without anesthesia**
3.15 4.49 FUD 010 T P3 80
AMA: 2002,Apr,13

28635 **requiring anesthesia**
3.81 5.04 FUD 010 J A2 80
AMA: 2002,Apr,13

28636 **Percutaneous skeletal fixation of metatarsophalangeal joint dislocation, with manipulation**
5.74 8.98 FUD 010 J A2
AMA: 2002,Apr,13

28645 **Open treatment of metatarsophalangeal joint dislocation, includes internal fixation, when performed**
14.0 18.9 FUD 090 J A2
AMA: 2018,Jan,8; 2017,Jan,8; 2016,Jan,13

28660 **Closed treatment of interphalangeal joint dislocation; without anesthesia**
2.56 3.38 FUD 010 T P3
AMA: 2002,Apr,13

28665 **requiring anesthesia**
3.72 4.41 FUD 010 T A2 80
AMA: 2002,Apr,13

28666 **Percutaneous skeletal fixation of interphalangeal joint dislocation, with manipulation**
4.79 4.79 FUD 010 J A2
AMA: 2002,Apr,13

28675 **Open treatment of interphalangeal joint dislocation, includes internal fixation, when performed**
11.6 16.4 FUD 090 J A2
AMA: 2002,Apr,13

28705-28760 Arthrodesis of Foot/Toe

28705 **Arthrodesis; pantalar**
35.4 35.4 FUD 090 J J8 80 50
AMA: 2020,May,13

28715 **triple**
27.1 27.1 FUD 090 J J8 80 50
AMA: 2020,May,13

28725 **subtalar**
INCLUDES Dunn arthrodesis
Grice arthrodesis
22.4 22.4 FUD 090 J J8 80 50
AMA: 2020,May,13; 2018,Jan,8; 2017,Jan,8; 2016,Jan,13

28730 **Arthrodesis, midtarsal or tarsometatarsal, multiple or transverse;**
INCLUDES Lambrinudi arthrodesis
21.2 21.2 FUD 090 J J8 80 50
AMA: 2020,May,13

28735 **with osteotomy (eg, flatfoot correction)**
22.4 22.4 FUD 090 J J8 80 50
AMA: 2020,May,13; 2019,May,10

28737 **Arthrodesis, with tendon lengthening and advancement, midtarsal, tarsal navicular-cuneiform (eg, Miller type procedure)**
19.8 19.8 FUD 090 J J8 80 50
AMA: 2020,May,13

28740 **Arthrodesis, midtarsal or tarsometatarsal, single joint**
17.9 24.3 FUD 090 J J8 80 50
AMA: 2020,May,13; 2018,Jan,8; 2017,Jan,8; 2016,Jan,13

28750 **Arthrodesis, great toe; metatarsophalangeal joint**
16.8 22.9 FUD 090 J J8 80 50
AMA: 2020,May,13; 2018,Jan,8; 2017,Jan,8; 2016,Dec,3; 2016,Jan,13

28755 **interphalangeal joint**
9.56 14.7 FUD 090 J A2 50
AMA: 2020,May,13

28760 **Arthrodesis, with extensor hallucis longus transfer to first metatarsal neck, great toe, interphalangeal joint (eg, Jones type procedure)**
INCLUDES Jones procedure
EXCLUDES *Hammer toe repair or interphalangeal fusion (28285)*
16.6 22.5 FUD 090 J A2 80 50
AMA: 2020,May,13

28800-28825 Amputation Foot/Toe

28800 Amputation, foot; midtarsal (eg, Chopart type procedure)
15.4 15.4 **FUD** 090 C 80 50
AMA: 2002,Apr,13; 1998,Nov,1

28805 transmetatarsal
20.9 20.9 **FUD** 090 J G2 80 50
AMA: 2002,Apr,13; 1997,May,4

28810 Amputation, metatarsal, with toe, single
12.3 12.3 **FUD** 090 J A2 80
AMA: 2002,Apr,13

28820 Amputation, toe; metatarsophalangeal joint
11.3 16.1 **FUD** 090 J A2
AMA: 2002,Apr,13; 1997,May,4

28825 interphalangeal joint
10.6 15.4 **FUD** 090 J A2
AMA: 2002,Apr,13

28890-28899 Other/Unlisted Procedures Foot/Toe

28890 Extracorporeal shock wave, high energy, performed by a physician or other qualified health care professional, requiring anesthesia other than local, including ultrasound guidance, involving the plantar fascia
EXCLUDES *Extracorporeal shock wave therapy integumentary system not otherwise specified, when performed on same treatment area ([0512T, 0513T])*
Extracorporeal shock wave therapy musculoskeletal system not otherwise specified (0101T-0102T)
6.38 9.18 **FUD** 090 J P3 50
AMA: 2018,Dec,5; 2018,Dec,5; 2018,Jan,8; 2017,Jan,8; 2016,Jan,13

28899 Unlisted procedure, foot or toes
0.00 0.00 **FUD** YYY T 80
AMA: 2018,Oct,11; 2018,Jan,8; 2017,Nov,10; 2017,Sep,14; 2017,Jan,8; 2016,Dec,3; 2016,Jun,8; 2016,Jan,13

29000-29086 Casting: Arm/Shoulder/Torso

INCLUDES Cast removal without replacement by same provider
Cast replacement during or after global period
EXCLUDES *Initial cast application performed with restorative treatment, report appropriate musculoskeletal system code*
Orthotic supervision and training (97760-97763)
Removal cast by different provider (29700, 29705, 29710)
Code also cast material

29000 Application of halo type body cast (see 20661-20663 for insertion)
5.57 9.69 **FUD** 000 T G2 80
AMA: 2018,Jan,8; 2018,Jan,3; 2017,Jan,8; 2016,Jan,13

29010 Application of Risser jacket, localizer, body; only
4.58 7.63 **FUD** 000 T P2 80
AMA: 2018,Jan,8; 2018,Jan,3; 2017,Jan,8; 2016,Jan,13

29015 including head
5.18 8.22 **FUD** 000 T P2 80
AMA: 2018,Jan,8; 2018,Jan,3; 2017,Jan,8; 2016,Jan,13

29035 Application of body cast, shoulder to hips;
4.08 7.13 **FUD** 000 T P2 80
AMA: 2018,Jan,8; 2018,Jan,3; 2017,Jan,8; 2016,Jan,13

29040 including head, Minerva type
4.95 8.17 **FUD** 000 T G2 80
AMA: 2018,Jan,8; 2018,Jan,3; 2017,Jan,8; 2016,Jan,13

29044 including 1 thigh
4.78 8.01 **FUD** 000 T P2 80
AMA: 2018,Jan,8; 2018,Jan,3; 2017,Jan,8; 2016,Jan,13

29046 including both thighs
5.37 8.78 **FUD** 000 T G2 80
AMA: 2018,Jan,8; 2018,Jan,3; 2017,Jan,8; 2016,Jan,13

29049 Application, cast; figure-of-eight
2.00 2.79 **FUD** 000 T P3 80
AMA: 2018,Jan,3; 2018,Jan,8; 2017,Jan,8; 2016,Jan,13

29055 shoulder spica
3.93 6.22 **FUD** 000 T P2 80
AMA: 2018,Jan,8; 2018,Jan,3; 2017,Jan,8; 2016,Jan,13

29058 plaster Velpeau
2.71 3.51 **FUD** 000 T P3 80
AMA: 2018,Jan,8; 2018,Jan,3; 2017,Jan,8; 2016,Jan,13

29065 shoulder to hand (long arm)
1.95 2.70 **FUD** 000 T P3 50
AMA: 2018,Jan,8; 2018,Jan,3; 2017,Jan,8; 2016,Jan,13

29075 elbow to finger (short arm)
1.76 2.43 **FUD** 000 T P3 50
AMA: 2018,Jan,8; 2018,Jan,3; 2017,Jan,8; 2016,Jan,13

29085 hand and lower forearm (gauntlet)
1.92 2.68 **FUD** 000 T P3 50
AMA: 2018,Jan,3; 2018,Jan,8; 2017,Jan,8; 2016,Jan,13

29086 finger (eg, contracture)
1.47 2.22 **FUD** 000 T P3 50
AMA: 2018,Jan,8; 2018,Jan,3; 2017,Jan,8; 2016,Jan,13

29105-29280 Splinting and Strapping: Torso/Upper Extremities

INCLUDES Replacement splint or strapping during or after global period
EXCLUDES *Initial splinting/strapping application performed with restorative treatment, report appropriate musculoskeletal system code*
Orthotic supervision and training (97760-97763)
Code also splint/strapping material

29105 Application of long arm splint (shoulder to hand)
1.38 2.33 **FUD** 000 T P3 50
AMA: 2018,Jan,3; 2018,Jan,8; 2017,Jan,8; 2016,Jan,13

29125 Application of short arm splint (forearm to hand); static
1.13 1.82 **FUD** 000 Q1 N1 50
AMA: 2018,Jan,8; 2018,Jan,3; 2017,Jan,8; 2016,Jan,13

29126 dynamic
1.40 2.18 **FUD** 000 Q1 N1 50
AMA: 2018,Jan,8; 2018,Jan,3; 2017,Jan,8; 2016,Jan,13

29130 Application of finger splint; static
0.85 1.18 **FUD** 000 Q1 N1 50
AMA: 2018,Jan,8; 2018,Jan,3; 2017,Jan,8; 2016,Jan,13

29131 dynamic
0.98 1.48 **FUD** 000 Q1 N1 50
AMA: 2018,Jan,8; 2018,Jan,3; 2017,Jan,8; 2016,Jan,13

29200 Strapping; thorax
EXCLUDES *Strapping of low back (29799)*
0.54 0.93 **FUD** 000 T P3
AMA: 2018,Jan,8; 2018,Jan,3; 2017,Jan,8; 2016,Jan,13

29240 shoulder (eg, Velpeau)
0.54 0.87 **FUD** 000 Q1 N1 50
AMA: 2018,Jan,3; 2018,Jan,8; 2017,Jan,8; 2016,Jan,13

29260 elbow or wrist
0.56 0.86 **FUD** 000 Q1 N1 50
AMA: 2018,Jan,8; 2018,Jan,3; 2017,Jan,8; 2016,Jan,13

29280 hand or finger
0.60 0.88 **FUD** 000 Q1 N1 50
AMA: 2018,Jan,8; 2018,Jan,3; 2017,Jan,8; 2016,Jan,13

29305-29450 Casting: Legs

INCLUDES Cast removal without replacement by same provider
Cast replacement during or after global period
EXCLUDES *Initial cast application performed with restorative treatment, report appropriate musculoskeletal system code*
Orthotic supervision and training (97760-97763)
Removal cast by different provider (29700, 29705, 29710)
Code also cast material

29305 Application of hip spica cast; 1 leg
EXCLUDES *Hip spica cast thighs only (29046)*
4.53 6.93 **FUD** 000 T P2 80
AMA: 2018,Jan,8; 2018,Jan,3; 2017,Jan,8; 2016,Jan,13

29325 **1 and one-half spica or both legs**
EXCLUDES *Hip spica cast thighs only (29046)*
5.11 7.75 FUD 000 T P2 80
AMA: 2018,Jan,8; 2018,Jan,3; 2017,Jan,8; 2016,Jan,13

29345 **Application of long leg cast (thigh to toes);**
2.87 3.85 FUD 000 T P3 50
AMA: 2018,Jan,3; 2018,Jan,8; 2017,Jan,8; 2016,Jan,13

29355 **walker or ambulatory type**
3.07 4.03 FUD 000 T P3 50
AMA: 2018,Jan,3; 2018,Jan,8; 2017,Jan,8; 2016,Jan,13

29358 **Application of long leg cast brace**
2.96 4.51 FUD 000 T P3 50
AMA: 2018,Jan,3; 2018,Jan,8; 2017,Jan,8; 2016,Jan,13

29365 **Application of cylinder cast (thigh to ankle)**
2.50 3.47 FUD 000 T P3 50
AMA: 2018,Jan,3; 2018,Jan,8; 2017,Jan,8; 2016,Jan,13

29405 **Application of short leg cast (below knee to toes);**
1.69 2.26 FUD 000 T P3 50
AMA: 2018,Jan,3; 2018,Jan,8; 2017,Jan,8; 2016,Jan,13

29425 **walking or ambulatory type**
1.59 2.17 FUD 000 T P3 50
AMA: 2018,Jan,3; 2018,Jan,8; 2017,Jan,8; 2016,Jan,13

29435 **Application of patellar tendon bearing (PTB) cast**
2.35 3.25 FUD 000 T P3 50
AMA: 2018,Jan,3; 2018,Jan,8; 2017,Jan,8; 2016,Jan,13

29440 **Adding walker to previously applied cast**
0.83 1.23 FUD 000 T P3 50
AMA: 2018,Jan,8; 2018,Jan,3; 2017,Jan,8; 2016,Jan,13

29445 **Application of rigid total contact leg cast**
2.94 3.72 FUD 000 T P3 50
AMA: 2018,Jan,3; 2018,Jan,8; 2017,Jan,8; 2016,Jan,13

29450 **Application of clubfoot cast with molding or manipulation, long or short leg**
3.26 4.11 FUD 000 T P3 50
AMA: 2018,Jan,8; 2018,Jan,3; 2017,Jan,8; 2016,Jan,13

29505-29584 Splinting and Strapping Ankle/Foot/Leg/Toes

INCLUDES Replacement splint or strapping during or after global period
EXCLUDES *Initial splinting/strapping application performed with restorative treatment, report appropriate musculoskeletal system code*
Orthotic supervision and training (97760-97763)
Code also splint/strapping material

29505 **Application of long leg splint (thigh to ankle or toes)**
1.45 2.41 FUD 000 T P3 50
AMA: 2018,Jan,3; 2018,Jan,8; 2017,Jan,8; 2016,Jan,13

29515 **Application of short leg splint (calf to foot)**
1.42 2.01 FUD 000 T P3 50
AMA: 2019,Oct,10; 2018,Jan,8; 2018,Jan,3; 2017,Jan,8; 2016,Jan,13

29520 **Strapping; hip**
EXCLUDES *For treatment in same extremity:*
Endovenous ablation therapy incompetent vein (36473-36479, [36482], [36483])
Sclerosal injection for incompetent vein(s) ([36465], [36466], 36468-36471)
0.55 1.00 FUD 000 Q1 N1 80 50
AMA: 2018,Jan,8; 2018,Jan,3; 2017,Jan,8; 2016,Jan,13

29530 **knee**
EXCLUDES *For treatment in same extremity:*
Endovenous ablation therapy incompetent vein (36473-36479, [36482], [36483])
Sclerosal injection for incompetent vein(s) ([36465], [36466], 36468-36471)
0.54 0.86 FUD 000 Q1 N1 50
AMA: 2018,Jan,3; 2018,Jan,8; 2017,Jan,8; 2016,Jan,13

29540 **ankle and/or foot**
EXCLUDES *For treatment in same extremity:*
Endovenous ablation therapy incompetent vein (36473-36479, [36482, 36483])
Multi-layer compression system (29581)
Sclerosal injection for incompetent vein(s) ([36465], [36466], 36468-36471)
Unna boot (29580)
0.51 0.81 FUD 000 T P3 50
AMA: 2018,Jan,3; 2018,Jan,8; 2017,Jan,8; 2016,Aug,3; 2016,Jan,13

29550 **toes**
EXCLUDES *For treatment in same extremity:*
Endovenous ablation therapy incompetent vein (36473-36479, [36482, 36483])
Sclerosal injection for incompetent vein(s) ([36465], [36466], 36468-36471)
0.33 0.54 FUD 000 Q1 N1 50
AMA: 2018,Jan,8; 2018,Jan,3; 2017,Jan,8; 2016,Jan,13

29580 **Unna boot**
EXCLUDES *Application multilayer compression system (29581)*
For treatment in same extremity:
Endovenous ablation therapy incompetent vein (36473-36479, [36482, 36483])
Sclerosal injection for incompetent vein(s) ([36465], [36466], 36468-36471)
Strapping ankle or foot (29540)
0.79 1.80 FUD 000 T P3 50
AMA: 2018,Jan,3; 2018,Jan,8; 2017,Jan,8; 2016,Aug,3; 2016,Jan,13

29581 **Application of multi-layer compression system; leg (below knee), including ankle and foot**
EXCLUDES *For treatment in same extremity:*
Endovenous ablation therapy incompetent vein (36473-36479, [36482, 36483])
Sclerosal injection for incompetent vein(s) ([36465], [36466], 36468-36471)
Strapping (29540, 29580)
0.80 2.54 FUD 000 T P3 80 50
AMA: 2018,Mar,3; 2018,Jan,8; 2018,Jan,3; 2017,Jan,8; 2016,Nov,3; 2016,Aug,3; 2016,Jan,13

29584 **upper arm, forearm, hand, and fingers**
EXCLUDES *For treatment in same extremity:*
Endovenous ablation therapy incompetent vein (36473-36479, [36482], [36483])
Sclerosal injection for incompetent vein(s) ([36465], [36466], 36468-36471)
0.47 2.37 FUD 000 T P2 80 50
AMA: 2018,Jan,3; 2018,Jan,8; 2017,Jan,8; 2016,Aug,3; 2016,Jan,13

29700-29799 Casting Services Other Than Application

INCLUDES Casts applied by treating individual
Removal casts applied by treating individual

29700 **Removal or bivalving; gauntlet, boot or body cast**
0.96 1.78 FUD 000 T P3
AMA: 2018,Jan,3; 2018,Jan,8; 2017,Jan,8; 2016,Jan,13

29705 **full arm or full leg cast**
1.31 1.82 FUD 000 T P3 50
AMA: 2018,Jan,3; 2018,Jan,8; 2017,Jan,8; 2016,Jan,13

29710 **shoulder or hip spica, Minerva, or Risser jacket, etc.**
2.41 3.48 FUD 000 T P3 80 50
AMA: 2018,Jan,3; 2018,Jan,8; 2017,Jan,8; 2016,Jan,13

29720 **Repair of spica, body cast or jacket**
1.26 2.38 FUD 000 T P3
AMA: 2018,Jan,3; 2018,Jan,8; 2017,Jan,8; 2016,Jan,13

29730 **Windowing of cast**
1.25 1.76 FUD 000 T P3
AMA: 2018,Jan,3; 2018,Jan,8; 2017,Jan,8; 2016,Jan,13

29740 Wedging of cast (except clubfoot casts)
2.02 2.82 FUD 000 T P3
AMA: 2018,Jan,3; 2018,Jan,8; 2017,Jan,8; 2016,Jan,13

29750 Wedging of clubfoot cast
2.26 3.07 FUD 000 T P3 80 50
AMA: 2018,Jan,3; 2018,Jan,8; 2017,Jan,8; 2016,Jan,13

29799 Unlisted procedure, casting or strapping
0.00 0.00 FUD YYY T 80
AMA: 2018,Jan,3; 2018,Jan,8; 2017,Jan,8; 2016,Aug,3; 2016,Jan,13

29800-29999 [29914, 29915, 29916] Arthroscopic Procedures

INCLUDES Diagnostic arthroscopy with surgical arthroscopy
EXCLUDES *Reporting removal foreign or loose body(ies) smaller than arthroscopic cannula diameter utilized for procedure*
Code also modifier 51 when arthroscopy performed with arthrotomy

29800 Arthroscopy, temporomandibular joint, diagnostic, with or without synovial biopsy (separate procedure)
15.2 15.2 FUD 090 J A2 80 50
AMA: 2018,Jan,8; 2017,Jan,8; 2016,Jan,13

29804 Arthroscopy, temporomandibular joint, surgical
EXCLUDES *Open surgery (21010)*
17.7 17.7 FUD 090 J A2 80 50
AMA: 2018,Jan,8; 2017,Jan,8; 2016,Jan,13

29805 Arthroscopy, shoulder, diagnostic, with or without synovial biopsy (separate procedure)
EXCLUDES *Open surgery (23065-23066, 23100-23101)*
13.5 13.5 FUD 090 J A2 50
AMA: 2018,Jan,8; 2017,Jan,8; 2016,Jan,13

29806 Arthroscopy, shoulder, surgical; capsulorrhaphy
EXCLUDES *Open surgery (23450-23466)*
Thermal capsulorrhaphy (29999)
30.5 30.5 FUD 090 J A2 50
AMA: 2020,Dec,8; 2018,Jun,11; 2018,Jan,8; 2017,Jan,8; 2016,Jan,13

29807 repair of SLAP lesion
29.8 29.8 FUD 090 J A2 50
AMA: 2018,Jan,8; 2017,Jan,8; 2016,Jan,13

29819 with removal of loose body or foreign body
EXCLUDES *Open surgery (23040-23044, 23107)*
16.9 16.9 FUD 090 J A2 50
AMA: 2020,Dec,8; 2020,Dec,13; 2018,Jun,11; 2018,Jan,8; 2017,Jan,8; 2016,Jan,13

29820 synovectomy, partial
EXCLUDES *Open surgery (23105)*
15.3 15.3 FUD 090 J A2 80 50
AMA: 2018,Jan,8; 2017,Jan,8; 2016,Jan,13

29821 synovectomy, complete
EXCLUDES *Open surgery (23105)*
17.1 17.1 FUD 090 J A2 80 50
AMA: 2018,Jan,8; 2017,Jan,8; 2016,Jan,13

29822 debridement, limited, 1 or 2 discrete structures (eg, humeral bone, humeral articular cartilage, glenoid bone, glenoid articular cartilage, biceps tendon, biceps anchor complex, labrum, articular capsule, articular side of the rotator cuff, bursal side of the rotator cuff, subacromial bursa, foreign body[ies])
EXCLUDES *Open surgery (see specific shoulder section)*
16.6 16.6 FUD 090 J A2 80 50
AMA: 2020,Dec,8; 2018,Jan,8; 2018,Jan,7; 2017,Jan,8; 2016,Jan,13

29823 debridement, extensive, 3 or more discrete structures (eg, humeral bone, humeral articular cartilage, glenoid bone, glenoid articular cartilage, biceps tendon, biceps anchor complex, labrum, articular capsule, articular side of the rotator cuff, bursal side of the rotator cuff, subacromial bursa, foreign body[ies])
EXCLUDES *Open surgery (see specific shoulder section)*
18.1 18.1 FUD 090 J A2 80 50
AMA: 2020,Dec,8; 2018,Jan,8; 2018,Jan,7; 2017,Jan,8; 2016,Dec,16; 2016,Jan,13

29824 distal claviculectomy including distal articular surface (Mumford procedure)
EXCLUDES *Open surgery (23120)*
19.4 19.4 FUD 090 J A2 80 50
AMA: 2018,Jan,8; 2017,Jan,8; 2016,Jan,13

29825 with lysis and resection of adhesions, with or without manipulation
EXCLUDES *Open surgery (see specific shoulder section)*
16.9 16.9 FUD 090 J A2 80 50
AMA: 2018,Jan,8; 2017,Jan,8; 2016,Jan,13

+ **29826 decompression of subacromial space with partial acromioplasty, with coracoacromial ligament (ie, arch) release, when performed (List separately in addition to code for primary procedure)**
EXCLUDES *Open surgery (23130, 23415)*
Code first (29806-29825, 29827-29828)
5.07 5.07 FUD ZZZ N N1 80 50
AMA: 2018,Jan,8; 2017,Jan,8; 2016,Jan,13

29827 with rotator cuff repair
EXCLUDES *Distal clavicle excision (29824)*
Open surgery or mini open repair (23412)
Subacromial decompression (29826)
30.9 30.9 FUD 090 J A2 80 50
AMA: 2018,Jan,8; 2017,Jan,8; 2016,Jul,8; 2016,Jan,13

29828 biceps tenodesis
EXCLUDES *Arthroscopy, shoulder, diagnostic, with or without synovial biopsy (29805)*
Arthroscopy, shoulder, surgical; debridement, limited (29822)
Arthroscopy, shoulder, surgical; synovectomy, partial (29820)
Tenodesis long tendon biceps (23430)
26.5 26.5 FUD 090 J G2 80 50
AMA: 2018,Jan,8; 2017,Jan,8; 2016,Jul,8; 2016,Jan,13

29830 Arthroscopy, elbow, diagnostic, with or without synovial biopsy (separate procedure)
13.1 13.1 FUD 090 J A2 50
AMA: 2018,Jan,8; 2017,Jan,8; 2016,Jan,13

29834 Arthroscopy, elbow, surgical; with removal of loose body or foreign body
14.1 14.1 FUD 090 J A2 80 50
AMA: 2020,Dec,8; 2018,Jan,8; 2017,Jan,8; 2016,Jan,13

29835 synovectomy, partial
14.6 14.6 FUD 090 J A2 80 50
AMA: 2018,Jan,8; 2017,Jan,8; 2016,Jan,13

29836 synovectomy, complete
16.8 16.8 FUD 090 J A2 80 50
AMA: 2018,Jan,8; 2017,Jan,8; 2016,Jan,13

29837 debridement, limited
15.2 15.2 FUD 090 J A2 80 50
AMA: 2018,Jan,8; 2017,Jan,8; 2016,Jan,13

29838 debridement, extensive
17.0 17.0 FUD 090 J A2 80 50
AMA: 2018,Jan,8; 2017,Jan,8; 2016,Jan,13

29840 Arthroscopy, wrist, diagnostic, with or without synovial biopsy (separate procedure)
12.9 12.9 FUD 090 J A2 50
AMA: 2018,Jan,8; 2017,Jan,8; 2016,Jan,13

29843 **Arthroscopy, wrist, surgical; for infection, lavage and drainage**
14.0 14.0 FUD 090 J A2 80 50
AMA: 2018,Jan,8; 2017,Jan,8; 2016,Jan,13

29844 **synovectomy, partial**
14.2 14.2 FUD 090 J A2 80 50
AMA: 2018,Jan,8; 2017,Jan,8; 2016,Jan,13

29845 **synovectomy, complete**
16.8 16.8 FUD 090 J A2 80 50
AMA: 2018,Jan,8; 2017,Jan,8; 2016,Jan,13

29846 **excision and/or repair of triangular fibrocartilage and/or joint debridement**
15.0 15.0 FUD 090 J A2 80 50
AMA: 2018,Jan,8; 2017,Jan,8; 2016,Jan,13

29847 **internal fixation for fracture or instability**
15.6 15.6 FUD 090 J A2 80 50
AMA: 2018,Jan,8; 2017,Jan,8; 2016,Jan,13

29848 **Endoscopy, wrist, surgical, with release of transverse carpal ligament**
EXCLUDES *Open surgery (64721)*
Tissue expander, other than breast (11960)
14.7 14.7 FUD 090 J A2 50
AMA: 2018,Apr,10; 2018,Jan,8; 2017,Jan,8; 2017,Jan,6; 2016,Jan,13

29850 **Arthroscopically aided treatment of intercondylar spine(s) and/or tuberosity fracture(s) of the knee, with or without manipulation; without internal or external fixation (includes arthroscopy)**
17.9 17.9 FUD 090 J A2 80
AMA: 2018,Jan,8; 2017,Jan,8; 2016,Jan,13

29851 **with internal or external fixation (includes arthroscopy)**
EXCLUDES *Bone graft (20900, 20902)*
26.8 26.8 FUD 090 J A2 80 50
AMA: 2018,Jan,8; 2017,Jan,8; 2016,Jan,13

29855 **Arthroscopically aided treatment of tibial fracture, proximal (plateau); unicondylar, includes internal fixation, when performed (includes arthroscopy)**
EXCLUDES *Bone graft (20900, 20902)*
22.5 22.5 FUD 090 J J8 80 50
AMA: 2019,Nov,13; 2018,Sep,14; 2018,Jan,8; 2017,Jan,8; 2016,Jan,13

29856 **bicondylar, includes internal fixation, when performed (includes arthroscopy)**
EXCLUDES *Bone graft (20900, 20902)*
28.6 28.6 FUD 090 J J8 80 50
AMA: 2018,Jan,8; 2017,Jan,8; 2016,Jan,13

29860 **Arthroscopy, hip, diagnostic with or without synovial biopsy (separate procedure)**
19.2 19.2 FUD 090 J A2 80 50
AMA: 2018,Jan,8; 2017,Jan,8; 2016,Jan,13

29861 **Arthroscopy, hip, surgical; with removal of loose body or foreign body**
20.8 20.8 FUD 090 J A2 80 50
AMA: 2020,Dec,8; 2018,Jan,8; 2017,Jan,8; 2016,Jan,13

29862 **with debridement/shaving of articular cartilage (chondroplasty), abrasion arthroplasty, and/or resection of labrum**
23.4 23.4 FUD 090 J A2 80 50
AMA: 2018,Jan,8; 2017,Jan,8; 2016,Jan,13

29863 **with synovectomy**
23.2 23.2 FUD 090 J A2 80 50
AMA: 2018,Jan,8; 2017,Jan,8; 2016,Jan,13

\# **29914** **with femoroplasty (ie, treatment of cam lesion)**
INCLUDES Chondroplasty (29862)
Synovectomy (29863)
28.7 28.7 FUD 090 J 62 80 50
AMA: 2018,Jan,8; 2017,Jan,8; 2016,Jan,13

\# **29915** **with acetabuloplasty (ie, treatment of pincer lesion)**
INCLUDES Chondroplasty (29862)
Synovectomy (29863)
29.5 29.5 FUD 090 J 62 80 50
AMA: 2018,Jan,8; 2017,Jan,8; 2016,Jan,13

\# **29916** **with labral repair**
INCLUDES Acetabuloplasty ([29915])
Chondroplasty (29862)
Synovectomy (29863)
29.5 29.5 FUD 090 J 62 80 50
AMA: 2018,Jan,8; 2017,Jan,8; 2016,Jan,13

29866 **Arthroscopy, knee, surgical; osteochondral autograft(s) (eg, mosaicplasty) (includes harvesting of the autograft[s])**
EXCLUDES *Open osteochondral autograft knee (27416)*
Procedures performed at same surgical session (29870-29871, 29875, 29884)
Procedures performed in same compartment (29874, 29877, 29879, 29885-29887)
30.3 30.3 FUD 090 J 62 80 50
AMA: 2018,Jan,8; 2017,Jan,8; 2016,Jan,13

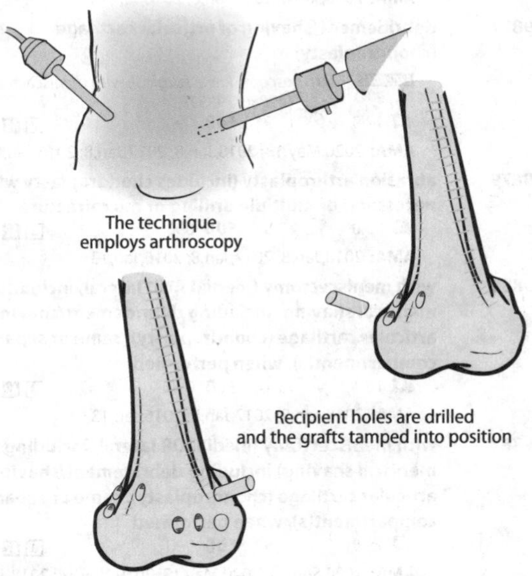
Cylindrical plugs of healthy bone are harvested, usually from a non-weight bearing area of the femur
The technique employs arthroscopy
Recipient holes are drilled and the grafts tamped into position

29867 **osteochondral allograft (eg, mosaicplasty)**
EXCLUDES *Procedures performed at same surgical session (27415, 27570, 29870-29871, 29875, 29884)*
Procedures performed in same compartment (29874, 29877, 29879, 29885-29887)
36.9 36.9 FUD 090 J J8 80 50
AMA: 2018,Jan,8; 2017,Jan,8; 2016,Jan,13

29868 **meniscal transplantation (includes arthrotomy for meniscal insertion), medial or lateral**
EXCLUDES *Procedures performed at same surgical session (29870-29871, 29875, 29880, 29883-29884)*
Procedures performed in same compartment (29874, 29877, 29881-29882)
48.4 48.4 FUD 090 J 62 80 50
AMA: 2018,Jan,8; 2017,Jan,8; 2016,Jan,13

29870 **Arthroscopy, knee, diagnostic, with or without synovial biopsy (separate procedure)**

EXCLUDES *Open procedure (27412)*

11.7 16.4 FUD 090 J A2 50

AMA: 2019,Nov,14; 2018,Jan,8; 2017,Jan,8; 2016,Jan,13

29871 **Arthroscopy, knee, surgical; for infection, lavage and drainage**

EXCLUDES *Injection contrast for knee arthrography (27369)*
Osteochondral graft (27412, 27415, 29866-29867)

14.8 14.8 FUD 090 J A2 50

AMA: 2019,Aug,7; 2018,Jan,8; 2017,Jan,8; 2016,Jan,13

29873 **with lateral release**

EXCLUDES *Open procedure (27425)*

15.2 15.2 FUD 090 J A2 50

AMA: 2018,Jan,8; 2017,Jan,8; 2016,Jan,13

29874 **for removal of loose body or foreign body (eg, osteochondritis dissecans fragmentation, chondral fragmentation)**

15.5 15.5 FUD 090 J A2 80 50

AMA: 2020,Dec,8; 2018,Jan,8; 2017,Jan,8; 2016,Jan,13

29875 **synovectomy, limited (eg, plica or shelf resection) (separate procedure)**

14.3 14.3 FUD 090 J A2 80 50

AMA: 2018,Jan,8; 2017,Jan,8; 2016,Jan,13; 2016,Jan,11

29876 **synovectomy, major, 2 or more compartments (eg, medial or lateral)**

18.8 18.8 FUD 090 J A2 50

AMA: 2018,Jan,8; 2017,Jan,8; 2016,Jan,13

29877 **debridement/shaving of articular cartilage (chondroplasty)**

EXCLUDES *Arthroscopy, knee, surgical; with meniscectomy (29880-29881)*

17.9 17.9 FUD 090 J A2 80 50

AMA: 2020,May,13; 2018,Jan,8; 2017,Jan,8; 2016,Jan,13

29879 **abrasion arthroplasty (includes chondroplasty where necessary) or multiple drilling or microfracture**

19.0 19.0 FUD 090 J A2 80 50

AMA: 2018,Jan,8; 2017,Jan,8; 2016,Jan,13

29880 **with meniscectomy (medial AND lateral, including any meniscal shaving) including debridement/shaving of articular cartilage (chondroplasty), same or separate compartment(s), when performed**

16.1 16.1 FUD 090 J A2 80 50

AMA: 2018,Jan,8; 2017,Jan,8; 2016,Jan,13

29881 **with meniscectomy (medial OR lateral, including any meniscal shaving) including debridement/shaving of articular cartilage (chondroplasty), same or separate compartment(s), when performed**

15.5 15.5 FUD 090 J A2 80 50

AMA: 2020,Sep,14; 2020,May,13; 2019,Nov,14; 2018,Jan,8; 2017,Jan,8; 2016,Jan,13; 2016,Jan,11

29882 **with meniscus repair (medial OR lateral)**

EXCLUDES *Meniscus transplant (29868)*

19.9 19.9 FUD 090 J A2 50

AMA: 2019,May,10; 2018,Jan,8; 2017,Jan,8; 2016,Jan,13

29883 **with meniscus repair (medial AND lateral)**

EXCLUDES *Meniscus transplant (29868)*

24.2 24.2 FUD 090 J A2 80 50

AMA: 2018,Jan,8; 2017,Jan,8; 2016,Jan,13

29884 **with lysis of adhesions, with or without manipulation (separate procedure)**

17.8 17.8 FUD 090 J A2 80 50

AMA: 2018,Jan,8; 2017,Jan,8; 2016,Jan,13

29885 **drilling for osteochondritis dissecans with bone grafting, with or without internal fixation (including debridement of base of lesion)**

21.7 21.7 FUD 090 J J8 80 50

AMA: 2018,Jan,8; 2017,Jan,8; 2016,Jan,13

29886 **drilling for intact osteochondritis dissecans lesion**

18.3 18.3 FUD 090 J A2 50

AMA: 2018,Jan,8; 2017,Jan,8; 2016,Jan,13

29887 **drilling for intact osteochondritis dissecans lesion with internal fixation**

21.6 21.6 FUD 090 J A2 80 50

AMA: 2018,Jan,8; 2017,Jan,8; 2016,Jan,13

29888 **Arthroscopically aided anterior cruciate ligament repair/augmentation or reconstruction**

28.3 28.3 FUD 090 J J8 80 50

AMA: 2018,Jan,8; 2017,Jan,8; 2016,Nov,9; 2016,Jan,13

29889 **Arthroscopically aided posterior cruciate ligament repair/augmentation or reconstruction**

35.3 35.3 FUD 090 J J8 80 50

AMA: 2018,Jan,8; 2017,Jan,8; 2016,Jan,13

29891 **Arthroscopy, ankle, surgical, excision of osteochondral defect of talus and/or tibia, including drilling of the defect**

19.3 19.3 FUD 090 J A2 80 50

AMA: 2018,Jan,8; 2017,Jan,8; 2016,Jan,13

29892 **Arthroscopically aided repair of large osteochondritis dissecans lesion, talar dome fracture, or tibial plafond fracture, with or without internal fixation (includes arthroscopy)**

18.7 18.7 FUD 090 J A2 80 50

AMA: 2018,Jan,8; 2017,Jan,8; 2016,Jan,13

29893 **Endoscopic plantar fasciotomy**

12.3 17.8 FUD 090 J A2 50

AMA: 2018,Jan,8; 2017,Jan,8; 2016,Jan,13

29894 **Arthroscopy, ankle (tibiotalar and fibulotalar joints), surgical; with removal of loose body or foreign body**

14.2 14.2 FUD 090 J A2 80 50

AMA: 2020,Dec,8; 2018,Jan,8; 2017,Jan,8; 2016,Jan,13

29895 **synovectomy, partial**

13.4 13.4 FUD 090 J A2 80 50

AMA: 2018,Jan,8; 2017,Jan,8; 2016,Jan,13

29897 **debridement, limited**

14.4 14.4 FUD 090 J A2 80 50

AMA: 2018,Jan,8; 2017,Jan,8; 2016,Jan,13

29898 **debridement, extensive**

16.1 16.1 FUD 090 J A2 80 50

AMA: 2018,Jan,8; 2017,Jan,8; 2016,Jan,13

29899 **with ankle arthrodesis**

EXCLUDES *Open procedure (27870)*

29.7 29.7 FUD 090 J J8 80 50

AMA: 2018,Jan,8; 2017,Jan,8; 2016,Jan,13

29900 **Arthroscopy, metacarpophalangeal joint, diagnostic, includes synovial biopsy**

EXCLUDES *Arthroscopy, metacarpophalangeal joint, surgical (29901-29902)*

14.3 14.3 FUD 090 J A2 80 50

AMA: 2018,Jan,8; 2017,Jan,8; 2016,Jan,13

29901 **Arthroscopy, metacarpophalangeal joint, surgical; with debridement**

15.4 15.4 FUD 090 J A2 80 50

AMA: 2018,Jan,8; 2017,Jan,8; 2016,Jan,13

29902 **with reduction of displaced ulnar collateral ligament (eg, Stenar lesion)**

16.4 16.4 FUD 090 J A2 80 50

AMA: 2018,Jan,8; 2017,Jan,8; 2016,Jan,13

29904 **Arthroscopy, subtalar joint, surgical; with removal of loose body or foreign body**
18.3 18.3 FUD 090 J G2 80 50
AMA: 2020,Dec,8; 2018,Jan,8; 2017,Jan,8; 2016,Jan,13

29905 **with synovectomy**
14.9 14.9 FUD 090 J G2 80 50
AMA: 2018,Jan,8; 2017,Jan,8; 2016,Jan,13

29906 **with debridement**
19.5 19.5 FUD 090 J G2 80 50
AMA: 2018,Jan,8; 2017,Jan,8; 2016,Jan,13

29907 **with subtalar arthrodesis**
25.3 25.3 FUD 090 J G2 80 50
AMA: 2018,Jan,8; 2017,Jan,8; 2016,Jan,13

29914 **Resequenced code. See code following 29863.**

29915 **Resequenced code. See code following 29863.**

29916 **Resequenced code. See code before 29866.**

29999 **Unlisted procedure, arthroscopy**
0.00 0.00 FUD YYY T 80 50
AMA: 2019,Dec,12; 2019,Nov,13; 2018,Jan,8; 2017,Apr,9; 2017,Jan,8; 2016,Dec,16; 2016,Jan,13

30000-30115 I&D, Biopsy, Excision Procedures of the Nose

30000 Drainage abscess or hematoma, nasal, internal approach

EXCLUDES *Incision and drainage (10060, 10140)*

3.38 | 7.18 | FUD 010 | T P2 80

AMA: 2005,May,13-14; 1994,Spr,24

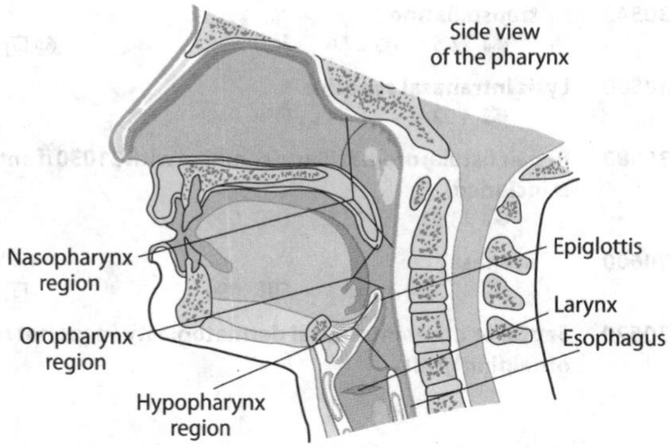

The nasopharynx is the membranous passage above the level of the soft palate; the oropharynx is the region between the soft palate and the upper edge of the epiglottis; the hypopharynx is the region of the epiglottis to the juncture of the larynx and esophagus; the three regions are collectively known as the pharynx

30020 Drainage abscess or hematoma, nasal septum

EXCLUDES *Lateral rhinotomy incision (30118, 30320)*

3.37 | 6.90 | FUD 010 | T P3

30100 Biopsy, intranasal

EXCLUDES *Superficial biopsy nose (11102-11107)*

1.91 | 4.03 | FUD 000 | T P3

AMA: 2019,Jan,9

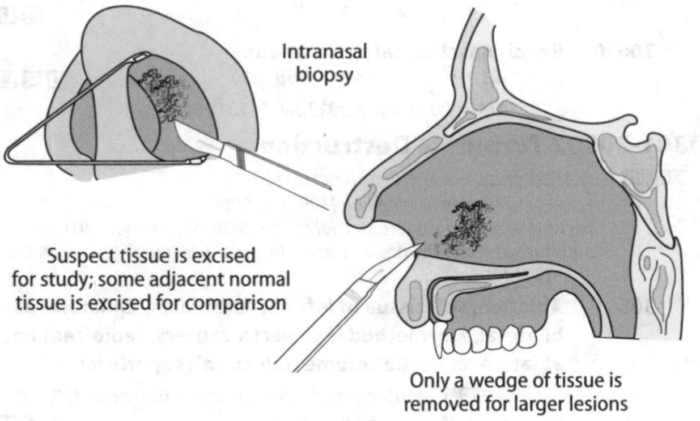

30110 Excision, nasal polyp(s), simple

3.70 | 6.82 | FUD 010 | T P3 50

30115 Excision, nasal polyp(s), extensive

12.7 | 12.7 | FUD 090 | J A2 50

30117-30118 Destruction Procedures Nose

CMS: 100-03,140.5 Laser Procedures

30117 Excision or destruction (eg, laser), intranasal lesion; internal approach

9.47 | 26.4 | FUD 090 | J A2

AMA: 2020,Sep,14; 2019,Nov,14; 2019,Jul,10

30118 external approach (lateral rhinotomy)

22.0 | 22.0 | FUD 090 | J A2

30120-30140 Excision Procedures Nose, Turbinate

30120 Excision or surgical planing of skin of nose for rhinophyma

12.3 | 14.6 | FUD 090 | J A2

AMA: 2018,Jan,8; 2017,Jan,8; 2016,Jan,13

30124 Excision dermoid cyst, nose; simple, skin, subcutaneous

8.19 | 8.19 | FUD 090 | T R2

30125 complex, under bone or cartilage

17.5 | 17.5 | FUD 090 | J A2 80

30130 Excision inferior turbinate, partial or complete, any method

EXCLUDES *Ablation, soft tissue inferior turbinates, unilateral or bilateral, any method (30801-30802)*
Excision middle/superior turbinate(s) (30999)
Fracture nasal inferior turbinate(s), therapeutic (30930)

11.2 | 11.2 | FUD 090 | J A2 50

AMA: 2018,Jan,8; 2017,Jan,8; 2016,Jan,13

30140 Submucous resection inferior turbinate, partial or complete, any method

EXCLUDES *Ablation, soft tissue inferior turbinates, unilateral or bilateral, any method (30801-30802)*
Endoscopic resection concha bullosa middle turbinate (31240)
Fracture nasal inferior turbinate(s), therapeutic (30930)
Submucous resection:
Nasal septum (30520)
Superior or middle turbinate (30999)

5.12 | 7.92 | FUD 000 | J A2 50

AMA: 2020,Jan,12; 2018,Jan,8; 2017,Jan,8; 2016,Jan,13

30150-30160 Surgical Removal: Nose

EXCLUDES *Reconstruction and/or closure (primary or delayed primary intention) (13151-13160, 14060-14302, 15120-15121, 15260-15261, 15760, 20900-20912)*

30150 Rhinectomy; partial

22.4 | 22.4 | FUD 090 | J A2

30160 total

22.6 | 22.6 | FUD 090 | J A2 80

30200-30320 Turbinate Injection, Removal Foreign Substance in the Nose

30200 Injection into turbinate(s), therapeutic

1.66 | 3.18 | FUD 000 | T P3

AMA: 2018,Jan,8; 2017,Jan,8; 2016,Jan,13

30210 Displacement therapy (Proetz type)

2.82 | 4.24 | FUD 010 | T P3

AMA: 2018,Jan,8; 2017,Jan,8; 2016,Jan,13

30220 Insertion, nasal septal prosthesis (button)

3.55 | 8.60 | FUD 010 | T A2

30300 Removal foreign body, intranasal; office type procedure

3.23 | 5.40 | FUD 010 | Q1 N1

AMA: 2018,Jan,8; 2017,Jan,8; 2016,Jan,13

30310 requiring general anesthesia

5.80 | 5.80 | FUD 010 | J A2 80

30320 by lateral rhinotomy

13.2 | 13.2 | FUD 090 | T A2 80

30400-30630 Reconstruction or Repair of Nose

EXCLUDES *Harvesting bone/tissue/fat grafts ([15769], 15773-15774, 20900-20924, 21210)*
Liposuction for autologous fat grafting (15773-15774)

30400 Rhinoplasty, primary; lateral and alar cartilages and/or elevation of nasal tip

INCLUDES Carpue's operation

EXCLUDES *Reconstruction columella (13151-13153)*

34.3 | 34.3 | FUD 090 | J A2 80

30410 complete, external parts including bony pyramid, lateral and alar cartilages, and/or elevation of nasal tip

39.8 | 39.8 | FUD 090 | J A2 80

30420 **including major septal repair**
40.3 | 40.3 | FUD 090 | J A2
AMA: 2018,Jan,8; 2017,Nov,11; 2017,Jan,8; 2016,Jul,8

30430 **Rhinoplasty, secondary; minor revision (small amount of nasal tip work)**
29.7 | 29.7 | FUD 090 | J A2 80

30435 **intermediate revision (bony work with osteotomies)**
37.6 | 37.6 | FUD 090 | J A2 80

30450 **major revision (nasal tip work and osteotomies)**
49.8 | 49.8 | FUD 090 | J A2 80

30460 **Rhinoplasty for nasal deformity secondary to congenital cleft lip and/or palate, including columellar lengthening; tip only**
23.5 | 23.5 | FUD 090 | J A2 80
AMA: 2018,Jan,8; 2017,Jan,8; 2016,Jan,13

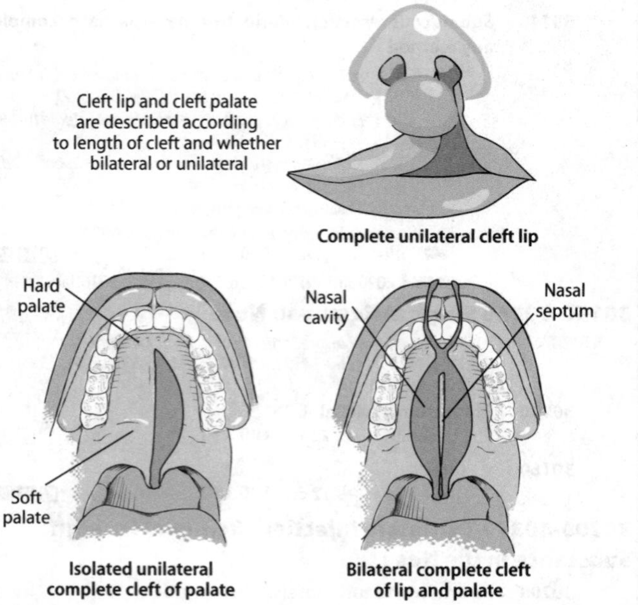

30462 **tip, septum, osteotomies**
45.1 | 45.1 | FUD 090 | J A2 80
AMA: 2018,Jan,8; 2017,Jan,8; 2016,Jan,13

30465 **Repair of nasal vestibular stenosis (eg, spreader grafting, lateral nasal wall reconstruction)**
INCLUDES Bilateral procedure
EXCLUDES *Harvesting ear cartilage graft, autogenous (21235)*
Repair nasal valve or vestibular lateral wall collapse with implants same side during same operative session (30468)
Repair nasal vestibular stenosis without graft, implant, or reconstruction lateral wall (30999)
Code also modifier 52 for unilateral procedure
28.5 | 28.5 | FUD 090 | J A2 80
AMA: 2020,Sep,14

30468 **Repair of nasal valve collapse with subcutaneous/submucosal lateral wall implant(s)**
INCLUDES Bilateral procedure
EXCLUDES *Repair nasal vestibular stenosis same side during same operative session (30465)*
Repair nasal vestibular stenosis without graft, implant, or reconstruction lateral wall (30999)
Code also modifier 52 for unilateral procedure
4.87 | 83.9 | FUD 000 | J8 50

30520 **Septoplasty or submucous resection, with or without cartilage scoring, contouring or replacement with graft**
EXCLUDES *Turbinate resection (30140)*
18.4 | 18.4 | FUD 090 | J A2
AMA: 2019,Jul,10; 2018,Jan,8; 2017,Jan,8; 2016,Jan,13

30540 **Repair choanal atresia; intranasal**
20.2 | 20.2 | FUD 090 | 63 J A2 80

30545 **transpalatine**
27.6 | 27.6 | FUD 090 | 63 J A2 80

30560 **Lysis intranasal synechia**
4.02 | 8.34 | FUD 010 | T A2

30580 **Repair fistula; oromaxillary (combine with 31030 if antrotomy is included)**
13.6 | 17.8 | FUD 090 | J A2

30600 **oronasal**
12.3 | 16.8 | FUD 090 | J A2 80

30620 **Septal or other intranasal dermatoplasty (does not include obtaining graft)**

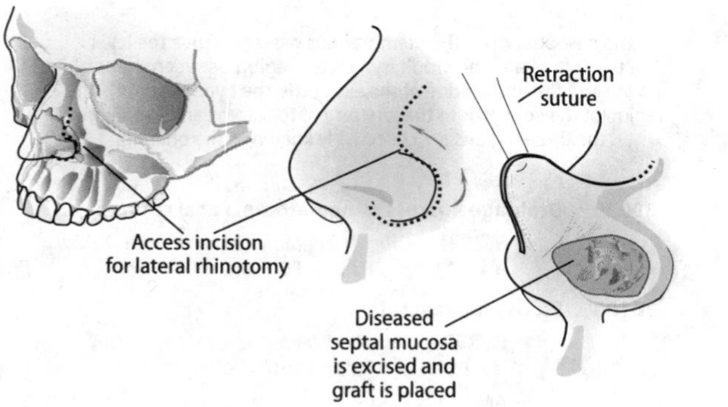

18.2 | 18.2 | FUD 090 | J A2

30630 **Repair nasal septal perforations**
18.0 | 18.0 | FUD 090 | J A2 80
AMA: 2018,Jan,8; 2017,Jan,8; 2016,Jan,13

30801-30802 Turbinate Destruction

EXCLUDES *Ablation middle/superior turbinates (30999)*
Cautery to stop nasal bleeding (30901-30906)
Excision inferior turbinate, partial or complete, any method (30130)
Submucous resection inferior turbinate, partial or complete, any method (30140)

30801 **Ablation, soft tissue of inferior turbinates, unilateral or bilateral, any method (eg, electrocautery, radiofrequency ablation, or tissue volume reduction); superficial**
EXCLUDES *Submucosal ablation inferior turbinates (30802)*
4.10 | 6.18 | FUD 010 | T A2
AMA: 2019,Jul,10

30802 **intramural (ie, submucosal)**
EXCLUDES *Superficial ablation inferior turbinates (30801)*
5.58 | 7.86 | FUD 010 | T A2
AMA: 2019,Jul,10; 2018,Jan,8; 2017,Jan,8; 2016,Jan,13

30901-30920 Control Nose Bleed

30901 **Control nasal hemorrhage, anterior, simple (limited cautery and/or packing) any method**
1.64 | 4.09 | FUD 000 | Q1 N1 50
AMA: 2020,Oct,13; 2020,Jul,13

30903 **Control nasal hemorrhage, anterior, complex (extensive cautery and/or packing) any method**
2.28 | 6.49 | FUD 000 | T A2 50
AMA: 1990,Win,4

30905 Control nasal hemorrhage, posterior, with posterior nasal packs and/or cautery, any method; initial
3.07 9.64 FUD 000 T A2
AMA: 2018,Jan,8; 2017,Jan,8; 2016,Jan,13

30906 subsequent
3.92 10.0 FUD 000 T A2
AMA: 2002,May,7

30915 Ligation arteries; ethmoidal
EXCLUDES *External carotid artery (37600)*
16.7 16.7 FUD 090 T A2

30920 internal maxillary artery, transantral
EXCLUDES *External carotid artery (37600)*
24.3 24.3 FUD 090 T A2

30930-30999 Other and Unlisted Procedures of Nose

30930 Fracture nasal inferior turbinate(s), therapeutic
EXCLUDES *Excision inferior turbinate, partial or complete, any method (30130)*
Fracture superior or middle turbinate(s) (30999)
Submucous resection inferior turbinate, partial or complete, any method (30140)
3.43 3.43 FUD 010 J A2
AMA: 2018,Jan,8; 2017,Nov,11; 2017,Jan,8; 2016,Jul,8; 2016,Jan,13

30999 Unlisted procedure, nose
0.00 0.00 FUD YYY T 80
AMA: 2020,Sep,14; 2019,Nov,14; 2018,Jan,8; 2017,Jan,8; 2016,Jan,13

31000-31230 Opening Sinuses

31000 Lavage by cannulation; maxillary sinus (antrum puncture or natural ostium)
3.02 5.17 FUD 010 T P2 50
AMA: 2018,Jan,8; 2017,Jan,8; 2016,Jan,13

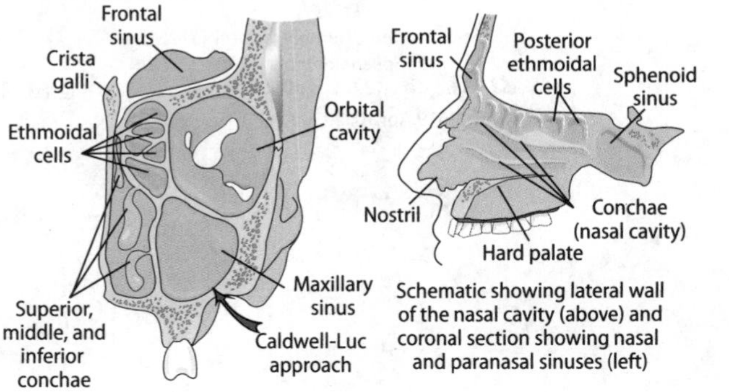

Schematic showing lateral wall of the nasal cavity (above) and coronal section showing nasal and paranasal sinuses (left)

31002 sphenoid sinus
5.39 5.39 FUD 010 T J8 80 50

31020 Sinusotomy, maxillary (antrotomy); intranasal
10.4 13.6 FUD 090 J A2 50

31030 radical (Caldwell-Luc) without removal of antrochoanal polyps
14.7 18.4 FUD 090 J A2 50

31032 radical (Caldwell-Luc) with removal of antrochoanal polyps
16.5 16.5 FUD 090 J A2 50

31040 Pterygomaxillary fossa surgery, any approach
EXCLUDES *Transantral ligation internal maxillary artery (30920)*
22.0 22.0 FUD 090 J R2 50

31050 Sinusotomy, sphenoid, with or without biopsy;
14.1 14.1 FUD 090 J A2 50

31051 with mucosal stripping or removal of polyp(s)
19.0 19.0 FUD 090 J A2 50

31070 Sinusotomy frontal; external, simple (trephine operation)
INCLUDES Killian operation
EXCLUDES *Intranasal frontal sinusotomy (31276)*
12.9 12.9 FUD 090 J A2 50

31075 transorbital, unilateral (for mucocele or osteoma, Lynch type)
22.8 22.8 FUD 090 J A2 80 50

31080 obliterative without osteoplastic flap, brow incision (includes ablation)
INCLUDES Ridell sinusotomy
30.0 30.0 FUD 090 J A2 80 50

31081 obliterative, without osteoplastic flap, coronal incision (includes ablation)
32.3 32.3 FUD 090 J A2 80 50

31084 obliterative, with osteoplastic flap, brow incision
33.5 33.5 FUD 090 J A2 80 50

31085 obliterative, with osteoplastic flap, coronal incision
34.6 34.6 FUD 090 J J8 80 50

31086 nonobliterative, with osteoplastic flap, brow incision
32.6 32.6 FUD 090 J A2 80 50

31087 nonobliterative, with osteoplastic flap, coronal incision
31.2 31.2 FUD 090 J A2 80 50

31090 Sinusotomy, unilateral, 3 or more paranasal sinuses (frontal, maxillary, ethmoid, sphenoid)
30.3 30.3 FUD 090 J A2 50
AMA: 1998,Nov,1; 1997,Nov,1

31200 Ethmoidectomy; intranasal, anterior
16.7 16.7 FUD 090 J A2 50
AMA: 2018,Jan,8; 2017,Jan,8; 2016,Feb,10

31201 intranasal, total
21.9 21.9 FUD 090 J A2 50
AMA: 2018,Jan,8; 2017,Jan,8; 2016,Feb,10

31205 extranasal, total
26.3 26.3 FUD 090 J A2 80 50
AMA: 2018,Jan,8; 2017,Jan,8; 2016,Feb,10

31225 Maxillectomy; without orbital exenteration
52.1 52.1 FUD 090 C 80 50

31230 with orbital exenteration (en bloc)
EXCLUDES *Orbital exenteration without maxillectomy (65110-65114)*
Skin grafts (15120-15121)
58.3 58.3 FUD 090 C 80 50

31231-31235 Nasal Endoscopy, Diagnostic

INCLUDES Complete sinus exam (e.g., nasal cavity, turbinates, sphenoethmoidal recess)

Code also stereotactic navigation, when performed (61782)

31231 Nasal endoscopy, diagnostic, unilateral or bilateral (separate procedure)
1.82 5.48 FUD 000 T P2
AMA: 2018,Apr,3; 2018,Jan,8; 2017,Jul,7; 2017,Jan,8; 2017,Jan,6; 2016,Dec,13; 2016,Feb,10; 2016,Jan,13

31233 Nasal/sinus endoscopy, diagnostic; with maxillary sinusoscopy (via inferior meatus or canine fossa puncture)
EXCLUDES *When performed on same side:*
Dilation of maxillary sinus ostium (31295)
Maxillary antrostomy (31256, 31267)
3.87 7.41 FUD 000 T A2 80 50
AMA: 2018,Apr,3; 2018,Jan,8; 2017,Jan,8; 2016,Jan,13

31235 **with sphenoid sinusoscopy (via puncture of sphenoidal face or cannulation of ostium)**

EXCLUDES *Insertion drug-eluting implant performed with biopsy, debridement, or polypectomy (31237)*
Insertion drug-eluting implant without other nasal/sinus endoscopic procedure (31299)
When performed on same side:
Sinus dilation (31297-31298)
Sphenoidotomy (31287-31288)
Total ethmoidectomy with sphenoidotomy ([31257, 31259])

4.54 | 8.49 | FUD 000 | J A2 80 50

AMA: 2018,Apr,3; 2018,Jan,8; 2017,Jan,8; 2016,Jan,13

31237-31253 [31253] Nasal Endoscopy, Surgical

INCLUDES Diagnostic nasal/sinus endoscopy

Code also stereotactic navigation, when performed (61782)

31237 **Nasal/sinus endoscopy, surgical; with biopsy, polypectomy or debridement (separate procedure)**

EXCLUDES *When performed on same side:*
Frontal sinus exploration (31276)
Maxillary antrostomy (31256, 31267)
Nasal hemorrhage control (31238)
Optic nerve decompression (31294)
Orbital wall decompression, medial and/or inferior (31292-31293)
Other total ethmoidectomy procedures ([31253], 31255, [31257], [31259])
Partial ethmoidectomy (31254)
Repair CSF leak (31290-31291)
Sphenoidotomy (31287-31288)

4.54 | 7.21 | FUD 000 | J A2 50

AMA: 2020,Jan,12; 2019,Jul,7; 2019,Apr,10; 2018,Apr,3; 2018,Jan,8; 2017,Jan,8; 2016,Feb,10; 2016,Jan,13

31238 **with control of nasal hemorrhage**

EXCLUDES *When performed on same side:*
Biopsy, polypectomy, or debridement (31237)
Sphenopalatine artery ligation (31241)

4.80 | 7.17 | FUD 000 | J A2 80 50

AMA: 2018,Apr,3; 2018,Jan,8; 2017,Jan,8; 2016,Jan,13

31239 **with dacryocystorhinostomy**

17.4 | 17.4 | FUD 010 | J A2 80 50

AMA: 2018,Apr,3; 2018,Jan,8; 2017,Jan,8; 2016,Jan,13

31240 **with concha bullosa resection**

4.52 | 4.52 | FUD 000 | J A2 80 50

AMA: 2018,Apr,3; 2018,Jan,8; 2017,Jan,8; 2016,Feb,10; 2016,Jan,13

31241 **with ligation of sphenopalatine artery**

EXCLUDES *When performed on same side:*
Nasal hemorrhage control (31238)

12.7 | 12.7 | FUD 000 | C G2 80 50

AMA: 2018,Apr,3

31253 **Resequenced code. See code following 31255.**

31254-31259 [31253, 31257, 31259] Nasal Endoscopy with Ethmoid Removal

INCLUDES Diagnostic nasal/sinus endoscopy
Sinusotomy, when applicable

EXCLUDES *When performed on same side:*
Biopsy, polypectomy, or debridement (31237)
Optic nerve decompression (31294)
Orbital wall decompression, medial, and/or inferior (31292-31293)
Repair CSF leak (31290-31291)

Code also stereotactic navigation, when performed (61782)

31254 **Nasal/sinus endoscopy, surgical with ethmoidectomy; partial (anterior)**

EXCLUDES *When performed on same side:*
Other total ethmoidectomy procedures (31253, 31255, [31257], [31259])

7.01 | 11.7 | FUD 000 | J A2 50

AMA: 2019,Apr,10; 2018,Apr,3; 2018,Jan,8; 2017,Jan,8; 2016,Feb,10; 2016,Jan,13

31255 **total (anterior and posterior)**

EXCLUDES *When performed on same side:*
Frontal sinus exploration (31276)
Other total ethmoidectomy procedures (31253, [31257], [31259])
Partial ethmoidectomy (31254)
Sphenoidotomy (31287-31288)

9.31 | 9.31 | FUD 000 | J A2 50

AMA: 2019,Apr,10; 2018,Apr,3; 2018,Apr,10; 2018,Jan,8; 2017,Jan,8; 2016,Feb,10; 2016,Jan,13

31253 **total (anterior and posterior), including frontal sinus exploration, with removal of tissue from frontal sinus, when performed**

EXCLUDES *When performed on same side:*
Dilation sinus (31296, 31298)
Frontal sinus exploration (31276)
Partial ethmoidectomy (31254)
Total ethmoidectomy (31255)

14.4 | 14.4 | FUD 000 | J G2 50

AMA: 2019,Apr,10; 2018,Apr,10; 2018,Apr,3

31257 **total (anterior and posterior), including sphenoidotomy**

EXCLUDES *When performed on same side:*
Diagnostic sphenoid sinusoscopy (31235)
Dilation sinus (31297-31298)
Other total ethmoidectomy procedures (31255, [31259])
Partial ethmoidectomy (31254)
Sphenoidotomy (31287-31288)

12.8 | 12.8 | FUD 000 | J G2 50

AMA: 2019,Apr,10; 2018,Apr,10; 2018,Apr,3

31259 **total (anterior and posterior), including sphenoidotomy, with removal of tissue from the sphenoid sinus**

EXCLUDES *When performed on same side:*
Diagnostic sphenoid sinusoscopy (31235)
Dilation sinus (31297-31298)
Other total ethmoidectomy procedures (31255, [31257])
Partial ethmoidectomy (31254)
Sphenoidotomy (31287-31288)

13.6 | 13.6 | FUD 000 | J G2 50

AMA: 2019,Apr,10; 2018,Apr,3

31256-31267 [31257, 31259] Nasal Endoscopy with Maxillary Procedures

INCLUDES Diagnostic nasal/sinus endoscopy
Sinusotomy, when applicable

EXCLUDES *When performed on same side:*
Biopsy, polypectomy, or debridement (31237)
Dilation maxillary sinus ostium (31295)
Maxillary sinusoscopy (31233)

Code also stereotactic navigation, when performed (61782)

31256 Nasal/sinus endoscopy, surgical, with maxillary antrostomy;

EXCLUDES *When performed on the same side:*
Maxillary antrostomy with removal of tissue from maxillary sinus (31267)

5.19 5.19 **FUD** 000 J A2 50

AMA: 2019,Apr,10; 2018,Apr,3; 2018,Apr,10; 2018,Jan,8; 2017,Jan,8; 2016,Jan,13

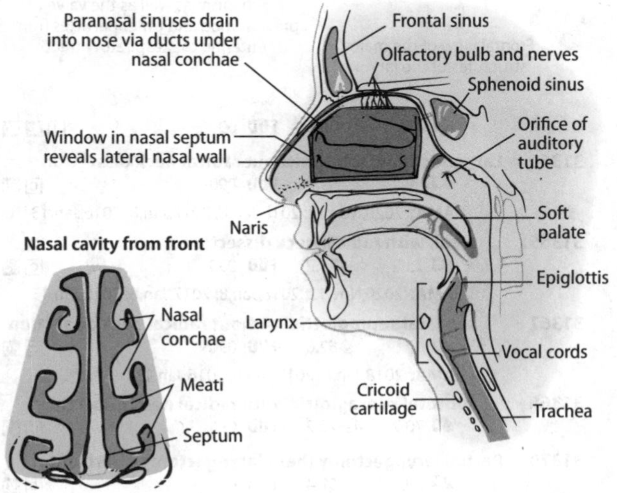

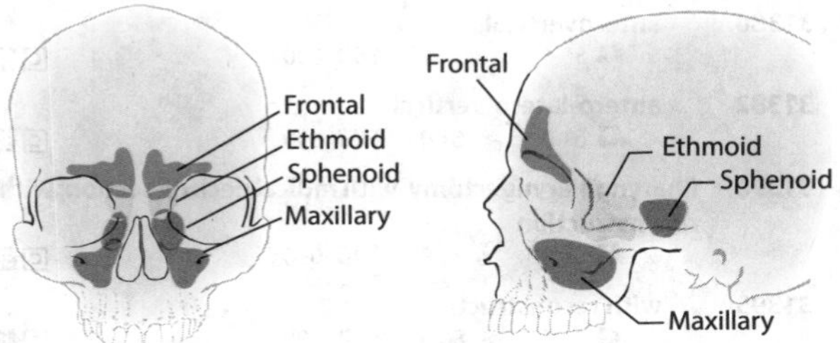

31257 **Resequenced code. See code following 31255.**

31259 **Resequenced code. See code following 31255.**

31267 with removal of tissue from maxillary sinus

EXCLUDES *When performed on same side:*
Maxillary antrostomy without removal tissue (31256)

7.61 7.61 **FUD** 000 J A2 50

AMA: 2019,Apr,10; 2018,Apr,3; 2018,Jan,8; 2017,Jan,8; 2016,Jan,13

31276 Nasal Endoscopy with Frontal Sinus Examination

INCLUDES Diagnostic nasal/sinus endoscopy
Sinusotomy, when applicable

EXCLUDES *When performed on same side:*
Biopsy, polypectomy, or debridement (31237)
Dilation frontal or frontal and sphenoid sinus (31296, 31298)
Other total ethmoidectomy procedures (31253, 31255)

Code also stereotactic navigation, when performed (61782)

31276 Nasal/sinus endoscopy, surgical, with frontal sinus exploration, including removal of tissue from frontal sinus, when performed

10.9 10.9 **FUD** 000 J A2 50

AMA: 2019,Apr,10; 2018,Apr,3; 2018,Apr,10; 2018,Jan,8; 2017,Jan,8; 2016,Jan,13

31287-31288 Nasal Endoscopy with Sphenoid Procedures

EXCLUDES *Sinus dilation (31297-31298)*
When performed on same side:
Biopsy, polypectomy, or debridement (31237)
Diagnostic sphenoid sinusoscopy (31235)
Optic nerve decompression (31294)
Other total ethmoidectomy procedures (31255, [31257], [31259])
Repair CSF leak (31291)

Code also stereotactic navigation, when performed (61782)

31287 Nasal/sinus endoscopy, surgical, with sphenoidotomy;

EXCLUDES *When performed on same side:*
Sphenoidotomy with removal tissue (31288)

5.78 5.78 **FUD** 000 J A2 80 50

AMA: 2019,Apr,10; 2018,Apr,3; 2018,Jan,8; 2017,Jan,8; 2016,Jan,13

31288 with removal of tissue from the sphenoid sinus

EXCLUDES *When performed on same side:*
Sphenoidotomy without removal tissue (31287)

6.71 6.71 **FUD** 000 J A2 80 50

AMA: 2019,Apr,10; 2018,Apr,3; 2018,Jan,8; 2017,Jan,8; 2016,Feb,10; 2016,Jan,13

31290-31294 Nasal Endoscopy with Repair and Decompression

INCLUDES Diagnostic nasal/sinus endoscopy
Sinusotomy, when applicable

EXCLUDES *When performed on same side: .*
Biopsy, polypectomy, or debridement (31237)
Other total ethmoidectomy procedures ([31253], 31255, [31257], [31259])
Partial ethmoidectomy (31254)

Code also stereotactic navigation, when performed (61782)

31290 Nasal/sinus endoscopy, surgical, with repair of cerebrospinal fluid leak; ethmoid region

32.7 32.7 **FUD** 010 C 80 50

AMA: 2018,Apr,3; 2018,Jan,8; 2017,Jan,8; 2016,Feb,10; 2016,Jan,13

31291 sphenoid region

EXCLUDES *When performed on same side:*
Sphenoidotomy (31287-31288)

34.9 34.9 **FUD** 010 C 80 50

AMA: 2018,Apr,3; 2018,Jan,8; 2017,Jan,8; 2016,Jan,13

31292 Nasal/sinus endoscopy, surgical, with orbital decompression; medial or inferior wall

EXCLUDES *When performed on same side:*
Dilation frontal sinus only (31296)
Orbital wall decompression, medial and inferior (31293)

28.4 28.4 **FUD** 010 J G2 80 50

AMA: 2018,Apr,3; 2018,Jan,8; 2017,Jan,8; 2016,Jan,13

31293 medial and inferior wall

EXCLUDES *When performed on same side:*
Orbital wall decompression, medial or inferior (31292)

30.8 30.8 **FUD** 010 J G2 80 50

AMA: 2018,Apr,3; 2018,Jan,8; 2017,Jan,8; 2016,Jan,13

31294 **Nasal/sinus endoscopy, surgical, with optic nerve decompression**

EXCLUDES *When performed on same side:*
Sphenoidotomy (31287-31288)

35.2 35.2 **FUD** 010 J G2 80 50

AMA: 2018,Apr,3; 2018,Jan,8; 2017,Jan,8; 2016,Jan,13

31295-31298 Nasal Endoscopy with Sinus Ostia Dilation

INCLUDES Any method tissue displacement
Fluoroscopy, when performed

Code also stereotactic navigation, when performed (61782)

31295 **Nasal/sinus endoscopy, surgical, with dilation (eg, balloon dilation); maxillary sinus ostium, transnasal or via canine fossa**

EXCLUDES *When performed on same side:*
Maxillary antrostomy (31256-31267)
Maxillary sinusoscopy (31233)

4.55 55.6 **FUD** 000 J P3 80 50

AMA: 2020,Jun,14; 2018,Apr,3; 2018,Jan,8; 2017,Jan,8; 2016,Jan,13

31296 **frontal sinus ostium**

EXCLUDES *When performed on same side:*
Frontal sinus exploration (31276)
Dilation frontal and sphenoid sinus (31298)
Dilation sphenoid sinus only (31297)
Total ethmoidectomy (31253)

5.15 54.2 **FUD** 000 J P3 80 50

AMA: 2020,Jun,14; 2018,Apr,3; 2018,Jan,8; 2017,Jan,8; 2016,Jan,13

31297 **sphenoid sinus ostium**

EXCLUDES *When performed on same side:*
Diagnostic sphenoid sinusoscopy (31235)
Dilation frontal and sphenoid sinus (31298)
Dilation frontal sinus only (31296)
Sphenoidotomy (31287-31288)
Total ethmoidectomy procedures ([31257], [31259])

4.12 53.1 **FUD** 000 J P3 80 50

AMA: 2020,Jun,14; 2018,Apr,3; 2018,Jan,8; 2017,Jan,8; 2016,Jan,13

31298 **frontal and sphenoid sinus ostia**

EXCLUDES *When performed on same side:*
Diagnostic sphenoid sinusoscopy (31235)
Dilation frontal sinus only (31296)
Dilation sphenoid sinus only (31297)
Frontal sinus exploration (31276)
Other total ethmoidectomy procedures (31253, [31257], [31259])
Sphenoidotomy (31287-31288)

7.34 102. **FUD** 000 J P2 80 50

AMA: 2020,Jun,14; 2018,Apr,3

31299 Unlisted Procedures of Accessory Sinuses

CMS: 100-04,4,180.3 Unlisted Service or Procedure

EXCLUDES *Hypophysectomy (61546, 61548)*

31299 **Unlisted procedure, accessory sinuses**

0.00 0.00 **FUD** YYY T 80

AMA: 2019,Jul,7; 2019,Apr,10; 2018,Jan,8; 2017,Nov,11; 2017,Jan,8; 2016,Feb,10; 2016,Jan,13

31300-31502 Procedures of the Larynx

31300 **Laryngotomy (thyrotomy, laryngofissure), with removal of tumor or laryngocele, cordectomy**

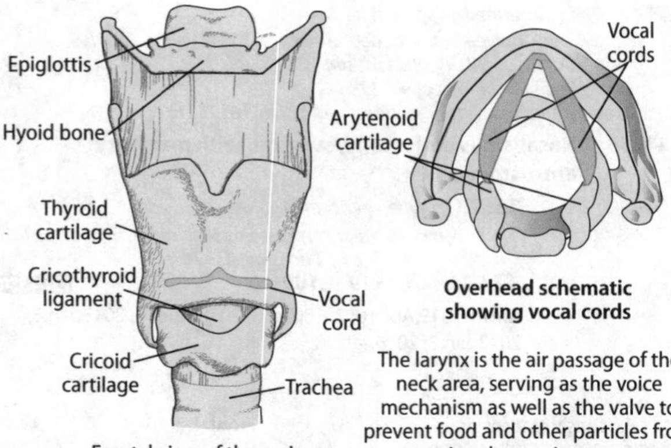

Frontal view of the major structures of the larynx

Overhead schematic showing vocal cords

The larynx is the air passage of the neck area, serving as the voice mechanism as well as the valve to prevent food and other particles from entering the respiratory tract

36.6 36.6 **FUD** 090 J A2 80

31360 **Laryngectomy; total, without radical neck dissection**

59.2 59.2 **FUD** 090 C 80

AMA: 2020,Nov,12; 2018,Jan,8; 2017,Jan,8; 2016,Jan,13

31365 **total, with radical neck dissection**

73.2 73.2 **FUD** 090 C 80

AMA: 2020,Nov,12; 2018,Jan,8; 2017,Jan,8; 2016,Jan,13

31367 **subtotal supraglottic, without radical neck dissection**

62.6 62.6 **FUD** 090 C 80

AMA: 2018,Jan,8; 2017,Jan,8; 2016,Jan,13

31368 **subtotal supraglottic, with radical neck dissection**

70.2 70.2 **FUD** 090 C 80

31370 **Partial laryngectomy (hemilaryngectomy); horizontal**

59.4 59.4 **FUD** 090 C 80

31375 **laterovertical**

55.8 55.8 **FUD** 090 C 80

31380 **anterovertical**

55.6 55.6 **FUD** 090 C 80

31382 **antero-latero-vertical**

61.0 61.0 **FUD** 090 C 80

31390 **Pharyngolaryngectomy, with radical neck dissection; without reconstruction**

81.0 81.0 **FUD** 090 C 80

31395 **with reconstruction**

86.5 86.5 **FUD** 090 C 80

31400 **Arytenoidectomy or arytenoidopexy, external approach**

EXCLUDES *Endoscopic arytenoidectomy (31560)*

28.0 28.0 **FUD** 090 J A2 80

31420 Epiglottidectomy

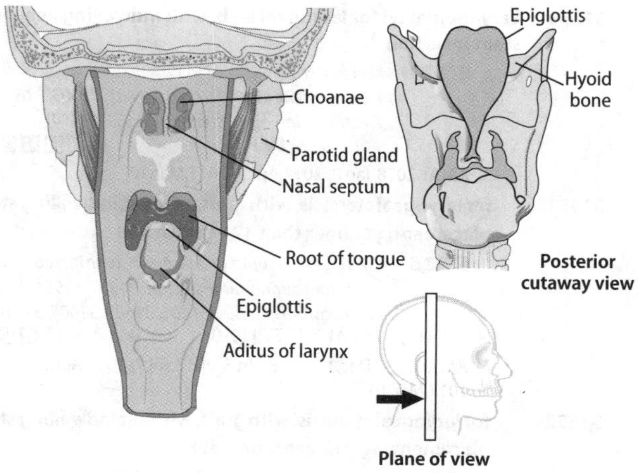

23.4 23.4 FUD 090 J A2 80

31500 Intubation, endotracheal, emergency procedure

EXCLUDES *Chest x-ray performed to confirm endotracheal tube position*

4.14 4.14 FUD 000 T G2

AMA: 2018,Jan,8; 2017,Jan,8; 2016,Oct,8; 2016,May,3; 2016,Jan,13

31502 Tracheotomy tube change prior to establishment of fistula tract

1.01 1.01 FUD 000 T G2

AMA: 2020,Dec,11

31505-31541 Endoscopy of the Larynx

31505 Laryngoscopy, indirect; diagnostic (separate procedure)

1.39 2.48 FUD 000 T P3

AMA: 2018,Jan,8; 2017,Jan,8; 2016,Jan,13

31510 with biopsy

3.46 6.01 FUD 000 J A2 80

AMA: 2018,Jan,8; 2017,Jan,8; 2016,Jan,13

31511 with removal of foreign body

3.79 6.04 FUD 000 T A2

AMA: 2018,Jan,8; 2017,Jan,8; 2016,Jan,13

31512 with removal of lesion

3.70 5.92 FUD 000 J A2 80

AMA: 2018,Jan,8; 2017,Jan,8; 2016,Jan,13

31513 with vocal cord injection

3.76 3.76 FUD 000 T A2 80

AMA: 2018,Jan,8; 2017,Jan,8; 2016,Jan,13

31515 Laryngoscopy direct, with or without tracheoscopy; for aspiration

3.12 5.79 FUD 000 T A2

AMA: 2020,Dec,11

31520 diagnostic, newborn A

4.44 4.44 FUD 000 63 T G2 80

AMA: 2020,Dec,11

31525 diagnostic, except newborn

4.56 7.15 FUD 000 J A2

AMA: 2020,Dec,11; 2018,Jan,8; 2017,Jan,8; 2016,Jan,13

31526 diagnostic, with operating microscope or telescope

INCLUDES Operating microscope (69990)

4.49 4.49 FUD 000 J A2

AMA: 2020,Dec,11; 2018,Jan,8; 2017,Jun,10; 2016,Feb,12

31527 with insertion of obturator

5.55 5.55 FUD 000 J A2 80

AMA: 2020,Dec,11

31528 with dilation, initial

4.09 4.09 FUD 000 J A2 80

AMA: 2020,Dec,11

31529 with dilation, subsequent

4.59 4.59 FUD 000 J A2 80

AMA: 2020,Dec,11

31530 Laryngoscopy, direct, operative, with foreign body removal;

5.70 5.70 FUD 000 J A2

AMA: 2020,Dec,11

31531 with operating microscope or telescope

INCLUDES Operating microscope (69990)

6.08 6.08 FUD 000 J A2 80

AMA: 2020,Dec,11; 2018,Jan,8; 2017,Jun,10; 2016,Feb,12

31535 Laryngoscopy, direct, operative, with biopsy;

5.39 5.39 FUD 000 J A2

AMA: 2020,Dec,11

31536 with operating microscope or telescope

INCLUDES Operating microscope (69990)

6.00 6.00 FUD 000 J A2

AMA: 2020,Dec,11; 2018,Jan,8; 2017,Jun,10; 2016,Feb,12

31540 Laryngoscopy, direct, operative, with excision of tumor and/or stripping of vocal cords or epiglottis;

6.89 6.89 FUD 000 J A2

AMA: 2020,Dec,11

31541 with operating microscope or telescope

INCLUDES Operating microscope (69990)

7.52 7.52 FUD 000 J A2

AMA: 2020,Dec,11; 2019,Sep,10; 2019,Jul,10; 2018,Jan,8; 2017,Jun,10; 2016,Feb,12

31545-31554 [31551, 31552, 31553, 31554] Endoscopy of Larynx with Reconstruction

INCLUDES Operating microscope (69990)

EXCLUDES *Laryngoscopy, direct, operative, with excision tumor and/or vocal cord or epiglottis stripping (31540-31541)*
Vocal cord reconstruction with allograft (31599)

31545 Laryngoscopy, direct, operative, with operating microscope or telescope, with submucosal removal of non-neoplastic lesion(s) of vocal cord; reconstruction with local tissue flap(s)

10.3 10.3 FUD 000 J A2 50

AMA: 2020,Dec,11; 2016,Feb,12

31546 reconstruction with graft(s) (includes obtaining autograft)

EXCLUDES *Autologous fat graft obtained by liposuction (15771-15774)*
Autologous soft tissue grafts obtained by direct excision ([15769])

15.7 15.7 FUD 000 J A2 50

AMA: 2020,Dec,11; 2018,Jan,8; 2017,Jan,8; 2016,Feb,12; 2016,Jan,13

31551 **Resequenced code. See code following 31580.**

31552 **Resequenced code. See code following 31580.**

31553 **Resequenced code. See code following 31580.**

31554 **Resequenced code. See code following 31580.**

31560-31571 Endoscopy of Larynx with Arytenoid Removal, Vocal Cord Injection

31560 Laryngoscopy, direct, operative, with arytenoidectomy;

8.97 8.97 FUD 000 J A2 80

AMA: 2020,Dec,11

31561 with operating microscope or telescope

INCLUDES Operating microscope (69990)

9.82 9.82 FUD 000 J A2 80

AMA: 2020,Dec,11; 2018,Jan,8; 2017,Jun,10; 2016,Feb,12

Respiratory System

31420 — 31561

● New Code ▲ Revised Code ○ Reinstated ● New Web Release ▲ Revised Web Release + Add-on Unlisted Not Covered # Resequenced
50 Optum Mod 50 Exempt ⊘ AMA Mod 51 Exempt 51 Optum Mod 51 Exempt 63 Mod 63 Exempt Non-FDA Drug ★ Telemedicine M Maternity A Age Edit

31570 **Laryngoscopy, direct, with injection into vocal cord(s), therapeutic;**
6.53 9.68 FUD 000 J A2
AMA: 2020,Dec,11; 2018,Jan,8; 2017,Jan,8; 2017,Jan,6; 2016,Jan,13

31571 **with operating microscope or telescope**
INCLUDES Operating microscope (69990)
7.14 7.14 FUD 000 J A2
AMA: 2020,Dec,11; 2018,Jan,8; 2017,Jun,10; 2017,Jan,8; 2017,Jan,6; 2016,Feb,12; 2016,Jan,13

31572-31579 [31572, 31573, 31574] Endoscopy of Larynx, Flexible Fiberoptic

EXCLUDES *Evaluation by flexible fiberoptic endoscope:*
Sensory assessment (92614-92615)
Swallowing (92612-92613)
Swallowing and sensory assessment (92616-92617)
Flexible fiberoptic endoscopic examination/testing by cine or video recording (92612-92617)

31572 **Resequenced code. See code following 31578.**

31573 **Resequenced code. See code following 31578.**

31574 **Resequenced code. See code following 31578.**

31575 **Laryngoscopy, flexible; diagnostic**
EXCLUDES *Diagnostic nasal endoscopy not through additional endoscope (31231)*
Procedure during same session ([31572, 31573, 31574], 31576-31578, 42975, 43197-43198, 92511, 92612, 92614, 92616)
1.90 3.49 FUD 000 T P2
AMA: 2020,Dec,11; 2018,Jan,8; 2017,Jul,7; 2017,Apr,8; 2017,Jan,8; 2016,Dec,13

31576 **with biopsy(ies)**
EXCLUDES *Destruction or excision lesion (31572, 31578)*
3.38 7.63 FUD 000 J A2
AMA: 2018,Jan,8; 2017,Jul,7; 2017,Apr,8; 2017,Jan,8; 2016,Dec,13

31577 **with removal of foreign body(s)**
3.82 7.93 FUD 000 T A2 80
AMA: 2018,Jan,8; 2017,Jul,7; 2017,Apr,8; 2017,Jan,8; 2016,Dec,13

31578 **with removal of lesion(s), non-laser**
4.27 8.59 FUD 000 J A2 80
AMA: 2018,Jan,8; 2017,Jul,7; 2017,Apr,8; 2017,Jan,8; 2016,Dec,13

31572 **with ablation or destruction of lesion(s) with laser, unilateral**
EXCLUDES *Biopsy or excision lesion (31576, 31578)*
5.15 14.7 FUD 000 J G2 80 50
AMA: 2020,Dec,11; 2019,Sep,10; 2018,Jan,8; 2017,Jul,7; 2017,Apr,8; 2017,Jan,8; 2016,Dec,13

31573 **with therapeutic injection(s) (eg, chemodenervation agent or corticosteroid, injected percutaneous, transoral, or via endoscope channel), unilateral**
4.27 7.61 FUD 000 J P3 80 50
AMA: 2020,Dec,11; 2018,May,7; 2018,Jan,8; 2017,Jul,7; 2017,Apr,8; 2017,Jan,8; 2016,Dec,13

31574 **with injection(s) for augmentation (eg, percutaneous, transoral), unilateral**
4.27 28.7 FUD 000 J G2 80 50
AMA: 2020,Dec,11; 2018,May,7; 2018,Jan,8; 2017,Jul,7; 2017,Apr,8; 2017,Jan,8; 2016,Dec,13

31579 **Laryngoscopy, flexible or rigid telescopic, with stroboscopy**
3.41 5.46 FUD 000 T P3
AMA: 2018,Jan,8; 2017,Jul,7; 2017,Apr,8; 2017,Jan,8; 2016,Dec,13

31580-31599 [31551, 31552, 31553, 31554] Larynx Reconstruction

31580 **Laryngoplasty; for laryngeal web, with indwelling keel or stent insertion**
EXCLUDES *Keel or stent removal (31599)*
Tracheostomy (31600-31601, 31603, 31605, 31610)
Treatment laryngeal stenosis (31551-31554)
35.7 35.7 FUD 090 J A2 80
AMA: 2018,Jan,8; 2017,Apr,5; 2017,Mar,10

31551 **for laryngeal stenosis, with graft, without indwelling stent placement, younger than 12 years of age** A
EXCLUDES *Cartilage graft obtained through same incision*
Procedure during same session (31552-31554, 31580)
Tracheostomy (31600-31601, 31603, 31605, 31610)
41.2 41.2 FUD 090 J G2 80
AMA: 2020,Dec,11; 2018,Jan,8; 2017,Jul,7; 2017,Apr,5; 2017,Mar,10

31552 **for laryngeal stenosis, with graft, without indwelling stent placement, age 12 years or older** A
EXCLUDES *Cartilage graft obtained through same incision*
Procedure during same session (31551, 31553-31554, 31580)
Tracheostomy (31600-31601, 31603, 31605, 31610)
42.0 42.0 FUD 090 J G2 80
AMA: 2020,Dec,11; 2018,Jan,8; 2017,Jul,7; 2017,Apr,5; 2017,Mar,10

31553 **for laryngeal stenosis, with graft, with indwelling stent placement, younger than 12 years of age** A
EXCLUDES *Cartilage graft obtained through same incision*
Procedure during same session (31551-31552, 31554, 31580)
Stent removal (31599)
Tracheostomy (31600-31601, 31603, 31605, 31610)
47.8 47.8 FUD 090 J G2 80
AMA: 2020,Dec,11; 2018,Jan,8; 2017,Jul,7; 2017,Apr,5; 2017,Mar,10

31554 **for laryngeal stenosis, with graft, with indwelling stent placement, age 12 years or older** A
EXCLUDES *Cartilage graft obtained through same incision*
Procedure during same session (31551-31553, 31580)
Stent removal (31599)
Tracheostomy (31600-31601, 31603, 31605, 31610)
47.8 47.8 FUD 090 J G2 80
AMA: 2020,Dec,11; 2018,Jan,8; 2017,Jul,7; 2017,Apr,5; 2017,Mar,10

31584 **with open reduction and fixation of (eg, plating) fracture, includes tracheostomy, if performed**
EXCLUDES *Cartilage graft obtained through same incision*
39.6 39.6 FUD 090 J G2 80
AMA: 2018,Jan,8; 2017,Apr,5; 2017,Mar,10

31587 **Laryngoplasty, cricoid split, without graft placement**
EXCLUDES *Tracheostomy (31600-31601, 31603, 31605, 31610)*
33.2 33.2 FUD 090 J G2 80
AMA: 2018,Jan,8; 2017,Apr,5; 2017,Mar,10

31590 **Laryngeal reinnervation by neuromuscular pedicle**
24.9 24.9 **FUD** 090 J A2 80
AMA: 2018,Jan,8; 2017,Mar,10

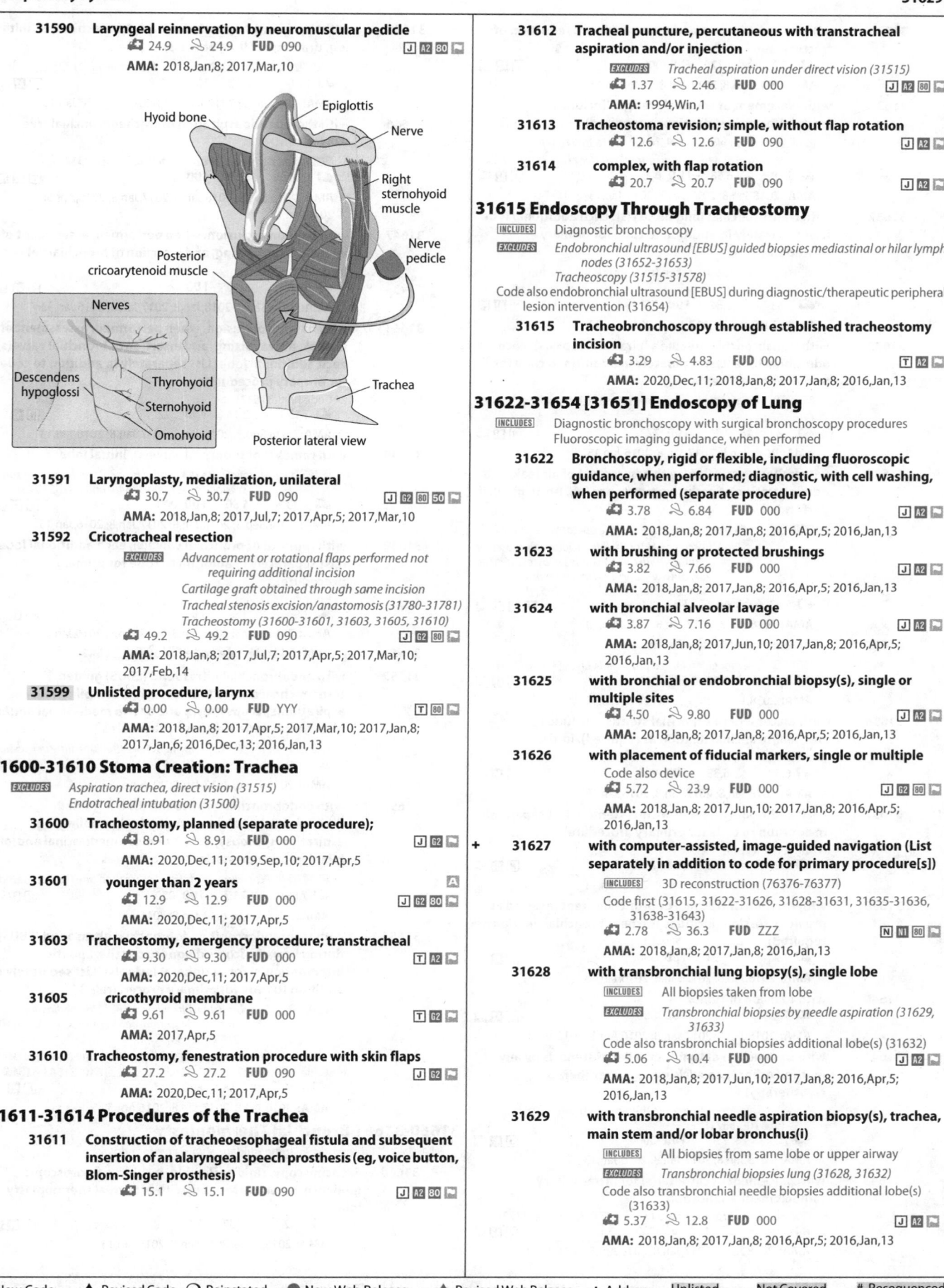

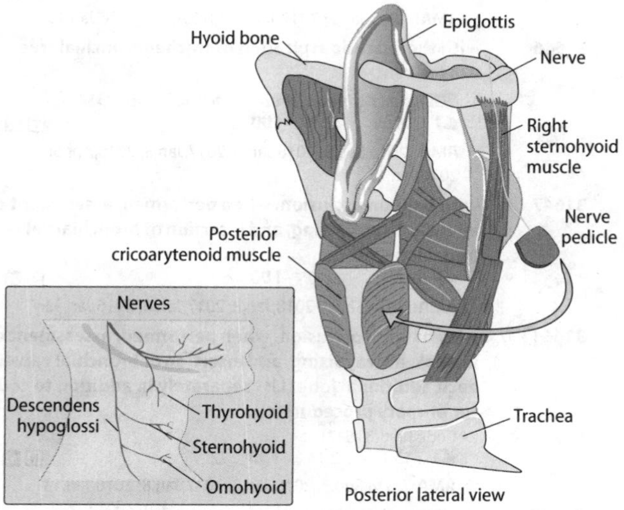

31591 **Laryngoplasty, medialization, unilateral**
30.7 30.7 **FUD** 090 J G2 80 50
AMA: 2018,Jan,8; 2017,Jul,7; 2017,Apr,5; 2017,Mar,10

31592 **Cricotracheal resection**
EXCLUDES *Advancement or rotational flaps performed not requiring additional incision*
Cartilage graft obtained through same incision
Tracheal stenosis excision/anastomosis (31780-31781)
Tracheostomy (31600-31601, 31603, 31605, 31610)
49.2 49.2 **FUD** 090 J G2 80
AMA: 2018,Jan,8; 2017,Jul,7; 2017,Apr,5; 2017,Mar,10; 2017,Feb,14

31599 **Unlisted procedure, larynx**
0.00 0.00 **FUD** YYY T 80
AMA: 2018,Jan,8; 2017,Apr,5; 2017,Mar,10; 2017,Jan,8; 2017,Jan,6; 2016,Dec,13; 2016,Jan,13

31600-31610 Stoma Creation: Trachea

EXCLUDES *Aspiration trachea, direct vision (31515)*
Endotracheal intubation (31500)

31600 **Tracheostomy, planned (separate procedure);**
8.91 8.91 **FUD** 000 J G2
AMA: 2020,Dec,11; 2019,Sep,10; 2017,Apr,5

31601 **younger than 2 years** A
12.9 12.9 **FUD** 000 J G2 80
AMA: 2020,Dec,11; 2017,Apr,5

31603 **Tracheostomy, emergency procedure; transtracheal**
9.30 9.30 **FUD** 000 T A2
AMA: 2020,Dec,11; 2017,Apr,5

31605 **cricothyroid membrane**
9.61 9.61 **FUD** 000 T G2
AMA: 2017,Apr,5

31610 **Tracheostomy, fenestration procedure with skin flaps**
27.2 27.2 **FUD** 090 J G2
AMA: 2020,Dec,11; 2017,Apr,5

31611-31614 Procedures of the Trachea

31611 **Construction of tracheoesophageal fistula and subsequent insertion of an alaryngeal speech prosthesis (eg, voice button, Blom-Singer prosthesis)**
15.1 15.1 **FUD** 090 J A2 80

31612 **Tracheal puncture, percutaneous with transtracheal aspiration and/or injection**
EXCLUDES *Tracheal aspiration under direct vision (31515)*
1.37 2.46 **FUD** 000 J A2 80
AMA: 1994,Win,1

31613 **Tracheostoma revision; simple, without flap rotation**
12.6 12.6 **FUD** 090 J A2

31614 **complex, with flap rotation**
20.7 20.7 **FUD** 090 J A2

31615 Endoscopy Through Tracheostomy

INCLUDES Diagnostic bronchoscopy
EXCLUDES *Endobronchial ultrasound [EBUS] guided biopsies mediastinal or hilar lymph nodes (31652-31653)*
Tracheoscopy (31515-31578)
Code also endobronchial ultrasound [EBUS] during diagnostic/therapeutic peripheral lesion intervention (31654)

31615 **Tracheobronchoscopy through established tracheostomy incision**
3.29 4.83 **FUD** 000 T A2
AMA: 2020,Dec,11; 2018,Jan,8; 2017,Jan,8; 2016,Jan,13

31622-31654 [31651] Endoscopy of Lung

INCLUDES Diagnostic bronchoscopy with surgical bronchoscopy procedures
Fluoroscopic imaging guidance, when performed

31622 **Bronchoscopy, rigid or flexible, including fluoroscopic guidance, when performed; diagnostic, with cell washing, when performed (separate procedure)**
3.78 6.84 **FUD** 000 J A2
AMA: 2018,Jan,8; 2017,Jan,8; 2016,Apr,5; 2016,Jan,13

31623 **with brushing or protected brushings**
3.82 7.66 **FUD** 000 J A2
AMA: 2018,Jan,8; 2017,Jan,8; 2016,Apr,5; 2016,Jan,13

31624 **with bronchial alveolar lavage**
3.87 7.16 **FUD** 000 J A2
AMA: 2018,Jan,8; 2017,Jun,10; 2017,Jan,8; 2016,Apr,5; 2016,Jan,13

31625 **with bronchial or endobronchial biopsy(s), single or multiple sites**
4.50 9.80 **FUD** 000 J A2
AMA: 2018,Jan,8; 2017,Jan,8; 2016,Apr,5; 2016,Jan,13

31626 **with placement of fiducial markers, single or multiple**
Code also device
5.72 23.9 **FUD** 000 J G2 80
AMA: 2018,Jan,8; 2017,Jun,10; 2017,Jan,8; 2016,Apr,5; 2016,Jan,13

+ **31627** **with computer-assisted, image-guided navigation (List separately in addition to code for primary procedure[s])**
INCLUDES 3D reconstruction (76376-76377)
Code first (31615, 31622-31626, 31628-31631, 31635-31636, 31638-31643)
2.78 36.3 **FUD** ZZZ N N1 80
AMA: 2018,Jan,8; 2017,Jan,8; 2016,Jan,13

31628 **with transbronchial lung biopsy(s), single lobe**
INCLUDES All biopsies taken from lobe
EXCLUDES *Transbronchial biopsies by needle aspiration (31629, 31633)*
Code also transbronchial biopsies additional lobe(s) (31632)
5.06 10.4 **FUD** 000 J A2
AMA: 2018,Jan,8; 2017,Jun,10; 2017,Jan,8; 2016,Apr,5; 2016,Jan,13

31629 **with transbronchial needle aspiration biopsy(s), trachea, main stem and/or lobar bronchus(i)**
INCLUDES All biopsies from same lobe or upper airway
EXCLUDES *Transbronchial biopsies lung (31628, 31632)*
Code also transbronchial needle biopsies additional lobe(s) (31633)
5.37 12.8 **FUD** 000 J A2
AMA: 2018,Jan,8; 2017,Jan,8; 2016,Apr,5; 2016,Jan,13

31630 **with tracheal/bronchial dilation or closed reduction of fracture**
5.72 5.72 FUD 000 J A2
AMA: 2018,Jan,8; 2017,Jan,8; 2016,Jan,13

31631 **with placement of tracheal stent(s) (includes tracheal/bronchial dilation as required)**
EXCLUDES *Bronchial stent placement (31636-31637)*
Revision bronchial or tracheal stent (31638)
6.58 6.58 FUD 000 J A2
AMA: 2018,Jan,8; 2017,Jan,8; 2016,Jan,13

+ **31632** **with transbronchial lung biopsy(s), each additional lobe (List separately in addition to code for primary procedure)**
INCLUDES All biopsies taken from additional lobe lung
Code first (31628)
1.43 1.82 FUD ZZZ N N1
AMA: 2018,Jan,8; 2017,Jan,8; 2016,Jan,13

+ **31633** **with transbronchial needle aspiration biopsy(s), each additional lobe (List separately in addition to code for primary procedure)**
INCLUDES All needle biopsies from another lobe or from trachea
Code first (31629)
1.82 2.26 FUD ZZZ N N1
AMA: 2018,Jan,8; 2017,Jan,8; 2016,Jan,13

31634 **with balloon occlusion, with assessment of air leak, with administration of occlusive substance (eg, fibrin glue), if performed**
EXCLUDES *When performed during same operative session:*
Bronchoscopy, rigid or flexible, including fluoroscopic guidance; with balloon occlusio, assessment air leak, airway sizing, and insertion bronchial valve(s), initial lobe (31647, [31651])
5.53 49.4 FUD 000 J G2 80
AMA: 2018,Jan,8; 2017,Jan,8; 2016,Jan,13

31635 **with removal of foreign body**
EXCLUDES *Removal implanted bronchial valves (31648-31649)*
5.06 8.03 FUD 000 J A2
AMA: 2018,Jan,8; 2017,Jan,8; 2016,Jan,13

31636 **with placement of bronchial stent(s) (includes tracheal/bronchial dilation as required), initial bronchus**
6.33 6.33 FUD 000 J J8
AMA: 2018,Jan,8; 2017,Jan,8; 2016,Jan,13

+ **31637** **each additional major bronchus stented (List separately in addition to code for primary procedure)**
Code first (31636)
2.22 2.22 FUD ZZZ N N1
AMA: 2018,Jan,8; 2017,Jan,8; 2016,Jan,13

31638 **with revision of tracheal or bronchial stent inserted at previous session (includes tracheal/bronchial dilation as required)**
7.21 7.21 FUD 000 J A2
AMA: 2018,Jan,8; 2017,Jan,8; 2016,Jan,13

31640 **with excision of tumor**
7.21 7.21 FUD 000 J A2
AMA: 2018,Jan,8; 2017,Jan,8; 2016,Apr,5; 2016,Jan,13

31641 **with destruction of tumor or relief of stenosis by any method other than excision (eg, laser therapy, cryotherapy)**
Code also any photodynamic therapy via bronchoscopy (96570-96571)
7.39 7.39 FUD 000 J A2
AMA: 2018,Jan,8; 2017,Jan,8; 2016,Jan,13

31643 **with placement of catheter(s) for intracavitary radioelement application**
Code also when appropriate (77761-77763, 77770-77772)
5.04 5.04 FUD 000 J A2
AMA: 2018,Jan,8; 2017,Jan,8; 2016,Apr,5; 2016,Jan,13

31645 **with therapeutic aspiration of tracheobronchial tree, initial (eg, drainage of lung abscess)**
EXCLUDES *Bedside aspiration trachea, bronchi (31725)*
4.21 7.42 FUD 000 J A2
AMA: 2018,Jan,8; 2017,Jan,8; 2016,Apr,5; 2016,Jan,13

31646 **with therapeutic aspiration of tracheobronchial tree, subsequent**
EXCLUDES *Bedside aspiration trachea, bronchi (31725)*
4.08 4.08 FUD 000 T A2
AMA: 2018,Sep,3; 2018,Jan,8; 2017,Jan,8; 2016,Apr,5; 2016,Jan,13

31647 **with balloon occlusion, when performed, assessment of air leak, airway sizing, and insertion of bronchial valve(s), initial lobe**
6.10 6.10 FUD 000 J J8
AMA: 2018,Sep,3; 2018,Jan,8; 2017,Jan,8; 2016,Jan,13

+ # **31651** **with balloon occlusion, when performed, assessment of air leak, airway sizing, and insertion of bronchial valve(s), each additional lobe (List separately in addition to code for primary procedure[s])**
Code first (31647)
2.13 2.13 FUD ZZZ N N1
AMA: 2018,Sep,3; 2018,Jan,8; 2017,Jan,8; 2016,Jan,13

31648 **with removal of bronchial valve(s), initial lobe**
EXCLUDES *Removal with reinsertion bronchial valve during same session (31647 and 31648) and ([31651])*
5.80 5.80 FUD 000 J G2
AMA: 2018,Sep,3; 2018,Jan,8; 2017,Jan,8; 2016,Jan,13

+ **31649** **with removal of bronchial valve(s), each additional lobe (List separately in addition to code for primary procedure)**
Code first (31648)
1.94 1.94 FUD ZZZ Q2 G2
AMA: 2018,Sep,3; 2018,Jan,8; 2017,Jan,8; 2016,Jan,13

31651 **Resequenced code. See code following 31647.**

31652 **with endobronchial ultrasound (EBUS) guided transtracheal and/or transbronchial sampling (eg, aspiration[s]/biopsy[ies]), one or two mediastinal and/or hilar lymph node stations or structures**
EXCLUDES *Procedures performed more than one time per session*
6.38 31.2 FUD 000 J G2
AMA: 2018,Jan,8; 2017,Jan,8; 2016,Apr,5

31653 **with endobronchial ultrasound (EBUS) guided transtracheal and/or transbronchial sampling (eg, aspiration[s]/biopsy[ies]), 3 or more mediastinal and/or hilar lymph node stations or structures**
EXCLUDES *Procedures performed more than one time per session*
7.08 28.7 FUD 000 J G2
AMA: 2018,Jan,8; 2017,Jan,8; 2016,Apr,5

+ **31654** **with transendoscopic endobronchial ultrasound (EBUS) during bronchoscopic diagnostic or therapeutic intervention(s) for peripheral lesion(s) (List separately in addition to code for primary procedure[s])**
EXCLUDES *Endobronchial ultrasound [EBUS] for mediastinal/hilar lymph node station/adjacent structure access (31652-31653)*
Procedures performed more than one time per session
Code first (31622-31626, 31628-31629, 31640, 31643-31646)
1.94 3.48 FUD ZZZ N N1
AMA: 2018,Jan,8; 2017,Jan,8; 2016,Apr,5

31660-31661 Bronchial Thermoplasty

INCLUDES Fluoroscopic imaging guidance, when performed

31660 **Bronchoscopy, rigid or flexible, including fluoroscopic guidance, when performed; with bronchial thermoplasty, 1 lobe**
5.62 5.62 FUD 000 J J8
AMA: 2018,Jan,8; 2017,Jan,8; 2016,Jan,13

31661 **with bronchial thermoplasty, 2 or more lobes**
5.93 5.93 **FUD** 000 J J8
AMA: 2018,Jan,8; 2017,Jan,8; 2016,Jan,13

31717-31899 Respiratory Procedures

EXCLUDES *Endotracheal intubation (31500)*
Tracheal aspiration under direct vision (31515)

31717 **Catheterization with bronchial brush biopsy**
3.18 7.98 **FUD** 000 T A2
AMA: 2018,Jan,8; 2017,Jan,8; 2016,Jan,13

31720 **Catheter aspiration (separate procedure); nasotracheal**
1.59 1.59 **FUD** 000 Q1 N1
AMA: 1994,Win,1

31725 **tracheobronchial with fiberscope, bedside**
2.27 2.27 **FUD** 000 C

31730 **Transtracheal (percutaneous) introduction of needle wire dilator/stent or indwelling tube for oxygen therapy**
4.33 33.8 **FUD** 000 J A2
AMA: 1992,Win,1

31750 **Tracheoplasty; cervical**
39.1 39.1 **FUD** 090 J A2 80

31755 **tracheopharyngeal fistulization, each stage**
49.1 49.1 **FUD** 090 J A2 80

31760 **intrathoracic**
39.6 39.6 **FUD** 090 C 80

31766 **Carinal reconstruction**
51.3 51.3 **FUD** 090 C 80

31770 **Bronchoplasty; graft repair**
EXCLUDES *Bronchoplasty done with lobectomy (32501)*
38.4 38.4 **FUD** 090 C 80

31775 **excision stenosis and anastomosis**
EXCLUDES *Bronchoplasty done with lobectomy (32501)*
40.4 40.4 **FUD** 090 C 80

31780 **Excision tracheal stenosis and anastomosis; cervical**
34.2 34.2 **FUD** 090 C 80
AMA: 2018,Jan,8; 2017,Apr,5; 2017,Feb,14

31781 **cervicothoracic**
39.8 39.8 **FUD** 090 C 80
AMA: 2018,Jan,8; 2017,Apr,5; 2017,Feb,14

31785 **Excision of tracheal tumor or carcinoma; cervical**
30.8 30.8 **FUD** 090 J G2 80
AMA: 2003,Jan,1

31786 **thoracic**
41.6 41.6 **FUD** 090 C 80

31800 **Suture of tracheal wound or injury; cervical**
20.3 20.3 **FUD** 090 C 80
AMA: 1994,Win,1

31805 **intrathoracic**
23.5 23.5 **FUD** 090 C 80

31820 **Surgical closure tracheostomy or fistula; without plastic repair**
EXCLUDES *Tracheoesophageal fistula repair (43305, 43312)*
9.35 12.3 **FUD** 090 J A2 80

31825 **with plastic repair**
EXCLUDES *Tracheoesophageal fistula repair (43305, 43312)*
13.6 17.1 **FUD** 090 J A2 80

31830 **Revision of tracheostomy scar**

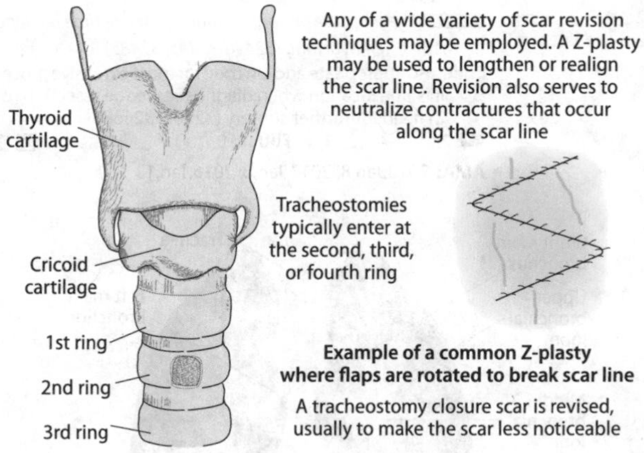
Any of a wide variety of scar revision techniques may be employed. A Z-plasty may be used to lengthen or realign the scar line. Revision also serves to neutralize contractures that occur along the scar line
Thyroid cartilage
Tracheostomies typically enter at the second, third, or fourth ring
Cricoid cartilage
1st ring
2nd ring
3rd ring
Example of a common Z-plasty where flaps are rotated to break scar line
A tracheostomy closure scar is revised, usually to make the scar less noticeable

10.0 13.2 **FUD** 090 J A2 80

31899 **Unlisted procedure, trachea, bronchi**
0.00 0.00 **FUD** YYY T 80
AMA: 2020,Dec,11; 2018,Jan,8; 2017,Jan,8; 2016,Jan,13

32035-32036 Procedures for Empyema

EXCLUDES *Wound exploration without thoracotomy for penetrating chest wound (20101)*

32035 **Thoracostomy; with rib resection for empyema**
21.0 21.0 **FUD** 090 C 80 50

32036 **with open flap drainage for empyema**
22.3 22.3 **FUD** 090 C 80 50

32096-32098 Open Biopsy of Chest and Pleura

INCLUDES Varying amounts lung tissue excised for analysis
Wedge technique with tissue obtained without precise margin consideration

EXCLUDES *Core needle biopsy, lung or mediastinum (32408)*
Percutaneous needle biopsy pleura (32400)
Thoracoscopy with:
Biopsy (32607-32609)
Diagnostic wedge resection resulting in anatomic lung resection (32507, 32668)

32096 **Thoracotomy, with diagnostic biopsy(ies) of lung infiltrate(s) (eg, wedge, incisional), unilateral**
EXCLUDES *Procedure performed more than one time per lung*
Removal lung (32440-32445, 32488)
Code also appropriate add-on code for more extensive procedure at same location when diagnostic wedge resection results in need for further surgery (32507, 32668)
23.1 23.1 **FUD** 090 C 80
AMA: 2018,Jan,8; 2017,Jan,8; 2016,Jan,13

32097 **Thoracotomy, with diagnostic biopsy(ies) of lung nodule(s) or mass(es) (eg, wedge, incisional), unilateral**

EXCLUDES *Procedure performed more than one time per lung*
Removal lung (32440-32445, 32488)

Code also appropriate add-on code for more extensive procedure in same location when diagnostic wedge resection results in need for further surgery (32507, 32668)

23.1 23.1 **FUD** 090 C 80

AMA: 2018,Jan,8; 2017,Jan,8; 2016,Jan,13

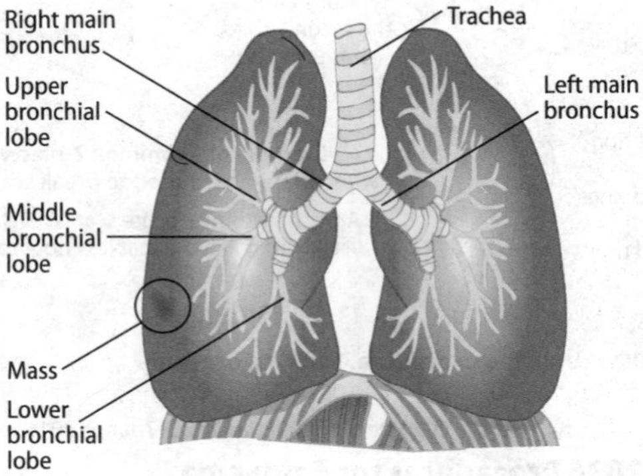

32098 **Thoracotomy, with biopsy(ies) of pleura**

21.9 21.9 **FUD** 090 C 80

AMA: 2018,Jan,8; 2017,Jan,8; 2016,Jan,13

32100-32160 Open Procedures: Chest

INCLUDES Exploration penetrating chest wound

EXCLUDES *Lung resection (32480-32504)*
Wound exploration without thoracotomy for penetrating chest wound (20101)

32100 **Thoracotomy; with exploration**

EXCLUDES *Excision chest wall tumor, when performed (21601-21603)*
Extracorporeal membrane oxygenation (ECMO)/extracorporeal life support (ECLS) (33955-33957, [33963, 33964])
Resection apical lung tumor (32503-32504)

23.3 23.3 **FUD** 090 C 80

AMA: 2019,Dec,5; 2019,Dec,4; 2018,Jan,8; 2017,Jan,8; 2016,Jan,13

32110 **with control of traumatic hemorrhage and/or repair of lung tear**

42.4 42.4 **FUD** 090 C 80

AMA: 2018,Jan,8; 2017,Jan,8; 2016,Jan,13

32120 **for postoperative complications**

25.2 25.2 **FUD** 090 C 80

32124 **with open intrapleural pneumonolysis**

26.7 26.7 **FUD** 090 C 80

AMA: 2018,Jan,8; 2017,Jan,8; 2016,Jan,13

32140 **with cyst(s) removal, includes pleural procedure when performed**

28.5 28.5 **FUD** 090 C 80

AMA: 2018,Jan,8; 2017,Jan,8; 2016,Jan,13

32141 **with resection-plication of bullae, includes any pleural procedure when performed**

EXCLUDES *Lung volume reduction (32491)*

44.0 44.0 **FUD** 090 C 80

AMA: 2018,Jan,8; 2017,Jan,8; 2016,Jan,13

32150 **with removal of intrapleural foreign body or fibrin deposit**

28.9 28.9 **FUD** 090 C 80

AMA: 2018,Jan,8; 2017,Jan,8; 2016,Jan,13

32151 **with removal of intrapulmonary foreign body**

29.0 29.0 **FUD** 090 C 80

32160 **with cardiac massage**

22.9 22.9 **FUD** 090 C 80

32200-32320 Open Procedures: Lung

32200 **Pneumonostomy, with open drainage of abscess or cyst**

EXCLUDES *Image-guided, percutaneous drainage (eg, abscess, cyst) of lungs/mediastinum via catheter (49405)*

(75989)

32.7 32.7 **FUD** 090 C 80

AMA: 2013,Nov,9; 1997,Nov,1

32215 **Pleural scarification for repeat pneumothorax**

23.0 23.0 **FUD** 090 C 80 50

32220 **Decortication, pulmonary (separate procedure); total**

45.9 45.9 **FUD** 090 C 80 50

32225 **partial**

28.7 28.7 **FUD** 090 C 80 50

32310 **Pleurectomy, parietal (separate procedure)**

26.3 26.3 **FUD** 090 C 80

AMA: 1994,Win,1

32320 **Decortication and parietal pleurectomy**

46.1 46.1 **FUD** 090 C 80

AMA: 1994,Fall,1

32400-32408 Lung Biopsy

EXCLUDES *Fine needle aspiration ([10004, 10005, 10006, 10007, 10008, 10009, 10010, 10011, 10012], 10021)*
Open lung biopsy (32096-32097)
Open mediastinal biopsy (39000-39010)
Thoracoscopic (VATS) biopsy lung, pericardium, pleural, or mediastinal space (32604-32609)

32400 **Biopsy, pleura, percutaneous needle**

(76942, 77002, 77012, 77021)

2.48 4.56 **FUD** 000 J A2

AMA: 2019,Apr,4; 2018,Jan,8; 2017,Jan,8; 2016,Jan,13

32408 **Core needle biopsy, lung or mediastinum, percutaneous, including imaging guidance, when performed**

INCLUDES Imaging guidance performed during tsame session on same lesion (76942, 77002, 77012, 77021)

Code also core needle biopsy performed during same operative session:
- Other anatomical site; report both codes and append modifier 59 on second code
- Same anatomical site, different lesion; report 32408 for each lesion biopsied and append modifier 59 on second code

Code also FNA biopsy and core needle biopsy performed during same operative session:
- Different lesion, utilizing same or different imaging guidance; report both codes and append modifier 59 on either code
- Same lesion, utilizing different imaging guidance; report both image-guided biopsy codes and append modifier 59 on either code
- Same lesion, utilizing same imaging guidance; report both codes and append modifier 52 on either code

4.44 27.7 **FUD** 000 G2

32440-32501 Lung Resection

32440 **Removal of lung, pneumonectomy;**

Code also excision chest wall tumor, when performed (21601-21603)

45.1 45.1 **FUD** 090 C 80

AMA: 2018,Jan,8; 2017,Jan,8; 2016,Jan,13

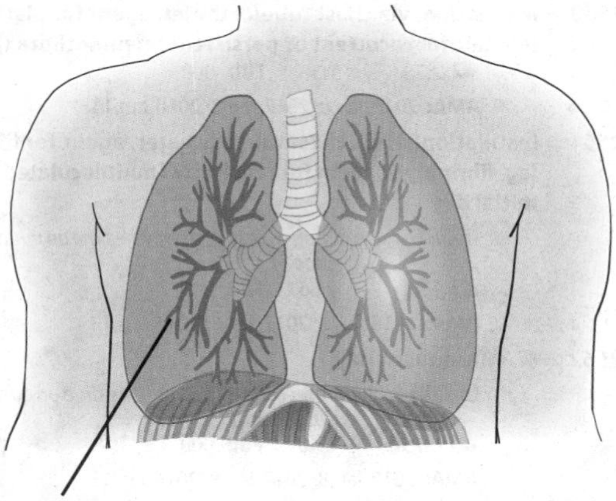

Removal of entire lung

32442 **with resection of segment of trachea followed by broncho-tracheal anastomosis (sleeve pneumonectomy)**

Code also excision chest wall tumor, when performed (21601-21603)

88.9 88.9 **FUD** 090 C 80

AMA: 2018,Jan,8; 2017,Jun,10; 2017,Jan,8; 2016,Jan,13

32445 **extrapleural**

Code also:

Empyemectomy with extrapleural pneumonectomy (32540)

Excision chest wall tumor, when performed (21601-21603)

102. 102. **FUD** 090 C 80

AMA: 2018,Jan,8; 2017,Jan,8; 2016,Jan,13

32480 **Removal of lung, other than pneumonectomy; single lobe (lobectomy)**

EXCLUDES *Lung removal with bronchoplasty (32501)*

Code also:

Decortication (32320)

Excision chest wall tumor, when performed (21601-21603)

42.6 42.6 **FUD** 090 C 80

AMA: 2018,Jan,8; 2017,Jan,8; 2016,Jan,13

32482 **2 lobes (bilobectomy)**

EXCLUDES *Lung removal with bronchoplasty (32501)*

Code also:

Decortication (32320)

Excision chest wall tumor, when performed (21601-21603)

45.8 45.8 **FUD** 090 C 80

AMA: 2018,Jan,8; 2017,Jan,8; 2016,Jan,13

32484 **single segment (segmentectomy)**

EXCLUDES *Lung removal with bronchoplasty (32501)*

Code also:

Decortication (32320)

Excision chest wall tumor, when performed (21601-21603)

41.3 41.3 **FUD** 090 C 80

AMA: 2018,Jan,8; 2017,Jan,8; 2016,Jan,13

32486 **with circumferential resection of segment of bronchus followed by broncho-bronchial anastomosis (sleeve lobectomy)**

Code also:

Decortication (32320)

Excision chest wall tumor, when performed (21601-21603)

68.1 68.1 **FUD** 090 C 80

AMA: 2018,Jan,8; 2017,Jun,10; 2017,Jan,8; 2016,Jan,13

32488 **with all remaining lung following previous removal of a portion of lung (completion pneumonectomy)**

Code also:

Decortication (32320)

Excision chest wall tumor, when performed (21601-21603)

69.1 69.1 **FUD** 090 C 80

AMA: 2018,Jan,8; 2017,Jan,8; 2016,Jan,13

32491 **with resection-plication of emphysematous lung(s) (bullous or non-bullous) for lung volume reduction, sternal split or transthoracic approach, includes any pleural procedure, when performed**

Code also:

Decortication (32320)

Excision chest wall tumor, when performed (21601-21603)

42.4 42.4 **FUD** 090 C 80 50

AMA: 2018,Jan,8; 2017,Jan,8; 2016,Jan,13

\+ **32501** **Resection and repair of portion of bronchus (bronchoplasty) when performed at time of lobectomy or segmentectomy (List separately in addition to code for primary procedure)**

INCLUDES Plastic closure bronchus, not closure resected bronchus

Code first (32480-32484)

7.04 7.04 **FUD** ZZZ C 80

AMA: 1995,Win,1

32503-32504 Excision of Lung Neoplasm

EXCLUDES *Excision chest wall tumor (21601-21603)*
Thoracentesis, needle or catheter, aspiration pleural space (32554-32555)
Thoracotomy; with exploration (32100)
Tube thoracostomy (32551)

32503 **Resection of apical lung tumor (eg, Pancoast tumor), including chest wall resection, rib(s) resection(s), neurovascular dissection, when performed; without chest wall reconstruction(s)**

51.9 51.9 **FUD** 090 C 80

AMA: 2019,Dec,4

32504 **with chest wall reconstruction**

59.1 59.1 **FUD** 090 C 80

AMA: 2019,Dec,4

32505-32507 Thoracotomy with Wedge Resection

INCLUDES Wedge technique with tissue obtained with precise consideration margins and complete resection

Code also resection chest wall tumor with lung resection, when performed (21601-21603)

32505 **Thoracotomy; with therapeutic wedge resection (eg, mass, nodule), initial**

EXCLUDES *Removal lung (32440, 32442, 32445, 32488)*

Code also more extensive procedure lung when performed on contralateral lung or different lobe with modifier 59 despite intraoperative pathology consultation

26.9 26.9 **FUD** 090 C 80

AMA: 2018,Jan,8; 2017,Jan,8; 2016,Jan,13

\+ **32506** **with therapeutic wedge resection (eg, mass or nodule), each additional resection, ipsilateral (List separately in addition to code for primary procedure)**

Code also more extensive procedure lung when performed on contralateral lung or different lobe with modifier 59 despite intraoperative pathology consultation

Code first (32505)

4.52 4.52 **FUD** ZZZ C 80

AMA: 2018,Jan,8; 2017,Jan,8; 2016,Jan,13

+ **32507** **with diagnostic wedge resection followed by anatomic lung resection (List separately in addition to code for primary procedure)**

INCLUDES Classification as diagnostic wedge resection when intraoperative pathology consultation dictates more extensive resection in same anatomical area

EXCLUDES *Diagnostic wedge resection by thoracoscopy (32668)*
Therapeutic wedge resection (32505-32506, 32666-32667)

Code first (32440, 32442, 32445, 32480-32488, 32503-32504)

4.52 4.52 **FUD** ZZZ C 80

AMA: 2018,Jan,8; 2017,Jan,8; 2016,Jan,13

32540 Removal of Empyema

32540 **Extrapleural enucleation of empyema (empyemectomy)**

Code also appropriate removal lung code when done with lobectomy (32480-32488)

50.1 50.1 **FUD** 090 C 80

AMA: 1994,Fall,1

32550-32552 Chest Tube/Catheter

32550 **Insertion of indwelling tunneled pleural catheter with cuff**

EXCLUDES *Procedures performed on same side chest with (32554-32557)*

(75989)

5.98 21.2 **FUD** 000 J G2

AMA: 2018,Jan,8; 2017,Jan,8; 2016,Jan,13

32551 **Tube thoracostomy, includes connection to drainage system (eg, water seal), when performed, open (separate procedure)**

EXCLUDES *Procedures performed on same side chest with (33020, 33025)*

4.56 4.56 **FUD** 000 T G2 50

AMA: 2019,Dec,4; 2018,Jul,7; 2018,Jan,8; 2017,Jun,10; 2017,Jan,8; 2016,Jan,13

32552 **Removal of indwelling tunneled pleural catheter with cuff**

4.55 5.28 **FUD** 010 Q2 G2 80

AMA: 2018,Jan,8; 2017,Jan,8; 2016,Jan,13

32553 Intrathoracic Placement Radiation Therapy Devices

EXCLUDES *Percutaneous placement interstitial device(s) for radiation therapy guidance: intra-abdominal, intrapelvic, and/or retroperitoneal (49411)*

Code also device

32553 **Placement of interstitial device(s) for radiation therapy guidance (eg, fiducial markers, dosimeter), percutaneous, intra-thoracic, single or multiple**

(76942, 77002, 77012, 77021)

5.17 15.1 **FUD** 000 S G2 80

AMA: 2018,Jan,8; 2017,Jan,8; 2016,Jun,3; 2016,Jan,13

32554-32557 Pleural Aspiration and Drainage

EXCLUDES *Chest x-ray performed to confirm chest tube position, complications, procedure adequacy*
Open tube thoracostomy (32551)
Placement indwelling tunneled pleural drainage catheter (cuffed) (32550)

32554 **Thoracentesis, needle or catheter, aspiration of the pleural space; without imaging guidance**

EXCLUDES *Radiologic guidance (75989, 76942, 77002, 77012, 77021)*

2.58 6.01 **FUD** 000 T G2 50

AMA: 2019,Dec,4; 2018,Jan,8; 2017,Jan,8; 2016,Jan,13

32555 **with imaging guidance**

INCLUDES Radiologic guidance (75989, 76942, 77002, 77012, 77021)

3.22 8.51 **FUD** 000 T G2 50

AMA: 2019,Dec,4; 2018,Jan,8; 2017,Jan,8; 2016,Jan,13

32556 **Pleural drainage, percutaneous, with insertion of indwelling catheter; without imaging guidance**

EXCLUDES *Radiologic guidance (75989, 76942, 77002, 77012, 77021)*

3.55 17.4 **FUD** 000 J G2 50

AMA: 2018,Jan,8; 2017,Jan,8; 2016,Jan,13

32557 **with imaging guidance**

INCLUDES Radiologic guidance (75989, 76942, 77002, 77012, 77021)

4.39 16.0 **FUD** 000 T G2 50

AMA: 2018,Jan,8; 2017,Jan,8; 2016,Jan,13

32560-32562 Instillation Drug/Chemical by Chest Tube

EXCLUDES *Insertion chest tube (32551)*

32560 **Instillation, via chest tube/catheter, agent for pleurodesis (eg, talc for recurrent or persistent pneumothorax)**

2.25 7.38 **FUD** 000 T G2

AMA: 2018,Jan,8; 2017,Jan,8; 2016,Jan,13

32561 **Instillation(s), via chest tube/catheter, agent for fibrinolysis (eg, fibrinolytic agent for break up of multiloculated effusion); initial day**

EXCLUDES *Reporting code more than one time on initial treatment date*

1.95 2.66 **FUD** 000 T G2 80

AMA: 2018,Jan,8; 2017,Jan,8; 2016,Jan,13

32562 **subsequent day**

EXCLUDES *Reporting code more than one time on each day subsequent treatment*

1.75 2.40 **FUD** 000 T G2 80

AMA: 2018,Jan,8; 2017,Jan,8; 2016,Jan,13

32601-32674 Thoracic Surgery: Video-Assisted (VATS)

INCLUDES Diagnostic thoracoscopy in surgical thoracoscopy

32601 **Thoracoscopy, diagnostic (separate procedure); lungs, pericardial sac, mediastinal or pleural space, without biopsy**

8.90 8.90 **FUD** 000 J G2 80

AMA: 2018,Jan,8; 2017,Jan,8; 2016,Jan,13

32604 **pericardial sac, with biopsy**

EXCLUDES *Open biopsy pericardium (39010)*

13.8 13.8 **FUD** 000 J G2 80

AMA: 2018,Jan,8; 2017,Jan,8; 2016,Jan,13

32606 **mediastinal space, with biopsy**

13.3 13.3 **FUD** 000 J G2 80

AMA: 2018,Jan,8; 2017,Jan,8; 2016,Jan,13

32607 **Thoracoscopy; with diagnostic biopsy(ies) of lung infiltrate(s) (eg, wedge, incisional), unilateral**

EXCLUDES *Removal lung (32440-32445, 32488)*
Thoracoscopy, surgical; with removal lung (32671)
Reporting code more than one time per lung

8.92 8.92 **FUD** 000 J G2 80

AMA: 2018,Jan,8; 2017,Jan,8; 2016,Jan,13

32608 **with diagnostic biopsy(ies) of lung nodule(s) or mass(es) (eg, wedge, incisional), unilateral**

EXCLUDES *Removal lung (32440-32445, 32488)*
Thoracoscopy, surgical; with removal lung (32671)
Reporting code more than one time per lung

10.9 10.9 **FUD** 000 J G2 80

AMA: 2018,Jan,8; 2017,Jan,8; 2016,Jan,13

32609 **with biopsy(ies) of pleura**

7.43 7.43 **FUD** 000 J G2 80

AMA: 2018,Jan,8; 2017,Jan,8; 2016,Jan,13

32650 **Thoracoscopy, surgical; with pleurodesis (eg, mechanical or chemical)**

19.1 19.1 **FUD** 090 C 80 50

AMA: 2018,Jan,8; 2017,Jan,8; 2016,Jan,13

32651 **with partial pulmonary decortication**

31.6 31.6 **FUD** 090 C 80 50

AMA: 2018,Jan,8; 2017,Jan,8; 2016,Jan,13

32652 **with total pulmonary decortication, including intrapleural pneumonolysis**

47.9 47.9 **FUD** 090 C 80 50

AMA: 2018,Jan,8; 2017,Jan,8; 2016,Jan,13

32653 **with removal of intrapleural foreign body or fibrin deposit**
30.6 30.6 FUD 090 C 80
AMA: 2018,Jan,8; 2017,Jan,8; 2016,Jan,13

32654 **with control of traumatic hemorrhage**
33.5 33.5 FUD 090 C 80 50
AMA: 2018,Jan,8; 2017,Jan,8; 2016,Jan,13

32655 **with resection-plication of bullae, includes any pleural procedure when performed**
EXCLUDES *Thoracoscopic lung volume reduction surgery (32672)*
27.5 27.5 FUD 090 C 80 50
AMA: 2018,Jan,8; 2017,Jan,8; 2016,Jan,13

32656 **with parietal pleurectomy**
23.1 23.1 FUD 090 C 80 50
AMA: 2018,Jan,8; 2017,Jan,8; 2016,Jan,13

32658 **with removal of clot or foreign body from pericardial sac**
20.6 20.6 FUD 090 C 80
AMA: 2018,Jan,8; 2017,Jan,8; 2016,Jan,13

32659 **with creation of pericardial window or partial resection of pericardial sac for drainage**
21.1 21.1 FUD 090 C 80
AMA: 2018,Jan,8; 2017,Jan,8; 2016,Jan,13

32661 **with excision of pericardial cyst, tumor, or mass**
23.0 23.0 FUD 090 C 80
AMA: 2018,Jan,8; 2017,Jan,8; 2016,Jan,13

32662 **with excision of mediastinal cyst, tumor, or mass**
25.7 25.7 FUD 090 C 80
AMA: 2018,Jan,8; 2017,Jan,8; 2016,Jan,13

32663 **with lobectomy (single lobe)**
EXCLUDES *Thoracoscopic segmentectomy (32669)*
40.4 40.4 FUD 090 C 80
AMA: 2018,Jan,8; 2017,Jan,8; 2016,Jan,13

32664 **with thoracic sympathectomy**
24.4 24.4 FUD 090 C 80 50
AMA: 2018,Jan,8; 2017,Jan,8; 2016,Jan,13

32665 **with esophagomyotomy (Heller type)**
EXCLUDES *Exploratory thoracoscopy with and without biopsy (32601-32609)*
Peroral endoscopic myotomy (POEM) (43497)
35.2 35.2 FUD 090 C 80
AMA: 2018,Jan,8; 2017,Jan,8; 2016,Jan,13

32666 **with therapeutic wedge resection (eg, mass, nodule), initial unilateral**
EXCLUDES *Removal lung (32440-32445, 32488)*
Thoracoscopy, surgical; with removal lung (32671)
Code also more extensive procedure lung when performed on contralateral lung or different lobe with modifier 59 despite pathology consultation
25.0 25.0 FUD 090 C 80 50
AMA: 2018,Jan,8; 2017,Jan,8; 2016,Jan,13

+ **32667** **with therapeutic wedge resection (eg, mass or nodule), each additional resection, ipsilateral (List separately in addition to code for primary procedure)**
EXCLUDES *Removal lung (32440-32445, 32488)*
Thoracoscopy, surgical; with removal lung (32671)
Code also more extensive procedure lung when performed on contralateral lung or different lobe with modifier 59 despite intraoperative pathology consultation
Code first (32666)
4.53 4.53 FUD ZZZ C 80
AMA: 2018,Jan,8; 2017,Jan,8; 2016,Jan,13

+ **32668** **with diagnostic wedge resection followed by anatomic lung resection (List separately in addition to code for primary procedure)**
INCLUDES Classification as diagnostic wedge resection when intraoperative pathology consultation dictates more extensive resection in same anatomical area
Code first (32440-32488, 32503-32504, 32663, 32669-32671)
4.54 4.54 FUD ZZZ C 80
AMA: 2018,Jan,8; 2017,Jan,8; 2016,Jan,13

32669 **with removal of a single lung segment (segmentectomy)**
38.8 38.8 FUD 090 C 80
AMA: 2018,Jan,8; 2017,Jan,8; 2016,Jan,13

32670 **with removal of two lobes (bilobectomy)**
46.2 46.2 FUD 090 C 80
AMA: 2018,Jan,8; 2017,Jan,8; 2016,Jan,13

32671 **with removal of lung (pneumonectomy)**
51.1 51.1 FUD 090 C 80
AMA: 2018,Jan,8; 2017,Jan,8; 2016,Jan,13

32672 **with resection-plication for emphysematous lung (bullous or non-bullous) for lung volume reduction (LVRS), unilateral includes any pleural procedure, when performed**
44.0 44.0 FUD 090 C 80
AMA: 2018,Jan,8; 2017,Jan,8; 2016,Jan,13

32673 **with resection of thymus, unilateral or bilateral**
EXCLUDES *Exploratory thoracoscopy with and without biopsy (32601-32609)*
Open excision mediastinal cyst (39200)
Open excision mediastinal tumor (39220)
Open thymectomy (60520-60522)
35.1 35.1 FUD 090 C 80
AMA: 2018,Jan,8; 2017,Jan,8; 2016,Jan,13

+ **32674** **with mediastinal and regional lymphadenectomy (List separately in addition to code for primary procedure)**

INCLUDES Mediastinal lymph nodes:
Left side:
Aortopulmonary window
Inferior pulmonary ligament
Paraesophageal
Subcarinal
Right side:
Inferior pulmonary ligament
Paraesophageal
Paratracheal
Subcarinal

EXCLUDES *Mediastinal and regional lymphadenectomy by thoracotomy (38746)*

Code first (21601, 31760, 31766, 31786, 32096-32200, 32220-32320, 32440-32491, 32503-32505, 32601-32663, 32666, 32669-32673, 32815, 33025, 33030, 33050-33130, 39200-39220, 39560-39561, 43101, 43112, 43117-43118, 43122-43123, 43287-43288, 43351, 60270, 60505)

6.23 6.23 FUD ZZZ C 80

AMA: 2018,Jan,8; 2017,Jan,8; 2016,Jan,13

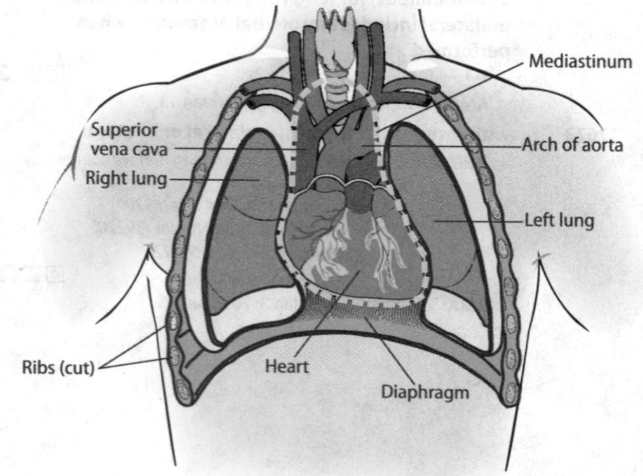

32701 Target Delineation for Stereotactic Radiation Therapy

INCLUDES Collaboration between radiation oncologist and surgeon
Correlation tumor and contiguous body structures
Determination borders and volume of tumor
Identification fiducial markers
Verification target when fiducial markers not used

EXCLUDES *Fiducial marker insertion (31626, 32553)*
Procedure performed by same physician as radiation treatment management (77427-77499)
Radiation oncology services (77295, 77331, 77370, 77373, 77435)
Therapeutic radiology (77261-77799 [77295, 77385, 77386, 77387, 77424, 77425])

32701 **Thoracic target(s) delineation for stereotactic body radiation therapy (SRS/SBRT), (photon or particle beam), entire course of treatment**

6.21 6.21 FUD XXX B 80 26

AMA: 2018,Jan,8; 2017,Jan,8; 2016,Jan,13

32800-32820 Chest Repair and Reconstruction Procedures

32800 **Repair lung hernia through chest wall**

27.0 27.0 FUD 090 C 80

32810 **Closure of chest wall following open flap drainage for empyema (Clagett type procedure)**

26.0 26.0 FUD 090 C 80

32815 **Open closure of major bronchial fistula**

81.0 81.0 FUD 090 C 80

32820 **Major reconstruction, chest wall (posttraumatic)**

38.3 38.3 FUD 090 C 80

32850-32856 Lung Transplant Procedures

INCLUDES Harvesting donor lung(s), cold preservation, preparation donor lung(s), transplantation into recipient

EXCLUDES *Assessment marginal cadaver donor lungs (0494T-0496T)*
Repairs or resection donor lung(s) (32491, 32505-32507, 35216, 35276)

32850 **Donor pneumonectomy(s) (including cold preservation), from cadaver donor**

0.00 0.00 FUD XXX C

AMA: 1993,Win,1

32851 **Lung transplant, single; without cardiopulmonary bypass**

94.8 94.8 FUD 090 C 80

AMA: 1993,Win,1

32852 **with cardiopulmonary bypass**

103. 103. FUD 090 C 80

AMA: 2017,Dec,3

32853 **Lung transplant, double (bilateral sequential or en bloc); without cardiopulmonary bypass**

133. 133. FUD 090 C 80

AMA: 1993,Win,1

32854 **with cardiopulmonary bypass**

141. 141. FUD 090 C 80

AMA: 2017,Dec,3

32855 **Backbench standard preparation of cadaver donor lung allograft prior to transplantation, including dissection of allograft from surrounding soft tissues to prepare pulmonary venous/atrial cuff, pulmonary artery, and bronchus; unilateral**

0.00 0.00 FUD XXX C 80

32856 **bilateral**

0.00 0.00 FUD XXX C 80

32900-32997 [32994] Chest and Respiratory Procedures

32900 **Resection of ribs, extrapleural, all stages**

41.0 41.0 FUD 090 C 80

32905 **Thoracoplasty, Schede type or extrapleural (all stages);**

38.5 38.5 FUD 090 C 80

32906 **with closure of bronchopleural fistula**

EXCLUDES *Open closure bronchial fistula (32815)*
Resection first rib for thoracic compression (21615-21616)

47.6 47.6 FUD 090 C 80

32940 **Pneumonolysis, extraperiosteal, including filling or packing procedures**

35.4 35.4 FUD 090 C 80

32960 **Pneumothorax, therapeutic, intrapleural injection of air**

2.62 3.61 FUD 000 T G2

32994 **Resequenced code. See code following 32998.**

32997 **Total lung lavage (unilateral)**

EXCLUDES *Broncho-alveolar lavage by bronchoscopy (31624)*

9.84 9.84 FUD 000 C 50

AMA: 2018,Jan,8; 2017,Jan,8; 2016,Jan,13

32998-32999 [32994] Destruction of Lung Neoplasm

32998 **Ablation therapy for reduction or eradication of 1 or more pulmonary tumor(s) including pleura or chest wall when involved by tumor extension, percutaneous, including imaging guidance when performed, unilateral; radiofrequency**

12.7 99.5 FUD 000 J G2 80 50

AMA: 2018,Jan,8; 2017,Nov,8

32994 **cryoablation**

12.8 155. FUD 000 J J8 80 50

AMA: 2018,Jan,8; 2017,Nov,8

32999 **Unlisted procedure, lungs and pleura**

0.00 0.00 FUD YYY T

AMA: 2018,Jan,8; 2017,Jan,8; 2016,Jan,13

33016-33050 Procedures of the Pericardial Sac

EXCLUDES *Surgical thoracoscopy (video-assisted thoracic surgery [VATS]) procedures pericardium (32601, 32604, 32658-32659, 32661)*

33016 Pericardiocentesis, including imaging guidance, when performed

INCLUDES Imaging guidance for needle placement:
Computed tomography (77012)
Fluoroscopy (77002)
Magnetic resonance (77021)
Ultrasound (76942)

EXCLUDES *Echocardiography for pericardiocentesis guidance (93303-93325)*

6.85 6.85 **FUD** 000 G2

AMA: 2020,Jan,7

33017 Pericardial drainage with insertion of indwelling catheter, percutaneous, including fluoroscopy and/or ultrasound guidance, when performed; 6 years and older without congenital cardiac anomaly

INCLUDES Catheters that remain in patient at procedure conclusion
Imaging guidance for needle placement:
Fluoroscopy (77002)
Magnetic resonance (77021)
Ultrasound (76942)

EXCLUDES *CT guided pericardial drainage (33019)*
Echocardiography for pericardiocentesis guidance (93303-93325)
Pericardial drainage for patients:
Any age with congenital cardiac anomaly (33018)
Younger than 6 years of age (33018)
Radiologically guided catheter placement for percutaneous drainage (75989)

7.10 7.10 **FUD** 000

AMA: 2020,Jan,7

33018 birth through 5 years of age or any age with congenital cardiac anomaly

INCLUDES Catheters that remain in patient at procedure conclusion
Imaging guidance for needle placement:
Fluoroscopy (77002)
Magnetic resonance (77021)
Ultrasound (76942)
Patient age birth to 5 years without congenital cardiac anomaly
Patient any age with congenital cardiac anomaly, such as heterotaxy, dextrocardia, mesocardia, or single ventricle anomaly, or 90 days following repair congenital cardiac anomaly

EXCLUDES *CT guided pericardial drainage (33019)*
Echocardiography for pericardiocentesis guidance (93303-93325)
Radiologically guided catheter placement for percutaneous drainage (75989)

8.09 8.09 **FUD** 000

AMA: 2020,Jan,7

33019 Pericardial drainage with insertion of indwelling catheter, percutaneous, including CT guidance

INCLUDES Catheters that remain in patient at procedure conclusion
Imaging guidance for needle placement:
Computed tomography (77012)
Fluoroscopy (77002)
Magnetic resonance (77021)
Ultrasound (76942)

EXCLUDES *Radiologically guided catheter placement for percutaneous drainage (75989)*

6.57 6.57 **FUD** 000

AMA: 2020,Jan,7

33020 Pericardiotomy for removal of clot or foreign body (primary procedure)

INCLUDES Tube thoracostomy when chest tube or pleural drain placed on same side (32551)

23.8 23.8 **FUD** 090 C 80

AMA: 1997,Nov,1

33025 Creation of pericardial window or partial resection for drainage

INCLUDES Tube thoracostomy when chest tube or pleural drain placed on same side (32551)

EXCLUDES *Surgical thoracoscopy (video-assisted thoracic surgery [VATS]) creation of pericardial window (32659)*

22.2 22.2 **FUD** 090 C 80

AMA: 1997,Nov,1

33030 Pericardiectomy, subtotal or complete; without cardiopulmonary bypass

INCLUDES Delorme pericardiectomy

57.8 57.8 **FUD** 090 C 80

AMA: 1997,Nov,1; 1994,Win,1

33031 with cardiopulmonary bypass

71.7 71.7 **FUD** 090 C 80

AMA: 2017,Dec,3

33050 Resection of pericardial cyst or tumor

EXCLUDES *Open biopsy pericardium (39010)*
Surgical thoracoscopy (video-assisted thoracic surgery [VATS]) resection of cyst, mass, or tumor pericardium (32661)

29.1 29.1 **FUD** 090 C 80

AMA: 1997,Nov,1

33120-33130 Neoplasms of Heart

Code also removal thrombus through separate heart incision, when performed (33310-33315); append modifier 59 to (33315)

33120 Excision of intracardiac tumor, resection with cardiopulmonary bypass

60.6 60.6 **FUD** 090 C 80

AMA: 2018,Jan,8; 2017,Dec,3; 2017,Jan,8; 2016,Jan,13

33130 Resection of external cardiac tumor

39.5 39.5 **FUD** 090 C 80

AMA: 2018,Jan,8; 2017,Jan,8; 2016,Jan,13

33140-33141 Transmyocardial Revascularization

33140 Transmyocardial laser revascularization, by thoracotomy; (separate procedure)

45.1 45.1 **FUD** 090 C 80

AMA: 2018,Jan,8; 2017,Jan,8; 2016,Jan,13

+ **33141 performed at the time of other open cardiac procedure(s) (List separately in addition to code for primary procedure)**

Code first (33390-33391, 33404-33496, 33510-33536, 33542)

3.80 3.80 **FUD** ZZZ C 80

AMA: 2018,Jan,8; 2017,Jan,8; 2016,Jan,13

33202-33203 Placement Epicardial Leads

CMS: 100-04,32,270 Implantable Cardiac Defibrillators (ICDs); 100-04,32,270.1 Coding Requirements for ICDs; 100-04,32,270.2 Special Editing for Inpatient Claims; 100-04,32,270.3 Denial Messaging

INCLUDES Imaging guidance:
Fluoroscopy (76000)
Ultrasound (76942, 76998, 93318)
Temporary pacemaker (33210-33211)

Code also insertion pulse generator when performed by same physician/same surgical session (33212-33213, [33221], 33230-33231, 33240)

33202 Insertion of epicardial electrode(s); open incision (eg, thoracotomy, median sternotomy, subxiphoid approach)
22.3 22.3 **FUD** 090 C
AMA: 2019,Mar,6; 2018,Jan,8; 2017,Jan,8; 2016,Aug,5; 2016,May,5; 2016,Jan,13

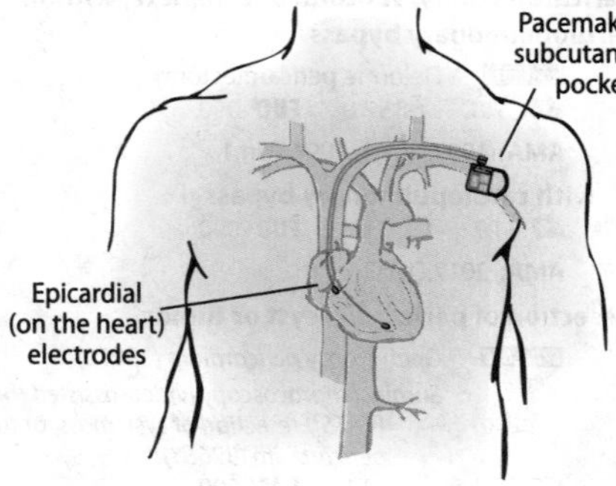

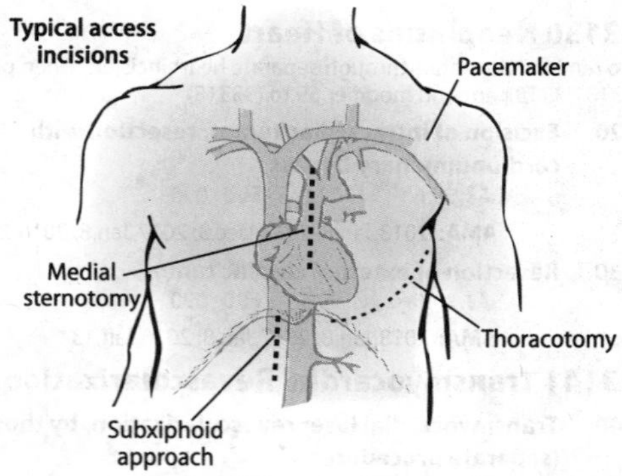

33203 endoscopic approach (eg, thoracoscopy, pericardioscopy)
23.3 23.3 **FUD** 090 C
AMA: 2019,Mar,6; 2018,Jan,8; 2017,Jan,8; 2016,Aug,5; 2016,May,5; 2016,Jan,13

33206-33214 [33221] Pacemakers

INCLUDES Device evaluation (93279-93298 [93260, 93261])
Dual lead: device that paces and senses in two heart chambers
Imaging guidance:
Fluoroscopy (76000)
Ultrasound (76942, 76998, 93318)
Multiple lead: device that paces and senses in three or more heart chambers
Radiological supervision and interpretation for pacemaker procedure
Single lead: device that paces and senses in one heart chamber
Skin pocket revision, when performed
Temporary pacemaker (33210-33211)

EXCLUDES *Electrode repositioning:*
Left ventricle (33226)
Pacemaker (33215)
Insertion lead for left ventricular (biventricular) pacing (33224-33225)
Leadless pacemaker systems ([33274, 33275])

Code also wound infection or hematoma incision/drainage, when performed (10140, 10180, 11042-11047 [11045, 11046])

33206 Insertion of new or replacement of permanent pacemaker with transvenous electrode(s); atrial
INCLUDES Pulse generator insertion/single transvenous electrode placement
EXCLUDES *Insertion transvenous electrode only (33216-33217)*
Removal with immediate replacement pacemaker pulse generator only, single lead system ([33227])
Code also removal old pacemaker pulse generator and electrode, when replacement entire system performed:
Electrode (33234)
Pulse generator (33233)
13.1 13.1 **FUD** 090 J J8
AMA: 2019,Oct,3; 2019,Mar,6; 2018,Jan,8; 2017,Jan,8; 2016,Aug,5; 2016,May,5; 2016,Jan,13

33207 ventricular
INCLUDES Pulse generator insertion/single transvenous electrode placement
EXCLUDES *Insertion transvenous electrode only (33216-33217)*
Removal with immediate replacement pacemaker pulse generator only, single lead system ([33227])
Code also removal old pacemaker pulse generator and electrode, when replacement entire system performed:
Electrode (33234)
Pulse generator (33233)
13.9 13.9 **FUD** 090 J J8
AMA: 2019,Oct,3; 2019,Mar,6; 2018,Jan,8; 2017,Jan,8; 2016,Aug,5; 2016,May,5; 2016,Jan,13

33208 atrial and ventricular
INCLUDES Pulse generator insertion/dual transvenous electrode placement
EXCLUDES *Insertion transvenous electrode(s) only (33216-33217)*
Removal with immediate replacement pacemaker pulse generator only, dual or multiple lead system ([33228, 33229])
Code also removal old pacemaker pulse generator and electrode, when replacement entire system performed:
Electrodes (33235)
Pulse generator (33233)
15.1 15.1 **FUD** 090 J J8
AMA: 2019,Oct,3; 2019,Mar,6; 2018,Jan,8; 2017,Jan,8; 2016,Aug,5; 2016,May,5; 2016,Jan,13

33210 Insertion or replacement of temporary transvenous single chamber cardiac electrode or pacemaker catheter (separate procedure)
4.74 4.74 **FUD** 000 J G2
AMA: 2019,Oct,3; 2019,Mar,6; 2018,Jan,8; 2017,Jan,8; 2016,Aug,5; 2016,May,5; 2016,Jan,13

33211 Insertion or replacement of temporary transvenous dual chamber pacing electrodes (separate procedure)
4.90 4.90 **FUD** 000 J J8
AMA: 2019,Oct,3; 2019,Mar,6; 2018,Jan,8; 2017,Jan,8; 2016,Aug,5; 2016,May,5; 2016,Jan,13

33212 Insertion of pacemaker pulse generator only; with existing single lead

EXCLUDES *Insertion for replacement single lead pacemaker pulse generator ([33227])*
Insertion transvenous electrode(s) (33216-33217)
Removal permanent pacemaker pulse generator only (33233)

Code also placement epicardial leads by same physician/same surgical session (33202-33203)

9.31 9.31 **FUD** 090 J J8

AMA: 2019,Oct,3; 2019,Mar,6; 2018,Jan,8; 2017,Jan,8; 2016,Aug,5; 2016,May,5; 2016,Jan,13

33213 with existing dual leads

EXCLUDES *Insertion for replacement dual lead pacemaker pulse generator ([33228])*
Insertion transvenous electrode(s) (33216-33217)
Removal permanent pacemaker pulse generator only (33233)

Code also placement epicardial leads by same physician/same surgical session (33202-33203)

9.73 9.73 **FUD** 090 J J8

AMA: 2019,Oct,3; 2019,Mar,6; 2018,Jan,8; 2017,Jan,8; 2016,Aug,5; 2016,May,5; 2016,Jan,13

33221 with existing multiple leads

EXCLUDES *Insertion for replacement multiple lead pacemaker pulse generator ([33229])*
Insertion transvenous electrode(s) (33216-33217)
Removal permanent pacemaker pulse generator only (33233)

Code also placement epicardial leads by same physician/same surgical session (33202-33203)

10.4 10.4 **FUD** 090 J J8

AMA: 2019,Oct,3; 2019,Mar,6; 2018,Jan,8; 2017,Jan,8; 2016,Aug,5; 2016,May,5; 2016,Jan,13

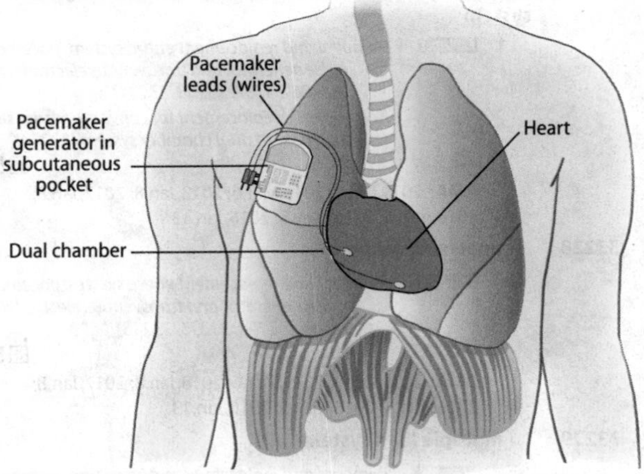

33214 Upgrade of implanted pacemaker system, conversion of single chamber system to dual chamber system (includes removal of previously placed pulse generator, testing of existing lead, insertion of new lead, insertion of new pulse generator)

EXCLUDES *Insertion transvenous electrode(s) (33216-33217)*
Removal and replacement pacemaker pulse generator (33227-33229)

13.8 13.8 **FUD** 090 J J8 80

AMA: 2019,Oct,3; 2019,Mar,6; 2018,Jan,8; 2017,Jan,8; 2016,Aug,5; 2016,May,5; 2016,Jan,13

33215-33249 [33221, 33227, 33228, 33229, 33230, 33231, 33262, 33263, 33264] Pacemakers/Implantable Defibrillator/Electrode Insertion/Replacement/Revision/Repair

INCLUDES Device evaluation (93279-93298 [93260, 93261])
Dual lead: device that paces and senses in two heart chambers
Imaging guidance:
  Fluoroscopy (76000)
  Ultrasound (76942, 76998, 93318)
Multiple lead: device that paces and senses in three or more heart chambers
Radiological supervision and interpretation for pacemaker or pacing cardioverter-defibrillator procedure
Single lead: device that paces and senses in one heart chamber
Skin pocket revision, when performed
Temporary pacemaker (33210-33211)

EXCLUDES *Electrode repositioning:*
  Left ventricle (33226)
  Pacemaker or implantable defibrillator (33215)
Insertion lead for left ventricular (biventricular) pacing (33224-33225)
Removal leadless pacemaker system ([33275])
Removal subcutaneous implantable defibrillator electrode ([33272])
Testing defibrillator threshold (DFT) during follow-up evaluation (93642-93644)
Testing defibrillator threshold (DFT) during insertion/replacement (93640-93641)

Code also wound infection or hematoma incision/drainage, when performed (10140, 10180, 11042-11047 [11045, 11046])

33215 Repositioning of previously implanted transvenous pacemaker or implantable defibrillator (right atrial or right ventricular) electrode

9.01 9.01 **FUD** 090 T G2

AMA: 2019,Oct,3; 2019,Mar,6; 2018,Jan,8; 2017,Jan,8; 2016,Aug,5; 2016,May,5; 2016,Jan,13

33216 Insertion of a single transvenous electrode, permanent pacemaker or implantable defibrillator

EXCLUDES *Insertion or replacement lead for cardiac venous system (33224-33225)*
Insertion or replacement permanent implantable defibrillator generator or system (33249)
Removal and replacement permanent pacemaker or implantable defibrillator (33206-33208, 33212-33213, [33221], 33227-33229, 33230-33231, 33240, [33262, 33263, 33264])

10.7 10.7 **FUD** 090 J J8

AMA: 2019,Oct,3; 2019,Mar,6; 2018,Jan,8; 2017,Jan,8; 2016,Aug,5; 2016,May,5; 2016,Jan,13

33217 Insertion of 2 transvenous electrodes, permanent pacemaker or implantable defibrillator

EXCLUDES *Insertion or replacement lead for cardiac venous system (33224-33225)*
Insertion or replacement permanent implantable defibrillator generator or system (33249)
Removal and replacement permanent pacemaker or implantable defibrillator (33206-33208, 33212-33213, [33221], 33227-33229, 33230-33231, 33240, [33262, 33263, 33264])

10.6 10.6 **FUD** 090 J J8

AMA: 2019,Oct,3; 2019,Mar,6; 2018,Jan,8; 2017,Jan,8; 2016,Aug,5; 2016,May,5; 2016,Jan,13

33218 Repair of single transvenous electrode, permanent pacemaker or implantable defibrillator

Code also removal old generator with insertion new generator replacement, when performed:
  Implantable defibrillator ([33262, 33263, 33264])
  Pacemaker ([33227, 33228, 33229])

11.2 11.2 **FUD** 090 T G2

AMA: 2019,Oct,3; 2019,Mar,6; 2018,Jan,8; 2017,Jan,8; 2016,Aug,5; 2016,May,5; 2016,Jan,13

33220 **Repair of 2 transvenous electrodes for permanent pacemaker or implantable defibrillator**

Code also modifier 52 Reduced services, when one electrode in two-chamber system repaired

Code also removal old generator with insertion new generator replacement, when performed:

Implantable defibrillator ([33263, 33264])

Pacemaker ([33228, 33229])

10.9 10.9 FUD 090 T J8

AMA: 2019,Oct,3; 2019,Mar,6; 2018,Jan,8; 2017,Jan,8; 2016,Aug,5; 2016,May,5; 2016,Jan,13

33221 **Resequenced code. See code following 33213.**

33222 **Relocation of skin pocket for pacemaker**

INCLUDES Formation new pocket

Procedures related to existing pocket:

Accessing pocket

Incision/drainage abscess or hematoma (10140, 10180)

Pocket closure (13100-13102)

EXCLUDES *Debridement, subcutaneous tissue (11042-11047 [11045, 11046])*

Code also removal and replacement existing generator

9.84 9.84 FUD 090 T A2

AMA: 2019,Oct,3; 2019,Mar,6; 2018,Jan,8; 2017,Jan,8; 2016,Aug,5; 2016,May,5; 2016,Jan,13

33223 **Relocation of skin pocket for implantable defibrillator**

INCLUDES Formation new pocket

Procedures related to existing pocket:

Accessing pocket

Incision/drainage abscess or hematoma (10140, 10180)

Pocket closure (13100-13102)

EXCLUDES *Debridement, subcutaneous tissue (11042-11047 [11045, 11046])*

Code also removal and replacement existing generator

11.8 11.8 FUD 090 T A2 80

AMA: 2019,Oct,3; 2019,Mar,6; 2018,Jan,8; 2017,Jan,8; 2016,Aug,5; 2016,Jan,13

33224 **Insertion of pacing electrode, cardiac venous system, for left ventricular pacing, with attachment to previously placed pacemaker or implantable defibrillator pulse generator (including revision of pocket, removal, insertion, and/or replacement of existing generator)**

Code also:

Body surface-activation mapping for optimization electrical synchrony when performed (0695T)

Placement epicardial electrode when appropriate (33202-33203)

14.9 14.9 FUD 000 J J8

AMA: 2019,Oct,3; 2019,Mar,6; 2018,Jan,8; 2017,Jan,8; 2016,Aug,5; 2016,May,5; 2016,Jan,13

+ **33225** **Insertion of pacing electrode, cardiac venous system, for left ventricular pacing, at time of insertion of implantable defibrillator or pacemaker pulse generator (eg, for upgrade to dual chamber system) (List separately in addition to code for primary procedure)**

Code also:

Body surface-activation mapping for optimization electrical synchrony when performed (0695T)

Placement epicardial electrode when appropriate (33202-33203)

Code first (33206-33208, 33212-33213, [33221], 33214, 33216-33217, 33223, 33228-33229, 33230-33231, 33233, 33234-33235, 33240, [33263, 33264], 33249)

Code first (33223) for relocation pocket for implantable defibrillator

Code first (33222) for relocation pocket for pacemaker pulse generator

13.6 13.6 FUD ZZZ N N1

AMA: 2019,Oct,3; 2019,Mar,6; 2018,Jan,8; 2017,Jan,8; 2016,Aug,5; 2016,May,5; 2016,Jan,13

33226 **Repositioning of previously implanted cardiac venous system (left ventricular) electrode (including removal, insertion and/or replacement of existing generator)**

Code also body surface-activation mapping for optimization electrical synchrony when performed (0695T)

14.4 14.4 FUD 000 T G2

AMA: 2019,Oct,3; 2019,Mar,6; 2018,Jan,8; 2017,Jan,8; 2016,Aug,5; 2016,May,5; 2016,Jan,13

33227 **Resequenced code. See code following 33233.**

33228 **Resequenced code. See code following 33233.**

33229 **Resequenced code. See code before 33234.**

33230 **Resequenced code. See code following 33240.**

33231 **Resequenced code. See code before 33241.**

33233 **Removal of permanent pacemaker pulse generator only**

EXCLUDES *Removal with immediate replacement pacemaker pulse generator, without replacement electrode(s):*

Dual lead system ([33228])

Multiple lead system ([33229])

Single lead system ([33227])

Code also insertion replacement pacemaker pulse generator with transvenous electrode(s) (total system), when performed:

Pacemaker and dual leads (33208)

Pacemaker and single atrial lead (33206)

Pacemaker and single ventricular lead (33207)

Code also removal electrode(s), when removal total system without replacement performed:

Dual leads (atrial and ventricular) (33235)

Single lead (atrial or ventricular) (33234)

6.68 6.68 FUD 090 02 J8

AMA: 2019,Oct,3; 2019,Mar,6; 2018,Jan,8; 2017,Jan,8; 2016,Aug,5; 2016,May,5; 2016,Jan,13

\# **33227** **Removal of permanent pacemaker pulse generator with replacement of pacemaker pulse generator; single lead system**

EXCLUDES *Removal and replacement entire system, pacemaker pulse generator and transvenous electrode, report (33206-33207, 33233, 33234)*

Removal and replacement for conversion from single chamber to dual chamber system (33214)

9.82 9.82 FUD 090 J J8

AMA: 2019,Oct,3; 2019,Mar,6; 2018,Jan,8; 2017,Jan,8; 2016,Aug,5; 2016,May,5; 2016,Jan,13

\# **33228** **dual lead system**

EXCLUDES *Removal and replacement entire system, pacemaker pulse generator and transvenous electrode(s), report (33208, 33233, 33235)*

10.2 10.2 FUD 090 J J8

AMA: 2019,Oct,3; 2019,Mar,6; 2018,Jan,8; 2017,Jan,8; 2016,Aug,5; 2016,May,5; 2016,Jan,13

\# **33229** **multiple lead system**

EXCLUDES *Removal and replacement entire system, pacemaker pulse generator and transvenous electrode(s), report (33208, 33233, 33235)*

10.8 10.8 FUD 090 J J8

AMA: 2019,Oct,3; 2019,Mar,6; 2018,Jan,8; 2017,Jan,8; 2016,Aug,5; 2016,May,5; 2016,Jan,13

33234 Removal of transvenous pacemaker electrode(s); single lead system, atrial or ventricular

Code also pacing electrode insertion in cardiac venous system for pacing left ventricle during insertion pulse generator (pacemaker or implantable defibrillator) when performed (33225)

Code also removal old pacemaker pulse generator and insertion replacement pacemaker pulse generator with transvenous electrode (total system), when performed:

Insertion pacemaker and atrial lead (33206) OR

Insertion pacemaker and ventricular lead (33207) AND

Removal generator (33233)

Code also thoracotomy to remove electrode, when performed, for unsuccessful transvenous removal (33238)

14.0 14.0 FUD 090 Q2 J8

AMA: 2019,Oct,3; 2019,Mar,6; 2018,Jan,8; 2017,Jan,8; 2016,Aug,5; 2016,May,5; 2016,Jan,13

33235 dual lead system

Code also pacing electrode insertion in cardiac venous system for pacing left ventricle during insertion pulse generator (pacemaker or implantable defibrillator) when performed (33225)

Code also removal old pacemaker pulse generator and insertion replacement pacemaker pulse generator with transvenous electrodes (total system), when performed:

Insertion generator and dual leads (33208) AND

Insertion pacemaker and atrial lead (33206) OR

Insertion pacemaker and ventricular lead (33207) AND

Removal generator (33233)

Code also thoracotomy to remove electrode, when performed, for unsuccessful transvenous removal (33238)

18.5 18.5 FUD 090 Q2 J8

AMA: 2019,Oct,3; 2019,Mar,6; 2018,Jan,8; 2017,Jan,8; 2016,Aug,5; 2016,May,5; 2016,Jan,13

33236 Removal of permanent epicardial pacemaker and electrodes by thoracotomy; single lead system, atrial or ventricular

EXCLUDES *Removal implantable defibrillator electrode(s) by thoracotomy (33243)*

Removal transvenous electrodes by thoracotomy (33238)

Removal transvenous pacemaker electrodes, single or dual lead system; without thoracotomy (33234, 33235)

22.5 22.5 FUD 090 C 80

AMA: 2019,Oct,3; 2019,Mar,6; 2018,Jan,8; 2017,Jan,8; 2016,Aug,5; 2016,May,5; 2016,Jan,13

33237 dual lead system

EXCLUDES *Removal implantable defibrillator electrode(s) by thoracotomy (33243)*

Removal transvenous electrodes by thoracotomy (33238)

Removal transvenous pacemaker electrodes, single or dual lead system; without thoracotomy (33234, 33235)

24.1 24.1 FUD 090 C 80

AMA: 2019,Oct,3; 2019,Mar,6; 2018,Jan,8; 2017,Jan,8; 2016,Aug,5; 2016,May,5; 2016,Jan,13

33238 Removal of permanent transvenous electrode(s) by thoracotomy

EXCLUDES *Removal implantable defibrillator electrode(s) by thoracotomy (33243)*

Removal transvenous pacemaker electrodes, single or dual lead system; without thoracotomy (33234, 33235)

27.0 27.0 FUD 090 C 80

AMA: 2019,Oct,3; 2018,Jan,8; 2017,Jan,8; 2016,Aug,5; 2016,May,5; 2016,Jan,13

33240 Insertion of implantable defibrillator pulse generator only; with existing single lead

EXCLUDES *Insertion electrode(s) (33216-33217, [33271])*

Removal and replacement implantable defibrillator pulse generator only ([33262, 33263, 33264])

Code also placement epicardial leads by same physician/same surgical session as generator insertion (33202-33203)

10.5 10.5 FUD 090 J J8

AMA: 2019,Oct,3; 2018,Jan,8; 2017,Jan,8; 2016,Aug,5; 2016,Jan,13

\# **33230 with existing dual leads**

EXCLUDES *Insertion single transvenous electrode, permanent pacemaker or implantable defibrillator (33216-33217)*

Removal and replacement implantable defibrillator pulse generator only ([33262, 33263, 33264])

Code also placement epicardial leads by same physician/same surgical session as generator insertion (33202-33203)

11.0 11.0 FUD 090 J J8

AMA: 2019,Oct,3; 2019,Mar,6; 2018,Jan,8; 2017,Jan,8; 2016,Aug,5; 2016,Jan,13

\# **33231 with existing multiple leads**

EXCLUDES *Insertion single transvenous electrode, permanent pacemaker or implantable defibrillator (33216-33217)*

Removal and replacement implantable defibrillator pulse generator only ([33262, 33263, 33264])

Code also placement epicardial leads by same physician/same surgical session as generator placement (33202-33203)

11.6 11.6 FUD 090 J J8

AMA: 2019,Oct,3; 2019,Mar,6; 2018,Jan,8; 2017,Jan,8; 2016,Aug,5; 2016,Jan,13

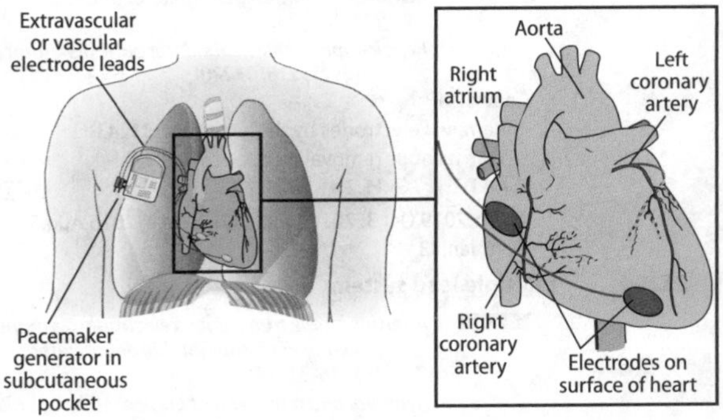

33241 Removal of implantable defibrillator pulse generator only

EXCLUDES *Removal substernal implantable defibrillator pulse generator only (0580T)*

Removal with immediate replacement implantable defibrillator pulse generator only ([33262, 33263, 33264])

Code also removal electrode(s) and insertion replacement defibrillator with electrode(s) (total system), when performed:

Removal electrode(s) (33243-33244) AND

Insertion defibrillator system, single or dual (33249) OR

Removal subcutaneous electrode ([33272]) AND

Insertion subcutaneous defibrillator system ([33270])

Code also removal electrode(s), when total system removed without replacement:

Subcutaneous electrode ([33272])

Transvenous electrode(s) (33243)

6.20 6.20 FUD 090 Q2 G2

AMA: 2019,Oct,3; 2018,Jan,8; 2017,Jan,8; 2016,Aug,5; 2016,Jan,13

 # 33262 Removal of implantable defibrillator pulse generator with replacement of implantable defibrillator pulse generator; single lead system

EXCLUDES *Insertion electrode(s) (33216-33217, [33271])*
Removal and replacement implantable defibrillator pulse generator and electrode(s) (total system) (33241, 33243-33244, 33249)
Removal and replacement subcutaneous defibrillator pulse generator and electrode(s) (total system) (33241, [33270], [33272])
Removal and replacement substernal implantable defibrillator pulse generator ([0614T])
Removal implantable defibrillator pulse generator only (33241)
Repair implantable defibrillator pulse generator and/or leads (33218, 33220)

Code also:
Electrode(s) removal by thoracotomy (33243)
Subcutaneous electrode removal ([33272])
Transvenous removal of electrode(s) (33244)

10.8 10.8 **FUD** 090 J J8

AMA: 2019,Oct,3; 2018,Jan,8; 2017,Jan,8; 2016,Aug,5; 2016,Jan,13

 # 33263 dual lead system

EXCLUDES *Insertion single transvenous electrode, permanent pacemaker or implantable defibrillator (33216-33217)*
Removal and replacement implantable defibrillator pulse generator and electrode(s) (total system) (33241, 33243-33244, 33249)
Removal and replacement subcutaneous defibrillator pulse generator and electrode (total system) (33241, [33270], [33272])
Removal implantable defibrillator pulse generator only (33241)
Repair implantable defibrillator pulse generator and/or leads (33218, 33220)

Code also:
Removal electrodes by thoracotomy (33243)
Transvenous removal electrodes (33244)

11.2 11.2 **FUD** 090 J J8

AMA: 2019,Oct,3; 2018,Jan,8; 2017,Jan,8; 2016,Aug,5; 2016,Jan,13

 # 33264 multiple lead system

EXCLUDES *Insertion single transvenous electrode, permanent pacemaker or implantable defibrillator (33216-33217)*
Removal and replacement implantable defibrillator pulse generator and electrode(s) (total system) (33241, 33243-33244, 33249)
Removal and replacement subcutaneous defibrillator pulse generator and electrode(s) (total system) (33241, [33270], [33272])
Removal implantable defibrillator pulse generator only (33241)
Repair implantable defibrillator pulse generator and/or leads (33218, 33220)

Code also:
Removal electrodes by thoracotomy (33243)
Transvenous removal electrodes (33244)

11.7 11.7 **FUD** 090 J J8

AMA: 2019,Oct,3; 2018,Jan,8; 2017,Jan,8; 2016,Aug,5; 2016,Jan,13

33243 Removal of single or dual chamber implantable defibrillator electrode(s); by thoracotomy

EXCLUDES *Transvenous removal defibrillator electrode(s) (33244)*

Code also removal implantable defibrillator pulse generator and insertion replacement defibrillator with electrodes (total system), when entire system replaced:
Insertion defibrillator system, single or dual (33249)
Removal generator (33241)

Code also removal implantable defibrillator pulse generator, when entire system removed without replacement (33241)

Code also replacement implantable defibrillator pulse generator, when performed:
Dual lead system ([33263])
Multiple lead system ([33264])
Single lead system ([33262])

39.6 39.6 **FUD** 090 C 80

AMA: 2019,Oct,3; 2018,Jan,8; 2017,Jan,8; 2016,Aug,5; 2016,Jan,13

33244 by transvenous extraction

Code also removal implantable defibrillator pulse generator and insertion replacement defibrillator with electrodes (total system), when entire system replaced:
Insertion defibrillator system, single or dual (33249)
Removal generator (33241)

Code also removal implantable defibrillator pulse generator, when entire system removed without replacement (33241)

Code also replacement implantable defibrillator pulse generator, when performed:
Dual lead system ([33263])
Multiple lead system ([33264])
Single lead system ([33262])

Code also thoracotomy to remove electrode, when performed, if transvenous removal unsuccessful (33238, 33243)

25.1 25.1 **FUD** 090 02 G2

AMA: 2019,Oct,3; 2018,Jan,8; 2017,Jan,8; 2016,Aug,5; 2016,Jan,13

33249 Insertion or replacement of permanent implantable defibrillator system, with transvenous lead(s), single or dual chamber

EXCLUDES *Insertion single transvenous electrode, permanent pacemaker or implantable defibrillator (33216-33217)*

Code also removal defibrillator generator when upgrading from single to dual-chamber system (33241)

Code also removal implantable defibrillator pulse generator and removal electrode(s), when entire system replaced:
Removal electrode(s) (33243-33244)
Removal generator (33241)

26.6 26.6 **FUD** 090 J J8

AMA: 2019,Oct,3; 2018,Jan,8; 2017,Jan,8; 2016,Aug,5; 2016,Jan,13

33270-33275 [33270, 33271, 33272, 33273, 33274, 33275] Subcutaneous Implantable Defibrillator

INCLUDES Programming and interrogation of:
Leadless pacemaker (93279, 93286, 93288, 93294, 93296)
Subcutaneous implantable defibrillator ([93260, 93261])

\# **33270** **Insertion or replacement of permanent subcutaneous implantable defibrillator system, with subcutaneous electrode, including defibrillation threshold evaluation, induction of arrhythmia, evaluation of sensing for arrhythmia termination, and programming or reprogramming of sensing or therapeutic parameters, when performed**

INCLUDES Electrophysiologic evaluation at initial insertion (93644)

EXCLUDES *Insertion subcutaneous implantable defibrillator electrode only ([33271])*
Insertion/replacement permanent implantable defibrillator system with substernal electrode (0571T)

Code also electrophysiologic evaluation following replacement subcutaneous implantable defibrillator, when performed (93644)

Code also removal subcutaneous implantable defibrillator and removal subcutaneous electrode, when entire system is being replaced:
Defibrillator (33241)
Electrode ([33272])

16.4 16.4 **FUD** 090 J J8

AMA: 2019,Oct,3; 2018,Jan,8; 2017,Jan,8; 2016,Aug,5; 2016,Jan,13

\# **33271** **Insertion of subcutaneous implantable defibrillator electrode**

EXCLUDES *Insertion implantable defibrillator pulse generator only, other than subcutaneous:*
Initial insertion (33240)
Removal/replacement ([33262])
Insertion subcutaneous implantable defibrillator and electrode (total system) ([33270])
Insertion substernal defibrillator electrode (0572T)

13.1 13.1 **FUD** 090 J J8

AMA: 2019,Oct,3; 2018,Jan,8; 2017,Jan,8; 2016,Aug,5; 2016,Jan,13

\# **33272** **Removal of subcutaneous implantable defibrillator electrode**

EXCLUDES *Removal substernal defibrillator electrode (0573T)*

Code also removal implantable defibrillator, when performed:
Removal with replacement ([33262])
Removal without replacement (33241)

Code also removal subcutaneous implantable defibrillator and insertion replacement implantable subcutaneous defibrillator with electrode (total system), when entire system is being replaced:
Insertion total system ([33270])
Removal defibrillator (33241)

10.0 10.0 **FUD** 090 Q2 G2

AMA: 2019,Oct,3; 2018,Jan,8; 2017,Jan,8; 2016,Aug,5; 2016,Jan,13

\# **33273** **Repositioning of previously implanted subcutaneous implantable defibrillator electrode**

EXCLUDES *Repositioning substernal defibrillator electrode (0574T)*

11.5 11.5 **FUD** 090 T G2

AMA: 2019,Oct,3; 2018,Jan,8; 2017,Jan,8; 2016,Aug,5; 2016,Jan,13

\# **33274** **Transcatheter insertion or replacement of permanent leadless pacemaker, right ventricular, including imaging guidance (eg, fluoroscopy, venous ultrasound, ventriculography, femoral venography) and device evaluation (eg, interrogation or programming), when performed**

INCLUDES Cardiac catheterization for insertion leadless pacemaker (93451, 93453, 93456-93457, 93460-93461, 93593-93594, 93596-93598)
Femoral venography (75820)
Imaging guidance (76000, 76937, 77002)
Right ventriculography (93566)

EXCLUDES *Removal permanent leadless pacemaker ([33275])*
Services for pacemakers with leads (33202-33203, 33206-33208, 33212-33214 [33221], 33215-33218, 33220, 33233-33237 [33227, 33228, 33229])

Code also intracardiac echocardiography, if performed (93662)

14.2 14.2 **FUD** 090 J8

AMA: 2019,Mar,6

\# **33275** **Transcatheter removal of permanent leadless pacemaker, right ventricular, including imaging guidance (eg, fluoroscopy, venous ultrasound, ventriculography, femoral venography), when performed**

INCLUDES Cardiac catheterization for insertion leadless pacemaker (93451, 93453, 93456-93457, 93460-93461, 93593-93594, 93596-93598)
Femoral venography (75820)
Imaging guidance (76000, 76937, 77002)
Right ventriculography (93566)

EXCLUDES *Insertion/replacement leadless pacemaker ([33274])*
Services for pacemakers with leads (33202-33203, 33206-33208, 33212-33214 [33221], 33215-33218, 33220, 33233-33237 [33227, 33228, 33229])

Code also intracardiac echocardiography, if performed (93662)

15.4 15.4 **FUD** 090 J8

AMA: 2019,Mar,6

33250-33251 Surgical Ablation Arrhythmogenic Foci, Supraventricular

INCLUDES Procedures using cryotherapy, laser, microwave, radiofrequency, and ultrasound

33250 **Operative ablation of supraventricular arrhythmogenic focus or pathway (eg, Wolff-Parkinson-White, atrioventricular node re-entry), tract(s) and/or focus (foci); without cardiopulmonary bypass**

EXCLUDES *Pacing and mapping during surgery by other provider (93631)*

42.4 42.4 **FUD** 090 C 80

AMA: 2018,Jan,8; 2017,Jan,8; 2016,Jan,13

33251 **with cardiopulmonary bypass**

47.0 47.0 **FUD** 090 C 80

AMA: 2018,Jan,8; 2017,Dec,3; 2017,Jan,8; 2016,Jan,13

33254-33256 Surgical Ablation Arrhythmogenic Foci, Atrial (e.g., Maze)

INCLUDES Excision or isolation left atrial appendage
Procedures using cryotherapy, laser, microwave, radiofrequency, and ultrasound

EXCLUDES *Any procedure involving median sternotomy or cardiopulmonary bypass*
Aortic valve procedures (33390-33391, 33404-33415)
Aortoplasty (33417)
Ascending aorta graft (33858-33859, 33863-33864)
Coronary artery bypass (33510-33516, 33517-33523, 33533-33536)
Excision intracardiac tumor, resection (33120)
Mitral valve procedures (33418-33430)
Outflow tract augmentation (33478)
Prosthetic valve repair (33496)
Pulmonary artery embolectomy (33910-33920)
Pulmonary valve procedures (33471-33477)
Repair aberrant coronary artery anatomy (33500-33507)
Repair aberrant heart anatomy (33600-33853)
Resection external cardiac tumor (33130)
Temporary pacemaker (33210-33211)
Thoracotomy; with exploration (32100)
Tricuspid valve procedures (33460-33468)
Tube thoracostomy, includes connection to drainage system (32551)
Ventricular reconstruction (33542-33548)
Ventriculomyotomy (33416)

33254 **Operative tissue ablation and reconstruction of atria, limited (eg, modified maze procedure)**
39.0 39.0 **FUD** 090 C 80
AMA: 2018,Jan,8; 2017,Jan,8; 2016,Jan,13

33255 **Operative tissue ablation and reconstruction of atria, extensive (eg, maze procedure); without cardiopulmonary bypass**
47.3 47.3 **FUD** 090 C 80
AMA: 2018,Jan,8; 2017,Jan,8; 2016,Jan,13

33256 **with cardiopulmonary bypass**
56.1 56.1 **FUD** 090 C 80
AMA: 2018,Jan,8; 2017,Dec,3; 2017,Jan,8; 2016,Jan,13

33257-33259 Surgical Ablation Arrhythmogenic Foci, Atrial, with Other Heart Procedure(s)

EXCLUDES *Operative tissue ablation and reconstruction atria (without other cardiac procedure), limited or extensive:*
Endoscopic (33265-33266)
Open (33254-33256)
Temporary pacemaker (33210-33211)
Tube thoracostomy, includes connection to drainage system (32551)

\+ **33257** **Operative tissue ablation and reconstruction of atria, performed at the time of other cardiac procedure(s), limited (eg, modified maze procedure) (List separately in addition to code for primary procedure)**
Code first (33120-33130, 33250-33251, 33261, 33300-33335, 33365, 33390-33391, 33404-33417 [33440], 33420-33430, 33460-33476, 33478, 33496, 33500-33507, 33510-33516, 33533-33548, 33600-33619, 33641-33697, 33702-33732, 33735-33767, 33770-33877, 33910-33922, 33925-33926, 33975-33983)
16.8 16.8 **FUD** ZZZ C 80

\+ **33258** **Operative tissue ablation and reconstruction of atria, performed at the time of other cardiac procedure(s), extensive (eg, maze procedure), without cardiopulmonary bypass (List separately in addition to code for primary procedure)**
Code first, when performed without cardiopulmonary bypass (33130, 33250, 33300, 33310, 33320-33321, 33330, 33365, 33420, 33471, 33501-33503, 33510-33516, 33533-33536, 33690, 33735, 33737, 33750-33766, 33800-33813, 33820-33824, 33840-33852, 33875, 33877, 33915, 33925, 33981, 33982)
18.7 18.7 **FUD** ZZZ C 80

\+ **33259** **Operative tissue ablation and reconstruction of atria, performed at the time of other cardiac procedure(s), extensive (eg, maze procedure), with cardiopulmonary bypass (List separately in addition to code for primary procedure)**
Code first, when performed with cardiopulmonary bypass (33120, 33251, 33261, 33305, 33315, 33322, 33335, 33390-33391, 33404-33410, 33411-33417, 33422-33430, 33460-33468, 33474-33478, 33496, 33500, 33504-33507, 33510-33516, 33533-33548, 33600-33688, 33692-33726, 33730, 33732, 33736, 33767, 33770, 33783, 33786-33788, 33814, 33853, 33858-33877, 33910, 33916-33922, 33926, 33975-33980, 33983)
24.3 24.3 **FUD** ZZZ C 80
AMA: 2017,Dec,3

33261-33264 [33262, 33263, 33264, 33267, 33268, 33269] Surgical Ablation Arrhythmogenic Foci, Ventricular

33261 **Operative ablation of ventricular arrhythmogenic focus with cardiopulmonary bypass**
46.7 46.7 **FUD** 090 C 80
AMA: 2018,Jan,8; 2017,Dec,3; 2017,Jan,8; 2016,Jan,13

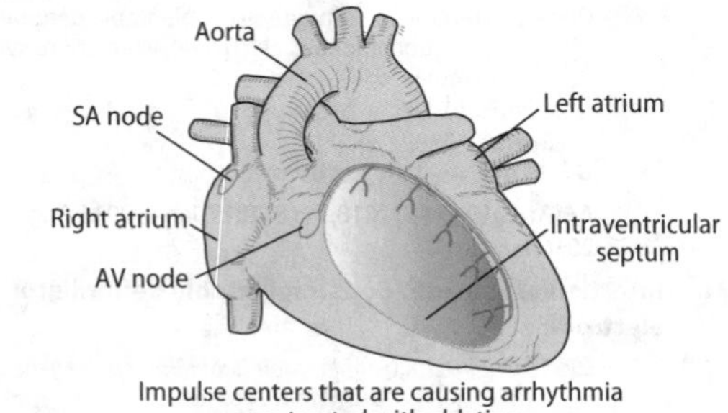

Impulse centers that are causing arrhythmia are treated with ablation

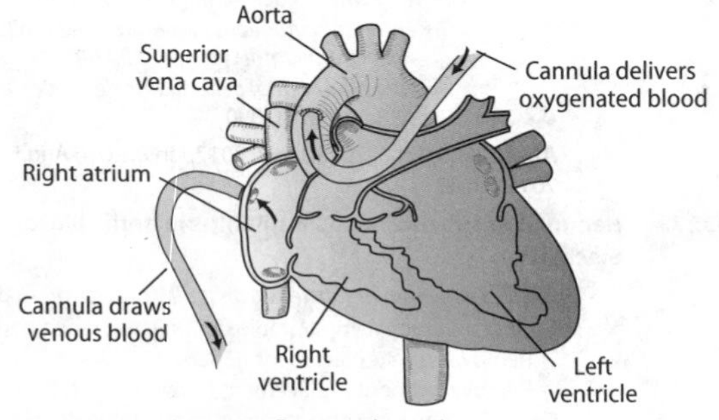

Bypass schematic

● # **33267** **Exclusion of left atrial appendage, open, any method (eg, excision, isolation via stapling, oversewing, ligation, plication, clip)**

EXCLUDES *Replacement, mitral valve (33430)*
Sternotomy/thoractomy procedures performed during same operative session
Tissue ablation/reconstruction atria (33254-33259, 33265-33266)
Valvotomy, mitral valve (33420, 33422)
Valvuloplasty, mitral valve (33425-33427)
0.00 0.00 **FUD** 000

● + # **33268** **Exclusion of left atrial appendage, open, performed at the time of other sternotomy or thoracotomy procedure(s), any method (eg, excision, isolation via stapling, oversewing, ligation, plication, clip) (List separately in addition to code for primary procedure)**

EXCLUDES *Replacement, mitral valve (33430)*
Tissue ablation/reconstruction atria (33254-33259, 33265-33266)
Valvotomy, mitral valve (33420, 33422)
Valvuloplasty, mitral valve (33425-33427)
Code first primary procedure requiring sternotomy/thoracotomy
0.00 0.00 **FUD** 000

26/TC PC/TC Only A2-Z3 ASC Payment 50 Bilateral ♂ Male Only ♀ Female Only Facility RVU Non-Facility RVU CCI CLIA
FUD Follow-up Days **CMS:** IOM **AMA:** CPT Asst A-Y OPPSI 80/80 Surg Assist Allowed / w/Doc Lab Crosswalk Radiology Crosswalk

● # **33269** **Exclusion of left atrial appendage, thoracoscopic, any method (eg, excision, isolation via stapling, oversewing, ligation, plication, clip)**

EXCLUDES *Replacement, mitral valve (33430)*
Tissue ablation/reconstruction atria (33254-33259, 33265-33266)
Valvotomy, mitral valve (33420, 33422)
Valvuloplasty, mitral valve (33425-33427)

0.00 0.00 FUD 000

33262 **Resequenced code. See code following 33241.**

33263 **Resequenced code. See code following 33241.**

33264 **Resequenced code. See code before 33243.**

33265-33275 [33267, 33268, 33269, 33270, 33271, 33272, 33273, 33274, 33275] Surgical Ablation Arrhythmogenic Foci, Endoscopic

EXCLUDES *Insertion or replacement temporary transvenous single chamber cardiac electrode or pacemaker catheter (separate procedure) (33210-33211)*
Tube thoracostomy, includes connection to drainage system (32551)

33265 **Endoscopy, surgical; operative tissue ablation and reconstruction of atria, limited (eg, modified maze procedure), without cardiopulmonary bypass**

39.3 39.3 FUD 090 C 80

AMA: 2018,Jan,8; 2017,Jan,8; 2016,Jan,13

33266 **operative tissue ablation and reconstruction of atria, extensive (eg, maze procedure), without cardiopulmonary bypass**

53.4 53.4 FUD 090 C 80

AMA: 2018,Jan,8; 2017,Jan,8; 2016,Jan,13

33267 **Resequenced code. See code following 33261.**

33268 **Resequenced code. See code following 33261.**

33269 **Resequenced code. See code following 33261.**

33270 **Resequenced code. See code following 33249.**

33271 **Resequenced code. See code following 33249.**

33272 **Resequenced code. See code following 33249.**

33273 **Resequenced code. See code following 33249.**

33274 **Resequenced code. See code following 33249.**

33275 **Resequenced code. See code following 33249.**

33285-33289 Cardiac Rhythm Monitor System

33285 **Insertion, subcutaneous cardiac rhythm monitor, including programming**

INCLUDES Implantation device into subcutaneous prepectoral pocket
Initial programming

EXCLUDES *Successive analysis and/or reprogramming (93285, 93291, 93298)*

2.57 142. FUD 000 J8

AMA: 2019,Oct,3; 2019,Apr,3

33286 **Removal, subcutaneous cardiac rhythm monitor**

2.54 3.80 FUD 000 G2

AMA: 2019,Apr,3

33289 **Transcatheter implantation of wireless pulmonary artery pressure sensor for long-term hemodynamic monitoring, including deployment and calibration of the sensor, right heart catheterization, selective pulmonary catheterization, radiological supervision and interpretation, and pulmonary artery angiography, when performed**

INCLUDES Device implantation into subcutaneous pocket
Fluoroscopy (76000)
Pulmonary artery angiography/injection (75741, 75743, 75746, 93568)
Pulmonary artery catheterization (36013-36015)
Radiologic supervision and interpretation
Remote monitoring (93264)
Right heart catheterization (93451, 93453, 93456-93457, 93460-93461, 93593-93594, 93596-93598)
Sensor deployment and calibration

9.55 9.55 FUD 000 80

AMA: 2019,Jun,3

33300-33315 Procedures for Injury of the Heart

INCLUDES Procedures with and without cardiopulmonary bypass

Code also transvascular ventricular support, when performed:
Balloon pump (33967, 33968, 33970-33974)
Extracorporeal membrane oxygenation (ECMO)/extracorporeal life support (ECLS) (33946-33949)
Ventricular assist device (33975-33983, [33995], 33990-33993 [33997])

33300 **Repair of cardiac wound; without bypass**

71.0 71.0 FUD 090 C 80

AMA: 1997,Nov,1

33305 **with cardiopulmonary bypass**

118. 118. FUD 090 C 80

AMA: 2017,Dec,3

33310 **Cardiotomy, exploratory (includes removal of foreign body, atrial or ventricular thrombus); without bypass**

EXCLUDES *Other cardiac procedures unless separate incision into heart necessary to remove thrombus*

33.7 33.7 FUD 090 C 80

AMA: 1997,Nov,1

33315 **with cardiopulmonary bypass**

EXCLUDES *Other cardiac procedures unless separate incision into heart necessary to remove thrombus*

Code also excision thrombus with cardiopulmonary bypass and append modifier 59 when separate incision required with (33120, 33130, 33420-33430, 33460-33468, 33496, 33542, 33545, 33641-33647, 33670, 33681, 33975-33980)

55.3 55.3 FUD 090 C 80

AMA: 2018,Jan,8; 2017,Dec,3; 2017,Jan,8; 2016,Jan,13

33320-33335 Procedures for Injury of the Aorta/Great Vessels

Code also transvascular ventricular support, when performed:
Balloon pump (33967, 33968, 33970-33974)
Extracorporeal membrane oxygenation (ECMO)/extracorporeal life support (ECLS) (33946-33949)
Ventricular assist device (33975-33983, [33995], 33990-33993 [33997])

33320 **Suture repair of aorta or great vessels; without shunt or cardiopulmonary bypass**

30.5 30.5 FUD 090 C 80

AMA: 2018,Jun,11; 2018,Jan,8; 2017,Jan,8; 2016,Jan,13

33321 **with shunt bypass**

34.3 34.3 FUD 090 C 80

AMA: 2018,Jun,11

33322 **with cardiopulmonary bypass**

40.2 40.2 FUD 090 C 80

AMA: 2018,Jun,11; 2018,Jan,8; 2017,Dec,3; 2017,Jan,8; 2016,Jan,13

33330 **Insertion of graft, aorta or great vessels; without shunt, or cardiopulmonary bypass**

41.2 41.2 FUD 090 C 80

AMA: 2018,Jun,11

33335 **with cardiopulmonary bypass**
54.6 54.6 FUD 090 C 80
AMA: 2018,Jun,11; 2017,Dec,3

33340 Closure Left Atrial Appendage

EXCLUDES *Cardiac catheterization except for reasons other than closure left atrial appendage (93451-93453, 93456, 93458-93461, 93462, 93593-93598)*
Code also intracardiac echocardiography, if performed (93662)
Code also transvascular ventricular support, when performed:
Balloon pump (33967, 33968, 33970-33974)
Extracorporeal membrane oxygenation (ECMO)/extracorporeal life support (ECLS) (33946-33949)
Ventricular assist device (33975-33983, [33995], 33990-33993 [33997])

33340 **Percutaneous transcatheter closure of the left atrial appendage with endocardial implant, including fluoroscopy, transseptal puncture, catheter placement(s), left atrial angiography, left atrial appendage angiography, when performed, and radiological supervision and interpretation**
22.9 22.9 FUD 000 C 80
AMA: 2018,Jan,8; 2017,Jul,3

33361-33369 Transcatheter Aortic Valve Replacement

CMS: 100-03,20.32 Transcatheter Aortic Valve Replacement (TAVR); 100-04,32,290.3 Claims Processing TAVR Inpatient; 100-04,32,290.4 Payment of TAVR for MA Plan Participants

INCLUDES
Access and implantation aortic valve (33361-33366)
Access sheath placement
Advancement valve delivery system
Arteriotomy closure
Balloon aortic valvuloplasty
Cardiac or open arterial approach
Deployment of valve
Percutaneous access
Radiology procedures:
Angiography during and after procedure
Assessment access site for closure
Documentation intervention completion
Guidance for valve placement
Supervision and interpretation
Temporary pacemaker
Valve repositioning when necessary

EXCLUDES *Cardiac catheterization procedures included in TAVR/TAVI service (93452-93453, 93458-93461, 93567)*
Percutaneous coronary interventional procedures

Code also cardiac catheterization services for purposes other than TAVR/TAVI
Code also diagnostic coronary angiography at different session from interventional procedure
Code also diagnostic coronary angiography same time as TAVR/TAVI when:
Previous study available, but documentation states patient's condition has changed since previous study, visualization anatomy/pathology inadequate, or change occurs during procedure warranting additional evaluation outside current target area
No previous catheter-based coronary angiography study available, and full diagnostic study performed, with decision to perform intervention based on that study
Code also modifier 59 when diagnostic coronary angiography procedures performed as separate and distinct procedural services on same day or session as TAVR/TAVI
Code also modifier 62 as all TAVI/TAVR procedures require work two physicians
Code also transvascular ventricular support, when performed:
Balloon pump (33967, 33970, 33973)
Ventricular assist device (33975-33976, [33995], 33990-33993 [33997])

33361 **Transcatheter aortic valve replacement (TAVR/TAVI) with prosthetic valve; percutaneous femoral artery approach**
Code also cardiopulmonary bypass when performed (33367-33369)
39.4 39.4 FUD 000 C 80
AMA: 2018,Jan,8; 2017,Jan,8; 2016,Jan,13

33362 **open femoral artery approach**
Code also cardiopulmonary bypass when performed (33367-33369)
43.1 43.1 FUD 000 C 80
AMA: 2018,Jan,8; 2017,Dec,3; 2017,Jan,8; 2016,Jan,13

33363 **open axillary artery approach**
Code also cardiopulmonary bypass when performed (33367-33369)
44.6 44.6 FUD 000 C 80
AMA: 2018,Jan,8; 2017,Dec,3; 2017,Jan,8; 2016,Jan,13

33364 **open iliac artery approach**
Code also cardiopulmonary bypass when performed (33367-33369)
46.1 46.1 FUD 000 C 80
AMA: 2018,Jan,8; 2017,Dec,3; 2017,Jan,8; 2016,Jan,13

33365 **transaortic approach (eg, median sternotomy, mediastinotomy)**
Code also cardiopulmonary bypass when performed (33367-33369)
51.8 51.8 FUD 000 C 80
AMA: 2018,Jan,8; 2017,Jan,8; 2016,Jan,13

33366 **transapical exposure (eg, left thoracotomy)**
Code also cardiopulmonary bypass when performed (33367-33369)
45.7 45.7 FUD 000 C 80
AMA: 2018,Jan,8; 2017,Jan,8; 2016,Jan,13

+ **33367** **cardiopulmonary bypass support with percutaneous peripheral arterial and venous cannulation (eg, femoral vessels) (List separately in addition to code for primary procedure)**
EXCLUDES *Cardiopulmonary bypass support with open or central arterial and venous cannulation (33368-33369)*
Cerebral embolic protection device (33370)
Code first (33361-33366, 33418, 33477, 0483T-0484T, 0544T, 0545T, [0643T], 0569T, 0570T, 0644T)
18.2 18.2 FUD ZZZ C 80
AMA: 2018,Jan,8; 2017,Jan,8; 2016,Mar,5; 2016,Jan,13

+ **33368** **cardiopulmonary bypass support with open peripheral arterial and venous cannulation (eg, femoral, iliac, axillary vessels) (List separately in addition to code for primary procedure)**
EXCLUDES *Cardiopulmonary bypass support with percutaneous or central arterial and venous cannulation (33367, 33369)*
Code first (33361-33366, 33418, 33477, 0483T-0484T, 0544T, 0545T, [0643T], 0569T, 0570T, 0644T)
21.7 21.7 FUD ZZZ C 80
AMA: 2018,Jan,8; 2017,Jan,8; 2016,Mar,5; 2016,Jan,13

+ **33369** **cardiopulmonary bypass support with central arterial and venous cannulation (eg, aorta, right atrium, pulmonary artery) (List separately in addition to code for primary procedure)**
EXCLUDES *Cardiopulmonary bypass support with percutaneous or open arterial and venous cannulation (33367-33368)*
Code first (33361-33366, 33418, 33477, 0483T-0484T, 0544T, 0545T, [0643T], 0569T-0570T, 0644T)
28.6 28.6 FUD ZZZ C 80
AMA: 2018,Jan,8; 2017,Jan,8; 2016,Mar,5; 2016,Jan,13

33370 Cerebral Embolic Protection Device

● + **33370** **Transcatheter placement and subsequent removal of cerebral embolic protection device(s), including arterial access, catheterization, imaging, and radiological supervision and interpretation, percutaneous (List separately in addition to code for primary procedure)**
INCLUDES
Angiography (75710)
Aortography (75600)
Ultrasound guidance (76937)
EXCLUDES *Additional or multiple filter placement*
Code first transcatheter aortic valve replacement (TAVR/TAVI) (33361-33366)
0.00 0.00 FUD 000

33390-33415 [33440] Aortic Valve Procedures

Code also transvascular ventricular support, when performed:
- Balloon pump (33967, 33968, 33970-33974)
- Extracorporeal membrane oxygenation (ECMO)/extracorporeal life support (ECLS) (33946-33949)
- Ventricular assist device (33975-33983, [33995], 33990-33993 [33997])

33390 Valvuloplasty, aortic valve, open, with cardiopulmonary bypass; simple (ie, valvotomy, debridement, debulking, and/or simple commissural resuspension)
55.8 55.8 **FUD** 090 C 80
AMA: 2018,Jan,8; 2017,Dec,3

33391 complex (eg, leaflet extension, leaflet resection, leaflet reconstruction, or annuloplasty)
INCLUDES Simple aortic valvuloplasty (33390)
66.4 66.4 **FUD** 090 C 80
AMA: 2018,Jan,8; 2017,Dec,3

33404 Construction of apical-aortic conduit
50.6 50.6 **FUD** 090 C 80
AMA: 2018,Jan,8; 2017,Dec,3; 2017,Jan,8; 2016,Jan,13

33405 Replacement, aortic valve, open, with cardiopulmonary bypass; with prosthetic valve other than homograft or stentless valve
65.7 65.7 **FUD** 090 C 80
AMA: 2019,Nov,9; 2019,Apr,6; 2018,Jan,8; 2017,Dec,3; 2017,Jan,8; 2016,Jan,13

33406 with allograft valve (freehand)
83.4 83.4 **FUD** 090 C 80
AMA: 2019,Nov,9; 2019,Apr,6; 2018,Jan,8; 2017,Dec,3; 2017,Jan,8; 2016,Jan,13

33410 with stentless tissue valve
73.6 73.6 **FUD** 090 C 80
AMA: 2019,Nov,9; 2019,Apr,6; 2018,Jan,8; 2017,Dec,3; 2017,Jan,8; 2016,Jan,13

33440 Replacement, aortic valve; by translocation of autologous pulmonary valve and transventricular aortic annulus enlargement of the left ventricular outflow tract with valved conduit replacement of pulmonary valve (Ross-Konno procedure)
INCLUDES Open replacement aortic valve with aortic annulus enlargement (33411-33412)
Open replacement aortic valve with translocation pulmonary valve (33413)
EXCLUDES *Aortoplasty for supravalvular stenosis (33417)*
Open replacement aortic valve (33405-33406, 33410)
Repair complex cardiac anomaly (except pulmonary atresia) (33608)
Repair left ventricular outlet obstruction (33414)
Repair pulmonary atresia (33920)
Replacement pulmonary valve (33475)
Resection/incision subvalvular tissue for aortic stenosis (33416)
98.1 98.1 **FUD** 090 80
AMA: 2019,Apr,6

33411 with aortic annulus enlargement, noncoronary sinus
97.4 97.4 **FUD** 090 C 80
AMA: 2019,Nov,9; 2019,Apr,6; 2018,Jan,8; 2017,Dec,3; 2017,Jan,8; 2016,Jan,13

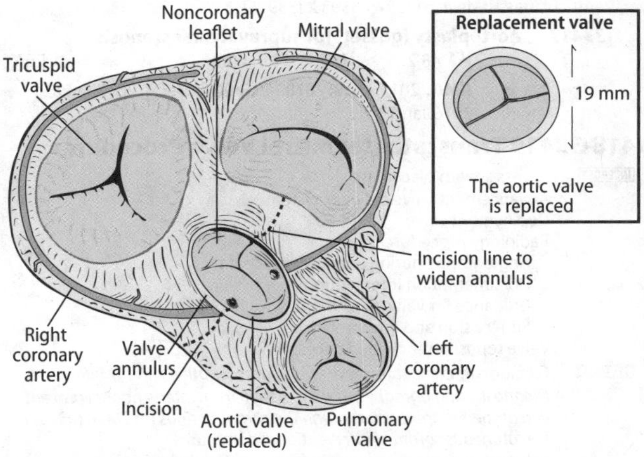

Overhead schematic of major heart valves

33412 with transventricular aortic annulus enlargement (Konno procedure)
EXCLUDES *Replacement aortic valve by translocation pulmonary valve, aortic annulus enlargement, valved conduit pulmonary valve replacement ([33440])*
Replacement aortic valve with translocation pulmonary valve (33413)
91.4 91.4 **FUD** 090 C 80
AMA: 2019,Nov,9; 2019,Apr,6; 2018,Jan,8; 2017,Dec,3; 2017,Jan,8; 2016,Jan,13

33413 by translocation of autologous pulmonary valve with allograft replacement of pulmonary valve (Ross procedure)
EXCLUDES *Replacement aortic valve by translocation pulmonary valve, aortic annulus enlargement, valved conduit pulmonary valve replacement ([33440])*
Replacement aortic valve with transventricular aortic annulus enlargement (33412)
92.7 92.7 **FUD** 090 C 80
AMA: 2019,Nov,9; 2019,Apr,6; 2018,Jan,8; 2017,Dec,3; 2017,Jan,8; 2016,Jan,13

33414 Repair of left ventricular outflow tract obstruction by patch enlargement of the outflow tract
62.2 62.2 **FUD** 090 C 80
AMA: 2019,Apr,6; 2018,Jan,8; 2017,Dec,3; 2017,Jan,8; 2016,Jan,13

33415 Resection or incision of subvalvular tissue for discrete subvalvular aortic stenosis
58.7 58.7 **FUD** 090 C 80
AMA: 2018,Jan,8; 2017,Dec,3; 2017,Jan,8; 2016,Jan,13

33416 Ventriculectomy

CMS: 100-03,20.26 Partial Ventriculectomy
EXCLUDES *Percutaneous transcatheter septal reduction therapy (93583)*
Code also transvascular ventricular support, when performed:
- Balloon pump (33967, 33968, 33970-33974)
- Extracorporeal membrane oxygenation (ECMO)/extracorporeal life support (ECLS) (33946-33949)
- Ventricular assist device (33975-33983, [33995], 33990-33993 [33997])

33416 Ventriculomyotomy (-myectomy) for idiopathic hypertrophic subaortic stenosis (eg, asymmetric septal hypertrophy)
58.5 58.5 **FUD** 090 C 80
AMA: 2019,Apr,6; 2018,Jan,8; 2017,Dec,3; 2017,Jan,8; 2016,Jan,13

33417 Repair of Supravalvular Stenosis by Aortoplasty

Code also transvascular ventricular support, when performed:
- Balloon pump (33967, 33968, 33970-33974)
- Extracorporeal membrane oxygenation (ECMO)/extracorporeal life support (ECLS) (33946-33949)
- Ventricular assist device (33975-33983, [33995], 33990-33993 [33997])

33417 **Aortoplasty (gusset) for supravalvular stenosis**
48.2 48.2 **FUD** 090 C 80
AMA: 2019,Apr,6; 2018,Jan,8; 2017,Dec,3; 2017,Jan,8; 2016,Jan,13

33418-33419 Transcatheter Mitral Valve Procedures

INCLUDES Access sheath placement
- Advancement valve delivery system
- Deployment valve
- Radiology procedures:
  - Angiography during and after procedure
  - Documentation intervention completion
  - Guidance for valve placement
  - Supervision and interpretation
- Valve repositioning when necessary

EXCLUDES *Cardiac catheterization services for purposes other than TMVR*
- *Diagnostic angiography different session from interventional procedure*
- *Percutaneous approach through the coronary sinus for TMVR (0345T)*
- *Percutaneous coronary interventional procedures*
- *Transcatheter mitral valve annulus reconstruction (0544T)*
- *Transcatheter TMVI by percutaneous or transthoracic approach (0483T-0484T)*

Code also cardiopulmonary bypass:
- Central (33369)
- Open peripheral (33368)
- Percutaneous peripheral (33367)

Code also diagnostic coronary angiography and cardiac catheterization procedures when:
- No previous study available and full diagnostic study performed
- Previous study inadequate or patient's clinical indication for study changed prior to or during procedure
- Report modifier 59 with cardiac catheterization procedures when on same day or same session as TMVR

Code also transvascular ventricular support, when performed:
- Balloon pump (33967, 33970, 33973)
- Ventricular assist device ([33995], 33990-33993 [33997])

33418 **Transcatheter mitral valve repair, percutaneous approach, including transseptal puncture when performed; initial prosthesis**
Code also left heart catheterization when performed by transapical puncture (93462)
52.1 52.1 **FUD** 090 C 80
AMA: 2018,Jan,8; 2017,Jan,8; 2016,Jan,13

\+ **33419** **additional prosthesis(es) during same session (List separately in addition to code for primary procedure)**
EXCLUDES *Procedures performed more than one time per session*
Code first (33418)
12.3 12.3 **FUD** ZZZ N N1 80
AMA: 2018,Jan,8; 2017,Jan,8; 2016,Jan,13

33420-33440 [33440] Mitral Valve Procedures

Code also thrombus removal through separate heart incision, when performed (33310-33315); append modifier 59 to (33315)
Code also transvascular ventricular support, when performed:
- Balloon pump (33967, 33968, 33970-33974)
- Extracorporeal membrane oxygenation (ECMO)/extracorporeal life support (ECLS) (33946-33949)
- Ventricular assist device (33975-33983, [33995], 33990-33993 [33997])

33420 **Valvotomy, mitral valve; closed heart**
42.3 42.3 **FUD** 090 C
AMA: 2018,Jan,8; 2017,Jan,8; 2016,Jan,13

33422 **open heart, with cardiopulmonary bypass**
48.1 48.1 **FUD** 090 C 80
AMA: 2018,Jan,8; 2017,Dec,3; 2017,Jan,8; 2016,Jan,13

33425 **Valvuloplasty, mitral valve, with cardiopulmonary bypass;**
79.1 79.1 **FUD** 090 C 80
AMA: 2018,Jan,8; 2017,Dec,3; 2017,Jan,8; 2016,Jan,13

33426 **with prosthetic ring**
69.0 69.0 **FUD** 090 C 80
AMA: 2018,Jan,8; 2017,Dec,3; 2017,Jan,8; 2016,Jan,13

33427 **radical reconstruction, with or without ring**
70.7 70.7 **FUD** 090 C 80
AMA: 2018,Jan,8; 2017,Dec,3; 2017,Jan,8; 2016,Jan,13

33430 **Replacement, mitral valve, with cardiopulmonary bypass**
81.1 81.1 **FUD** 090 C 80
AMA: 2018,Jan,8; 2017,Dec,3; 2017,Jan,8; 2016,Jan,13

33440 **Resequenced code. See code following 33410.**

33460-33468 Tricuspid Valve Procedures

EXCLUDES *Transcatheter tricuspid valve annulus reconstruction (0545T)*
- *Transcatheter tricuspid valve implantation (TTVI)/replacement ([0646T])*
- *Transcatheter tricuspid valve repair (0569T-0570T)*

Code also thrombus removal through separate heart incision, when performed (33310-33315); append modifier 59 to (33315)
Code also transvascular ventricular support, when performed:
- Balloon pump (33967, 33968, 33970-33974)
- Extracorporeal membrane oxygenation (ECMO)/extracorporeal life support (ECLS) (33946-33949)
- Ventricular assist device (33975-33983, [33995], 33990-33993 [33997])

33460 **Valvectomy, tricuspid valve, with cardiopulmonary bypass**
69.6 69.6 **FUD** 090 C 80
AMA: 2018,Jan,8; 2017,Dec,3; 2017,Jan,8; 2016,Jan,13

33463 **Valvuloplasty, tricuspid valve; without ring insertion**
89.4 89.4 **FUD** 090 C 80
AMA: 2018,Jan,8; 2017,Dec,3; 2017,Jan,8; 2016,Jan,13

33464 **with ring insertion**
70.7 70.7 **FUD** 090 C 80
AMA: 2018,Jan,8; 2017,Dec,3; 2017,Jan,8; 2016,Jan,13

33465 **Replacement, tricuspid valve, with cardiopulmonary bypass**
79.9 79.9 **FUD** 090 C 80
AMA: 2018,Jan,8; 2017,Dec,3; 2017,Jan,8; 2016,Jan,13

33468 **Tricuspid valve repositioning and plication for Ebstein anomaly**
71.0 71.0 **FUD** 090 C 80
AMA: 2018,Jan,8; 2017,Dec,3; 2017,Jan,8; 2016,Jan,13

33470-33474 Pulmonary Valvotomy

INCLUDES Brock's operation

Code also concurrent systemic-to-pulmonary artery shunt ligation/takedown (33924)
Code also transvascular ventricular support, when performed:
- Balloon pump (33967, 33968, 33970-33974)
- Extracorporeal membrane oxygenation (ECMO)/extracorporeal life support (ECLS) (33946-33949)
- Ventricular assist device (33975-33983, [33995], 33990-33993 [33997])

33470 ~~**Valvotomy, pulmonary valve, closed heart; transventricular**~~

▲ **33471** **Valvotomy, pulmonary valve, closed heart, via pulmonary artery**
EXCLUDES *Percutaneous valvuloplasty pulmonary valve (92990)*
38.3 38.3 **FUD** 090 C 80
AMA: 2018,Jan,8; 2017,Jan,8; 2016,Jan,13

33474 **Valvotomy, pulmonary valve, open heart, with cardiopulmonary bypass**
63.0 63.0 **FUD** 090 C 80
AMA: 2017,Dec,3

33475-33476 Other Procedures Pulmonary Valve

Code also concurrent systemic-to-pulmonary artery shunt ligation/takedown (33924)
Code also transvascular ventricular support, when performed:
- Balloon pump (33967, 33968, 33970-33974)
- Extracorporeal membrane oxygenation (ECMO)/extracorporeal life support (ECLS) (33946-33949)
- Ventricular assist device (33975-33983, [33995], 33990-33993 [33997])

33475 **Replacement, pulmonary valve**
67.5 67.5 **FUD** 090 C 80
AMA: 2019,Apr,6; 2018,Jan,8; 2017,Dec,3; 2017,Jan,8; 2016,Jan,13

33476 **Right ventricular resection for infundibular stenosis, with or without commissurotomy**

INCLUDES Brock's operation

44.0 44.0 FUD 090 C 80

AMA: 2018,Jan,8; 2017,Dec,3; 2017,Jan,8; 2016,Jan,13

33477 Transcatheter Pulmonary Valve Implantation

INCLUDES Procedures integral to TPVI:

Cardiac catheterization/angiography procedures (93451, 93453-93461, 93593-93594, 93596-93568)

Fluoroscopy (76000)

Injection procedures during cardiac catheterization (93563, 93566-93568)

Pulmonary artery angioplasty/valvuloplasty within treatment area (92997-92998)

Pulmonary artery stenting within treatment area (37236-37237)

EXCLUDES *Procedures performed at a separate session from TPVI:*

Diagnostic coronary angiography, when performed

Percutaneous coronary interventional procedures, when performed

Percutaneous interventions pulmonary artery branch, when performed

Procedures performed more than one time per session

Code also, when performed:

Balloon pump (33967, 33970, 33973)

Concurrent systemic-to-pulmonary artery shunt ligation/takedown (33924)

Diagnostic cardiac catheterization/angiography procedures, when performed distinctly separate from TPVI, if patient's condition (clinical indication) changed since intervention or prior study, no available prior catheter-based diagnostic study in treatment zone, or prior study not adequate (93451-93461, 93563-93564, 93568, 93593-93598)

Diagnostic cardiac catheterization procedures when performed distinctly separate from TPVI during same day/session, and append modifier 59 (93451-93461, 93593-93598)

Extracorporeal membrane oxygenation (ECMO)/extracorporeal life support (ECLS) (33946-33959, [33962], [33963], [33964], [33965], [33966], [33969], [33984], [33985], [33986], [33987], [33988], [33989])

Ventricular assist device ([33995], 33990-33993 [33997])

33477 **Transcatheter pulmonary valve implantation, percutaneous approach, including pre-stenting of the valve delivery site, when performed**

39.4 39.4 FUD 000 C 80

AMA: 2018,Jan,8; 2017,Jan,8; 2016,Aug,9; 2016,Mar,5

33478 Outflow Tract Augmentation

Code also for cavopulmonary anastomosis to second superior vena cava (33768)

Code also concurrent ligation/takedown systemic-to-pulmonary artery shunt (33924)

Code also transvascular ventricular support, when performed:

Balloon pump (33967, 33968, 33970-33974)

Extracorporeal membrane oxygenation (ECMO)/extracorporeal life support (ECLS) (33946-33949)

Ventricular assist device (33975-33983, [33995], 33990-33993 [33997])

33478 **Outflow tract augmentation (gusset), with or without commissurotomy or infundibular resection**

45.4 45.4 FUD 090 C 80

AMA: 2018,Jan,8; 2017,Dec,3; 2017,Jan,8; 2016,Jan,13

33496 Prosthetic Valve Repair

Code also thrombus removal through separate heart incision, when performed (33310-33315); append modifier 59 to (33315)

Code also reoperation if performed (33530)

33496 **Repair of non-structural prosthetic valve dysfunction with cardiopulmonary bypass (separate procedure)**

48.5 48.5 FUD 090 C 80

AMA: 2018,Jan,8; 2017,Dec,3; 2017,Jan,8; 2016,Jan,13

33500-33507 Repair Aberrant Coronary Artery Anatomy

INCLUDES Angioplasty and/or endarterectomy

33500 **Repair of coronary arteriovenous or arteriocardiac chamber fistula; with cardiopulmonary bypass**

45.0 45.0 FUD 090 C 80

AMA: 2017,Dec,3

33501 **without cardiopulmonary bypass**

32.2 32.2 FUD 090 C 80

AMA: 2007,Mar,1-3; 1997,Nov,1

33502 **Repair of anomalous coronary artery from pulmonary artery origin; by ligation**

36.9 36.9 FUD 090 63 C 80

AMA: 2017,Dec,3

33503 **by graft, without cardiopulmonary bypass**

38.3 38.3 FUD 090 63 C 80

AMA: 2007,Mar,1-3; 1997,Nov,1

33504 **by graft, with cardiopulmonary bypass**

42.3 42.3 FUD 090 C 80

AMA: 2017,Dec,3

33505 **with construction of intrapulmonary artery tunnel (Takeuchi procedure)**

59.8 59.8 FUD 090 63 C 80

AMA: 2017,Dec,3

33506 **by translocation from pulmonary artery to aorta**

57.8 57.8 FUD 090 63 C 80

AMA: 2017,Dec,3

33507 **Repair of anomalous (eg, intramural) aortic origin of coronary artery by unroofing or translocation**

49.8 49.8 FUD 090 C 80

AMA: 2018,Jan,8; 2017,Dec,3; 2017,Jan,8; 2016,Jan,13

33508-33509 Endoscopic Harvesting Bypass Grafts

INCLUDES Diagnostic endoscopy

+ **33508** **Endoscopy, surgical, including video-assisted harvest of vein(s) for coronary artery bypass procedure (List separately in addition to code for primary procedure)**

EXCLUDES *Harvesting upper extremity vein, open (35500)*

Harvesting femoropopliteal vein (35572)

Code first (33510-33523)

0.48 0.48 FUD ZZZ N N1 80

AMA: 1997,Nov,1

● **33509** **Harvest of upper extremity artery, 1 segment, for coronary artery bypass procedure, endoscopic**

EXCLUDES *Harvesting upper extremity artery, open (35600)*

0.00 0.00 FUD 000 ⊘ 50

33510-33523 Coronary Artery Bypass: Venous Grafts

INCLUDES Obtaining saphenous vein grafts

EXCLUDES *Percutaneous ventricular assist devices ([33995], 33990-33993 [33997])*

Code also:

Modifier 80 when assistant at surgery obtains grafts

Vein graft harvest (33508, 35500, 35572)

33510 **Coronary artery bypass, vein only; single coronary venous graft**

55.9 55.9 FUD 090 C 80

AMA: 2018,Jan,8; 2017,Dec,3; 2017,Jan,8; 2016,Jan,13

33511 **2 coronary venous grafts**

61.4 61.4 FUD 090 C 80

AMA: 2018,Jan,8; 2017,Dec,3; 2017,Jan,8; 2016,Jan,13

33512 **3 coronary venous grafts**

70.0 70.0 FUD 090 C 80

AMA: 2018,Jan,8; 2017,Dec,3; 2017,Jan,8; 2016,Jan,13

33513 **4 coronary venous grafts**

71.9 71.9 FUD 090 C 80

AMA: 2018,Jan,8; 2017,Dec,3; 2017,Jan,8; 2016,Jan,13

33514 **5 coronary venous grafts**

75.6 75.6 FUD 090 C 80

AMA: 2018,Jan,8; 2017,Dec,3; 2017,Jan,8; 2016,Jan,13

33516 **6 or more coronary venous grafts**

78.4 78.4 FUD 090 C 80

AMA: 2018,Jan,8; 2017,Dec,3; 2017,Jan,8; 2016,Jan,13

+ **33517** **Coronary artery bypass, using venous graft(s) and arterial graft(s); single vein graft (List separately in addition to code for primary procedure)**

Code first (33533-33536)

5.44 5.44 FUD ZZZ C 80

AMA: 2018,Jan,8; 2017,Jan,8; 2016,Jan,13

\+ **33518** **2 venous grafts (List separately in addition to code for primary procedure)**

Code first (33533-33536)

11.9 11.9 FUD ZZZ C 80

AMA: 2018,Jan,8; 2017,Jan,8; 2016,Jan,13

\+ **33519** **3 venous grafts (List separately in addition to code for primary procedure)**

Code first (33533-33536)

15.8 15.8 FUD ZZZ C 80

AMA: 2018,Jan,8; 2017,Jan,8; 2016,Jan,13

\+ **33521** **4 venous grafts (List separately in addition to code for primary procedure)**

Code first (33533-33536)

18.9 18.9 FUD ZZZ C 80

AMA: 2018,Jan,8; 2017,Jan,8; 2016,Jan,13

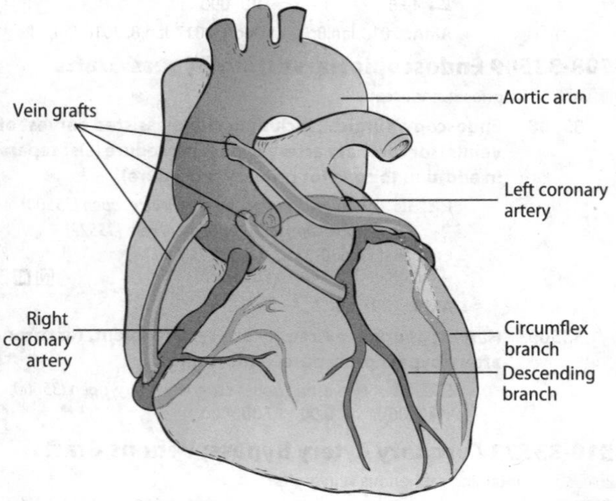

\+ **33522** **5 venous grafts (List separately in addition to code for primary procedure)**

Code first (33533-33536)

21.2 21.2 FUD ZZZ C 80

AMA: 2018,Jan,8; 2017,Jan,8; 2016,Jan,13

\+ **33523** **6 or more venous grafts (List separately in addition to code for primary procedure)**

Code first (33533-33536)

24.0 24.0 FUD ZZZ C 80

AMA: 2018,Jan,8; 2017,Jan,8; 2016,Jan,13

33530 Reoperative Coronary Artery Bypass Graft or Valve Procedure

EXCLUDES *Percutaneous ventricular assist devices (33990-33993)*

Code first (33390-33391, 33404-33496, 33510-33536, 33863)

\+ **33530** **Reoperation, coronary artery bypass procedure or valve procedure, more than 1 month after original operation (List separately in addition to code for primary procedure)**

15.2 15.2 FUD ZZZ C 80

AMA: 2018,Jan,8; 2017,Jan,8; 2016,Jan,13

33533-33536 Coronary Artery Bypass: Arterial Grafts

INCLUDES Arterial grafts obtained from all sites except upper extremity (eg, epigastric, internal mammary, gastroepiploic and others)

EXCLUDES *Percutaneous ventricular assist devices ([33995], 33990-33993 [33997])*
Venous bypass (33510-33516)

Code also:

Arterial graft harvest, upper extremity (eg, radial artery): (33509, 35600)
Combined arterial-venous grafts (33517-33523)
Modifier 80 when assistant at surgery obtains grafts

33533 **Coronary artery bypass, using arterial graft(s); single arterial graft**

54.1 54.1 FUD 090 C 80

AMA: 2018,Jan,8; 2017,Dec,3; 2017,Jan,8; 2016,Jan,13

33534 **2 coronary arterial grafts**

63.6 63.6 FUD 090 C 80

AMA: 2018,Jan,8; 2017,Dec,3; 2017,Jan,8; 2016,Jan,13

33535 **3 coronary arterial grafts**

70.9 70.9 FUD 090 C 80

AMA: 2018,Jan,8; 2017,Dec,3; 2017,Jan,8; 2016,Jan,13

33536 **4 or more coronary arterial grafts**

76.1 76.1 FUD 090 C 80

AMA: 2018,Jan,8; 2017,Dec,3; 2017,Jan,8; 2016,Jan,13

33542-33548 Ventricular Reconstruction

EXCLUDES *Percutaneous ventricular assist devices ([33995], 33990-33993 [33997])*

33542 **Myocardial resection (eg, ventricular aneurysmectomy)**

Code also thrombus removal through separate heart incision, when performed (33310-33315); append modifier 59 to (33315)

76.1 76.1 FUD 090 C 80

AMA: 2018,Jan,8; 2017,Dec,3; 2017,Jan,8; 2016,Jan,13

33545 **Repair of postinfarction ventricular septal defect, with or without myocardial resection**

Code also thrombus removal through separate heart incision, when performed (33310-33315); append modifier 59 to (33315)

89.0 89.0 FUD 090 C 80

AMA: 2018,Jan,8; 2017,Dec,3; 2017,Jan,8; 2016,Jan,13

33548 **Surgical ventricular restoration procedure, includes prosthetic patch, when performed (eg, ventricular remodeling, SVR, SAVER, Dor procedures)**

EXCLUDES *Batista procedure or pachopexy (33999)*
Cardiotomy, exploratory (33310, 33315)
Implantation transcatheter left ventricular restoration device ([0643T])
Temporary pacemaker (33210-33211)
Tube thoracostomy (32551)

85.8 85.8 FUD 090 C 80

AMA: 2018,Jan,8; 2017,Dec,3; 2017,Jan,8; 2016,Jan,13

33572 Endarterectomy with CABG (LAD, RCA, Cx)

Code first (33510-33516, 33533-33536)

\+ **33572** **Coronary endarterectomy, open, any method, of left anterior descending, circumflex, or right coronary artery performed in conjunction with coronary artery bypass graft procedure, each vessel (List separately in addition to primary procedure)**

6.67 6.67 FUD ZZZ C 80

AMA: 1997,Nov,1; 1994,Win,1

33600-33622 Repair Aberrant Heart Anatomy

33600 **Closure of atrioventricular valve (mitral or tricuspid) by suture or patch**

49.8 49.8 FUD 090 C 80

AMA: 2018,Jan,8; 2017,Dec,3; 2017,Jan,8; 2016,Jan,13

33602 **Closure of semilunar valve (aortic or pulmonary) by suture or patch**

Code also concurrent systemic-to-pulmonary artery shunt ligation/takedown (33924)

48.2 48.2 FUD 090 C 80

AMA: 2017,Dec,3

33606 **Anastomosis of pulmonary artery to aorta (Damus-Kaye-Stansel procedure)**

Code also concurrent systemic-to-pulmonary artery shunt ligation/takedown (33924)

51.4 51.4 FUD 090 C 80

AMA: 2017,Dec,3

33608 Repair of complex cardiac anomaly other than pulmonary atresia with ventricular septal defect by construction or replacement of conduit from right or left ventricle to pulmonary artery

EXCLUDES *Unifocalization arborization anomalies pulmonary artery (33925, 33926)*

Code also concurrent systemic-to-pulmonary artery shunt ligation/takedown (33924)

52.2 52.2 FUD 090 C 80

AMA: 2019,Apr,6; 2017,Dec,3

33610 Repair of complex cardiac anomalies (eg, single ventricle with subaortic obstruction) by surgical enlargement of ventricular septal defect

Code also concurrent systemic-to-pulmonary artery shunt ligation/takedown (33924)

51.5 51.5 FUD 090 63 C 80

AMA: 2017,Dec,3

33611 Repair of double outlet right ventricle with intraventricular tunnel repair;

Code also concurrent systemic-to-pulmonary artery shunt ligation/takedown (33924)

56.5 56.5 FUD 090 63 C 80

AMA: 2017,Dec,3

33612 with repair of right ventricular outflow tract obstruction

Code also concurrent systemic-to-pulmonary artery shunt ligation/takedown (33924)

58.2 58.2 FUD 090 C 80

AMA: 2017,Dec,3

33615 Repair of complex cardiac anomalies (eg, tricuspid atresia) by closure of atrial septal defect and anastomosis of atria or vena cava to pulmonary artery (simple Fontan procedure)

Code also concurrent systemic-to-pulmonary artery shunt ligation/takedown (33924)

58.0 58.0 FUD 090 C 80

AMA: 2017,Dec,3

33617 Repair of complex cardiac anomalies (eg, single ventricle) by modified Fontan procedure

Code also:

Cavopulmonary anastomosis to second superior vena cava (33768)

Concurrent systemic-to-pulmonary artery shunt ligation/takedown (33924)

62.6 62.6 FUD 090 C 80

AMA: 2017,Dec,3

33619 Repair of single ventricle with aortic outflow obstruction and aortic arch hypoplasia (hypoplastic left heart syndrome) (eg, Norwood procedure)

79.3 79.3 FUD 090 63 C 80

AMA: 2018,Jan,8; 2017,Dec,3; 2017,Jan,8; 2016,Jul,3; 2016,Jan,13

33620 Application of right and left pulmonary artery bands (eg, hybrid approach stage 1)

EXCLUDES *Banding main pulmonary artery related to septal defect (33690)*

Code also transthoracic insertion catheter for stent placement with catheter removal and closure when performed during same session (33621)

47.7 47.7 FUD 090 C 80

AMA: 2018,Jan,8; 2017,Dec,3; 2017,Jan,8; 2016,Jul,3; 2016,Jan,13

33621 Transthoracic insertion of catheter for stent placement with catheter removal and closure (eg, hybrid approach stage 1)

Code also:

Application right and left pulmonary artery bands when performed during same session (33620)

Stent placement (37236)

26.9 26.9 FUD 090 C 80

AMA: 2018,Jan,8; 2017,Dec,3; 2017,Jan,8; 2016,Jul,3; 2016,Jan,13

33622 Reconstruction of complex cardiac anomaly (eg, single ventricle or hypoplastic left heart) with palliation of single ventricle with aortic outflow obstruction and aortic arch hypoplasia, creation of cavopulmonary anastomosis, and removal of right and left pulmonary bands (eg, hybrid approach stage 2, Norwood, bidirectional Glenn, pulmonary artery debanding)

EXCLUDES *Excision coarctation aorta (33840, 33845, 33851)*
Repair hypoplastic or interrupted aortic arch (33853)
Repair patent ductus arteriosus (33822)
Repair pulmonary artery stenosis by reconstruction with patch or graft (33917)
Repair single ventricle with aortic outflow obstruction and aortic arch hypoplasia (33619)
Shunt; superior vena cava to pulmonary artery for flow to both lungs (33767)

Code also:

Anastomosis, cavopulmonary, second superior vena cava for bilateral bidirectional Glenn procedure (33768)

Concurrent systemic-to-pulmonary artery shunt ligation/takedown (33924)

100. 100. FUD 090 C 80

AMA: 2018,Jan,8; 2017,Dec,3; 2017,Jan,8; 2016,Jul,3; 2016,Jan,13

33641-33645 Closure of Defect: Atrium

Code also thrombus removal through separate heart incision, when performed (33310-33315); append modifier 59 to (33315)

33641 Repair atrial septal defect, secundum, with cardiopulmonary bypass, with or without patch

47.3 47.3 FUD 090 C 80

AMA: 2018,Jan,8; 2017,Dec,3; 2017,Jan,8; 2016,Jan,13

33645 Direct or patch closure, sinus venosus, with or without anomalous pulmonary venous drainage

EXCLUDES *Repair isolated partial anomalous pulmonary venous return (33724)*
Repair pulmonary venous stenosis (33726)

49.8 49.8 FUD 090 C 80

AMA: 2017,Dec,3

33647 Closure of Septal Defect: Atrium AND Ventricle

EXCLUDES *Tricuspid atresia repair procedures (33615)*

Code also thrombus removal through separate heart incision, when performed (33310-33315); append modifier 59 to (33315)

33647 Repair of atrial septal defect and ventricular septal defect, with direct or patch closure

52.6 52.6 FUD 090 63 C 80

AMA: 2017,Dec,3

33660-33670 Closure of Defect: Atrioventricular Canal

33660 Repair of incomplete or partial atrioventricular canal (ostium primum atrial septal defect), with or without atrioventricular valve repair

50.8 50.8 FUD 090 C 80

AMA: 2017,Dec,3

33665 Repair of intermediate or transitional atrioventricular canal, with or without atrioventricular valve repair

55.6 55.6 FUD 090 C 80

AMA: 2017,Dec,3

33670 Repair of complete atrioventricular canal, with or without prosthetic valve

Code also thrombus removal through separate heart incision, when performed (33310-33315); append modifier 59 to (33315)

57.4 57.4 FUD 090 63 C 80

AMA: 2017,Dec,3

33675-33677 Closure of Multiple Septal Defects: Ventricle

EXCLUDES *Closure single ventricular septal defect (33681, 33684, 33688)*
Insertion or replacement temporary transvenous single chamber cardiac electrode or pacemaker catheter (33210)
Percutaneous closure (93581)
Thoracentesis (32554-32555)
Thoracotomy (32100)
Tube thoracostomy (32551)

33675 Closure of multiple ventricular septal defects;
57.1 57.1 **FUD** 090 C 80
AMA: 2018,Jan,8; 2017,Dec,3; 2017,Jan,8; 2016,Jan,13

33676 with pulmonary valvotomy or infundibular resection (acyanotic)
58.6 58.6 **FUD** 090 C 80
AMA: 2018,Jan,8; 2017,Dec,3; 2017,Jan,8; 2016,Jan,13

33677 with removal of pulmonary artery band, with or without gusset
60.9 60.9 **FUD** 090 C 80
AMA: 2018,Jan,8; 2017,Dec,3; 2017,Jan,8; 2016,Jan,13

33681-33688 Closure of Septal Defect: Ventricle

EXCLUDES *Repair pulmonary vein that requires creating an atrial septal defect (33724)*

33681 Closure of single ventricular septal defect, with or without patch;
Code also thrombus removal through separate heart incision, when performed (33310-33315); append modifier 59 to (33315)
53.0 53.0 **FUD** 090 C 80
AMA: 2018,Jan,8; 2017,Dec,3; 2017,Jan,8; 2016,Jan,13

33684 with pulmonary valvotomy or infundibular resection (acyanotic)
Code also concurrent systemic-to-pulmonary artery shunt ligation/takedown, if performed (33924)
54.8 54.8 **FUD** 090 C 80
AMA: 2017,Dec,3

33688 with removal of pulmonary artery band, with or without gusset
Code also concurrent systemic-to-pulmonary artery shunt ligation/takedown, if performed (33924)
54.8 54.8 **FUD** 090 C 80
AMA: 2017,Dec,3

33690 Reduce Pulmonary Overcirculation in Septal Defects

EXCLUDES *Left and right pulmonary artery banding in single ventricle (33620)*

33690 Banding of pulmonary artery
34.7 34.7 **FUD** 090 63 C 80
AMA: 2018,Jan,8; 2017,Jan,8; 2016,Jan,13

33692-33697 Repair of Defects of Tetralogy of Fallot

Code also concurrent systemic-to-pulmonary artery shunt ligation/takedown, when performed (33924)

33692 Complete repair tetralogy of Fallot without pulmonary atresia;
56.6 56.6 **FUD** 090 C 80
AMA: 2017,Dec,3

33694 with transannular patch
56.5 56.5 **FUD** 090 63 C 80
AMA: 2017,Dec,3

33697 Complete repair tetralogy of Fallot with pulmonary atresia including construction of conduit from right ventricle to pulmonary artery and closure of ventricular septal defect
59.7 59.7 **FUD** 090 C 80
AMA: 2018,Jan,8; 2017,Dec,3; 2017,Jan,8; 2016,Jan,13

33702-33722 Repair Anomalies Sinus of Valsalva

33702 Repair sinus of Valsalva fistula, with cardiopulmonary bypass;
44.8 44.8 **FUD** 090 C 80
AMA: 2018,Jan,8; 2017,Dec,3; 2017,Jan,8; 2016,Jan,13

33710 with repair of ventricular septal defect
59.6 59.6 **FUD** 090 C 80
AMA: 2017,Dec,3

33720 Repair sinus of Valsalva aneurysm, with cardiopulmonary bypass
44.7 44.7 **FUD** 090 C 80
AMA: 2017,Dec,3

33722 ~~**Closure of aortico-left ventricular tunnel**~~

33724-33732 Repair Aberrant Pulmonary Venous Connection

33724 Repair of isolated partial anomalous pulmonary venous return (eg, Scimitar Syndrome)
EXCLUDES *Temporary pacemaker (33210-33211)*
Tube thoracostomy (32551)
44.6 44.6 **FUD** 090 C 80
AMA: 2018,Jan,8; 2017,Dec,3; 2017,Jan,8; 2016,Jan,13

33726 Repair of pulmonary venous stenosis
EXCLUDES *Temporary pacemaker (33210-33211)*
Tube thoracostomy (32551)
58.8 58.8 **FUD** 090 C 80
AMA: 2018,Jan,8; 2017,Dec,3; 2017,Jan,8; 2016,Jan,13

33730 Complete repair of anomalous pulmonary venous return (supracardiac, intracardiac, or infracardiac types)
EXCLUDES *Partial anomalous pulmonary venous return (33724)*
Repair pulmonary venous stenosis (33726)
58.0 58.0 **FUD** 090 63 C 80
AMA: 2018,Jan,8; 2017,Dec,3; 2017,Jan,8; 2016,Jan,13

33732 Repair of cor triatriatum or supravalvular mitral ring by resection of left atrial membrane
47.6 47.6 **FUD** 090 63 C 80
AMA: 2018,Jan,8; 2017,Dec,3; 2017,Jan,8; 2016,Jan,13

33735-33737 Creation of Atrial Septal Defect

Code also concurrent systemic-to-pulmonary artery shunt ligation/takedown, when performed (33924)

33735 Atrial septectomy or septostomy; closed heart (Blalock-Hanlon type operation)
37.4 37.4 **FUD** 090 63 C 80
AMA: 2018,Jan,8; 2017,Jan,8; 2016,Jan,13

33736 open heart with cardiopulmonary bypass
40.7 40.7 **FUD** 090 63 C 80
AMA: 2017,Dec,3

33737 open heart, with inflow occlusion
37.6 37.6 **FUD** 090 C 80
AMA: 2020,Nov,7

33741-33746 Transcatheter Procedures

33741 Transcatheter atrial septostomy (TAS) for congenital cardiac anomalies to create effective atrial flow, including all imaging guidance by the proceduralist, when performed, any method (eg, Rashkind, Sang-Park, balloon, cutting balloon, blade)

INCLUDES Angiography to carry out procedure
Fluoroscopic and ultrasound guidance for access and intervention
Percutaneous access, access sheath placement, advancement transcatheter delivery system, creation effective intracardiac blood flow

EXCLUDES *Left heart catheterization via transseptal puncture (93462)*
Septostomy performed for noncongenital indications (93799)

Code also:
Diagnostic congenital cardiac catheterization procedures when patient's condition (clinical indication) changed since intervention or prior study, no available prior catheter-based diagnostic study in treatment zone, or prior study not adequate, and append modifier 59 (93593-93597)
Injection, diagnostic angiography, when performed separate from shunt creation and append modifier 59 (93563, 93565-93568)

22.1 22.1 FUD 000 63 80

33745 Transcatheter intracardiac shunt (TIS) creation by stent placement for congenital cardiac anomalies to establish effective intracardiac flow, including all imaging guidance by the proceduralist, when performed, left and right heart diagnostic cardiac catheterization for congenital cardiac anomalies, and target zone angioplasty, when performed (eg, atrial septum, Fontan fenestration, right ventricular outflow tract, Mustard/Senning/Warden baffles); initial intracardiac shunt

INCLUDES Angiography to carry out procedure
Balloon angioplasty(ies) and dilation(s) performed in target lesion
Diagnostic cardiac catheterization (93451-93453, 93456, 93458, 93460)
Fluoroscopic and ultrasound guidance for access and intervention
Intracardiac stent(s), including angioplasty before and after placement
Percutaneous access, access sheath placement, advancement transcatheter delivery system, creation effective intracardiac blood flow

EXCLUDES *Heart catheterization for congenital cardiac anomalies (93593-93597)*

Code also injection, diagnostic angiography when performed distinctly separate from shunt creation and append modifier 59 (93563, 93565-93568)

31.2 31.2 FUD 000 80

\+ **33746 each additional intracardiac shunt location (List separately in addition to code for primary procedure)**

INCLUDES Balloon angioplasty(ies) and dilation(s) performed in target lesion
Intracardiac stent(s), including angioplasty before and after placement

EXCLUDES *Heart catheterization for congenital cardiac anomalies (93593-93597)*

Code also angioplasty performed in distinctly separate cardiac lesion
Code first (33745)

12.3 12.3 FUD ZZZ 80

33750-33767 Systemic Vessel to Pulmonary Artery Shunts

Code also concurrent systemic-to-pulmonary artery shunt ligation/takedown, when performed (33924)

33750 Shunt; subclavian to pulmonary artery (Blalock-Taussig type operation)
36.5 36.5 FUD 090 63 C 80
AMA: 2017,Dec,3

33755 ascending aorta to pulmonary artery (Waterston type operation)
38.0 38.0 FUD 090 63 C 80
AMA: 2017,Dec,3

33762 descending aorta to pulmonary artery (Potts-Smith type operation)
37.1 37.1 FUD 090 63 C 80
AMA: 2017,Dec,3

33764 central, with prosthetic graft
38.0 38.0 FUD 090 C 80
AMA: 2017,Dec,3

33766 superior vena cava to pulmonary artery for flow to 1 lung (classical Glenn procedure)
38.6 38.6 FUD 090 C 80
AMA: 2017,Dec,3

33767 superior vena cava to pulmonary artery for flow to both lungs (bidirectional Glenn procedure)
41.1 41.1 FUD 090 C 80
AMA: 2018,Jan,8; 2017,Dec,3; 2017,Jan,8; 2016,Jul,3

33768 Cavopulmonary Anastomosis to Decrease Volume Load

EXCLUDES *Temporary pacemaker (33210-33211)*
Tube thoracostomy (32551)

Code first (33478, 33617, 33622, 33767)

\+ **33768 Anastomosis, cavopulmonary, second superior vena cava (List separately in addition to primary procedure)**
12.0 12.0 FUD ZZZ C 80
AMA: 2018,Jan,8; 2017,Jan,8; 2016,Jul,3; 2016,Jan,13

33770-33783 Repair Aberrant Anatomy: Transposition Great Vessels

Code also concurrent systemic-to-pulmonary artery shunt ligation/takedown, when performed (33924)

33770 Repair of transposition of the great arteries with ventricular septal defect and subpulmonary stenosis; without surgical enlargement of ventricular septal defect
61.3 61.3 FUD 090 C 80
AMA: 2018,Jan,8; 2017,Dec,3; 2017,Jan,8; 2016,Jan,13

33771 with surgical enlargement of ventricular septal defect
63.1 63.1 FUD 090 C 80
AMA: 2017,Dec,3

33774 Repair of transposition of the great arteries, atrial baffle procedure (eg, Mustard or Senning type) with cardiopulmonary bypass;
52.0 52.0 FUD 090 C 80
AMA: 2017,Dec,3

33775 with removal of pulmonary band
53.6 53.6 FUD 090 C 80
AMA: 2017,Dec,3

33776 with closure of ventricular septal defect
56.7 56.7 FUD 090 C 80
AMA: 2017,Dec,3

33777 with repair of subpulmonic obstruction
54.9 54.9 FUD 090 C 80
AMA: 2017,Dec,3

33778 Repair of transposition of the great arteries, aortic pulmonary artery reconstruction (eg, Jatene type);
68.0 68.0 FUD 090 63 C 80
AMA: 2017,Dec,3

33779 with removal of pulmonary band
67.4 67.4 FUD 090 C 80
AMA: 2017,Dec,3

33780 with closure of ventricular septal defect
68.6 68.6 FUD 090 C 80
AMA: 2017,Dec,3

33781 **with repair of subpulmonic obstruction**
67.0 67.0 FUD 090 C 80
AMA: 2018,Jan,8; 2017,Dec,3; 2017,Jan,8; 2016,Jan,13

33782 **Aortic root translocation with ventricular septal defect and pulmonary stenosis repair (ie, Nikaidoh procedure); without coronary ostium reimplantation**
EXCLUDES *Closure single ventricular septal defect (33681)*
Repair complex cardiac anomaly other than pulmonary atresia (33608)
Repair pulmonary atresia with ventricular septal defect (33920)
Repair transposition great arteries (33770-33771, 33778, 33780)
Replacement, aortic valve (33412-33413)
94.0 94.0 FUD 090 C 80
AMA: 2017,Dec,3

33783 **with reimplantation of 1 or both coronary ostia**
101. 101. FUD 090 C 80
AMA: 2017,Dec,3

33786-33788 Repair Aberrant Anatomy: Truncus Arteriosus

33786 **Total repair, truncus arteriosus (Rastelli type operation)**
Code also concurrent systemic-to-pulmonary artery shunt ligation/takedown, when performed (33924)
66.0 66.0 FUD 090 63 C 80
AMA: 2018,Jan,8; 2017,Dec,3; 2017,Jan,8; 2016,Jan,13

33788 **Reimplantation of an anomalous pulmonary artery**
EXCLUDES *Pulmonary artery banding (33690)*
44.3 44.3 FUD 090 C 80
AMA: 2018,Jan,8; 2017,Dec,3; 2017,Jan,8; 2016,Jan,13

33800-33853 Repair Aberrant Anatomy: Aorta

33800 **Aortic suspension (aortopexy) for tracheal decompression (eg, for tracheomalacia) (separate procedure)**
28.6 28.6 FUD 090 C 80
AMA: 2018,Jan,8; 2017,Jan,8; 2016,Jan,13

33802 **Division of aberrant vessel (vascular ring);**
31.4 31.4 FUD 090 C 80
AMA: 2017,Dec,3

33803 **with reanastomosis**
33.4 33.4 FUD 090 C 80
AMA: 2017,Dec,3

33813 **Obliteration of aortopulmonary septal defect; without cardiopulmonary bypass**
35.8 35.8 FUD 090 C 80
AMA: 2007,Mar,1-3; 1997,Nov,1

33814 **with cardiopulmonary bypass**
44.1 44.1 FUD 090 C 80
AMA: 2017,Dec,3

33820 **Repair of patent ductus arteriosus; by ligation**
EXCLUDES *Percutaneous transcatheter closure patent ductus arteriosus (93582)*
27.9 27.9 FUD 090 C 80
AMA: 2018,Jan,8; 2017,Dec,3; 2017,Jan,8; 2016,Jan,13

33822 **by division, younger than 18 years** A
EXCLUDES *Percutaneous transcatheter closure patent ductus arteriosus (93582)*
29.6 29.6 FUD 090 C 80
AMA: 2018,Jan,8; 2017,Dec,3; 2017,Jan,8; 2016,Jul,3; 2016,Jan,13

33824 **by division, 18 years and older**
EXCLUDES *Percutaneous closure patent ductus arteriosus (93582)*
34.2 34.2 FUD 090 C 80
AMA: 2017,Dec,3

33840 **Excision of coarctation of aorta, with or without associated patent ductus arteriosus; with direct anastomosis**
35.8 35.8 FUD 090 C 80
AMA: 2018,Jan,8; 2017,Dec,3; 2017,Jan,8; 2016,Jul,3

33845 **with graft**
38.5 38.5 FUD 090 C 80
AMA: 2018,Jan,8; 2017,Dec,3; 2017,Jan,8; 2016,Jul,3

33851 **repair using either left subclavian artery or prosthetic material as gusset for enlargement**
36.8 36.8 FUD 090 C 80
AMA: 2018,Jan,8; 2017,Dec,3; 2017,Jan,8; 2016,Jul,3

33852 **Repair of hypoplastic or interrupted aortic arch using autogenous or prosthetic material; without cardiopulmonary bypass**
EXCLUDES *Hypoplastic left heart syndrome repair by excision coarctation of aorta (33619)*
38.5 38.5 FUD 090 C 80
AMA: 2007,Mar,1-3; 1997,Nov,1

33853 **with cardiopulmonary bypass**
EXCLUDES *Hypoplastic left heart syndrome repair by excision coarctation of aorta (33619)*
53.0 53.0 FUD 090 C 80
AMA: 2018,Jan,8; 2017,Dec,3; 2017,Jan,8; 2016,Jul,3; 2016,Jan,13

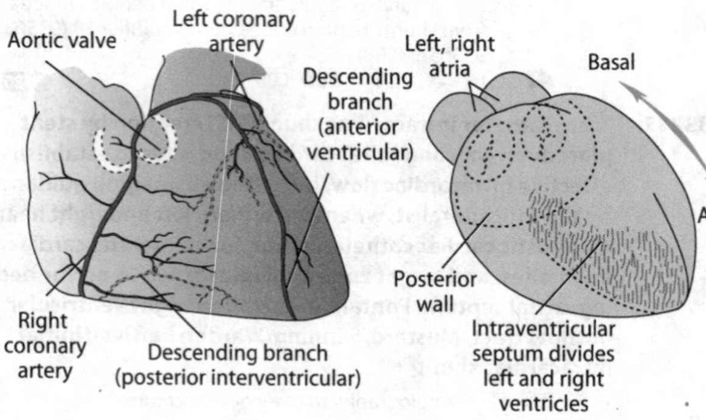

33858-33877 Aortic Graft Procedures

33858 **Ascending aorta graft, with cardiopulmonary bypass, includes valve suspension, when performed; for aortic dissection**
INCLUDES Treatment for aortic dissection
EXCLUDES *Ascending aorta graft:*
Treatment other aortic disease(s), such as aneurysm (33859)
With remodeling aortic root (33864)
With replacement aortic root (33863)
98.5 98.5 FUD 090 80

33859 **for aortic disease other than dissection (eg, aneurysm)**
INCLUDES Treatment of aortic disease(s) other than dissection, such as aneurysm
EXCLUDES *Ascending aorta graft:*
Treatment other aortic dissection (33858)
With remodeling aortic root (33864)
With replacement aortic root (33863)
70.7 70.7 FUD 090 80

33863 **Ascending aorta graft, with cardiopulmonary bypass, with aortic root replacement using valved conduit and coronary reconstruction (eg, Bentall)**
EXCLUDES *Ascending aorta graft:*
With remodeling aortic root (33864)
Without aortic root replacement or remodeling (33858-33859)
Replacement, aortic valve, with cardiopulmonary bypass (33405-33406, 33410-33413)
91.4 91.4 FUD 090 C 80
AMA: 2019,Nov,9; 2018,Jan,8; 2017,Dec,3; 2017,Jan,8; 2016,Jan,13

33864 **Ascending aorta graft, with cardiopulmonary bypass with valve suspension, with coronary reconstruction and valve-sparing aortic root remodeling (eg, David Procedure, Yacoub Procedure)**

EXCLUDES *Ascending aorta graft:*
With replacement aortic root (33863)
Without aortic root replacement or remodeling (33858-33859)

93.3 93.3 **FUD** 090 C 80

AMA: 2019,Nov,9; 2018,Jan,8; 2017,Dec,3; 2017,Jan,8; 2016,Jan,13

\+ **33866** **Aortic hemiarch graft including isolation and control of the arch vessels, beveled open distal aortic anastomosis extending under one or more of the arch vessels, and total circulatory arrest or isolated cerebral perfusion (List separately in addition to code for primary procedure)**

INCLUDES Procedure includes:
Extension ascending aortic graft by beveled anastomosis creation to distal ascending aorta and aortic arch without crossclamp (open anastamosis)
Incision into transverse arch that extends under one or more arch vessels (e.g., left common carotid, left subclavian, innominate artery)
Total circulatory arrest or isolated cerebral perfusion (antegrade or retrograde)

EXCLUDES *Complete transverse arch graft (33871)*

Code first (33858-33859, 33863-33864)

26.7 26.7 **FUD** ZZZ N1 80

AMA: 2019,Nov,9

33871 **Transverse aortic arch graft, with cardiopulmonary bypass, with profound hypothermia, total circulatory arrest and isolated cerebral perfusion with reimplantation of arch vessel(s) (eg, island pedicle or individual arch vessel reimplantation)**

EXCLUDES *Ascending aortic graft (33858-33859, 33863-33864)*
Hemiarch aortic graft performed in addition to ascending aorta graft (33866)

94.7 94.7 **FUD** 090 80

33875 **Descending thoracic aorta graft, with or without bypass**

79.5 79.5 **FUD** 090 C 80

AMA: 2017,Dec,3

33877 **Repair of thoracoabdominal aortic aneurysm with graft, with or without cardiopulmonary bypass**

105. 105. **FUD** 090 C 80

AMA: 2017,Dec,3

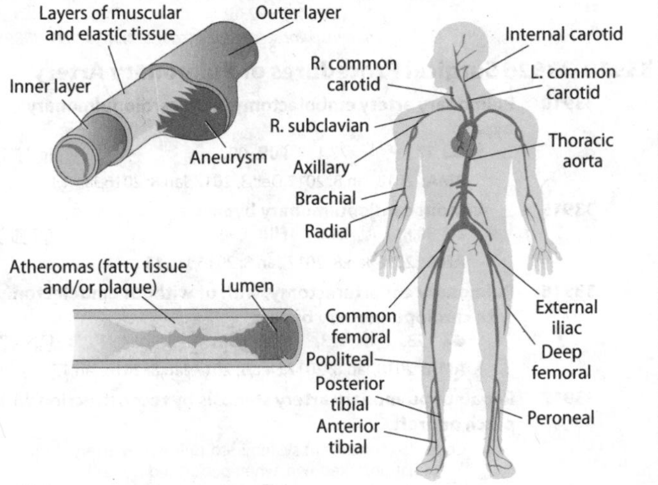

33880-33891 Endovascular Repair Aortic Aneurysm: Thoracic

INCLUDES Balloon angioplasty
Introduction, manipulation, placement, and device deployment
Stent deployment

EXCLUDES *Additional interventional procedures provided during endovascular repair*
Carotid-carotid bypass (33891)
Guidewire and catheter insertion (36140, 36200-36218)
Open exposure artery/subsequent closure ([34812], 34714-34716 [34820, 34833, 34834])
Stent deployment or balloon angioplasty, congenital coarctation or postsurgical recoarctation aorta (33894-33895, 33897)
Subclavian to carotid artery transposition (33889)
Substantial artery repair/replacement (35226, 35286)

33880 **Endovascular repair of descending thoracic aorta (eg, aneurysm, pseudoaneurysm, dissection, penetrating ulcer, intramural hematoma, or traumatic disruption); involving coverage of left subclavian artery origin, initial endoprosthesis plus descending thoracic aortic extension(s), if required, to level of celiac artery origin**

INCLUDES Placement distal extensions in distal thoracic aorta

EXCLUDES *Proximal extensions*

(75956)

52.0 52.0 **FUD** 090 C 80

AMA: 2018,Jan,8; 2017,Dec,3; 2017,Jan,8; 2016,Jan,13

33881 **not involving coverage of left subclavian artery origin, initial endoprosthesis plus descending thoracic aortic extension(s), if required, to level of celiac artery origin**

INCLUDES Placement distal extensions in distal thoracic aorta

EXCLUDES *Procedure where extension placement includes coverage left subclavian artery origin (33880)*
Proximal extensions

(75957)

44.6 44.6 **FUD** 090 C 80

AMA: 2018,Jan,8; 2017,Dec,3; 2017,Jan,8; 2016,Jan,13

33883 **Placement of proximal extension prosthesis for endovascular repair of descending thoracic aorta (eg, aneurysm, pseudoaneurysm, dissection, penetrating ulcer, intramural hematoma, or traumatic disruption); initial extension**

EXCLUDES *Procedure where extension placement includes coverage left subclavian artery origin (33880)*

(75958)

32.3 32.3 **FUD** 090 C 80

AMA: 2018,Jan,8; 2017,Dec,3; 2017,Jan,8; 2016,Jan,13

\+ **33884** **each additional proximal extension (List separately in addition to code for primary procedure)**

Code first (33883)

(75958)

11.5 11.5 **FUD** ZZZ C 80

AMA: 2018,Jan,8; 2017,Dec,3; 2017,Jan,8; 2016,Jan,13

33886 Placement of distal extension prosthesis(s) delayed after endovascular repair of descending thoracic aorta

INCLUDES All modules deployed

EXCLUDES *Endovascular repair descending thoracic aorta (33880, 33881)*

(75959)

27.7 27.7 FUD 090 C 80

AMA: 2018,Jan,8; 2017,Dec,3; 2017,Jan,8; 2016,Jan,13

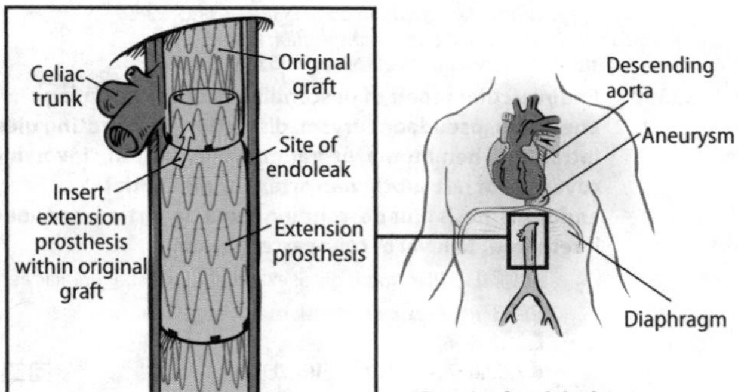

Repair of endoleak in descending thoracic aorta

33889 Open subclavian to carotid artery transposition performed in conjunction with endovascular repair of descending thoracic aorta, by neck incision, unilateral

EXCLUDES *Transposition and/or reimplantation; subclavian to carotid artery (35694)*

22.9 22.9 FUD 000 C 80 50

AMA: 2018,Jan,8; 2017,Jan,8; 2016,Jan,13

33891 Bypass graft, with other than vein, transcervical retropharyngeal carotid-carotid, performed in conjunction with endovascular repair of descending thoracic aorta, by neck incision

EXCLUDES *Bypass graft (35509, 35601)*

28.0 28.0 FUD 000 C 80 50

AMA: 2018,Jan,8; 2017,Jan,8; 2016,Jan,13

33894-33897 Repair Coarctation Aorta

INCLUDES Balloon angioplasty within targeted treatment area
Fluoroscopic guidance for all diagnostic and interventional procedures across the targeted treatment area
Temporay pacemaker insertion (33210)

EXCLUDES *Angiography other vascular structures*
Aortography (75600, 75605, 75625)
Endovascular repair infrarenal aorta and/or iliac artery(ies) by deployment of:
Aorto-aortic tube endograft (34701-34702)
Aorto-uni-iliac or aorto-bi-iliac endograft (34703-34706)
Heart catheterization for congenital heart defect(s) (93595-93597)
Injection during cardiac catheterization (93567)
Introduction catheter, aorta (36200)
Right heart catheterization for congenital heart defect(s), during same operative session (93593-93594)

Code also balloon angioplasty aorta, other than coarctation during same operative session, when performed (37246)

● **33894 Endovascular stent repair of coarctation of the ascending, transverse, or descending thoracic or abdominal aorta, involving stent placement; across major side branches**

INCLUDES Stent(s) deployed over target and as extension from target area
Treatment across one or more major side branches of aorta: brachiocephalic, carotid, celiac, inferior/superior mesenteric, subclavian, and renal arteries

EXCLUDES *Balloon angioplasty within the same treatment area (33897, [37246], 37236)*
Injection during cardiac catheterization (93563-93566, 93568)

Code also interventions performed on other vessels (i.e., carotid, iliac, innomiante, pulmonary, subclavian, visceral), including balloon angioplasty, embolization, and stenting, during same operative session, when performed

● **33895 not crossing major side branches**

INCLUDES Stent(s) deployed over target and as extension from target area

EXCLUDES *Balloon angioplasty within the same treatment area (33897, [37246], 37236)*
Injection during cardiac catheterization (93563-93566, 93568)

Code also interventions performed on other vessels (i.e., carotid, iliac, innominate, pulmonary, subclavian, visceral), including balloon angioplasty, embolization, and stenting, during same operative session, when performed

● **33897 Percutaneous transluminal angioplasty of native or recurrent coarctation of the aorta**

INCLUDES Dilation coarctation utilizing balloon angioplasty without stent deployment

EXCLUDES *Balloon angioplasty within the same treatment area ([37246], 37236)*
Endovascular stent repair, coarctation (33894-33895)

33910-33926 Surgical Procedures of Pulmonary Artery

33910 Pulmonary artery embolectomy; with cardiopulmonary bypass

77.1 77.1 FUD 090 C 80

AMA: 2018,Jan,8; 2017,Dec,3; 2017,Jan,8; 2016,Jan,13

33915 without cardiopulmonary bypass

39.8 39.8 FUD 090 C 80

AMA: 2018,Jan,8; 2017,Jan,8; 2016,Jan,13

33916 Pulmonary endarterectomy, with or without embolectomy, with cardiopulmonary bypass

123. 123. FUD 090 C 80

AMA: 2018,Jan,8; 2017,Dec,3; 2017,Jan,8; 2016,Jan,13

33917 Repair of pulmonary artery stenosis by reconstruction with patch or graft

Code also concurrent systemic-to-pulmonary artery shunt ligation/takedown, when performed (33924)

42.1 42.1 FUD 090 C 80

AMA: 2018,Jan,8; 2017,Dec,3; 2017,Jan,8; 2016,Jul,3; 2016,Jan,13

33920 Repair of pulmonary atresia with ventricular septal defect, by construction or replacement of conduit from right or left ventricle to pulmonary artery

EXCLUDES *Repair complicated cardiac anomalies by creating/replacing conduit from ventricle to pulmonary artery (33608)*

Code also concurrent systemic-to-pulmonary artery shunt ligation/takedown, when performed (33924)

52.4 52.4 FUD 090 C 80

AMA: 2019,Apr,6; 2018,Jan,8; 2017,Dec,3; 2017,Jan,8; 2016,Jan,13

33922 Transection of pulmonary artery with cardiopulmonary bypass

Code also concurrent systemic-to-pulmonary artery shunt ligation/takedown, when performed (33924)

40.1 40.1 FUD 090 63 C 80

AMA: 2017,Dec,3

\+ **33924 Ligation and takedown of a systemic-to-pulmonary artery shunt, performed in conjunction with a congenital heart procedure (List separately in addition to code for primary procedure)**

Code first (33471-33478, 33600-33617, 33622, 33684-33688, 33692-33697, 33735-33767, 33770-33783, 33786, 33917, 33920-33922, 33925-33926, 33935, 33945)

8.29 8.29 FUD ZZZ C 80

AMA: 1997,Nov,1; 1995,Win,1

33925 Repair of pulmonary artery arborization anomalies by unifocalization; without cardiopulmonary bypass

Code also concurrent systemic-to-pulmonary artery shunt ligation/takedown, when performed (33924)

49.7 49.7 FUD 090 C 80

33926 with cardiopulmonary bypass

Code also concurrent systemic-to-pulmonary artery shunt ligation/takedown, when performed (33924)

70.0 70.0 FUD 090 C 80

AMA: 2017,Dec,3

33927-33945 Heart and Heart-Lung Transplants

INCLUDES Backbench work to prepare donor heart and/or lungs for transplantation (33933, 33944)
Harvesting donor organs with cold preservation (33930, 33940)
Transplantation heart and/or lungs into recipient (33935, 33945)

33927 Implantation of a total replacement heart system (artificial heart) with recipient cardiectomy

EXCLUDES *Implantation ventricular assist device:*
Extracorporeal (33975-33976)
Intracorporeal (33979)
Percutaneous ([33995], 33990-33991)

74.2 74.2 FUD XXX C 80

AMA: 2018,Jun,3

33928 Removal and replacement of total replacement heart system (artificial heart)

EXCLUDES *Replacement or revision elements artificial heart (33999)*

0.00 0.00 FUD XXX C 80

AMA: 2018,Jun,3

\+ **33929 Removal of a total replacement heart system (artificial heart) for heart transplantation (List separately in addition to code for primary procedure)**

Code first (33945)

0.00 0.00 FUD ZZZ C 80

AMA: 2018,Jun,3

33930 Donor cardiectomy-pneumonectomy (including cold preservation)

0.00 0.00 FUD XXX C

AMA: 1997,Nov,1

33933 Backbench standard preparation of cadaver donor heart/lung allograft prior to transplantation, including dissection of allograft from surrounding soft tissues to prepare aorta, superior vena cava, inferior vena cava, and trachea for implantation

0.00 0.00 FUD XXX C 80

AMA: 1997,Nov,1

33935 Heart-lung transplant with recipient cardiectomy-pneumonectomy

Code also concurrent systemic-to-pulmonary artery shunt ligation/takedown, when performed (33924)

143. 143. FUD 090 C 80

AMA: 2017,Dec,3

33940 Donor cardiectomy (including cold preservation)

0.00 0.00 FUD XXX C

AMA: 2018,Jan,8; 2017,Jan,8; 2016,Jan,13

33944 Backbench standard preparation of cadaver donor heart allograft prior to transplantation, including dissection of allograft from surrounding soft tissues to prepare aorta, superior vena cava, inferior vena cava, pulmonary artery, and left atrium for implantation

EXCLUDES *Procedures performed on donor heart (33300, 33310, 33320, 33390, 33463-33464, 33510, 33641, 35216, 35276, 35685)*

0.00 0.00 FUD XXX C 80

AMA: 1997,Nov,1

33945 Heart transplant, with or without recipient cardiectomy

Code also concurrent systemic-to-pulmonary artery shunt ligation/takedown, when performed (33924)

141. 141. FUD 090 C 80

AMA: 2018,Jun,3; 2017,Dec,3

33946-33989 [33962, 33963, 33964, 33965, 33966, 33969, 33984, 33985, 33986, 33987, 33988, 33989] Extracorporeal Circulatory and Respiratory Support

INCLUDES Cannula repositioning and cannula insertion performed during same procedure
Multiple physician and nonphysician team collaboration
Veno-arterial ECMO/ECLS for heart and lung support
Veno-venous ECMO/ECLS for lung support

Code also:
Extensive arterial repair/replacement (35266, 35286, 35371, 35665)
Overall daily management services needed to manage patient; report appropriate observation, hospital inpatient, or critical care E/M codes

33946 Extracorporeal membrane oxygenation (ECMO)/extracorporeal life support (ECLS) provided by physician; initiation, veno-venous

EXCLUDES *Daily ECMO/ECLS veno-venous management initial service date (33948)*
Repositioning ECMO/ECLS cannula initial service date (33957-33959 [33962, 33963, 33964])

Code also cannula insertion (33951-33956)

8.95 8.95 FUD XXX 63 C

AMA: 2018,Jan,8; 2017,Jan,8; 2016,Mar,5; 2016,Jan,13

33947 initiation, veno-arterial

EXCLUDES *Daily ECMO/ECLS veno-venous management initial service date (33948)*
Repositioning ECMO/ECLS cannula initial service date (33957-33959 [33962, 33963, 33964])

Code also cannula insertion (33951-33956)

9.99 9.99 FUD XXX 63 C

AMA: 2018,Jan,8; 2017,Jan,8; 2016,Mar,5; 2016,Jan,13

33948 daily management, each day, veno-venous

EXCLUDES *ECMO/ECLS initiation, veno-venous (33946)*

6.94 6.94 FUD XXX 63 C

AMA: 2018,Jan,8; 2017,Jan,8; 2016,Mar,5; 2016,Jan,13

33949 daily management, each day, veno-arterial

EXCLUDES *ECMO/ECLS initiation, veno-arterial (33947)*

6.73 6.73 FUD XXX 63 C

AMA: 2018,Jan,8; 2017,Jan,8; 2016,Mar,5; 2016,Jan,13

33951 insertion of peripheral (arterial and/or venous) cannula(e), percutaneous, birth through 5 years of age (includes fluoroscopic guidance, when performed) A

INCLUDES Cannula replacement same vessel
Cannula repositioning during same episode care

Code also:
Cannula removal when new cannula inserted in different vessel with ([33965, 33966, 33969, 33984, 33985, 33986])
ECMO/ECLS initiation or daily management (33946-33947, 33948-33949)

12.3 12.3 **FUD** 000 C 80

AMA: 2018,Jan,8; 2017,Jan,8; 2016,Mar,5; 2016,Jan,13

33952 insertion of peripheral (arterial and/or venous) cannula(e), percutaneous, 6 years and older (includes fluoroscopic guidance, when performed) A

INCLUDES Cannula replacement same vessel
Cannula repositioning during same episode care

Code also:
Cannula removal when new cannula inserted in different vessel with ([33965, 33966, 33969, 33984, 33985, 33986])
ECMO/ECLS initiation or daily management (33946-33947, 33948-33949)

12.4 12.4 **FUD** 000 C 80

AMA: 2018,Jan,8; 2017,Jan,8; 2016,Mar,5; 2016,Jan,13

33953 insertion of peripheral (arterial and/or venous) cannula(e), open, birth through 5 years of age A

INCLUDES Cannula replacement same vessel
Cannula repositioning during same episode care

EXCLUDES *Open artery exposure for delivery/deployment endovascular prosthesis ([34812], 34714-34716 [34820, 34833, 34834], [34820])*

Code also:
Cannula removal when new cannula inserted in different vessel with ([33965, 33966, 33969, 33984, 33985, 33986])
ECMO/ECLS initiation or daily management (33946-33947, 33948-33949)

13.8 13.8 **FUD** 000 C 80

AMA: 2018,Jan,8; 2017,Dec,3; 2017,Jan,8; 2016,Mar,5; 2016,Jan,13

33954 insertion of peripheral (arterial and/or venous) cannula(e), open, 6 years and older A

INCLUDES Cannula replacement same vessel
Cannula repositioning during same episode care

EXCLUDES *Open artery exposure for delivery/deployment endovascular prosthesis ([34812], 34714-34716 [34820, 34833, 34834])*

Code also:
Cannula removal when new cannula inserted in different vessel with ([33965, 33966, 33969, 33984, 33985, 33986])
ECMO/ECLS initiation or daily management (33946-33947, 33948-33949)

13.8 13.8 **FUD** 000 C 80

AMA: 2018,Jan,8; 2017,Dec,3; 2017,Jan,8; 2016,Mar,5; 2016,Jan,13

33955 insertion of central cannula(e) by sternotomy or thoracotomy, birth through 5 years of age A

INCLUDES Cannula replacement same vessel
Cannula repositioning during same episode care

EXCLUDES *Mediastinotomy (39010)*
Thoracotomy (32100)

Code also:
Cannula removal when new cannula inserted in different vessel with ([33965, 33966, 33969, 33984, 33985, 33986])
ECMO/ECLS initiation or daily management (33946-33947, 33948-33949)

24.0 24.0 **FUD** 000 C 80

AMA: 2018,Jan,8; 2017,Jan,8; 2016,Mar,5; 2016,Jan,13

33956 insertion of central cannula(e) by sternotomy or thoracotomy, 6 years and older A

INCLUDES Cannula replacement same vessel
Cannula repositioning during same episode care

EXCLUDES *Mediastinotomy (39010)*
Thoracotomy (32100)

Code also:
Cannula removal when new cannula inserted in different vessel with ([33965, 33966, 33969, 33984, 33985, 33986])
ECMO/ECLS initiation or daily management (33946-33947, 33948-33949)

24.2 24.2 **FUD** 000 C 80

AMA: 2018,Jan,8; 2017,Jan,8; 2016,Mar,5; 2016,Jan,13

33957 reposition peripheral (arterial and/or venous) cannula(e), percutaneous, birth through 5 years of age (includes fluoroscopic guidance, when performed) A

INCLUDES Fluoroscopic guidance

EXCLUDES *ECMO/ECLS initiation, veno-arterial (33947)*
ECMO/ECLS initiation, veno-venous (33946)
ECMO/ECLS insertion cannula (33951-33956)
Percutaneous access and closure femoral artery for endograft delivery (34713)

5.36 5.36 **FUD** 000 C 80

AMA: 2018,Jan,8; 2017,Jan,8; 2016,Mar,5; 2016,Jan,13

33958 reposition peripheral (arterial and/or venous) cannula(e), percutaneous, 6 years and older (includes fluoroscopic guidance, when performed) A

INCLUDES Fluoroscopic guidance

EXCLUDES *ECMO/ECLS initiation, veno-arterial (33947)*
ECMO/ECLS initiation, veno-venous (33946)
ECMO/ECLS insertion of cannula (33951-33956)
Percutaneous access and closure femoral artery for endograft delivery (34713)

5.36 5.36 **FUD** 000 C 80

AMA: 2018,Jan,8; 2017,Jan,8; 2016,Mar,5; 2016,Jan,13

33959 reposition peripheral (arterial and/or venous) cannula(e), open, birth through 5 years of age (includes fluoroscopic guidance, when performed) A

INCLUDES Fluoroscopic guidance

EXCLUDES *ECMO/ECLS initiation, veno-arterial (33947)*
ECMO/ECLS initiation, veno-venous (33946)
ECMO/ECLS insertion of cannula (33951-33956)
Open artery exposure for delivery/deployment endovascular prosthesis ([34812], 34714-34716 [34820, 34833, 34834])

6.84 6.84 **FUD** 000 C 80

AMA: 2018,Jan,8; 2017,Dec,3; 2017,Jan,8; 2016,Mar,5; 2016,Jan,13

33962 reposition peripheral (arterial and/or venous) cannula(e), open, 6 years and older (includes fluoroscopic guidance, when performed) A

INCLUDES Fluoroscopic guidance

EXCLUDES *ECMO/ECLS initiation, veno-arterial (33947)*
ECMO/ECLS initiation, veno-venous (33946)
ECMO/ECLS insertion of cannula (33951-33956)
Open artery exposure for delivery/deployment endovascular prosthesis ([34812], 34714-34716 [34820, 34833, 34834])

6.79 6.79 **FUD** 000 C 80

AMA: 2018,Jan,8; 2017,Dec,3; 2017,Jan,8; 2016,Mar,5; 2016,Jan,13

33963 **reposition of central cannula(e) by sternotomy or thoracotomy, birth through 5 years of age (includes fluoroscopic guidance, when performed)** A

INCLUDES Fluoroscopic guidance

EXCLUDES *ECMO/ECLS initiation, veno-arterial (33947)*
ECMO/ECLS initiation, veno-venous (33946)
ECMO/ECLS insertion of cannula (33951-33956)
Open artery exposure for delivery/deployment endovascular prosthesis ([34812], 34714-34716 [34820, 34833, 34834])

13.5 13.5 FUD 000 C 80

AMA: 2018,Jan,8; 2017,Jan,8; 2016,Mar,5; 2016,Jan,13

33964 **reposition central cannula(e) by sternotomy or thoracotomy, 6 years and older (includes fluoroscopic guidance, when performed)** A

INCLUDES Fluoroscopic guidance

EXCLUDES *ECMO/ECLS initiation, veno-arterial (33947)*
ECMO/ECLS initiation, veno-venous (33946)
ECMO/ECLS insertion cannula (33951-33956)
Mediastinotomy (39010)
Thoracotomy (32100)

14.3 14.3 FUD 000 C 80

AMA: 2018,Jan,8; 2017,Jan,8; 2016,Mar,5; 2016,Jan,13

33965 **removal of peripheral (arterial and/or venous) cannula(e), percutaneous, birth through 5 years of age** A

Code also:
Extensive arterial repair/replacement, when performed (35266, 35286, 35371, 35665)
New cannula insertion into different vessel (33951-33956)

5.36 5.36 FUD 000 C 80

AMA: 2018,Jan,8; 2017,Jan,8; 2016,Mar,5; 2016,Jan,13

33966 **removal of peripheral (arterial and/or venous) cannula(e), percutaneous, 6 years and older** A

Code also:
Extensive arterial repair/replacement, when performed (35266, 35286, 35371, 35665)
New cannula insertion into different vessel (33951-33956)

6.87 6.87 FUD 000 C 80

AMA: 2018,Jan,8; 2017,Jan,8; 2016,Mar,5; 2016,Jan,13

33969 **removal of peripheral (arterial and/or venous) cannula(e), open, birth through 5 years of age** A

EXCLUDES *Open artery exposure for delivery/deployment endovascular prosthesis ([34812], 34714-34716 [34820, 34833, 34834])*
Repair blood vessel (35201, 35206, 35211, 35216, 35226)

Code also:
Extensive arterial repair/replacement, when performed (35266, 35286, 35371, 35665)
New cannula insertion into different vessel (33951-33956)

7.98 7.98 FUD 000 C 80

AMA: 2018,Jan,8; 2017,Dec,3; 2017,Jan,8; 2016,Mar,5; 2016,Jan,13

33984 **removal of peripheral (arterial and/or venous) cannula(e), open, 6 years and older** A

EXCLUDES *Open artery exposure for delivery/deployment endovascular prosthesis ([34812], 34714-34716 [34820, 34833, 34834])*
Repair blood vessel (35201, 35206, 35211, 35216, 35226)

8.25 8.25 FUD 000 C 80

AMA: 2018,Jan,8; 2017,Dec,3; 2017,Jan,8; 2016,Mar,5; 2016,Jan,13

33985 **removal of central cannula(e) by sternotomy or thoracotomy, birth through 5 years of age** A

EXCLUDES *Repair blood vessel (35201, 35206, 35211, 35216, 35226)*

Code also:
Extensive arterial repair/replacement, when performed (35266, 35286, 35371, 35665)
New cannula insertion into different vessel (33951-33956)

14.9 14.9 FUD 000 C 80

AMA: 2018,Jan,8; 2017,Jan,8; 2016,Mar,5; 2016,Jan,13

33986 **removal of central cannula(e) by sternotomy or thoracotomy, 6 years and older** A

EXCLUDES *Repair blood vessel (35201, 35206, 35211, 35216, 35226)*

Code also:
Extensive arterial repair/replacement, when performed (35266, 35286, 35371, 35665)
New cannula insertion into different vessel (33951-33956)

15.1 15.1 FUD 000 C 80

AMA: 2018,Jan,8; 2017,Jan,8; 2016,Mar,5; 2016,Jan,13

+ # 33987 **Arterial exposure with creation of graft conduit (eg, chimney graft) to facilitate arterial perfusion for ECMO/ECLS (List separately in addition to code for primary procedure)**

EXCLUDES *Open artery exposure for delivery/deployment endovascular prosthesis ([34812], 34714-34716 [34820, 34833, 34834])*

Code first (33953-33956)

6.09 6.09 FUD ZZZ C 80

AMA: 2018,Jan,8; 2017,Dec,3; 2017,Jan,8; 2016,Mar,5; 2016,Jan,13

33988 **Insertion of left heart vent by thoracic incision (eg, sternotomy, thoracotomy) for ECMO/ECLS**

22.5 22.5 FUD 000 C 80

AMA: 2018,Jan,8; 2017,Jan,8; 2016,Mar,5; 2016,Jan,13

33989 **Removal of left heart vent by thoracic incision (eg, sternotomy, thoracotomy) for ECMO/ECLS**

14.3 14.3 FUD 000 C 80

AMA: 2018,Jan,8; 2017,Jan,8; 2016,Mar,5; 2016,Jan,13

33962-33999 [33962, 33963, 33964, 33965, 33966, 33969, 33984, 33985, 33986, 33987, 33988, 33989, 33995, 33997] Mechanical Circulatory Support

EXCLUDES *Insertion, removal, replacement, or repositioning permanently implantable aortic counterpulsation ventricular assist system (33999)*

33962 **Resequenced code. See code following 33959.**

33963 **Resequenced code. See code following 33959.**

33964 **Resequenced code. See code following 33959.**

33965 **Resequenced code. See code following 33959.**

33966 **Resequenced code. See code following 33959.**

33967 **Insertion of intra-aortic balloon assist device, percutaneous**

7.51 7.51 FUD 000 C 80

AMA: 2018,Jan,8; 2017,Jan,8; 2016,Mar,5; 2016,Jan,13

33968 **Removal of intra-aortic balloon assist device, percutaneous**

0.98 0.98 FUD 000 C

AMA: 2018,Jan,8; 2017,Jan,8; 2016,Mar,5; 2016,Jan,13

33969 **Resequenced code. See code following 33959.**

33970 **Insertion of intra-aortic balloon assist device through the femoral artery, open approach**

EXCLUDES *Percutaneous insertion intra-aortic balloon assist device (33967)*

10.2 10.2 FUD 000 C 80

AMA: 2018,Jan,8; 2017,Jan,8; 2016,Mar,5; 2016,Jan,13

33971 **Removal of intra-aortic balloon assist device including repair of femoral artery, with or without graft**

20.3 20.3 FUD 090 C

AMA: 2018,Jan,8; 2017,Jan,8; 2016,Mar,5; 2016,Jan,13

33973 **Insertion of intra-aortic balloon assist device through the ascending aorta**

14.8 14.8 FUD 000 C 80

AMA: 2018,Jan,8; 2017,Jan,8; 2016,Mar,5; 2016,Jan,13

33974 **Removal of intra-aortic balloon assist device from the ascending aorta, including repair of the ascending aorta, with or without graft**

25.7 25.7 FUD 090 C

AMA: 2018,Jan,8; 2017,Jan,8; 2016,Mar,5; 2016,Jan,13

33975 Insertion of ventricular assist device; extracorporeal, single ventricle

INCLUDES Insertion new pump with de-airing, connection, and initiation
Removal old pump with replacement entire ventricular assist device system, including pump(s) and cannulas
Transthoracic approach

EXCLUDES *Percutaneous approach ([33995], 33990-33991)*

Code also removal thrombus through separate heart incision, when performed (33310-33315); append modifier 59 to (33315)

37.8 37.8 **FUD** XXX C 80

AMA: 2018,Jun,3; 2018,Jan,8; 2017,Dec,3; 2017,Jan,8; 2016,Mar,5; 2016,Jan,13

33976 extracorporeal, biventricular

INCLUDES Insertion new pump with de-airing, connection, and initiation
Removal with replacement entire ventricular assist device system, including pump(s) and cannulas
Transthoracic approach

EXCLUDES *Percutaneous approach ([33995], 33990-33991)*

Code also removal thrombus through separate heart incision, when performed (33310-33315); append modifier 59 to (33315)

46.0 46.0 **FUD** XXX C 80

AMA: 2018,Jun,3; 2018,Jan,8; 2017,Dec,3; 2017,Jan,8; 2016,Mar,5; 2016,Jan,13

33977 Removal of ventricular assist device; extracorporeal, single ventricle

INCLUDES Removal entire device and cannulas

EXCLUDES *Removal ventricular assist device when performed same time as new device insertion*

Code also thrombus removal through separate heart incision, when performed (33310-33315); append modifier 59 to (33315)

32.6 32.6 **FUD** XXX C 80

AMA: 2018,Jan,8; 2017,Dec,3; 2017,Jan,8; 2016,Mar,5; 2016,Jan,13

33978 extracorporeal, biventricular

INCLUDES Removal entire device and cannulas

EXCLUDES *Removal ventricular assist device when performed same time as new device insertion*

Code also thrombus removal through separate heart incision, when performed (33310-33315); append modifier 59 to (33315)

38.5 38.5 **FUD** XXX C 80

AMA: 2018,Jan,8; 2017,Dec,3; 2017,Jan,8; 2016,Mar,5; 2016,Jan,13

33979 Insertion of ventricular assist device, implantable intracorporeal, single ventricle

INCLUDES New pump insertion with connection, de-airing, and initiation
Removal with replacement entire ventricular assist device system, including pump(s) and cannulas
Transthoracic approach

EXCLUDES *Percutaneous approach ([33995], 33990-33991)*

Code also thrombus removal through separate heart incision, when performed (33310-33315); append modifier 59 to (33315)

56.5 56.5 **FUD** XXX C 80

AMA: 2018,Jun,3; 2018,Jan,8; 2017,Dec,3; 2017,Jan,8; 2016,Mar,5; 2016,Jan,13

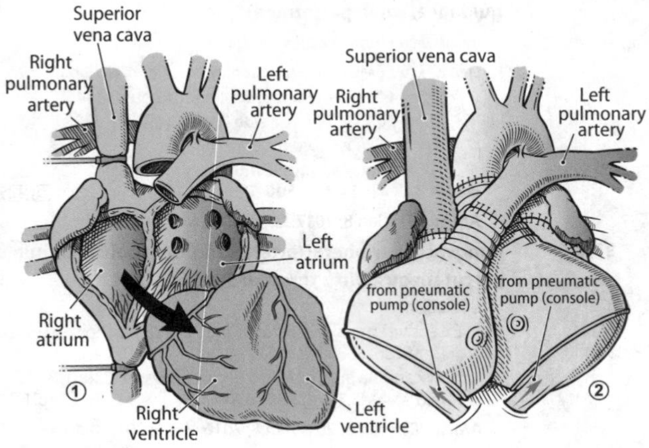

33980 Removal of ventricular assist device, implantable intracorporeal, single ventricle

INCLUDES Removal entire device and cannulas

EXCLUDES *Removal ventricular assist device when performed same time as new device insertion*

Code also thrombus removal through separate heart incision, when performed (33310-33315); append modifier 59 to (33315)

51.5 51.5 **FUD** XXX C 80

AMA: 2018,Jan,8; 2017,Dec,3; 2017,Jan,8; 2016,Mar,5; 2016,Jan,13

33981 Replacement of extracorporeal ventricular assist device, single or biventricular, pump(s), single or each pump

INCLUDES New pump insertion with de-airing, connection, and initiation
Removal old pump

24.3 24.3 **FUD** XXX C 80

AMA: 2018,Jan,8; 2017,Jan,8; 2016,Mar,5; 2016,Jan,13

33982 Replacement of ventricular assist device pump(s); implantable intracorporeal, single ventricle, without cardiopulmonary bypass

INCLUDES New pump insertion with connection, de-airing, and initiation
Removal old pump

57.1 57.1 **FUD** XXX C 80

AMA: 2018,Jan,8; 2017,Jan,8; 2016,Mar,5; 2016,Jan,13

33983 implantable intracorporeal, single ventricle, with cardiopulmonary bypass

INCLUDES Removal old pump

EXCLUDES *Percutaneous transseptal approach (33999)*

67.0 67.0 **FUD** XXX C 80

AMA: 2018,Jan,8; 2017,Dec,3; 2017,Jan,8; 2016,Mar,5; 2016,Jan,13

33984 **Resequenced code. See code following 33959.**

33985 **Resequenced code. See code following 33959.**

33986 **Resequenced code. See code following 33959.**

33987 **Resequenced code. See code following 33959.**

33988 **Resequenced code. See code following 33959.**

33989 **Resequenced code. See code following 33959.**

\# **33995** **Insertion of ventricular assist device, percutaneous, including radiological supervision and interpretation; right heart, venous access only**

INCLUDES Initial insertion and replacement percutaneous ventricular assist device

EXCLUDES *Extensive artery repair/replacement (35226, 35286)*
Open arterial approach to aid insertion percutaneous ventricular assist device, when used ([34812], 34714-34716 [34820, 34833, 34834])
Removal percutaneous ventricular assist device with entire system replacement (33992)
Transthoracic approach (33975-33976, 33979)

10.6 10.6 **FUD** 000 80

AMA: 2020,Dec,4

33990 **left heart, arterial access only**

INCLUDES Initial insertion and replacement percutaneous ventricular assist device

EXCLUDES *Extensive artery repair/replacement (35226, 35286)*
Open arterial approach to aid insertion percutaneous ventricular assist device, when used ([34812], 34714-34716 [34820, 34833, 34834])
Removal percutaneous ventricular assist device with entire system replacement (33992)
Transthoracic approach (33975-33976, 33979)

12.4 12.4 **FUD** XXX C 80

AMA: 2020,Dec,4; 2018,Jun,3; 2018,Jan,8; 2017,Dec,3; 2017,Jan,8; 2016,Mar,5; 2016,Jan,13

33991 **left heart, both arterial and venous access, with transseptal puncture**

INCLUDES Initial insertion and replacement percutaneous ventricular assist device

EXCLUDES *Extensive artery repair/replacement (35226, 35286)*
Open arterial approach to aid with insertion percutaneous ventricular assist device, when performed (34812 [34812], 34714-34716 [34820, 34833, 34834])
Removal percutaneous ventricular assist device with entire system replacement (33992)
Transthoracic approach (33975-33976, 33979)

18.1 18.1 **FUD** XXX C 80

AMA: 2020,Dec,4; 2018,Jun,3; 2018,Jan,8; 2017,Dec,3; 2017,Jan,8; 2016,Mar,5; 2016,Jan,13

33992 **Removal of percutaneous left heart ventricular assist device, arterial or arterial and venous cannula(s), at separate and distinct session from insertion**

INCLUDES Removal device and cannulas

Code also modifier 59 when percutaneous ventricular assist device removed on same day as insertion, but different session

5.80 5.80 **FUD** XXX C 80

AMA: 2020,Dec,4; 2018,Jan,8; 2017,Jan,8; 2016,Mar,5; 2016,Jan,13

\# **33997** **Removal of percutaneous right heart ventricular assist device, venous cannula, at separate and distinct session from insertion**

4.72 4.72 **FUD** 000 80

AMA: 2020,Dec,4

33993 **Repositioning of percutaneous right or left heart ventricular assist device with imaging guidance at separate and distinct session from insertion**

EXCLUDES *Repositioning percutaneous ventricular assist device without image guidance*
Repositioning percutaneous ventricular assist device same session as insertion (33990-33991)

Code also modifier 59 when percutaneous ventricular assist device repositioned using imaging guidance on same day as insertion, but different session

5.09 5.09 **FUD** XXX C 80

AMA: 2020,Dec,4; 2018,Jan,8; 2017,Jan,8; 2016,Mar,5; 2016,Jan,13

33995 **Resequenced code. See code following 33983.**

33997 **Resequenced code. See code following 33992.**

33999 **Unlisted procedure, cardiac surgery**

0.00 0.00 **FUD** YYY T 80

AMA: 2019,Apr,10; 2019,Jan,14; 2018,Jun,3; 2018,Jan,8; 2017,Jan,8; 2016,May,5; 2016,Jan,13

34001-34530 Surgical Revascularization: Veins and Arteries

INCLUDES Repair blood vessel
Surgeon's component operative arteriogram

34001 **Embolectomy or thrombectomy, with or without catheter; carotid, subclavian or innominate artery, by neck incision**

27.8 27.8 **FUD** 090 C 80 50

AMA: 1997,Nov,1

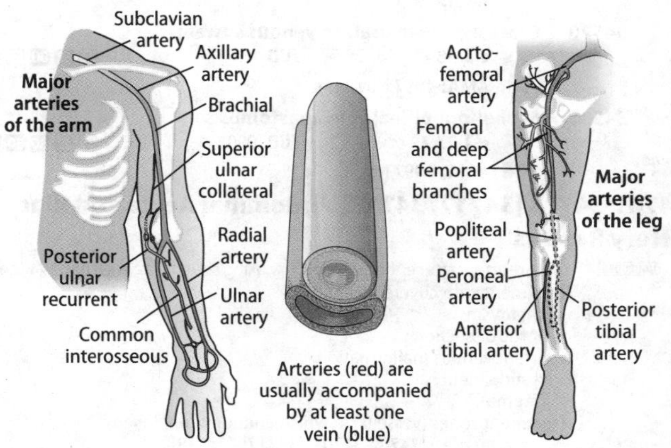

34051 **innominate, subclavian artery, by thoracic incision**

28.6 28.6 **FUD** 090 C 80 50

AMA: 1997,Nov,1

34101 **axillary, brachial, innominate, subclavian artery, by arm incision**

17.3 17.3 **FUD** 090 T 62 80 50

AMA: 1997,Nov,1

34111 **radial or ulnar artery, by arm incision**

17.3 17.3 **FUD** 090 T 62 80 50

AMA: 1997,Nov,1

34151 **renal, celiac, mesentery, aortoiliac artery, by abdominal incision**

40.4 40.4 **FUD** 090 C 80 50

AMA: 1997,Nov,1

34201 **femoropopliteal, aortoiliac artery, by leg incision**

29.8 29.8 **FUD** 090 T 62 80 50

AMA: 2018,Jan,8; 2017,Jan,8; 2016,Jan,13

34203 **popliteal-tibio-peroneal artery, by leg incision**

27.6 27.6 **FUD** 090 T 62 80 50

AMA: 1997,Nov,1

34401 Thrombectomy, direct or with catheter; vena cava, iliac vein, by abdominal incision
42.4 42.4 FUD 090 C 80 50
AMA: 1997,Nov,1

34421 vena cava, iliac, femoropopliteal vein, by leg incision
21.5 21.5 FUD 090 T G2 80 50
AMA: 2018,Jan,8; 2017,Jan,8; 2016,Jan,13

34451 vena cava, iliac, femoropopliteal vein, by abdominal and leg incision
41.7 41.7 FUD 090 C 80 50
AMA: 1997,Nov,1

34471 subclavian vein, by neck incision
31.1 31.1 FUD 090 T G2 50
AMA: 1997,Nov,1

34490 axillary and subclavian vein, by arm incision
18.5 18.5 FUD 090 T G2 50
AMA: 1997,Nov,1

34501 Valvuloplasty, femoral vein
25.8 25.8 FUD 090 T G2 80 50
AMA: 1997,Nov,1

34502 Reconstruction of vena cava, any method
44.7 44.7 FUD 090 C 80
AMA: 1997,Nov,1

34510 Venous valve transposition, any vein donor
29.6 29.6 FUD 090 T G2 80 50
AMA: 1997,Nov,1

34520 Cross-over vein graft to venous system
28.7 28.7 FUD 090 T G2 80 50
AMA: 1997,Nov,1

34530 Saphenopopliteal vein anastomosis
27.2 27.2 FUD 090 T G2 80 50
AMA: 1997,Nov,1

34701-34713 [34717, 34718] Abdominal Aorta and Iliac Artery Repairs

INCLUDES Closure artery after endograft delivery using sheath size less than 12 French
Treatment with covered stent for:
- Aneurysm
- Aortic dissection
- Arteriovenous malformation
- Pseudoaneurysm
- Trauma

Treatment zones (vessel(s) in which endograft deployed):
- Iliac artery(ies) (34707-34708, [34717], [34718])
- Infrarenal aorta (34701-34702)
- Infrarenal aorta and both common iliac arteries (34705-34706)
- Infrarenal aorta and ipsilateral common iliac artery (34703-34704)

EXCLUDES *Treatment atherosclerotic occlusive disease with covered stent:*
- *Aorta (37236-37237)*
- *Iliac artery(ies) (37221, 37223)*

Code also:
- Open arterial exposure, when appropriate ([34812], 34714 [34820, 34833, 34834], 34715-34716)
- Percutaneous closure artery when endograft delivered through sheath 12 French or larger (34713)
- Selective catheterization arteries outside target treatment zone

34701 Endovascular repair of infrarenal aorta by deployment of an aorto-aortic tube endograft including pre-procedure sizing and device selection, all nonselective catheterization(s), all associated radiological supervision and interpretation, all endograft extension(s) placed in the aorta from the level of the renal arteries to the aortic bifurcation, and all angioplasty/stenting performed from the level of the renal arteries to the aortic bifurcation; for other than rupture (eg, for aneurysm, pseudoaneurysm, dissection, penetrating ulcer)
INCLUDES Nonselective catheterization
Code also intravascular ultrasound when performed (37252-37253)
36.1 36.1 FUD 090 C 80
AMA: 2019,Nov,6; 2018,Jan,8; 2017,Dec,3

34702 for rupture including temporary aortic and/or iliac balloon occlusion, when performed (eg, for aneurysm, pseudoaneurysm, dissection, penetrating ulcer, traumatic disruption)
INCLUDES Nonselective catheterization
Code also:
- Decompressive laparotomy for treatment abdominal compartment syndrome (49000)
- Intravascular ultrasound when performed (37252-37253)

53.9 53.9 FUD 090 C 80
AMA: 2019,Nov,6; 2018,Jan,8; 2017,Dec,3

34703 Endovascular repair of infrarenal aorta and/or iliac artery(ies) by deployment of an aorto-uni-iliac endograft including pre-procedure sizing and device selection, all nonselective catheterization(s), all associated radiological supervision and interpretation, all endograft extension(s) placed in the aorta from the level of the renal arteries to the iliac bifurcation, and all angioplasty/stenting performed from the level of the renal arteries to the iliac bifurcation; for other than rupture (eg, for aneurysm, pseudoaneurysm, dissection, penetrating ulcer)
INCLUDES Endograft extensions ending in common iliac arteries
Nonselective catheterization
Code also intravascular ultrasound when performed (37252-37253)
39.8 39.8 FUD 090 C 80
AMA: 2019,Nov,6; 2018,Jan,8; 2017,Dec,3

34704 for rupture including temporary aortic and/or iliac balloon occlusion, when performed (eg, for aneurysm, pseudoaneurysm, dissection, penetrating ulcer, traumatic disruption)
INCLUDES Endograft extensions ending in common iliac arteries
Nonselective catheterization
Code also:
- Decompressive laparotomy for treatment abdominal compartment syndrome (49000)
- Intravascular ultrasound when performed (37252-37253)

66.4 66.4 FUD 090 C 80
AMA: 2019,Nov,6; 2018,Jan,8; 2017,Dec,3

34705 Endovascular repair of infrarenal aorta and/or iliac artery(ies) by deployment of an aorto-bi-iliac endograft including pre-procedure sizing and device selection, all nonselective catheterization(s), all associated radiological supervision and interpretation, all endograft extension(s) placed in the aorta from the level of the renal arteries to the iliac bifurcation, and all angioplasty/stenting performed from the level of the renal arteries to the iliac bifurcation; for other than rupture (eg, for aneurysm, pseudoaneurysm, dissection, penetrating ulcer)
INCLUDES Endograft extensions ending in common iliac arteries
Nonselective catheterization
Code also intravascular ultrasound when performed (37252-37253)
44.5 44.5 FUD 090 C 80
AMA: 2019,Nov,6; 2018,Jan,8; 2017,Dec,3

34706 for rupture including temporary aortic and/or iliac balloon occlusion, when performed (eg, for aneurysm, pseudoaneurysm, dissection, penetrating ulcer, traumatic disruption)
INCLUDES Endograft extensions ending in common iliac arteries
Nonselective catheterization
Code also:
- Decompressive laparotomy for treatment abdominal compartment syndrome (49000)
- Intravascular ultrasound when performed (37252-37253)

67.1 67.1 FUD 090 C 80
AMA: 2019,Nov,6; 2018,Jan,8; 2017,Dec,3

34707 Endovascular repair of iliac artery by deployment of an ilio-iliac tube endograft including pre-procedure sizing and device selection, all nonselective catheterization(s), all associated radiological supervision and interpretation, and all endograft extension(s) proximally to the aortic bifurcation and distally to the iliac bifurcation, and treatment zone angioplasty/stenting, when performed, unilateral; for other than rupture (eg, for aneurysm, pseudoaneurysm, dissection, arteriovenous malformation)

INCLUDES Endograft extensions ending in common iliac arteries
Nonselective catheterization

EXCLUDES *Deployment iliac branched endograft:*
At same time as aorto-iliac graft placement ([34717])
Delayed/separate from aorto-iliac endograft deployment ([34718])

Code also intravascular ultrasound when performed (37252-37253)

33.7 33.7 FUD 090 C 80 50

AMA: 2019,Nov,6; 2018,Jan,8; 2017,Dec,3

34708 for rupture including temporary aortic and/or iliac balloon occlusion, when performed (eg, for aneurysm, pseudoaneurysm, dissection, arteriovenous malformation, traumatic disruption)

INCLUDES Endograft extensions ending in common iliac arteries
Nonselective catheterization

EXCLUDES *Deployment iliac branched endograft:*
At same time as aorto-iliac graft placement ([34717])
Delayed/separate from aorto-iliac endograft deployment ([34718])

Code also:
Decompressive laparotomy for treatment abdominal compartment syndrome (49000)
Intravascular ultrasound when performed (37252-37253)

53.8 53.8 FUD 090 C 80 50

AMA: 2019,Nov,6; 2018,Jan,8; 2017,Dec,3

+ # 34717 Endovascular repair of iliac artery at the time of aorto-iliac artery endograft placement by deployment of an iliac branched endograft including pre-procedure sizing and device selection, all ipsilateral selective iliac artery catheterization(s), all associated radiological supervision and interpretation, and all endograft extension(s) proximally to the aortic bifurcation and distally in the internal iliac, external iliac, and common femoral artery(ies), and treatment zone angioplasty/stenting, when performed, for rupture or other than rupture (eg, for aneurysm, pseudoaneurysm, dissection, arteriovenous malformation, penetrating ulcer, traumatic disruption), unilateral (List separately in addition to code for primary procedure)

INCLUDES Endograft extensions into internal and external iliac, and/or common femoral arteries

EXCLUDES *Delayed deployment branched iliac endograft, separate from aorto-iliac endograft placement ([34718])*
Placement prosthesis extensions on same side (34709, 34710-34711)
Reporting with modifier 50. Report once for each side when performed bilaterally

Code first (34703-34706)

12.9 12.9 FUD ZZZ 80

+ 34709 Placement of extension prosthesis(es) distal to the common iliac artery(ies) or proximal to the renal artery(ies) for endovascular repair of infrarenal abdominal aortic or iliac aneurysm, false aneurysm, dissection, penetrating ulcer, including pre-procedure sizing and device selection, all nonselective catheterization(s), all associated radiological supervision and interpretation, and treatment zone angioplasty/stenting, when performed, per vessel treated (List separately in addition to code for primary procedure)

EXCLUDES *Placement covered stent (37236-37237)*
Placement iliac branched endograft ([34717], [34718])
Reporting code more than one time for each vessel treated

Code first (34701-34708, 34845-34848)

9.42 9.42 FUD ZZZ C 80

AMA: 2019,Nov,6; 2018,Jan,8; 2017,Dec,3

 # 34718 Endovascular repair of iliac artery, not associated with placement of an aorto-iliac artery endograft at the same session, by deployment of an iliac branched endograft, including pre-procedure sizing and device selection, all ipsilateral selective iliac artery catheterization(s), all associated radiological supervision and interpretation, and all endograft extension(s) proximally to the aortic bifurcation and distally in the internal iliac, external iliac, and common femoral artery(ies), and treatment zone angioplasty/stenting, when performed, for other than rupture (eg, for aneurysm, pseudoaneurysm, dissection, arteriovenous malformation, penetrating ulcer), unilateral

INCLUDES Endograft extensions into internal and external iliac, and/or common femoral arteries

EXCLUDES *Branched iliac endograft deployed same session as aorto-iliac endograft placement (34703-34706, [34717])*
Placement isolated iliac branched endograft, for rupture (37799)
Placement prosthesis extensions on same side (34709, 34710-34711)

36.0 36.0 FUD 090 80

34710 Delayed placement of distal or proximal extension prosthesis for endovascular repair of infrarenal abdominal aortic or iliac aneurysm, false aneurysm, dissection, endoleak, or endograft migration, including pre-procedure sizing and device selection, all nonselective catheterization(s), all associated radiological supervision and interpretation, and treatment zone angioplasty/stenting, when performed; initial vessel treated

EXCLUDES *Fenestrated endograft repair (34841-34848)*
Initial endovascular repair by endograft (34701-34709)
Reporting code more than one time per procedure

Code also decompressive laparotomy for treatment abdominal compartment syndrome (49000)

23.3 23.3 FUD 090 C 80

AMA: 2019,Nov,6; 2018,Jan,8; 2017,Dec,3

+ 34711 each additional vessel treated (List separately in addition to code for primary procedure)

EXCLUDES *Fenestrated endograft repair (34841-34848)*
Initial endovascular repair by endograft (34701-34709)
Reporting code more than one time per procedure

Code first (34710)

8.68 8.68 FUD ZZZ C 80

AMA: 2019,Nov,6; 2018,Jan,8; 2017,Dec,3

34712 Transcatheter delivery of enhanced fixation device(s) to the endograft (eg, anchor, screw, tack) and all associated radiological supervision and interpretation

EXCLUDES *Reporting code more than one time per procedure*

19.2 19.2 FUD 090 C 80

AMA: 2018,Jan,8; 2017,Dec,3

+ 34713 Percutaneous access and closure of femoral artery for delivery of endograft through a large sheath (12 French or larger), including ultrasound guidance, when performed, unilateral (List separately in addition to code for primary procedure)

INCLUDES Ultrasound imaging guidance
Unilateral procedure through large sheath 12 French or larger

EXCLUDES *Reporting with modifier 50. Report once for each side when performed bilaterally*

Code first (33880-33881, 33883-33884, 33886, 34701-34708, [34718], 34710, 34712, 34841-34848)

3.63 3.63 FUD ZZZ N NI 80

AMA: 2018,Jan,8; 2017,Dec,3

34812-34834 [34717, 34718, 34812, 34820, 34833, 34834] Open Exposure for Endovascular Prosthesis Delivery

INCLUDES Balloon angioplasty/stent deployment within target treatment zone
Introduction, manipulation, placement, and device deployment
Open exposure femoral or iliac artery/subsequent closure
Thromboendarterectomy at site of aneurysm

EXCLUDES *Additional interventional procedures outside target treatment zone*
Guidewire and catheter insertion (36140, 36200, 36245-36248)
Substantial artery repair/replacement (35226, 35286)

+ # 34812 Open femoral artery exposure for delivery of endovascular prosthesis, by groin incision, unilateral (List separately in addition to code for primary procedure)

EXCLUDES *ECMO/ECLS insertion, removal or repositioning (33953-33954, 33959, [33962], [33969], [33984], [33987])*
Extensive repair femoral artery (35226, 35286, 35371)
Reporting with modifier 50. Report once for each side when performed bilaterally

Code first (33880-33881, 33883-33884, 33886, 33990-33991, 34701-34708, [34718], 34710, 34712, 34841-34848)

6.01 6.01 FUD ZZZ C 80

AMA: 2018,Jan,8; 2017,Dec,3; 2017,Jan,8; 2016,Jan,13

+ 34714 Open femoral artery exposure with creation of conduit for delivery of endovascular prosthesis or for establishment of cardiopulmonary bypass, by groin incision, unilateral (List separately in addition to code for primary procedure)

EXCLUDES *Delivery endovascular prosthesis via open femoral artery ([34812])*
ECMO/ECLS insertion, removal or repositioning on same side (33953-33954, 33959, [33962], [33969], [33984])
Reporting with modifier 50. Report once for each side when performed bilaterally
Transcatheter aortic valve replacement via open axillary artery (33362)

Code first (32852, 32854, 33031, 33120, 33251, 33256, 33259, 33261, 33305, 33315, 33322, 33335, 33390-33391, 33404-33406, 33410, 33440 [33440], 33411-33417, 33422, 33425-33427, 33430, 33460, 33463-33465, 33468, 33474-33476, 33478, 33496, 33500, 33502, 33504-33507, 33510-33516, 33533-33536, 33542, 33545, 33548, 33600-33688, 33692, 33694, 33697, 33702, 33710, 33720, 33724, 33726, 33730, 33732, 33736, 33750, 33755, 33762, 33764, 33766-33767, 33770-33783, 33786, 33788, 33802-33803, 33814, 33820, 33822, 33824, 33840, 33845, 33851, 33853, 33858-33859, 33863-33864, 33871, 33875, 33877, 33880-33881, 33883-33884, 33886, 33910, 33916-33917, 33920, 33922, 33926, 33935, 33945, 33975-33980, 33983, 33990-33991, 34701-34708, 34718 [34718], 34710, 34712, 34841-34848)

7.87 7.87 FUD ZZZ N NI 80

AMA: 2018,Jan,8; 2017,Dec,3

+ # 34820 Open iliac artery exposure for delivery of endovascular prosthesis or iliac occlusion during endovascular therapy, by abdominal or retroperitoneal incision, unilateral (List separately in addition to code for primary procedure)

EXCLUDES *ECMO/ECLS insertion, removal or repositioning (33953-33954, 33959, [33962], [33969], [33984])*
Reporting with modifier 50. Report once for each side when performed bilaterally

Code first (33880-33881, 33883-33884, 33886, 33990-33991, 34701-34708, [34718], 34710, 34712, 34841-34848)

10.1 10.1 FUD ZZZ C 80

AMA: 2018,Jan,8; 2017,Dec,3; 2017,Jan,8; 2016,Jan,13

+ # 34833 Open iliac artery exposure with creation of conduit for delivery of endovascular prosthesis or for establishment of cardiopulmonary bypass, by abdominal or retroperitoneal incision, unilateral (List separately in addition to code for primary procedure)

EXCLUDES *Delivery endovascular prosthesis via open iliac artery ([34820])*
ECMO/ECLS insertion, removal or repositioning on same side (33953-33954, 33959, [33962], [33969], [33984])
Reporting with modifier 50. Report once for each side when performed bilaterally
Transcatheter aortic valve replacement via open iliac artery (33364)

Code first (32852, 32854, 33031, 33256, 33259, 33261, 33305, 33315, 33322, 33335, 33390-33391, 33404-33406, 33410, [33440], 33411-33417, 33422, 33425-33427, 33430, 33460, 33463-33465, 33468, 33474-33476, 33478, 33496, 33500, 33502, 33504-33514, 33516, 33533-33536, 33542, 33545, 33548, 33600-33688, 33692, 33694, 33697, 33702, 33710, 33720, 33724, 33726, 33730, 33732, 33736, 33750, 33755, 33762, 33764, 33766-33767, 33770-33783, 33786, 33788, 33802-33803, 33814, 33820, 33822, 33824, 33840, 33845, 33851, 33853, 33858-33859, 33863-33864, 33871, 33875, 33877, 33880-33881, 33883-33884, 33886, 33910, 33916-33917, 33920, 33922, 33926, 33935, 33945, 33975-33980, 33983, 33990-33991, 34701-34708, [34718], 34710, 34712, 34841-34848)

11.7 11.7 FUD ZZZ C 80

AMA: 2018,Jan,8; 2017,Dec,3; 2017,Jan,8; 2016,Jan,13

+ # 34834 Open brachial artery exposure for delivery of endovascular prosthesis, unilateral (List separately in addition to code for primary procedure)

EXCLUDES *ECMO/ECLS insertion, removal or repositioning (33953-33954, 33959, [33962], [33969], [33984])*
Reporting with modifier 50. Report once for each side when performed bilaterally

Code first (33880-33881, 33883-33884, 33886, 33990-33991, 34701-34708, [34718], 34710, 34712, 34841-34848)

3.75 3.75 FUD ZZZ C 80

AMA: 2018,Jan,8; 2017,Dec,3; 2017,Jan,8; 2016,Jan,13

+ 34715 Open axillary/subclavian artery exposure for delivery of endovascular prosthesis by infraclavicular or supraclavicular incision, unilateral (List separately in addition to code for primary procedure)

EXCLUDES *ECMO/ECLS insertion, removal or repositioning on same side (33953-33954, 33959, [33962], [33969], [33984])*
Reporting with modifier 50. Report once for each side when performed bilaterally
Transcatheter aortic valve replacement via open axillary artery (33363)

Code first (33880-33881, 33883-33884, 33886, 33990-33991, 34701-34708, [34718], 34710, 34712, 34841-34848)

8.72 8.72 FUD ZZZ N NI 80

AMA: 2018,Jan,8; 2017,Dec,3

+ **34716** **Open axillary/subclavian artery exposure with creation of conduit for delivery of endovascular prosthesis or for establishment of cardiopulmonary bypass, by infraclavicular or supraclavicular incision, unilateral (List separately in addition to code for primary procedure)**

EXCLUDES *Reporting with modifier 50. Report once for each side when performed bilaterally*

Code first (32852, 32854, 33031, 33120, 33251, 33256, 33259, 33261, 33305, 33315, 33322, 33335, 33390-33391, 33404-33406, 33410, [33440], 33411-33417, 33422, 33425-33427, 33430, 33460, 33463-33465, 33468, 33474-33476, 33478, 33496, 33500, 33502, 33504-33514, 33516, 33533-33536, 33542, 33545, 33548, 33600-33688, 33692, 33694, 33697, 33702, 33710, 33720, 33724, 33726, 33730, 33732, 33736, 33750, 33755, 33762, 33764, 33766-33767, 33770-33783, 33786, 33788, 33802-33803, 33814, 33820, 33822, 33824, 33840, 33845, 33851, 33853, 33858-33859, 33863-33864, 33871, 33875, 33877, 33880-33881, 33883-33884, 33886, 33910, 33916-33917, 33920, 33922, 33926, 33935, 33945, 33975-33980, 33983, 33990-33991, 34701-34708, [34718], 34710, 34712, 34841-34848)

10.8 10.8 **FUD** ZZZ N N1 80

AMA: 2018,Jan,8; 2017,Dec,3

34717 **Resequenced code. See code following 34708.**

34718 **Resequenced code. See code following 34709.**

+ **34808** **Endovascular placement of iliac artery occlusion device (List separately in addition to code for primary procedure)**

Code first (34701-34704, 34707-34708, 34709, 34710, 34813, 34841-34844)

5.81 5.81 **FUD** ZZZ C 80

AMA: 2018,Jan,8; 2017,Jan,8; 2016,Jan,13

34812 **Resequenced code. See code following 34713.**

+ **34813** **Placement of femoral-femoral prosthetic graft during endovascular aortic aneurysm repair (List separately in addition to code for primary procedure)**

EXCLUDES *Grafting femoral artery (35521, 35533, 35539, 35540, 35556, 35558, 35566, 35621, 35646, 35654-35661, 35666, 35700)*

Code first ([34812])

6.85 6.85 **FUD** ZZZ C 80

AMA: 2018,Jan,8; 2017,Jan,8; 2016,Jan,13

34820 **Resequenced code. See code following 34714.**

34830 **Open repair of infrarenal aortic aneurysm or dissection, plus repair of associated arterial trauma, following unsuccessful endovascular repair; tube prosthesis**

51.2 51.2 **FUD** 090 C 80

AMA: 2018,Jan,8; 2017,Jan,8; 2016,Jan,13

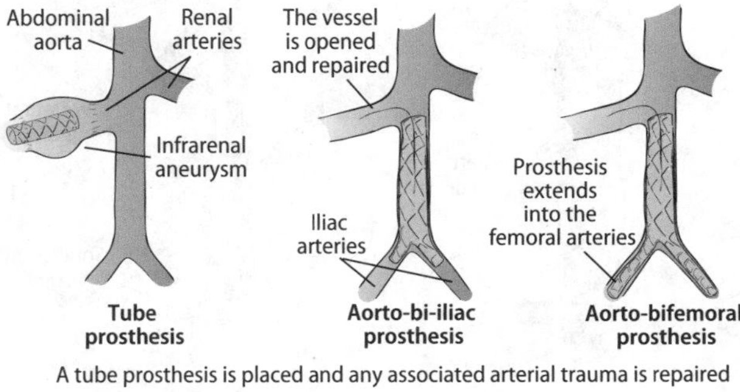

A tube prosthesis is placed and any associated arterial trauma is repaired

34831 **aorto-bi-iliac prosthesis**

56.0 56.0 **FUD** 090 C 80

AMA: 2018,Jan,8; 2017,Jan,8; 2016,Jan,13

34832 **aorto-bifemoral prosthesis**

54.7 54.7 **FUD** 090 C 80

AMA: 2018,Jan,8; 2017,Jan,8; 2016,Jan,13

34833 **Resequenced code. See code following 34714.**

34834 **Resequenced code. See code following 34714.**

34839-34848 Repair Visceral Aorta with Fenestrated Endovascular Grafts

INCLUDES Angiography
Balloon angioplasty before and after graft deployment
Fluoroscopic guidance
Guidewire and catheter insertion vessels in target treatment zone
Radiologic supervision and interpretation
Visceral aorta (34841-34844)
Visceral aorta and associated infrarenal abdominal aorta (34845-34848)

EXCLUDES *Catheterization:*
Arterial families outside treatment zone
Hypogastric arteries
Distal extension prosthesis terminating in common femoral, external iliac, or internal iliac artery (34709-34711 [34718])
Insertion bare metal or covered intravascular stents in visceral branches in target treatment zone (37236-37237)
Interventional procedures outside treatment zone
Open exposure access vessels (34713-34716 [34812, 34820, 34833, 34834])
Placement distal extension prosthesis into internal/external iliac or common femoral artery (34709, [34718], 34710-34711)
Repair abdominal aortic aneurysm without fenestrated graft (34701-34708)
Substantial artery repair (35226, 35286)

Code also associated endovascular repair descending thoracic aorta (33880-33886, 75956-75959)

34839 **Physician planning of a patient-specific fenestrated visceral aortic endograft requiring a minimum of 90 minutes of physician time**

EXCLUDES *3D rendering with interpretation and image reporting (76376-76377)*
Endovascular repair procedure on day of or day after planning (34701-34706, 34841-34848)
Planning on day of or day before endovascular repair procedure
Total planning time less than 90 minutes

0.00 0.00 **FUD** YYY B 80

34841 **Endovascular repair of visceral aorta (eg, aneurysm, pseudoaneurysm, dissection, penetrating ulcer, intramural hematoma, or traumatic disruption) by deployment of a fenestrated visceral aortic endograft and all associated radiological supervision and interpretation, including target zone angioplasty, when performed; including one visceral artery endoprosthesis (superior mesenteric, celiac or renal artery)**

EXCLUDES *Endovascular repair aorta (34701-34706, 34845-34848)*
Physician planning patient-specific fenestrated visceral aortic endograft (34839)

0.00 0.00 **FUD** YYY C 80

AMA: 2018,Jan,8; 2017,Dec,3; 2017,Jul,3; 2017,Jan,8; 2016,Jan,13

34842 **including two visceral artery endoprostheses (superior mesenteric, celiac and/or renal artery[s])**

INCLUDES Repairs extending from visceral aorta to one or more four visceral artery origins to infrarenal aorta level

EXCLUDES *Endovascular repair aorta (34701-34706, 34845-34848)*
Physician planning patient-specific fenestrated visceral aortic endograft (34839)

0.00 0.00 **FUD** YYY C 80

AMA: 2018,Jan,8; 2017,Dec,3; 2017,Jul,3; 2017,Jan,8; 2016,Jan,13

34843 **including three visceral artery endoprostheses (superior mesenteric, celiac and/or renal artery[s])**

INCLUDES Repairs extending from visceral aorta to one or more four visceral artery origins to infrarenal aorta level

EXCLUDES *Endovascular repair aorta (34701-34706, 34845-34848)*
Physician planning patient-specific fenestrated visceral aortic endograft (34839)

0.00 0.00 **FUD** YYY C 80

AMA: 2018,Jan,8; 2017,Dec,3; 2017,Jul,3; 2017,Jan,8; 2016,Jan,13

34844 **including four or more visceral artery endoprostheses (superior mesenteric, celiac and/or renal artery[s])**

INCLUDES Repairs extending from visceral aorta to one or more four visceral artery origins to infrarenal aorta level

EXCLUDES *Endovascular repair aorta (34701-34706, 34845-34848)*
Physician planning patient-specific fenestrated visceral aortic endograft (34839)

Facility RVU 0.00 Non-Facility RVU 0.00 **FUD** YYY C 80

AMA: 2018,Jan,8; 2017,Dec,3; 2017,Jul,3; 2017,Jan,8; 2016,Jan,13

34845 **Endovascular repair of visceral aorta and infrarenal abdominal aorta (eg, aneurysm, pseudoaneurysm, dissection, penetrating ulcer, intramural hematoma, or traumatic disruption) with a fenestrated visceral aortic endograft and concomitant unibody or modular infrarenal aortic endograft and all associated radiological supervision and interpretation, including target zone angioplasty, when performed; including one visceral artery endoprosthesis (superior mesenteric, celiac or renal artery)**

INCLUDES Placement device and extensions into common iliac arteries
Repairs extending from visceral aorta to one or more four visceral artery origins to infrarenal aorta level

EXCLUDES *Direct repair aneurysm (35081, 35102)*
Endovascular repair aorta (34701-34706, 34845-34848)
Physician planning patient-specific fenestrated visceral aortic endograft (34839)

Code also iliac artery revascularization when performed outside target treatment zone (37220-37223)

Facility RVU 0.00 Non-Facility RVU 0.00 **FUD** YYY C 80

AMA: 2018,Jan,8; 2017,Dec,3; 2017,Jul,3; 2017,Jan,8; 2016,Jan,13

34846 **including two visceral artery endoprostheses (superior mesenteric, celiac and/or renal artery[s])**

INCLUDES Placement device and extensions into common iliac arteries
Repairs extending from visceral aorta to one or more four visceral artery origins to infrarenal aorta level

EXCLUDES *Direct repair aneurysm (35081, 35102)*
Endovascular repair aorta (34701-34706, 34841-34844)
Physician planning patient-specific fenestrated visceral aortic endograft (34839)

Code also iliac artery revascularization when performed outside target treatment zone (37220-37223)

Facility RVU 0.00 Non-Facility RVU 0.00 **FUD** YYY C 80

AMA: 2018,Jan,8; 2017,Dec,3; 2017,Jul,3; 2017,Jan,8; 2016,Jan,13

34847 **including three visceral artery endoprostheses (superior mesenteric, celiac and/or renal artery[s])**

INCLUDES Placement device and extensions into common iliac arteries
Repairs extending from visceral aorta to one or more four visceral artery origins to infrarenal aorta level

EXCLUDES *Direct repair aneurysm (35081, 35102)*
Endovascular repair aorta (34701-34706, 34841-34844)
Physician planning patient-specific fenestrated visceral aortic endograft (34839)

Code also iliac artery revascularization when performed outside target treatment zone (37220-37223)

Facility RVU 0.00 Non-Facility RVU 0.00 **FUD** YYY C 80

AMA: 2018,Jan,8; 2017,Dec,3; 2017,Jul,3; 2017,Jan,8; 2016,Jan,13

34848 **including four or more visceral artery endoprostheses (superior mesenteric, celiac and/or renal artery[s])**

INCLUDES Placement device and extensions into common iliac arteries
Repairs extending from visceral aorta to one or more four visceral artery origins to infrarenal aorta level

EXCLUDES *Direct repair aneurysm (35081, 35102)*
Endovascular repair aorta (34701-34706, 34841-34844)
Physician planning patient-specific fenestrated visceral aortic endograft (34839)

Code also iliac artery revascularization when performed outside target treatment zone (37220-37223)

Facility RVU 0.00 Non-Facility RVU 0.00 **FUD** YYY C 80

AMA: 2018,Jan,8; 2017,Dec,3; 2017,Aug,9; 2017,Jul,3; 2017,Jan,8; 2016,Jul,6; 2016,Jan,13

35001-35152 Repair Aneurysm, False Aneurysm, Related Arterial Disease

INCLUDES Endarterectomy procedures

EXCLUDES *Endovascular repairs:*
Abdominal aortic aneurysm (34701-34716 [34717, 34718, 34812, 34820, 34833, 34834])
Thoracic aortic aneurysm (33858-33859, 33863-33875)
Intracranial aneurysms (61697-61710)
Repairs related to occlusive disease only (35201-35286)

35001 **Direct repair of aneurysm, pseudoaneurysm, or excision (partial or total) and graft insertion, with or without patch graft; for aneurysm and associated occlusive disease, carotid, subclavian artery, by neck incision**

Facility RVU 32.6 Non-Facility RVU 32.6 **FUD** 090 C 80 50

AMA: 2002,May,7; 2000,Dec,1

35002 **for ruptured aneurysm, carotid, subclavian artery, by neck incision**

Facility RVU 33.0 Non-Facility RVU 33.0 **FUD** 090 C 80 50

AMA: 2002,May,7; 1997,Nov,1

35005 **for aneurysm, pseudoaneurysm, and associated occlusive disease, vertebral artery**

Facility RVU 28.6 Non-Facility RVU 28.6 **FUD** 090 C 80 50

AMA: 2002,May,7; 1997,Nov,1

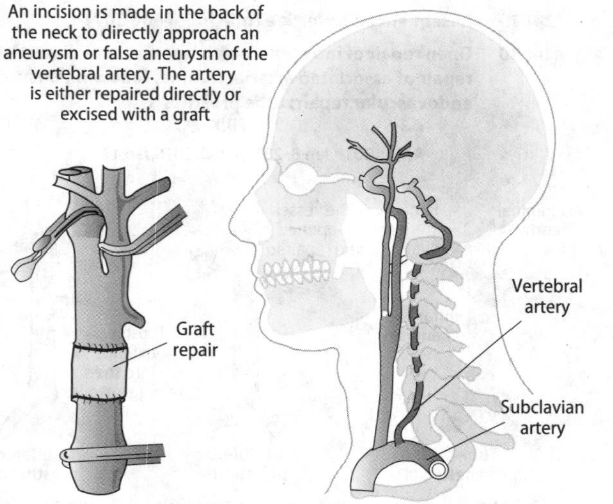
An incision is made in the back of the neck to directly approach an aneurysm or false aneurysm of the vertebral artery. The artery is either repaired directly or excised with a graft
Graft repair
Vertebral artery
Subclavian artery

35011 **for aneurysm and associated occlusive disease, axillary-brachial artery, by arm incision**

Facility RVU 29.0 Non-Facility RVU 29.0 **FUD** 090 T G2 80 50

AMA: 2002,May,7; 1997,Nov,1

35013 **for ruptured aneurysm, axillary-brachial artery, by arm incision**

Facility RVU 36.6 Non-Facility RVU 36.6 **FUD** 090 C 80 50

AMA: 2002,May,7; 1997,Nov,1

35021 **for aneurysm, pseudoaneurysm, and associated occlusive disease, innominate, subclavian artery, by thoracic incision**
36.4 36.4 FUD 090 C 80 50
AMA: 2002,May,7; 1997,Nov,1

35022 **for ruptured aneurysm, innominate, subclavian artery, by thoracic incision**
41.9 41.9 FUD 090 C 80 50
AMA: 2002,May,7; 1997,Nov,1

35045 **for aneurysm, pseudoaneurysm, and associated occlusive disease, radial or ulnar artery**
28.4 28.4 FUD 090 T G2 80 50
AMA: 2002,May,7; 1997,Nov,1

35081 **for aneurysm, pseudoaneurysm, and associated occlusive disease, abdominal aorta**
50.3 50.3 FUD 090 C 80
AMA: 2018,Jan,8; 2017,Jan,8; 2016,Jan,13

35082 **for ruptured aneurysm, abdominal aorta**
63.4 63.4 FUD 090 C 80
AMA: 2002,May,7; 1997,Nov,1

35091 **for aneurysm, pseudoaneurysm, and associated occlusive disease, abdominal aorta involving visceral vessels (mesenteric, celiac, renal)**
52.0 52.0 FUD 090 C 80 50
AMA: 2018,Jan,8; 2017,Jan,8; 2016,Jan,13

35092 **for ruptured aneurysm, abdominal aorta involving visceral vessels (mesenteric, celiac, renal)**
75.7 75.7 FUD 090 C 80 50
AMA: 2002,May,7; 1997,Nov,1

35102 **for aneurysm, pseudoaneurysm, and associated occlusive disease, abdominal aorta involving iliac vessels (common, hypogastric, external)**
54.6 54.6 FUD 090 C 80 50
AMA: 2018,Jan,8; 2017,Jan,8; 2016,Jan,13

35103 **for ruptured aneurysm, abdominal aorta involving iliac vessels (common, hypogastric, external)**
65.0 65.0 FUD 090 C 80 50
AMA: 2002,May,7; 1997,Nov,1

35111 **for aneurysm, pseudoaneurysm, and associated occlusive disease, splenic artery**
38.5 38.5 FUD 090 C 80 50
AMA: 2002,May,7; 1997,Nov,1

35112 **for ruptured aneurysm, splenic artery**
47.4 47.4 FUD 090 C 80 50
AMA: 2002,May,7; 1997,Nov,1

35121 **for aneurysm, pseudoaneurysm, and associated occlusive disease, hepatic, celiac, renal, or mesenteric artery**
45.9 45.9 FUD 090 C 80 50
AMA: 2002,May,7; 1997,Nov,1

35122 **for ruptured aneurysm, hepatic, celiac, renal, or mesenteric artery**
54.9 54.9 FUD 090 C 80 50
AMA: 2002,May,7; 1997,Nov,1

35131 **for aneurysm, pseudoaneurysm, and associated occlusive disease, iliac artery (common, hypogastric, external)**
40.2 40.2 FUD 090 C 80 50
AMA: 2018,Jan,8; 2017,Jan,8; 2016,Jan,13

35132 **for ruptured aneurysm, iliac artery (common, hypogastric, external)**
47.4 47.4 FUD 090 C 80 50
AMA: 2002,May,7; 1997,Nov,1

35141 **for aneurysm, pseudoaneurysm, and associated occlusive disease, common femoral artery (profunda femoris, superficial femoral)**
31.9 31.9 FUD 090 C 80 50
AMA: 2002,May,7; 1997,Nov,1

35142 **for ruptured aneurysm, common femoral artery (profunda femoris, superficial femoral)**
38.6 38.6 FUD 090 C 80 50
AMA: 2002,May,7; 1997,Nov,1

35151 **for aneurysm, pseudoaneurysm, and associated occlusive disease, popliteal artery**
35.9 35.9 FUD 090 C 80 50
AMA: 2002,May,7; 1997,Nov,1

35152 **for ruptured aneurysm, popliteal artery**
40.5 40.5 FUD 090 C 80 50
AMA: 2002,May,7; 1997,Nov,1

35180-35190 Surgical Repair Arteriovenous Fistula

35180 **Repair, congenital arteriovenous fistula; head and neck**
25.4 25.4 FUD 090 T G2 80
AMA: 2018,Jan,8; 2017,Jan,8; 2016,Jan,13

35182 **thorax and abdomen**
51.9 51.9 FUD 090 C 80
AMA: 2018,Jan,8; 2017,Jan,8; 2016,Jan,13

35184 **extremities**
27.9 27.9 FUD 090 T G2 80
AMA: 2018,Jan,8; 2017,Jan,8; 2016,Jan,13

35188 **Repair, acquired or traumatic arteriovenous fistula; head and neck**
36.9 36.9 FUD 090 T A2 80
AMA: 2018,Jan,8; 2017,Jan,8; 2016,Jan,13

35189 **thorax and abdomen**
43.8 43.8 FUD 090 C 80
AMA: 2018,Jan,8; 2017,Jan,8; 2016,Jan,13

35190 **extremities**
22.0 22.0 FUD 090 T G2 80
AMA: 2018,Jan,8; 2017,Jan,8; 2016,Jan,13

35201-35286 Surgical Repair Artery or Vein

EXCLUDES *Arteriovenous fistula repair (35180-35190)*
Primary open vascular procedures

35201 **Repair blood vessel, direct; neck**
EXCLUDES *Removal ECMO/ECLS cannula ([33969, 33984, 33985, 33986])*
27.3 27.3 FUD 090 T G2 80 50
AMA: 2019,Dec,5; 2018,Jan,8; 2017,Jan,8; 2016,Jan,13

35206 **upper extremity**
EXCLUDES *Removal ECMO/ECLS cannula ([33969, 33984, 33985, 33986])*
22.6 22.6 FUD 090 T G2 80 50
AMA: 2020,Dec,4; 2019,Dec,5; 2018,Jan,8; 2017,Jan,8; 2016,Jan,13

35207 **hand, finger**
21.7 21.7 FUD 090 T A2 50
AMA: 2019,Dec,5

35211 **intrathoracic, with bypass**
EXCLUDES *Removal ECMO/ECLS cannula ([33969, 33984, 33985, 33986])*
40.0 40.0 FUD 090 C 80 50
AMA: 2015,Jul,3; 2012,Apr,3-9

35216 **intrathoracic, without bypass**
EXCLUDES *Removal ECMO/ECLS cannula ([33969, 33984, 33985, 33986])*
60.0 60.0 FUD 090 C 80 50
AMA: 2018,Jan,8; 2017,Jan,8; 2016,Jan,13

35221 **intra-abdominal**
42.6 42.6 FUD 090 C 80 50
AMA: 2012,Apr,3-9; 2003,Feb,1

35226 **lower extremity**

EXCLUDES *Removal ECMO/ECLS cannula ([33969, 33984, 33985, 33986])*

24.1 24.1 **FUD** 090 T G2 80 50

AMA: 2020,Dec,4; 2019,Jul,10; 2018,Jan,8; 2017,Aug,10; 2017,Jul,3; 2017,Jan,8; 2016,Jul,6; 2016,Jan,13

35231 **Repair blood vessel with vein graft; neck**

36.3 36.3 **FUD** 090 T G2 80 50

AMA: 2019,Dec,5

35236 **upper extremity**

29.1 29.1 **FUD** 090 T G2 80 50

AMA: 2019,Dec,5; 2018,Jan,8; 2017,Jan,8; 2016,Jan,13

35241 **intrathoracic, with bypass**

41.5 41.5 **FUD** 090 C 80 50

AMA: 2012,Apr,3-9; 2003,Feb,1

35246 **intrathoracic, without bypass**

45.2 45.2 **FUD** 090 C 80 50

AMA: 2012,Apr,3-9; 2003,Feb,1

35251 **intra-abdominal**

50.7 50.7 **FUD** 090 C 80 50

AMA: 2012,Apr,3-9; 2003,Feb,1

35256 **lower extremity**

29.7 29.7 **FUD** 090 T G2 80 50

AMA: 2019,Dec,5

35261 **Repair blood vessel with graft other than vein; neck**

28.4 28.4 **FUD** 090 T G2 80 50

AMA: 2019,Dec,5

35266 **upper extremity**

25.1 25.1 **FUD** 090 T G2 80 50

AMA: 2019,Dec,5; 2018,Jan,8; 2017,Jan,8; 2016,Jan,13

35271 **intrathoracic, with bypass**

39.9 39.9 **FUD** 090 C 80 50

AMA: 2012,Apr,3-9; 2003,Feb,1

35276 **intrathoracic, without bypass**

42.1 42.1 **FUD** 090 C 80 50

AMA: 2012,Apr,3-9; 2003,Feb,1

35281 **intra-abdominal**

47.3 47.3 **FUD** 090 C 80 50

AMA: 2012,Apr,3-9; 2003,Feb,1

35286 **lower extremity**

26.9 26.9 **FUD** 090 T G2 80 50

AMA: 2020,Dec,4; 2019,Dec,5; 2019,Jul,10; 2018,Jan,8; 2017,Aug,10; 2017,Jul,3; 2017,Jan,8; 2016,Jul,6; 2016,Jan,13

35301-35372 Surgical Thromboendarterectomy Peripheral and Visceral Arteries

INCLUDES Obtaining saphenous or arm vein for graft
Thrombectomy/embolectomy

EXCLUDES *Coronary artery bypass procedures (33510-33536, 33572)*
Thromboendarterectomy for vascular occlusion on different vessel during same session

35301 **Thromboendarterectomy, including patch graft, if performed; carotid, vertebral, subclavian, by neck incision**

32.7 32.7 **FUD** 090 C 80 50

AMA: 2018,Jan,8; 2017,Jan,8; 2016,Jan,13

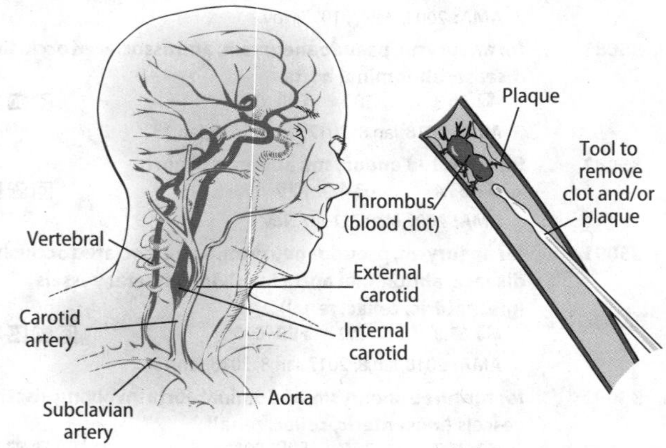

35302 **superficial femoral artery**

EXCLUDES *Revascularization, endovascular, open or percutaneous, femoral, popliteal artery(s) (37225, 37227)*

32.6 32.6 **FUD** 090 C 80 50

AMA: 2018,Jan,8; 2017,Jan,8; 2016,Jan,13

35303 **popliteal artery**

EXCLUDES *Revascularization, endovascular, open or percutaneous, femoral, popliteal artery(s) (37225, 37227)*

36.0 36.0 **FUD** 090 C 80 50

AMA: 2018,Jan,8; 2017,Jan,8; 2016,Jan,13

35304 **tibioperoneal trunk artery**

EXCLUDES *Revascularization, endovascular, open or percutaneous, tibial/peroneal artery (37229, 37231, 37233, 37235)*

37.0 37.0 **FUD** 090 C 80 50

AMA: 2018,Jan,8; 2017,Jan,8; 2016,Jan,13

35305 **tibial or peroneal artery, initial vessel**

EXCLUDES *Revascularization, endovascular, open or percutaneous, tibial/peroneal artery (37229, 37231, 37233, 37235)*

35.6 35.6 **FUD** 090 C 80 50

AMA: 2018,Jan,8; 2017,Jan,8; 2016,Jan,13

\+ **35306** **each additional tibial or peroneal artery (List separately in addition to code for primary procedure)**

EXCLUDES *Revascularization, endovascular, open or percutaneous, tibial/peroneal artery (37229, 37231, 37233, 37235)*

Code first (35305)

12.9 12.9 **FUD** ZZZ C 80

AMA: 2018,Jan,8; 2017,Jan,8; 2016,Jan,13

35311 **subclavian, innominate, by thoracic incision**

45.1 45.1 **FUD** 090 C 80 50

AMA: 1997,Nov,1

35321 **axillary-brachial**

25.9 25.9 **FUD** 090 T G2 80 50

AMA: 1997,Nov,1

35331 **abdominal aorta**

42.2 42.2 **FUD** 090 C 80 50

AMA: 1997,Nov,1

35341 **mesenteric, celiac, or renal**
39.9 39.9 FUD 090 C 80 50
AMA: 1997,Nov,1

35351 **iliac**
37.3 37.3 FUD 090 C 80 50
AMA: 1997,Nov,1

35355 **iliofemoral**
29.9 29.9 FUD 090 C 80 50
AMA: 1997,Nov,1

35361 **combined aortoiliac**
44.2 44.2 FUD 090 C 80 50
AMA: 1997,Nov,1

35363 **combined aortoiliofemoral**
47.1 47.1 FUD 090 C 80 50
AMA: 1997,Nov,1

35371 **common femoral**
23.7 23.7 FUD 090 C 80 50
AMA: 2020,Dec,4; 2018,Jan,8; 2017,Aug,10; 2017,Jul,3; 2017,Jan,8; 2016,Jan,13

35372 **deep (profunda) femoral**
28.4 28.4 FUD 090 C 80 50
AMA: 2018,Jan,8; 2017,Jan,8; 2016,Jan,13

35390 Surgical Thromboendarterectomy: Carotid Reoperation

Code first (35301)

\+ **35390** **Reoperation, carotid, thromboendarterectomy, more than 1 month after original operation (List separately in addition to code for primary procedure)**
4.65 4.65 FUD ZZZ C 80
AMA: 1997,Nov,1; 1993,Win,1

35400 Endoscopic Visualization of Vessels

Code first therapeutic intervention

\+ **35400** **Angioscopy (noncoronary vessels or grafts) during therapeutic intervention (List separately in addition to code for primary procedure)**
4.32 4.32 FUD ZZZ C 80
AMA: 1997,Dec,1; 1997,Nov,1

35500 Obtain Arm Vein for Graft

EXCLUDES *Endoscopic harvest (33508)*
Harvesting multiple vein segments (35682, 35683)

Code first (33510-33536, 35556, 35566, 35570-35571, 35583-35587)

\+ **35500** **Harvest of upper extremity vein, 1 segment, for lower extremity or coronary artery bypass procedure (List separately in addition to code for primary procedure)**
9.29 9.29 FUD ZZZ N 80
AMA: 2018,Jan,8; 2017,Jan,8; 2016,Jan,13

35501-35571 Arterial Bypass Using Vein Grafts

INCLUDES Obtaining saphenous vein grafts

EXCLUDES *Obtaining multiple vein segments (35682, 35683)*
Obtaining vein grafts, upper extremity or femoropopliteal (35500, 35572)
Treatment different sites with different bypass procedures during same operative session

35501 **Bypass graft, with vein; common carotid-ipsilateral internal carotid**
42.4 42.4 FUD 090 C 80 50
AMA: 2018,Jan,8; 2017,Jan,8; 2016,Jan,13

35506 **carotid-subclavian or subclavian-carotid**
37.0 37.0 FUD 090 C 80 50
AMA: 2018,Jan,8; 2017,Jan,8; 2016,Jan,13

35508 **carotid-vertebral**
INCLUDES Endoscopic procedure
38.5 38.5 FUD 090 C 80 50
AMA: 1999,Mar,6; 1999,Apr,11

35509 **carotid-contralateral carotid**
40.6 40.6 FUD 090 C 80 50
AMA: 2018,Jan,8; 2017,Jan,8; 2016,Jan,13

35510 **carotid-brachial**
35.7 35.7 FUD 090 C 80 50
AMA: 2018,Jan,8; 2017,Jan,8; 2016,Jan,13

35511 **subclavian-subclavian**
32.5 32.5 FUD 090 C 80 50
AMA: 2018,Jan,8; 2017,Jan,8; 2016,Jan,13

35512 **subclavian-brachial**
35.0 35.0 FUD 090 C 80 50
AMA: 2018,Jan,8; 2017,Jan,8; 2016,Jan,13

35515 **subclavian-vertebral**
38.5 38.5 FUD 090 C 80 50
AMA: 1999,Mar,6; 1999,Apr,11

35516 **subclavian-axillary**
35.4 35.4 FUD 090 C 80 50
AMA: 1999,Mar,6; 1999,Apr,11

35518 **axillary-axillary**
33.1 33.1 FUD 090 C 80 50
AMA: 2018,Jan,8; 2017,Jan,8; 2016,Jan,13

35521 **axillary-femoral**
EXCLUDES *Synthetic graft (35621)*
35.6 35.6 FUD 090 C 80 50
AMA: 2018,Jan,8; 2017,Jan,8; 2016,Jan,13

35522 **axillary-brachial**
35.3 35.3 FUD 090 C 80 50
AMA: 2018,Jan,8; 2017,Jan,8; 2016,Jan,13

35523 **brachial-ulnar or -radial**
EXCLUDES *Bypass graft using synthetic conduit (37799)*
Bypass graft, with vein; brachial-brachial (35525)
Distal revascularization and interval ligation (DRIL), upper extremity hemodialysis access (steal syndrome) (36838)
Harvest upper extremity vein, 1 segment, for lower extremity or coronary artery bypass procedure (35500)
Repair blood vessel, direct; upper extremity (35206)
37.1 37.1 FUD 090 C 80 50

35525 **brachial-brachial**
33.0 33.0 FUD 090 C 80 50
AMA: 2018,Jan,8; 2017,Jan,8; 2016,Jan,13

35526 **aortosubclavian, aortoinnominate, or aortocarotid**
EXCLUDES *Synthetic graft (35626)*
50.1 50.1 FUD 090 C 80 50
AMA: 1999,Mar,6; 1999,Apr,11

35531 **aortoceliac or aortomesenteric**
56.6 56.6 FUD 090 C 80 50
AMA: 1999,Mar,6; 1999,Apr,11

35533 **axillary-femoral-femoral**
EXCLUDES *Synthetic graft (35654)*
43.7 43.7 FUD 090 C 80 50
AMA: 2012,Apr,3-9; 1999,Mar,6

35535 **hepatorenal**
EXCLUDES *Bypass graft (35536, 35560, 35631, 35636)*
Harvest upper extremity vein, 1 segment, for lower extremity or coronary artery bypass procedure (35500)
Repair blood vessel (35221, 35251, 35281)
55.3 55.3 FUD 090 C 80 50

35536 **splenorenal**
49.1 49.1 FUD 090 C 80 50
AMA: 2018,Jan,8; 2017,Jan,8; 2016,Jan,13

35537 **aortoiliac**
EXCLUDES *Bypass graft, with vein; aortobi-iliac (35538)*
Synthetic graft (35637)
60.6 60.6 FUD 090 C 80
AMA: 2018,Jan,8; 2017,Jan,8; 2016,Jan,13

Cardiovascular, Hemic, and Lymphatic 35341 — 35537

35538 **aortobi-iliac**

EXCLUDES *Bypass graft, with vein; aortoiliac (35537)*
Synthetic graft (35638)

67.9 67.9 **FUD** 090 C 80

AMA: 2018,Jan,8; 2017,Jan,8; 2016,Jan,13

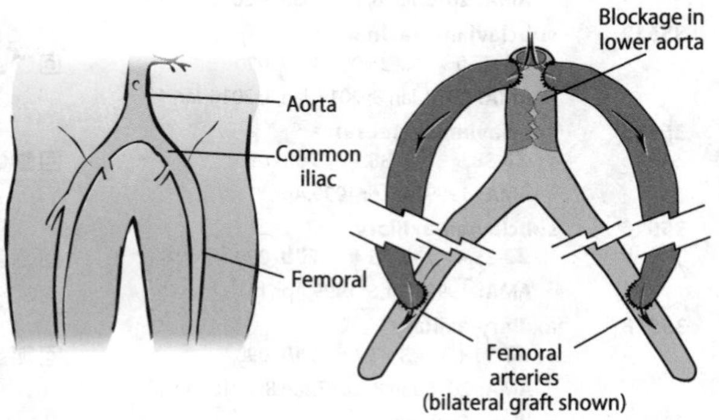

35539 **aortofemoral**

EXCLUDES *Bypass graft, with vein; aortobifemoral (35540)*
Synthetic graft (35647)

63.7 63.7 **FUD** 090 C 80 50

AMA: 2018,Jan,8; 2017,Jan,8; 2016,Jan,13

35540 **aortobifemoral**

EXCLUDES *Bypass graft, with vein; aortofemoral (35539)*
Synthetic graft (35646)

70.6 70.6 **FUD** 090 C 50

AMA: 2018,Jan,8; 2017,Jan,8; 2016,Jan,13

35556 **femoral-popliteal**

40.7 40.7 **FUD** 090 C 80 50

AMA: 2018,Jan,8; 2017,Jan,8; 2016,Jan,13

35558 **femoral-femoral**

35.7 35.7 **FUD** 090 C 80 50

AMA: 2012,Apr,3-9; 1999,Mar,6

35560 **aortorenal**

49.2 49.2 **FUD** 090 C 80 50

AMA: 2018,Jan,8; 2017,Jan,8; 2016,Jan,13

35563 **ilioiliac**

38.4 38.4 **FUD** 090 C 80 50

AMA: 1999,Mar,6; 1999,Apr,11

35565 **iliofemoral**

38.1 38.1 **FUD** 090 C 80 50

AMA: 2012,Apr,3-9; 2004,Oct,6

35566 **femoral-anterior tibial, posterior tibial, peroneal artery or other distal vessels**

48.6 48.6 **FUD** 090 C 80 50

AMA: 2018,Jan,8; 2017,Jan,8; 2016,Jan,13

35570 **tibial-tibial, peroneal-tibial, or tibial/peroneal trunk-tibial**

EXCLUDES *Repair blood vessel with graft (35256, 35286)*

42.8 42.8 **FUD** 090 C 80 50

AMA: 2018,Jan,8; 2017,Jan,8; 2016,Jan,13

35571 **popliteal-tibial, -peroneal artery or other distal vessels**

38.5 38.5 **FUD** 090 C 80 50

AMA: 2018,Jan,8; 2017,Jan,8; 2016,Jan,13

35572 Obtain Femoropopliteal Vein for Graft

EXCLUDES *Reporting with modifier 50. Report once for each side when performed bilaterally*

Code first (33510-33523, 33533-33536, 34502, 34520, 35001-35002, 35011-35022, 35102-35103, 35121-35152, 35231-35256, 35501-35587, 35879-35907)

\+ **35572** **Harvest of femoropopliteal vein, 1 segment, for vascular reconstruction procedure (eg, aortic, vena caval, coronary, peripheral artery) (List separately in addition to code for primary procedure)**

10.0 10.0 **FUD** ZZZ N N1 80

AMA: 2018,Jan,8; 2017,Jan,8; 2016,Jan,13

35583-35587 Lower Extremity Revascularization: In-situ Vein Bypass

INCLUDES Obtaining saphenous vein grafts

EXCLUDES *Obtaining multiple vein segments (35682, 35683)*
Obtaining vein graft, upper extremity or femoropopliteal (35500, 35572)

35583 **In-situ vein bypass; femoral-popliteal**

Code also:

Aortobifemoral bypass graft other than vein for aortobifemoral bypass using synthetic conduit and femoral-popliteal bypass with vein conduit in situ (35646)

Concurrent aortofemoral bypass for aortofemoral bypass graft with synthetic conduit and femoral-popliteal bypass with vein conduit in-situ (35647)

Concurrent aortofemoral bypass (vein) for aortofemoral bypass using vein conduit or femoral-popliteal bypass with vein conduit in-situ (35539)

41.8 41.8 **FUD** 090 C 80 50

AMA: 2018,Jan,8; 2017,Jan,8; 2016,Jan,13

35585 **femoral-anterior tibial, posterior tibial, or peroneal artery**

48.6 48.6 **FUD** 090 C 80 50

AMA: 2018,Jan,8; 2017,Jan,8; 2016,Jan,13

35587 **popliteal-tibial, peroneal**

39.6 39.6 **FUD** 090 C 80 50

AMA: 2018,Jan,8; 2017,Jan,8; 2016,Jan,13

35600 Obtain Arm Artery for Coronary Bypass

EXCLUDES *Transposition and/or reimplantation arteries (35691-35695)*

▲ **35600** **Harvest of upper extremity artery, 1 segment, for coronary artery bypass procedure, open**

EXCLUDES *Endoscopic approach (33508-33509, 37500)*

7.43 7.43 **FUD** ZZZ ⊘ C 80 50

AMA: 2018,Jan,8; 2017,Jan,8; 2016,Jan,13

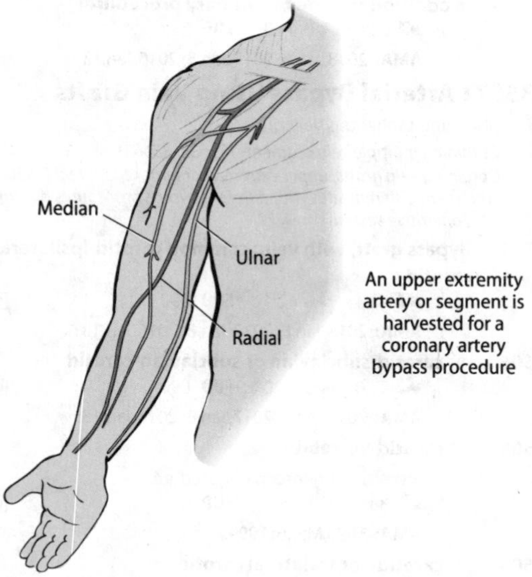

35601-35671 Arterial Bypass: Grafts Other Than Veins

EXCLUDES *Transposition and/or reimplantation arteries (35691-35695)*

35601 **Bypass graft, with other than vein; common carotid-ipsilateral internal carotid**
EXCLUDES *Open transcervical common carotid-common carotid bypass with endovascular repair descending thoracic aorta (33891)*
40.4 40.4 FUD 090 C 80 50
AMA: 2018,Jan,8; 2017,Jan,8; 2016,Jan,13

35606 **carotid-subclavian**
EXCLUDES *Open subclavian to carotid artery transposition performed with endovascular thoracic aneurysm repair via neck incision (33889)*
34.0 34.0 FUD 090 C 80 50
AMA: 1997,Nov,1

35612 **subclavian-subclavian**
30.3 30.3 FUD 090 C 80 50
AMA: 1997,Nov,1

35616 **subclavian-axillary**
32.0 32.0 FUD 090 C 80 50
AMA: 1997,Nov,1

35621 **axillary-femoral**
31.8 31.8 FUD 090 C 80 50
AMA: 2018,Jan,8; 2017,Jan,8; 2016,Jan,13

35623 **axillary-popliteal or -tibial**
38.1 38.1 FUD 090 C 80 50
AMA: 2012,Apr,3-9; 1997,Nov,1

35626 **aortosubclavian, aortoinnominate, or aortocarotid**
46.1 46.1 FUD 090 C 80 50
AMA: 1997,Nov,1

35631 **aortoceliac, aortomesenteric, aortorenal**
53.8 53.8 FUD 090 C 80 50
AMA: 1997,Nov,1

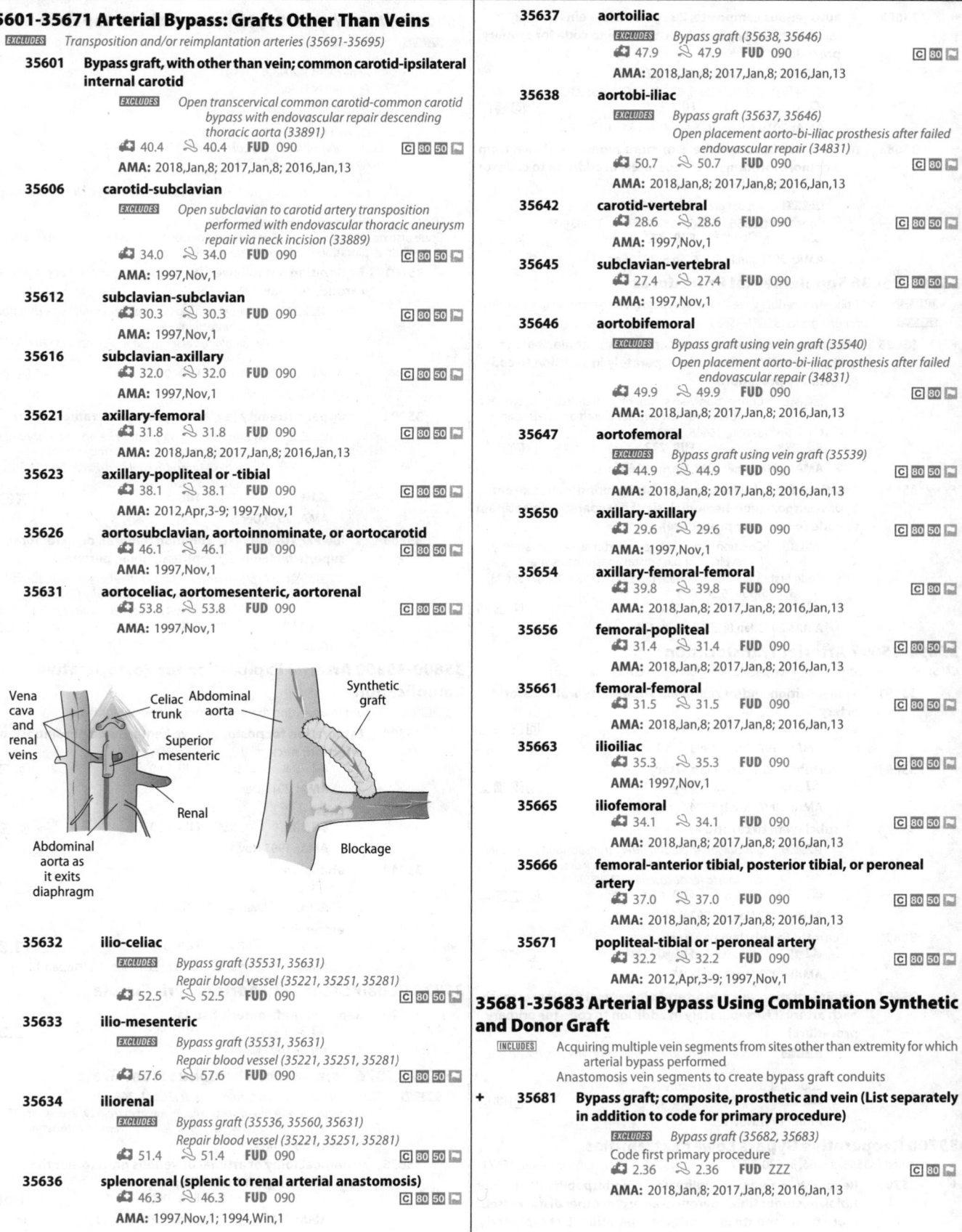

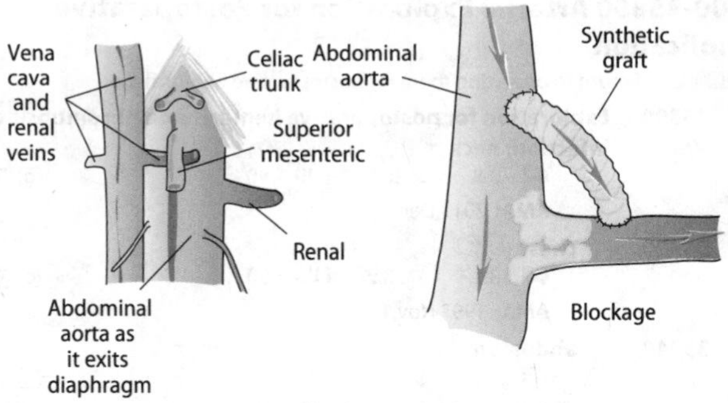

35632 **ilio-celiac**
EXCLUDES *Bypass graft (35531, 35631)*
Repair blood vessel (35221, 35251, 35281)
52.5 52.5 FUD 090 C 80 50

35633 **ilio-mesenteric**
EXCLUDES *Bypass graft (35531, 35631)*
Repair blood vessel (35221, 35251, 35281)
57.6 57.6 FUD 090 C 80 50

35634 **iliorenal**
EXCLUDES *Bypass graft (35536, 35560, 35631)*
Repair blood vessel (35221, 35251, 35281)
51.4 51.4 FUD 090 C 80 50

35636 **splenorenal (splenic to renal arterial anastomosis)**
46.3 46.3 FUD 090 C 80 50
AMA: 1997,Nov,1; 1994,Win,1

35637 **aortoiliac**
EXCLUDES *Bypass graft (35638, 35646)*
47.9 47.9 FUD 090 C 80
AMA: 2018,Jan,8; 2017,Jan,8; 2016,Jan,13

35638 **aortobi-iliac**
EXCLUDES *Bypass graft (35637, 35646)*
Open placement aorto-bi-iliac prosthesis after failed endovascular repair (34831)
50.7 50.7 FUD 090 C 80
AMA: 2018,Jan,8; 2017,Jan,8; 2016,Jan,13

35642 **carotid-vertebral**
28.6 28.6 FUD 090 C 80 50
AMA: 1997,Nov,1

35645 **subclavian-vertebral**
27.4 27.4 FUD 090 C 80 50
AMA: 1997,Nov,1

35646 **aortobifemoral**
EXCLUDES *Bypass graft using vein graft (35540)*
Open placement aorto-bi-iliac prosthesis after failed endovascular repair (34831)
49.9 49.9 FUD 090 C 80
AMA: 2018,Jan,8; 2017,Jan,8; 2016,Jan,13

35647 **aortofemoral**
EXCLUDES *Bypass graft using vein graft (35539)*
44.9 44.9 FUD 090 C 80 50
AMA: 2018,Jan,8; 2017,Jan,8; 2016,Jan,13

35650 **axillary-axillary**
29.6 29.6 FUD 090 C 80 50
AMA: 1997,Nov,1

35654 **axillary-femoral-femoral**
39.8 39.8 FUD 090 C 80
AMA: 2018,Jan,8; 2017,Jan,8; 2016,Jan,13

35656 **femoral-popliteal**
31.4 31.4 FUD 090 C 80 50
AMA: 2018,Jan,8; 2017,Jan,8; 2016,Jan,13

35661 **femoral-femoral**
31.5 31.5 FUD 090 C 80 50
AMA: 2018,Jan,8; 2017,Jan,8; 2016,Jan,13

35663 **ilioiliac**
35.3 35.3 FUD 090 C 80 50
AMA: 1997,Nov,1

35665 **iliofemoral**
34.1 34.1 FUD 090 C 80 50
AMA: 2018,Jan,8; 2017,Jan,8; 2016,Jan,13

35666 **femoral-anterior tibial, posterior tibial, or peroneal artery**
37.0 37.0 FUD 090 C 80 50
AMA: 2018,Jan,8; 2017,Jan,8; 2016,Jan,13

35671 **popliteal-tibial or -peroneal artery**
32.2 32.2 FUD 090 C 80 50
AMA: 2012,Apr,3-9; 1997,Nov,1

35681-35683 Arterial Bypass Using Combination Synthetic and Donor Graft

INCLUDES Acquiring multiple vein segments from sites other than extremity for which arterial bypass performed
Anastomosis vein segments to create bypass graft conduits

+ **35681** **Bypass graft; composite, prosthetic and vein (List separately in addition to code for primary procedure)**
EXCLUDES *Bypass graft (35682, 35683)*
Code first primary procedure
2.36 2.36 FUD ZZZ C 80
AMA: 2018,Jan,8; 2017,Jan,8; 2016,Jan,13

+ **35682** **autogenous composite, 2 segments of veins from 2 locations (List separately in addition to code for primary procedure)**

EXCLUDES *Bypass graft (35681, 35683)*

Code first (35556, 35566, 35570-35571, 35583-35587)

10.2 | 10.2 | FUD ZZZ | C 80

AMA: 2018,Jan,8; 2017,Jan,8; 2016,Jan,13

+ **35683** **autogenous composite, 3 or more segments of vein from 2 or more locations (List separately in addition to code for primary procedure)**

EXCLUDES *Bypass graft (35681-35682)*

Code first (35556, 35566, 35570-35571, 35583-35587)

11.8 | 11.8 | FUD ZZZ | C 80

AMA: 2018,Jan,8; 2017,Jan,8; 2016,Jan,13

35685-35686 Supplemental Procedures

INCLUDES Additional procedures needed with bypass graft to increase graft patency

EXCLUDES *Composite grafts (35681-35683)*

+ **35685** **Placement of vein patch or cuff at distal anastomosis of bypass graft, synthetic conduit (List separately in addition to code for primary procedure)**

INCLUDES Connection vein segment (cuff or patch) between distal portion synthetic graft and native artery

Code first (35656, 35666, 35671)

5.78 | 5.78 | FUD ZZZ | N 80

AMA: 2018,Jan,8; 2017,Jan,8; 2016,Jan,13

+ **35686** **Creation of distal arteriovenous fistula during lower extremity bypass surgery (non-hemodialysis) (List separately in addition to code for primary procedure)**

INCLUDES Creation fistula between peroneal or tibial artery and vein at or past distal anastomosis site

Code first (35556, 35566, 35570-35571, 35583-35587, 35623, 35656, 35666, 35671)

4.68 | 4.68 | FUD ZZZ | N 80

AMA: 2018,Jan,8; 2017,Jan,8; 2016,Jan,13

35691-35697 Arterial Translocation

CMS: 100-03,160.8 Electroencephalographic Monitoring During Cerebral Vasculature Surgery

35691 **Transposition and/or reimplantation; vertebral to carotid artery**

27.2 | 27.2 | FUD 090 | C 80 50

AMA: 1997,Nov,1; 1993,Win,1

35693 **vertebral to subclavian artery**

23.6 | 23.6 | FUD 090 | C 80 50

AMA: 1997,Nov,1; 1994,Sum,29

35694 **subclavian to carotid artery**

EXCLUDES *Subclavian to carotid artery transposition procedure (open) with concurrent repair descending thoracic aorta (endovascular) (33889)*

28.4 | 28.4 | FUD 090 | C 80 50

AMA: 1997,Nov,1; 1993,Win,1

35695 **carotid to subclavian artery**

29.7 | 29.7 | FUD 090 | C 80 50

AMA: 1997,Nov,1; 1993,Win,1

+ **35697** **Reimplantation, visceral artery to infrarenal aortic prosthesis, each artery (List separately in addition to code for primary procedure)**

EXCLUDES *Repair thoracoabdominal aortic aneurysm with graft (33877)*

Code first primary procedure

4.29 | 4.29 | FUD ZZZ | C 80

AMA: 1997,Nov,1

35700 Reoperative Bypass Lower Extremities

Code first (35556, 35566, 35570-35571, 35583, 35585, 35587, 35656, 35666, 35671)

+ **35700** **Reoperation, femoral-popliteal or femoral (popliteal)-anterior tibial, posterior tibial, peroneal artery, or other distal vessels, more than 1 month after original operation (List separately in addition to code for primary procedure)**

4.44 | 4.44 | FUD ZZZ | C 80

AMA: 2018,Jan,8; 2017,Jan,8; 2016,Jan,13

35701-35703 Arterial Exploration without Repair

EXCLUDES *Exploration to identify recipient artery for microvascular free graft/flap anastomosis:*
- *Bone (20955-20962)*
- *Jejunum (43496)*
- *Muscle, skin or fascia (15756-15758)*
- *Omentum (49906)*
- *Osteocutaneous (20969-20973)*

Exploration without surgical repair:
- *Abdominal artery (49000)*
- *Chest artery (32100)*
- *Other arteries not in neck, upper or lower extremities, chest, abdomen, or retroperitoneum (37799)*
- *Retroperitoneal artery (49010)*

Code also nonvascular surgical procedures performed in addition to exploration when exploration through separate incision

35701 **Exploration not followed by surgical repair, artery; neck (eg, carotid, subclavian)**

EXCLUDES *Exploration for postoperative hemorrhage, thrombosis or infection (35800)*

Repair blood vessel on same side neck (35201, 35231, 35261)

12.6 | 12.6 | FUD 090 | C 80 50

AMA: 2019,Dec,5

35702 **upper extremity (eg, axillary, brachial, radial, ulnar)**

EXCLUDES *Exploration for postoperative hemorrhage, thrombosis or infection in same extremity (35860)*

Repair blood vessel in same extremity (35206-35207, 35236, 35266)

11.9 | 11.9 | FUD 090 | 80 50

AMA: 2019,Dec,5

35703 **lower extremity (eg, common femoral, deep femoral, superficial femoral, popliteal, tibial, peroneal)**

EXCLUDES *Exploration for postoperative hemorrhage, thrombosis or infection in same extremity (35860)*

Repair blood vessel in same extremity (35256, 35286)

12.0 | 12.0 | FUD 090 | 80 50

AMA: 2019,Dec,5

35800-35860 Arterial Exploration for Postoperative Complication

INCLUDES Return to operating room for postoperative hemorrhage

35800 **Exploration for postoperative hemorrhage, thrombosis or infection; neck**

20.8 | 20.8 | FUD 090 | C 80

AMA: 2019,Dec,5

35820 **chest**

58.2 | 58.2 | FUD 090 | C 80

AMA: 1997,Nov,1

35840 **abdomen**

34.8 | 34.8 | FUD 090 | C 80

AMA: 1997,May,4; 1997,Nov,1

35860 **extremity**

24.2 | 24.2 | FUD 090 | T G2 80

AMA: 2019,Dec,5; 2018,Jan,8; 2017,Jan,8; 2016,Jan,13

35870 Repair Secondary Aortoenteric Fistula

35870 **Repair of graft-enteric fistula**

36.1 | 36.1 | FUD 090 | C 80

AMA: 1997,Nov,1

35875-35876 Removal of Thrombus from Graft

EXCLUDES *Thrombectomy dialysis fistula or graft (36831, 36833)*

Thrombectomy with blood vessel repair, lower extremity, vein graft (35256)

Thrombectomy with blood vessel repair, lower extremity, with/without patch angioplasty (35226)

35875 **Thrombectomy of arterial or venous graft (other than hemodialysis graft or fistula);**

17.3 | 17.3 | FUD 090 | T A2

AMA: 2018,Jan,8; 2017,Jan,8; 2016,Jan,13

35876 **with revision of arterial or venous graft**

27.5 | 27.5 | FUD 090 | T A2 80

AMA: 1999,Mar,6; 1999,Nov,1

35879-35884 Revision Lower Extremity Bypass Graft

EXCLUDES *Removal infected graft (35901-35907)*
Revascularization following removal infected graft(s)
Thrombectomy dialysis fistula or graft (36831, 36833)
Thrombectomy with blood vessel repair, lower extremity, vein graft (35256)
Thrombectomy with blood vessel repair, lower extremity, with/without patch angioplasty (35226)
Thrombectomy with graft revision (35876)

35879 **Revision, lower extremity arterial bypass, without thrombectomy, open; with vein patch angioplasty**
26.8 26.8 **FUD** 090 T G2 80 50
AMA: 2018,Jan,8; 2017,Jan,8; 2016,Jan,13

35881 **with segmental vein interposition**
EXCLUDES *Revision femoral anastomosis synthetic arterial bypass graft (35883-35884)*
29.6 29.6 **FUD** 090 T G2 80 50
AMA: 2018,Jan,8; 2017,Jan,8; 2016,Jan,13

35883 **Revision, femoral anastomosis of synthetic arterial bypass graft in groin, open; with nonautogenous patch graft (eg, Dacron, ePTFE, bovine pericardium)**
EXCLUDES *Reoperation, femoral-popliteal or femoral (popliteal)-anterior tibial, posterior tibial, peroneal artery, or other distal vessels (35700)*
Revision, femoral anastomosis synthetic arterial bypass graft in groin, open; with autogenous vein patch graft (35884)
Thrombectomy arterial or venous graft (35875)
34.8 34.8 **FUD** 090 T G2 80 50
AMA: 2018,Jan,8; 2017,Jan,8; 2016,Jan,13

35884 **with autogenous vein patch graft**
EXCLUDES *Reoperation, femoral-popliteal or femoral (popliteal)-anterior tibial, posterior tibial, peroneal artery, or other distal vessels (35700)*
Revision, femoral anastomosis synthetic arterial bypass graft in groin, open; with autogenous vein patch graft (35883)
Thrombectomy arterial or venous graft (35875-35876)
36.0 36.0 **FUD** 090 T G2 80 50
AMA: 2018,Jan,8; 2017,Jan,8; 2016,Jan,13

35901-35907 Removal of Infected Graft

35901 **Excision of infected graft; neck**
13.6 13.6 **FUD** 090 C 80
AMA: 1997,Nov,1; 1993,Win,1

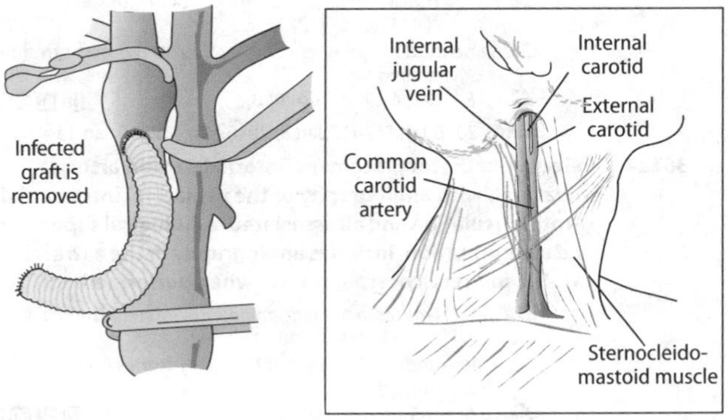

The physician removes an infected graft from the neck and repairs the blood vessel. If a new graft is placed, report the appropriate revascularization code

35903 **extremity**
16.4 16.4 **FUD** 090 T G2 80
AMA: 2018,Aug,10

35905 **thorax**
48.5 48.5 **FUD** 090 C 80
AMA: 1997,Nov,1; 1993,Win,1

35907 **abdomen**
55.3 55.3 **FUD** 090 C 80
AMA: 1997,Nov,1; 1993,Win,1

36000 Intravenous Access Established

INCLUDES Venous access for phlebotomy, prophylactic intravenous access, infusion therapy, chemotherapy, hydration, transfusion, drug administration, etc., included in primary procedure work value

36000 **Introduction of needle or intracatheter, vein**
0.26 0.79 **FUD** XXX N N1
AMA: 2019,Aug,8; 2018,Mar,3; 2018,Jan,8; 2017,Jan,8; 2016,Nov,3; 2016,Jan,13

36002 Injection Treatment of Pseudoaneurysm

INCLUDES Insertion needle or catheter, local anesthesia, contrast injection, power injections, and all pre- and postinjection care provided
EXCLUDES *Arteriotomy site sealant*
Compression repair pseudoaneurysm, ultrasound guided (76936)
Medications, contrast material, catheters

36002 **Injection procedures (eg, thrombin) for percutaneous treatment of extremity pseudoaneurysm**
(76942, 77002, 77012, 77021)
3.04 4.43 **FUD** 000 T G2 50
AMA: 2018,Mar,3; 2018,Jan,8; 2017,Jan,8; 2016,Nov,3; 2016,Jan,13

36005-36015 Insertion Needle or Intracatheter: Venous

INCLUDES Insertion needle or catheter, local anesthesia, contrast injection, power injections, and all pre- and postinjection care provided
EXCLUDES *Medications, contrast materials, catheters*

Code also:
Catheterization second order vessels (or higher) supplied by same first order branch, same vascular family (36012)
Each vascular family (e.g., bilateral procedures are separate vascular families)

36005 **Injection procedure for extremity venography (including introduction of needle or intracatheter)**
(75820, 75822)
1.38 8.44 **FUD** 000 N N1 80 50
AMA: 2018,Mar,3; 2018,Jan,8; 2017,Jan,8; 2016,Nov,3; 2016,Jul,6; 2016,Jan,13

36010 **Introduction of catheter, superior or inferior vena cava**
3.19 15.0 **FUD** XXX N N1 50
AMA: 2018,Jan,8; 2017,Feb,14; 2017,Jan,8; 2016,Jul,6; 2016,Jan,13

36011 **Selective catheter placement, venous system; first order branch (eg, renal vein, jugular vein)**
4.54 24.0 **FUD** XXX N N1 50
AMA: 2018,Jan,8; 2017,Jan,8; 2016,Jul,6; 2016,Jan,13

36012 **second order, or more selective, branch (eg, left adrenal vein, petrosal sinus)**
5.04 25.0 **FUD** XXX N N1 50
AMA: 2018,Oct,3; 2018,Jan,8; 2017,Jan,8; 2016,Jul,6; 2016,Jan,13

36013 **Introduction of catheter, right heart or main pulmonary artery**
3.53 22.7 **FUD** XXX N N1
AMA: 2019,Jun,3; 2018,Jan,8; 2017,Jan,8; 2016,Jul,6; 2016,Jan,13

36014 **Selective catheter placement, left or right pulmonary artery**
4.41 23.7 **FUD** XXX N N1 50
AMA: 2019,Jun,3; 2018,Jan,8; 2017,Jan,8; 2016,Jul,6; 2016,Jan,13

36015 **Selective catheter placement, segmental or subsegmental pulmonary artery**
EXCLUDES *Placement Swan Ganz/other flow directed catheter for monitoring (93503)*
Selective blood sampling, specific organs (36500)
5.00 25.7 **FUD** XXX N N1 50
AMA: 2019,Jun,3; 2018,Jan,8; 2017,Jan,8; 2016,Jul,6; 2016,Jan,13

36100-36218 Insertion Needle or Intracatheter: Arterial

INCLUDES Introduction catheter and catheterization all lesser order vessels used for approach
Local anesthesia, placement catheter/needle, contrast injection, power injections, all pre- and postinjection care

EXCLUDES *Angiography (36222-36228, 75600-75774)*
Angioplasty ([37246, 37247])
Chemotherapy injections (96401-96549)
Injection procedures for cardiac catheterizations (93454-93461, 93564, 93593-93597)
Internal mammary artery angiography without left heart catheterization (36216, 36217)
Medications, contrast, catheters
Transcatheter interventions (37200, 37211, 37213-37214, 37241-37244, 61624, 61626)

Code also:
Additional first order or higher catheterization for vascular families when vascular family supplied by first order vessel different from one already coded
Catheterization second and third order vessels supplied by same first order branch, same vascular family (36218, 36248)

36100 Introduction of needle or intracatheter, carotid or vertebral artery
4.54 14.8 **FUD** XXX N N1 50
AMA: 2000,Oct,4; 1998,Apr,1

36140 Introduction of needle or intracatheter, upper or lower extremity artery
EXCLUDES *Arteriovenous cannula insertion (36810-36821)*
2.60 13.6 **FUD** XXX N N1
AMA: 2018,Jan,8; 2017,Jan,8; 2016,Jan,13

36160 Introduction of needle or intracatheter, aortic, translumbar
3.59 14.6 **FUD** XXX N N1
AMA: 2018,Jan,8; 2017,Jan,8; 2016,Jan,13

36200 Introduction of catheter, aorta
EXCLUDES *Nonselective angiography extracranial carotid and/or cerebral vessels and cervicocerebral arch (36221)*
4.06 16.8 **FUD** 000 N N1 50
AMA: 2018,Jan,8; 2017,Mar,3; 2017,Jan,8; 2016,Jul,6; 2016,Jan,13

36215 Selective catheter placement, arterial system; each first order thoracic or brachiocephalic branch, within a vascular family
INCLUDES Introduction catheter into aorta (36200)
EXCLUDES *Placement catheter for coronary angiography (93454-93461)*
6.13 30.7 **FUD** 000 N N1
AMA: 2018,Jan,8; 2017,Mar,3; 2017,Jan,8; 2016,Jul,6; 2016,Jan,13

36216 initial second order thoracic or brachiocephalic branch, within a vascular family
7.90 32.5 **FUD** 000 N N1
AMA: 2018,Jan,8; 2017,Jan,8; 2016,Jul,6; 2016,Jan,13

36217 initial third order or more selective thoracic or brachiocephalic branch, within a vascular family
9.52 53.9 **FUD** 000 N N1
AMA: 2018,Jan,8; 2017,Jan,8; 2016,Jul,6; 2016,Jan,13

\+ **36218 additional second order, third order, and beyond, thoracic or brachiocephalic branch, within a vascular family (List in addition to code for initial second or third order vessel as appropriate)**
Code also transcatheter therapy procedures (37200, 37211, 37213-37214, 37236-37239, 37241-37244, 61624, 61626)
Code first (36216-36217, 36225-36226)
1.51 6.89 **FUD** ZZZ N N1
AMA: 2018,Oct,3; 2018,Jan,8; 2017,Jan,8; 2016,Jul,6; 2016,Jan,13

36221-36228 Diagnostic Studies: Aortic Arch/Carotid/Vertebral Arteries

INCLUDES Accessing vessel
Arterial contrast injection including arterial, capillary, and venous phase imaging, when performed
Arteriotomy closure (pressure or closure device)
Catheter placement
Radiologic supervision and interpretation
Reporting selective catheter placement based on service intensity in following hierarchy:
36226>36225
36224>36223>36222

EXCLUDES *3D rendering when performed (76376-76377)*
Interventional procedures
Ultrasound guidance (76937)

Code also diagnostic angiography upper extremities/other vascular beds during same session, when performed (75774)

36221 Non-selective catheter placement, thoracic aorta, with angiography of the extracranial carotid, vertebral, and/or intracranial vessels, unilateral or bilateral, and all associated radiological supervision and interpretation, includes angiography of the cervicocerebral arch, when performed
EXCLUDES *Selective catheter placement, common carotid or innominate artery (36222-36226)*
Transcatheter intravascular stent placement common carotid or innominate artery on same side (37217)
5.80 29.3 **FUD** 000 Q2 N1
AMA: 2018,Jan,8; 2017,Jan,8; 2016,Mar,3; 2016,Jan,13

36222 Selective catheter placement, common carotid or innominate artery, unilateral, any approach, with angiography of the ipsilateral extracranial carotid circulation and all associated radiological supervision and interpretation, includes angiography of the cervicocerebral arch, when performed
EXCLUDES *Transcatheter placement intravascular stent(s) (37215-37218)*
Code also modifier 59 when different territories on both sides body studied
8.22 34.7 **FUD** 000 Q2 N1 50
AMA: 2018,Jan,8; 2017,Jan,8; 2016,Mar,3; 2016,Jan,13

36223 Selective catheter placement, common carotid or innominate artery, unilateral, any approach, with angiography of the ipsilateral intracranial carotid circulation and all associated radiological supervision and interpretation, includes angiography of the extracranial carotid and cervicocerebral arch, when performed
EXCLUDES *Transcatheter placement intravascular stent(s) (37215-37218)*
Code also modifier 59 when different territories on both sides body studied
9.18 43.9 **FUD** 000 Q2 N1 50
AMA: 2018,Jan,8; 2017,Jan,8; 2016,Mar,3; 2016,Jan,13

36224 Selective catheter placement, internal carotid artery, unilateral, with angiography of the ipsilateral intracranial carotid circulation and all associated radiological supervision and interpretation, includes angiography of the extracranial carotid and cervicocerebral arch, when performed
EXCLUDES *Transcatheter placement intravascular stent(s) (37215-37218)*
Code also modifier 59 when different territories on both sides body studied
10.4 56.8 **FUD** 000 Q2 N1 50
AMA: 2018,Jan,8; 2017,Jan,8; 2016,Mar,3; 2016,Jan,13

36225 Selective catheter placement, subclavian or innominate artery, unilateral, with angiography of the ipsilateral vertebral circulation and all associated radiological supervision and interpretation, includes angiography of the cervicocerebral arch, when performed
EXCLUDES *Transcatheter placement intravascular stent(s) (37217)*
9.16 42.3 **FUD** 000 Q2 N1 50
AMA: 2018,Jan,8; 2017,Jan,8; 2016,Mar,3; 2016,Jan,13

36226 Selective catheter placement, vertebral artery, unilateral, with angiography of the ipsilateral vertebral circulation and all associated radiological supervision and interpretation, includes angiography of the cervicocerebral arch, when performed

EXCLUDES *Transcatheter placement intravascular stent(s) (37217)*

10.3 53.7 **FUD** 000 Q2 N1 50

AMA: 2018,Jan,8; 2017,Jan,8; 2016,Mar,3; 2016,Jan,13

+ **36227 Selective catheter placement, external carotid artery, unilateral, with angiography of the ipsilateral external carotid circulation and all associated radiological supervision and interpretation (List separately in addition to code for primary procedure)**

EXCLUDES *Reporting with modifier 50. Report once for each side when performed bilaterally*
Transcatheter placement intravascular stent(s) (37217)

Code first (36222-36224)

3.41 7.23 **FUD** ZZZ N N1 50

AMA: 2018,Jan,8; 2017,Jan,8; 2016,Jan,13

+ **36228 Selective catheter placement, each intracranial branch of the internal carotid or vertebral arteries, unilateral, with angiography of the selected vessel circulation and all associated radiological supervision and interpretation (eg, middle cerebral artery, posterior inferior cerebellar artery) (List separately in addition to code for primary procedure)**

EXCLUDES *Procedure performed more than two times per side*
Reporting with modifier 50. Report once for each side when performed bilaterally

Code first (36223-36226)

7.03 37.6 **FUD** ZZZ N N1 50

AMA: 2018,Jan,8; 2017,Jan,8; 2016,Jan,13

36245-36254 Catheter Placement: Arteries of the Lower Body

INCLUDES Introduction catheter and catheterization all lesser order vessels used for approach
Local anesthesia, placement catheter/needle, contrast injection, power injections

EXCLUDES *Angiography (36222-36228, 75600-75774)*
Chemotherapy injections (96401-96549)
Injection procedures for cardiac catheterizations (93454-93461, 93564, 93593-93597)
Internal mammary artery angiography without left heart catheterization (36216-36217)
Medications, contrast, catheters
Transcatheter procedures (37200, 37211, 37213-37214, 37236-37239, 37241-37244, 61624, 61626)

Code also:
Additional first order or higher catheterization for vascular families when vascular family supplied by first order vessel different from one already coded
Catheterization second and third order vessels supplied by same first order branch, same vascular family (36218, 36248)

(75600-75774)

36245 Selective catheter placement, arterial system; each first order abdominal, pelvic, or lower extremity artery branch, within a vascular family

6.89 38.1 **FUD** XXX N N1 50

AMA: 2018,Jan,8; 2017,Jan,8; 2016,Jul,6; 2016,Jan,13

36246 initial second order abdominal, pelvic, or lower extremity artery branch, within a vascular family

7.35 24.5 **FUD** 000 N N1 50

AMA: 2018,Jan,8; 2017,Jan,8; 2016,Jul,6; 2016,Jan,13

36247 initial third order or more selective abdominal, pelvic, or lower extremity artery branch, within a vascular family

8.75 43.2 **FUD** 000 N N1 50

AMA: 2020,Sep,14; 2018,Jan,8; 2017,Jan,8; 2016,Jul,6; 2016,Jan,13

+ **36248 additional second order, third order, and beyond, abdominal, pelvic, or lower extremity artery branch, within a vascular family (List in addition to code for initial second or third order vessel as appropriate)**

Code first (36246, 36247)

1.41 3.92 **FUD** ZZZ N N1

AMA: 2018,Oct,3; 2018,Jan,8; 2017,Jan,8; 2016,Jul,6; 2016,Jan,13

36251 Selective catheter placement (first-order), main renal artery and any accessory renal artery(s) for renal angiography, including arterial puncture and catheter placement(s), fluoroscopy, contrast injection(s), image postprocessing, permanent recording of images, and radiological supervision and interpretation, including pressure gradient measurements when performed, and flush aortogram when performed; unilateral

INCLUDES Closure device placement at vascular access site

EXCLUDES *Transcatheter renal sympathetic denervation, percutaneous approach (0338T-0339T)*

7.51 39.7 **FUD** 000 Q2 N1

AMA: 2018,Jan,8; 2017,Jan,8; 2016,Jan,13

36252 bilateral

INCLUDES Closure device placement at vascular access site

EXCLUDES *Transcatheter renal sympathetic denervation, percutaneous approach (0338T-0339T)*

10.4 42.8 **FUD** 000 Q2 N1

AMA: 2018,Jan,8; 2017,Jan,8; 2016,Jan,13

36253 Superselective catheter placement (one or more second order or higher renal artery branches) renal artery and any accessory renal artery(s) for renal angiography, including arterial puncture, catheterization, fluoroscopy, contrast injection(s), image postprocessing, permanent recording of images, and radiological supervision and interpretation, including pressure gradient measurements when performed, and flush aortogram when performed; unilateral

INCLUDES Closure device placement at vascular access site

EXCLUDES *Procedure performed on same kidney with (36251)*
Transcatheter renal sympathetic denervation, percutaneous approach (0338T-0339T)

10.3 62.9 **FUD** 000 Q2 N1

AMA: 2018,Jan,8; 2017,Jan,8; 2016,Jan,13

36254 bilateral

INCLUDES Closure device placement at vascular access site

EXCLUDES *Selective catheter placement (first-order), main renal artery and any accessory renal artery(s) for renal angiography (36252)*
Transcatheter renal sympathetic denervation, percutaneous approach (0338T-0339T)

12.0 61.6 **FUD** 000 Q2 N1

AMA: 2018,Jan,8; 2017,Jan,8; 2016,Jan,13

36260-36299 Implanted Infusion Pumps: Intra-arterial

36260 Insertion of implantable intra-arterial infusion pump (eg, for chemotherapy of liver)

18.8 18.8 **FUD** 090 T A2

AMA: 2018,Jan,8; 2017,Jan,8; 2016,Jan,13

36261 Revision of implanted intra-arterial infusion pump

11.7 11.7 **FUD** 090 T J8 80

AMA: 2000,Oct,4; 1997,Nov,1

36262 Removal of implanted intra-arterial infusion pump

8.96 8.96 **FUD** 090 Q2 G2

AMA: 2000,Oct,4; 1997,Nov,1

36299 Unlisted procedure, vascular injection

0.00 0.00 **FUD** YYY N 80

AMA: 2000,Oct,4; 1997,Nov,1

36400-36425 Specimen Collection: Phlebotomy

EXCLUDES *Specimen collection from:*
Completely implantable device (36591)
Established catheter (36592)

36400 Venipuncture, younger than age 3 years, necessitating the skill of a physician or other qualified health care professional, not to be used for routine venipuncture; femoral or jugular vein A
0.53 0.75 FUD XXX N N1
AMA: 2018,Jan,8; 2017,Jan,8; 2016,Jan,13

36405 scalp vein A
0.44 0.66 FUD XXX N N1
AMA: 2018,Jan,8; 2017,Jan,8; 2016,Jan,13

36406 other vein A
0.25 0.47 FUD XXX N N1
AMA: 2018,Jan,8; 2017,Jan,8; 2016,Jan,13

36410 Venipuncture, age 3 years or older, necessitating the skill of a physician or other qualified health care professional (separate procedure), for diagnostic or therapeutic purposes (not to be used for routine venipuncture) A
0.27 0.49 FUD XXX N N1
AMA: 2019,Aug,8; 2018,Mar,3; 2018,Jan,8; 2017,Jan,8; 2016,Nov,3; 2016,Jan,13

36415 Collection of venous blood by venipuncture
0.00 0.00 FUD XXX 63 Q
AMA: 2019,Aug,8; 2018,Jan,8; 2017,Jan,8; 2016,Jan,13

36416 Collection of capillary blood specimen (eg, finger, heel, ear stick)
0.00 0.00 FUD XXX N N1
AMA: 2008,Apr,-9; 2003,Feb,7

36420 Venipuncture, cutdown; younger than age 1 year A
1.35 1.35 FUD XXX 63 Q1 N1 80
AMA: 2018,Jan,8; 2017,Jan,8; 2016,Jan,13

36425 age 1 or over A
EXCLUDES *Endovenous ablation therapy incompetent vein, extremity (36475-36476, 36478-36479)*
1.15 1.15 FUD XXX Q1 N1
AMA: 2018,Mar,3; 2018,Jan,8; 2017,Jan,8; 2016,Nov,3; 2016,Jan,13

36430-36460 Transfusions

CMS: 100-01,3,20.5 Blood Deductibles; 100-03,110.16 Transfusion in Kidney Transplants; 100-03,110.7 Blood Transfusions; 100-03,110.8 Blood Platelet Transfusions

36430 Transfusion, blood or blood components
EXCLUDES *Infant partial exchange transfusion (36456)*
0.99 0.99 FUD XXX S P3
AMA: 2020,Jun,14; 2019,Jun,5; 2018,Jan,8; 2017,Jul,3; 2017,Jan,8; 2016,Jan,13

36440 Push transfusion, blood, 2 years or younger A
EXCLUDES *Infant partial exchange transfusion (36456)*
1.46 1.46 FUD XXX S R2 80
AMA: 2018,Jan,8; 2017,Jul,3; 2017,Jan,8; 2016,Jan,13

36450 Exchange transfusion, blood; newborn A
EXCLUDES *Automated red cell exchange (36512)*
Infant partial exchange transfusion (36456)
4.93 4.93 FUD XXX 63 S R2 80
AMA: 2018,Jan,8; 2017,Jul,3

36455 other than newborn A
EXCLUDES *Automated red cell exchange (36512)*
3.68 3.68 FUD XXX S G2
AMA: 2003,Apr,7; 1997,Nov,1

36456 Partial exchange transfusion, blood, plasma or crystalloid necessitating the skill of a physician or other qualified health care professional, newborn A
EXCLUDES *Automated red cell exchange (36512)*
Transfusions other types (36430-36450)
2.93 2.93 FUD XXX 63 S 80
AMA: 2018,Jan,8; 2017,Jul,3

36460 Transfusion, intrauterine, fetal A ♀
(76941)
10.1 10.1 FUD XXX 63 S G2 80
AMA: 2003,Apr,7; 1997,Nov,1

36465-36466 [36465, 36466] Destruction Spider Veins

INCLUDES All supplies, equipment, compression stockings or bandages when performed in physician office

EXCLUDES *Multi-layer compression system applied to leg (29581, 29584)*
Strapping leg: ankle, foot, hip, knee, toes same extremity (29520, 29530, 29540, 29550)
Unna boot (29580)
Reporting code more than one time for each extremity treated
Vascular embolization and occlusion (37241-37244)
Vascular embolization vein in same operative field (37241)

36465 **Resequenced code. See code following 36471.**

36466 **Resequenced code. See code following 36471.**

36468 Injection(s) of sclerosant for spider veins (telangiectasia), limb or trunk
(76942)
0.00 0.00 FUD 000 Q1 N1 80
AMA: 2018,Mar,3; 2018,Jan,8; 2017,Jan,8; 2016,Nov,3; 2016,Jan,13

36470 Injection of sclerosant; single incompetent vein (other than telangiectasia)
EXCLUDES *Injection foam sclerosant with ultrasound guidance for compression maneuvers (36465-36466)*
(76942)
1.10 3.10 FUD 000 T P3 50
AMA: 2018,Dec,10; 2018,Dec,10; 2018,Mar,3; 2018,Jan,8; 2017,Jan,8; 2016,Nov,3; 2016,Jan,13

36471 multiple incompetent veins (other than telangiectasia), same leg
EXCLUDES *Injection foam sclerosant with ultrasound guidance for compression maneuvers (36465-36466)*
(76942)
2.22 5.59 FUD 000 T P3 50
AMA: 2018,Dec,10; 2018,Dec,10; 2018,Mar,3; 2018,Jan,8; 2017,Jan,8; 2016,Nov,3; 2016,Jan,13

36465 Injection of non-compounded foam sclerosant with ultrasound compression maneuvers to guide dispersion of the injectate, inclusive of all imaging guidance and monitoring; single incompetent extremity truncal vein (eg, great saphenous vein, accessory saphenous vein)
EXCLUDES *Ablation vein using chemical adhesive ([36482, 36483])*
Injection foam sclerosant with ultrasound guidance for compression maneuvers (36465-36466)
3.48 42.9 FUD 000 T P2 50
AMA: 2019,Feb,9; 2018,Dec,10; 2018,Dec,10; 2018,Mar,3

36466 multiple incompetent truncal veins (eg, great saphenous vein, accessory saphenous vein), same leg
EXCLUDES *Ablation vein using chemical adhesive ([36482, 36483])*
Injection foam sclerosant with ultrasound guidance for compression maneuvers (36465-36466)
4.46 47.6 FUD 000 T P2 50
AMA: 2019,Feb,9; 2018,Dec,10; 2018,Dec,10; 2018,Mar,3

36473-36483 [36482, 36483] Vein Ablation

INCLUDES Multi-layer compression system applied to leg (29581, 29584)
Patient monitoring
Radiological guidance (76000, 76937, 76942, 76998, 77002)
Venous access/injections (36000-36005, 36410, 36425)

EXCLUDES *Duplex scans (93970-93971)*
Strapping leg: ankle, foot, hip, knee, toes same extremity (29520, 29530, 29540, 29550)
Transcatheter embolization (75894)
Unna boot (29580)
Vascular embolization vein in same operative field (37241)

36473 Endovenous ablation therapy of incompetent vein, extremity, inclusive of all imaging guidance and monitoring, percutaneous, mechanochemical; first vein treated

INCLUDES Local anesthesia

EXCLUDES *Laser ablation incompetent vein (36478-36479)*
Radiofrequency ablation incompetent vein (36475-36476)

5.18 40.4 FUD 000 T P3 50

AMA: 2019,Feb,9; 2018,Mar,3; 2018,Jan,8; 2017,Jan,8; 2016,Nov,3

\+ **36474 subsequent vein(s) treated in a single extremity, each through separate access sites (List separately in addition to code for primary procedure)**

INCLUDES Local anesthesia

EXCLUDES *Laser ablation incompetent vein (36478-36479)*
Radiofrequency ablation incompetent vein (36475-36476)
Reporting code more than one time per extremity

Code first (36473)

2.60 8.23 FUD ZZZ N N1 50

AMA: 2019,Feb,9; 2018,Mar,3; 2018,Jan,8; 2017,Jan,8; 2016,Nov,3

36475 Endovenous ablation therapy of incompetent vein, extremity, inclusive of all imaging guidance and monitoring, percutaneous, radiofrequency; first vein treated

INCLUDES Tumescent anesthesia

EXCLUDES *Ablation vein using chemical adhesive ([36482, 36483])*
Endovenous ablation therapy incompetent vein (36478-36479)

8.09 38.9 FUD 000 T A2 50

AMA: 2018,Mar,3; 2018,Jan,8; 2017,Jan,8; 2016,Nov,3; 2016,Aug,3; 2016,Jan,13

\+ **36476 subsequent vein(s) treated in a single extremity, each through separate access sites (List separately in addition to code for primary procedure)**

INCLUDES Tumescent anesthesia

EXCLUDES *Ablation vein using chemical adhesive ([36482, 36483])*
Endovenous ablation therapy incompetent vein (36478-36479)
Reporting code more than one time per extremity
Vascular embolization or occlusion (37242-37244)

Code first (36475)

3.92 8.81 FUD ZZZ N N1 50

AMA: 2018,Mar,3; 2018,Jan,8; 2017,Jan,8; 2016,Nov,3; 2016,Aug,3; 2016,Jan,13

36478 Endovenous ablation therapy of incompetent vein, extremity, inclusive of all imaging guidance and monitoring, percutaneous, laser; first vein treated

INCLUDES Tumescent anesthesia

EXCLUDES *Ablation vein using chemical adhesive ([36482, 36483])*
Endovenous ablation therapy incompetent vein (36478-36479)

8.06 30.2 FUD 000 T A2 50

AMA: 2020,May,13; 2018,Mar,3; 2018,Jan,8; 2017,Jan,8; 2016,Nov,3; 2016,Aug,3; 2016,Jan,13

\+ **36479 subsequent vein(s) treated in a single extremity, each through separate access sites (List separately in addition to code for primary procedure)**

INCLUDES Tumescent anesthesia

EXCLUDES *Ablation vein using chemical adhesive ([36482, 36483])*
Endovenous ablation therapy incompetent vein (36478-36479)
Vascular embolization or occlusion (37241)

Code first (36478)

3.96 9.28 FUD ZZZ N N1 50

AMA: 2020,May,13; 2018,Mar,3; 2018,Jan,8; 2017,Jan,8; 2016,Nov,3; 2016,Aug,3; 2016,Jan,13

\# **36482 Endovenous ablation therapy of incompetent vein, extremity, by transcatheter delivery of a chemical adhesive (eg, cyanoacrylate) remote from the access site, inclusive of all imaging guidance and monitoring, percutaneous; first vein treated**

INCLUDES Local anesthesia

EXCLUDES *Laser ablation incompetent vein (36478-36479)*
Radiofrequency ablation incompetent vein (36475-36476)

5.20 54.0 FUD 000 T P3 50

AMA: 2019,Feb,9; 2018,Mar,3

\+ # **36483 subsequent vein(s) treated in a single extremity, each through separate access sites (List separately in addition to code for primary procedure)**

INCLUDES Local anesthesia

EXCLUDES *Laser ablation incompetent vein (36478-36479)*
Radiofrequency ablation incompetent vein (36475-36476)
Reporting code more than one time per extremity

Code first ([36482])

2.61 4.45 FUD ZZZ N N1 50

AMA: 2019,Feb,9; 2018,Mar,3

36481-36510 [36482, 36483] Other Venous Catheterization Procedures

EXCLUDES *Specimen collection from:*
Completely implantable device (36591)
Established catheter (36592)

36481 Percutaneous portal vein catheterization by any method

(75885, 75887)

9.56 54.6 FUD 000 N N1

AMA: 2018,Jan,8; 2017,Jan,8; 2016,Jan,13

36482 **Resequenced code. See code following 36479.**

36483 **Resequenced code. See code following 36479.**

36500 Venous catheterization for selective organ blood sampling

EXCLUDES *Inferior or superior vena cava catheterization (36010)*

(75893)

5.30 5.30 FUD 000 N N1

AMA: 2014,Jan,11; 1997,Nov,1

36510 Catheterization of umbilical vein for diagnosis or therapy, newborn A

EXCLUDES *Specimen collection from:*
Capillary blood (36416)
Venipuncture (36415)

1.55 2.36 FUD 000 63 N N1 80

AMA: 2018,Jan,8; 2017,Jan,8; 2016,May,3; 2016,Jan,13

36511-36516 Apheresis

CMS: 100-03,110.14 Apheresis (Therapeutic Pheresis); 100-04,4,231.9 Billing for Pheresis and Apheresis Services

EXCLUDES *Specimen collection for therapeutic treatment from:*
Completely implantable device (36591)
Established catheter (36592)

36511 Therapeutic apheresis; for white blood cells

3.15 3.15 FUD 000 S 62

AMA: 2018,Jan,8; 2017,Jan,8; 2016,Jan,13

36512 **for red blood cells**

EXCLUDES *Manual red cell exchange (36450, 36455, 36456)*

3.12 3.12 FUD 000 S G2

AMA: 2018,Jan,8; 2017,Jan,8; 2016,Jan,13

36513 **for platelets**

EXCLUDES *Collection platelets from donors*

3.15 3.15 FUD 000 S R2

AMA: 2018,Jan,8; 2017,Jan,8; 2016,Jan,13

36514 **for plasma pheresis**

2.75 19.1 FUD 000 S G2

AMA: 2018,May,10; 2018,Jan,8; 2017,Jan,8; 2016,Jan,13

36516 **with extracorporeal immunoadsorption, selective adsorption or selective filtration and plasma reinfusion**

Code also modifier 26 for professional evaluation

2.44 55.4 FUD 000 S P3

AMA: 2018,Jan,8; 2017,Jan,8; 2016,Jan,13

36522 Extracorporeal Photopheresis

CMS: 100-03,110.4 Extracorporeal Photopheresis; 100-04,32,190 Billing for Extracorporeal Photopheresis; 100-04,32,190.2 Healthcare Common Procedural Coding System (HCPCS), Applicable Diagnosis Codes and Procedure Code; 100-04,32,190.3 Medicare Summary Notices (MSNs), Remittance Advice Remark Codes (RAs) and Claim Adjustment Reason Code; 100-04,4,231.9 Billing for Pheresis and Apheresis Services

EXCLUDES *Dialysis (90935-90999)*
Therapeutic apheresis (36511-36514, 36516)
Therapeutic ultrafiltration (0692T)

36522 **Photopheresis, extracorporeal**

2.79 61.2 FUD 000 S G2

AMA: 2018,May,10; 2018,Jan,8; 2017,Jan,8; 2016,Jan,13

36555-36573 [36572, 36573] Placement of Implantable Venous Access Device

INCLUDES Devices accessed by exposed catheter, or subcutaneous port or pump
Devices inserted via cutdown or percutaneous access:
Centrally (eg, femoral, jugular, subclavian veins, or inferior vena cava)
Peripherally (e.g., basilic, cephalic, saphenous vein)
Devices terminating in brachiocephalic (innominate), iliac, subclavian veins, vena cava, or right atrium

EXCLUDES *Insertion midline catheter (36400, 36406, 36410)*
Maintenance/refilling implantable pump/reservoir (96522)

Code also removal central venous access device (if code available) when new device placed through separate venous access

36555 **Insertion of non-tunneled centrally inserted central venous catheter; younger than 5 years of age** A

EXCLUDES *Peripheral insertion (36568)*

(76937, 77001)

2.44 5.35 FUD 000 T A2

AMA: 2019,May,3; 2018,Jan,8; 2017,Jan,8; 2016,Jan,13

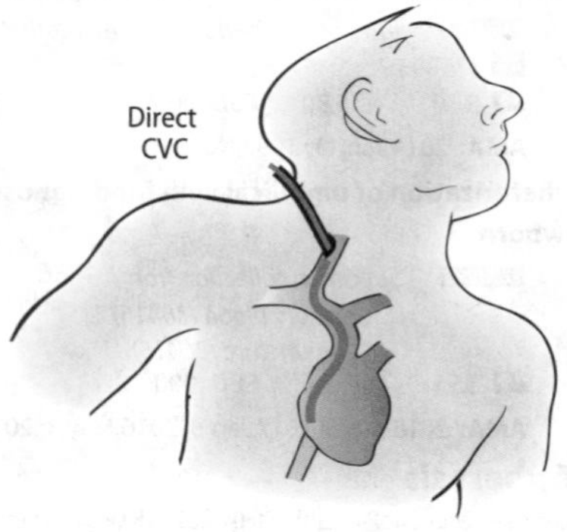

A non-tunneled centrally inserted CVC is inserted

36556 **age 5 years or older** A

EXCLUDES *Peripheral insertion (36569)*

(76937, 77001)

2.46 6.08 FUD 000 T A2

AMA: 2019,May,3; 2018,Nov,11; 2018,Jan,8; 2017,Jan,8; 2016,Jan,13

36557 **Insertion of tunneled centrally inserted central venous catheter, without subcutaneous port or pump; younger than 5 years of age** A

(76937, 77001)

9.25 31.3 FUD 010 T A2 80 50

AMA: 2018,Jan,8; 2017,Jan,8; 2016,Jan,13

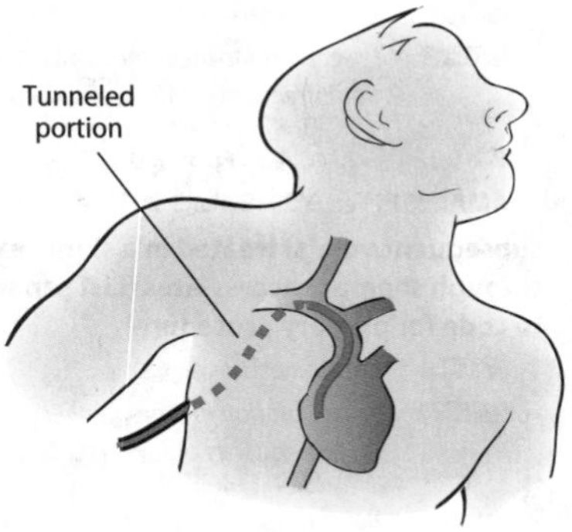

A tunneled centrally inserted CVC is inserted

36558 **age 5 years or older** A

EXCLUDES *Peripheral insertion (36571)*

(76937, 77001)

7.55 23.1 FUD 010 T A2 80 50

AMA: 2018,Jan,8; 2017,Jan,8; 2016,Jan,13

36560 **Insertion of tunneled centrally inserted central venous access device, with subcutaneous port; younger than 5 years of age** A

EXCLUDES *Peripheral insertion (36570)*

(76937, 77001)

11.0 37.4 FUD 010 T G2 80 50

AMA: 2018,Jan,8; 2017,Jan,8; 2016,Jan,13

36561 **age 5 years or older** A

EXCLUDES *Peripheral insertion (36571)*

(76937, 77001)

9.74 30.6 FUD 010 T A2 80 50

AMA: 2018,Jan,8; 2017,Jan,8; 2016,Jan,13

36563 **Insertion of tunneled centrally inserted central venous access device with subcutaneous pump**

(76937, 77001)

10.6 33.9 FUD 010 T A2 80

AMA: 2018,Jan,8; 2017,Jan,8; 2016,Jan,13

36565 **Insertion of tunneled centrally inserted central venous access device, requiring 2 catheters via 2 separate venous access sites; without subcutaneous port or pump (eg, Tesio type catheter)**

(76937, 77001)

9.71 25.0 FUD 010 T A2 80 50

AMA: 2018,Jan,8; 2017,Jan,8; 2016,Jan,13

36566 **with subcutaneous port(s)**

(76937, 77001)

10.4 132. FUD 010 T A2 80 50

AMA: 2018,Jan,8; 2017,Jan,8; 2016,Jan,13

36568 Insertion of peripherally inserted central venous catheter (PICC), without subcutaneous port or pump, without imaging guidance; younger than 5 years of age A

EXCLUDES *Centrally inserted placement (36555)*
Imaging guidance (76937, 77001)
Peripherally inserted ([36572])
PICC line removal with codes for removal tunneled central venous catheters; report appropriate E/M code

2.65 2.65 FUD 000 T A2

AMA: 2019,May,3; 2018,Jan,8; 2017,Jan,8; 2016,Jan,13

36569 age 5 years or older A

EXCLUDES *Centrally inserted placement (36556)*
Imaging guidance (76937, 77001)
Peripherally inserted ([36573])
PICC line removal with codes for removal tunneled central venous catheters; report appropriate E/M code

2.73 2.73 FUD 000 T A2

AMA: 2019,May,3; 2018,Jan,8; 2017,Jan,8; 2016,Jan,13

\# **36572 Insertion of peripherally inserted central venous catheter (PICC), without subcutaneous port or pump, including all imaging guidance, image documentation, and all associated radiological supervision and interpretation required to perform the insertion; younger than 5 years of age** A

INCLUDES Verification site catheter tip (71045-71048)

EXCLUDES *Centrally inserted placement (36555)*
Imaging guidance (76937, 77001)
Peripherally inserted without imaging guidance (36568)

2.62 12.3 FUD 000 G2

AMA: 2019,May,3; 2019,Mar,10

\# **36573 age 5 years or older** A

INCLUDES Verification site catheter tip (71045-71048)

EXCLUDES *Centrally inserted placement (36556)*
Imaging guidance (76937, 77001)
Peripherally inserted without imaging guidance (36569)

2.45 11.3 FUD 000 G2

AMA: 2019,May,3; 2019,Mar,10

36570 Insertion of peripherally inserted central venous access device, with subcutaneous port; younger than 5 years of age A

EXCLUDES *Centrally inserted placement (36560)*

9.61 42.3 FUD 010 T A2 80 50

AMA: 2018,Jan,8; 2017,Jan,8; 2016,Jan,13

36571 age 5 years or older A

EXCLUDES *Centrally inserted placement (36561)*

9.03 37.0 FUD 010 T A2 80 50

AMA: 2018,Jan,8; 2017,Jan,8; 2016,Jan,13

36572 **Resequenced code. See code following 36569.**

36573 **Resequenced code. See code following 36569.**

36575-36590 Repair, Removal, and Replacement Implantable Venous Access Device

EXCLUDES *Mechanical removal obstructive material, pericatheter/intraluminal (36595, 36596)*

Code also frequency of two for procedures involving both catheters from multicatheter device

36575 Repair of tunneled or non-tunneled central venous access catheter, without subcutaneous port or pump, central or peripheral insertion site

INCLUDES Repair device without replacing any parts

1.01 4.57 FUD 000 T A2 80

AMA: 2018,Jan,8; 2017,Jan,8; 2016,Jan,13

36576 Repair of central venous access device, with subcutaneous port or pump, central or peripheral insertion site

INCLUDES Repair device without replacing any parts

5.33 9.31 FUD 010 T A2 80

AMA: 2018,Jan,8; 2017,Jan,8; 2016,Jan,13

36578 Replacement, catheter only, of central venous access device, with subcutaneous port or pump, central or peripheral insertion site

INCLUDES Partial replacement (catheter only)

EXCLUDES *Total replacement entire device using same venous access sites (36582-36583)*

5.89 13.4 FUD 010 T A2 80

AMA: 2018,Jan,8; 2017,Jan,8; 2016,Jan,13

36580 Replacement, complete, of a non-tunneled centrally inserted central venous catheter, without subcutaneous port or pump, through same venous access

INCLUDES Complete replacement (replace all components/same access site)

1.91 6.22 FUD 000 T J8

AMA: 2018,Jan,8; 2017,Jan,8; 2016,Jan,13

36581 Replacement, complete, of a tunneled centrally inserted central venous catheter, without subcutaneous port or pump, through same venous access

INCLUDES Complete replacement (replace all components/same access site)

EXCLUDES *Removal old device and insertion new device using separate venous access site*

5.30 22.9 FUD 010 T A2 80

AMA: 2018,Jan,8; 2017,Jan,8; 2016,Jan,13

36582 Replacement, complete, of a tunneled centrally inserted central venous access device, with subcutaneous port, through same venous access

INCLUDES Complete replacement (replace all components/same access site)

EXCLUDES *Removal old device and insertion new device using separate venous access site*

8.40 28.2 FUD 010 T A2 80

AMA: 2018,Jan,8; 2017,Jan,8; 2016,Jan,13

36583 Replacement, complete, of a tunneled centrally inserted central venous access device, with subcutaneous pump, through same venous access

INCLUDES Complete replacement (replace all components/same access site)

EXCLUDES *Removal old device and insertion new device using separate venous access site*

9.45 35.9 FUD 010 T G2 80

AMA: 2018,Jan,8; 2017,Jan,8; 2016,Jan,13

36584 Replacement, complete, of a peripherally inserted central venous catheter (PICC), without subcutaneous port or pump, through same venous access, including all imaging guidance, image documentation, and all associated radiological supervision and interpretation required to perform the replacement

INCLUDES Complete replacement (replace all components/same access site)
Imaging guidance (76937, 77001)
Verification site catheter tip (71045-71048)

EXCLUDES *Replacement PICC line without imaging guidance (37799)*

1.73 9.92 FUD 000 T A2

AMA: 2019,May,3; 2019,Mar,10; 2018,Jan,8; 2017,Jan,8; 2016,Jan,13

36585 Replacement, complete, of a peripherally inserted central venous access device, with subcutaneous port, through same venous access

INCLUDES Complete replacement (replace all components/same access site)

7.86 31.4 FUD 010 T A2 80

AMA: 2018,Jan,8; 2017,Jan,8; 2016,Jan,13

36589 **Removal of tunneled central venous catheter, without subcutaneous port or pump**
INCLUDES Complete removal/all components
EXCLUDES *Non-tunneled central venous catheter removal; report appropriate E/M code*
3.97 | 4.76 | FUD 010 | Q2 A2 80
AMA: 2018,Jan,8; 2017,Jan,8; 2016,Jan,13

36590 **Removal of tunneled central venous access device, with subcutaneous port or pump, central or peripheral insertion**
INCLUDES Complete removal/all components
EXCLUDES *Non-tunneled central venous catheter removal; report appropriate E/M code*
5.51 | 6.40 | FUD 010 | Q2 A2 80
AMA: 2018,Jan,8; 2017,Jan,8; 2016,Jan,13

36591-36592 Obtain Blood Specimen from Implanted Device or Catheter

EXCLUDES *Reporting code with any other service except laboratory services*

36591 **Collection of blood specimen from a completely implantable venous access device**
EXCLUDES *Collection:*
Capillary blood specimen (36416)
Venous blood specimen by venipuncture (36415)
0.70 | 0.70 | FUD XXX | Q1 N1 80 TC
AMA: 2019,Aug,8; 2018,Jan,8; 2017,Jan,8; 2016,Jan,13

36592 **Collection of blood specimen using established central or peripheral catheter, venous, not otherwise specified**
EXCLUDES *Collection blood from established arterial catheter (37799)*
0.77 | 0.77 | FUD XXX | Q1 N1 80 TC
AMA: 2018,Jan,8; 2017,Jan,8; 2016,Jan,13

36593-36596 Restore Patency of Occluded Catheter or Device

EXCLUDES *Venous catheterization (36010-36012)*

36593 **Declotting by thrombolytic agent of implanted vascular access device or catheter**
0.89 | 0.89 | FUD XXX | T P3 80 TC
AMA: 2018,Jan,8; 2017,Jan,8; 2016,Jan,13

36595 **Mechanical removal of pericatheter obstructive material (eg, fibrin sheath) from central venous device via separate venous access**
EXCLUDES *Declotting by thrombolytic agent (36593)*
(75901)
5.30 | 17.3 | FUD 000 | T J8
AMA: 2018,Jan,8; 2017,Jan,8; 2016,Jan,13

36596 **Mechanical removal of intraluminal (intracatheter) obstructive material from central venous device through device lumen**
EXCLUDES *Declotting by thrombolytic agent (36593)*
(75902)
1.26 | 3.47 | FUD 000 | T G2
AMA: 2018,Jan,8; 2017,Jan,8; 2016,Jan,13

36597-36598 Repositioning or Assessment of In Situ Venous Access Device

36597 **Repositioning of previously placed central venous catheter under fluoroscopic guidance**
(76000)
1.75 | 3.79 | FUD 000 | T G2
AMA: 2018,Jan,8; 2017,Jan,8; 2016,Jan,13

36598 **Contrast injection(s) for radiologic evaluation of existing central venous access device, including fluoroscopy, image documentation and report**
EXCLUDES *Complete venography studies (75820, 75825, 75827)*
Fluoroscopy (76000)
Mechanical removal pericatheter obstructive material (36595-36596)
1.07 | 3.44 | FUD 000 | T P3 80 50
AMA: 2014,Jan,11

36600-36660 Insertion Needle or Catheter: Artery

36600 **Arterial puncture, withdrawal of blood for diagnosis**
EXCLUDES *Critical care services*
0.45 | 0.86 | FUD XXX | Q1 N1
AMA: 2019,Aug,8; 2018,Jan,8; 2017,Jan,8; 2016,Jan,13

36620 **Arterial catheterization or cannulation for sampling, monitoring or transfusion (separate procedure); percutaneous**
1.28 | 1.28 | FUD 000 | N N1
AMA: 2018,Jan,8; 2017,Jan,8; 2016,Jan,13

36625 **cutdown**
3.06 | 3.06 | FUD 000 | N N1
AMA: 2018,Jan,8; 2017,Jan,8; 2016,Jan,13

36640 **Arterial catheterization for prolonged infusion therapy (chemotherapy), cutdown**
EXCLUDES *Intra-arterial chemotherapy (96420-96425)*
Transcatheter embolization (75894)
3.31 | 3.31 | FUD 000 | T A2
AMA: 2018,Jan,8; 2017,Jan,8; 2016,Jan,13

36660 **Catheterization, umbilical artery, newborn, for diagnosis or therapy** A
1.97 | 1.97 | FUD 000 | 63 C 80
AMA: 2018,Jan,8; 2017,Jan,8; 2016,Jan,13

36680 Percutaneous Placement of Catheter/Needle into Bone Marrow Cavity

36680 **Placement of needle for intraosseous infusion**
1.74 | 1.74 | FUD 000 | Q1 N1 80
AMA: 2018,Jan,8; 2017,Jan,8; 2016,Jan,13

36800-36821 Vascular Access for Hemodialysis

36800 **Insertion of cannula for hemodialysis, other purpose (separate procedure); vein to vein**
3.55 | 3.55 | FUD 000 | T G2
AMA: 2018,Jan,8; 2017,Jan,8; 2016,Jan,13

36810 **arteriovenous, external (Scribner type)**
6.11 | 6.11 | FUD 000 | T A2
AMA: 2018,Jan,8; 2017,Jan,8; 2016,Jan,13

36815 **arteriovenous, external revision, or closure**
3.91 | 3.91 | FUD 000 | T A2
AMA: 2018,Jan,8; 2017,Jan,8; 2016,Jan,13

36818 **Arteriovenous anastomosis, open; by upper arm cephalic vein transposition**
INCLUDES Two incisions in upper arm: medial incision over brachial artery and lateral incision for exposure to portion of cephalic vein
EXCLUDES *When performed unilaterally with:*
Arteriovenous anastomosis, open (36819-36820)
Creation arteriovenous fistula by other than direct arteriovenous anastomosis (36830)
Code also modifier 50 or 59, as appropriate, for bilateral procedure
20.1 | 20.1 | FUD 090 | T A2 80
AMA: 2018,Jan,8; 2017,Mar,3; 2017,Jan,8; 2016,Mar,10; 2016,Jan,13

36819 **by upper arm basilic vein transposition**

EXCLUDES *When performed unilaterally with:*
Arteriovenous anastomosis, open (36818, 36820-36821)
Creation arteriovenous fistula by other than direct arteriovenous anastomosis (36830)

Code also modifier 50 or 59, as appropriate, for bilateral procedure

21.2 21.2 **FUD** 090 T A2 80

AMA: 2018,Jan,8; 2017,Mar,3; 2017,Jan,8; 2016,Jan,13

36820 **by forearm vein transposition**

21.2 21.2 **FUD** 090 T A2 80 50

AMA: 2018,Jan,8; 2017,Mar,3; 2017,Jan,8; 2016,Jan,13

36821 **direct, any site (eg, Cimino type) (separate procedure)**

19.3 19.3 **FUD** 090 T A2 80

AMA: 2018,Jan,8; 2017,Mar,3; 2017,Jan,8; 2016,Jan,13

36823 Vascular Access for Extracorporeal Circulation

INCLUDES Chemotherapy perfusion

EXCLUDES *Chemotherapy administration (96409-96425)*
Maintenance for extracorporeal circulation (33946-33949)

36823 **Insertion of arterial and venous cannula(s) for isolated extracorporeal circulation including regional chemotherapy perfusion to an extremity, with or without hyperthermia, with removal of cannula(s) and repair of arteriotomy and venotomy sites**

40.5 40.5 **FUD** 090 C

AMA: 2018,Jan,8; 2017,Mar,3

36825-36835 Permanent Vascular Access Procedures

36825 **Creation of arteriovenous fistula by other than direct arteriovenous anastomosis (separate procedure); autogenous graft**

EXCLUDES *Direct arteriovenous (AV) anastomosis (36821)*

23.0 23.0 **FUD** 090 T A2 80

AMA: 2018,Jan,8; 2017,Mar,3; 2017,Jan,8; 2016,Jan,13

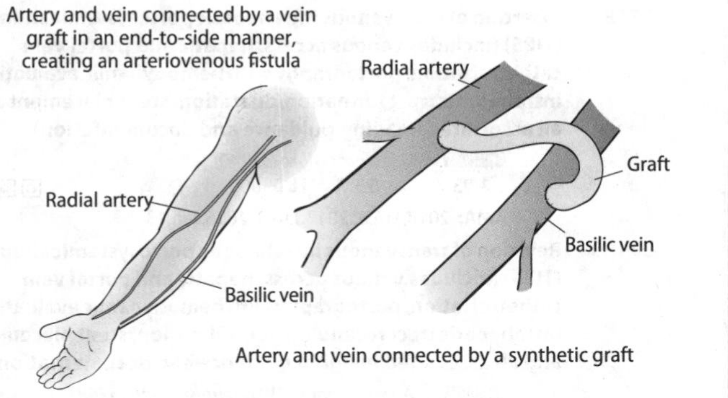

Artery and vein connected by a vein graft in an end-to-side manner, creating an arteriovenous fistula
Radial artery
Graft
Radial artery
Basilic vein
Basilic vein
Artery and vein connected by a synthetic graft

36830 **nonautogenous graft (eg, biological collagen, thermoplastic graft)**

EXCLUDES *Direct arteriovenous (AV) anastomosis (36821)*

19.4 19.4 **FUD** 090 T A2 80

AMA: 2018,Jan,8; 2017,Mar,3; 2017,Jan,8; 2016,Jan,13

36831 **Thrombectomy, open, arteriovenous fistula without revision, autogenous or nonautogenous dialysis graft (separate procedure)**

17.9 17.9 **FUD** 090 T A2 80

AMA: 2018,Jan,8; 2017,Mar,3; 2017,Jan,8; 2016,Jan,13

36832 **Revision, open, arteriovenous fistula; without thrombectomy, autogenous or nonautogenous dialysis graft (separate procedure)**

INCLUDES Revision arteriovenous access fistula or graft

21.9 21.9 **FUD** 090 T A2 80

AMA: 2018,Jan,8; 2017,Mar,3; 2017,Jan,8; 2016,Jan,13

36833 **with thrombectomy, autogenous or nonautogenous dialysis graft (separate procedure)**

EXCLUDES *Hemodialysis circuit procedures (36901-36906)*

23.5 23.5 **FUD** 090 T A2 80

AMA: 2018,Jan,8; 2017,Mar,3; 2017,Jan,8; 2016,Jan,13

36835 **Insertion of Thomas shunt (separate procedure)**

13.8 13.8 **FUD** 090 T J8

AMA: 2014,Jan,11; 1997,Nov,1

36838 DRIL Procedure for Ischemic Steal Syndrome

EXCLUDES *Bypass graft, with vein (35512, 35522-35523)*
Ligation (37607, 37618)
Revision, open, arteriovenous fistula (36832)

36838 **Distal revascularization and interval ligation (DRIL), upper extremity hemodialysis access (steal syndrome)**

33.3 33.3 **FUD** 090 T G2 80 50

AMA: 2014,Jan,11; 1997,Nov,1

36860-36861 Restore Patency of Occluded Cannula or Arteriovenous Fistula

36860 **External cannula declotting (separate procedure); without balloon catheter**

(76000)

3.23 7.05 **FUD** 000 T A2

AMA: 2018,Jan,8; 2017,Jan,8; 2016,Jan,13

36861 **with balloon catheter**

(76000)

4.05 4.05 **FUD** 000 T A2

AMA: 2018,Jan,8; 2017,Jan,8; 2016,Jan,13

36901-36909 Hemodialysis Circuit Procedures

EXCLUDES *Arteriography to assess inflow to hemodialysis circuit when performed (76937)*

36901 **Introduction of needle(s) and/or catheter(s), dialysis circuit, with diagnostic angiography of the dialysis circuit, including all direct puncture(s) and catheter placement(s), injection(s) of contrast, all necessary imaging from the arterial anastomosis and adjacent artery through entire venous outflow including the inferior or superior vena cava, fluoroscopic guidance, radiological supervision and interpretation and image documentation and report;**

INCLUDES Access
Catheter advancement (e.g., imaging of accessory veins, assess all circuit sections)
Contrast injection

EXCLUDES *Balloon angioplasty peripheral segment (36902)*
Open revision with thrombectomy arteriovenous fistula (36833)
Percutaneous transluminal procedures peripheral segment (36904-36906)
Stent placement in peripheral segment (36903)
Reporting code more than one time per procedure

4.88 18.3 **FUD** 000 T P2

AMA: 2018,Jan,8; 2017,Mar,3

36902 **with transluminal balloon angioplasty, peripheral dialysis segment, including all imaging and radiological supervision and interpretation necessary to perform the angioplasty**

EXCLUDES *Open revision with thrombectomy arteriovenous fistula (36833)*
Percutaneous transluminal procedures peripheral segment (36904-36906)
Stent placement in peripheral segment (36903)
Reporting code more than one time per procedure

6.94 36.9 **FUD** 000 J G2

AMA: 2018,Jan,8; 2017,Jul,3; 2017,Mar,3

36903 with transcatheter placement of intravascular stent(s), peripheral dialysis segment, including all imaging and radiological supervision and interpretation necessary to perform the stenting, and all angioplasty within the peripheral dialysis segment

INCLUDES Balloon angioplasty peripheral segment (36902)

EXCLUDES *Central hemodialysis circuit procedures (36907-36908)*

Open revision with thrombectomy arteriovenous fistula (36833)

Percutaneous transluminal procedures peripheral segment (36904-36906)

Reporting code more than one time per procedure

9.20 146. FUD 000 J J8

AMA: 2018,Jan,8; 2017,Jul,3; 2017,Mar,3

36904 Percutaneous transluminal mechanical thrombectomy and/or infusion for thrombolysis, dialysis circuit, any method, including all imaging and radiological supervision and interpretation, diagnostic angiography, fluoroscopic guidance, catheter placement(s), and intraprocedural pharmacological thrombolytic injection(s);

EXCLUDES *Open thrombectomy arteriovenous fistula with/without revision (36831, 36833)*

Reporting code more than one time per procedure

10.7 54.7 FUD 000 J G2

AMA: 2018,Jan,8; 2017,Jul,3; 2017,Mar,3

36905 with transluminal balloon angioplasty, peripheral dialysis segment, including all imaging and radiological supervision and interpretation necessary to perform the angioplasty

INCLUDES Percutaneous mechanical thrombectomy (36904)

EXCLUDES *Reporting code more than one time per procedure*

12.8 68.7 FUD 000 J G2

AMA: 2018,Jan,8; 2017,Jul,3; 2017,Mar,3

36906 with transcatheter placement of intravascular stent(s), peripheral dialysis segment, including all imaging and radiological supervision and interpretation necessary to perform the stenting, and all angioplasty within the peripheral dialysis circuit

INCLUDES Percutaneous transluminal balloon angioplasty (36905)

Percutaneous transluminal thrombectomy (36904)

EXCLUDES *Hemodialysis circuit procedures provided by catheter or needle access (36901-36903)*

Reporting code more than one time per procedure

Code also:

Balloon angioplasty central veins, when performed (36907)

Stent placement in central veins, when performed (36908)

14.9 186. FUD 000 J J8

AMA: 2018,Jan,8; 2017,Jul,3; 2017,Mar,3

+ **36907 Transluminal balloon angioplasty, central dialysis segment, performed through dialysis circuit, including all imaging and radiological supervision and interpretation required to perform the angioplasty (List separately in addition to code for primary procedure)**

INCLUDES All central hemodialysis segment angiography

EXCLUDES *Angiography with stent placement (36908)*

Code first (36818-36833, 36901-36906)

4.25 19.6 FUD ZZZ N N1

AMA: 2018,Jan,8; 2017,Jul,3; 2017,Mar,3

+ **36908 Transcatheter placement of intravascular stent(s), central dialysis segment, performed through dialysis circuit, including all imaging and radiological supervision and interpretation required to perform the stenting, and all angioplasty in the central dialysis segment (List separately in addition to code for primary procedure)**

INCLUDES All central hemodialysis segment stent(s) placed

Balloon angioplasty central dialysis segment (36907)

Code first when performed (36818-36833, 36901-36906)

6.02 59.6 FUD ZZZ N N1

AMA: 2018,Jan,8; 2017,Jul,3; 2017,Mar,3

+ **36909 Dialysis circuit permanent vascular embolization or occlusion (including main circuit or any accessory veins), endovascular, including all imaging and radiological supervision and interpretation necessary to complete the intervention (List separately in addition to code for primary procedure)**

INCLUDES All embolization/occlusion procedures performed in hemodialysis circuit

EXCLUDES *Banding/ligation arteriovenous fistula (37607)*

Reporting code more than one time per day

Code first (36901-36906)

5.83 56.8 FUD ZZZ N N1

AMA: 2018,Jan,8; 2017,Mar,3

37140-37181 Open Decompression of Portal Circulation

EXCLUDES *Peritoneal-venous shunt (49425)*

37140 Venous anastomosis, open; portocaval

67.7 67.7 FUD 090 C

AMA: 2014,Jan,11; 1997,Nov,1

37145 renoportal

62.7 62.7 FUD 090 C 80

AMA: 2014,Jan,11; 1997,Nov,1

37160 caval-mesenteric

64.4 64.4 FUD 090 C 80

AMA: 2014,Jan,11; 1997,Nov,1

37180 splenorenal, proximal

61.9 61.9 FUD 090 C 80

AMA: 2014,Jan,11; 1997,Nov,1

37181 splenorenal, distal (selective decompression of esophagogastric varices, any technique)

EXCLUDES *Percutaneous procedure (37182)*

67.7 67.7 FUD 090 C 80

AMA: 2014,Jan,11; 1997,Nov,1

37182-37183 Transvenous Decompression of Portal Circulation

INCLUDES Percutaneous transhepatic portography (75885, 75887)

37182 Insertion of transvenous intrahepatic portosystemic shunt(s) (TIPS) (includes venous access, hepatic and portal vein catheterization, portography with hemodynamic evaluation, intrahepatic tract formation/dilatation, stent placement and all associated imaging guidance and documentation)

EXCLUDES *Open procedure (37140)*

23.7 23.7 FUD 000 C 80

AMA: 2018,Jan,8; 2017,Jan,8; 2016,Jan,13

37183 Revision of transvenous intrahepatic portosystemic shunt(s) (TIPS) (includes venous access, hepatic and portal vein catheterization, portography with hemodynamic evaluation, intrahepatic tract recanulization/dilatation, stent placement and all associated imaging guidance and documentation)

EXCLUDES *Arteriovenous (AV) aneurysm repair (36832)*

10.8 176. FUD 000 J J8 80

AMA: 2018,Jan,8; 2017,Jan,8; 2016,Jan,13

37184-37188 Removal of Thrombus from Vessel: Percutaneous

INCLUDES Fluoroscopic guidance (76000)
Injection(s) thrombolytics during procedure
Postprocedure evaluation
Pretreatment planning

EXCLUDES *Catheter placement*
Continuous infusion thrombolytics prior to and after procedure (37211-37214)
Diagnostic studies
Intracranial arterial mechanical thrombectomy or infusion (61645)
Mechanical thrombectomy, coronary (92973)
Other interventions performed percutaneously (e.g., balloon angioplasty)
Radiological supervision/interpretation

37184 Primary percutaneous transluminal mechanical thrombectomy, noncoronary, non-intracranial, arterial or arterial bypass graft, including fluoroscopic guidance and intraprocedural pharmacological thrombolytic injection(s); initial vessel

EXCLUDES *Intracranial arterial mechanical thrombectomy (61645)*
Mechanical thrombectomy another vascular family/separate access site, append modifier 59 to primary service
Mechanical thrombectomy for embolus/thrombus complicating another percutaneous interventional procedure (37186)
Therapeutic, prophylactic, or diagnostic injection (96374)

12.9 60.2 **FUD** 000 J J8 50

AMA: 2019,Sep,5; 2018,Jan,8; 2017,Jan,8; 2016,Jul,6; 2016,Mar,3; 2016,Jan,13

+ **37185 second and all subsequent vessel(s) within the same vascular family (List separately in addition to code for primary mechanical thrombectomy procedure)**

INCLUDES Treatment second and all succeeding vessel(s) in same vascular family

EXCLUDES *Intravenous drug injections administered subsequent to initial service*
Mechanical thrombectomy another vascular family/separate access site, append modifier 59 to primary service
Therapeutic, prophylactic, or diagnostic injection (96375)

Code first (37184)

4.77 16.9 **FUD** ZZZ N N1

AMA: 2019,Sep,5; 2018,Jan,8; 2017,Jan,8; 2016,Jul,6; 2016,Jan,13

+ **37186 Secondary percutaneous transluminal thrombectomy (eg, nonprimary mechanical, snare basket, suction technique), noncoronary, non-intracranial, arterial or arterial bypass graft, including fluoroscopic guidance and intraprocedural pharmacological thrombolytic injections, provided in conjunction with another percutaneous intervention other than primary mechanical thrombectomy (List separately in addition to code for primary procedure)**

INCLUDES Removal small emboli/thrombi prior to or after another percutaneous procedure

EXCLUDES *Primary percutaneous transluminal mechanical thrombectomy, noncoronary, non-intracranial (37184-37185)*
Therapeutic, prophylactic, or diagnostic injection (96375)

Code first primary procedure

7.10 37.4 **FUD** ZZZ N N1

AMA: 2019,Sep,5; 2018,Jan,8; 2017,Jan,8; 2016,Jul,6; 2016,Jan,13

37187 Percutaneous transluminal mechanical thrombectomy, vein(s), including intraprocedural pharmacological thrombolytic injections and fluoroscopic guidance

INCLUDES Secondary or subsequent intravenous injection after another initial service

EXCLUDES *Therapeutic, prophylactic, or diagnostic injection (96375)*

11.4 55.0 **FUD** 000 J J8 50

AMA: 2018,Jan,8; 2017,Jan,8; 2016,Jul,6; 2016,Mar,3; 2016,Jan,13

37188 Percutaneous transluminal mechanical thrombectomy, vein(s), including intraprocedural pharmacological thrombolytic injections and fluoroscopic guidance, repeat treatment on subsequent day during course of thrombolytic therapy

EXCLUDES *Therapeutic, prophylactic, or diagnostic injection (96375)*

8.10 46.3 **FUD** 000 T G2 50

AMA: 2018,Jan,8; 2017,Jan,8; 2016,Jul,6; 2016,Mar,3; 2016,Jan,13

37191-37193 Vena Cava Filters

37191 Insertion of intravascular vena cava filter, endovascular approach including vascular access, vessel selection, and radiological supervision and interpretation, intraprocedural roadmapping, and imaging guidance (ultrasound and fluoroscopy), when performed

EXCLUDES *Open ligation inferior vena cava via laparotomy or retroperitoneal approach (37619)*

6.48 68.0 **FUD** 000 T J8

AMA: 2018,Jan,8; 2017,Feb,14; 2017,Jan,8; 2016,May,11; 2016,Jan,13

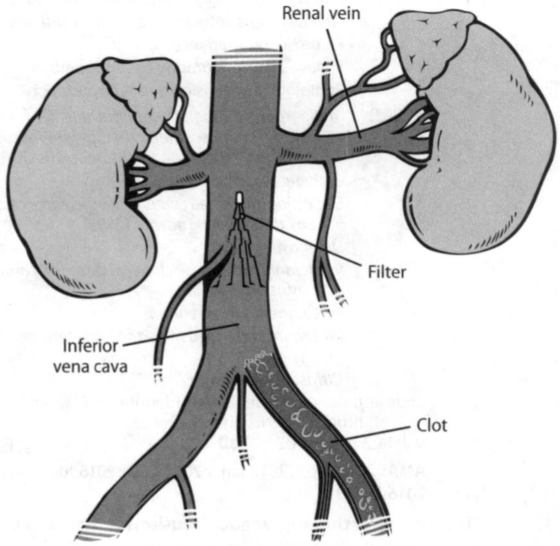

37192 Repositioning of intravascular vena cava filter, endovascular approach including vascular access, vessel selection, and radiological supervision and interpretation, intraprocedural roadmapping, and imaging guidance (ultrasound and fluoroscopy), when performed

EXCLUDES *Insertion intravascular vena cava filter (37191)*

10.0 38.2 **FUD** 000 T J8

AMA: 2018,Jan,8; 2017,Jan,8; 2016,May,11; 2016,Jan,13

37193 Retrieval (removal) of intravascular vena cava filter, endovascular approach including vascular access, vessel selection, and radiological supervision and interpretation, intraprocedural roadmapping, and imaging guidance (ultrasound and fluoroscopy), when performed

EXCLUDES *Transcatheter retrieval intravascular foreign body, percutaneous (37197)*

10.1 44.0 **FUD** 000 T G2

AMA: 2018,Jan,8; 2017,Jan,8; 2016,May,11; 2016,Jan,13

37195 Intravenous Cerebral Thrombolysis

37195 Thrombolysis, cerebral, by intravenous infusion

0.00 0.00 **FUD** XXX T G2 80

AMA: 2020,Jan,12

37197-37214 Transcatheter Procedures: Infusions, Biopsy, Foreign Body Removal

37197 Transcatheter retrieval, percutaneous, of intravascular foreign body (eg, fractured venous or arterial catheter), includes radiological supervision and interpretation, and imaging guidance (ultrasound or fluoroscopy), when performed

EXCLUDES *Percutaneous vena cava filter retrieval (37193)*
Removal leadless pacemaker system ([33275])

Facility RVU 8.78 Non-Facility RVU 43.4 **FUD** 000 T G2 CCI

AMA: 2018,Jan,8; 2017,Feb,14; 2017,Jan,8; 2016,May,11; 2016,Jan,13

37200 Transcatheter biopsy

Radiology Crosswalk (75970)

Facility RVU 6.30 Non-Facility RVU 6.30 **FUD** 000 T G2 CCI

AMA: 2014,Jan,11; 1998,Nov,1

37211 Transcatheter therapy, arterial infusion for thrombolysis other than coronary or intracranial, any method, including radiological supervision and interpretation, initial treatment day

INCLUDES Catheter change or position change
E/M services on day of and related to thrombolysis
First day transcatheter thrombolytic infusion
Fluoroscopic guidance
Follow-up arteriography or venography
Radiologic supervision and interpretation

EXCLUDES *Angiography through existing catheter for follow-up study for transcatheter therapy, embolization, or infusion, other than for thrombolysis (75898)*
Catheter placement
Declotting implanted catheter or vascular access device by thrombolytic agent (36593)
Diagnostic studies
Intracranial arterial mechanical thrombectomy or infusion (61645)
Percutaneous interventions
Procedure performed more than one time per date of service
Ultrasound guidance (76937)

Code also significant, separately identifiable E/M service on day of thrombolysis using modifier 25

Facility RVU 11.2 Non-Facility RVU 11.2 **FUD** 000 T G2 50 CCI

AMA: 2019,Sep,6; 2018,Jan,8; 2017,Jan,8; 2016,Jul,6; 2016,Mar,3; 2016,Jan,13

37212 Transcatheter therapy, venous infusion for thrombolysis, any method, including radiological supervision and interpretation, initial treatment day

INCLUDES Catheter change or position change
E/M services on day of and related to thrombolysis
First day transcatheter thrombolytic infusion
Fluoroscopic guidance
Follow-up arteriography or venography
Initiation and completion thrombolysis on same date of service
Radiologic supervision and interpretation

EXCLUDES *Angiography through existing catheter for follow-up study for transcatheter therapy, embolization, or infusion, other than for thrombolysis (75898)*
Catheter placement
Declotting implanted catheter or vascular access device by thrombolytic agent (36593)
Diagnostic studies
Percutaneous interventions
Procedure performed more than one time per date of service
Ultrasound guidance (76937)

Code also significant, separately identifiable E/M service on day of thrombolysis using modifier 25

Facility RVU 9.81 Non-Facility RVU 9.81 **FUD** 000 T G2 50 CCI

AMA: 2019,Sep,6; 2018,Jan,8; 2017,Jan,8; 2016,Jul,6; 2016,Mar,3; 2016,Jan,13

37213 Transcatheter therapy, arterial or venous infusion for thrombolysis other than coronary, any method, including radiological supervision and interpretation, continued treatment on subsequent day during course of thrombolytic therapy, including follow-up catheter contrast injection, position change, or exchange, when performed;

INCLUDES Continued thrombolytic infusions on subsequent days besides initial and last days of treatment
E/M services on day of and related to thrombolysis
Fluoroscopic guidance
Radiologic supervision and interpretation

EXCLUDES *Angiography through existing catheter for follow-up study for transcatheter therapy, embolization, or infusion, other than for thrombolysis (75898)*
Catheter placement
Declotting implanted catheter or vascular access device by thrombolytic agent (36593)
Diagnostic studies
Percutaneous interventions
Procedure performed more than one time per date of service
Ultrasound guidance (76937)

Code also significant, separately identifiable E/M service on day of thrombolysis using modifier 25

Facility RVU 6.76 Non-Facility RVU 6.76 **FUD** 000 T G2 CCI

AMA: 2019,Sep,6; 2018,Jan,8; 2017,Jan,8; 2016,Jul,6; 2016,Mar,3; 2016,Jan,13

37214 cessation of thrombolysis including removal of catheter and vessel closure by any method

INCLUDES E/M services on day of and related to thrombolysis
Fluoroscopic guidance
Last day transcatheter thrombolytic infusions
Radiologic supervision and interpretation

EXCLUDES *Angiography through existing catheter for follow-up study for transcatheter therapy, embolization, or infusion, other than for thrombolysis (75898)*
Catheter placement
Declotting implanted catheter or vascular access device by thrombolytic agent (36593)
Diagnostic studies
Percutaneous interventions
Procedure performed more than one time per date of service
Ultrasound guidance (76937)

Code also significant, separately identifiable E/M service on day of thrombolysis using modifier 25

Facility RVU 3.57 Non-Facility RVU 3.57 **FUD** 000 T G2 CCI

AMA: 2019,Sep,6; 2018,Jan,8; 2017,Jan,8; 2016,Jul,6; 2016,Mar,3; 2016,Jan,13

37215-37216 Stenting of Cervical Carotid Artery with/without Insertion Distal Embolic Protection Device

INCLUDES Carotid stenting, if required
Ipsilateral cerebral and cervical carotid diagnostic imaging/supervision and interpretation
Ipsilateral selective carotid catheterization

EXCLUDES *Carotid catheterization and imaging, if carotid stenting not required*
Selective catheter placement, common carotid or innominate artery (36222-36224)
Transcatheter placement extracranial vertebral artery stents, open or percutaneous (0075T, 0076T)

37215 **Transcatheter placement of intravascular stent(s), cervical carotid artery, open or percutaneous, including angioplasty, when performed, and radiological supervision and interpretation; with distal embolic protection**

29.0 29.0 **FUD** 090 C 80 50

AMA: 2018,Jan,8; 2017,Jul,3; 2017,Jan,8; 2016,Jan,13

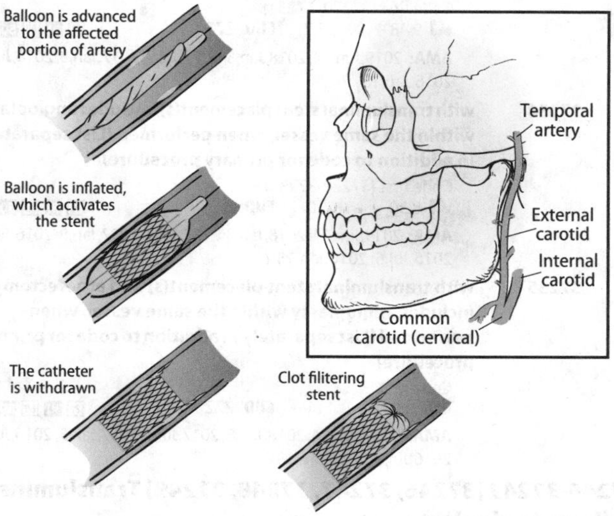
Balloon is advanced to the affected portion of artery
Balloon is inflated, which activates the stent
The catheter is withdrawn
Clot filitering stent
Temporal artery
External carotid
Internal carotid
Common carotid (cervical)

37216 **without distal embolic protection**

28.2 28.2 **FUD** 090 E

AMA: 2018,Jan,8; 2017,Jul,3; 2017,Jan,8; 2016,Jan,13

37217-37218 Stenting of Intrathoracic Carotid Artery/Innominate Artery

INCLUDES Access to vessel (open)
Arteriotomy closure by suture
Catheterization vessel (selective) (36222-36227)
Imaging during and after procedure
Radiological supervision and interpretation

EXCLUDES *Carotid artery revascularization procedures when performed during same session*
Transcatheter insertion extracranial vertebral artery stents, open or percutaneous (0075T-0076T)
Transcatheter insertion intracranial stents (61635)
Transcatheter insertion intravascular cervical carotid artery stents, open or percutaneous (37215-37216)

37217 **Transcatheter placement of intravascular stent(s), intrathoracic common carotid artery or innominate artery by retrograde treatment, open ipsilateral cervical carotid artery exposure, including angioplasty, when performed, and radiological supervision and interpretation**

INCLUDES When performed on same side:
Direct repair blood vessel, neck (35201)
Nonselective catheterization, thoracic aorta (36221)
Transluminal balloon angioplasty (37246-37247 [37246, 37247])

31.3 31.3 **FUD** 090 C 80 50

AMA: 2018,Jan,8; 2017,Jul,3; 2017,Jan,8; 2016,Jan,13

37218 **Transcatheter placement of intravascular stent(s), intrathoracic common carotid artery or innominate artery, open or percutaneous antegrade approach, including angioplasty, when performed, and radiological supervision and interpretation**

EXCLUDES *Selective catheter placement, common carotid or innominate artery (36222-36224)*

23.7 23.7 **FUD** 090 C 80 50

AMA: 2018,Jan,8; 2017,Jul,3; 2017,Jan,8; 2016,Jan,13

37220-37235 Endovascular Revascularization Lower Extremities

INCLUDES Percutaneous and open interventional and associated procedures for lower extremity occlusive disease; unilateral
Accessing vessel
Arteriotomy closure by suturing puncture or pressure with arterial closure device application
Atherectomy (e.g., directional, laser, rotational)
Balloon angioplasty (e.g., cryoplasty, cutting balloon, low-profile)
Catheterization vessel (selective)
Embolic protection
Imaging once procedure complete
Radiological supervision and interpretation
Stenting (e.g., bare metal, balloon-expandable, covered, drug-eluting, self-expanding)
Traversing lesion
Reporting most comprehensive treatment in given vessel according to following hierarchy:
1. Stent and atherectomy
2. Atherectomy
3. Stent
4. PTA
Revascularization procedures for three arterial vascular territories:
Femoral/popliteal vascular territory including common, deep, and superficial femoral arteries, and popliteal artery (one extremity = a single vessel) (37224-37227)
Iliac vascular territory: common iliac, external iliac, internal iliac (37220-37223)
Tibial/peroneal territory: includes anterior tibial, peroneal artery, posterior tibial (37228-37235)

EXCLUDES *Assignment more than one code from this family for each lower extremity vessel treated*
Assignment more than one code when multiple vessels are treated in femoral/popliteal territory (report most complex service for more than one lesion in territory); when contiguous lesion that spans from one territory to another can be opened with single procedure; or when more than one stent deployed in same vessel
Extensive repair or replacement artery (35226, 35286)
Mechanical thrombectomy and/or thrombolysis

Code also:
Add-on codes for different vessels, but not different lesions in same vessel; and for multiple territories in same leg
Modifier 59 if same territory(ies) both legs are treated during same surgical session
Code first one primary code for initial service in each leg

37220 **Revascularization, endovascular, open or percutaneous, iliac artery, unilateral, initial vessel; with transluminal angioplasty**

Code also only when transluminal angioplasty performed outside treatment target zone of (34701-34708, 34709, [34718], 34710-34711, 34845-34848)

11.6 82.1 **FUD** 000 J G2 50

AMA: 2019,Jun,14; 2018,Jan,8; 2017,Jul,3; 2017,Jan,8; 2016,Jul,8; 2016,Jan,13

37221 **with transluminal stent placement(s), includes angioplasty within the same vessel, when performed**

Code also only when transluminal angioplasty performed outside treatment target zone of (34701-34708, 34709, [34718], 34710-34711, 34845-34848)

14.4 118. **FUD** 000 J J8 80 50

AMA: 2019,Jun,14; 2018,Jan,8; 2017,Dec,3; 2017,Jul,3; 2017,Jan,8; 2016,Jul,6; 2016,Jul,8; 2016,Jan,13

+ **37222 Revascularization, endovascular, open or percutaneous, iliac artery, each additional ipsilateral iliac vessel; with transluminal angioplasty (List separately in addition to code for primary procedure)**

Code also only when transluminal angioplasty performed outside treatment target zone of (34701-34708, 34709, [34718], 34710-34711, 34845-34848)

Code first (37220-37221)

5.42 21.2 **FUD** ZZZ N N1 80 50

AMA: 2019,Jun,14; 2018,Jan,8; 2017,Jul,3; 2017,Jan,8; 2016,Jul,8; 2016,Jan,13

+ **37223 with transluminal stent placement(s), includes angioplasty within the same vessel, when performed (List separately in addition to code for primary procedure)**

Code also only when transluminal angioplasty performed outside treatment target zone of (34701-34708, 34709, [34718], 34710-34711, 34845-34848)

Code first (37221)

6.20 62.6 **FUD** ZZZ N N1 80 50

AMA: 2019,Jun,14; 2018,Jan,8; 2017,Dec,3; 2017,Jul,3; 2017,Jan,8; 2016,Jul,8; 2016,Jul,6; 2016,Jan,13

37224 Revascularization, endovascular, open or percutaneous, femoral, popliteal artery(s), unilateral; with transluminal angioplasty

EXCLUDES *Revascularization with intravascular stent grafts in femoral-popliteal segment (0505T)*

12.9 97.6 **FUD** 000 J J8 80 50

AMA: 2019,Jun,14; 2018,Jan,8; 2017,Jul,3; 2017,Jan,8; 2016,Jul,8; 2016,Jan,13

37225 with atherectomy, includes angioplasty within the same vessel, when performed

EXCLUDES *Revascularization with intravascular stent grafts in femoral-popliteal segment (0505T)*

17.5 320. **FUD** 000 J J8 80 50

AMA: 2019,Jun,14; 2018,Jan,8; 2017,Jul,3; 2017,Jan,8; 2016,Jul,8; 2016,Jan,13

37226 with transluminal stent placement(s), includes angioplasty within the same vessel, when performed

EXCLUDES *Revascularization with intravascular stent grafts in femoral-popliteal segment (0505T)*

15.1 285. **FUD** 000 J J8 80 50

AMA: 2019,Jun,14; 2018,Jan,8; 2017,Jul,3; 2017,Jan,8; 2016,Jul,6; 2016,Jul,8; 2016,Jan,13

37227 with transluminal stent placement(s) and atherectomy, includes angioplasty within the same vessel, when performed

EXCLUDES *Revascularization with intravascular stent grafts in femoral-popliteal segment (0505T)*

21.1 444. **FUD** 000 J J8 80 50

AMA: 2019,Jun,14; 2018,Jan,8; 2017,Jul,3; 2017,Jan,8; 2016,Jul,6; 2016,Jul,8; 2016,Jan,13

37228 Revascularization, endovascular, open or percutaneous, tibial, peroneal artery, unilateral, initial vessel; with transluminal angioplasty

15.7 140. **FUD** 000 J J8 80 50

AMA: 2019,Jun,14; 2018,Jan,8; 2017,Jul,3; 2017,Jan,8; 2016,Jul,8; 2016,Jan,13

37229 with atherectomy, includes angioplasty within the same vessel, when performed

20.4 322. **FUD** 000 J J8 80 50

AMA: 2019,Jun,14; 2018,Jan,8; 2017,Jul,3; 2017,Jan,8; 2016,Jul,8; 2016,Jan,13

37230 with transluminal stent placement(s), includes angioplasty within the same vessel, when performed

20.3 289. **FUD** 000 J J8 80 50

AMA: 2020,Jul,13; 2019,Jun,14; 2018,Jan,8; 2017,Jul,3; 2017,Jan,8; 2016,Jul,6; 2016,Jul,8; 2016,Jan,13

37231 with transluminal stent placement(s) and atherectomy, includes angioplasty within the same vessel, when performed

22.0 401. **FUD** 000 J J8 80 50

AMA: 2019,Jun,14; 2018,Jan,8; 2017,Jul,3; 2017,Jan,8; 2016,Jul,8; 2016,Jul,6; 2016,Jan,13

+ **37232 Revascularization, endovascular, open or percutaneous, tibial/peroneal artery, unilateral, each additional vessel; with transluminal angioplasty (List separately in addition to code for primary procedure)**

Code first (37228-37231)

5.83 29.0 **FUD** ZZZ N N1 80 50

AMA: 2019,Jun,14; 2018,Jan,8; 2017,Jul,3; 2017,Jan,8; 2016,Jul,8; 2016,Jan,13

+ **37233 with atherectomy, includes angioplasty within the same vessel, when performed (List separately in addition to code for primary procedure)**

Code first (37229, 37231)

9.48 35.7 **FUD** ZZZ N N1 80 50

AMA: 2019,Jun,14; 2018,Jan,8; 2017,Jul,3; 2017,Jan,8; 2016,Jul,8; 2016,Jan,13

+ **37234 with transluminal stent placement(s), includes angioplasty within the same vessel, when performed (List separately in addition to code for primary procedure)**

Code first (37229-37231)

8.30 110. **FUD** ZZZ N N1 80 50

AMA: 2019,Jun,14; 2018,Jan,8; 2017,Jul,3; 2017,Jan,8; 2016,Jul,8; 2016,Jul,6; 2016,Jan,13

+ **37235 with transluminal stent placement(s) and atherectomy, includes angioplasty within the same vessel, when performed (List separately in addition to code for primary procedure)**

Code first (37231)

11.7 116. **FUD** ZZZ N N1 80 50

AMA: 2019,Jun,14; 2018,Jan,8; 2017,Jul,3; 2017,Jan,8; 2016,Jul,6; 2016,Jul,8; 2016,Jan,13

37246-37249 [37246, 37247, 37248, 37249] Transluminal Balloon Angioplasty

INCLUDES Open and percutaneous balloon angioplasty
Radiological supervision and interpretation (37220-37235)

EXCLUDES *Angioplasty other vessels:*
Aortic/visceral arteries (with endovascular repair) (34841-34848)
Coronary artery (92920-92944)
Intracranial artery (61630, 61635)
Performed in hemodialysis circuit (36901-36909)
Infusion thrombolytics (37211-37214)
Mechanical thrombectomy (37184-37188)
Pulmonary artery (92997-92998)
Reporting codes more than one time for all services performed in single vessel or treatable with one angioplasty procedure

Code also:
Angioplasty different vessel, when performed ([37247], [37249])
Extensive artery repair or replacement, when performed (35226, 35286)
Intravascular ultrasound, when performed (37252-37253)

37246 Transluminal balloon angioplasty (except lower extremity artery(ies) for occlusive disease, intracranial, coronary, pulmonary, or dialysis circuit), open or percutaneous, including all imaging and radiological supervision and interpretation necessary to perform the angioplasty within the same artery; initial artery

EXCLUDES *Intravascular stent placement except lower extremities (37236-37237)*
Revascularization lower extremities (37220-37235)
Stent placement:
Cervical carotid artery (37215-37216)
Intrathoracic carotid or innominate artery (37217-37218)

10.1 58.3 **FUD** 000 J G2 50

AMA: 2018,Jan,8; 2017,Aug,10; 2017,Jul,3

+ # **37247** **each additional artery (List separately in addition to code for primary procedure)**

EXCLUDES *Intravascular stent placement except lower extremities (37236-37237)*
Revascularization lower extremities (37220-37235)
Stent placement:
Cervical carotid artery (37215-37216)
Intrathoracic carotid or innominate artery (37217-37218)

Code first ([37246])
4.97 20.5 **FUD** ZZZ N N1 50

AMA: 2018,Jan,8; 2017,Aug,10; 2017,Jul,3

37248 **Transluminal balloon angioplasty (except dialysis circuit), open or percutaneous, including all imaging and radiological supervision and interpretation necessary to perform the angioplasty within the same vein; initial vein**

EXCLUDES *Endovascular venous arterialization with intravascular stent graft(s) in tibial-peroneal segment (0620T)*
Placement intravascular (venous) stent in same vein, same session as (37238-37239)
Revascularization with intravascular stent grafts in femoral-popliteal segment (0505T)

8.64 42.9 **FUD** 000 J G2 50

AMA: 2018,Jan,8; 2017,Aug,10; 2017,Jul,3; 2017,Mar,3

+ # **37249** **each additional vein (List separately in addition to code for primary procedure)**

EXCLUDES *Endovascular venous arterialization with intravascular stent graft(s) in tibial-peroneal segment (0620T)*
Placement intravascular (venous) stent in same vein, same session as (37238-37239)
Revascularization with intravascular stent grafts in femoral-popliteal segment (0505T)

Code first ([37248])
4.24 15.6 **FUD** ZZZ N N1 50

AMA: 2018,Jan,8; 2017,Aug,10; 2017,Jul,3; 2017,Mar,3

37236-37239 Endovascular Revascularization Excluding Lower Extremities

INCLUDES Arteriotomy closure by suturing puncture, pressure, or arterial closure device application
Balloon angioplasty
Post-dilation after stent deployment
Predilation performed as primary or secondary angioplasty
Treatment lesion inside same vessel but outside stented portion
Treatment using different-sized balloons to accomplish procedure
Endovascular revascularization arteries and veins other than carotid, coronary, extracranial, intracranial, lower extremities
Imaging once procedure complete
Radiological supervision and interpretation
Stent placement provided as only treatment

EXCLUDES *Angioplasty in unrelated vessel*
Extensive repair or replacement artery (35226, 35286)
Insertion multiple stents in single vessel using more than one code
Intravascular ultrasound (37252-37253)
Mechanical thrombectomy (37184-37188)
Selective and nonselective catheterization (36005, 36010-36015, 36200, 36215-36218, 36245-36248)
Stent placement in:
Cervical carotid artery (37215-37216)
Extracranial vertebral (0075T-0076T)
Hemodialysis circuit (36903, 36905, 36908)
Intracoronary (92928-92929, 92933-92934, 92937-92938, 92941, 92943-92944)
Intracranial (61635)
Intrathoracic common carotid or innominate artery, retrograde or antegrade approach (37218)
Lower extremity arteries for occlusive disease (37221, 37223, 37226-37227, 37230-37231, 37234-37235)
Visceral arteries with fenestrated aortic repair (34841-34848)
Thrombolytic therapy (37211-37214)
Ultrasound guidance (76937)

Code also add-on codes for different vessels treated during same operative session

37236 **Transcatheter placement of an intravascular stent(s) (except lower extremity artery(s) for occlusive disease, cervical carotid, extracranial vertebral or intrathoracic carotid, intracranial, or coronary), open or percutaneous, including radiological supervision and interpretation and including all angioplasty within the same vessel, when performed; initial artery**

EXCLUDES *Procedures in same target treatment zone with (34841-34848)*

12.9 101. **FUD** 000 J J8 80 50

AMA: 2018,Jan,8; 2017,Dec,3; 2017,Jul,3; 2017,Jan,8; 2016,Jul,3; 2016,Jul,6; 2016,Mar,5; 2016,Jan,13

+ **37237** **each additional artery (List separately in addition to code for primary procedure)**

EXCLUDES *Procedures in same target treatment zone with (34841-34848)*

Code first (37236)
6.18 53.2 **FUD** ZZZ N N1 80 50

AMA: 2018,Jan,8; 2017,Dec,3; 2017,Jul,3; 2017,Jan,8; 2016,Jul,6; 2016,Mar,5; 2016,Jan,13

37238 **Transcatheter placement of an intravascular stent(s), open or percutaneous, including radiological supervision and interpretation and including angioplasty within the same vessel, when performed; initial vein**

EXCLUDES *Endovascular venous arterialization with intravascular stent graft(s) in tibial-peroneal segment (0620T)*
Revascularization with intravascular stent grafts in femoral-popliteal segment (0505T)

8.88 90.3 **FUD** 000 J J8 80 50

AMA: 2018,Jan,8; 2017,Jul,3; 2017,Mar,3; 2017,Jan,8; 2016,Jul,6; 2016,Jun,8

+ **37239** **each additional vein (List separately in addition to code for primary procedure)**

EXCLUDES *Endovascular venous arterialization with intravascular stent graft(s) in tibial-peroneal segment (0620T)*
Revascularization with intravascular stent grafts in femoral-popliteal segment (0505T)

Code first (37238)

4.43 41.8 FUD ZZZ N N1 80 50

AMA: 2018,Jan,8; 2017,Jul,3; 2017,Mar,3; 2017,Jan,8; 2016,Jul,6

37241-37249 [37246, 37247, 37248, 37249] Therapeutic Vascular Embolization/Occlusion

INCLUDES Embolization or occlusion arteries, lymphatics, and veins except for head/neck and central nervous system
Imaging once procedure complete
Intraprocedural guidance
Radiological supervision and interpretation
Roadmapping
Stent placement provided as support for embolization

EXCLUDES *Embolization code assigned more than once per operative field*
Head, neck, or central nervous system embolization (61624, 61626, 61710)
Multiple codes for indications that overlap, code only indication needing most immediate attention
Stent deployment as primary aneurysm management, pseudoaneurysm, or vascular extravasation
Vein destruction with sclerosing solution (36468-36471)

Code also:
Additional embolization procedure(s) and appropriate modifiers (e.g., modifier 59) when embolization procedures performed in multiple operative fields
Diagnostic angiography and catheter placement; append modifier 59 when appropriate

37241 **Vascular embolization or occlusion, inclusive of all radiological supervision and interpretation, intraprocedural roadmapping, and imaging guidance necessary to complete the intervention; venous, other than hemorrhage (eg, congenital or acquired venous malformations, venous and capillary hemangiomas, varices, varicoceles)**

EXCLUDES *Embolization side branch(es) outflow vein from hemodialysis access (36909)*
Procedure in same operative field with:
Endovenous ablation therapy incompetent vein (36475-36479)
Injection sclerosing solution; single vein (36470-36471)
Transcatheter embolization procedures (75894, 75898)
Vein destruction (36468-36479 [36465, 36466])

12.7 140. FUD 000 J P2

AMA: 2019,Sep,6; 2018,Mar,3; 2018,Jan,8; 2017,Mar,3; 2017,Jan,8; 2016,Nov,3; 2016,Jan,13

37242 **arterial, other than hemorrhage or tumor (eg, congenital or acquired arterial malformations, arteriovenous malformations, arteriovenous fistulas, aneurysms, pseudoaneurysms)**

EXCLUDES *Percutaneous treatment pseudoaneurysm extremity (36002)*

13.8 211. FUD 000 J J8

AMA: 2019,Sep,6; 2018,Jul,14; 2018,Mar,3; 2018,Jan,8; 2017,Jan,8; 2016,Jan,13

37243 **for tumors, organ ischemia, or infarction**

INCLUDES Embolization uterine fibroids (37244)

EXCLUDES *Procedure in same operative field:*
Angiography (75898)
Transcatheter embolization in same operative field (75894)

Code also:
Chemotherapy when provided with embolization procedure (96420-96425)
Injection radioisotopes when provided with embolization procedure (79445)

16.3 273. FUD 000 J G2

AMA: 2019,Sep,6; 2018,Mar,3; 2018,Jan,8; 2017,Jan,8; 2016,Jan,13

37244 **for arterial or venous hemorrhage or lymphatic extravasation**

INCLUDES Embolization uterine arteries for hemorrhage

19.3 200. FUD 000 J J8

AMA: 2019,Sep,6; 2018,Jul,14; 2018,Mar,3; 2018,Jan,8; 2017,Oct,9; 2017,Jan,8; 2016,Jan,13

37246 **Resequenced code. See code following 37235.**

37247 **Resequenced code. See code following 37235.**

37248 **Resequenced code. See code following 37235.**

37249 **Resequenced code. See code following 37235.**

37252-37253 Intravascular Ultrasound: Noncoronary

INCLUDES Manipulation and repositioning transducer prior to and after therapeutic interventional procedures

EXCLUDES *Selective or non-selective catheter placement for access (36005-36248)*
Transcatheter procedures (37200, 37236-37239, 37241-37244, 61624, 61626)
Vena cava filter procedures (37191-37193, 37197)

Code first (33361-33369, 33477, 33880-33886, 34701-34708, 34709, [34718], 34710-34711, 34712, 34841-34848, 36010-36015, 36100-36218, 36221-36228, 36245-36248, 36251-36254, 36481, 36555-36571 [36572, 36573], 36578, 36580-36585, 36595, 36901-36909, 37184-37188, 37200, 37211-37218, 37220-37239 [37246, 37247, 37248, 37249], 37241-37244, 61623, 75600-75635, 75705-75774, 75805, 75807, 75810, 75820-75833, 75860-75872, 75885-75898, 75901-75902, 75956-75959, 75970, 76000, 77001, 0075T-0076T, 0234T-0238T, 0338T)

+ **37252** **Intravascular ultrasound (noncoronary vessel) during diagnostic evaluation and/or therapeutic intervention, including radiological supervision and interpretation; initial noncoronary vessel (List separately in addition to code for primary procedure)**

Code first primary procedure

2.63 33.2 FUD ZZZ N N1 80

AMA: 2019,Nov,6; 2018,Jan,8; 2017,Dec,3; 2017,Aug,10; 2017,Mar,3; 2017,Jan,8; 2016,Jul,6; 2016,May,11

+ **37253** **each additional noncoronary vessel (List separately in addition to code for primary procedure)**

Code first (37252)

2.11 5.38 FUD ZZZ N N1 80

AMA: 2019,Nov,6; 2018,Jan,8; 2017,Dec,3; 2017,Aug,10; 2017,Mar,3; 2017,Jan,8; 2016,Jul,6; 2016,May,11

37500-37501 Vascular Endoscopic Procedures

INCLUDES Diagnostic endoscopy

EXCLUDES *Open procedure (37760)*

37500 **Vascular endoscopy, surgical, with ligation of perforator veins, subfascial (SEPS)**

18.3 18.3 FUD 090 T A2 50

AMA: 2018,Jan,8; 2017,Jan,8; 2016,Jan,13

37501 **Unlisted vascular endoscopy procedure**

0.00 0.00 FUD YYY T 50

AMA: 2014,Jan,11; 1997,Nov,1

37565-37606 Ligation Procedures: Jugular Vein, Carotid Arteries

CMS: 100-03,160.8 Electroencephalographic Monitoring During Cerebral Vasculature Surgery

EXCLUDES *Arterial balloon occlusion, endovascular, temporary (61623)*
Suture arteries and veins (35201-35286)
Transcatheter arterial embolization/occlusion, permanent (61624-61626)
Treatment intracranial aneurysm (61703)

37565 **Ligation, internal jugular vein**

20.7 20.7 FUD 090 T G2 80 50

AMA: 2014,Jan,11; 1997,Nov,1

37600 Ligation; external carotid artery
21.2 21.2 **FUD** 090 T G2 80
AMA: 2014,Jan,11; 1997,Nov,1

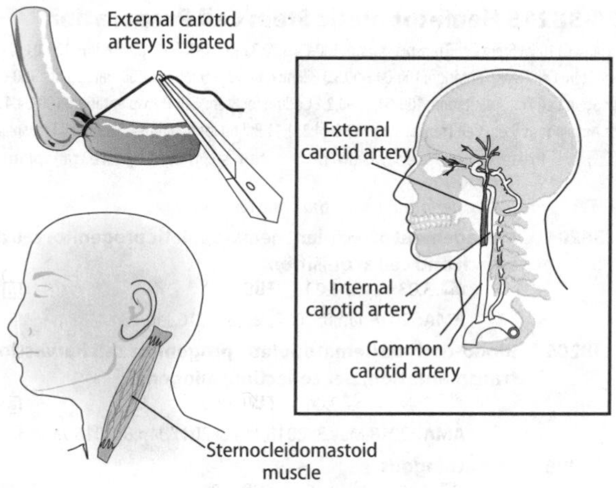

37605 internal or common carotid artery
21.4 21.4 **FUD** 090 T G2 80
AMA: 2014,Jan,11; 1997,Nov,1

37606 internal or common carotid artery, with gradual occlusion, as with Selverstone or Crutchfield clamp
20.7 20.7 **FUD** 090 T G2 80
AMA: 2014,Jan,11; 1997,Nov,1

37607-37609 Ligation Hemodialysis Angioaccess or Temporal Artery

EXCLUDES *Suture arteries and veins (35201-35286)*

37607 Ligation or banding of angioaccess arteriovenous fistula
10.8 10.8 **FUD** 090 T A2
AMA: 2014,Jan,11; 1997,Nov,1

37609 Ligation or biopsy, temporal artery
5.94 8.94 **FUD** 010 J A2 50
AMA: 2014,Jan,11; 1997,Nov,1

37615-37618 Arterial Ligation, Major Vessel, for Injury/Rupture

EXCLUDES *Suture arteries and veins (35201-35286)*

37615 Ligation, major artery (eg, post-traumatic, rupture); neck
INCLUDES Touroff ligation
15.3 15.3 **FUD** 090 T G2 80
AMA: 2014,Jan,11; 1997,Nov,1

37616 chest
INCLUDES Bardenheurer operation
32.0 32.0 **FUD** 090 C 80
AMA: 2014,Jan,11; 1997,Nov,1

37617 abdomen
38.6 38.6 **FUD** 090 C 80
AMA: 2018,Jan,8; 2017,Jan,8; 2016,Jan,13

37618 extremity
11.2 11.2 **FUD** 090 C 80
AMA: 2014,Jan,11; 1997,Nov,1

37619 Ligation Inferior Vena Cava

EXCLUDES *Suture arteries and veins (35201-35286)*
Endovascular delivery inferior vena cava filter (37191)

37619 Ligation of inferior vena cava
50.0 50.0 **FUD** 090 T G2 80
AMA: 2018,Jan,8; 2017,Jan,8; 2016,Jan,13

37650-37660 Venous Ligation, Femoral and Common Iliac

EXCLUDES *Suture arteries and veins (35201-35286)*

37650 Ligation of femoral vein
13.2 13.2 **FUD** 090 T A2 50
AMA: 2014,Jan,11; 1997,Nov,1

37660 Ligation of common iliac vein
38.3 38.3 **FUD** 090 C 80 50
AMA: 2014,Jan,11; 1997,Nov,1

37700-37785 Treatment of Varicose Veins of Legs

EXCLUDES *Suture arteries and veins (35201-35286)*

37700 Ligation and division of long saphenous vein at saphenofemoral junction, or distal interruptions
INCLUDES Babcock operation
EXCLUDES *Ligation, division, and stripping vein (37718, 37722)*
7.08 7.08 **FUD** 090 T A2 50
AMA: 2018,Mar,3; 2018,Jan,8; 2017,Jan,8; 2016,Jan,13

37718 Ligation, division, and stripping, short saphenous vein
EXCLUDES *Ligation, division, and stripping vein (37700, 37735, 37780)*
12.2 12.2 **FUD** 090 T A2 50
AMA: 2018,Mar,3; 2018,Jan,8; 2017,Jan,8

37722 Ligation, division, and stripping, long (greater) saphenous veins from saphenofemoral junction to knee or below
EXCLUDES *Ligation, division, and stripping vein (37700, 37718, 37735)*
13.6 13.6 **FUD** 090 T A2 50
AMA: 2018,Mar,3; 2018,Jan,8; 2017,Jan,8

37735 Ligation and division and complete stripping of long or short saphenous veins with radical excision of ulcer and skin graft and/or interruption of communicating veins of lower leg, with excision of deep fascia
EXCLUDES *Ligation, division, and stripping vein (37700, 37718, 37722, 37780)*
16.8 16.8 **FUD** 090 T A2 50
AMA: 2018,Mar,3; 2018,Jan,8; 2017,Jan,8; 2016,Jan,13

37760 Ligation of perforator veins, subfascial, radical (Linton type), including skin graft, when performed, open,1 leg
EXCLUDES *Duplex scan extremity veins (93971)*
Ligation subfascial perforator veins, endoscopic (37500)
Ultrasonic guidance (76937, 76942, 76998)
18.1 18.1 **FUD** 090 T A2 50
AMA: 2018,Mar,3; 2018,Jan,8; 2017,Jan,8; 2016,Jan,13

37761 Ligation of perforator vein(s), subfascial, open, including ultrasound guidance, when performed, 1 leg
INCLUDES Ultrasonic guidance (76937, 76942, 76998)
EXCLUDES *Duplex scan extremity veins (93971)*
Ligation subfascial perforator veins, endoscopic (37500)
15.7 15.7 **FUD** 090 T R2 80 50
AMA: 2018,Mar,3; 2018,Jan,8; 2017,Jan,8; 2016,Jan,13

37765 Stab phlebectomy of varicose veins, 1 extremity; 10-20 stab incisions
EXCLUDES *Fewer than 10 incisions (37799)*
More than 20 incisions (37766)
7.88 12.6 **FUD** 010 T P3 50
AMA: 2018,Mar,3; 2018,Jan,8; 2017,Jan,8; 2016,Nov,3; 2016,Jan,13

37766 more than 20 incisions
EXCLUDES *Fewer than 10 incisions (37799)*
10-20 incisions (37765)
9.65 14.8 **FUD** 010 T P3 50
AMA: 2018,Mar,3; 2018,Jan,8; 2017,Jan,8; 2016,Nov,3; 2016,Jan,13

37780 Ligation and division of short saphenous vein at saphenopopliteal junction (separate procedure)
6.75 6.75 **FUD** 090 T A2 50
AMA: 2018,Jan,8; 2017,Jan,8; 2016,Jan,13

37785 **Ligation, division, and/or excision of varicose vein cluster(s), 1 leg**
7.45 10.0 FUD 090 T A2 50
AMA: 2018,Jan,8; 2017,Jan,8; 2016,Jan,13

37788-37790 Treatment of Vascular Disease of the Penis

37788 **Penile revascularization, artery, with or without vein graft** ♂
36.5 36.5 FUD 090 C 80
AMA: 2014,Jan,11; 1997,Nov,1

37790 **Penile venous occlusive procedure**
14.0 14.0 FUD 090 J A2 80
AMA: 2014,Jan,11; 1997,Nov,1

37799 Unlisted Vascular Surgery Procedures

CMS: 100-04,32,161 Intracranial Percutaneous Transluminal Angioplasty (PTA) With Stenting; 100-04,4,180.3 Unlisted Service or Procedure

37799 **Unlisted procedure, vascular surgery**
0.00 0.00 FUD YYY T 80
AMA: 2019,Dec,5; 2019,Nov,6; 2018,Nov,11; 2018,Jan,8; 2017,Jan,8; 2016,Nov,3; 2016,Jan,13

38100-38200 Splenic Procedures

38100 **Splenectomy; total (separate procedure)**
33.5 33.5 FUD 090 C 80
AMA: 2018,Jan,8; 2017,Jan,8; 2016,Jan,13

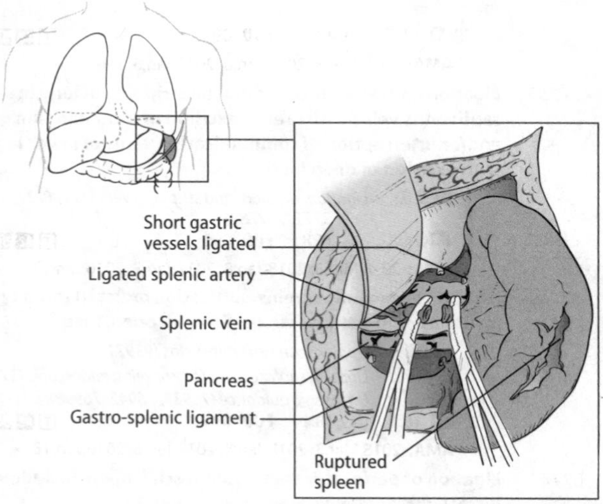

38101 **partial (separate procedure)**
33.5 33.5 FUD 090 C 80
AMA: 2018,Jan,8; 2017,Jan,8; 2016,Jan,13

+ **38102** **total, en bloc for extensive disease, in conjunction with other procedure (List in addition to code for primary procedure)**
Code first primary procedure
7.63 7.63 FUD ZZZ C 80
AMA: 2018,Jan,8; 2017,Jan,8; 2016,Jan,13

38115 **Repair of ruptured spleen (splenorrhaphy) with or without partial splenectomy**
37.1 37.1 FUD 090 C 80
AMA: 2018,Jan,8; 2017,Jan,8; 2016,Jan,13

38120 **Laparoscopy, surgical, splenectomy**
INCLUDES Diagnostic laparoscopy (49320)
30.6 30.6 FUD 090 J G2 80
AMA: 2018,Jan,8; 2017,Jan,8; 2016,Jan,13

38129 **Unlisted laparoscopy procedure, spleen**
0.00 0.00 FUD YYY J 80
AMA: 2018,Jan,8; 2017,Jan,8; 2016,Jan,13

38200 **Injection procedure for splenoportography**
(75810)
3.85 3.85 FUD 000 N N1 80
AMA: 2014,Jan,11

38204-38215 Hematopoietic Stem Cell Preparation

CMS: 100-03,110.23 Stem Cell Transplantation; 100-04,3,90.3 Stem Cell Transplantation; 100-04,3,90.3.1 Allogeneic Stem Cell Transplantation; 100-04,3,90.3.3 Billing for Allogeneic Stem Cell Transplants; 100-04,32,90 Billing for Stem Cell Transplantation; 100-04,32,90.2.1 Coding for Stem Cell Transplantation; 100-04,4,231.10 Billing for Autologous Stem Cell Transplants; 100-04,4,231.11 Billing for Allogeneic Stem Cell Transplants

INCLUDES Preservation, preparation, purification stem cells before transplant or reinfusion
EXCLUDES *Procedure performed more than one time per day*

38204 **Management of recipient hematopoietic progenitor cell donor search and cell acquisition**
3.03 3.03 FUD XXX N N1
AMA: 2018,Jan,8; 2017,Jan,8; 2016,Jan,13

38205 **Blood-derived hematopoietic progenitor cell harvesting for transplantation, per collection; allogeneic**
2.44 2.44 FUD 000 B 80
AMA: 2018,May,3; 2018,Jan,8; 2017,Jan,8; 2016,Jan,13

38206 **autologous**
2.39 2.39 FUD 000 S G2 80
AMA: 2018,May,3; 2018,Jan,8; 2017,Jan,8; 2016,Jan,13

38207 **Transplant preparation of hematopoietic progenitor cells; cryopreservation and storage**
EXCLUDES *Flow cytometry (88182, 88184-88189)*
(88240)
1.31 1.31 FUD XXX S G2
AMA: 2018,Jan,8; 2017,Jan,8; 2016,Jan,13

38208 **thawing of previously frozen harvest, without washing, per donor**
EXCLUDES *Flow cytometry (88182, 88184-88189)*
(88241)
0.83 0.83 FUD XXX S G2
AMA: 2018,Jan,8; 2017,Jan,8; 2016,Jan,13

38209 **thawing of previously frozen harvest, with washing, per donor**
EXCLUDES *Flow cytometry (88182, 88184-88189)*
0.35 0.35 FUD XXX S G2
AMA: 2018,Jan,8; 2017,Jan,8; 2016,Jan,13

38210 **specific cell depletion within harvest, T-cell depletion**
EXCLUDES *Flow cytometry (88182, 88184-88189)*
2.29 2.29 FUD XXX S G2
AMA: 2018,Jan,8; 2017,Jan,8; 2016,Jan,13

38211 **tumor cell depletion**
EXCLUDES *Flow cytometry (88182, 88184-88189)*
2.08 2.08 FUD XXX S G2
AMA: 2018,Jan,8; 2017,Jan,8; 2016,Jan,13

38212 **red blood cell removal**
EXCLUDES *Flow cytometry (88182, 88184-88189)*
1.39 1.39 FUD XXX S G2
AMA: 2018,Jan,8; 2017,Jan,8; 2016,Jan,13

38213 **platelet depletion**
EXCLUDES *Flow cytometry (88182, 88184-88189)*
0.35 0.35 FUD XXX S G2
AMA: 2018,Jan,8; 2017,Jan,8; 2016,Jan,13

38214 **plasma (volume) depletion**
EXCLUDES *Flow cytometry (88182, 88184-88189)*
1.23 1.23 FUD XXX S G2
AMA: 2018,Jan,8; 2017,Jan,8; 2016,Jan,13

38215 **cell concentration in plasma, mononuclear, or buffy coat layer**
EXCLUDES *Flow cytometry (88182, 88184-88189)*
1.39 1.39 FUD XXX S G2
AMA: 2018,Jan,8; 2017,Jan,8; 2016,Jan,13

37785 — 38215

38220-38232 Bone Marrow Procedures

CMS: 100-03,110.23 Stem Cell Transplantation; 100-04,3,90.3 Stem Cell Transplantation; 100-04,32,90 Billing for Stem Cell Transplantation; 100-04,4,231.11 Billing for Allogeneic Stem Cell Transplants

38220 Diagnostic bone marrow; aspiration(s)

EXCLUDES *Aspiration bone marrow for spinal graft (20939)*
Bone marrow biopsy (38221)
Bone marrow for platelet rich stem cell injection (0232T)

Code also biopsy bone marrow during same session (38222)

1.99 4.71 **FUD** XXX J P3 80 50

AMA: 2018,May,3; 2018,Jan,8; 2017,Jan,8; 2016,Jan,13

38221 biopsy(ies)

EXCLUDES *Aspiration and biopsy during same session (38222)*
Aspiration bone marrow (38220)

(88305)

2.00 4.47 **FUD** XXX J P3 80 50

AMA: 2018,May,3; 2018,Jan,8; 2017,Jan,8; 2016,Jan,13

38222 biopsy(ies) and aspiration(s)

EXCLUDES *Aspiration bone marrow only (38221)*
Biopsy bone marrow only (38220)

(88305)

2.24 4.94 **FUD** XXX J G2 80 50

AMA: 2018,May,3

38230 Bone marrow harvesting for transplantation; allogeneic

EXCLUDES *Aspiration bone marrow for platelet rich stem cell injection (0232T)*
Harvesting blood-derived hematopoietic progenitor cells for transplant (allogeneic) (38205)

5.92 5.92 **FUD** 000 S G2 80

AMA: 2018,Jan,8; 2017,Jan,8; 2016,Jan,13

38232 autologous

EXCLUDES *Aspiration bone marrow (38220, 38222)*
Aspiration bone marrow for platelet rich stem cell injection (0232T)
Aspiration bone marrow for spinal graft (20939)
Harvesting blood-derived peripheral stem cells for transplant (allogenic/autologous) (38205-38206)

5.76 5.76 **FUD** 000 S G2 80

AMA: 2018,Jan,8; 2017,Jan,8; 2016,Jan,13

38240-38243 [38243] Hematopoietic Progenitor Cell Transplantation

CMS: 100-03,110.23 Stem Cell Transplantation; 100-04,3,90.3 Stem Cell Transplantation; 100-04,3,90.3.1 Allogeneic Stem Cell Transplantation; 100-04,3,90.3.2 Autologous Stem Cell Transplantation (AuSCT); 100-04,90.3.3 Billing for Allogeneic Stem Cell Transplants; 100-04,32,90 Billing for Stem Cell Transplantation; 100-04,32,90.2 Allogeneic Stem Cell Transplantation; 100-04,32,90.2.1 Coding for Stem Cell Transplantation; 100-04,32,90.3 Autologous Stem Cell Transplantation; 100-04,32,90.4 Edits Stem Cell Transplant; 100-04,32,90.6 Clinical Trials for Stem Cell Transplant for Myelodysplastic Syndrome (; 100-04,4,231.10 Billing for Autologous Stem Cell Transplants; 100-04,4,231.11 Billing for Allogeneic Stem Cell Transplants

INCLUDES Evaluation patient prior to, during, and after infusion
Management uncomplicated adverse reactions such as hives or nausea
Monitoring physiological parameters
Physician presence during infusion
Supervision clinical staff

EXCLUDES *Administration fluids for transplant or incidental hydration separately*
Concurrent administration medications with infusion for transplant
Cryopreservation, freezing, and storage hematopoietic progenitor cells for transplant (38207)
Human leukocyte antigen (HLA) testing (81379-81383, 86812-86821)
Modification, treatment, processing hematopoietic progenitor cell specimens for transplant (38210-38215)
Thawing and expansion hematopoietic progenitor cells for transplant (38208-38209)

Code also:
Administration medications and/or fluids not related to transplant, append modifier 59
E/M service for treatment more complicated adverse reactions after infusion, as appropriate
Separately identifiable E/M service on same date, appending modifier 25 as appropriate (99211-99215, 99217-99220, [99224, 99225, 99226], 99221-99223, 99231-99239, 99471-99472, 99475-99476)

38240 Hematopoietic progenitor cell (HPC); allogeneic transplantation per donor

EXCLUDES *Allogeneic lymphocyte infusions on same date of service with (38242)*
Hematopoietic progenitor cell (HPC); HPC boost on same date of service with ([38243])

6.78 6.78 **FUD** XXX J G2 80

AMA: 2018,Jan,8; 2017,Jan,8; 2016,Jan,13

38241 autologous transplantation

5.02 5.02 **FUD** XXX S G2 80

AMA: 2018,Jan,8; 2017,Jan,8; 2016,Jan,13

\# **38243 HPC boost**

EXCLUDES *Allogeneic lymphocyte infusions on same date of service with (38242)*
Hematopoietic progenitor cell (HPC); allogeneic transplantation per donor on same date of service with (38240)

3.47 3.47 **FUD** 000 S R2 80

AMA: 2018,Jan,8; 2017,Jan,8; 2016,Jan,13

38242 Allogeneic lymphocyte infusions

EXCLUDES *Aspiration bone marrow (38220, 38222)*
Aspiration bone marrow for platelet rich stem cell injection (0232T)
Aspiration bone marrow for spinal graft (20939)
Hematopoietic progenitor cell (HPC); allogeneic transplantation per donor on same date of service with (38240)
Hematopoietic progenitor cell (HPC); HPC boost on same service date with ([38243])

(81379-81383, 86812-86813, 86816-86817, 86821)

3.63 3.63 **FUD** 000 S R2 80

AMA: 2018,Jan,8; 2017,Jan,8; 2016,Jan,13

38243 **Resequenced code. See code following 38241.**

38300-38382 Incision Lymphatic Vessels

38300 Drainage of lymph node abscess or lymphadenitis; simple

5.91 9.40 **FUD** 010 J A2

AMA: 2014,Jan,11

38305 extensive

14.1 14.1 **FUD** 090 J A2

AMA: 2014,Jan,11

38308 **Lymphangiotomy or other operations on lymphatic channels**
13.0 13.0 FUD 090 J A2 80
AMA: 2014,Jan,11

38380 **Suture and/or ligation of thoracic duct; cervical approach**
16.3 16.3 FUD 090 C 80
AMA: 2014,Jan,11

38381 **thoracic approach**
23.2 23.2 FUD 090 C 80
AMA: 2014,Jan,11

38382 **abdominal approach**
19.4 19.4 FUD 090 C 80
AMA: 2014,Jan,11

38500-38555 Biopsy/Excision Lymphatic Vessels

EXCLUDES *Injection for sentinel node identification (38792)*
Percutaneous needle biopsy retroperitoneal mass (49180)

38500 **Biopsy or excision of lymph node(s); open, superficial**
EXCLUDES *Lymphadenectomy (38700-38780)*
7.38 9.68 FUD 010 J A2 50
AMA: 2019,Feb,8; 2018,Jan,8; 2017,Jan,8; 2016,Jan,13

38505 **by needle, superficial (eg, cervical, inguinal, axillary)**
EXCLUDES *Fine needle aspiration (10004-10012, 10021)*
(88172-88173)
(76942, 77002, 77012, 77021)
2.02 3.55 FUD 000 J A2 50
AMA: 2019,Feb,8; 2018,Jan,8; 2017,Jan,8; 2016,Jan,13

38510 **open, deep cervical node(s)**
12.0 14.9 FUD 010 J A2 50
AMA: 2020,Dec,11; 2019,Feb,8; 2018,Jan,8; 2017,Jan,8; 2016,Jan,13

38520 **open, deep cervical node(s) with excision scalene fat pad**
13.4 13.4 FUD 090 J A2 50
AMA: 2019,Feb,8; 2018,Jan,8; 2017,Jan,8; 2016,Jan,13

38525 **open, deep axillary node(s)**
12.6 12.6 FUD 090 J A2 50
AMA: 2019,Feb,8; 2018,Jan,8; 2017,Jan,8; 2016,Jan,13

38530 **open, internal mammary node(s)**
EXCLUDES *Fine needle aspiration (10005-10012)*
Lymphadenectomy (38720-38746)
16.3 16.3 FUD 090 J A2 80 50
AMA: 2019,Feb,8; 2018,Jan,8; 2017,Jan,8; 2016,Jan,13

38531 **open, inguinofemoral node(s)**
12.5 12.5 FUD 090 G2 80 50
AMA: 2019,Feb,8

38542 **Dissection, deep jugular node(s)**
EXCLUDES *Complete cervical lymphadenectomy (38720)*
14.8 14.8 FUD 090 J A2 80 50
AMA: 2019,Feb,8; 2018,Jan,8; 2017,Jan,8; 2016,Jan,13

38550 **Excision of cystic hygroma, axillary or cervical; without deep neurovascular dissection**
14.7 14.7 FUD 090 J A2 80
AMA: 2014,Jan,11; 1994,Win,1

38555 **with deep neurovascular dissection**
29.5 29.5 FUD 090 J A2 80
AMA: 2014,Jan,11; 1994,Win,1

38562-38564 Limited Lymphadenectomy: Staging

38562 **Limited lymphadenectomy for staging (separate procedure); pelvic and para-aortic**
EXCLUDES *Prostatectomy (55812, 55842)*
Radioactive substance inserted into prostate (55862)
20.4 20.4 FUD 090 C 80
AMA: 2019,Feb,8; 2018,Jan,8; 2017,Jan,8; 2016,Jan,13

38564 **retroperitoneal (aortic and/or splenic)**
20.4 20.4 FUD 090 C 80
AMA: 2019,Feb,8

38570-38589 Laparoscopic Lymph Node Procedures

INCLUDES Diagnostic laparoscopy (49320)
EXCLUDES *Laparoscopy with draining lymphocele to peritoneal cavity (49323)*
Limited lymphadenectomy:
Pelvic (38562)
Retroperitoneal (38564)

38570 **Laparoscopy, surgical; with retroperitoneal lymph node sampling (biopsy), single or multiple**
14.7 14.7 FUD 010 J A2 80
AMA: 2019,Feb,8; 2018,Jan,8; 2017,Jan,8; 2016,Jan,13

38571 **with bilateral total pelvic lymphadenectomy**
19.1 19.1 FUD 010 J A2 80
AMA: 2019,Feb,8; 2018,Jan,8; 2017,Jan,8; 2016,Jan,13

38572 **with bilateral total pelvic lymphadenectomy and peri-aortic lymph node sampling (biopsy), single or multiple**
EXCLUDES *Lymphocele drainage into peritoneal cavity (49323)*
26.3 26.3 FUD 010 J A2 80
AMA: 2019,Feb,8; 2018,Jan,8; 2017,Jan,8; 2016,Jan,13

38573 **with bilateral total pelvic lymphadenectomy and peri-aortic lymph node sampling, peritoneal washings, peritoneal biopsy(ies), omentectomy, and diaphragmatic washings, including diaphragmatic and other serosal biopsy(ies), when performed**
EXCLUDES *Laparoscopic hysterectomy procedures (58541-58554)*
Laparoscopic omentopexy (separate procedure) (49326)
Laparoscopy abdomen, diagnostic (separate procedure)(49320)
Laparoscopy unlisted (38589)
Laparoscopy without omentectomy (38570-38572)
Lymphadenectomy for staging (38562-38564)
Omentectomy (separate procedure) (49255)
Pelvic lymphadenectomy external iliac, hypogastric, and obturator nodes (38770)
Retroperitoneal lymphadenectomy aortic, pelvic, and renal nodes (separate procedure) (38780)
33.5 33.5 FUD 010 J G2 80
AMA: 2019,Mar,5; 2018,Apr,10

38589 **Unlisted laparoscopy procedure, lymphatic system**
0.00 0.00 FUD YYY J 80 50
AMA: 2018,Apr,10; 2018,Jan,8; 2017,Jan,8; 2016,Jan,13

38700-38780 Lymphadenectomy Procedures

INCLUDES Lymph node biopsy/excision (38500)
EXCLUDES *Excision lymphedematous skin and subcutaneous tissue (15004-15005)*
Limited lymphadenectomy
Pelvic (38562)
Retroperitoneal (38564)
Repair lymphedematous skin and tissue (15570-15650)

38700 **Suprahyoid lymphadenectomy**
23.1 23.1 FUD 090 J G2 80 50
AMA: 2020,Dec,11; 2019,Feb,8; 2018,Jan,8; 2017,Jan,8; 2016,Jan,13

38720 **Cervical lymphadenectomy (complete)**
38.5 38.5 FUD 090 J G2 80 50
AMA: 2020,Apr,10; 2019,Feb,8; 2018,Jan,8; 2017,Jan,8; 2016,Jan,13

38724 **Cervical lymphadenectomy (modified radical neck dissection)**
41.5 41.5 FUD 090 C 80 50
AMA: 2020,Dec,11; 2019,Mar,10; 2019,Feb,8; 2018,Jan,8; 2017,Jan,8; 2016,Jan,13

38740 **Axillary lymphadenectomy; superficial**
20.2 20.2 FUD 090 J A2 80 50
AMA: 2019,Feb,8; 2018,Jan,8; 2017,Jan,8; 2016,Jan,13

38745 **complete**
25.4 25.4 FUD 090 J A2 80 50
AMA: 2019,Feb,8

\+ **38746** **Thoracic lymphadenectomy by thoracotomy, mediastinal and regional lymphadenectomy (List separately in addition to code for primary procedure)**
INCLUDES Left side
Aortopulmonary window
Inferior pulmonary ligament
Paraesophageal
Subcarinal
Right side
Inferior pulmonary ligament
Paraesophageal
Paratracheal
Subcarinal
EXCLUDES *Thoracoscopic mediastinal and regional lymphadenectomy (32674)*
Code first (21601, 31760, 31766, 31786, 32096-32200, 32220-32320, 32440-32491, 32503-32505, 33025, 33030, 33050-33130, 39200-39220, 39560-39561, 43101, 43112, 43117-43118, 43122-43123, 43351, 60270, 60505)
6.22 6.22 FUD ZZZ C 80
AMA: 2019,Feb,8; 2018,Jan,8; 2017,Jan,8; 2016,Jan,13

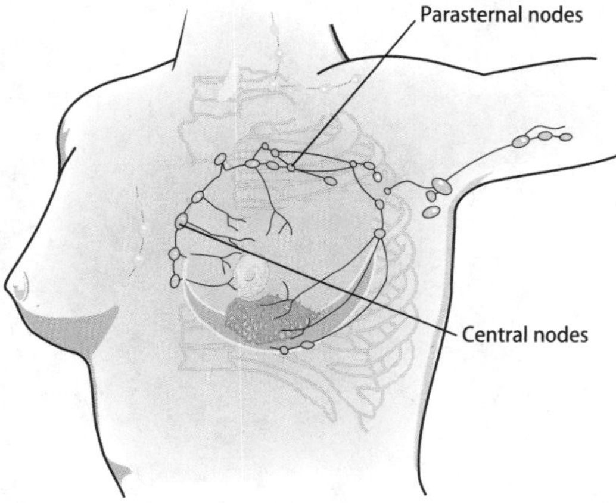

\+ **38747** **Abdominal lymphadenectomy, regional, including celiac, gastric, portal, peripancreatic, with or without para-aortic and vena caval nodes (List separately in addition to code for primary procedure)**
Code first primary procedure
7.77 7.77 FUD ZZZ C 80
AMA: 2020,Apr,10; 2019,Feb,8

38760 **Inguinofemoral lymphadenectomy, superficial, including Cloquet's node (separate procedure)**
24.2 24.2 FUD 090 J A2 80 50
AMA: 2019,Feb,8; 2018,Jan,8; 2017,Jan,8; 2016,Jan,13

38765 **Inguinofemoral lymphadenectomy, superficial, in continuity with pelvic lymphadenectomy, including external iliac, hypogastric, and obturator nodes (separate procedure)**
37.7 37.7 FUD 090 C 80 50
AMA: 2019,Feb,8; 2018,Jan,8; 2017,Jan,8; 2016,Jan,13

38770 **Pelvic lymphadenectomy, including external iliac, hypogastric, and obturator nodes (separate procedure)**
23.2 23.2 FUD 090 C 80 50
AMA: 2019,Feb,8

38780 **Retroperitoneal transabdominal lymphadenectomy, extensive, including pelvic, aortic, and renal nodes (separate procedure)**
29.9 29.9 FUD 090 C 80
AMA: 2019,Feb,8

38790-38999 Cannulation/Injection/Other Procedures

38790 **Injection procedure; lymphangiography**
(75801-75807)
2.36 2.36 FUD 000 N N1 50
AMA: 2014,Jan,11; 1999,Jul,6

38792 **radioactive tracer for identification of sentinel node**
EXCLUDES *Sentinel node excision (38500-38542)*
Sentinel node(s) identification (mapping) intraoperative with nonradioactive dye injection (38900)
(78195)
0.97 2.37 FUD 000 Q1 N1 50
AMA: 2019,Feb,8; 2018,Jan,8; 2017,Jan,8; 2016,Jan,13

38794 **Cannulation, thoracic duct**
8.52 8.52 FUD 090 N N1 80
AMA: 2014,Jan,11

\+ **38900** **Intraoperative identification (eg, mapping) of sentinel lymph node(s) includes injection of non-radioactive dye, when performed (List separately in addition to code for primary procedure)**
EXCLUDES *Injection tracer for sentinel node identification (38792)*
Code first (19302, 19307, 38500, 38510, 38520, 38525, 38530-38531, 38542, 38562-38564, 38570-38572, 38740, 38745, 38760, 38765, 38770, 38780, 56630-56634, 56637, 56640)
4.03 4.03 FUD ZZZ N N1 80 50
AMA: 2019,Feb,8; 2018,Jan,8; 2017,Jan,8; 2016,Jan,13

38999 **Unlisted procedure, hemic or lymphatic system**
0.00 0.00 FUD YYY S 80
AMA: 2020,Dec,11; 2018,Jan,8; 2017,Jan,8; 2016,Jan,13

39000-39499 Surgical Procedures: Mediastinum

39000 **Mediastinotomy with exploration, drainage, removal of foreign body, or biopsy; cervical approach**
14.3 14.3 FUD 090 C 80
AMA: 2014,Jan,11; 1994,Win,1

39010 **transthoracic approach, including either transthoracic or median sternotomy**
EXCLUDES *ECMO/ECLS insertion or reposition cannula (33955-33956, [33963, 33964])*
Video-assisted thoracic surgery (VATS) pericardial biopsy (32604)
22.7 22.7 FUD 090 C 80
AMA: 2018,Jan,8; 2017,Jan,8; 2016,Jan,13

39200 **Resection of mediastinal cyst**
25.2 25.2 FUD 090 C 80
AMA: 2014,Jan,11; 2012,Oct,9-11

39220 **Resection of mediastinal tumor**
EXCLUDES *Thymectomy (60520)*
Thyroidectomy, substernal (60270)
Video-assisted thoracic surgery (VATS) resection cyst, mass, or tumor of mediastinum (32662)
32.7 32.7 FUD 090 C 80
AMA: 2014,Jan,11; 2012,Oct,9-11

39401 **Mediastinoscopy; includes biopsy(ies) of mediastinal mass (eg, lymphoma), when performed**
8.93 8.93 FUD 000 J G2
AMA: 2018,Jan,8; 2017,Jan,8; 2016,Jun,4

39402 **with lymph node biopsy(ies) (eg, lung cancer staging)**
11.7 11.7 FUD 000 J G2
AMA: 2018,Jan,8; 2017,Jan,8; 2016,Jun,4

39499 **Unlisted procedure, mediastinum**
0.00 0.00 FUD YYY C 80
AMA: 2014,Jan,11

39501-39599 Surgical Procedures: Diaphragm

EXCLUDES *Esophagogastric fundoplasty, with fundic patch (43325)*
Repair diaphragmatic (esophageal) hernias:
Laparoscopic with fundoplication (43280-43282)
Laparotomy (43332-43333)
Thoracoabdominal (43336-43337)
Thoracotomy (43334-43335)

39501 Repair, laceration of diaphragm, any approach
24.6 24.6 **FUD** 090 C 80
AMA: 2018,Jan,8; 2017,Jan,8; 2016,Jan,13

39503 Repair, neonatal diaphragmatic hernia, with or without chest tube insertion and with or without creation of ventral hernia A
173. 173. **FUD** 090 63 C 80
AMA: 2018,Jan,8; 2017,Jan,8; 2016,Jan,13

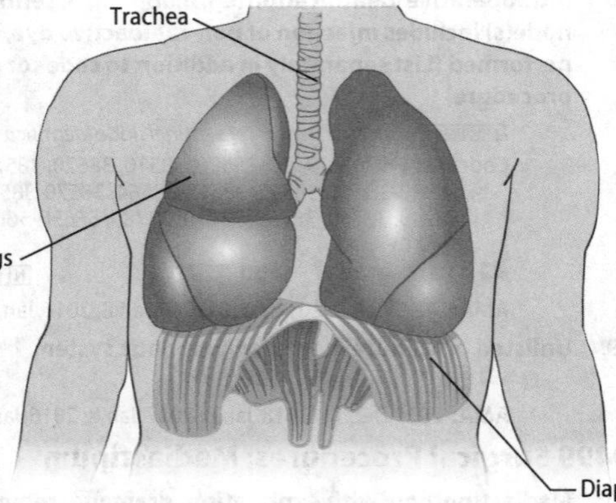

A defect of the diaphragm can allow abdominal contents to herniate into the thoracic cavity

39540 Repair, diaphragmatic hernia (other than neonatal), traumatic; acute
25.3 25.3 **FUD** 090 C 80
AMA: 2018,Jan,8; 2017,Jan,8; 2016,Jan,13

39541 chronic
27.3 27.3 **FUD** 090 C 80
AMA: 2018,Jan,8; 2017,Jan,8; 2016,Jan,13

39545 Imbrication of diaphragm for eventration, transthoracic or transabdominal, paralytic or nonparalytic
25.8 25.8 **FUD** 090 C 80
AMA: 2018,Jan,8; 2017,Jan,8; 2016,Jan,13

39560 Resection, diaphragm; with simple repair (eg, primary suture)
23.1 23.1 **FUD** 090 C 80
AMA: 2018,Jan,8; 2017,Jan,8; 2016,Jan,13

39561 with complex repair (eg, prosthetic material, local muscle flap)
35.9 35.9 **FUD** 090 C 80
AMA: 2018,Jan,8; 2017,Jan,8; 2016,Jan,13

39599 Unlisted procedure, diaphragm
EXCLUDES *Insertion/replacement diaphragmatic stimulation system (0674T-0675T, 0680T)*
0.00 0.00 **FUD** YYY C 80
AMA: 2014,Jan,11

26/TC PC/TC Only A2-Z3 ASC Payment 50 Bilateral ♂ Male Only ♀ Female Only Facility RVU Non-Facility RVU CCI CLIA
FUD Follow-up Days CMS: IOM AMA: CPT Asst A-Y OPPSI 80/80 Surg Assist Allowed / w/Doc Lab Crosswalk Radiology Crosswalk

40490-40799 Resection and Repair Procedures of the Lips

EXCLUDES *Procedures on skin of lips — see integumentary section codes*

40490 Biopsy of lip
2.03 3.55 **FUD** 000 T P3
AMA: 2019,Jan,9

40500 Vermilionectomy (lip shave), with mucosal advancement
10.4 14.7 **FUD** 090 J A2
AMA: 2014,Jan,11; 2000,Sep,11

40510 Excision of lip; transverse wedge excision with primary closure
EXCLUDES *Excision mucous lesions (40810-40816)*
10.0 13.9 **FUD** 090 J A2
AMA: 2014,Jan,11

40520 V-excision with primary direct linear closure
EXCLUDES *Excision mucous lesions (40810-40816)*
10.2 14.2 **FUD** 090 J A2
AMA: 2014,Jan,11; 2000,Sep,11

40525 full thickness, reconstruction with local flap (eg, Estlander or fan)
15.8 15.8 **FUD** 090 J A2
AMA: 2014,Jan,11

40527 full thickness, reconstruction with cross lip flap (Abbe-Estlander)
INCLUDES Cleft lip repair with cross lip pedicle flap (Abbe-Estlander type), without pedicle sectioning and insertion
EXCLUDES *Cleft lip repair with cross lip pedicle flap (Abbe-Estlander type), with pedicle sectioning and insertion (40761)*
17.7 17.7 **FUD** 090 J A2 80
AMA: 2014,Jan,11

40530 Resection of lip, more than one-fourth, without reconstruction
EXCLUDES *Reconstruction (13131-13153)*
11.4 15.6 **FUD** 090 J A2
AMA: 2014,Jan,11

40650 Repair lip, full thickness; vermilion only
8.79 13.2 **FUD** 090 T A2 80
AMA: 2018,Jan,8; 2017,Jan,8; 2016,Nov,7; 2016,Jan,13

40652 up to half vertical height
10.2 14.5 **FUD** 090 T A2 80
AMA: 2018,Jan,8; 2017,Jan,8; 2016,Nov,7; 2016,Jan,13

40654 over one-half vertical height, or complex
12.1 16.5 **FUD** 090 T A2
AMA: 2018,Jan,8; 2017,Jan,8; 2016,Nov,7

40700 Plastic repair of cleft lip/nasal deformity; primary, partial or complete, unilateral
EXCLUDES *Cleft lip repair with cross lip pedicle flap (Abbe-Estlander type):*
With pedicle sectioning and insertion (40761)
Without pedicle sectioning and insertion (40527)
Rhinoplasty for nasal deformity secondary to congenital cleft lip (30460, 30462)
29.2 29.2 **FUD** 090 J A2 80
AMA: 2018,Jan,8; 2017,Jan,8; 2016,Jan,13

40701 primary bilateral, 1-stage procedure
EXCLUDES *Cleft lip repair with cross lip pedicle flap (Abbe-Estlander type):*
With pedicle sectioning and insertion (40761)
Without pedicle sectioning and insertion (40527)
Rhinoplasty for nasal deformity secondary to congenital cleft lip (30460, 30462)
34.6 34.6 **FUD** 090 J A2 80
AMA: 2018,Jan,8; 2017,Jan,8; 2016,Jan,13

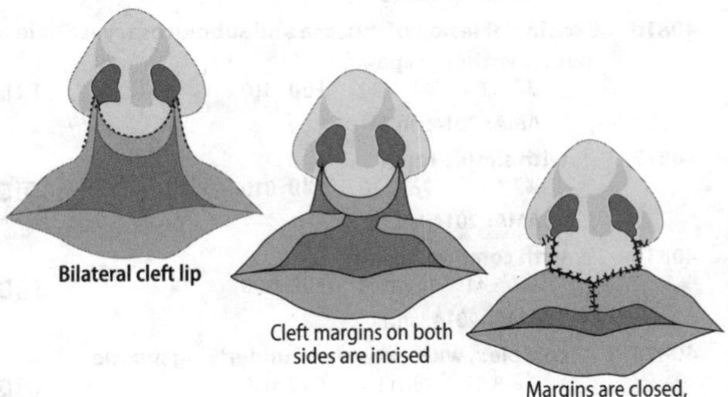
Bilateral cleft lip
Cleft margins on both sides are incised
Margins are closed, correcting cleft

40702 primary bilateral, 1 of 2 stages
EXCLUDES *Cleft lip repair with cross lip pedicle flap (Abbe-Estlander type):*
With pedicle sectioning and insertion (40761)
Without pedicle sectioning and insertion (40527)
Rhinoplasty for nasal deformity secondary to congenital cleft lip (30460, 30462)
29.0 29.0 **FUD** 090 J R2 80
AMA: 2018,Jan,8; 2017,Jan,8; 2016,Jan,13

40720 secondary, by recreation of defect and reclosure
EXCLUDES *Cleft lip repair with cross lip pedicle flap (Abbe-Estlander type):*
With pedicle sectioning and insertion (40761)
Without pedicle sectioning and insertion (40527)
Rhinoplasty for nasal deformity secondary to congenital cleft lip (30460, 30462)
29.8 29.8 **FUD** 090 J A2 80 50
AMA: 2018,Jan,8; 2017,Jan,8; 2016,Jan,13

40761 with cross lip pedicle flap (Abbe-Estlander type), including sectioning and inserting of pedicle
EXCLUDES *Cleft lip repair with cross lip pedicle flap (Abbe-Estlander type) without sectioning and insertion pedicle (40527)*
Cleft palate repair (42200-42225)
Other reconstructive procedures (14060-14061, 15120-15261, 15574, 15576, 15630)
31.3 31.3 **FUD** 090 J A2
AMA: 2014,Jan,11

40799 Unlisted procedure, lips
0.00 0.00 **FUD** YYY T 80
AMA: 2014,Jan,11

40800-40819 Incision and Resection of Buccal Cavity

INCLUDES Mucosal/submucosal tissue of lips/cheeks
Oral cavity outside dentoalveolar structures

40800 Drainage of abscess, cyst, hematoma, vestibule of mouth; simple
3.56 5.96 **FUD** 010 T P3
AMA: 2014,Jan,11

40801 complicated
5.96 8.59 **FUD** 010 T A2
AMA: 2014,Jan,11

40804 Removal of embedded foreign body, vestibule of mouth; simple
3.37 5.48 **FUD** 010 Q1 N1 80
AMA: 2014,Jan,11

40805 complicated
6.43 8.91 **FUD** 010 T P3 80
AMA: 2014,Jan,11

40806 **Incision of labial frenum (frenotomy)**
0.87 2.84 **FUD** 000 T P3 80
AMA: 2014,Jan,11

40808 **Biopsy, vestibule of mouth**
2.47 4.54 **FUD** 010 T P3
AMA: 2019,Jan,9

40810 **Excision of lesion of mucosa and submucosa, vestibule of mouth; without repair**
3.64 5.99 **FUD** 010 J P3
AMA: 2014,Jan,11

40812 with simple repair
5.63 8.30 **FUD** 010 J P3
AMA: 2014,Jan,11

40814 with complex repair
8.41 10.8 **FUD** 090 J A2
AMA: 2014,Jan,11

40816 complex, with excision of underlying muscle
8.81 11.4 **FUD** 090 J A2
AMA: 2014,Jan,11

40818 **Excision of mucosa of vestibule of mouth as donor graft**
7.78 10.4 **FUD** 090 T A2 80
AMA: 2014,Jan,11

40819 **Excision of frenum, labial or buccal (frenumectomy, frenulectomy, frenectomy)**
6.79 9.05 **FUD** 090 T A2 80
AMA: 2020,Aug,14

40820 Destruction of Lesion of Buccal Cavity

CMS: 100-03,140.5 Laser Procedures

INCLUDES Mucosal/submucosal tissue lips/cheeks
Oral cavity outside dentoalveolar structures

40820 **Destruction of lesion or scar of vestibule of mouth by physical methods (eg, laser, thermal, cryo, chemical)**
4.78 7.42 **FUD** 010 J P3
AMA: 2014,Jan,11; 1997,Nov,1

40830-40899 Repair Procedures of the Buccal Cavity

INCLUDES Mucosal/submucosal tissue lips/cheeks
Oral cavity outside dentoalveolar structures

EXCLUDES *Skin grafts (15002-15630)*

40830 **Closure of laceration, vestibule of mouth; 2.5 cm or less**
4.84 7.98 **FUD** 010 T G2 80
AMA: 2014,Jan,11

40831 over 2.5 cm or complex
6.64 10.1 **FUD** 010 T A2 80
AMA: 2014,Jan,11

40840 **Vestibuloplasty; anterior**
18.0 23.5 **FUD** 090 J A2 80
AMA: 2014,Jan,11

40842 posterior, unilateral
19.5 26.2 **FUD** 090 J A2 80
AMA: 2014,Jan,11

40843 posterior, bilateral
23.6 30.1 **FUD** 090 J A2 80
AMA: 2014,Jan,11

40844 entire arch
34.2 42.9 **FUD** 090 J A2 80
AMA: 2014,Jan,11

40845 complex (including ridge extension, muscle repositioning)
35.2 42.2 **FUD** 090 J A2 80
AMA: 2014,Jan,11

40899 **Unlisted procedure, vestibule of mouth**
0.00 0.00 **FUD** YYY T 80
AMA: 2014,Jan,11

41000-41018 Surgical Incision of Floor of Mouth or Tongue

EXCLUDES *Frenoplasty (41520)*

41000 **Intraoral incision and drainage of abscess, cyst, or hematoma of tongue or floor of mouth; lingual**
3.13 4.54 **FUD** 010 T P3
AMA: 2014,Jan,11

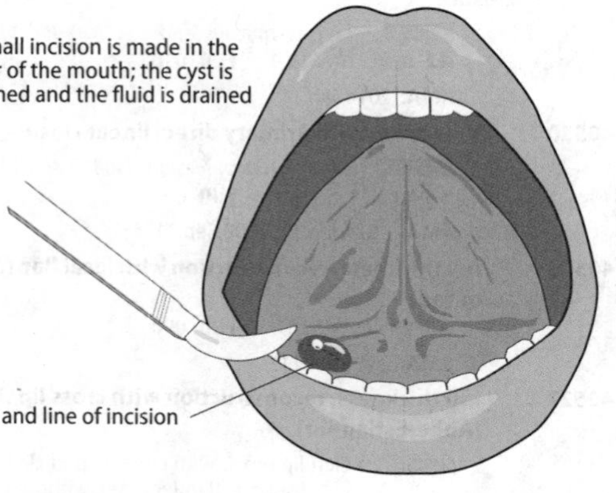
A small incision is made in the floor of the mouth; the cyst is opened and the fluid is drained
Cyst and line of incision

41005 sublingual, superficial
3.30 6.20 **FUD** 010 T A2 80
AMA: 2014,Jan,11

41006 sublingual, deep, supramylohyoid
6.85 9.81 **FUD** 090 T A2 80
AMA: 2014,Jan,11

41007 submental space
6.64 9.63 **FUD** 090 T A2 80
AMA: 2014,Jan,11

41008 submandibular space
7.45 10.9 **FUD** 090 J A2 80
AMA: 2014,Jan,11

41009 masticator space
8.19 11.8 **FUD** 090 T A2 80
AMA: 2014,Jan,11

41010 **Incision of lingual frenum (frenotomy)**
3.09 5.97 **FUD** 010 T A2 80
AMA: 2020,Aug,14; 2018,Jan,8; 2017,Nov,10; 2017,Sep,14

41015 **Extraoral incision and drainage of abscess, cyst, or hematoma of floor of mouth; sublingual**
8.92 11.6 **FUD** 090 T A2 80
AMA: 2014,Jan,11

41016 submental
9.92 13.0 **FUD** 090 J A2 80
AMA: 2014,Jan,11

41017 submandibular
9.86 12.9 **FUD** 090 J A2 80
AMA: 2014,Jan,11

41018 masticator space
11.4 14.5 **FUD** 090 T A2 80
AMA: 2014,Jan,11

41019 Placement of Devices for Brachytherapy

EXCLUDES *Application interstitial radioelements (77770-77772, 77778)*
Intracranial brachytherapy radiation sources with stereotactic insertion (61770)

41019 **Placement of needles, catheters, or other device(s) into the head and/or neck region (percutaneous, transoral, or transnasal) for subsequent interstitial radioelement application**
(76942, 77002, 77012, 77021)
13.9 13.9 FUD 000 J G2 80
AMA: 2018,Jan,8; 2017,Jan,8; 2016,Jan,13

41100-41599 Resection and Repair of the Tongue

41100 **Biopsy of tongue; anterior two-thirds**
3.07 4.94 FUD 010 T P3
AMA: 2019,Jan,9

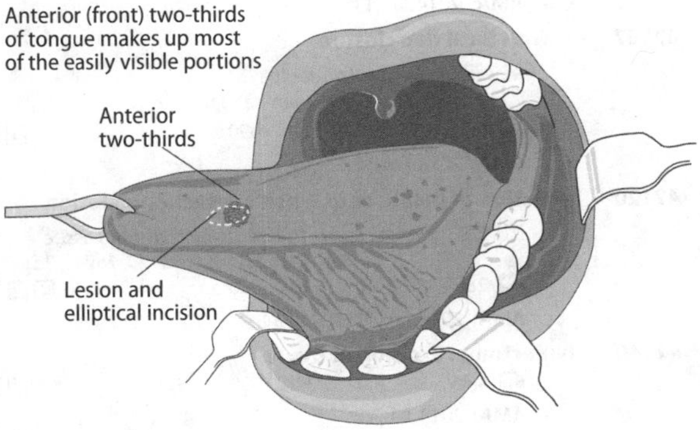
Anterior (front) two-thirds of tongue makes up most of the easily visible portions
Anterior two-thirds
Lesion and elliptical incision

41105 **posterior one-third**
3.11 5.05 FUD 010 J P3
AMA: 2014,Jan,11

41108 **Biopsy of floor of mouth**
2.52 4.43 FUD 010 J P3
AMA: 2019,Jan,9

41110 **Excision of lesion of tongue without closure**
3.73 6.29 FUD 010 J P3
AMA: 2014,Jan,11

41112 **Excision of lesion of tongue with closure; anterior two-thirds**
7.03 9.57 FUD 090 J A2
AMA: 2014,Jan,11

41113 **posterior one-third**
7.98 10.5 FUD 090 J A2
AMA: 2014,Jan,11

41114 **with local tongue flap**
INCLUDES Excision lesion tongue with closure anterior/posterior two-thirds (41112-41113)
17.7 17.7 FUD 090 J A2 80
AMA: 2014,Jan,11

41115 **Excision of lingual frenum (frenectomy)**
4.16 7.25 FUD 010 T P3 80
AMA: 2018,Jan,8; 2017,Nov,10; 2017,Sep,14

41116 **Excision, lesion of floor of mouth**
6.18 9.50 FUD 090 J A2
AMA: 2014,Jan,11

41120 **Glossectomy; less than one-half tongue**
30.3 30.3 FUD 090 J A2 80
AMA: 2018,Jan,8; 2017,Jan,8; 2016,Jan,13

41130 **hemiglossectomy**
38.0 38.0 FUD 090 C 80
AMA: 2018,Jan,8; 2017,Jan,8; 2016,Jan,13

41135 **partial, with unilateral radical neck dissection**
62.0 62.0 FUD 090 C 80
AMA: 2018,Jan,8; 2017,Jan,8; 2016,Jan,13

41140 **complete or total, with or without tracheostomy, without radical neck dissection**
INCLUDES Regnoli's excision
62.3 62.3 FUD 090 C 80
AMA: 2018,Jan,8; 2017,Jan,8; 2016,Jan,13

41145 **complete or total, with or without tracheostomy, with unilateral radical neck dissection**
78.9 78.9 FUD 090 C 80
AMA: 2018,Jan,8; 2017,Jan,8; 2016,Jan,13

41150 **composite procedure with resection floor of mouth and mandibular resection, without radical neck dissection**
62.8 62.8 FUD 090 C 80
AMA: 2018,Jan,8; 2017,Jan,8; 2016,Jan,13

41153 **composite procedure with resection floor of mouth, with suprahyoid neck dissection**
68.8 68.8 FUD 090 C 80
AMA: 2018,Jan,8; 2017,Jan,8; 2016,Jan,13

41155 **composite procedure with resection floor of mouth, mandibular resection, and radical neck dissection (Commando type)**
86.1 86.1 FUD 090 C 80
AMA: 2018,Jan,8; 2017,Jan,8; 2016,Jan,13

41250 **Repair of laceration 2.5 cm or less; floor of mouth and/or anterior two-thirds of tongue**
4.43 7.98 FUD 010 Q1 N1 80
AMA: 2014,Jan,11

41251 **posterior one-third of tongue**
5.27 8.83 FUD 010 T A2 80
AMA: 2014,Jan,11

41252 **Repair of laceration of tongue, floor of mouth, over 2.6 cm or complex**
6.01 9.18 FUD 010 T A2 80
AMA: 2014,Jan,11

41510 **Suture of tongue to lip for micrognathia (Douglas type procedure)**
13.0 13.0 FUD 090 J A2 80
AMA: 2018,Jan,8; 2017,Jan,8; 2016,Jan,13

41512 **Tongue base suspension, permanent suture technique**
EXCLUDES *Suture tongue to lip for micrognathia (41510)*
18.8 18.8 FUD 090 J G2 80
AMA: 2018,Jan,8; 2017,Jan,8; 2016,Jan,13

41520 **Frenoplasty (surgical revision of frenum, eg, with Z-plasty)**
EXCLUDES *Frenotomy (40806, 41010)*
7.11 10.1 FUD 090 J A2 80
AMA: 2020,Aug,14; 2018,Jan,8; 2017,Nov,10; 2017,Sep,14

41530 **Submucosal ablation of the tongue base, radiofrequency, 1 or more sites, per session**
10.7 27.4 FUD 000 J P3 80
AMA: 2018,Jan,8; 2017,Jan,8; 2016,Jan,13

41599 **Unlisted procedure, tongue, floor of mouth**
0.00 0.00 FUD YYY T 80
AMA: 2018,Jan,8; 2017,Jan,8; 2016,Jan,13

41800-41899 Procedures of the Teeth and Supporting Structures

41800 **Drainage of abscess, cyst, hematoma from dentoalveolar structures**
4.35 8.29 FUD 010 Q1 N1
AMA: 2014,Jan,11

41805 **Removal of embedded foreign body from dentoalveolar structures; soft tissues**
5.42 8.45 FUD 010 T P3 80
AMA: 2014,Jan,11

41806 **bone**
7.86 11.4 FUD 010 T P3 80
AMA: 2014,Jan,11

41820 **Gingivectomy, excision gingiva, each quadrant**
0.00 0.00 **FUD** 000 J R2 80
AMA: 2014,Jan,11

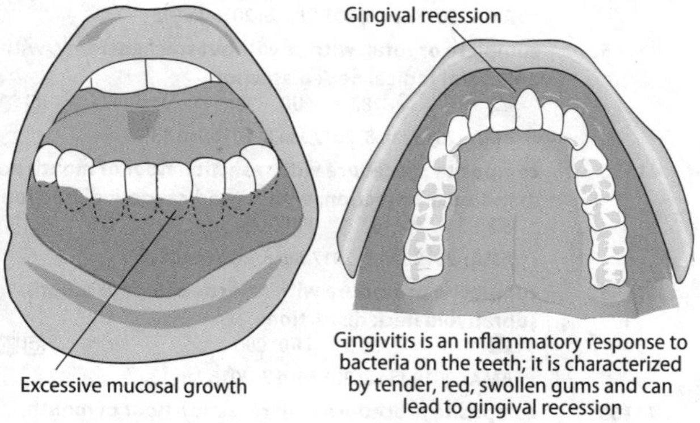

Gingivitis is an inflammatory response to bacteria on the teeth; it is characterized by tender, red, swollen gums and can lead to gingival recession

41821 **Operculectomy, excision pericoronal tissues**
0.00 0.00 **FUD** 000 T G2 80
AMA: 2014,Jan,11

41822 **Excision of fibrous tuberosities, dentoalveolar structures**
5.71 9.88 **FUD** 010 T P3 80
AMA: 2014,Jan,11

41823 **Excision of osseous tuberosities, dentoalveolar structures**
10.2 14.5 **FUD** 090 J P3 80
AMA: 2014,Jan,11

41825 **Excision of lesion or tumor (except listed above), dentoalveolar structures; without repair**
EXCLUDES *Lesion destruction nonexcisional (41850)*
3.43 6.19 **FUD** 010 J P3
AMA: 2014,Jan,11

41826 **with simple repair**
EXCLUDES *Lesion destruction nonexcisional (41850)*
5.88 8.96 **FUD** 010 J P3
AMA: 2014,Jan,11

41827 **with complex repair**
EXCLUDES *Lesion destruction nonexcisional (41850)*
8.59 12.7 **FUD** 090 J A2
AMA: 2014,Jan,11

41828 **Excision of hyperplastic alveolar mucosa, each quadrant (specify)**
6.43 9.95 **FUD** 010 J P3 80
AMA: 2014,Jan,11; 1994,Win,1

41830 **Alveolectomy, including curettage of osteitis or sequestrectomy**
8.91 13.0 **FUD** 010 J P3 80
AMA: 2014,Jan,11

41850 **Destruction of lesion (except excision), dentoalveolar structures**
0.00 0.00 **FUD** 000 T R2 80
AMA: 2014,Jan,11

41870 **Periodontal mucosal grafting**
0.00 0.00 **FUD** 000 J G2 80
AMA: 2014,Jan,11

41872 **Gingivoplasty, each quadrant (specify)**
8.54 12.8 **FUD** 090 J P3 80
AMA: 2014,Jan,11; 1994,Win,1

41874 **Alveoloplasty, each quadrant (specify)**
EXCLUDES *Fracture reduction (21421-21490)*
Laceration closure (40830-40831)
Maxilla osteotomy, segmental (21206)
7.21 11.2 **FUD** 090 J P3 80
AMA: 2014,Jan,11; 1994,Win,1

41899 **Unlisted procedure, dentoalveolar structures**
0.00 0.00 **FUD** YYY T 80
AMA: 2014,Jan,11

42000-42299 Procedures of the Palate and Uvula

42000 **Drainage of abscess of palate, uvula**
2.98 4.49 **FUD** 010 T A2 80
AMA: 2014,Jan,11

42100 **Biopsy of palate, uvula**
3.08 4.22 **FUD** 010 T P3
AMA: 2014,Jan,11

42104 **Excision, lesion of palate, uvula; without closure**
3.90 6.20 **FUD** 010 J P3
AMA: 2014,Jan,11

42106 **with simple primary closure**
4.86 7.62 **FUD** 010 J P3
AMA: 2014,Jan,11

42107 **with local flap closure**
EXCLUDES *Mucosal graft (40818)*
Skin graft (14040-14302)
9.73 13.2 **FUD** 090 J A2
AMA: 2014,Jan,11

42120 **Resection of palate or extensive resection of lesion**
EXCLUDES *Palate reconstruction using extraoral tissue (14040-14302, 15050, 15120, 15240, 15576)*
28.7 28.7 **FUD** 090 J A2 80
AMA: 2014,Jan,11; 1991,Fall,1

42140 **Uvulectomy, excision of uvula**
4.46 8.04 **FUD** 090 J A2
AMA: 2014,Jan,11

42145 **Palatopharyngoplasty (eg, uvulopalatopharyngoplasty, uvulopharyngoplasty)**
EXCLUDES *Excision maxillary torus palatinus (21032)*
Excision torus mandibularis (21031)
19.8 19.8 **FUD** 090 J A2
AMA: 2018,Jan,8; 2017,Jan,8; 2016,Jan,13

42160 **Destruction of lesion, palate or uvula (thermal, cryo or chemical)**
4.15 6.71 **FUD** 010 J P3 80
AMA: 2018,Jan,8; 2017,Jan,8; 2016,Jan,13

42180 **Repair, laceration of palate; up to 2 cm**
5.28 7.17 **FUD** 010 T A2 80
AMA: 2014,Jan,11

42182 **over 2 cm or complex**
7.34 9.34 **FUD** 010 J A2 80
AMA: 2014,Jan,11

42200 **Palatoplasty for cleft palate, soft and/or hard palate only**
27.2 27.2 **FUD** 090 J A2 80
AMA: 2018,Jan,8; 2017,Jan,8; 2016,Jan,13

42205 **Palatoplasty for cleft palate, with closure of alveolar ridge; soft tissue only**
28.4 28.4 **FUD** 090 J A2 80
AMA: 2014,Jan,11

42210 **with bone graft to alveolar ridge (includes obtaining graft)**
31.7 31.7 **FUD** 090 J J8 80
AMA: 2014,Jan,11

42215 **Palatoplasty for cleft palate; major revision**
20.7 20.7 **FUD** 090 J A2 80
AMA: 2014,Jan,11

42220 **secondary lengthening procedure**
17.0 17.0 **FUD** 090 J A2 80
AMA: 2014,Jan,11

42225 **attachment pharyngeal flap**
28.2 28.2 **FUD** 090 J G2 80
AMA: 2018,Jan,8; 2017,Jan,8; 2016,Jan,13

42226 **Lengthening of palate, and pharyngeal flap**
25.3 25.3 FUD 090 J A2 80
AMA: 2014,Jan,11

42227 **Lengthening of palate, with island flap**
23.6 23.6 FUD 090 J G2 80
AMA: 2014,Jan,11

42235 **Repair of anterior palate, including vomer flap**
EXCLUDES *Oronasal fistula repair (30600)*
20.7 20.7 FUD 090 J A2 80
AMA: 2018,Jan,8; 2017,Jan,8; 2016,Jan,13

42260 **Repair of nasolabial fistula**
EXCLUDES *Cleft lip repair (40700-40761)*
18.9 23.8 FUD 090 J A2 80
AMA: 2014,Jan,11

42280 **Maxillary impression for palatal prosthesis**
3.12 5.08 FUD 010 T P3 80
AMA: 2014,Jan,11

42281 **Insertion of pin-retained palatal prosthesis**
4.64 6.51 FUD 010 J G2 80
AMA: 2014,Jan,11

42299 **Unlisted procedure, palate, uvula**
0.00 0.00 FUD YYY T 80
AMA: 2018,Jan,8; 2017,Jan,8; 2016,Jan,13

42300-42699 Procedures of the Salivary Ducts and Glands

42300 **Drainage of abscess; parotid, simple**
4.39 6.10 FUD 010 T A2
AMA: 2014,Jan,11

42305 **parotid, complicated**
12.2 12.2 FUD 090 J A2 80
AMA: 2014,Jan,11

42310 **Drainage of abscess; submaxillary or sublingual, intraoral**
3.81 4.99 FUD 010 T A2 80
AMA: 2014,Jan,11

42320 **submaxillary, external**
5.03 7.31 FUD 010 T A2 80
AMA: 2014,Jan,11

42330 **Sialolithotomy; submandibular (submaxillary), sublingual or parotid, uncomplicated, intraoral**
4.69 6.63 FUD 010 J P3
AMA: 2014,Jan,11

42335 **submandibular (submaxillary), complicated, intraoral**
7.37 11.5 FUD 090 J P3
AMA: 2014,Jan,11

42340 **parotid, extraoral or complicated intraoral**
9.65 14.1 FUD 090 J A2 80 50
AMA: 2014,Jan,11

42400 **Biopsy of salivary gland; needle**
EXCLUDES *Fine needle aspiration (10021, [10004, 10005, 10006, 10007, 10008, 10009, 10010, 10011, 10012])*
(76942, 77002, 77012, 77021)
(88172-88173)
1.54 2.95 FUD 000 T P3
AMA: 2019,Apr,4

42405 **incisional**
(76942, 77002, 77012, 77021)
6.48 8.61 FUD 010 J A2
AMA: 2014,Jan,11

42408 **Excision of sublingual salivary cyst (ranula)**
10.0 15.0 FUD 090 J A2 80
AMA: 2014,Jan,11

42409 **Marsupialization of sublingual salivary cyst (ranula)**
6.42 10.4 FUD 090 J A2 80
AMA: 2014,Jan,11

42410 **Excision of parotid tumor or parotid gland; lateral lobe, without nerve dissection**
EXCLUDES *Facial nerve suture or graft (64864, 64865, 69740, 69745)*
17.9 17.9 FUD 090 J A2 80 50
AMA: 2014,Jan,11

42415 **lateral lobe, with dissection and preservation of facial nerve**
EXCLUDES *Facial nerve suture or graft (64864, 64865, 69740, 69745)*
30.2 30.2 FUD 090 J A2 80 50
AMA: 2014,Jan,11

42420 **total, with dissection and preservation of facial nerve**
EXCLUDES *Facial nerve suture or graft (64864, 64865, 69740, 69745)*
33.9 33.9 FUD 090 J A2 80 50
AMA: 2014,Jan,11; 2010,Aug,3-7

42425 **total, en bloc removal with sacrifice of facial nerve**
EXCLUDES *Facial nerve suture or graft (64864, 64865, 69740, 69745)*
23.9 23.9 FUD 090 J A2 80 50
AMA: 2014,Jan,11

42426 **total, with unilateral radical neck dissection**
EXCLUDES *Facial nerve suture or graft (64864, 64865, 69740, 69745)*
38.8 38.8 FUD 090 C 80 50
AMA: 2018,Jan,8; 2017,Jan,8; 2016,Jan,13

42440 **Excision of submandibular (submaxillary) gland**
11.8 11.8 FUD 090 J A2 80 50
AMA: 2014,Jan,11

42450 **Excision of sublingual gland**
10.3 13.1 FUD 090 J A2 80
AMA: 2014,Jan,11

42500 **Plastic repair of salivary duct, sialodochoplasty; primary or simple**
9.71 12.4 FUD 090 J A2 80
AMA: 2014,Jan,11

42505 **secondary or complicated**
12.9 15.9 FUD 090 J A2
AMA: 2014,Jan,11

42507 **Parotid duct diversion, bilateral (Wilke type procedure);**
14.4 14.4 FUD 090 J A2 80
AMA: 2014,Jan,11

42509 **with excision of both submandibular glands**
23.6 23.6 FUD 090 J A2 80
AMA: 2014,Jan,11

42510 **with ligation of both submandibular (Wharton's) ducts**
17.5 17.5 FUD 090 J A2 80
AMA: 2014,Jan,11

42550 **Injection procedure for sialography**
(70390)
1.83 4.39 FUD 000 N N1
AMA: 2014,Jan,11

42600 **Closure salivary fistula**
9.99 14.5 FUD 090 J A2 80
AMA: 2014,Jan,11

42650 **Dilation salivary duct**
1.65 2.25 FUD 000 T P3
AMA: 2014,Jan,11

42660 **Dilation and catheterization of salivary duct, with or without injection**
2.52 3.52 FUD 000 T P3 80
AMA: 2014,Jan,11

42665 **Ligation salivary duct, intraoral**
5.97 9.82 FUD 090 J A2 80
AMA: 2014,Jan,11

42699 **Unlisted procedure, salivary glands or ducts**
0.00 | 0.00 | FUD YYY | T 80
AMA: 2014,Jan,11

42700-42999 Procedures of the Adenoids/Throat/Tonsils

42700 **Incision and drainage abscess; peritonsillar**
3.88 | 5.43 | FUD 010 | T A2
AMA: 2014,Jan,11

42720 **retropharyngeal or parapharyngeal, intraoral approach**
11.1 | 12.9 | FUD 010 | J A2 80
AMA: 2014,Jan,11

42725 **retropharyngeal or parapharyngeal, external approach**
23.0 | 23.0 | FUD 090 | J A2 80
AMA: 2014,Jan,11

42800 **Biopsy; oropharynx**
EXCLUDES *Laryngoscopy with biopsy (31510, 31535-31536)*
3.22 | 4.49 | FUD 010 | J P3
AMA: 2014,Jan,11

42804 **nasopharynx, visible lesion, simple**
EXCLUDES *Laryngoscopy with biopsy (31510, 31535-31536)*
3.27 | 5.65 | FUD 010 | J A2
AMA: 2014,Jan,11

42806 **nasopharynx, survey for unknown primary lesion**
EXCLUDES *Laryngoscopy with biopsy (31510, 31535-31536)*
3.81 | 6.33 | FUD 010 | J A2
AMA: 2014,Jan,11

42808 **Excision or destruction of lesion of pharynx, any method**
4.66 | 6.53 | FUD 010 | J A2
AMA: 2014,Jan,11

42809 **Removal of foreign body from pharynx**
3.56 | 5.76 | FUD 010 | Q1 N1
AMA: 2014,Jan,11

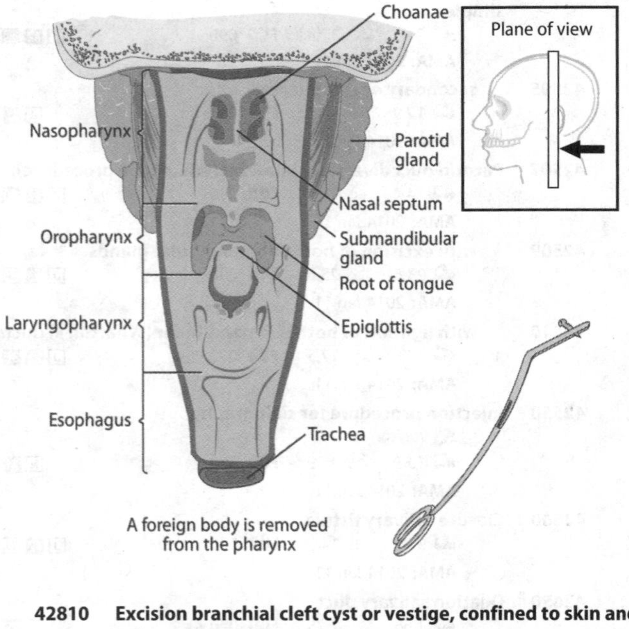

A foreign body is removed from the pharynx

42810 **Excision branchial cleft cyst or vestige, confined to skin and subcutaneous tissues**
8.10 | 11.0 | FUD 090 | J A2 80 50
AMA: 2014,Jan,11

42815 **Excision branchial cleft cyst, vestige, or fistula, extending beneath subcutaneous tissues and/or into pharynx**
15.6 | 15.6 | FUD 090 | J A2 80 50
AMA: 2014,Jan,11

42820 **Tonsillectomy and adenoidectomy; younger than age 12** A
8.26 | 8.26 | FUD 090 | J A2 80
AMA: 2018,Jan,8; 2017,Jan,8; 2016,Jan,13

42821 **age 12 or over** A
8.62 | 8.62 | FUD 090 | J A2 80
AMA: 2018,Jan,8; 2017,Jan,8; 2016,Jan,13

42825 **Tonsillectomy, primary or secondary; younger than age 12** A
7.52 | 7.52 | FUD 090 | J A2 80
AMA: 2018,Jan,8; 2017,Jan,8; 2016,Jan,13

42826 **age 12 or over** A
7.20 | 7.20 | FUD 090 | J A2
AMA: 2018,Jan,8; 2017,Jan,8; 2016,Jan,13

42830 **Adenoidectomy, primary; younger than age 12** A
5.95 | 5.95 | FUD 090 | J A2 80
AMA: 2018,Jan,8; 2017,Jan,8; 2016,Jan,13

42831 **age 12 or over** A
6.44 | 6.44 | FUD 090 | J A2 80
AMA: 2018,Jan,8; 2017,Jan,8; 2016,Jan,13

42835 **Adenoidectomy, secondary; younger than age 12** A
5.51 | 5.51 | FUD 090 | J A2 80
AMA: 2018,Jan,8; 2017,Jan,8; 2016,Jan,13

42836 **age 12 or over** A
6.89 | 6.89 | FUD 090 | J A2 80
AMA: 2018,Jan,8; 2017,Jan,8; 2016,Jan,13

42842 **Radical resection of tonsil, tonsillar pillars, and/or retromolar trigone; without closure**
28.7 | 28.7 | FUD 090 | J G2 80
AMA: 2018,Jan,8; 2017,Jan,8; 2016,Jan,13

42844 **closure with local flap (eg, tongue, buccal)**
39.9 | 39.9 | FUD 090 | J G2 80
AMA: 2018,Jan,8; 2017,Jan,8; 2016,Jan,13

42845 **closure with other flap**
Code also:
Closure with other flap(s)
Radical neck dissection when combined (38720)
63.9 | 63.9 | FUD 090 | C 80
AMA: 2018,Jan,8; 2017,Jan,8; 2016,Jan,13

42860 **Excision of tonsil tags**
5.40 | 5.40 | FUD 090 | J A2 80
AMA: 2014,Jan,11

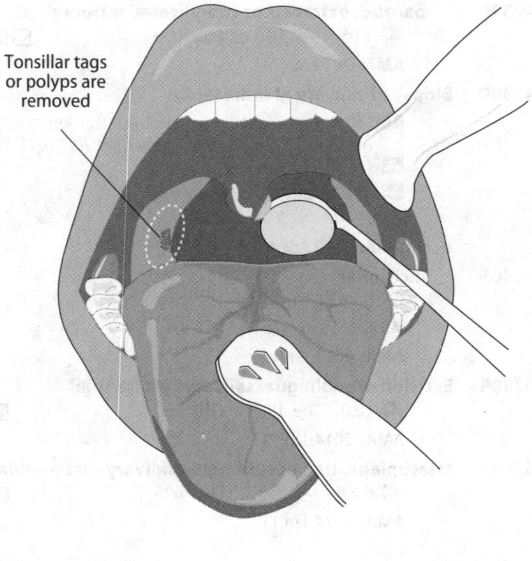

42870 Excision or destruction lingual tonsil, any method (separate procedure)

EXCLUDES *Nasopharynx resection (juvenile angiofibroma) by transzygomatic/bicoronal approach (61586, 61600)*

17.0 17.0 FUD 090 J A2 80

AMA: 2014,Jan,11

42890 Limited pharyngectomy

Code also radical neck dissection when combined (38720)

40.7 40.7 FUD 090 J A2 80

AMA: 2014,Jan,11; 2010,Aug,3-7

42892 Resection of lateral pharyngeal wall or pyriform sinus, direct closure by advancement of lateral and posterior pharyngeal walls

Code also radical neck dissection when combined (38720)

53.6 53.6 FUD 090 J A2 80

AMA: 2018,Jan,8; 2017,Jan,8; 2016,Jan,13

42894 Resection of pharyngeal wall requiring closure with myocutaneous or fasciocutaneous flap or free muscle, skin, or fascial flap with microvascular anastomosis

EXCLUDES *Flap used for reconstruction (15730, 15733-15734, 15756-15758)*

Code also radical neck dissection when combined (38720)

67.7 67.7 FUD 090 C 80

AMA: 2018,Jan,8; 2017,Jan,8; 2016,Jan,13

42900 Suture pharynx for wound or injury

9.56 9.56 FUD 010 T J8 80

AMA: 2014,Jan,11

42950 Pharyngoplasty (plastic or reconstructive operation on pharynx)

EXCLUDES *Pharyngeal flap (42225)*

22.8 22.8 FUD 090 J A2 80

AMA: 2019,Oct,10; 2018,Jan,8; 2017,Jan,8; 2016,Apr,8

42953 Pharyngoesophageal repair

Code also closure using myocutaneous or other flap

27.3 27.3 FUD 090 C 80

AMA: 2014,Jan,11

42955 Pharyngostomy (fistulization of pharynx, external for feeding)

21.7 21.7 FUD 090 T A2 80

AMA: 2014,Jan,11

42960 Control oropharyngeal hemorrhage, primary or secondary (eg, post-tonsillectomy); simple

4.83 4.83 FUD 010 T A2 80

AMA: 2014,Jan,11

42961 complicated, requiring hospitalization

11.9 11.9 FUD 090 C 80

AMA: 2014,Jan,11

42962 with secondary surgical intervention

14.7 14.7 FUD 090 J A2

AMA: 2014,Jan,11

42970 Control of nasopharyngeal hemorrhage, primary or secondary (eg, postadenoidectomy); simple, with posterior nasal packs, with or without anterior packs and/or cautery

11.7 11.7 FUD 090 T R2

AMA: 2014,Jan,11; 2002,May,7

42971 complicated, requiring hospitalization

12.9 12.9 FUD 090 C 80

AMA: 2014,Jan,11

42972 with secondary surgical intervention

14.5 14.5 FUD 090 J A2 80

AMA: 2014,Jan,11

● **42975 Drug-induced sleep endoscopy, with dynamic evaluation of velum, pharynx, tongue base, and larynx for evaluation of sleep-disordered breathing, flexible, diagnostic**

EXCLUDES *Diagnostic flexible laryngoscopy (31575)*

Nasal endoscopy, diagnostic, unless different type endoscope used and for different condition (31231)

Nasopharyngoscopy with endoscope (92511)

42999 Unlisted procedure, pharynx, adenoids, or tonsils

0.00 0.00 FUD YYY T 80

AMA: 2018,Jan,8; 2017,Jan,8; 2016,Jan,13

43020-43135 Incision/Resection of Esophagus

43020 Esophagotomy, cervical approach, with removal of foreign body

EXCLUDES *Laparotomy with esophageal intubation (43510)*

16.2 16.2 FUD 090 T G2 80

AMA: 2014,Jan,11

43030 Cricopharyngeal myotomy

EXCLUDES *Laparotomy with esophageal intubation (43510)*

14.8 14.8 FUD 090 J G2 80

AMA: 2020,Nov,12; 2020,Jul,13

43045 Esophagotomy, thoracic approach, with removal of foreign body

EXCLUDES *Laparotomy with esophageal intubation (43510)*

37.6 37.6 FUD 090 C 80

AMA: 2014,Jan,11; 1994,Win,1

43100 Excision of lesion, esophagus, with primary repair; cervical approach

EXCLUDES *Gastrointestinal reconstruction for previous esophagectomy (43360-43361)*

Wide excision malignant lesion cervical esophagus, with total laryngectomy:

With radical neck dissection (31365, 43107, 43116, 43124)

Without radical neck dissection (31360, 43107, 43116, 43124)

18.0 18.0 FUD 090 C 80

AMA: 2014,Jan,11; 1994,Win,1

43101 thoracic or abdominal approach

EXCLUDES *Gastrointestinal reconstruction for previous esophagectomy (43360-43361)*

Wide excision malignant lesion cervical esophagus, with total laryngectomy:

With radical neck dissection (31365, 43107, 43116, 43124)

Without radical neck dissection (31360, 43107, 43116, 43124)

29.1 29.1 FUD 090 C 80

AMA: 2018,Jan,8; 2017,Jan,8; 2016,Jan,13

43107 Total or near total esophagectomy, without thoracotomy; with pharyngogastrostomy or cervical esophagogastrostomy, with or without pyloroplasty (transhiatal)

EXCLUDES *Gastrointestinal reconstruction for previous esophagectomy (43360-43361)*

86.5 86.5 FUD 090 C 80

AMA: 2014,Jan,11; 2010,Aug,3-7

43108 with colon interposition or small intestine reconstruction, including intestine mobilization, preparation and anastomosis(es)

EXCLUDES *Gastrointestinal reconstruction for previous esophagectomy (43360-43361)*

129. 129. FUD 090 C 80

AMA: 2014,Jan,11; 2002,May,7

Digestive System

42870 — 43108

43112 **Total or near total esophagectomy, with thoracotomy; with pharyngogastrostomy or cervical esophagogastrostomy, with or without pyloroplasty (ie, McKeown esophagectomy or tri-incisional esophagectomy)**

EXCLUDES *Gastrointestinal reconstruction for previous esophagectomy (43360-43361)*

101. 101. FUD 090 C 80

AMA: 2018,Jul,7; 2018,Jan,8; 2017,Jan,8; 2016,Jan,13

43113 **with colon interposition or small intestine reconstruction, including intestine mobilization, preparation, and anastomosis(es)**

EXCLUDES *Gastrointestinal reconstruction for previous esophagectomy (43360-43361)*

126. 126. FUD 090 C 80

AMA: 2014,Jan,11; 2002,May,7

43116 **Partial esophagectomy, cervical, with free intestinal graft, including microvascular anastomosis, obtaining the graft and intestinal reconstruction**

INCLUDES Operating microscope (69990)

EXCLUDES *Free jejunal graft with microvascular anastomosis performed by different physician (43496)*

Gastrointestinal reconstruction for previous esophagectomy (43360-43361)

Code also modifier 52 when intestinal or free jejunal graft with microvascular anastomosis performed by another physician

145. 145. FUD 090 C 80

AMA: 2016,Feb,12

43117 **Partial esophagectomy, distal two-thirds, with thoracotomy and separate abdominal incision, with or without proximal gastrectomy; with thoracic esophagogastrostomy, with or without pyloroplasty (Ivor Lewis)**

EXCLUDES *Esophagogastrectomy (lower third) and vagotomy (43122)*

Gastrointestinal reconstruction for previous esophagectomy (43360-43361)

Total esophagectomy with gastropharyngostomy (43107, 43124)

94.3 94.3 FUD 090 C 80

AMA: 2014,Jan,11; 1994,Win,1

43118 **with colon interposition or small intestine reconstruction, including intestine mobilization, preparation, and anastomosis(es)**

EXCLUDES *Esophagogastrectomy (lower third) and vagotomy (43122)*

Gastrointestinal reconstruction for previous esophagectomy (43360-43361)

Total esophagectomy with gastropharyngostomy (43107, 43124)

105. 105. FUD 090 C 80

AMA: 2014,Jan,11; 2002,May,7

43121 **Partial esophagectomy, distal two-thirds, with thoracotomy only, with or without proximal gastrectomy, with thoracic esophagogastrostomy, with or without pyloroplasty**

EXCLUDES *Gastrointestinal reconstruction for previous esophagectomy (43360-43361)*

82.8 82.8 FUD 090 C 80

AMA: 2014,Jan,11; 1994,Win,1

43122 **Partial esophagectomy, thoracoabdominal or abdominal approach, with or without proximal gastrectomy; with esophagogastrostomy, with or without pyloroplasty**

EXCLUDES *Gastrointestinal reconstruction for previous esophagectomy (43360-43361)*

74.3 74.3 FUD 090 C 80

AMA: 2014,Jan,11; 1994,Win,1

43123 **with colon interposition or small intestine reconstruction, including intestine mobilization, preparation, and anastomosis(es)**

EXCLUDES *Gastrointestinal reconstruction for previous esophagectomy (43360-43361)*

131. 131. FUD 090 C 80

AMA: 2014,Jan,11; 2002,May,7

43124 **Total or partial esophagectomy, without reconstruction (any approach), with cervical esophagostomy**

EXCLUDES *Gastrointestinal reconstruction for previous esophagectomy (43360-43361)*

110. 110. FUD 090 C 80

AMA: 2018,Jan,8; 2017,Jan,8; 2016,Jan,13

43130 **Diverticulectomy of hypopharynx or esophagus, with or without myotomy; cervical approach**

EXCLUDES *Diverticulectomy hypopharynx or cervical esophagus, endoscopic (43180)*

Gastrointestinal reconstruction for previous esophagectomy (43360-43361)

22.6 22.6 FUD 090 J G2 80

AMA: 2018,Jan,8; 2017,Jan,8; 2016,Jan,13

43135 **thoracic approach**

EXCLUDES *Diverticulectomy hypopharynx or cervical esophagus, endoscopic (43180)*

Gastrointestinal reconstruction for previous esophagectomy (43360-43361)

42.6 42.6 FUD 090 C 80

AMA: 2018,Jan,8; 2017,Jan,8; 2016,Jan,13

43180-43233 [43210, 43211, 43212, 43213, 43214, 43233] Endoscopic Procedures: Esophagus

INCLUDES Control bleeding due to endoscopic procedure during same operative session

Diagnostic endoscopy with surgical endoscopy

Examination upper esophageal sphincter (cricopharyngeus muscle) to/including gastroesophageal junction

Retroflexion examination proximal region stomach

43180 **Esophagoscopy, rigid, transoral with diverticulectomy of hypopharynx or cervical esophagus (eg, Zenker's diverticulum), with cricopharyngeal myotomy, includes use of telescope or operating microscope and repair, when performed**

INCLUDES Operating microscope (69990)

EXCLUDES *Esophagogastroduodenoscopy, flexible, transoral; with esophagogastric fundoplasty (43210)*

Open diverticulectomy hypopharynx or esophagus (43130-43135)

15.6 15.6 FUD 090 J G2

AMA: 2018,Jan,8; 2017,Jan,8; 2016,Feb,12; 2016,Jan,13

43191 **Esophagoscopy, rigid, transoral; diagnostic, including collection of specimen(s) by brushing or washing when performed (separate procedure)**

EXCLUDES *Esophagogastroduodenoscopy, flexible, transoral; with esophagogastric fundoplasty (43210)*

Esophagoscopy:

Flexible, transnasal (43197-43198)

Flexible, transoral (43200)

Rigid, transoral (43192-43196)

Myotomy, transoral lower esophageal (43497)

4.45 4.45 FUD 000 J G2

AMA: 2018,Jan,8; 2017,Jan,8; 2016,Jan,13

43192 **with directed submucosal injection(s), any substance**

EXCLUDES *Esophagoscopy:*

Flexible, transnasal (43197-43198)

Flexible, transoral (43201)

Rigid, transoral (43191)

Injection sclerosis of esophageal varices:

Flexible, transoral (43204)

Rigid, transoral (43499)

4.88 4.88 FUD 000 J G2

AMA: 2018,Jan,8; 2017,Jan,8; 2016,Jan,13

43193 **with biopsy, single or multiple**

EXCLUDES *Esophagoscopy:*

Flexible, transnasal (43197-43198)

Flexible, transoral (43202)

Rigid, transoral (43191)

4.85 4.85 FUD 000 J G2

AMA: 2018,Jan,8; 2017,Jan,8; 2016,Jan,13

43194 **with removal of foreign body(s)**

EXCLUDES *Esophagoscopy:*
Flexible, transnasal (43197-43198)
Flexible, transoral (43215)
Rigid, transoral (43191)

(76000)

5.55 5.55 FUD 000 J G2

AMA: 2018,Jan,8; 2017,Jan,8; 2016,Jan,13

43195 **with balloon dilation (less than 30 mm diameter)**

EXCLUDES *Dilation of esophagus:*
Flexible, with balloon diameter 30 mm or larger (43214, 43233)
Flexible, with balloon diameter less than 30 mm (43220)
Without endoscopic visualization (43450-43453)
Esophagoscopy:
Flexible, transnasal (43197-43198)
Rigid, transoral (43191)

(74360)

5.28 5.28 FUD 000 J G2

AMA: 2018,Jan,8; 2017,Jan,8; 2016,Jan,13

43196 **with insertion of guide wire followed by dilation over guide wire**

EXCLUDES *Esophagoscopy:*
Flexible, transnasal (43197-43198)
Flexible, transoral (43226)
Rigid, transoral (43191)

(74360)

5.63 5.63 FUD 000 J G2

AMA: 2018,Jan,8; 2017,Jan,8; 2016,Jan,13

43197 **Esophagoscopy, flexible, transnasal; diagnostic, including collection of specimen(s) by brushing or washing, when performed (separate procedure)**

EXCLUDES *Esophagogastroduodenoscopy, flexible, transnasal (0652T-0654T)*
Esophagogastroduodenoscopy, flexible, transoral (43235-43259 [43233, 43266, 43270])
Esophagoscopy:
Flexible, transnasal; with biopsy, single or multiple (43198)
Flexible, transoral (43200-43232 [43211, 43212, 43213, 43214])
Rigid, transoral (43191-43196)
Laryngoscopy, flexible fiberoptic; diagnostic (31575)
Myotomy, transoral lower esophageal (43497)
Nasal endoscopy, diagnostic, unless different type endoscope used (31231)
Nasopharyngoscopy with endoscope (92511)

2.40 5.34 FUD 000 T P3

AMA: 2018,Jan,8; 2017,Jul,7; 2017,Jan,8; 2016,Dec,13; 2016,Sep,6; 2016,Jan,13

43198 **with biopsy, single or multiple**

EXCLUDES *Esophagogastroduodenoscopy, flexible, transnasal (0652T-0654T)*
Esophagogastroduodenoscopy, flexible, transoral (43235-43259 [43233, 43266, 43270])
Esophagoscopy:
Flexible, transnasal (43197)
Flexible, transoral (43200-43232 [43211, 43212, 43213, 43214])
Rigid, transoral (43191-43196)
Laryngoscopy, flexible fiberoptic; diagnostic (31575)
Nasal endoscopy, diagnostic, unless different type endoscope used (31231)
Nasopharyngoscopy with endoscope (92511)

2.86 6.08 FUD 000 T P3

AMA: 2018,Jan,8; 2017,Jul,7; 2017,Jan,8; 2016,Dec,13; 2016,Sep,6; 2016,Jan,13

43200 **Esophagoscopy, flexible, transoral; diagnostic, including collection of specimen(s) by brushing or washing, when performed (separate procedure)**

EXCLUDES *Esophagogastroduodenoscopy, flexible, transoral (43235)*
Esophagoscopy:
Flexible, transnasal (43197-43198)
Flexible, transoral (43201-43232 [43211, 43212, 43213, 43214])
Rigid, transoral (43191)
Myotomy, transoral lower esophageal (43497)

2.53 6.50 FUD 000 T A2

AMA: 2018,Jan,8; 2017,Jan,8; 2016,Jan,13

43201 **with directed submucosal injection(s), any substance**

EXCLUDES *Esophagoscopy:*
Flexible, transnasal (43197-43198)
Flexible, transoral, on same lesion (43200, 43204, 43211, 43227)
Injection sclerosis esophageal varices:
Flexible, transoral (43204)
Rigid, transoral (43192, 43499)

2.98 6.89 FUD 000 J A2

AMA: 2018,Jan,8; 2017,Jan,8; 2016,Jan,13

43202 **with biopsy, single or multiple**

EXCLUDES *Esophagoscopy:*
Flexible, transnasal (43197-43198)
Flexible, transoral; diagnostic (43200)
Flexible, transoral, on same lesion (43211)
Rigid, transoral (43193)

2.97 9.64 FUD 000 J A2

AMA: 2018,Jan,8; 2017,Jan,8; 2016,Jan,13

43204 **with injection sclerosis of esophageal varices**

EXCLUDES *Band ligation non-variceal bleeding (43227)*
Esophagoscopy:
Flexible, transnasal or transoral; diagnostic (43197-43198, 43200)
Flexible, transoral; with control bleeding, any method, on same lesion (43227)
Flexible, transoral; with directed submucosal injection(s), any substance, on same lesion (43201)
Rigid, transoral, with injection esophageal varices (43499)

3.90 3.90 FUD 000 J A2

AMA: 2018,Jan,8; 2017,Jan,8; 2016,Jan,13

43205 **with band ligation of esophageal varices**

EXCLUDES *Band ligation non-variceal bleeding on same lesion (43227)*
Esophagoscopy, flexible, transnasal or transoral; diagnostic (43197-43198, 43200)

4.07 4.07 FUD 000 J A2

AMA: 2018,Jan,8; 2017,Jan,8; 2016,Jan,13

43206 **with optical endomicroscopy**

EXCLUDES *Esophagoscopy, flexible, transnasal or transoral; diagnostic (43197-43198, 43200)*
Optical endomicroscopic image(s), interpretation and report (88375)

Code also contrast agent

3.90 7.85 FUD 000 J G2

AMA: 2018,Jan,8; 2017,Nov,10; 2017,Jan,8; 2016,Jan,13

43210 **Resequenced code. See code following 43259.**

43211 **Resequenced code. See code following 43217.**

43212 **Resequenced code. See code following 43217.**

43213 **Resequenced code. See code following 43220.**

43214 **Resequenced code. See code following 43220.**

43215 **with removal of foreign body(s)**

Esophagoscopy:
Flexible, transnasal or transoral; diagnostic (43197-43198, 43200)
Rigid, transoral (43194)

(76000)

4.14 10.5 FUD 000 J A2

AMA: 2018,Jan,8; 2017,Jan,8; 2016,Jan,13

43216 **with removal of tumor(s), polyp(s), or other lesion(s) by hot biopsy forceps**

EXCLUDES *Esophagoscopy, flexible, transnasal or transoral; diagnostic (43197-43198, 43200)*

3.86 11.1 FUD 000 J A2

AMA: 2018,Jan,8; 2017,Jan,8; 2016,Jan,13

43217 **with removal of tumor(s), polyp(s), or other lesion(s) by snare technique**

EXCLUDES *Esophagogastroduodenoscopy, flexible, transoral (43251)*
Esophagoscopy:
Flexible, transnasal or transoral; diagnostic (43197-43198, 43200)
Flexible, transoral; with endoscopic mucosal resection, on same lesion (43211)

4.62 11.4 FUD 000 J A2

AMA: 2020,May,13; 2018,Jan,8; 2017,Jan,8; 2016,Jan,13

\# **43211** **with endoscopic mucosal resection**

EXCLUDES *Esophagoscopy:*
Flexible, transnasal or transoral; diagnostic (43197-43198, 43200)
Flexible, transoral; with directed submucosal injection(s), on same lesion (43201-43202)
Flexible, transoral; with removal tumor(s), polyp(s), or other lesion(s) by snare technique, on same lesion (43217)

6.77 6.77 FUD 000 J G2

AMA: 2019,Dec,14; 2018,Jan,8; 2017,Nov,10; 2017,Jan,8; 2016,Jan,13

\# **43212** **with placement of endoscopic stent (includes pre- and post-dilation and guide wire passage, when performed)**

EXCLUDES *Esophagogastroduodenoscopy, flexible, transoral; with insertion of intraluminal tube or catheter (43241)*
Esophagoscopy:
Flexible, transnasal or transoral; diagnostic (43197-43198, 43200)
Flexible, transoral; with insertion guide wire followed by passage dilator(s) over guide wire (43226)
Flexible, transoral; with transendoscopic balloon dilation (43220)

(74360)

5.48 5.48 FUD 000 J J8

AMA: 2018,Jan,8; 2017,Jan,8; 2016,Jan,13

43220 **with transendoscopic balloon dilation (less than 30 mm diameter)**

EXCLUDES *Dilation esophagus:*
Rigid, with balloon diameter 30 mm or larger (43214)
Rigid, with balloon diameter less than 30mm (43195)
Without endoscopic visualization (43450, 43453)
Esophagoscopy:
Flexible, transnasal; diagnostic (43197-43198)
Flexible, transoral (43200, 43212, 43226, 43229)

(74360)

3.43 29.5 FUD 000 J A2

AMA: 2018,Jan,8; 2017,Jan,8; 2016,Jan,13

\# **43213** **with dilation of esophagus, by balloon or dilator, retrograde (includes fluoroscopic guidance, when performed)**

INCLUDES Fluoroscopy (76000)

EXCLUDES *Esophagoscopy, flexible, transnasal or transoral; diagnostic (43197-43198, 43200)*
Intraluminal dilation of strictures and/or obstructions (eg, esophagus), radiological supervision and interpretation (74360)

Code also each additional stricture treated in same operative session with modifier 59 and (43213)

7.48 34.9 FUD 000 J G2

AMA: 2018,Jan,8; 2017,Jan,8; 2016,Jan,13

\# **43214** **with dilation of esophagus with balloon (30 mm diameter or larger) (includes fluoroscopic guidance, when performed)**

INCLUDES Fluoroscopy (76000)

EXCLUDES *Esophagoscopy, flexible, transnasal or transoral; diagnostic (43197-43198, 43200)*
Intraluminal dilation strictures and/or obstructions (eg, esophagus), radiological supervision and interpretation (74360)

5.61 5.61 FUD 000 J G2

AMA: 2018,Jan,8; 2017,Jan,8; 2016,Jan,13

43226 **with insertion of guide wire followed by passage of dilator(s) over guide wire**

EXCLUDES *Esophagoscopy:*
Flexible, transnasal or transoral; diagnostic (43197-43198, 43200)
Flexible, transoral; with ablation tumor(s), polyp(s), or other lesion(s), on same lesion (43229)
Flexible, transoral; with placement endoscopic stent (43212)
Flexible, transoral; with transendoscopic balloon dilation (43220)
Rigid, transoral (43196)

(74360)

3.75 10.1 FUD 000 J A2

AMA: 2018,Jan,8; 2017,Jan,8; 2016,Jan,13

43227 **with control of bleeding, any method**

EXCLUDES *Esophagoscopy:*
Flexible, transnasal or transoral; diagnostic (43197-43198, 43200)
Flexible, transoral; with directed submucosal injection(s), on same lesion (43201)
Flexible, transoral; with injection sclerosis esophageal varices, on same lesion (43204-43205)

4.75 17.6 FUD 000 J A2

AMA: 2018,Jan,8; 2017,Jan,8; 2016,Jan,13

43229 **with ablation of tumor(s), polyp(s), or other lesion(s) (includes pre- and post-dilation and guide wire passage, when performed)**

EXCLUDES *Esophagoscopy:*
Flexible, transnasal or transoral; diagnostic (43197-43198, 43200)
Flexible, transoral; with insertion guide wire followed by passage dilator(s) over guide wire, on same lesion (43226)
Flexible, transoral; with transendoscopic balloon dilation, on same lesion (43220)

Code also esophagoscopic photodynamic therapy, when performed (96570-96571)

5.70 19.8 FUD 000 J J8

AMA: 2018,Jan,8; 2017,Jan,8; 2016,Jan,13

26/TC PC/TC Only A2-Z3 ASC Payment 50 Bilateral ♂ Male Only ♀ Female Only Facility RVU Non-Facility RVU CCI CLIA
FUD Follow-up Days CMS: IOM AMA: CPT Asst A-Y OPPSI 80/80 Surg Assist Allowed / w/Doc Lab Crosswalk Radiology Crosswalk

43231 with endoscopic ultrasound examination

INCLUDES Gastrointestinal endoscopic ultrasound, supervision, and interpretation (76975)

EXCLUDES *Esophagoscopy:*

Flexible, transnasal or transoral; diagnostic (43197-43198, 43200)

Flexible, transoral; with transendoscopic ultrasound-guided intramural or transmural fine needle aspiration/biopsy(s) (43232)

Procedure performed more than one time per operative session

4.59 4.59 FUD 000 J A2

AMA: 2018,Jan,8; 2017,Jan,8; 2016,Jan,13

43232 with transendoscopic ultrasound-guided intramural or transmural fine needle aspiration/biopsy(s)

INCLUDES Gastrointestinal endoscopic ultrasound, supervision and interpretation (76975)

Ultrasonic guidance (76942)

EXCLUDES *Esophagoscopy:*

Flexible, transnasal or transoral; diagnostic (43197-43198, 43200)

Flexible, transoral; with endoscopic ultrasound examination (43231)

Procedure performed more than one time per operative session

5.75 5.75 FUD 000 J A2

AMA: 2018,Jan,8; 2017,Jan,8; 2016,Jan,13

43233 **Resequenced code. See code following 43249.**

43235-43210 [43210, 43233, 43266, 43270] Endoscopic Procedures: Esophagogastroduodenoscopy (EGD)

INCLUDES Control bleeding due to endoscopic procedure during same operative session

Diagnostic endoscopy with surgical endoscopy

Exam jejunum distal to anastomosis in surgically altered stomach, including post-gastroenterostomy (Billroth II) and gastric bypass (43235-43259 [43233, 43266, 43270])

EXCLUDES *Exam upper esophageal sphincter (cricopharyngeus muscle) to/including gastroesophageal junction and/or retroflexion exam proximal region stomach (43197-43232 [43211, 43212, 43213, 43214])*

Code also:

Modifier 52 when duodenum not examined either deliberately or due to significant issues and repeat procedure will not be performed

Modifier 53 when duodenum not examined either deliberately or due to significant issues and repeat procedure is planned

43235 Esophagogastroduodenoscopy, flexible, transoral; diagnostic, including collection of specimen(s) by brushing or washing, when performed (separate procedure)

EXCLUDES *Endoscopy small intestine (44360-44379)*

Esophagogastroduodenoscopy, flexible, transoral; with esophagogastric fundoplasty (43210)

Esophagoscopy, flexible, transnasal; diagnostic (43197-43198)

Myotomy, transoral lower esophageal (43497)

Procedure performed with surgical endoscopy (43236-43259 [43233, 43266, 43270])

3.54 7.98 FUD 000 T A2

AMA: 2019,Oct,10; 2018,Jul,14; 2018,Jan,8; 2017,Jul,10; 2017,Jan,8; 2016,Jan,13

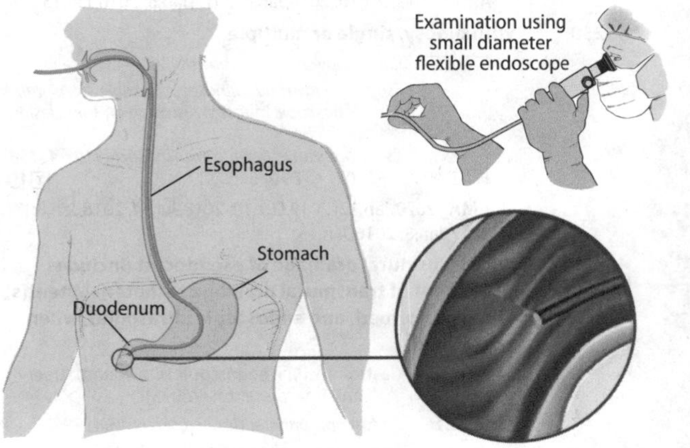

43236 with directed submucosal injection(s), any substance

EXCLUDES *Endoscopy small intestine (44360-44379)*

Esophagogastroduodenoscopy, on same lesion:

Flexible, transoral; with control bleeding, any method (43255)

Flexible, transoral; with endoscopic mucosal resection (43254)

Flexible, transoral; with injection sclerosis esophageal/gastric varices (43243)

Esophagoscopy, flexible, transnasal or transoral; diagnostic (43197-43198, 43235)

Injection sclerosis varices, esophageal/gastric (43243)

4.05 10.0 FUD 000 T A2

AMA: 2019,Oct,10; 2018,Jan,8; 2017,Jan,8; 2016,Jan,13

43237 **with endoscopic ultrasound examination limited to the esophagus, stomach or duodenum, and adjacent structures**

INCLUDES Ultrasonic guidance (76942, 76975)

EXCLUDES *Endoscopy of small intestine (44360-44379)*
Esophagogastroduodenoscopy, flexible, transoral (43238, 43242, 43253, 43259)
Esophagoscopy, flexible, transnasal; diagnostic (43197-43198)
Procedure performed more than one time per operative session

5.73 5.73 **FUD** 000 J A2

AMA: 2019,Oct,10; 2018,Jan,8; 2017,Jan,8; 2016,Jan,13; 2016,Jan,11

43238 **with transendoscopic ultrasound-guided intramural or transmural fine needle aspiration/biopsy(s), (includes endoscopic ultrasound examination limited to the esophagus, stomach or duodenum, and adjacent structures)**

INCLUDES Gastrointestinal endoscopic ultrasound, supervision and interpretation (76975)
Ultrasonic guidance (76942)

EXCLUDES *Endoscopy small intestine (44360-44379)*
Esophagogastroduodenoscopy, flexible, transoral (43237, 43242)
Esophagoscopy, flexible, transnasal (43197-43198)
Procedure performed more than one time per operative session

6.70 6.70 **FUD** 000 J A2

AMA: 2019,Oct,10; 2018,Jan,8; 2017,Jan,8; 2016,Jan,13

43239 **with biopsy, single or multiple**

EXCLUDES *Endoscopy small intestine (44360-44379)*
Esophagogastroduodenoscopy, flexible, transoral; with endoscopic mucosal resection on same lesion (43254)
Esophagoscopy, flexible, transnasal (43197-43198)

3.99 10.6 **FUD** 000 T A2

AMA: 2020,Jan,12; 2019,Oct,10; 2018,Jul,14; 2018,Jan,8; 2017,Jan,8; 2016,Jan,13

43240 **with transmural drainage of pseudocyst (includes placement of transmural drainage catheter[s]/stent[s], when performed, and endoscopic ultrasound, when performed)**

INCLUDES Gastrointestinal endoscopic ultrasound, supervision and interpretation (76975)

EXCLUDES *Endoscopic pancreatic necrosectomy (48999)*
Endoscopy small intestine (44360-44379)
Esophagogastroduodenoscopy:
Flexible, transoral (43242, [43266], 43259)
Flexible, transoral; with transendoscopic ultrasound-guided transmural injection diagnostic or therapeutic substance(s), on same lesion (43253)
Esophagoscopy, flexible, transnasal (43197-43198)
Procedure performed more than one time per operative session

11.5 11.5 **FUD** 000 J J8

AMA: 2019,Oct,10; 2018,Jan,8; 2017,Jan,8; 2016,Jan,13

43241 **with insertion of intraluminal tube or catheter**

EXCLUDES *Endoscopy small intestine (44360-44379)*
Esophagogastroduodenoscopy, flexible, transoral ([43266])
Esophagoscopy, flexible, transnasal or transoral (43197-43198, 43212)
Insertion long gastrointestinal tube (44500, 74340)
Naso or oro-gastric requiring professional skill and fluoroscopic guidance (43752)

4.17 4.17 **FUD** 000 J A2

AMA: 2019,Oct,10; 2018,Jan,8; 2017,Jan,8; 2016,Jan,13

43242 **with transendoscopic ultrasound-guided intramural or transmural fine needle aspiration/biopsy(s) (includes endoscopic ultrasound examination of the esophagus, stomach, and either the duodenum or a surgically altered stomach where the jejunum is examined distal to the anastomosis)**

INCLUDES Gastrointestinal endoscopic ultrasound, supervision and interpretation (76975)
Ultrasonic guidance (76942)

EXCLUDES *Endoscopy small intestine (44360-44379)*
Esophagogastroduodenoscopy, flexible, transoral (43237-43238, 43240, 43259)
Esophagoscopy, flexible, transnasal (43197-43198)
Procedure performed more than one time per operative session
Transmural fine needle biopsy/aspiration with ultrasound guidance, transendoscopic, esophagus/stomach/duodenum/neighboring structure (43238)

88172-88173

7.58 7.58 **FUD** 000 J A2

AMA: 2019,Oct,10; 2018,Jan,8; 2017,Jan,8; 2016,Jan,13

43243 **with injection sclerosis of esophageal/gastric varices**

EXCLUDES *Endoscopy small intestine (44360-44379)*
Esophagogastroduodenoscopy, flexible, transoral on same lesion (43236, 43255)
Esophagoscopy, flexible, transnasal (43197-43198)

6.85 6.85 **FUD** 000 J A2

AMA: 2019,Oct,10; 2018,Jan,8; 2017,Jan,8; 2016,Jan,13

43244 **with band ligation of esophageal/gastric varices**

EXCLUDES *Band ligation, non-variceal bleeding (43255)*
Endoscopy small intestine (44360-44379)
Esophagoscopy, flexible, transnasal (43197-43198)

7.08 7.08 **FUD** 000 J A2

AMA: 2019,Oct,10; 2018,Jan,8; 2017,Jan,8; 2016,Jan,13

43245 **with dilation of gastric/duodenal stricture(s) (eg, balloon, bougie)**

EXCLUDES *Endoscopy small intestine (44360-44379)*
Esophagogastroduodenoscopy, flexible, transoral ([43266])
Esophagoscopy, flexible, transnasal (43197-43198)

(74360)

5.08 16.7 **FUD** 000 J A2

AMA: 2019,Oct,10; 2018,Jan,8; 2017,Jan,8; 2016,Jan,13

43246 **with directed placement of percutaneous gastrostomy tube**

EXCLUDES *Endoscopy small intestine (44360-44372, 44376-44379)*
Esophagoscopy, flexible, transnasal (43197-43198)
Gastrostomy tube replacement without endoscopy or imaging (43762-43763)
Percutaneous insertion gastrostomy tube (49440)

5.86 5.86 FUD 000 J A2 80

AMA: 2019,Oct,10; 2019,Feb,5; 2018,Jan,8; 2017,Jan,8; 2016,Jan,13

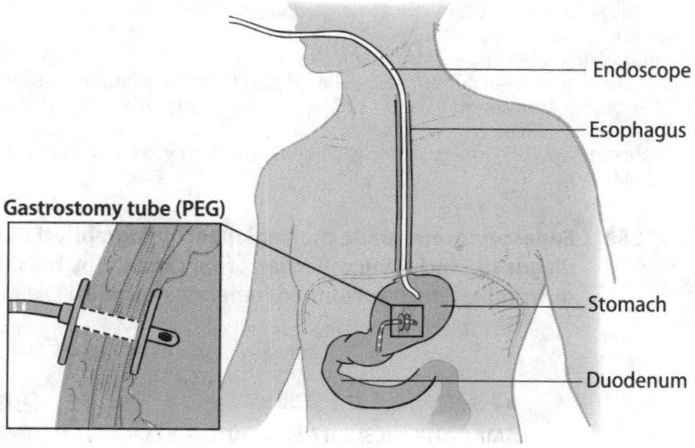

43247 **with removal of foreign body(s)**

EXCLUDES *Endoscopy small intestine (44360-44379)*
Esophagoscopy, flexible, transnasal (43197-43198)

(76000)

5.11 10.5 FUD 000 T A2

AMA: 2019,Oct,10; 2018,Jan,8; 2017,Jan,8; 2016,Jan,13

43248 **with insertion of guide wire followed by passage of dilator(s) through esophagus over guide wire**

EXCLUDES *Endoscopy small intestine (44360-44379)*
Esophagogastroduodenoscopy, flexible, transoral ([43266], [43270])
Esophagoscopy, flexible, transnasal (43197-43198)

(74360)

4.78 11.0 FUD 000 T A2

AMA: 2019,Oct,10; 2018,Jan,8; 2017,Jul,10; 2017,Jan,8; 2016,Jan,13

43249 **with transendoscopic balloon dilation of esophagus (less than 30 mm diameter)**

EXCLUDES *Endoscopy small intestine (44360-44379)*
Esophagogastroduodenoscopy:
Ablation lesion/tumor/polyp, when performed on same lesion ([43270])
With placement endoscopic stent ([43266])
Esophagoscopy, flexible, transnasal (43197-43198)

(74360)

4.42 31.0 FUD 000 J A2

AMA: 2019,Oct,10; 2018,Jul,14; 2018,Jan,8; 2017,Jan,8; 2016,Jan,13

\# **43233** **with dilation of esophagus with balloon (30 mm diameter or larger) (includes fluoroscopic guidance, when performed)**

INCLUDES Fluoroscopy (76000)

EXCLUDES *Endoscopy small intestine (44360-44379)*
Esophagoscopy, flexible, transnasal (43197-43198)
Intraluminal dilation strictures and/or obstructions (e.g., esophagus), radiological supervision and interpretation (74360)

6.62 6.62 FUD 000 J G2

AMA: 2019,Oct,10; 2018,Jan,8; 2017,Jan,8; 2016,Jan,13

43250 **with removal of tumor(s), polyp(s), or other lesion(s) by hot biopsy forceps**

EXCLUDES *Endoscopy small intestine (44360-44379)*
Esophagoscopy, flexible, transnasal (43197-43198)

4.97 11.8 FUD 000 J A2

AMA: 2019,Oct,10; 2018,Jan,8; 2017,Jan,8; 2016,Jan,13

43251 **with removal of tumor(s), polyp(s), or other lesion(s) by snare technique**

EXCLUDES *Endoscopic mucosal resection when performed on same lesion (43254)*
Endoscopy small intestine (44360-44379)
Esophagoscopy, flexible, transnasal (43197-43198)

5.66 13.5 FUD 000 J A2

AMA: 2019,Oct,10; 2018,Jan,8; 2017,Jan,8; 2016,Jan,13

43252 **with optical endomicroscopy**

EXCLUDES *Endoscopy small intestine (44360-44379)*
Esophagoscopy, flexible, transnasal (43197-43198)
Optical endomicroscopic image(s), interpretation and report (88375)

Code also contrast agent

4.95 8.96 FUD 000 J G2

AMA: 2019,Oct,10; 2018,Jan,8; 2017,Jan,8; 2016,Jan,13

43253 **with transendoscopic ultrasound-guided transmural injection of diagnostic or therapeutic substance(s) (eg, anesthetic, neurolytic agent) or fiducial marker(s) (includes endoscopic ultrasound examination of the esophagus, stomach, and either the duodenum or a surgically altered stomach where the jejunum is examined distal to the anastomosis)**

INCLUDES Gastrointestinal endoscopic ultrasound, supervision and interpretation (76975)
Ultrasonic guidance (76942)

EXCLUDES *Endoscopy small intestine (44360-44379)*
Esophagogastroduodenoscopy:
Flexible, transoral (43237, 43259)
Flexible, transoral; with transmural drainage pseudocyst on same lesion with (43240)
Esophagoscopy, flexible, transnasal (43197-43198)
Procedure performed more than one time per operative session
Transmural fine needle biopsy/aspiration with ultrasound guidance, transendoscopic, esophagus/stomach/duodenum/neighboring structures (43238, 43242)

7.70 7.70 FUD 000 J G2

AMA: 2019,Oct,10; 2018,Apr,10; 2018,Jan,8; 2017,Jan,8; 2016,Jan,13

43254 **with endoscopic mucosal resection**

EXCLUDES *Endoscopy small intestine (44360-44379)*
Esophagogastroduodenoscopy, flexible, transoral, on same lesion (43236, 43239, 43251)
Esophagoscopy, flexible, transnasal (43197-43198)

7.80 7.80 FUD 000 J G2

AMA: 2019,Dec,14; 2019,Oct,10; 2018,Jan,8; 2017,Jan,8; 2016,Jan,13

43255 **with control of bleeding, any method**

EXCLUDES *Endoscopy small intestine (44360-44379)*
Esophagogastroduodenoscopy, flexible, transoral, on same lesion (43236, 43243-43244)
Esophagoscopy, flexible, transnasal (43197-43198)

5.79 18.6 FUD 000 J A2

AMA: 2019,Oct,10; 2018,Jan,8; 2017,Jan,8; 2016,Jan,13

\# **43266** **with placement of endoscopic stent (includes pre- and post-dilation and guide wire passage, when performed)**

INCLUDES When performed:
Balloon dilation esophagus (43249)
Dilation gastric/duodenal stricture (43245)
Insertion guidewire/dilator (43248)

EXCLUDES *Endoscopy small intestine (44360-44379)*
Esophagogastroduodenoscopy:
Insertion intraluminal tube or catheter (43241)
Transmural drainage pseudocyst (43240)
Esophagoscopy, flexible, transnasal (43197-43198)

(74360)

6.39 6.39 **FUD** 000 J J8

AMA: 2019,Oct,10; 2018,Jan,8; 2017,Jan,8; 2016,Jan,13

43257 **with delivery of thermal energy to the muscle of lower esophageal sphincter and/or gastric cardia, for treatment of gastroesophageal reflux disease**

EXCLUDES *Endoscopy small intestine (44360-44379)*
Esophageal lesion ablation (43229, [43270])
Esophagoscopy, flexible, transnasal (43197-43198)

6.74 6.74 **FUD** 000 J A2

AMA: 2019,Oct,10; 2018,Jan,8; 2017,Jan,8; 2016,Jan,13

\# **43270** **with ablation of tumor(s), polyp(s), or other lesion(s) (includes pre- and post-dilation and guide wire passage, when performed)**

INCLUDES Endoscopic dilation performed on same lesion (43248-43249)

EXCLUDES *Endoscopy small intestine (44360-44379)*
Esophagoscopy, flexible, transnasal (43197-43198)

Code also photodynamic therapy, when performed (96570-96571)

6.48 20.3 **FUD** 000 J G2

AMA: 2019,Oct,10; 2018,Jan,8; 2017,Jan,8; 2016,Jan,13

43259 **with endoscopic ultrasound examination, including the esophagus, stomach, and either the duodenum or a surgically altered stomach where the jejunum is examined distal to the anastomosis**

INCLUDES Gastrointestinal endoscopic ultrasound, supervision and interpretation (76975)

EXCLUDES *Endoscopy small intestine (44360-44379)*
Esophagogastroduodenoscopy, flexible, transoral (43237, 43240, 43242, 43253)
Esophagoscopy, flexible, transnasal (43197-43198)
Procedure performed more than one time per operative session

6.53 6.53 **FUD** 000 J A2

AMA: 2019,Oct,10; 2018,Jan,8; 2017,Jan,8; 2016,Jan,13; 2016,Jan,11

\# **43210** **with esophagogastric fundoplasty, partial or complete, includes duodenoscopy when performed**

EXCLUDES *Esophagogastroduodenoscopy:*
Flexible, transnasal (43197)
Rigid, transoral (43180, 43191)
Esophagoscopy, flexible, transoral (43200)

12.5 12.5 **FUD** 000 J G2

AMA: 2018,Jan,8; 2017,Jan,8; 2016,Jan,13

43260-43278 [43266, 43270, 43274, 43275, 43276, 43277, 43278] Endoscopic Procedures: ERCP

INCLUDES Diagnostic endoscopy with surgical endoscopy
Pancreaticobiliary system:
Biliary tree (right and left hepatic ducts, cystic duct/gallbladder, and common bile ducts)
Pancreas (major and minor ducts)

EXCLUDES *ERCP via Roux-en-Y anatomy (for instance post-gastric or bariatric bypass or post total gastrectomy) or via gastrostomy (open or laparoscopic) (47999, 48999)*
Optical endomicroscopy biliary tract and pancreas, report one time per session (0397T)
Percutaneous biliary catheter procedures (47490-47544)

Code also:
Appropriate endoscopy each anatomic site examined
ERCP procedure when performed on altered postoperative anatomy (i.e., Billroth II gastroenterostomy) (43260, 43262-43265, [43274], [43275], [43276], [43277], [43278], 43273)
Sphincteroplasty or ductal stricture dilation, when necessary to access debris/stones ([43277])

(74328-74330)

43260 **Endoscopic retrograde cholangiopancreatography (ERCP); diagnostic, including collection of specimen(s) by brushing or washing, when performed (separate procedure)**

EXCLUDES *Endoscopic retrograde cholangiopancreatography (ERCP), therapeutic (43261-43265, 43274-43278 [43274, 43275, 43276, 43277, 43278])*

9.31 9.31 **FUD** 000 J A2

AMA: 2018,Jan,8; 2017,Jan,8; 2016,Jan,13

43261 **with biopsy, single or multiple**

INCLUDES Endoscopic retrograde cholangiopancreatography (ERCP); diagnostic (43260)

EXCLUDES *Percutaneous endoluminal biopsy biliary tree (47543)*

9.92 9.92 **FUD** 000 J A2

AMA: 2018,Jan,8; 2017,Jan,8; 2016,Jan,13

43262 **with sphincterotomy/papillotomy**

INCLUDES Endoscopic retrograde cholangiopancreatography (ERCP), diagnostic (43260)

EXCLUDES *Endoscopic retrograde cholangiopancreatography (ERCP):*
With exchange/insertion/removal stent in same location ([43274], [43276])
With trans-endoscopic balloon dilation ampulla/biliary or pancreatic ducts ([43277])
Percutaneous balloon dilation biliary duct or ampulla (47542)

Code also procedure performed with sphincterotomy (43261, 43263-43265, [43275], [43278])

10.3 10.3 **FUD** 000 J A2

AMA: 2018,Jan,8; 2017,Jan,8; 2016,Jan,13

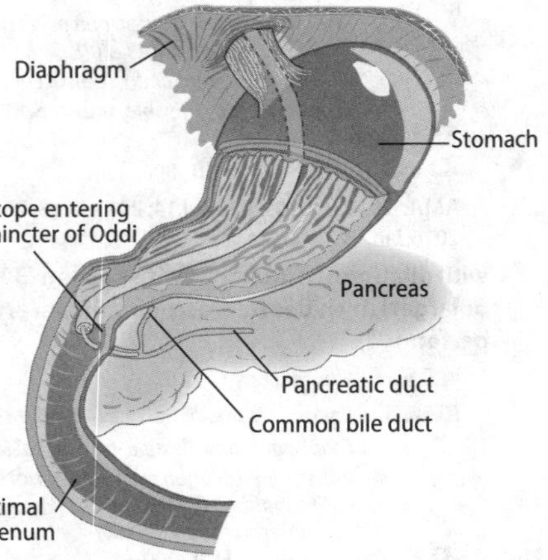

An endoscope is fed through the stomach and into the duodenum Usually a smaller sub-scope is fed up the sphincter of Oddi and into the ducts that drain the pancreas and the gallbladder (common bile)

43263 **with pressure measurement of sphincter of Oddi**

INCLUDES Endoscopic retrograde cholangiopancreatography (ERCP); diagnostic (43260)

EXCLUDES *Procedure performed more than one time per session*

10.4 10.4 FUD 000 J A2

AMA: 2018,Jan,8; 2017,Jan,8; 2016,Jan,13

43264 **with removal of calculi/debris from biliary/pancreatic duct(s)**

INCLUDES Endoscopic retrograde cholangiopancreatography (ERCP); diagnostic (43260)
Incidental dilation due to instrument passage

EXCLUDES *Endoscopic retrograde cholangiopancreatography (ERCP) with calculi destruction (43265)*
Findings without debris or calculi, even when balloon used
Percutaneous calculus/debris removal (47544)

Code also sphincteroplasty when dilation necessary to access debris/stones ([43277])

10.4 10.4 FUD 000 J A2

AMA: 2018,Jan,8; 2017,Jan,8; 2016,Jan,13

43265 **with destruction of calculi, any method (eg, mechanical, electrohydraulic, lithotripsy)**

INCLUDES Endoscopic retrograde cholangiopancreatography (ERCP); diagnostic (43260)
Incidental dilation due to instrument passage
Stone removal in same ductal system

EXCLUDES *Endoscopic retrograde cholangiopancreatography (ERCP) with removal of calculi/debris from biliary/pancreatic duct(s) (43264)*
Findings without debris or calculi, even when balloon used
Percutaneous calculus/debris removal (47544)

Code also sphincteroplasty when dilation necessary to access debris/stones ([43277])

12.5 12.5 FUD 000 J A2

AMA: 2018,Jan,8; 2017,Jan,8; 2016,Jan,13

43266 **Resequenced code. See code following 43255.**

43270 **Resequenced code. See code following 43257.**

43274 **with placement of endoscopic stent into biliary or pancreatic duct, including pre- and post-dilation and guide wire passage, when performed, including sphincterotomy, when performed, each stent**

INCLUDES Balloon dilation in same duct
Endoscopic retrograde cholangiopancreatography (ERCP); diagnostic (43260)
Tube placement for naso-pancreatic or naso-biliary drainage

EXCLUDES *Percutaneous placement biliary stent (47538-47540)*
Procedures for stent placement or exchange in same duct (43262, [43275], [43276], [43277])

Code also for each additional stent placement in different ducts or side by side in same duct same session/day, using modifier 59 with ([43274])

13.3 13.3 FUD 000 J G2

AMA: 2018,Jan,8; 2017,Jan,8; 2016,Jan,13

43275 **with removal of foreign body(s) or stent(s) from biliary/pancreatic duct(s)**

INCLUDES Endoscopic retrograde cholangiopancreatography (ERCP); diagnostic (43260)

EXCLUDES *Endoscopic retrograde cholangiopancreatography (ERCP) with exchange, placement, or removal of stent ([43274], [43276])*
Pancreatic or biliary duct stent removal without ERCP (43247)
Percutaneous calculus/debris removal (47544)
Procedure performed more than one time per session

11.0 11.0 FUD 000 J G2

AMA: 2018,Jan,8; 2017,Jan,8; 2016,Jan,13

43276 **with removal and exchange of stent(s), biliary or pancreatic duct, including pre- and post-dilation and guide wire passage, when performed, including sphincterotomy, when performed, each stent exchanged**

INCLUDES Balloon dilation in same duct
Endoscopic retrograde cholangiopancreatography (ERCP); diagnostic (43260)
Stent placement or exchange one stent

EXCLUDES *Endoscopic retrograde cholangiopancreatography (ERCP) with removal foreign body(s) or stent(s) ([43275])*
Procedures for stent insertion or exchange stent in same duct (43262, [43274])

Code also each additional stent exchanged same session/day, using modifier 59 with ([43276])

13.9 13.9 FUD 000 J G2

AMA: 2018,Jan,8; 2017,Jan,8; 2016,Jan,13

43277 **with trans-endoscopic balloon dilation of biliary/pancreatic duct(s) or of ampulla (sphincteroplasty), including sphincterotomy, when performed, each duct**

INCLUDES Endoscopic retrograde cholangiopancreatography (ERCP); diagnostic (43260)

EXCLUDES *Endoscopic retrograde cholangiopancreatography (ERCP):*
With ablation tumor(s), polyp(s), or other lesion(s) for same lesion ([43278])
With sphincterotomy/papillotomy (43262)
With stent exchange/removal same biliary/pancreatic duct ([43276])
With stent placement into same biliary/pancreatic duct ([43274])
Percutaneous dilation biliary duct/ampulla (47542)
Removal stone/debris, dilation incidental to instrument passage (43264-43265)

Code also:
Both right and left hepatic duct (bilateral) balloon dilation, using ([43277]); append modifier 59 to second procedure
Each additional balloon dilation in different ducts or side by side in same duct same session/day, appending modifier 59 to ([43277])
Sphincterotomy without sphincteroplasty during same operative session in different duct, appending modifier 59 to (43262)

10.9 10.9 FUD 000 J G2

AMA: 2018,Jan,8; 2017,Jan,8; 2016,Jan,13

43278 **with ablation of tumor(s), polyp(s), or other lesion(s), including pre- and post-dilation and guide wire passage, when performed**

INCLUDES Endoscopic retrograde cholangiopancreatography (ERCP); diagnostic (43260)

EXCLUDES *Ampullectomy (43254)*
Endoscopic retrograde cholangiopancreatography (ERCP); with trans-endoscopic balloon dilation biliary/pancreatic duct(s) or ampulla (sphincteroplasty) in same lesion with ([43277])

12.5 12.5 FUD 000 J G2

AMA: 2018,Jan,8; 2017,Jan,8; 2016,Jan,13

+ **43273** **Endoscopic cannulation of papilla with direct visualization of pancreatic/common bile duct(s) (List separately in addition to code(s) for primary procedure)**

EXCLUDES *Procedure performed more than one time per session*

Code first (43260-43265, [43274], [43275], [43276], [43277], [43278])

3.47 3.47 FUD ZZZ N N1 80

AMA: 2018,Jan,8; 2017,Jan,8; 2016,Jan,13

43274 **Resequenced code. See code following code 43270.**

43275 **Resequenced code. See code following code 43270.**

43276 **Resequenced code. See code following code 43270.**

43277 **Resequenced code. See code following code 43270.**

43278 **Resequenced code. See code following code 43270.**

43279-43289 Laparoscopic Procedures of Esophagus

INCLUDES Diagnostic laparoscopy with surgical laparoscopy (49320)

43279 Laparoscopy, surgical, esophagomyotomy (Heller type), with fundoplasty, when performed

EXCLUDES *Esophagomyotomy, open method (43330-43331)*
Laparoscopy, surgical, esophagogastric fundoplasty (43280)

37.5 37.5 FUD 090 C 80

AMA: 2018,Jan,8; 2017,Aug,6; 2017,Jan,8; 2016,Jan,13

43280 Laparoscopy, surgical, esophagogastric fundoplasty (eg, Nissen, Toupet procedures)

EXCLUDES *Esophagogastric fundoplasty, open method (43327-43328)*
Esophagogastroduodenoscopy fundoplasty, transoral (43210)
Laparoscopy, surgical, esophageal sphincter augmentation (43284-43285)
Laparoscopy, surgical, esophagomyotomy (43279)
Laparoscopy, surgical, fundoplasty (43281-43282)

31.4 31.4 FUD 090 J G2 80

AMA: 2018,Jan,8; 2017,Aug,6; 2017,Jan,8; 2016,Jan,13

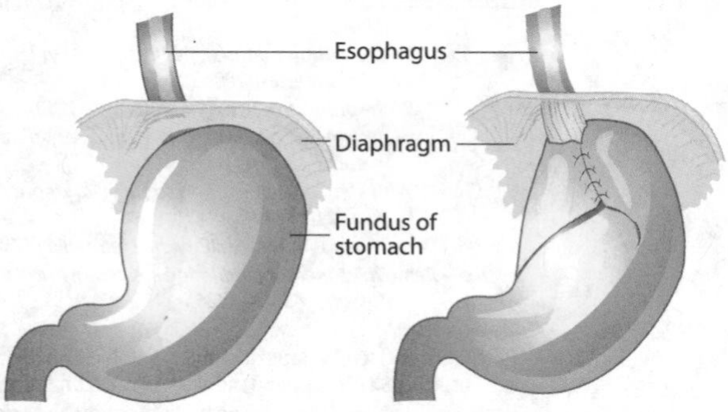

43281 Laparoscopy, surgical, repair of paraesophageal hernia, includes fundoplasty, when performed; without implantation of mesh

EXCLUDES *Dilation esophagus (43450, 43453)*
Implantation mesh or other prosthesis (49568)
Laparoscopy, surgical, esophagogastric fundoplasty (43280)
Transabdominal repair paraesophageal hiatal hernia (43332-43333)
Transthoracic repair diaphragmatic hernia (43334-43335)

44.7 44.7 FUD 090 J G2 80

AMA: 2018,Nov,11; 2018,Sep,14; 2018,Jan,8; 2017,Aug,6; 2017,Jan,8; 2016,Jan,13

43282 with implantation of mesh

EXCLUDES *Dilation esophagus (43450, 43453)*
Laparoscopy, surgical, esophagogastric fundoplasty (43280)
Transabdominal paraesophageal hernia repair (43332-43333)
Transthoracic paraesophageal hernia repair (43334-43335)

50.6 50.6 FUD 090 J G2 80

AMA: 2018,Jan,8; 2017,Aug,6; 2017,Jan,8; 2016,Aug,9; 2016,Jan,13

+ **43283 Laparoscopy, surgical, esophageal lengthening procedure (eg, Collis gastroplasty or wedge gastroplasty) (List separately in addition to code for primary procedure)**

Code first (43280-43282)

4.60 4.60 FUD ZZZ C 80

AMA: 2018,Jan,8; 2017,Jan,8; 2016,Jan,13

43284 Laparoscopy, surgical, esophageal sphincter augmentation procedure, placement of sphincter augmentation device (ie, magnetic band), including cruroplasty when performed

EXCLUDES *Performed during same session (43279-43282)*

18.9 18.9 FUD 090 J J8 80

AMA: 2019,Apr,10; 2018,Sep,14; 2018,Jan,8; 2017,Aug,6

43285 Removal of esophageal sphincter augmentation device

19.5 19.5 FUD 090 Q2 G2 80

AMA: 2018,Jan,8; 2017,Aug,6

43286 Esophagectomy, total or near total, with laparoscopic mobilization of the abdominal and mediastinal esophagus and proximal gastrectomy, with laparoscopic pyloric drainage procedure if performed, with open cervical pharyngogastrostomy or esophagogastrostomy (ie, laparoscopic transhiatal esophagectomy)

90.9 90.9 FUD 090 C 80

AMA: 2018,Jul,7

43287 Esophagectomy, distal two-thirds, with laparoscopic mobilization of the abdominal and lower mediastinal esophagus and proximal gastrectomy, with laparoscopic pyloric drainage procedure if performed, with separate thoracoscopic mobilization of the middle and upper mediastinal esophagus and thoracic esophagogastrostomy (ie, laparoscopic thoracoscopic esophagectomy, Ivor Lewis esophagectomy)

EXCLUDES *Right tube thoracostomy (32551)*

104. 104. FUD 090 C 80

AMA: 2018,Jul,7

43288 Esophagectomy, total or near total, with thoracoscopic mobilization of the upper, middle, and lower mediastinal esophagus, with separate laparoscopic proximal gastrectomy, with laparoscopic pyloric drainage procedure if performed, with open cervical pharyngogastrostomy or esophagogastrostomy (ie, thoracoscopic, laparoscopic and cervical incision esophagectomy, McKeown esophagectomy, tri-incisional esophagectomy)

EXCLUDES *Right tube thoracostomy (32551)*

109. 109. FUD 090 C 80

AMA: 2018,Jul,7

43289 Unlisted laparoscopy procedure, esophagus

0.00 0.00 FUD YYY J 80 50

AMA: 2018,Jul,7; 2018,Jan,8; 2017,Jan,8; 2016,Jan,13

43300-43425 Open Esophageal Repair Procedures

43300 **Esophagoplasty (plastic repair or reconstruction), cervical approach; without repair of tracheoesophageal fistula**
17.6 17.6 FUD 090 C 80
AMA: 2014,Jan,11; 2013,Jan,11-12

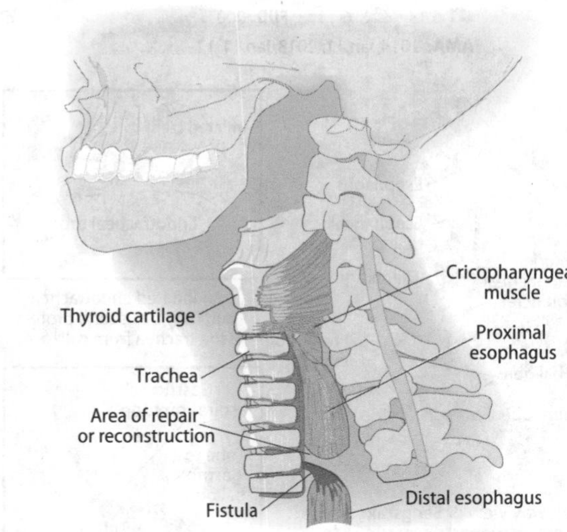

Example of esophageal atresia where the proximal esophagus fails to communicate with the lower portion; note that a fistula has developed from the trachea

43305 **with repair of tracheoesophageal fistula**
31.3 31.3 FUD 090 C 80
AMA: 2014,Jan,11; 2013,Jan,11-12

43310 **Esophagoplasty (plastic repair or reconstruction), thoracic approach; without repair of tracheoesophageal fistula**
42.9 42.9 FUD 090 C 80
AMA: 2014,Jan,11; 2013,Jan,11-12

43312 **with repair of tracheoesophageal fistula**
46.1 46.1 FUD 090 C 80
AMA: 2014,Jan,11; 2013,Jan,11-12

43313 **Esophagoplasty for congenital defect (plastic repair or reconstruction), thoracic approach; without repair of congenital tracheoesophageal fistula**
79.3 79.3 FUD 090 63 C 80
AMA: 2014,Jan,11; 2013,Jan,11-12

43314 **with repair of congenital tracheoesophageal fistula**
85.2 85.2 FUD 090 63 C 80
AMA: 2014,Jan,11; 2013,Jan,11-12

43320 **Esophagogastrostomy (cardioplasty), with or without vagotomy and pyloroplasty, transabdominal or transthoracic approach**
EXCLUDES *Laparoscopic approach (43280)*
40.7 40.7 FUD 090 C 80
AMA: 2014,Jan,11; 2013,Jan,11-12

43325 **Esophagogastric fundoplasty, with fundic patch (Thal-Nissen procedure)**
EXCLUDES *Myotomy, cricopharyngeal (43030)*
39.6 39.6 FUD 090 C 80
AMA: 2014,Jan,11; 2013,Jan,11-12

43327 **Esophagogastric fundoplasty partial or complete; laparotomy**
23.9 23.9 FUD 090 C 80
AMA: 2018,Jan,8; 2017,Jan,8; 2016,Jan,13

43328 **thoracotomy**
EXCLUDES *Esophagogastroduodenoscopy fundoplasty, transoral (43210)*
32.6 32.6 FUD 090 C 80
AMA: 2018,Jan,8; 2017,Jan,8; 2016,Jan,13

43330 **Esophagomyotomy (Heller type); abdominal approach**
EXCLUDES *Esophagomyotomy, laparoscopic method (43279)*
38.9 38.9 FUD 090 C 80
AMA: 2018,Jan,8; 2017,Jan,8; 2016,Jan,13

43331 **thoracic approach**
EXCLUDES *Thoracoscopy with esophagomyotomy (32665)*
38.7 38.7 FUD 090 C 80
AMA: 2018,Jan,8; 2017,Jan,8; 2016,Jan,13

43332 **Repair, paraesophageal hiatal hernia (including fundoplication), via laparotomy, except neonatal; without implantation of mesh or other prosthesis**
EXCLUDES *Neonatal diaphragmatic hernia repair (39503)*
33.7 33.7 FUD 090 C 80
AMA: 2018,Jan,8; 2017,Jan,8; 2016,Jan,13

43333 **with implantation of mesh or other prosthesis**
EXCLUDES *Neonatal diaphragmatic hernia repair (39503)*
36.8 36.8 FUD 090 C 80
AMA: 2018,Jan,8; 2017,Jan,8; 2016,Jan,13

43334 **Repair, paraesophageal hiatal hernia (including fundoplication), via thoracotomy, except neonatal; without implantation of mesh or other prosthesis**
EXCLUDES *Neonatal diaphragmatic hernia repair (39503)*
36.2 36.2 FUD 090 C 80
AMA: 2018,Jan,8; 2017,Jan,8; 2016,Jan,13

43335 **with implantation of mesh or other prosthesis**
EXCLUDES *Neonatal diaphragmatic hernia repair (39503)*
38.7 38.7 FUD 090 C 80
AMA: 2018,Jan,8; 2017,Jan,8; 2016,Jan,13

43336 **Repair, paraesophageal hiatal hernia, (including fundoplication), via thoracoabdominal incision, except neonatal; without implantation of mesh or other prosthesis**
EXCLUDES *Neonatal diaphragmatic hernia repair (39503)*
42.0 42.0 FUD 090 C 80
AMA: 2018,Jan,8; 2017,Jan,8; 2016,Jan,13

43337 **with implantation of mesh or other prosthesis**
EXCLUDES *Neonatal diaphragmatic hernia repair (39503)*
44.8 44.8 FUD 090 C 80
AMA: 2018,Jan,8; 2017,Jan,8; 2016,Jan,13

\+ **43338** **Esophageal lengthening procedure (eg, Collis gastroplasty or wedge gastroplasty) (List separately in addition to code for primary procedure)**
Code first (43280, 43327-43337)
3.37 3.37 FUD ZZZ C 80
AMA: 2018,Jan,8; 2017,Jan,8; 2016,Jan,13

43340 **Esophagojejunostomy (without total gastrectomy); abdominal approach**
40.0 40.0 FUD 090 C 80
AMA: 2014,Jan,11; 2013,Jan,11-12

43341 **thoracic approach**
40.5 40.5 FUD 090 C 80
AMA: 2014,Jan,11; 2013,Jan,11-12

43351 **Esophagostomy, fistulization of esophagus, external; thoracic approach**
38.0 38.0 FUD 090 C 80
AMA: 2014,Jan,11; 2013,Jan,11-12

43352 **cervical approach**
30.8 30.8 FUD 090 C 80
AMA: 2014,Jan,11; 2013,Jan,11-12

43360 **Gastrointestinal reconstruction for previous esophagectomy, for obstructing esophageal lesion or fistula, or for previous esophageal exclusion; with stomach, with or without pyloroplasty**
65.3 65.3 FUD 090 C 80
AMA: 2014,Jan,11; 2013,Jan,11-12

43361 **with colon interposition or small intestine reconstruction, including intestine mobilization, preparation, and anastomosis(es)**
Facility RVU 78.6 | Non-Facility RVU 78.6 | **FUD** 090 | C 80 CCI
AMA: 2014,Jan,11; 2013,Jan,11-12

43400 **Ligation, direct, esophageal varices**
Facility RVU 44.4 | Non-Facility RVU 44.4 | **FUD** 090 | C 80 CCI
AMA: 2014,Jan,11; 2013,Jan,11-12

43405 **Ligation or stapling at gastroesophageal junction for pre-existing esophageal perforation**
Facility RVU 42.1 | Non-Facility RVU 42.1 | **FUD** 090 | C 80 CCI
AMA: 2014,Jan,11; 2013,Jan,11-12

43410 **Suture of esophageal wound or injury; cervical approach**
Facility RVU 29.3 | Non-Facility RVU 29.3 | **FUD** 090 | C 80 CCI
AMA: 2018,Jan,8; 2017,Jan,8; 2016,Jan,13

43415 **transthoracic or transabdominal approach**
Facility RVU 74.5 | Non-Facility RVU 74.5 | **FUD** 090 | C 80 CCI
AMA: 2014,Jan,11; 2013,Jan,11-12

43420 **Closure of esophagostomy or fistula; cervical approach**
EXCLUDES *Paraesophageal hiatal hernia repair:*
Transabdominal (43332-43333)
Transthoracic (43334-43335)
Facility RVU 29.1 | Non-Facility RVU 29.1 | **FUD** 090 | J G2 80 CCI
AMA: 2014,Jan,11; 2013,Jan,11-12

43425 **transthoracic or transabdominal approach**
EXCLUDES *Paraesophageal hiatal hernia repair:*
Transabdominal (43332-43333)
Transthoracic (43334-43335)
Facility RVU 41.8 | Non-Facility RVU 41.8 | **FUD** 090 | C 80 CCI
AMA: 2014,Jan,11; 2013,Jan,11-12

43450-43453 Esophageal Dilation

43450 **Dilation of esophagus, by unguided sound or bougie, single or multiple passes**
Radiology Crosswalk (74220, 74360)
Facility RVU 2.27 | Non-Facility RVU 4.87 | **FUD** 000 | T A2 CCI
AMA: 2018,Jan,8; 2017,Jul,10; 2017,Jan,8; 2016,Jan,13

43453 **Dilation of esophagus, over guide wire**
EXCLUDES *Dilation performed with endoscopic visualization (43195, 43226)*
Endoscopic dilation by dilator or balloon:
Balloon diameter 30 mm or larger (43214, 43233)
Balloon diameter less than 30 mm (43195, 43220, 43249)
Radiology Crosswalk (74220, 74360)
Facility RVU 2.50 | Non-Facility RVU 25.4 | **FUD** 000 | J A2 CCI
AMA: 2018,Jan,8; 2017,Jan,8; 2016,Jan,13

43460-43499 Other/Unlisted Esophageal Procedures

43460 **Esophagogastric tamponade, with balloon (Sengstaken type)**
EXCLUDES *Removal foreign body esophagus with balloon catheter (43499, 74235)*
Radiology Crosswalk (74220)
Facility RVU 6.13 | Non-Facility RVU 6.13 | **FUD** 000 | C CCI
AMA: 2014,Jan,11; 2013,Jan,11-12

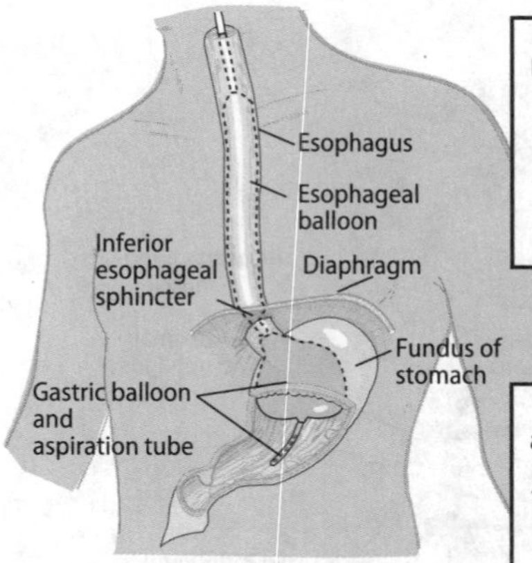

Cutaway view of Sengstaken-type esophagogastric tamponade with balloons inflated

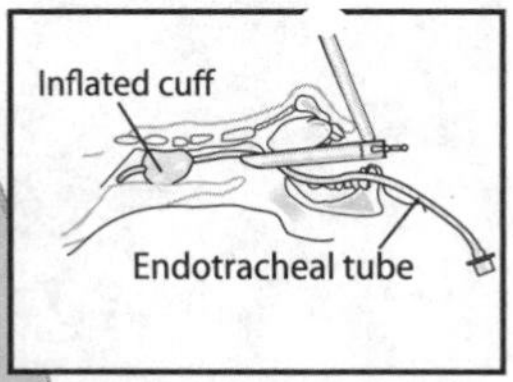

An inflated endotracheal cuff may be used to protect the trachea from collapse

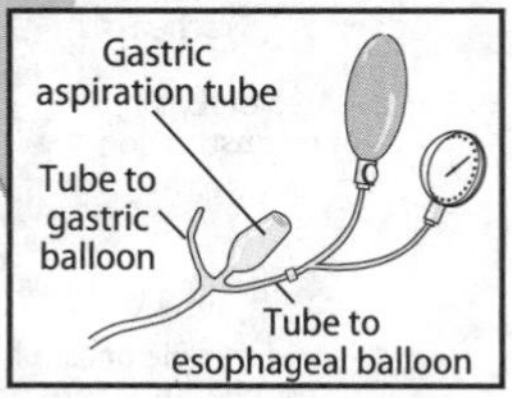

43496 **Free jejunum transfer with microvascular anastomosis**
INCLUDES Operating microscope (69990)
Facility RVU 0.00 | Non-Facility RVU 0.00 | **FUD** 090 | C 80 CCI
AMA: 2019,Dec,5; 2018,Jan,8; 2017,Jan,8; 2016,Feb,12; 2016,Jan,13

● **43497** **Lower esophageal myotomy, transoral (ie, peroral endoscopic myotomy [POEM])**
EXCLUDES *Esophagogastroduodenoscopy, flexible, transoral (43235)*
Esophagoscopy:
Flexible, transnasal (43197)
Flexible, transoral (43200)
Rigid, transoral (43191)
Thoracoscopy with esophagomyotomy (32665)

43499 **Unlisted procedure, esophagus**
Facility RVU 0.00 | Non-Facility RVU 0.00 | **FUD** YYY | T CCI
AMA: 2018,Jul,7; 2018,Jan,8; 2017,Jan,8; 2016,Jan,13

43500-43641 Open Gastric Incisional and Resection Procedures

43500 **Gastrotomy; with exploration or foreign body removal**
Facility RVU 22.7 | Non-Facility RVU 22.7 | **FUD** 090 | C 80 CCI
AMA: 2014,Jan,11; 2013,Jan,11-12

43501 **with suture repair of bleeding ulcer**
Facility RVU 39.2 | Non-Facility RVU 39.2 | **FUD** 090 | C 80 CCI
AMA: 2014,Jan,11; 2013,Jan,11-12

43502 **with suture repair of pre-existing esophagogastric laceration (eg, Mallory-Weiss)**
Facility RVU 44.5 | Non-Facility RVU 44.5 | **FUD** 090 | C 80 CCI
AMA: 2014,Jan,11; 2013,Jan,11-12

43510 **with esophageal dilation and insertion of permanent intraluminal tube (eg, Celestin or Mousseaux-Barbin)**
Facility RVU 27.6 | Non-Facility RVU 27.6 | **FUD** 090 | T G2 80 CCI
AMA: 2014,Jan,11; 2013,Jan,11-12

43520 **Pyloromyotomy, cutting of pyloric muscle (Fredet-Ramstedt type operation)**
Facility RVU 19.9 | Non-Facility RVU 19.9 | **FUD** 090 | 63 C 80 CCI
AMA: 2014,Jan,11; 2013,Jan,11-12

43605 **Biopsy of stomach, by laparotomy**
24.4 24.4 FUD 090 C 80
AMA: 2014,Jan,11; 2013,Jan,11-12

43610 **Excision, local; ulcer or benign tumor of stomach**
28.5 28.5 FUD 090 C 80
AMA: 2014,Jan,11; 2013,Jan,11-12

43611 **malignant tumor of stomach**
35.6 35.6 FUD 090 C 80
AMA: 2014,Jan,11; 2013,Jan,11-12

43620 **Gastrectomy, total; with esophagoenterostomy**
57.8 57.8 FUD 090 C 80
AMA: 2014,Jan,11; 2013,Jan,11-12

43621 **with Roux-en-Y reconstruction**
66.2 66.2 FUD 090 C 80
AMA: 2014,Jan,11; 2013,Jan,11-12

43622 **with formation of intestinal pouch, any type**
67.5 67.5 FUD 090 C 80
AMA: 2014,Jan,11; 2013,Jan,11-12

43631 **Gastrectomy, partial, distal; with gastroduodenostomy**
INCLUDES Billroth operation
42.0 42.0 FUD 090 C 80
AMA: 2014,Jan,11; 2013,Jan,11-12

43632 **with gastrojejunostomy**
INCLUDES Polya anastomosis
59.3 59.3 FUD 090 C 80
AMA: 2014,Jan,11; 2013,Jan,11-12

43633 **with Roux-en-Y reconstruction**
56.1 56.1 FUD 090 C 80
AMA: 2014,Jan,11; 2013,Jan,11-12

43634 **with formation of intestinal pouch**
62.0 62.0 FUD 090 C 80
AMA: 2014,Jan,11; 2013,Jan,11-12

+ **43635** **Vagotomy when performed with partial distal gastrectomy (List separately in addition to code[s] for primary procedure)**
Code first as appropriate (43631-43634)
3.29 3.29 FUD ZZZ C 80
AMA: 2014,Jan,11; 2013,Jan,11-12

43640 **Vagotomy including pyloroplasty, with or without gastrostomy; truncal or selective**
EXCLUDES *Pyloroplasty (43800)*
Vagotomy (64755, 64760)
34.1 34.1 FUD 090 C 80
AMA: 2014,Jan,11; 2013,Jan,11-12

43641 **parietal cell (highly selective)**
EXCLUDES *Upper gastrointestinal endoscopy (43235-43259 [43233, 43266, 43270])*
34.9 34.9 FUD 090 C 80
AMA: 2014,Jan,11; 2013,Jan,11-12

43644-43645 Laparoscopic Gastric Bypass with Small Bowel Resection

CMS: 100-03,100.1 Bariatric Surgery for Treatment Co-morbid Conditions Due to Morbid Obesity; 100-04,32,150.1 Bariatric Surgery: Treatment of Co-Morbid Conditions Due to Morbid Obesity; 100-04,32,150.2 HCPCS Procedure Codes for Bariatric Surgery; 100-04,32,150.5 ICD Diagnosis Codes for BMI ≥35; 100-04,32,150.6 Bariatric Surgery Claims Guidance

INCLUDES Diagnostic laparoscopy (49320)
EXCLUDES *Endoscopy, upper gastrointestinal, (esophagus/stomach/duodenum/jejunum) (43235-43259 [43233, 43266, 43270])*

43644 **Laparoscopy, surgical, gastric restrictive procedure; with gastric bypass and Roux-en-Y gastroenterostomy (roux limb 150 cm or less)**
EXCLUDES *Roux limb less than 150 cm (43846)*
Roux limb greater than 150 cm (43645)
50.6 50.6 FUD 090 C 80
AMA: 2014,Jan,11; 2013,Jan,11-12

43645 **with gastric bypass and small intestine reconstruction to limit absorption**
EXCLUDES *Roux limb less than 150 cm (43847)*
53.9 53.9 FUD 090 C 80
AMA: 2018,Jan,8; 2017,Jan,8; 2016,Jan,13

43647-43659 Other and Unlisted Laparoscopic Gastric Procedures

INCLUDES Diagnostic laparoscopy (49320)
EXCLUDES *Endoscopy, upper gastrointestinal, (esophagus/stomach/duodenum/jejunum) (43235-43259 [43233, 43266, 43270])*

43647 **Laparoscopy, surgical; implantation or replacement of gastric neurostimulator electrodes, antrum**
EXCLUDES *Electronic analysis/programming gastric neurostimulator (95980-95982)*
Insertion gastric neurostimulator pulse generator, incisional (64590)
Laparoscopy with implantation, removal, or revision gastric neurostimulator electrodes on lesser curvature stomach (43659)
Open method (43881)
Vagus nerve blocking pulse generator and/or neurostimulator electrode array implantation, reprogramming, replacement, revision, or removal at esophagogastric junction performed laparoscopically (0312T-0317T)
0.00 0.00 FUD YYY J J8 80
AMA: 2019,Feb,6; 2018,Jan,8; 2017,Jan,8; 2016,Jan,13

43648 **revision or removal of gastric neurostimulator electrodes, antrum**
EXCLUDES *Electronic analysis/programming gastric neurostimulator (95980-95982)*
Laparoscopy with implantation, removal, or revision gastric neurostimulator electrodes on lesser curvature stomach (43659)
Open method (43882)
Removal or revision gastric neurostimulator pulse generator (64595)
Vagus nerve blocking pulse generator and/or neurostimulator electrode array implantation, reprogramming, replacement, revision, or removal at esophagogastric junction performed laparoscopically (0312T-0317T)
0.00 0.00 FUD YYY J G2 80
AMA: 2019,Feb,6; 2018,Jan,8; 2017,Jan,8; 2016,Jan,13

43651 **Laparoscopy, surgical; transection of vagus nerves, truncal**
19.0 19.0 FUD 090 J G2 80
AMA: 2018,Jan,8; 2017,Jan,8; 2016,Jan,13

43652 **transection of vagus nerves, selective or highly selective**
22.2 22.2 FUD 090 J G2 80
AMA: 2018,Jan,8; 2017,Jan,8; 2016,Jan,13

43653 **gastrostomy, without construction of gastric tube (eg, Stamm procedure) (separate procedure)**
16.6 16.6 FUD 090 J A2 80
AMA: 2018,Jan,8; 2017,Jan,8; 2016,Jan,13

43659 **Unlisted laparoscopy procedure, stomach**
0.00 0.00 FUD YYY J 80 50
AMA: 2018,Jul,7; 2018,Jan,8; 2017,Jan,8; 2016,Jan,13

43752-43763 Nonsurgical Gastric Tube Procedures

43752 Naso- or oro-gastric tube placement, requiring physician's skill and fluoroscopic guidance (includes fluoroscopy, image documentation and report)

EXCLUDES *Critical care services (99291-99292)*
Initial inpatient neonatal/pediatric critical care, per day (99468-99469, 99471-99472)
Insertion long gastrointestinal tube (44500, 74340)
Percutaneous insertion gastrostomy tube (43246, 49440)
Subsequent intensive care, per day, for low birth weight infant (99478-99479)

1.18 1.18 FUD 000 Q1 G2

AMA: 2019,Aug,8; 2018,Mar,11; 2018,Jan,8; 2017,Jan,8; 2016,Jan,13

43753 Gastric intubation and aspiration(s) therapeutic, necessitating physician's skill (eg, for gastrointestinal hemorrhage), including lavage if performed

0.63 0.63 FUD 000 Q1 N1 80

AMA: 2019,Aug,8; 2018,Jan,8; 2017,Jan,8; 2016,Jan,13

43754 Gastric intubation and aspiration, diagnostic; single specimen (eg, acid analysis)

EXCLUDES *Analysis gastric acid (82930)*
Naso- or oro-gastric tube placement using fluoroscopic guidance (43752)

1.03 5.18 FUD 000 Q1 N1 80

AMA: 2018,Jan,8; 2017,Jan,8; 2016,Jan,13

43755 collection of multiple fractional specimens with gastric stimulation, single or double lumen tube (gastric secretory study) (eg, histamine, insulin, pentagastrin, calcium, secretin), includes drug administration

EXCLUDES *Analysis gastric acid (82930)*
Naso- or oro-gastric tube placement using fluoroscopic guidance (43752)

Code also drugs or substances administered

1.74 4.43 FUD 000 S G2 80

AMA: 2018,Jan,8; 2017,Jan,8; 2016,Jan,13

43756 Duodenal intubation and aspiration, diagnostic, includes image guidance; single specimen (eg, bile study for crystals or afferent loop culture)

Code also drugs or substances administered

(89049-89240)

1.46 7.11 FUD 000 Q1 G2 80

AMA: 2018,Jan,8; 2017,Jan,8; 2016,Jan,13

43757 collection of multiple fractional specimens with pancreatic or gallbladder stimulation, single or double lumen tube, includes drug administration

Code also drugs or substances administered

(89049-89240)

2.20 9.76 FUD 000 T G2 80

AMA: 2018,Jan,8; 2017,Jan,8; 2016,Jan,13

43761 Repositioning of a naso- or oro-gastric feeding tube, through the duodenum for enteric nutrition

EXCLUDES *Conversion gastrostomy tube to gastro-jejunostomy tube, percutaneous (49446)*
Gastrostomy tube converted endoscopically to jejunostomy tube (44373)
Insertion long gastrointestinal tube (44500, 74340)

(76000)

3.01 3.50 FUD 000 T A2

AMA: 2018,Jan,8; 2017,Jan,8; 2016,Jan,13

43762 Replacement of gastrostomy tube, percutaneous, includes removal, when performed, without imaging or endoscopic guidance; not requiring revision of gastrostomy tract

1.10 6.45 FUD 000 G2

AMA: 2019,Feb,5

43763 requiring revision of gastrostomy tract

EXCLUDES *Gastrostomy tube replacement using fluoroscopy (49450)*
Percutaneous insertion gastrostomy tube (43246)

2.44 9.64 FUD 000 G2

AMA: 2019,Oct,10; 2019,Feb,5

43770-43775 Laparoscopic Bariatric Procedures

CMS: 100-03,100.1 Bariatric Surgery for Treatment Co-morbid Conditions Due to Morbid Obesity; 100-04,32,150.1 Bariatric Surgery: Treatment of Co-Morbid Conditions Due to Morbid Obesity; 100-04,32,150.2 HCPCS Procedure Codes for Bariatric Surgery; 100-04,32,150.5 ICD Diagnosis Codes for BMI ≥35; 100-04,32,150.6 Bariatric Surgery Claims Guidance

INCLUDES Diagnostic laparoscopy (49320)
Stomach/duodenum/jejunum/ileum
Subsequent band adjustments (change gastric band component diameter by injection/aspiration fluid through subcutaneous port component) during postoperative period

43770 Laparoscopy, surgical, gastric restrictive procedure; placement of adjustable gastric restrictive device (eg, gastric band and subcutaneous port components)

Code also modifier 52 for placement individual component

32.8 32.8 FUD 090 J J8 80

AMA: 2018,Jan,8; 2017,Jan,8; 2016,Jan,13

43771 revision of adjustable gastric restrictive device component only

37.2 37.2 FUD 090 C 80

AMA: 2018,Jan,8; 2017,Jan,8; 2016,Jan,13

43772 removal of adjustable gastric restrictive device component only

27.4 27.4 FUD 090 J G2 80

AMA: 2018,Jan,8; 2017,Jan,8; 2016,Jan,13

43773 removal and replacement of adjustable gastric restrictive device component only

EXCLUDES *Laparoscopy, surgical, gastric restrictive procedure; removal adjustable gastric restrictive device component only (43772)*

37.2 37.2 FUD 090 J G2 80

AMA: 2018,Jan,8; 2017,Jan,8; 2016,Jan,13

43774 removal of adjustable gastric restrictive device and subcutaneous port components

EXCLUDES *Removal/replacement subcutaneous port components and gastric band (43659)*

28.0 28.0 FUD 090 J G2 80

AMA: 2018,Jan,8; 2017,Jan,8; 2016,Jan,13

43775 longitudinal gastrectomy (ie, sleeve gastrectomy)

EXCLUDES *Open gastric restrictive procedure for morbid obesity, without gastric bypass, other than vertical-banded gastroplasty (43843)*
Vagus nerve blocking pulse generator and/or neurostimulator electrode array implantation, reprogramming, replacement, revision, or removal at esophagogastric junction performed laparoscopically (0312T-0317T)

32.5 32.5 FUD 090 C 80

AMA: 2019,Oct,10

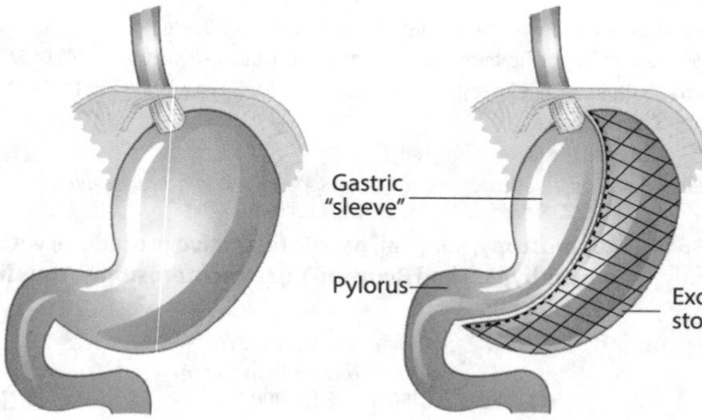

43800-43840 Open Gastric Incisional/Repair/Resection Procedures

43800 Pyloroplasty

EXCLUDES *Vagotomy with pyloroplasty (43640)*

27.2 | 27.2 | FUD 090 | C 80

AMA: 2014,Jan,11; 2013,Jan,11-12

43810 Gastroduodenostomy

29.7 | 29.7 | FUD 090 | C 80

AMA: 2014,Jan,11; 2013,Jan,11-12

43820 Gastrojejunostomy; without vagotomy

39.1 | 39.1 | FUD 090 | C 80

AMA: 2014,Jan,11; 2013,Jan,11-12

43825 with vagotomy, any type

38.0 | 38.0 | FUD 090 | C 80

AMA: 2014,Jan,11; 2013,Jan,11-12

43830 Gastrostomy, open; without construction of gastric tube (eg, Stamm procedure) (separate procedure)

20.4 | 20.4 | FUD 090 | J G2 80

AMA: 2019,Feb,5; 2018,Jan,8; 2017,Jan,8; 2016,Jan,13

43831 neonatal, for feeding A

EXCLUDES *Change gastrostomy tube (43762-43763)*
Gastrostomy tube replacement using fluoroscopy (49450)

17.5 | 17.5 | FUD 090 | 63 T G2 80

AMA: 2019,Feb,5; 2018,Jan,8; 2017,Jan,8; 2016,Jan,13

43832 with construction of gastric tube (eg, Janeway procedure)

EXCLUDES *Endoscopic placement percutaneous gastrostomy tube (43246)*

30.3 | 30.3 | FUD 090 | C 80

AMA: 2018,Jan,8; 2017,Jan,8; 2016,Jan,13

43840 Gastrorrhaphy, suture of perforated duodenal or gastric ulcer, wound, or injury

39.4 | 39.4 | FUD 090 | C 80

AMA: 2014,Jan,11; 2013,Jan,11-12

43842-43848 Open Bariatric Procedures for Morbid Obesity

CMS: 100-03,100.1 Bariatric Surgery for Treatment Co-morbid Conditions Due to Morbid Obesity; 100-04,32,150.1 Bariatric Surgery: Treatment of Co-Morbid Conditions Due to Morbid Obesity; 100-04,32,150.2 HCPCS Procedure Codes for Bariatric Surgery; 100-04,32,150.5 ICD Diagnosis Codes for BMI ≥35; 100-04,32,150.6 Bariatric Surgery Claims Guidance

43842 Gastric restrictive procedure, without gastric bypass, for morbid obesity; vertical-banded gastroplasty

33.4 | 33.4 | FUD 090 | E

AMA: 2018,Jan,8; 2017,Jan,8; 2016,Jan,13

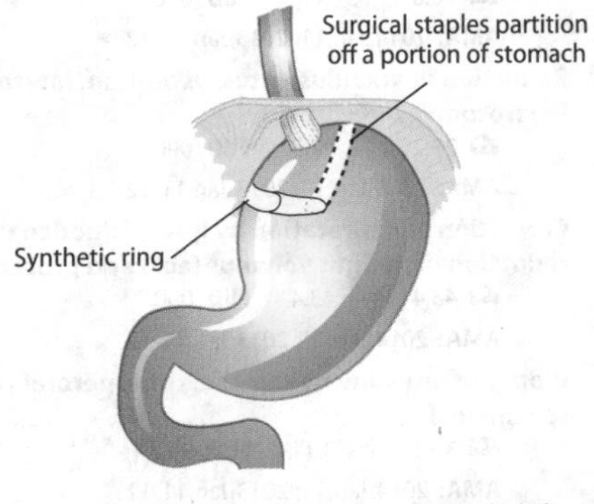

The stomach is surgically restricted to treat morbid obesity; a vertical-banded partitioning technique gives the patient a sensation of fullness, thus decreasing daily caloric intake

43843 other than vertical-banded gastroplasty

EXCLUDES *Laparoscopic longitudinal gastrectomy (e.g., sleeve gastrectomy) (43775)*

37.4 | 37.4 | FUD 090 | C 80

AMA: 2018,Jan,8; 2017,Jan,8; 2016,Jan,13

43845 Gastric restrictive procedure with partial gastrectomy, pylorus-preserving duodenoileostomy and ileoileostomy (50 to 100 cm common channel) to limit absorption (biliopancreatic diversion with duodenal switch)

EXCLUDES *Enteroenterostomy, anastomosis intestine (44130)*
Exploratory laparotomy, exploratory celiotomy (49000)
Gastrectomy, partial, distal; with Roux-en-Y reconstruction (43633)
Gastric restrictive procedure, with gastric bypass for morbid obesity; with small intestine reconstruction (43847)

56.8 | 56.8 | FUD 090 | C 80

AMA: 2018,Jan,8; 2017,Jan,8; 2016,Jan,13

43846 Gastric restrictive procedure, with gastric bypass for morbid obesity; with short limb (150 cm or less) Roux-en-Y gastroenterostomy

EXCLUDES *Performed laparoscopically (43644)*
Roux limb more than 150 cm (43847)

47.3 | 47.3 | FUD 090 | C 80

AMA: 2018,Jan,8; 2017,Jan,8; 2016,Jan,13

43847 with small intestine reconstruction to limit absorption

EXCLUDES *Performed laparoscopically (43645)*

52.1 | 52.1 | FUD 090 | C 80

AMA: 2018,Jan,8; 2017,Jan,8; 2016,Jan,13

43848 Revision, open, of gastric restrictive procedure for morbid obesity, other than adjustable gastric restrictive device (separate procedure)

EXCLUDES *Gastric restrictive port procedures (43886-43888)*
Procedures for adjustable gastric restrictive devices (43770-43774)

55.9 | 55.9 | FUD 090 | C 80

AMA: 2018,Jan,8; 2017,Jan,8; 2016,Jan,13

43850-43882 Open Gastric Procedures: Closure/Implantation/Replacement/Revision

43850 ~~Revision of gastroduodenal anastomosis (gastroduodenostomy) with reconstruction; without vagotomy~~

43855 ~~with vagotomy~~

43860 Revision of gastrojejunal anastomosis (gastrojejunostomy) with reconstruction, with or without partial gastrectomy or intestine resection; without vagotomy

47.7 | 47.7 | FUD 090 | C 80

AMA: 2014,Jan,11; 2013,Jan,11-12

43865 with vagotomy

49.9 | 49.9 | FUD 090 | C 80

AMA: 2014,Jan,11; 2013,Jan,11-12

43870 Closure of gastrostomy, surgical

20.6 | 20.6 | FUD 090 | J A2 80

AMA: 2018,Jul,14

43880 Closure of gastrocolic fistula

46.1 | 46.1 | FUD 090 | C 80

AMA: 2014,Jan,11; 2013,Jan,11-12

43881 **Implantation or replacement of gastric neurostimulator electrodes, antrum, open**

EXCLUDES *Electronic analysis and programming (95980-95982)*
Implantation/removal/revision gastric neurostimulator electrodes, lesser curvature or vagal trunk (EGJ):
Laparoscopically (43659)
Open, lesser curvature (43999)
Implantation/replacement performed laparoscopically (43647)
Insertion gastric neurostimulator pulse generator (64590)
Vagus nerve blocking pulse generator and/or neurostimulator electrode array implantation, reprogramming, replacement, revision, or removal at esophagogastric junction performed laparoscopically (0312T-0317T)

Facility RVU 0.00 Non-Facility RVU 0.00 **FUD** YYY C 80

AMA: 2019,Feb,6; 2018,Jan,8; 2017,Jan,8; 2016,Jan,13

43882 **Revision or removal of gastric neurostimulator electrodes, antrum, open**

EXCLUDES *Electronic analysis and programming (95980-95982)*
Implantation/removal/revision gastric neurostimulator electrodes, lesser curvature or vagal trunk (EGJ):
Laparoscopic (43659)
Open, lesser curvature (43999)
Revision/removal gastric neurostimulator electrodes, antrum, performed laparoscopically (43648)
Revision/removal gastric neurostimulator pulse generator (64595)
Vagus nerve blocking pulse generator and/or neurostimulator electrode array implantation, reprogramming, replacement, revision, or removal at esophagogastric junction performed laparoscopically (0312T-0317T)

Facility RVU 0.00 Non-Facility RVU 0.00 **FUD** YYY C 80

AMA: 2019,Feb,6; 2018,Jan,8; 2017,Jan,8; 2016,Jan,13

43886-43999 Bariatric Procedures: Removal/Replacement/Revision Port Components

CMS: 100-04,32,150.1 Bariatric Surgery: Treatment of Co-Morbid Conditions Due to Morbid Obesity; 100-04,32,150.2 HCPCS Procedure Codes for Bariatric Surgery; 100-04,32,150.5 ICD Diagnosis Codes for BMI ≥35; 100-04,32,150.6 Bariatric Surgery Claims Guidance

43886 **Gastric restrictive procedure, open; revision of subcutaneous port component only**

Facility RVU 10.5 Non-Facility RVU 10.5 **FUD** 090 T G2 80

AMA: 2018,Jan,8; 2017,Jan,8; 2016,Jan,13

43887 **removal of subcutaneous port component only**

EXCLUDES *Gastric band and subcutaneous port components:*
Removal and replacement performed laparoscopically (43659)
Removal performed laparoscopically (43774)

Facility RVU 9.52 Non-Facility RVU 9.52 **FUD** 090 02 G2 80

AMA: 2018,Jan,8; 2017,Jan,8; 2016,Jan,13

43888 **removal and replacement of subcutaneous port component only**

EXCLUDES *Gastric band and subcutaneous port components:*
Removal and replacement performed laparoscopically (43659)
Removal performed laparoscopically (43774)
Gastric restrictive procedure, open; removal subcutaneous port component only (43887)

Facility RVU 13.4 Non-Facility RVU 13.4 **FUD** 090 T G2 80

AMA: 2018,Jan,8; 2017,Jan,8; 2016,Jan,13

43999 **Unlisted procedure, stomach**

Facility RVU 0.00 Non-Facility RVU 0.00 **FUD** YYY T 80

AMA: 2018,Dec,10; 2018,Dec,10; 2018,Jul,14; 2018,Jan,8; 2017,Jan,8; 2016,Jan,13

44005-44130 Incisional and Resection Procedures of Bowel

44005 **Enterolysis (freeing of intestinal adhesion) (separate procedure)**

EXCLUDES *Enterolysis performed laparoscopically (44180)*
Excision ileoanal reservoir with ileostomy (45136)

Facility RVU 31.7 Non-Facility RVU 31.7 **FUD** 090 C 80

AMA: 2018,Feb,11; 2018,Jan,8; 2017,Jan,8; 2016,Jan,13

44010 **Duodenotomy, for exploration, biopsy(s), or foreign body removal**

Facility RVU 24.8 Non-Facility RVU 24.8 **FUD** 090 C 80

AMA: 2014,Jan,11; 2013,Jan,11-12

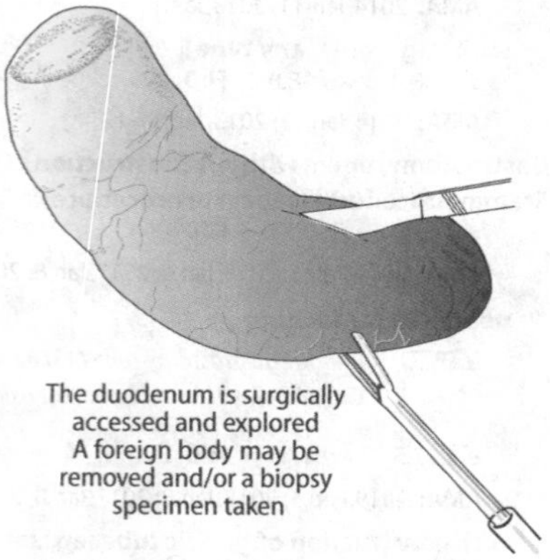

The duodenum is surgically accessed and explored A foreign body may be removed and/or a biopsy specimen taken

+ **44015** **Tube or needle catheter jejunostomy for enteral alimentation, intraoperative, any method (List separately in addition to primary procedure)**

Code first primary procedure

Facility RVU 4.15 Non-Facility RVU 4.15 **FUD** ZZZ C 80

AMA: 2018,Jan,8; 2017,Jan,8; 2016,Jan,13

44020 **Enterotomy, small intestine, other than duodenum; for exploration, biopsy(s), or foreign body removal**

Facility RVU 28.2 Non-Facility RVU 28.2 **FUD** 090 C 80

AMA: 2014,Jan,11; 2013,Jan,11-12

44021 **for decompression (eg, Baker tube)**

Facility RVU 28.3 Non-Facility RVU 28.3 **FUD** 090 C 80

AMA: 2014,Jan,11; 2013,Jan,11-12

44025 **Colotomy, for exploration, biopsy(s), or foreign body removal**

INCLUDES Amussat's operation

EXCLUDES *Intestine exteriorization (Mikulicz resection with crushing of spur) (44602-44605)*

Facility RVU 28.6 Non-Facility RVU 28.6 **FUD** 090 C 80

AMA: 2014,Jan,11; 2013,Jan,11-12

44050 **Reduction of volvulus, intussusception, internal hernia, by laparotomy**

Facility RVU 27.2 Non-Facility RVU 27.2 **FUD** 090 C 80

AMA: 2014,Jan,11; 2013,Jan,11-12

44055 **Correction of malrotation by lysis of duodenal bands and/or reduction of midgut volvulus (eg, Ladd procedure)**

Facility RVU 43.4 Non-Facility RVU 43.4 **FUD** 090 63 C 80

AMA: 2014,Jan,11; 2013,Jan,11-12

44100 **Biopsy of intestine by capsule, tube, peroral (1 or more specimens)**

Facility RVU 3.11 Non-Facility RVU 3.11 **FUD** 000 T A2

AMA: 2014,Jan,11; 2013,Jan,11-12

44110 **Excision of 1 or more lesions of small or large intestine not requiring anastomosis, exteriorization, or fistulization; single enterotomy**

Facility RVU 24.6 Non-Facility RVU 24.6 **FUD** 090 C 80

AMA: 2014,Jan,11; 2013,Jan,11-12

44111 **multiple enterotomies**
28.5 28.5 FUD 090 C 80
AMA: 2014,Jan,11; 2013,Jan,11-12

44120 **Enterectomy, resection of small intestine; single resection and anastomosis**
35.6 35.6 FUD 090 C 80
AMA: 2018,Nov,11; 2018,Jan,8; 2017,Jan,8; 2016,Jan,13

+ **44121** **each additional resection and anastomosis (List separately in addition to code for primary procedure)**
Code first (44120)
7.04 7.04 FUD ZZZ C 80
AMA: 2014,Jan,11; 2013,Jan,11-12

44125 **with enterostomy**
34.3 34.3 FUD 090 C 80
AMA: 2014,Jan,11; 2013,Jan,11-12

44126 **Enterectomy, resection of small intestine for congenital atresia, single resection and anastomosis of proximal segment of intestine; without tapering**
71.7 71.7 FUD 090 63 C 80
AMA: 2014,Jan,11; 2013,Jan,11-12

44127 **with tapering**
83.3 83.3 FUD 090 63 C 80
AMA: 2014,Jan,11; 2013,Jan,11-12

+ **44128** **each additional resection and anastomosis (List separately in addition to code for primary procedure)**
Code first single resection small intestine (44126, 44127)
7.10 7.10 FUD ZZZ 63 C 80
AMA: 2014,Jan,11; 2013,Jan,11-12

44130 **Enteroenterostomy, anastomosis of intestine, with or without cutaneous enterostomy (separate procedure)**
38.2 38.2 FUD 090 C 80
AMA: 2014,Jan,11; 2013,Jan,11-12

44132-44137 Intestine Transplant Procedures

CMS: 100-03,260.5 Intestinal and Multi-Visceral Transplantation; 100-04,3,90.6 Intestinal and Multi-Visceral Transplants

44132 **Donor enterectomy (including cold preservation), open; from cadaver donor**
INCLUDES Graft:
Cold preservation
Harvest
EXCLUDES *Preparation/reconstruction backbench intestinal graft (44715, 44720-44721)*
0.00 0.00 FUD XXX C 80
AMA: 2014,Jan,11; 2013,Jan,11-12

44133 **partial, from living donor**
INCLUDES Donor care
Graft:
Cold preservation
Harvest
EXCLUDES *Preparation/reconstruction backbench intestinal graft (44715, 44720-44721)*
0.00 0.00 FUD XXX C 80
AMA: 2014,Jan,11; 2013,Jan,11-12

44135 **Intestinal allotransplantation; from cadaver donor**
INCLUDES Allograft transplantation
Recipient care
0.00 0.00 FUD XXX C 80
AMA: 2014,Jan,11; 2013,Jan,11-12

44136 **from living donor**
INCLUDES Allograft transplantation
Recipient care
0.00 0.00 FUD XXX C 80
AMA: 2014,Jan,11; 2013,Jan,11-12

44137 **Removal of transplanted intestinal allograft, complete**
EXCLUDES *Partial removal transplant allograft (44120-44121, 44140)*
0.00 0.00 FUD XXX C 80
AMA: 2014,Jan,11; 2013,Jan,11-12

44139-44160 Colon Resection Procedures

+ **44139** **Mobilization (take-down) of splenic flexure performed in conjunction with partial colectomy (List separately in addition to primary procedure)**
Code first partial colectomy (44140-44147)
3.52 3.52 FUD ZZZ C 80
AMA: 2014,Jan,11; 2013,Jan,11-12

44140 **Colectomy, partial; with anastomosis**
EXCLUDES *Laparoscopic method (44204)*
39.0 39.0 FUD 090 C 80
AMA: 2020,Apr,10; 2018,Jan,8; 2017,Jan,8; 2016,Jan,13

44141 **with skin level cecostomy or colostomy**
52.9 52.9 FUD 090 C 80
AMA: 2018,Jan,8; 2017,Jan,8; 2016,Jan,13

44143 **with end colostomy and closure of distal segment (Hartmann type procedure)**
EXCLUDES *Laparoscopic method (44206)*
48.4 48.4 FUD 090 C 80
AMA: 2018,Jan,8; 2017,Jan,8; 2016,Jan,13

44144 **with resection, with colostomy or ileostomy and creation of mucofistula**
51.4 51.4 FUD 090 C 80
AMA: 2018,Jan,8; 2017,Jan,8; 2016,Jan,13

44145 **with coloproctostomy (low pelvic anastomosis)**
EXCLUDES *Laparoscopic method (44207)*
48.0 48.0 FUD 090 C 80
AMA: 2014,Jan,11; 2013,Jan,11-12

44146 **with coloproctostomy (low pelvic anastomosis), with colostomy**
EXCLUDES *Laparoscopic method (44208)*
61.2 61.2 FUD 090 C 80
AMA: 2018,Jun,11; 2018,Jan,8; 2017,Jan,8; 2016,Jan,13

44147 **abdominal and transanal approach**
56.3 56.3 FUD 090 C 80
AMA: 2018,Jan,8; 2017,Jan,8; 2016,Jan,13

44150 **Colectomy, total, abdominal, without proctectomy; with ileostomy or ileoproctostomy**
INCLUDES Lane's operation
EXCLUDES *Laparoscopic method (44210)*
54.0 54.0 FUD 090 C 80
AMA: 2014,Jan,11; 2013,Jan,11-12

44151 **with continent ileostomy**
62.9 62.9 FUD 090 C 80
AMA: 2014,Jan,11; 2013,Jan,11-12

44155 **Colectomy, total, abdominal, with proctectomy; with ileostomy**
INCLUDES Miles' colectomy
EXCLUDES *Laparoscopic method (44212)*
60.0 60.0 FUD 090 C 80
AMA: 2014,Jan,11; 2013,Jan,11-12

44156 **with continent ileostomy**
67.4 67.4 FUD 090 C 80
AMA: 2014,Jan,11; 2013,Jan,11-12

44157 **with ileoanal anastomosis, includes loop ileostomy, and rectal mucosectomy, when performed**
63.9 63.9 FUD 090 C 80
AMA: 2014,Jan,11; 2013,Jan,11-12

44158 **with ileoanal anastomosis, creation of ileal reservoir (S or J), includes loop ileostomy, and rectal mucosectomy, when performed**

EXCLUDES *Laparoscopic method (44211)*

65.5 65.5 FUD 090

AMA: 2014,Jan,11; 2013,Jan,11-12

44160 **Colectomy, partial, with removal of terminal ileum with ileocolostomy**

EXCLUDES *Laparoscopic method (44205)*

36.0 36.0 FUD 090

AMA: 2018,Jan,8; 2017,Jan,8; 2016,Jan,13

44180 Laparoscopic Enterolysis

INCLUDES Diagnostic laparoscopy (49320)

EXCLUDES *Laparoscopic salpingolysis/ovariolysis (58660)*

44180 **Laparoscopy, surgical, enterolysis (freeing of intestinal adhesion) (separate procedure)**

26.6 26.6 FUD 090

AMA: 2018,Feb,11; 2018,Jan,8; 2017,Jan,8; 2016,Jan,13

44186-44238 Laparoscopic Enterostomy Procedures

INCLUDES Diagnostic laparoscopy (49320)

44186 **Laparoscopy, surgical; jejunostomy (eg, for decompression or feeding)**

18.9 18.9 FUD 090

AMA: 2018,Jan,8; 2017,Jan,8; 2016,Jan,13

44187 **ileostomy or jejunostomy, non-tube**

EXCLUDES *Open method (44310)*

31.8 31.8 FUD 090

AMA: 2019,Sep,10; 2018,Jan,8; 2017,Jan,8; 2016,Jan,13

44188 **Laparoscopy, surgical, colostomy or skin level cecostomy**

EXCLUDES *Laparoscopy, surgical, appendectomy (44970)*
Open method (44320)

35.4 35.4 FUD 090

AMA: 2018,Jan,8; 2017,Jan,8; 2016,Jan,13

44202 **Laparoscopy, surgical; enterectomy, resection of small intestine, single resection and anastomosis**

EXCLUDES *Open method (44120)*

40.1 40.1 FUD 090

AMA: 2020,Jul,13; 2018,Jan,8; 2017,Jan,8; 2016,Jan,13

\+ **44203** **each additional small intestine resection and anastomosis (List separately in addition to code for primary procedure)**

EXCLUDES *Open method (44121)*

Code first single resection small intestine (44202)

7.00 7.00 FUD ZZZ

AMA: 2018,Jan,8; 2017,Jan,8; 2016,Jan,13

44204 **colectomy, partial, with anastomosis**

EXCLUDES *Open method (44140)*

44.7 44.7 FUD 090

AMA: 2018,Jan,8; 2017,Dec,14; 2017,Jan,8; 2016,Jan,13

44205 **colectomy, partial, with removal of terminal ileum with ileocolostomy**

EXCLUDES *Open method (44160)*

38.8 38.8 FUD 090

AMA: 2018,Jan,8; 2017,Jan,8; 2016,Jan,13

44206 **colectomy, partial, with end colostomy and closure of distal segment (Hartmann type procedure)**

EXCLUDES *Open method (44143)*

50.7 50.7 FUD 090

AMA: 2018,Jan,8; 2017,Jan,8; 2016,Jan,13

44207 **colectomy, partial, with anastomosis, with coloproctostomy (low pelvic anastomosis)**

EXCLUDES *Open method (44145)*

52.6 52.6 FUD 090

AMA: 2018,Jan,8; 2017,Jan,8; 2016,Jan,13

44208 **colectomy, partial, with anastomosis, with coloproctostomy (low pelvic anastomosis) with colostomy**

EXCLUDES *Open method (44146)*

57.4 57.4 FUD 090

AMA: 2018,Jan,8; 2017,Jan,8; 2016,Jan,13

44210 **colectomy, total, abdominal, without proctectomy, with ileostomy or ileoproctostomy**

EXCLUDES *Open method (44150)*

51.3 51.3 FUD 090

AMA: 2018,Jan,8; 2017,Jan,8; 2016,Jan,13

44211 **colectomy, total, abdominal, with proctectomy, with ileoanal anastomosis, creation of ileal reservoir (S or J), with loop ileostomy, includes rectal mucosectomy, when performed**

EXCLUDES *Open method (44157-44158)*

61.2 61.2 FUD 090

AMA: 2018,Jan,8; 2017,Jan,8; 2016,Jan,13

44212 **colectomy, total, abdominal, with proctectomy, with ileostomy**

EXCLUDES *Open method (44155)*

59.0 59.0 FUD 090

AMA: 2018,Jan,8; 2017,Jan,8; 2016,Jan,13

\+ **44213** **Laparoscopy, surgical, mobilization (take-down) of splenic flexure performed in conjunction with partial colectomy (List separately in addition to primary procedure)**

EXCLUDES *Open method (44139)*

Code first partial colectomy (44204-44208)

5.43 5.43 FUD ZZZ

AMA: 2018,Jan,8; 2017,Jan,8; 2016,Jan,13

44227 **Laparoscopy, surgical, closure of enterostomy, large or small intestine, with resection and anastomosis**

EXCLUDES *Open method (44625-44626)*

48.4 48.4 FUD 090

AMA: 2018,Jan,8; 2017,Jan,8; 2016,Jan,13

44238 **Unlisted laparoscopy procedure, intestine (except rectum)**

0.00 0.00 FUD YYY

AMA: 2020,Jul,13; 2019,Oct,10; 2018,Jan,8; 2017,Jul,10; 2017,Jan,8; 2016,Jan,13

44300-44346 Open Enterostomy Procedures

44300 **Placement, enterostomy or cecostomy, tube open (eg, for feeding or decompression) (separate procedure)**

EXCLUDES *Intraoperative lavage, colon (44701)*
Other gastrointestinal tube(s) placed percutaneously with fluoroscopic imaging guidance (49441-49442)

24.5 24.5 FUD 090

AMA: 2018,Jan,8; 2017,Jan,8; 2016,Jan,13

44310 **Ileostomy or jejunostomy, non-tube**

EXCLUDES *Colectomy, partial; with resection, with colostomy or ileostomy and creation mucofistula (44144)*
Colectomy, total, abdominal (44150-44151, 44155-44156)
Excision ileoanal reservoir with ileostomy (45136)
Laparoscopic method (44187)
Proctectomy (45113, 45119)

30.2 30.2 FUD 090

AMA: 2018,Jan,8; 2017,Jan,8; 2016,Jan,13

44312 **Revision of ileostomy; simple (release of superficial scar) (separate procedure)**

17.1 17.1 FUD 090

AMA: 2014,Jan,11; 2013,Jan,11-12

44314 **complicated (reconstruction in-depth) (separate procedure)**

29.1 29.1 FUD 090

AMA: 2014,Jan,11; 2013,Jan,11-12

44316 **Continent ileostomy (Kock procedure) (separate procedure)**

EXCLUDES *Fiberoptic evaluation (44385)*

41.2 41.2 FUD 090 C 80

AMA: 2014,Jan,11; 2013,Jan,11-12

44320 **Colostomy or skin level cecostomy;**

EXCLUDES *Closure fistula (45805, 45825, 57307)*
Colectomy, partial (44141, 44144, 44146)
Exploration, repair, and presacral drainage (45563)
Laparoscopic method (44188)
Pelvic exenteration (45126, 51597, 58240)
Proctectomy (45110, 45119)
Suture large intestine (44605)
Ureterosigmoidostomy (50810)

34.9 34.9 FUD 090 C 80

AMA: 2018,Jan,8; 2017,Jan,8; 2016,Jan,13

44322 **with multiple biopsies (eg, for congenital megacolon) (separate procedure)**

29.2 29.2 FUD 090 C 80

AMA: 2014,Jan,11; 2013,Jan,11-12

44340 **Revision of colostomy; simple (release of superficial scar) (separate procedure)**

18.0 18.0 FUD 090 T A2

AMA: 2014,Jan,11; 2013,Jan,11-12

44345 **complicated (reconstruction in-depth) (separate procedure)**

30.4 30.4 FUD 090 C 80

AMA: 2014,Jan,11; 2013,Jan,11-12

44346 **with repair of paracolostomy hernia (separate procedure)**

34.2 34.2 FUD 090 C 80

AMA: 2018,Jan,8; 2017,Jan,8; 2016,Jan,13

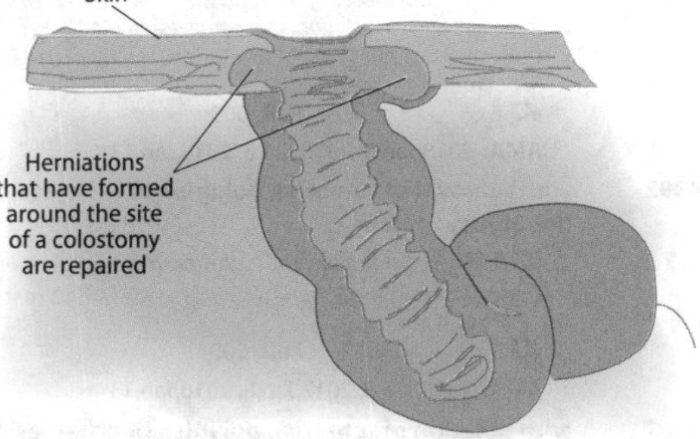

The colon is mobilized, trimmed if necessary, and a new stoma is often created

44360-44379 Endoscopy of Small Intestine

INCLUDES Control bleeding due to endoscopic procedure during same operative session

44360 **Small intestinal endoscopy, enteroscopy beyond second portion of duodenum, not including ileum; diagnostic, including collection of specimen(s) by brushing or washing, when performed (separate procedure)**

EXCLUDES *Esophagogastroduodenoscopy, flexible, transoral (43235-43259 [43233, 43266, 43270])*

4.14 4.14 FUD 000 J A2

AMA: 2019,Oct,10; 2018,Jan,8; 2017,Jan,8; 2016,Jan,13

44361 **with biopsy, single or multiple**

EXCLUDES *Esophagogastroduodenoscopy, flexible, transoral (43235-43259 [43233, 43266, 43270])*

4.65 4.65 FUD 000 J A2

AMA: 2019,Oct,10

44363 **with removal of foreign body(s)**

EXCLUDES *Esophagogastroduodenoscopy, flexible, transoral (43235-43259 [43233, 43266, 43270])*

5.54 5.54 FUD 000 J A2 80

AMA: 2019,Oct,10

44364 **with removal of tumor(s), polyp(s), or other lesion(s) by snare technique**

EXCLUDES *Esophagogastroduodenoscopy, flexible, transoral (43235-43259 [43233, 43266, 43270])*

5.90 5.90 FUD 000 J A2 80

AMA: 2019,Oct,10

44365 **with removal of tumor(s), polyp(s), or other lesion(s) by hot biopsy forceps or bipolar cautery**

EXCLUDES *Esophagogastroduodenoscopy, flexible, transoral (43235-43259 [43233, 43266, 43270])*

5.24 5.24 FUD 000 J A2 80

AMA: 2019,Oct,10

44366 **with control of bleeding (eg, injection, bipolar cautery, unipolar cautery, laser, heater probe, stapler, plasma coagulator)**

EXCLUDES *Esophagogastroduodenoscopy, flexible, transoral (43235-43259 [43233, 43266, 43270])*

6.93 6.93 FUD 000 J A2

AMA: 2019,Oct,10; 2018,Jan,8; 2017,Jan,8; 2016,Jan,13

44369 **with ablation of tumor(s), polyp(s), or other lesion(s) not amenable to removal by hot biopsy forceps, bipolar cautery or snare technique**

EXCLUDES *Esophagogastroduodenoscopy, flexible, transoral (43235-43259 [43233, 43266, 43270])*

7.10 7.10 FUD 000 J A2 80

AMA: 2019,Oct,10

44370 **with transendoscopic stent placement (includes predilation)**

EXCLUDES *Esophagogastroduodenoscopy, flexible, transoral (43235-43259 [43233, 43266, 43270])*

7.80 7.80 FUD 000 J J8 80

AMA: 2019,Oct,10; 2018,Jan,8; 2017,Jan,8; 2016,Jan,13

44372 **with placement of percutaneous jejunostomy tube**

EXCLUDES *Esophagogastroduodenoscopy, flexible, transoral (43235-43259 [43233, 43266, 43270])*

7.02 7.02 FUD 000 J A2

AMA: 2019,Oct,10; 2018,Jan,8; 2017,Jan,8; 2016,Jan,13

44373 **with conversion of percutaneous gastrostomy tube to percutaneous jejunostomy tube**

EXCLUDES *Esophagogastroduodenoscopy, flexible, transoral (43235-43259 [43233, 43266, 43270])*

5.62 5.62 FUD 000 J A2

AMA: 2019,Oct,10; 2018,Jan,8; 2017,Jan,8; 2016,Jan,13

44376 **Small intestinal endoscopy, enteroscopy beyond second portion of duodenum, including ileum; diagnostic, with or without collection of specimen(s) by brushing or washing (separate procedure)**

EXCLUDES *Small intestinal endoscopy, enteroscopy (44360-44373)*

8.33 8.33 FUD 000 J A2 80

AMA: 2018,Jan,8; 2017,Jan,8; 2016,Jan,13

44377 **with biopsy, single or multiple**

EXCLUDES *Small intestinal endoscopy, enteroscopy (44360-44373)*

8.63 8.63 FUD 000 J A2 80

AMA: 2018,Jan,8; 2017,Jan,8; 2016,Jan,13

44378 **with control of bleeding (eg, injection, bipolar cautery, unipolar cautery, laser, heater probe, stapler, plasma coagulator)**

EXCLUDES *Small intestinal endoscopy, enteroscopy (44360-44373)*

11.2 11.2 FUD 000 J A2 80

AMA: 2018,Jan,8; 2017,Jan,8; 2016,Jan,13

44379 **with transendoscopic stent placement (includes predilation)**

EXCLUDES *Small intestinal endoscopy, enteroscopy (44360-44373)*

Facility RVU 11.8 Non-Facility RVU 11.8 FUD 000 J A2 80 CCI

AMA: 2018,Jan,8; 2017,Jan,8; 2016,Jan,13

44380-44384 [44381] Ileoscopy Via Stoma

INCLUDES Control bleeding due to endoscopic procedure during same operative session

EXCLUDES *Computed tomographic colonography (74261-74263)*

Code also exam nonfunctional distal colon/rectum, when performed, with:
Anoscopy (46600, 46604-46606, 46608-46615)
Proctosigmoidoscopy (45300-45327)
Sigmoidoscopy (45330-45347 [45346])

44380 **Ileoscopy, through stoma; diagnostic, including collection of specimen(s) by brushing or washing, when performed (separate procedure)**

EXCLUDES *Ileoscopy, through stoma (44382-44384 [44381])*

Facility RVU 1.61 Non-Facility RVU 5.20 FUD 000 T A2 CCI

AMA: 2018,Jan,8; 2017,Jan,8; 2016,Jan,13

44381 **Resequenced code. See code following 44382.**

44382 **with biopsy, single or multiple**

EXCLUDES *Ileoscopy, through stoma; diagnostic (44380)*

Facility RVU 2.10 Non-Facility RVU 8.14 FUD 000 T A2 CCI

AMA: 2018,Jan,8; 2017,Jan,8; 2016,Jan,13

\# **44381** **with transendoscopic balloon dilation**

EXCLUDES *Ileoscopy, through stoma (44380, 44384)*

Code also each additional stricture dilated in same session, using modifier 59 with (44381)

Radiology Crosswalk (74360)

Facility RVU 2.46 Non-Facility RVU 26.3 FUD 000 J G2 CCI

AMA: 2018,Jan,8; 2017,Jan,8; 2016,Jan,13

44384 **with placement of endoscopic stent (includes pre- and post-dilation and guide wire passage, when performed)**

EXCLUDES *Ileoscopy, through stoma (44380-44381)*

Radiology Crosswalk (74360)

Facility RVU 4.44 Non-Facility RVU 4.44 FUD 000 J G2 CCI

AMA: 2018,Jan,8; 2017,Jan,8; 2016,Jan,13

44385-44386 Endoscopy of Small Intestinal Pouch

INCLUDES Control bleeding due to endoscopic procedure during same operative session

EXCLUDES *Computed tomographic colonography (74261-74263)*

44385 **Endoscopic evaluation of small intestinal pouch (eg, Kock pouch, ileal reservoir [S or J]); diagnostic, including collection of specimen(s) by brushing or washing, when performed (separate procedure)**

EXCLUDES *Endoscopic evaluation small intestinal pouch (44386)*

Facility RVU 2.09 Non-Facility RVU 5.60 FUD 000 T A2 CCI

AMA: 2018,Jan,8; 2017,Jan,8; 2016,Jan,13

44386 **with biopsy, single or multiple**

EXCLUDES *Endoscopic evaluation small intestinal pouch (44385)*

Facility RVU 2.57 Non-Facility RVU 8.54 FUD 000 T A2 CCI

AMA: 2018,Jan,8; 2017,Jan,8; 2016,Jan,13

44388-44408 [44401] Colonoscopy Via Stoma

INCLUDES Control bleeding due to endoscopic procedure during same operative session

EXCLUDES *Colonoscopy via rectum (45378, 45392-45393 [45390, 45398])*
Computed tomographic colonography (74261-74263)

Code also exam nonfunctional distal colon/rectum, when performed, with:
Anoscopy (46600, 46604-46606, 46608-46615)
Proctosigmoidoscopy (45300-45327)
Sigmoidoscopy (45330-45347 [45346])

44388 **Colonoscopy through stoma; diagnostic, including collection of specimen(s) by brushing or washing, when performed (separate procedure)**

EXCLUDES *Colonoscopy through stoma (44389-44408 [44401])*

Code also modifier 53 when planned total colonoscopy cannot be completed

Facility RVU 4.56 Non-Facility RVU 8.42 FUD 000 T A2 CCI

AMA: 2018,Jan,8; 2017,Jan,8; 2016,Jan,13

44389 **with biopsy, single or multiple**

EXCLUDES *Colonoscopy through stoma; diagnostic (44388)*
Colonoscopy through stoma; with endoscopic mucosal resection on same lesion (44403)

Code also modifier 52 when colonoscope fails to reach junction small intestine

Facility RVU 4.97 Non-Facility RVU 11.4 FUD 000 T A2 CCI

AMA: 2018,Jan,8; 2017,Jan,8; 2016,Jan,13

44390 **with removal of foreign body(s)**

EXCLUDES *Colonoscopy through stoma; diagnostic (44388)*

Code also modifier 52 when colonoscope fails to reach junction small intestine

Radiology Crosswalk (76000)

Facility RVU 6.07 Non-Facility RVU 11.2 FUD 000 T A2 CCI

AMA: 2018,Jan,8; 2017,Jan,8; 2016,Jan,13

44391 **with control of bleeding, any method**

EXCLUDES *Colonoscopy through stoma; diagnostic (44388)*
Colonoscopy through stoma; with directed submucosal injection(s) in same lesion (44404)

Code also modifier 52 when colonoscope fails to reach junction small intestine

Facility RVU 6.65 Non-Facility RVU 19.2 FUD 000 T A2 CCI

AMA: 2018,Jan,8; 2017,Jan,8; 2016,Jan,13

44392 **with removal of tumor(s), polyp(s), or other lesion(s) by hot biopsy forceps**

EXCLUDES *Colonoscopy through stoma; diagnostic (44388)*

Code also modifier 52 when colonoscope fails to reach junction small intestine

Facility RVU 5.82 Non-Facility RVU 10.2 FUD 000 T A2 CCI

AMA: 2018,Jan,8; 2017,Jan,8; 2016,Jan,13

\# **44401** **with ablation of tumor(s), polyp(s), or other lesion(s) (includes pre-and post-dilation and guide wire passage, when performed)**

EXCLUDES *Colonoscopy through stoma; diagnostic (44388)*
Colonoscopy through stoma; with transendoscopic balloon dilation for same lesion (44405)

Code also modifier 52 when colonoscope fails to reach junction small intestine

Facility RVU 7.00 Non-Facility RVU 80.2 FUD 000 T G2 CCI

AMA: 2018,Jan,8; 2017,Jan,8; 2016,Jan,13

44394 **with removal of tumor(s), polyp(s), or other lesion(s) by snare technique**

EXCLUDES *Colonoscopy through stoma; diagnostic (44388)*
Colonoscopy through stoma; with directed submucosal injection(s) same lesion (44403)

Code also modifier 52 when colonoscope fails to reach junction small intestine

Facility RVU 6.60 Non-Facility RVU 11.7 FUD 000 T A2 CCI

AMA: 2018,Jan,8; 2017,Jan,8; 2016,Jan,13

44401 **Resequenced code. See code following 44392.**

44402 **with endoscopic stent placement (including pre- and post-dilation and guide wire passage, when performed)**

EXCLUDES *Colonoscopy through stoma (44388, 44405)*

Code also modifier 52 when colonoscope fails to reach junction small intestine

(74360)

7.56 7.56 FUD 000 J J8

AMA: 2018,Jan,8; 2017,Jan,8; 2016,Jan,13

44403 **with endoscopic mucosal resection**

EXCLUDES *Colonoscopy through stoma; diagnostic (44388)*

Colonoscopy through stoma for same lesion (44389, 44394, 44404)

Code also modifier 52 when colonoscope fails to reach junction small intestine

8.77 8.77 FUD 000 T G2

AMA: 2019,Dec,14; 2018,Jan,8; 2017,Jan,8; 2016,Jan,13

44404 **with directed submucosal injection(s), any substance**

EXCLUDES *Colonoscopy through stoma; diagnostic (44388)*

Colonoscopy through stoma for same lesion (44391, 44403)

Code also modifier 52 when colonoscope fails to reach small intestine junction

4.97 11.3 FUD 000 T G2

AMA: 2018,Jan,8; 2017,Jan,8; 2016,Jan,13

44405 **with transendoscopic balloon dilation**

EXCLUDES *Colonoscopy through stoma (44388, [44401], 44402)*

Code also:

Each additional stricture dilated same session, appending modifier 59 to (44405)

Modifier 52 when colonoscope fails to reach small intestine junction

(74360)

5.28 15.9 FUD 000 T G2

AMA: 2018,Jan,8; 2017,Jan,8; 2016,Jan,13

44406 **with endoscopic ultrasound examination, limited to the sigmoid, descending, transverse, or ascending colon and cecum and adjacent structures**

INCLUDES Gastrointestinal endoscopic ultrasound, supervision and interpretation (76975)

EXCLUDES *Colonoscopy through stoma (44388, 44407)*

Procedure performed more than one time per operative session

Code also modifier 52 when colonoscope fails to reach small intestine junction

6.62 6.62 FUD 000 T G2

AMA: 2018,Jan,8; 2017,Jan,8; 2016,Jan,13

44407 **with transendoscopic ultrasound guided intramural or transmural fine needle aspiration/biopsy(s), includes endoscopic ultrasound examination limited to the sigmoid, descending, transverse, or ascending colon and cecum and adjacent structures**

INCLUDES Gastrointestinal endoscopic ultrasound, supervision and interpretation (76975)

Ultrasonic guidance (76942)

EXCLUDES *Colonoscopy through stoma (44388, 44406)*

Procedure performed more than one time per operative session

Code also modifier 52 when colonoscope fails to reach small intestine junction

8.11 8.11 FUD 000 T G2

AMA: 2018,Jan,8; 2017,Jan,8; 2016,Jan,13

44408 **with decompression (for pathologic distention) (eg, volvulus, megacolon), including placement of decompression tube, when performed**

EXCLUDES *Colonoscopy through stoma; diagnostic (44388)*

Procedure performed more than one time per operative session

6.68 6.68 FUD 000 T R2

AMA: 2018,Jan,8; 2017,Jan,8; 2016,Jan,13

44500 Gastrointestinal Intubation

44500 **Introduction of long gastrointestinal tube (eg, Miller-Abbott) (separate procedure)**

EXCLUDES *Placement oro- or naso-gastric tube (43752)*

(74340)

0.56 0.56 FUD 000 ⊘ T G2 80

AMA: 2020,Aug,9; 2018,Jan,8; 2017,Jan,8; 2016,Sep,9; 2016,Jan,13

44602-44680 Open Repair Procedures of Intestines

44602 **Suture of small intestine (enterorrhaphy) for perforated ulcer, diverticulum, wound, injury or rupture; single perforation**

41.0 41.0 FUD 090 C 80

AMA: 2020,Feb,13

44603 **multiple perforations**

47.1 47.1 FUD 090 C 80

AMA: 2014,Jan,11; 2013,Dec,3

44604 **Suture of large intestine (colorrhaphy) for perforated ulcer, diverticulum, wound, injury or rupture (single or multiple perforations); without colostomy**

30.7 30.7 FUD 090 C 80

AMA: 2014,Jan,11; 2013,Dec,3

44605 **with colostomy**

37.7 37.7 FUD 090 C 80

AMA: 2014,Jan,11; 2013,Dec,3

44615 **Intestinal stricturoplasty (enterotomy and enterorrhaphy) with or without dilation, for intestinal obstruction**

31.1 31.1 FUD 090 C 80

AMA: 2014,Jan,11; 2013,Dec,3

44620 **Closure of enterostomy, large or small intestine;**

EXCLUDES *Laparoscopic method (44227)*

25.1 25.1 FUD 090 C 80

AMA: 2014,Jan,11; 2013,Dec,3

44625 **with resection and anastomosis other than colorectal**

EXCLUDES *Laparoscopic method (44227)*

29.3 29.3 FUD 090 C 80

AMA: 2014,Jan,11; 2013,Dec,3

44626 **with resection and colorectal anastomosis (eg, closure of Hartmann type procedure)**

EXCLUDES *Laparoscopic method (44227)*

46.5 46.5 FUD 090 C 80

AMA: 2014,Jan,11; 2013,Dec,3

44640 **Closure of intestinal cutaneous fistula**

40.6 40.6 FUD 090 C 80

AMA: 2014,Jan,11; 2013,Dec,3

44650 **Closure of enteroenteric or enterocolic fistula**

42.0 42.0 FUD 090 C 80

AMA: 2014,Jan,11; 2013,Dec,3

44660 **Closure of enterovesical fistula; without intestinal or bladder resection**

EXCLUDES *Closure fistula:*

Gastrocolic (43880)

Rectovesical (45800, 45805)

Renocolic (50525-50526)

38.7 38.7 FUD 090 C 80

AMA: 2014,Jan,11; 2013,Dec,3

44661 **with intestine and/or bladder resection**

EXCLUDES *Closure fistula:*

Gastrocolic (43880)

Rectovesical (45800, 45805)

Renocolic (50525-50526)

45.0 45.0 FUD 090 C 80

AMA: 2014,Jan,11; 2013,Dec,3

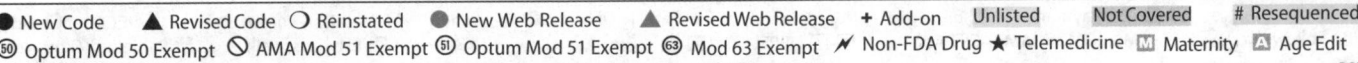

44680 **Intestinal plication (separate procedure)**
INCLUDES Noble intestinal plication
30.8 30.8 FUD 090 C 80
AMA: 2014,Jan,11; 2013,Dec,3

44700-44705 Other Intestinal Procedures

44700 **Exclusion of small intestine from pelvis by mesh or other prosthesis, or native tissue (eg, bladder or omentum)**
EXCLUDES *Therapeutic radiation clinical treatment (77261-77799 [77295, 77385, 77386, 77387, 77424, 77425])*
29.1 29.1 FUD 090 C 80
AMA: 2014,Jan,11; 2013,Dec,3

+ 44701 **Intraoperative colonic lavage (List separately in addition to code for primary procedure)**
EXCLUDES *Appendectomy (44950-44960)*
Code first as appropriate (44140, 44145, 44150, 44604)
4.94 4.94 FUD ZZZ N N1 80
AMA: 2014,Jan,11; 2013,Dec,3

44705 **Preparation of fecal microbiota for instillation, including assessment of donor specimen**
EXCLUDES *Fecal instillation by enema or oro-nasogastric tube (44799)*
Therapeutic enema (74283)
2.16 3.25 FUD XXX B
AMA: 2018,Jan,8; 2017,Jan,8; 2016,Jan,13

44715-44799 Backbench Transplant Procedures

CMS: 100-04,3,90.6 Intestinal and Multi-Visceral Transplants

44715 **Backbench standard preparation of cadaver or living donor intestine allograft prior to transplantation, including mobilization and fashioning of the superior mesenteric artery and vein**
INCLUDES Mobilization/fashioning of superior mesenteric vein/artery
0.00 0.00 FUD XXX C 80
AMA: 2014,Jan,11; 2013,Dec,3

44720 **Backbench reconstruction of cadaver or living donor intestine allograft prior to transplantation; venous anastomosis, each**
8.02 8.02 FUD XXX C 80
AMA: 2014,Jan,11; 2013,Dec,3

44721 **arterial anastomosis, each**
11.2 11.2 FUD XXX C 80
AMA: 2018,Jan,8; 2017,Jan,8; 2016,Jan,13

44799 **Unlisted procedure, small intestine**
EXCLUDES *Unlisted colon procedure (45399)*
Unlisted intestinal procedure performed laparoscopically (44238)
Unlisted rectal procedure (45499, 45999)
0.00 0.00 FUD YYY T
AMA: 2018,Jan,8; 2017,Jan,8; 2016,Jan,13

44800-44899 Meckel's Diverticulum and Mesentery Procedures

44800 **Excision of Meckel's diverticulum (diverticulectomy) or omphalomesenteric duct**
22.3 22.3 FUD 090 C 80
AMA: 2014,Jan,11; 2013,Dec,3

44820 **Excision of lesion of mesentery (separate procedure)**
EXCLUDES *Resection intestine (44120-44128, 44140-44160)*
24.3 24.3 FUD 090 C 80
AMA: 2014,Jan,11; 2013,Dec,3

44850 **Suture of mesentery (separate procedure)**
EXCLUDES *Internal hernia repair/reduction (44050)*
21.7 21.7 FUD 090 C 80
AMA: 2014,Jan,11; 2013,Dec,3

44899 **Unlisted procedure, Meckel's diverticulum and the mesentery**
0.00 0.00 FUD YYY C 80
AMA: 2020,Jul,13

44900-44979 Open and Endoscopic Appendix Procedures

44900 **Incision and drainage of appendiceal abscess, open**
EXCLUDES *Image guided percutaneous catheter drainage (49406)*
22.4 22.4 FUD 090 C 80
AMA: 2014,Jan,11; 2013,Nov,9

44950 **Appendectomy;**
INCLUDES Battle's operation
EXCLUDES *Procedure performed with other intra-abdominal procedure(s) when appendectomy incidental*
18.7 18.7 FUD 090 J G2 80
AMA: 2018,Jan,8; 2017,Jan,8; 2016,Jan,13

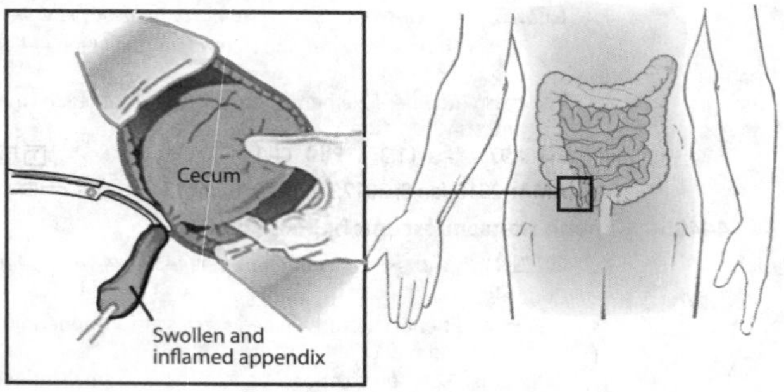

+ 44955 **when done for indicated purpose at time of other major procedure (not as separate procedure) (List separately in addition to code for primary procedure)**
Code first primary procedure
2.45 2.45 FUD ZZZ N N1 80
AMA: 2018,Jan,8; 2017,Jan,8; 2016,Jan,13

44960 **for ruptured appendix with abscess or generalized peritonitis**
INCLUDES Battle's operation
25.5 25.5 FUD 090 C 80
AMA: 2019,Dec,12; 2018,Jan,8; 2017,Jan,8; 2016,Jan,13

44970 **Laparoscopy, surgical, appendectomy**
INCLUDES Diagnostic laparoscopy
17.4 17.4 FUD 090 J G2 80
AMA: 2019,Dec,12; 2018,Jan,8; 2017,Jan,8; 2016,Jan,13

44979 **Unlisted laparoscopy procedure, appendix**
0.00 0.00 FUD YYY J 80 50
AMA: 2018,Jan,8; 2017,Jan,8; 2016,Jan,13

45000-45190 Open and Transrectal Procedures of Rectum

45000 **Transrectal drainage of pelvic abscess**
EXCLUDES *Image guided transrectal catheter drainage (49407)*
12.2 12.2 FUD 090 T A2
AMA: 2014,Jan,11; 2013,Nov,9

45005 **Incision and drainage of submucosal abscess, rectum**
4.69 8.38 FUD 010 T A2
AMA: 2014,Jan,11; 2013,Dec,3

45020 **Incision and drainage of deep supralevator, pelvirectal, or retrorectal abscess**
EXCLUDES *Incision and drainage perianal, ischiorectal, intramural abscess (46050, 46060)*
16.5 16.5 FUD 090 J A2
AMA: 2014,Jan,11; 2013,Dec,3

45100 **Biopsy of anorectal wall, anal approach (eg, congenital megacolon)**
EXCLUDES *Biopsy performed endoscopically (45305)*
8.65 8.65 FUD 090 J A2
AMA: 2014,Jan,11; 2013,Dec,3

45108 **Anorectal myomectomy**
10.7 10.7 FUD 090 J A2
AMA: 2014,Jan,11; 2013,Dec,3

45110 **Proctectomy; complete, combined abdominoperineal, with colostomy**
EXCLUDES *Laparoscopic method (45395)*
53.1 53.1 FUD 090 C 80
AMA: 2014,Jan,11; 2013,Dec,3

45111 **partial resection of rectum, transabdominal approach**
31.4 31.4 FUD 090 C 80
AMA: 2014,Jan,11; 2013,Dec,3

45112 **Proctectomy, combined abdominoperineal, pull-through procedure (eg, colo-anal anastomosis)**
EXCLUDES *Proctectomy for colo-anal anastomosis with colonic pouch or reservoir creation (45119)*
53.9 53.9 FUD 090 C 80
AMA: 2014,Jan,11; 2013,Dec,3

45113 **Proctectomy, partial, with rectal mucosectomy, ileoanal anastomosis, creation of ileal reservoir (S or J), with or without loop ileostomy**
54.7 54.7 FUD 090 C 80
AMA: 2014,Jan,11; 2013,Dec,3

45114 **Proctectomy, partial, with anastomosis; abdominal and transsacral approach**
53.0 53.0 FUD 090 C 80
AMA: 2014,Jan,11; 2013,Dec,3

45116 **transsacral approach only (Kraske type)**
45.1 45.1 FUD 090 C 80
AMA: 2014,Jan,11; 2013,Dec,3

45119 **Proctectomy, combined abdominoperineal pull-through procedure (eg, colo-anal anastomosis), with creation of colonic reservoir (eg, J-pouch), with diverting enterostomy when performed**
EXCLUDES *Laparoscopic method (45397)*
55.9 55.9 FUD 090 C 80
AMA: 2018,Jan,8; 2017,Jan,8; 2016,Jan,13

45120 **Proctectomy, complete (for congenital megacolon), abdominal and perineal approach; with pull-through procedure and anastomosis (eg, Swenson, Duhamel, or Soave type operation)**
46.5 46.5 FUD 090 C 80
AMA: 2014,Jan,11; 2013,Dec,3

45121 **with subtotal or total colectomy, with multiple biopsies**
50.5 50.5 FUD 090 C 80
AMA: 2014,Jan,11; 2013,Dec,3

45123 **Proctectomy, partial, without anastomosis, perineal approach**
32.4 32.4 FUD 090 C 80
AMA: 2014,Jan,11; 2013,Dec,3

45126 **Pelvic exenteration for colorectal malignancy, with proctectomy (with or without colostomy), with removal of bladder and ureteral transplantations, and/or hysterectomy, or cervicectomy, with or without removal of tube(s), with or without removal of ovary(s), or any combination thereof**
80.1 80.1 FUD 090 C 80
AMA: 2014,Jan,11; 2013,Dec,3

45130 **Excision of rectal procidentia, with anastomosis; perineal approach**
INCLUDES Altemeier procedure
31.3 31.3 FUD 090 C 80
AMA: 2014,Jan,11; 2013,Dec,3

45135 **abdominal and perineal approach**
INCLUDES Altemeier procedure
37.6 37.6 FUD 090 C 80
AMA: 2014,Jan,11; 2013,Dec,3

45136 **Excision of ileoanal reservoir with ileostomy**
EXCLUDES *Enterolysis (44005)*
Ileostomy or jejunostomy, non-tube (44310)
51.8 51.8 FUD 090 C 80
AMA: 2014,Jan,11; 2013,Dec,3

45150 **Division of stricture of rectum**
12.1 12.1 FUD 090 T A2 80
AMA: 2014,Jan,11; 2013,Dec,3

45160 **Excision of rectal tumor by proctotomy, transsacral or transcoccygeal approach**
29.7 29.7 FUD 090 J A2 80
AMA: 2014,Jan,11; 2013,Dec,3

45171 **Excision of rectal tumor, transanal approach; not including muscularis propria (ie, partial thickness)**
EXCLUDES *Transanal destruction rectal tumor (45190)*
Transanal endoscopic microsurgical tumor excision (TEMS) (0184T)
17.5 17.5 FUD 090 J G2 80
AMA: 2018,Jan,8; 2017,Jan,8; 2016,Jan,13

45172 **including muscularis propria (ie, full thickness)**
EXCLUDES *Transanal destruction rectal tumor (45190)*
Transanal endoscopic microsurgical tumor excision (TEMS) (0184T)
23.5 23.5 FUD 090 J G2 80
AMA: 2018,Feb,11; 2018,Jan,8; 2017,Jan,8; 2016,Jan,13

45190 **Destruction of rectal tumor (eg, electrodesiccation, electrosurgery, laser ablation, laser resection, cryosurgery) transanal approach**
EXCLUDES *Transanal endoscopic microsurgical tumor excision (TEMS) (0184T)*
Transanal excision rectal tumor (45171-45172)
20.2 20.2 FUD 090 J A2
AMA: 2018,Jan,8; 2017,Jan,8; 2016,Jan,13

45300-45327 Rigid Proctosigmoidoscopy Procedures

INCLUDES Control bleeding due to endoscopic procedure during same operative session
Exam:
Entire rectum
Portion sigmoid colon

EXCLUDES *Computed tomographic colonography (74261-74263)*

Code also examination colon through stoma:
Colonoscopy via stoma (44388-44408 [44401])
Ileoscopy via stoma (44380-44384 [44381])

45300 **Proctosigmoidoscopy, rigid; diagnostic, with or without collection of specimen(s) by brushing or washing (separate procedure)**
(74360)
1.38 3.52 FUD 000 T P3
AMA: 2018,Jan,8; 2017,Jan,8; 2016,Jan,13

45303 **with dilation (eg, balloon, guide wire, bougie)**
(74360)
2.45 27.2 FUD 000 T P2
AMA: 2018,Jan,8; 2017,Jan,8; 2016,Jan,13

45305 **with biopsy, single or multiple**
2.10 4.63 FUD 000 T A2
AMA: 2018,Jan,8; 2017,Jan,8; 2016,Jan,13

45307 **with removal of foreign body**
2.81 5.33 FUD 000 J A2 80
AMA: 2018,Jan,8; 2017,Jan,8; 2016,Jan,13

45308 **with removal of single tumor, polyp, or other lesion by hot biopsy forceps or bipolar cautery**
2.44 5.25 FUD 000 J A2
AMA: 2018,Jan,8; 2017,Jan,8; 2016,Jan,13

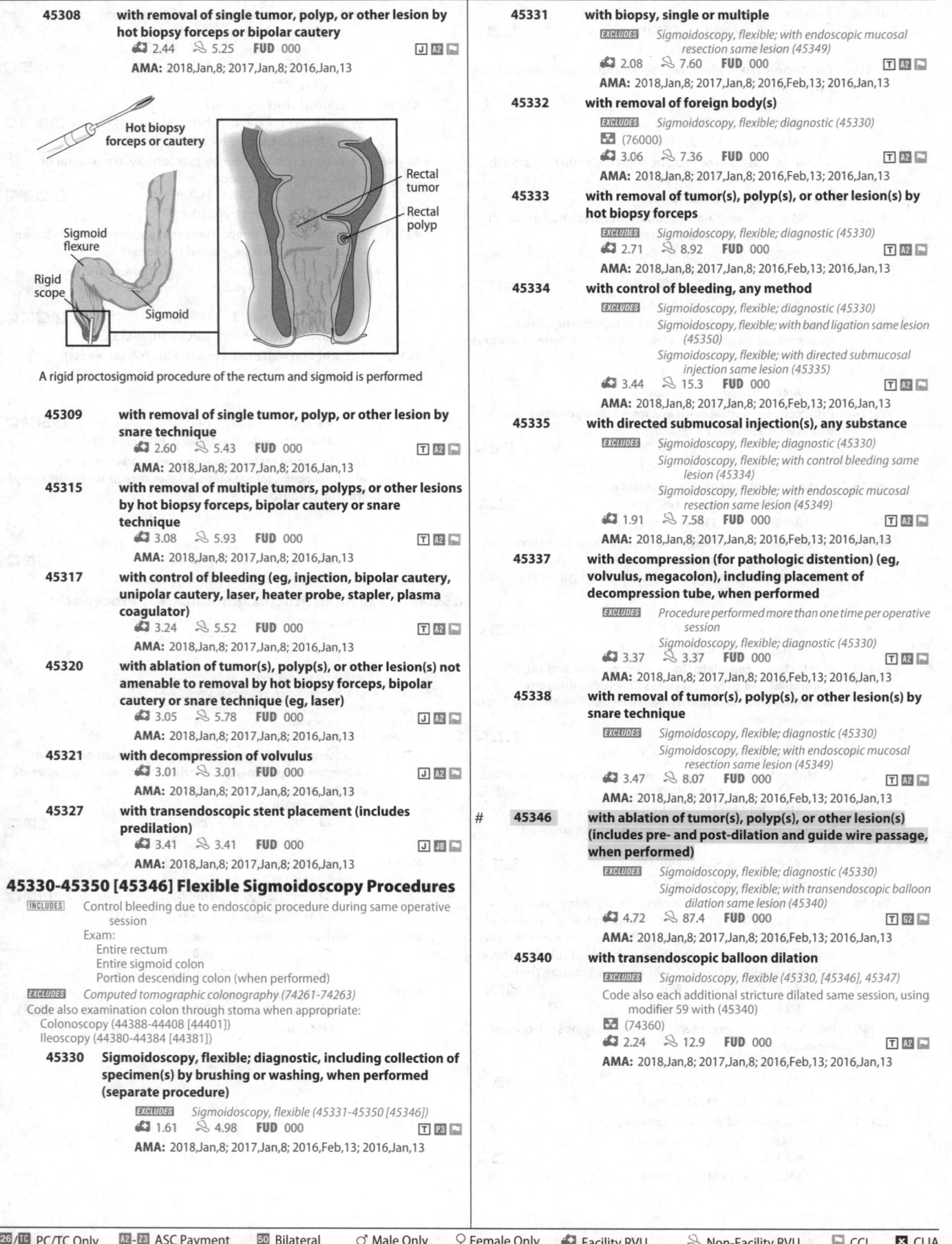

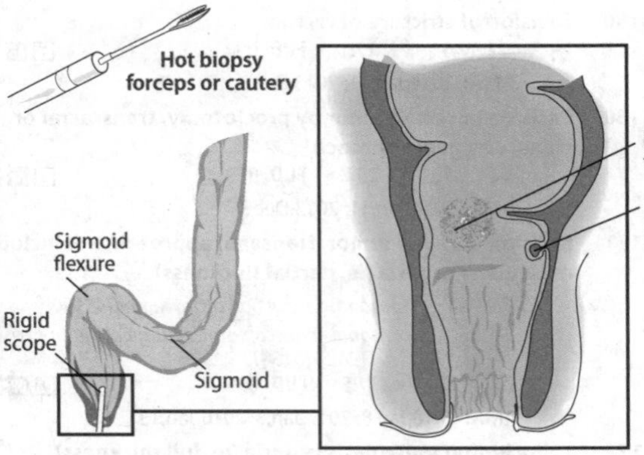

A rigid proctosigmoid procedure of the rectum and sigmoid is performed

45309 **with removal of single tumor, polyp, or other lesion by snare technique**
2.60 5.43 FUD 000 T A2
AMA: 2018,Jan,8; 2017,Jan,8; 2016,Jan,13

45315 **with removal of multiple tumors, polyps, or other lesions by hot biopsy forceps, bipolar cautery or snare technique**
3.08 5.93 FUD 000 T A2
AMA: 2018,Jan,8; 2017,Jan,8; 2016,Jan,13

45317 **with control of bleeding (eg, injection, bipolar cautery, unipolar cautery, laser, heater probe, stapler, plasma coagulator)**
3.24 5.52 FUD 000 T A2
AMA: 2018,Jan,8; 2017,Jan,8; 2016,Jan,13

45320 **with ablation of tumor(s), polyp(s), or other lesion(s) not amenable to removal by hot biopsy forceps, bipolar cautery or snare technique (eg, laser)**
3.05 5.78 FUD 000 J A2
AMA: 2018,Jan,8; 2017,Jan,8; 2016,Jan,13

45321 **with decompression of volvulus**
3.01 3.01 FUD 000 J A2
AMA: 2018,Jan,8; 2017,Jan,8; 2016,Jan,13

45327 **with transendoscopic stent placement (includes predilation)**
3.41 3.41 FUD 000 J J8
AMA: 2018,Jan,8; 2017,Jan,8; 2016,Jan,13

45330-45350 [45346] Flexible Sigmoidoscopy Procedures

INCLUDES Control bleeding due to endoscopic procedure during same operative session
Exam:
- Entire rectum
- Entire sigmoid colon
- Portion descending colon (when performed)

EXCLUDES *Computed tomographic colonography (74261-74263)*

Code also examination colon through stoma when appropriate:
- Colonoscopy (44388-44408 [44401])
- Ileoscopy (44380-44384 [44381])

45330 **Sigmoidoscopy, flexible; diagnostic, including collection of specimen(s) by brushing or washing, when performed (separate procedure)**
EXCLUDES *Sigmoidoscopy, flexible (45331-45350 [45346])*
1.61 4.98 FUD 000 T P3
AMA: 2018,Jan,8; 2017,Jan,8; 2016,Feb,13; 2016,Jan,13

45331 **with biopsy, single or multiple**
EXCLUDES *Sigmoidoscopy, flexible; with endoscopic mucosal resection same lesion (45349)*
2.08 7.60 FUD 000 T A2
AMA: 2018,Jan,8; 2017,Jan,8; 2016,Feb,13; 2016,Jan,13

45332 **with removal of foreign body(s)**
EXCLUDES *Sigmoidoscopy, flexible; diagnostic (45330)*
(76000)
3.06 7.36 FUD 000 T A2
AMA: 2018,Jan,8; 2017,Jan,8; 2016,Feb,13; 2016,Jan,13

45333 **with removal of tumor(s), polyp(s), or other lesion(s) by hot biopsy forceps**
EXCLUDES *Sigmoidoscopy, flexible; diagnostic (45330)*
2.71 8.92 FUD 000 T A2
AMA: 2018,Jan,8; 2017,Jan,8; 2016,Feb,13; 2016,Jan,13

45334 **with control of bleeding, any method**
EXCLUDES *Sigmoidoscopy, flexible; diagnostic (45330)*
Sigmoidoscopy, flexible; with band ligation same lesion (45350)
Sigmoidoscopy, flexible; with directed submucosal injection same lesion (45335)
3.44 15.3 FUD 000 T A2
AMA: 2018,Jan,8; 2017,Jan,8; 2016,Feb,13; 2016,Jan,13

45335 **with directed submucosal injection(s), any substance**
EXCLUDES *Sigmoidoscopy, flexible; diagnostic (45330)*
Sigmoidoscopy, flexible; with control bleeding same lesion (45334)
Sigmoidoscopy, flexible; with endoscopic mucosal resection same lesion (45349)
1.91 7.58 FUD 000 T A2
AMA: 2018,Jan,8; 2017,Jan,8; 2016,Feb,13; 2016,Jan,13

45337 **with decompression (for pathologic distention) (eg, volvulus, megacolon), including placement of decompression tube, when performed**
EXCLUDES *Procedure performed more than one time per operative session*
Sigmoidoscopy, flexible; diagnostic (45330)
3.37 3.37 FUD 000 T A2
AMA: 2018,Jan,8; 2017,Jan,8; 2016,Feb,13; 2016,Jan,13

45338 **with removal of tumor(s), polyp(s), or other lesion(s) by snare technique**
EXCLUDES *Sigmoidoscopy, flexible; diagnostic (45330)*
Sigmoidoscopy, flexible; with endoscopic mucosal resection same lesion (45349)
3.47 8.07 FUD 000 T A2
AMA: 2018,Jan,8; 2017,Jan,8; 2016,Feb,13; 2016,Jan,13

45346 **with ablation of tumor(s), polyp(s), or other lesion(s) (includes pre- and post-dilation and guide wire passage, when performed)**
EXCLUDES *Sigmoidoscopy, flexible; diagnostic (45330)*
Sigmoidoscopy, flexible; with transendoscopic balloon dilation same lesion (45340)
4.72 87.4 FUD 000 T G2
AMA: 2018,Jan,8; 2017,Jan,8; 2016,Feb,13; 2016,Jan,13

45340 **with transendoscopic balloon dilation**
EXCLUDES *Sigmoidoscopy, flexible (45330, [45346], 45347)*
Code also each additional stricture dilated same session, using modifier 59 with (45340)
(74360)
2.24 12.9 FUD 000 T A2
AMA: 2018,Jan,8; 2017,Jan,8; 2016,Feb,13; 2016,Jan,13

45341 **with endoscopic ultrasound examination**

INCLUDES Gastrointestinal endoscopic ultrasound, supervision, and interpretation (76975)
Ultrasound, transrectal (76872)

EXCLUDES *Procedure performed more than one time per operative session*
Sigmoidoscopy, flexible (45330, 45342)

3.57 3.57 FUD 000 T A2

AMA: 2018,Jan,8; 2017,Jan,8; 2016,Feb,13; 2016,Jan,13

45342 **with transendoscopic ultrasound guided intramural or transmural fine needle aspiration/biopsy(s)**

INCLUDES Gastrointestinal endoscopic ultrasound, supervision and interpretation (76975)
Ultrasonic guidance (76942)
Ultrasound, transrectal (76872)

EXCLUDES *Procedure performed more than one time per operative session*
Sigmoidoscopy, flexible (45330, 45341)

4.89 4.89 FUD 000 T A2

AMA: 2018,Jan,8; 2017,Jan,8; 2016,Feb,13; 2016,Jan,13

45346 **Resequenced code. See code following 45338.**

45347 **with placement of endoscopic stent (includes pre- and post-dilation and guide wire passage, when performed)**

EXCLUDES *Sigmoidoscopy, flexible (45330, 45340)*
(74360)

4.44 4.44 FUD 000 J J8

AMA: 2018,Jan,8; 2017,Jan,8; 2016,Feb,13; 2016,Jan,13

45349 **with endoscopic mucosal resection**

EXCLUDES *Procedure performed same lesion with (45331, 45335, 45338, 45350)*
Sigmoidoscopy, flexible; diagnostic (45330)

5.73 5.73 FUD 000 T G2

AMA: 2020,May,13; 2019,Dec,14; 2018,Jan,8; 2017,Jan,8; 2016,Jan,13

45350 **with band ligation(s) (eg, hemorrhoids)**

EXCLUDES *Hemorrhoidectomy, internal, by rubber band ligation (46221)*
Procedure performed more than one time per operative session
Sigmoidoscopy, flexible; diagnostic (45330)
Sigmoidoscopy, flexible; with control bleeding same lesion (45334)
Sigmoidoscopy, flexible; with endoscopic mucosal resection (45349)

2.92 17.8 FUD 000 T G2

AMA: 2020,Feb,11; 2018,Jan,8; 2017,Jan,8; 2016,Jan,13

45378-45398 [45388, 45390, 45398] Flexible and Rigid Colonoscopy Procedures

INCLUDES Control bleeding due to endoscopic procedure during same operative session
Exam:
Entire colon (rectum to cecum)
Terminal ileum (when performed)

EXCLUDES *Computed tomographic colonography (74261-74263)*

Code also modifier 53 (physician), or 73, 74 (facility) for incomplete colonoscopy

45378 **Colonoscopy, flexible; diagnostic, including collection of specimen(s) by brushing or washing, when performed (separate procedure)**

EXCLUDES *Colonoscopy, flexible (45379-45393 [45388, 45390, 45398])*
Decompression for pathological distention (45393)

5.35 9.42 FUD 000 T A2

AMA: 2018,Jan,7; 2018,Jan,8; 2017,Sep,14; 2017,Jan,8; 2016,Jan,13

45379 **with removal of foreign body(s)**

EXCLUDES *Colonoscopy, flexible; diagnostic (45378)*

Code also modifier 52 when colonoscope fails to reach small intestine junction
(76000)

6.91 12.1 FUD 000 T A2

AMA: 2018,Jan,8; 2017,Jan,8; 2016,Jan,13

45380 **with biopsy, single or multiple**

EXCLUDES *Colonoscopy, flexible; diagnostic (45378)*
Colonoscopy, flexible; with endoscopic mucosal resection same lesion (45390)

Code also modifier 52 when colonoscope fails to reach small intestine junction

5.87 11.7 FUD 000 T A2

AMA: 2018,Jan,8; 2017,Jan,8; 2016,Jan,13

45381 **with directed submucosal injection(s), any substance**

EXCLUDES *Colonoscopy, flexible; diagnostic (45378)*
Colonoscopy, flexible; with control bleeding same lesion (45382)
Colonoscopy, flexible; with endoscopic mucosal resection same lesion (45390)

Code also modifier 52 when colonoscope fails to reach small intestine junction

5.87 11.5 FUD 000 T A2

AMA: 2018,Jan,8; 2017,Jan,8; 2017,Jan,6; 2016,Jan,13

45382 **with control of bleeding, any method**

EXCLUDES *Colonoscopy, flexible; diagnostic (45378)*
Colonoscopy, flexible; with band ligation same lesion ([45398])
Colonoscopy, flexible; with directed submucosal injection same lesion (45381)

Code also modifier 52 when colonoscope fails to reach small intestine junction

7.48 20.0 FUD 000 T A2

AMA: 2018,Jan,8; 2017,Jan,8; 2016,Jan,13

\# **45388** **with ablation of tumor(s), polyp(s), or other lesion(s) (includes pre- and post-dilation and guide wire passage, when performed)**

EXCLUDES *Colonoscopy, flexible (45378, 45386)*

7.83 82.9 FUD 000 T G2

AMA: 2018,Jan,8; 2017,Jan,8; 2016,Jan,13

45384 **with removal of tumor(s), polyp(s), or other lesion(s) by hot biopsy forceps**

EXCLUDES *Colonoscopy, flexible; diagnostic (45378)*

Code also modifier 52 when colonoscope fails to reach small intestine junction

6.68 13.1 FUD 000 T A2

AMA: 2018,Jan,8; 2017,Jan,8; 2016,Jan,13

45385 **with removal of tumor(s), polyp(s), or other lesion(s) by snare technique**

EXCLUDES *Colonoscopy, flexible; diagnostic (45378)*
Colonoscopy, flexible; with endoscopic mucosal resection same lesion (45390)

7.35 12.6 FUD 000 T A2

AMA: 2018,Jan,8; 2017,Jan,8; 2017,Jan,6; 2016,Jan,13

45386 **with transendoscopic balloon dilation**

EXCLUDES *Colonoscopy, flexible (45378, [45388], 45389)*

Code also each additional stricture dilated same operative session, using modifier 59 with (45386)
(74360)

6.20 17.0 FUD 000 T A2

AMA: 2018,Jan,8; 2017,Jan,8; 2016,Jan,13

45388 **Resequenced code. See code following 45382.**

45389 **with endoscopic stent placement (includes pre- and post-dilation and guide wire passage, when performed)**

EXCLUDES *Colonoscopy, flexible (45378, 45386)*
(74360)

8.37 8.37 FUD 000 J J8

AMA: 2018,Jan,8; 2017,Jan,8; 2016,Jan,13

45390 **Resequenced code. See code following 45392.**

Digestive System
45341 — 45390

● New Code ▲ Revised Code ○ Reinstated ● New Web Release ▲ Revised Web Release + Add-on Unlisted Not Covered # Resequenced
Optum Mod 50 Exempt ⊘ AMA Mod 51 Exempt Optum Mod 51 Exempt Mod 63 Exempt Non-FDA Drug ★ Telemedicine Maternity Age Edit

45391 **with endoscopic ultrasound examination limited to the rectum, sigmoid, descending, transverse, or ascending colon and cecum, and adjacent structures**

INCLUDES Gastrointestinal endoscopic ultrasound, supervision and interpretation (76975)
Ultrasound, transrectal (76872)

EXCLUDES *Colonoscopy, flexible (45378, 45392)*
Procedure performed more than one time per operative session

7.43 7.43 FUD 000 T A2

AMA: 2018,Jan,8; 2017,Jan,8; 2016,Jan,13

45392 **with transendoscopic ultrasound guided intramural or transmural fine needle aspiration/biopsy(s), includes endoscopic ultrasound examination limited to the rectum, sigmoid, descending, transverse, or ascending colon and cecum, and adjacent structures**

INCLUDES Gastrointestinal endoscopic ultrasound, supervision and interpretation (76975)
Ultrasonic guidance (76942)
Ultrasound, transrectal (76872)

EXCLUDES *Colonoscopy, flexible (45378, 45391)*
Procedure performed more than one time per operative session

8.78 8.78 FUD 000 T A2

AMA: 2018,Jan,8; 2017,Jan,8; 2016,Jan,13

\# **45390** **with endoscopic mucosal resection**

EXCLUDES *Colonoscopy, flexible; diagnostic (45378)*
Colonoscopy, flexible; with band ligation same lesion ([45398])
Colonoscopy, flexible; with biopsy same lesion (45380-45381)
Colonoscopy, flexible; with removal tumor(s), polyp(s), or other lesion(s) by snare technique same lesion (45385)

9.79 9.79 FUD 000 T G2

AMA: 2020,May,13; 2019,Dec,14; 2018,Jan,8; 2017,Jan,6; 2017,Jan,8; 2016,Jan,13

45393 **with decompression (for pathologic distention) (eg, volvulus, megacolon), including placement of decompression tube, when performed**

EXCLUDES *Colonoscopy, flexible; diagnostic (45378)*
Procedure performed more than one time per operative session

7.31 7.31 FUD 000 T G2

AMA: 2018,Jan,8; 2017,Jan,8; 2016,Jan,13

\# **45398** **with band ligation(s) (eg, hemorrhoids)**

EXCLUDES *Bleeding control by band ligation (45382)*
Colonoscopy, flexible (45378, 45390)
Hemorrhoidectomy, internal, by rubber band ligation (46221)
Procedure performed more than one time per operative session

Code also modifier 52 when colonoscope fails to reach small intestine junction

6.83 22.3 FUD 000 T G2

AMA: 2020,Feb,11; 2018,Jan,8; 2018,Jan,7; 2017,Sep,14; 2017,Jan,8; 2016,Jan,13

45395-45499 [45398, 45399] Laparoscopic Procedures of Rectum

INCLUDES Diagnostic laparoscopy

45395 **Laparoscopy, surgical; proctectomy, complete, combined abdominoperineal, with colostomy**

EXCLUDES *Open method (45110)*

56.8 56.8 FUD 090 C 80

AMA: 2018,Jan,8; 2017,Jan,8; 2016,Jan,13

45397 **proctectomy, combined abdominoperineal pull-through procedure (eg, colo-anal anastomosis), with creation of colonic reservoir (eg, J-pouch), with diverting enterostomy, when performed**

EXCLUDES *Open method (45119)*

61.8 61.8 FUD 090 C 80

AMA: 2018,Jan,8; 2017,Jan,8; 2016,Jan,13

45398 **Resequenced code. See code following 45393.**

45399 **Resequenced code. See code before 45990.**

45400 **Laparoscopy, surgical; proctopexy (for prolapse)**

EXCLUDES *Open method (45540-45541)*

32.8 32.8 FUD 090 C 80

AMA: 2018,Jan,8; 2017,Jan,8; 2016,Jan,13

45402 **proctopexy (for prolapse), with sigmoid resection**

EXCLUDES *Open method (45550)*

43.8 43.8 FUD 090 C 80

AMA: 2018,Jan,8; 2017,Jan,8; 2016,Jan,13

45499 **Unlisted laparoscopy procedure, rectum**

EXCLUDES *Unlisted rectal procedure performed via open technique (45999)*

0.00 0.00 FUD YYY J 80

AMA: 2014,Jan,11; 2013,Jan,11-12

45500-45825 Open Repairs of Rectum

45500 **Proctoplasty; for stenosis**

16.3 16.3 FUD 090 J A2 80

AMA: 2014,Jan,11; 2013,Jan,11-12

45505 **for prolapse of mucous membrane**

17.2 17.2 FUD 090 J A2

AMA: 2018,Jan,8; 2017,Jan,8; 2016,Jan,13

45520 **Perirectal injection of sclerosing solution for prolapse**

1.16 4.41 FUD 000 Q1 N1

AMA: 2018,Jan,8; 2017,Jan,8; 2016,Jan,13

45540 **Proctopexy (eg, for prolapse); abdominal approach**

EXCLUDES *Laparoscopic method (45400)*

30.6 30.6 FUD 090 C 80

AMA: 2014,Jan,11; 2013,Jan,11-12

45541 **perineal approach**

27.3 27.3 FUD 090 J G2 80

AMA: 2014,Jan,11; 2013,Jan,11-12

45550 **with sigmoid resection, abdominal approach**

INCLUDES Frickman proctopexy

EXCLUDES *Laparoscopic method (45402)*

42.3 42.3 FUD 090 C 80

AMA: 2014,Jan,11; 2013,Jan,11-12

45560 **Repair of rectocele (separate procedure)**

EXCLUDES *Posterior colporrhaphy with rectocele repair (57250)*

19.7 19.7 FUD 090 J A2 80

AMA: 2014,Jan,11; 2013,Jan,11-12

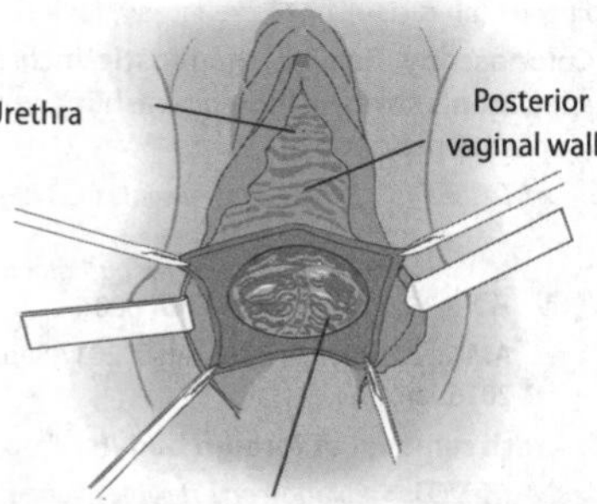

The posterior wall of the vagina is opened directly over the rectocele; the walls of both structures are repaired; a rectocele is a herniated protrusion of part of the rectum into the vagina

45562 **Exploration, repair, and presacral drainage for rectal injury;**
32.7 32.7 FUD 090 C 80
AMA: 2014,Jan,11; 2013,Jan,11-12

45563 **with colostomy**
INCLUDES Maydl colostomy
48.3 48.3 FUD 090 C 80
AMA: 2014,Jan,11; 2013,Jan,11-12

45800 **Closure of rectovesical fistula;**
36.7 36.7 FUD 090 C 80
AMA: 2014,Jan,11; 2013,Jan,11-12

45805 **with colostomy**
42.8 42.8 FUD 090 C 80
AMA: 2014,Jan,11; 2013,Jan,11-12

45820 **Closure of rectourethral fistula;**
EXCLUDES *Closure fistula, rectovaginal (57300-57308)*
37.0 37.0 FUD 090 C 80
AMA: 2014,Jan,11; 2013,Jan,11-12

45825 **with colostomy**
EXCLUDES *Closure fistula, rectovaginal (57300-57308)*
44.4 44.4 FUD 090 C 80
AMA: 2014,Jan,11; 2013,Jan,11-12

45900-45999 [45399] Closed Procedures of Rectum With Anesthesia

45900 **Reduction of procidentia (separate procedure) under anesthesia**
6.14 6.14 FUD 010 T A2 80
AMA: 2014,Jan,11; 2013,Jan,11-12

45905 **Dilation of anal sphincter (separate procedure) under anesthesia other than local**
4.86 4.86 FUD 010 T A2
AMA: 2014,Jan,11; 2013,Jan,11-12

45910 **Dilation of rectal stricture (separate procedure) under anesthesia other than local**
5.54 5.54 FUD 010 T A2
AMA: 2014,Jan,11; 2013,Jan,11-12

45915 **Removal of fecal impaction or foreign body (separate procedure) under anesthesia**
6.65 9.90 FUD 010 T A2
AMA: 2018,Jan,8; 2017,Jan,8; 2016,Jan,13

45399 **Unlisted procedure, colon**
0.00 0.00 FUD YYY T
AMA: 2018,Jan,8; 2017,Jan,8; 2016,Jan,13

45990 **Anorectal exam, surgical, requiring anesthesia (general, spinal, or epidural), diagnostic**
INCLUDES Diagnostic:
Anoscopy
Proctoscopy, rigid
Exam:
Pelvic (when performed)
Perineal, external
Rectal, digital
EXCLUDES *Anogenital examination (99170)*
Anoscopy; diagnostic (46600)
Pelvic examination under anesthesia (57410)
Proctosigmoidoscopy, rigid (45300-45327)
3.09 3.09 FUD 000 J A2 80
AMA: 2018,Jan,8; 2017,Jan,8; 2016,Jan,13

45999 **Unlisted procedure, rectum**
EXCLUDES *Unlisted rectal procedure performed laparoscopically (45499)*
0.00 0.00 FUD YYY T 80
AMA: 2018,Jan,8; 2017,Jan,8; 2016,Jan,13

46020-46083 Surgical Incision of Anus

EXCLUDES *Cryosurgical destruction hemorrhoid(s) (46999)*
Fistulotomy, subcutaneous (46270)
Hemorrhoidopexy ([46947])
Injection hemorrhoid(s) (46500)
Thermal energy destruction internal hemorrhoid(s) (46930)

46020 **Placement of seton**
EXCLUDES *Anoscopy; diagnostic (46600)*
Incision and drainage ischiorectal or intramural abscess (46060)
Surgical anal fistula treatment (46280)
6.82 8.10 FUD 010 J A2
AMA: 2014,Jan,11; 2013,Jan,11-12

46030 **Removal of anal seton, other marker**
2.59 4.13 FUD 010 T A2 80
AMA: 2014,Jan,11; 2013,Jan,11-12

46040 **Incision and drainage of ischiorectal and/or perirectal abscess (separate procedure)**
12.1 15.7 FUD 090 T A2
AMA: 2014,Jan,11; 2013,Jan,11-12

46045 **Incision and drainage of intramural, intramuscular, or submucosal abscess, transanal, under anesthesia**
12.6 12.6 FUD 090 J A2
AMA: 2014,Jan,11; 2013,Jan,11-12

46050 **Incision and drainage, perianal abscess, superficial**
EXCLUDES *Incision and drainage abscess:*
Ischiorectal/intramural (46060)
Supralevator/pelvirectal/retrorectal (45020)
2.85 6.27 FUD 010 T A2
AMA: 2014,Jan,11; 2013,Jan,11-12

46060 **Incision and drainage of ischiorectal or intramural abscess, with fistulectomy or fistulotomy, submuscular, with or without placement of seton**
EXCLUDES *Incision and drainage abscess:*
Supralevator/pelvirectal/retrorectal (45020)
Placement seton (46020)
13.8 13.8 FUD 090 J A2
AMA: 2014,Jan,11; 2013,Jan,11-12

46070 **Incision, anal septum (infant)** A
EXCLUDES *Anoplasty (46700-46705)*
7.52 7.52 FUD 090 63 J G2 80
AMA: 2014,Jan,11; 2013,Jan,11-12

46080 **Sphincterotomy, anal, division of sphincter (separate procedure)**
4.59 7.41 FUD 010 J A2
AMA: 2014,Jan,11; 2013,Jan,11-12

46083 **Incision of thrombosed hemorrhoid, external**
3.08 5.24 FUD 010 T P2
AMA: 2018,Jan,8; 2017,Jan,8; 2016,Jan,13

46200-46262 [46220, 46320, 46945, 46946, 46948] Anal Resection and Hemorrhoidectomies

EXCLUDES *Cryosurgical destruction hemorrhoid(s) (46999)*
Hemorrhoidopexy ([46947])
Injection hemorrhoid(s) (46500)
Thermal energy destruction internal hemorrhoid(s) (46930)

46200 **Fissurectomy, including sphincterotomy, when performed**
9.45 13.0 FUD 090 J A2
AMA: 2014,Jan,11; 2013,Jan,11-12

46220 **Resequenced code. See code before 46230.**

46221 **Hemorrhoidectomy, internal, by rubber band ligation(s)**
EXCLUDES *Colonoscopy or sigmoidoscopy, flexible; with band ligation (45350, [45398])*
Transanal hemorrhoidal dearterialization, two or more columns/groups ([46948])
5.51 7.77 FUD 010 T P3
AMA: 2020,Feb,11; 2018,Jan,8; 2018,Jan,7; 2017,Sep,14; 2017,Jan,8; 2016,Jan,13

Digestive System

45562 — 46221

 # 46945 Hemorrhoidectomy, internal, by ligation other than rubber band; single hemorrhoid column/group, without imaging guidance

EXCLUDES *Transanal hemorrhoidal dearterialization, two or more columns/groups ([46948])*
Ultrasonic guidance (76942)
Ultrasonic guidance, intraoperative (76998)
Ultrasound, transrectal (76872)

6.54 9.08 **FUD** 090 J R2

AMA: 2020,Feb,11; 2018,Jan,8; 2017,Jan,8; 2016,Jan,13

 # 46946 2 or more hemorrhoid columns/groups, without imaging guidance

EXCLUDES *Transanal hemorrhoidal dearterialization, two or more columns/groups ([46948])*
Ultrasonic guidance (76942)
Ultrasonic guidance, intraoperative (76998)
Ultrasound, transrectal (76872)

6.50 9.17 **FUD** 090 J A2

AMA: 2020,Feb,11; 2018,Jan,8; 2017,Jan,8; 2016,Jan,13

 # 46948 Hemorrhoidectomy, internal, by transanal hemorrhoidal dearterialization, 2 or more hemorrhoid columns/groups, including ultrasound guidance, with mucopexy, when performed

INCLUDES Ultrasonic guidance (76872, 76942, 76998)

EXCLUDES *Transanal hemorrhoidal dearterialization, single column/group (46999)*

12.7 12.7 **FUD** 090 G2

AMA: 2020,Feb,11

 # 46220 Excision of single external papilla or tag, anus

3.43 6.54 **FUD** 010 T A2

AMA: 2014,Jan,11; 2013,Jan,11-12

46230 Excision of multiple external papillae or tags, anus

5.00 8.43 **FUD** 010 J A2

AMA: 2014,Jan,11; 2013,Jan,11-12

 # 46320 Excision of thrombosed hemorrhoid, external

3.22 5.65 **FUD** 010 T P3

AMA: 2014,Jan,11; 2013,Jan,11-12

46250 Hemorrhoidectomy, external, 2 or more columns/groups

EXCLUDES *Hemorrhoidectomy, external, single column/group (46999)*
Transanal hemorrhoidal dearterialization, two or more columns/groups ([46948])

9.19 13.6 **FUD** 090 J A2

AMA: 2014,Jan,11; 2013,Jan,11-12

46255 Hemorrhoidectomy, internal and external, single column/group;

EXCLUDES *Transanal hemorrhoidal dearterialization, two or more columns/groups ([46948])*

10.3 14.8 **FUD** 090 J A2

AMA: 2018,Jan,8; 2017,Jan,8; 2016,Jan,13

46257 with fissurectomy

EXCLUDES *Transanal hemorrhoidal dearterialization, two or more columns/groups ([46948])*

12.3 12.3 **FUD** 090 J A2

AMA: 2014,Jan,11; 2013,Jan,11-12

46258 with fistulectomy, including fissurectomy, when performed

EXCLUDES *Transanal hemorrhoidal dearterialization, two or more columns/groups ([46948])*

13.7 13.7 **FUD** 090 J A2 80

AMA: 2014,Jan,11; 2013,Jan,11-12

46260 Hemorrhoidectomy, internal and external, 2 or more columns/groups;

INCLUDES Whitehead hemorrhoidectomy

EXCLUDES *Transanal hemorrhoidal dearterialization, two or more columns/groups ([46948])*

13.8 13.8 **FUD** 090 J A2

AMA: 2014,Jan,11; 2013,Jan,11-12

46261 with fissurectomy

EXCLUDES *Transanal hemorrhoidal dearterialization, two or more columns/groups ([46948])*

15.1 15.1 **FUD** 090 J A2

AMA: 2014,Jan,11; 2013,Jan,11-12

46262 with fistulectomy, including fissurectomy, when performed

EXCLUDES *Transanal hemorrhoidal dearterialization, two or more columns/groups ([46948])*

16.0 16.0 **FUD** 090 J A2

AMA: 2018,Jan,8; 2017,Jan,8; 2016,Jan,13

46270-46320 [46320] Resection of Anal Fistula

46270 Surgical treatment of anal fistula (fistulectomy/fistulotomy); subcutaneous

11.3 14.8 **FUD** 090 J A2

AMA: 2014,Jan,11; 2013,Jan,11-12

46275 intersphincteric

11.9 15.6 **FUD** 090 J A2

AMA: 2014,Jan,11; 2013,Jan,11-12

46280 transsphincteric, suprasphincteric, extrasphincteric or multiple, including placement of seton, when performed

EXCLUDES *Placement seton (46020)*

13.7 13.7 **FUD** 090 J A2

AMA: 2014,Jan,11; 2013,Jan,11-12

46285 second stage

12.0 15.7 **FUD** 090 J A2

AMA: 2014,Jan,11; 2013,Jan,11-12

46288 Closure of anal fistula with rectal advancement flap

15.8 15.8 **FUD** 090 J A2

AMA: 2014,Jan,11; 2013,Jan,11-12

46320 **Resequenced code. See code following 46230.**

46500 Other Hemorrhoid Procedures

EXCLUDES *Anoscopic injection bulking agent, submucosal, for fecal incontinence (46999)*

46500 Injection of sclerosing solution, hemorrhoids

5.20 8.54 **FUD** 010 T P3

AMA: 2018,Jan,8; 2017,Jan,8; 2016,Jan,13

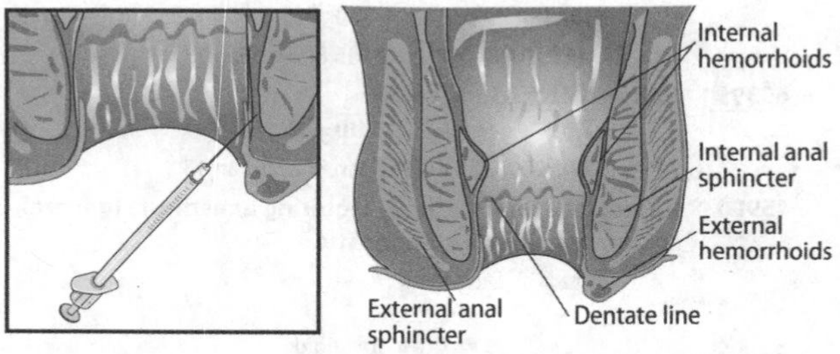

A sclerosing agent is injected into the tissues underlying hemorrhoids

46505 Chemodenervation Anal Sphincter

EXCLUDES *Chemodenervation:*
Extremity muscles (64642-64645)
Muscles/facial nerve (64612)
Neck muscles (64616)
Other peripheral nerve/branch (64640)
Pudendal nerve (64630)
Trunk muscles (64646-64647)

Code also drug(s)/substance(s) given

46505 Chemodenervation of internal anal sphincter

7.00 8.55 **FUD** 010 T G2 50

AMA: 2019,Apr,9; 2018,Jan,8; 2017,Jan,8; 2016,Jan,13

46600-46615 Anoscopic Procedures

EXCLUDES *Delivery thermal energy via anoscope to anal canal muscle (46999)*
Injection bulking agent, submucosal, for fecal incontinence (46999)

46600 Anoscopy; diagnostic, including collection of specimen(s) by brushing or washing, when performed (separate procedure)

EXCLUDES *Excision rectal tumor, transanal endoscopic microsurgical approach (i.e., TEMS) (0184T)*
High-resolution anoscopy (HRA), diagnostic (46601)
Surgical incision anus (46020-46761 [46220, 46320, 46320, 46945, 46946, 46947, 46948])

1.17 2.94 FUD 000 Q1 N1

AMA: 2018,Jan,7; 2018,Jan,8; 2017,Jan,8; 2016,Jan,13

46601 diagnostic, with high-resolution magnification (HRA) (eg, colposcope, operating microscope) and chemical agent enhancement, including collection of specimen(s) by brushing or washing, when performed

INCLUDES Operating microscope (69990)

2.72 3.88 FUD 000 Q1 N1

AMA: 2018,Oct,11; 2016,Feb,12

46604 with dilation (eg, balloon, guide wire, bougie)

1.90 18.3 FUD 000 T P2

AMA: 2018,Jan,8; 2017,Jan,8; 2016,Jan,13

46606 with biopsy, single or multiple

EXCLUDES *High resolution anoscopy (HRA) with biopsy (46607)*

2.17 7.31 FUD 000 T P3

AMA: 2019,Sep,10; 2018,Jan,8; 2017,Jan,8; 2016,Jan,13

46607 with high-resolution magnification (HRA) (eg, colposcope, operating microscope) and chemical agent enhancement, with biopsy, single or multiple

INCLUDES Operating microscope (69990)

3.65 5.75 FUD 000 T G2

AMA: 2019,Dec,12; 2018,Oct,11; 2016,Feb,12

46608 with removal of foreign body

2.44 7.68 FUD 000 T A2

AMA: 2018,Jan,8; 2017,Jan,8; 2016,Jan,13

46610 with removal of single tumor, polyp, or other lesion by hot biopsy forceps or bipolar cautery

2.34 7.30 FUD 000 J A2

AMA: 2018,Jan,8; 2017,Jan,8; 2016,Jan,13

46611 with removal of single tumor, polyp, or other lesion by snare technique

2.31 5.78 FUD 000 T A2

AMA: 2018,Jan,8; 2017,Jan,8; 2016,Jan,13

46612 with removal of multiple tumors, polyps, or other lesions by hot biopsy forceps, bipolar cautery or snare technique

2.76 8.90 FUD 000 J A2

AMA: 2018,Jan,8; 2017,Jan,8; 2016,Jan,13

46614 with control of bleeding (eg, injection, bipolar cautery, unipolar cautery, laser, heater probe, stapler, plasma coagulator)

1.85 4.21 FUD 000 T P3

AMA: 2018,Jan,8; 2017,Jan,8; 2016,Jan,13

46615 with ablation of tumor(s), polyp(s), or other lesion(s) not amenable to removal by hot biopsy forceps, bipolar cautery or snare technique

2.64 4.34 FUD 000 J A2

AMA: 2018,Jan,8; 2017,Jan,8; 2016,Jan,13

46700-46947 [46947] Anal Repairs and Stapled Hemorrhoidopexy

46700 Anoplasty, plastic operation for stricture; adult

18.9 18.9 FUD 090 J A2

AMA: 2014,Jan,11; 2013,Jan,11-12

46705 infant A

EXCLUDES *Anal septum incision (46070)*

16.1 16.1 FUD 090 63 C 80

AMA: 2014,Jan,11; 2013,Jan,11-12

46706 Repair of anal fistula with fibrin glue

5.14 5.14 FUD 010 J A2

AMA: 2014,Jan,11; 2013,Jan,11-12

46707 Repair of anorectal fistula with plug (eg, porcine small intestine submucosa [SIS])

14.4 14.4 FUD 090 J J8 80

AMA: 2018,Jan,8; 2017,Jan,8; 2016,Jan,13

46710 Repair of ileoanal pouch fistula/sinus (eg, perineal or vaginal), pouch advancement; transperineal approach

32.3 32.3 FUD 090 C 80

AMA: 2018,Jan,8; 2017,Jan,8; 2016,Jan,13

46712 combined transperineal and transabdominal approach

65.0 65.0 FUD 090 C 80

AMA: 2018,Jan,8; 2017,Jan,8; 2016,Jan,13

46715 Repair of low imperforate anus; with anoperineal fistula (cut-back procedure)

15.9 15.9 FUD 090 63 C 80

AMA: 2014,Jan,11; 2013,Jan,11-12

46716 with transposition of anoperineal or anovestibular fistula

35.4 35.4 FUD 090 63 C 80

AMA: 2014,Jan,11; 2013,Jan,11-12

46730 Repair of high imperforate anus without fistula; perineal or sacroperineal approach

57.4 57.4 FUD 090 63 C 80

AMA: 2014,Jan,11; 2013,Jan,11-12

46735 combined transabdominal and sacroperineal approaches

66.2 66.2 FUD 090 63 C 80

AMA: 2014,Jan,11; 2013,Jan,11-12

46740 Repair of high imperforate anus with rectourethral or rectovaginal fistula; perineal or sacroperineal approach

62.7 62.7 FUD 090 63 C 80

AMA: 2014,Jan,11; 2013,Jan,11-12

46742 combined transabdominal and sacroperineal approaches

72.7 72.7 FUD 090 63 C 80

AMA: 2014,Jan,11; 2013,Jan,11-12

46744 Repair of cloacal anomaly by anorectovaginoplasty and urethroplasty, sacroperineal approach ♀

103. 103. FUD 090 63 C 80

AMA: 2014,Jan,11; 2013,Jan,11-12

46746 Repair of cloacal anomaly by anorectovaginoplasty and urethroplasty, combined abdominal and sacroperineal approach; ♀

113. 113. FUD 090 C 80

AMA: 2014,Jan,11; 2013,Jan,11-12

46748 with vaginal lengthening by intestinal graft or pedicle flaps ♀

122. 122. FUD 090 C 80

AMA: 2014,Jan,11; 2013,Jan,11-12

46750 Sphincteroplasty, anal, for incontinence or prolapse; adult

21.7 21.7 FUD 090 J A2 80

AMA: 2014,Jan,11; 2013,Jan,11-12

46751 child A

19.2 19.2 FUD 090 C 80

AMA: 2014,Jan,11; 2013,Jan,11-12

46753 Graft (Thiersch operation) for rectal incontinence and/or prolapse

17.7 17.7 FUD 090 J A2

AMA: 2014,Jan,11; 2013,Jan,11-12

Digestive System

46600 — 46753

46754 **Removal of Thiersch wire or suture, anal canal**
6.76 9.30 FUD 010 J A2 80
AMA: 2014,Jan,11; 2013,Jan,11-12

46760 **Sphincteroplasty, anal, for incontinence, adult; muscle transplant**
31.6 31.6 FUD 090 J A2 80
AMA: 2014,Jan,11; 2013,Jan,11-12

46761 **levator muscle imbrication (Park posterior anal repair)**
26.6 26.6 FUD 090 J A2 80
AMA: 2014,Jan,11; 2013,Jan,11-12

\# **46947** **Hemorrhoidopexy (eg, for prolapsing internal hemorrhoids) by stapling**
11.1 11.1 FUD 090 J A2
AMA: 2018,Jan,8; 2017,Jan,8; 2016,Jan,13

46900-46999 [46945, 46946, 46947, 46948] Destruction Procedures: Anus

46900 **Destruction of lesion(s), anus (eg, condyloma, papilloma, molluscum contagiosum, herpetic vesicle), simple; chemical**
3.92 6.76 FUD 010 T P3
AMA: 2014,Jan,11; 2013,Jan,11-12

46910 **electrodesiccation**
3.84 7.39 FUD 010 T P3
AMA: 2019,Dec,12

46916 **cryosurgery**
4.06 7.00 FUD 010 T P2
AMA: 2014,Jan,11; 2013,Jan,11-12

46917 **laser surgery**
3.68 11.9 FUD 010 J A2
AMA: 2014,Jan,11; 2013,Jan,11-12

46922 **surgical excision**
3.92 8.00 FUD 010 J A2
AMA: 2014,Jan,11; 2013,Jan,11-12

46924 **Destruction of lesion(s), anus (eg, condyloma, papilloma, molluscum contagiosum, herpetic vesicle), extensive (eg, laser surgery, electrosurgery, cryosurgery, chemosurgery)**
5.21 15.1 FUD 010 J A2
AMA: 2014,Jan,11; 2013,Jan,11-12

46930 **Destruction of internal hemorrhoid(s) by thermal energy (eg, infrared coagulation, cautery, radiofrequency)**
EXCLUDES *Other hemorrhoid procedures:*
Cryosurgery destruction (46999)
Excision ([46320], 46250-46262)
Hemorrhoidopexy ([46947])
Incision (46083)
Injection sclerosing solution (46500)
Ligation (46221, [46945, 46946])
4.33 6.12 FUD 090 T P3 80
AMA: 2018,Jan,8; 2017,Jan,8; 2016,Jul,8; 2016,Jan,13

46940 **Curettage or cautery of anal fissure, including dilation of anal sphincter (separate procedure); initial**
4.20 6.79 FUD 010 J P3
AMA: 2014,Jan,11; 2013,Jan,11-12

46942 **subsequent**
3.74 6.72 FUD 010 T P3 80
AMA: 2014,Jan,11; 2013,Jan,11-12

46945 **Resequenced code. See code following 46221.**

46946 **Resequenced code. See code following resequenced code 46945.**

46947 **Resequenced code. See code following 46761.**

46948 **Resequenced code. See code before resequenced code 46220.**

46999 **Unlisted procedure, anus**
0.00 0.00 FUD YYY T 80
AMA: 2020,Feb,11; 2018,Oct,11; 2018,Jan,8; 2017,Jan,8; 2016,Jan,13

47000-47001 Needle Biopsy of Liver

EXCLUDES *Fine needle aspiration (10021, [10004, 10005, 10006, 10007, 10008, 10009, 10010, 10011, 10012])*

47000 **Biopsy of liver, needle; percutaneous**
(76942, 77002, 77012, 77021)
(88172-88173)
2.56 8.85 FUD 000 J A2
AMA: 2019,Apr,4; 2018,Jan,8; 2017,Jan,8; 2016,Jan,13

\+ **47001** **when done for indicated purpose at time of other major procedure (List separately in addition to code for primary procedure)**
Code first primary procedure
(76942, 77002)
(88172-88173)
3.04 3.04 FUD ZZZ N N1
AMA: 2018,Jan,8; 2017,Jan,8; 2016,Jan,13

47010-47130 Open Incisional and Resection Procedures of Liver

47010 **Hepatotomy, for open drainage of abscess or cyst, 1 or 2 stages**
EXCLUDES *Image guided percutaneous catheter drainage (49505)*
35.2 35.2 FUD 090 C 80
AMA: 2014,Jan,11; 2013,Nov,9

47015 **Laparotomy, with aspiration and/or injection of hepatic parasitic (eg, amoebic or echinococcal) cyst(s) or abscess(es)**
33.9 33.9 FUD 090 C 80
AMA: 2014,Jan,11; 2013,Jan,11-12

47100 **Biopsy of liver, wedge**
24.6 24.6 FUD 090 C 80
AMA: 2014,Jan,11; 2013,Jan,11-12

47120 **Hepatectomy, resection of liver; partial lobectomy**
68.0 68.0 FUD 090 C 80
AMA: 2018,Jan,8; 2017,Jan,8; 2016,Oct,11; 2016,Jan,13

47122 **trisegmentectomy**
100. 100. FUD 090 C 80
AMA: 2014,Jan,11; 2013,Jan,11-12

47125 **total left lobectomy**
89.8 89.8 FUD 090 C 80
AMA: 2014,Jan,11; 2013,Jan,11-12

47130 **total right lobectomy**
96.4 96.4 FUD 090 C 80
AMA: 2014,Jan,11; 2013,Jan,11-12

47133-47147 Liver Transplant Procedures

CMS: 100-03,260.1 Adult Liver Transplantation; 100-03,260.2 Pediatric Liver Transplantation; 100-04,3,90.4 Liver Transplants; 100-04,3,90.4.1 Standard Liver Acquisition Charge; 100-04,3,90.4.2 Billing for Liver Transplant and Acquisition Services; 100-04,3,90.6 Intestinal and Multi-Visceral Transplants

47133 **Donor hepatectomy (including cold preservation), from cadaver donor**
INCLUDES Graft:
Cold preservation
Harvest
0.00 0.00 FUD XXX C
AMA: 2014,Jan,11; 2013,Jan,11-12

47135 **Liver allotransplantation, orthotopic, partial or whole, from cadaver or living donor, any age**
INCLUDES Partial/whole recipient hepatectomy
Partial/whole transplant allograft
Recipient care
157. 157. FUD 090 C 80
AMA: 2018,Jan,8; 2017,Jan,8; 2016,Jan,13

47140 **Donor hepatectomy (including cold preservation), from living donor; left lateral segment only (segments II and III)**

INCLUDES Donor care
Graft:
Cold preservation
Harvest

103. 103. FUD 090 C 80

AMA: 2018,Jan,8; 2017,Jan,8; 2016,Jan,13

47141 **total left lobectomy (segments II, III and IV)**

INCLUDES Donor care
Graft:
Cold preservation
Harvest

124. 124. FUD 090 C 80

AMA: 2014,Jan,11; 2013,Jan,11-12

47142 **total right lobectomy (segments V, VI, VII and VIII)**

INCLUDES Donor care
Graft:
Cold preservation
Harvest

136. 136. FUD 090 C 80

AMA: 2014,Jan,11; 2013,Jan,11-12

47143 **Backbench standard preparation of cadaver donor whole liver graft prior to allotransplantation, including cholecystectomy, if necessary, and dissection and removal of surrounding soft tissues to prepare the vena cava, portal vein, hepatic artery, and common bile duct for implantation; without trisegment or lobe split**

EXCLUDES *Cholecystectomy (47600, 47610)*
Hepatectomy (47120-47125)

0.00 0.00 FUD XXX C 80

AMA: 2018,Jan,8; 2017,Jan,8; 2016,Jan,13

47144 **with trisegment split of whole liver graft into 2 partial liver grafts (ie, left lateral segment [segments II and III] and right trisegment [segments I and IV through VIII])**

EXCLUDES *Cholecystectomy (47600, 47610)*
Hepatectomy (47120-47125)

0.00 0.00 FUD XXX C 80

AMA: 2014,Jan,11; 2013,Jan,11-12

47145 **with lobe split of whole liver graft into 2 partial liver grafts (ie, left lobe [segments II, III, and IV] and right lobe [segments I and V through VIII])**

EXCLUDES *Cholecystectomy (47600, 47610)*
Hepatectomy (47120-47125)

0.00 0.00 FUD XXX C 80

AMA: 2014,Jan,11; 2013,Jan,11-12

47146 **Backbench reconstruction of cadaver or living donor liver graft prior to allotransplantation; venous anastomosis, each**

EXCLUDES *Cholecystectomy (47600, 47610)*
Hepatectomy (47120-47125)

9.57 9.57 FUD XXX C 80

AMA: 2014,Jan,11; 2013,Jan,11-12

47147 **arterial anastomosis, each**

EXCLUDES *Cholecystectomy (47600, 47610)*
Hepatectomy (47120-47125)

11.1 11.1 FUD XXX C 80

AMA: 2014,Jan,11; 2013,Jan,11-12

47300-47362 Open Repair of Liver

47300 **Marsupialization of cyst or abscess of liver**

32.9 32.9 FUD 090 C 80

AMA: 2014,Jan,11; 2013,Jan,11-12

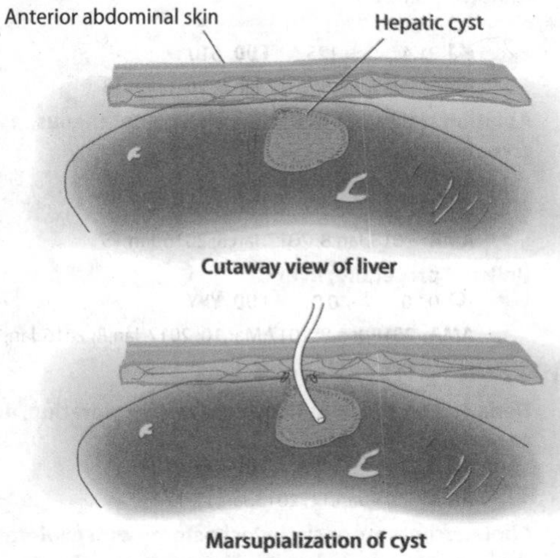

A liver cyst or abscess is marsupialized; this method involves surgical access to the cyst and making an incision into it; the edges of the cyst are sutured to the abdominal wall and drainage, open or closed, is placed into the cyst

47350 **Management of liver hemorrhage; simple suture of liver wound or injury**

39.7 39.7 FUD 090 C 80

AMA: 2020,Oct,14

47360 **complex suture of liver wound or injury, with or without hepatic artery ligation**

54.8 54.8 FUD 090 C 80

AMA: 2020,Oct,14

47361 **exploration of hepatic wound, extensive debridement, coagulation and/or suture, with or without packing of liver**

88.0 88.0 FUD 090 C 80

AMA: 2020,Oct,14

47362 **re-exploration of hepatic wound for removal of packing**

42.1 42.1 FUD 090 C 80

AMA: 2020,Jan,6

47370-47379 Laparoscopic Ablation Liver Tumors

INCLUDES Diagnostic laparoscopy (49320)

47370 **Laparoscopy, surgical, ablation of 1 or more liver tumor(s); radiofrequency**

(76940)

36.4 36.4 FUD 090 J 62 80

AMA: 2018,Jan,8; 2017,Jan,8; 2016,Jan,13

47371 **cryosurgical**

(76940)

36.5 36.5 FUD 090 J 62 80

AMA: 2014,Jan,11; 2013,Jan,11-12

47379 **Unlisted laparoscopic procedure, liver**

0.00 0.00 FUD YYY J 80

AMA: 2018,Aug,10; 2018,Jan,8; 2017,Jan,8; 2016,Jan,13

47380-47399 Open/Percutaneous Ablation Liver Tumors

47380 **Ablation, open, of 1 or more liver tumor(s); radiofrequency**

(76940)

42.1 42.1 FUD 090 C 80

AMA: 2018,Jan,8; 2017,Jan,8; 2016,Jan,13

47381 **cryosurgical**
(76940)
43.2 43.2 **FUD** 090 C 80
AMA: 2014,Jan,11; 2013,Jan,11-12

47382 **Ablation, 1 or more liver tumor(s), percutaneous, radiofrequency**
(76940, 77013, 77022)
21.4 125. **FUD** 010 J G2
AMA: 2018,Jan,8; 2017,Jan,8; 2016,Jan,13

47383 **Ablation, 1 or more liver tumor(s), percutaneous, cryoablation**
(76940, 77013, 77022)
13.1 195. **FUD** 010 J J8
AMA: 2018,Jan,8; 2017,Jan,8; 2016,Jan,13

47399 **Unlisted procedure, liver**
0.00 0.00 **FUD** YYY T
AMA: 2018,Jan,8; 2017,Mar,10; 2017,Jan,8; 2016,Jan,13

47400-47490 Biliary Tract Procedures

47400 **Hepaticotomy or hepaticostomy with exploration, drainage, or removal of calculus**
62.9 62.9 **FUD** 090 C 80
AMA: 2014,Jan,11; 2013,Jan,11-12

47420 **Choledochotomy or choledochostomy with exploration, drainage, or removal of calculus, with or without cholecystotomy; without transduodenal sphincterotomy or sphincteroplasty**
39.1 39.1 **FUD** 090 C 80
AMA: 2014,Jan,11; 2013,Jan,11-12

47425 **with transduodenal sphincterotomy or sphincteroplasty**
39.9 39.9 **FUD** 090 C 80
AMA: 2014,Jan,11; 2013,Jan,11-12

47460 **Transduodenal sphincterotomy or sphincteroplasty, with or without transduodenal extraction of calculus (separate procedure)**
37.0 37.0 **FUD** 090 C 80
AMA: 2014,Jan,11; 2013,Jan,11-12

47480 **Cholecystotomy or cholecystostomy, open, with exploration, drainage, or removal of calculus (separate procedure)**
EXCLUDES *Percutaneous cholecystostomy (47490)*
25.4 25.4 **FUD** 090 C 80
AMA: 2018,Jan,8; 2017,Jan,8; 2016,Jan,13

47490 **Cholecystostomy, percutaneous, complete procedure, including imaging guidance, catheter placement, cholecystogram when performed, and radiological supervision and interpretation**
INCLUDES Radiological guidance (75989, 76942, 77002, 77012, 77021)
EXCLUDES *Injection procedure for cholangiography (47531-47532)*
Open cholecystostomy (47480)
9.56 9.56 **FUD** 010 J G2
AMA: 2018,Jan,8; 2017,Jan,8; 2016,Jan,13

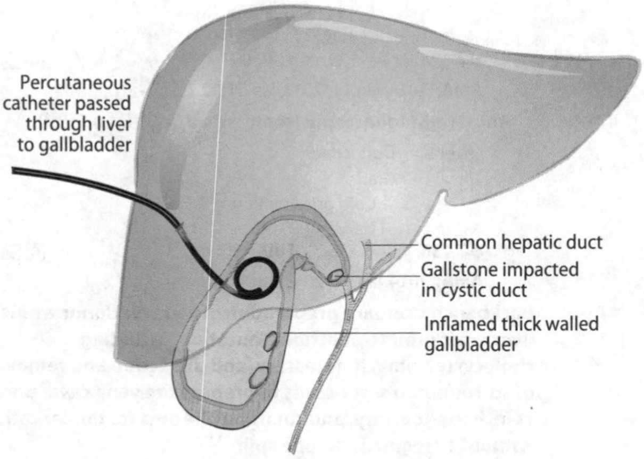

47531-47532 Injection/Insertion Procedures of Biliary Tract

INCLUDES Contrast material injection
Radiologic supervision and interpretation
EXCLUDES *Intraoperative cholangiography (74300-74301)*
Procedures performed via same access (47490, 47533-47541)

47531 **Injection procedure for cholangiography, percutaneous, complete diagnostic procedure including imaging guidance (eg, ultrasound and/or fluoroscopy) and all associated radiological supervision and interpretation; existing access**
2.06 9.89 **FUD** 000 Q2 N1
AMA: 2018,Jan,8; 2017,Jan,8

47532 **new access (eg, percutaneous transhepatic cholangiogram)**
6.18 23.2 **FUD** 000 Q2 N1
AMA: 2018,Jan,8; 2017,Jan,8

47533-47544 Percutaneous Procedures of the Biliary Tract

47533 **Placement of biliary drainage catheter, percutaneous, including diagnostic cholangiography when performed, imaging guidance (eg, ultrasound and/or fluoroscopy), and all associated radiological supervision and interpretation; external**
EXCLUDES *Conversion to internal-external drainage catheter (47535)*
Percutaneous placement stent bile duct (47538)
Placement stent bile duct, new access (47540)
Replacement existing internal drainage catheter (47536)
7.74 35.2 **FUD** 000 J G2
AMA: 2018,Jan,8; 2017,Jan,8

47534 **internal-external**
EXCLUDES *Conversion to external only drainage catheter (47536)*
Percutaneous placement stent bile duct (47538)
Placement stent bile duct, new access (47540)
10.8 41.8 **FUD** 000 J G2
AMA: 2018,Jan,8; 2017,Jan,8

47535 Conversion of external biliary drainage catheter to internal-external biliary drainage catheter, percutaneous, including diagnostic cholangiography when performed, imaging guidance (eg, fluoroscopy), and all associated radiological supervision and interpretation

5.75 28.4 FUD 000 J G2

AMA: 2018,Jan,8; 2017,Jan,8

47536 Exchange of biliary drainage catheter (eg, external, internal-external, or conversion of internal-external to external only), percutaneous, including diagnostic cholangiography when performed, imaging guidance (eg, fluoroscopy), and all associated radiological supervision and interpretation

INCLUDES Exchange one drainage catheter

EXCLUDES *Placement stent(s) into bile duct, percutaneous (47538)*

Code also exchange additional catheters same session with modifier 59 (47536)

3.84 19.5 FUD 000 J G2

AMA: 2018,Jan,8; 2017,Jan,8

47537 Removal of biliary drainage catheter, percutaneous, requiring fluoroscopic guidance (eg, with concurrent indwelling biliary stents), including diagnostic cholangiography when performed, imaging guidance (eg, fluoroscopy), and all associated radiological supervision and interpretation

EXCLUDES *Placement stent(s) into bile duct via same access (47538)*

Removal without fluoroscopic guidance; report with appropriate E/M service code

2.79 11.5 FUD 000 Q2 G2

AMA: 2018,Jan,8; 2017,Jan,8

47538 Placement of stent(s) into a bile duct, percutaneous, including diagnostic cholangiography, imaging guidance (eg, fluoroscopy and/or ultrasound), balloon dilation, catheter exchange(s) and catheter removal(s) when performed, and all associated radiological supervision and interpretation; existing access

EXCLUDES *Drainage catheter inserted following stent placement (47536)*

Procedures performed via same access (47536-47537)

Treatment same lesion same operative session ([43277], 47542, 47555-47556)

Code also multiple stents placed during same session when: (47538-47540)

Serial stents placed within same bile duct

Stent placement via two or more percutaneous access sites or space between two other stents

Two or more stents inserted through same percutaneous access

6.88 122. FUD 000 J J8

AMA: 2018,Jan,8; 2017,Jan,8; 2016,Mar,10

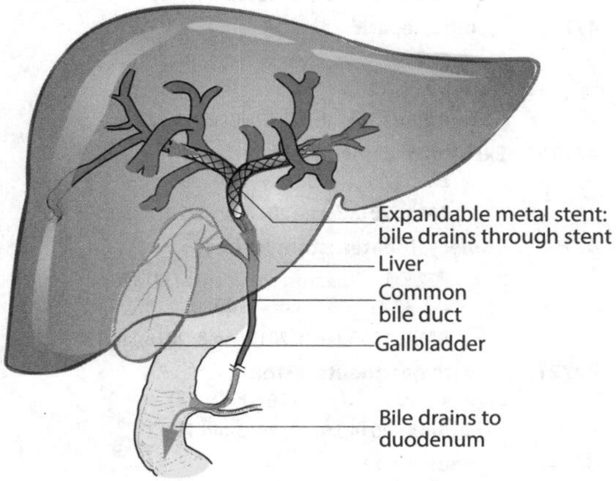

47539 new access, without placement of separate biliary drainage catheter

EXCLUDES *Treatment same lesion same operative session ([43277], 47542, 47555-47556)*

Code also multiple stents placed during same session when: (47538-47540)

Serial stents placed within same bile duct

Stent placement via two or more percutaneous access sites or space between two other stents

Two or more stents inserted through same percutaneous access

12.4 136. FUD 000 J G2

AMA: 2018,Jan,8; 2017,Jan,8; 2016,Mar,10

47540 new access, with placement of separate biliary drainage catheter (eg, external or internal-external)

EXCLUDES *Procedures performed via same access (47533-47534)*

Treatment same lesion same operative session ([43277], 47542, 47555-47556)

Code also multiple stents placed during same session when: (47538-47540)

Serial stents placed within same bile duct

Stent placement via two or more percutaneous access sites or space between two other stents

Two or more stents inserted through same percutaneous access

12.8 137. FUD 000 J J8

AMA: 2018,Jan,8; 2017,Jan,8; 2016,Mar,10

47541 Placement of access through the biliary tree and into small bowel to assist with an endoscopic biliary procedure (eg, rendezvous procedure), percutaneous, including diagnostic cholangiography when performed, imaging guidance (eg, ultrasound and/or fluoroscopy), and all associated radiological supervision and interpretation, new access

EXCLUDES *Access through biliary tree into small bowel for endoscopic biliary procedure (47535-47537)*

Conversion, exchange, or removal external biliary drainage catheter (47535-47537)

Injection procedure for cholangiography (47531-47532)

Placement biliary drainage catheter (47533-47534)

Placement stent(s) into bile duct (47538-47540)

Procedure performed when previous catheter access exists

9.64 33.8 FUD 000 J G2

AMA: 2018,Jan,8; 2017,Jan,8

+ **47542 Balloon dilation of biliary duct(s) or of ampulla (sphincteroplasty), percutaneous, including imaging guidance (eg, fluoroscopy), and all associated radiological supervision and interpretation, each duct (List separately in addition to code for primary procedure)**

EXCLUDES *Biliary endoscopy, with dilation of biliary duct stricture (47555-47556)*

Endoscopic balloon dilation ([43277], 47555-47556)

Endoscopic retrograde cholangiopancreatography (ERCP) (43262, [43277])

Placement stent(s) into a bile duct (47538-47540)

Procedure performed with balloon to remove calculi, debris, sludge without dilation (47544)

Code also one additional dilation code when more than one dilation performed same session, using modifier 59 with (47542)

Code first (47531-47537, 47541)

3.94 13.9 FUD ZZZ N N1

AMA: 2018,Jan,8; 2017,Jan,8

+ **47543** **Endoluminal biopsy(ies) of biliary tree, percutaneous, any method(s) (eg, brush, forceps, and/or needle), including imaging guidance (eg, fluoroscopy), and all associated radiological supervision and interpretation, single or multiple (List separately in addition to code for primary procedure)**

EXCLUDES *Endoscopic biopsy (46261, 47553)*
Endoscopic brushings (43260, 47552)
Procedure performed more than one time per session

Code first (47531-47540)
4.20 13.3 FUD ZZZ N N1
AMA: 2018,Jan,8; 2017,Jan,8

+ **47544** **Removal of calculi/debris from biliary duct(s) and/or gallbladder, percutaneous, including destruction of calculi by any method (eg, mechanical, electrohydraulic, lithotripsy) when performed, imaging guidance (eg, fluoroscopy), and all associated radiological supervision and interpretation (List separately in addition to code for primary procedure)**

EXCLUDES *Device deployment without finding calculi/debris*
Endoscopic calculi removal/destruction (43264-43265, 47554)
Endoscopic retrograde cholangiopancreatography (ERCP); with removal calculi/debris from biliary/pancreatic duct(s) (43264)
Procedures with removal incidental debris (47531-47543)

Code first when debris removal not incidental, as appropriate (47531-47540)
4.65 30.5 FUD ZZZ N N1
AMA: 2018,Jan,8; 2017,Jan,8

47550-47556 Endoscopic Procedures of the Biliary Tract

INCLUDES Diagnostic endoscopy (49320)
EXCLUDES *Endoscopic retrograde cholangiopancreatography (ERCP) (43260-43265, [43274], [43275], [43276], [43277], [43278], 74328-74330, 74363)*

+ **47550** **Biliary endoscopy, intraoperative (choledochoscopy) (List separately in addition to code for primary procedure)**

Code first primary procedure
4.80 4.80 FUD ZZZ C 80
AMA: 2014,Jan,11; 2013,Jan,11-12

47552 **Biliary endoscopy, percutaneous via T-tube or other tract; diagnostic, with collection of specimen(s) by brushing and/or washing, when performed (separate procedure)**
9.01 9.01 FUD 000 J A2
AMA: 2018,Jan,8; 2017,Jan,8; 2016,Jan,13

47553 **with biopsy, single or multiple**
8.91 8.91 FUD 000 J A2
AMA: 2018,Jan,8; 2017,Jan,8; 2016,Jan,13

47554 **with removal of calculus/calculi**
14.9 14.9 FUD 000 J A2
AMA: 2018,Jan,8; 2017,Jan,8; 2016,Jan,13

47555 **with dilation of biliary duct stricture(s) without stent**
(74363)
9.46 9.46 FUD 000 J A2
AMA: 2018,Jan,8; 2017,Jan,8; 2016,Jan,13

47556 **with dilation of biliary duct stricture(s) with stent**
(74363)
10.7 10.7 FUD 000 J J8
AMA: 2018,Jan,8; 2017,Jan,8; 2016,Jan,13

47562-47579 Laparoscopic Gallbladder Procedures

INCLUDES Diagnostic laparoscopy (49320)

47562 **Laparoscopy, surgical; cholecystectomy**
19.0 19.0 FUD 090 J G2 80
AMA: 2020,Aug,14; 2018,Jan,8; 2017,Jan,8; 2016,Jan,13

47563 **cholecystectomy with cholangiography**

EXCLUDES *Percutaneous cholangiography (47531-47532)*

Code also intraoperative radiology supervision and interpretation (74300-74301)
20.7 20.7 FUD 090 J G2 80
AMA: 2019,Mar,10; 2018,Jan,8; 2017,Jan,8; 2016,Jan,13

47564 **cholecystectomy with exploration of common duct**
32.2 32.2 FUD 090 J G2 80
AMA: 2018,Jan,8; 2017,Jan,8; 2016,Jan,13

47570 **cholecystoenterostomy**
22.5 22.5 FUD 090 C 80
AMA: 2018,Jan,8; 2017,Jan,8; 2016,Jan,13

47579 **Unlisted laparoscopy procedure, biliary tract**
0.00 0.00 FUD YYY J 80 50
AMA: 2018,Jan,8; 2017,Jan,8; 2016,Jan,13

47600-47620 Open Gallbladder Procedures

47600 **Cholecystectomy;**

EXCLUDES *Laparoscopic method (47562-47564)*
30.9 30.9 FUD 090 C 80
AMA: 2018,Jan,8; 2017,Jan,8; 2016,Jan,13

47605 **with cholangiography**

EXCLUDES *Laparoscopic method (47563-47564)*
32.6 32.6 FUD 090 C 80
AMA: 2018,Jan,8; 2017,Jan,8; 2016,Jan,13

47610 **Cholecystectomy with exploration of common duct;**

EXCLUDES *Laparoscopic method (47564)*

Code also biliary endoscopy when performed in conjunction with cholecystectomy with exploration common duct (47550)
36.3 36.3 FUD 090 C 80
AMA: 2018,Jan,8; 2017,Jan,8; 2016,Jan,13

47612 **with choledochoenterostomy**
36.6 36.6 FUD 090 C 80
AMA: 2014,Jan,11; 2013,Jan,11-12

47620 **with transduodenal sphincterotomy or sphincteroplasty, with or without cholangiography**
40.0 40.0 FUD 090 C 80
AMA: 2014,Jan,11; 2013,Jan,11-12

47700-47999 Open Resection and Repair of Biliary Tract

47700 **Exploration for congenital atresia of bile ducts, without repair, with or without liver biopsy, with or without cholangiography**
30.6 30.6 FUD 090 63 C 80
AMA: 2014,Jan,11; 2013,Jan,11-12

47701 **Portoenterostomy (eg, Kasai procedure)**
50.4 50.4 FUD 090 63 C 80
AMA: 2014,Jan,11; 2013,Jan,11-12

47711 **Excision of bile duct tumor, with or without primary repair of bile duct; extrahepatic**

EXCLUDES *Anastomosis (47760-47800)*
45.1 45.1 FUD 090 C 80
AMA: 2014,Jan,11; 2013,Jan,11-12

47712 **intrahepatic**

EXCLUDES *Anastomosis (47760-47800)*
58.1 58.1 FUD 090 C 80
AMA: 2014,Jan,11; 2013,Jan,11-12

47715 **Excision of choledochal cyst**
38.6 38.6 FUD 090 C 80
AMA: 2018,Jan,8; 2017,Jan,8; 2016,Jan,13

47720 **Cholecystoenterostomy; direct**

EXCLUDES *Laparoscopic method (47570)*
33.4 33.4 FUD 090 C 80
AMA: 2018,Jan,8; 2017,Jan,8; 2016,Jan,13

47721 **with gastroenterostomy**
39.3 39.3 FUD 090 C 80
AMA: 2014,Jan,11; 2013,Jan,11-12

47740 **Roux-en-Y**
37.7 37.7 FUD 090 C 80
AMA: 2014,Jan,11; 2013,Jan,11-12

47741 **Roux-en-Y with gastroenterostomy**
42.8 42.8 FUD 090 C 80
AMA: 2014,Jan,11; 2013,Jan,11-12

47760 **Anastomosis, of extrahepatic biliary ducts and gastrointestinal tract**
65.4 65.4 FUD 090 C 80
AMA: 2014,Jan,11; 2013,Jan,11-12

47765 **Anastomosis, of intrahepatic ducts and gastrointestinal tract**
INCLUDES Longmire anastomosis
87.9 87.9 FUD 090 C 80
AMA: 2014,Jan,11; 2013,Jan,11-12

47780 **Anastomosis, Roux-en-Y, of extrahepatic biliary ducts and gastrointestinal tract**
71.8 71.8 FUD 090 C 80
AMA: 2014,Jan,11; 2013,Jan,11-12

47785 **Anastomosis, Roux-en-Y, of intrahepatic biliary ducts and gastrointestinal tract**
94.4 94.4 FUD 090 C 80
AMA: 2014,Jan,11; 2013,Jan,11-12

47800 **Reconstruction, plastic, of extrahepatic biliary ducts with end-to-end anastomosis**
45.5 45.5 FUD 090 C 80
AMA: 2014,Jan,11; 2013,Jan,11-12

47801 **Placement of choledochal stent**
32.3 32.3 FUD 090 C 80
AMA: 2018,Jan,8; 2017,Jan,8; 2016,Jan,13

47802 **U-tube hepaticoenterostomy**
44.3 44.3 FUD 090 C 80
AMA: 2014,Jan,11; 2013,Jan,11-12

47900 **Suture of extrahepatic biliary duct for pre-existing injury (separate procedure)**
39.7 39.7 FUD 090 C 80
AMA: 2014,Jan,11; 2013,Jan,11-12

47999 **Unlisted procedure, biliary tract**
0.00 0.00 FUD YYY T
AMA: 2018,Jan,8; 2017,Jan,8; 2016,Jan,13

48000-48548 Open Procedures of the Pancreas

EXCLUDES *Peroral pancreatic procedures performed endoscopically (43260-43265, [43274], [43275], [43276], [43277], [43278])*

48000 **Placement of drains, peripancreatic, for acute pancreatitis;**
54.7 54.7 FUD 090 C 80
AMA: 2014,Jan,11; 2013,Jan,11-12

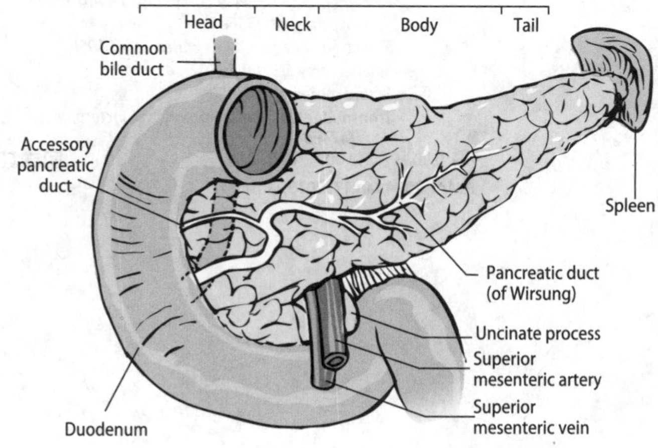

48001 **with cholecystostomy, gastrostomy, and jejunostomy**
67.1 67.1 FUD 090 C 80
AMA: 2014,Jan,11; 2013,Jan,11-12

48020 **Removal of pancreatic calculus**
34.1 34.1 FUD 090 C 80
AMA: 2014,Jan,11; 2013,Jan,11-12

48100 **Biopsy of pancreas, open (eg, fine needle aspiration, needle core biopsy, wedge biopsy)**
25.8 25.8 FUD 090 C 80
AMA: 2014,Jan,11; 2013,Jan,11-12

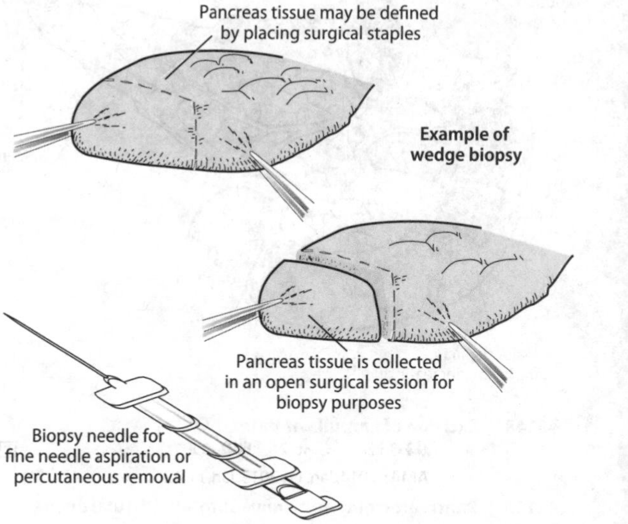

48102 **Biopsy of pancreas, percutaneous needle**
EXCLUDES *Fine needle aspiration ([10005, 10006, 10007, 10008, 10009, 10010, 10011, 10012])*
(76942, 77002, 77012, 77021)
(88172-88173)
6.97 15.1 FUD 010 J A2
AMA: 2019,Apr,4

48105 **Resection or debridement of pancreas and peripancreatic tissue for acute necrotizing pancreatitis**
82.4 82.4 FUD 090 C 80
AMA: 2014,Jan,11; 2013,Jan,11-12

48120 **Excision of lesion of pancreas (eg, cyst, adenoma)**
32.0 32.0 FUD 090 C 80
AMA: 2014,Jan,11; 2013,Jan,11-12

48140 **Pancreatectomy, distal subtotal, with or without splenectomy; without pancreaticojejunostomy**
45.4 45.4 FUD 090 C 80
AMA: 2018,Jan,8; 2017,Jul,10

48145 **with pancreaticojejunostomy**
47.4 47.4 FUD 090 C 80
AMA: 2014,Jan,11; 2013,Jan,11-12

48146 **Pancreatectomy, distal, near-total with preservation of duodenum (Child-type procedure)**
54.5 54.5 **FUD** 090 C 80
AMA: 2014,Jan,11; 2013,Jan,11-12

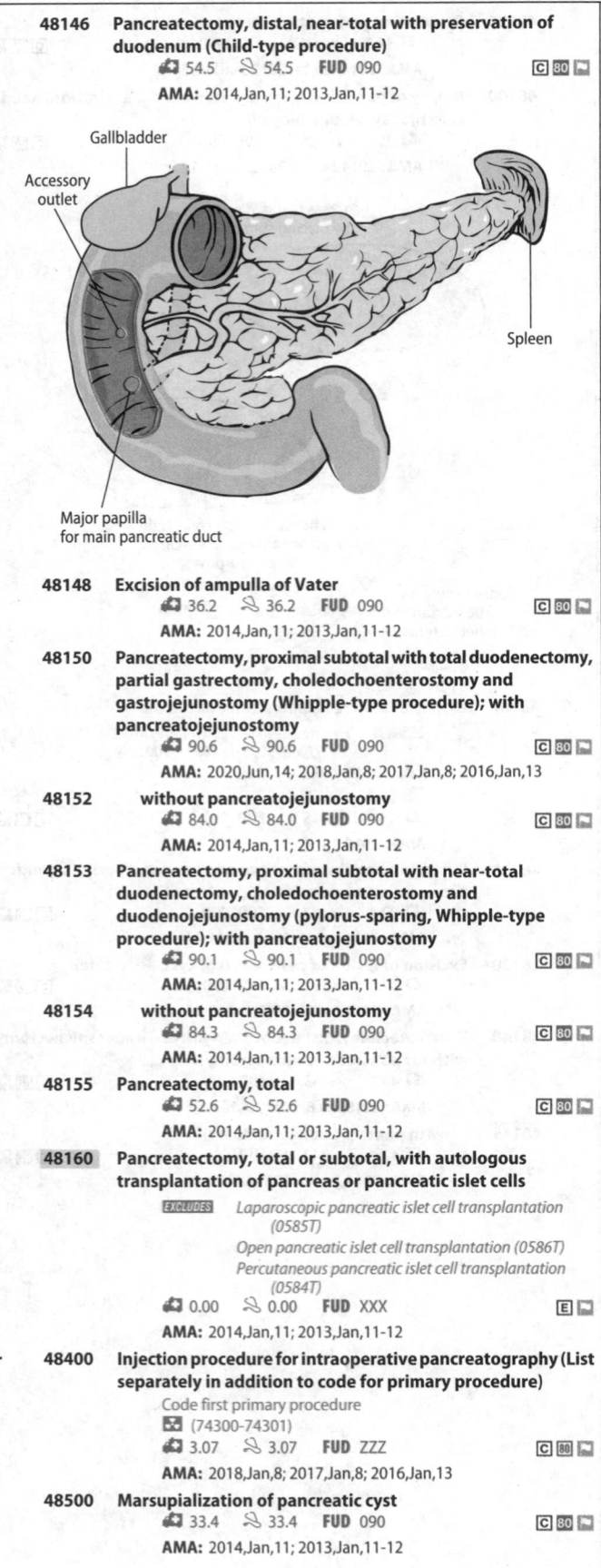

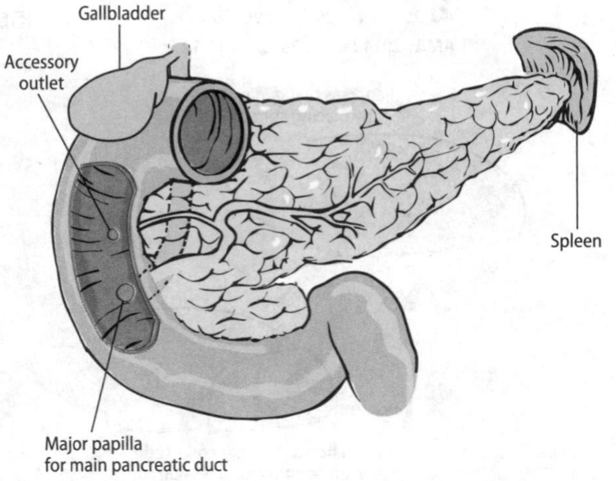

48148 **Excision of ampulla of Vater**
36.2 36.2 **FUD** 090 C 80
AMA: 2014,Jan,11; 2013,Jan,11-12

48150 **Pancreatectomy, proximal subtotal with total duodenectomy, partial gastrectomy, choledochoenterostomy and gastrojejunostomy (Whipple-type procedure); with pancreatojejunostomy**
90.6 90.6 **FUD** 090 C 80
AMA: 2020,Jun,14; 2018,Jan,8; 2017,Jan,8; 2016,Jan,13

48152 **without pancreatojejunostomy**
84.0 84.0 **FUD** 090 C 80
AMA: 2014,Jan,11; 2013,Jan,11-12

48153 **Pancreatectomy, proximal subtotal with near-total duodenectomy, choledochoenterostomy and duodenojejunostomy (pylorus-sparing, Whipple-type procedure); with pancreatojejunostomy**
90.1 90.1 **FUD** 090 C 80
AMA: 2014,Jan,11; 2013,Jan,11-12

48154 **without pancreatojejunostomy**
84.3 84.3 **FUD** 090 C 80
AMA: 2014,Jan,11; 2013,Jan,11-12

48155 **Pancreatectomy, total**
52.6 52.6 **FUD** 090 C 80
AMA: 2014,Jan,11; 2013,Jan,11-12

48160 **Pancreatectomy, total or subtotal, with autologous transplantation of pancreas or pancreatic islet cells**
EXCLUDES *Laparoscopic pancreatic islet cell transplantation (0585T)*
Open pancreatic islet cell transplantation (0586T)
Percutaneous pancreatic islet cell transplantation (0584T)
0.00 0.00 **FUD** XXX E
AMA: 2014,Jan,11; 2013,Jan,11-12

\+ **48400** **Injection procedure for intraoperative pancreatography (List separately in addition to code for primary procedure)**
Code first primary procedure
(74300-74301)
3.07 3.07 **FUD** ZZZ C 80
AMA: 2018,Jan,8; 2017,Jan,8; 2016,Jan,13

48500 **Marsupialization of pancreatic cyst**
33.4 33.4 **FUD** 090 C 80
AMA: 2014,Jan,11; 2013,Jan,11-12

48510 **External drainage, pseudocyst of pancreas, open**
EXCLUDES *Image guided percutaneous catheter drainage (49405)*
31.7 31.7 **FUD** 090 C 80
AMA: 2014,Jan,11; 2013,Nov,9

48520 **Internal anastomosis of pancreatic cyst to gastrointestinal tract; direct**
31.5 31.5 **FUD** 090 C 80
AMA: 2014,Jan,11; 2013,Jan,11-12

48540 **Roux-en-Y**
37.8 37.8 **FUD** 090 C 80
AMA: 2014,Jan,11; 2013,Jan,11-12

48545 **Pancreatorrhaphy for injury**
38.9 38.9 **FUD** 090 C 80
AMA: 2014,Jan,11; 2013,Jan,11-12

48547 **Duodenal exclusion with gastrojejunostomy for pancreatic injury**
52.1 52.1 **FUD** 090 C 80
AMA: 2014,Jan,11; 2013,Jan,11-12

48548 **Pancreaticojejunostomy, side-to-side anastomosis (Puestow-type operation)**
48.2 48.2 **FUD** 090 C 80
AMA: 2014,Jan,11; 2013,Jan,11-12

48550-48999 Pancreas Transplant Procedures

CMS: 100-03,260.3 Pancreas Transplants; 100-04,3,90.5 Pancreas Transplants with Kidney Transplants; 100-04,3,90.5.1 Pancreas Transplants Alone

48550 **Donor pancreatectomy (including cold preservation), with or without duodenal segment for transplantation**
INCLUDES Graft:
Cold preservation
Harvest (with or without duodenal segment)
0.00 0.00 **FUD** XXX E
AMA: 2018,Jan,8; 2017,Jan,8; 2016,Jan,13

48551 **Backbench standard preparation of cadaver donor pancreas allograft prior to transplantation, including dissection of allograft from surrounding soft tissues, splenectomy, duodenotomy, ligation of bile duct, ligation of mesenteric vessels, and Y-graft arterial anastomoses from iliac artery to superior mesenteric artery and to splenic artery**
EXCLUDES *Biopsy pancreas (48100-48102)*
Bypass graft, with vein (35531, 35563)
Duodenotomy (44010)
Endoscopic procedures biliary tract (47550-47556)
Excision lesion mesentery (44820)
Excision lesion pancreas (48120)
Pancreatorrhaphy for injury (48545)
Placement vein patch or cuff at distal anastomosis bypass graft (35685)
Resection or debridement pancreas (48105)
Splenectomy (38100-38102)
Suture mesentery (44850)
Transduodenal sphincterotomy, sphincteroplasty (47460)
0.00 0.00 **FUD** XXX C 80
AMA: 2014,Jan,11; 2013,Jan,11-12

48552 Backbench reconstruction of cadaver donor pancreas allograft prior to transplantation, venous anastomosis, each

EXCLUDES *Biopsy pancreas (48100-48102)*
Bypass graft, with vein (35531, 35563)
Duodenotomy (44010)
Endoscopic procedures biliary tract (47550-47556)
Excision lesion mesentery (44820)
Excision lesion pancreas (48120)
Pancreatorrhaphy for injury (48545)
Placement vein patch or cuff at distal anastomosis bypass graft (35685)
Resection or debridement pancreas (48105)
Splenectomy (38100-38102)
Suture mesentery (44850)
Transduodenal sphincterotomy, sphincteroplasty (47460)

6.87 6.87 **FUD** XXX C 80

AMA: 2014,Jan,11; 2013,Jan,11-12

48554 Transplantation of pancreatic allograft

INCLUDES Allograft transplant
Recipient care

74.4 74.4 **FUD** 090 C 80

AMA: 2014,Jan,11; 2013,Jan,11-12

48556 Removal of transplanted pancreatic allograft

37.1 37.1 **FUD** 090 C 80

AMA: 2014,Jan,11; 2013,Jan,11-12

48999 Unlisted procedure, pancreas

0.00 0.00 **FUD** YYY T 80

AMA: 2018,Jan,8; 2017,Jan,8; 2016,Jan,13

49000-49084 Exploratory and Drainage Procedures: Abdomen/Peritoneum

49000 Exploratory laparotomy, exploratory celiotomy with or without biopsy(s) (separate procedure)

EXCLUDES *Exploration penetrating wound without laparotomy (20102)*

22.3 22.3 **FUD** 090 C 80

AMA: 2020,Jan,6; 2019,Dec,5; 2018,Jan,8; 2017,Dec,3; 2017,Jan,8; 2016,Jan,13

49002 Reopening of recent laparotomy

EXCLUDES *Hepatic wound re-exploration for packing removal (47362)*
Pelvic wound re-exploration for packing removal/repacking (49014)

30.4 30.4 **FUD** 090 C 80

AMA: 2020,Jan,6; 2018,Jan,8; 2017,Jan,8; 2016,Jan,13

49010 Exploration, retroperitoneal area with or without biopsy(s) (separate procedure)

EXCLUDES *Exploration penetrating wound without laparotomy (20102)*

26.8 26.8 **FUD** 090 C 80

AMA: 2020,Jan,6; 2019,Dec,5

49013 Preperitoneal pelvic packing for hemorrhage associated with pelvic trauma, including local exploration

12.7 12.7 **FUD** 000

AMA: 2020,Jan,6

49014 Re-exploration of pelvic wound with removal of preperitoneal pelvic packing, including repacking, when performed

10.5 10.5 **FUD** 000

AMA: 2020,Jan,6

49020 Drainage of peritoneal abscess or localized peritonitis, exclusive of appendiceal abscess, open

EXCLUDES *Appendiceal abscess (44900)*
Image-guided percutaneous catheter drainage abscess/peritonitis via catheter (49406)
Image-guided transrectal/transvaginal drainage peritoneal abscess via catheter (49407)

46.3 46.3 **FUD** 090 C 80

AMA: 2014,Jan,11; 2013,Nov,9

49040 Drainage of subdiaphragmatic or subphrenic abscess, open

EXCLUDES *Image-guided percutaneous drainage subdiaphragmatic/subphrenic abscess via catheter (49406)*

29.1 29.1 **FUD** 090 C 80

AMA: 2014,Jan,11; 2013,Nov,9

49060 Drainage of retroperitoneal abscess, open

EXCLUDES *Image-guided percutaneous drainage retroperitoneal abscess via catheter (49406)*
Transrectal/transvaginal image-guided drainage retroperitoneal abscess via catheter (49407)

32.0 32.0 **FUD** 090 C

AMA: 2018,Jan,8; 2017,Jan,8; 2016,Jan,13

49062 Drainage of extraperitoneal lymphocele to peritoneal cavity, open

EXCLUDES *Drainage lymphocele to peritoneal cavity, laparoscopic (49323)*
Image-guided percutaneous drainage retroperitoneal lymphocele via catheter (49406)

21.3 21.3 **FUD** 090 C 80

AMA: 2018,Jan,8; 2017,Jan,8; 2016,Jan,13

49082 Abdominal paracentesis (diagnostic or therapeutic); without imaging guidance

2.12 5.67 **FUD** 000 T G2

AMA: 2018,Jan,8; 2017,Jan,8; 2016,Jan,13

49083 with imaging guidance

INCLUDES Radiological guidance (76942, 77002, 77012, 77021)

EXCLUDES *Image-guided percutaneous drainage retroperitoneal abscess via catheter (49406)*

3.11 8.44 **FUD** 000 T G2

AMA: 2018,Jan,8; 2017,Jan,8; 2016,Jan,13

49084 Peritoneal lavage, including imaging guidance, when performed

INCLUDES Radiological guidance (76942, 77002, 77012, 77021)

EXCLUDES *Image-guided percutaneous drainage retroperitoneal abscess via catheter (49406)*

3.16 3.16 **FUD** 000 T G2

AMA: 2018,Jan,8; 2017,Jan,8; 2016,Jan,13

49180 Biopsy of Mass: Abdomen/Retroperitoneum

EXCLUDES *Fine needle aspiration (10021, [10004, 10005, 10006, 10007, 10008, 10009, 10010, 10011, 10012])*
Lysis intestinal adhesions (44005)

49180 Biopsy, abdominal or retroperitoneal mass, percutaneous needle

(76942, 77002, 77012, 77021)
(88172-88173)

2.43 4.86 **FUD** 000 J A2

AMA: 2019,Feb,8; 2019,Apr,4; 2018,Jan,8; 2017,Jan,8; 2016,Jan,13

Digestive System

48552 — 49180

49185 Sclerotherapy of a Fluid Collection

49185 Sclerotherapy of a fluid collection (eg, lymphocele, cyst, or seroma), percutaneous, including contrast injection(s), sclerosant injection(s), diagnostic study, imaging guidance (eg, ultrasound, fluoroscopy) and radiological supervision and interpretation when performed

INCLUDES Multiple lesions treated via same access

EXCLUDES *Contrast injection for assessment abscess or cyst (49424)*
Pleurodesis (32560)
Radiologic examination, abscess, fistula or sinus tract stud (76080)
Sclerosis veins/endovenous ablation incompetent veins extremity (36468, 36470-36471, 36475-36476, 36478-36479)
Sclerotherapy lymphatic/vascular malformation (37241)

Code also:
Access or drainage via needle or catheter (10030, 10160, 49405-49407, 50390)
Existing catheter exchange pre- or post-sclerosant injection (49423, 75984)
Modifier 59 for treatment multiple lesions same session via separate access

3.47 | 33.4 | FUD 000 | T G2

AMA: 2018,Jan,8; 2017,Jan,8; 2016,Mar,10

49203-49205 Open Destruction or Excision: Abdominal Tumors

EXCLUDES *Ablation, open, one or more renal mass lesion(s), cryosurgical*
Biopsy kidney or ovary (50205, 58900)
Cryoablation renal tumor (50250, 50593)
Excision perinephric cyst (50290)
Excision presacral or sacrococcygeal tumor (49215)
Exploration, renal or retroperitoneal area (49010, 50010)
Exploratory laparotomy (49000)
Laparotomy, for staging or restaging ovarian, tubal, or primary peritoneal malignancy (58960)
Nephrectomy (50225, 50236)
Oophorectomy (58940-58958)
Ovarian cystectomy (58925)
Pelvic or retroperitoneal lymphadenectomy (38770, 38780)
Primary, recurrent ovarian, uterine, or tubal resection (58957-58958)
Wedge resection or bisection ovary (58920)

Code also:
Colectomy (44140)
Nephrectomy (50220, 50240)
Small bowel resection (44120)
Vena caval resection with reconstruction (37799)

49203 Excision or destruction, open, intra-abdominal tumors, cysts or endometriomas, 1 or more peritoneal, mesenteric, or retroperitoneal primary or secondary tumors; largest tumor 5 cm diameter or less

34.7 | 34.7 | FUD 090 | C 80

AMA: 2018,Jan,8; 2017,Jan,8; 2016,Jan,13

49204 largest tumor 5.1-10.0 cm diameter

44.2 | 44.2 | FUD 090 | C 80

AMA: 2018,Jan,8; 2017,Jan,8; 2016,Jan,13

49205 largest tumor greater than 10.0 cm diameter

50.6 | 50.6 | FUD 090 | C 80

AMA: 2018,Jan,8; 2017,Jan,8; 2016,Jan,13

49215 Resection Presacral/Sacrococcygeal Tumor

49215 Excision of presacral or sacrococcygeal tumor

64.2 | 64.2 | FUD 090 | 63 C 80

AMA: 2014,Jan,11; 2013,Jan,11-12

49250-49255 Other Open Abdominal Procedures

EXCLUDES *Lysis intestinal adhesions (44005)*

49250 Umbilectomy, omphalectomy, excision of umbilicus (separate procedure)

17.0 | 17.0 | FUD 090 | J A2

AMA: 2014,Jan,11; 2013,Jan,11-12

49255 Omentectomy, epiploectomy, resection of omentum (separate procedure)

22.8 | 22.8 | FUD 090 | C 80

AMA: 2018,Mar,11; 2018,Jan,8; 2017,Jan,8; 2016,Jan,13

49320-49329 Laparoscopic Procedures of the Abdomen/Peritoneum/Omentum

INCLUDES Diagnostic laparoscopy (49320)

EXCLUDES *Fulguration/excision lesions ovary/pelvic viscera/peritoneal surface, performed laparoscopically (58662)*

49320 Laparoscopy, abdomen, peritoneum, and omentum, diagnostic, with or without collection of specimen(s) by brushing or washing (separate procedure)

9.54 | 9.54 | FUD 010 | J A2 80

AMA: 2018,Jan,8; 2017,Apr,7; 2017,Jan,8; 2016,Jan,13

49321 Laparoscopy, surgical; with biopsy (single or multiple)

10.0 | 10.0 | FUD 010 | J A2 80

AMA: 2018,Aug,10; 2018,Jan,8; 2017,Jan,8; 2016,Jan,13

49322 with aspiration of cavity or cyst (eg, ovarian cyst) (single or multiple)

10.8 | 10.8 | FUD 010 | J A2 80

AMA: 2018,Jan,8; 2017,Jan,8; 2016,Jan,13

49323 with drainage of lymphocele to peritoneal cavity

EXCLUDES *Open drainage lymphocele to peritoneal cavity (49062)*

18.3 | 18.3 | FUD 090 | J G2 80

AMA: 2018,Jan,8; 2017,Jan,8; 2016,Jan,13

49324 with insertion of tunneled intraperitoneal catheter

EXCLUDES *Open approach (49421)*

Code also insertion subcutaneous extension to intraperitoneal cannula with remote chest exit site, when appropriate (49435)

11.3 | 11.3 | FUD 010 | J G2 80

AMA: 2014,Jan,11; 2013,Jan,11-12

49325 with revision of previously placed intraperitoneal cannula or catheter, with removal of intraluminal obstructive material if performed

12.1 | 12.1 | FUD 010 | J G2 80

AMA: 2014,Jan,11; 2013,Jan,11-12

+ **49326 with omentopexy (omental tacking procedure) (List separately in addition to code for primary procedure)**

Code first laparoscopy with permanent intraperitoneal cannula or catheter insertion or revision previously placed catheter/cannula (49324, 49325)

5.52 | 5.52 | FUD ZZZ | N N1 80

AMA: 2014,Jan,11; 2013,Jan,11-12

+ **49327 with placement of interstitial device(s) for radiation therapy guidance (eg, fiducial markers, dosimeter), intra-abdominal, intrapelvic, and/or retroperitoneum, including imaging guidance, if performed, single or multiple (List separately in addition to code for primary procedure)**

EXCLUDES *Open approach (49412)*
Percutaneous approach (49411)

Code first laparoscopic abdominal, pelvic or retroperitoneal procedures

3.81 | 3.81 | FUD ZZZ | N N1 80

AMA: 2014,Jan,11; 2013,Jan,11-12

49329 Unlisted laparoscopy procedure, abdomen, peritoneum and omentum

0.00 | 0.00 | FUD YYY | J 80 50

AMA: 2020,Feb,13; 2019,Mar,10; 2018,Jan,8; 2017,Jan,8; 2016,Jan,13

49400-49436 Peritoneal and Visceral Procedures: Drainage/Insertion/Modifications/Removal

49400 **Injection of air or contrast into peritoneal cavity (separate procedure)**

(74190)

2.68 3.93 FUD 000 N N1

AMA: 2018,Jan,8; 2017,Jan,8; 2016,Jan,13

49402 **Removal of peritoneal foreign body from peritoneal cavity**

EXCLUDES *Enterolysis (44005)*

Percutaneous or open drainage or lavage (49020, 49040, 49082-49084, 49406)

Percutaneous tunneled intraperitoneal catheter insertion without subcutaneous port (49418)

24.9 24.9 FUD 090 J A2

AMA: 2014,Jan,11; 2013,Jan,11-12

49405 **Image-guided fluid collection drainage by catheter (eg, abscess, hematoma, seroma, lymphocele, cyst); visceral (eg, kidney, liver, spleen, lung/mediastinum), percutaneous**

INCLUDES Radiological guidance (75989, 76942, 77002-77003, 77012, 77021)

EXCLUDES *Open drainage (47010, 48510, 50020)*

Percutaneous cholecystostomy (47490)

Percutaneous pleural drainage (32556-32557)

Pneumonostomy (32200)

Thoracentesis (32554-32555)

Code also each individual collection drained per separate catheter

5.71 25.1 FUD 000 J G2

AMA: 2020,Feb,13; 2018,Jan,8; 2017,Jan,8; 2016,Jan,13

49406 **peritoneal or retroperitoneal, percutaneous**

INCLUDES Radiological guidance (75989, 76942, 77002-77003, 77012, 77021)

EXCLUDES *Diagnostic or therapeutic percutaneous abdominal paracentesis (49082-49083)*

Open peritoneal/retroperitoneal drainage (44900, 49020-49062, 49084, 50020, 58805, 58822)

Open transrectal drainage pelvic abscess (45000)

Percutaneous tunneled intraperitoneal catheter insertion without subcutaneous port (49418)

Transrectal/transvaginal image-guided peritoneal/retroperitoneal drainage via catheter (49407)

Code also each individual collection drained per separate catheter

5.70 25.1 FUD 000 J G2

AMA: 2020,Feb,13; 2018,Jan,8; 2017,Jan,8; 2016,Jan,13

49407 **peritoneal or retroperitoneal, transvaginal or transrectal**

INCLUDES Radiological guidance (75989, 76942, 77002-77003, 77012, 77021)

EXCLUDES *Image-guided percutaneous catheter drainage soft tissue (eg, abdominal wall, neck, extremity) (10030)*

Open transrectal/transvaginal drainage (45000, 58800, 58820)

Percutaneous pleural drainage (32556-32557)

Peritoneal drainage or lavage, open or percutaneous (49020, 49040, 49060)

Thoracentesis (32554-32555)

Code also each individual collection drained per separate catheter

6.05 20.6 FUD 000 J G2

AMA: 2018,Jan,8; 2017,Jan,8; 2016,Jan,13

49411 **Placement of interstitial device(s) for radiation therapy guidance (eg, fiducial markers, dosimeter), percutaneous, intra-abdominal, intra-pelvic (except prostate), and/or retroperitoneum, single or multiple**

EXCLUDES *Placement (percutaneous) interstitial device(s) for intrathoracic radiation therapy guidance (32553)*

Code also supply device

(76942, 77002, 77012, 77021)

5.33 13.9 FUD 000 S P3 80

AMA: 2018,Jan,8; 2017,Jan,8; 2016,Jun,3; 2016,Jan,13

+ **49412** **Placement of interstitial device(s) for radiation therapy guidance (eg, fiducial markers, dosimeter), open, intra-abdominal, intrapelvic, and/or retroperitoneum, including image guidance, if performed, single or multiple (List separately in addition to code for primary procedure)**

EXCLUDES *Laparoscopic approach (49327)*

Percutaneous approach (49411)

Code first open abdominal, pelvic or retroperitoneal procedure(s)

2.41 2.41 FUD ZZZ C 80

AMA: 2014,Jan,11; 2013,Jan,11-12

49418 **Insertion of tunneled intraperitoneal catheter (eg, dialysis, intraperitoneal chemotherapy instillation, management of ascites), complete procedure, including imaging guidance, catheter placement, contrast injection when performed, and radiological supervision and interpretation, percutaneous**

5.88 34.1 FUD 000 J G2 80

AMA: 2014,Jan,11; 2013,Nov,9

49419 **Insertion of tunneled intraperitoneal catheter, with subcutaneous port (ie, totally implantable)**

EXCLUDES *Removal catheter/cannula (49422)*

12.5 12.5 FUD 090 T A2

AMA: 2014,Jan,11; 2013,Jan,11-12

49421 **Insertion of tunneled intraperitoneal catheter for dialysis, open**

EXCLUDES *Laparoscopic approach (49324)*

Code also insertion subcutaneous extension to intraperitoneal cannula with remote chest exit site, when appropriate (49435)

6.65 6.65 FUD 000 J G2

AMA: 2018,Jan,8; 2017,Jan,8; 2016,Jan,13

49422 **Removal of tunneled intraperitoneal catheter**

EXCLUDES *Removal temporary catheter or cannula (Report appropriate E/M code)*

6.46 6.46 FUD 000 Q2 A2

AMA: 2014,Jan,11; 2013,Jan,11-12

49423 **Exchange of previously placed abscess or cyst drainage catheter under radiological guidance (separate procedure)**

(75984)

2.05 16.9 FUD 000 J G2 80

AMA: 2018,Jan,8; 2017,Jan,8; 2016,Jan,13

49424 **Contrast injection for assessment of abscess or cyst via previously placed drainage catheter or tube (separate procedure)**

(76080)

1.10 4.35 FUD 000 N N1 80

AMA: 2018,Jan,8; 2017,Jan,8; 2016,Jan,13

49425 **Insertion of peritoneal-venous shunt**

20.7 20.7 FUD 090 C 80

AMA: 2014,Jan,11; 2013,Jan,11-12

49426 **Revision of peritoneal-venous shunt**

EXCLUDES *Shunt patency test (78291)*

19.4 19.4 FUD 090 J A2

AMA: 2014,Jan,11; 2013,Jan,11-12

49427 **Injection procedure (eg, contrast media) for evaluation of previously placed peritoneal-venous shunt**

(75809, 78291)

1.13 1.13 FUD 000 N N1 80

AMA: 2014,Jan,11; 2013,Jan,11-12

Digestive System

49400 — 49427

49428 **Ligation of peritoneal-venous shunt**
12.5 | 12.5 | FUD 010 | C
AMA: 2014,Jan,11; 2013,Jan,11-12

49429 **Removal of peritoneal-venous shunt**
13.3 | 13.3 | FUD 010 | Q2 G2
AMA: 2014,Jan,11; 2013,Jan,11-12

\+ **49435** **Insertion of subcutaneous extension to intraperitoneal cannula or catheter with remote chest exit site (List separately in addition to code for primary procedure)**
Code first permanent insertion intraperitoneal catheter/cannula (49324, 49421)
3.50 | 3.50 | FUD ZZZ | N N1 80
AMA: 2014,Jan,11; 2013,Jan,11-12

49436 **Delayed creation of exit site from embedded subcutaneous segment of intraperitoneal cannula or catheter**
5.42 | 5.42 | FUD 010 | J G2 80
AMA: 2014,Jan,11; 2013,Jan,11-12

49440-49442 Insertion of Percutaneous Gastrointestinal Tube

EXCLUDES *Naso- or oro-gastric tube placement (43752)*

49440 **Insertion of gastrostomy tube, percutaneous, under fluoroscopic guidance including contrast injection(s), image documentation and report**
INCLUDES Needle placement with fluoroscopic guidance (77002)
Code also gastrostomy to gastro-jejunostomy tube conversion with initial gastrostomy tube insertion, when performed (49446)
5.93 | 26.6 | FUD 010 | J G2 80
AMA: 2018,Jan,8; 2017,Jan,8; 2016,Jan,13

49441 **Insertion of duodenostomy or jejunostomy tube, percutaneous, under fluoroscopic guidance including contrast injection(s), image documentation and report**
EXCLUDES *Gastrostomy tube to gastrojejunostomy tube conversion (49446)*
7.00 | 30.6 | FUD 010 | J G2 80
AMA: 2018,Jan,8; 2017,Jan,8; 2016,Jan,13

49442 **Insertion of cecostomy or other colonic tube, percutaneous, under fluoroscopic guidance including contrast injection(s), image documentation and report**
6.00 | 25.2 | FUD 010 | T G2 80
AMA: 2018,Jan,8; 2017,Jan,8; 2016,Jan,13

49446 Percutaneous Conversion: Gastrostomy to Gastro-jejunostomy Tube

EXCLUDES *Code also initial gastrostomy tube insertion (49440) when conversion performed same time*

49446 **Conversion of gastrostomy tube to gastro-jejunostomy tube, percutaneous, under fluoroscopic guidance including contrast injection(s), image documentation and report**
4.30 | 25.6 | FUD 000 | J G2 80
AMA: 2018,Jan,8; 2017,Jan,8; 2016,Jan,13

49450-49452 Replacement Gastrointestinal Tube

EXCLUDES *Placement new tube whether gastrostomy, jejunostomy, duodenostomy, gastro-jejunostomy, or cecostomy different percutaneous site (49440-49442)*

49450 **Replacement of gastrostomy or cecostomy (or other colonic) tube, percutaneous, under fluoroscopic guidance including contrast injection(s), image documentation and report**
EXCLUDES *Change gastrostomy tube, percutaneous, without imaging or endoscopic guidance (43762-43763)*
1.91 | 18.7 | FUD 000 | T G2 80
AMA: 2019,Feb,5; 2018,Jan,8; 2017,Jan,8; 2016,Jan,13

49451 **Replacement of duodenostomy or jejunostomy tube, percutaneous, under fluoroscopic guidance including contrast injection(s), image documentation and report**
2.61 | 20.3 | FUD 000 | T G2 80
AMA: 2018,Jan,8; 2017,Jan,8; 2016,Jan,13

49452 **Replacement of gastro-jejunostomy tube, percutaneous, under fluoroscopic guidance including contrast injection(s), image documentation and report**
4.01 | 25.1 | FUD 000 | T G2 80
AMA: 2018,Jan,8; 2017,Jan,8; 2016,Jan,13

49460-49465 Removal of Obstruction/Injection for Contrast Through Gastrointestinal Tube

49460 **Mechanical removal of obstructive material from gastrostomy, duodenostomy, jejunostomy, gastro-jejunostomy, or cecostomy (or other colonic) tube, any method, under fluoroscopic guidance including contrast injection(s), if performed, image documentation and report**
INCLUDES Contrast injection (49465)
EXCLUDES *Replacement gastrointestinal tube (49450-49452)*
1.39 | 20.4 | FUD 000 | T G2 80
AMA: 2018,Jan,8; 2017,Jan,8; 2016,Jan,13

49465 **Contrast injection(s) for radiological evaluation of existing gastrostomy, duodenostomy, jejunostomy, gastro-jejunostomy, or cecostomy (or other colonic) tube, from a percutaneous approach including image documentation and report**
EXCLUDES *Mechanical removal obstructive material from gastrointestinal tube (49460)*
Replacement gastrointestinal tube (49450-49452)
0.89 | 4.48 | FUD 000 | Q1 G2 80
AMA: 2018,Jan,8; 2017,Jan,8; 2016,Jan,13

49491-49492 Inguinal Hernia Repair on Premature Infant

INCLUDES Hernia repairs done on preterm infants younger than or equal to 50 weeks postconception age and younger than 6 months
Initial repair: no previous repair required
Mesh or other prosthesis
EXCLUDES *Abdominal wall debridement (11042, 11043)*
Intra-abdominal hernia repair/reduction (44050)
Code also repair or excision testicle(s), intestine, ovaries, when performed (44120, 54520, 58940)

49491 **Repair, initial inguinal hernia, preterm infant (younger than 37 weeks gestation at birth), performed from birth up to 50 weeks postconception age, with or without hydrocelectomy; reducible** A
23.2 | 23.2 | FUD 090 | 63 J G2 80 50
AMA: 2018,Jan,8; 2017,Jan,8; 2016,Jan,13

49492 **incarcerated or strangulated** A
27.9 | 27.9 | FUD 090 | 63 J G2 80 50
AMA: 2018,Jan,8; 2017,Jan,8; 2016,Jan,13

49495-49557 Hernia Repair: Femoral/Inguinal /Lumbar

INCLUDES Initial repair: no previous repair required
Mesh or other prosthesis
Recurrent repair: required previous repair(s)
EXCLUDES *Abdominal wall debridement (11042, 11043)*
Intra-abdominal hernia repair/reduction (44050)
Code also repair or excision testicle(s), intestine, ovaries, when performed (44120, 54520, 58940)

49495 **Repair, initial inguinal hernia, full term infant younger than age 6 months, or preterm infant older than 50 weeks postconception age and younger than age 6 months at the time of surgery, with or without hydrocelectomy; reducible** A
INCLUDES Hernia repairs done on preterm infants older than 50 weeks postconception age and younger than 6 months
11.8 | 11.8 | FUD 090 | 63 J A2 80 50
AMA: 2018,Jan,8; 2017,Jan,8; 2016,Jan,13

49496 **incarcerated or strangulated** A
INCLUDES Hernia repairs done on preterm infants older than 50 weeks postconception age and younger than 6 months
17.7 | 17.7 | FUD 090 | 63 J A2 80 50
AMA: 2018,Jan,8; 2017,Jan,8; 2016,Jan,13

49500 Repair initial inguinal hernia, age 6 months to younger than 5 years, with or without hydrocelectomy; reducible A

INCLUDES Repairs performed on patients 6 months to younger than 5 years old

11.9 11.9 **FUD** 090 J A2 80 50

AMA: 2018,Jan,8; 2017,Jan,8; 2016,Jan,13

49501 incarcerated or strangulated A

INCLUDES Repairs performed on patients 6 months to younger than 5 years old

17.6 17.6 **FUD** 090 J A2 80 50

AMA: 2018,Jan,8; 2017,Jan,8; 2016,Jan,13

49505 Repair initial inguinal hernia, age 5 years or older; reducible A

INCLUDES MacEwen hernia repair

Code also when performed:

Excision hydrocele (55040)

Excision spermatocele (54840)

Simple orchiectomy (54520)

15.0 15.0 **FUD** 090 J A2 80 50

AMA: 2018,Jan,8; 2017,Jan,8; 2016,Jan,13

49507 incarcerated or strangulated A

Code also when performed:

Excision hydrocele (55040)

Excision spermatocele (54840)

Simple orchiectomy (54520)

17.0 17.0 **FUD** 090 J A2 80 50

AMA: 2018,Jan,8; 2017,Jan,8; 2016,Jan,13

49520 Repair recurrent inguinal hernia, any age; reducible

18.3 18.3 **FUD** 090 J A2 80 50

AMA: 2018,Jan,8; 2017,Jan,8; 2016,Jan,13

49521 incarcerated or strangulated

20.8 20.8 **FUD** 090 J A2 80 50

AMA: 2018,Jan,8; 2017,Jan,8; 2016,Jan,13

49525 Repair inguinal hernia, sliding, any age

EXCLUDES *Inguinal hernia repair, incarcerated/strangulated (49496, 49501, 49507, 49521)*

16.7 16.7 **FUD** 090 J A2 80 50

AMA: 2018,Jan,8; 2017,Jan,8; 2016,Jan,13

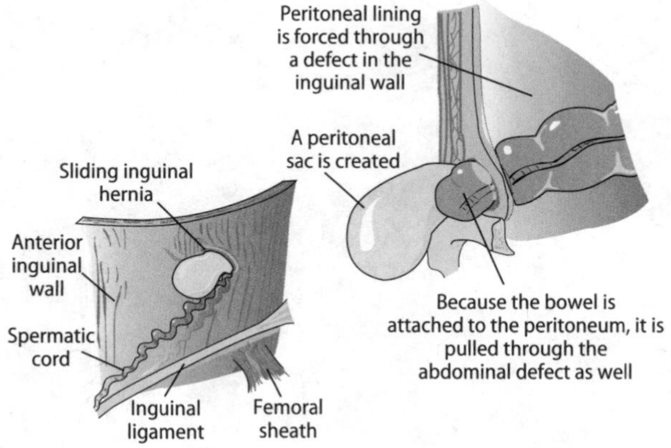

Peritoneal lining is forced through a defect in the inguinal wall
A peritoneal sac is created
Sliding inguinal hernia
Anterior inguinal wall
Spermatic cord
Inguinal ligament
Femoral sheath
Because the bowel is attached to the peritoneum, it is pulled through the abdominal defect as well

49540 Repair lumbar hernia

19.5 19.5 **FUD** 090 J A2 80 50

AMA: 2018,Jan,8; 2017,Jan,8; 2016,Jan,13

49550 Repair initial femoral hernia, any age; reducible

16.7 16.7 **FUD** 090 J A2 80 50

AMA: 2018,Jan,8; 2017,Jan,8; 2016,Jan,13

49553 incarcerated or strangulated

18.3 18.3 **FUD** 090 J A2 80 50

AMA: 2018,Jan,8; 2017,Jan,8; 2016,Jan,13

49555 Repair recurrent femoral hernia; reducible

17.5 17.5 **FUD** 090 J A2 80 50

AMA: 2018,Jan,8; 2017,Jan,8; 2016,Jan,13

49557 incarcerated or strangulated

21.0 21.0 **FUD** 090 J A2 80 50

AMA: 2018,Jan,8; 2017,Jan,8; 2016,Jan,13

49560-49568 Hernia Repair: Incisional/Ventral

INCLUDES Initial repair: no previous repair required

Recurrent repair: required previous repair(s)

EXCLUDES *Abdominal wall debridement (11042, 11043)*

Intra-abdominal hernia repair/reduction (44050)

Code also repair or excision testicle(s), intestine, ovaries, when performed (44120, 54520, 58940)

49560 Repair initial incisional or ventral hernia; reducible

Code also implantation mesh or other prosthesis, when performed (49568)

21.5 21.5 **FUD** 090 J A2 80 50

AMA: 2019,Nov,14; 2018,Jan,8; 2017,Jan,8; 2016,Jan,13

49561 incarcerated or strangulated

Code also implantation mesh or other prosthesis, when performed (49568)

27.0 27.0 **FUD** 090 J A2 80 50

AMA: 2019,Nov,14; 2018,Jul,14; 2018,Mar,11; 2018,Jan,8; 2017,Jan,8; 2016,Jan,13

49565 Repair recurrent incisional or ventral hernia; reducible

Code also implantation mesh or other prosthesis, when performed (49568)

22.3 22.3 **FUD** 090 J A2 80 50

AMA: 2019,Nov,14; 2018,Jan,8; 2017,Jan,8; 2016,Jan,13

49566 incarcerated or strangulated

Code also implantation mesh or other prosthesis, when performed (49568)

27.3 27.3 **FUD** 090 J A2 80 50

AMA: 2019,Nov,14; 2018,Jan,8; 2017,Jan,8; 2016,Jan,13

\+ **49568 Implantation of mesh or other prosthesis for open incisional or ventral hernia repair or mesh for closure of debridement for necrotizing soft tissue infection (List separately in addition to code for the incisional or ventral hernia repair)**

EXCLUDES *Reporting with modifier 50. Report once for each side when performed bilaterally*

Code first (11004-11006, 49560-49566)

7.77 7.77 **FUD** ZZZ N N1 80

AMA: 2019,Nov,14; 2018,Jan,8; 2017,Jan,8; 2016,Jan,13

49570-49590 Hernia Repair: Epigastric/Lateral Ventral/Umbilical

INCLUDES Mesh or other prosthesis

EXCLUDES *Abdominal wall debridement (11042, 11043)*

Intra-abdominal hernia repair/reduction (44050)

Code also repair or excision testicle(s), intestine, ovaries, when performed (44120, 54520, 58940)

49570 Repair epigastric hernia (eg, preperitoneal fat); reducible (separate procedure)

12.1 12.1 **FUD** 090 J A2 80 50

AMA: 2018,Jan,8; 2017,Jan,8; 2016,Jan,13

49572 incarcerated or strangulated

14.9 14.9 **FUD** 090 J A2 80 50

AMA: 2018,Jan,8; 2017,Jan,8; 2016,Jan,13

49580 Repair umbilical hernia, younger than age 5 years; reducible A

9.69 9.69 **FUD** 090 J A2 80

AMA: 2018,Jan,8; 2017,Jan,8; 2016,Jan,13

49582 incarcerated or strangulated A

14.0 14.0 **FUD** 090 J A2 80

AMA: 2018,Jan,8; 2017,Jan,8; 2016,Jan,13

49585 Repair umbilical hernia, age 5 years or older; reducible A

INCLUDES Mayo hernia repair

12.9 12.9 **FUD** 090 J A2 80

AMA: 2018,Jan,8; 2017,Jan,8; 2016,Jan,13

49587 incarcerated or strangulated A

13.7 13.7 **FUD** 090 J A2 80

AMA: 2018,Jan,8; 2017,Jan,8; 2016,Jan,13

49590 **Repair spigelian hernia**
16.5 16.5 FUD 090 J A2 80 50
AMA: 2018,Jan,8; 2017,Jan,8; 2016,Jan,13

49600-49611 Repair Birth Defect Abdominal Wall: Omphalocele/Gastroschisis

INCLUDES Mesh or other prosthesis
EXCLUDES *Abdominal wall debridement (11042, 11043)*
Intra-abdominal hernia repair/reduction (44050)
Repair:
Diaphragmatic or hiatal hernia (39503, 43332-43337)
Omentum (49999)

49600 **Repair of small omphalocele, with primary closure**
21.0 21.0 FUD 090 63 J A2 80
AMA: 2018,Jan,8; 2017,Jan,8; 2016,Jan,13

49605 **Repair of large omphalocele or gastroschisis; with or without prosthesis**
144. 144. FUD 090 63 C 80
AMA: 2018,Jan,8; 2017,Jan,8; 2016,Jan,13

49606 **with removal of prosthesis, final reduction and closure, in operating room**
32.9 32.9 FUD 090 63 C 80
AMA: 2018,Jan,8; 2017,Jan,8; 2016,Jan,13

49610 **Repair of omphalocele (Gross type operation); first stage**
20.1 20.1 FUD 090 63 C 80
AMA: 2018,Jan,8; 2017,Jan,8; 2016,Jan,13

49611 **second stage**
17.7 17.7 FUD 090 63 C 80
AMA: 2018,Jan,8; 2017,Jan,8; 2016,Jan,13

49650-49659 Laparoscopic Hernia Repair

INCLUDES Diagnostic laparoscopy (49320)
Mesh or other prosthesis (49568)

49650 **Laparoscopy, surgical; repair initial inguinal hernia**
12.5 12.5 FUD 090 J A2 80 50
AMA: 2018,Jan,8; 2017,Jan,8; 2016,Jan,13

49651 **repair recurrent inguinal hernia**
16.2 16.2 FUD 090 J A2 80 50
AMA: 2018,Jan,8; 2017,Jan,8; 2016,Jan,13

49652 **Laparoscopy, surgical, repair, ventral, umbilical, spigelian or epigastric hernia (includes mesh insertion, when performed); reducible**
INCLUDES Laparoscopy, surgical, enterolysis (44180)
21.5 21.5 FUD 090 J G2 80 50
AMA: 2014,Jan,11; 2013,Jan,11-12

49653 **incarcerated or strangulated**
INCLUDES Laparoscopy, surgical, enterolysis (44180)
27.0 27.0 FUD 090 J G2 80 50
AMA: 2014,Jan,11; 2013,Jan,11-12

49654 **Laparoscopy, surgical, repair, incisional hernia (includes mesh insertion, when performed); reducible**
INCLUDES Laparoscopy, surgical, enterolysis (44180)
24.6 24.6 FUD 090 J G2 80 50
AMA: 2018,Jan,7

49655 **incarcerated or strangulated**
INCLUDES Laparoscopy, surgical, enterolysis (44180)
29.9 29.9 FUD 090 J G2 80 50
AMA: 2018,Jan,7

49656 **Laparoscopy, surgical, repair, recurrent incisional hernia (includes mesh insertion, when performed); reducible**
INCLUDES Laparoscopy, surgical, enterolysis (44180)
26.7 26.7 FUD 090 J G2 80 50
AMA: 2014,Jan,11; 2013,Jan,11-12

49657 **incarcerated or strangulated**
INCLUDES Laparoscopy, surgical, enterolysis (44180)
38.2 38.2 FUD 090 J G2 80 50
AMA: 2014,Jan,11; 2013,Jan,11-12

49659 **Unlisted laparoscopy procedure, hernioplasty, herniorrhaphy, herniotomy**
0.00 0.00 FUD YYY J 80 50
AMA: 2018,Jan,8; 2017,Jul,10; 2017,Jan,8; 2016,Jan,13

49900 Surgical Repair Abdominal Wall

EXCLUDES *Abdominal wall debridement (11042, 11043)*
Suture ruptured diaphragm (39540-39541)

49900 **Suture, secondary, of abdominal wall for evisceration or dehiscence**
23.7 23.7 FUD 090 C 80
AMA: 2018,Jan,8; 2017,Jan,8; 2016,Jan,13

49904-49999 Harvesting of Omental Flap

49904 **Omental flap, extra-abdominal (eg, for reconstruction of sternal and chest wall defects)**
INCLUDES Harvest and transfer
EXCLUDES *Omental flap harvest by second surgeon: both surgeons report code with modifier 62*
40.5 40.5 FUD 090 C
AMA: 2014,Jan,11; 2013,Jan,11-12

+ **49905** **Omental flap, intra-abdominal (List separately in addition to code for primary procedure)**
EXCLUDES *Exclusion small intestine from pelvis by mesh, other prosthesis, or native tissue (44700)*
Code first primary procedure
10.3 10.3 FUD ZZZ C 80
AMA: 2020,Feb,13; 2018,Jan,8; 2017,Jan,8; 2016,Jan,13

49906 **Free omental flap with microvascular anastomosis**
INCLUDES Operating microscope (69990)
0.00 0.00 FUD 090 C
AMA: 2019,Dec,5; 2018,Jan,8; 2017,Jan,8; 2016,Feb,12; 2016,Jan,13

49999 **Unlisted procedure, abdomen, peritoneum and omentum**
0.00 0.00 FUD YYY T
AMA: 2020,Jun,14; 2019,Nov,14; 2018,Jan,8; 2017,Jan,8; 2016,Jan,13

50010-50045 Kidney Procedures for Exploration or Drainage

EXCLUDES Donor nephrectomy performed laparoscopically (50547)
Retroperitoneal
Abscess drainage (49060)
Exploration (49010)
Tumor/cyst excision (49203-49205)

50010 Renal exploration, not necessitating other specific procedures

EXCLUDES *Laparoscopic ablation mass lesions of kidney (50542)*
21.2 21.2 FUD 090 C 80 50
AMA: 2014,Jan,11; 2008,Aug,7-9

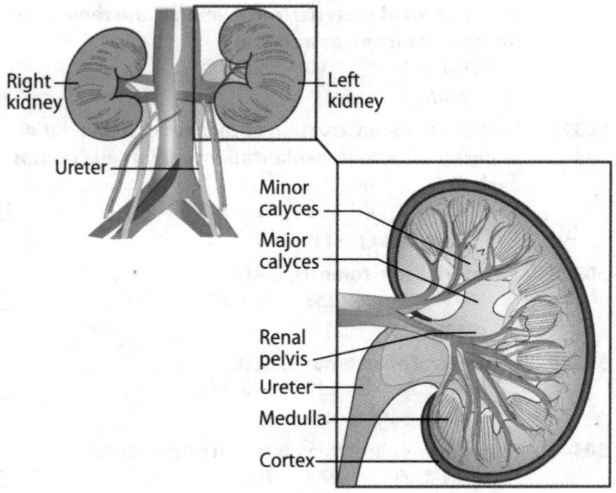

50020 Drainage of perirenal or renal abscess, open

EXCLUDES *Image-guided percutaneous drainage perirenal or renal abscess (49405)*
29.2 29.2 FUD 090 J 62
AMA: 2018,Jan,8; 2017,Jan,8; 2016,Jan,13

50040 Nephrostomy, nephrotomy with drainage

26.6 26.6 FUD 090 C 50
AMA: 2018,Jan,8; 2017,Jan,8; 2016,Jan,13

50045 Nephrotomy, with exploration

EXCLUDES *Renal endoscopy through nephrotomy (50570-50580)*
26.9 26.9 FUD 090 C 80 50
AMA: 2018,Jan,8; 2017,Jan,8; 2016,Jan,13

50060-50081 Treatment of Kidney Stones

CMS: 100-03,230.1 NCD for Treatment of Kidney Stones

EXCLUDES *Retroperitoneal:*
Abscess drainage (49060)
Exploration (49010)
Tumor/cyst excision (49203-49205)

50060 Nephrolithotomy; removal of calculus

32.9 32.9 FUD 090 C 80 50
AMA: 2018,Jan,8; 2017,Jan,8; 2016,Jan,13

50065 secondary surgical operation for calculus

34.9 34.9 FUD 090 C 80 50
AMA: 2018,Jan,8; 2017,Jan,8; 2016,Jan,13

50070 complicated by congenital kidney abnormality

34.2 34.2 FUD 090 C 80 50
AMA: 2018,Jan,8; 2017,Jan,8; 2016,Jan,13

50075 removal of large staghorn calculus filling renal pelvis and calyces (including anatrophic pyelolithotomy)

42.1 42.1 FUD 090 C 80 50
AMA: 2018,Jan,8; 2017,Jan,8; 2016,Jan,13

50080 Percutaneous nephrostolithotomy or pyelostolithotomy, with or without dilation, endoscopy, lithotripsy, stenting, or basket extraction; up to 2 cm

EXCLUDES *Dilation existing tract by same provider ([50436, 50437])*
Nephrostomy without nephrostolithotomy (50040, [50432, 50433], 52334)
(76000)
25.0 25.0 FUD 090 J 62 50
AMA: 2018,Jan,8; 2017,Jan,8; 2016,Jan,13

50081 over 2 cm

EXCLUDES *Dilation existing tract by same provider ([50436, 50437])*
Nephrostomy without nephrostolithotomy (50040, [50432, 50433], 52334)
(76000)
36.9 36.9 FUD 090 J 62 80 50
AMA: 2018,Jan,8; 2017,Jan,8; 2016,Jan,13

50100 Repair of Anomalous Vessels of the Kidney

EXCLUDES *Retroperitoneal:*
Abscess drainage (49060)
Exploration (49010)
Tumor/cyst excision (49203-49205)

50100 Transection or repositioning of aberrant renal vessels (separate procedure)

31.4 31.4 FUD 090 C 80 50
AMA: 2018,Jan,8; 2017,Jan,8; 2016,Jan,13

50120-50135 Procedures of Renal Pelvis

EXCLUDES *Retroperitoneal:*
Abscess drainage (49060)
Exploration (49010)
Tumor/cyst excision (49203-49205)

50120 Pyelotomy; with exploration

INCLUDES Gol-Vernet pyelotomy
EXCLUDES *Renal endoscopy through pyelotomy (50570-50580)*
27.4 27.4 FUD 090 C 80 50
AMA: 2018,Jan,8; 2017,Jan,8; 2016,Jan,13

50125 with drainage, pyelostomy

28.3 28.3 FUD 090 C 80 50
AMA: 2018,Jan,8; 2017,Jan,8; 2016,Jan,13

50130 with removal of calculus (pyelolithotomy, pelviolithotomy, including coagulum pyelolithotomy)

29.8 29.8 FUD 090 C 80 50
AMA: 2018,Jan,8; 2017,Jan,8; 2016,Jan,13

50135 complicated (eg, secondary operation, congenital kidney abnormality)

32.4 32.4 FUD 090 C 80 50
AMA: 2018,Jan,8; 2017,Jan,8; 2016,Jan,13

50200-50205 Biopsy of Kidney

EXCLUDES *Laparoscopic renal mass lesion ablation (50542)*
Retroperitoneal tumor/cyst excision (49203-49205)

50200 Renal biopsy; percutaneous, by trocar or needle

EXCLUDES *Fine needle aspiration ([10005, 10006, 10007, 10008, 10009, 10010, 10011, 10012])*
(76942, 77002, 77012, 77021)
(88172-88173)
3.70 15.4 FUD 000 J A2 50
AMA: 2019,Apr,4; 2018,Jan,8; 2017,Jan,8; 2016,Jan,13

50205 by surgical exposure of kidney

21.9 21.9 FUD 090 C 80 50
AMA: 2018,Jan,8; 2017,Jan,8; 2016,Jan,13

50220-50240 Nephrectomy Procedures

EXCLUDES *Laparoscopic renal mass lesion ablation (50542)*
Retroperitoneal tumor/cyst excision (49203-49205)

50220 Nephrectomy, including partial ureterectomy, any open approach including rib resection;

30.3 30.3 FUD 090 C 80 50
AMA: 2018,Jan,8; 2017,Jan,8; 2016,Jan,13

Urinary System
50010 — 50220

● New Code ▲ Revised Code ○ Reinstated ● New Web Release ▲ Revised Web Release + Add-on Unlisted Not Covered # Resequenced
50 Optum Mod 50 Exempt ⊘ AMA Mod 51 Exempt 51 Optum Mod 51 Exempt 63 Mod 63 Exempt Non-FDA Drug ★ Telemedicine M Maternity A Age Edit

50225 **complicated because of previous surgery on same kidney**
34.7 34.7 FUD 090 C 80 50
AMA: 2018,Jan,8; 2017,Jan,8; 2016,Jan,13

50230 **radical, with regional lymphadenectomy and/or vena caval thrombectomy**
EXCLUDES *Vena caval resection with reconstruction (37799)*
37.0 37.0 FUD 090 C 80 50
AMA: 2018,Jan,8; 2017,Jan,8; 2016,Jan,13

50234 **Nephrectomy with total ureterectomy and bladder cuff; through same incision**
37.6 37.6 FUD 090 C 80 50
AMA: 2018,Jan,8; 2017,Jan,8; 2016,Jan,13

50236 **through separate incision**
42.3 42.3 FUD 090 C 80 50
AMA: 2018,Jan,8; 2017,Jan,8; 2016,Jan,13

50240 **Nephrectomy, partial**
EXCLUDES *Laparoscopic partial nephrectomy (50543)*
38.2 38.2 FUD 090 C 80 50
AMA: 2018,Jan,8; 2017,Jan,8; 2016,Jan,13

50250-50290 Open Removal Kidney Lesions

EXCLUDES *Open destruction or excision intra-abdominal tumors (49203-49205)*

50250 **Ablation, open, 1 or more renal mass lesion(s), cryosurgical, including intraoperative ultrasound guidance and monitoring, if performed**
EXCLUDES *Laparoscopic renal mass lesion ablation (50542)*
Percutaneous renal tumor ablation (50592-50593)
35.1 35.1 FUD 090 C 80
AMA: 2018,Jan,8; 2017,Jan,8; 2016,Jan,13

50280 **Excision or unroofing of cyst(s) of kidney**
EXCLUDES *Renal cyst laparoscopic ablation (50541)*
27.6 27.6 FUD 090 C 80 50
AMA: 2018,Jan,8; 2017,Jan,8; 2016,Jan,13

50290 **Excision of perinephric cyst**
25.9 25.9 FUD 090 C 80
AMA: 2018,Jan,8; 2017,Jan,8; 2016,Jan,13

50300-50380 Kidney Transplant Procedures

CMS: 100-04,3,90.1 Kidney Transplant - General; 100-04,3,90.1.1 Standard Kidney Acquisition Charge; 100-04,3,90.1.2 Billing for Kidney Transplant and Acquisition Services; 100-04,3,90.5 Pancreas Transplants with Kidney Transplants

EXCLUDES *Dialysis procedures (90935-90999)*
Lymphocele drainage to peritoneal cavity performed laparoscopically (49323)

50300 **Donor nephrectomy (including cold preservation); from cadaver donor, unilateral or bilateral**
INCLUDES Graft:
Cold preservation
Harvesting
EXCLUDES *Donor nephrectomy performed laparoscopically (50547)*
0.00 0.00 FUD XXX C
AMA: 2018,Jan,8; 2017,Jan,8; 2016,Jan,13

50320 **open, from living donor**
INCLUDES Donor care
Graft:
Cold preservation
Harvesting
EXCLUDES *Donor nephrectomy performed laparoscopically (50547)*
43.7 43.7 FUD 090 C 80 50
AMA: 2018,Jan,8; 2017,Jan,8; 2016,Jan,13

50323 **Backbench standard preparation of cadaver donor renal allograft prior to transplantation, including dissection and removal of perinephric fat, diaphragmatic and retroperitoneal attachments, excision of adrenal gland, and preparation of ureter(s), renal vein(s), and renal artery(s), ligating branches, as necessary**
EXCLUDES *Adrenalectomy (60540, 60545)*
0.00 0.00 FUD XXX C 80
AMA: 2018,Jan,8; 2017,Jan,8; 2016,Jan,13

50325 **Backbench standard preparation of living donor renal allograft (open or laparoscopic) prior to transplantation, including dissection and removal of perinephric fat and preparation of ureter(s), renal vein(s), and renal artery(s), ligating branches, as necessary**
0.00 0.00 FUD XXX C 80
AMA: 2014,Jan,11

50327 **Backbench reconstruction of cadaver or living donor renal allograft prior to transplantation; venous anastomosis, each**
6.29 6.29 FUD XXX C 80
AMA: 2014,Jan,11

50328 **arterial anastomosis, each**
5.53 5.53 FUD XXX C 80
AMA: 2014,Jan,11

50329 **ureteral anastomosis, each**
5.24 5.24 FUD XXX C 80
AMA: 2014,Jan,11

50340 **Recipient nephrectomy (separate procedure)**
27.4 27.4 FUD 090 C 80 50
AMA: 2014,Jan,11

50360 **Renal allotransplantation, implantation of graft; without recipient nephrectomy**
INCLUDES Allograft transplantation
Recipient care
Code also:
Backbench work (50323, 50325, 50327-50329)
Donor nephrectomy (cadaver or living donor) (50300, 50320, 50547)
70.0 70.0 FUD 090 C 80
AMA: 2014,Jan,11; 1994,Win,1

50365 **with recipient nephrectomy**
INCLUDES Allograft transplantation
Recipient care
83.5 83.5 FUD 090 C 80 50
AMA: 2018,Jan,8; 2017,Jan,8; 2016,Jan,13

50370 **Removal of transplanted renal allograft**
35.0 35.0 FUD 090 C 80
AMA: 2014,Jan,11; 2002,Oct,5

50380 **Renal autotransplantation, reimplantation of kidney**
INCLUDES Reimplantation autograft
EXCLUDES *Secondary procedures:*
Nephrolithotomy (50060-50075)
Partial nephrectomy (50240, 50543)
58.4 58.4 FUD 090 C 80
AMA: 2019,Sep,10; 2018,Jan,8; 2017,Jan,8; 2016,Jan,13

50382-50386 Removal With/Without Replacement Internal Ureteral Stent

INCLUDES Radiological supervision and interpretation

50382 **Removal (via snare/capture) and replacement of internally dwelling ureteral stent via percutaneous approach, including radiological supervision and interpretation**
EXCLUDES *Dilation existing tract, percutaneous for endourologic procedure ([50436, 50437])*
Removal and replacement internally dwelling ureteral stent using transurethral approach (50385)
7.46 31.3 FUD 000 J G2 50
AMA: 2018,Jan,8; 2017,Jan,8; 2016,Jan,13; 2016,Jan,3

50384 **Removal (via snare/capture) of internally dwelling ureteral stent via percutaneous approach, including radiological supervision and interpretation**

EXCLUDES *Dilation existing tract, percutaneous for endourologic procedure ([50436, 50437])*

Removal internally dwelling ureteral stent using transurethral approach (50386)

6.68 25.0 **FUD** 000 Q2 G2 50

AMA: 2018,Jan,8; 2017,Jan,8; 2016,Jan,13; 2016,Jan,3

50385 **Removal (via snare/capture) and replacement of internally dwelling ureteral stent via transurethral approach, without use of cystoscopy, including radiological supervision and interpretation**

6.34 30.7 **FUD** 000 J G2 80 50

AMA: 2018,Jan,8; 2017,Jan,8; 2016,Jan,13; 2016,Jan,3

50386 **Removal (via snare/capture) of internally dwelling ureteral stent via transurethral approach, without use of cystoscopy, including radiological supervision and interpretation**

4.70 20.3 **FUD** 000 Q2 P3 80 50

AMA: 2018,Jan,8; 2017,Jan,8; 2016,Jan,3; 2016,Jan,13

50387 Remove/Replace Accessible Ureteral Stent

EXCLUDES *Removal and replacement ureteral stent through ureterostomy tube or ileal conduit (50688)*

Removal without replacement externally accessible ureteral stent without fluoroscopic guidance, report with appropriate E/M code

50387 **Removal and replacement of externally accessible nephroureteral catheter (eg, external/internal stent) requiring fluoroscopic guidance, including radiological supervision and interpretation**

2.43 14.6 **FUD** 000 J G2 80 50

AMA: 2018,Jan,8; 2017,Jan,8; 2016,Mar,10; 2016,Jan,13; 2016,Jan,3

50389-50435 [50430, 50431, 50432, 50433, 50434, 50435, 50436, 50437] Percutaneous and Injection Procedures With/Without Indwelling Tube/Catheter Access

50389 **Removal of nephrostomy tube, requiring fluoroscopic guidance (eg, with concurrent indwelling ureteral stent)**

EXCLUDES *Nephrostomy tube removal without fluoroscopic guidance, report with appropriate E/M code*

1.56 9.49 **FUD** 000 Q2 G2 50

AMA: 2018,Jan,8; 2017,Jan,8; 2016,Jan,13; 2016,Jan,3

50390 **Aspiration and/or injection of renal cyst or pelvis by needle, percutaneous**

EXCLUDES *Antegrade nephrostogram/pyelogram ([50430, 50431])*

(74425, 74470, 76942, 77002, 77012, 77021)

2.78 2.78 **FUD** 000 T A2 50

AMA: 2018,Jan,8; 2017,Jan,8; 2016,Jan,13

50391 **Instillation(s) of therapeutic agent into renal pelvis and/or ureter through established nephrostomy, pyelostomy or ureterostomy tube (eg, anticarcinogenic or antifungal agent)**

Code also therapeutic agent

2.84 3.52 **FUD** 000 T P3 50

AMA: 2018,Jan,8; 2017,Jan,8; 2016,Jan,13

50436 **Dilation of existing tract, percutaneous, for an endourologic procedure including imaging guidance (eg, ultrasound and/or fluoroscopy) and all associated radiological supervision and interpretation, with postprocedure tube placement, when performed**

EXCLUDES *Percutaneous nephrostolithotomy (50080-50081)*

Procedure performed for same renal collecting system/ureter ([50430, 50431, 50432, 50433], 52334, 74485)

Removal, replacement internally dwelling ureteral stent (50382, 50384)

4.35 4.35 **FUD** 000 G2 50

50437 **including new access into the renal collecting system**

EXCLUDES *Percutaneous nephrostolithotomy (50080-50081)*

Procedure performed for same renal collecting system/ureter ([50430, 50431, 50432, 50433], 52334, 74485)

Removal, replacement internally dwelling ureteral stent (50382, 50384)

7.29 7.29 **FUD** 000 G2 50

50396 **Manometric studies through nephrostomy or pyelostomy tube, or indwelling ureteral catheter**

(74425)

3.38 3.38 **FUD** 000 J A2 80 50

AMA: 2018,Jan,8; 2017,Jan,8; 2016,Jan,13

50430 **Injection procedure for antegrade nephrostogram and/or ureterogram, complete diagnostic procedure including imaging guidance (eg, ultrasound and fluoroscopy) and all associated radiological supervision and interpretation; new access**

INCLUDES Renal pelvis and associated ureter as single element

EXCLUDES *Procedure performed for same renal collecting system/ureter ([50432, 50433, 50434, 50435], 50693-50695, 74425)*

4.46 14.5 **FUD** 000 Q2 N1 80 50

AMA: 2018,Jan,8; 2017,Jan,8; 2016,Jan,3; 2016,Jan,13

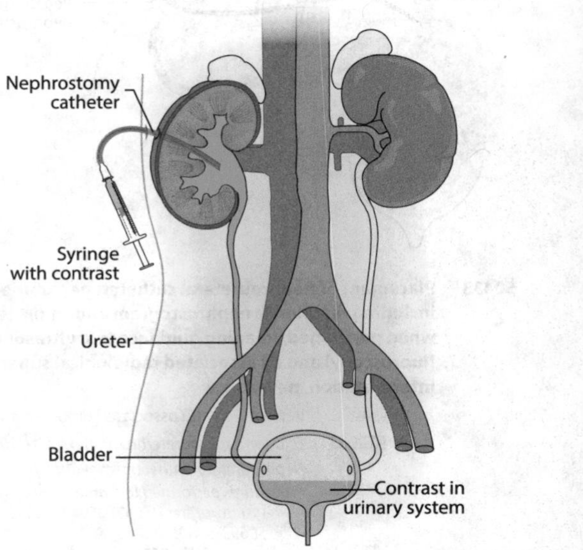

50431 **existing access**

INCLUDES Renal pelvis and associated ureter as single element

EXCLUDES *Procedure performed for same renal collecting system/ureter ([50432, 50433, 50434, 50435], 50693-50695, 74425)*

1.91 4.64 **FUD** 000 Q2 N1 50

AMA: 2018,Jan,8; 2017,Jan,8; 2016,Jan,3; 2016,Jan,13

Urinary System

50384 — 50431

\# **50432** **Placement of nephrostomy catheter, percutaneous, including diagnostic nephrostogram and/or ureterogram when performed, imaging guidance (eg, ultrasound and/or fluoroscopy) and all associated radiological supervision and interpretation**

INCLUDES Renal pelvis and associated ureter as single element

EXCLUDES *Dilation nephroureteral catheter tract ([50436, 50437])*
Procedure performed for same renal collecting system/ureter ([50430, 50431], [50433], 50694-50695, 74425)

5.98 23.5 FUD 000 J G2 50

AMA: 2018,Mar,11; 2018,Jan,8; 2017,Jan,8; 2016,Jan,3; 2016,Jan,13

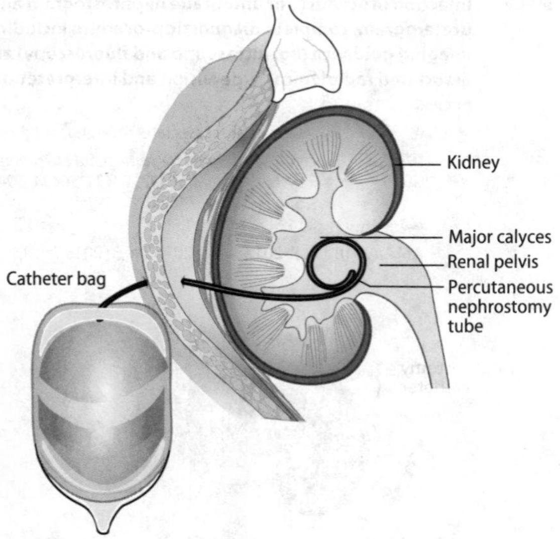

\# **50433** **Placement of nephroureteral catheter, percutaneous, including diagnostic nephrostogram and/or ureterogram when performed, imaging guidance (eg, ultrasound and/or fluoroscopy) and all associated radiological supervision and interpretation, new access**

INCLUDES Renal pelvis and associated ureter as single element

EXCLUDES *Dilation nephroureteral catheter tract ([50436, 50437])*
Nephroureteral catheter removal/replacement (50387)
Procedures performed for same renal collecting system/ureter ([50430, 50431, 50432], 50693-50695, 74425)

7.44 31.2 FUD 000 J G2 50

AMA: 2018,Mar,11; 2018,Jan,8; 2017,Jan,8; 2016,Jan,3; 2016,Jan,13

\# **50434** **Convert nephrostomy catheter to nephroureteral catheter, percutaneous, including diagnostic nephrostogram and/or ureterogram when performed, imaging guidance (eg, ultrasound and/or fluoroscopy) and all associated radiological supervision and interpretation, via pre-existing nephrostomy tract**

INCLUDES Renal pelvis and associated ureter as single element

EXCLUDES *Procedure performed for same renal collecting system/ureter ([50430, 50431], [50435], 50684, 50693, 74425)*

5.60 24.6 FUD 000 J G2 50

AMA: 2018,Jan,8; 2017,Jan,8; 2016,Jan,3; 2016,Jan,13

\# **50435** **Exchange nephrostomy catheter, percutaneous, including diagnostic nephrostogram and/or ureterogram when performed, imaging guidance (eg, ultrasound and/or fluoroscopy) and all associated radiological supervision and interpretation**

INCLUDES Renal pelvis and associated ureter as single element

EXCLUDES *Procedure performed for same renal collecting system/ureter ([50430, 50431], [50434], 50693, 74425)*
Removal nephrostomy catheter requiring fluoroscopic guidance (50389)

2.90 14.6 FUD 000 J G2 50

AMA: 2018,Mar,11; 2018,Jan,8; 2017,Jan,8; 2016,Jan,3; 2016,Jan,13

50400-50540 [50430, 50431, 50432, 50433, 50434, 50435, 50436, 50437] Open Surgical Procedures of Kidney

50400 **Pyeloplasty (Foley Y-pyeloplasty), plastic operation on renal pelvis, with or without plastic operation on ureter, nephropexy, nephrostomy, pyelostomy, or ureteral splinting; simple**

EXCLUDES *Laparoscopic pyeloplasty (50544)*

33.5 33.5 FUD 090 C 80 50

AMA: 2018,Jan,8; 2017,Jan,8; 2016,Jan,13

50405 **complicated (congenital kidney abnormality, secondary pyeloplasty, solitary kidney, calycoplasty)**

EXCLUDES *Laparoscopic pyeloplasty (50544)*

40.3 40.3 FUD 090 C 80 50

AMA: 2018,Jan,8; 2017,Jan,8; 2016,Jan,13

50430 **Resequenced code. See code following 50396.**

50431 **Resequenced code. See code following 50396.**

50432 **Resequenced code. See code following 50396.**

50433 **Resequenced code. See code following 50396.**

50434 **Resequenced code. See code following 50396.**

50435 **Resequenced code. See code following 50396.**

50436 **Resequenced code. See code following 50391.**

50437 **Resequenced code. See code following 50391.**

50500 **Nephrorrhaphy, suture of kidney wound or injury**

37.3 37.3 FUD 090 C 80

AMA: 2014,Jan,11

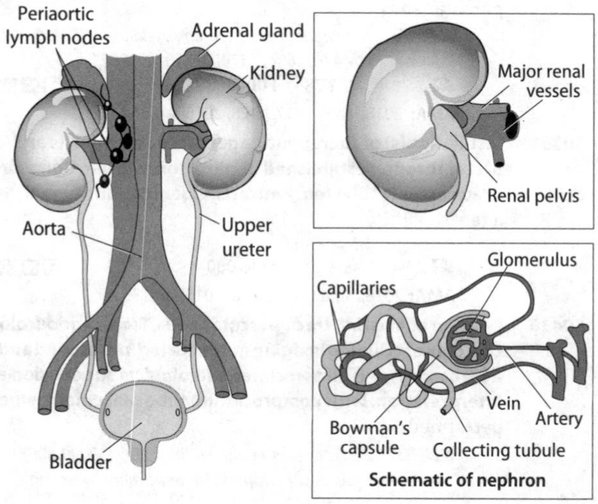

50520 **Closure of nephrocutaneous or pyelocutaneous fistula**

33.6 33.6 FUD 090 C 80

AMA: 2014,Jan,11; 2000,Oct,8

50525 **Closure of nephrovisceral fistula (eg, renocolic), including visceral repair; abdominal approach**
42.6 42.6 FUD 090 C 80
AMA: 2014,Jan,11

50526 **thoracic approach**
45.9 45.9 FUD 090 C 80
AMA: 2014,Jan,11

50540 **Symphysiotomy for horseshoe kidney with or without pyeloplasty and/or other plastic procedure, unilateral or bilateral (1 operation)**
33.1 33.1 FUD 090 C 80
AMA: 2014,Jan,11; 2000,Oct,8

50541-50549 Laparoscopic Surgical Procedures of the Kidney

INCLUDES Diagnostic laparoscopy (49320)

EXCLUDES *Laparoscopic drainage lymphocele to peritoneal cavity (49323)*

50541 **Laparoscopy, surgical; ablation of renal cysts**
26.5 26.5 FUD 090 J G2 80 50
AMA: 2018,Jan,8; 2017,Jan,8; 2016,Jan,13

50542 **ablation of renal mass lesion(s), including intraoperative ultrasound guidance and monitoring, when performed**
EXCLUDES *Open ablation renal mass lesions (50250)*
Percutaneous ablation renal tumors (50592-50593)
33.7 33.7 FUD 090 J G2 80 50
AMA: 2018,Jan,8; 2017,Jan,8; 2016,Jan,13

50543 **partial nephrectomy**
EXCLUDES *Partial nephrectomy, open approach (50240)*
43.0 43.0 FUD 090 J G2 80 50
AMA: 2018,Jan,8; 2017,Jan,8; 2016,Jan,13

50544 **pyeloplasty**
36.0 36.0 FUD 090 J G2 80 50
AMA: 2018,Jan,8; 2017,Jan,8; 2016,Jan,13

50545 **radical nephrectomy (includes removal of Gerota's fascia and surrounding fatty tissue, removal of regional lymph nodes, and adrenalectomy)**
EXCLUDES *Radical nephrectomy, open approach (50230)*
38.7 38.7 FUD 090 C 80 50
AMA: 2018,Jan,8; 2017,Jan,8; 2016,Jan,13

50546 **nephrectomy, including partial ureterectomy**
34.7 34.7 FUD 090 C 80 50
AMA: 2018,Jan,8; 2017,Jan,8; 2016,Jan,13

50547 **donor nephrectomy (including cold preservation), from living donor**
INCLUDES Donor care
Graft:
Cold preservation
Harvesting
EXCLUDES *Backbench reconstruction renal allograft prior to transplantation (50327-50329)*
Backbench standard preparation living donor renal allograft prior to transplantation (50325)
Donor nephrectomy, open approach (50320)
46.4 46.4 FUD 090 C 80 50
AMA: 2018,Jan,8; 2017,Jan,8; 2016,Jan,13

50548 **nephrectomy with total ureterectomy**
EXCLUDES *Nephrectomy, open approach (50234, 50236)*
38.9 38.9 FUD 090 C 80 50
AMA: 2018,Jan,8; 2017,Jan,8; 2016,Jan,13

50549 **Unlisted laparoscopy procedure, renal**
0.00 0.00 FUD YYY J 80 50
AMA: 2018,Jan,8; 2017,Jan,8; 2016,Jan,13

50551-50562 Endoscopic Procedures of Kidney via Established Nephrostomy/Pyelostomy Access

50551 **Renal endoscopy through established nephrostomy or pyelostomy, with or without irrigation, instillation, or ureteropyelography, exclusive of radiologic service;**
8.54 10.4 FUD 000 J A2 80 50
AMA: 2018,Jan,8; 2017,Jan,8; 2016,Jan,13

50553 **with ureteral catheterization, with or without dilation of ureter**
EXCLUDES *Image-guided ureter dilation without endoscopic guidance (50706)*
9.09 11.1 FUD 000 J A2 50
AMA: 2018,Jan,8; 2017,Jan,8; 2016,Jan,3; 2016,Jan,13

50555 **with biopsy**
EXCLUDES *Image-guided biopsy ureter/renal pelvis without endoscopic guidance (50606)*
9.88 11.9 FUD 000 J A2 80 50
AMA: 2018,Jan,8; 2017,Jan,8; 2016,Jan,3; 2016,Jan,13

50557 **with fulguration and/or incision, with or without biopsy**
10.0 12.1 FUD 000 J A2 80 50
AMA: 2018,Jan,8; 2017,Jan,8; 2016,Jan,13

50561 **with removal of foreign body or calculus**
11.3 13.6 FUD 000 J A2 80 50
AMA: 2018,Jan,8; 2017,Jan,8; 2016,Jan,13

50562 **with resection of tumor**
16.8 16.8 FUD 090 J G2 80
AMA: 2018,Jan,8; 2017,Jan,8; 2016,Jan,13

50570-50580 Endoscopic Procedures of Kidney via Nephrotomy/Pyelotomy Access

Code also when provided service significant and identifiable (50045, 50120)

50570 **Renal endoscopy through nephrotomy or pyelotomy, with or without irrigation, instillation, or ureteropyelography, exclusive of radiologic service;**
14.2 14.2 FUD 000 J G2 80 50
AMA: 2018,Jan,8; 2017,Jan,8; 2016,Jan,13

50572 **with ureteral catheterization, with or without dilation of ureter**
EXCLUDES *Image-guided ureter dilation without endoscopic guidance (50706)*
15.4 15.4 FUD 000 T G2 80 50
AMA: 2018,Jan,8; 2017,Jan,8; 2016,Jan,3; 2016,Jan,13

50574 **with biopsy**
EXCLUDES *Image-guide ureter/renal pelvis biopsy without endoscopic guidance (50606)*
16.3 16.3 FUD 000 J G2 80 50
AMA: 2018,Jan,8; 2017,Jan,8; 2016,Jan,3; 2016,Jan,13

50575 **with endopyelotomy (includes cystoscopy, ureteroscopy, dilation of ureter and ureteral pelvic junction, incision of ureteral pelvic junction and insertion of endopyelotomy stent)**
20.6 20.6 FUD 000 J G2 50
AMA: 2018,Jan,8; 2017,Jan,8; 2016,Jan,13

50576 **with fulguration and/or incision, with or without biopsy**
16.3 16.3 FUD 000 J G2 80 50
AMA: 2018,Jan,8; 2017,Jan,8; 2016,Jan,13

50580 **with removal of foreign body or calculus**
17.5 17.5 FUD 000 J G2 80 50
AMA: 2018,Jan,8; 2017,Jan,8; 2016,Jan,13

50590-50593 Noninvasive and Minimally Invasive Procedures of the Kidney

50590 Lithotripsy, extracorporeal shock wave
Facility RVU 16.4 Non-Facility RVU 20.8 FUD 090 J G2 50
AMA: 2018,Jan,8; 2017,Jan,8; 2016,Jan,13

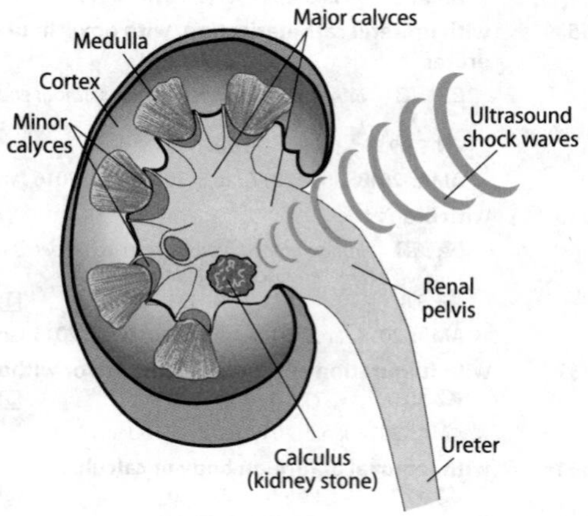

50592 Ablation, 1 or more renal tumor(s), percutaneous, unilateral, radiofrequency
Radiology Crosswalk (76940, 77013, 77022)
Facility RVU 9.93 Non-Facility RVU 92.3 FUD 010 J G2 50
AMA: 2014,Jan,11

50593 Ablation, renal tumor(s), unilateral, percutaneous, cryotherapy
Radiology Crosswalk (76940, 77013, 77022)
Facility RVU 13.3 Non-Facility RVU 125. FUD 010 J J8 80 50
AMA: 2018,Jan,8

50600-50940 Open and Injection Procedures of Ureter

50600 Ureterotomy with exploration or drainage (separate procedure)
Code also ureteral endoscopy through ureterotomy when procedures constitute significant identifiable service (50970-50980)
Facility RVU 27.1 Non-Facility RVU 27.1 FUD 090 C 80 50
AMA: 2014,Jan,11; 2000,Oct,8

50605 Ureterotomy for insertion of indwelling stent, all types
Facility RVU 28.6 Non-Facility RVU 28.6 FUD 090 C 80 50
AMA: 2018,Jan,8; 2017,Jan,8; 2016,Jan,13

+ **50606 Endoluminal biopsy of ureter and/or renal pelvis, non-endoscopic, including imaging guidance (eg, ultrasound and/or fluoroscopy) and all associated radiological supervision and interpretation (List separately in addition to code for primary procedure)**
INCLUDES Renal pelvis and associated ureter as single element
EXCLUDES *Procedure performed for same renal collecting system/associated ureter with (50555, 50574, 50955, 50974, 52007, 74425)*
Code first (50382-50389, [50430, 50431, 50432, 50433, 50434, 50435], 50684, 50688, 50690, 50693-50695, 51610)
Facility RVU 4.43 Non-Facility RVU 18.8 FUD ZZZ N N1 50
AMA: 2018,Jan,8; 2017,Jan,8; 2016,Jan,3

50610 Ureterolithotomy; upper one-third of ureter
EXCLUDES *Cystotomy with calculus basket extraction ureteral calculus (51065)*
Transvesical ureterolithotomy (51060)
Ureteral calculus manipulation/extraction performed endoscopically (50080-50081, 50561, 50961, 50980, 52320-52330, 52352-52353, [52356])
Ureterolithotomy performed laparoscopically (50945)
Facility RVU 27.3 Non-Facility RVU 27.3 FUD 090 C 80 50
AMA: 2018,Jan,8; 2017,Jan,8; 2016,Jan,13

50620 middle one-third of ureter
EXCLUDES *Cystotomy with calculus basket extraction ureteral calculus (51065)*
Transvesical ureterolithotomy (51060)
Ureteral calculus manipulation/extraction performed endoscopically (50080-50081, 50561, 50961, 50980, 52320-52330, 52352-52353, [52356])
Ureterolithotomy performed laparoscopically (50945)
Facility RVU 26.1 Non-Facility RVU 26.1 FUD 090 C 80 50
AMA: 2018,Jan,8; 2017,Jan,8; 2016,Jan,13

50630 lower one-third of ureter
EXCLUDES *Cystotomy with calculus basket extraction ureteral calculus (51065)*
Transvesical ureterolithotomy (51060)
Ureteral calculus manipulation/extraction performed endoscopically (50080-50081, 50561, 50961, 50980, 52320-52330, 52352-52353, [52356])
Ureterolithotomy performed laparoscopically (50945)
Facility RVU 25.8 Non-Facility RVU 25.8 FUD 090 C 80 50
AMA: 2018,Jan,8; 2017,Jan,8; 2016,Jan,13

50650 Ureterectomy, with bladder cuff (separate procedure)
EXCLUDES *Ureterocele (51535, 52300)*
Facility RVU 30.0 Non-Facility RVU 30.0 FUD 090 C 80 50
AMA: 2014,Jan,11

50660 Ureterectomy, total, ectopic ureter, combination abdominal, vaginal and/or perineal approach
EXCLUDES *Ureterocele (51535, 52300)*
Facility RVU 33.0 Non-Facility RVU 33.0 FUD 090 C 80
AMA: 2014,Jan,11

50684 Injection procedure for ureterography or ureteropyelography through ureterostomy or indwelling ureteral catheter
EXCLUDES *Placement nephroureteral catheter ([50433, 50434])*
Placement ureteral stent (50693-50695)
Radiology Crosswalk (74425)
Facility RVU 1.45 Non-Facility RVU 3.10 FUD 000 N N1 50
AMA: 2018,Jan,8; 2017,Jan,8; 2016,Jan,3

50686 Manometric studies through ureterostomy or indwelling ureteral catheter
Facility RVU 2.54 Non-Facility RVU 4.03 FUD 000 S P2 80
AMA: 2014,Jan,11

50688 Change of ureterostomy tube or externally accessible ureteral stent via ileal conduit
Radiology Crosswalk (75984)
Facility RVU 2.25 Non-Facility RVU 2.25 FUD 010 J A2
AMA: 2018,Jan,8; 2017,Jan,8; 2016,Jan,3

50690 Injection procedure for visualization of ileal conduit and/or ureteropyelography, exclusive of radiologic service
Radiology Crosswalk (74420, 74425)
Facility RVU 2.02 Non-Facility RVU 2.87 FUD 000 N N1
AMA: 2018,Jan,8; 2017,Jan,8; 2016,Jan,3

50693 Placement of ureteral stent, percutaneous, including diagnostic nephrostogram and/or ureterogram when performed, imaging guidance (eg, ultrasound and/or fluoroscopy), and all associated radiological supervision and interpretation; pre-existing nephrostomy tract

INCLUDES Renal pelvis and associated ureter as single element

EXCLUDES *Procedure performed for same renal collecting system/ureter ([50430, 50431, 50432, 50433, 50434, 50435], 50684, 74425)*

5.94 28.7 FUD 000 J 62 50

AMA: 2018,Jan,8; 2017,Jan,8; 2016,Jan,3; 2016,Jan,13

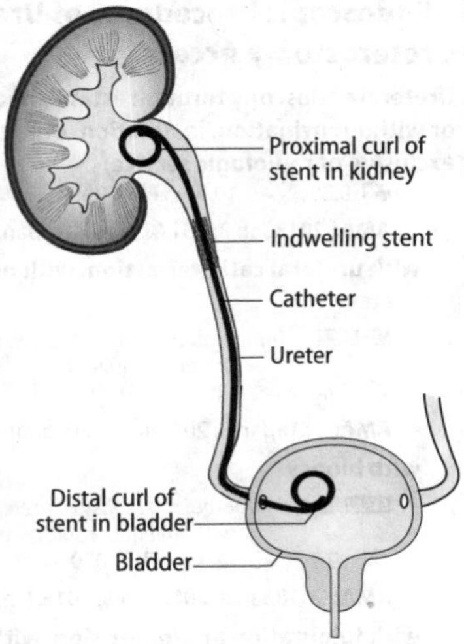

50694 new access, without separate nephrostomy catheter

INCLUDES Renal pelvis and associated ureter as single element

EXCLUDES *Procedure performed for same renal collecting system/ureter ([50430, 50431, 50432, 50433, 50434, 50435], 50684, 74425)*

7.77 31.7 FUD 000 J 62 50

AMA: 2018,Jan,8; 2017,Jan,8; 2016,Jan,3; 2016,Jan,13

50695 new access, with separate nephrostomy catheter

INCLUDES Placement separate ureteral stent and nephrostomy catheter into ureter/associated renal pelvis through new access

Renal pelvis and associated ureter as single element

EXCLUDES *Procedure performed for same renal collecting system/ureter ([50430, 50431, 50432, 50433, 50434, 50435], 50684, 74425)*

9.96 37.8 FUD 000 J 62 50

AMA: 2018,Jan,8; 2017,Jan,8; 2016,Jan,3; 2016,Jan,13

50700 Ureteroplasty, plastic operation on ureter (eg, stricture)

26.7 26.7 FUD 090 C 80 50

AMA: 2014,Jan,11

\+ **50705 Ureteral embolization or occlusion, including imaging guidance (eg, ultrasound and/or fluoroscopy) and all associated radiological supervision and interpretation (List separately in addition to code for primary procedure)**

INCLUDES Renal pelvis and associated ureter as single element

Code also when performed:
- Additional catheter insertions
- Diagnostic pyelography/ureterography
- Other interventions

Code first (50382-50389, [50430, 50431, 50432, 50433, 50434, 50435], 50684, 50688, 50690, 50693-50695, 51610)

5.69 56.8 FUD ZZZ N N1 50

AMA: 2018,Jan,8; 2017,Jan,8; 2016,Jan,3

\+ **50706 Balloon dilation, ureteral stricture, including imaging guidance (eg, ultrasound and/or fluoroscopy) and all associated radiological supervision and interpretation (List separately in addition to code for primary procedure)**

INCLUDES Dilation nephrostomy, ureters, or urethra (74485)

Renal pelvis and associated ureter as single element

EXCLUDES *Cystourethroscopy (52341, 52344-52345)*

Renal endoscopy (50553, 50572)

Ureteral endoscopy (50953, 50972)

Code also when performed:
- Additional catheter insertions
- Diagnostic pyelography/ureterography
- Other interventions

Code first (50382-50389, [50430, 50431, 50432, 50433, 50434, 50435], 50684, 50688, 50690, 50693-50695, 51610)

5.31 27.4 FUD ZZZ N N1 50

AMA: 2018,Jan,8; 2017,Jan,8; 2016,Jan,3

50715 Ureterolysis, with or without repositioning of ureter for retroperitoneal fibrosis

35.2 35.2 FUD 090 C 80 50

AMA: 2014,Jan,11

50722 Ureterolysis for ovarian vein syndrome ♀

29.8 29.8 FUD 090 C 80

AMA: 2014,Jan,11

50725 Ureterolysis for retrocaval ureter, with reanastomosis of upper urinary tract or vena cava

31.9 31.9 FUD 090 C 80

AMA: 2014,Jan,11

50727 Revision of urinary-cutaneous anastomosis (any type urostomy);

14.7 14.7 FUD 090 J 62 80

AMA: 2014,Jan,11; 1992,Win,1

50728 with repair of fascial defect and hernia

21.2 21.2 FUD 090 C 80

AMA: 2014,Jan,11; 1992,Win,1

50740 Ureteropyelostomy, anastomosis of ureter and renal pelvis

35.4 35.4 FUD 090 C 80 50

AMA: 2018,Jan,8; 2017,Jan,8; 2016,Jan,13

50750 Ureterocalycostomy, anastomosis of ureter to renal calyx

33.3 33.3 FUD 090 C 80 50

AMA: 2018,Jan,8; 2017,Jan,8; 2016,Jan,13

50760 Ureteroureterostomy

32.6 32.6 FUD 090 C 80 50

AMA: 2018,Jan,8; 2017,Jan,8; 2016,Jan,13

50770 Transureteroureterostomy, anastomosis of ureter to contralateral ureter

33.3 33.3 FUD 090 C 80

AMA: 2014,Jan,11

50780 Ureteroneocystostomy; anastomosis of single ureter to bladder

INCLUDES Minor procedures to prevent vesicoureteral reflux

EXCLUDES *Cystourethroplasty with ureteroneocystostomy (51820)*

31.9 31.9 FUD 090 C 80 50

AMA: 2018,Feb,11; 2018,Jan,8; 2017,Jan,8; 2016,Jan,13

50782 anastomosis of duplicated ureter to bladder

INCLUDES Minor procedures to prevent vesicoureteral reflux

31.1 31.1 FUD 090 C 80 50

AMA: 2018,Jan,8; 2017,Jan,8; 2016,Jan,13

50783 with extensive ureteral tailoring

INCLUDES Minor procedures to prevent vesicoureteral reflux

32.6 32.6 FUD 090 C 80 50

AMA: 2018,Jan,8; 2017,Jan,8; 2016,Jan,13

50785 with vesico-psoas hitch or bladder flap

INCLUDES Minor procedures to prevent vesicoureteral reflux

35.1 35.1 FUD 090 C 80 50

AMA: 2018,Jan,8; 2017,Jan,8; 2016,Jan,13

50800 **Ureteroenterostomy, direct anastomosis of ureter to intestine**
EXCLUDES *Cystectomy with ureterosigmoidostomy/ureteroileal conduit (51580-51595)*
26.8 26.8 FUD 090 C 80 50
AMA: 2018,Jan,8; 2017,Jan,8; 2016,Jan,13

50810 **Ureterosigmoidostomy, with creation of sigmoid bladder and establishment of abdominal or perineal colostomy, including intestine anastomosis**
EXCLUDES *Cystectomy with ureterosigmoidostomy/ureteroileal conduit (51580-51595)*
40.8 40.8 FUD 090 C 80
AMA: 2018,Jan,8; 2017,Jan,8; 2016,Jan,13

50815 **Ureterocolon conduit, including intestine anastomosis**
EXCLUDES *Cystectomy with ureterosigmoidostomy/ureteroileal conduit (51580-51595)*
35.3 35.3 FUD 090 C 80 50
AMA: 2018,Jan,8; 2017,Jan,8; 2016,Jan,13

50820 **Ureteroileal conduit (ileal bladder), including intestine anastomosis (Bricker operation)**
EXCLUDES *Cystectomy with ureterosigmoidostomy/ureteroileal conduit (51580-51595)*
38.0 38.0 FUD 090 C 80 50
AMA: 2018,Jan,8; 2017,Jan,8; 2016,Jan,13

50825 **Continent diversion, including intestine anastomosis using any segment of small and/or large intestine (Kock pouch or Camey enterocystoplasty)**
47.8 47.8 FUD 090 C 80
AMA: 2018,Jan,8; 2017,Jan,8; 2016,Jan,13

50830 **Urinary undiversion (eg, taking down of ureteroileal conduit, ureterosigmoidostomy or ureteroenterostomy with ureteroureterostomy or ureteroneocystostomy)**
52.1 52.1 FUD 090 C 80
AMA: 2018,Jan,8; 2017,Jan,8; 2016,Jan,13

50840 **Replacement of all or part of ureter by intestine segment, including intestine anastomosis**
35.5 35.5 FUD 090 C 80 50
AMA: 2018,Jan,8; 2017,Jan,8; 2016,Jan,13

50845 **Cutaneous appendico-vesicostomy**
INCLUDES Mitrofanoff operation
36.1 36.1 FUD 090 C 80
AMA: 2014,Jan,11; 1993,Win,1

50860 **Ureterostomy, transplantation of ureter to skin**
27.3 27.3 FUD 090 C 80 50
AMA: 2014,Jan,11; 2001,Oct,8

50900 **Ureterorrhaphy, suture of ureter (separate procedure)**
24.3 24.3 FUD 090 C 80 50
AMA: 2014,Jan,11; 2001,Oct,8

50920 **Closure of ureterocutaneous fistula**
25.5 25.5 FUD 090 C 80
AMA: 2014,Jan,11; 2001,Oct,8

50930 **Closure of ureterovisceral fistula (including visceral repair)**
31.8 31.8 FUD 090 C 80
AMA: 2014,Jan,11; 2001,Oct,8

50940 **Deligation of ureter**
EXCLUDES *Ureteroplasty/ureterolysis (50700-50860)*
25.6 25.6 FUD 090 C 80 50
AMA: 2014,Jan,11; 2001,Oct,8

50945-50949 Laparoscopic Procedures of Ureter

INCLUDES Diagnostic laparoscopy (49320)
EXCLUDES *Ureteroneocystostomy, open approach (50780-50785)*

50945 **Laparoscopy, surgical; ureterolithotomy**
28.1 28.1 FUD 090 J G2 80 50
AMA: 2018,Jan,8; 2017,Jan,8; 2016,Jan,13

50947 **ureteroneocystostomy with cystoscopy and ureteral stent placement**
40.1 40.1 FUD 090 J A2 80 50
AMA: 2018,Jan,8; 2017,Jan,8; 2016,Jan,13

50948 **ureteroneocystostomy without cystoscopy and ureteral stent placement**
36.7 36.7 FUD 090 J A2 80 50
AMA: 2018,Jan,8; 2017,Jan,8; 2016,Jan,13

50949 **Unlisted laparoscopy procedure, ureter**
0.00 0.00 FUD YYY J 80 50
AMA: 2018,Jan,8; 2017,Jan,8; 2016,Jan,13

50951-50961 Endoscopic Procedures of Ureter via Established Ureterostomy Access

50951 **Ureteral endoscopy through established ureterostomy, with or without irrigation, instillation, or ureteropyelography, exclusive of radiologic service;**
8.89 10.9 FUD 000 J A2 80 50
AMA: 2018,Jan,8; 2017,Jan,8; 2016,Jan,13

50953 **with ureteral catheterization, with or without dilation of ureter**
EXCLUDES *Image-guided ureter dilation without endoscopic guidance (50706)*
9.46 11.5 FUD 000 J A2 80 50
AMA: 2018,Jan,8; 2017,Jan,8; 2016,Jan,13; 2016,Jan,3

50955 **with biopsy**
EXCLUDES *Image-guided biopsy of ureter and/or renal pelvis without endoscopic guidance (50606)*
10.2 12.3 FUD 000 J A2 80 50
AMA: 2018,Jan,8; 2017,Jan,8; 2016,Jan,13; 2016,Jan,3

50957 **with fulguration and/or incision, with or without biopsy**
10.2 12.4 FUD 000 J A2 80 50
AMA: 2018,Jan,8; 2017,Jan,8; 2016,Jan,13

50961 **with removal of foreign body or calculus**
9.17 11.1 FUD 000 J A2 80 50
AMA: 2018,Jan,8; 2017,Jan,8; 2016,Jan,13

50970-50980 Endoscopic Procedures of Ureter via Ureterotomy

EXCLUDES *Ureterotomy (50600)*

50970 **Ureteral endoscopy through ureterotomy, with or without irrigation, instillation, or ureteropyelography, exclusive of radiologic service;**
10.7 10.7 FUD 000 J A2 80 50
AMA: 2018,Jan,8; 2017,Jan,8; 2016,Jan,13

50972 **with ureteral catheterization, with or without dilation of ureter**
EXCLUDES *Image-guided ureter dilation without endoscopic guidance (50706)*
10.3 10.3 FUD 000 J A2 80 50
AMA: 2018,Jan,8; 2017,Jan,8; 2016,Jan,3; 2016,Jan,13

50974 **with biopsy**
EXCLUDES *Image-guided biopsy of ureter and/or renal pelvis without endoscopic guidance (50606)*
13.6 13.6 FUD 000 J A2 80 50
AMA: 2018,Jan,8; 2017,Jan,8; 2016,Jan,3; 2016,Jan,13

50976 **with fulguration and/or incision, with or without biopsy**
13.5 13.5 FUD 000 J A2 80 50
AMA: 2018,Jan,8; 2017,Jan,8; 2016,Jan,13

50980 **with removal of foreign body or calculus**
10.3 10.3 FUD 000 J A2 80 50
AMA: 2018,Jan,8; 2017,Jan,8; 2016,Jan,13

51020-51080 Open Incisional Procedures of Bladder

51020 **Cystotomy or cystostomy; with fulguration and/or insertion of radioactive material**
13.5 13.5 FUD 090 J A2 80
AMA: 2014,Jan,11

26/TC PC/TC Only · A2-Z3 ASC Payment · 50 Bilateral · ♂ Male Only · ♀ Female Only · Facility RVU · Non-Facility RVU · CCI · CLIA
FUD Follow-up Days · CMS: IOM · AMA: CPT Asst · A-Y OPPSI · 80/80 Surg Assist Allowed / w/Doc · Lab Crosswalk · Radiology Crosswalk

51030 **with cryosurgical destruction of intravesical lesion**
13.6 13.6 FUD 090 J A2 80
AMA: 2014,Jan,11

51040 **Cystostomy, cystotomy with drainage**
8.36 8.36 FUD 090 J A2 80
AMA: 2014,Jan,11

51045 **Cystotomy, with insertion of ureteral catheter or stent (separate procedure)**
14.4 14.4 FUD 090 J A2 80
AMA: 2014,Jan,11

51050 **Cystolithotomy, cystotomy with removal of calculus, without vesical neck resection**
13.6 13.6 FUD 090 J A2 80
AMA: 2014,Jan,11

51060 **Transvesical ureterolithotomy**
16.8 16.8 FUD 090 J G2 80
AMA: 2014,Jan,11

51065 **Cystotomy, with calculus basket extraction and/or ultrasonic or electrohydraulic fragmentation of ureteral calculus**
16.7 16.7 FUD 090 J A2 80
AMA: 2014,Jan,11; 2002,May,7

51080 **Drainage of perivesical or prevesical space abscess**
EXCLUDES *Image-guided percutaneous catheter drainage (49406)*
11.8 11.8 FUD 090 J A2 80
AMA: 2014,Jan,11

51100-51102 Bladder Aspiration Procedures

51100 **Aspiration of bladder; by needle**
(76942, 77002, 77012)
1.13 1.84 FUD 000 T P3
AMA: 2018,Jan,8; 2017,Jan,8; 2016,Jan,13

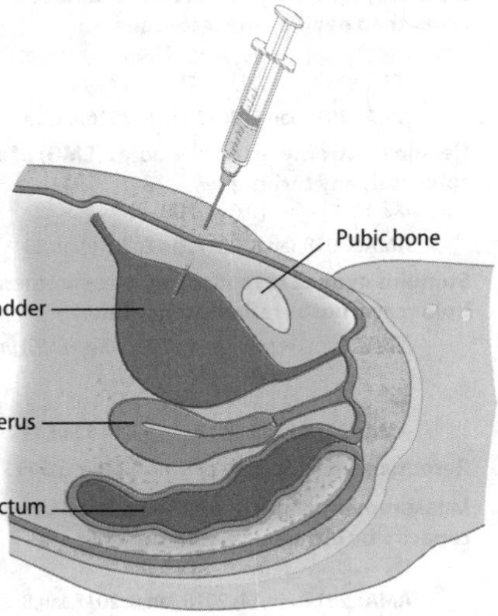

51101 **by trocar or intracatheter**
(76942, 77002, 77012)
1.50 3.79 FUD 000 S P3
AMA: 2018,Jan,8; 2017,Jan,8; 2016,Jan,13

51102 **with insertion of suprapubic catheter**
(76942, 77002, 77012)
4.20 6.78 FUD 000 J A2
AMA: 2018,Jan,8; 2017,Jan,8; 2016,Jan,13

51500-51597 Open Excisional Procedures of Bladder

51500 **Excision of urachal cyst or sinus, with or without umbilical hernia repair**
18.4 18.4 FUD 090 J A2 80
AMA: 2014,Jan,11

51520 **Cystotomy; for simple excision of vesical neck (separate procedure)**
17.1 17.1 FUD 090 J A2 80
AMA: 2014,Jan,11

51525 **for excision of bladder diverticulum, single or multiple (separate procedure)**
EXCLUDES *Transurethral resection (52305)*
24.8 24.8 FUD 090 C 80
AMA: 2014,Jan,11

51530 **for excision of bladder tumor**
EXCLUDES *Transurethral resection (52234-52240, 52305)*
22.2 22.2 FUD 090 C 80
AMA: 2014,Jan,11

51535 **Cystotomy for excision, incision, or repair of ureterocele**
EXCLUDES *Transurethral excision (52300)*
22.5 22.5 FUD 090 J G2 80 50
AMA: 2014,Jan,11; 1993,Sum,25

51550 **Cystectomy, partial; simple**
27.9 27.9 FUD 090 C 80
AMA: 2014,Jan,11

51555 **complicated (eg, postradiation, previous surgery, difficult location)**
36.6 36.6 FUD 090 C 80
AMA: 2014,Jan,11

51565 **Cystectomy, partial, with reimplantation of ureter(s) into bladder (ureteroneocystostomy)**
37.5 37.5 FUD 090 C 80
AMA: 2014,Jan,11

51570 **Cystectomy, complete; (separate procedure)**
42.6 42.6 FUD 090 C 80
AMA: 2014,Jan,11; 1993,Spr,34

51575 **with bilateral pelvic lymphadenectomy, including external iliac, hypogastric, and obturator nodes**
52.7 52.7 FUD 090 C 80
AMA: 2014,Jan,11; 1993,Spr,34

51580 **Cystectomy, complete, with ureterosigmoidostomy or ureterocutaneous transplantations;**
54.7 54.7 FUD 090 C 80
AMA: 2014,Jan,11; 1993,Spr,34

51585 **with bilateral pelvic lymphadenectomy, including external iliac, hypogastric, and obturator nodes**
61.1 61.1 FUD 090 C 80
AMA: 2014,Jan,11; 1993,Spr,34

51590 **Cystectomy, complete, with ureteroileal conduit or sigmoid bladder, including intestine anastomosis;**
55.9 55.9 FUD 090 C 80
AMA: 2014,Jan,11; 2002,May,7

51595 **with bilateral pelvic lymphadenectomy, including external iliac, hypogastric, and obturator nodes**
63.3 63.3 FUD 090 C 80
AMA: 2014,Jan,11; 2002,May,7

51596 **Cystectomy, complete, with continent diversion, any open technique, using any segment of small and/or large intestine to construct neobladder**
68.1 68.1 FUD 090 C 80
AMA: 2014,Jan,11; 2002,May,7

51597 **Pelvic exenteration, complete, for vesical, prostatic or urethral malignancy, with removal of bladder and ureteral transplantations, with or without hysterectomy and/or abdominoperineal resection of rectum and colon and colostomy, or any combination thereof**
EXCLUDES *Pelvic exenteration for gynecologic malignancy (58240)*
66.2 66.2 FUD 090 C 80
AMA: 2014,Jan,11

51600-51720 Injection/Insertion/Instillation Procedures of Bladder

51600 Injection procedure for cystography or voiding urethrocystography
(74430, 74455)
1.29 5.57 FUD 000 N N1
AMA: 2019,Oct,10

51605 Injection procedure and placement of chain for contrast and/or chain urethrocystography
(74430)
1.11 1.11 FUD 000 N N1
AMA: 2014,Jan,11

51610 Injection procedure for retrograde urethrocystography
(74450)
1.85 3.21 FUD 000 N N1
AMA: 2019,Oct,10; 2018,Jan,8; 2017,Jan,8; 2016,Jan,3

51700 Bladder irrigation, simple, lavage and/or instillation
0.87 2.12 FUD 000 T P3
AMA: 2014,Jan,11

51701 Insertion of non-indwelling bladder catheter (eg, straight catheterization for residual urine)
EXCLUDES *Catheterization for specimen collection (P9612)*
Insertion catheter as another procedure component
0.73 1.27 FUD 000 Q1 N1
AMA: 2018,Jan,8; 2017,Jan,8; 2016,Jan,13

51702 Insertion of temporary indwelling bladder catheter; simple (eg, Foley)
EXCLUDES *Focused ultrasound ablation uterine leiomyomata (0071T-0072T)*
Insertion catheter as another procedure component
0.74 1.74 FUD 000 Q1 N1
AMA: 2018,Jan,8; 2017,Jan,8; 2016,Jan,13

51703 complicated (eg, altered anatomy, fractured catheter/balloon)
2.23 3.98 FUD 000 S P2
AMA: 2018,Jan,8; 2017,Jan,8; 2016,Jan,13

51705 Change of cystostomy tube; simple
1.50 2.67 FUD 000 T P3
AMA: 2018,Jan,8; 2017,Jan,8; 2016,Jan,13

51710 complicated
(75984)
2.28 3.77 FUD 000 T A2
AMA: 2018,Jan,8; 2017,Jan,8; 2016,Jan,13

51715 Endoscopic injection of implant material into the submucosal tissues of the urethra and/or bladder neck
EXCLUDES *Injection bulking agent (submucosal) for fecal incontinence, via anoscope (46999)*
5.79 9.78 FUD 000 J J8 80
AMA: 2014,Jan,11; 1993,Win,1

51720 Bladder instillation of anticarcinogenic agent (including retention time)
Code also bacillus Calmette-Guerin vaccine (BCG) (90586)
1.27 2.40 FUD 000 T P3
AMA: 2020,NovSE,1; 2020,Jan,11; 2018,Jan,8; 2017,Jan,8; 2016,Jan,13

51725-51798 [51797] Uroflowmetric Evaluations

INCLUDES Equipment
Fees for technician services
Medications
Supplies
Code also modifier 26 when physician/other qualified health care professional provides only interpretation results and/or operates equipment

51725 Simple cystometrogram (CMG) (eg, spinal manometer)
6.04 6.04 FUD 000 T P2 80
AMA: 2018,Jan,8; 2017,Jan,8; 2016,Jan,13

51726 Complex cystometrogram (ie, calibrated electronic equipment);
8.23 8.23 FUD 000 T A2
AMA: 2018,Jan,8; 2017,Jan,8; 2016,Jan,13

51727 with urethral pressure profile studies (ie, urethral closure pressure profile), any technique
9.39 9.39 FUD 000 T P3 80
AMA: 2018,Jan,8; 2017,Jan,8; 2016,Jan,13

51728 with voiding pressure studies (ie, bladder voiding pressure), any technique
10.0 10.0 FUD 000 T P3 80
AMA: 2018,Jan,8; 2017,Jan,8; 2016,Jan,13

51729 with voiding pressure studies (ie, bladder voiding pressure) and urethral pressure profile studies (ie, urethral closure pressure profile), any technique
10.6 10.6 FUD 000 T P3 80
AMA: 2018,Jan,8; 2017,Jan,8; 2016,Jan,13

+ # 51797 Voiding pressure studies, intra-abdominal (ie, rectal, gastric, intraperitoneal) (List separately in addition to code for primary procedure)
Code first (51728-51729)
4.61 4.61 FUD ZZZ N N1 80
AMA: 2018,Jan,8; 2017,Jan,8; 2016,Jan,13

51736 Simple uroflowmetry (UFR) (eg, stop-watch flow rate, mechanical uroflowmeter)
0.39 0.39 FUD XXX Q1 N1 80
AMA: 2018,Jan,8; 2017,Jan,8; 2016,Jan,13

51741 Complex uroflowmetry (eg, calibrated electronic equipment)
0.41 0.41 FUD XXX Q1 N1
AMA: 2018,Jan,8; 2017,Jan,8; 2016,Jan,13

51784 Electromyography studies (EMG) of anal or urethral sphincter, other than needle, any technique
EXCLUDES *Stimulus evoked response (51792)*
1.92 1.92 FUD XXX S P3
AMA: 2018,Jan,8; 2017,Jan,8; 2016,Jan,13

51785 Needle electromyography studies (EMG) of anal or urethral sphincter, any technique
10.6 10.6 FUD XXX T A2 80
AMA: 2018,Jan,8; 2017,Jan,8; 2016,Jan,13

51792 Stimulus evoked response (eg, measurement of bulbocavernosus reflex latency time)
EXCLUDES *Electromyography studies (EMG) anal or urethral sphincter (51784)*
7.04 7.04 FUD 000 Q1 N1 80
AMA: 2018,Jan,8; 2017,Jan,8; 2016,Jan,13

51797 **Resequenced code. See code following 51729.**

51798 Measurement of post-voiding residual urine and/or bladder capacity by ultrasound, non-imaging
0.36 0.36 FUD XXX Q1 N1 80 TC
AMA: 2018,Jun,11; 2018,Jan,8; 2017,Jan,8; 2016,Jan,13

51800-51980 Open Repairs Urinary System

51800 Cystoplasty or cystourethroplasty, plastic operation on bladder and/or vesical neck (anterior Y-plasty, vesical fundus resection), any procedure, with or without wedge resection of posterior vesical neck
30.3 30.3 FUD 090 C 80
AMA: 2014,Jan,11

51820 Cystourethroplasty with unilateral or bilateral ureteroneocystostomy
31.3 31.3 FUD 090 C 80
AMA: 2014,Jan,11

51840 Anterior vesicourethropexy, or urethropexy (eg, Marshall-Marchetti-Krantz, Burch); simple

EXCLUDES *Pereyra type urethropexy (57289)*

19.3 19.3 FUD 090 C 80

AMA: 2018,Jan,8; 2017,Jan,8; 2016,Jan,13

51841 complicated (eg, secondary repair)

EXCLUDES *Pereyra type urethropexy (57289)*

22.4 22.4 FUD 090 C 80

AMA: 2018,Jan,8; 2017,Jan,8; 2016,Jan,13

51845 Abdomino-vaginal vesical neck suspension, with or without endoscopic control (eg, Stamey, Raz, modified Pereyra) ♀

16.8 16.8 FUD 090 J G2 80

AMA: 2018,Jan,8; 2017,Jan,8; 2016,Jan,13

51860 Cystorrhaphy, suture of bladder wound, injury or rupture; simple

21.5 21.5 FUD 090 J G2 80

AMA: 2014,Jan,11

51865 complicated

25.9 25.9 FUD 090 C 80

AMA: 2014,Jan,11

51880 Closure of cystostomy (separate procedure)

13.5 13.5 FUD 090 J A2 80

AMA: 2014,Jan,11

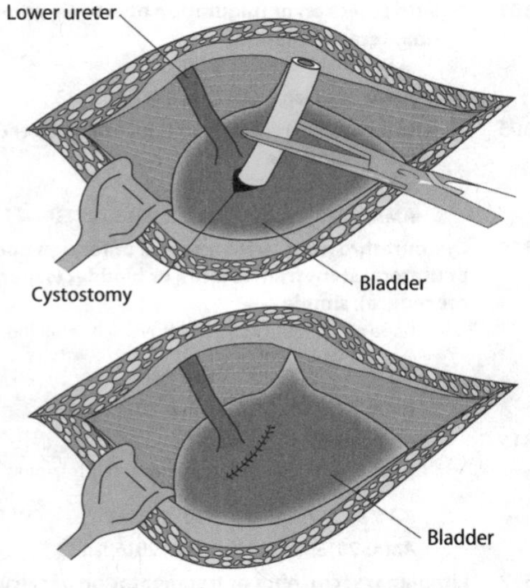

Physician removes a cystostomy tube

51900 Closure of vesicovaginal fistula, abdominal approach ♀

EXCLUDES *Vesicovaginal fistula closure, vaginal approach (57320-57330)*

23.8 23.8 FUD 090 C 80

AMA: 2014,Jan,11

51920 Closure of vesicouterine fistula; ♀

EXCLUDES *Enterovesical fistula closure (44660-44661)*
Rectovesical fistula closure (45800-45805)

22.0 22.0 FUD 090 C 80

AMA: 2014,Jan,11

51925 with hysterectomy ♀

EXCLUDES *Enterovesical fistula closure (44660-44661)*
Rectovesical fistula closure (45800-45805)

29.5 29.5 FUD 090 C 80

AMA: 2014,Jan,11

51940 Closure, exstrophy of bladder

EXCLUDES *Epispadias reconstruction with exstrophy bladder (54390)*

47.5 47.5 FUD 090 C 80

AMA: 2014,Jan,11; 2002,May,7

51960 Enterocystoplasty, including intestinal anastomosis

40.0 40.0 FUD 090 C 80

AMA: 2014,Jan,11; 2002,May,7

51980 Cutaneous vesicostomy

20.6 20.6 FUD 090 C 80

AMA: 2014,Jan,11

51990-51999 Laparoscopic Procedures of Urinary System

CMS: 100-03,230.10 Incontinence Control Devices

INCLUDES Diagnostic laparoscopy (49320)

51990 Laparoscopy, surgical; urethral suspension for stress incontinence

21.6 21.6 FUD 090 J G2 80

AMA: 2019,Feb,10; 2018,Jan,8; 2017,Jan,8; 2016,Jan,13

51992 sling operation for stress incontinence (eg, fascia or synthetic)

EXCLUDES *Removal/revision sling for stress incontinence (57287)*
Sling operation for stress incontinence, open approach (57288)

24.0 24.0 FUD 090 J J8 80

AMA: 2019,Feb,10; 2018,Jan,8; 2017,Jan,8; 2016,Jan,13

51999 Unlisted laparoscopy procedure, bladder

0.00 0.00 FUD YYY J 80

AMA: 2018,Jan,8; 2017,Dec,14

52000-52318 Endoscopic Procedures via Urethra: Bladder and Urethra

INCLUDES Diagnostic and therapeutic endoscopy bowel segments utilized as replacements for native bladder

52000 Cystourethroscopy (separate procedure)

EXCLUDES *Cystourethroscopy (52001, 52320, 52325, 52327, 52330, 52332, 52334, 52341-52343, [52356], 57240,. 57260, 57265)*

2.34 5.39 FUD 000 T A2

AMA: 2019,Feb,10; 2018,Nov,10; 2018,Jan,8; 2017,Oct,9; 2017,Jan,8; 2016,Jan,13

52001 Cystourethroscopy with irrigation and evacuation of multiple obstructing clots

INCLUDES Cystourethroscopy (separate procedure) (52000)

8.31 11.3 FUD 000 J A2

AMA: 2014,Jan,11; 2001,May,5

52005 Cystourethroscopy, with ureteral catheterization, with or without irrigation, instillation, or ureteropyelography, exclusive of radiologic service;

INCLUDES Howard test

3.84 8.05 FUD 000 J A2

AMA: 2019,Mar,10; 2018,Jan,8; 2017,Jan,8; 2016,Jan,13

52007 with brush biopsy of ureter and/or renal pelvis

EXCLUDES *Image-guided ureter/renal pelvis biopsy without endoscopic guidance (50606)*

4.80 13.1 FUD 000 J A2 50

AMA: 2018,Jan,8; 2017,Jan,8; 2016,Jan,13; 2016,Jan,3

52010 Cystourethroscopy, with ejaculatory duct catheterization, with or without irrigation, instillation, or duct radiography, exclusive of radiologic service ♂

(74440)

4.79 10.9 FUD 000 T A2

AMA: 2018,Jan,8; 2017,Jan,8; 2016,Jan,13

52204 Cystourethroscopy, with biopsy(s)

4.08 10.8 FUD 000 J A2

AMA: 2018,Jan,8; 2017,Jan,8; 2016,May,12; 2016,Jan,13

52214 **Cystourethroscopy, with fulguration (including cryosurgery or laser surgery) of trigone, bladder neck, prostatic fossa, urethra, or periurethral glands**

Code also modifier 78 when performed by same physician:
- During postoperative period (52601, 52630)
- During postoperative period related surgical procedure
- For postoperative bleeding

5.10 | 20.0 | **FUD** 000 | J A2

AMA: 2018,Jan,8; 2017,Jan,8; 2016,May,12; 2016,Jan,13

52224 **Cystourethroscopy, with fulguration (including cryosurgery or laser surgery) or treatment of MINOR (less than 0.5 cm) lesion(s) with or without biopsy**

5.89 | 20.9 | **FUD** 000 | J A2

AMA: 2018,Jan,8; 2017,Jan,8; 2016,May,12; 2016,Jan,13

52234 **Cystourethroscopy, with fulguration (including cryosurgery or laser surgery) and/or resection of; SMALL bladder tumor(s) (0.5 up to 2.0 cm)**

EXCLUDES *Bladder tumor excision through cystotomy (51530)*

7.12 | 7.12 | **FUD** 000 | J A2

AMA: 2018,Jan,8; 2017,Jan,8; 2016,May,12; 2016,Jan,13

52235 **MEDIUM bladder tumor(s) (2.0 to 5.0 cm)**

EXCLUDES *Bladder tumor excision through cystotomy (51530)*

8.34 | 8.34 | **FUD** 000 | J A2

AMA: 2018,Jan,8; 2017,Jan,8; 2016,May,12; 2016,Jan,13

52240 **LARGE bladder tumor(s)**

EXCLUDES *Bladder tumor excision through cystotomy (51530)*

11.3 | 11.3 | **FUD** 000 | J A2

AMA: 2018,Jan,8; 2017,Jan,8; 2016,May,12; 2016,Jan,13

52250 **Cystourethroscopy with insertion of radioactive substance, with or without biopsy or fulguration**

6.92 | 6.92 | **FUD** 000 | J A2

AMA: 2018,Jan,8; 2017,Jan,8; 2016,Jan,13

52260 **Cystourethroscopy, with dilation of bladder for interstitial cystitis; general or conduction (spinal) anesthesia**

6.07 | 6.07 | **FUD** 000 | J A2

AMA: 2018,Jan,8; 2017,Jan,8; 2016,Jan,13

52265 **local anesthesia**

4.67 | 10.6 | **FUD** 000 | J P3

AMA: 2018,Jan,8; 2017,Jan,8; 2016,Jan,13

52270 **Cystourethroscopy, with internal urethrotomy; female** ♀

5.27 | 10.9 | **FUD** 000 | J A2

AMA: 2018,Jan,8; 2017,Jan,8; 2016,Jan,13

52275 **male** ♂

7.19 | 14.4 | **FUD** 000 | J A2

AMA: 2018,Jan,8; 2017,Jan,8; 2016,Jan,13

52276 **Cystourethroscopy with direct vision internal urethrotomy**

7.65 | 7.65 | **FUD** 000 | J A2

AMA: 2019,Feb,10; 2018,Jan,8; 2017,Jan,8; 2016,Jan,13

52277 **Cystourethroscopy, with resection of external sphincter (sphincterotomy)**

9.35 | 9.35 | **FUD** 000 | J A2 80

AMA: 2018,Jan,8; 2017,Jan,8; 2016,Jan,13

52281 **Cystourethroscopy, with calibration and/or dilation of urethral stricture or stenosis, with or without meatotomy, with or without injection procedure for cystography, male or female**

EXCLUDES *Urethral delivery therapeutic drug (0499T)*

4.40 | 8.53 | **FUD** 000 | J A2

AMA: 2018,Jan,8; 2017,Oct,9; 2017,Jan,8; 2016,Jan,13

52282 **Cystourethroscopy, with insertion of permanent urethral stent**

EXCLUDES *Placement temporary prostatic urethral stent (53855)*

9.76 | 9.76 | **FUD** 000 | J A2

AMA: 2018,Jan,8; 2017,Jan,8; 2016,Jan,13

52283 **Cystourethroscopy, with steroid injection into stricture**

5.83 | 8.68 | **FUD** 000 | J A2

AMA: 2019,Feb,10; 2018,Jan,8; 2017,Jan,8; 2016,Jan,13

52285 **Cystourethroscopy for treatment of the female urethral syndrome with any or all of the following: urethral meatotomy, urethral dilation, internal urethrotomy, lysis of urethrovaginal septal fibrosis, lateral incisions of the bladder neck, and fulguration of polyp(s) of urethra, bladder neck, and/or trigone** ♀

5.66 | 8.66 | **FUD** 000 | J A2

AMA: 2018,Jan,8; 2017,Jan,8; 2016,Jan,13

52287 **Cystourethroscopy, with injection(s) for chemodenervation of the bladder**

Code also supply chemodenervation agent

4.89 | 9.65 | **FUD** 000 | J G2

AMA: 2019,Apr,9

52290 **Cystourethroscopy; with ureteral meatotomy, unilateral or bilateral**

7.07 | 7.07 | **FUD** 000 | J A2

AMA: 2018,Jan,8; 2017,Jan,8; 2016,Jan,13

52300 **with resection or fulguration of orthotopic ureterocele(s), unilateral or bilateral**

8.09 | 8.09 | **FUD** 000 | J A2 80

AMA: 2018,Jan,8; 2017,Jan,8; 2016,Jan,13

52301 **with resection or fulguration of ectopic ureterocele(s), unilateral or bilateral**

8.38 | 8.38 | **FUD** 000 | J A2 80

AMA: 2018,Jan,8; 2017,Jan,8; 2016,Jan,13

52305 **with incision or resection of orifice of bladder diverticulum, single or multiple**

8.06 | 8.06 | **FUD** 000 | J A2

AMA: 2018,Jan,8; 2017,Jan,8; 2016,Jan,13

52310 **Cystourethroscopy, with removal of foreign body, calculus, or ureteral stent from urethra or bladder (separate procedure); simple**

Code also modifier 58 for removal self-retaining, indwelling ureteral stent

4.38 | 7.68 | **FUD** 000 | J A2

AMA: 2018,Jan,8; 2017,Jan,8; 2016,Jan,13

52315 **complicated**

Code also modifier 58 for removal self-retaining, indwelling ureteral stent

7.94 | 12.6 | **FUD** 000 | J A2

AMA: 2018,Jan,8; 2017,Jan,8; 2016,Jan,13

52317 **Litholapaxy: crushing or fragmentation of calculus by any means in bladder and removal of fragments; simple or small (less than 2.5 cm)**

10.0 | 24.1 | **FUD** 000 | J A2

AMA: 2018,Jan,8; 2017,Jan,8; 2016,Jan,13

52318 **complicated or large (over 2.5 cm)**

13.7 | 13.7 | **FUD** 000 | J A2

AMA: 2018,Jan,8; 2017,Jan,8; 2016,Jan,13

52320-52356 [52356] Endoscopic Procedures via Urethra: Renal Pelvis and Ureter

INCLUDES Diagnostic cystourethroscopy when performed with therapeutic cystourethroscopy

Insertion/removal temporary ureteral catheter (52005)

EXCLUDES *Self-retaining/indwelling ureteral stent removal by cystourethroscope, with modifier 58 when appropriate (52310, 52315)*

Code also insertion indwelling stent performed in addition to other procedures within this section (52332)

52320 **Cystourethroscopy (including ureteral catheterization); with removal of ureteral calculus**

INCLUDES Cystourethroscopy (separate procedure) (52000)

7.13 | 7.13 | **FUD** 000 | J A2 50

AMA: 2018,Jan,8; 2017,Jan,8; 2016,Jan,13

26/TC PC/TC Only | A2-Z3 ASC Payment | 50 Bilateral | ♂ Male Only | ♀ Female Only | Facility RVU | Non-Facility RVU | CCI | CLIA

FUD Follow-up Days | **CMS:** IOM | **AMA:** CPT Asst | A-Y OPPSI | 80/80 Surg Assist Allowed / w/Doc | Lab Crosswalk | Radiology Crosswalk

52325 **with fragmentation of ureteral calculus (eg, ultrasonic or electro-hydraulic technique)**

INCLUDES Cystourethroscopy (separate procedure) (52000)

9.27 9.27 FUD 000 J A2 50

AMA: 2018,Jan,8; 2017,Jan,8; 2016,Jan,13

52327 **with subureteric injection of implant material**

INCLUDES Cystourethroscopy (separate procedure) (52000)

7.59 7.59 FUD 000 J J8 50

AMA: 2018,Jan,8; 2017,Jan,8; 2016,Jan,13

52330 **with manipulation, without removal of ureteral calculus**

INCLUDES Cystourethroscopy (separate procedure) (52000)

7.63 15.4 FUD 000 J A2 50

AMA: 2018,Jan,8; 2017,Jan,8; 2016,Jan,13

52332 **Cystourethroscopy, with insertion of indwelling ureteral stent (eg, Gibbons or double-J type)**

INCLUDES Cystourethroscopy (separate procedure) (52000)

EXCLUDES *Cystourethroscopy, with ureteroscopy and/or pyeloscopy; with lithotripsy when performed on same side with (52353, [52356])*

4.50 13.5 FUD 000 J A2 50

AMA: 2019,Dec,12; 2018,Jan,8; 2017,Jan,8; 2016,Jan,13

52334 **Cystourethroscopy with insertion of ureteral guide wire through kidney to establish a percutaneous nephrostomy, retrograde**

INCLUDES Cystourethroscopy (separate procedure) (52000)

EXCLUDES *Cystourethroscopy with incision/fulguration/resection congenital posterior urethral valves/obstructive hypertrophic mucosal folds (52400)*
Cystourethroscopy with pyeloscopy and/or ureteroscopy (52351-52353 [52356])
Dilation nephroureteral catheter tract ([50436], [50437])
Nephrostomy tract establishment only ([50432, 50433])
Percutaneous nephrostolithotomy (50080, 50081)

5.30 5.30 FUD 000 J A2

AMA: 2018,Jan,8; 2017,Jan,8; 2016,Jan,13

52341 **Cystourethroscopy; with treatment of ureteral stricture (eg, balloon dilation, laser, electrocautery, and incision)**

INCLUDES Diagnostic cystourethroscopy (52351)

EXCLUDES *Balloon dilation with imaging guidance (50706)*
Cystourethroscopy, separate procedure (52000)

(74485)

8.21 8.21 FUD 000 J A2 50

AMA: 2018,Jan,8; 2017,Jan,8; 2016,Jan,13; 2016,Jan,3

52342 **with treatment of ureteropelvic junction stricture (eg, balloon dilation, laser, electrocautery, and incision)**

INCLUDES Diagnostic cystourethroscopy (52351)

EXCLUDES *Balloon dilation with imaging guidance (50706)*
Cystourethroscopy (separate procedure) (52000)

(74485)

8.93 8.93 FUD 000 J A2 50

AMA: 2018,Jan,8; 2017,Jan,8; 2016,Jan,13

52343 **with treatment of intra-renal stricture (eg, balloon dilation, laser, electrocautery, and incision)**

INCLUDES Diagnostic cystourethroscopy (52351)

EXCLUDES *Balloon dilation with imaging guidance (50706)*
Cystourethroscopy (separate procedure) (52000)

(74485)

9.96 9.96 FUD 000 J A2 50

AMA: 2018,Jan,8; 2017,Jan,8; 2016,Jan,13

52344 **Cystourethroscopy with ureteroscopy; with treatment of ureteral stricture (eg, balloon dilation, laser, electrocautery, and incision)**

INCLUDES Diagnostic cystourethroscopy (52351)

EXCLUDES *Balloon dilation, ureteral stricture (50706)*
Cystourethroscopy with transurethral resection or incision ejaculatory ducts (52402)

(74485)

10.6 10.6 FUD 000 J A2 50

AMA: 2018,Jan,8; 2017,Jan,8; 2016,Jan,13; 2016,Jan,3

52345 **with treatment of ureteropelvic junction stricture (eg, balloon dilation, laser, electrocautery, and incision)**

INCLUDES Diagnostic cystourethroscopy (52351)

EXCLUDES *Balloon dilation, ureteral stricture (50706)*
Cystourethroscopy with transurethral resection or incision ejaculatory ducts (52402)

(74485)

11.4 11.4 FUD 000 J A2 80 50

AMA: 2018,Jan,8; 2017,Jan,8; 2016,Jan,13; 2016,Jan,3

52346 **with treatment of intra-renal stricture (eg, balloon dilation, laser, electrocautery, and incision)**

INCLUDES Diagnostic cystourethroscopy (52351)

EXCLUDES *Balloon dilation with imaging guidance (50706)*
Cystourethroscopy with transurethral resection or incision ejaculatory ducts (52402)

(74485)

12.9 12.9 FUD 000 J A2 80 50

AMA: 2018,Jan,8; 2017,Jan,8; 2016,Jan,13

52351 **Cystourethroscopy, with ureteroscopy and/or pyeloscopy; diagnostic**

EXCLUDES *Cystourethroscopy (52341-52346, 52352-52353 [52356])*

8.75 8.75 FUD 000 J A2

AMA: 2018,Jan,8; 2017,Jan,8; 2016,Jan,13

52352 **with removal or manipulation of calculus (ureteral catheterization is included)**

INCLUDES Diagnostic cystourethroscopy (52351)

10.2 10.2 FUD 000 J A2 50

AMA: 2018,Jan,8; 2017,Jan,8; 2016,Jan,13

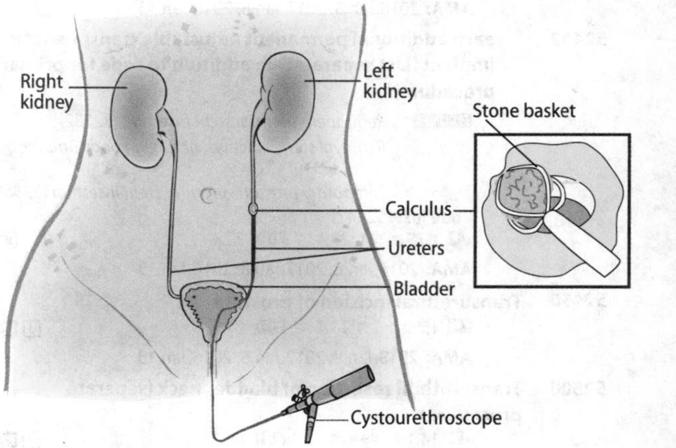

52353 **with lithotripsy (ureteral catheterization is included)**

INCLUDES Diagnostic cystourethroscopy (52351)

EXCLUDES *Cystourethroscopy when performed on same side (52332, [52356])*

11.3 11.3 FUD 000 J A2 50

AMA: 2019,Dec,12; 2018,Jan,8; 2017,Jan,8; 2016,Jan,13

\# **52356** **with lithotripsy including insertion of indwelling ureteral stent (eg, Gibbons or double-J type)**

INCLUDES Diagnostic cystourethroscopy (52351)

EXCLUDES *Cystourethroscopy (separate procedure) (52000)*

When performed on same side:

Cystourethroscopy, with insertion indwelling ureteral stent (e.g., Gibbons or double-J type) (52332)

Cystourethroscopy, with ureteroscopy and/or pyeloscopy; with lithotripsy (ureteral catheterization is included) (52353)

12.0 12.0 FUD 000 J G2 50

AMA: 2019,Dec,12; 2018,Jan,8; 2017,Jan,8; 2016,Jan,13

52354 **with biopsy and/or fulguration of ureteral or renal pelvic lesion**

INCLUDES Diagnostic cystourethroscopy (52351)

EXCLUDES *Image guided biopsy without endoscopic guidance (50606)*

12.0 12.0 FUD 000 J A2 50

AMA: 2018,Jan,8; 2017,Jan,8; 2016,Jan,13

52355 **with resection of ureteral or renal pelvic tumor**

INCLUDES Diagnostic cystourethroscopy (52351)

13.5 13.5 FUD 000 J A2 50

AMA: 2018,Jan,8; 2017,Jan,8; 2016,Jan,13

52356 **Resequenced code. See code following 52353.**

52400-52700 Endoscopic Procedures via Urethra: Prostate and Vesical Neck

52400 **Cystourethroscopy with incision, fulguration, or resection of congenital posterior urethral valves, or congenital obstructive hypertrophic mucosal folds**

13.8 13.8 FUD 090 J A2

AMA: 2018,Jan,8; 2017,Jan,8; 2016,Jan,13

52402 **Cystourethroscopy with transurethral resection or incision of ejaculatory ducts** ♂

7.73 7.73 FUD 000 J A2

AMA: 2014,Jan,11; 2001,Apr,4

52441 **Cystourethroscopy, with insertion of permanent adjustable transprostatic implant; single implant**

6.58 35.7 FUD 000 B

AMA: 2018,Jan,8; 2017,Jan,8; 2016,Jan,13

\+ **52442** **each additional permanent adjustable transprostatic implant (List separately in addition to code for primary procedure)**

EXCLUDES *Permanent urethral stent insertion (52282)*

Removal stent, calculus, or foreign body (implant) (52310)

Temporary prostatic urethral stent insertion (53855)

Code first (52441)

1.75 27.4 FUD ZZZ B

AMA: 2018,Jan,8; 2017,Jan,8; 2016,Jan,13

52450 **Transurethral incision of prostate** ♂

13.5 13.5 FUD 090 J A2

AMA: 2018,Jan,8; 2017,Jan,8; 2016,Jan,13

52500 **Transurethral resection of bladder neck (separate procedure)**

14.1 14.1 FUD 090 J A2

AMA: 2018,Jan,8; 2017,Jan,8; 2016,Jan,13

52601 **Transurethral electrosurgical resection of prostate, including control of postoperative bleeding, complete (vasectomy, meatotomy, cystourethroscopy, urethral calibration and/or dilation, and internal urethrotomy are included)** ♂

INCLUDES Stage 1 partial transurethral resection prostate

EXCLUDES *Ablation by waterjet (0421T)*

Excision prostate (55801-55845)

Transurethral fulguration prostate (52214)

Code also modifier 58 for stage 2 partial transurethral resection prostate

21.0 21.0 FUD 090 J A2

AMA: 2018,Jan,8; 2017,Jan,8; 2016,Jan,13

52630 **Transurethral resection; residual or regrowth of obstructive prostate tissue including control of postoperative bleeding, complete (vasectomy, meatotomy, cystourethroscopy, urethral calibration and/or dilation, and internal urethrotomy are included)** ♂

EXCLUDES *Ablation by waterjet (0421T)*

Excision prostate (55801-55845)

Code also modifier 78 when performed by same physician within postoperative period related procedure

11.5 11.5 FUD 090 J A2

AMA: 2018,Jan,8; 2017,Jan,8; 2016,Jan,13

52640 **of postoperative bladder neck contracture**

EXCLUDES *Excision prostate (55801-55845)*

9.12 9.12 FUD 090 J A2

AMA: 2018,Jan,8; 2017,Jan,8; 2016,Jan,13

52647 **Laser coagulation of prostate, including control of postoperative bleeding, complete (vasectomy, meatotomy, cystourethroscopy, urethral calibration and/or dilation, and internal urethrotomy are included if performed)** ♂

18.7 46.2 FUD 090 J A2

AMA: 2018,Jan,8; 2017,Jan,8; 2016,Jan,13

52648 **Laser vaporization of prostate, including control of postoperative bleeding, complete (vasectomy, meatotomy, cystourethroscopy, urethral calibration and/or dilation, internal urethrotomy and transurethral resection of prostate are included if performed)** ♂

19.9 47.7 FUD 090 J A2

AMA: 2018,Jan,8; 2017,Jan,8; 2016,Jan,13

52649 **Laser enucleation of the prostate with morcellation, including control of postoperative bleeding, complete (vasectomy, meatotomy, cystourethroscopy, urethral calibration and/or dilation, internal urethrotomy and transurethral resection of prostate are included if performed)** ♂

INCLUDES Cystourethroscopy (52000, 52276, 52281)

Laser coagulation prostate (52647-52648)

Meatotomy (53020)

Transurethral resection of prostate (52601)

Vasectomy (55250)

23.8 23.8 FUD 090 J G2 80

AMA: 2018,Jan,8; 2017,Jan,8; 2016,Jan,13

52700 **Transurethral drainage of prostatic abscess** ♂
EXCLUDES *Litholapaxy (52317, 52318)*
12.7 12.7 **FUD** 090 J A2 80
AMA: 2018,Jan,8; 2017,Jan,8; 2016,Jan,13

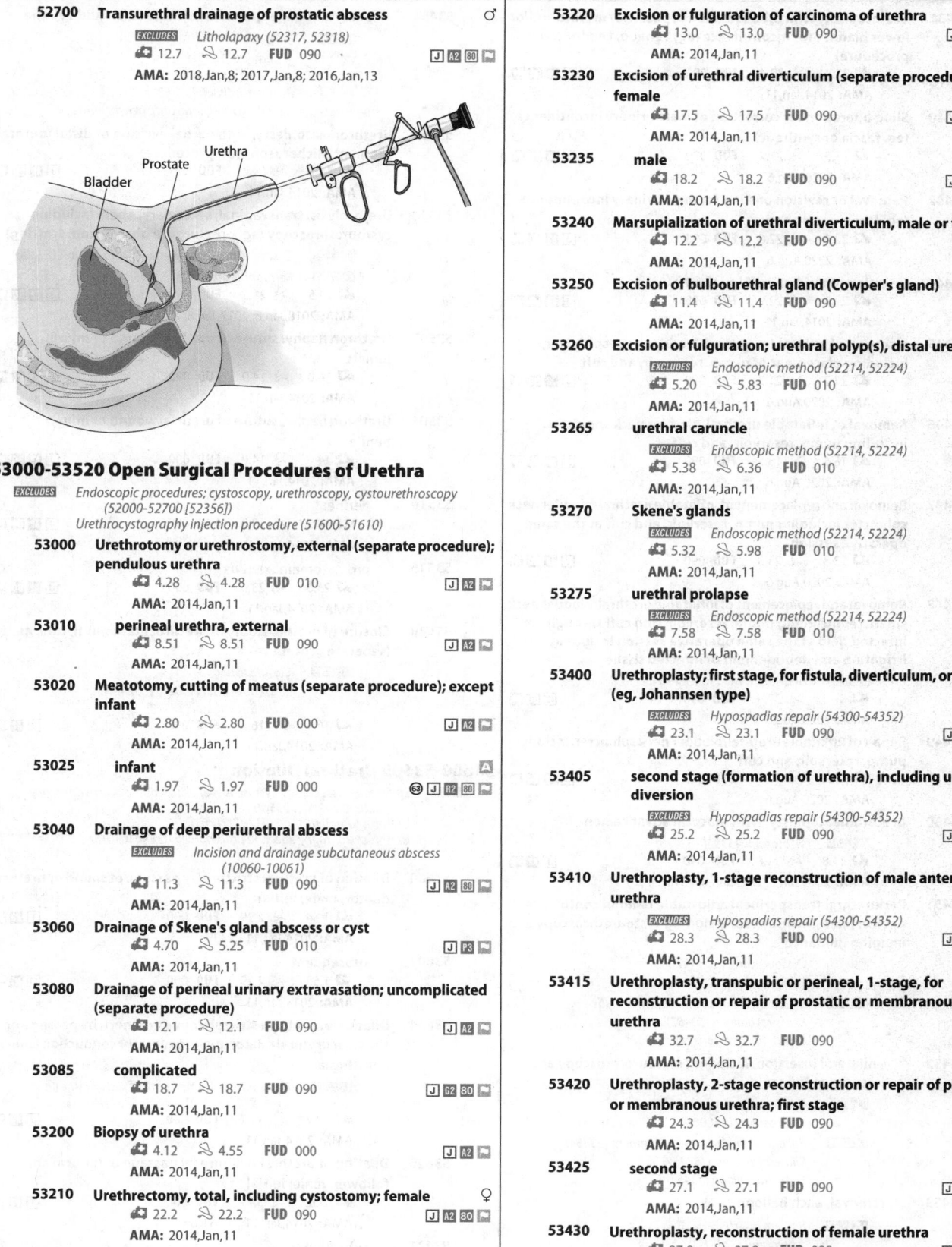

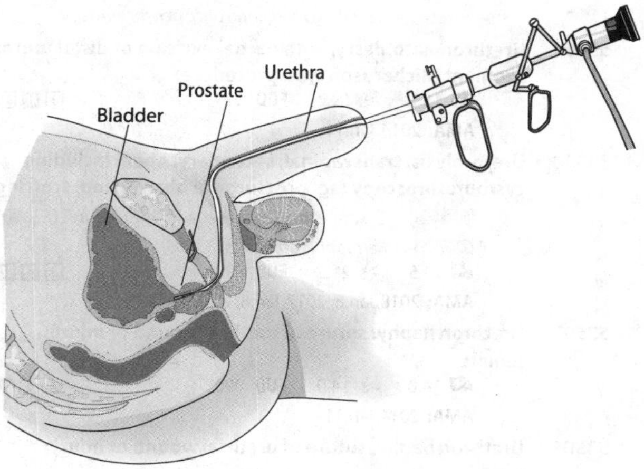

53000-53520 Open Surgical Procedures of Urethra

EXCLUDES *Endoscopic procedures; cystoscopy, urethroscopy, cystourethroscopy (52000-52700 [52356])*
Urethrocystography injection procedure (51600-51610)

53000 **Urethrotomy or urethrostomy, external (separate procedure); pendulous urethra**
4.28 4.28 **FUD** 010 J A2
AMA: 2014,Jan,11

53010 **perineal urethra, external**
8.51 8.51 **FUD** 090 J A2
AMA: 2014,Jan,11

53020 **Meatotomy, cutting of meatus (separate procedure); except infant**
2.80 2.80 **FUD** 000 J A2
AMA: 2014,Jan,11

53025 **infant** A
1.97 1.97 **FUD** 000 63 J R2 80
AMA: 2014,Jan,11

53040 **Drainage of deep periurethral abscess**
EXCLUDES *Incision and drainage subcutaneous abscess (10060-10061)*
11.3 11.3 **FUD** 090 J A2 80
AMA: 2014,Jan,11

53060 **Drainage of Skene's gland abscess or cyst**
4.70 5.25 **FUD** 010 J P3
AMA: 2014,Jan,11

53080 **Drainage of perineal urinary extravasation; uncomplicated (separate procedure)**
12.1 12.1 **FUD** 090 J A2
AMA: 2014,Jan,11

53085 **complicated**
18.7 18.7 **FUD** 090 J G2 80
AMA: 2014,Jan,11

53200 **Biopsy of urethra**
4.12 4.55 **FUD** 000 J A2
AMA: 2014,Jan,11

53210 **Urethrectomy, total, including cystostomy; female** ♀
22.2 22.2 **FUD** 090 J A2 80
AMA: 2014,Jan,11

53215 **male** ♂
26.8 26.8 **FUD** 090 J A2 80
AMA: 2014,Jan,11

53220 **Excision or fulguration of carcinoma of urethra**
13.0 13.0 **FUD** 090 J A2 80
AMA: 2014,Jan,11

53230 **Excision of urethral diverticulum (separate procedure); female** ♀
17.5 17.5 **FUD** 090 J A2 80
AMA: 2014,Jan,11

53235 **male** ♂
18.2 18.2 **FUD** 090 J A2 80
AMA: 2014,Jan,11

53240 **Marsupialization of urethral diverticulum, male or female**
12.2 12.2 **FUD** 090 J A2
AMA: 2014,Jan,11

53250 **Excision of bulbourethral gland (Cowper's gland)**
11.4 11.4 **FUD** 090 J A2
AMA: 2014,Jan,11

53260 **Excision or fulguration; urethral polyp(s), distal urethra**
EXCLUDES *Endoscopic method (52214, 52224)*
5.20 5.83 **FUD** 010 J A2
AMA: 2014,Jan,11

53265 **urethral caruncle**
EXCLUDES *Endoscopic method (52214, 52224)*
5.38 6.36 **FUD** 010 J A2
AMA: 2014,Jan,11

53270 **Skene's glands**
EXCLUDES *Endoscopic method (52214, 52224)*
5.32 5.98 **FUD** 010 J A2
AMA: 2014,Jan,11

53275 **urethral prolapse**
EXCLUDES *Endoscopic method (52214, 52224)*
7.58 7.58 **FUD** 010 J A2
AMA: 2014,Jan,11

53400 **Urethroplasty; first stage, for fistula, diverticulum, or stricture (eg, Johannsen type)**
EXCLUDES *Hypospadias repair (54300-54352)*
23.1 23.1 **FUD** 090 J A2 80
AMA: 2014,Jan,11

53405 **second stage (formation of urethra), including urinary diversion**
EXCLUDES *Hypospadias repair (54300-54352)*
25.2 25.2 **FUD** 090 J A2 80
AMA: 2014,Jan,11

53410 **Urethroplasty, 1-stage reconstruction of male anterior urethra** ♂
EXCLUDES *Hypospadias repair (54300-54352)*
28.3 28.3 **FUD** 090 J A2 80
AMA: 2014,Jan,11

53415 **Urethroplasty, transpubic or perineal, 1-stage, for reconstruction or repair of prostatic or membranous urethra** ♂
32.7 32.7 **FUD** 090 C 80
AMA: 2014,Jan,11

53420 **Urethroplasty, 2-stage reconstruction or repair of prostatic or membranous urethra; first stage** ♂
24.3 24.3 **FUD** 090 J A2
AMA: 2014,Jan,11

53425 **second stage** ♂
27.1 27.1 **FUD** 090 J A2 80
AMA: 2014,Jan,11

53430 **Urethroplasty, reconstruction of female urethra** ♀
27.9 27.9 **FUD** 090 J A2 80
AMA: 2014,Jan,11

53431 **Urethroplasty with tubularization of posterior urethra and/or lower bladder for incontinence (eg, Tenago, Leadbetter procedure)**
33.4 33.4 FUD 090 J A2 80
AMA: 2014,Jan,11

53440 **Sling operation for correction of male urinary incontinence (eg, fascia or synthetic)** ♂
21.7 21.7 FUD 090 J J8 80
AMA: 2020,Aug,6

53442 **Removal or revision of sling for male urinary incontinence (eg, fascia or synthetic)** ♂
22.6 22.6 FUD 090 J A2 80
AMA: 2020,Aug,6

53444 **Insertion of tandem cuff (dual cuff)**
22.9 22.9 FUD 090 J J8 80
AMA: 2014,Jan,11

53445 **Insertion of inflatable urethral/bladder neck sphincter, including placement of pump, reservoir, and cuff**
21.7 21.7 FUD 090 J J8 80
AMA: 2020,Aug,6

53446 **Removal of inflatable urethral/bladder neck sphincter, including pump, reservoir, and cuff**
18.5 18.5 FUD 090 Q2 A2 80
AMA: 2020,Aug,6

53447 **Removal and replacement of inflatable urethral/bladder neck sphincter including pump, reservoir, and cuff at the same operative session**
23.3 23.3 FUD 090 J J8 80
AMA: 2020,Aug,6

53448 **Removal and replacement of inflatable urethral/bladder neck sphincter including pump, reservoir, and cuff through an infected field at the same operative session including irrigation and debridement of infected tissue**
INCLUDES Debridement (11042, 11043)
37.0 37.0 FUD 090 C 80
AMA: 2020,Aug,6

53449 **Repair of inflatable urethral/bladder neck sphincter, including pump, reservoir, and cuff**
17.6 17.6 FUD 090 J A2 80
AMA: 2020,Aug,6

53450 **Urethromeatoplasty, with mucosal advancement**
EXCLUDES *Meatotomy (53020, 53025)*
11.8 11.8 FUD 090 J A2
AMA: 2018,Jan,8; 2017,Jan,8; 2016,Jan,13

● **53451** **Periurethral transperineal adjustable balloon continence device; bilateral insertion, including cystourethroscopy and imaging guidance**
INCLUDES Cystourethroscopy (52000)
Fluoroscopy (76000)
EXCLUDES *Balloon(s) fluid volume adjustment (53454)*
Removal balloon (53453)
Unilateral insertion only (53452)

● **53452** **unilateral insertion, including cystourethroscopy and imaging guidance**
INCLUDES Cystourethroscopy (52000)
Fluoroscopy (76000)
EXCLUDES *Balloon(s) fluid volume adjustment (53454)*
Bilateral insertion (53452)
Removal balloon (53453)

● **53453** **removal, each balloon**
EXCLUDES *Balloon insertion:*
Bilateral (53451)
Unilateral (53452)
Balloon(s) fluid volume adjustment (53454)

● **53454** **percutaneous adjustment of balloon(s) fluid volume**
EXCLUDES *Balloon insertion:*
Bilateral (53451)
Unilateral (53452)
Removal balloon (53453)
Reporting more than once per encounter

53460 **Urethromeatoplasty, with partial excision of distal urethral segment (Richardson type procedure)**
13.2 13.2 FUD 090 J A2 80
AMA: 2014,Jan,11

53500 **Urethrolysis, transvaginal, secondary, open, including cystourethroscopy (eg, postsurgical obstruction, scarring)**
INCLUDES Cystourethroscopy (separate procedure) (52000)
EXCLUDES *Retropubic approach (53899)*
21.5 21.5 FUD 090 J G2 80
AMA: 2018,Jan,8; 2017,Jan,8; 2016,Jan,13

53502 **Urethrorrhaphy, suture of urethral wound or injury, female** ♀
14.0 14.0 FUD 090 J A2
AMA: 2014,Jan,11

53505 **Urethrorrhaphy, suture of urethral wound or injury; penile** ♂
14.0 14.0 FUD 090 J A2 80
AMA: 2014,Jan,11

53510 **perineal** ♂
18.2 18.2 FUD 090 J A2 80
AMA: 2014,Jan,11

53515 **prostatomembranous** ♂
23.0 23.0 FUD 090 J A2 80
AMA: 2014,Jan,11

53520 **Closure of urethrostomy or urethrocutaneous fistula, male (separate procedure)** ♂
EXCLUDES *Closure fistula:*
Urethrorectal (45820, 45825)
Urethrovaginal (57310)
16.1 16.1 FUD 090 J A2
AMA: 2014,Jan,11

53600-53665 Urethral Dilation

EXCLUDES *Endoscopic procedures; cystoscopy, urethroscopy, cystourethroscopy (52000-52700 [52356])*
Urethral catheterization (51701-51703)
Urethrocystography injection procedure (51600-51610)
(74485)

53600 **Dilation of urethral stricture by passage of sound or urethral dilator, male; initial** ♂
1.84 2.39 FUD 000 T P3
AMA: 2014,Jan,11

53601 **subsequent** ♂
1.55 2.29 FUD 000 Q1 N1
AMA: 2014,Jan,11

53605 **Dilation of urethral stricture or vesical neck by passage of sound or urethral dilator, male, general or conduction (spinal) anesthesia** ♂
EXCLUDES *Procedure performed under local anesthesia (53600-53601, 53620-53621)*
1.87 1.87 FUD 000 J A2
AMA: 2014,Jan,11

53620 **Dilation of urethral stricture by passage of filiform and follower, male; initial** ♂
2.52 3.79 FUD 000 T P3
AMA: 2014,Jan,11; 1996,Nov,1

53621 **subsequent** ♂
2.09 3.56 FUD 000 T P3
AMA: 2014,Jan,11

53660 **Dilation of female urethra including suppository and/or instillation; initial** ♀
1.20 1.99 FUD 000 S P3
AMA: 2014,Jan,11

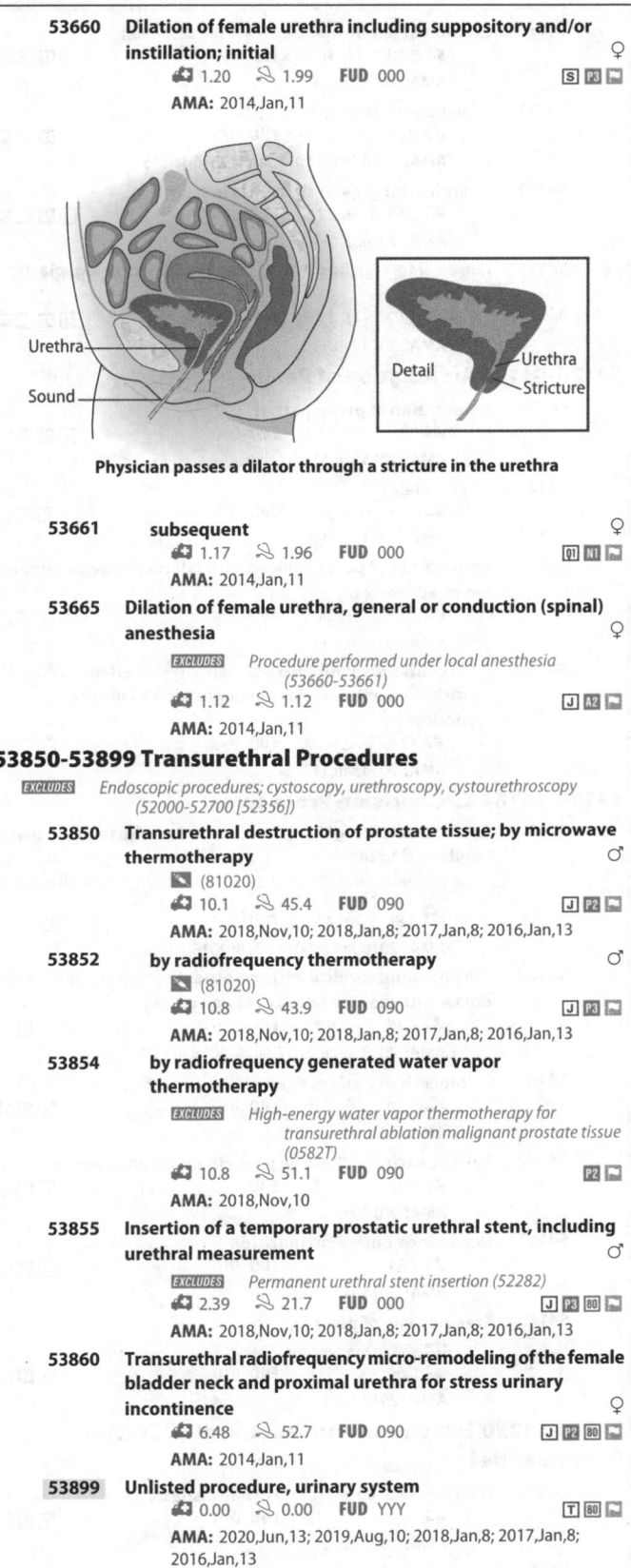

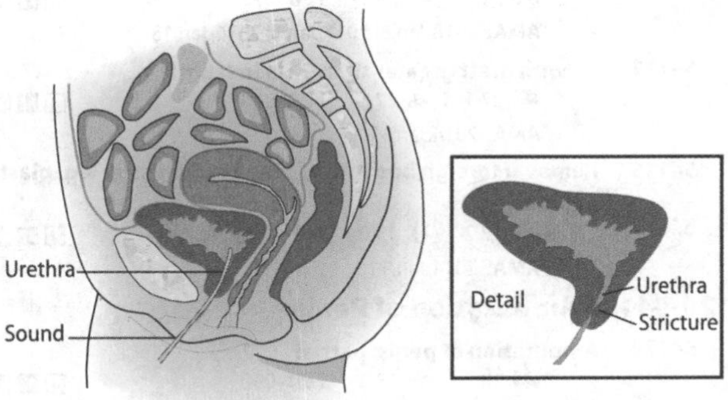

Physician passes a dilator through a stricture in the urethra

53661 **subsequent** ♀
1.17 1.96 FUD 000 Q1 N1
AMA: 2014,Jan,11

53665 **Dilation of female urethra, general or conduction (spinal) anesthesia** ♀
EXCLUDES *Procedure performed under local anesthesia (53660-53661)*
1.12 1.12 FUD 000 J A2
AMA: 2014,Jan,11

53850-53899 Transurethral Procedures

EXCLUDES *Endoscopic procedures; cystoscopy, urethroscopy, cystourethroscopy (52000-52700 [52356])*

53850 **Transurethral destruction of prostate tissue; by microwave thermotherapy** ♂
(81020)
10.1 45.4 FUD 090 J P2
AMA: 2018,Nov,10; 2018,Jan,8; 2017,Jan,8; 2016,Jan,13

53852 **by radiofrequency thermotherapy** ♂
(81020)
10.8 43.9 FUD 090 J P3
AMA: 2018,Nov,10; 2018,Jan,8; 2017,Jan,8; 2016,Jan,13

53854 **by radiofrequency generated water vapor thermotherapy**
EXCLUDES *High-energy water vapor thermotherapy for transurethral ablation malignant prostate tissue (0582T)*
10.8 51.1 FUD 090 P2
AMA: 2018,Nov,10

53855 **Insertion of a temporary prostatic urethral stent, including urethral measurement** ♂
EXCLUDES *Permanent urethral stent insertion (52282)*
2.39 21.7 FUD 000 J P3 80
AMA: 2018,Nov,10; 2018,Jan,8; 2017,Jan,8; 2016,Jan,13

53860 **Transurethral radiofrequency micro-remodeling of the female bladder neck and proximal urethra for stress urinary incontinence** ♀
6.48 52.7 FUD 090 J P2 80
AMA: 2014,Jan,11

53899 **Unlisted procedure, urinary system**
0.00 0.00 FUD YYY T 80
AMA: 2020,Jun,13; 2019,Aug,10; 2018,Jan,8; 2017,Jan,8; 2016,Jan,13

54000-54015 Procedures of Penis: Incisional

EXCLUDES *Debridement abdominal perineal gangrene (11004-11006)*

54000 **Slitting of prepuce, dorsal or lateral (separate procedure); newborn** A ♂
3.14 4.40 FUD 010 63 J A2 80
AMA: 2014,Jan,11

54001 **except newborn** ♂
4.02 5.44 FUD 010 J A2
AMA: 2014,Jan,11

54015 **Incision and drainage of penis, deep** ♂
EXCLUDES *Abscess, skin/subcutaneous (10060-10160)*
8.92 8.92 FUD 010 J A2 80
AMA: 2014,Jan,11

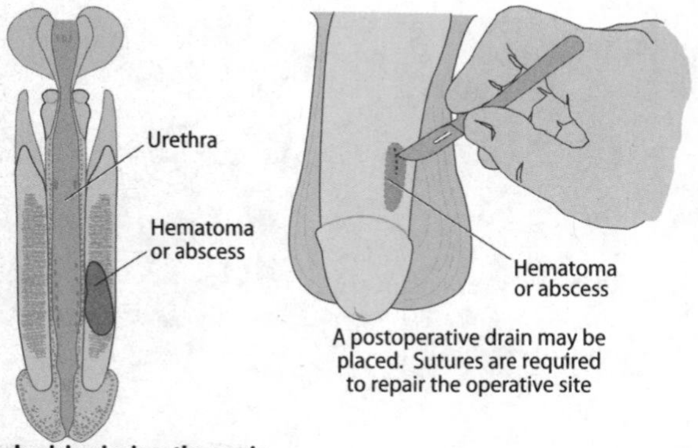
Urethra
Hematoma or abscess
Hematoma or abscess
A postoperative drain may be placed. Sutures are required to repair the operative site

The physician incises the penis to drain an abscess or hematoma

54050-54065 Destruction of Penis Lesions: Multiple Methods

EXCLUDES *Excision/destruction other lesions (11420-11426, 11620-11626, 17000-17250, 17270-17276)*

54050 **Destruction of lesion(s), penis (eg, condyloma, papilloma, molluscum contagiosum, herpetic vesicle), simple; chemical** ♂
3.05 3.80 FUD 010 Q1 N1
AMA: 2014,Jan,11; 1997,Nov,1

54055 **electrodesiccation** ♂
2.69 3.49 FUD 010 T P3
AMA: 2014,Jan,11; 1997,Nov,1

54056 **cryosurgery** ♂
3.18 4.03 FUD 010 Q1 N1
AMA: 2014,Jan,11; 1997,Nov,1

54057 **laser surgery** ♂
2.72 3.94 FUD 010 T A2
AMA: 2014,Jan,11; 1997,Nov,1

54060 **surgical excision** ♂
3.76 5.29 FUD 010 T A2
AMA: 2014,Jan,11

54065 **Destruction of lesion(s), penis (eg, condyloma, papilloma, molluscum contagiosum, herpetic vesicle), extensive (eg, laser surgery, electrosurgery, cryosurgery, chemosurgery)** ♂
4.97 6.31 FUD 010 T A2
AMA: 2014,Jan,11; 1997,Nov,1

54100-54115 Procedures of Penis: Excisional

54100 **Biopsy of penis; (separate procedure)** ♂
3.64 5.71 FUD 000 J A2
AMA: 2019,Jan,9; 2018,Jan,8; 2017,Jan,8; 2016,Jan,13

54105 **deep structures** ♂
6.16 7.68 FUD 010 J A2
AMA: 2014,Jan,11

54110 **Excision of penile plaque (Peyronie disease);** ♂
18.0 18.0 FUD 090 J A2 80
AMA: 2014,Jan,11

54111 **with graft to 5 cm in length** ♂
23.1 23.1 FUD 090 J A2 80
AMA: 2018,Jan,8; 2017,Jan,8; 2016,Jan,13

54112 **with graft greater than 5 cm in length** ♂
27.1 27.1 FUD 090 J A2 80
AMA: 2014,Jan,11

54115 **Removal foreign body from deep penile tissue (eg, plastic implant)** ♂
12.2 13.0 FUD 090 J A2 80
AMA: 2014,Jan,11

54120-54135 Amputation of Penis

54120 **Amputation of penis; partial** ♂
18.2 18.2 FUD 090 J A2 80
AMA: 2014,Jan,11

54125 **complete** ♂
23.5 23.5 FUD 090 C 80
AMA: 2014,Jan,11

54130 **Amputation of penis, radical; with bilateral inguinofemoral lymphadenectomy** ♂
34.5 34.5 FUD 090 C 80
AMA: 2014,Jan,11

54135 **in continuity with bilateral pelvic lymphadenectomy, including external iliac, hypogastric and obturator nodes** ♂
43.7 43.7 FUD 090 C 80
AMA: 2014,Jan,11

54150-54164 Circumcision Procedures

54150 **Circumcision, using clamp or other device with regional dorsal penile or ring block** ♂
Code also modifier 52 when performed without dorsal penile or ring block
2.83 4.42 FUD 000 63 J A2 80
AMA: 2018,Jan,8; 2017,Jan,8; 2016,Jan,13

54160 **Circumcision, surgical excision other than clamp, device, or dorsal slit; neonate (28 days of age or less)** A ♂
4.17 6.32 FUD 010 63 J A2
AMA: 2018,Jan,8; 2017,Jan,8; 2016,Jan,13

54161 **older than 28 days of age** A ♂
5.70 5.70 FUD 010 J A2
AMA: 2018,Jan,8; 2017,Jan,8; 2016,Jan,13

54162 **Lysis or excision of penile post-circumcision adhesions** ♂
5.77 7.42 FUD 010 J A2
AMA: 2014,Jan,11

54163 **Repair incomplete circumcision** ♂
6.31 6.31 FUD 010 J A2
AMA: 2014,Jan,11

54164 **Frenulotomy of penis** ♂
EXCLUDES *Circumcision (54150-54163)*
5.60 5.60 FUD 010 J A2
AMA: 2014,Jan,11

54200-54250 Evaluation and Treatment of Erectile Abnormalities

54200 **Injection procedure for Peyronie disease;** ♂
2.42 3.13 FUD 010 T P3
AMA: 2014,Jan,11

54205 **with surgical exposure of plaque** ♂
15.4 15.4 FUD 090 J A2 80
AMA: 2014,Jan,11

54220 **Irrigation of corpora cavernosa for priapism** ♂
3.87 5.97 **FUD** 000 T A2
AMA: 2014,Jan,11

54230 **Injection procedure for corpora cavernosography** ♂
(74445)
2.30 2.82 **FUD** 000 N N1
AMA: 2014,Jan,11

54231 **Dynamic cavernosometry, including intracavernosal injection of vasoactive drugs (eg, papaverine, phentolamine)** ♂
3.36 4.08 **FUD** 000 J P3
AMA: 2014,Jan,11; 1994,Sum,29

54235 **Injection of corpora cavernosa with pharmacologic agent(s) (eg, papaverine, phentolamine)** ♂
2.11 2.56 **FUD** 000 T P3
AMA: 2018,Jan,8; 2017,Jan,8; 2016,Jan,13

54240 **Penile plethysmography** ♂
2.94 2.94 **FUD** 000 S P3 80
AMA: 2014,Jan,11

54250 **Nocturnal penile tumescence and/or rigidity test** ♂
3.50 3.50 **FUD** 000 T P3 80
AMA: 2014,Jan,11

54300-54390 Hypospadias Repair and Related Procedures

EXCLUDES *Other urethroplasties (53400-53430)*
Revascularization penis (37788)

54300 **Plastic operation of penis for straightening of chordee (eg, hypospadias), with or without mobilization of urethra** ♂
18.6 18.6 **FUD** 090 J A2 80
AMA: 2018,Jan,8; 2017,Jan,8; 2016,Jan,13

54304 **Plastic operation on penis for correction of chordee or for first stage hypospadias repair with or without transplantation of prepuce and/or skin flaps** ♂
21.6 21.6 **FUD** 090 J A2 80
AMA: 2014,Jan,11

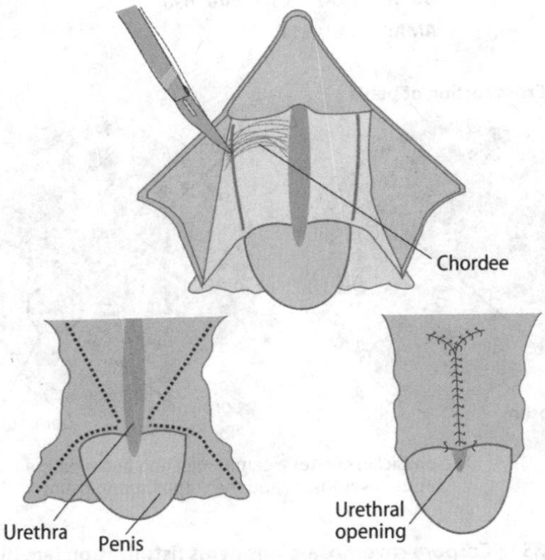

The foreskin is used in either a free graft or a flap graft to cover the ventral skin defects created to correct the chordee

54308 **Urethroplasty for second stage hypospadias repair (including urinary diversion); less than 3 cm** ♂
20.6 20.6 **FUD** 090 J A2 80
AMA: 2014,Jan,11

54312 **greater than 3 cm** ♂
23.6 23.6 **FUD** 090 J A2 80
AMA: 2014,Jan,11

54316 **Urethroplasty for second stage hypospadias repair (including urinary diversion) with free skin graft obtained from site other than genitalia** ♂
28.8 28.8 **FUD** 090 J A2 80
AMA: 2014,Jan,11

54318 **Urethroplasty for third stage hypospadias repair to release penis from scrotum (eg, third stage Cecil repair)** ♂
20.5 20.5 **FUD** 090 J A2 80
AMA: 2014,Jan,11

54322 **1-stage distal hypospadias repair (with or without chordee or circumcision); with simple meatal advancement (eg, Magpi, V-flap)** ♂
22.6 22.6 **FUD** 090 J A2 80
AMA: 2014,Jan,11

54324 **with urethroplasty by local skin flaps (eg, flip-flap, prepucial flap)** ♂
INCLUDES Browne's operation
28.0 28.0 **FUD** 090 J A2 80
AMA: 2014,Jan,11

54326 **with urethroplasty by local skin flaps and mobilization of urethra** ♂
27.3 27.3 **FUD** 090 J A2 80
AMA: 2014,Jan,11

54328 **with extensive dissection to correct chordee and urethroplasty with local skin flaps, skin graft patch, and/or island flap** ♂
EXCLUDES *Urethroplasty/straightening chordee (54308)*
27.1 27.1 **FUD** 090 J A2 80
AMA: 2018,Jan,8; 2017,Jan,8; 2016,Jan,13

54332 **1-stage proximal penile or penoscrotal hypospadias repair requiring extensive dissection to correct chordee and urethroplasty by use of skin graft tube and/or island flap** ♂
29.3 29.3 **FUD** 090 J G2 80
AMA: 2018,Jan,8; 2017,Jan,8; 2016,Jan,13

54336 **1-stage perineal hypospadias repair requiring extensive dissection to correct chordee and urethroplasty by use of skin graft tube and/or island flap** ♂
34.4 34.4 **FUD** 090 J G2 80
AMA: 2018,Jan,8; 2017,Jan,8; 2016,Jan,13

▲ **54340** **Repair of hypospadias complication(s) (ie, fistula, stricture, diverticula); by closure, incision, or excision, simple** ♂
16.4 16.4 **FUD** 090 J A2 80
AMA: 2014,Jan,11

▲ **54344** **requiring mobilization of skin flaps and urethroplasty with flap or patch graft** ♂
27.4 27.4 **FUD** 090 J A2 80
AMA: 2014,Jan,11

▲ **54348** **requiring extensive dissection, and urethroplasty with flap, patch or tubed graft (including urinary diversion, when performed)** ♂
29.3 29.3 **FUD** 090 J A2 80
AMA: 2014,Jan,11

▲ **54352 Revision of prior hypospadias repair requiring extensive dissection and excision of previously constructed structures including re-release of chordee and reconstruction of urethra and penis by use of local skin as grafts and island flaps and skin brought in as flaps or grafts** ♂

EXCLUDES *Application skin substitute graft (15275)*
Excision urethral diverticulum (53235)
Hypospadias repair:
Complications (54340, 54344, 54348)
Extensive dissection to correct chordee and urethroplasty, 1-stage perineal (54336)
Island pedicle flap (15740)
Plastic repair:
Angulation (54360)
Chordee (54300)
Tubed pedicle formation (15574)
Urethroplasty, 1-stage reconstruction male anterior urethra (53410)

41.0 41.0 **FUD** 090 J A2 80

AMA: 2014,Jan,11

54360 Plastic operation on penis to correct angulation ♂

20.8 20.8 **FUD** 090 J A2 80

AMA: 2014,Jan,11

54380 Plastic operation on penis for epispadias distal to external sphincter; ♂

INCLUDES Lowsley's operation

23.1 23.1 **FUD** 090 J A2 80

AMA: 2014,Jan,11

54385 with incontinence ♂

26.8 26.8 **FUD** 090 J A2 80

AMA: 2014,Jan,11

54390 with exstrophy of bladder ♂

35.9 35.9 **FUD** 090 C 80

AMA: 2014,Jan,11

54400-54417 Procedures to Treat Impotence

CMS: 100-03,230.4 Diagnosis and Treatment of Impotence

EXCLUDES *Other urethroplasties (53400-53430)*
Revascularization penis (37788)

54400 Insertion of penile prosthesis; non-inflatable (semi-rigid) ♂

EXCLUDES *Replacement/removal penile prosthesis (54415, 54416)*

15.3 15.3 **FUD** 090 J J8

AMA: 2014,Jan,11

54401 inflatable (self-contained) ♂

EXCLUDES *Replacement/removal penile prosthesis (54415, 54416)*

18.9 18.9 **FUD** 090 J J8

AMA: 2014,Jan,11

54405 Insertion of multi-component, inflatable penile prosthesis, including placement of pump, cylinders, and reservoir ♂

Code also modifier 52 for reduced services

23.4 23.4 **FUD** 090 J J8 80

AMA: 2014,Jan,11

54406 Removal of all components of a multi-component, inflatable penile prosthesis without replacement of prosthesis ♂

Code also modifier 52 for reduced services

21.1 21.1 **FUD** 090 Q2 A2 80

AMA: 2014,Jan,11

54408 Repair of component(s) of a multi-component, inflatable penile prosthesis ♂

22.8 22.8 **FUD** 090 J A2 80

AMA: 2014,Jan,11

54410 Removal and replacement of all component(s) of a multi-component, inflatable penile prosthesis at the same operative session ♂

24.8 24.8 **FUD** 090 J J8 80

AMA: 2014,Jan,11

54411 Removal and replacement of all components of a multi-component inflatable penile prosthesis through an infected field at the same operative session, including irrigation and debridement of infected tissue ♂

INCLUDES Debridement (11042, 11043)

Code also modifier 52 for reduced services

29.7 29.7 **FUD** 090 J J8 80

AMA: 2014,Jan,11

54415 Removal of non-inflatable (semi-rigid) or inflatable (self-contained) penile prosthesis, without replacement of prosthesis ♂

15.3 15.3 **FUD** 090 Q2 A2 80

AMA: 2014,Jan,11

54416 Removal and replacement of non-inflatable (semi-rigid) or inflatable (self-contained) penile prosthesis at the same operative session ♂

20.5 20.5 **FUD** 090 J J8 80

AMA: 2014,Jan,11

54417 Removal and replacement of non-inflatable (semi-rigid) or inflatable (self-contained) penile prosthesis through an infected field at the same operative session, including irrigation and debridement of infected tissue ♂

INCLUDES Debridement (11042, 11043)

26.0 26.0 **FUD** 090 J J8 80

AMA: 2014,Jan,11

54420-54450 Other Procedures of the Penis

EXCLUDES *Other urethroplasties (53400-53430)*
Revascularization penis (37788)

54420 Corpora cavernosa-saphenous vein shunt (priapism operation), unilateral or bilateral ♂

20.3 20.3 **FUD** 090 J A2 80

AMA: 2014,Jan,11

54430 Corpora cavernosa-corpus spongiosum shunt (priapism operation), unilateral or bilateral ♂

18.5 18.5 **FUD** 090 C 80

AMA: 2014,Jan,11

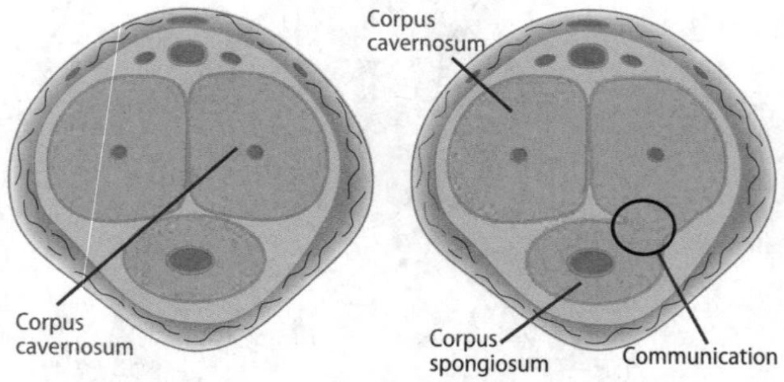

The physician creates a communication between the corpus cavernosum and the corpus spongiosum

54435 Corpora cavernosa-glans penis fistulization (eg, biopsy needle, Winter procedure, rongeur, or punch) for priapism ♂

12.0 12.0 **FUD** 090 J A2

AMA: 2014,Jan,11

54437 Repair of traumatic corporeal tear(s) ♂

EXCLUDES *Urethral repair (53410, 53415)*

19.4 19.4 **FUD** 090 J G2 80

54438 **Replantation, penis, complete amputation including urethral repair** ♂

EXCLUDES *Replantation/repair corporeal tear in incomplete amputation penis (54437)*

Replantation/urethral repair in incomplete amputation penis (53410-53415)

38.7 38.7 FUD 090 C 80

54440 **Plastic operation of penis for injury** ♂

0.00 0.00 FUD 090 J A2 80

AMA: 2014,Jan,11

54450 **Foreskin manipulation including lysis of preputial adhesions and stretching** ♂

1.67 1.99 FUD 000 T A2

AMA: 2014,Jan,11

54500-54560 Testicular Procedures: Incisional

EXCLUDES *Debridement abdominal perineal gangrene (11004-11006)*

54500 **Biopsy of testis, needle (separate procedure)** ♂

EXCLUDES *Fine needle aspiration (10021, [10004, 10005, 10006, 10007, 10008, 10009, 10010, 10011, 10012])*

(88172-88173)

2.16 2.16 FUD 000 J A2 80 50

AMA: 2019,Apr,4

54505 **Biopsy of testis, incisional (separate procedure)** ♂

Code also when combined with epididymogram, seminal vesiculogram or vasogram (55300)

6.07 6.07 FUD 010 J A2 80 50

AMA: 2018,Jan,8; 2017,Jan,8; 2016,Jan,13

54512 **Excision of extraparenchymal lesion of testis** ♂

15.6 15.6 FUD 090 J A2 50

AMA: 2018,Jan,8; 2017,Jan,8; 2016,Jan,13

54520 **Orchiectomy, simple (including subcapsular), with or without testicular prosthesis, scrotal or inguinal approach** ♂

INCLUDES Huggins' orchiectomy

EXCLUDES *Lymphadenectomy, radical retroperitoneal (38780)*

Code also hernia repair, when performed (49505, 49507)

9.45 9.45 FUD 090 J A2 50

AMA: 2018,Jan,8; 2017,Jan,8; 2016,Jan,13

54522 **Orchiectomy, partial** ♂

EXCLUDES *Lymphadenectomy, radical retroperitoneal (38780)*

17.0 17.0 FUD 090 J A2 80 50

AMA: 2018,Jan,8; 2017,Jan,8; 2016,Jan,13

54530 **Orchiectomy, radical, for tumor; inguinal approach** ♂

EXCLUDES *Lymphadenectomy, radical retroperitoneal (38780)*

14.6 14.6 FUD 090 J A2 80 50

AMA: 2018,Jan,8; 2017,Jan,8; 2016,Jan,13

54535 **with abdominal exploration** ♂

EXCLUDES *Lymphadenectomy, radical retroperitoneal (38780)*

21.5 21.5 FUD 090 J G2 80 50

AMA: 2018,Jan,8; 2017,Jan,8; 2016,Jan,13

54550 **Exploration for undescended testis (inguinal or scrotal area)** ♂

14.2 14.2 FUD 090 J A2 80 50

AMA: 2018,Jan,8; 2017,Mar,10; 2017,Jan,8; 2016,Jan,13

54560 **Exploration for undescended testis with abdominal exploration** ♂

19.8 19.8 FUD 090 J G2 80 50

AMA: 2018,Jan,8; 2017,Jan,8; 2016,Jan,13

54600-54699 Open and Laparoscopic Testicular Procedures

54600 **Reduction of torsion of testis, surgical, with or without fixation of contralateral testis** ♂

13.1 13.1 FUD 090 J A2 50

AMA: 2018,Jan,8; 2017,Jan,8; 2016,Jan,13

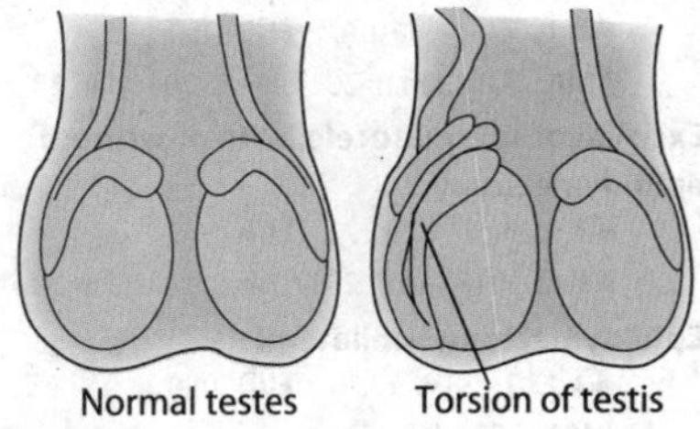

54620 **Fixation of contralateral testis (separate procedure)** ♂

8.66 8.66 FUD 010 J A2 50

AMA: 2014,Jan,11

54640 **Orchiopexy, inguinal or scrotal approach** ♂

INCLUDES Bevan's operation

Koop inguinal orchiopexy

Prentice orchiopexy

EXCLUDES *Repair inguinal hernia with inguinal orchiopexy (49495-49525)*

13.8 13.8 FUD 090 J A2 80 50

AMA: 2018,Jan,8; 2017,Mar,10; 2017,Jan,8; 2016,Jan,13

54650 **Orchiopexy, abdominal approach, for intra-abdominal testis (eg, Fowler-Stephens)** ♂

EXCLUDES *Laparoscopic orchiopexy (54692)*

20.5 20.5 FUD 090 J G2 80 50

AMA: 2018,Jan,8; 2017,Jan,8; 2016,Jan,13

54660 **Insertion of testicular prosthesis (separate procedure)** ♂

10.3 10.3 FUD 090 J J8 80 50

AMA: 2018,Jan,8; 2017,Jan,8; 2016,Jan,13

54670 **Suture or repair of testicular injury** ♂

11.7 11.7 FUD 090 J A2 80 50

AMA: 2018,Jan,8; 2017,Jan,8; 2016,Jan,13

54680 **Transplantation of testis(es) to thigh (because of scrotal destruction)** ♂

22.7 22.7 FUD 090 J A2 80 50

AMA: 2018,Jan,8; 2017,Jan,8; 2016,Jan,13

54690 **Laparoscopy, surgical; orchiectomy** ♂

INCLUDES Diagnostic laparoscopy (49320)

19.0 19.0 FUD 090 J A2 80 50

AMA: 2019,Feb,10; 2018,Jan,8; 2017,Jan,8; 2016,Jan,13

54692 **orchiopexy for intra-abdominal testis** ♂

INCLUDES Diagnostic laparoscopy (49320)

21.9 21.9 FUD 090 J G2 50

AMA: 2018,Jan,8; 2017,Jan,8; 2016,Jan,13

54699 **Unlisted laparoscopy procedure, testis** ♂

0.00 0.00 FUD YYY J 80 50

AMA: 2018,Jan,8; 2017,Jan,8; 2016,Jan,13

54700-54901 Open Procedures of the Epididymis

54700 **Incision and drainage of epididymis, testis and/or scrotal space (eg, abscess or hematoma)** ♂

EXCLUDES *Debridement genitalia for necrotizing soft tissue infection (11004-11006)*

6.16 6.16 FUD 010 J A2 50

AMA: 2018,Jan,8; 2017,Jan,8; 2016,Jan,13

54800 **Biopsy of epididymis, needle** ♂
EXCLUDES *Fine needle aspiration (10021, [10004, 10005, 10006, 10007, 10008, 10009, 10010, 10011, 10012])*
88172-88173
3.64 3.64 **FUD** 000 J A2 80 50
AMA: 2019,Apr,4; 2018,Jan,8; 2017,Jan,8; 2016,Jan,13

54830 **Excision of local lesion of epididymis** ♂
10.7 10.7 **FUD** 090 J A2 80 50
AMA: 2018,Jan,8; 2017,Jan,8; 2016,Jan,13

54840 **Excision of spermatocele, with or without epididymectomy** ♂
9.29 9.29 **FUD** 090 J A2 50
AMA: 2018,Jan,8; 2017,Jan,8; 2016,Jan,13

54860 **Epididymectomy; unilateral** ♂
12.1 12.1 **FUD** 090 J A2
AMA: 2014,Jan,11

54861 **bilateral** ♂
16.3 16.3 **FUD** 090 J A2 80
AMA: 2014,Jan,11

54865 **Exploration of epididymis, with or without biopsy** ♂
10.3 10.3 **FUD** 090 J A2 80
AMA: 2014,Jan,11; 2007,Jul,5

54900 **Epididymovasostomy, anastomosis of epididymis to vas deferens; unilateral** ♂
EXCLUDES *Operating microscope (69990)*
23.1 23.1 **FUD** 090 J A2 80
AMA: 2018,Jan,8; 2017,Jan,8; 2016,Jan,13

54901 **bilateral** ♂
EXCLUDES *Operating microscope (69990)*
30.5 30.5 **FUD** 090 J A2 80
AMA: 2018,Jan,8; 2017,Jan,8; 2016,Jan,13

55000-55180 Procedures of the Tunica Vaginalis and Scrotum

55000 **Puncture aspiration of hydrocele, tunica vaginalis, with or without injection of medication** ♂
2.44 3.39 **FUD** 000 T P3 50
AMA: 2014,Jan,11

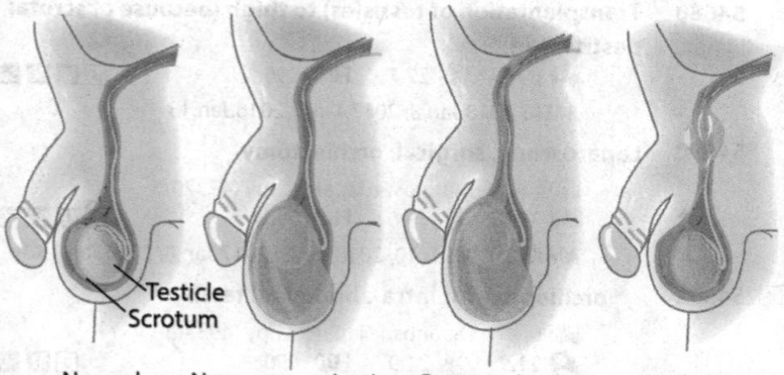

Normal | Noncommunicating hydrocele | Communicating hydrocele | Hydrocele of the cord

55040 **Excision of hydrocele; unilateral** ♂
EXCLUDES *Repair hernia with hydrocelectomy (49495-49501)*
9.77 9.77 **FUD** 090 J A2
AMA: 2018,Jan,8; 2017,Nov,10; 2017,Jan,8; 2016,Jan,13

55041 **bilateral** ♂
EXCLUDES *Repair hernia with hydrocelectomy (49495-49501)*
14.7 14.7 **FUD** 090 J A2
AMA: 2014,Jan,11

55060 **Repair of tunica vaginalis hydrocele (Bottle type)** ♂
11.0 11.0 **FUD** 090 J A2 80 50
AMA: 2018,Jan,8; 2017,Jan,8; 2016,Jan,13

55100 **Drainage of scrotal wall abscess** ♂
EXCLUDES *Debridement genitalia for necrotizing soft tissue infection (11004-11006)*
Incision and drainage scrotal space (54700)
4.80 6.43 **FUD** 010 J A2
AMA: 2014,Jan,11

55110 **Scrotal exploration** ♂
11.1 11.1 **FUD** 090 J A2
AMA: 2014,Jan,11

55120 **Removal of foreign body in scrotum** ♂
10.1 10.1 **FUD** 090 J A2 80
AMA: 2014,Jan,11

55150 **Resection of scrotum** ♂
EXCLUDES *Lesion excision skin, scrotum (11420-11426, 11620-11626)*
14.2 14.2 **FUD** 090 J A2 80
AMA: 2014,Jan,11

55175 **Scrotoplasty; simple** ♂
10.5 10.5 **FUD** 090 J A2 80
AMA: 2018,Jan,8; 2017,Jan,8; 2016,Jan,13

55180 **complicated** ♂
20.0 20.0 **FUD** 090 J A2 80
AMA: 2014,Jan,11

55200-55680 Procedures of Other Male Genital Ducts and Glands

55200 **Vasotomy, cannulization with or without incision of vas, unilateral or bilateral (separate procedure)** ♂
8.00 11.7 **FUD** 090 J A2 80
AMA: 2014,Jan,11

55250 **Vasectomy, unilateral or bilateral (separate procedure), including postoperative semen examination(s)** ♂
6.58 10.6 **FUD** 090 J A2
AMA: 2018,Jan,8; 2017,Jan,8; 2016,Jan,13

55300 **Vasotomy for vasograms, seminal vesiculograms, or epididymograms, unilateral or bilateral** ♂
Code also biopsy testis and modifier 51 when combined (54505)
(74440)
5.39 5.39 **FUD** 000 N N1 80
AMA: 2014,Jan,11

55400 **Vasovasostomy, vasovasorrhaphy** ♂
EXCLUDES *Operating microscope (69990)*
14.4 14.4 **FUD** 090 J A2 80 50
AMA: 2018,Jan,8; 2017,Jan,8; 2016,Jan,13

55500 **Excision of hydrocele of spermatic cord, unilateral (separate procedure)** ♂
11.3 11.3 **FUD** 090 J A2 80 50
AMA: 2018,Jan,8; 2017,Jan,8; 2016,Jan,13

55520 **Excision of lesion of spermatic cord (separate procedure)** ♂
13.2 13.2 **FUD** 090 J A2 80 50
AMA: 2018,Jan,8; 2017,Jan,8; 2016,Jan,13

55530 **Excision of varicocele or ligation of spermatic veins for varicocele; (separate procedure)** ♂
10.1 10.1 **FUD** 090 J A2 50
AMA: 2018,Jan,8; 2017,Jan,8; 2016,Jan,13

55535 **abdominal approach** ♂
12.4 12.4 **FUD** 090 J A2 80 50
AMA: 2018,Jan,8; 2017,Jan,8; 2016,Jan,13

55540 **with hernia repair** ♂
16.0 16.0 **FUD** 090 J A2 50
AMA: 2018,Jan,8; 2017,Jan,8; 2016,Jan,13

55550 **Laparoscopy, surgical, with ligation of spermatic veins for varicocele** ♂
INCLUDES Diagnostic laparoscopy (49320)
12.3 12.3 FUD 090 J A2 80 50
AMA: 2018,Jan,8; 2017,Jan,8; 2016,Jan,13

55559 **Unlisted laparoscopy procedure, spermatic cord** ♂
0.00 0.00 FUD YYY J 80 50
AMA: 2018,Jan,8; 2017,Jan,8; 2016,Jan,13

55600 **Vesiculotomy;** ♂
12.1 12.1 FUD 090 J R2 80 50
AMA: 2014,Jan,11

55605 **complicated** ♂
15.0 15.0 FUD 090 C 80 50
AMA: 2014,Jan,11

55650 **Vesiculectomy, any approach** ♂
20.7 20.7 FUD 090 C 80 50
AMA: 2014,Jan,11

55680 **Excision of Mullerian duct cyst** ♂
EXCLUDES *Injection procedure (52010, 55300)*
9.99 9.99 FUD 090 J A2 80 50
AMA: 2014,Jan,11

55700-55725 Procedures of Prostate: Incisional

55700 **Biopsy, prostate; needle or punch, single or multiple, any approach** ♂
EXCLUDES *Fine needle aspiration (10021, [10004, 10005, 10006, 10007, 10008, 10009, 10010, 10011, 10012])*
Needle biopsy prostate, saturation sampling for prostate mapping (55706)
(76942, 77002, 77012, 77021)
(88172-88173)
3.77 7.12 FUD 000 J A2
AMA: 2018,Jul,11; 2018,Jan,8; 2017,Jan,8; 2016,Jan,13

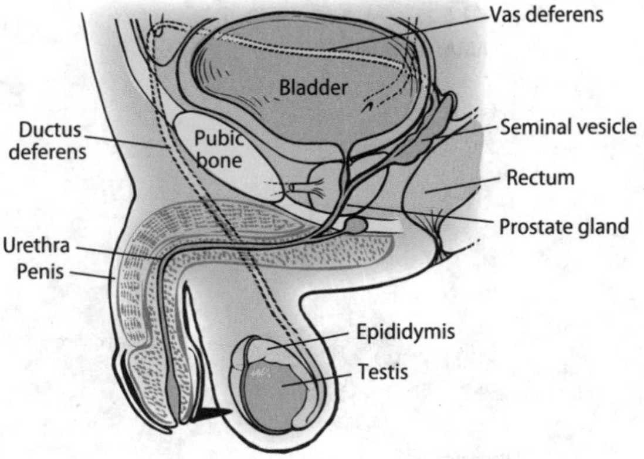

55705 **incisional, any approach** ♂
7.67 7.67 FUD 010 J A2
AMA: 2014,Jan,11

55706 **Biopsies, prostate, needle, transperineal, stereotactic template guided saturation sampling, including imaging guidance** ♂
EXCLUDES *Biopsy, prostate; needle or punch (55700)*
10.7 10.7 FUD 010 J G2 80
AMA: 2018,Jan,8; 2017,Jan,8; 2016,Jan,13

55720 **Prostatotomy, external drainage of prostatic abscess, any approach; simple** ♂
EXCLUDES *Drainage prostatic abscess, transurethral (52700)*
13.0 13.0 FUD 090 J A2 80
AMA: 2014,Jan,11

55725 **complicated** ♂
EXCLUDES *Drainage prostatic abscess, transurethral (52700)*
17.1 17.1 FUD 090 J A2 80
AMA: 2014,Jan,11

55801-55845 Open Prostatectomy

EXCLUDES *Limited pelvic lymphadenectomy for staging (separate procedure) (38562)*
Node dissection, independent (38770-38780)
Transurethral prostate:
Destruction (53850-53852)
Resection (52601-52640)

55801 **Prostatectomy, perineal, subtotal (including control of postoperative bleeding, vasectomy, meatotomy, urethral calibration and/or dilation, and internal urethrotomy)** ♂
31.6 31.6 FUD 090 C 80
AMA: 2014,Jan,11; 2003,Jun,6

55810 **Prostatectomy, perineal radical;** ♂
INCLUDES Walsh modified radical prostatectomy
37.8 37.8 FUD 090 C 80
AMA: 2014,Jan,11; 2003,Jun,6

55812 **with lymph node biopsy(s) (limited pelvic lymphadenectomy)** ♂
46.4 46.4 FUD 090 C 80
AMA: 2014,Jan,11

55815 **with bilateral pelvic lymphadenectomy, including external iliac, hypogastric and obturator nodes** ♂
EXCLUDES *When performed on separate days, report:*
Pelvic lymphadenectomy, bilateral, and append modifier 50 (38770)
Perineal radical prostatectomy (55810)
50.9 50.9 FUD 090 C 80
AMA: 2014,Jan,11

55821 **Prostatectomy (including control of postoperative bleeding, vasectomy, meatotomy, urethral calibration and/or dilation, and internal urethrotomy); suprapubic, subtotal, 1 or 2 stages** ♂
25.2 25.2 FUD 090 C 80
AMA: 2014,Jan,11; 2003,Jun,6

55831 **retropubic, subtotal** ♂
27.3 27.3 FUD 090 C 80
AMA: 2014,Jan,11; 2003,Jun,6

55840 **Prostatectomy, retropubic radical, with or without nerve sparing;** ♂
EXCLUDES *Prostatectomy, radical retropubic, performed laparoscopically (55866)*
33.8 33.8 FUD 090 C 80
AMA: 2014,Jan,11; 2003,Jun,6

55842 **with lymph node biopsy(s) (limited pelvic lymphadenectomy)** ♂
EXCLUDES *Prostatectomy, retropubic radical, performed laparoscopically (55866)*
33.8 33.8 FUD 090 C 80
AMA: 2014,Jan,11; 2003,Jun,6

55845 **with bilateral pelvic lymphadenectomy, including external iliac, hypogastric, and obturator nodes** ♂
EXCLUDES *Prostatectomy, retropubic radical, performed laparoscopically (55866)*
When performed on separate days, report:
Pelvic lymphadenectomy, bilateral, and append modifier 50 (38770)
Radical prostatectomy, retropubic, with or without nerve sparing (55840)
39.3 39.3 FUD 090 C 80
AMA: 2014,Jan,11; 2003,Jun,6

55860-55865 Prostate Exposure for Radiation Source Application

55860 Exposure of prostate, any approach, for insertion of radioactive substance; ♂
EXCLUDES *Interstitial radioelement application (77770-77772, 77778)*
25.2 25.2 FUD 090 J G2
AMA: 2014,Jan,11

55862 with lymph node biopsy(s) (limited pelvic lymphadenectomy) ♂
31.6 31.6 FUD 090 C 80
AMA: 2014,Jan,11

55865 with bilateral pelvic lymphadenectomy, including external iliac, hypogastric and obturator nodes ♂
38.5 38.5 FUD 090 C 80
AMA: 2014,Jan,11

55866 Laparoscopic Prostatectomy

55866 Laparoscopy, surgical prostatectomy, retropubic radical, including nerve sparing, includes robotic assistance, when performed ♂
INCLUDES Diagnostic laparoscopy (49320)
EXCLUDES *Open method (55840)*
41.6 41.6 FUD 090 J G2 80
AMA: 2018,Jan,8; 2017,Jan,8; 2016,Jan,13

55870-55899 Miscellaneous Prostate Procedures

55870 Electroejaculation ♂
EXCLUDES *Artificial insemination (58321-58322)*
4.10 5.04 FUD 000 T P3
AMA: 2014,Jan,11; 1991,Win,1

55873 Cryosurgical ablation of the prostate (includes ultrasonic guidance and monitoring) ♂
22.0 175. FUD 090 J J8
AMA: 2019,Sep,10; 2018,Jan,8; 2017,Jan,8; 2016,Jan,13

55874 Transperineal placement of biodegradable material, peri-prostatic, single or multiple injection(s), including image guidance, when performed ♂
INCLUDES Ultrasound guidance (76942)
4.77 87.0 FUD 000 T J8

55875 Transperineal placement of needles or catheters into prostate for interstitial radioelement application, with or without cystoscopy ♂
EXCLUDES *Placement needles/catheters for interstitial radioelement application, pelvic organs/genitalia, except prostate (55920)*
Code also interstitial radioelement application (77770-77772, 77778)
(76965)
22.2 22.2 FUD 090 J A2 80
AMA: 2018,Jan,8; 2017,Jan,8; 2016,Jan,13

55876 Placement of interstitial device(s) for radiation therapy guidance (eg, fiducial markers, dosimeter), prostate (via needle, any approach), single or multiple ♂
Code also supply device
(76942, 77002, 77012, 77021)
2.91 4.16 FUD 000 S P3
AMA: 2018,Jan,8; 2017,Jan,8; 2016,Jun,3; 2016,Jan,13

55880 Ablation of malignant prostate tissue, transrectal, with high intensity-focused ultrasound (HIFU), including ultrasound guidance ♂
28.5 28.5 FUD 090 G2

55899 Unlisted procedure, male genital system ♂
0.00 0.00 FUD YYY T 80
AMA: 2020,Aug,6; 2019,Dec,12; 2019,Jun,14; 2018,Jan,8; 2017,Jan,8; 2017,Jan,6; 2016,Jan,13

55920 Insertion Brachytherapy Catheters/Needles Pelvis/Genitalia, Male/Female

55920 Placement of needles or catheters into pelvic organs and/or genitalia (except prostate) for subsequent interstitial radioelement application
EXCLUDES *Insertion Heyman capsules for brachytherapy (58346)*
Insertion vaginal ovoids and/or uterine tandems for brachytherapy (57155)
Placement catheters or needles, prostate (55875)
13.0 13.0 FUD 000 J G2 80
AMA: 2018,Jan,8; 2017,Jan,8; 2016,Jan,13

55970-55980 Transsexual Surgery

CMS: 100-02,16,10 Exclusions from Coverage; 100-02,16,180 Services Related to Noncovered Procedures

55970 Intersex surgery; male to female ♂
0.00 0.00 FUD YYY J G2
AMA: 2014,Jan,11

55980 female to male ♀
0.00 0.00 FUD YYY J G2
AMA: 2014,Jan,11

56405-56420 Incision and Drainage of Abscess

EXCLUDES *Incision and drainage Skene's gland cyst/abscess (53060)*
Incision and drainage subcutaneous abscess/cyst/furuncle (10040, 10060, 10061)

56405 Incision and drainage of vulva or perineal abscess ♀
3.43 3.69 FUD 010 T P3
AMA: 2019,Jul,6

56420 Incision and drainage of Bartholin's gland abscess ♀
2.97 4.47 FUD 010 T P2
AMA: 2019,Jul,6

56440-56442 Other Female Genital Incisional Procedures

EXCLUDES *Incision and drainage subcutaneous abscess/cyst/furuncle (10040, 10060, 10061)*

56440 Marsupialization of Bartholin's gland cyst ♀
5.25 5.25 FUD 010 J A2
AMA: 2019,Jul,6

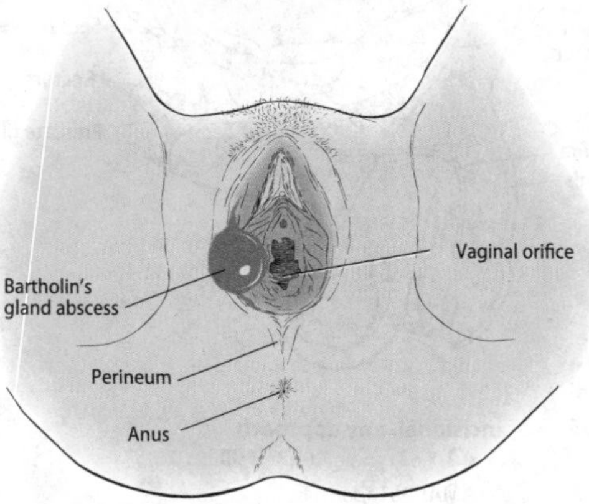

56441 Lysis of labial adhesions ♀
4.09 4.33 FUD 010 J A2 80
AMA: 2019,Jul,6

56442 Hymenotomy, simple incision ♀
1.36 1.36 FUD 000 J A2 80
AMA: 2019,Jul,6

56501-56515 Destruction of Vulvar Lesions, Any Method

EXCLUDES *Excision/fulguration/destruction:*
Skene's glands (53270)
Urethral caruncle (53265)

56501 Destruction of lesion(s), vulva; simple (eg, laser surgery, electrosurgery, cryosurgery, chemosurgery) ♀
3.60 4.69 FUD 010 T P3
AMA: 2019,Aug,10; 2019,Jul,6

56515 extensive (eg, laser surgery, electrosurgery, cryosurgery, chemosurgery) ♀
5.97 7.25 FUD 010 T A2
AMA: 2019,Aug,10; 2019,Jul,6

56605-56606 Vulvar and Perineal Biopsies

EXCLUDES *Excision local lesion (11420-11426, 11620-11626)*

56605 Biopsy of vulva or perineum (separate procedure); 1 lesion ♀
1.71 2.43 FUD 000 T P3
AMA: 2019,Jul,6; 2019,Jan,9; 2018,Jan,8; 2017,Jan,8; 2016,Jan,13

+ **56606 each separate additional lesion (List separately in addition to code for primary procedure)** ♀
Code first (56605)
0.86 1.11 FUD ZZZ N N1
AMA: 2019,Jul,6; 2019,Jan,9

56620-56640 Vulvectomy Procedures

INCLUDES Removal:
Greater than 80% vulvar area - complete procedure
Less than 80% vulvar area - partial procedure
Skin and deep subcutaneous tissue - radical procedure
Skin and superficial subcutaneous tissues - simple procedure

EXCLUDES *Skin graft (15004-15005, 15120-15121, 15240-15241)*

56620 Vulvectomy simple; partial ♀
15.9 15.9 FUD 090 J A2 80
AMA: 2019,Jul,6; 2019,Jan,14; 2018,Jan,8; 2017,Jan,8; 2016,Jan,13

56625 complete ♀
18.6 18.6 FUD 090 J A2 80
AMA: 2019,Jul,6

56630 Vulvectomy, radical, partial; ♀
Code also lymph node biopsy/excision when partial radical vulvectomy with inguinofemoral lymph node biopsy without inguinofemoral lymphadenectomy performed (38531)
27.0 27.0 FUD 090 C 80
AMA: 2019,Jul,6; 2019,Feb,8

56631 with unilateral inguinofemoral lymphadenectomy ♀
INCLUDES Bassett's operation
34.4 34.4 FUD 090 C 80
AMA: 2019,Jul,6; 2019,Feb,8

56632 with bilateral inguinofemoral lymphadenectomy ♀
INCLUDES Bassett's operation
40.2 40.2 FUD 090 C 80
AMA: 2019,Jul,6; 2019,Feb,8

56633 Vulvectomy, radical, complete; ♀
INCLUDES Bassett's operation
34.9 34.9 FUD 090 C 80
AMA: 2019,Jul,6; 2019,Feb,8

56634 with unilateral inguinofemoral lymphadenectomy ♀
INCLUDES Bassett's operation
36.8 36.8 FUD 090 C 80
AMA: 2019,Jul,6; 2019,Feb,8

56637 with bilateral inguinofemoral lymphadenectomy ♀
INCLUDES Bassett's operation
Code also lymph node biopsy/excision when complete radical vulvectomy with inguinofemoral lymph node biopsy without inguinofemoral lymphadenectomy performed (38531)
43.9 43.9 FUD 090 C 80
AMA: 2019,Jul,6; 2019,Feb,8

56640 Vulvectomy, radical, complete, with inguinofemoral, iliac, and pelvic lymphadenectomy ♀
INCLUDES Bassett's operation
EXCLUDES *Lymphadenectomy (38760-38780)*
43.3 43.3 FUD 090 C 80 50
AMA: 2019,Jul,6; 2019,Feb,8

56700-56740 Other Excisional Procedures: External Female Genitalia

56700 Partial hymenectomy or revision of hymenal ring ♀
5.38 5.38 FUD 010 J A2 80
AMA: 2019,Jul,6

56740 Excision of Bartholin's gland or cyst ♀
EXCLUDES *Excision/fulguration/marsupialization:*
Skene's glands (53270)
Urethral carcinoma (53220)
Urethral caruncle (53265)
Urethral diverticulum (53230, 53240)
8.92 8.92 FUD 010 J A2 50
AMA: 2019,Jul,6

56800-56810 Repair/Reconstruction External Female Genitalia

EXCLUDES *Repair urethra for mucosal prolapse (53275)*

56800 Plastic repair of introitus ♀
INCLUDES Emmet's operation
7.17 7.17 FUD 010 J A2 80
AMA: 2019,Jul,6

56805 Clitoroplasty for intersex state ♀
33.6 33.6 FUD 090 J G2 80
AMA: 2019,Jul,6

56810 Perineoplasty, repair of perineum, nonobstetrical (separate procedure) ♀
INCLUDES Emmet's operation
EXCLUDES *Genitalia wound repair (12001-12007, 12041-12047, 13131-13133)*
Introitus plastic repair (56800)
Sphincteroplasty, anal (46750-46751)
Vaginal/perineum recent injury repair, nonobstetrical (57210)
7.72 7.72 FUD 010 J A2 80
AMA: 2019,Jul,6

56820-56821 Vulvar Colposcopy with/without Biopsy

EXCLUDES *Colposcopic procedures and/or examinations:*
Cervix (57452-57461)
Vagina (57420-57421)

56820 Colposcopy of the vulva; ♀
2.46 3.28 FUD 000 T P3
AMA: 2019,Jul,6; 2018,Jan,8; 2017,Jan,8; 2016,Jan,13

56821 with biopsy(s) ♀
3.28 4.36 FUD 000 T P3
AMA: 2019,Jul,6; 2018,Jan,8; 2017,Jan,8; 2016,Jan,13

57000-57023 Incisional Procedures: Vagina

57000 Colpotomy; with exploration ♀
5.44 5.44 FUD 010 J A2 80
AMA: 2019,Jul,6; 2018,Jan,8; 2017,Jan,8; 2016,Jan,13

57010 **with drainage of pelvic abscess** ♀
INCLUDES Laroyenne operation
12.4 12.4 FUD 090 J A2 80
AMA: 2019,Jul,6

57020 **Colpocentesis (separate procedure)** ♀
2.29 2.77 FUD 000 J A2 80
AMA: 2019,Jul,6

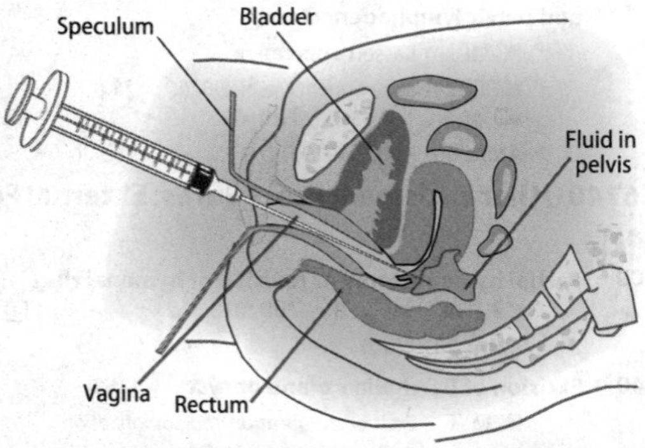

The physician aspirates matter from the pelvis through a needle inserted through the vaginal wall

57022 **Incision and drainage of vaginal hematoma; obstetrical/postpartum** ♀
4.86 4.86 FUD 010 J R2 80
AMA: 2019,Jul,6

57023 **non-obstetrical (eg, post-trauma, spontaneous bleeding)** ♀
8.83 8.83 FUD 010 J A2 80
AMA: 2019,Jul,6

57061-57065 Destruction of Vaginal Lesions, Any Method

CMS: 100-03,140.5 Laser Procedures

57061 **Destruction of vaginal lesion(s); simple (eg, laser surgery, electrosurgery, cryosurgery, chemosurgery)** ♀
2.92 3.52 FUD 010 J P3
AMA: 2019,Jul,6; 2018,Jan,8; 2017,Jan,8; 2016,Jan,13

57065 **extensive (eg, laser surgery, electrosurgery, cryosurgery, chemosurgery)** ♀
5.08 5.88 FUD 010 J A2
AMA: 2019,Jul,6; 2018,Jan,8; 2017,Jan,8; 2016,Jan,13

57100-57135 Excisional Procedures: Vagina

57100 **Biopsy of vaginal mucosa; simple (separate procedure)** ♀
1.91 2.64 FUD 000 T P3
AMA: 2019,Jul,6

57105 **extensive, requiring suture (including cysts)** ♀
3.75 4.19 FUD 010 J A2
AMA: 2019,Jul,6

57106 **Vaginectomy, partial removal of vaginal wall;** ♀
14.5 14.5 FUD 090 J G2 80
AMA: 2019,Jul,6; 2018,Jan,8; 2017,Jan,8; 2016,Jan,13

57107 **with removal of paravaginal tissue (radical vaginectomy)** ♀
41.9 41.9 FUD 090 J G2 80
AMA: 2019,Jul,6; 2018,Jan,8; 2017,Jan,8; 2016,Jan,13

57109 **with removal of paravaginal tissue (radical vaginectomy) with bilateral total pelvic lymphadenectomy and para-aortic lymph node sampling (biopsy)** ♀
51.1 51.1 FUD 090 J G2 80
AMA: 2019,Jul,6; 2018,Jan,8; 2017,Jan,8; 2016,Jan,13

57110 **Vaginectomy, complete removal of vaginal wall;** ♀
25.3 25.3 FUD 090 C 80
AMA: 2019,Jul,6; 2018,Jan,8; 2017,Jan,8; 2016,Jan,13

57111 **with removal of paravaginal tissue (radical vaginectomy)** ♀
51.1 51.1 FUD 090 C 80
AMA: 2019,Jul,6; 2018,Jan,8; 2017,Jan,8; 2016,Jan,13

57120 **Colpocleisis (Le Fort type)** ♀
14.6 14.6 FUD 090 J G2 80
AMA: 2019,Jul,6

57130 **Excision of vaginal septum** ♀
4.60 5.32 FUD 010 J A2 80
AMA: 2019,Jul,6

57135 **Excision of vaginal cyst or tumor** ♀
5.05 5.80 FUD 010 J A2
AMA: 2019,Jul,6

57150-57180 Irrigation/Insertion/Introduction Vaginal Medication or Supply

57150 **Irrigation of vagina and/or application of medicament for treatment of bacterial, parasitic, or fungoid disease** ♀
0.75 1.38 FUD 000 Q1 N1
AMA: 2019,Jul,6

57155 **Insertion of uterine tandem and/or vaginal ovoids for clinical brachytherapy** ♀
EXCLUDES *Insertion radioelement sources or ribbons (77761-77763, 77770-77772)*
Placement needles or catheters into pelvic organs and/or genitalia (except prostate) for interstitial radioelement application (55920)
8.09 10.6 FUD 000 J A2
AMA: 2019,Jul,6; 2018,Jan,8; 2017,Jan,8; 2016,Jan,13

57156 **Insertion of a vaginal radiation afterloading apparatus for clinical brachytherapy** ♀
4.27 5.92 FUD 000 T G2 80
AMA: 2019,Jul,6

57160 **Fitting and insertion of pessary or other intravaginal support device** ♀
1.33 1.79 FUD 000 T P3
AMA: 2019,Jul,6; 2018,Jan,8; 2017,Jan,8; 2016,Jan,13

57170 **Diaphragm or cervical cap fitting with instructions** ♀
1.37 1.85 FUD 000 T P3 80
AMA: 2019,Jul,6

57180 **Introduction of any hemostatic agent or pack for spontaneous or traumatic nonobstetrical vaginal hemorrhage (separate procedure)** ♀
3.11 4.37 FUD 010 T A2
AMA: 2019,Jul,6; 2018,Jan,8; 2017,Jan,8; 2016,Jan,13

57200-57335 Vaginal Repair and Reconstruction

EXCLUDES *Marshall-Marchetti-Kranz type urethral suspension, abdominal approach (51840-51841)*
Urethral suspension performed laparoscopically (51990)

57200 **Colporrhaphy, suture of injury of vagina (nonobstetrical)** ♀
8.87 8.87 FUD 090 J A2 80
AMA: 2019,Jul,6

57210 **Colpoperineorrhaphy, suture of injury of vagina and/or perineum (nonobstetrical)** ♀
10.6 10.6 FUD 090 J A2 80
AMA: 2019,Jul,6

57220 **Plastic operation on urethral sphincter, vaginal approach (eg, Kelly urethral plication)** ♀
9.24 9.24 FUD 090 J A2 80
AMA: 2019,Jul,6

57230 **Plastic repair of urethrocele** ♀
11.3 11.3 FUD 090 J A2 80
AMA: 2019,Jul,6

57240 Anterior colporrhaphy, repair of cystocele with or without repair of urethrocele, including cystourethroscopy, when performed ♀

INCLUDES Cystourethroscopy (52000)

17.0 17.0 FUD 090 J A2 80

AMA: 2019,Jul,6; 2018,Jan,8; 2017,Jan,8; 2016,Jan,13

57250 Posterior colporrhaphy, repair of rectocele with or without perineorrhaphy ♀

INCLUDES Rectocele repair (separate procedure) without posterior colporrhaphy (45560)

17.0 17.0 FUD 090 J A2 80

AMA: 2019,Jul,6; 2018,Jan,8; 2017,Jan,8; 2016,Jan,13

57260 Combined anteroposterior colporrhaphy, including cystourethroscopy, when performed; ♀

INCLUDES Cystourethroscopy (52000)

21.7 21.7 FUD 090 J A2 80

AMA: 2019,Jul,6; 2018,Jan,8; 2017,Jan,8; 2016,Jan,13

57265 with enterocele repair ♀

INCLUDES Cystourethroscopy (52000)

24.4 24.4 FUD 090 J A2 80

AMA: 2019,Jul,6; 2018,Jan,8; 2017,Jan,8; 2016,Jan,13

+ **57267 Insertion of mesh or other prosthesis for repair of pelvic floor defect, each site (anterior, posterior compartment), vaginal approach (List separately in addition to code for primary procedure)** ♀

Code first (45560, 57240-57265, 57285)

7.25 7.25 FUD ZZZ N N1 80

AMA: 2019,Jul,6; 2018,Jan,8; 2017,Jan,8; 2016,Jan,13

57268 Repair of enterocele, vaginal approach (separate procedure) ♀

13.9 13.9 FUD 090 J A2 80

AMA: 2019,Jul,6; 2018,Jan,8; 2017,Jan,8; 2016,Jan,13

57270 Repair of enterocele, abdominal approach (separate procedure) ♀

23.0 23.0 FUD 090 C 80

AMA: 2019,Jul,6; 2018,Jan,8; 2017,Jan,8; 2016,Jan,13

57280 Colpopexy, abdominal approach ♀

27.2 27.2 FUD 090 C 80

AMA: 2019,Jul,6; 2018,Jan,8; 2017,Jan,8; 2016,Jan,13

57282 Colpopexy, vaginal; extra-peritoneal approach (sacrospinous, iliococcygeus) ♀

15.1 15.1 FUD 090 J G2 80

AMA: 2019,Jul,6; 2018,Jan,8; 2017,Jan,8; 2016,Jan,13

57283 intra-peritoneal approach (uterosacral, levator myorrhaphy) ♀

EXCLUDES *Excision cervical stump (57556)*

Vaginal hysterectomy (58263, 58270, 58280, 58292, 58294)

19.6 19.6 FUD 090 J G2 80

AMA: 2019,Jul,6; 2018,Jan,8; 2017,Jan,8; 2016,Jan,13

57284 Paravaginal defect repair (including repair of cystocele, if performed); open abdominal approach ♀

EXCLUDES *Anterior colporrhaphy (57240)*

Anterior vesicourethropexy (51840-51841)

Combined anteroposterior colporrhaphy (57260-57265)

Hysterectomy (58152, 58267)

Laparoscopy, surgical; urethral suspension for stress incontinence (51990)

23.8 23.8 FUD 090 J G2 80

AMA: 2019,Jul,6; 2018,Jan,8; 2017,Jan,8; 2016,Jan,13

57285 vaginal approach ♀

EXCLUDES *Anterior colporrhaphy (57240)*

Combined anteroposterior colporrhaphy (57260-57265)

Laparoscopy, surgical; urethral suspension for stress incontinence (51990)

Vaginal hysterectomy (58267)

19.8 19.8 FUD 090 J G2 80

AMA: 2019,Jul,6; 2018,Jan,8; 2017,Jan,8; 2016,Jan,13

57287 Removal or revision of sling for stress incontinence (eg, fascia or synthetic) ♀

20.6 20.6 FUD 090 Q2 G2 80

AMA: 2019,Jul,6; 2018,Jan,8; 2017,Jan,8; 2016,Jan,13

57288 Sling operation for stress incontinence (eg, fascia or synthetic) ♀

INCLUDES Millin-Read operation

EXCLUDES *Sling operation for stress incontinence performed laparoscopically (51992)*

21.1 21.1 FUD 090 J J8 80

AMA: 2019,Jul,6; 2019,Feb,10; 2018,Jan,8; 2017,Jan,8; 2016,Jan,13

57289 Pereyra procedure, including anterior colporrhaphy ♀

22.6 22.6 FUD 090 J A2 80

AMA: 2019,Jul,6; 2018,Jan,8; 2017,Jan,8; 2016,Jan,13

57291 Construction of artificial vagina; without graft ♀

INCLUDES McIndoe vaginal construction

15.6 15.6 FUD 090 J A2 80

AMA: 2019,Jul,6

57292 with graft ♀

23.9 23.9 FUD 090 J G2 80

AMA: 2019,Jul,6

57295 Revision (including removal) of prosthetic vaginal graft; vaginal approach ♀

EXCLUDES *Laparoscopic approach (57426)*

14.2 14.2 FUD 090 J G2 80

AMA: 2019,Jul,6

57296 open abdominal approach ♀

EXCLUDES *Laparoscopic approach (57426)*

27.4 27.4 FUD 090 C 80

AMA: 2019,Jul,6

57300 Closure of rectovaginal fistula; vaginal or transanal approach ♀

17.0 17.0 FUD 090 J A2 80

AMA: 2019,Jul,6

57305 abdominal approach ♀

27.9 27.9 FUD 090 C 80

AMA: 2019,Jul,6

57307 abdominal approach, with concomitant colostomy ♀

30.3 30.3 FUD 090 C 80

AMA: 2019,Jul,6

57308 transperineal approach, with perineal body reconstruction, with or without levator plication ♀

19.0 19.0 FUD 090 C 80

AMA: 2019,Jul,6

57310 Closure of urethrovaginal fistula; ♀

13.8 13.8 FUD 090 J G2 80

AMA: 2019,Jul,6

57311 with bulbocavernosus transplant ♀

15.6 15.6 FUD 090 C 80

AMA: 2019,Jul,6

57320 Closure of vesicovaginal fistula; vaginal approach ♀

EXCLUDES *Cystostomy, concomitant (51020-51040, 51101-51102)*

15.8 15.8 FUD 090 J G2 80

AMA: 2019,Jul,6

Genital System 57240 — 57320

57330 **transvesical and vaginal approach** ♀

EXCLUDES *Vesicovaginal fistula closure, abdominal approach (51900)*

21.8 21.8 FUD 090 J G2 80

AMA: 2019,Jul,6

57335 **Vaginoplasty for intersex state** ♀

33.9 33.9 FUD 090 J G2 80

AMA: 2019,Jul,6

57400-57415 Treatment of Vaginal Disorders Under Anesthesia

57400 **Dilation of vagina under anesthesia (other than local)** ♀

3.78 3.78 FUD 000 J A2 80

AMA: 2019,Jul,6

57410 **Pelvic examination under anesthesia (other than local)** ♀

3.05 3.05 FUD 000 J A2

AMA: 2019,Jul,6; 2018,Jan,8; 2017,Jan,8; 2016,Jan,13

57415 **Removal of impacted vaginal foreign body (separate procedure) under anesthesia (other than local)** ♀

EXCLUDES *Removal impacted vaginal foreign body without anesthesia, report with appropriate E/M code*

4.89 4.89 FUD 010 J A2 80

AMA: 2019,Jul,6

57420-57426 Endoscopic Vaginal Procedures

57420 **Colposcopy of the entire vagina, with cervix if present;** ♀

EXCLUDES *Colposcopic procedures and/or examinations:*
Cervix (57452-57461)
Vulva (56820-56821)

Code also:
Computer-aided cervical mapping during colposcopy (57465)
Endometrial sampling (biopsy) performed same time as colposcopy (58110)
Modifier 51 for colposcopic procedures different sites, as appropriate

2.62 3.61 FUD 000 T P3

AMA: 2020,Dec,10; 2019,Jul,6; 2018,Jan,8; 2017,Jan,8; 2016,Jan,13

57421 **with biopsy(s) of vagina/cervix** ♀

EXCLUDES *Colposcopic procedures and/or examinations:*
Cervix (57452-57461)
Vulva (56820-56821)

Code also:
Computer-aided cervical mapping during colposcopy (57465)
Endometrial sampling (biopsy) performed same time as colposcopy (58110)
Modifier 51 for colposcopic procedures different sites, as appropriate

3.55 4.86 FUD 000 T P3

AMA: 2020,Dec,10; 2019,Jul,6; 2018,Jan,8; 2017,Jan,8; 2016,Jan,13

57423 **Paravaginal defect repair (including repair of cystocele, if performed), laparoscopic approach** ♀

EXCLUDES *Anterior colporrhaphy (57240)*
Anterior vesicourethropexy (51840-51841)
Combined anteroposterior colporrhaphy (57260)
Diagnostic laparoscopy (49320)
Hysterectomy (58152, 58267)
Laparoscopy, surgical; urethral suspension for stress incontinence (51990)

26.8 26.8 FUD 090 J G2 80

AMA: 2019,Jul,6; 2018,Jan,8; 2017,Jan,8; 2016,Jan,13

57425 **Laparoscopy, surgical, colpopexy (suspension of vaginal apex)** ♀

27.6 27.6 FUD 090 J G2 80

AMA: 2019,Jul,6

57426 **Revision (including removal) of prosthetic vaginal graft, laparoscopic approach** ♀

EXCLUDES *Open abdominal approach (57296)*
Vaginal approach (57295)

24.8 24.8 FUD 090 J G2 80

AMA: 2019,Jul,6

57452-57465 Endoscopic Cervical Procedures

EXCLUDES *Colposcopic procedures and/or examinations:*
Vagina (57420-57421)
Vulva (56820-56821)

Code also endometrial sampling (biopsy) performed same time as colposcopy (58110)

57452 **Colposcopy of the cervix including upper/adjacent vagina;** ♀

Code also computer-aided cervical mapping during colposcopy (57465)

2.64 3.45 FUD 000 T P3

AMA: 2020,Dec,10; 2019,Jul,6; 2018,Jan,8; 2017,Jan,8; 2016,Jan,13

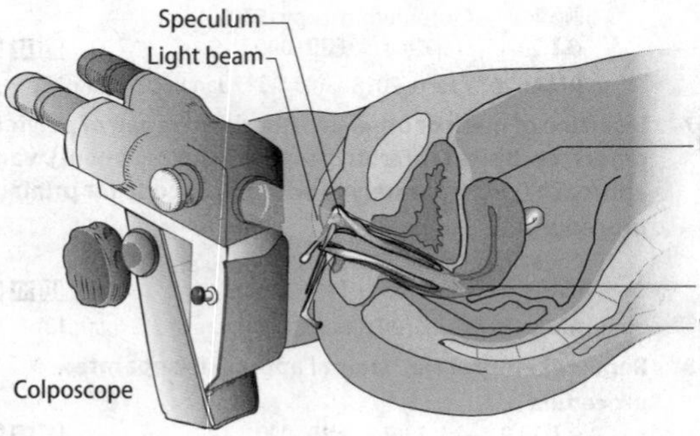

57454 **with biopsy(s) of the cervix and endocervical curettage** ♀

INCLUDES Colposcopy cervix (57452)

Code also computer-aided cervical mapping during colposcopy (57465)

3.89 4.71 FUD 000 T P3

AMA: 2020,Dec,10; 2019,Jul,6; 2018,Jan,8; 2017,Jan,8; 2016,Jan,13

57455 **with biopsy(s) of the cervix** ♀

INCLUDES Colposcopy cervix (57452)

Code also computer-aided cervical mapping during colposcopy (57465)

3.19 4.44 FUD 000 T P3

AMA: 2020,Dec,10; 2019,Jul,6; 2018,Jan,8; 2017,Jan,8; 2016,Jan,13

57456 **with endocervical curettage** ♀

INCLUDES Colposcopy cervix (57452)

EXCLUDES *Colposcopy cervix including upper/adjacent vagina; with loop electrode conization cervix (57461)*

Code also computer-aided cervical mapping during colposcopy (57465)

2.90 3.95 FUD 000 T P3

AMA: 2020,Dec,10; 2019,Jul,6; 2018,Jan,8; 2017,Jan,8; 2016,Jan,13

57460 **with loop electrode biopsy(s) of the cervix** ♀

INCLUDES Colposcopy cervix (57452)

Code also computer-aided cervical mapping during colposcopy (57465)

4.66 8.78 FUD 000 J P3

AMA: 2020,Dec,10; 2019,Jul,6; 2018,Jan,8; 2017,Jan,8; 2016,Jan,13

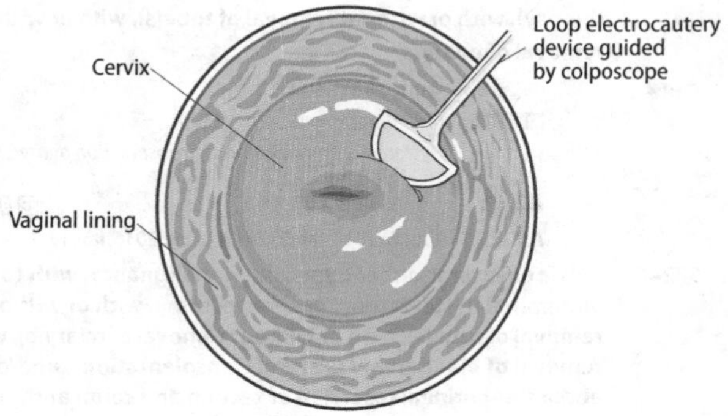

57461 **with loop electrode conization of the cervix** ♀

INCLUDES Colposcopy cervix (57452)

EXCLUDES *Colposcopy cervix including upper/adjacent vagina; with endocervical curettage (57456)*

Code also computer-aided cervical mapping during colposcopy (57465)

5.39 9.85 FUD 000 J P3

AMA: 2020,Dec,10; 2019,Jul,6; 2018,Jan,8; 2017,Jan,8; 2016,Jan,13

\+ **57465** **Computer-aided mapping of cervix uteri during colposcopy, including optical dynamic spectral imaging and algorithmic quantification of the acetowhitening effect (List separately in addition to code for primary procedure)** ♀

Code first (57420-57421, 57452-57461)

1.27 1.66 FUD ZZZ 80

AMA: 2020,Dec,10

57500-57556 Cervical Procedures: Multiple Techniques

EXCLUDES *Radical surgical procedures (58200-58240)*

57500 **Biopsy of cervix, single or multiple, or local excision of lesion, with or without fulguration (separate procedure)** ♀

2.17 4.11 FUD 000 T P3

AMA: 2019,Jul,6

57505 **Endocervical curettage (not done as part of a dilation and curettage)** ♀

2.90 3.69 FUD 010 T P3

AMA: 2019,Jul,6; 2018,Jan,8; 2017,Jan,8; 2016,Jan,13

57510 **Cautery of cervix; electro or thermal** ♀

3.29 4.33 FUD 010 J P3

AMA: 2019,Jul,6

57511 **cryocautery, initial or repeat** ♀

3.73 4.12 FUD 010 T P3

AMA: 2019,Jul,6

57513 **laser ablation** ♀

4.05 5.08 FUD 010 J A2

AMA: 2019,Jul,6

57520 **Conization of cervix, with or without fulguration, with or without dilation and curettage, with or without repair; cold knife or laser** ♀

EXCLUDES *Dilation and curettage, diagnostic/therapeutic, nonobstetrical (58120)*

8.23 9.59 FUD 090 J A2

AMA: 2019,Jul,6; 2018,Jan,8; 2017,Jan,8; 2016,Jan,13

57522 **loop electrode excision** ♀

7.21 8.25 FUD 090 J A2

AMA: 2019,Jul,6; 2018,Jan,8; 2017,Jan,8; 2016,Jan,13

57530 **Trachelectomy (cervicectomy), amputation of cervix (separate procedure)** ♀

10.0 10.0 FUD 090 J A2 80

AMA: 2019,Jul,6

57531 **Radical trachelectomy, with bilateral total pelvic lymphadenectomy and para-aortic lymph node sampling biopsy, with or without removal of tube(s), with or without removal of ovary(s)** ♀

EXCLUDES *Radical hysterectomy (58210)*

52.9 52.9 FUD 090 C 80

AMA: 2019,Jul,6

57540 **Excision of cervical stump, abdominal approach;** ♀

22.8 22.8 FUD 090 C 80

AMA: 2019,Jul,6

57545 **with pelvic floor repair** ♀

24.0 24.0 FUD 090 C 80

AMA: 2019,Jul,6

57550 **Excision of cervical stump, vaginal approach;** ♀

12.1 12.1 FUD 090 J A2 80

AMA: 2019,Jul,6

57555 **with anterior and/or posterior repair** ♀

17.7 17.7 FUD 090 J G2 80

AMA: 2019,Jul,6

57556 **with repair of enterocele** ♀

EXCLUDES *Insertion hemostatic agent/pack for spontaneous/traumatic nonobstetrical vaginal hemorrhage (57180)*

Intrauterine device insertion (58300)

16.8 16.8 FUD 090 J A2 80

AMA: 2019,Jul,6

57558-57800 Cervical Procedures: Dilation, Suturing, or Instrumentation

57558 **Dilation and curettage of cervical stump** ♀

EXCLUDES *Radical surgical procedures (58200-58240)*

3.33 3.80 FUD 010 J A2

AMA: 2019,Jul,6

57700 **Cerclage of uterine cervix, nonobstetrical** ♀

INCLUDES McDonald cerclage

Shirodker operation

9.13 9.13 FUD 090 J A2 80

AMA: 2019,Jul,6

57720 **Trachelorrhaphy, plastic repair of uterine cervix, vaginal approach** ♀

INCLUDES Emmet operation

9.33 9.33 FUD 090 J A2 80

AMA: 2019,Jul,6

57800 **Dilation of cervical canal, instrumental (separate procedure)** ♀

1.39 2.01 FUD 000 J P3

AMA: 2019,Jul,6

58100-58120 Procedures Involving the Endometrium

58100 **Endometrial sampling (biopsy) with or without endocervical sampling (biopsy), without cervical dilation, any method (separate procedure)** ♀

EXCLUDES *Endocervical curettage only (57505)*

Endometrial sampling (biopsy) performed in conjunction with colposcopy (58110)

1.86 2.80 FUD 000 T P3

AMA: 2019,Jul,6

Genital System

58110 — 58267

\+ **58110 Endometrial sampling (biopsy) performed in conjunction with colposcopy (List separately in addition to code for primary procedure)** ♀

Code first colposcopy (57420-57421, 57452-57461)

1.19 1.46 FUD ZZZ N N1 80

AMA: 2019,Jul,6; 2018,Jan,8; 2017,Jan,8; 2016,Jan,13

58120 Dilation and curettage, diagnostic and/or therapeutic (nonobstetrical) ♀

EXCLUDES *Postpartum hemorrhage (59160)*

6.35 7.66 FUD 010 J A2

AMA: 2019,Jul,6; 2018,Jan,8; 2017,Jan,8; 2016,Jan,13

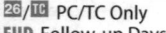

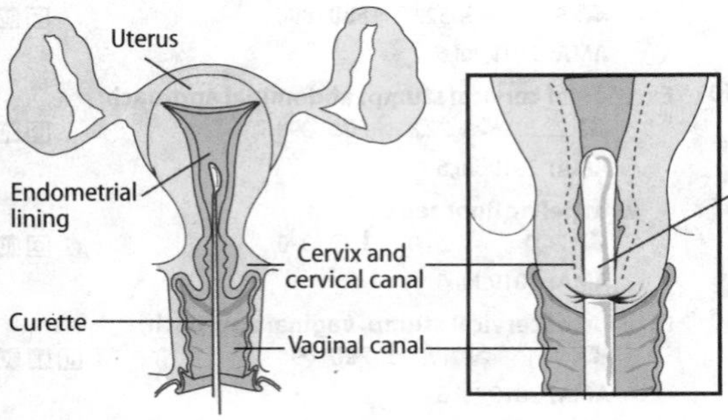

58140-58146 Myomectomy Procedures

58140 Myomectomy, excision of fibroid tumor(s) of uterus, 1 to 4 intramural myoma(s) with total weight of 250 g or less and/or removal of surface myomas; abdominal approach ♀

26.9 26.9 FUD 090 C 80

AMA: 2019,Jul,6; 2018,Jan,8; 2017,Jan,8; 2016,Jan,13

58145 vaginal approach ♀

16.2 16.2 FUD 090 J A2 80

AMA: 2019,Jul,6

58146 Myomectomy, excision of fibroid tumor(s) of uterus, 5 or more intramural myomas and/or intramural myomas with total weight greater than 250 g, abdominal approach ♀

EXCLUDES *Hysterectomy (58150-58240)*

Myomectomy procedures (58140-58145)

33.5 33.5 FUD 090 C 80

AMA: 2019,Jul,6; 2018,Jan,8; 2017,Jan,8; 2016,Jan,13

58150-58294 Abdominal and Vaginal Hysterectomies

CMS: 100-03,230.3 Sterilization

EXCLUDES *Destruction/excision endometriomas, open method (49203-49205, 58957-58958)*

Paracentesis (49082-49083)

Pelvic laparotomy (49000)

Secondary closure disruption evisceration abdominal wall (49900)

58150 Total abdominal hysterectomy (corpus and cervix), with or without removal of tube(s), with or without removal of ovary(s); ♀

29.2 29.2 FUD 090 C 80

AMA: 2019,Jul,6; 2018,Jan,8; 2017,Jan,8; 2016,Jan,13

58152 with colpo-urethrocystopexy (eg, Marshall-Marchetti-Krantz, Burch) ♀

EXCLUDES *Urethrocystopexy without hysterectomy (51840-51841)*

36.3 36.3 FUD 090 C 80

AMA: 2019,Jul,6; 2018,Jan,8; 2017,Jan,8; 2016,Jan,13

58180 Supracervical abdominal hysterectomy (subtotal hysterectomy), with or without removal of tube(s), with or without removal of ovary(s) ♀

27.3 27.3 FUD 090 C 80

AMA: 2019,Jul,6

58200 Total abdominal hysterectomy, including partial vaginectomy, with para-aortic and pelvic lymph node sampling, with or without removal of tube(s), with or without removal of ovary(s) ♀

39.0 39.0 FUD 090 C 80

AMA: 2019,Jul,6

58210 Radical abdominal hysterectomy, with bilateral total pelvic lymphadenectomy and para-aortic lymph node sampling (biopsy), with or without removal of tube(s), with or without removal of ovary(s) ♀

INCLUDES Wertheim hysterectomy

EXCLUDES *Chemotherapy (96401-96549)*

Hysterectomy, radical, with transposition ovary(s) (58825)

53.4 53.4 FUD 090 C 80

AMA: 2019,Jul,6; 2018,Jan,8; 2017,Jan,8; 2016,Jan,13

58240 Pelvic exenteration for gynecologic malignancy, with total abdominal hysterectomy or cervicectomy, with or without removal of tube(s), with or without removal of ovary(s), with removal of bladder and ureteral transplantations, and/or abdominoperineal resection of rectum and colon and colostomy, or any combination thereof ♀

EXCLUDES *Chemotherapy (96401-96549)*

Pelvic exenteration for male genital malignancy or lower urinary tract (51597)

83.8 83.8 FUD 090 C 80

AMA: 2019,Jul,6

58260 Vaginal hysterectomy, for uterus 250 g or less; ♀

24.2 24.2 FUD 090 J G2 80

AMA: 2019,Jul,6; 2018,Jan,8; 2017,Jan,8; 2016,Jan,13

58262 with removal of tube(s), and/or ovary(s) ♀

26.1 26.1 FUD 090 J G2 80

AMA: 2019,Jul,6

58263 with removal of tube(s), and/or ovary(s), with repair of enterocele ♀

28.8 28.8 FUD 090 J G2 80

AMA: 2019,Jul,6

58267 with colpo-urethrocystopexy (Marshall-Marchetti-Krantz type, Pereyra type) with or without endoscopic control ♀

30.9 30.9 FUD 090 C 80

AMA: 2019,Jul,6; 2018,Jan,8; 2017,Jan,8; 2016,Jan,13

58270 **with repair of enterocele** ♀

EXCLUDES *Vaginal hysterectomy with repair enterocele and removal tubes and/or ovaries (58263)*

25.8 25.8 **FUD** 090 J G2 80

AMA: 2019,Jul,6

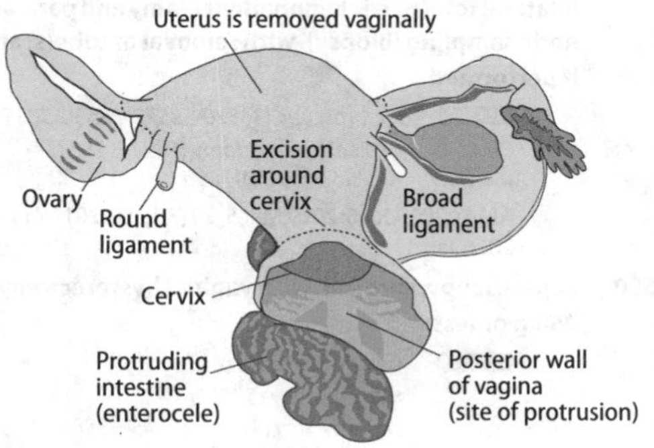

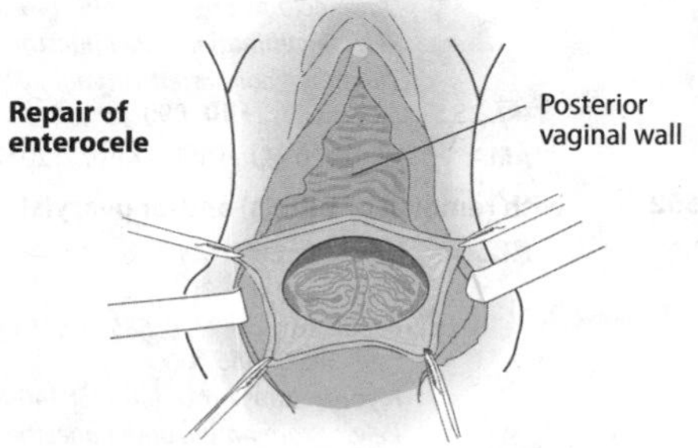

58275 **Vaginal hysterectomy, with total or partial vaginectomy;** ♀

28.6 28.6 **FUD** 090 C 80

AMA: 2019,Jul,6

58280 **with repair of enterocele** ♀

29.7 29.7 **FUD** 090 C 80

AMA: 2019,Jul,6

58285 **Vaginal hysterectomy, radical (Schauta type operation)** ♀

41.8 41.8 **FUD** 090 C 80

AMA: 2019,Jul,6; 2018,Jan,8; 2017,Jan,8; 2016,Jan,13

58290 **Vaginal hysterectomy, for uterus greater than 250 g;** ♀

33.4 33.4 **FUD** 090 J G2 80

AMA: 2019,Jul,6

58291 **with removal of tube(s) and/or ovary(s)** ♀

36.2 36.2 **FUD** 090 J G2 80

AMA: 2019,Jul,6

58292 **with removal of tube(s) and/or ovary(s), with repair of enterocele** ♀

38.2 38.2 **FUD** 090 J G2 80

AMA: 2019,Jul,6

58294 **with repair of enterocele** ♀

34.3 34.3 **FUD** 090 J G2 80

AMA: 2019,Jul,6

58300-58323 Contraception and Reproduction Procedures

58300 **Insertion of intrauterine device (IUD)** ♀

EXCLUDES *Insertion and/or removal implantable contraceptive capsules (11976, 11981-11983)*

1.49 2.60 **FUD** XXX E

AMA: 2019,Jul,6; 2018,Jan,8; 2017,Jan,8; 2016,Jan,13

58301 **Removal of intrauterine device (IUD)** ♀

EXCLUDES *Insertion and/or removal implantable contraceptive capsules (11976, 11981-11983)*

1.95 2.91 **FUD** 000 Q2 P3 80

AMA: 2019,Jul,6; 2018,Jan,8; 2017,Jan,8; 2016,Jan,13

58321 **Artificial insemination; intra-cervical** ♀

1.40 2.26 **FUD** 000 T P3 80

AMA: 2019,Jul,6

58322 **intra-uterine** ♀

1.70 2.56 **FUD** 000 T P3 80

AMA: 2019,Jul,6

58323 **Sperm washing for artificial insemination** ♀

0.37 0.45 **FUD** 000 T P3 80

AMA: 2019,Jul,6

58340-58350 Fallopian Tube Patency and Brachytherapy Procedures

58340 **Catheterization and introduction of saline or contrast material for saline infusion sonohysterography (SIS) or hysterosalpingography** ♀

(74740, 76831)

1.65 5.53 **FUD** 000 N N1

AMA: 2019,Jul,6; 2018,Jan,8; 2017,Jan,8; 2016,Jan,13

58345 **Transcervical introduction of fallopian tube catheter for diagnosis and/or re-establishing patency (any method), with or without hysterosalpingography** ♀

(74742)

8.27 8.27 **FUD** 010 J A2 80 50

AMA: 2019,Jul,6; 2018,Jan,8; 2017,Jan,8; 2016,Jan,13

58346 **Insertion of Heyman capsules for clinical brachytherapy** ♀

EXCLUDES *Insertion radioelement sources or ribbons (77761-77763, 77770-77772)*

Placement needles or catheters into pelvic organs and/or genitalia (except prostate) for interstitial radioelement application (55920)

13.2 13.2 **FUD** 090 J A2

AMA: 2019,Jul,6; 2018,Jan,8; 2017,Jan,8; 2016,Jan,13

58350 **Chromotubation of oviduct, including materials** ♀

2.51 3.62 **FUD** 010 J A2 50

AMA: 2019,Jul,6; 2018,Jan,8; 2017,Jan,8; 2016,Jan,13

58353-58356 Ablation of Endometrium

EXCLUDES *Destruction/excision endometriomas, open method (49203-49205)*

58353 **Endometrial ablation, thermal, without hysteroscopic guidance** ♀

EXCLUDES *Endometrial ablation performed hysteroscopically (58563)*

6.54 28.5 **FUD** 010 J A2

AMA: 2019,Jul,6; 2018,Jan,8; 2017,Jan,8; 2016,Jan,13

58356 **Endometrial cryoablation with ultrasonic guidance, including endometrial curettage, when performed** ♀

EXCLUDES *Dilation and curettage (58120)*

Endometrial biopsy (58100)

Hysterosalpingography (58340)

Ultrasound (76700, 76856)

10.2 52.0 **FUD** 010 J P3 80

AMA: 2019,Jul,6

58400-58540 Uterine Repairs: Vaginal and Abdominal

58400 **Uterine suspension, with or without shortening of round ligaments, with or without shortening of sacrouterine ligaments; (separate procedure)** ♀

INCLUDES Alexander's operation

Baldy-Webster operation

Manchester colporrhaphy

EXCLUDES *Anastomosis tubes to uterus (58752)*

13.1 13.1 **FUD** 090 C 80

AMA: 2019,Jul,6

58410 **with presacral sympathectomy** ♀

INCLUDES Alexander's operation

EXCLUDES *Anastomosis tubes to uterus (58752)*

23.5 23.5 **FUD** 090 C 80

AMA: 2019,Jul,6; 2018,Jan,8; 2017,Jan,8; 2016,Jan,13

58520 **Hysterorrhaphy, repair of ruptured uterus (nonobstetrical)** ♀

23.0 23.0 **FUD** 090 C 80

AMA: 2019,Jul,6

58540 **Hysteroplasty, repair of uterine anomaly (Strassman type)** ♀

INCLUDES Strassman type

EXCLUDES *Vesicouterine fistula closure (51920)*

26.5 26.5 **FUD** 090 C 80

AMA: 2019,Jul,6

58674-58554 [58674] Laparoscopic Procedures of the Uterus

INCLUDES Diagnostic laparoscopy

EXCLUDES *Hysteroscopy (58555-58565)*

58674 **Laparoscopy, surgical, ablation of uterine fibroid(s) including intraoperative ultrasound guidance and monitoring, radiofrequency** ♀

INCLUDES Intraoperative ultrasound (76998)

EXCLUDES *Laparoscopy (49320, 58541-58554, 58570-58573)*

23.6 23.6 **FUD** 090 J G2 80

AMA: 2019,Jul,6; 2018,Jan,8; 2017,Apr,7; 2017,Feb,14

58541 **Laparoscopy, surgical, supracervical hysterectomy, for uterus 250 g or less;** ♀

EXCLUDES *Colpotomy (57000)*
Hysteroscopy (58561)
Laparoscopy (49320, 58545-58546, 58661, 58670-58671)
Myomectomy procedures (58140-58146)
Pelvic examination under anesthesia (57410)
Treatment nonobstetrical vaginal hemorrhage (57180)

21.0 21.0 **FUD** 090 J G2 80

AMA: 2019,Jul,6; 2018,Jan,8; 2017,Apr,7; 2017,Jan,8; 2016,Jan,13

58542 **with removal of tube(s) and/or ovary(s)** ♀

EXCLUDES *Colpotomy (57000)*
Hysteroscopy (58561)
Laparoscopy (49320, 58545-58546, 58661, 58670-58671)
Myomectomy procedures (58140-58146)
Pelvic examination under anesthesia (57410)
Treatment nonobstetrical vaginal hemorrhage (57180)

23.9 23.9 **FUD** 090 J G2 80

AMA: 2019,Jul,6; 2018,Jan,8; 2017,Apr,7; 2017,Jan,8; 2016,Jan,13

58543 **Laparoscopy, surgical, supracervical hysterectomy, for uterus greater than 250 g;** ♀

EXCLUDES *Colpotomy (57000)*
Hysteroscopy (58561)
Laparoscopy (49320, 58545-58546, 58661, 58670-58671)
Myomectomy procedures (58140-58146)
Pelvic examination under anesthesia (57410)
Treatment nonobstetrical vaginal hemorrhage (57180)

24.3 24.3 **FUD** 090 J G2 80

AMA: 2019,Jul,6; 2018,Jan,8; 2017,Apr,7; 2017,Jan,8; 2016,Jan,13

58544 **with removal of tube(s) and/or ovary(s)** ♀

EXCLUDES *Colpotomy (57000)*
Hysteroscopy (58561)
Laparoscopy (49320, 58545-58546, 58661, 58670-58671)
Myomectomy procedures (58140-58146)
Pelvic examination under anesthesia (57410)
Treatment nonobstetrical vaginal hemorrhage (57180)

26.2 26.2 **FUD** 090 J G2 80

AMA: 2019,Jul,6; 2018,Jan,8; 2017,Apr,7; 2017,Jan,8; 2016,Jan,13

58545 **Laparoscopy, surgical, myomectomy, excision; 1 to 4 intramural myomas with total weight of 250 g or less and/or removal of surface myomas** ♀

26.0 26.0 **FUD** 090 J A2 80

AMA: 2019,Jul,6; 2017,Apr,7

58546 **5 or more intramural myomas and/or intramural myomas with total weight greater than 250 g** ♀

31.6 31.6 **FUD** 090 J A2 80

AMA: 2019,Jul,6; 2018,Jan,8; 2017,Apr,7; 2017,Jan,8; 2016,Jan,13

58548 **Laparoscopy, surgical, with radical hysterectomy, with bilateral total pelvic lymphadenectomy and para-aortic lymph node sampling (biopsy), with removal of tube(s) and ovary(s), if performed** ♀

EXCLUDES *Laparoscopy (38570-38572, 58550-58554)*
Radical hysterectomy (58210, 58285)

53.9 53.9 **FUD** 090 C 80

AMA: 2019,Jul,6; 2019,Mar,5; 2018,Jan,8; 2017,Apr,7; 2017,Jan,8; 2016,Jan,13

58550 **Laparoscopy, surgical, with vaginal hysterectomy, for uterus 250 g or less;** ♀

EXCLUDES *Colpotomy (57000)*
Hysteroscopy (58561)
Laparoscopy (49320, 58545-58546, 58661, 58670-58671)
Myomectomy procedures (58140-58146)
Pelvic examination under anesthesia (57410)
Treatment nonobstetrical vaginal hemorrhage (57180)

25.5 25.5 **FUD** 090 J A2 80

AMA: 2019,Jul,6; 2018,Jan,8; 2017,Apr,7; 2017,Jan,8; 2016,Jan,13

58552 **with removal of tube(s) and/or ovary(s)** ♀

EXCLUDES *Colpotomy (57000)*
Hysteroscopy (58561)
Laparoscopy (49320, 58545-58546, 58661, 58670-58671)
Myomectomy procedures (58140-58146)
Pelvic examination under anesthesia (57410)
Treatment nonobstetrical vaginal hemorrhage (57180)

28.0 28.0 **FUD** 090 J G2 80

AMA: 2019,Jul,6; 2018,Jan,8; 2017,Apr,7; 2017,Jan,8; 2016,Jan,13

58553 **Laparoscopy, surgical, with vaginal hysterectomy, for uterus greater than 250 g;** ♀

EXCLUDES *Colpotomy (57000)*
Hysteroscopy (58561)
Laparoscopy (49320, 58545-58546, 58661, 58670-58671)
Myomectomy procedures (58140-58146)
Pelvic examination under anesthesia (57410)
Treatment nonobstetrical vaginal hemorrhage (57180)

31.8 31.8 **FUD** 090 J G2 80

AMA: 2019,Jul,6; 2018,Jan,8; 2017,Apr,7

58554 **with removal of tube(s) and/or ovary(s)** ♀

EXCLUDES *Colpotomy (57000)*
Hysteroscopy (58561)
Laparoscopy (49320, 58545-58546, 58661, 58670-58671)
Myomectomy procedures (58140-58146)
Pelvic examination under anesthesia (57410)
Treatment nonobstetrical vaginal hemorrhage (57180)

38.1 38.1 **FUD** 090 J G2 80

AMA: 2019,Jul,6; 2018,Jan,8; 2017,Apr,7

58555-58565 Hysteroscopy

INCLUDES Diagnostic hysteroscopy (58555)
EXCLUDES *Laparoscopy (58541-58554, 58570-58578)*

58555 Hysteroscopy, diagnostic (separate procedure) ♀
4.35 | 8.40 | **FUD** 000 | J A2 80
AMA: 2019,Jul,6; 2018,Jan,8; 2017,Jan,8; 2016,Jan,13

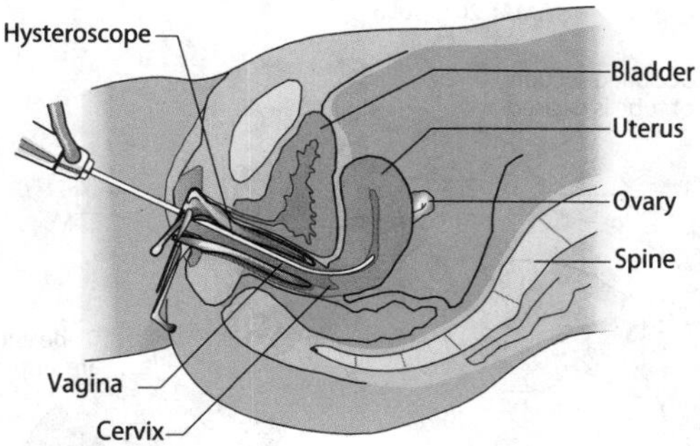

58558 Hysteroscopy, surgical; with sampling (biopsy) of endometrium and/or polypectomy, with or without D & C ♀
6.74 | 39.6 | **FUD** 000 | J A2
AMA: 2019,Jul,6; 2018,Jan,8; 2017,Jan,8; 2016,Jan,13

58559 with lysis of intrauterine adhesions (any method) ♀
8.33 | 8.33 | **FUD** 000 | J A2
AMA: 2019,Jul,6; 2018,Jan,8; 2017,Jan,8; 2016,Jan,13

58560 with division or resection of intrauterine septum (any method) ♀
9.16 | 9.16 | **FUD** 000 | J A2 80
AMA: 2019,Jul,6; 2018,Jan,8; 2017,Jan,8; 2016,Jan,13

58561 with removal of leiomyomata ♀
10.4 | 10.4 | **FUD** 000 | J A2 80
AMA: 2019,Jul,6; 2018,Jan,8; 2017,Jan,8; 2016,Jan,13

58562 with removal of impacted foreign body ♀
6.34 | 10.3 | **FUD** 000 | J A2
AMA: 2019,Jul,6; 2018,Jan,8; 2017,Jan,8; 2016,Jan,13

58563 with endometrial ablation (eg, endometrial resection, electrosurgical ablation, thermoablation) ♀
7.18 | 55.6 | **FUD** 000 | J A2 80
AMA: 2019,Jul,6; 2018,Jan,8; 2017,Jan,8; 2016,Jan,13

58565 with bilateral fallopian tube cannulation to induce occlusion by placement of permanent implants ♀
EXCLUDES *Diagnostic hysteroscopy (58555)*
Dilation cervical canal (57800)
Code also modifier 52 when unilateral procedure performed
12.9 | 51.6 | **FUD** 090 | J A2
AMA: 2019,Jul,6; 2018,Jan,8; 2017,Jan,8; 2016,Jan,13

58570-58579 Other Uterine Endoscopy

INCLUDES Diagnostic laparoscopy
EXCLUDES *Hysteroscopy (58555-58565)*

58570 Laparoscopy, surgical, with total hysterectomy, for uterus 250 g or less; ♀
EXCLUDES *Colpotomy (57000)*
Hysteroscopy (58561)
Laparoscopy (49320, 58545-58546, 58661, 58670-58671)
Myomectomy procedures (58140-58146)
Pelvic examination under anesthesia (57410)
Total abdominal hysterectomy (58150)
Treatment nonobstetrical vaginal hemorrhage (57180)
22.9 | 22.9 | **FUD** 090 | J G2 80
AMA: 2019,Jul,6; 2018,Jan,8; 2017,Apr,7

58571 with removal of tube(s) and/or ovary(s) ♀
EXCLUDES *Colpotomy (57000)*
Hysteroscopy (58561)
Laparoscopy (49320, 58545-58546, 58661, 58670-58671)
Myomectomy procedures (58140-58146)
Pelvic examination under anesthesia (57410)
Total abdominal hysterectomy (58150)
Treatment nonobstetrical vaginal hemorrhage (57180)
25.9 | 25.9 | **FUD** 090 | J G2 80
AMA: 2019,Jul,6; 2018,Feb,11; 2018,Jan,8; 2017,Apr,7; 2017,Jan,8; 2016,Jan,13

58572 Laparoscopy, surgical, with total hysterectomy, for uterus greater than 250 g; ♀
EXCLUDES *Colpotomy (57000)*
Hysteroscopy (58561)
Laparoscopy (49320, 58545-58546, 58661, 58670-58671)
Myomectomy procedures (58140-58146)
Pelvic examination under anesthesia (57410)
Total abdominal hysterectomy (58150)
Treatment nonobstetrical vaginal hemorrhage (57180)
29.3 | 29.3 | **FUD** 090 | J G2 80
AMA: 2019,Jul,6; 2018,Jan,8; 2017,Apr,7

58573 with removal of tube(s) and/or ovary(s) ♀
EXCLUDES *Colpotomy (57000)*
Hysteroscopy (58561)
Laparoscopy (49320, 58545-58546, 58661, 58670-58671)
Myomectomy procedures (58140-58146)
Pelvic examination under anesthesia (57410)
Total abdominal hysterectomy (58150)
Treatment nonobstetrical vaginal hemorrhage (57180)
35.0 | 35.0 | **FUD** 090 | J G2 80
AMA: 2019,Jul,6; 2019,Mar,5; 2018,Apr,10; 2018,Feb,11; 2018,Jan,8; 2017,Apr,7; 2017,Jan,8; 2016,Jan,13

58575 Laparoscopy, surgical, total hysterectomy for resection of malignancy (tumor debulking), with omentectomy including salpingo-oophorectomy, unilateral or bilateral, when performed ♀
EXCLUDES *Laparoscopy (49320-49321, 58570-58573, 58661)*
Omentectomy (49255)
54.9 | 54.9 | **FUD** 090 | C 80
AMA: 2019,Jul,6; 2019,Mar,5

58578 Unlisted laparoscopy procedure, uterus ♀
0.00 | 0.00 | **FUD** YYY | J 80 50
AMA: 2019,Jul,6; 2018,Jan,8; 2017,Jan,8; 2016,Jan,13

58579 Unlisted hysteroscopy procedure, uterus ♀
0.00 | 0.00 | **FUD** YYY | T 80 50
AMA: 2019,Jul,6; 2018,Jan,8; 2017,Jan,8; 2016,Jan,13

58600-58615 Sterilization by Tubal Interruption

CMS: 100-03,230.3 Sterilization
EXCLUDES *Destruction/excision endometriomas, open method (49203-49205)*

58600 Ligation or transection of fallopian tube(s), abdominal or vaginal approach, unilateral or bilateral ♀
INCLUDES Madlener operation
10.6 | 10.6 | **FUD** 090 | J G2 80
AMA: 2019,Jul,6; 2018,Jan,8; 2017,Jan,8; 2016,Jan,13

58605 Ligation or transection of fallopian tube(s), abdominal or vaginal approach, postpartum, unilateral or bilateral, during same hospitalization (separate procedure) ♀
EXCLUDES *Laparoscopic methods (58670-58671)*
9.65 | 9.65 | **FUD** 090 | C 80
AMA: 2019,Jul,6; 2018,Jan,8; 2017,Jan,8; 2016,Jan,13

+ 58611 Ligation or transection of fallopian tube(s) when done at the time of cesarean delivery or intra-abdominal surgery (not a separate procedure) (List separately in addition to code for primary procedure) ♀

Code first primary procedure

2.24 2.24 FUD ZZZ C 80

AMA: 2019,Jul,6

58615 Occlusion of fallopian tube(s) by device (eg, band, clip, Falope ring) vaginal or suprapubic approach ♀

EXCLUDES *Laparoscopic method (58671)*
Lysis adnexal adhesions (58740)

7.24 7.24 FUD 010 J G2 80

AMA: 2019,Jul,6; 2018,Jan,8; 2017,Jan,8; 2016,Jan,13

58660-58679 [58674] Endoscopic Procedures Fallopian Tubes and/or Ovaries

CMS: 100-03,230.3 Sterilization

INCLUDES Diagnostic laparoscopy (49320)

EXCLUDES *Laparoscopy with biopsy fallopian tube or ovary (49321)*
Laparoscopy with ovarian cyst aspiration (49322)

58660 Laparoscopy, surgical; with lysis of adhesions (salpingolysis, ovariolysis) (separate procedure) ♀

19.6 19.6 FUD 090 J A2 80

AMA: 2019,Jul,6; 2018,Jan,8; 2017,Jan,8; 2016,Jan,13

58661 with removal of adnexal structures (partial or total oophorectomy and/or salpingectomy) ♀

18.8 18.8 FUD 010 J A2 80 50

AMA: 2020,Jan,12; 2019,Jul,6; 2018,Jan,8; 2017,Jan,8; 2016,Jan,13

58662 with fulguration or excision of lesions of the ovary, pelvic viscera, or peritoneal surface by any method ♀

20.6 20.6 FUD 090 J A2 80

AMA: 2019,Jul,6; 2018,Jan,8; 2017,Dec,14; 2017,Jan,8; 2016,Jan,13

58670 with fulguration of oviducts (with or without transection) ♀

10.3 10.3 FUD 090 J A2

AMA: 2019,Jul,6; 2018,Jan,8; 2017,Jan,8; 2016,Jan,13

58671 with occlusion of oviducts by device (eg, band, clip, or Falope ring) ♀

10.6 10.6 FUD 090 J A2

AMA: 2019,Jul,6; 2018,Jan,8; 2017,Jan,8; 2016,Jan,13

58672 with fimbrioplasty ♀

21.3 21.3 FUD 090 J A2 80 50

AMA: 2019,Jul,6; 2018,Jan,8; 2017,Jan,8; 2016,Jan,13

58673 with salpingostomy (salpingoneostomy) ♀

23.1 23.1 FUD 090 J A2 80 50

AMA: 2019,Jul,6; 2018,Jan,8; 2017,Jan,8; 2016,Jan,13

58674 **Resequenced code. See code before 58541.**

58679 Unlisted laparoscopy procedure, oviduct, ovary ♀

0.00 0.00 FUD YYY J 80 50

AMA: 2019,Jul,6; 2018,Jan,8; 2017,Jan,8; 2016,Jan,13

58700-58770 Open Procedures Fallopian Tubes, with/without Ovaries

EXCLUDES *Destruction/excision endometriomas, open method (49203-49205)*

58700 Salpingectomy, complete or partial, unilateral or bilateral (separate procedure) ♀

22.3 22.3 FUD 090 C 80

AMA: 2019,Jul,6; 2018,Sep,14

58720 Salpingo-oophorectomy, complete or partial, unilateral or bilateral (separate procedure) ♀

21.5 21.5 FUD 090 C 80

AMA: 2019,Jul,6; 2018,Jan,8; 2017,Jan,8; 2016,Jan,13

58740 Lysis of adhesions (salpingolysis, ovariolysis) ♀

EXCLUDES *Excision/fulguration lesions performed laparoscopically (58662)*
Laparoscopic method (58660)

25.9 25.9 FUD 090 C 80

AMA: 2019,Jul,6; 2018,Jan,8; 2017,Jan,8; 2016,Jan,13

58750 Tubotubal anastomosis ♀

26.3 26.3 FUD 090 C 80 50

AMA: 2019,Jul,6

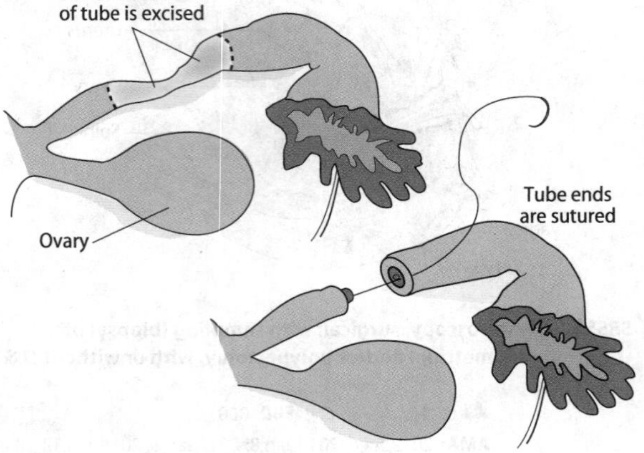

58752 Tubouterine implantation ♀

25.4 25.4 FUD 090 C 80 50

AMA: 2019,Jul,6

58760 Fimbrioplasty ♀

EXCLUDES *Laparoscopic method (58672)*

23.7 23.7 FUD 090 C 80 50

AMA: 2019,Jul,6; 2018,Jan,8; 2017,Jan,8; 2016,Jan,13

58770 Salpingostomy (salpingoneostomy) ♀

EXCLUDES *Laparoscopic method (58673)*

24.9 24.9 FUD 090 J G2 80 50

AMA: 2019,Jul,6; 2018,Jan,8; 2017,Jan,8; 2016,Jan,13

58800-58925 Open Procedures: Ovary

CMS: 100-03,230.3 Sterilization

EXCLUDES *Destruction/excision endometriomas, open method (49203-49205)*

58800 Drainage of ovarian cyst(s), unilateral or bilateral (separate procedure); vaginal approach ♀

8.92 9.96 FUD 090 J A2

AMA: 2019,Jul,6

58805 abdominal approach ♀

12.1 12.1 FUD 090 J G2 80

AMA: 2019,Jul,6

58820 Drainage of ovarian abscess; vaginal approach, open ♀

EXCLUDES *Transrectal fluid drainage using catheter, image guided (49407)*

9.02 9.02 FUD 090 J A2 80 50

AMA: 2019,Jul,6

58822 abdominal approach ♀

EXCLUDES *Transrectal fluid drainage using catheter, image guided (49407)*

19.8 19.8 FUD 090 C 80 50

AMA: 2019,Jul,6

58825 Transposition, ovary(s) ♀

20.4 20.4 FUD 090 C 80

AMA: 2019,Jul,6

58900 **Biopsy of ovary, unilateral or bilateral (separate procedure)** ♀

EXCLUDES *Laparoscopy with biopsy fallopian tube or ovary (49321)*

11.8 11.8 **FUD** 090 J A2 80

AMA: 2019,Jul,6; 2018,Jan,8; 2017,Jan,8; 2016,Jan,13

58920 **Wedge resection or bisection of ovary, unilateral or bilateral** ♀

19.8 19.8 **FUD** 090 J G2 80

AMA: 2019,Jul,6

58925 **Ovarian cystectomy, unilateral or bilateral** ♀

21.9 21.9 **FUD** 090 J G2 80

AMA: 2019,Jul,6

58940-58960 Removal Ovary(s) with/without Multiple Procedures for Malignancy

CMS: 100-03,230.3 Sterilization

EXCLUDES *Chemotherapy (96401-96549)*
Destruction/excision tumors, cysts, or endometriomas, open method (49203-49205)

58940 **Oophorectomy, partial or total, unilateral or bilateral;** ♀

EXCLUDES *Oophorectomy with tumor debulking for ovarian malignancy (58952)*

15.3 15.3 **FUD** 090 C 80

AMA: 2019,Jul,6; 2018,Jan,8; 2017,Jan,8; 2016,Jan,13

58943 **for ovarian, tubal or primary peritoneal malignancy, with para-aortic and pelvic lymph node biopsies, peritoneal washings, peritoneal biopsies, diaphragmatic assessments, with or without salpingectomy(s), with or without omentectomy** ♀

33.6 33.6 **FUD** 090 C 80

AMA: 2019,Jul,6

58950 **Resection (initial) of ovarian, tubal or primary peritoneal malignancy with bilateral salpingo-oophorectomy and omentectomy;** ♀

EXCLUDES *Resection/tumor debulking recurrent ovarian/tubal/primary peritoneal/uterine malignancy (58957-58958)*

32.6 32.6 **FUD** 090 C 80

AMA: 2019,Jul,6

58951 **with total abdominal hysterectomy, pelvic and limited para-aortic lymphadenectomy** ♀

EXCLUDES *Resection/tumor debulking recurrent ovarian/tubal/primary peritoneal/uterine malignancy (58957-58958)*

42.1 42.1 **FUD** 090 C 80

AMA: 2019,Jul,6; 2018,Jan,8; 2017,Jan,8; 2016,Jan,13

58952 **with radical dissection for debulking (ie, radical excision or destruction, intra-abdominal or retroperitoneal tumors)** ♀

EXCLUDES *Resection/tumor debulking recurrent ovarian/tubal/primary peritoneal/uterine malignancy (58957-58958)*

46.9 46.9 **FUD** 090 C 80

AMA: 2019,Jul,6; 2018,Jan,8; 2017,Jan,8; 2016,Jan,13

58953 **Bilateral salpingo-oophorectomy with omentectomy, total abdominal hysterectomy and radical dissection for debulking;** ♀

58.7 58.7 **FUD** 090 C 80

AMA: 2019,Jul,6; 2018,Jan,8; 2017,Jan,8; 2016,Jan,13

58954 **with pelvic lymphadenectomy and limited para-aortic lymphadenectomy** ♀

62.4 62.4 **FUD** 090 C 80

AMA: 2019,Jul,6; 2018,Jan,8; 2017,Jan,8; 2016,Jan,13

58956 **Bilateral salpingo-oophorectomy with total omentectomy, total abdominal hysterectomy for malignancy** ♀

EXCLUDES *Biopsy ovary (58900)*
Hysterectomy (58150, 58180, 58262-58263)
Laparoscopy (58550, 58661)
Omentectomy (49255)
Oophorectomy (58940)
Ovarian cystectomy (58925)
Resection malignancy (58957-58958)
Salpingectomy salpingo-oophorectomy, (58700, 58720)

39.1 39.1 **FUD** 090 C 80

AMA: 2019,Jul,6; 2018,Jan,8; 2017,Jan,8; 2016,Jan,13

58957 **Resection (tumor debulking) of recurrent ovarian, tubal, primary peritoneal, uterine malignancy (intra-abdominal, retroperitoneal tumors), with omentectomy, if performed;** ♀

EXCLUDES *Biopsy ovary (58900)*
Destruction, excision cysts, endometriomas, or tumors (49203-49215)
Enterolysis (44005)
Exploratory laparotomy (49000)
Lymphadenectomy (38770, 38780)
Omentectomy (49255)

46.2 46.2 **FUD** 090 C 80

AMA: 2019,Jul,6

58958 **with pelvic lymphadenectomy and limited para-aortic lymphadenectomy** ♀

EXCLUDES *Biopsy ovary (58900)*
Destruction, excision cysts, endometriomas, or tumors (49203-49215)
Enterolysis (44005)
Exploratory laparotomy (49000)
Lymphadenectomy (38770, 38780)
Omentectomy (49255)

51.2 51.2 **FUD** 090 C 80

AMA: 2019,Jul,6

58960 **Laparotomy, for staging or restaging of ovarian, tubal, or primary peritoneal malignancy (second look), with or without omentectomy, peritoneal washing, biopsy of abdominal and pelvic peritoneum, diaphragmatic assessment with pelvic and limited para-aortic lymphadenectomy** ♀

EXCLUDES *Resection malignancy (58957-58958)*

27.9 27.9 **FUD** 090 C 80

AMA: 2019,Jul,6

58970-58999 Procedural Components: In Vitro Fertilization

58970 **Follicle puncture for oocyte retrieval, any method** M ♀

(76948)

5.74 6.75 **FUD** 000 T A2 80

AMA: 2019,Jul,6

58974 **Embryo transfer, intrauterine** M ♀

0.00 0.00 **FUD** 000 T A2 80

AMA: 2019,Jul,6

58976 **Gamete, zygote, or embryo intrafallopian transfer, any method** M ♀

EXCLUDES *Adnexal procedures performed laparoscopically (58660-58673)*

6.20 7.33 **FUD** 000 T A2 80

AMA: 2019,Jul,6; 2018,Jan,8; 2017,Jan,8; 2016,Jan,13

58999 **Unlisted procedure, female genital system (nonobstetrical)** ♀

0.00 0.00 **FUD** YYY T

AMA: 2019,Jul,6; 2018,Jan,8; 2017,Jan,8; 2016,Jan,13

59000-59001 Aspiration of Amniotic Fluid

EXCLUDES *Intrauterine fetal transfusion (36460)*
Unlisted fetal invasive procedure (59897)

59000 Amniocentesis; diagnostic M ♀
(76946)
Facility RVU 2.33 Non-Facility RVU 3.47 **FUD** 000 T P3
AMA: 2019,Jul,6; 2018,Jan,8; 2017,Jan,8; 2016,Jan,13

59001 therapeutic amniotic fluid reduction (includes ultrasound guidance) M ♀
Facility RVU 5.18 Non-Facility RVU 5.18 **FUD** 000 T R2
AMA: 2019,Jul,6; 2018,Jan,8; 2017,Jan,8; 2016,Jan,13

59012-59076 Fetal Testing and Treatment

EXCLUDES *Intrauterine fetal transfusion (36460)*
Unlisted fetal invasive procedures (59897)

59012 Cordocentesis (intrauterine), any method M ♀
(76941)
Facility RVU 5.87 Non-Facility RVU 5.87 **FUD** 000 T G2 80
AMA: 2019,Jul,6

59015 Chorionic villus sampling, any method M ♀
(76945)
Facility RVU 3.82 Non-Facility RVU 4.51 **FUD** 000 T P3 80
AMA: 2019,Jul,6; 2018,Jan,8; 2017,Jan,8; 2016,Jan,13

59020 Fetal contraction stress test M ♀
Facility RVU 2.00 Non-Facility RVU 2.00 **FUD** 000 T P3 80
AMA: 2019,Jul,6; 2018,Jan,8; 2017,Jan,8; 2016,Jan,13

59025 Fetal non-stress test M ♀
Facility RVU 1.37 Non-Facility RVU 1.37 **FUD** 000 T P3 80
AMA: 2019,Jul,6; 2018,Jan,8; 2017,Jan,8; 2016,Jan,13

59030 Fetal scalp blood sampling M ♀
Code also modifier 76 or 77, as appropriate, for repeat fetal scalp blood sampling
Facility RVU 3.28 Non-Facility RVU 3.28 **FUD** 000 T G2 80
AMA: 2019,Jul,6

59050 Fetal monitoring during labor by consulting physician (ie, non-attending physician) with written report; supervision and interpretation M ♀
Facility RVU 1.49 Non-Facility RVU 1.49 **FUD** XXX M 80
AMA: 2019,Jul,6

59051 interpretation only M ♀
Facility RVU 1.23 Non-Facility RVU 1.23 **FUD** XXX B 80
AMA: 2019,Jul,6

59070 Transabdominal amnioinfusion, including ultrasound guidance M ♀
Facility RVU 8.99 Non-Facility RVU 11.6 **FUD** 000 T G2 80
AMA: 2019,Jul,6; 2018,Jan,8; 2017,Jan,8; 2016,Jan,13

59072 Fetal umbilical cord occlusion, including ultrasound guidance M ♀
Facility RVU 15.2 Non-Facility RVU 15.2 **FUD** 000 T J8
AMA: 2019,Jul,6; 2018,Jan,8; 2017,Jan,8; 2016,Jan,13

59074 Fetal fluid drainage (eg, vesicocentesis, thoracocentesis, paracentesis), including ultrasound guidance M ♀
Facility RVU 8.92 Non-Facility RVU 11.1 **FUD** 000 T G2 80
AMA: 2019,Jul,6; 2018,Jan,8; 2017,Jan,8; 2016,Jan,13

59076 Fetal shunt placement, including ultrasound guidance M ♀
Facility RVU 15.2 Non-Facility RVU 15.2 **FUD** 000 T G2 80
AMA: 2019,Jul,6; 2018,Jan,8; 2017,Jan,8; 2016,Jan,13

59100-59151 Tubal Pregnancy/Hysterotomy Procedures

CMS: 100-03,230.3 Sterilization

59100 Hysterotomy, abdominal (eg, for hydatidiform mole, abortion) M ♀
Code also ligation fallopian tubes when performed same time as hysterotomy (58611)
Facility RVU 24.1 Non-Facility RVU 24.1 **FUD** 090 J R2 80
AMA: 2019,Jul,6

59120 Surgical treatment of ectopic pregnancy; tubal or ovarian, requiring salpingectomy and/or oophorectomy, abdominal or vaginal approach M ♀
Facility RVU 23.4 Non-Facility RVU 23.4 **FUD** 090 C 80
AMA: 2019,Jul,6

59121 tubal or ovarian, without salpingectomy and/or oophorectomy M ♀
Facility RVU 23.0 Non-Facility RVU 23.0 **FUD** 090 C 80
AMA: 2019,Jul,6

59130 abdominal pregnancy M ♀
Facility RVU 26.8 Non-Facility RVU 26.8 **FUD** 090 C 80
AMA: 2019,Jul,6

~~**59135 interstitial, uterine pregnancy requiring total hysterectomy**~~

59136 interstitial, uterine pregnancy with partial resection of uterus M ♀
Facility RVU 25.9 Non-Facility RVU 25.9 **FUD** 090 C 80
AMA: 2019,Jul,6

59140 cervical, with evacuation M ♀
Facility RVU 11.9 Non-Facility RVU 11.9 **FUD** 090 C 80
AMA: 2019,Jul,6

59150 Laparoscopic treatment of ectopic pregnancy; without salpingectomy and/or oophorectomy M ♀
Facility RVU 22.7 Non-Facility RVU 22.7 **FUD** 090 J G2 80
AMA: 2019,Jul,6; 2018,Jan,8; 2017,Jan,8; 2016,Jan,13

59151 with salpingectomy and/or oophorectomy M ♀
Facility RVU 21.7 Non-Facility RVU 21.7 **FUD** 090 J G2 80
AMA: 2019,Jul,6

59160-59200 Procedures of Uterus Prior To/After Delivery

59160 Curettage, postpartum M ♀
Facility RVU 5.11 Non-Facility RVU 6.21 **FUD** 010 J A2 80
AMA: 2019,Jul,6; 2018,Jan,8; 2017,Jan,8; 2016,Jan,13

59200 Insertion of cervical dilator (eg, laminaria, prostaglandin) (separate procedure) M ♀
EXCLUDES *Fetal transfusion, intrauterine (36460)*
Hypertonic solution/prostaglandin introduction for labor initiation (59850-59857)
Facility RVU 1.30 Non-Facility RVU 2.56 **FUD** 000 T P3
AMA: 2019,Jul,6; 2018,Jan,8; 2017,Dec,14; 2017,Jan,8; 2016,Jan,13

59300-59350 Postpartum Vaginal/Cervical/Uterine Repairs

EXCLUDES *Nonpregnancy-related cerclage (57700)*

59300 Episiotomy or vaginal repair, by other than attending M ♀
Facility RVU 4.26 Non-Facility RVU 6.15 **FUD** 000 J P3 80
AMA: 2019,Jul,6

59320 **Cerclage of cervix, during pregnancy; vaginal** M ♀
4.37 4.37 FUD 000 J A2 80
AMA: 2019,Jul,6; 2018,Jan,8; 2017,Jan,8; 2016,Jan,13

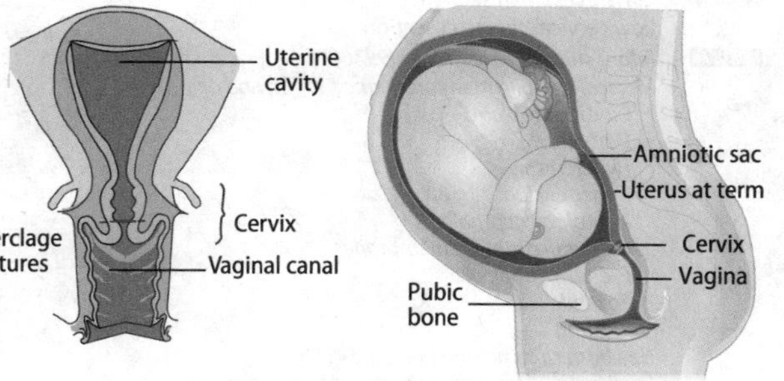

59325 **abdominal** M ♀
6.96 6.96 FUD 000 C 80
AMA: 2019,Jul,6; 2018,Jan,8; 2017,Jan,8; 2016,Jan,13

59350 **Hysterorrhaphy of ruptured uterus** M ♀
8.08 8.08 FUD 000 C 80
AMA: 2019,Jul,6

59400-59410 Vaginal Delivery: Comprehensive and Component Services

CMS: 100-02,15,180 Nurse-Midwife (CNM) Services; 100-02,15,20.1 Physician Expense for Surgery, Childbirth, and Treatment for Infertility

INCLUDES Care provided for uncomplicated pregnancy including delivery, antepartum, and postpartum care:
- Admission history
- Admission to hospital
- Artificial rupture membranes
- Management uncomplicated labor
- Physical exam
- Vaginal delivery with or without episiotomy or forceps

EXCLUDES *Medical complications pregnancy, labor, and delivery:*
- *Cardiac problems*
- *Diabetes*
- *Hyperemesis*
- *Hypertension*
- *Neurological problems*
- *Premature rupture membranes*
- *Pre-term labor*
- *Toxemia*
- *Trauma*

Newborn circumcision (54150, 54160)
Services incidental to or unrelated to pregnancy

59400 **Routine obstetric care including antepartum care, vaginal delivery (with or without episiotomy, and/or forceps) and postpartum care** M ♀

INCLUDES Fetal heart tones
- Hospital/office visits following cesarean section or vaginal delivery
- Initial/subsequent history
- Physical exams
- Recording weight/blood pressures
- Routine chemical urinalysis
- Routine prenatal visits:
  - Each month up to 28 weeks gestation
  - Every other week from 29 to 36 weeks gestation
  - Weekly from 36 weeks until delivery

60.4 60.4 FUD MMM B
AMA: 2019,Jul,6; 2018,Jan,8; 2017,Jan,8; 2016,Jan,13

59409 **Vaginal delivery only (with or without episiotomy and/or forceps);** M ♀
Code also inpatient management after delivery/discharge services (99217-99239 [99224, 99225, 99226])
23.3 23.3 FUD MMM J G2 80
AMA: 2019,Jul,6; 2018,Jan,8; 2017,Jan,8; 2016,Jan,13

59410 **including postpartum care** M ♀
INCLUDES Hospital/office visits following cesarean section or vaginal delivery
29.9 29.9 FUD MMM B
AMA: 2019,Jul,6

59412-59414 Other Maternity Services

CMS: 100-02,15,180 Nurse-Midwife (CNM) Services; 100-02,15,20.1 Physician Expense for Surgery, Childbirth, and Treatment for Infertility

59412 **External cephalic version, with or without tocolysis** M ♀
Code also delivery code(s)
2.95 2.95 FUD MMM J G2 80
AMA: 2019,Jul,6

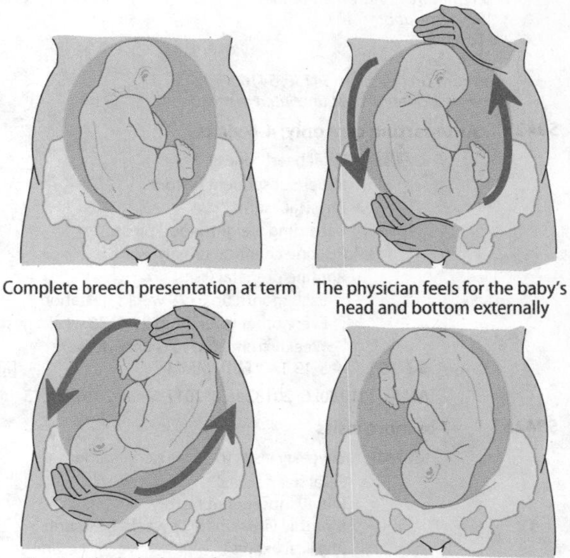
Complete breech presentation at term
The physician feels for the baby's head and bottom externally
Turning the baby by applying external pressure
Baby is in cephalic presentation, engaged for normal delivery

59414 **Delivery of placenta (separate procedure)** M ♀
2.65 2.65 FUD MMM J G2 80
AMA: 2019,Jul,6; 2018,Jan,8; 2017,Jan,8; 2016,Jan,13

59425-59430 Prenatal and Postpartum Visits

CMS: 100-02,15,180 Nurse-Midwife (CNM) Services; 100-02,15,20.1 Physician Expense for Surgery, Childbirth, and Treatment for Infertility

INCLUDES Physician/other qualified health care professional providing all or portion antepartum/postpartum care, but no delivery due to:
- Referral to another physician for delivery
- Termination pregnancy by abortion

EXCLUDES *Antepartum care, one to three visits, report with appropriate E/M service code*
Medical complications pregnancy, labor, and delivery:
- *Cardiac problems*
- *Diabetes*
- *Hyperemesis*
- *Hypertension*
- *Neurological problems*
- *Premature rupture membranes*
- *Pre-term labor*
- *Toxemia*
- *Trauma*

Newborn circumcision (54150, 54160)
Services incidental to or unrelated to pregnancy

59425 Antepartum care only; 4-6 visits M ♀

INCLUDES Fetal heart tones
Initial/subsequent history
Physical exams
Recording weight/blood pressures
Routine chemical urinalysis
Routine prenatal visits:
- Each month up to 28 weeks gestation
- Every other week from 29 to 36 weeks gestation
- Weekly from 36 weeks until delivery

10.2 | 13.1 **FUD** MMM B 80

AMA: 2019,Jul,6; 2018,Jan,8; 2017,Jan,8; 2016,Jan,13

59426 7 or more visits M ♀

INCLUDES Biweekly visits to 36 weeks gestation
Fetal heart tones
Initial/subsequent history
Monthly visits up to 28 weeks gestation
Physical exams
Recording weight/blood pressures
Routine chemical urinalysis
Weekly visits until delivery

17.9 | 23.5 **FUD** MMM B 80

AMA: 2019,Jul,6; 2018,Jan,8; 2017,Jan,8; 2016,Jan,13

59430 Postpartum care only (separate procedure) M ♀

INCLUDES Office/other outpatient visits following cesarean section or vaginal delivery

3.97 | 5.57 **FUD** MMM B

AMA: 2019,Jul,6; 2018,Jan,8; 2017,Jan,8; 2016,Jan,13

59510-59525 Cesarean Section Delivery: Comprehensive and Components of Care

CMS: 100-02,15,20.1 Physician Expense for Surgery, Childbirth, and Treatment for Infertility

INCLUDES Classic cesarean section
Low cervical cesarean section

EXCLUDES *Infant standby attendance (99360)*
Medical complications pregnancy, labor, and delivery:
- *Cardiac problems*
- *Diabetes*
- *Hyperemesis*
- *Hypertension*
- *Neurological problems*
- *Premature rupture membranes*
- *Pre-term labor*
- *Toxemia*
- *Trauma*

Newborn circumcision (54150, 54160)
Services incidental to or unrelated to pregnancy
Vaginal delivery after prior cesarean section (59610-59614)

59510 Routine obstetric care including antepartum care, cesarean delivery, and postpartum care M ♀

INCLUDES Admission history
Admission to hospital
Cesarean delivery
Fetal heart tones
Hospital/office visits following cesarean section
Initial/subsequent history
Management uncomplicated labor
Physical exam
Recording weight/blood pressures
Routine chemical urinalysis
Routine prenatal visits:
- Each month up to 28 weeks gestation
- Every other week 29 to 36 weeks gestation
- Weekly from 36 weeks until delivery

67.0 | 67.0 **FUD** MMM B

AMA: 2019,Jul,6; 2018,Jan,8; 2017,Jan,8; 2016,Jan,13

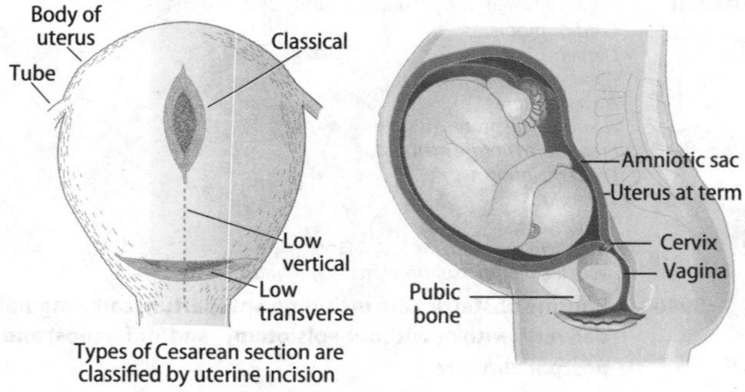

Types of Cesarean section are classified by uterine incision

59514 Cesarean delivery only; M ♀

INCLUDES Admission history
Admission to hospital
Cesarean delivery
Management uncomplicated labor
Physical exam

Code also inpatient management after delivery/discharge services (99217-99239 [99224, 99225, 99226])

26.3 | 26.3 **FUD** MMM C 80

AMA: 2019,Jul,6; 2018,Jan,8; 2017,Jan,8; 2016,Jan,13

59515 including postpartum care M ♀

INCLUDES Admission history
Admission to hospital
Cesarean delivery
Hospital/office visits following cesarean section or vaginal delivery
Management uncomplicated labor
Physical exam

36.4 | 36.4 **FUD** MMM B

AMA: 2019,Jul,6; 2018,Jan,8; 2017,Jan,8; 2016,Jan,13

+ **59525 Subtotal or total hysterectomy after cesarean delivery (List separately in addition to code for primary procedure)** M ♀

Code first cesarean delivery (59510, 59514, 59515, 59618, 59620, 59622)

13.9 13.9 FUD ZZZ C 80

AMA: 2019,Jul,6

59610-59614 Vaginal Delivery After Prior Cesarean Section: Comprehensive and Components of Care

CMS: 100-02,15,180 Nurse-Midwife (CNM) Services; 100-02,15,20.1 Physician Expense for Surgery, Childbirth, and Treatment for Infertility

INCLUDES Admission history
Admission to hospital
Management uncomplicated labor
Patients with previous cesarean delivery who present with vaginal delivery expectation
Physical exam
Successful vaginal delivery after previous cesarean delivery (VBAC)
Vaginal delivery with or without episiotomy or forceps

EXCLUDES *Elective cesarean delivery (59510, 59514, 59515)*
Medical complications pregnancy, labor, and delivery:
Cardiac problems
Diabetes
Hyperemesis
Hypertension
Neurological problems
Premature rupture membranes
Pre-term labor
Toxemia
Trauma
Newborn circumcision (54150, 54160)
Services incidental to or unrelated to pregnancy

59610 Routine obstetric care including antepartum care, vaginal delivery (with or without episiotomy, and/or forceps) and postpartum care, after previous cesarean delivery M ♀

INCLUDES Fetal heart tones
Hospital/office visits following cesarean section or vaginal delivery
Initial/subsequent history
Physical exams
Recording weight/blood pressures
Routine chemical urinalysis
Routine prenatal visits:
Each month up to 28 weeks gestation
Every other week 29 to 36 weeks gestation
Weekly from 36 weeks until delivery

63.4 63.4 FUD MMM B 80

AMA: 2019,Jul,6; 2018,Jan,8; 2017,Jan,8; 2016,Jan,13

59612 Vaginal delivery only, after previous cesarean delivery (with or without episiotomy and/or forceps); M ♀

Code also inpatient management after delivery/discharge services (99217-99239 [99224, 99225, 99226])

26.3 26.3 FUD MMM J G2 80

AMA: 2019,Jul,6; 2018,Jan,8; 2017,Jan,8; 2016,Jan,13

59614 including postpartum care M ♀

INCLUDES Hospital/office visits following cesarean section or vaginal delivery

32.7 32.7 FUD MMM B 80

AMA: 2019,Jul,6; 2018,Jan,8; 2017,Jan,8; 2016,Jan,13

59618-59622 Cesarean Section After Attempted Vaginal Birth/Prior C-Section

CMS: 100-02,15,20.1 Physician Expense for Surgery, Childbirth, and Treatment for Infertility

INCLUDES Admission history
Admission to hospital
Cesarean delivery
Cesarean delivery following unsuccessful vaginal delivery attempt after previous cesarean delivery
Management uncomplicated labor
Patients with previous cesarean delivery who present with vaginal delivery expectation
Physical exam

EXCLUDES *Elective cesarean delivery (59510, 59514, 59515)*
Medical complications of pregnancy, labor, and delivery:
Cardiac problems
Diabetes
Hyperemesis
Hypertension
Neurological problems
Premature rupture of membranes
Pre-term labor
Toxemia
Trauma
Newborn circumcision (54150, 54160)
Services incidental to or unrelated to the pregnancy

59618 Routine obstetric care including antepartum care, cesarean delivery, and postpartum care, following attempted vaginal delivery after previous cesarean delivery M ♀

INCLUDES Fetal heart tones
Hospital/office visits following cesarean section or vaginal delivery
Initial/subsequent history
Physical exams
Recording weight/blood pressures
Routine chemical urinalysis
Routine prenatal visits:
Each month up to 28 weeks gestation
Every two weeks 29 to 36 weeks gestation
Weekly from 36 weeks until delivery

67.8 67.8 FUD MMM B 80

AMA: 2019,Jul,6; 2018,Jan,8; 2017,Jan,8; 2016,Jan,13

59620 Cesarean delivery only, following attempted vaginal delivery after previous cesarean delivery; M ♀

Code also inpatient management after delivery/discharge services (99217-99239 [99224, 99225, 99226])

27.2 27.2 FUD MMM C 80

AMA: 2019,Jul,6; 2018,Jan,8; 2017,Jan,8; 2016,Jan,13

59622 including postpartum care M ♀

INCLUDES Hospital/office visits following cesarean section or vaginal delivery

37.4 37.4 FUD MMM B 80

AMA: 2019,Jul,6; 2018,Jan,8; 2017,Jan,8; 2016,Jan,13

59812-59830 Treatment of Miscarriage

CMS: 100-02,15,20.1 Physician Expense for Surgery, Childbirth, and Treatment for Infertility

EXCLUDES *Medical treatment spontaneous complete abortion, any trimester (99202-99233 [99224, 99225, 99226])*

59812 Treatment of incomplete abortion, any trimester, completed surgically M ♀

INCLUDES Surgical treatment spontaneous abortion

8.59 9.37 FUD 090 J A2

AMA: 2019,Jul,6; 2018,Jan,8; 2017,Jan,8; 2016,Jan,13

59820 Treatment of missed abortion, completed surgically; first trimester M ♀

10.4 11.2 FUD 090 J A2

AMA: 2019,Jul,6; 2018,Jan,8; 2017,Jan,8; 2016,Jan,13

59821 second trimester M ♀

10.3 11.2 FUD 090 J A2 80

AMA: 2019,Jul,6; 2018,Jan,8; 2017,Jan,8; 2016,Jan,13

59830 Treatment of septic abortion, completed surgically M ♀

13.1 13.1 FUD 090 C 80

AMA: 2019,Jul,6; 2018,Jan,8; 2017,Jan,8; 2016,Jan,13

59840-59866 Elective Abortions

CMS: 100-02,1,90 Termination of Pregnancy; 100-02,15,20.1 Physician Expense for Surgery, Childbirth, and Treatment for Infertility; 100-03,140.1 Abortion; 100-04,3,100.1 Billing for Abortion Services

59840 **Induced abortion, by dilation and curettage** M ♀
6.08 6.50 **FUD** 010 J A2 80
AMA: 2019,Jul,6; 2018,Jan,8; 2017,Jan,8; 2016,Jan,13

59841 **Induced abortion, by dilation and evacuation** M ♀
10.4 11.2 **FUD** 010 J A2 80
AMA: 2019,Jul,6; 2018,Jan,8; 2017,Jan,8; 2016,Jan,13

59850 **Induced abortion, by 1 or more intra-amniotic injections (amniocentesis-injections), including hospital admission and visits, delivery of fetus and secundines;** M ♀
EXCLUDES *Cervical dilator insertion (59200)*
10.1 10.1 **FUD** 090 C 80
AMA: 2019,Jul,6; 2018,Jan,8; 2017,Jan,8; 2016,Jan,13

59851 **with dilation and curettage and/or evacuation** M ♀
EXCLUDES *Cervical dilator insertion (59200)*
10.9 10.9 **FUD** 090 C 80
AMA: 2019,Jul,6; 2018,Jan,8; 2017,Jan,8; 2016,Jan,13

59852 **with hysterotomy (failed intra-amniotic injection)** M ♀
EXCLUDES *Cervical dilator insertion (59200)*
16.5 16.5 **FUD** 090 C 80
AMA: 2019,Jul,6; 2018,Jan,8; 2017,Jan,8; 2016,Jan,13

59855 **Induced abortion, by 1 or more vaginal suppositories (eg, prostaglandin) with or without cervical dilation (eg, laminaria), including hospital admission and visits, delivery of fetus and secundines;** M ♀
12.2 12.2 **FUD** 090 C 80
AMA: 2019,Jul,6

59856 **with dilation and curettage and/or evacuation** M ♀
14.3 14.3 **FUD** 090 C 80
AMA: 2019,Jul,6

59857 **with hysterotomy (failed medical evacuation)** M ♀
16.8 16.8 **FUD** 090 C 80
AMA: 2019,Jul,6

59866 **Multifetal pregnancy reduction(s) (MPR)** M ♀
6.22 6.22 **FUD** 000 T G2 80
AMA: 2019,Jul,6

59870-59899 Miscellaneous Obstetrical Procedures

CMS: 100-02,15,20.1 Physician Expense for Surgery, Childbirth, and Treatment for Infertility

59870 **Uterine evacuation and curettage for hydatidiform mole** M ♀
14.7 14.7 **FUD** 090 J A2 80
AMA: 2019,Jul,6; 2018,Jan,8; 2017,Jan,8; 2016,Jan,13

59871 **Removal of cerclage suture under anesthesia (other than local)** M ♀
3.83 3.83 **FUD** 000 Q2 A2 80
AMA: 2019,Jul,6; 2018,Jan,8; 2017,Jan,8; 2016,Jan,13

59897 **Unlisted fetal invasive procedure, including ultrasound guidance, when performed** M ♀
0.00 0.00 **FUD** YYY T
AMA: 2019,Jul,6

59898 **Unlisted laparoscopy procedure, maternity care and delivery** M ♀
0.00 0.00 **FUD** YYY J 80 50
AMA: 2019,Jul,6; 2018,Jan,8; 2017,Jan,8; 2016,Jan,13

59899 **Unlisted procedure, maternity care and delivery** M ♀
0.00 0.00 **FUD** YYY T 80
AMA: 2019,Jul,6; 2018,Jan,8; 2017,Jan,8; 2016,Jan,13

60000 I&D of Infected Thyroglossal Cyst

60000 Incision and drainage of thyroglossal duct cyst, infected
4.37 4.99 FUD 010 T A2 80
AMA: 2014,Jan,11; 2002,May,7

60100 Core Needle Biopsy: Thyroid

EXCLUDES *Fine needle aspiration (10021, [10004, 10005, 10006, 10007, 10008, 10009, 10010, 10011, 10012])*

60100 Biopsy thyroid, percutaneous core needle
(76942, 77002, 77012, 77021)
(88172-88173)
2.25 3.18 FUD 000 T P3
AMA: 2019,Apr,4; 2018,Jan,8; 2017,Jan,8; 2016,Jan,13

60200 Surgical Removal Thyroid Cyst or Mass; Division of Isthmus

60200 Excision of cyst or adenoma of thyroid, or transection of isthmus
19.0 19.0 FUD 090 J A2 80
AMA: 2018,Jan,8; 2017,Jan,8; 2016,Jan,13

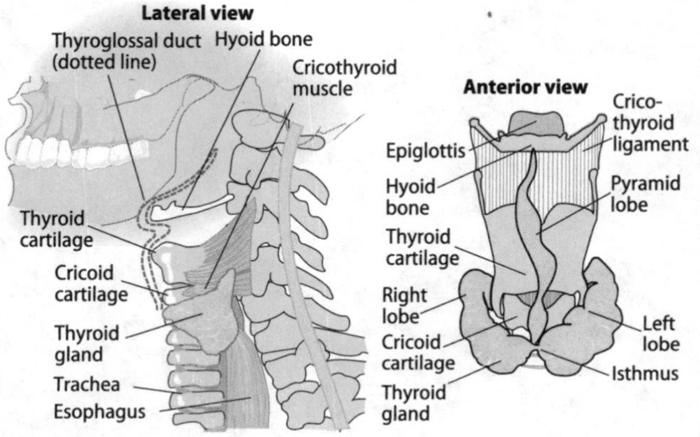

60210-60225 Subtotal Thyroidectomy

60210 Partial thyroid lobectomy, unilateral; with or without isthmusectomy
20.3 20.3 FUD 090 J G2 80
AMA: 2018,Jan,8; 2017,Jan,8; 2016,Jan,13

60212 with contralateral subtotal lobectomy, including isthmusectomy
29.0 29.0 FUD 090 J G2 80
AMA: 2018,Jan,8; 2017,Jan,8; 2016,Jan,13

60220 Total thyroid lobectomy, unilateral; with or without isthmusectomy
20.3 20.3 FUD 090 J G2 80
AMA: 2020,Aug,14; 2018,Jan,8; 2017,Jan,8; 2016,Jan,13

60225 with contralateral subtotal lobectomy, including isthmusectomy
26.8 26.8 FUD 090 J G2 80
AMA: 2018,Jan,8; 2017,Jan,8; 2016,Jan,13

60240-60271 Complete Thyroidectomy Procedures

60240 Thyroidectomy, total or complete
EXCLUDES *Subtotal or partial thyroidectomy (60271)*
26.4 26.4 FUD 090 J G2 80
AMA: 2018,Jan,8; 2017,Jan,8; 2016,Jan,13

60252 Thyroidectomy, total or subtotal for malignancy; with limited neck dissection
38.0 38.0 FUD 090 J G2 80
AMA: 2018,Jan,8; 2017,Jan,8; 2016,Jan,13

60254 with radical neck dissection
48.2 48.2 FUD 090 C 80
AMA: 2018,Jan,8; 2017,Jan,8; 2016,Jan,13

60260 Thyroidectomy, removal of all remaining thyroid tissue following previous removal of a portion of thyroid
31.4 31.4 FUD 090 J G2 80 50
AMA: 2018,Jan,8; 2017,Jan,8; 2016,Jan,13

60270 Thyroidectomy, including substernal thyroid; sternal split or transthoracic approach
39.4 39.4 FUD 090 C 80
AMA: 2018,Jan,8; 2017,Jan,8; 2016,Jan,13

60271 cervical approach
30.4 30.4 FUD 090 J G2 80
AMA: 2020,Aug,14; 2018,Jan,8; 2017,Jan,8; 2016,Jan,13

60280-60300 Treatment of Cyst/Sinus of Thyroid

60280 Excision of thyroglossal duct cyst or sinus;
EXCLUDES *Thyroid ultrasound (76536)*
12.6 12.6 FUD 090 J A2 80
AMA: 2014,Jan,11

60281 recurrent
EXCLUDES *Thyroid ultrasound (76536)*
16.8 16.8 FUD 090 J A2 80
AMA: 2014,Jan,11; 1994,Win,1

60300 Aspiration and/or injection, thyroid cyst
EXCLUDES *Fine needle aspiration (10021, [10004, 10005, 10006, 10007, 10008, 10009, 10010, 10011, 10012])*
(76942, 77012)
1.42 3.24 FUD 000 T P3
AMA: 2014,Jan,11

60500-60512 Parathyroid Procedures

60500 Parathyroidectomy or exploration of parathyroid(s);
27.9 27.9 FUD 090 J G2 80
AMA: 2018,Jan,8; 2017,Jan,8; 2016,Jan,13

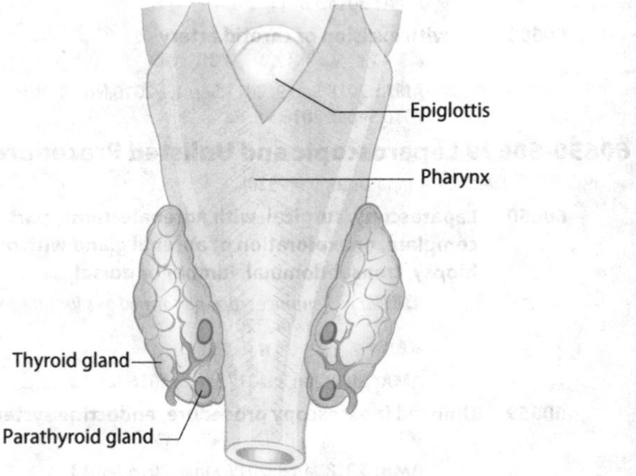

Posterior view of pharynx, thyroid glands, and parathyroid glands

60502 re-exploration
37.5 37.5 FUD 090 J G2 80
AMA: 2018,Jan,8; 2017,Jan,8; 2016,Jan,13

60505 with mediastinal exploration, sternal split or transthoracic approach
40.1 40.1 FUD 090 C 80
AMA: 2018,Jan,8; 2017,Jan,8; 2016,Jan,13

\+ **60512 Parathyroid autotransplantation (List separately in addition to code for primary procedure)**
Code first (60212, 60225, 60240, 60252, 60254, 60260, 60270-60271, 60500, 60502, 60505)
7.03 7.03 FUD ZZZ N N1 80
AMA: 2018,Jan,8; 2017,Jan,8; 2017,Jan,6; 2016,Jan,13

60520-60522 Thymus Procedures

EXCLUDES *Surgical thoracoscopy (video-assisted thoracic surgery (VATS) thymectomy (32673)*

60520 Thymectomy, partial or total; transcervical approach (separate procedure)
30.4 30.4 **FUD** 090 J 62 80
AMA: 2019,Mar,10

60521 sternal split or transthoracic approach, without radical mediastinal dissection (separate procedure)
32.4 32.4 **FUD** 090 C 80
AMA: 2018,Jan,8; 2017,Jan,8; 2016,Jan,13

60522 sternal split or transthoracic approach, with radical mediastinal dissection (separate procedure)
39.5 39.5 **FUD** 090 C 80
AMA: 2014,Jan,11; 2012,Oct,9-11

60540-60545 Adrenal Gland Procedures

EXCLUDES *Laparoscopic approach (60650)*
Removal remote or disseminated pheochromocytoma (49203-49205)
Standard backbench preparation cadaver donor (50323)

60540 Adrenalectomy, partial or complete, or exploration of adrenal gland with or without biopsy, transabdominal, lumbar or dorsal (separate procedure);
31.0 31.0 **FUD** 090 C 80 50
AMA: 2014,Jan,11; 1998,Nov,1

60545 with excision of adjacent retroperitoneal tumor
35.7 35.7 **FUD** 090 C 80 50
AMA: 2014,Jan,11; 1998,Nov,1

60600-60605 Carotid Body Procedures

60600 Excision of carotid body tumor; without excision of carotid artery
39.7 39.7 **FUD** 090 C 80
AMA: 2014,Jan,11

60605 with excision of carotid artery
47.9 47.9 **FUD** 090 C 80
AMA: 2018,Sep,9; 2017,Sep,13; 2016,Nov,8; 2016,Oct,10; 2016,Sep,8; 2016,Jul,10

60650-60699 Laparoscopic and Unlisted Procedures

INCLUDES Diagnostic laparoscopy (49320)

60650 Laparoscopy, surgical, with adrenalectomy, partial or complete, or exploration of adrenal gland with or without biopsy, transabdominal, lumbar or dorsal
EXCLUDES *Peritoneoscopy performed as separate procedure (49320)*
34.6 34.6 **FUD** 090 C 80 50
AMA: 2018,Jan,8; 2017,Jan,8; 2016,Jan,13

60659 Unlisted laparoscopy procedure, endocrine system
0.00 0.00 **FUD** YYY J 80 50
AMA: 2018,Jan,8; 2017,Jan,8; 2016,Jan,13

60699 Unlisted procedure, endocrine system
0.00 0.00 **FUD** YYY J 80
AMA: 2018,Jan,8; 2017,Jan,8; 2016,Jan,13

61000-61253 Transcranial Access via Puncture, Burr Hole, Twist Hole, or Trephine

EXCLUDES *Injection for cerebral angiography (36100-36218)*

61000 Subdural tap through fontanelle, or suture, infant, unilateral or bilateral; initial A

EXCLUDES *Injection for:*
Pneumoencephalography (61055)
Ventriculography (61026, 61120)

3.25 3.25 FUD 000 T R2

AMA: 2014,Jan,11

Overhead view of newborn skull

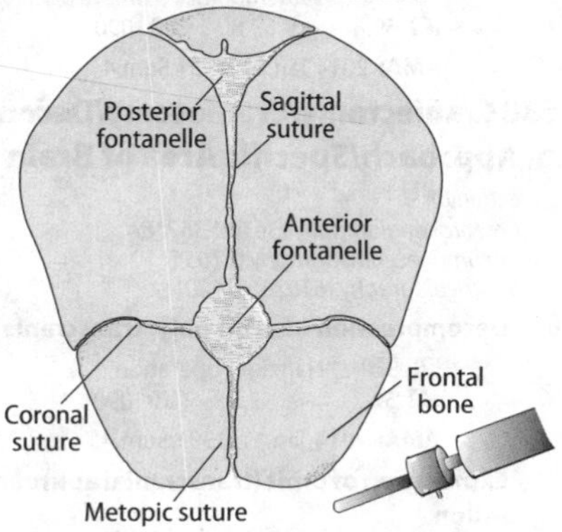

An initial tap through to the subdural level is performed on an infant via a fontanelle or suture, either unilateral or bilateral

61001 subsequent taps A

3.09 3.09 FUD 000 T R2

AMA: 2014,Jan,11

61020 Ventricular puncture through previous burr hole, fontanelle, suture, or implanted ventricular catheter/reservoir; without injection

2.87 2.87 FUD 000 T A2

AMA: 2014,Jan,11

61026 with injection of medication or other substance for diagnosis or treatment

INCLUDES Injection for ventriculography

3.05 3.05 FUD 000 T A2

AMA: 2014,Jan,11; 2002,May,7

61050 Cisternal or lateral cervical (C1-C2) puncture; without injection (separate procedure)

2.44 2.44 FUD 000 T A2 80

AMA: 2014,Jan,11; 1991,Win,1

61055 with injection of medication or other substance for diagnosis or treatment

INCLUDES Injection for pneumoencephalography

EXCLUDES *Myelography via lumbar injection (62302-62305)*
Radiology procedures except when furnished by different provider

3.62 3.62 FUD 000 T A2

AMA: 2020,Oct,3

61070 Puncture of shunt tubing or reservoir for aspiration or injection procedure

(75809)

1.63 1.63 FUD 000 T A2

AMA: 2020,Oct,3; 2018,Jan,8; 2017,Jan,8; 2016,Jan,13

61105 Twist drill hole for subdural or ventricular puncture

13.5 13.5 FUD 090 C 80

AMA: 2014,Jan,11

61107 Twist drill hole(s) for subdural, intracerebral, or ventricular puncture; for implanting ventricular catheter, pressure recording device, or other intracerebral monitoring device

Code also intracranial neuroendoscopic ventricular catheter insertion or reinsertion, when performed (62160)

9.08 9.08 FUD 000 ⊘ C

AMA: 2014,Jan,11; 2007,Jun,10-11

61108 for evacuation and/or drainage of subdural hematoma

25.8 25.8 FUD 090 C

AMA: 2014,Jan,11

61120 Burr hole(s) for ventricular puncture (including injection of gas, contrast media, dye, or radioactive material)

INCLUDES Injection for ventriculography

21.8 21.8 FUD 090 C 80

AMA: 2014,Jan,11

61140 Burr hole(s) or trephine; with biopsy of brain or intracranial lesion

36.9 36.9 FUD 090 C 80

AMA: 2014,Jan,11

61150 with drainage of brain abscess or cyst

39.0 39.0 FUD 090 C

AMA: 2014,Jan,11

61151 with subsequent tapping (aspiration) of intracranial abscess or cyst

29.1 29.1 FUD 090 C

AMA: 2014,Jan,11

61154 Burr hole(s) with evacuation and/or drainage of hematoma, extradural or subdural

36.6 36.6 FUD 090 C 80 50

AMA: 2014,Jan,11

61156 Burr hole(s); with aspiration of hematoma or cyst, intracerebral

36.5 36.5 FUD 090 C 80

AMA: 2014,Jan,11

61210 for implanting ventricular catheter, reservoir, EEG electrode(s), pressure recording device, or other cerebral monitoring device (separate procedure)

Code also intracranial neuroendoscopic ventricular catheter insertion or reinsertion, when performed (62160)

10.6 10.6 FUD 000 C

AMA: 2018,Jan,8; 2017,Jan,8; 2016,Jan,13

61215 Insertion of subcutaneous reservoir, pump or continuous infusion system for connection to ventricular catheter

EXCLUDES *Chemotherapy (96450)*
Refilling and maintenance implantable infusion pump (95990)

14.8 14.8 FUD 090 J A2

AMA: 2018,Jan,8; 2017,Jan,8; 2016,Jan,13

61250 Burr hole(s) or trephine, supratentorial, exploratory, not followed by other surgery

EXCLUDES *Burr hole or trephine followed by craniotomy same operative session (61304-61321)*

25.4 25.4 FUD 090 C 80 50

AMA: 2014,Jan,11

61253 Burr hole(s) or trephine, infratentorial, unilateral or bilateral

EXCLUDES *Burr hole or trephine followed by craniotomy same operative session (61304-61321)*

29.1 29.1 FUD 090 C 80

AMA: 2018,Jan,8; 2017,Jan,8; 2016,Jan,13

61304-61323 Craniectomy/Craniotomy: By Indication/Specific Area of Brain

EXCLUDES *Injection for:*
Cerebral angiography (36100-36218)
Pneumoencephalography (61055)
Ventriculography (61026, 61120)

61304 Craniectomy or craniotomy, exploratory; supratentorial
EXCLUDES *Other craniectomy/craniotomy procedures when performed same anatomical site and during same surgical encounter*
48.1 48.1 FUD 090 C 80
AMA: 2014,Jan,11; 2002,Sep,10

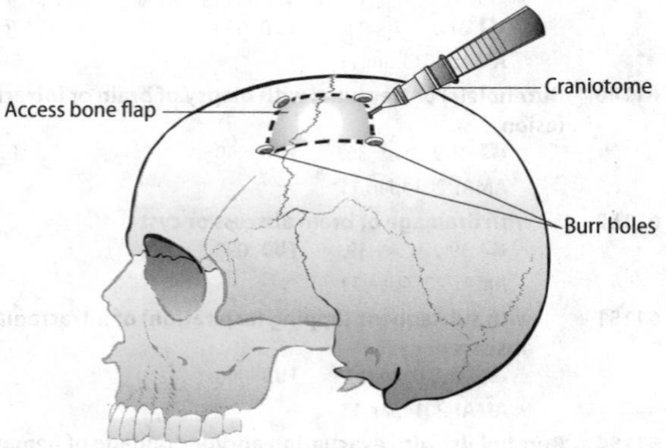

61305 infratentorial (posterior fossa)
EXCLUDES *Other craniectomy/craniotomy procedures when performed same anatomical site and during same surgical encounter*
58.6 58.6 FUD 090 C 80
AMA: 2014,Jan,11; 2002,Sep,10

61312 Craniectomy or craniotomy for evacuation of hematoma, supratentorial; extradural or subdural
60.8 60.8 FUD 090 C 80
AMA: 2018,Jan,8; 2017,Jan,8; 2016,Jan,13

61313 intracerebral
57.2 57.2 FUD 090 C 80
AMA: 2014,Jan,11; 2002,Sep,10

61314 Craniectomy or craniotomy for evacuation of hematoma, infratentorial; extradural or subdural
53.2 53.2 FUD 090 C 80
AMA: 2014,Jan,11; 2002,Sep,10

61315 intracerebellar
60.4 60.4 FUD 090 C 80
AMA: 2014,Jan,11; 2002,Sep,10

+ **61316 Incision and subcutaneous placement of cranial bone graft (List separately in addition to code for primary procedure)**
Code first (61304, 61312-61313, 61322-61323, 61340, 61570-61571, 61680-61705)
2.54 2.54 FUD ZZZ C
AMA: 2014,Jan,11; 2002,Sep,10

61320 Craniectomy or craniotomy, drainage of intracranial abscess; supratentorial
54.8 54.8 FUD 090 C 80
AMA: 2014,Jan,11; 2002,Sep,10

61321 infratentorial
62.7 62.7 FUD 090 C 80
AMA: 2014,Jan,11; 2002,Sep,10

61322 Craniectomy or craniotomy, decompressive, with or without duraplasty, for treatment of intracranial hypertension, without evacuation of associated intraparenchymal hematoma; without lobectomy
EXCLUDES *Craniectomy or craniotomy for evacuation hematoma (61313)*
Subtemporal decompression (61340)
69.7 69.7 FUD 090 C 80
AMA: 2020,May,13; 2018,Aug,10

61323 with lobectomy
EXCLUDES *Craniectomy or craniotomy for evacuation hematoma (61313)*
Subtemporal decompression (61340)
69.8 69.8 FUD 090 C 80
AMA: 2014,Jan,11; 1991,Sum,4

61330-61530 Craniectomy/Craniotomy/Decompression Brain By Surgical Approach/Specific Area of Brain

EXCLUDES *Injection for:*
Cerebral angiography (36100-36218)
Pneumoencephalography (61055)
Ventriculography (61026, 61120)

61330 Decompression of orbit only, transcranial approach
INCLUDES Naffziger operation
52.2 52.2 FUD 090 J 62 80 50
AMA: 2014,Jan,11; 1991,Sum,4

61333 Exploration of orbit (transcranial approach); with removal of lesion
59.6 59.6 FUD 090 C 80 50
AMA: 2014,Jan,11; 1991,Sum,4

61340 Subtemporal cranial decompression (pseudotumor cerebri, slit ventricle syndrome)
EXCLUDES *Decompression craniotomy or craniectomy for intracranial hypertension, without hematoma removal (61322-61323)*
41.4 41.4 FUD 090 C 80 50
AMA: 2020,May,13

61343 Craniectomy, suboccipital with cervical laminectomy for decompression of medulla and spinal cord, with or without dural graft (eg, Arnold-Chiari malformation)
63.4 63.4 FUD 090 C 80
AMA: 2014,Jan,11; 1991,Sum,4

61345 Other cranial decompression, posterior fossa
EXCLUDES *Kroenlein procedure*
Orbital decompression using lateral wall approach (67445)
60.1 60.1 FUD 090 C 80
AMA: 2014,Jan,11; 1991,Sum,4

61450 Craniectomy, subtemporal, for section, compression, or decompression of sensory root of gasserian ganglion
INCLUDES Frazier-Spiller procedure
Hartley-Krause
Krause decompression
Taarnhoj procedure
56.6 56.6 FUD 090 C 80
AMA: 2014,Jan,11; 1991,Sum,4

61458 Craniectomy, suboccipital; for exploration or decompression of cranial nerves
INCLUDES Jannetta decompression
58.8 58.8 FUD 090 C 80
AMA: 2014,Jan,11; 1991,Sum,4

61460 **for section of 1 or more cranial nerves**
61.7 61.7 **FUD** 090 C 80
AMA: 2014,Jan,11; 1991,Sum,4

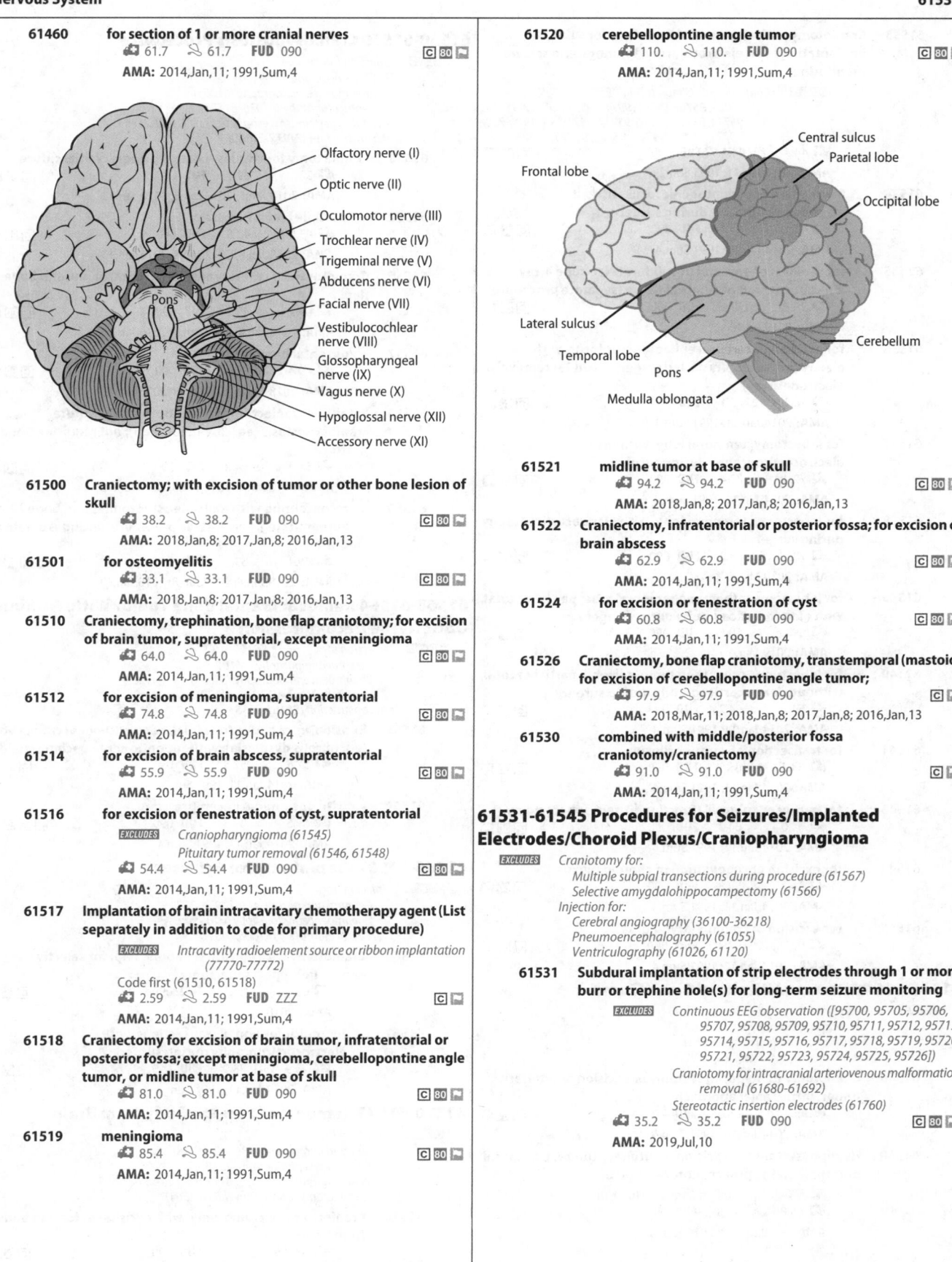

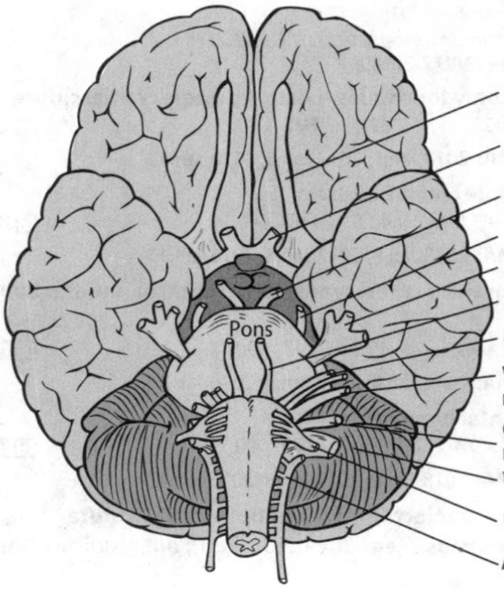

61500 **Craniectomy; with excision of tumor or other bone lesion of skull**
38.2 38.2 **FUD** 090 C 80
AMA: 2018,Jan,8; 2017,Jan,8; 2016,Jan,13

61501 **for osteomyelitis**
33.1 33.1 **FUD** 090 C 80
AMA: 2018,Jan,8; 2017,Jan,8; 2016,Jan,13

61510 **Craniectomy, trephination, bone flap craniotomy; for excision of brain tumor, supratentorial, except meningioma**
64.0 64.0 **FUD** 090 C 80
AMA: 2014,Jan,11; 1991,Sum,4

61512 **for excision of meningioma, supratentorial**
74.8 74.8 **FUD** 090 C 80
AMA: 2014,Jan,11; 1991,Sum,4

61514 **for excision of brain abscess, supratentorial**
55.9 55.9 **FUD** 090 C 80
AMA: 2014,Jan,11; 1991,Sum,4

61516 **for excision or fenestration of cyst, supratentorial**
EXCLUDES *Craniopharyngioma (61545)*
Pituitary tumor removal (61546, 61548)
54.4 54.4 **FUD** 090 C 80
AMA: 2014,Jan,11; 1991,Sum,4

\+ **61517** **Implantation of brain intracavitary chemotherapy agent (List separately in addition to code for primary procedure)**
EXCLUDES *Intracavity radioelement source or ribbon implantation (77770-77772)*
Code first (61510, 61518)
2.59 2.59 **FUD** ZZZ C
AMA: 2014,Jan,11; 1991,Sum,4

61518 **Craniectomy for excision of brain tumor, infratentorial or posterior fossa; except meningioma, cerebellopontine angle tumor, or midline tumor at base of skull**
81.0 81.0 **FUD** 090 C 80
AMA: 2014,Jan,11; 1991,Sum,4

61519 **meningioma**
85.4 85.4 **FUD** 090 C 80
AMA: 2014,Jan,11; 1991,Sum,4

61520 **cerebellopontine angle tumor**
110. 110. **FUD** 090 C 80
AMA: 2014,Jan,11; 1991,Sum,4

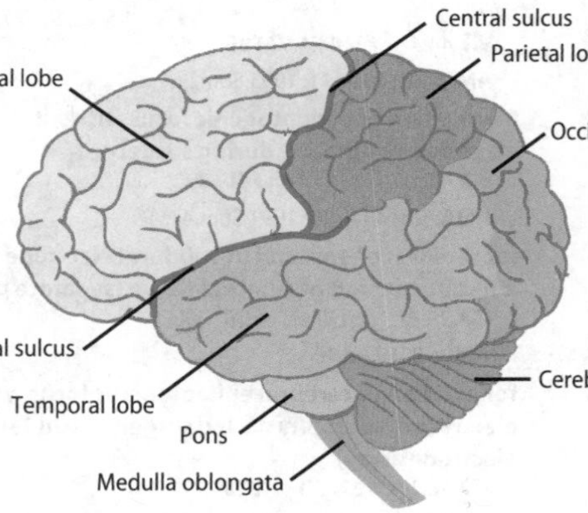

61521 **midline tumor at base of skull**
94.2 94.2 **FUD** 090 C 80
AMA: 2018,Jan,8; 2017,Jan,8; 2016,Jan,13

61522 **Craniectomy, infratentorial or posterior fossa; for excision of brain abscess**
62.9 62.9 **FUD** 090 C 80
AMA: 2014,Jan,11; 1991,Sum,4

61524 **for excision or fenestration of cyst**
60.8 60.8 **FUD** 090 C 80
AMA: 2014,Jan,11; 1991,Sum,4

61526 **Craniectomy, bone flap craniotomy, transtemporal (mastoid) for excision of cerebellopontine angle tumor;**
97.9 97.9 **FUD** 090 C
AMA: 2018,Mar,11; 2018,Jan,8; 2017,Jan,8; 2016,Jan,13

61530 **combined with middle/posterior fossa craniotomy/craniectomy**
91.0 91.0 **FUD** 090 C
AMA: 2014,Jan,11; 1991,Sum,4

61531-61545 Procedures for Seizures/Implanted Electrodes/Choroid Plexus/Craniopharyngioma

EXCLUDES *Craniotomy for:*
Multiple subpial transections during procedure (61567)
Selective amygdalohippocampectomy (61566)
Injection for:
Cerebral angiography (36100-36218)
Pneumoencephalography (61055)
Ventriculography (61026, 61120)

61531 **Subdural implantation of strip electrodes through 1 or more burr or trephine hole(s) for long-term seizure monitoring**
EXCLUDES *Continuous EEG observation ([95700, 95705, 95706, 95707, 95708, 95709, 95710, 95711, 95712, 95713, 95714, 95715, 95716, 95717, 95718, 95719, 95720, 95721, 95722, 95723, 95724, 95725, 95726])*
Craniotomy for intracranial arteriovenous malformation removal (61680-61692)
Stereotactic insertion electrodes (61760)
35.2 35.2 **FUD** 090 C 80
AMA: 2019,Jul,10

61533 **Craniotomy with elevation of bone flap; for subdural implantation of an electrode array, for long-term seizure monitoring**

EXCLUDES *Continuous EEG monitoring ([95700, 95705, 95706, 95707, 95708, 95709, 95710, 95711, 95712, 95713, 95714, 95715, 95716, 95717, 95718, 95719, 95720, 95721, 95722, 95723, 95724, 95725, 95726])*

44.4 44.4 **FUD** 090 C 80

AMA: 2014,Jan,11; 1993,Sum,25

61534 **for excision of epileptogenic focus without electrocorticography during surgery**

47.4 47.4 **FUD** 090 C 80

AMA: 2014,Jan,11; 1991,Sum,4

61535 **for removal of epidural or subdural electrode array, without excision of cerebral tissue (separate procedure)**

29.1 29.1 **FUD** 090 C 80

AMA: 2019,Jul,10

61536 **for excision of cerebral epileptogenic focus, with electrocorticography during surgery (includes removal of electrode array)**

76.1 76.1 **FUD** 090 C 80

AMA: 2014,Jan,11; 1991,Sum,4

61537 **for lobectomy, temporal lobe, without electrocorticography during surgery**

72.4 72.4 **FUD** 090 C 80

AMA: 2014,Jan,11; 1991,Sum,4

61538 **for lobectomy, temporal lobe, with electrocorticography during surgery**

78.2 78.2 **FUD** 090 C 80

AMA: 2019,Mar,6

61539 **for lobectomy, other than temporal lobe, partial or total, with electrocorticography during surgery**

69.6 69.6 **FUD** 090 C 80

AMA: 2019,Mar,6

61540 **for lobectomy, other than temporal lobe, partial or total, without electrocorticography during surgery**

64.2 64.2 **FUD** 090 C 80

AMA: 2014,Jan,11; 1991,Sum,4

61541 **for transection of corpus callosum**

63.3 63.3 **FUD** 090 C 80

AMA: 2014,Jan,11; 1991,Sum,4

61543 **for partial or subtotal (functional) hemispherectomy**

64.0 64.0 **FUD** 090 C 80

AMA: 2014,Jan,11; 1991,Sum,4

61544 **for excision or coagulation of choroid plexus**

54.8 54.8 **FUD** 090 C 80

AMA: 2014,Jan,11; 1991,Sum,4

61545 **for excision of craniopharyngioma**

92.3 92.3 **FUD** 090 C 80

AMA: 2014,Jan,11; 1991,Sum,4

61546-61548 Removal Pituitary Gland/Tumor

EXCLUDES *Injection for:*
Cerebral angiography (36100-36218)
Pneumoencephalography (61055)
Ventriculography (61026, 61120)

61546 **Craniotomy for hypophysectomy or excision of pituitary tumor, intracranial approach**

66.6 66.6 **FUD** 090 C 80

AMA: 2014,Jan,11; 1991,Sum,4

61548 **Hypophysectomy or excision of pituitary tumor, transnasal or transseptal approach, nonstereotactic**

INCLUDES Operating microscope (69990)

45.8 45.8 **FUD** 090 C 80

AMA: 2019,Dec,12; 2016,Feb,12

61550-61559 Craniosynostosis Procedures

EXCLUDES *Injection for:*
Cerebral angiography (36100-36218)
Pneumoencephalography (61055)
Ventriculography (61026, 61120)
Orbital hypertelorism reconstruction (21260-21263)
Reconstruction (21172-21180)

61550 **Craniectomy for craniosynostosis; single cranial suture**

32.1 32.1 **FUD** 090 C 80

AMA: 2018,Jan,8; 2017,Jan,8; 2016,Jan,13

61552 **multiple cranial sutures**

43.5 43.5 **FUD** 090 C 80

AMA: 2018,Jan,8; 2017,Jan,8; 2016,Jan,13

61556 **Craniotomy for craniosynostosis; frontal or parietal bone flap**

49.2 49.2 **FUD** 090 C 80

AMA: 2018,Jan,8; 2017,Jan,8; 2016,Jan,13

61557 **bifrontal bone flap**

49.4 49.4 **FUD** 090 C 80

AMA: 2018,Jan,8; 2017,Jan,8; 2016,Jan,13

61558 **Extensive craniectomy for multiple cranial suture craniosynostosis (eg, cloverleaf skull); not requiring bone grafts**

54.2 54.2 **FUD** 090 C 80

AMA: 2018,Jan,8; 2017,Jan,8; 2016,Jan,13

61559 **recontouring with multiple osteotomies and bone autografts (eg, barrel-stave procedure) (includes obtaining grafts)**

69.1 69.1 **FUD** 090 C 80

AMA: 2018,Jan,8; 2017,Jan,8; 2016,Jan,13

61563-61564 Removal Cranial Bone Tumor With/Without Optic Nerve Decompression

EXCLUDES *Injection for:*
Cerebral angiography (36100-36218)
Pneumoencephalography (61055)
Ventriculography (61026, 61120)
Reconstruction (21181-21183)

61563 **Excision, intra and extracranial, benign tumor of cranial bone (eg, fibrous dysplasia); without optic nerve decompression**

57.5 57.5 **FUD** 090 C 80

AMA: 2014,Jan,11; 1991,Sum,4

61564 **with optic nerve decompression**

69.5 69.5 **FUD** 090 C 80 50

AMA: 2014,Jan,11; 1991,Sum,4

61566-61567 Craniotomy for Seizures

EXCLUDES *Injection for:*
Cerebral angiography (36100-36218)
Pneumoencephalography (61055)
Ventriculography (61026, 61120)

61566 **Craniotomy with elevation of bone flap; for selective amygdalohippocampectomy**

66.1 66.1 **FUD** 090 C 80

AMA: 2018,Nov,7

61567 **for multiple subpial transections, with electrocorticography during surgery**

73.9 73.9 **FUD** 090 C 80

AMA: 2014,Jan,11; 1991,Sum,4

61570-61571 Removal of Foreign Body from Brain

EXCLUDES *Injection for:*
Cerebral angiography (36100-36218)
Pneumoencephalography (61055)
Ventriculography (61026, 61120)
Sequestrectomy for osteomyelitis (61501)

61570 **Craniectomy or craniotomy; with excision of foreign body from brain**

53.9 53.9 **FUD** 090 C 80

AMA: 2014,Jan,11; 1991,Sum,4

61571 **with treatment of penetrating wound of brain**
57.4 57.4 FUD 090 C 80
AMA: 2014,Jan,11; 1991,Sum,4

61575-61576 Transoral Approach Posterior Cranial Fossa/Upper Cervical Cord

EXCLUDES *Arthrodesis (22548)*
Injection for:
Cerebral angiography (36100-36218)
Pneumoencephalography (61055)
Ventriculography (61026, 61120)

61575 **Transoral approach to skull base, brain stem or upper spinal cord for biopsy, decompression or excision of lesion;**
72.4 72.4 FUD 090 C 80
AMA: 2014,Jan,11; 1991,Sum,4

61576 **requiring splitting of tongue and/or mandible (including tracheostomy)**
121. 121. FUD 090 C 80
AMA: 2014,Jan,11; 1991,Sum,4

61580-61598 Surgical Approach: Cranial Fossae

EXCLUDES *Definitive surgery (61600-61616)*
Dural repair and/or reconstruction (61618-61619)
Injection for:
Cerebral angiography (36100-36218)
Pneumoencephalography (61055)
Ventriculography (61026, 61120)
Primary closure (15730, 15733, 15756-15758)

61580 **Craniofacial approach to anterior cranial fossa; extradural, including lateral rhinotomy, ethmoidectomy, sphenoidectomy, without maxillectomy or orbital exenteration**
70.5 70.5 FUD 090 C 50
AMA: 2018,Jan,8; 2017,Jan,8; 2016,Jan,13

61581 **extradural, including lateral rhinotomy, orbital exenteration, ethmoidectomy, sphenoidectomy and/or maxillectomy**
76.6 76.6 FUD 090 C 50
AMA: 2018,Jan,8; 2017,Jan,8; 2016,Jan,13

61582 **extradural, including unilateral or bifrontal craniotomy, elevation of frontal lobe(s), osteotomy of base of anterior cranial fossa**
88.5 88.5 FUD 090 C 80
AMA: 2018,Jan,8; 2017,Jan,8; 2016,Jan,13

61583 **intradural, including unilateral or bifrontal craniotomy, elevation or resection of frontal lobe, osteotomy of base of anterior cranial fossa**
84.2 84.2 FUD 090 C 80
AMA: 2018,Jan,8; 2017,Dec,13; 2017,Jan,8; 2016,Jan,13

61584 **Orbitocranial approach to anterior cranial fossa, extradural, including supraorbital ridge osteotomy and elevation of frontal and/or temporal lobe(s); without orbital exenteration**
83.7 83.7 FUD 090 C 80 50
AMA: 2018,Jan,8; 2017,Jan,8; 2016,Jan,13

61585 **with orbital exenteration**
95.1 95.1 FUD 090 C 80 50
AMA: 2018,Jan,8; 2017,Jan,8; 2016,Jan,13

61586 **Bicoronal, transzygomatic and/or LeFort I osteotomy approach to anterior cranial fossa with or without internal fixation, without bone graft**
71.2 71.2 FUD 090 C 80
AMA: 2014,Jan,11; 1997,Nov,1

61590 **Infratemporal pre-auricular approach to middle cranial fossa (parapharyngeal space, infratemporal and midline skull base, nasopharynx), with or without disarticulation of the mandible, including parotidectomy, craniotomy, decompression and/or mobilization of the facial nerve and/or petrous carotid artery**
87.6 87.6 FUD 090 C 80 50
AMA: 2020,Apr,10; 2018,Jan,8; 2017,Jan,8; 2016,Jan,13

61591 **Infratemporal post-auricular approach to middle cranial fossa (internal auditory meatus, petrous apex, tentorium, cavernous sinus, parasellar area, infratemporal fossa) including mastoidectomy, resection of sigmoid sinus, with or without decompression and/or mobilization of contents of auditory canal or petrous carotid artery**
89.1 89.1 FUD 090 C 80 50
AMA: 2018,Jan,8; 2017,Jan,8; 2016,Jan,13

61592 **Orbitocranial zygomatic approach to middle cranial fossa (cavernous sinus and carotid artery, clivus, basilar artery or petrous apex) including osteotomy of zygoma, craniotomy, extra- or intradural elevation of temporal lobe**
91.7 91.7 FUD 090 C 80 50
AMA: 2018,Jan,8; 2017,Jan,8; 2016,Jan,13

61595 **Transtemporal approach to posterior cranial fossa, jugular foramen or midline skull base, including mastoidectomy, decompression of sigmoid sinus and/or facial nerve, with or without mobilization**
68.1 68.1 FUD 090 C 50
AMA: 2018,Mar,11; 2018,Jan,8; 2017,Jan,8; 2016,Jan,13

61596 **Transcochlear approach to posterior cranial fossa, jugular foramen or midline skull base, including labyrinthectomy, decompression, with or without mobilization of facial nerve and/or petrous carotid artery**
70.0 70.0 FUD 090 C 80 50
AMA: 2018,Jan,8; 2017,Jan,8; 2016,Jan,13

61597 **Transcondylar (far lateral) approach to posterior cranial fossa, jugular foramen or midline skull base, including occipital condylectomy, mastoidectomy, resection of C1-C3 vertebral body(s), decompression of vertebral artery, with or without mobilization**
84.9 84.9 FUD 090 C 80 50
AMA: 2018,Jan,8; 2017,Jan,8; 2016,Jan,13

61598 **Transpetrosal approach to posterior cranial fossa, clivus or foramen magnum, including ligation of superior petrosal sinus and/or sigmoid sinus**
82.4 82.4 FUD 090 C 80
AMA: 2018,Jan,8; 2017,Jan,8; 2016,Jan,13

61600-61616 Definitive Procedures: Cranial Fossae

EXCLUDES *Dural repair and/or reconstruction (61618-61619)*
Injection for:
Cerebral angiography (36100-36218)
Pneumoencephalography (61055)
Ventriculography (61026, 61120)
Primary closure (15730, 15733, 15756-15758)
Surgical approach (61580-61598)

61600 **Resection or excision of neoplastic, vascular or infectious lesion of base of anterior cranial fossa; extradural**
61.5 61.5 FUD 090 C 80
AMA: 2018,Jan,8; 2017,Jan,8; 2016,Jan,13

61601 **intradural, including dural repair, with or without graft**
69.6 69.6 FUD 090 C 80
AMA: 2018,Jan,8; 2017,Jan,8; 2016,Jan,13

61605 **Resection or excision of neoplastic, vascular or infectious lesion of infratemporal fossa, parapharyngeal space, petrous apex; extradural**
62.2 62.2 FUD 090 C 80
AMA: 2020,Apr,10; 2018,Jan,8; 2017,Jan,8; 2016,Jan,13

61606 **intradural, including dural repair, with or without graft**
84.8 84.8 FUD 090 C 80
AMA: 2018,Jan,8; 2017,Jan,8; 2016,Jan,13

61607 **Resection or excision of neoplastic, vascular or infectious lesion of parasellar area, cavernous sinus, clivus or midline skull base; extradural**
77.8 77.8 FUD 090 C 80
AMA: 2018,Jan,8; 2017,Jan,8; 2016,Jan,13

61608 **intradural, including dural repair, with or without graft**
95.7 95.7 FUD 090 C 80
AMA: 2018,Jan,8; 2017,Jan,8; 2016,Jan,13

\+ **61611** **Transection or ligation, carotid artery in petrous canal; without repair (List separately in addition to code for primary procedure)**
Code first (61605-61608)
13.8 13.8 FUD ZZZ C 80
AMA: 2018,Jan,8; 2017,Jan,8; 2016,Jan,13

61613 **Obliteration of carotid aneurysm, arteriovenous malformation, or carotid-cavernous fistula by dissection within cavernous sinus**
96.9 96.9 FUD 090 C 80 50
AMA: 2018,Jan,8; 2017,Jan,8; 2016,Jan,13

61615 **Resection or excision of neoplastic, vascular or infectious lesion of base of posterior cranial fossa, jugular foramen, foramen magnum, or C1-C3 vertebral bodies; extradural**
82.3 82.3 FUD 090 C 80
AMA: 2018,Jan,8; 2017,Jan,8; 2016,Jan,13

61616 **intradural, including dural repair, with or without graft**
97.3 97.3 FUD 090 C 80
AMA: 2018,Mar,11; 2018,Jan,8; 2017,Jan,8; 2016,Jan,13

61618-61619 Reconstruction Post-Surgical Cranial Fossae Defects

EXCLUDES *Definitive surgery (61600-61616)*
Injection for:
Cerebral angiography (36100-36218)
Pneumoencephalography (61055)
Ventriculography (61026, 61120)
Primary closure (15730, 15733, 15756-15758)
Surgical approach (61580-61598)

61618 **Secondary repair of dura for cerebrospinal fluid leak, anterior, middle or posterior cranial fossa following surgery of the skull base; by free tissue graft (eg, pericranium, fascia, tensor fascia lata, adipose tissue, homologous or synthetic grafts)**
37.5 37.5 FUD 090 C 80
AMA: 2018,Jan,8; 2017,Jan,8; 2016,Jan,13

61619 **by local or regionalized vascularized pedicle flap or myocutaneous flap (including galea, temporalis, frontalis or occipitalis muscle)**
41.3 41.3 FUD 090 C 80
AMA: 2018,Jan,8; 2017,Jan,8; 2016,Jan,13

61623-61651 Neurovascular Interventional Procedures

61623 **Endovascular temporary balloon arterial occlusion, head or neck (extracranial/intracranial) including selective catheterization of vessel to be occluded, positioning and inflation of occlusion balloon, concomitant neurological monitoring, and radiologic supervision and interpretation of all angiography required for balloon occlusion and to exclude vascular injury post occlusion**
EXCLUDES *Diagnostic angiography target artery just before temporary occlusion; report only radiological supervision and interpretation*
Selective catheterization and angiography artery besides the target artery; report catheterization and radiological supervision and interpretation codes as appropriate
16.6 16.6 FUD 000 J J8
AMA: 2018,Jan,8; 2017,Jan,8; 2016,Jan,13

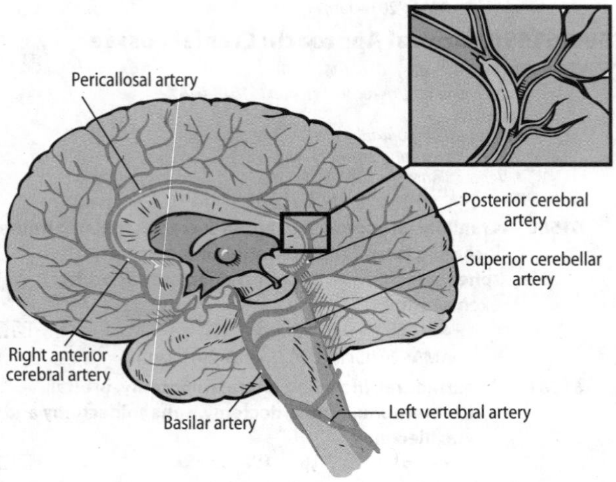

61624 **Transcatheter permanent occlusion or embolization (eg, for tumor destruction, to achieve hemostasis, to occlude a vascular malformation), percutaneous, any method; central nervous system (intracranial, spinal cord)**
EXCLUDES *Non-central nervous system transcatheter occlusion or embolization other than head or neck (37241-37244)*
(75894)
33.7 33.7 FUD 000 C
AMA: 2019,Sep,6; 2018,Jan,8; 2017,Jan,8; 2016,Jan,13

61626 **non-central nervous system, head or neck (extracranial, brachiocephalic branch)**
EXCLUDES *Non-central nervous system transcatheter occlusion or embolization other than head or neck (37241-37244)*
(75894)
25.5 25.5 FUD 000 J J8
AMA: 2019,Sep,6; 2018,Jan,8; 2017,Jan,8; 2016,Jan,13

61630 **Balloon angioplasty, intracranial (eg, atherosclerotic stenosis), percutaneous**
INCLUDES Diagnostic arteriogram when stent or angioplasty necessary
Radiology services for arteriography target vascular territory
Selective catheterization target vascular territory
EXCLUDES *Diagnostic arteriogram when stent or angioplasty not necessary (report applicable code for selective catheterization and radiology services)*
Percutaneous arterial transluminal mechanical thrombectomy and/or infusion for thrombolysis performed same vascular territory (61645)
40.6 40.6 FUD XXX C 80
AMA: 2018,Jan,8; 2017,Jul,3; 2017,Apr,9; 2017,Jan,8; 2016,Mar,3; 2016,Jan,13

61635 Transcatheter placement of intravascular stent(s), intracranial (eg, atherosclerotic stenosis), including balloon angioplasty, if performed

INCLUDES Diagnostic arteriogram when stent or angioplasty necessary
Radiology services for arteriography target vascular territory
Selective catheterization target vascular territory

EXCLUDES *Diagnostic arteriogram when stent or angioplasty not necessary (report applicable code for selective catheterization and radiology services)*
Percutaneous arterial transluminal mechanical thrombectomy and/or infusion for thrombolysis performed same vascular territory (61645)

42.6 42.6 FUD XXX C 80

AMA: 2018,Jan,8; 2017,Jul,3; 2017,Jan,8; 2016,Mar,3; 2016,Jan,13

61640 Balloon dilatation of intracranial vasospasm, percutaneous; initial vessel

INCLUDES Angiography after dilation vessel
Fluoroscopic guidance
Injection contrast material
Roadmapping
Selective catheterization target vessel
Vessel analysis

EXCLUDES *Endovascular intracranial prolonged administration pharmacologic agent performed same vascular territory (61650-61651)*

14.0 14.0 FUD 000 E

AMA: 2018,Jan,8; 2017,Jan,8; 2016,Mar,3; 2016,Jan,13

+ **61641 each additional vessel in same vascular territory (List separately in addition to code for primary procedure)**

INCLUDES Angiography after dilation vessel
Fluoroscopic guidance
Injection contrast material
Roadmapping
Selective catheterization target vessel
Vessel analysis

EXCLUDES *Endovascular intracranial prolonged administration pharmacologic agent performed same vascular territory (61640)*

Code first (61640)

4.92 4.92 FUD ZZZ E

AMA: 2018,Jan,8; 2017,Jan,8; 2016,Mar,3; 2016,Jan,13

+ **61642 each additional vessel in different vascular territory (List separately in addition to code for primary procedure))**

INCLUDES Angiography after dilation vessel
Fluoroscopic guidance
Injection contrast material
Roadmapping
Selective catheterization target vessel
Vessel analysis

EXCLUDES *Endovascular intracranial prolonged administration pharmacologic agent performed same vascular territory (61650-61651)*

Code first (61640)

9.84 9.84 FUD ZZZ E

AMA: 2018,Jan,8; 2017,Jan,8; 2016,Mar,3; 2016,Jan,13

61645 Percutaneous arterial transluminal mechanical thrombectomy and/or infusion for thrombolysis, intracranial, any method, including diagnostic angiography, fluoroscopic guidance, catheter placement, and intraprocedural pharmacological thrombolytic injection(s)

INCLUDES Interventions performed in intracranial artery including:
Angiography with radiologic supervision and interpretation (diagnostic and subsequent)
Closure arteriotomy by any method
Fluoroscopy
Patient monitoring
Procedures performed in vascular territories:
Left carotid
Right carotid
Vertebro-basilar

EXCLUDES *Procedure performed same vascular target area:*
Balloon angioplasty, intracranial (61630)
Diagnostic studies: aortic arch, carotid, and vertebral arteries (36221-36226)
Endovascular intracranial prolonged administration pharmacologic agent (61650-61651)
Transcatheter placement intravascular stent (61635)
Transluminal thrombectomy (37184, 37186)
Reporting code more than one time for treatment each intracranial vascular territory
Venous thrombectomy or thrombolysis (37187-37188, 37212, 37214)

24.3 24.3 FUD 000 C 80 50

AMA: 2019,Sep,6; 2019,Sep,5; 2018,Jan,8; 2017,Jan,8; 2016,Mar,3; 2016,Jan,13

61650 Endovascular intracranial prolonged administration of pharmacologic agent(s) other than for thrombolysis, arterial, including catheter placement, diagnostic angiography, and imaging guidance; initial vascular territory

INCLUDES Interventions performed in intracranial artery, including:
Angiography with radiologic supervision and interpretation (diagnostic and subsequent)
Closure arteriotomy by any method
Fluoroscopy
Patient monitoring
Procedures performed in vascular territories:
Left carotid
Right carotid
Vertebro-basilar
Prolonged (at least 10 minutes) arterial administration nonthrombolytic agents

EXCLUDES *Procedure performed same vascular target area:*
Balloon dilatation intracranial vasospasm (61640-61642)
Chemotherapy administration (96420-96425)
Diagnostic studies: aortic arch, carotid, and vertebral arteries (36221-36228)
Transluminal thrombectomy (37184, 37186, 61645)
Reporting code more than one time for treatment each intracranial vascular territory
Treatment iatrogenic condition
Venous thrombectomy or thrombolysis

16.1 16.1 FUD 000 C

AMA: 2019,Sep,6; 2018,Jan,8; 2017,Jan,8; 2016,Mar,3; 2016,Jan,13

\+ **61651** **each additional vascular territory (List separately in addition to code for primary procedure)**

INCLUDES Interventions performed in intracranial artery, including:
- Angiography with radiologic supervision and interpretation (diagnostic and subsequent)
- Closure arteriotomy by any method
- Fluoroscopy
- Patient monitoring
- Procedures performed in vascular territories:
  - Left carotid
  - Right carotid
  - Vertebro-basilar

Prolonged (at least 10 minutes) arterial administration nonthrombolytic agents

EXCLUDES *Procedure performed same vascular target area:*
- *Balloon dilatation intracranial vasospasm (61640-61642)*
- *Chemotherapy administration (96420-96425)*
- *Diagnostic studies: aortic arch, carotid, and vertebral arteries (36221-36228)*
- *Transluminal thrombectomy (37184, 37186, 61645)*

Reporting code more than one time for treatment each intracranial vascular territory
Treatment iatrogenic condition
Venous thrombectomy or thrombolysis

Code first (61650)

7.01 7.01 **FUD** ZZZ C

AMA: 2019,Sep,6; 2018,Jan,8; 2017,Jan,8; 2016,Mar,3; 2016,Jan,13

61680-61692 Surgical Treatment of Arteriovenous Malformation of the Brain

INCLUDES Craniotomy

61680 **Surgery of intracranial arteriovenous malformation; supratentorial, simple**
66.1 66.1 **FUD** 090 C 80
AMA: 2014,Jan,11

61682 **supratentorial, complex**
123. 123. **FUD** 090 C 80
AMA: 2018,Jan,8; 2017,Jan,8; 2016,Jan,13

61684 **infratentorial, simple**
83.1 83.1 **FUD** 090 C 80
AMA: 2014,Jan,11

61686 **infratentorial, complex**
136. 136. **FUD** 090 C 80
AMA: 2018,Jan,8; 2017,Jan,8; 2016,Jan,13

61690 **dural, simple**
63.6 63.6 **FUD** 090 C 80
AMA: 2014,Jan,11

61692 **dural, complex**
108. 108. **FUD** 090 C 80
AMA: 2018,Jan,8; 2017,Jan,8; 2016,Jan,13

61697-61703 Surgical Treatment Brain Aneurysm

INCLUDES Craniotomy

61697 **Surgery of complex intracranial aneurysm, intracranial approach; carotid circulation**

INCLUDES Aneurysms bigger than 15 mm
- Calcification aneurysm neck
- Inclusion normal vessels in aneurysm neck
- Surgery needing temporary vessel occlusion, trapping, or cardiopulmonary bypass to treat aneurysm

125. 125. **FUD** 090 C 80
AMA: 2018,Jan,8; 2017,Dec,13

61698 **vertebrobasilar circulation**

INCLUDES Aneurysm bigger than 15 mm
- Calcification aneurysm neck
- Inclusion normal vessels in aneurysm neck
- Surgery needing temporary vessel occlusion, trapping, or cardiopulmonary bypass to treat aneurysm

140. 140. **FUD** 090 C 80
AMA: 2014,Jan,11

61700 **Surgery of simple intracranial aneurysm, intracranial approach; carotid circulation**
100. 100. **FUD** 090 C 80
AMA: 2018,Jan,8; 2017,Dec,13; 2017,Jan,8; 2016,Jan,13

61702 **vertebrobasilar circulation**
118. 118. **FUD** 090 C 80
AMA: 2014,Jan,11

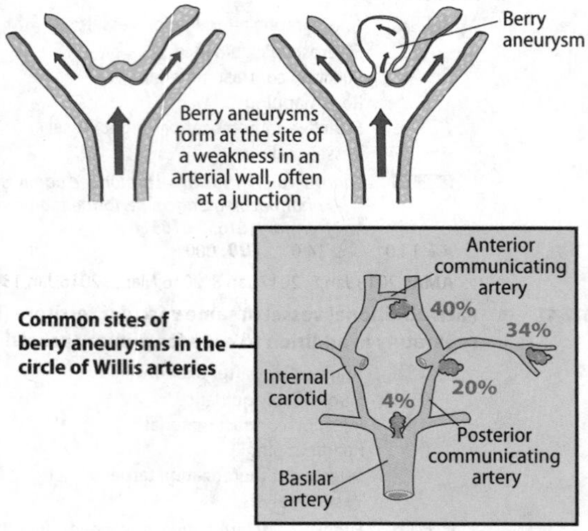

61703 **Surgery of intracranial aneurysm, cervical approach by application of occluding clamp to cervical carotid artery (Selverstone-Crutchfield type)**

EXCLUDES *Cervical approach for direct ligation carotid artery (37600-37606)*

39.9 39.9 **FUD** 090 C 80
AMA: 2014,Jan,11

61705-61710 Other Procedures for Aneurysm, Arteriovenous Malformation, and Carotid-Cavernous Fistula

INCLUDES Craniotomy

61705 **Surgery of aneurysm, vascular malformation or carotid-cavernous fistula; by intracranial and cervical occlusion of carotid artery**
73.6 73.6 **FUD** 090 C 80
AMA: 2014,Jan,11

61708 **by intracranial electrothrombosis**

EXCLUDES *Ligation or gradual occlusion internal or common carotid artery (37605-37606)*

75.1 75.1 **FUD** 090 C 80
AMA: 2014,Jan,11; 2000,Sep,11

61710 **by intra-arterial embolization, injection procedure, or balloon catheter**
62.0 62.0 **FUD** 090 C 80
AMA: 2018,Jan,8; 2017,Jan,8; 2016,Jan,13

61711 Extracranial-Intracranial Bypass

CMS: 100-02,16,10 Exclusions from Coverage; 100-03,20.2 Extracranial-intracranial (EC-IC) Arterial Bypass Surgery

INCLUDES Craniotomy

EXCLUDES *Carotid or vertebral thromboendarterectomy (35301)*

Code also operating microscope when appropriate (69990)

61711 **Anastomosis, arterial, extracranial-intracranial (eg, middle cerebral/cortical) arteries**
74.9 74.9 **FUD** 090 C 80
AMA: 2014,Jan,11

61720-61791 Stereotactic Procedures of the Brain

61720 **Creation of lesion by stereotactic method, including burr hole(s) and localizing and recording techniques, single or multiple stages; globus pallidus or thalamus**
37.3 37.3 **FUD** 090 J G2
AMA: 2018,Jan,8; 2017,Jan,8; 2016,Jan,13

61735 **subcortical structure(s) other than globus pallidus or thalamus**
46.8 46.8 **FUD** 090 C
AMA: 2014,Jul,8; 2014,Jan,11

● **61736** **Laser interstitial thermal therapy (LITT) of lesion, intracranial, including burr hole(s), with magnetic resonance imaging guidance, when performed; single trajectory for 1 simple lesion**

INCLUDES MRI (70551-70553, 70557-70559, 77021-77022)

EXCLUDES *Application cranial tongs, caliper, or stereotactic frame (20660)*
Laser interstitial thermal therapy (LITT), multiple trajectories (61737)
Stereotactic computer-assisted navigation, cranial/intradural (61781)

● **61737** **multiple trajectories for multiple or complex lesion(s)**

INCLUDES MRI (70551-70553, 70557-70559, 77021-77022)

EXCLUDES *Application cranial tongs, caliper, stereotactic frame (20660)*
Laser interstitial thermal therapy (LITT), single trajectory (61736)
Stereotactic computer-assisted navigation, cranial/intradural (61781)

61750 **Stereotactic biopsy, aspiration, or excision, including burr hole(s), for intracranial lesion;**
41.4 41.4 **FUD** 090 C
AMA: 2018,Jan,8; 2017,Jan,8; 2016,Jan,13

61751 **with computed tomography and/or magnetic resonance guidance**
(70450, 70460, 70470, 70551-70553)
39.7 39.7 **FUD** 090 C
AMA: 2018,Jan,8; 2017,Jan,8; 2016,Jan,13

61760 **Stereotactic implantation of depth electrodes into the cerebrum for long-term seizure monitoring**
46.0 46.0 **FUD** 090 C
AMA: 2014,Jul,8; 2014,Jan,11

61770 **Stereotactic localization, including burr hole(s), with insertion of catheter(s) or probe(s) for placement of radiation source**
47.7 47.7 **FUD** 090 J G2
AMA: 2018,Jan,8; 2017,Jan,8; 2016,Jan,13

\+ **61781** **Stereotactic computer-assisted (navigational) procedure; cranial, intradural (List separately in addition to code for primary procedure)**

EXCLUDES *Creation lesion by stereotactic method (61720-61791)*
Extradural stereotactic computer-assisted procedure for same surgical session by same individual (61782)
Radiation treatment delivery, stereotactic radiosurgery (SRS) (77371-77373)
Stereotactic implantation neurostimulator electrode array (61863-61868)
Stereotactic radiation treatment management (77432)
Stereotactic radiosurgery (61796-61799)
Ventriculocisternostomy (62201)

Code first primary procedure
6.94 6.94 **FUD** ZZZ N N1 80
AMA: 2018,Jan,8; 2017,Jan,8; 2016,Jan,13

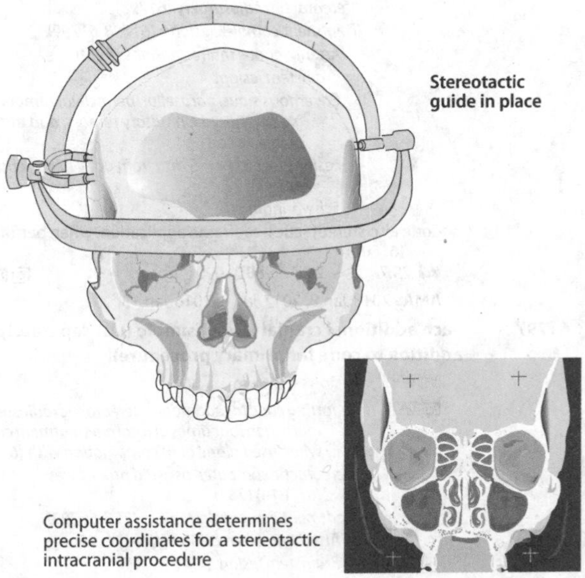
Stereotactic guide in place
Computer assistance determines precise coordinates for a stereotactic intracranial procedure
CT or MRI scan

\+ **61782** **cranial, extradural (List separately in addition to code for primary procedure)**

EXCLUDES *Intradural stereotactic computer-assisted procedure for same surgical session by same individual (61781)*
Stereotactic radiosurgery (61796-61799)

Code first primary procedure
5.02 5.02 **FUD** ZZZ N N1 80
AMA: 2018,Apr,3; 2018,Jan,8; 2017,Jan,8; 2016,Jan,13

\+ **61783** **spinal (List separately in addition to code for primary procedure)**

EXCLUDES *Stereotactic radiosurgery (61796-61799, 63620-63621)*

Code first primary procedure
6.80 6.80 **FUD** ZZZ N N1 80
AMA: 2018,Jan,8; 2017,Jan,8; 2016,Jan,13

61790 **Creation of lesion by stereotactic method, percutaneous, by neurolytic agent (eg, alcohol, thermal, electrical, radiofrequency); gasserian ganglion**
25.7 25.7 **FUD** 090 J A2 50
AMA: 2014,Jul,8; 2014,Jan,11

61791 **trigeminal medullary tract**
33.0 33.0 **FUD** 090 J A2 80 50
AMA: 2018,Jan,8; 2017,Jan,8; 2016,Jan,13

61796-61800 Stereotactic Radiosurgery (SRS): Brain

INCLUDES Planning, dosimetry, targeting, positioning, or blocking performed by neurosurgeon

EXCLUDES *Application cranial tongs, caliper, or stereotactic frame (20660)*
Intensity modulated beam delivery plan and treatment (77301, 77385-77386)
Radiation treatment management and radiosurgery by same provider (77427-77435)
Stereotactic body radiation therapy (77373, 77435)
Stereotactic radiosurgery more than once per lesion per treatment course
Treatment planning, physics and dosimetry, and treatment delivery performed by radiation oncologist

61796 Stereotactic radiosurgery (particle beam, gamma ray, or linear accelerator); 1 simple cranial lesion

INCLUDES Lesions < 3.5 cm

EXCLUDES *Reporting code more than one time per treatment course*
Stereotactic computer-assisted procedures (61781-61783)
Stereotactic radiosurgery (61798)
Treatment complex lesions: (61798-61799)
Arteriovenous malformations (AVM)
Brainstem lesions
Cavernous sinus/parasellar/petroclival tumors, glomus tumors, pituitary tumors, and tumors pineal region
Lesions located <= 5 mm from optic nerve, chasm, or tract
Schwannomas

Code also stereotactic headframe application, when performed (61800)

Facility RVU 29.7 Non-Facility RVU 29.7 **FUD** 090 B 80 CCI

AMA: 2018,Jan,8; 2017,Jan,8; 2016,Jan,13

+ **61797 each additional cranial lesion, simple (List separately in addition to code for primary procedure)**

INCLUDES Lesions < 3.5 cm

EXCLUDES *Reporting code for additional stereotactic radiosurgery more than four times in total per treatment course when used alone or in combination with (61799)*
Stereotactic computer-assisted procedures (61781-61783)
Treatment complex lesions: (61798-61799)
Arteriovenous malformations (AVM)
Brainstem lesion
Cavernous sinus/parasellar/petroclival tumors, glomus tumors, pituitary tumors, and tumors pineal region
Lesions located <= 5 mm from optic nerve, chasm, or tract
Schwannomas

Code first (61796, 61798)

Facility RVU 6.52 Non-Facility RVU 6.52 **FUD** ZZZ B 80 CCI

AMA: 2018,Jan,8; 2017,Jan,8; 2016,Jan,13

61798 1 complex cranial lesion

INCLUDES All therapeutic lesion creation procedures
Treatment complex lesions:
Arteriovenous malformations (AVM)
Brainstem lesions
Cavernous sinus, parasellar, petroclival, glomus, pineal region, and pituitary tumors
Lesions located <= 5 mm from optic nerve, chasm, or tract
Lesions >= 3.5 cm
Schwannomas
Treatment multiple lesions when at least one considered complex

EXCLUDES *Reporting code more than one time per treatment course*
Stereotactic computer-assisted procedures (61781-61783)
Stereotactic radiosurgery (61796)

Code also stereotactic headframe application, when performed (61800)

Facility RVU 40.5 Non-Facility RVU 40.5 **FUD** 090 B 80 CCI

AMA: 2018,Jan,8; 2017,Jan,8; 2016,Jan,13

+ **61799 each additional cranial lesion, complex (List separately in addition to code for primary procedure)**

INCLUDES All therapeutic lesion creation procedures
Treatment complex lesions:
Arteriovenous malformations (AVM)
Brainstem lesions
Cavernous sinus, parasellar, petroclival, glomus, pineal region, and pituitary tumors
Lesions located <= 5 mm from optic nerve, chasm, or tract
Lesions >= 3.5 cm
Schwannomas

EXCLUDES *Reporting code for additional stereotactic radiosurgery more than four times in total per treatment course when used alone or in combination with (61797)*
Stereotactic computer-assisted procedures (61781-61783)

Code first (61798)

Facility RVU 8.98 Non-Facility RVU 8.98 **FUD** ZZZ B 80 CCI

AMA: 2018,Jan,8; 2017,Jan,8; 2016,Jan,13

+ **61800 Application of stereotactic headframe for stereotactic radiosurgery (List separately in addition to code for primary procedure)**

Code first (61796, 61798)

Facility RVU 4.40 Non-Facility RVU 4.40 **FUD** ZZZ B 80 CCI

AMA: 2018,Jan,8; 2017,Jan,8; 2016,Jan,13

61850-61888 Intracranial Neurostimulation

INCLUDES Analysis system at implantation (95970)
Microelectrode recording by operating surgeon

EXCLUDES *Electronic analysis and reprogramming neurostimulator pulse generator (95970, 95976-95977, [95983, 95984])*
Neurophysiological mapping by another physician/qualified health care professional (95961-95962)

61850 Twist drill or burr hole(s) for implantation of neurostimulator electrodes, cortical

Facility RVU 28.8 Non-Facility RVU 28.8 **FUD** 090 C 80 CCI

AMA: 2019,Feb,6; 2018,Jan,8; 2017,Jan,8; 2016,Jan,13

61860 Craniectomy or craniotomy for implantation of neurostimulator electrodes, cerebral, cortical

Facility RVU 45.7 Non-Facility RVU 45.7 **FUD** 090 C 80 CCI

AMA: 2019,Feb,6; 2018,Jan,8; 2017,Jan,8; 2016,Jan,13

61863 Twist drill, burr hole, craniotomy, or craniectomy with stereotactic implantation of neurostimulator electrode array in subcortical site (eg, thalamus, globus pallidus, subthalamic nucleus, periventricular, periaqueductal gray), without use of intraoperative microelectrode recording; first array

Facility RVU 43.9 Non-Facility RVU 43.9 **FUD** 090 C 80 50 CCI

AMA: 2019,Feb,6; 2018,Jan,8; 2017,Jan,8; 2016,Jan,13

+ **61864 each additional array (List separately in addition to primary procedure)**

Code first (61863)

Facility RVU 8.36 Non-Facility RVU 8.36 **FUD** ZZZ C 80 CCI

AMA: 2019,Feb,6

61867 Twist drill, burr hole, craniotomy, or craniectomy with stereotactic implantation of neurostimulator electrode array in subcortical site (eg, thalamus, globus pallidus, subthalamic nucleus, periventricular, periaqueductal gray), with use of intraoperative microelectrode recording; first array

Facility RVU 66.8 Non-Facility RVU 66.8 **FUD** 090 C 80 50 CCI

AMA: 2019,Feb,6

+ **61868 each additional array (List separately in addition to primary procedure)**

Code first (61867)

Facility RVU 14.7 Non-Facility RVU 14.7 **FUD** ZZZ C 80 CCI

AMA: 2019,Feb,6; 2018,Jan,8; 2017,Jan,8; 2016,Jan,13

61880 Revision or removal of intracranial neurostimulator electrodes

Facility RVU 16.6 Non-Facility RVU 16.6 **FUD** 090 Q2 G2 80 50 CCI

AMA: 2019,Feb,6

61885 **Insertion or replacement of cranial neurostimulator pulse generator or receiver, direct or inductive coupling; with connection to a single electrode array**

EXCLUDES *Percutaneous procedure to place cranial nerve neurostimulator electrode(s) (64553)*
Revision or replacement cranial nerve neurostimulator electrode array (64569)

14.9 14.9 FUD 090 J J8 80 50

AMA: 2019,Feb,6; 2018,Jan,8; 2017,Jan,8; 2016,Jan,13

61886 **with connection to 2 or more electrode arrays**

EXCLUDES *Percutaneous procedure to place cranial nerve neurostimulator electrode(s) (64553)*
Revision or replacement cranial nerve neurostimulator electrode array (64569)

24.5 24.5 FUD 090 J J8 80

AMA: 2019,Feb,6; 2018,Jan,8; 2017,Jan,8; 2016,Jan,13

61888 **Revision or removal of cranial neurostimulator pulse generator or receiver**

EXCLUDES *Insertion or replacement cranial neurostimulator pulse generator or receiver (61885-61886)*

11.3 11.3 FUD 010 J J8 50

AMA: 2019,Feb,6; 2018,Jan,8; 2017,Jan,8; 2016,Jan,13

62000-62148 Repair of Skull and/or Cerebrospinal Fluid Leaks

62000 **Elevation of depressed skull fracture; simple, extradural**

30.2 30.2 FUD 090 J 62

AMA: 2014,Jan,11

62005 **compound or comminuted, extradural**

37.2 37.2 FUD 090 C 80

AMA: 2014,Jan,11

62010 **with repair of dura and/or debridement of brain**

44.7 44.7 FUD 090 C 80

AMA: 2014,Jan,11

62100 **Craniotomy for repair of dural/cerebrospinal fluid leak, including surgery for rhinorrhea/otorrhea**

EXCLUDES *Repair spinal fluid leak (63707, 63709)*

45.6 45.6 FUD 090 C 80

AMA: 2014,Jan,11; 2002,May,7

62115 **Reduction of craniomegalic skull (eg, treated hydrocephalus); not requiring bone grafts or cranioplasty**

49.2 49.2 FUD 090 C 80

AMA: 2014,Jan,11

62117 **requiring craniotomy and reconstruction with or without bone graft (includes obtaining grafts)**

57.8 57.8 FUD 090 C 80

AMA: 2014,Jan,11

62120 **Repair of encephalocele, skull vault, including cranioplasty**

61.9 61.9 FUD 090 C 80

AMA: 2014,Jan,11

62121 **Craniotomy for repair of encephalocele, skull base**

45.7 45.7 FUD 090 C 80

AMA: 2014,Jan,11

62140 **Cranioplasty for skull defect; up to 5 cm diameter**

29.9 29.9 FUD 090 C 80

AMA: 2018,Jan,8; 2017,Jan,8; 2016,Jan,13

62141 **larger than 5 cm diameter**

33.1 33.1 FUD 090 C 80

AMA: 2018,Jan,8; 2017,Jan,8; 2016,Jan,13

62142 **Removal of bone flap or prosthetic plate of skull**

25.8 25.8 FUD 090 C 80

AMA: 2018,Jan,8; 2017,Jan,8; 2016,Jan,13

62143 **Replacement of bone flap or prosthetic plate of skull**

30.3 30.3 FUD 090 C 80

AMA: 2018,Jan,8; 2017,Jan,8; 2016,Jan,13

62145 **Cranioplasty for skull defect with reparative brain surgery**

41.0 41.0 FUD 090 C 80

AMA: 2018,Jan,8; 2017,Jan,8; 2016,Jan,13

62146 **Cranioplasty with autograft (includes obtaining bone grafts); up to 5 cm diameter**

34.2 34.2 FUD 090 C 80

AMA: 2018,Jan,8; 2017,Jan,8; 2016,Jan,13

62147 **larger than 5 cm diameter**

41.0 41.0 FUD 090 C 80

AMA: 2018,Jan,8; 2017,Jan,8; 2016,Jan,13

\+ **62148** **Incision and retrieval of subcutaneous cranial bone graft for cranioplasty (List separately in addition to code for primary procedure)**

Code first (62140-62147)

3.73 3.73 FUD ZZZ C

AMA: 2014,Jan,11

62160-62165 Neuroendoscopic Brain Procedures

INCLUDES Diagnostic endoscopy

\+ **62160** **Neuroendoscopy, intracranial, for placement or replacement of ventricular catheter and attachment to shunt system or external drainage (List separately in addition to code for primary procedure)**

Code first (61107, 61210, 62220-62230, 62258)

5.61 5.61 FUD ZZZ N N1

AMA: 2018,Jan,8; 2017,Jan,8; 2016,Jan,13

62161 **Neuroendoscopy, intracranial; with dissection of adhesions, fenestration of septum pellucidum or intraventricular cysts (including placement, replacement, or removal of ventricular catheter)**

44.1 44.1 FUD 090 C 80

AMA: 2014,Jan,11

62162 **with fenestration or excision of colloid cyst, including placement of external ventricular catheter for drainage**

55.3 55.3 FUD 090 C 80

AMA: 2014,Jan,11

62164 **with excision of brain tumor, including placement of external ventricular catheter for drainage**

60.3 60.3 FUD 090 C 80

AMA: 2014,Jan,11

62165 **with excision of pituitary tumor, transnasal or trans-sphenoidal approach**

44.6 44.6 FUD 090 C 80

AMA: 2019,Dec,12; 2018,Jan,8; 2017,Dec,14

62180-62258 Cerebrospinal Fluid Diversion Procedures

62180 **Ventriculocisternostomy (Torkildsen type operation)**

47.0 47.0 FUD 090 C 80

AMA: 2014,Jan,11

62190 Creation of shunt; subarachnoid/subdural-atrial, -jugular, -auricular

26.6 | 26.6 | FUD 090 | C

AMA: 2014,Jan,11; 2000,Dec,12

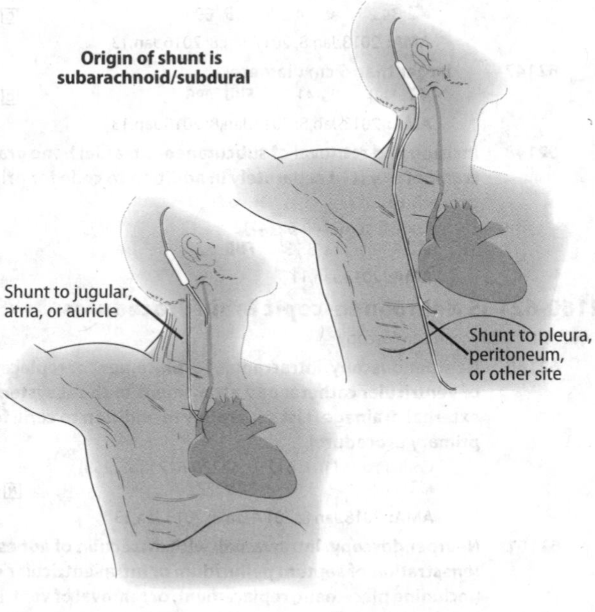

62192 subarachnoid/subdural-peritoneal, -pleural, other terminus

28.3 | 28.3 | FUD 090 | C 80

AMA: 2014,Jan,11

62194 Replacement or irrigation, subarachnoid/subdural catheter

14.2 | 14.2 | FUD 010 | J A2 80

AMA: 2018,Jan,8; 2017,Jan,8; 2016,Jan,13

62200 Ventriculocisternostomy, third ventricle;

INCLUDES Dandy ventriculocisternostomy

39.7 | 39.7 | FUD 090 | C 80

AMA: 2014,Jan,11

62201 stereotactic, neuroendoscopic method

EXCLUDES *Intracranial neuroendoscopic surgery (62161-62165)*

34.8 | 34.8 | FUD 090 | C

AMA: 2018,Jan,8; 2017,Jan,8; 2016,Jan,13

62220 Creation of shunt; ventriculo-atrial, -jugular, -auricular

Code also intracranial neuroendoscopic ventricular catheter insertion, when performed (62160)

28.4 | 28.4 | FUD 090 | C 80

AMA: 2014,Jan,11; 2007,Jun,10-11

62223 ventriculo-peritoneal, -pleural, other terminus

Code also intracranial neuroendoscopic ventricular catheter insertion, when performed (62160)

30.0 | 30.0 | FUD 090 | C 80

AMA: 2014,Jan,11; 2007,Jun,10-11

62225 Replacement or irrigation, ventricular catheter

Code also intracranial neuroendoscopic ventricular catheter insertion, when performed (62160)

15.1 | 15.1 | FUD 090 | J A2

AMA: 2018,Jan,8; 2017,Jan,8; 2016,Jan,13

62230 Replacement or revision of cerebrospinal fluid shunt, obstructed valve, or distal catheter in shunt system

Code also:

Intracranial neuroendoscopic ventricular catheter insertion, when performed (62160)

Proximal catheter and valve replacement, when performed (62225)

24.2 | 24.2 | FUD 090 | J A2 80

AMA: 2018,Jan,8; 2017,Jan,8; 2016,Jan,13

62252 Reprogramming of programmable cerebrospinal shunt

2.31 | 2.31 | FUD XXX | S P3 80

AMA: 2014,Jan,11; 2002,May,7

62256 Removal of complete cerebrospinal fluid shunt system; without replacement

EXCLUDES *Reprogramming cerebrospinal fluid (CSF) shunt (62252)*

17.5 | 17.5 | FUD 090 | C 80

AMA: 2014,Jan,11; 2002,May,7

62258 with replacement by similar or other shunt at same operation

EXCLUDES *Aspiration or irrigation shunt reservoir (61070)*

Reprogramming cerebrospinal fluid (CSF) shunt (62252)

Code also intracranial neuroendoscopic ventricular catheter insertion, when performed (62160)

32.0 | 32.0 | FUD 090 | C 80

AMA: 2018,Jan,8; 2017,Jan,8; 2016,Jan,13

62263-62264 Lysis of Epidural Lesions with Injection of Solution/Mechanical Methods

INCLUDES Fluoroscopic guidance (77003)

Percutaneous mechanical lysis

62263 Percutaneous lysis of epidural adhesions using solution injection (eg, hypertonic saline, enzyme) or mechanical means (eg, catheter) including radiologic localization (includes contrast when administered), multiple adhesiolysis sessions; 2 or more days

INCLUDES All adhesiolysis treatments, injections, and infusions during treatment course

Percutaneous epidural catheter insertion and removal for neurolytic agent injections during treatment sessions series

EXCLUDES *Procedure performed more than one time for complete series spanning two or more treatment days*

8.92 | 17.1 | FUD 010 | T A2

AMA: 2018,Jan,8; 2017,Jan,8; 2016,Jan,13

62264 1 day

INCLUDES Multiple treatment sessions performed same day

EXCLUDES *Percutaneous lysis epidural adhesions using solution injection,two or more treatment days (62263)*

6.89 | 12.2 | FUD 010 | T A2

AMA: 2018,Jan,8; 2017,Jan,8; 2016,Jan,13

62267-62269 Percutaneous Procedures of Spinal Cord

62267 Percutaneous aspiration within the nucleus pulposus, intervertebral disc, or paravertebral tissue for diagnostic purposes

EXCLUDES *Bone biopsy (20225)*

Decompression intervertebral disc (62287)

Fine needle aspiration ([10005, 10006, 10007, 10008, 10009, 10010, 10011, 10012])

Injection for discography (62290-62291)

Code also fluoroscopic guidance (77003)

4.55 | 7.34 | FUD 000 | T G2 80

AMA: 2019,Apr,4; 2018,Jan,8; 2017,Feb,12; 2017,Jan,8; 2016,Jan,13

62268 Percutaneous aspiration, spinal cord cyst or syrinx

(76942, 77002, 77012)

7.44 | 7.44 | FUD 000 | T A2

AMA: 2018,Jan,8; 2017,Dec,13

62269 Biopsy of spinal cord, percutaneous needle

EXCLUDES *Fine needle aspiration [(10005, 1006, 1007, 1008, 1009, 10010, 10011, 10012)]*

(76942, 77002, 77012)

(88172-88173)

7.66 | 7.66 | FUD 000 | J A2 80

AMA: 2019,Apr,4

62270-62329 [62328, 62329] Spinal Puncture, Subarachnoid Space, Diagnostic/Therapeutic

62270 **Spinal puncture, lumbar, diagnostic;**
EXCLUDES *Radiological guidance (77003, 77012)*
Code also ultrasound or MRI guidance (76942, 77021)
1.79 3.97 **FUD** 000 T A2
AMA: 2020,Jun,10; 2018,Jan,8; 2017,Jan,8; 2016,Jan,13

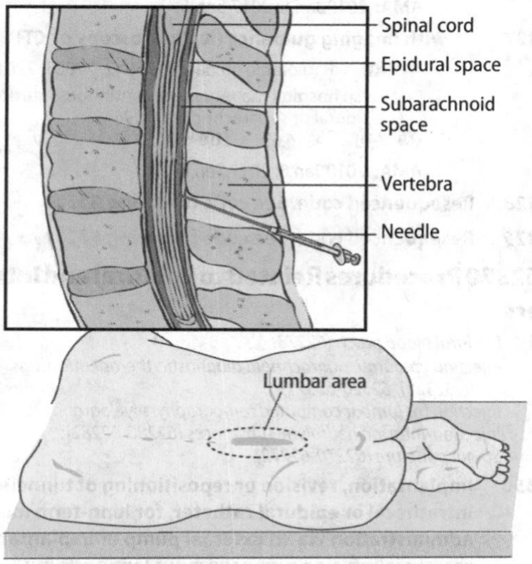

Common position to access vertebral interspace

\# **62328** **with fluoroscopic or CT guidance**
INCLUDES Radiological guidance (77003, 77012)
Code also ultrasound or MRI guidance (76942, 77021)
2.59 7.40 **FUD** 000 G2
AMA: 2020,Jun,10

62272 **Spinal puncture, therapeutic, for drainage of cerebrospinal fluid (by needle or catheter);**
EXCLUDES *Radiological guidance (77003, 77012)*
Code also ultrasound or MRI guidance (76942, 77021)
2.54 5.22 **FUD** 000 T A2
AMA: 2020,Jun,10; 2018,Jan,8; 2017,Jan,8; 2016,Jan,13

\# **62329** **with fluoroscopic or CT guidance**
INCLUDES Radiological guidance (77003, 77012)
Code also ultrasound or MRI guidance (76942, 77021)
3.26 9.19 **FUD** 000 G2
AMA: 2020,Jul,15; 2020,Jun,10

62273 Epidural Blood Patch

CMS: 100-03,10.5 NCD for Autogenous Epidural Blood Graft (10.5)
EXCLUDES *Injection diagnostic or therapeutic material (62320-62327)*
Code also fluoroscopic guidance (77003)

62273 **Injection, epidural, of blood or clot patch**
3.26 4.93 **FUD** 000 T A2
AMA: 2018,Jan,8; 2017,Jan,8; 2016,Jan,13

62280-62282 Neurolysis

INCLUDES Contrast injection during fluoroscopic guidance/localization
EXCLUDES *Injection diagnostic or therapeutic material only (62320-62327)*
Code also fluoroscopic guidance and localization unless formal contrast study performed (77003)

62280 **Injection/infusion of neurolytic substance (eg, alcohol, phenol, iced saline solutions), with or without other therapeutic substance; subarachnoid**
4.76 9.45 **FUD** 010 T A2
AMA: 2018,Jan,8; 2017,Jan,8; 2016,Jan,13

62281 **epidural, cervical or thoracic**
4.58 6.83 **FUD** 010 T A2
AMA: 2018,Jan,8; 2017,Jan,8; 2016,Jan,13

62282 **epidural, lumbar, sacral (caudal)**
4.13 8.76 **FUD** 010 T A2
AMA: 2018,Jan,8; 2017,Jan,8; 2016,Jan,13

62284-62294 Injection/Aspiration of Spine, Diagnostic/Therapeutic

62284 **Injection procedure for myelography and/or computed tomography, lumbar**
EXCLUDES *Injection C1-C2 (61055)*
Myelography (62302-62305, 72240, 72255, 72265, 72270)
Code also fluoroscopic guidance (77003)
2.50 5.66 **FUD** 000 N N1
AMA: 2018,Jan,8; 2017,Jan,8; 2016,Jan,13

62287 **Decompression procedure, percutaneous, of nucleus pulposus of intervertebral disc, any method utilizing needle based technique to remove disc material under fluoroscopic imaging or other form of indirect visualization, with discography and/or epidural injection(s) at the treated level(s), when performed, single or multiple levels, lumbar**
INCLUDES Endoscopic approach
EXCLUDES *Injection for discography (62290)*
Injection diagnostic or therapeutic substance(s) (62322)
Lumbar discography (72295)
Percutaneous aspiration, diagnostic (62267)
Percutaneous decompression nucleus pulposus intervertebral disc, non-needle based technique (0274T-0275T)
Radiological guidance (77003, 77012)
16.7 16.7 **FUD** 090 J A2
AMA: 2019,Dec,12; 2018,Jan,8; 2017,Feb,12; 2017,Jan,8; 2016,Jan,13

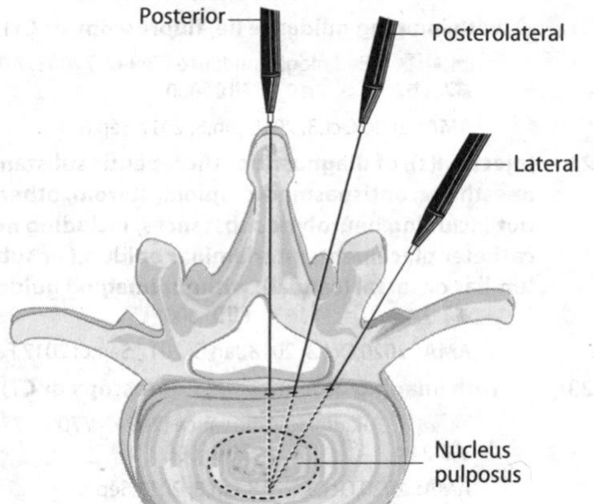

62290 **Injection procedure for discography, each level; lumbar**
(72295)
4.81 9.62 **FUD** 000 N N1
AMA: 2018,Jan,8; 2017,Feb,12; 2017,Jan,8; 2016,Jan,13

62291 **cervical or thoracic**
(72285)
4.57 9.55 **FUD** 000 N N1
AMA: 2018,Jan,8; 2017,Jan,8; 2016,Jan,13

62292 **Injection procedure for chemonucleolysis, including discography, intervertebral disc, single or multiple levels, lumbar**
16.6 16.6 **FUD** 090 J R2 80
AMA: 2018,Jan,8; 2017,Jan,8; 2016,Jan,13

62294 **Injection procedure, arterial, for occlusion of arteriovenous malformation, spinal**
27.3 27.3 **FUD** 090 T A2
AMA: 2014,Jan,11; 2000,Jan,1

62302-62305 Myelography

EXCLUDES *Injection C1-C2 (61055)*
Lumbar myelogram furnished by other providers (62284, 72240, 72255, 72265, 72270)

62302 Myelography via lumbar injection, including radiological supervision and interpretation; cervical
EXCLUDES *Myelography (62303-62305)*
3.53 6.91 FUD 000 Q2 N1

62303 thoracic
EXCLUDES *Myelography (62302, 62304-62305)*
3.53 7.07 FUD 000 Q2 N1

62304 lumbosacral
EXCLUDES *Myelography (62302-62303, 62305)*
3.46 6.82 FUD 000 Q2 N1

62305 2 or more regions (eg, lumbar/thoracic, cervical/thoracic, lumbar/cervical, lumbar/thoracic/cervical)
EXCLUDES *Myelography (62302-62305)*
3.60 7.65 FUD 000 Q2 N1

62320-62329 [62328, 62329] Injection/Infusion Diagnostic/Therapeutic Material

EXCLUDES *Reporting code more than one time even when catheter tip or injected drug travels into different spinal area*
Transforaminal epidural injection (64479-64484)

62320 Injection(s), of diagnostic or therapeutic substance(s) (eg, anesthetic, antispasmodic, opioid, steroid, other solution), not including neurolytic substances, including needle or catheter placement, interlaminar epidural or subarachnoid, cervical or thoracic; without imaging guidance
2.85 4.68 FUD 000 T G2
AMA: 2020,Oct,3; 2018,Jan,8; 2017,Sep,6

62321 with imaging guidance (ie, fluoroscopy or CT)
INCLUDES Radiologic guidance (76942, 77003, 77012)
3.07 7.19 FUD 000 T G2
AMA: 2020,Oct,3; 2018,Jan,8; 2017,Sep,6

62322 Injection(s), of diagnostic or therapeutic substance(s) (eg, anesthetic, antispasmodic, opioid, steroid, other solution), not including neurolytic substances, including needle or catheter placement, interlaminar epidural or subarachnoid, lumbar or sacral (caudal); without imaging guidance
2.46 4.36 FUD 000 T G2
AMA: 2020,Oct,3; 2018,Jan,8; 2017,Sep,6; 2017,Feb,12

62323 with imaging guidance (ie, fluoroscopy or CT)
INCLUDES Radiologic guidance (76942, 77003, 77012)
2.84 7.11 FUD 000 T G2
AMA: 2020,Oct,3; 2018,Jan,8; 2017,Sep,6

62324 Injection(s), including indwelling catheter placement, continuous infusion or intermittent bolus, of diagnostic or therapeutic substance(s) (eg, anesthetic, antispasmodic, opioid, steroid, other solution), not including neurolytic substances, interlaminar epidural or subarachnoid, cervical or thoracic; without imaging guidance
Code also hospital management continuous infusion drug, epidural or subarachnoid (01996)
2.60 4.12 FUD 000 T G2
AMA: 2018,Jan,8; 2017,Sep,6

62325 with imaging guidance (ie, fluoroscopy or CT)
INCLUDES Radiologic guidance (76942, 77003, 77012)
Code also hospital management continuous infusion drug, epidural or subarachnoid (01996)
3.08 6.67 FUD 000 T G2
AMA: 2018,Jan,8; 2017,Sep,6

62326 Injection(s), including indwelling catheter placement, continuous infusion or intermittent bolus, of diagnostic or therapeutic substance(s) (eg, anesthetic, antispasmodic, opioid, steroid, other solution), not including neurolytic substances, interlaminar epidural or subarachnoid, lumbar or sacral (caudal); without imaging guidance
Code also hospital management continuous infusion drug, epidural or subarachnoid (01996)
2.56 4.28 FUD 000 T G2
AMA: 2018,Jan,8; 2017,Sep,6

62327 with imaging guidance (ie, fluoroscopy or CT)
INCLUDES Radiologic guidance (76942, 77003, 77012)
Code also hospital management continuous infusion drug, epidural or subarachnoid (01996)
2.78 6.69 FUD 000 T G2
AMA: 2018,Jan,8; 2017,Sep,6

62328 **Resequenced code. See code following 62270.**

62329 **Resequenced code. See code following 62272.**

62350-62370 Procedures Related to Epidural and Intrathecal Catheters

EXCLUDES *Epidural blood patch (62273)*
Injection epidural/subarachnoid diagnostic/therapeutic drugs ([62328], [62329], 62320-62327)
Injection for lumbar computed tomography/myelography (62284)
Injection/infusion neurolytic substances (62280-62282)
Spinal puncture (62270-62272)

62350 Implantation, revision or repositioning of tunneled intrathecal or epidural catheter, for long-term medication administration via an external pump or implantable reservoir/infusion pump; without laminectomy
EXCLUDES *Maintenance and refilling infusion pumps for CNS drug therapy (95990-95991)*
11.5 11.5 FUD 010 J J8
AMA: 2018,Jan,8; 2017,Jan,8; 2016,Jan,13

62351 with laminectomy
EXCLUDES *Maintenance and refilling infusion pumps for CNS drug therapy (95990-95991)*
25.1 25.1 FUD 090 J G2 80
AMA: 2018,Jan,8; 2017,Jan,8; 2016,Jan,13

62355 Removal of previously implanted intrathecal or epidural catheter
7.79 7.79 FUD 010 Q2 A2 80
AMA: 2014,Jan,11; 1995,Win,1

62360 Implantation or replacement of device for intrathecal or epidural drug infusion; subcutaneous reservoir
9.13 9.13 FUD 010 J J8 80
AMA: 2014,Jan,11; 1995,Win,1

62361 nonprogrammable pump
12.5 12.5 FUD 010 J J8 80
AMA: 2014,Jan,11; 1995,Win,1

62362 programmable pump, including preparation of pump, with or without programming
11.0 11.0 FUD 010 J J8 80
AMA: 2018,Jan,8; 2017,Jan,8; 2016,Jan,13

62365 Removal of subcutaneous reservoir or pump, previously implanted for intrathecal or epidural infusion
8.48 8.48 FUD 010 Q2 A2 80
AMA: 2014,Jan,11; 1995,Win,1

62367 Electronic analysis of programmable, implanted pump for intrathecal or epidural drug infusion (includes evaluation of reservoir status, alarm status, drug prescription status); without reprogramming or refill
EXCLUDES *Maintenance and refilling infusion pumps for CNS drug therapy (95990-95991)*
0.72 1.14 FUD XXX S P3
AMA: 2018,Jan,8; 2017,Jan,8; 2016,Jan,13

62368 **with reprogramming**

EXCLUDES *Maintenance and refilling infusion pumps for CNS drug therapy (95990-95991)*

1.01 1.57 FUD XXX S P3

AMA: 2018,Jan,8; 2017,Jan,8; 2016,Jan,13

62369 **with reprogramming and refill**

EXCLUDES *Maintenance and refilling infusion pumps for CNS drug therapy (95990-95991)*

1.01 3.34 FUD XXX S P3

AMA: 2018,Jan,8; 2017,Jan,8; 2016,Jan,13

62370 **with reprogramming and refill (requiring skill of a physician or other qualified health care professional)**

EXCLUDES *Maintenance and refilling infusion pumps for CNS drug therapy (95990-95991)*

1.33 3.47 FUD XXX S P3

AMA: 2018,Jan,8; 2017,Jan,8; 2016,Jan,13

62380 Endoscopic Decompression/Laminectomy/Laminotomy

EXCLUDES *Open decompression (63030, 63056)*
Percutaneous decompression (62267, 0274T-0275T)

62380 **Endoscopic decompression of spinal cord, nerve root(s), including laminotomy, partial facetectomy, foraminotomy, discectomy and/or excision of herniated intervertebral disc, 1 interspace, lumbar**

0.00 0.00 FUD 090 J G2 80 50

AMA: 2018,Jan,8; 2017,Feb,12

63001-63053 [63052, 63053] Posterior Midline Approach: Laminectomy/Laminotomy/Decompression

INCLUDES Endoscopic assistance through open and direct visualization

EXCLUDES *Arthrodesis (22590-22614)*
Percutaneous decompression (62287, 0274T, 0275T)

63001 **Laminectomy with exploration and/or decompression of spinal cord and/or cauda equina, without facetectomy, foraminotomy or discectomy (eg, spinal stenosis), 1 or 2 vertebral segments; cervical**

35.7 35.7 FUD 090 J G2 80

AMA: 2018,Jan,8; 2017,Mar,7; 2017,Jan,8; 2016,Jan,13

63003 **thoracic**

35.7 35.7 FUD 090 J G2 80

AMA: 2018,Jan,8; 2017,Mar,7; 2017,Jan,8; 2016,Jan,13

63005 **lumbar, except for spondylolisthesis**

34.4 34.4 FUD 090 J G2 80

AMA: 2018,Jan,8; 2017,Mar,7; 2017,Feb,9; 2017,Jan,8; 2016,Jan,13

63011 **sacral**

31.6 31.6 FUD 090 J G2 80

AMA: 2018,Jan,8; 2017,Mar,7; 2017,Jan,8; 2016,Jan,13

63012 **Laminectomy with removal of abnormal facets and/or pars inter-articularis with decompression of cauda equina and nerve roots for spondylolisthesis, lumbar (Gill type procedure)**

34.6 34.6 FUD 090 J G2 80

AMA: 2019,Dec,12; 2018,Jan,8; 2017,Mar,7; 2017,Feb,9; 2017,Jan,8; 2016,Jan,13

63015 **Laminectomy with exploration and/or decompression of spinal cord and/or cauda equina, without facetectomy, foraminotomy or discectomy (eg, spinal stenosis), more than 2 vertebral segments; cervical**

42.7 42.7 FUD 090 J G2 80

AMA: 2018,Jan,8; 2017,Mar,7; 2017,Jan,8; 2016,Jan,13

63016 **thoracic**

44.3 44.3 FUD 090 J G2 80

AMA: 2018,Jan,8; 2017,Mar,7; 2017,Jan,8; 2016,Jan,13

63017 **lumbar**

36.7 36.7 FUD 090 J G2 80

AMA: 2018,Jan,8; 2017,Mar,7; 2017,Feb,9; 2017,Jan,8; 2016,Jan,13

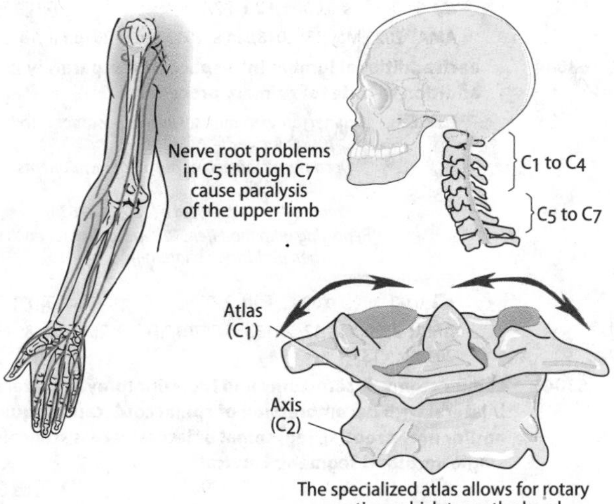

The specialized atlas allows for rotary motion, which turns the head

63020 **Laminotomy (hemilaminectomy), with decompression of nerve root(s), including partial facetectomy, foraminotomy and/or excision of herniated intervertebral disc; 1 interspace, cervical**

33.4 33.4 FUD 090 J G2 80 50

AMA: 2018,Jan,8; 2017,Mar,7; 2017,Jan,8; 2016,Jan,13

63030 **1 interspace, lumbar**

EXCLUDES *Laminectomy at same session as posterior interbody fusion for:*
Decompression nerves or spinal components ([63052])
Preparation of interspace (22630, 22633)

28.2 28.2 FUD 090 J G2 80 50

AMA: 2020,May,13; 2019,Nov,14; 2018,Jan,8; 2017,Mar,7; 2017,Feb,12; 2017,Feb,9; 2017,Jan,8; 2016,May,13; 2016,Jan,13

+ **63035** **each additional interspace, cervical or lumbar (List separately in addition to code for primary procedure)**

EXCLUDES *Laminectomy at same session as posterior interbody fusion for:*
Decompression nerves or spinal components ([63053])
Preparation of interspace (22632, 22634)
Reporting with modifier 50. Report once for each side when performed bilaterally

Code first (63020-63030)

5.55 5.55 FUD ZZZ N N1 80

AMA: 2018,Jan,8; 2017,Feb,9; 2017,Jan,8; 2016,Jan,13

63040 **Laminotomy (hemilaminectomy), with decompression of nerve root(s), including partial facetectomy, foraminotomy and/or excision of herniated intervertebral disc, reexploration, single interspace; cervical**

40.4 40.4 FUD 090 J G2 80 50

AMA: 2020,May,13; 2018,Jan,8; 2017,Mar,7; 2017,Jan,8; 2016,Jan,13

63042 **lumbar**

EXCLUDES *Laminectomy at same session as posterior interbody fusion for:*
Decompression nerves or spinal components ([63052])
Preparation of interspace (22630, 22633)

37.5 37.5 FUD 090 J G2 80 50

AMA: 2020,May,13; 2018,Jan,8; 2017,Mar,7; 2017,Feb,9; 2017,Jan,8; 2016,Jan,13

+ **63043** **each additional cervical interspace (List separately in addition to code for primary procedure)**

EXCLUDES *Reporting with modifier 50. Report once for each side when performed bilaterally*

Code first (63040)

0.00 0.00 FUD ZZZ N N1 80

AMA: 2020,May,13; 2018,Jan,8; 2017,Jan,8; 2016,Jan,13

+ **63044** **each additional lumbar interspace (List separately in addition to code for primary procedure)**

EXCLUDES *Laminectomy at same session as posterior interbody fusion for:*
Decompression nerves or spinal components ([63053])
Preparation of interspace (22632, 22634)
Reporting with modifier 50. Report once for each side when performed bilaterally

Code first (63042)

0.00 0.00 FUD ZZZ N N1 80

AMA: 2020,May,13; 2018,Jan,8; 2017,Feb,9; 2017,Jan,8; 2016,Jan,13

63045 **Laminectomy, facetectomy and foraminotomy (unilateral or bilateral with decompression of spinal cord, cauda equina and/or nerve root[s], [eg, spinal or lateral recess stenosis]), single vertebral segment; cervical**

37.1 37.1 FUD 090 J G2 80

AMA: 2018,Jan,8; 2017,Mar,7; 2017,Jan,8; 2016,Jan,13

63046 **thoracic**

35.4 35.4 FUD 090 J G2 80

AMA: 2018,Jan,8; 2017,Mar,7; 2017,Jan,8; 2016,Jan,13

63047 **lumbar**

EXCLUDES *Laminectomy, facetectomy or foraminotomy at same session as posterior interbody fusion for:*
Decompression nerves or spinal components ([63052])
Preparation of interspace (22630, 22633)

31.9 31.9 FUD 090 J G2 80

AMA: 2020,May,13; 2019,Dec,12; 2018,May,10; 2018,May,9; 2018,Jan,8; 2017,Mar,7; 2017,Feb,9; 2017,Feb,12; 2017,Jan,8; 2016,Oct,11; 2016,Jan,13

▲ + **63048** **each additional vertebral segment, cervical, thoracic, or lumbar (List separately in addition to code for primary procedure)**

EXCLUDES *Laminectomy, facetectomy or foraminotomy at same session as posterior interbody fusion for:*
Decompression nerves or spinal components ([63053])
Preparation of interspace (22632, 22634)

Code first (63045-63047)

6.13 6.13 FUD ZZZ N N1 80

AMA: 2018,Jan,8; 2017,Feb,9; 2017,Jan,8; 2016,Jan,13

● + # **63052** **Laminectomy, facetectomy, or foraminotomy (unilateral or bilateral with decompression of spinal cord, cauda equina and/or nerve root[s] [eg, spinal or lateral recess stenosis]), during posterior interbody arthrodesis, lumbar; single vertebral segment (List separately in addition to code for primary procedure)**

Code first (22630-22634)

0.00 0.00 FUD 000

● + # **63053** **each additional segment (List separately in addition to code for primary procedure)**

Code first (22630-22634, [63052])

0.00 0.00 FUD 000

63050-63051 Cervical Laminoplasty: Posterior Midline Approach

EXCLUDES *Procedure performed on same vertebral segment(s) (22600, 22614, 22840-22842, 63001, 63015, 63045, 63048, 63295)*

63050 **Laminoplasty, cervical, with decompression of the spinal cord, 2 or more vertebral segments;**

43.5 43.5 FUD 090 C 80

AMA: 2018,Jan,8; 2017,Mar,7; 2017,Jan,8; 2016,Jan,13

63051 **with reconstruction of the posterior bony elements (including the application of bridging bone graft and non-segmental fixation devices [eg, wire, suture, mini-plates], when performed)**

49.3 49.3 FUD 090 C 80

AMA: 2018,Jan,8; 2017,Mar,7; 2017,Jan,8; 2016,Jan,13

63052-63066 [63052, 63053] Spinal Cord/Nerve Root Decompression: Costovertebral or Transpedicular Approach

63052 **Resequenced code. See code following 63048.**

63053 **Resequenced code. See code following 63048.**

63055 **Transpedicular approach with decompression of spinal cord, equina and/or nerve root(s) (eg, herniated intervertebral disc), single segment; thoracic**

47.0 47.0 FUD 090 J G2 80

AMA: 2018,Jan,8; 2017,Mar,7; 2017,Jan,8; 2016,Jan,13

63056 **lumbar (including transfacet, or lateral extraforaminal approach) (eg, far lateral herniated intervertebral disc)**

EXCLUDES *Discectomy at same session as posterior interbody fusion for:*
Decompression nerves or spinal components ([63052])
Preparation of interspace (22630, 22633)

43.0 43.0 FUD 090 J G2 80

AMA: 2019,Nov,14; 2018,Jan,8; 2017,Mar,7; 2017,Feb,12; 2017,Jan,8; 2016,Jan,13

+ **63057** **each additional segment, thoracic or lumbar (List separately in addition to code for primary procedure)**

EXCLUDES *Discectomy at same session as posterior interbody fusion for:*
Decompression nerves or spinal components ([63053])
Preparation of interspace (22632, 22634)

Code first (63055-63056)

9.28 9.28 FUD ZZZ N N1 80

AMA: 2018,Jan,8; 2017,Jan,8; 2016,Jan,13

63064 **Costovertebral approach with decompression of spinal cord or nerve root(s) (eg, herniated intervertebral disc), thoracic; single segment**

EXCLUDES *Laminectomy with intraspinal thoracic lesion removal (63266, 63271, 63276, 63281, 63286)*

51.5 51.5 FUD 090 J G2 80

AMA: 2018,Jan,8; 2017,Mar,7; 2017,Jan,8; 2016,Jan,13

+ **63066** **each additional segment (List separately in addition to code for primary procedure)**

EXCLUDES *Laminectomy with intraspinal thoracic lesion removal (63266, 63271, 63276, 63281, 63286)*

Code first (63064)

5.97 5.97 FUD ZZZ N N1 80

AMA: 2014,Jan,11; 1996,Feb,6

63075-63078 Discectomy: Anterior or Anterolateral Approach

INCLUDES Operating microscope (69990)

63075 **Discectomy, anterior, with decompression of spinal cord and/or nerve root(s), including osteophytectomy; cervical, single interspace**

EXCLUDES *Anterior cervical discectomy and anterior interbody fusion at same level during same operative session (22551)*
Anterior interbody arthrodesis (even by another provider) (22554)

39.1 39.1 FUD 090 J G2 80

AMA: 2018,Jan,8; 2017,Mar,7; 2017,Jan,8; 2016,Feb,12; 2016,Jan,13

\+ **63076** **cervical, each additional interspace (List separately in addition to code for primary procedure)**

EXCLUDES *Anterior cervical discectomy and anterior interbody fusion at same level during same operative session (22552)*

Anterior interbody arthrodesis (even by another provider) (22554)

Code first (63075)

7.20 7.20 **FUD** ZZZ N N1 80

AMA: 2018,Jan,8; 2017,Jan,8; 2016,Feb,12; 2016,Jan,13

63077 **thoracic, single interspace**

44.2 44.2 **FUD** 090 C 80

AMA: 2018,Jan,8; 2017,Mar,7; 2017,Jan,8; 2016,Feb,12; 2016,Jan,13

\+ **63078** **thoracic, each additional interspace (List separately in addition to code for primary procedure)**

Code first (63077)

6.01 6.01 **FUD** ZZZ C 80

AMA: 2018,Jan,8; 2017,Jan,8; 2016,Feb,12; 2016,Jan,13

63081-63091 Vertebral Corpectomy, All Levels, Anterior Approach

INCLUDES Disc removal level below and/or above vertebral segment

Partial removal:

Cervical: Removal ≥ 1/2 vertebral body

Lumbar: Removal ≥ 1/3 vertebral body

Thoracic: Removal ≥ 1/3 vertebral body

EXCLUDES *Arthrodesis (22548-22812)*

Code also reconstruction (20930-20938, 22548-22812, 22840-22855 [22859])

63081 **Vertebral corpectomy (vertebral body resection), partial or complete, anterior approach with decompression of spinal cord and/or nerve root(s); cervical, single segment**

EXCLUDES *Transoral approach (61575-61576)*

50.9 50.9 **FUD** 090 C 80

AMA: 2018,Jan,8; 2017,Mar,7; 2017,Jan,8; 2016,Apr,8; 2016,Jan,13

\+ **63082** **cervical, each additional segment (List separately in addition to code for primary procedure)**

EXCLUDES *Transoral approach (61575-61576)*

Code first (63081)

7.72 7.72 **FUD** ZZZ C 80

AMA: 2018,Jan,8; 2017,Jan,8; 2016,Apr,8; 2016,Jan,13

63085 **Vertebral corpectomy (vertebral body resection), partial or complete, transthoracic approach with decompression of spinal cord and/or nerve root(s); thoracic, single segment**

55.7 55.7 **FUD** 090 C 80

AMA: 2018,Jan,8; 2017,Mar,7; 2017,Jan,8; 2016,Apr,8; 2016,Jan,13

\+ **63086** **thoracic, each additional segment (List separately in addition to code for primary procedure)**

Code first (63085)

5.53 5.53 **FUD** ZZZ C 80

AMA: 2018,Jan,8; 2017,Jan,8; 2016,Apr,8; 2016,Jan,13

63087 **Vertebral corpectomy (vertebral body resection), partial or complete, combined thoracolumbar approach with decompression of spinal cord, cauda equina or nerve root(s), lower thoracic or lumbar; single segment**

69.8 69.8 **FUD** 090 C 80

AMA: 2018,Jan,8; 2017,Mar,7; 2017,Jan,8; 2016,Apr,8; 2016,Jan,13

\+ **63088** **each additional segment (List separately in addition to code for primary procedure)**

Code first (63087)

7.43 7.43 **FUD** ZZZ C 80

AMA: 2018,Jan,8; 2017,Jan,8; 2016,Apr,8; 2016,Jan,13

63090 **Vertebral corpectomy (vertebral body resection), partial or complete, transperitoneal or retroperitoneal approach with decompression of spinal cord, cauda equina or nerve root(s), lower thoracic, lumbar, or sacral; single segment**

56.8 56.8 **FUD** 090 C 80

AMA: 2018,Jan,8; 2017,Mar,7; 2017,Jan,8; 2016,Apr,8; 2016,Jan,13

\+ **63091** **each additional segment (List separately in addition to code for primary procedure)**

Code first (63090)

5.18 5.18 **FUD** ZZZ C 80

AMA: 2018,Jan,8; 2017,Jan,8; 2016,Apr,8; 2016,Jan,13

63101-63103 Corpectomy: Lateral Extracavitary Approach

INCLUDES Partial removal:

Cervical: Removal ≥ 1/2 vertebral body

Lumbar: Removal ≥ 1/3 vertebral body

Thoracic: Removal ≥ 1/3 vertebral body

63101 **Vertebral corpectomy (vertebral body resection), partial or complete, lateral extracavitary approach with decompression of spinal cord and/or nerve root(s) (eg, for tumor or retropulsed bone fragments); thoracic, single segment**

67.2 67.2 **FUD** 090 C 80

AMA: 2018,Jan,8; 2017,Mar,7; 2017,Jan,8; 2016,Jan,13

63102 **lumbar, single segment**

65.5 65.5 **FUD** 090 C 80

AMA: 2018,Jan,8; 2017,Mar,7; 2017,Jan,8; 2016,Jan,13

\+ **63103** **thoracic or lumbar, each additional segment (List separately in addition to code for primary procedure)**

Code first (63101-63102)

8.53 8.53 **FUD** ZZZ C 80

AMA: 2014,Jan,11

63170-63295 Laminectomies

63170 **Laminectomy with myelotomy (eg, Bischof or DREZ type), cervical, thoracic, or thoracolumbar**

45.9 45.9 **FUD** 090 C 80

AMA: 2018,Jan,8; 2017,Mar,7; 2017,Jan,8; 2016,Jan,13

63172 **Laminectomy with drainage of intramedullary cyst/syrinx; to subarachnoid space**

40.0 40.0 **FUD** 090 C 80

AMA: 2018,Jan,8; 2017,Mar,7; 2017,Jan,8; 2016,Jan,13

63173 **to peritoneal or pleural space**

49.7 49.7 **FUD** 090 C 80

AMA: 2018,Jan,8; 2017,Mar,7; 2017,Jan,8; 2016,Jan,13

63185 **Laminectomy with rhizotomy; 1 or 2 segments**

INCLUDES Dana rhizotomy

Stoffel rhizotomy

33.1 33.1 **FUD** 090 C 80

AMA: 2018,Jan,8; 2017,Mar,7; 2017,Jan,8; 2016,Jan,13

63190 **more than 2 segments**

36.0 36.0 **FUD** 090 C 80

AMA: 2018,Jan,8; 2017,Mar,7; 2017,Jan,8; 2016,Jan,13

63191 **Laminectomy with section of spinal accessory nerve**

EXCLUDES *Division sternocleidomastoid muscle for torticollis (21720)*

39.7 39.7 **FUD** 090 C 80 50

AMA: 2018,Jan,8; 2017,Mar,7; 2017,Jan,8; 2016,Jan,13

~~**63194** **Laminectomy with cordotomy, with section of 1 spinothalamic tract, 1 stage; cervical**~~

~~**63195** **thoracic**~~

~~**63196** **Laminectomy with cordotomy, with section of both spinothalamic tracts, 1 stage; cervical**~~

▲ **63197** **Laminectomy with cordotomy, with section of both spinothalamic tracts, 1 stage, thoracic**

49.3 49.3 **FUD** 090 C 80

AMA: 2018,Jan,8; 2017,Mar,7; 2017,Jan,8; 2016,Jan,13

~~**63198 Laminectomy with cordotomy with section of both spinothalamic tracts, 2 stages within 14 days; cervical**~~

63199 thoracic

63200 Laminectomy, with release of tethered spinal cord, lumbar
44.1 44.1 **FUD** 090 C 80
AMA: 2018,Jan,8; 2017,Mar,7; 2017,Jan,8; 2016,Jan,13

63250 Laminectomy for excision or occlusion of arteriovenous malformation of spinal cord; cervical
87.8 87.8 **FUD** 090 C 80
AMA: 2018,Jan,8; 2017,Mar,7; 2017,Jan,8; 2016,Jan,13

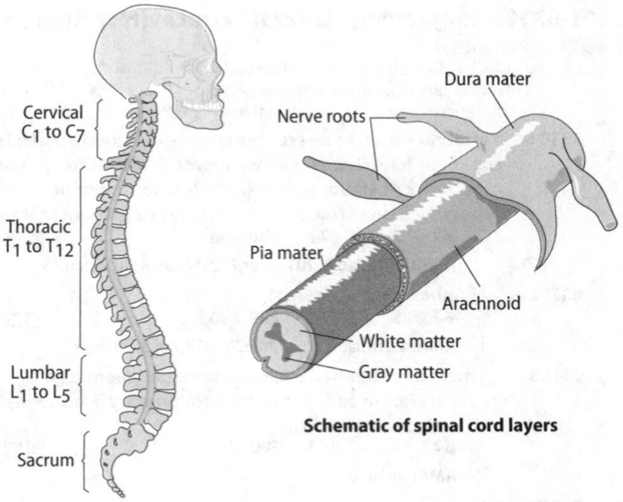

Schematic of spinal cord layers

63251 thoracic
87.8 87.8 **FUD** 090 C 80
AMA: 2018,Jan,8; 2017,Mar,7; 2017,Jan,8; 2016,Jan,13

63252 thoracolumbar
87.8 87.8 **FUD** 090 C 80
AMA: 2018,Jan,8; 2017,Mar,7; 2017,Jan,8; 2016,Jan,13

63265 Laminectomy for excision or evacuation of intraspinal lesion other than neoplasm, extradural; cervical
48.2 48.2 **FUD** 090 C 80
AMA: 2018,Jan,8; 2017,Mar,7; 2017,Jan,8; 2016,Jan,13

63266 thoracic
49.7 49.7 **FUD** 090 C 80
AMA: 2017,Mar,7

63267 lumbar
39.6 39.6 **FUD** 090 C 80
AMA: 2018,Jan,8; 2017,Mar,7; 2017,Jan,8; 2016,Jan,13

63268 sacral
40.9 40.9 **FUD** 090 C 80
AMA: 2018,Jan,8; 2017,Mar,7; 2017,Jan,8; 2016,Jan,13

63270 Laminectomy for excision of intraspinal lesion other than neoplasm, intradural; cervical
60.4 60.4 **FUD** 090 C 80
AMA: 2018,Jan,8; 2017,Mar,7; 2017,Jan,8; 2016,Jan,13

63271 thoracic
59.8 59.8 **FUD** 090 C 80
AMA: 2018,Jan,8; 2017,Mar,7; 2017,Jan,8; 2016,Jan,13

63272 lumbar
54.5 54.5 **FUD** 090 C 80
AMA: 2018,Jan,8; 2017,Mar,7; 2017,Jan,8; 2016,Jan,13

63273 sacral
53.8 53.8 **FUD** 090 C 80
AMA: 2018,Jan,8; 2017,Mar,7; 2017,Jan,8; 2016,Jan,13

63275 Laminectomy for biopsy/excision of intraspinal neoplasm; extradural, cervical
52.1 52.1 **FUD** 090 C 80
AMA: 2018,Jan,8; 2017,Mar,7; 2017,Jan,8; 2016,Jan,13

63276 extradural, thoracic
51.7 51.7 **FUD** 090 C 80
AMA: 2018,Jan,8; 2017,Mar,7; 2017,Jan,8; 2016,Jan,13

63277 extradural, lumbar
45.0 45.0 **FUD** 090 C 80
AMA: 2018,Jan,8; 2017,Mar,7; 2017,Jan,8; 2016,Jan,13

63278 extradural, sacral
45.9 45.9 **FUD** 090 C 80
AMA: 2018,Jan,8; 2017,Mar,7; 2017,Jan,8; 2016,Jan,13

63280 intradural, extramedullary, cervical
61.2 61.2 **FUD** 090 C 80
AMA: 2018,Jan,8; 2017,Mar,7; 2017,Jan,8; 2016,Jan,13

63281 intradural, extramedullary, thoracic
60.5 60.5 **FUD** 090 C 80
AMA: 2018,Jan,8; 2017,Mar,7; 2017,Jan,8; 2016,Jan,13

63282 intradural, extramedullary, lumbar
57.7 57.7 **FUD** 090 C 80
AMA: 2018,Jan,8; 2017,Mar,7; 2017,Jan,8; 2016,Jan,13

63283 intradural, sacral
55.3 55.3 **FUD** 090 C 80
AMA: 2018,Jan,8; 2017,Mar,7; 2017,Jan,8; 2016,Jan,13

63285 intradural, intramedullary, cervical
77.2 77.2 **FUD** 090 C 80
AMA: 2018,Jan,8; 2017,Mar,7; 2017,Jan,8; 2016,Jan,13

63286 intradural, intramedullary, thoracic
74.7 74.7 **FUD** 090 C 80
AMA: 2018,Jan,8; 2017,Mar,7; 2017,Jan,8; 2016,Jan,13

63287 intradural, intramedullary, thoracolumbar
80.1 80.1 **FUD** 090 C 80
AMA: 2018,Jan,8; 2017,Mar,7; 2017,Jan,8; 2016,Jan,13

63290 combined extradural-intradural lesion, any level
EXCLUDES *Drainage intramedullary cyst or syrinx (63172-63173)*
80.7 80.7 **FUD** 090 C 80
AMA: 2018,Jan,8; 2017,Mar,7; 2017,Jan,8; 2016,Jan,13

\+ **63295 Osteoplastic reconstruction of dorsal spinal elements, following primary intraspinal procedure (List separately in addition to code for primary procedure)**
EXCLUDES *Procedure performed same vertebral segment(s) (22590-22614, 22840-22844, 63050-63051)*
Code first (63172-63173, 63185, 63190, 63200-63290)
9.76 9.76 **FUD** ZZZ C 80
AMA: 2014,Jan,11

63300-63308 Vertebral Corpectomy for Intraspinal Lesion: Anterior/Anterolateral Approach

INCLUDES Partial removal:
- Cervical: Removal ≥ 1/2 vertebral body
- Lumbar: Removal ≥ 1/3 vertebral body
- Thoracic: Removal ≥ 1/3 vertebral body

EXCLUDES *Arthrodesis (22548-22585)*
Spinal reconstruction (20930-20938)

63300 Vertebral corpectomy (vertebral body resection), partial or complete, for excision of intraspinal lesion, single segment; extradural, cervical
53.1 53.1 **FUD** 090 C 80
AMA: 2018,Jan,8; 2017,Mar,7; 2017,Jan,8; 2016,Jan,13

63301 extradural, thoracic by transthoracic approach
63.7 63.7 **FUD** 090 C 80
AMA: 2018,Jan,8; 2017,Mar,7; 2017,Jan,8; 2016,Jan,13

63302 extradural, thoracic by thoracolumbar approach
62.9 62.9 **FUD** 090 C 80
AMA: 2018,Jan,8; 2017,Mar,7; 2017,Jan,8; 2016,Jan,13

63303 **extradural, lumbar or sacral by transperitoneal or retroperitoneal approach**
63.1 63.1 FUD 090 C 80
AMA: 2018,Jan,8; 2017,Mar,7; 2017,Jan,8; 2016,Jan,13

63304 **intradural, cervical**
67.8 67.8 FUD 090 C 80
AMA: 2018,Jan,8; 2017,Mar,7; 2017,Jan,8; 2016,Jan,13

63305 **intradural, thoracic by transthoracic approach**
73.7 73.7 FUD 090 C 80
AMA: 2018,Jan,8; 2017,Mar,7; 2017,Jan,8; 2016,Jan,13

63306 **intradural, thoracic by thoracolumbar approach**
71.0 71.0 FUD 090 C 80
AMA: 2018,Jan,8; 2017,Mar,7; 2017,Jan,8; 2016,Jan,13

63307 **intradural, lumbar or sacral by transperitoneal or retroperitoneal approach**
69.5 69.5 FUD 090 C 80
AMA: 2018,Jan,8; 2017,Mar,7; 2017,Jan,8; 2016,Jan,13

\+ **63308** **each additional segment (List separately in addition to codes for single segment)**
Code first (63300-63307)
9.37 9.37 FUD ZZZ C 80
AMA: 2014,Jan,11; 2002,Feb,4

63600-63610 Stereotactic Procedures of the Spinal Cord

63600 **Creation of lesion of spinal cord by stereotactic method, percutaneous, any modality (including stimulation and/or recording)**
32.0 32.0 FUD 090 J A2 80
AMA: 2014,Jan,11; 2000,Dec,12

63610 **Stereotactic stimulation of spinal cord, percutaneous, separate procedure not followed by other surgery**
17.1 17.1 FUD 000 J J8 80
AMA: 2014,Jan,11

63620-63621 Stereotactic Radiosurgery (SRS): Spine

INCLUDES Computer assisted planning
Planning dosimetry, targeting, positioning, or blocking by neurosurgeon

EXCLUDES *Arteriovenous malformations (see Radiation Oncology Section)*
Intensity modulated beam delivery plan and treatment (77301, 77385-77386)
Radiation treatment management by same provider (77427-77432)
Stereotactic body radiation therapy (77373, 77435)
Stereotactic computer-assisted procedures (61781-61783)
Treatment planning, physics, dosimetry, treatment delivery and management provided by radiation oncologist (77261-77790 [77295, 77385, 77386, 77387, 77424, 77425])

63620 **Stereotactic radiosurgery (particle beam, gamma ray, or linear accelerator); 1 spinal lesion**
EXCLUDES *Reporting code more than one time per entire treatment course*
32.2 32.2 FUD 090 B 80
AMA: 2018,Jan,8; 2017,Jan,8; 2016,Jan,13

\+ **63621** **each additional spinal lesion (List separately in addition to code for primary procedure)**
EXCLUDES *Reporting code more than one time per lesion*
Reporting code more than two times per entire treatment course
Code first (63620)
7.30 7.30 FUD ZZZ B 80
AMA: 2018,Jan,8; 2017,Jan,8; 2016,Jan,13

63650-63688 Spinal Neurostimulation

INCLUDES Analysis system at implantation (95970)
Complex and simple neurostimulators

EXCLUDES *Analysis and programming neurostimulator pulse generator (95970-95972)*

63650 **Percutaneous implantation of neurostimulator electrode array, epidural**
INCLUDES Neurostimulator system components:
Multiple contacts which four or more provide electrical stimulation in epidural space
Contacts on catheter-type lead (array)
Extension
External controller
Implanted neurostimulator
11.9 54.1 FUD 010 J J8
AMA: 2019,Feb,6; 2018,Oct,11; 2018,Jan,8; 2017,Dec,13; 2017,Jan,8; 2016,Jan,13; 2016,Jan,11

63655 **Laminectomy for implantation of neurostimulator electrodes, plate/paddle, epidural**
INCLUDES Neurostimulator system components:
Multiple contacts which four or more provide electrical stimulation in epidural space
Contacts on catheter-type lead (array)
Extension
External controller
Implanted neurostimulator
24.0 24.0 FUD 090 J J8 80
AMA: 2020,Dec,13; 2019,Feb,6; 2018,Jan,8; 2017,Jan,8; 2016,Jan,13

63661 **Removal of spinal neurostimulator electrode percutaneous array(s), including fluoroscopy, when performed**
INCLUDES Neurostimulator system components:
Multiple contacts which four or more provide electrical stimulation in epidural space
Contacts on catheter-type lead (array)
Extension
External controller
Implanted neurostimulator
EXCLUDES *Reporting code when removing or replacing temporary array placed percutaneously for external generator*
9.33 18.3 FUD 010 Q2 G2 80
AMA: 2019,Feb,6; 2018,Jan,8; 2017,Jan,8; 2016,Jan,13

63662 **Removal of spinal neurostimulator electrode plate/paddle(s) placed via laminotomy or laminectomy, including fluoroscopy, when performed**
INCLUDES Neurostimulator system components:
Multiple contacts which four or more provide electrical stimulation in epidural space
Contacts on catheter-type lead (array)
Extension
External controller
Implanted neurostimulator
24.3 24.3 FUD 090 Q2 G2 80
AMA: 2020,Dec,13; 2019,Feb,6; 2018,Jan,8; 2017,Jan,8; 2016,Jan,13

63663 **Revision including replacement, when performed, of spinal neurostimulator electrode percutaneous array(s), including fluoroscopy, when performed**
INCLUDES Neurostimulator system components:
Multiple contacts which four or more provide electrical stimulation in epidural space
Contacts on catheter-type lead (array)
Extension
External controller
Implanted neurostimulator
EXCLUDES *Removal of spinal neurostimulator electrode percutaneous array(s), plate/paddle(s) at same level (63661-63662)*
Reporting code when removing or replacing temporary array placed percutaneously for external generator
12.9 23.4 FUD 010 J J8 80
AMA: 2019,Feb,6; 2018,Jan,8; 2017,Jan,8; 2016,Jan,13

63664 **Revision including replacement, when performed, of spinal neurostimulator electrode plate/paddle(s) placed via laminotomy or laminectomy, including fluoroscopy, when performed**

INCLUDES Neurostimulator system components:
- Multiple contacts which four or more provide electrical stimulation in epidural space
- Contacts on catheter-type lead (array)
- Extension
- External controller
- Implanted neurostimulator

EXCLUDES *Removal spinal neurostimulator electrode percutaneous array(s), plate/paddle(s) at same level (63661-63662)*

25.2 25.2 **FUD** 090 J J8 80

AMA: 2019,Feb,6; 2018,Jan,8; 2017,Jan,8; 2016,Jan,13

63685 **Insertion or replacement of spinal neurostimulator pulse generator or receiver, direct or inductive coupling**

EXCLUDES *Reporting code for insertion/replacement with code for revision/removal (63688)*

10.3 10.3 **FUD** 010 J J8 80

AMA: 2019,Feb,6; 2018,Jan,8; 2017,Dec,13; 2017,Jan,8; 2016,Jan,13

63688 **Revision or removal of implanted spinal neurostimulator pulse generator or receiver**

EXCLUDES *Reporting code for revision/removal with code for insertion/replacement (63685)*

10.7 10.7 **FUD** 010 Q2 A2 80

AMA: 2019,Feb,6; 2018,Jan,8; 2017,Jan,8; 2016,Jan,13

63700-63706 Repair Congenital Neural Tube Defects

EXCLUDES *Complex skin repair (see appropriate integumentary closure code)*

63700 **Repair of meningocele; less than 5 cm diameter**

37.6 37.6 **FUD** 090 63 C 80

AMA: 2014,Jan,11

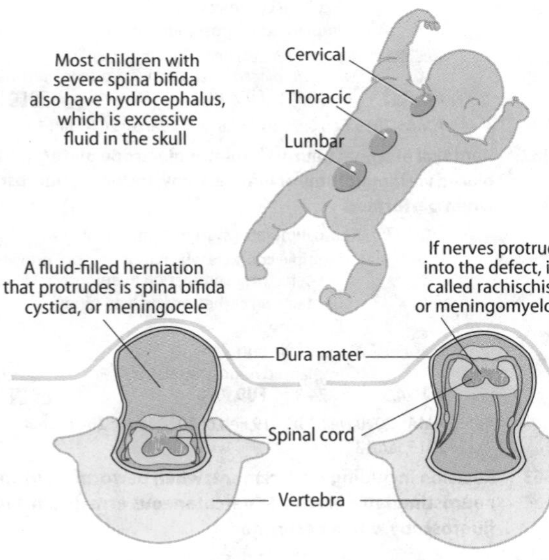
Most children with severe spina bifida also have hydrocephalus, which is excessive fluid in the skull
Cervical
Thoracic
Lumbar
A fluid-filled herniation that protrudes is spina bifida cystica, or meningocele
If nerves protrude into the defect, it is called rachischisis, or meningomyelocele
Dura mater
Spinal cord
Vertebra

63702 **larger than 5 cm diameter**

41.8 41.8 **FUD** 090 63 C 80

AMA: 2014,Jan,11

63704 **Repair of myelomeningocele; less than 5 cm diameter**

47.7 47.7 **FUD** 090 63 C 80

AMA: 2014,Jan,11

63706 **larger than 5 cm diameter**

53.1 53.1 **FUD** 090 63 C 80

AMA: 2014,Jan,11

63707-63710 Repair Dural Cerebrospinal Fluid Leak

63707 **Repair of dural/cerebrospinal fluid leak, not requiring laminectomy**

26.8 26.8 **FUD** 090 C 80

AMA: 2014,Jan,11; 2002,May,7

63709 **Repair of dural/cerebrospinal fluid leak or pseudomeningocele, with laminectomy**

32.0 32.0 **FUD** 090 C 80

AMA: 2014,Jan,11; 2002,May,7

63710 **Dural graft, spinal**

31.6 31.6 **FUD** 090 C 80

AMA: 2014,Jan,11

63740-63746 Cerebrospinal Fluid (CSF) Shunt: Lumbar

EXCLUDES *Placement subarachnoid catheter with reservoir and/or pump:*
- *Not requiring laminectomy (62350, 62360-62362)*
- *With laminectomy (62351, 62360-62362)*

63740 **Creation of shunt, lumbar, subarachnoid-peritoneal, -pleural, or other; including laminectomy**

28.1 28.1 **FUD** 090 C 80

AMA: 2014,Jan,11; 2000,Dec,12

63741 **percutaneous, not requiring laminectomy**

19.7 19.7 **FUD** 090 J J8 80

AMA: 2014,Jan,11; 1990,Win,4

63744 **Replacement, irrigation or revision of lumbosubarachnoid shunt**

19.5 19.5 **FUD** 090 J J8 80

AMA: 2014,Jan,11

63746 **Removal of entire lumbosubarachnoid shunt system without replacement**

17.3 17.3 **FUD** 090 Q2 A2 80

AMA: 2014,Jan,11

64400-64484 [64461, 64462, 64463] Nerve Blocks and Transforaminal Injections

EXCLUDES *Epidural or subarachnoid injection (62320-62327)*
Nerve destruction (62280-62282, 64600-64681 [64624, 64625, 64633, 64634, 64635, 64636])
Reporting code more than one time per encounter when multiple injections required to block nerve and branches

Code also imaging guidance and localization, when performed, except with (64451, 64454, 64479-64480, 64483-64484)

64400 **Injection(s), anesthetic agent(s) and/or steroid; trigeminal nerve, each branch (ie, ophthalmic, maxillary, mandibular)**

1.44 3.05 **FUD** 000 T P3 50

AMA: 2018,Jan,8; 2017,Jan,8; 2016,Jan,13

64405 **greater occipital nerve**

1.55 2.07 **FUD** 000 T P3 50

AMA: 2018,Jan,8; 2017,Jan,8; 2016,Oct,11; 2016,Jan,13

64408 **vagus nerve**

2.44 3.35 **FUD** 000 T P3 80 50

AMA: 2018,Jan,8; 2017,Jan,8; 2016,Jan,13

64415 **brachial plexus**

1.83 3.22 **FUD** 000 T A2 50

AMA: 2018,Jan,8; 2017,Jan,8; 2016,Jan,13

64416 **brachial plexus, continuous infusion by catheter (including catheter placement)**

EXCLUDES *Management epidural or subarachnoid continuous drug administration (01996)*

1.85 1.85 **FUD** 000 T G2 50

AMA: 2018,Jan,8; 2017,Jan,8; 2016,Jan,13

64417 **axillary nerve**

2.02 3.76 **FUD** 000 T A2 50

AMA: 2018,Jan,8; 2017,Jan,8; 2016,Jan,13

64418 **suprascapular nerve**

1.64 2.42 **FUD** 000 T P3 50

AMA: 2018,Jan,8; 2017,Jan,8; 2016,Jan,13

64420 **intercostal nerve, single level**
1.72 | 2.85 | FUD 000 | T A2 50
AMA: 2018,Jan,8; 2017,Jan,8; 2016,Jan,9; 2016,Jan,13

+ **64421** **intercostal nerve, each additional level (List separately in addition to code for primary procedure)**
EXCLUDES *Reporting with modifier 50. Report once for each side when performed bilaterally*
Code first (64420)
0.73 | 0.97 | FUD ZZZ | T A2
AMA: 2018,Jan,8; 2017,Jan,8; 2016,Jan,9; 2016,Jan,13

64425 **ilioinguinal, iliohypogastric nerves**
1.60 | 3.19 | FUD 000 | T P3 50
AMA: 2018,Jan,8; 2017,Jan,8; 2016,Jan,13

64430 **pudendal nerve**
2.30 | 4.14 | FUD 000 | T A2 50
AMA: 2018,Jan,8; 2017,Jan,8; 2016,Jan,13

64435 **paracervical (uterine) nerve** ♀
1.26 | 2.09 | FUD 000 | T P3 50
AMA: 2018,Jan,8; 2017,Jan,8; 2016,Jan,13

64445 **sciatic nerve**
2.09 | 3.89 | FUD 000 | T P3 50
AMA: 2018,Jan,8; 2017,Jan,8; 2016,Jan,13

64446 **sciatic nerve, continuous infusion by catheter (including catheter placement)**
EXCLUDES *Management epidural or subarachnoid continuous drug administration (01996)*
2.28 | 2.28 | FUD 000 | T G2 50
AMA: 2018,Jan,8; 2017,Jan,8; 2016,Jan,13

64447 **femoral nerve**
EXCLUDES *Injection genicular nerve branches (64454)*
Management epidural or subarachnoid continuous drug administration (01996)
1.91 | 3.46 | FUD 000 | T P3 50
AMA: 2018,Jan,8; 2017,Jan,8; 2016,Jan,13

64448 **femoral nerve, continuous infusion by catheter (including catheter placement)**
EXCLUDES *Injection genicular nerve branches (64454)*
Management epidural or subarachnoid continuous drug administration (01996)
2.05 | 2.05 | FUD 000 | T G2 50
AMA: 2018,Jan,8; 2017,Jan,8; 2016,Jan,13

64449 **lumbar plexus, posterior approach, continuous infusion by catheter (including catheter placement)**
EXCLUDES *Management epidural or subarachnoid continuous drug administration (01996)*
1.79 | 1.79 | FUD 000 | T G2 50
AMA: 2018,Jan,8; 2017,Jan,8; 2016,Jan,13

64450 **other peripheral nerve or branch**
EXCLUDES *Injection genicular nerve branches (64454)*
Injection nerves innervating the sacroiliac joint (64451)
1.28 | 2.19 | FUD 000 | T P3 50
AMA: 2019,Nov,14; 2018,Nov,10; 2018,Jan,8; 2017,Jan,8; 2016,Oct,11; 2016,Jan,13

64451 **nerves innervating the sacroiliac joint, with image guidance (ie, fluoroscopy or computed tomography)**
INCLUDES Imaging guidance and any contrast injection
EXCLUDES *Injection nerves innervating paravertebral facet joint (64493-64495)*
Injection with ultrasound (76999)
2.29 | 5.99 | FUD 000 | G2 50
AMA: 2020,Jul,13

64454 **genicular nerve branches, including imaging guidance, when performed**
INCLUDES Articular branches of the following innervating the knee joint:
Common peroneal
Femoral
Obturator
Saphenous
Tibial
Imaging guidance and any contrast injection
Code also modifier 52 for injection fewer than following all genicular nerve branches: superolateral, superomedial, and inferomedial
2.36 | 6.05 | FUD 000 | P3 50
AMA: 2020,Dec,13; 2019,Dec,8

64455 **plantar common digital nerve(s) (eg, Morton's neuroma)**
INCLUDES Single or multiple injections on the same site
EXCLUDES *Destruction by neurolytic agent; plantar common digital nerve (64632)*
Code also imaging guidance and localization, when performed
1.00 | 1.36 | FUD 000 | T P3 80 50
AMA: 2018,Jan,8; 2017,Jan,8; 2016,Jan,13

64461 **Resequenced code. See code following 64484.**

64462 **Resequenced code. See code following 64484.**

64463 **Resequenced code. See code following 64484.**

64479 **transforaminal epidural, with imaging guidance (fluoroscopy or CT), cervical or thoracic, single level**
INCLUDES Imaging guidance (fluoroscopy or CT) and contrast injection
Single or multiple injections same site
Transforaminal epidural injection T12-L1 level
3.76 | 6.95 | FUD 000 | T A2 50
AMA: 2018,Jan,8; 2017,Jan,8; 2016,Jan,13; 2016,Jan,9

Thoracic vertebra (superior view)

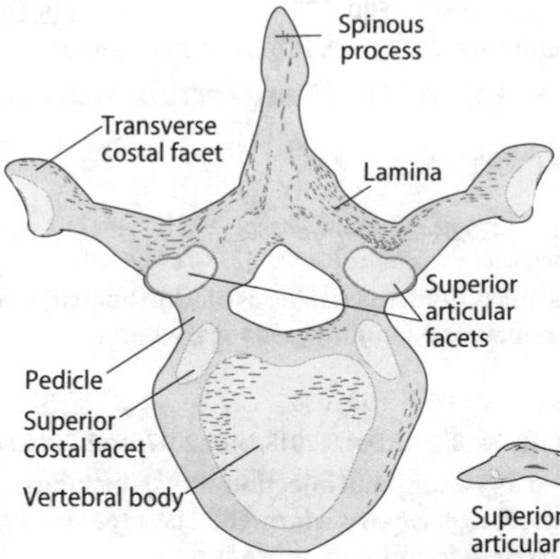

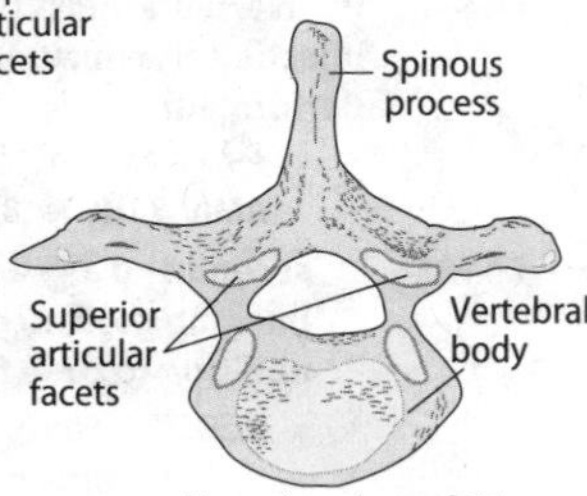

Superior view of C7

\+ 64480 **transforaminal epidural, with imaging guidance (fluoroscopy or CT), cervical or thoracic, each additional level (List separately in addition to code for primary procedure)**

INCLUDES Imaging guidance (fluoroscopy or CT) and contrast injection
Single or multiple injections same site

EXCLUDES *Destruction genicular nerve branches ([64624])*
Injection genicular nerve branches (64454)
Reporting with modifier 50. Report once for each side when performed bilaterally
Transforaminal epidural injection T12-L1 level

Code first (64479)

1.80 | 3.42 | FUD ZZZ | N N1

AMA: 2018,Jan,8; 2017,Jan,8; 2016,Jan,9; 2016,Jan,13

64483 **transforaminal epidural, with imaging guidance (fluoroscopy or CT), lumbar or sacral, single level**

INCLUDES Imaging guidance (fluoroscopy or CT) and contrast injection
Single or multiple injections same site

EXCLUDES *Destruction genicular nerve branches ([64624])*
Injection genicular nerve branches (64454)

3.19 | 6.44 | FUD 000 | T A2 50

AMA: 2018,Jan,8; 2017,Jan,8; 2016,Oct,11; 2016,Jan,13; 2016,Jan,9

\+ 64484 **transforaminal epidural, with imaging guidance (fluoroscopy or CT), lumbar or sacral, each additional level (List separately in addition to code for primary procedure)**

INCLUDES Imaging guidance (fluoroscopy or CT) and contrast injection
Single or multiple injections same site

EXCLUDES *Destruction genicular nerve branches ([64624])*
Injection genicular nerve branches (64454)
Reporting with modifier 50. Report once for each side when performed bilaterally

Code first (64483)

1.49 | 2.62 | FUD ZZZ | N N1

AMA: 2018,Jan,8; 2017,Jan,8; 2016,Jan,9; 2016,Jan,13

64461-64463 [64461, 64462, 64463] Paravertebral Blocks

INCLUDES Contrast injection
Imaging guidance (76942, 77002-77003)

EXCLUDES *Injection:*
Anesthetic agent (64420-64421, 64479-64480)
Diagnostic or therapeutic substance (62320, 62324, 64490-64492)

\# 64461 **Paravertebral block (PVB) (paraspinous block), thoracic; single injection site (includes imaging guidance, when performed)**

2.33 | 3.96 | FUD 000 | T G2 50

AMA: 2018,Dec,8; 2018,Dec,8; 2018,Jan,8; 2017,Jan,8; 2016,Jan,9

\+ # 64462 **second and any additional injection site(s) (includes imaging guidance, when performed) (List separately in addition to code for primary procedure)**

EXCLUDES *Procedure performed more than one time per day*
Reporting with modifier 50. Report once for each side when performed bilaterally

Code first (64461)

1.47 | 2.20 | FUD ZZZ | N N1 50

AMA: 2018,Dec,8; 2018,Dec,8; 2018,Jan,8; 2017,Jan,8; 2016,Jan,9

\# 64463 **continuous infusion by catheter (includes imaging guidance, when performed)**

2.42 | 5.13 | FUD 000 | T G2 50

AMA: 2018,Dec,8; 2018,Dec,8; 2018,Jan,8; 2017,Jan,8; 2016,Jan,9

64486-64489 Transversus Abdominis Plane (TAP) Block

INCLUDES Imaging guidance and any contrast injection

64486 **Transversus abdominis plane (TAP) block (abdominal plane block, rectus sheath block) unilateral; by injection(s) (includes imaging guidance, when performed)**

1.61 | 3.12 | FUD 000 | N N1 50

AMA: 2018,Jan,8; 2017,Jan,8; 2016,Jan,13

64487 **by continuous infusion(s) (includes imaging guidance, when performed)**

1.91 | 3.80 | FUD 000 | N N1 50

AMA: 2018,Jan,8; 2017,Jan,8; 2016,Jan,13

64488 **Transversus abdominis plane (TAP) block (abdominal plane block, rectus sheath block) bilateral; by injections (includes imaging guidance, when performed)**

2.05 | 3.83 | FUD 000 | N N1

AMA: 2018,Jan,8; 2017,Jan,8; 2016,Jan,13

64489 **by continuous infusions (includes imaging guidance, when performed)**

2.28 | 5.19 | FUD 000 | N N1

AMA: 2018,Jan,8; 2017,Jan,8; 2016,Jan,13

64490-64495 Paraspinal Nerve Injections

INCLUDES Image guidance (CT or fluoroscopy) and any contrast injection

EXCLUDES *Injection without imaging (20552-20553)*
Ultrasonic guidance (0213T-0218T)

64490 **Injection(s), diagnostic or therapeutic agent, paravertebral facet (zygapophyseal) joint (or nerves innervating that joint) with image guidance (fluoroscopy or CT), cervical or thoracic; single level**

INCLUDES Injection T12-L1 joint and nerves that innervate joint

3.04 | 5.38 | FUD 000 | T G2 80 50

AMA: 2018,Jan,8; 2017,Jan,8; 2016,Jan,9; 2016,Jan,13

\+ 64491 **second level (List separately in addition to code for primary procedure)**

EXCLUDES *Reporting with modifier 50. Report once for each side when performed bilaterally*

Code first (64490)

1.72 | 2.68 | FUD ZZZ | N N1 80

AMA: 2018,Jan,8; 2017,Jan,8; 2016,Jan,9; 2016,Jan,13

\+ 64492 **third and any additional level(s) (List separately in addition to code for primary procedure)**

EXCLUDES *Procedure performed more than one time per day*
Reporting with modifier 50. Report once for each side when performed bilaterally

Code also when appropriate (64491)

Code first (64490)

1.74 | 2.70 | FUD ZZZ | N N1 80

AMA: 2018,Jan,8; 2017,Jan,8; 2016,Jan,9; 2016,Jan,13

64493 **Injection(s), diagnostic or therapeutic agent, paravertebral facet (zygapophyseal) joint (or nerves innervating that joint) with image guidance (fluoroscopy or CT), lumbar or sacral; single level**

EXCLUDES *Injection nerves innervating sacroiliac joint (64451)*

2.58 | 4.91 | FUD 000 | T G2 80 50

AMA: 2020,Jul,13; 2018,May,10; 2018,Jan,8; 2017,Jan,8; 2016,Jan,13

\+ 64494 **second level (List separately in addition to code for primary procedure)**

EXCLUDES *Reporting with modifier 50. Report once for each side when performed bilaterally*

Code first (64493)

1.49 | 2.49 | FUD ZZZ | N N1 80

AMA: 2020,Jul,13; 2018,May,10; 2018,Jan,8; 2017,Jan,8; 2016,Jan,13

\+ 64495 **third and any additional level(s) (List separately in addition to code for primary procedure)**

EXCLUDES *Procedure performed more than one time per day*
Reporting with modifier 50. Report once for each side when performed bilaterally

Code also when appropriate (64494)

Code first (64493)

1.51 | 2.49 | FUD ZZZ | N N1 80

AMA: 2018,May,10; 2018,Jan,8; 2017,Jan,8; 2016,Jan,13

64505-64530 Sympathetic Nerve Blocks

64505 Injection, anesthetic agent; sphenopalatine ganglion
2.69 3.36 FUD 000 T P3 50
AMA: 2018,Jan,8; 2017,Jan,8; 2016,Jan,13

64510 stellate ganglion (cervical sympathetic)
2.13 3.78 FUD 000 T A2 50
AMA: 2018,Jan,8; 2017,Jan,8; 2016,Jan,13

64517 superior hypogastric plexus
3.60 5.47 FUD 000 T A2
AMA: 2018,Jan,8; 2017,Jan,8; 2016,Jan,13

64520 lumbar or thoracic (paravertebral sympathetic)
2.34 5.75 FUD 000 T A2 50
AMA: 2018,Jan,8; 2017,Jan,8; 2016,Jan,13

64530 celiac plexus, with or without radiologic monitoring
EXCLUDES *Transmural anesthetic injection with transendoscopic ultrasound-guidance (43253)*
2.63 5.73 FUD 000 T A2
AMA: 2018,Jan,8; 2017,Jan,8; 2016,Jan,13

64553-64570 Electrical Nerve Stimulation: Insertion/Replacement/Removal/Revision

INCLUDES Analysis system at implantation (95970)
Simple and complex neurostimulators
EXCLUDES *Analysis and programming neurostimulator pulse generator (95970-95972, 0589T-0590T)*
TENS therapy (97014, 97032)

64553 Percutaneous implantation of neurostimulator electrode array; cranial nerve
INCLUDES Temporary and permanent percutaneous array placement
EXCLUDES *Open procedure (61885-61886)*
Percutaneous electrical stimulation peripheral nerve with needle or needle electrodes (64999)
10.1 48.8 FUD 010 J J8 80
AMA: 2019,Feb,6; 2018,Oct,8; 2018,Jan,8; 2017,Jan,8; 2016,Jan,13

64555 peripheral nerve (excludes sacral nerve)
INCLUDES Temporary and permanent percutaneous array placement
EXCLUDES *Percutaneous electrical stimulation cranial nerve with needle or needle electrodes (64999)*
Posterior tibial neurostimulation (64566, 0587T-0588T)
9.85 44.3 FUD 010 J J8
AMA: 2019,Feb,6; 2018,Oct,8; 2018,Aug,10; 2018,Jan,8; 2017,Dec,13; 2017,Jan,8; 2016,Feb,13; 2016,Jan,13

64561 sacral nerve (transforaminal placement) including image guidance, if performed
INCLUDES Temporary and permanent percutaneous array placement
EXCLUDES *Percutaneous electrical stimulation or neuromodulation with needle or needle electrodes (64999)*
8.75 20.9 FUD 010 J J8 50
AMA: 2019,Feb,6; 2018,Oct,8; 2018,Jan,8; 2017,Jan,8; 2016,Jan,13

64566 Posterior tibial neurostimulation, percutaneous needle electrode, single treatment, includes programming
EXCLUDES *Electronic analysis implanted neurostimulator pulse generator system (95970-95972)*
Percutaneous implantation neurostimulator electrode array; peripheral nerve (64555)
Posterior tibial neurostimulation (0587T-0588T)
0.87 3.62 FUD 000 T P3 80
AMA: 2019,Feb,6; 2018,Oct,8; 2018,Jan,8; 2017,Jan,8; 2016,Jan,13

▲ **64568 Open implantation of cranial nerve (eg, vagus nerve) neurostimulator electrode array and pulse generator**
EXCLUDES *Insertion, replacement cranial neurostimulator pulse generator or receiver (61885-61886)*
Removal neurostimulator electrode array and pulse generator (64570)
18.4 18.4 FUD 090 J J8 80 50
AMA: 2019,Feb,6; 2018,Mar,9; 2018,Jan,8; 2017,Jan,8; 2016,Nov,6; 2016,Jan,13

64569 Revision or replacement of cranial nerve (eg, vagus nerve) neurostimulator electrode array, including connection to existing pulse generator
EXCLUDES *Removal neurostimulator electrode array and pulse generator (64570)*
Replacement pulse generator (61885)
Revision, removal pulse generator (61888)
22.1 22.1 FUD 090 J J8 80 50
AMA: 2019,Feb,6; 2018,Mar,9; 2018,Jan,8; 2017,Jan,8; 2016,Nov,6; 2016,Jan,13

64570 Removal of cranial nerve (eg, vagus nerve) neurostimulator electrode array and pulse generator
EXCLUDES *Laparoscopic revision, replacement, removal, or implantation vagus nerve blocking neurostimulator pulse generator and/or electrode array at esophagogastric junction (0312T-0317T)*
Revision, removal pulse generator (61888)
21.4 21.4 FUD 090 02 G2 80 50
AMA: 2019,Feb,6; 2018,Mar,9; 2018,Jan,8; 2017,Jan,8; 2016,Nov,6; 2016,Jan,13

64575-64595 Implantation/Revision/Removal Neurostimulators: Incisional

INCLUDES Simple and complex neurostimulators
EXCLUDES *Analysis and programming neurostimulator pulse generator (95970-95972, 0589T-0590T)*

▲ **64575 Open implantation of neurostimulator electrode array; peripheral nerve (excludes sacral nerve)**
EXCLUDES *Posterior tibial neurostimulation (0587T-0588T)*
9.80 9.80 FUD 090 J J8
AMA: 2019,Feb,6

▲ **64580 neuromuscular**
8.97 8.97 FUD 090 J J8 80
AMA: 2019,Feb,6

▲ **64581 sacral nerve (transforaminal placement)**
19.0 19.0 FUD 090 J J8
AMA: 2019,Feb,6; 2018,Jan,8; 2017,Jan,8; 2016,Jan,13

● **64582 Open implantation of hypoglossal nerve neurostimulator array, pulse generator, and distal respiratory sensor electrode or electrode array**

● **64583 Revision or replacement of hypoglossal nerve neurostimulator array and distal respiratory sensor electrode or electrode array, including connection to existing pulse generator**
EXCLUDES *Implantation neurostimulator array (64582)*
Removal neurostimulator array, pulse generator, and distal respiratory sensor (64584)
Replacement pulse generator (61886)
Code also modifier 52 for revision or replacement of neurostimulator array or distal respiratory sensor only

● **64584 Removal of hypoglossal nerve neurostimulator array, pulse generator, and distal respiratory sensor electrode or electrode array**
Code also modifier 52 for removal of only one or two components

64585 Revision or removal of peripheral neurostimulator electrode array
4.14 7.03 FUD 010 02 A2
AMA: 2019,Feb,6

64590 Insertion or replacement of peripheral or gastric neurostimulator pulse generator or receiver, direct or inductive coupling

EXCLUDES *Posterior tibial neurostimulation (0587T-0588T)*
Revision, removal neurostimulator pulse generator (64595)

4.64 7.60 **FUD** 010 J J8

AMA: 2019,Feb,6; 2018,Aug,10; 2018,Jan,8; 2017,Dec,13; 2017,Jan,8; 2016,Jan,13

64595 Revision or removal of peripheral or gastric neurostimulator pulse generator or receiver

EXCLUDES *Insertion, replacement neurostimulator pulse generator (64590)*

3.63 6.89 **FUD** 010 Q2 A2

AMA: 2019,Feb,6; 2018,Jan,8; 2017,Jan,8; 2016,Jan,13

64600-64610 Chemical Denervation Trigeminal Nerve

INCLUDES Injection therapeutic medication

EXCLUDES *Electromyography or muscle electric stimulation guidance (95873-95874)*
Nerve destruction:
Anal sphincter (46505)
Bladder (52287)
Strabismus involving extraocular muscles (67345)
Treatments that do not destroy target nerve (64999)

Code also chemodenervation agent

64600 Destruction by neurolytic agent, trigeminal nerve; supraorbital, infraorbital, mental, or inferior alveolar branch

6.66 12.3 **FUD** 010 T A2

AMA: 2020,Dec,13; 2019,Apr,9; 2018,Jan,8; 2017,Jan,8; 2016,Jan,13

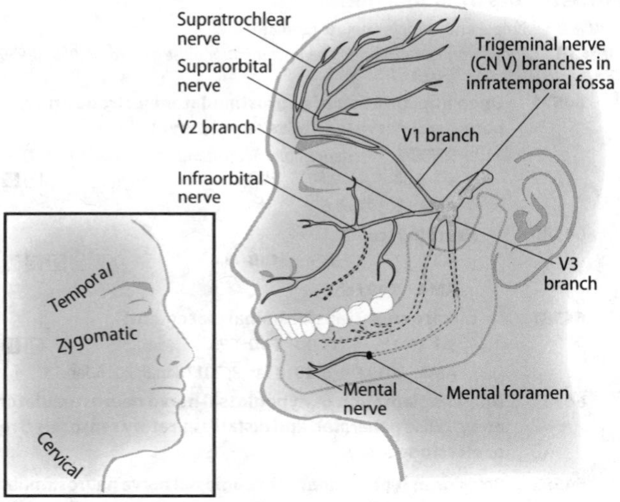

64605 second and third division branches at foramen ovale

10.0 16.8 **FUD** 010 J A2 80 50

AMA: 2020,Dec,13; 2019,Apr,9; 2018,Jan,8; 2017,Jan,8; 2016,Jan,13

64610 second and third division branches at foramen ovale under radiologic monitoring

14.2 22.0 **FUD** 010 J A2 50

AMA: 2020,Dec,13; 2019,Apr,9; 2018,Jan,8; 2017,Apr,9; 2017,Jan,8; 2016,Jan,13

64624 [64624] Chemical Denervation Genicular Nerve Branches

\# **64624 Destruction by neurolytic agent, genicular nerve branches including imaging guidance, when performed**

EXCLUDES *Injection genicular nerve branches (64454)*

Code also modifier 52 for destruction fewer than all genicular nerve branches: superolateral, superomedial, and inferomedial

4.23 11.5 **FUD** 010 G2 80 50

AMA: 2020,Dec,13; 2019,Dec,8

64625-64629 [64625, 64628, 64629] Radiofrequency Ablation Sacroiliac Joint Nerves

\# **64625 Radiofrequency ablation, nerves innervating the sacroiliac joint, with image guidance (ie, fluoroscopy or computed tomography)**

INCLUDES CT needle guidance (77012)
Electrical stimulation or needle electromyelograph for guidance (95873-95874)
Fluoroscopic needle guidance or localization (77002-77003)

EXCLUDES *Destruction by neurolytic agent, paravertebral facet joint nerve ([64635])*
Radiofrequency ablation with ultrasound (76999)

5.59 14.1 **FUD** 010 G2 50

AMA: 2020,Dec,13; 2020,Jun,14; 2019,Dec,8

● # **64628 Thermal destruction of intraosseous basivertebral nerve, including all imaging guidance; first 2 vertebral bodies, lumbar or sacral**

INCLUDES CT needle guidance (77012)
Fluoroscopic needle guidance and localization (77003)

0.00 0.00 **FUD** 000

● + # **64629 each additional vertebral body, lumbar or sacral (List separately in addition to code for primary procedure)**

INCLUDES CT needle guidance (77012)
Fluoroscopic needle guidance and localization (77003)

Code first ([64628])

0.00 0.00 **FUD** 000

64611-64617 Chemical Denervation Procedures Head and Neck

INCLUDES Injection therapeutic medication

EXCLUDES *Electromyography or muscle electric stimulation guidance (95873-95874)*
Nerve destruction:
Anal sphincter (46505)
Bladder (52287)
Extraocular muscles to treat strabismus (67345)
Treatments that do not destroy target nerve (64999)

64611 Chemodenervation of parotid and submandibular salivary glands, bilateral

Code also modifier 52 for injection of fewer than four salivary glands

3.03 3.45 **FUD** 010 T P3 80

AMA: 2020,Dec,13; 2019,Apr,9; 2018,Jan,8; 2017,Jan,8; 2016,Jan,13

64612 Chemodenervation of muscle(s); muscle(s) innervated by facial nerve, unilateral (eg, for blepharospasm, hemifacial spasm)

3.39 3.83 **FUD** 010 T P3 50

AMA: 2020,Dec,13; 2019,Apr,9; 2018,Jan,8; 2017,Jan,8; 2016,Jan,13

64615 **muscle(s) innervated by facial, trigeminal, cervical spinal and accessory nerves, bilateral (eg, for chronic migraine)**

EXCLUDES *Chemodenervation (64612, 64616-64617, 64642-64647)*
Procedure performed more than one time per session
Code also any guidance by muscle electrical stimulation or needle electromyography but report only once (95873-95874)
3.58 4.27 FUD 010 T P3
AMA: 2020,Dec,13; 2019,Apr,9; 2018,Jan,8; 2017,Jan,8; 2016,Jan,13

64616 **neck muscle(s), excluding muscles of the larynx, unilateral (eg, for cervical dystonia, spasmodic torticollis)**

Code also guidance by muscle electrical stimulation or needle electromyography, but report only once (95873-95874)
3.18 3.80 FUD 010 T P3 50
AMA: 2020,Dec,13; 2019,Apr,9; 2018,Jan,8; 2017,Jan,8; 2016,Jan,13

64617 **larynx, unilateral, percutaneous (eg, for spasmodic dysphonia), includes guidance by needle electromyography, when performed**

EXCLUDES *Chemodenervation larynx via direct laryngoscopy (31570-31571)*
Diagnostic needle electromyography larynx (95865)
Electrical stimulation guidance for chemodenervation (95873-95874)
3.14 4.62 FUD 010 T P3 50
AMA: 2020,Dec,13; 2019,Apr,9; 2018,Jan,8; 2017,Jan,8; 2016,Jan,13

64620-64640 [64624, 64625, 64628, 64629, 64633, 64634, 64635, 64636] Chemical Denervation Intercostal, Facet Joint, Plantar, and Pudendal Nerve(s)

INCLUDES Injection therapeutic medication

64620 **Destruction by neurolytic agent, intercostal nerve**
5.00 5.91 FUD 010 T A2
AMA: 2020,Dec,13; 2019,Nov,14; 2019,Apr,9; 2018,Jan,8; 2017,Jan,8; 2016,Jan,13

64624 **Resequenced code. See code following 64610.**

64625 **Resequenced code. See code before 64611.**

64628 **Resequenced code. See code before 64611.**

64629 **Resequenced code. See code before 64611.**

\# **64633** **Destruction by neurolytic agent, paravertebral facet joint nerve(s), with imaging guidance (fluoroscopy or CT); cervical or thoracic, single facet joint**

INCLUDES Paravertebral facet destruction T12-L1 joint or nerve(s) that innervate joint
Radiological guidance (77003, 77012)
EXCLUDES *Denervation performed using chemical, low grade thermal, or pulsed radiofrequency methods (64999)*
Destruction paravertebral facet joint nerve(s) without imaging guidance (64999)
6.43 11.8 FUD 010 J G2 50
AMA: 2020,Dec,13; 2019,Apr,9; 2018,Jan,8; 2017,Jan,8; 2016,Jan,13

\+ # **64634** **cervical or thoracic, each additional facet joint (List separately in addition to code for primary procedure)**

INCLUDES Radiological guidance (77003, 77012)
EXCLUDES *Denervation performed using chemical, low grade thermal, or pulsed radiofrequency methods (64999)*
Destruction paravertebral facet joint nerve(s) without imaging guidance (64999)
Reporting with modifier 50. Report once for each side when performed bilaterally
Code first ([64633])
1.95 5.34 FUD ZZZ N N1
AMA: 2020,Dec,13; 2019,Apr,9; 2018,Jan,8; 2017,Jan,8; 2016,Jan,13

\# **64635** **lumbar or sacral, single facet joint**

INCLUDES Radiological guidance (77003, 77012)
EXCLUDES *Denervation performed using chemical, low grade thermal, or pulsed radiofrequency methods (64999)*
Destruction individual nerves, sacroiliac joint, by neurolytic agent (64640)
Destruction paravertebral facet joint nerve(s) without imaging guidance (64999)
6.34 11.7 FUD 010 J G2 50
AMA: 2020,Dec,13; 2020,May,13; 2019,Dec,8; 2019,Apr,9; 2018,Jan,8; 2017,Jan,8; 2016,Jan,13

\+ # **64636** **lumbar or sacral, each additional facet joint (List separately in addition to code for primary procedure)**

INCLUDES Radiological guidance (77003, 77012)
EXCLUDES *Denervation performed using chemical, low grade thermal, or pulsed radiofrequency methods (64999)*
Destruction individual nerves, sacroiliac joint, by neurolytic agent (64640)
Destruction paravertebral facet joint nerve(s) without imaging guidance (64999)
Radiofrequency ablation nerves innervating sacroiliac joint with imaging ([64625])
Reporting with modifier 50. Report once for each side when performed bilaterally
Code first ([64635])
1.71 4.85 FUD ZZZ N N1
AMA: 2020,Dec,13; 2020,May,13; 2019,Apr,9; 2018,Jan,8; 2017,Jan,8; 2016,Jan,13

64630 **Destruction by neurolytic agent; pudendal nerve**
5.47 6.77 FUD 010 T A2 80
AMA: 2020,Dec,13; 2019,Apr,9; 2018,Jan,8; 2017,Oct,9; 2017,Jan,8; 2016,Jan,13

64632 **plantar common digital nerve**

EXCLUDES *Injection(s), anesthetic agent and/or steroid (64455)*
1.96 2.45 FUD 010 T P3 80 50
AMA: 2020,Dec,13; 2019,Apr,9; 2018,Jan,8; 2017,Oct,9; 2017,Jan,8; 2016,Jan,13

64633 **Resequenced code. See code following 64620.**

64634 **Resequenced code. See code following 64620.**

64635 **Resequenced code. See code following 64620.**

64636 **Resequenced code. See code before 64630.**

64640 **other peripheral nerve or branch**

INCLUDES Neurolytic destruction of nerves of sacroiliac joint
2.69 3.86 FUD 010 T P3 50
AMA: 2020,Dec,13; 2019,Apr,9; 2018,Jan,8; 2018,Jan,7; 2017,Oct,9; 2017,Jan,8; 2016,Jan,13

64642-64645 Chemical Denervation Extremity Muscles

INCLUDES Somatic muscles except the erector spinae, paraspinal, rectus abdominus, or oblique trunk muscles
EXCLUDES *Chemodenervation with needle-guided electromyography or with guidance provided by muscle electrical stimulation (95873-95874)*
Procedure performed more than once per extremity
Code also other extremities when appropriate, up to total four units per patient (when all extremities injected) (64642-64645)

64642 **Chemodenervation of one extremity; 1-4 muscle(s)**

EXCLUDES *Reporting more than one base code per session (64642)*
3.12 4.15 FUD 000 T P3
AMA: 2019,Aug,10; 2019,Apr,9; 2018,Jan,8; 2017,Jan,8; 2016,Jan,13

\+ **64643** **each additional extremity, 1-4 muscle(s) (List separately in addition to code for primary procedure)**

Code first (64642, 64644)
2.08 2.65 FUD ZZZ N N1
AMA: 2019,Aug,10; 2019,Apr,9; 2018,Jan,8; 2017,Jan,8; 2016,Jan,13

64644 **Chemodenervation of one extremity; 5 or more muscles**
EXCLUDES *Reporting more than one base code per session (64644)*
Facility RVU 3.42 Non-Facility RVU 4.82 FUD 000 T P3
AMA: 2019,Aug,10; 2019,Apr,9; 2018,Jan,8; 2017,Jan,8; 2016,Jan,13

+ **64645** **each additional extremity, 5 or more muscles (List separately in addition to code for primary procedure)**
Code first (64644)
Facility RVU 2.40 Non-Facility RVU 3.33 FUD ZZZ N N1
AMA: 2019,Aug,10; 2019,Apr,9; 2018,Jan,8; 2017,Jan,8; 2016,Jan,13

64646-64647 Chemical Denervation Trunk Muscles

INCLUDES Trunk muscles include erector spinae, paraspinal, rectus abdominus and oblique muscles
EXCLUDES *Procedure performed more than once per session*

64646 **Chemodenervation of trunk muscle(s); 1-5 muscle(s)**
Facility RVU 3.34 Non-Facility RVU 4.35 FUD 000 T P3
AMA: 2019,Apr,9; 2018,Jan,8; 2017,Jan,8; 2016,Jan,13

64647 **6 or more muscles**
Facility RVU 3.96 Non-Facility RVU 5.12 FUD 000 T P3
AMA: 2019,Apr,9; 2018,Jan,8; 2017,Jan,8; 2016,Jan,13

64650-64653 Chemical Denervation Eccrine Glands

INCLUDES Injection therapeutic medication
EXCLUDES *Bladder chemodenervation (52287)*
Chemodenervation extremities (64999)
Code also drugs or other substances used

64650 **Chemodenervation of eccrine glands; both axillae**
Facility RVU 1.21 Non-Facility RVU 2.25 FUD 000 T P3 80
AMA: 2019,Apr,9; 2018,Jan,8; 2017,Jan,8; 2016,Jan,13

64653 **other area(s) (eg, scalp, face, neck), per day**
Facility RVU 1.55 Non-Facility RVU 2.76 FUD 000 T P3 80
AMA: 2019,Apr,9; 2018,Jan,8; 2017,Jan,8; 2016,Jan,13

64680-64681 Neurolysis: Celiac Plexus, Superior Hypogastric Plexus

INCLUDES Injection therapeutic medication

64680 **Destruction by neurolytic agent, with or without radiologic monitoring; celiac plexus**
EXCLUDES *Transmural neurolytic agent injection with transendoscopic ultrasound guidance (43253)*
Facility RVU 4.66 Non-Facility RVU 9.07 FUD 010 T A2
AMA: 2019,Apr,9; 2018,Jan,8; 2017,Jan,8; 2016,Jan,13

64681 **superior hypogastric plexus**
Facility RVU 7.87 Non-Facility RVU 16.4 FUD 010 T A2
AMA: 2019,Apr,9; 2018,Jan,8; 2017,Jan,8; 2016,Jan,13

64702-64727 Decompression and/or Transposition of Nerve

INCLUDES External neurolysis and/or transposition to repair or restore nerve
Neuroplasty with nerve wrapping
Surgical decompression/freeing nerve from scar tissue
EXCLUDES *Facial nerve decompression (69720)*
Percutaneous neurolysis (62263-62264, 62280-62282)
Reporting with tissue expander insertion (11960)

64702 **Neuroplasty; digital, 1 or both, same digit**
Facility RVU 14.3 Non-Facility RVU 14.3 FUD 090 J A2
AMA: 2018,Jan,8; 2017,Jan,8; 2016,Jan,13

64704 **nerve of hand or foot**
Facility RVU 9.23 Non-Facility RVU 9.23 FUD 090 J A2 80
AMA: 2018,Jan,8; 2017,Jan,8; 2016,Jan,13

64708 **Neuroplasty, major peripheral nerve, arm or leg, open; other than specified**
Facility RVU 14.4 Non-Facility RVU 14.4 FUD 090 J G2 80
AMA: 2018,Jan,8; 2017,Nov,10; 2017,Jan,8; 2016,Jan,13

64712 **sciatic nerve**
Facility RVU 16.7 Non-Facility RVU 16.7 FUD 090 J G2 80 50
AMA: 2018,Jan,8; 2017,Jan,8; 2016,Jan,13

64713 **brachial plexus**
Facility RVU 22.1 Non-Facility RVU 22.1 FUD 090 J G2 80 50
AMA: 2018,Jan,8; 2017,Jan,8; 2016,Jan,13

64714 **lumbar plexus**
Facility RVU 20.8 Non-Facility RVU 20.8 FUD 090 J G2 80 50
AMA: 2018,Jan,8; 2017,Jan,8; 2016,Jan,13

64716 **Neuroplasty and/or transposition; cranial nerve (specify)**
Facility RVU 15.0 Non-Facility RVU 15.0 FUD 090 J A2 80
AMA: 2018,Jan,8; 2017,Jan,8; 2016,Jan,13

64718 **ulnar nerve at elbow**
Facility RVU 17.0 Non-Facility RVU 17.0 FUD 090 J A2 80 50
AMA: 2020,Jun,14; 2018,Jan,8; 2017,Jan,8; 2016,Jan,13

64719 **ulnar nerve at wrist**
Facility RVU 11.5 Non-Facility RVU 11.5 FUD 090 J A2 50
AMA: 2018,Jan,8; 2017,Jan,8; 2016,Jan,13

64721 **median nerve at carpal tunnel**
EXCLUDES *Endoscopic procedure (29848)*
Facility RVU 12.3 Non-Facility RVU 12.4 FUD 090 J A2 50
AMA: 2018,Jan,8; 2017,Jan,8; 2016,Jan,13

64722 **Decompression; unspecified nerve(s) (specify)**
Facility RVU 10.3 Non-Facility RVU 10.3 FUD 090 J A2 80
AMA: 2018,Jan,8; 2017,Jan,8; 2016,Jan,13

64726 **plantar digital nerve**
Facility RVU 7.80 Non-Facility RVU 7.80 FUD 090 J A2
AMA: 2018,Jan,8; 2017,Jan,8; 2016,Jan,13

+ **64727** **Internal neurolysis, requiring use of operating microscope (List separately in addition to code for neuroplasty) (Neuroplasty includes external neurolysis)**
INCLUDES Operating microscope (69990)
Code first neuroplasty (64702-64721)
Facility RVU 5.31 Non-Facility RVU 5.31 FUD ZZZ N N1
AMA: 2018,Jan,8; 2017,Jan,8; 2016,Feb,12; 2016,Jan,13

64732-64772 Surgical Avulsion/Transection of Nerve

EXCLUDES *Stereotactic lesion gasserian ganglion (61790)*

64732 **Transection or avulsion of; supraorbital nerve**
Facility RVU 12.8 Non-Facility RVU 12.8 FUD 090 J A2 80 50
AMA: 2018,Jan,8; 2017,Jan,8; 2016,Jan,13

64734 **infraorbital nerve**
Facility RVU 14.5 Non-Facility RVU 14.5 FUD 090 J A2 80 50
AMA: 2014,Jan,11

64736 **mental nerve**
Facility RVU 10.0 Non-Facility RVU 10.0 FUD 090 J A2 80 50
AMA: 2014,Jan,11

64738 **inferior alveolar nerve by osteotomy**
Facility RVU 13.3 Non-Facility RVU 13.3 FUD 090 J A2 80 50
AMA: 2014,Jan,11

64740 **lingual nerve**
Facility RVU 14.0 Non-Facility RVU 14.0 FUD 090 J A2 80 50
AMA: 2014,Jan,11

64742 **facial nerve, differential or complete**
Facility RVU 14.1 Non-Facility RVU 14.1 FUD 090 J A2 80 50
AMA: 2014,Jan,11

64744 **greater occipital nerve**
Facility RVU 14.2 Non-Facility RVU 14.2 FUD 090 J A2 80 50
AMA: 2014,Jan,11

64746 **phrenic nerve**
Facility RVU 12.4 Non-Facility RVU 12.4 FUD 090 J A2 80 50
AMA: 2014,Jan,11

64755 **vagus nerves limited to proximal stomach (selective proximal vagotomy, proximal gastric vagotomy, parietal cell vagotomy, supra- or highly selective vagotomy)**
EXCLUDES *Laparoscopic procedure (43652)*
Facility RVU 26.3 Non-Facility RVU 26.3 FUD 090 C 80
AMA: 2018,Jan,8; 2017,Jan,8; 2016,Jan,13

64760 **vagus nerve (vagotomy), abdominal**
EXCLUDES *Laparoscopic procedure (43651)*
Facility RVU 14.9 Non-Facility RVU 14.9 FUD 090 C 80
AMA: 2018,Jan,8; 2017,Jan,8; 2016,Jan,13

64763 **Transection or avulsion of obturator nerve, extrapelvic, with or without adductor tenotomy**
14.7 | 14.7 | FUD 090 | J G2 80 50
AMA: 2014,Jan,11

64766 **Transection or avulsion of obturator nerve, intrapelvic, with or without adductor tenotomy**
17.8 | 17.8 | FUD 090 | J G2 80 50
AMA: 2014,Jan,11

64771 **Transection or avulsion of other cranial nerve, extradural**
17.0 | 17.0 | FUD 090 | J A2 80
AMA: 2014,Jan,11

64772 **Transection or avulsion of other spinal nerve, extradural**
EXCLUDES *Removal tender scar and soft tissue including neuroma when necessary (11400-11446, 13100-13153)*
16.2 | 16.2 | FUD 090 | J A2 80
AMA: 2018,Jan,8; 2017,Jan,8; 2016,Jan,13

64774-64823 Excisional Nerve Procedures

EXCLUDES *Morton neuroma excision (28080)*

64774 **Excision of neuroma; cutaneous nerve, surgically identifiable**
11.7 | 11.7 | FUD 090 | J A2
AMA: 2014,Jan,11

64776 **digital nerve, 1 or both, same digit**
11.1 | 11.1 | FUD 090 | J A2 80
AMA: 2014,Jan,11

+ **64778** **digital nerve, each additional digit (List separately in addition to code for primary procedure)**
Code first (64776)
5.30 | 5.30 | FUD ZZZ | N N1
AMA: 2014,Jan,11

64782 **hand or foot, except digital nerve**
13.2 | 13.2 | FUD 090 | J A2
AMA: 2014,Jan,11

+ **64783** **hand or foot, each additional nerve, except same digit (List separately in addition to code for primary procedure)**
Code first (64782)
6.33 | 6.33 | FUD ZZZ | N N1
AMA: 2014,Jan,11

64784 **major peripheral nerve, except sciatic**
20.9 | 20.9 | FUD 090 | J A2 80
AMA: 2014,Jan,11

64786 **sciatic nerve**
28.9 | 28.9 | FUD 090 | J A2 80 50
AMA: 2014,Jan,11

+ **64787** **Implantation of nerve end into bone or muscle (List separately in addition to neuroma excision)**
Code also, when appropriate (64774-64786)
6.96 | 6.96 | FUD ZZZ | N N1 80
AMA: 2014,Jan,11

64788 **Excision of neurofibroma or neurolemmoma; cutaneous nerve**
11.5 | 11.5 | FUD 090 | J A2
AMA: 2018,Jan,8; 2017,Jan,8; 2016,Apr,3

64790 **major peripheral nerve**
24.1 | 24.1 | FUD 090 | J A2 80
AMA: 2018,Jan,8; 2017,Jan,8; 2016,Apr,3

64792 **extensive (including malignant type)**
EXCLUDES *Destruction neurofibroma skin (0419T-0420T)*
31.4 | 31.4 | FUD 090 | J A2 80
AMA: 2018,Jan,8; 2017,Jan,8; 2016,Apr,3

64795 **Biopsy of nerve**
5.64 | 5.64 | FUD 000 | J A2
AMA: 2014,Jan,11

64802 **Sympathectomy, cervical**
24.3 | 24.3 | FUD 090 | J A2 80 50
AMA: 2014,Jan,11

64804 **Sympathectomy, cervicothoracic**
34.1 | 34.1 | FUD 090 | J G2 80 50
AMA: 2014,Jan,11

64809 **Sympathectomy, thoracolumbar**
INCLUDES Leriche sympathectomy
31.0 | 31.0 | FUD 090 | C 80 50
AMA: 2014,Jan,11

64818 **Sympathectomy, lumbar**
22.5 | 22.5 | FUD 090 | C 80 50
AMA: 2014,Jan,11

64820 **Sympathectomy; digital arteries, each digit**
INCLUDES Operating microscope (69990)
20.5 | 20.5 | FUD 090 | J G2
AMA: 2018,Jan,8; 2017,Jan,8; 2016,Feb,12; 2016,Jan,13

64821 **radial artery**
INCLUDES Operating microscope (69990)
20.0 | 20.0 | FUD 090 | J A2 50
AMA: 2016,Feb,12

64822 **ulnar artery**
INCLUDES Operating microscope (69990)
20.0 | 20.0 | FUD 090 | J G2 50
AMA: 2016,Feb,12

64823 **superficial palmar arch**
INCLUDES Operating microscope (69990)
22.7 | 22.7 | FUD 090 | J G2 50
AMA: 2016,Feb,12

64831-64907 Nerve Repair: Suture and Nerve Grafts

64831 **Suture of digital nerve, hand or foot; 1 nerve**
19.7 | 19.7 | FUD 090 | J A2 50
AMA: 2018,Jan,8; 2017,Jan,8; 2016,Jan,13

+ **64832** **each additional digital nerve (List separately in addition to code for primary procedure)**
Code first (64831)
9.73 | 9.73 | FUD ZZZ | N N1 80
AMA: 2018,Jan,8; 2017,Jan,8; 2016,Jan,13

64834 **Suture of 1 nerve; hand or foot, common sensory nerve**
21.3 | 21.3 | FUD 090 | J A2 80 50
AMA: 2014,Jan,11

64835 **median motor thenar**
23.5 | 23.5 | FUD 090 | J A2 80 50
AMA: 2014,Jan,11

64836 **ulnar motor**
23.5 | 23.5 | FUD 090 | J A2 80 50
AMA: 2014,Jan,11

+ **64837** **Suture of each additional nerve, hand or foot (List separately in addition to code for primary procedure)**
Code first (64834-64836)
10.6 | 10.6 | FUD ZZZ | N N1 80
AMA: 2014,Jan,11

64840 **Suture of posterior tibial nerve**
27.8 | 27.8 | FUD 090 | J A2 80 50
AMA: 2014,Jan,11

64856 **Suture of major peripheral nerve, arm or leg, except sciatic; including transposition**
29.2 | 29.2 | FUD 090 | J A2
AMA: 2014,Jan,11

64857 **without transposition**
30.4 | 30.4 | FUD 090 | J A2 80
AMA: 2014,Jan,11

64858 **Suture of sciatic nerve**
34.0 | 34.0 | FUD 090 | J J8 80 50
AMA: 2014,Jan,11

+ **64859** **Suture of each additional major peripheral nerve (List separately in addition to code for primary procedure)**
Code first (64856-64857)
7.23 7.23 FUD ZZZ N N1 80
AMA: 2014,Jan,11

64861 **Suture of; brachial plexus**
44.5 44.5 FUD 090 J A2 80 50
AMA: 2014,Jan,11

64862 **lumbar plexus**
39.8 39.8 FUD 090 J A2 80 50
AMA: 2014,Jan,11

64864 **Suture of facial nerve; extracranial**
24.8 24.8 FUD 090 J A2 80
AMA: 2014,Jan,11

64865 **infratemporal, with or without grafting**
31.4 31.4 FUD 090 J A2 80
AMA: 2014,Jan,11

64866 **Anastomosis; facial-spinal accessory**
36.7 36.7 FUD 090 C 80
AMA: 2014,Jan,11

64868 **facial-hypoglossal**
INCLUDES Korte-Ballance anastomosis
28.8 28.8 FUD 090 C 80
AMA: 2014,Jan,11

+ **64872** **Suture of nerve; requiring secondary or delayed suture (List separately in addition to code for primary neurorrhaphy)**
Code first (64831-64865)
3.39 3.39 FUD ZZZ N N1 80
AMA: 2014,Jan,11

+ **64874** **requiring extensive mobilization, or transposition of nerve (List separately in addition to code for nerve suture)**
Code first (64831-64865)
5.05 5.05 FUD ZZZ N N1 80
AMA: 2014,Jan,11

+ **64876** **requiring shortening of bone of extremity (List separately in addition to code for nerve suture)**
Code first (64831-64865)
5.71 5.71 FUD ZZZ N N1 80
AMA: 2014,Jan,11; 2003,Jan,1

64885 **Nerve graft (includes obtaining graft), head or neck; up to 4 cm in length**
32.1 32.1 FUD 090 J A2 80
AMA: 2018,Jan,8; 2017,Dec,12; 2017,Jan,8; 2016,Jan,13

64886 **more than 4 cm length**
37.2 37.2 FUD 090 J J8 80
AMA: 2018,Jan,8; 2017,Dec,12; 2017,Jan,8; 2016,Jan,13

64890 **Nerve graft (includes obtaining graft), single strand, hand or foot; up to 4 cm length**
31.2 31.2 FUD 090 J A2 80
AMA: 2018,Jan,8; 2017,Dec,12; 2017,Jan,8; 2016,Jan,13

64891 **more than 4 cm length**
33.2 33.2 FUD 090 J J8 80
AMA: 2018,Jan,8; 2017,Dec,12

64892 **Nerve graft (includes obtaining graft), single strand, arm or leg; up to 4 cm length**
30.4 30.4 FUD 090 J A2 80
AMA: 2018,Jan,8; 2017,Dec,12

64893 **more than 4 cm length**
32.4 32.4 FUD 090 J G2 80
AMA: 2018,Jan,8; 2017,Dec,12

64895 **Nerve graft (includes obtaining graft), multiple strands (cable), hand or foot; up to 4 cm length**
38.4 38.4 FUD 090 J A2 80
AMA: 2018,Jan,8; 2017,Dec,12; 2017,Jan,8; 2016,Jan,13

64896 **more than 4 cm length**
41.4 41.4 FUD 090 J A2 80
AMA: 2018,Jan,8; 2017,Dec,12; 2017,Jan,8; 2016,Jan,13

64897 **Nerve graft (includes obtaining graft), multiple strands (cable), arm or leg; up to 4 cm length**
36.7 36.7 FUD 090 J G2 80
AMA: 2018,Jan,8; 2017,Dec,12; 2017,Jan,8; 2016,Jan,13

64898 **more than 4 cm length**
39.7 39.7 FUD 090 J A2 80
AMA: 2018,Jan,8; 2017,Dec,12; 2017,Jan,8; 2016,Jan,13

+ **64901** **Nerve graft, each additional nerve; single strand (List separately in addition to code for primary procedure)**
Code first (64885-64893)
17.4 17.4 FUD ZZZ N N1 80
AMA: 2018,Jan,8; 2017,Dec,12; 2017,Jan,8; 2016,Jan,13

+ **64902** **multiple strands (cable) (List separately in addition to code for primary procedure)**
Code first (64885-64886, 64895-64898)
20.1 20.1 FUD ZZZ N N1 80
AMA: 2018,Jan,8; 2017,Dec,12; 2017,Jan,8; 2016,Jan,13

64905 **Nerve pedicle transfer; first stage**
29.4 29.4 FUD 090 J A2 80
AMA: 2018,Jan,8; 2017,Dec,12

64907 **second stage**
37.7 37.7 FUD 090 J A2 80
AMA: 2018,Jan,8; 2017,Dec,12

64910-64999 Nerve Repair: Synthetic and Vein Grafts

64910 **Nerve repair; with synthetic conduit or vein allograft (eg, nerve tube), each nerve**
INCLUDES Operating microscope (69990)
22.7 22.7 FUD 090 J J8 80
AMA: 2018,Jan,8; 2017,Dec,12; 2017,Jan,8; 2016,Jan,13

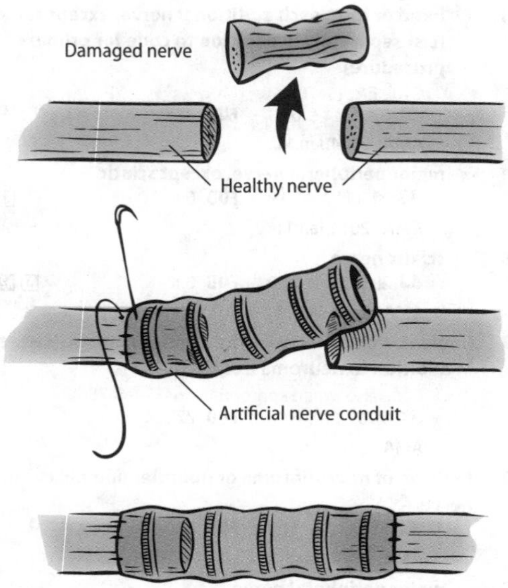

A synthetic "bridge" is affixed to each end of a severed nerve with sutures
The procedure is performed using an operating microscope

64911 **with autogenous vein graft (includes harvest of vein graft), each nerve**
INCLUDES Operating microscope (69990)
29.5 29.5 FUD 090 J G2 80
AMA: 2018,Jan,8; 2017,Dec,12; 2017,Jan,8; 2016,Jan,13

64912 **with nerve allograft, each nerve, first strand (cable)**

INCLUDES Operating microscope (69990)

26.3 26.3 FUD 090 J J8 80

AMA: 2018,Jan,8; 2017,Dec,12

\+ **64913** **with nerve allograft, each additional strand (List separately in addition to code for primary procedure)**

INCLUDES Operating microscope (69990)

Code first (64912)

5.16 5.16 FUD ZZZ N N1 80

AMA: 2018,Jan,8; 2017,Dec,12

64999 **Unlisted procedure, nervous system**

0.00 0.00 FUD YYY T 80

AMA: 2020,Dec,13; 2020,Jun,14; 2020,Feb,13; 2019,Dec,12; 2019,Jul,10; 2019,May,10; 2019,Apr,9; 2018,Dec,8; 2018,Dec,8; 2018,Oct,8; 2018,Oct,11; 2018,Aug,10; 2018,Mar,9; 2018,Jan,8; 2018,Jan,7; 2017,Dec,14; 2017,Dec,12; 2017,Dec,13; 2017,Jan,8; 2016,Nov,6; 2016,Oct,11; 2016,Feb,13; 2016,Jan,13

65091-65093 Surgical Removal of Eyeball Contents

INCLUDES Operating microscope (69990)

65091 **Evisceration of ocular contents; without implant**
18.4 18.4 FUD 090 J A2 80 50
AMA: 2016,Feb,12

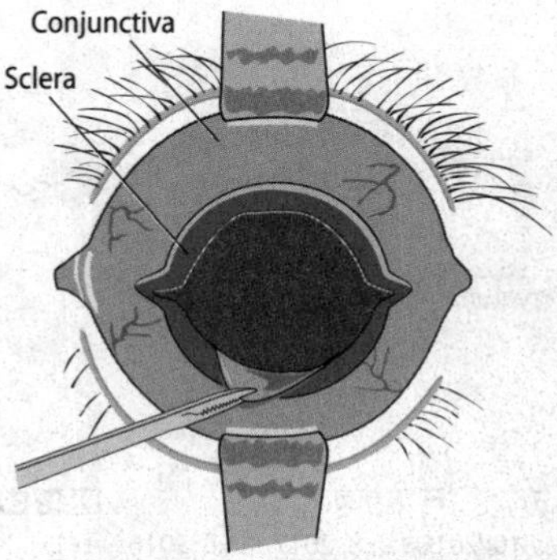

Evisceration involves removal of the contents of the eyeball: the vitreous; retina; choroid; lens; iris; and ciliary muscle. Only the scleral shell remains. A temporary or permanent implant is usually inserted

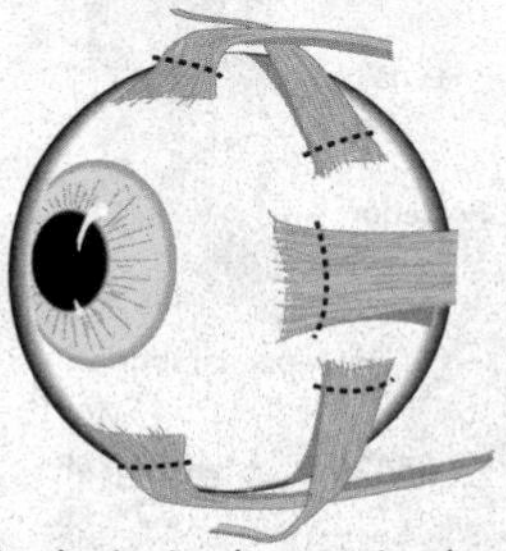

Enucleation involves severing the extraorbital muscles and optic nerve with removal of the eyeball. An implant is usually inserted and, if permanent, may involve attachment to the severed extraorbital muscles

65093 **with implant**
19.3 19.3 FUD 090 J A2 50
AMA: 2016,Feb,12

65101-65105 Surgical Removal of Eyeball

INCLUDES Operating microscope (69990)
EXCLUDES *Conjunctivoplasty following enucleation (68320-68328)*

65101 **Enucleation of eye; without implant**
21.3 21.3 FUD 090 J A2 50
AMA: 2016,Feb,12

65103 **with implant, muscles not attached to implant**
23.3 23.3 FUD 090 J A2 50
AMA: 2016,Feb,12

65105 **with implant, muscles attached to implant**
24.4 24.4 FUD 090 J A2 80 50
AMA: 2016,Feb,12

65110-65114 Surgical Removal of Orbital Contents

INCLUDES Operating microscope (69990)
EXCLUDES *Free full thickness graft (15260-15261)*
Repair more extensive than skin (67930-67975)
Skin graft (15120-15121)

65110 **Exenteration of orbit (does not include skin graft), removal of orbital contents; only**
36.0 36.0 FUD 090 J A2 80 50
AMA: 2016,Feb,12

65112 **with therapeutic removal of bone**
41.5 41.5 FUD 090 J A2 80 50
AMA: 2016,Feb,12

65114 **with muscle or myocutaneous flap**
43.4 43.4 FUD 090 J A2 80 50
AMA: 2016,Feb,12

65125-65175 Implant Procedures: Insertion, Removal, and Revision

INCLUDES Ocular implant procedures (inside muscle cone)
Operating microscope (69990)
EXCLUDES *Orbital implant insertion (outside muscle cone) (67550)*
Orbital implant removal or revision (outside muscle cone) (67560)

65125 **Modification of ocular implant with placement or replacement of pegs (eg, drilling receptacle for prosthesis appendage) (separate procedure)**
8.26 12.9 FUD 090 J G2 50
AMA: 2016,Feb,12

65130 **Insertion of ocular implant secondary; after evisceration, in scleral shell**
21.1 21.1 FUD 090 J A2 50
AMA: 2016,Feb,12

65135 **after enucleation, muscles not attached to implant**
21.4 21.4 FUD 090 J A2 50
AMA: 2016,Feb,12

65140 **after enucleation, muscles attached to implant**
23.3 23.3 FUD 090 J A2 50
AMA: 2016,Feb,12

65150 **Reinsertion of ocular implant; with or without conjunctival graft**
18.0 18.0 FUD 090 J A2 80 50
AMA: 2016,Feb,12

65155 **with use of foreign material for reinforcement and/or attachment of muscles to implant**
25.6 25.6 FUD 090 J A2 50
AMA: 2016,Feb,12

65175 **Removal of ocular implant**
19.0 19.0 FUD 090 J A2 50
AMA: 2016,Feb,12

65205-65265 Foreign Body Removal By Area of Eye

INCLUDES Operating microscope (69990)
EXCLUDES *Removal foreign body:*
Eyelid (67938)
Lacrimal system (68530)
Orbit:
Frontal approach (67413)
Lateral approach (67430)
Removal implant:
Anterior segment (65920)
Ocular (65175)
Orbital (67560)
Posterior segment (67120)

65205 **Removal of foreign body, external eye; conjunctival superficial**
(70030, 76529)
1.02 1.31 FUD 000 Q1 N1 50
AMA: 2018,Jan,8; 2017,Jan,8; 2016,Feb,12; 2016,Jan,13

65210 **conjunctival embedded (includes concretions), subconjunctival, or scleral nonperforating**
(70030, 76529)
1.04 1.30 FUD 000 Q1 N1 50
AMA: 2016,Feb,12

65220 **corneal, without slit lamp**
EXCLUDES *Repair corneal wound with foreign body (65275)*
(70030, 76529)
1.19 1.70 FUD 000 Q1 N1 50
AMA: 2018,Jan,8; 2017,Jan,8; 2016,Feb,12; 2016,Jan,13

65222 **corneal, with slit lamp**
EXCLUDES *Repair corneal wound with foreign body (65275)*
(70030, 76529)
1.46 1.93 FUD 000 Q1 N1 50
AMA: 2018,Jan,8; 2017,Jan,8; 2016,Feb,12; 2016,Jan,13

65235 **Removal of foreign body, intraocular; from anterior chamber of eye or lens**
EXCLUDES *Removal implanted material from anterior segment (65920)*
(70030, 76529)
20.2 20.2 FUD 090 J A2 80 50
AMA: 2018,Jan,8; 2017,Jan,8; 2016,Feb,12; 2016,Jan,13

65260 **from posterior segment, magnetic extraction, anterior or posterior route**
EXCLUDES *Removal implanted material from posterior segment (67120)*
(70030, 76529)
27.5 27.5 FUD 090 J A2 80 50
AMA: 2016,Feb,12

65265 **from posterior segment, nonmagnetic extraction**
EXCLUDES *Removal implanted material from posterior segment (67120)*
(70030, 76529)
30.9 30.9 FUD 090 J A2 80 50
AMA: 2016,Feb,12

65270-65290 Laceration Repair External Eye

INCLUDES Conjunctival flap
Operating microscope (69990)
Restoration anterior chamber with air or saline injection

EXCLUDES *Repair:*
Ciliary body or iris (66680)
Eyelid laceration (12011-12018, 12051-12057, 13151-13160, 67930, 67935)
Lacrimal system injury (68700)
Surgical wound (66250)
Treatment orbit fracture (21385-21408)

65270 **Repair of laceration; conjunctiva, with or without nonperforating laceration sclera, direct closure**
3.99 7.94 FUD 010 J A2 80 50
AMA: 2018,Jan,8; 2017,Jan,8; 2016,Feb,12; 2016,Jan,13

65272 **conjunctiva, by mobilization and rearrangement, without hospitalization**
10.0 14.5 FUD 090 J A2 50
AMA: 2016,Feb,12

65273 **conjunctiva, by mobilization and rearrangement, with hospitalization**
10.8 10.8 FUD 090 C 50
AMA: 2016,Feb,12

65275 **cornea, nonperforating, with or without removal foreign body**
13.1 16.5 FUD 090 J A2 80 50
AMA: 2016,Feb,12

65280 **cornea and/or sclera, perforating, not involving uveal tissue**
EXCLUDES *Procedure performed for surgical wound repair*
19.1 19.1 FUD 090 J A2 80 50
AMA: 2018,Jan,8; 2017,Jan,8; 2016,Feb,12; 2016,Jan,13

65285 **cornea and/or sclera, perforating, with reposition or resection of uveal tissue**
EXCLUDES *Procedure performed for surgical wound repair*
31.4 31.4 FUD 090 J A2 50
AMA: 2018,Jan,8; 2017,Jan,8; 2016,Feb,12; 2016,Jan,13

65286 **application of tissue glue, wounds of cornea and/or sclera**
14.1 20.0 FUD 090 J P3 50
AMA: 2018,Jan,8; 2017,Jan,8; 2016,Feb,12; 2016,Jan,13

65290 **Repair of wound, extraocular muscle, tendon and/or Tenon's capsule**
13.9 13.9 FUD 090 J A2 50
AMA: 2016,Feb,12

65400-65600 Removal Corneal Lesions

INCLUDES Operating microscope (69990)

65400 **Excision of lesion, cornea (keratectomy, lamellar, partial), except pterygium**
17.0 19.4 FUD 090 T A2 50
AMA: 2018,Jan,8; 2017,Jan,8; 2016,Feb,12; 2016,Jan,13

65410 **Biopsy of cornea**
2.96 4.11 FUD 000 J A2 80 50
AMA: 2018,Jan,8; 2017,Jan,8; 2016,Feb,12; 2016,Jan,13

65420 **Excision or transposition of pterygium; without graft**
10.6 15.0 FUD 090 J A2 50
AMA: 2018,Jan,8; 2017,Jan,8; 2016,Feb,12; 2016,Jan,13

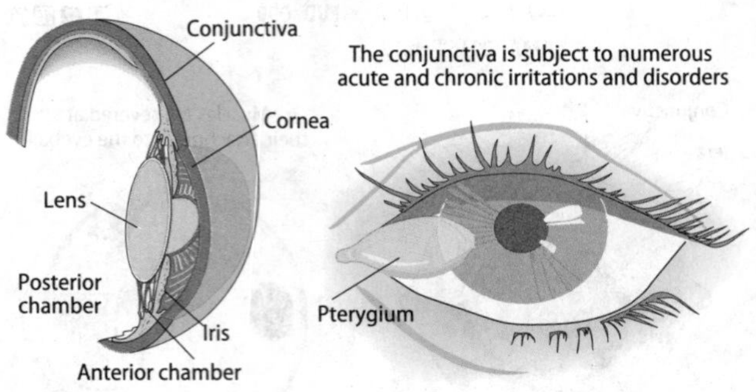

65426 **with graft**
13.6 18.7 FUD 090 J A2 50
AMA: 2018,May,10; 2018,Jan,8; 2017,Jan,8; 2016,Feb,12; 2016,Jan,13

65430 **Scraping of cornea, diagnostic, for smear and/or culture**
2.90 3.28 FUD 000 01 N1 50
AMA: 2016,Feb,12

65435 **Removal of corneal epithelium; with or without chemocauterization (abrasion, curettage)**
EXCLUDES *Collagen cross-linking, cornea (0402T)*
1.98 2.33 FUD 000 T P3 50
AMA: 2018,Jan,8; 2017,Jan,8; 2016,Feb,12; 2016,Jan,13

65436 **with application of chelating agent (eg, EDTA)**
10.5 11.0 FUD 090 J P3 50
AMA: 2016,Feb,12

65450 **Destruction of lesion of cornea by cryotherapy, photocoagulation or thermocauterization**
9.15 9.30 FUD 090 T G2 50
AMA: 2016,Feb,12

65600 **Multiple punctures of anterior cornea (eg, for corneal erosion, tattoo)**
9.61 11.7 FUD 090 J P3 50
AMA: 2016,Feb,12

65710-65757 Corneal Transplants

CMS: 100-03,80.7 Refractive Keratoplasty

INCLUDES Operating microscope (69990)

EXCLUDES *Computerized corneal topography (92025)*
Processing, preserving, and transporting corneal tissue (V2785)

65710 **Keratoplasty (corneal transplant); anterior lamellar**
INCLUDES Use and preparation fresh or preserved graft
EXCLUDES *Refractive keratoplasty surgery (65760-65767)*
31.7 31.7 FUD 090 J A2 80 50
AMA: 2018,Jan,8; 2017,Jan,8; 2016,Feb,12; 2016,Jan,13

65730 **penetrating (except in aphakia or pseudophakia)**
INCLUDES Use and preparation fresh or preserved graft
EXCLUDES *Refractive keratoplasty surgery (65760-65767)*
35.1 35.1 FUD 090 J A2 80 50
AMA: 2018,Jan,8; 2017,Jan,8; 2016,Feb,12; 2016,Jan,13

65750 **penetrating (in aphakia)**
INCLUDES Use and preparation fresh or preserved graft
EXCLUDES *Refractive keratoplasty surgery (65760-65767)*
35.3 35.3 FUD 090 J A2 80 50
AMA: 2018,Jan,8; 2017,Jan,8; 2016,Feb,12; 2016,Jan,13

65755 **penetrating (in pseudophakia)**
INCLUDES Use and preparation fresh or preserved graft
EXCLUDES *Refractive keratoplasty surgery (65760-65767)*
35.1 35.1 FUD 090 J A2 80 50
AMA: 2018,Jan,8; 2017,Jan,8; 2016,Feb,12; 2016,Jan,13

65756 **endothelial**

EXCLUDES *Refractive keratoplasty surgery (65760-65767)*

Code also:
Backbench preparation, when appropriate (65757)
Donor material

33.4 | 33.4 | FUD 090 | J G2 80 50

AMA: 2018,Jan,8; 2017,Jan,8; 2016,Feb,12; 2016,Jan,13

\+ **65757** **Backbench preparation of corneal endothelial allograft prior to transplantation (List separately in addition to code for primary procedure)**

Code first (65756)

0.00 | 0.00 | FUD ZZZ | N N1 80

AMA: 2018,Jan,8; 2017,Jan,8; 2016,Feb,12; 2016,Jan,13

65760-65785 Corneal Refractive Procedures

CMS: 100-03,80.7 Refractive Keratoplasty

INCLUDES Operating microscope (69990)

EXCLUDES *Unlisted corneal procedures (66999)*

65760 **Keratomileusis**

EXCLUDES *Computerized corneal topography (92025)*

0.00 | 0.00 | FUD XXX | E

AMA: 2016,Feb,12

65765 **Keratophakia**

EXCLUDES *Computerized corneal topography (92025)*

0.00 | 0.00 | FUD XXX | E

AMA: 2016,Feb,12

65767 **Epikeratoplasty**

EXCLUDES *Computerized corneal topography (92025)*

0.00 | 0.00 | FUD XXX | E

AMA: 2016,Feb,12

65770 **Keratoprosthesis**

EXCLUDES *Computerized corneal topography (92025)*

39.5 | 39.5 | FUD 090 | J J8 80 50

AMA: 2016,Feb,12

65771 **Radial keratotomy**

EXCLUDES *Computerized corneal topography (92025)*

0.00 | 0.00 | FUD XXX | E

AMA: 2016,Feb,12

65772 **Corneal relaxing incision for correction of surgically induced astigmatism**

11.5 | 12.8 | FUD 090 | T A2 50

AMA: 2016,Feb,12

65775 **Corneal wedge resection for correction of surgically induced astigmatism**

EXCLUDES *Fitting contact lens to treat disease (92071-92072)*

15.8 | 15.8 | FUD 090 | J A2 50

AMA: 2018,Jan,8; 2017,Jan,8; 2016,Feb,12; 2016,Jan,13

65778 **Placement of amniotic membrane on the ocular surface; without sutures**

EXCLUDES *Ocular surface reconstruction (65780)*
Removal corneal epithelium (65435)
Scraping cornea, diagnostic (65430)
Using tissue glue to place amniotic membrane (66999)

1.58 | 40.0 | FUD 000 | Q2 N1 80 50

AMA: 2018,Feb,11; 2018,Jan,8; 2017,Jan,8; 2016,Feb,12; 2016,Jan,13

65779 **single layer, sutured**

EXCLUDES *Ocular surface reconstruction (65780)*
Removal corneal epithelium (65435)
Scraping cornea, diagnostic (65430)
Using tissue glue to place amniotic membrane (66999)

4.32 | 34.5 | FUD 000 | Q2 N1 80 50

AMA: 2018,Feb,11; 2018,Jan,8; 2017,Jan,8; 2016,Feb,12; 2016,Jan,13

65780 **Ocular surface reconstruction; amniotic membrane transplantation, multiple layers**

EXCLUDES *Placement amniotic membrane without reconstruction without sutures or single layer sutures (65778-65779)*

18.9 | 18.9 | FUD 090 | J A2 50

AMA: 2018,Feb,11; 2018,Jan,8; 2017,Jan,8; 2016,Feb,12; 2016,Jan,13

65781 **limbal stem cell allograft (eg, cadaveric or living donor)**

37.9 | 37.9 | FUD 090 | J J8 80 50

AMA: 2018,Jan,8; 2017,Jan,8; 2016,Feb,12; 2016,Jan,13

65782 **limbal conjunctival autograft (includes obtaining graft)**

EXCLUDES *Conjunctival allograft harvest from living donor (68371)*

32.6 | 32.6 | FUD 090 | J A2 50

AMA: 2018,Jan,8; 2017,Jan,8; 2016,Feb,12; 2016,Jan,13

65785 **Implantation of intrastromal corneal ring segments**

12.5 | 69.5 | FUD 090 | J P2 50

AMA: 2016,Feb,12

65800-66030 Anterior Segment Procedures

INCLUDES Operating microscope (69990)

EXCLUDES *Unlisted procedures anterior segment (66999)*

65800 **Paracentesis of anterior chamber of eye (separate procedure); with removal of aqueous**

EXCLUDES *Insertion ocular telescope prosthesis (0308T)*

2.59 | 3.42 | FUD 000 | J A2 50

AMA: 2018,Jan,8; 2017,Jan,8; 2016,Feb,12; 2016,Jan,13

65810 **with removal of vitreous and/or discission of anterior hyaloid membrane, with or without air injection**

EXCLUDES *Insertion ocular telescope prosthesis (0308T)*

13.2 | 13.2 | FUD 090 | J A2 50

AMA: 2018,Jan,8; 2017,Jan,8; 2016,Feb,12; 2016,Jan,13

65815 **with removal of blood, with or without irrigation and/or air injection**

EXCLUDES *Injection only (66020-66030)*
Insertion ocular telescope prosthesis (0308T)
Removal blood clot only (65930)

13.5 | 18.2 | FUD 090 | J A2 50

AMA: 2018,Jan,8; 2017,Jan,8; 2016,Feb,12; 2016,Jan,13

65820 **Goniotomy**

INCLUDES Barkan's operation

Code also ophthalmic endoscope if used (66990)

21.5 | 21.5 | FUD 090 | 63 J A2 80 50

AMA: 2019,Sep,10; 2018,Dec,8; 2018,Dec,8; 2018,Jul,3; 2018,Jan,8; 2017,Jan,8; 2016,Feb,12; 2016,Jan,13

65850 **Trabeculotomy ab externo**

23.8 | 23.8 | FUD 090 | J A2 50

AMA: 2016,Feb,12

65855 **Trabeculoplasty by laser surgery**

EXCLUDES *Severing adhesions anterior segment (65860-65880)*
Trabeculectomy ab externo (66170)

5.91 | 7.01 | FUD 010 | T P3 50

AMA: 2018,Jan,8; 2017,Jan,8; 2016,Feb,12; 2016,Jan,13

65860 **Severing adhesions of anterior segment, laser technique (separate procedure)**

7.18 | 8.81 | FUD 090 | T P3 80 50

AMA: 2016,Feb,12

65865 **Severing adhesions of anterior segment of eye, incisional technique (with or without injection of air or liquid) (separate procedure); goniosynechiae**

EXCLUDES *Laser trabeculectomy (65855)*

13.4 | 13.4 | FUD 090 | J A2 50

AMA: 2016,Feb,12

65870 **anterior synechiae, except goniosynechiae**

16.7 | 16.7 | FUD 090 | J A2 50

AMA: 2016,Feb,12

65875 **posterior synechiae**
Code also ophthalmic endoscope when used (66990)
Facility RVU 17.9 Non-Facility RVU 17.9 FUD 090 J A2 50
AMA: 2018,Jan,8; 2017,Jan,8; 2016,Feb,12; 2016,Jan,13

65880 **corneovitreal adhesions**
EXCLUDES *Laser procedure (66821)*
Facility RVU 18.8 Non-Facility RVU 18.8 FUD 090 J A2 50
AMA: 2016,Feb,12

65900 **Removal of epithelial downgrowth, anterior chamber of eye**
Facility RVU 27.6 Non-Facility RVU 27.6 FUD 090 J A2 80 50
AMA: 2016,Feb,12

65920 **Removal of implanted material, anterior segment of eye**
Code also ophthalmic endoscope when used (66990)
Facility RVU 22.3 Non-Facility RVU 22.3 FUD 090 J A2 50
AMA: 2018,Jan,8; 2017,Jan,8; 2016,Feb,12; 2016,Jan,13

65930 **Removal of blood clot, anterior segment of eye**
Facility RVU 18.0 Non-Facility RVU 18.0 FUD 090 J A2 50
AMA: 2016,Feb,12

66020 **Injection, anterior chamber of eye (separate procedure); air or liquid**
EXCLUDES *Insertion ocular telescope prosthesis (0308T)*
Facility RVU 3.74 Non-Facility RVU 5.43 FUD 010 J A2 50
AMA: 2018,Jan,8; 2017,Jan,8; 2016,Feb,12; 2016,Jan,13

66030 **medication**
EXCLUDES *Insertion ocular telescope prosthesis (0308T)*
Facility RVU 3.16 Non-Facility RVU 4.87 FUD 010 J A2 50
AMA: 2016,Feb,12

66130 Excision Scleral Lesion

INCLUDES Operating microscope (69990)
EXCLUDES *Removal intraocular foreign body (65235)*
Surgery on posterior sclera (67250, 67255)

66130 **Excision of lesion, sclera**
Facility RVU 16.1 Non-Facility RVU 19.9 FUD 090 J A2 80 50
AMA: 2016,Feb,12

66150-66185 Procedures for Glaucoma

INCLUDES Operating microscope (69990)
EXCLUDES *Removal intraocular foreign body (65235)*
Surgery on posterior sclera (67250, 67255)

66150 **Fistulization of sclera for glaucoma; trephination with iridectomy**
Facility RVU 24.9 Non-Facility RVU 24.9 FUD 090 J A2 50
AMA: 2018,Jul,3; 2016,Feb,12

66155 **thermocauterization with iridectomy**
Facility RVU 24.9 Non-Facility RVU 24.9 FUD 090 J A2 50
AMA: 2018,Jul,3; 2016,Feb,12

66160 **sclerectomy with punch or scissors, with iridectomy**
INCLUDES Knapp's operation
Facility RVU 27.9 Non-Facility RVU 27.9 FUD 090 J A2 50
AMA: 2018,Jul,3; 2016,Feb,12

66170 **trabeculectomy ab externo in absence of previous surgery**
EXCLUDES *Repair surgical wound (66250)*
Trabeculectomy ab externo (65850)
Facility RVU 31.1 Non-Facility RVU 31.1 FUD 090 J A2 80 50
AMA: 2018,Dec,8; 2018,Dec,10; 2018,Dec,8; 2018,Dec,10; 2018,Jul,3; 2018,Jan,8; 2017,Jan,8; 2016,Feb,12; 2016,Jan,13

66172 **trabeculectomy ab externo with scarring from previous ocular surgery or trauma (includes injection of antifibrotic agents)**
Facility RVU 33.9 Non-Facility RVU 33.9 FUD 090 J A2 80 50
AMA: 2019,Apr,7; 2018,Dec,10; 2018,Dec,10; 2018,Jul,3; 2018,Jan,8; 2017,Jan,8; 2016,Feb,12; 2016,Jan,13

66174 **Transluminal dilation of aqueous outflow canal; without retention of device or stent**
EXCLUDES *Goniotomy (65820)*
Facility RVU 26.9 Non-Facility RVU 26.9 FUD 090 J A2 80 50
AMA: 2019,Sep,10; 2018,Dec,8; 2018,Dec,8; 2016,Feb,12

66175 **with retention of device or stent**
Facility RVU 28.2 Non-Facility RVU 28.2 FUD 090 J A2 80 50
AMA: 2016,Feb,12

66179 **Aqueous shunt to extraocular equatorial plate reservoir, external approach; without graft**
Facility RVU 30.6 Non-Facility RVU 30.6 FUD 090 J G2 80 50
AMA: 2018,Jul,3; 2018,Jan,8; 2017,Jan,8; 2016,Feb,12; 2016,Jan,13

66180 **with graft**
EXCLUDES *Scleral reinforcement (67255)*
Facility RVU 32.3 Non-Facility RVU 32.3 FUD 090 J J8 80 50
AMA: 2018,Jul,3; 2018,Jan,8; 2017,Jan,8; 2016,Feb,12; 2016,Jan,13

66183 **Insertion of anterior segment aqueous drainage device, without extraocular reservoir, external approach**
Facility RVU 29.2 Non-Facility RVU 29.2 FUD 090 J J8 80 50
AMA: 2020,Jun,14; 2018,Jul,3; 2018,Jan,8; 2017,Jan,8; 2016,Feb,12; 2016,Jan,13

66184 **Revision of aqueous shunt to extraocular equatorial plate reservoir; without graft**
Facility RVU 22.3 Non-Facility RVU 22.3 FUD 090 J G2 80 50
AMA: 2018,Jan,8; 2017,Jan,8; 2016,Feb,12; 2016,Jan,13

66185 **with graft**
EXCLUDES *Removal implanted shunt (67120)*
Scleral reinforcement (67255)
Facility RVU 24.0 Non-Facility RVU 24.0 FUD 090 J A2 80 50
AMA: 2018,Jan,8; 2017,Jan,8; 2016,Feb,12; 2016,Jan,13

66225 Staphyloma Repair

INCLUDES Operating microscope (69990)
EXCLUDES *Scleral procedures with retinal procedures (67101-67228)*
Scleral reinforcement (67250, 67255)

66225 **Repair of scleral staphyloma; with graft**
Facility RVU 26.4 Non-Facility RVU 26.4 FUD 090 J G2 50
AMA: 2016,Feb,12

66250 Anterior Segment Operative Wound Revision or Repair

INCLUDES Operating microscope (69990)
EXCLUDES *Unlisted procedures anterior sclera (66999)*

66250 **Revision or repair of operative wound of anterior segment, any type, early or late, major or minor procedure**
Facility RVU 15.8 Non-Facility RVU 21.4 FUD 090 J A2 50
AMA: 2018,Dec,8; 2018,Dec,8; 2018,Jan,8; 2017,Jan,8; 2016,Feb,12; 2016,Jan,13

66500-66505 Iridotomy With/Without Transfixion

INCLUDES Operating microscope (69990)
EXCLUDES *Photocoagulation iridotomy (66761)*

66500 **Iridotomy by stab incision (separate procedure); except transfixion**
Facility RVU 10.2 Non-Facility RVU 10.2 FUD 090 J A2 50
AMA: 2016,Feb,12

66505 **with transfixion as for iris bombe**
Facility RVU 11.1 Non-Facility RVU 11.1 FUD 090 J A2 50
AMA: 2016,Feb,12

66600-66635 Iridectomy Procedures

INCLUDES Operating microscope (69990)
EXCLUDES *Insertion ocular telescope prosthesis (0308T)*
Photocoagulation coreoplasty (66762)

66600 **Iridectomy, with corneoscleral or corneal section; for removal of lesion**
Facility RVU 23.9 Non-Facility RVU 23.9 FUD 090 J A2 50
AMA: 2016,Feb,12

66605 **with cyclectomy**
30.3 30.3 FUD 090 J A2 50
AMA: 2016,Feb,12

66625 **peripheral for glaucoma (separate procedure)**
12.2 12.2 FUD 090 J A2 50
AMA: 2016,Feb,12

66630 **sector for glaucoma (separate procedure)**
16.1 16.1 FUD 090 J A2 50
AMA: 2016,Feb,12

66635 **optical (separate procedure)**
16.3 16.3 FUD 090 J A2 50
AMA: 2016,Feb,12

66680-66770 Other Procedures of the Uveal Tract

INCLUDES Operating microscope (69990)
EXCLUDES *Unlisted procedures ciliary body or iris (66999)*

66680 **Repair of iris, ciliary body (as for iridodialysis)**
EXCLUDES *Resection/repositioning uveal tissue for perforating laceration, cornea and/or sclera (65285)*
14.7 14.7 FUD 090 J A2 50
AMA: 2016,Feb,12

66682 **Suture of iris, ciliary body (separate procedure) with retrieval of suture through small incision (eg, McCannel suture)**
18.3 18.3 FUD 090 J A2 50
AMA: 2016,Feb,12

66700 **Ciliary body destruction; diathermy**
INCLUDES Heine's operation
11.1 12.8 FUD 090 J A2 80 50
AMA: 2016,Feb,12

66710 **cyclophotocoagulation, transscleral**
11.1 12.6 FUD 090 J A2 50
AMA: 2018,Jan,8; 2017,Jan,8; 2016,Feb,12; 2016,Jan,13

66711 **cyclophotocoagulation, endoscopic, without concomitant removal of crystalline lens**
EXCLUDES *Endoscopic cyclophotocoagulation performed in conjunction with extracapsular cataract removal with insertion lens ([66987], [66988])*
18.2 18.2 FUD 090 J A2 50
AMA: 2019,Dec,6; 2018,Jan,8; 2017,Jan,8; 2016,Feb,12; 2016,Jan,13

66720 **cryotherapy**
11.6 13.1 FUD 090 J A2 50
AMA: 2016,Feb,12

66740 **cyclodialysis**
11.1 12.5 FUD 090 J A2 50
AMA: 2016,Feb,12

66761 **Iridotomy/iridectomy by laser surgery (eg, for glaucoma) (per session)**
EXCLUDES *Insertion ocular telescope prosthesis (0308T)*
6.68 8.49 FUD 010 T P3 50
AMA: 2018,Jan,8; 2017,Jan,8; 2016,Feb,12; 2016,Jan,13

66762 **Iridoplasty by photocoagulation (1 or more sessions) (eg, for improvement of vision, for widening of anterior chamber angle)**
12.0 13.5 FUD 090 T P2 50
AMA: 2018,Jan,8; 2017,Jan,8; 2016,Feb,12; 2016,Jan,13

66770 **Destruction of cyst or lesion iris or ciliary body (nonexcisional procedure)**
EXCLUDES *Excision:*
Epithelial downgrowth (65900)
Iris, ciliary body lesion (66600-66605)
13.7 15.0 FUD 090 T P2 50
AMA: 2016,Feb,12

66820-66825 Post-Cataract Surgery Procedures

INCLUDES Operating microscope (69990)

66820 **Discission of secondary membranous cataract (opacified posterior lens capsule and/or anterior hyaloid); stab incision technique (Ziegler or Wheeler knife)**
11.4 11.4 FUD 090 J G2 50
AMA: 2016,Feb,12

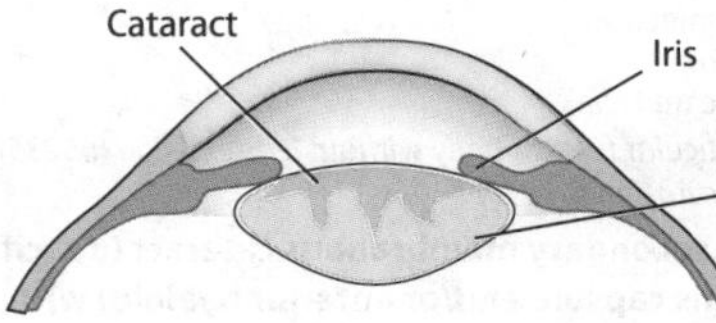

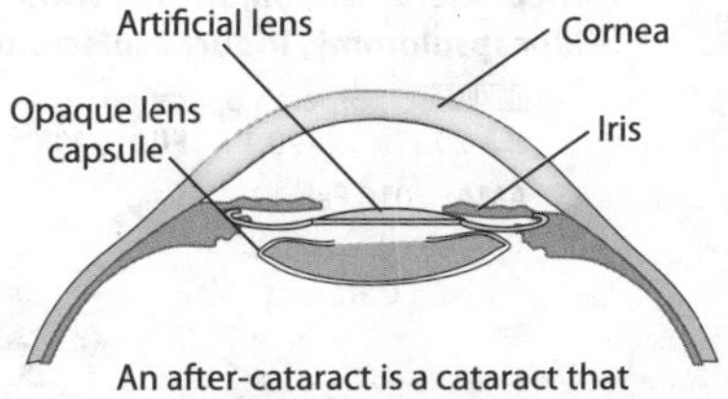

An after-cataract is a cataract that develops in a lens tissue that remains after most of the lens has already been removed

66821 **laser surgery (eg, YAG laser) (1 or more stages)**
8.85 9.42 FUD 090 T A2 50
AMA: 2016,Feb,12

66825 **Repositioning of intraocular lens prosthesis, requiring an incision (separate procedure)**
EXCLUDES *Insertion ocular telescope prosthesis (0308T)*
21.8 21.8 FUD 090 J A2 80 50
AMA: 2016,Feb,12

Eye, Ocular Adnexa, and Ear

66605 — 66825

66830-66940 Cataract Extraction; Without Insertion Intraocular Lens

CMS: 100-03,80.10 Phacoemulsification Procedure--Cataract Extraction

INCLUDES Anterior and/or posterior capsulotomy
Enzymatic zonulysis
Iridectomy/iridotomy
Lateral canthotomy
Medications
Operating microscope (69990)
Subconjunctival injection
Subtenon injection
Using viscoelastic material

EXCLUDES *Removal intralenticular foreign body without lens excision (65235)*
Repair surgical laceration (66250)

66830 Removal of secondary membranous cataract (opacified posterior lens capsule and/or anterior hyaloid) with corneo-scleral section, with or without iridectomy (iridocapsulotomy, iridocapsulectomy)

INCLUDES Graefe's operation

20.1 20.1 **FUD** 090 J A2 50

AMA: 2016,Feb,12

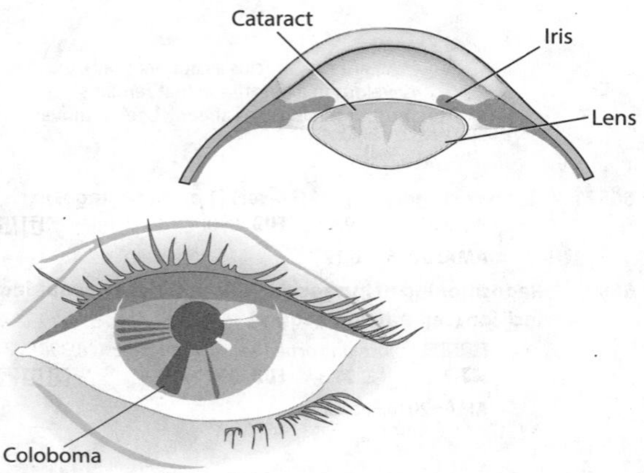

A congenital keyhole pupil is also called a coloboma of the iris

66840 Removal of lens material; aspiration technique, 1 or more stages

INCLUDES Fukala's operation

19.7 19.7 **FUD** 090 J A2 50

AMA: 2018,Jan,8; 2017,Jan,8; 2016,Sep,9; 2016,Jun,6; 2016,Apr,8; 2016,Feb,12; 2016,Jan,13

66850 phacofragmentation technique (mechanical or ultrasonic) (eg, phacoemulsification), with aspiration

22.5 22.5 **FUD** 090 J A2 50

AMA: 2018,Jan,8; 2017,Jan,8; 2016,Jun,6; 2016,Feb,12; 2016,Jan,13

66852 pars plana approach, with or without vitrectomy

23.9 23.9 **FUD** 090 J A2 80 50

AMA: 2018,Jan,8; 2017,Jan,8; 2016,Jun,6; 2016,Feb,12; 2016,Jan,13

66920 intracapsular

21.4 21.4 **FUD** 090 J A2 80 50

AMA: 2018,Jan,8; 2017,Jan,8; 2016,Feb,12; 2016,Jan,13

66930 intracapsular, for dislocated lens

24.3 24.3 **FUD** 090 J A2 80 50

AMA: 2018,Jan,8; 2017,Jan,8; 2016,Feb,12; 2016,Jan,13

66940 extracapsular (other than 66840, 66850, 66852)

22.2 22.2 **FUD** 090 J A2 80 50

AMA: 2018,Jan,8; 2017,Jan,8; 2016,Jun,6; 2016,Feb,12; 2016,Jan,13

66982-66988 [66987, 66988, 66989, 66991] Cataract Extraction: With Insertion Intraocular Lens

INCLUDES Anterior or posterior capsulotomy
Enzymatic zonulysis
Iridectomy/iridotomy
Lateral canthotomy
Medications
Operating microscope (69990)
Subconjunctival injection
Subtenon injection
Using viscoelastic material

EXCLUDES *Implanted material removal from anterior segment (65920)*
Insertion ocular telescope prosthesis (0308T)
Secondary fixation (66682)
Supply intraocular lens

66982 Extracapsular cataract removal with insertion of intraocular lens prosthesis (1-stage procedure), manual or mechanical technique (eg, irrigation and aspiration or phacoemulsification), complex, requiring devices or techniques not generally used in routine cataract surgery (eg, iris expansion device, suture support for intraocular lens, or primary posterior capsulorrhexis) or performed on patients in the amblyogenic developmental stage; without endoscopic cyclophotocoagulation

EXCLUDES *Complex extracapsular cataract removal in conjunction with aqueous drainage device insertion ([66989])*
Complex extracapsular cataract removal in conjunction with endoscopic cyclophotocoagulation ([66987])

(76519)

22.5 22.5 **FUD** 090 J A2 50

AMA: 2019,Dec,6; 2018,Dec,6; 2018,Dec,6; 2018,Jan,8; 2017,Dec,14; 2017,Jan,8; 2016,Mar,10; 2016,Feb,12; 2016,Jan,13

● # **66989 with insertion of intraocular (eg, trabecular meshwork, supraciliary, suprachoroidal) anterior segment aqueous drainage device, without extraocular reservoir, internal approach, one or more**

EXCLUDES *Complex extracapsular cataract removal without aqueous drainage device insertion during same operative session (66982)*
Insertion anterior segment aqueous drainage device only ([0671T])

0.00 0.00 **FUD** 000

66987 with endoscopic cyclophotocoagulation

EXCLUDES *Complex extracapsular cataract removal without endoscopic cyclophotocoagulation (66982)*

0.00 0.00 **FUD** 090 J8 80 50

AMA: 2019,Dec,6

66983 Intracapsular cataract extraction with insertion of intraocular lens prosthesis (1 stage procedure)

(76519)

21.0 21.0 **FUD** 090 J A2 50

AMA: 2019,Dec,6; 2018,Jan,8; 2017,Jan,8; 2016,Feb,12; 2016,Jan,13

66984 Extracapsular cataract removal with insertion of intraocular lens prosthesis (1 stage procedure), manual or mechanical technique (eg, irrigation and aspiration or phacoemulsification); without endoscopic cyclophotocoagulation

EXCLUDES *Complex extracapsular cataract removal (66982)*
Complex extracapsular cataract removal in conjunction with aqueous drainage device insertion ([66989])
Extracapsular cataract removal in conjunction with endoscopic cyclophotocoagulation ([66988])
Insertion anterior segment aqueous drainage device only ([0671T])

(76519)

18.1 18.1 **FUD** 090 J A2 50

AMA: 2020,Dec,13; 2019,Dec,6; 2018,Dec,6; 2018,Dec,6; 2018,Jan,8; 2017,Jan,8; 2016,Feb,12; 2016,Jan,13

● # **66991** **with insertion of intraocular (eg, trabecular meshwork, supraciliary, suprachoroidal) anterior segment aqueous drainage device, without extraocular reservoir, internal approach, one or more**

EXCLUDES *Extracapsular cataract removal without aqueous drainage device insertion during same operative session (66984)*
Insertion anterior segment aqueous drainage device only ([0671T])

0.00 0.00 FUD 000

66988 **with endoscopic cyclophotocoagulation**

EXCLUDES *Complex extracapsular cataract removal in conjunction with endoscopic cyclophotocoagulation ([66987])*
Extracapsular cataract removal without endoscopic cyclophotocoagulation (66984)

0.00 0.00 FUD 090 J8 80 50

AMA: 2019,Dec,6

66985-66989 [66987, 66988, 66989] Secondary Insertion or Replacement of Intraocular Lens

INCLUDES Operating microscope (69990)

EXCLUDES *Implanted material removal from anterior segment (65920)*
Insertion ocular telescope prosthesis (0308T)
Secondary fixation (66682)
Supply intraocular lens

Code also ophthalmic endoscope if used (66990)

66985 **Insertion of intraocular lens prosthesis (secondary implant), not associated with concurrent cataract removal**

EXCLUDES *Implanted material removal from anterior segment (65920)*
Insertion lens at time of cataract procedure (66982-66984)
Insertion ocular telescope prosthesis (0308T)
Secondary fixation (66682)
Supply intraocular lens

(76519)

21.8 21.8 FUD 090 J A2 50

AMA: 2018,Jan,8; 2017,Jan,8; 2016,Feb,12; 2016,Jan,13

66986 **Exchange of intraocular lens**

(76519)

25.8 25.8 FUD 090 J A2 50

AMA: 2018,Jan,8; 2017,Jan,8; 2016,Feb,12; 2016,Jan,13

66987 **Resequenced code. See code following resequenced code 66989.**

66988 **Resequenced code. See code following resequenced code 66991.**

66989 **Resequenced code. See code following 66982.**

66990-66999 [66991] Ophthalmic Endoscopy

INCLUDES Operating microscope (69990)

\+ **66990** **Use of ophthalmic endoscope (List separately in addition to code for primary procedure)**

Code first (65820, 65875, 65920, 66985-66986, 67036, 67039-67043, 67113)

2.56 2.56 FUD ZZZ N N1

AMA: 2018,Jul,3; 2018,Jan,8; 2017,Jan,8; 2016,Sep,5; 2016,Feb,12; 2016,Jan,13

66991 **Resequenced code. See code following 66984.**

66999 **Unlisted procedure, anterior segment of eye**

0.00 0.00 FUD YYY J 80 50

AMA: 2018,Jan,8; 2017,Jan,8; 2016,Apr,8; 2016,Feb,12; 2016,Jan,13

67005-67015 Vitrectomy: Partial and Subtotal

INCLUDES Operating microscope (69990)

67005 **Removal of vitreous, anterior approach (open sky technique or limbal incision); partial removal**

EXCLUDES *Anterior chamber vitrectomy by paracentesis (65810)*
Severing corneovitreal adhesions (65880)

13.4 13.4 FUD 090 J A2 50

AMA: 2018,Jan,8; 2017,Jan,8; 2016,Feb,12; 2016,Jan,13

67010 **subtotal removal with mechanical vitrectomy**

EXCLUDES *Anterior chamber vitrectomy by paracentesis (65810)*
Severing corneovitreal adhesions (65880)

15.4 15.4 FUD 090 J A2 50

AMA: 2018,Jan,8; 2017,Jan,8; 2016,Feb,12; 2016,Jan,13

67015 **Aspiration or release of vitreous, subretinal or choroidal fluid, pars plana approach (posterior sclerotomy)**

16.5 16.5 FUD 090 J A2 50

AMA: 2018,Jan,8; 2017,Jan,8; 2016,Sep,5; 2016,Jun,6; 2016,Feb,12

67025-67028 Intravitreal Injection/Implantation

INCLUDES Operating microscope (69990)

67025 **Injection of vitreous substitute, pars plana or limbal approach (fluid-gas exchange), with or without aspiration (separate procedure)**

17.9 20.8 FUD 090 J A2 50

AMA: 2019,Aug,10; 2018,Feb,3; 2016,Feb,12

67027 **Implantation of intravitreal drug delivery system (eg, ganciclovir implant), includes concomitant removal of vitreous**

EXCLUDES *Removal drug delivery system (67121)*

24.2 24.2 FUD 090 J A2 80 50

AMA: 2018,Feb,3; 2018,Jan,8; 2017,Jan,8; 2016,Feb,12; 2016,Jan,13

67028 **Intravitreal injection of a pharmacologic agent (separate procedure)**

2.79 2.86 FUD 000 S P3 50

AMA: 2018,Feb,3; 2018,Jan,8; 2017,Jan,8; 2016,Feb,12; 2016,Jan,13

67030-67031 Incision of Vitreous Strands/Membranes

INCLUDES Operating microscope (69990)

67030 **Discission of vitreous strands (without removal), pars plana approach**

15.2 15.2 FUD 090 J A2 50

AMA: 2016,Feb,12

67031 **Severing of vitreous strands, vitreous face adhesions, sheets, membranes or opacities, laser surgery (1 or more stages)**

10.1 11.1 FUD 090 T A2 50

AMA: 2016,Feb,12

67036-67043 Pars Plana Mechanical Vitrectomy

INCLUDES Operating microscope (69990)

EXCLUDES *Lens removal (66850)*
Removal foreign body (65260, 65265)
Unlisted vitreal procedures (67299)
Vitrectomy in retinal detachment (67108, 67113)

Code also ophthalmic endoscope if used (66990)

67036 **Vitrectomy, mechanical, pars plana approach;**

25.6 25.6 FUD 090 J A2 80 50

AMA: 2018,Jan,8; 2017,Jan,8; 2016,Sep,5; 2016,Feb,12; 2016,Jan,13

67039 **with focal endolaser photocoagulation**

27.4 27.4 FUD 090 J A2 80 50

AMA: 2018,Jan,8; 2017,Jan,8; 2016,Sep,5; 2016,Feb,12; 2016,Jan,13

67040 **with endolaser panretinal photocoagulation**

29.6 29.6 FUD 090 J A2 80 50

AMA: 2018,Jan,8; 2017,Jan,8; 2016,Sep,5; 2016,Feb,12; 2016,Jan,13

67041 **with removal of preretinal cellular membrane (eg, macular pucker)**

32.7 32.7 FUD 090 J G2 80 50

AMA: 2018,Jan,8; 2017,Jan,8; 2016,Sep,5; 2016,Feb,12; 2016,Jan,13

67042 **with removal of internal limiting membrane of retina (eg, for repair of macular hole, diabetic macular edema), includes, if performed, intraocular tamponade (ie, air, gas or silicone oil)**
32.7 32.7 FUD 090 J G2 80 50
AMA: 2018,Jan,8; 2017,Jan,8; 2016,Sep,5; 2016,Feb,12; 2016,Jan,13

67043 **with removal of subretinal membrane (eg, choroidal neovascularization), includes, if performed, intraocular tamponade (ie, air, gas or silicone oil) and laser photocoagulation**
34.3 34.3 FUD 090 J G2 80 50
AMA: 2018,Jan,8; 2017,Jan,8; 2016,Sep,5; 2016,Feb,12; 2016,Jan,13

67101-67115 Detached Retina Repair

INCLUDES Operating microscope (69990)
Primary technique when cryotherapy and/or diathermy and/or photocoagulation are used in combination

67101 **Repair of retinal detachment, including drainage of subretinal fluid when performed; cryotherapy**
8.10 9.40 FUD 010 J P3 50
AMA: 2018,Jan,8; 2017,Feb,14; 2017,Jan,8; 2016,Sep,5; 2016,Jun,6; 2016,Feb,12; 2016,Jan,13

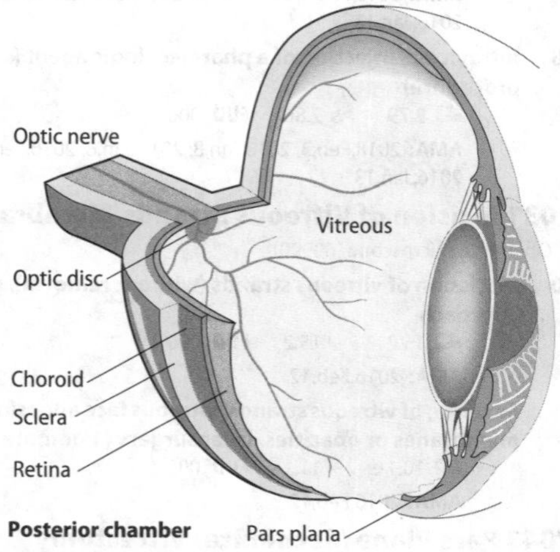

67105 **photocoagulation**
7.82 8.45 FUD 010 T P3 50
AMA: 2018,Jan,8; 2017,Feb,14; 2017,Jan,8; 2016,Sep,5; 2016,Jun,6; 2016,Feb,12; 2016,Jan,13

67107 **Repair of retinal detachment; scleral buckling (such as lamellar scleral dissection, imbrication or encircling procedure), including, when performed, implant, cryotherapy, photocoagulation, and drainage of subretinal fluid**
INCLUDES Gonin's operation
31.9 31.9 FUD 090 J G2 80 50
AMA: 2019,Aug,10; 2018,Jan,8; 2017,Jan,8; 2016,Sep,5; 2016,Jun,6; 2016,Feb,12

67108 **with vitrectomy, any method, including, when performed, air or gas tamponade, focal endolaser photocoagulation, cryotherapy, drainage of subretinal fluid, scleral buckling, and/or removal of lens by same technique**
34.1 34.1 FUD 090 J G2 80 50
AMA: 2018,Jan,8; 2017,Jan,8; 2016,Sep,5; 2016,Jun,6; 2016,Feb,12; 2016,Jan,13

67110 **by injection of air or other gas (eg, pneumatic retinopexy)**
23.1 25.0 FUD 090 J P3 50
AMA: 2018,Jan,8; 2017,Jan,8; 2016,Sep,5; 2016,Jun,6; 2016,Feb,12

67113 **Repair of complex retinal detachment (eg, proliferative vitreoretinopathy, stage C-1 or greater, diabetic traction retinal detachment, retinopathy of prematurity, retinal tear of greater than 90 degrees), with vitrectomy and membrane peeling, including, when performed, air, gas, or silicone oil tamponade, cryotherapy, endolaser photocoagulation, drainage of subretinal fluid, scleral buckling, and/or removal of lens**
EXCLUDES *Vitrectomy for other than retinal detachment, pars plana approach (67036-67043)*
Code also ophthalmic endoscope if used (66990)
38.0 38.0 FUD 090 J G2 80 50
AMA: 2018,Jan,8; 2017,Jan,8; 2016,Sep,5; 2016,Jun,6; 2016,Feb,12; 2016,Jan,13

67115 **Release of encircling material (posterior segment)**
14.1 14.1 FUD 090 J A2 50
AMA: 2016,Feb,12

67120-67121 Removal of Previously Implanted Prosthetic Device

INCLUDES Operating microscope (69990)
EXCLUDES *Foreign body removal (65260, 65265)*
Removal implanted material anterior segment (65920)

67120 **Removal of implanted material, posterior segment; extraocular**
15.8 18.8 FUD 090 J A2 50
AMA: 2016,Feb,12

67121 **intraocular**
25.6 25.6 FUD 090 J A2 80 50
AMA: 2016,Feb,12

67141-67145 Retinal Detachment: Preventative Procedures

INCLUDES Operating microscope (69990)
Treatment at one or more sessions that may occur at different encounters
EXCLUDES *Procedure performed more than one time during defined period of treatment*

▲ **67141** **Prophylaxis of retinal detachment (eg, retinal break, lattice degeneration) without drainage; cryotherapy, diathermy**
13.8 14.9 FUD 090 T A2 50
AMA: 2018,Jan,8; 2017,Jan,8; 2016,Sep,5; 2016,Feb,12; 2016,Jan,13

▲ **67145** **photocoagulation**
14.1 15.0 FUD 090 T P2 50
AMA: 2018,Jan,8; 2017,Jan,8; 2016,Sep,5; 2016,Feb,12; 2016,Jan,13

67208-67218 Destruction of Retinal Lesions

INCLUDES Operating microscope (69990)
Treatment at one or more sessions that may occur at different encounters
EXCLUDES *Procedure performed more than one time during defined period of treatment*
Unlisted retinal procedures (67299)

67208 **Destruction of localized lesion of retina (eg, macular edema, tumors), 1 or more sessions; cryotherapy, diathermy**
16.4 17.0 FUD 090 T P2 50
AMA: 2018,Jan,8; 2017,Jan,8; 2016,Feb,12; 2016,Jan,13

67210 **photocoagulation**
14.1 14.6 FUD 090 T P2 50
AMA: 2018,Jan,8; 2017,Jan,8; 2016,Feb,12; 2016,Jan,13

67218 **radiation by implantation of source (includes removal of source)**
39.4 39.4 FUD 090 J A2 50
AMA: 2018,Jan,8; 2017,Jan,8; 2016,Feb,12; 2016,Jan,13

67220-67225 Destruction of Choroidal Lesions

INCLUDES Operating microscope (69990)

67220 **Destruction of localized lesion of choroid (eg, choroidal neovascularization); photocoagulation (eg, laser), 1 or more sessions**

INCLUDES Treatment at one or more sessions that may occur at different encounters

EXCLUDES *Procedure performed more than one time during defined period of treatment*

14.1 15.0 FUD 090 T P2 50

AMA: 2018,Jan,8; 2017,Jan,8; 2016,Feb,12; 2016,Jan,13

67221 **photodynamic therapy (includes intravenous infusion)**

6.05 8.07 FUD 000 T P3

AMA: 2018,Feb,10; 2018,Jan,8; 2017,Jan,8; 2016,Feb,12; 2016,Jan,13

\+ **67225** **photodynamic therapy, second eye, at single session (List separately in addition to code for primary eye treatment)**

Code first (67221)

0.81 0.85 FUD ZZZ N N1

AMA: 2018,Jan,8; 2017,Jan,8; 2016,Feb,12; 2016,Jan,13

67227-67229 Destruction Retinopathy

INCLUDES Operating microscope (69990)

EXCLUDES *Unlisted retinal procedures (67299)*

67227 **Destruction of extensive or progressive retinopathy (eg, diabetic retinopathy), cryotherapy, diathermy**

7.24 8.33 FUD 010 J P3 50

AMA: 2018,Jan,8; 2017,Jan,8; 2016,Feb,12; 2016,Jan,13

67228 **Treatment of extensive or progressive retinopathy (eg, diabetic retinopathy), photocoagulation**

8.64 9.67 FUD 010 T P3 50

AMA: 2018,Jan,8; 2017,Jan,8; 2016,Feb,12; 2016,Jan,13

67229 **Treatment of extensive or progressive retinopathy, 1 or more sessions, preterm infant (less than 37 weeks gestation at birth), performed from birth up to 1 year of age (eg, retinopathy of prematurity), photocoagulation or cryotherapy**

INCLUDES Treatment at one or more sessions that may occur at different encounters

EXCLUDES *Procedure performed more than one time during defined period of treatment*

33.1 33.1 FUD 090 T R2 50

AMA: 2018,Jan,8; 2017,Jan,8; 2016,Feb,12; 2016,Jan,13

67250-67255 Reinforcement of Posterior Sclera

INCLUDES Operating microscope (69990)

EXCLUDES *Removal scleral lesion (66130)*
Repair scleral staphyloma (66225)

67250 **Scleral reinforcement (separate procedure); without graft**

22.6 22.6 FUD 090 J A2 50

AMA: 2016,Feb,12

67255 **with graft**

EXCLUDES *Aqueous shunt to extraocular equatorial plate reservoir (66180)*
Revision aqueous shunt to extraocular equatorial plate reservoir; with graft (66185)

19.3 19.3 FUD 090 J A2 80 50

AMA: 2018,Jan,8; 2017,Jan,8; 2016,Feb,12; 2016,Jan,13

67299 Unlisted Posterior Segment Procedure

CMS: 100-04,4,180.3 Unlisted Service or Procedure

INCLUDES Operating microscope (69990)

67299 **Unlisted procedure, posterior segment**

0.00 0.00 FUD YYY J 80 50

AMA: 2018,Jan,8; 2017,Jan,8; 2016,Feb,12; 2016,Jan,13

67311-67334 Strabismus Procedures on Extraocular Muscles

INCLUDES Operating microscope (69990)

Code also adjustable sutures (67335)

67311 **Strabismus surgery, recession or resection procedure; 1 horizontal muscle**

16.8 16.8 FUD 090 J A2 50

AMA: 2018,Jan,8; 2017,Jan,8; 2017,Jan,6; 2016,Feb,12; 2016,Jan,13

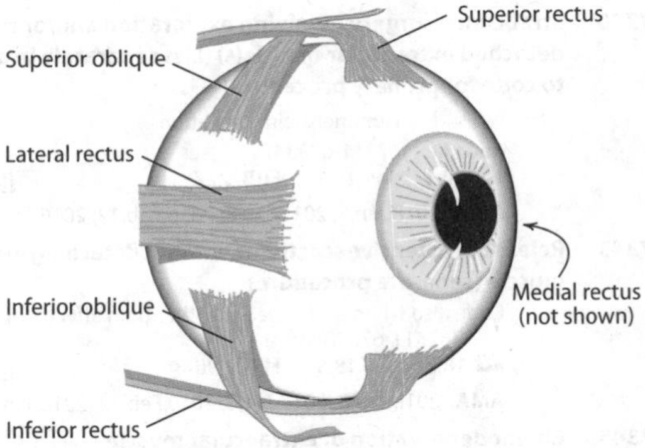

Muscles of the eyeball (right eye shown)

67312 **2 horizontal muscles**

20.3 20.3 FUD 090 J A2 50

AMA: 2018,Jan,8; 2017,Jan,8; 2016,Feb,12; 2016,Jan,13

67314 **1 vertical muscle (excluding superior oblique)**

19.1 19.1 FUD 090 J A2 50

AMA: 2018,Jan,8; 2017,Jan,8; 2016,Feb,12; 2016,Jan,13

67316 **2 or more vertical muscles (excluding superior oblique)**

22.7 22.7 FUD 090 J A2 80 50

AMA: 2018,Jan,8; 2017,Jan,8; 2016,Feb,12; 2016,Jan,13

67318 **Strabismus surgery, any procedure, superior oblique muscle**

20.0 20.0 FUD 090 J A2 50

AMA: 2018,Jan,8; 2017,Jan,8; 2016,Feb,12; 2016,Jan,13

\+ **67320** **Transposition procedure (eg, for paretic extraocular muscle), any extraocular muscle (specify) (List separately in addition to code for primary procedure)**

Code first (67311-67318)

9.17 9.17 FUD ZZZ N N1

AMA: 2018,Jan,8; 2017,Jan,8; 2016,Feb,12; 2016,Jan,13

\+ **67331** **Strabismus surgery on patient with previous eye surgery or injury that did not involve the extraocular muscles (List separately in addition to code for primary procedure)**

Code first (67311-67318)

8.70 8.70 FUD ZZZ N N1 50

AMA: 2018,Jan,8; 2017,Jan,8; 2016,Feb,12; 2016,Jan,13

\+ **67332** **Strabismus surgery on patient with scarring of extraocular muscles (eg, prior ocular injury, strabismus or retinal detachment surgery) or restrictive myopathy (eg, dysthyroid ophthalmopathy) (List separately in addition to code for primary procedure)**

Code first (67311-67318)

9.37 9.37 FUD ZZZ N N1 50

AMA: 2018,Jan,8; 2017,Jan,8; 2016,Feb,12; 2016,Jan,13

\+ **67334** **Strabismus surgery by posterior fixation suture technique, with or without muscle recession (List separately in addition to code for primary procedure)**

Code first (67311-67318)

8.52 8.52 FUD ZZZ N N1 50

AMA: 2018,Jan,8; 2017,Jan,8; 2016,Feb,12; 2016,Jan,13

67335-67399 Other Procedures of Extraocular Muscles

INCLUDES Operating microscope (69990)

+ **67335** **Placement of adjustable suture(s) during strabismus surgery, including postoperative adjustment(s) of suture(s) (List separately in addition to code for specific strabismus surgery)**

Code first (67311-67334)

4.21 4.21 FUD ZZZ N N1 50

AMA: 2018,Jan,8; 2017,Jan,8; 2016,Feb,12; 2016,Jan,13

+ **67340** **Strabismus surgery involving exploration and/or repair of detached extraocular muscle(s) (List separately in addition to code for primary procedure)**

INCLUDES Hummelsheim operation

Code first (67311-67334)

10.1 10.1 FUD ZZZ N N1 80

AMA: 2018,Jan,8; 2017,Jan,8; 2016,Feb,12; 2016,Jan,13

67343 **Release of extensive scar tissue without detaching extraocular muscle (separate procedure)**

Code also when performed on other than affected muscle (67311-67340)

18.5 18.5 FUD 090 J A2 50

AMA: 2018,Jan,8; 2017,Jan,8; 2016,Feb,12; 2016,Jan,13

67345 **Chemodenervation of extraocular muscle**

EXCLUDES *Nerve destruction for blepharospasm and other neurological disorders (64612, 64616)*

6.22 6.96 FUD 010 T P3 50

AMA: 2019,Apr,9; 2018,Jan,8; 2017,Jan,8; 2016,Feb,12; 2016,Jan,13

67346 **Biopsy of extraocular muscle**

EXCLUDES *Repair laceration extraocular muscle, tendon, or Tenon's capsule (65290)*

5.50 5.50 FUD 000 J A2 80 50

AMA: 2016,Feb,12

67399 **Unlisted procedure, extraocular muscle**

0.00 0.00 FUD YYY T 80 50

AMA: 2018,Jan,8; 2017,Jul,10; 2016,Feb,12

67400-67415 Frontal Orbitotomy

INCLUDES Operating microscope (69990)

67400 **Orbitotomy without bone flap (frontal or transconjunctival approach); for exploration, with or without biopsy**

26.7 26.7 FUD 090 J A2 50

AMA: 2016,Feb,12

67405 **with drainage only**

22.8 22.8 FUD 090 J A2 50

AMA: 2018,Jan,8; 2017,Jan,8; 2016,Feb,12; 2016,Jan,13

67412 **with removal of lesion**

26.1 26.1 FUD 090 J A2 50

AMA: 2016,Feb,12

67413 **with removal of foreign body**

25.8 25.8 FUD 090 J A2 80 50

AMA: 2016,Feb,12

67414 **with removal of bone for decompression**

38.1 38.1 FUD 090 J G2 80 50

AMA: 2018,Jan,8; 2017,Jan,8; 2016,Feb,12; 2016,Jan,13

67415 **Fine needle aspiration of orbital contents**

EXCLUDES *Decompression optic nerve (67570)*
Exenteration, enucleation, and repair (65101-65175)

2.97 2.97 FUD 000 J A2 80 50

AMA: 2016,Feb,12

67420-67450 Lateral Orbitotomy

INCLUDES Operating microscope (69990)

EXCLUDES *Orbital implant (67550, 67560)*
Surgical removal all or some orbital contents or repair after removal (65091-65175)
Transcranial approach orbitotomy (61330, 61333)

67420 **Orbitotomy with bone flap or window, lateral approach (eg, Kroenlein); with removal of lesion**

47.5 47.5 FUD 090 J A2 80 50

AMA: 2016,Feb,12

67430 **with removal of foreign body**

37.3 37.3 FUD 090 J A2 80 50

AMA: 2016,Feb,12

67440 **with drainage**

36.1 36.1 FUD 090 J A2 80 50

AMA: 2016,Feb,12

67445 **with removal of bone for decompression**

EXCLUDES *Decompression optic nerve sheath (67570)*

41.6 41.6 FUD 090 J A2 80 50

AMA: 2019,Dec,14; 2016,Feb,12

67450 **for exploration, with or without biopsy**

36.1 36.1 FUD 090 J A2 80 50

AMA: 2016,Feb,12

67500-67515 Eye Injections

INCLUDES Operating microscope (69990)

67500 **Retrobulbar injection; medication (separate procedure, does not include supply of medication)**

1.74 2.07 FUD 000 T P3 50

AMA: 2018,Jan,8; 2017,Jan,8; 2016,Feb,12; 2016,Jan,13

67505 **alcohol**

2.03 2.38 FUD 000 T P3 50

AMA: 2016,Feb,12

67515 **Injection of medication or other substance into Tenon's capsule**

EXCLUDES *Subconjunctival injection (68200)*

2.06 2.24 FUD 000 T P3 50

AMA: 2018,Jan,8; 2017,Jan,8; 2016,Feb,12; 2016,Jan,13

67550-67560 Orbital Implant

INCLUDES Operating microscope (69990)

EXCLUDES *Fracture repair malar area, orbit (21355-21408)*
Ocular implant inside muscle cone (65093-65105, 65130-65175)

67550 **Orbital implant (implant outside muscle cone); insertion**

29.0 29.0 FUD 090 J A2 50

AMA: 2016,Feb,12

67560 **removal or revision**

28.5 28.5 FUD 090 J A2 80 50

AMA: 2016,Feb,12

67570-67599 Other and Unlisted Orbital Procedures

INCLUDES Operating microscope (69990)

67570 **Optic nerve decompression (eg, incision or fenestration of optic nerve sheath)**

35.6 35.6 FUD 090 J A2 80 50

AMA: 2016,Feb,12

67599 **Unlisted procedure, orbit**

0.00 0.00 FUD YYY T 80 50

AMA: 2016,Feb,12

67700-67810 [67810] Incisional Procedures of Eyelids

INCLUDES Operating microscope (69990)

67700 **Blepharotomy, drainage of abscess, eyelid**

3.31 7.82 FUD 010 T P2 50

AMA: 2018,Jan,8; 2017,Jan,8; 2016,Feb,12; 2016,Jan,13

67710 **Severing of tarsorrhaphy**

2.75 6.68 FUD 010 T P3 50

AMA: 2018,Jan,8; 2017,Jan,8; 2016,Feb,12; 2016,Jan,13

67715 **Canthotomy (separate procedure)**

EXCLUDES *Canthoplasty (67950)*
Symblepharon division (68340)

3.08 7.07 FUD 010 J A2 50

AMA: 2018,Jan,8; 2017,Jan,8; 2016,Feb,12; 2016,Jan,13

\# **67810** **Incisional biopsy of eyelid skin including lid margin**

EXCLUDES *Biopsy eyelid skin (11102-11107)*

2.03 4.99 FUD 000 T P2 50

AMA: 2019,Jan,9; 2018,Jan,8; 2017,Jan,8; 2016,Feb,12; 2016,Jan,13

67800-67808 Excision of Chalazion (Meibomian Cyst)

INCLUDES Lesion removal requiring more than skin:
Lid margin
Palpebral conjunctiva
Tarsus
Operating microscope (69990)

EXCLUDES *Blepharoplasty, graft, or reconstructive procedures (67930-67975)*
Excision/destruction skin lesion eyelid (11310-11313, 11440-11446, 11640-11646, 17000-17004)

67800 **Excision of chalazion; single**

2.91 3.64 FUD 010 T P3

AMA: 2018,Jan,8; 2017,Jan,8; 2016,Feb,12; 2016,Jan,13

67801 **multiple, same lid**

3.74 4.61 FUD 010 T P3

AMA: 2016,Feb,12

67805 **multiple, different lids**

4.63 5.72 FUD 010 T P3

AMA: 2018,Jan,8; 2017,Jan,8; 2016,Feb,12; 2016,Jan,13

67808 **under general anesthesia and/or requiring hospitalization, single or multiple**

10.4 10.4 FUD 090 J A2

AMA: 2016,Feb,12

67810-67850 [67810] Other Eyelid Procedures

INCLUDES Operating microscope (69990)

67810 **Resequenced code. See code following 67715.**

67820 **Correction of trichiasis; epilation, by forceps only**

0.99 0.93 FUD 000 Q1 N1 50

AMA: 2018,Jan,8; 2017,Jan,8; 2016,Feb,12; 2016,Jan,13

67825 **epilation by other than forceps (eg, by electrosurgery, cryotherapy, laser surgery)**

3.46 3.71 FUD 010 T P3 50

AMA: 2018,Jan,8; 2017,Jan,8; 2016,Feb,12; 2016,Jan,13

67830 **incision of lid margin**

3.92 7.64 FUD 010 T A2 50

AMA: 2016,Feb,12

67835 **incision of lid margin, with free mucous membrane graft**

12.4 12.4 FUD 090 J A2 80 50

AMA: 2016,Feb,12

67840 **Excision of lesion of eyelid (except chalazion) without closure or with simple direct closure**

EXCLUDES *Eyelid resection and reconstruction (67961, 67966)*

4.49 7.91 FUD 010 T P3 50

AMA: 2019,Jan,14; 2016,Feb,12

67850 **Destruction of lesion of lid margin (up to 1 cm)**

EXCLUDES *Mohs micro procedures (17311-17315)*
Topical chemotherapy (99202-99215)

3.75 6.12 FUD 010 T P3 50

AMA: 2016,Feb,12

67875-67882 Suturing of the Eyelids

INCLUDES Operating microscope (69990)

EXCLUDES *Canthoplasty (67950)*
Canthotomy (67715)
Severing of tarsorrhaphy (67710)

67875 **Temporary closure of eyelids by suture (eg, Frost suture)**

2.75 4.96 FUD 000 T G2 50

AMA: 2016,Feb,12

67880 **Construction of intermarginal adhesions, median tarsorrhaphy, or canthorrhaphy;**

10.4 13.1 FUD 090 J A2 50

AMA: 2016,Feb,12

67882 **with transposition of tarsal plate**

13.3 16.1 FUD 090 J A2 50

AMA: 2016,Feb,12

67900-67912 Repair of Ptosis/Retraction Eyelids, Eyebrows

INCLUDES Operating microscope (69990)

67900 **Repair of brow ptosis (supraciliary, mid-forehead or coronal approach)**

EXCLUDES *Forehead rhytidectomy (15824)*

14.4 18.2 FUD 090 J A2 50

AMA: 2018,Jan,8; 2017,Jan,8; 2016,Feb,12; 2016,Jan,13

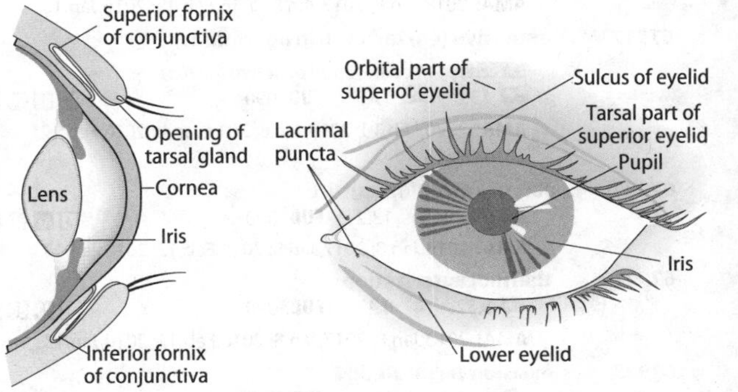

67901 **Repair of blepharoptosis; frontalis muscle technique with suture or other material (eg, banked fascia)**

16.5 21.9 FUD 090 J A2 50

AMA: 2018,Jan,8; 2017,Jul,10; 2017,Jan,8; 2016,Feb,12; 2016,Jan,13

67902 **frontalis muscle technique with autologous fascial sling (includes obtaining fascia)**

20.5 20.5 FUD 090 J A2 50

AMA: 2018,Jan,8; 2017,Jan,8; 2016,Feb,12; 2016,Jan,13

67903 **(tarso) levator resection or advancement, internal approach**

13.7 16.9 FUD 090 J A2 50

AMA: 2018,Jan,8; 2017,Jan,8; 2016,Feb,12; 2016,Jan,13

67904 **(tarso) levator resection or advancement, external approach**

INCLUDES Everbusch's operation

16.9 20.9 FUD 090 J A2 50

AMA: 2018,Jan,8; 2017,Jan,8; 2016,Feb,12; 2016,Jan,13

67906 **superior rectus technique with fascial sling (includes obtaining fascia)**

14.4 14.4 FUD 090 J A2 50

AMA: 2018,Jan,8; 2017,Jan,8; 2016,Feb,12; 2016,Jan,13

67908 **conjunctivo-tarso-Muller's muscle-levator resection (eg, Fasanella-Servat type)**

12.1 14.1 FUD 090 J A2 50

AMA: 2018,Jan,8; 2017,Jan,8; 2016,Feb,12; 2016,Jan,13

67909 **Reduction of overcorrection of ptosis**

12.4 15.3 FUD 090 J A2 50

AMA: 2018,Jan,8; 2017,Jan,8; 2016,Feb,12; 2016,Jan,13

67911 **Correction of lid retraction**

EXCLUDES *Autologous graft harvest ([15769], 20920, 20922)*
Lid defect correction using fat obtained via liposuction (15773-15774)
Mucous membrane graft repair trichiasis (67835)

15.9 15.9 FUD 090 J A2 50

AMA: 2018,Jan,8; 2017,Jan,8; 2016,Feb,12; 2016,Jan,13

67912 **Correction of lagophthalmos, with implantation of upper eyelid lid load (eg, gold weight)**

13.8 25.4 FUD 090 J A2 50

AMA: 2018,Jan,8; 2017,Jan,8; 2016,Feb,12; 2016,Jan,13

67914-67924 Repair Ectropion/Entropion

INCLUDES Operating microscope (69990)

EXCLUDES *Cicatricial ectropion or entropion with scar excision or graft (67961-67966)*

67914 **Repair of ectropion; suture**

INCLUDES Canthoplasty (67950)

9.29 13.5 FUD 090 J A2 50

AMA: 2018,Jan,8; 2017,Jan,8; 2016,Feb,12; 2016,Jan,13

67915 **thermocauterization**

5.62 8.52 FUD 090 J P3 50

AMA: 2018,Jan,8; 2017,Jan,8; 2016,Feb,12; 2016,Jan,13

67916 **excision tarsal wedge**

12.2 17.0 FUD 090 J A2 50

AMA: 2018,Jan,8; 2017,Jan,8; 2016,Feb,12; 2016,Jan,13

67917 **extensive (eg, tarsal strip operations)**

EXCLUDES *Repair everted punctum (68705)*

13.0 17.3 FUD 090 J A2 50

AMA: 2020,Feb,13; 2018,Jan,8; 2017,Jan,8; 2016,Feb,12; 2016,Jan,13

67921 **Repair of entropion; suture**

8.82 13.2 FUD 090 J A2 50

AMA: 2018,Jan,8; 2017,Jan,8; 2016,Feb,12; 2016,Jan,13

67922 **thermocauterization**

5.52 8.42 FUD 090 J P3 50

AMA: 2018,Jan,8; 2017,Jan,8; 2016,Feb,12; 2016,Jan,13

67923 **excision tarsal wedge**

12.1 17.1 FUD 090 J A2 50

AMA: 2018,Jan,8; 2017,Jan,8; 2016,Feb,12; 2016,Jan,13

67924 **extensive (eg, tarsal strip or capsulopalpebral fascia repairs operation)**

INCLUDES Canthoplasty (67950)

12.9 18.2 FUD 090 J A2 50

AMA: 2018,Jan,8; 2017,Jan,8; 2016,Feb,12; 2016,Jan,13

67930-67935 Repair Eyelid Wound

INCLUDES Operating microscope (69990)
Repairs involving more than skin:
- Lid margin
- Palpebral conjunctiva
- Tarsus

EXCLUDES *Blepharoplasty for entropion or ectropion (67916-67917, 67923-67924)*
Correction lid retraction and blepharoptosis (67901-67911)
Free graft (15120-15121, 15260-15261)
Graft preparation (15004)
Plastic repair lacrimal canaliculi (68700)
Removal eyelid lesion (67800 [67810], 67840-67850)
Repair blepharochalasis (15820-15823)
Repair involving eyelid skin (12011-12018, 12051-12057, 13151-13153)
Skin adjacent tissue transfer (14060-14061)
Tarsorrhaphy, canthorrhaphy (67880, 67882)

67930 **Suture of recent wound, eyelid, involving lid margin, tarsus, and/or palpebral conjunctiva direct closure; partial thickness**

6.78 10.4 FUD 010 J P3 50

AMA: 2016,Feb,12

67935 **full thickness**

12.5 16.9 FUD 090 J A2 50

AMA: 2016,Feb,12

67938-67999 Eyelid Reconstruction/Repair/Removal Deep Foreign Body

INCLUDES Operating microscope (69990)

EXCLUDES *Blepharoplasty for entropion or ectropion (67916-67917, 67923-67924)*
Correction lid retraction and blepharoptosis (67901-67911)
Free graft (15120-15121, 15260-15261)
Graft preparation (15004)
Plastic repair lacrimal canaliculi (68700)
Removal eyelid lesion (67800-67808, 67840-67850)
Repair blepharochalasis (15820-15823)
Repair involving eyelid skin (12011-12018, 12051-12057, 13151-13153)
Skin adjacent tissue transfer (14060-14061)
Tarsorrhaphy, canthorrhaphy (67880, 67882)

67938 **Removal of embedded foreign body, eyelid**

3.28 7.36 FUD 010 T P2 50

AMA: 2018,Jan,8; 2017,Jan,8; 2016,Feb,12; 2016,Jan,13

67950 **Canthoplasty (reconstruction of canthus)**

13.1 16.4 FUD 090 J A2 50

AMA: 2016,Feb,12

67961 **Excision and repair of eyelid, involving lid margin, tarsus, conjunctiva, canthus, or full thickness, may include preparation for skin graft or pedicle flap with adjacent tissue transfer or rearrangement; up to one-fourth of lid margin**

INCLUDES Canthoplasty (67950)

EXCLUDES *Delay flap (15630)*
Flap attachment (15650)
Free skin grafts (15120-15121, 15260-15261)
Tubed pedicle flap preparation (15576)

12.9 16.4 FUD 090 J A2 80 50

AMA: 2018,Jan,8; 2017,Jan,8; 2016,Feb,12; 2016,Jan,13

67966 **over one-fourth of lid margin**

INCLUDES Canthoplasty (67950)

EXCLUDES *Delay flap (15630)*
Flap attachment (15650)
Free skin grafts (15120-15121, 15260-15261)
Tubed pedicle flap preparation (15576)

18.7 21.9 FUD 090 J A2 50

AMA: 2018,Jan,8; 2017,Jan,8; 2016,Feb,12; 2016,Jan,13

67971 **Reconstruction of eyelid, full thickness by transfer of tarsoconjunctival flap from opposing eyelid; up to two-thirds of eyelid, 1 stage or first stage**

INCLUDES Dupuy-Dutemp reconstruction
Landboldt's operation

20.4 20.4 FUD 090 J A2 50

AMA: 2016,Feb,12

67973 **total eyelid, lower, 1 stage or first stage**

INCLUDES Landboldt's operation

26.3 26.3 FUD 090 J A2 80 50

AMA: 2016,Feb,12

67974 **total eyelid, upper, 1 stage or first stage**

INCLUDES Landboldt's operation

26.2 26.2 FUD 090 J A2 80 50

AMA: 2016,Feb,12

67975 **second stage**

INCLUDES Landboldt's operation

19.4 19.4 FUD 090 J A2 50

AMA: 2016,Feb,12

67999 **Unlisted procedure, eyelids**

0.00 0.00 FUD YYY T 80 50

AMA: 2018,Jan,8; 2017,Jul,10; 2017,Jan,8; 2016,Feb,12; 2016,Jan,13

68020-68200 Conjunctival Biopsy/Injection/Treatment of Lesions

INCLUDES Operating microscope (69990)
EXCLUDES *Foreign body removal (65205-65265)*

68020 Incision of conjunctiva, drainage of cyst
3.11 | 3.41 | FUD 010 | T P3 50
AMA: 2016,Feb,12

68040 Expression of conjunctival follicles (eg, for trachoma)
EXCLUDES *Automated evacuation meibomian glands with heat/pressure (0207T)*
Manual evacuation meibomian glands ([0563T])
1.40 | 1.78 | FUD 000 | T P3 50
AMA: 2018,Jan,8; 2017,Jan,8; 2016,Feb,12; 2016,Jan,13

68100 Biopsy of conjunctiva
2.75 | 4.97 | FUD 000 | J P3 50
AMA: 2019,Jan,9; 2016,Feb,12

68110 Excision of lesion, conjunctiva; up to 1 cm
4.18 | 6.63 | FUD 010 | J P3 50
AMA: 2018,Feb,11; 2018,Jan,8; 2017,Jan,6; 2016,Feb,12

68115 over 1 cm
5.18 | 9.19 | FUD 010 | J A2 50
AMA: 2018,Feb,11; 2016,Feb,12

68130 with adjacent sclera
11.6 | 15.5 | FUD 090 | J A2 50
AMA: 2016,Feb,12

68135 Destruction of lesion, conjunctiva
4.24 | 4.46 | FUD 010 | J P3 50
AMA: 2016,Feb,12

68200 Subconjunctival injection
EXCLUDES *Retrobulbar or Tenon's capsule injection (67500-67515)*
0.99 | 1.19 | FUD 000 | Q1 N1 50
AMA: 2018,Jan,8; 2017,Jan,8; 2016,Feb,12; 2016,Jan,13

68320-68340 Conjunctivoplasty Procedures

INCLUDES Operating microscope (69990)
EXCLUDES *Conjunctival foreign body removal (65205, 65210)*
Laceration repair (65270-65273)

68320 Conjunctivoplasty; with conjunctival graft or extensive rearrangement
15.3 | 20.8 | FUD 090 | J A2 50
AMA: 2018,Jan,8; 2017,Jan,8; 2016,Feb,12; 2016,Jan,13

68325 with buccal mucous membrane graft (includes obtaining graft)
18.5 | 18.5 | FUD 090 | J A2 50
AMA: 2016,Feb,12

68326 Conjunctivoplasty, reconstruction cul-de-sac; with conjunctival graft or extensive rearrangement
18.2 | 18.2 | FUD 090 | J A2 50
AMA: 2016,Feb,12

68328 with buccal mucous membrane graft (includes obtaining graft)
20.1 | 20.1 | FUD 090 | J A2 80 50
AMA: 2016,Feb,12

68330 Repair of symblepharon; conjunctivoplasty, without graft
13.0 | 17.4 | FUD 090 | J A2 80 50
AMA: 2016,Feb,12

68335 with free graft conjunctiva or buccal mucous membrane (includes obtaining graft)
18.2 | 18.2 | FUD 090 | J A2 50
AMA: 2016,Feb,12

68340 division of symblepharon, with or without insertion of conformer or contact lens
11.2 | 16.4 | FUD 090 | J A2 80 50
AMA: 2016,Feb,12

68360-68399 Conjunctival Flaps and Unlisted Procedures

INCLUDES Operating microscope (69990)

68360 Conjunctival flap; bridge or partial (separate procedure)
EXCLUDES *Conjunctival flap for injury (65280, 65285)*
Conjunctival foreign body removal (65205, 65210)
Surgical wound repair (66250)
11.7 | 15.3 | FUD 090 | J A2 50
AMA: 2016,Feb,12

68362 total (such as Gunderson thin flap or purse string flap)
EXCLUDES *Conjunctival flap for injury (65280, 65285)*
Conjunctival foreign body removal (65205, 65210)
Surgical wound repair (66250)
18.5 | 18.5 | FUD 090 | J A2 50
AMA: 2018,Jan,8; 2017,Jan,8; 2016,Feb,12; 2016,Jan,13

68371 Harvesting conjunctival allograft, living donor
11.7 | 11.7 | FUD 010 | J A2 50
AMA: 2018,Jan,8; 2017,Jan,8; 2016,Feb,12; 2016,Jan,13

68399 Unlisted procedure, conjunctiva
0.00 | 0.00 | FUD YYY | T 80 50
AMA: 2018,Jan,8; 2017,Jan,8; 2016,Feb,12; 2016,Jan,13

68400-68899 Nasolacrimal System Procedures

INCLUDES Operating microscope (69990)

68400 Incision, drainage of lacrimal gland
3.71 | 8.30 | FUD 010 | T P3 50
AMA: 2016,Feb,12

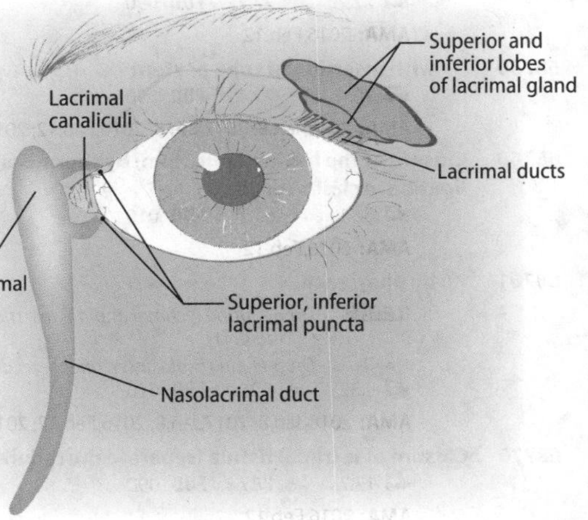

68420 Incision, drainage of lacrimal sac (dacryocystotomy or dacryocystostomy)
4.78 | 9.28 | FUD 010 | J P3 50
AMA: 2016,Feb,12

68440 Snip incision of lacrimal punctum
2.80 | 2.92 | FUD 010 | T P3 50
AMA: 2016,Feb,12

68500 Excision of lacrimal gland (dacryoadenectomy), except for tumor; total
28.6 | 28.6 | FUD 090 | J A2 50
AMA: 2016,Feb,12

68505 partial
28.5 | 28.5 | FUD 090 | J A2 50
AMA: 2016,Feb,12

68510 Biopsy of lacrimal gland
8.26 | 12.9 | FUD 000 | J A2 80 50
AMA: 2016,Feb,12

68520 Excision of lacrimal sac (dacryocystectomy)
20.0 | 20.0 | FUD 090 | J A2 80 50
AMA: 2016,Feb,12

68525 Biopsy of lacrimal sac
7.52 7.52 FUD 000 J A2 50
AMA: 2016,Feb,12

68530 Removal of foreign body or dacryolith, lacrimal passages
INCLUDES Meller's excision
7.23 12.2 FUD 010 T P2 50
AMA: 2016,Feb,12

68540 Excision of lacrimal gland tumor; frontal approach
27.0 27.0 FUD 090 J A2 50
AMA: 2016,Feb,12

68550 involving osteotomy
33.3 33.3 FUD 090 J A2 50
AMA: 2016,Feb,12

68700 Plastic repair of canaliculi
17.0 17.0 FUD 090 J A2 50
AMA: 2016,Feb,12

68705 Correction of everted punctum, cautery
4.68 7.19 FUD 010 T P2 50
AMA: 2020,Feb,13; 2018,Jan,8; 2017,Jan,8; 2016,Feb,12; 2016,Jan,13

68720 Dacryocystorhinostomy (fistulization of lacrimal sac to nasal cavity)
22.1 22.1 FUD 090 J A2 80 50
AMA: 2018,Jan,8; 2017,Jan,8; 2016,Feb,12; 2016,Jan,13

68745 Conjunctivorhinostomy (fistulization of conjunctiva to nasal cavity); without tube
22.2 22.2 FUD 090 J A2 80 50
AMA: 2016,Feb,12

68750 with insertion of tube or stent
22.4 22.4 FUD 090 J A2 80 50
AMA: 2018,Jan,8; 2017,Jan,8; 2016,Feb,12; 2016,Jan,13

68760 Closure of the lacrimal punctum; by thermocauterization, ligation, or laser surgery
4.11 6.07 FUD 010 T P2 50
AMA: 2016,Feb,12

68761 by plug, each
EXCLUDES *Drug-eluting lacrimal implant insertion or removal (68841)*
Drug-eluting ocular insert under eyelid(s) (0444T-0445T)
3.32 4.20 FUD 010 T P3 80 50
AMA: 2018,Jan,8; 2017,Jan,8; 2016,Feb,12; 2016,Jan,13

68770 Closure of lacrimal fistula (separate procedure)
17.7 17.7 FUD 090 J A2 80 50
AMA: 2016,Feb,12

68801 Dilation of lacrimal punctum, with or without irrigation
2.18 2.60 FUD 010 Q1 N1 50
AMA: 2016,Feb,12

68810 Probing of nasolacrimal duct, with or without irrigation;
EXCLUDES *Ophthalmological exam under anesthesia (92018)*
3.64 4.47 FUD 010 T A2 50
AMA: 2018,Jan,8; 2017,Jan,8; 2016,Feb,12; 2016,Jan,13

68811 requiring general anesthesia
EXCLUDES *Ophthalmological exam under anesthesia (92018)*
3.82 3.82 FUD 010 J A2 50
AMA: 2018,Jan,8; 2017,Jan,8; 2016,Feb,12; 2016,Jan,13

68815 with insertion of tube or stent
EXCLUDES *Drug-eluting lacrimal implant insertion or removal (68841)*
Drug-eluting ocular insert under eyelid(s) (0444T-0445T)
Ophthalmological exam under anesthesia (92018)
6.27 11.0 FUD 010 J A2 50
AMA: 2018,Jan,8; 2017,Jan,8; 2016,Feb,12; 2016,Jan,13

68816 with transluminal balloon catheter dilation
EXCLUDES *Probing nasolacrimal duct (68810-68811, 68815)*
4.45 22.2 FUD 010 J G2 50
AMA: 2018,Jan,8; 2017,Jan,8; 2016,Feb,12; 2016,Jan,13

68840 Probing of lacrimal canaliculi, with or without irrigation
3.27 3.70 FUD 010 T P3 50
AMA: 2016,Feb,12

● **68841 Insertion of drug-eluting implant, including punctal dilation when performed, into lacrimal canaliculus, each**
EXCLUDES *Drug-eluting ocular insert under eyelid(s) (0444T-0445T)*
Code also drug-eluting implant with 99070 or other appropriate supply code

68850 Injection of contrast medium for dacryocystography
(70170, 78660)
1.59 1.80 FUD 000 N N1 50
AMA: 2018,Jan,8; 2017,Jan,8; 2016,Feb,12; 2016,Jan,13

68899 Unlisted procedure, lacrimal system
0.00 0.00 FUD YYY T 80 50
AMA: 2014,Jan,11; 1991,Sum,17

69000-69020 Treatment External Abscess/Hematoma

69000 Drainage external ear, abscess or hematoma; simple
3.47 5.34 FUD 010 T P3 50
AMA: 2018,Jan,8; 2017,Jan,8; 2016,Jan,13

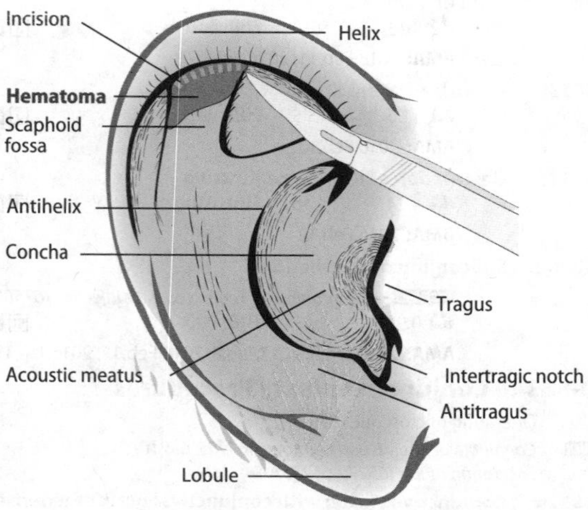

An incision is made to drain the contents of an abscess or hematoma

69005 complicated
4.50 6.13 FUD 010 J P3 50
AMA: 2014,Jan,11; 1999,Oct,10

69020 Drainage external auditory canal, abscess
4.03 6.57 FUD 010 T P3 50
AMA: 2018,Jan,8; 2017,Jan,8; 2016,Jan,13

69090 Cosmetic Ear Piercing

CMS: 100-02,16,10 Exclusions from Coverage; 100-02,16,120 Cosmetic Procedures

69090 Ear piercing
0.00 0.00 FUD XXX E
AMA: 2014,Jan,11; 1999,Oct,10

69100-69222 External Ear/Auditory Canal Procedures

EXCLUDES *Reconstruction ear (see integumentary section codes)*

69100 Biopsy external ear
1.37 2.79 FUD 000 T P3
AMA: 2019,Jan,9

69105 Biopsy external auditory canal
1.78 4.00 FUD 000 T P3 50
AMA: 2014,Jan,11; 1999,Oct,10

69110 Excision external ear; partial, simple repair
9.28 13.1 FUD 090 J A2 50
AMA: 2014,Jan,11; 1999,Oct,10

69120 complete amputation
11.1 11.1 FUD 090 J A2
AMA: 2014,Jan,11; 1999,Oct,10

69140 Excision exostosis(es), external auditory canal
24.8 24.8 FUD 090 J A2 80 50
AMA: 2014,Jan,11; 1999,Oct,10

69145 Excision soft tissue lesion, external auditory canal
7.04 11.1 FUD 090 J A2 50
AMA: 2019,Dec,14

69150 Radical excision external auditory canal lesion; without neck dissection
EXCLUDES *Skin graft (15004-15261)*
Temporal bone resection (69535)
29.5 29.5 FUD 090 J A2
AMA: 2014,Jan,11; 2003,Jan,1

69155 with neck dissection
EXCLUDES *Skin graft (15004-15261)*
Temporal bone resection (69535)
47.0 47.0 FUD 090 C 80
AMA: 2014,Jan,11; 1999,Oct,10

69200 Removal foreign body from external auditory canal; without general anesthesia
1.35 2.31 FUD 000 Q1 N1 50
AMA: 2014,Jan,11; 1999,Oct,10

69205 with general anesthesia
2.77 2.77 FUD 010 J A2 50
AMA: 2018,Jan,8; 2017,Jan,8; 2016,Jan,13

69209 Removal impacted cerumen using irrigation/lavage, unilateral
EXCLUDES *Removal impacted cerumen using instrumentation (69210)*
Removal nonimpacted cerumen (see appropriate E/M code(s)) (99202-99233 [99224, 99225, 99226], 99241-99255, 99281-99285, 99304-99318, 99324-99337, 99341-99350)
0.40 0.40 FUD 000 Q1 N1 50
AMA: 2018,Jan,8; 2017,Jan,8; 2016,Mar,10; 2016,Feb,13; 2016,Jan,7

69210 Removal impacted cerumen requiring instrumentation, unilateral
EXCLUDES *Removal impacted cerumen using irrigation or lavage (69209)*
Removal nonimpacted cerumen (see appropriate E/M code(s)) (99202-99233 [99224, 99225, 99226], 99241-99255, 99281-99285, 99304-99318, 99324-99337, 99341-99350)
0.96 1.36 FUD 000 Q1 N1
AMA: 2018,Jan,8; 2017,Jan,8; 2016,Mar,10; 2016,Feb,13; 2016,Jan,13; 2016,Jan,7

69220 Debridement, mastoidectomy cavity, simple (eg, routine cleaning)
1.46 2.25 FUD 000 Q1 N1 50
AMA: 2014,Jan,11; 1999,Oct,10

69222 Debridement, mastoidectomy cavity, complex (eg, with anesthesia or more than routine cleaning)
3.81 6.02 FUD 010 T P3 50
AMA: 2014,Jan,11; 1999,Oct,10

69300 Plastic Surgery for Prominent Ears

CMS: 100-02,16,120 Cosmetic Procedures; 100-02,16,180 Services Related to Noncovered Procedures
EXCLUDES *Suture laceration external ear (12011-14302)*

69300 Otoplasty, protruding ear, with or without size reduction
13.1 17.6 FUD YYY J A2 80 50
AMA: 2014,Jan,11; 1999,Oct,10

69310-69399 Reconstruction Auditory Canal: Postaural Approach

EXCLUDES *Suture laceration external ear (12011-14302)*

69310 Reconstruction of external auditory canal (meatoplasty) (eg, for stenosis due to injury, infection) (separate procedure)
30.9 30.9 FUD 090 J A2 50
AMA: 2018,Jan,8; 2017,Jan,8; 2016,Jan,13

69320 Reconstruction external auditory canal for congenital atresia, single stage
EXCLUDES *Other reconstruction surgery with graft (13151-15760, 21230-21235)*
Tympanoplasty (69631, 69641)
43.4 43.4 FUD 090 J A2 80 50
AMA: 2014,Jan,11; 1999,Oct,10

69399 Unlisted procedure, external ear
EXCLUDES *Otoscopy under general anesthesia (92502)*
0.00 0.00 FUD YYY T 80
AMA: 2014,Jan,11; 1999,Oct,10

69420-69450 Ear Drum Procedures

69420 Myringotomy including aspiration and/or eustachian tube inflation
3.39 5.31 FUD 010 T P2 50
AMA: 2018,Jan,8; 2017,Jan,8; 2016,Jan,13

69421 Myringotomy including aspiration and/or eustachian tube inflation requiring general anesthesia
4.21 4.21 FUD 010 J A2 50
AMA: 2018,Jan,8; 2017,Jan,8; 2016,Jan,13

69424 Ventilating tube removal requiring general anesthesia
EXCLUDES *Cochlear device implantation (69930)*
Eardrum repair (69610-69646)
Foreign body removal (69205)
Implantation, replacement electromagnetic bone conduction hearing device in temporal bone (69710-69745)
Labyrinth procedures (69801-69915)
Mastoid obliteration (69670)
Myringotomy (69420-69421)
Polyp, glomus tumor removal (69535-69554)
Removal impacted cerumen requiring instrumentation (69210)
Repair window (69666-69667)
Revised mastoidectomy (69601-69604)
Stapes procedures (69650-69662)
Transmastoid excision (69501-69530)
Tympanic neurectomy (69676)
Tympanostomy, tympanolysis (69433-69450)
1.73 3.62 FUD 000 Q2 P3 50
AMA: 2018,Jan,8; 2017,Jan,8; 2016,Jan,13

69433 Tympanostomy (requiring insertion of ventilating tube), local or topical anesthesia

EXCLUDES *Tympanostomy with tube insertion using iontophoresis and automated tube delivery system (0583T)*

3.72 5.62 **FUD** 010 T P3 50

AMA: 2018,Feb,11; 2018,Jan,8; 2017,Jan,8; 2016,Jan,13

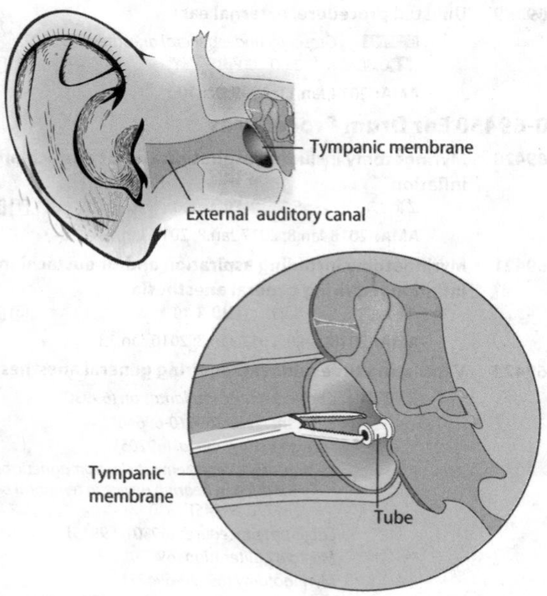

69436 Tympanostomy (requiring insertion of ventilating tube), general anesthesia

4.51 4.51 **FUD** 010 T A2 50

AMA: 2018,Feb,11; 2018,Jan,8; 2017,Jan,8; 2016,Jan,13

69440 Middle ear exploration through postauricular or ear canal incision

EXCLUDES *Atticotomy (69601-69604)*

19.5 19.5 **FUD** 090 J A2 50

AMA: 2014,Jan,11; 2008,Sep,10-11

69450 Tympanolysis, transcanal

15.4 15.4 **FUD** 090 J A2 80 50

AMA: 2014,Jan,11; 2008,Sep,10-11

69501-69530 Transmastoid Excision

EXCLUDES *Mastoidectomy cavity debridement (69220, 69222)*
Skin graft (15004-15770)

69501 Transmastoid antrotomy (simple mastoidectomy)

20.3 20.3 **FUD** 090 J A2 50

AMA: 2018,Jan,8; 2017,Jan,8; 2016,Jan,13

69502 Mastoidectomy; complete

27.3 27.3 **FUD** 090 J A2 80 50

AMA: 2018,Jan,8; 2017,Jan,8; 2016,Jan,13

69505 modified radical

34.2 34.2 **FUD** 090 J A2 80 50

AMA: 2018,Jan,8; 2017,Jan,8; 2016,Jan,13

69511 radical

35.0 35.0 **FUD** 090 J A2 80 50

AMA: 2018,Jan,8; 2017,Jan,8; 2016,Jan,13

69530 Petrous apicectomy including radical mastoidectomy

47.1 47.1 **FUD** 090 J A2 80 50

AMA: 2014,Jan,11; 1999,Oct,10

69535-69554 Polyp and Glomus Tumor Removal

69535 Resection temporal bone, external approach

EXCLUDES *Middle fossa approach (69950-69970)*

75.4 75.4 **FUD** 090 C 50

AMA: 2014,Jan,11; 1999,Oct,10

69540 Excision aural polyp

3.58 5.83 **FUD** 010 T P3 50

AMA: 2014,Jan,11; 1999,Oct,10

69550 Excision aural glomus tumor; transcanal

29.5 29.5 **FUD** 090 J A2 80 50

AMA: 2014,Jan,11; 1999,Oct,10

69552 transmastoid

44.6 44.6 **FUD** 090 J A2 80 50

AMA: 2014,Jan,11; 1999,Oct,10

69554 extended (extratemporal)

71.5 71.5 **FUD** 090 C 80 50

AMA: 2014,Jan,11; 1999,Oct,10

69601-69604 Revised Mastoidectomy

EXCLUDES *Skin graft (15120-15121, 15260-15261)*

69601 Revision mastoidectomy; resulting in complete mastoidectomy

29.5 29.5 **FUD** 090 J A2 80 50

AMA: 2018,Jan,8; 2017,Jan,8; 2016,Jan,13

69602 resulting in modified radical mastoidectomy

30.8 30.8 **FUD** 090 J A2 80 50

AMA: 2018,Jan,8; 2017,Jan,8; 2016,Jan,13

69603 resulting in radical mastoidectomy

35.9 35.9 **FUD** 090 J A2 80 50

AMA: 2018,Jan,8; 2017,Jan,8; 2016,Jan,13

69604 resulting in tympanoplasty

EXCLUDES *Secondary tympanoplasty following mastoidectomy (69631-69632)*

31.5 31.5 **FUD** 090 J A2 50

AMA: 2018,Jan,8; 2017,Jan,8; 2016,Jan,13

69610-69646 Eardrum Repair with/without Other Procedures

69610 Tympanic membrane repair, with or without site preparation of perforation for closure, with or without patch

8.27 10.8 **FUD** 010 J P3 50

AMA: 2018,Jan,8; 2017,Jan,8; 2016,Jan,13

69620 Myringoplasty (surgery confined to drumhead and donor area)

13.9 20.0 **FUD** 090 J A2 50

AMA: 2018,Jan,8; 2017,Jan,8; 2016,Jan,13

69631 Tympanoplasty without mastoidectomy (including canalplasty, atticotomy and/or middle ear surgery), initial or revision; without ossicular chain reconstruction

25.0 25.0 **FUD** 090 J A2 50

AMA: 2018,Jan,8; 2017,Jan,8; 2016,Jan,13

69632 with ossicular chain reconstruction (eg, postfenestration)

30.5 30.5 **FUD** 090 J A2 50

AMA: 2018,Jan,8; 2017,Jan,8; 2016,Jan,13

69633 with ossicular chain reconstruction and synthetic prosthesis (eg, partial ossicular replacement prosthesis [PORP], total ossicular replacement prosthesis [TORP])

29.6 29.6 **FUD** 090 J A2 50

AMA: 2018,Jan,8; 2017,Jan,8; 2016,Jan,13

69635 **Tympanoplasty with antrotomy or mastoidotomy (including canalplasty, atticotomy, middle ear surgery, and/or tympanic membrane repair); without ossicular chain reconstruction**
35.3 35.3 FUD 090 J A2 50
AMA: 2018,Jan,8; 2017,Jan,8; 2016,Jan,13

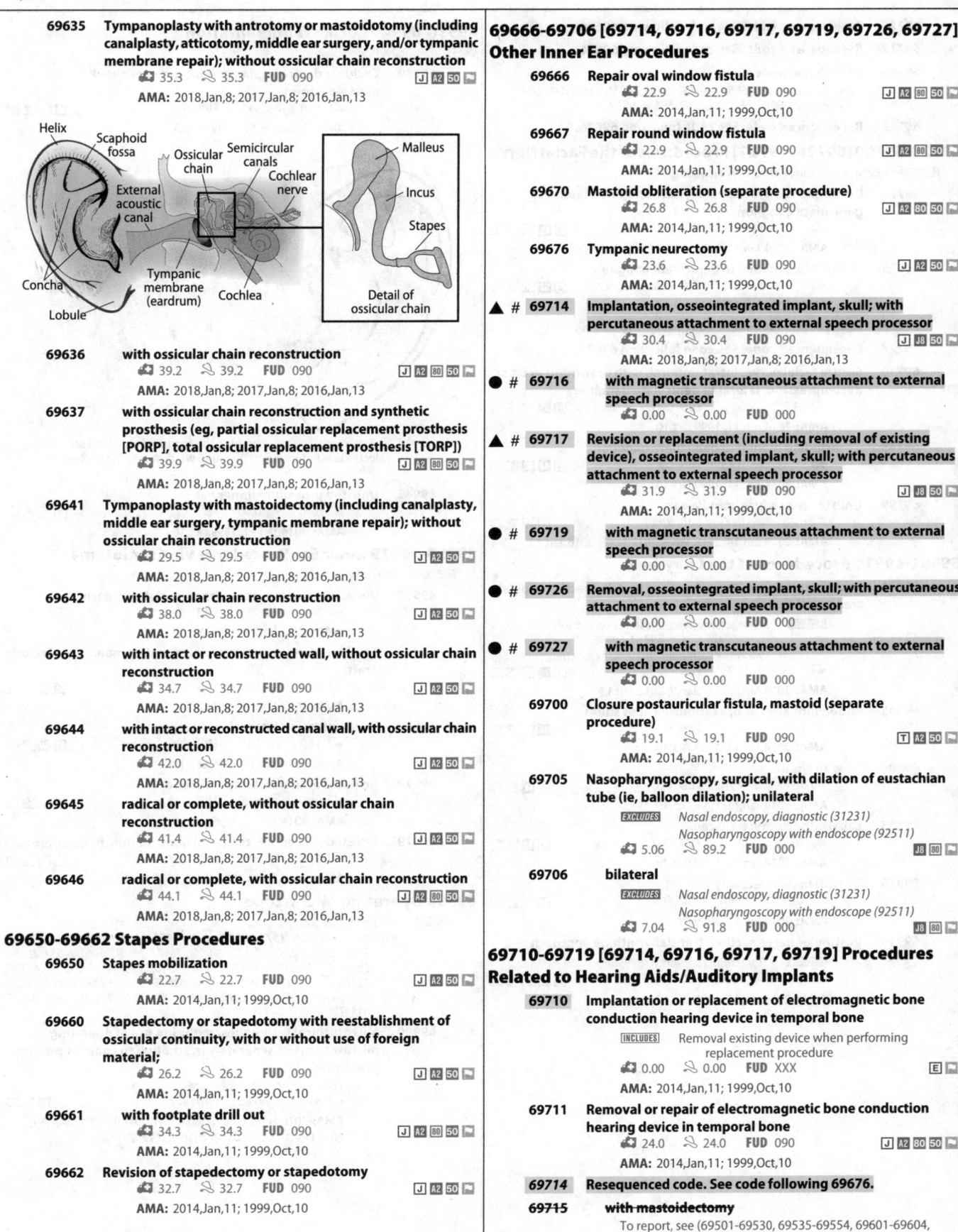

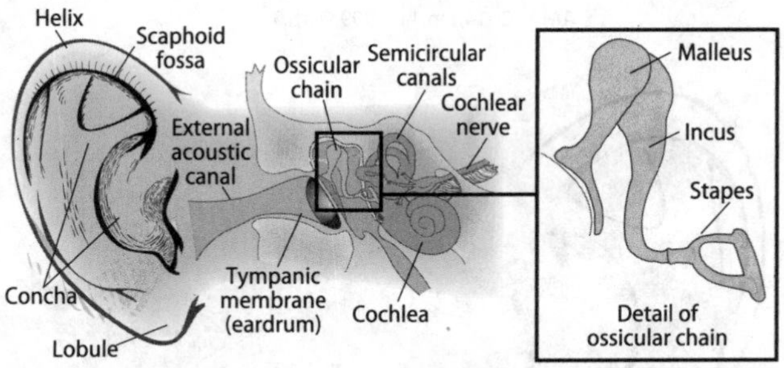

69636 **with ossicular chain reconstruction**
39.2 39.2 FUD 090 J A2 80 50
AMA: 2018,Jan,8; 2017,Jan,8; 2016,Jan,13

69637 **with ossicular chain reconstruction and synthetic prosthesis (eg, partial ossicular replacement prosthesis [PORP], total ossicular replacement prosthesis [TORP])**
39.9 39.9 FUD 090 J A2 80 50
AMA: 2018,Jan,8; 2017,Jan,8; 2016,Jan,13

69641 **Tympanoplasty with mastoidectomy (including canalplasty, middle ear surgery, tympanic membrane repair); without ossicular chain reconstruction**
29.5 29.5 FUD 090 J A2 50
AMA: 2018,Jan,8; 2017,Jan,8; 2016,Jan,13

69642 **with ossicular chain reconstruction**
38.0 38.0 FUD 090 J A2 50
AMA: 2018,Jan,8; 2017,Jan,8; 2016,Jan,13

69643 **with intact or reconstructed wall, without ossicular chain reconstruction**
34.7 34.7 FUD 090 J A2 50
AMA: 2018,Jan,8; 2017,Jan,8; 2016,Jan,13

69644 **with intact or reconstructed canal wall, with ossicular chain reconstruction**
42.0 42.0 FUD 090 J A2 50
AMA: 2018,Jan,8; 2017,Jan,8; 2016,Jan,13

69645 **radical or complete, without ossicular chain reconstruction**
41.4 41.4 FUD 090 J A2 50
AMA: 2018,Jan,8; 2017,Jan,8; 2016,Jan,13

69646 **radical or complete, with ossicular chain reconstruction**
44.1 44.1 FUD 090 J A2 80 50
AMA: 2018,Jan,8; 2017,Jan,8; 2016,Jan,13

69650-69662 Stapes Procedures

69650 **Stapes mobilization**
22.7 22.7 FUD 090 J A2 50
AMA: 2014,Jan,11; 1999,Oct,10

69660 **Stapedectomy or stapedotomy with reestablishment of ossicular continuity, with or without use of foreign material;**
26.2 26.2 FUD 090 J A2 50
AMA: 2014,Jan,11; 1999,Oct,10

69661 **with footplate drill out**
34.3 34.3 FUD 090 J A2 80 50
AMA: 2014,Jan,11; 1999,Oct,10

69662 **Revision of stapedectomy or stapedotomy**
32.7 32.7 FUD 090 J A2 50
AMA: 2014,Jan,11; 1999,Oct,10

69666-69706 [69714, 69716, 69717, 69719, 69726, 69727] Other Inner Ear Procedures

69666 **Repair oval window fistula**
22.9 22.9 FUD 090 J A2 80 50
AMA: 2014,Jan,11; 1999,Oct,10

69667 **Repair round window fistula**
22.9 22.9 FUD 090 J A2 80 50
AMA: 2014,Jan,11; 1999,Oct,10

69670 **Mastoid obliteration (separate procedure)**
26.8 26.8 FUD 090 J A2 80 50
AMA: 2014,Jan,11; 1999,Oct,10

69676 **Tympanic neurectomy**
23.6 23.6 FUD 090 J A2 50
AMA: 2014,Jan,11; 1999,Oct,10

▲ # **69714** **Implantation, osseointegrated implant, skull; with percutaneous attachment to external speech processor**
30.4 30.4 FUD 090 J J8 50
AMA: 2018,Jan,8; 2017,Jan,8; 2016,Jan,13

● # **69716** **with magnetic transcutaneous attachment to external speech processor**
0.00 0.00 FUD 000

▲ # **69717** **Revision or replacement (including removal of existing device), osseointegrated implant, skull; with percutaneous attachment to external speech processor**
31.9 31.9 FUD 090 J J8 50
AMA: 2014,Jan,11; 1999,Oct,10

● # **69719** **with magnetic transcutaneous attachment to external speech processor**
0.00 0.00 FUD 000

● # **69726** **Removal, osseointegrated implant, skull; with percutaneous attachment to external speech processor**
0.00 0.00 FUD 000

● # **69727** **with magnetic transcutaneous attachment to external speech processor**
0.00 0.00 FUD 000

69700 **Closure postauricular fistula, mastoid (separate procedure)**
19.1 19.1 FUD 090 T A2 50
AMA: 2014,Jan,11; 1999,Oct,10

69705 **Nasopharyngoscopy, surgical, with dilation of eustachian tube (ie, balloon dilation); unilateral**
EXCLUDES *Nasal endoscopy, diagnostic (31231)*
Nasopharyngoscopy with endoscope (92511)
5.06 89.2 FUD 000 J8 80

69706 **bilateral**
EXCLUDES *Nasal endoscopy, diagnostic (31231)*
Nasopharyngoscopy with endoscope (92511)
7.04 91.8 FUD 000 J8 80

69710-69719 [69714, 69716, 69717, 69719] Procedures Related to Hearing Aids/Auditory Implants

69710 **Implantation or replacement of electromagnetic bone conduction hearing device in temporal bone**
INCLUDES Removal existing device when performing replacement procedure
0.00 0.00 FUD XXX E
AMA: 2014,Jan,11; 1999,Oct,10

69711 **Removal or repair of electromagnetic bone conduction hearing device in temporal bone**
24.0 24.0 FUD 090 J A2 80 50
AMA: 2014,Jan,11; 1999,Oct,10

69714 **Resequenced code. See code following 69676.**

69715 **~~with mastoidectomy~~**
To report, see (69501-69530, 69535-69554, 69601-69604, 69610-69646, 69650-69662, 69666-69676)

69716 **Resequenced code. See code following 69676.**

69717 **Resequenced code. See code following 69676.**

69718 **with mastoidectomy**
To report, see (69501-69530, 69535-69554, 69601-69604, 69610-69646, 69650-69662, 69666-69676)

69719 **Resequenced code. See code following 69676.**

69720-69799 [69726, 69727] Procedures of the Facial Nerve

EXCLUDES *Extracranial suture facial nerve (64864)*

69720 **Decompression facial nerve, intratemporal; lateral to geniculate ganglion**
34.1 34.1 FUD 090 J A2 80 50
AMA: 2014,Jan,11; 1999,Oct,10

69725 **including medial to geniculate ganglion**
53.5 53.5 FUD 090 J G2 80 50
AMA: 2014,Jan,11; 1999,Oct,10

69726 **Resequenced code. See code following 69676.**

69727 **Resequenced code. See code following 69676.**

69740 **Suture facial nerve, intratemporal, with or without graft or decompression; lateral to geniculate ganglion**
33.2 33.2 FUD 090 J A2 80 50
AMA: 2014,Jan,11; 1999,Oct,10

69745 **including medial to geniculate ganglion**
35.3 35.3 FUD 090 J A2 80 50
AMA: 2014,Jan,11; 1999,Oct,10

69799 **Unlisted procedure, middle ear**
0.00 0.00 FUD YYY T 80 50
AMA: 2019,Jan,14; 2018,Jan,8; 2017,Jan,8; 2016,Jan,13

69801-69915 Procedures of the Labyrinth

69801 **Labyrinthotomy, with perfusion of vestibuloactive drug(s), transcanal**
EXCLUDES *Myringotomy, tympanostomy on same ear (69420-69421, 69433, 69436)*
Procedure performed more than one time per day
3.58 5.83 FUD 000 T P3 80 50
AMA: 2018,Jan,8; 2017,Jan,8; 2016,Jan,13

69805 **Endolymphatic sac operation; without shunt**
29.8 29.8 FUD 090 J A2 80 50
AMA: 2014,Jan,11; 1999,Oct,10

69806 **with shunt**
26.6 26.6 FUD 090 J A2 50
AMA: 2014,Jan,11; 1999,Oct,10

69905 **Labyrinthectomy; transcanal**
26.0 26.0 FUD 090 J A2 50
AMA: 2014,Jan,11; 1999,Oct,10

69910 **with mastoidectomy**
28.7 28.7 FUD 090 J A2 80 50
AMA: 2014,Jan,11; 1999,Oct,10

69915 **Vestibular nerve section, translabyrinthine approach**
EXCLUDES *Transcranial approach (69950)*
43.6 43.6 FUD 090 J A2 80 50
AMA: 2014,Jan,11; 1999,Oct,10

69930-69949 Cochlear Implantation

CMS: 100-02,16,100 Hearing Devices

69930 **Cochlear device implantation, with or without mastoidectomy**
34.8 34.8 FUD 090 J J8 80 50
AMA: 2014,Jan,11; 1999,Oct,10

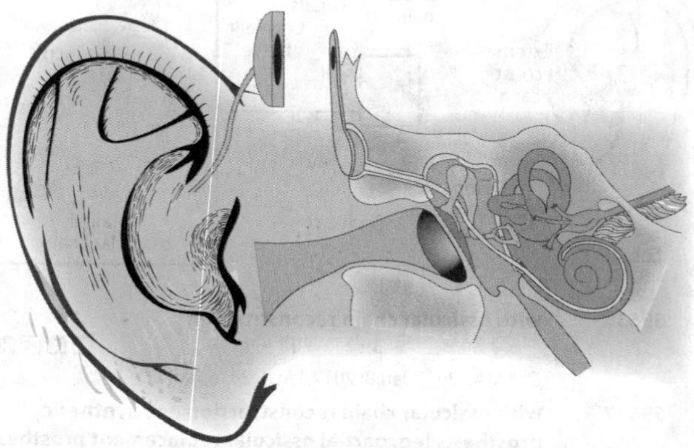

The internal coil is secured to the temporal bone and an electrode is fed through the round window into the cochlea

69949 **Unlisted procedure, inner ear**
0.00 0.00 FUD YYY T 80 50
AMA: 2014,Jan,11; 1999,Oct,10

69950-69979 Inner Ear Procedures via Craniotomy

EXCLUDES *External approach (69535)*

69950 **Vestibular nerve section, transcranial approach**
50.6 50.6 FUD 090 C 80 50
AMA: 2014,Jan,11; 1999,Oct,10

69955 **Total facial nerve decompression and/or repair (may include graft)**
56.2 56.2 FUD 090 J G2 80 50
AMA: 2014,Jan,11; 1999,Oct,10

69960 **Decompression internal auditory canal**
54.2 54.2 FUD 090 J G2 80 50
AMA: 2014,Jan,11; 1999,Oct,10

69970 **Removal of tumor, temporal bone**
61.0 61.0 FUD 090 J G2 80 50
AMA: 2014,Jan,11; 1999,Oct,10

69979 **Unlisted procedure, temporal bone, middle fossa approach**
0.00 0.00 FUD YYY T 80 50
AMA: 2018,Jan,8; 2017,Jan,8; 2016,Jan,13

69990 Operating Microscope

EXCLUDES *Magnifying loupes*
Reporting code with (15756-15758, 15842, 19364, 19368, 20955-20962, 20969-20973, 22551-22552, 22856-22857 [22858], 22861, 26551-26554, 26556, 31526, 31531, 31536, 31541-31546, 31561, 31571, 43116, 43180, 43496, 46601, 46607, 49906, 61548, 63075-63078, 64727, 64820-64823, 64912-64913, 65091-68850 [66987, 66988, 67810], 0184T, 0308T, 0402T, 0583T)

\+ **69990** **Microsurgical techniques, requiring use of operating microscope (List separately in addition to code for primary procedure)**
Code first primary procedure
6.40 6.40 FUD ZZZ N N1 80
AMA: 2018,Feb,11; 2018,Jan,8; 2017,Dec,12; 2017,Dec,13; 2017,Dec,14; 2017,Jan,8; 2016,Feb,12; 2016,Jan,13

70010-70015 Radiography: Neurodiagnostic

70010 **Myelography, posterior fossa, radiological supervision and interpretation**
1.73 1.73 FUD XXX Q2 N1 80
AMA: 2018,Jan,8; 2017,Jan,8; 2016,Jan,13

70015 **Cisternography, positive contrast, radiological supervision and interpretation**
4.60 4.60 FUD XXX Q2 N1 80
AMA: 2014,Jan,11; 2012,Feb,9-10

70030-70390 Radiography: Head, Neck, Orofacial Structures

INCLUDES Minimum number views or more views when needed to adequately complete study
Radiographs repeated during encounter due to substandard quality; only one unit reported

EXCLUDES *Obtaining more films after initial film review, based on radiologist discretion, order for test, and change in patient's condition*

70030 **Radiologic examination, eye, for detection of foreign body**
0.87 0.87 FUD XXX Q1 N1 80
AMA: 2014,Jan,11; 2012,Feb,9-10

70100 **Radiologic examination, mandible; partial, less than 4 views**
1.03 1.03 FUD XXX Q1 N1 80
AMA: 2014,Jan,11; 2012,Feb,9-10

70110 **complete, minimum of 4 views**
1.19 1.19 FUD XXX Q1 N1 80
AMA: 2014,Jan,11; 2012,Feb,9-10

70120 **Radiologic examination, mastoids; less than 3 views per side**
0.97 0.97 FUD XXX Q1 N1 80
AMA: 2014,Jan,11; 2012,Feb,9-10

70130 **complete, minimum of 3 views per side**
1.68 1.68 FUD XXX Q1 N1 80
AMA: 2014,Jan,11; 2012,Feb,9-10

70134 **Radiologic examination, internal auditory meati, complete**
1.59 1.59 FUD XXX Q1 N1 80
AMA: 2014,Jan,11; 2012,Feb,9-10

70140 **Radiologic examination, facial bones; less than 3 views**
0.88 0.88 FUD XXX Q1 N1 80
AMA: 2014,Jan,11; 2012,Feb,9-10

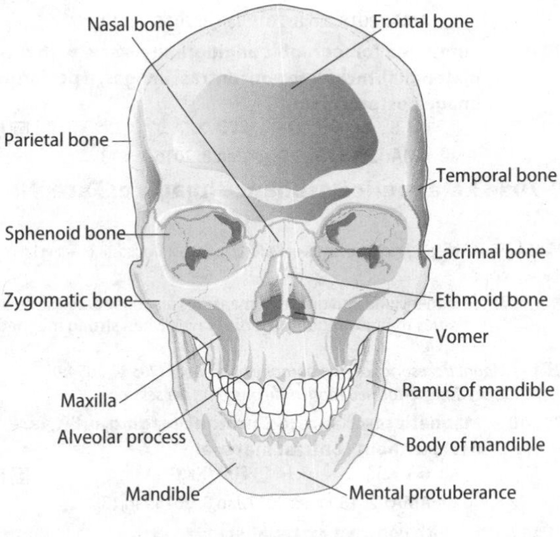

70150 **complete, minimum of 3 views**
1.29 1.29 FUD XXX Q1 N1 80
AMA: 2014,Jan,11; 2012,Feb,9-10

70160 **Radiologic examination, nasal bones, complete, minimum of 3 views**
1.02 1.02 FUD XXX Q1 N1 80
AMA: 2014,Jan,11; 2012,Feb,9-10

70170 **Dacryocystography, nasolacrimal duct, radiological supervision and interpretation**
EXCLUDES *Injection contrast (68850)*
0.00 0.00 FUD XXX Q2 N1 80
AMA: 2014,Jan,11; 2012,Feb,9-10

70190 **Radiologic examination; optic foramina**
1.08 1.08 FUD XXX Q1 N1 80
AMA: 2014,Jan,11; 2012,Feb,9-10

70200 **orbits, complete, minimum of 4 views**
1.31 1.31 FUD XXX Q1 N1 80
AMA: 2014,Jan,11; 2012,Feb,9-10

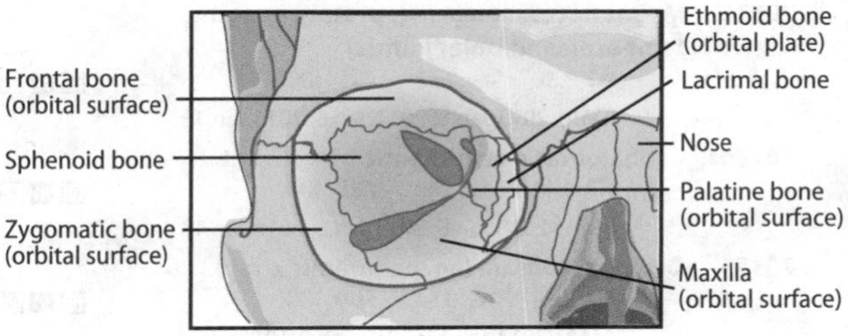

70210 **Radiologic examination, sinuses, paranasal, less than 3 views**
0.87 0.87 FUD XXX Q1 N1 80
AMA: 2014,Jan,11; 2012,Feb,9-10

70220 **Radiologic examination, sinuses, paranasal, complete, minimum of 3 views**
1.10 1.10 FUD XXX Q1 N1 80
AMA: 2014,Jan,11; 2012,Feb,9-10

70240 **Radiologic examination, sella turcica**
0.94 0.94 FUD XXX Q1 N1 80
AMA: 2014,Jan,11; 2012,Feb,9-10

70250 **X-ray of skull, fewer than 4 views**
1.00 1.00 FUD XXX Q1 N1 80
AMA: 2014,Jan,11; 2012,Feb,9-10

70260 **complete, minimum of 4 views**
1.24 1.24 FUD XXX Q1 N1 80
AMA: 2014,Jan,11; 2012,Feb,9-10

70300 **Radiologic examination, teeth; single view**
0.39 0.39 FUD XXX Q1 N1 80
AMA: 2014,Jan,11; 2012,Feb,9-10

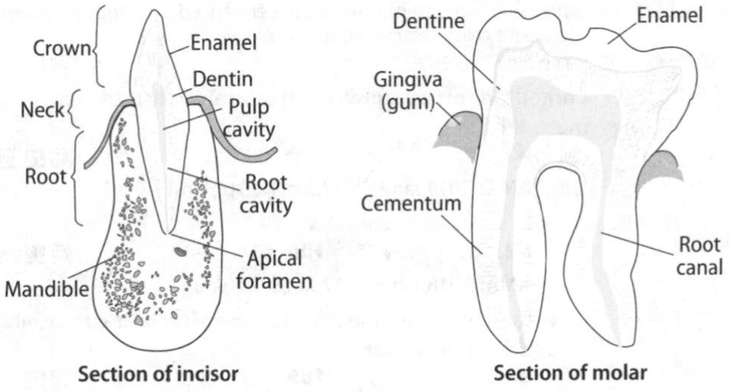

70310 **partial examination, less than full mouth**
1.06 1.06 FUD XXX Q1 N1 80
AMA: 2014,Jan,11; 2012,Feb,9-10

70320 **complete, full mouth**
1.53 1.53 FUD XXX Q1 N1 80
AMA: 2014,Jan,11; 2012,Feb,9-10

70328 Radiologic examination, temporomandibular joint, open and closed mouth; unilateral
🎥 0.94   📐 0.94   **FUD** XXX   01 N1 80 💻
AMA: 2014,Jan,11; 2012,Feb,9-10

70330 bilateral
🎥 1.45   📐 1.45   **FUD** XXX   01 N1 80 💻
AMA: 2018,Jan,8; 2017,Jan,8; 2016,Jan,13

70332 Temporomandibular joint arthrography, radiological supervision and interpretation
INCLUDES Fluoroscopic guidance (77002)
🎥 2.15   📐 2.15   **FUD** XXX   02 N1 80 💻
AMA: 2018,Jan,8; 2017,Jan,8; 2016,Jan,13

70336 Magnetic resonance (eg, proton) imaging, temporomandibular joint(s)
🎥 8.68   📐 8.68   **FUD** XXX   03 Z2 80 💻
AMA: 2018,Jan,8; 2017,Jan,8; 2016,Jan,13

70350 Cephalogram, orthodontic
🎥 0.49   📐 0.49   **FUD** XXX   01 N1 80 💻
AMA: 2018,Jan,8; 2017,Jan,8; 2016,Jan,13

70355 Orthopantogram (eg, panoramic x-ray)
🎥 0.54   📐 0.54   **FUD** XXX   01 N1 80 💻
AMA: 2014,Jan,11; 2012,Feb,9-10

70360 Radiologic examination; neck, soft tissue
🎥 0.86   📐 0.86   **FUD** XXX   01 N1 80 💻
AMA: 2014,Jan,11; 2012,Feb,9-10

70370 pharynx or larynx, including fluoroscopy and/or magnification technique
🎥 2.49   📐 2.49   **FUD** XXX   01 N1 80 💻
AMA: 2014,Jan,11; 2012,Feb,9-10

70371 Complex dynamic pharyngeal and speech evaluation by cine or video recording
EXCLUDES Laryngeal computed tomography (70490-70492)
🎥 3.03   📐 3.03   **FUD** XXX   01 N1 80 💻
AMA: 2018,Jan,8; 2017,Jan,8; 2016,Jan,13

70380 Radiologic examination, salivary gland for calculus
🎥 1.01   📐 1.01   **FUD** XXX   01 N1 80 💻
AMA: 2014,Jan,11; 2012,Feb,9-10

70390 Sialography, radiological supervision and interpretation
🎥 3.16   📐 3.16   **FUD** XXX   02 N1 80 💻
AMA: 2014,Jan,11; 2012,Feb,9-10

70450-70492 Computerized Tomography: Head, Neck, Face

CMS: 100-04,4,250.16 Multiple Procedure Payment Reduction: Certain Diagnostic Imaging Procedures Rendered by Physicians
INCLUDES Imaging using tomographic technique enhanced by computer imaging to create cross-sectional body plane view
EXCLUDES 3D rendering (76376-76377)

70450 Computed tomography, head or brain; without contrast material
🎥 3.25   📐 3.25   **FUD** XXX   03 Z2 80 💻
AMA: 2018,Jan,8; 2017,Jan,8; 2016,Jan,13

70460 with contrast material(s)
🎥 4.61   📐 4.61   **FUD** XXX   03 Z2 80 💻
AMA: 2018,Jan,8; 2017,Jan,8; 2016,Jan,13

70470 without contrast material, followed by contrast material(s) and further sections
🎥 5.38   📐 5.38   **FUD** XXX   03 Z2 80 💻
AMA: 2018,Jan,8; 2017,Jan,8; 2016,Jan,13

70480 Computed tomography, orbit, sella, or posterior fossa or outer, middle, or inner ear; without contrast material
🎥 5.64   📐 5.64   **FUD** XXX   03 Z2 80 💻
AMA: 2018,Jan,8; 2017,Jan,8; 2016,Jan,13

70481 with contrast material(s)
🎥 6.29   📐 6.29   **FUD** XXX   03 Z2 80 💻
AMA: 2018,Jan,8; 2017,Jan,8; 2016,Jan,13

70482 without contrast material, followed by contrast material(s) and further sections
🎥 6.97   📐 6.97   **FUD** XXX   03 Z2 80 💻
AMA: 2014,Jan,11; 2012,Feb,9-10

70486 Computed tomography, maxillofacial area; without contrast material
🎥 3.92   📐 3.92   **FUD** XXX   03 Z2 80 💻
AMA: 2018,Jan,8; 2017,Jan,8; 2016,Jan,13

70487 with contrast material(s)
🎥 4.70   📐 4.70   **FUD** XXX   03 Z2 80 💻
AMA: 2014,Jan,11; 2012,Feb,9-10

70488 without contrast material, followed by contrast material(s) and further sections
🎥 5.73   📐 5.73   **FUD** XXX   03 Z2 80 💻
AMA: 2014,Jan,11; 2012,Feb,9-10

70490 Computed tomography, soft tissue neck; without contrast material
EXCLUDES CT cervical spine (72125)
🎥 4.63   📐 4.63   **FUD** XXX   03 Z2 80 💻
AMA: 2014,Jan,11; 2012,Feb,9-10

70491 with contrast material(s)
EXCLUDES CT cervical spine (72125)
🎥 5.70   📐 5.70   **FUD** XXX   03 Z2 80 💻
AMA: 2014,Jan,11; 2012,Feb,9-10

70492 without contrast material followed by contrast material(s) and further sections
EXCLUDES CT cervical spine (72125)
🎥 6.89   📐 6.89   **FUD** XXX   03 Z2 80 💻
AMA: 2014,Jan,11; 2012,Feb,9-10

70496-70498 Computerized Tomographic Angiography: Head and Neck

CMS: 100-04,4,250.16 Multiple Procedure Payment Reduction: Certain Diagnostic Imaging Procedures Rendered by Physicians
INCLUDES Computed tomography to visualize arterial and venous vessels
EXCLUDES Noninvasive arterial plaque analysis non-coronary computerized tomography angiography (0710T-0713T)

70496 Computed tomographic angiography, head, with contrast material(s), including noncontrast images, if performed, and image postprocessing
🎥 8.35   📐 8.35   **FUD** XXX   03 Z2 80 💻
AMA: 2018,Jan,8; 2017,Jan,8; 2016,Jan,13

70498 Computed tomographic angiography, neck, with contrast material(s), including noncontrast images, if performed, and image postprocessing
🎥 8.34   📐 8.34   **FUD** XXX   03 Z2 80 💻
AMA: 2018,Jan,8; 2017,Jan,8; 2016,Jan,13

70540-70543 Magnetic Resonance Imaging: Face, Neck, Orbits

CMS: 100-04,4,250.16 Multiple Procedure Payment Reduction: Certain Diagnostic Imaging Procedures Rendered by Physicians
INCLUDES Three-dimensional imaging that measures response oatomic nuclei in soft tissues to high-frequency radio waves when strong magnetic field applied
EXCLUDES Magnetic resonance angiography head/neck (70544-70549)
Procedure performed more than one time per session

70540 Magnetic resonance (eg, proton) imaging, orbit, face, and/or neck; without contrast material(s)
🎥 7.34   📐 7.34   **FUD** XXX   03 Z2 80 💻
AMA: 2018,Jan,8; 2017,Jan,8; 2016,Jan,13

70542 with contrast material(s)
🎥 8.72   📐 8.72   **FUD** XXX   03 Z2 80 💻
AMA: 2018,Jan,8; 2017,Jan,8; 2016,Jan,13

70543 without contrast material(s), followed by contrast material(s) and further sequences
🎥 11.1   📐 11.1   **FUD** XXX   03 Z2 80 💻
AMA: 2018,Jan,8; 2017,Jan,8; 2016,Jan,13

26/TC PC/TC Only   A2-Z3 ASC Payment   50 Bilateral   ♂ Male Only   ♀ Female Only   🎥 Facility RVU   📐 Non-Facility RVU   💻 CCI   ❌ CLIA
FUD Follow-up Days   CMS: IOM   AMA: CPT Asst   A-Y OPPSI   80/80 Surg Assist Allowed / w/Doc   📋 Lab Crosswalk   📷 Radiology Crosswalk

320   CPT © 2021 American Medical Association. All Rights Reserved.   © 2021 Optum360, LLC

70544-70549 Magnetic Resonance Angiography: Head and Neck

CMS: 100-04,13,40.1.1 Magnetic Resonance Angiography; 100-04,13,40.1.2 HCPCS Coding Requirements; 100-04,4,250.16 Multiple Procedure Payment Reduction: Certain Diagnostic Imaging Procedures Rendered by Physicians

INCLUDES Magnetic fields and radio waves to produce detailed cross-sectional internal body structure images

EXCLUDES *Reporting code with following unless separate diagnostic MRI performed (70551-70553)*

70544 **Magnetic resonance angiography, head; without contrast material(s)**
6.90 6.90 **FUD** XXX Q3 Z2 80
AMA: 2018,Jan,8; 2017,Jan,8; 2016,Jan,13

70545 **with contrast material(s)**
7.21 7.21 **FUD** XXX Q3 Z2 80
AMA: 2018,Jan,8; 2017,Jan,8; 2016,Jan,13

70546 **without contrast material(s), followed by contrast material(s) and further sequences**
10.4 10.4 **FUD** XXX Q3 Z2 80
AMA: 2018,Jan,8; 2017,Jan,8; 2016,Jan,13

70547 **Magnetic resonance angiography, neck; without contrast material(s)**
6.93 6.93 **FUD** XXX Q3 Z2 80
AMA: 2018,Jan,8; 2017,Jan,8; 2016,Jan,13

70548 **with contrast material(s)**
7.74 7.74 **FUD** XXX Q3 Z2 80
AMA: 2018,Jan,8; 2017,Jan,8; 2016,Jan,13

70549 **without contrast material(s), followed by contrast material(s) and further sequences**
10.9 10.9 **FUD** XXX Q3 Z2 80
AMA: 2018,Jan,8; 2017,Jan,8; 2016,Jan,13

70551-70553 Magnetic Resonance Imaging: Brain and Brain Stem

CMS: 100-04,4,200.3.2 Multi-Source Photon Stereotactic RadiosurgeryPlanning and Delivery; 100-04,4,250.16 Multiple Procedure Payment Reduction: Certain Diagnostic Imaging Procedures Rendered by Physicians

INCLUDES Three-dimensional imaging that measures response oatomic nuclei in soft tissues to high-frequency radio waves when strong magnetic field applied

EXCLUDES *Magnetic spectroscopy (76390)*

70551 **Magnetic resonance (eg, proton) imaging, brain (including brain stem); without contrast material**
6.28 6.28 **FUD** XXX Q3 Z2 80
AMA: 2018,Jan,8; 2017,Jan,8; 2016,Jan,13

70552 **with contrast material(s)**
8.69 8.69 **FUD** XXX Q3 Z2 80
AMA: 2018,Jan,8; 2017,Jan,8; 2016,Jan,13

70553 **without contrast material, followed by contrast material(s) and further sequences**
10.2 10.2 **FUD** XXX Q3 Z2 80
AMA: 2018,Jan,8; 2017,Jan,8; 2016,Jan,13

70554-70555 Magnetic Resonance Imaging: Brain Mapping

INCLUDES Neuroimaging technique using MRI to identify and map signals related to brain activity

EXCLUDES *Reporting code with following unless separate diagnostic MRI performed (70551-70553)*

70554 **Magnetic resonance imaging, brain, functional MRI; including test selection and administration of repetitive body part movement and/or visual stimulation, not requiring physician or psychologist administration**
EXCLUDES *Functional brain mapping (96020)*
Testing performed by physician or psychologist (70555)
12.1 12.1 **FUD** XXX Q3 Z2 80
AMA: 2018,Jan,8; 2017,Jan,8; 2016,Jan,13

70555 **requiring physician or psychologist administration of entire neurofunctional testing**
EXCLUDES *Testing performed by technologist, nonphysician, or nonpsychologist (70554)*
Code also (96020)
0.00 0.00 **FUD** XXX S Z2 80
AMA: 2018,Jan,8; 2017,Jan,8; 2016,Jan,13

70557-70559 Magnetic Resonance Imaging: Intraoperative

EXCLUDES *Intracranial lesion stereotaxic biopsy with magnetic resonance guidance (61751, 77021-77022)*
Procedures performed more than one time per surgical encounter
Reporting codes unless separate report generated

Code also stereotactic biopsy, aspiration, or excision, when performed with MRI (61751)

70557 **Magnetic resonance (eg, proton) imaging, brain (including brain stem and skull base), during open intracranial procedure (eg, to assess for residual tumor or residual vascular malformation); without contrast material**
0.00 0.00 **FUD** XXX S Z2 80
AMA: 2014,Jan,11; 2012,Feb,9-10

70558 **with contrast material(s)**
0.00 0.00 **FUD** XXX S Z2 80
AMA: 2014,Jan,11; 2012,Feb,9-10

70559 **without contrast material(s), followed by contrast material(s) and further sequences**
0.00 0.00 **FUD** XXX S Z2 80
AMA: 2014,Jan,11; 2012,Feb,9-10

71045-71130 Radiography: Thorax

71045 **Radiologic examination, chest; single view**
EXCLUDES *Acute abdomen series, complete (2 or more views) including chest view (74022)*
Remotely performed CAD (0175T)
Code also concurrent computer-aided detection (CAD) (0174T)
0.72 0.72 **FUD** XXX Q3 Z3 80
AMA: 2019,Aug,8; 2019,May,10; 2019,Mar,10; 2018,Apr,7

71046 **2 views**
EXCLUDES *Acute abdomen series, complete (2 or more views) including chest view (74022)*
Remotely performed CAD (0175T)
Code also concurrent computer-aided detection (CAD) (0174T)
0.89 0.89 **FUD** XXX Q3 Z3 80
AMA: 2019,Aug,8; 2019,Mar,10; 2018,Apr,7

71047 **3 views**
EXCLUDES *Acute abdomen series, complete (2 or more views) including chest view (74022)*
Remotely performed CAD (0175T)
Code also concurrent computer-aided detection (CAD) (0174T)
1.16 1.16 **FUD** XXX Q1 N1 80
AMA: 2019,Mar,10; 2018,Apr,7

71048 **4 or more views**
EXCLUDES *Acute abdomen series, complete (2 or more views) including chest view (74022)*
Remotely performed CAD (0175T)
Code also concurrent computer-aided detection (CAD) (0174T)
1.21 1.21 **FUD** XXX Q1 N1 80
AMA: 2019,Mar,10; 2018,Apr,7

71100 **Radiologic examination, ribs, unilateral; 2 views**
1.00 1.00 FUD XXX Q1 N1 80
AMA: 2014,Jan,11; 2012,Feb,9-10

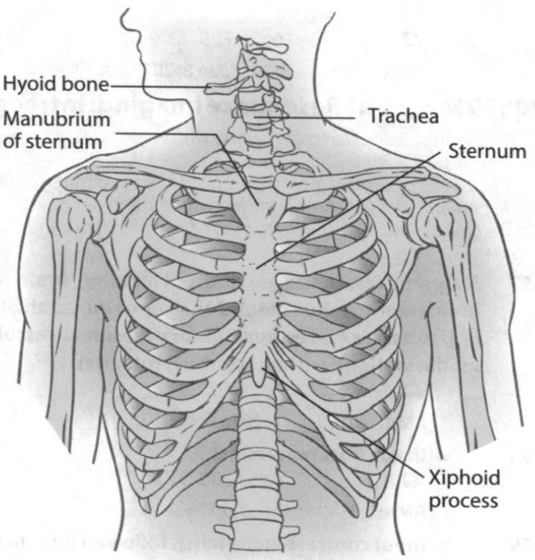

71101 **including posteroanterior chest, minimum of 3 views**
1.15 1.15 FUD XXX Q1 N1 80
AMA: 2014,Jan,11; 2012,Feb,9-10

71110 **Radiologic examination, ribs, bilateral; 3 views**
1.21 1.21 FUD XXX Q1 N1 80
AMA: 2014,Jan,11; 2012,Feb,9-10

71111 **including posteroanterior chest, minimum of 4 views**
1.44 1.44 FUD XXX Q1 N1 80
AMA: 2014,Jan,11; 2012,Feb,9-10

71120 **Radiologic examination; sternum, minimum of 2 views**
0.92 0.92 FUD XXX Q1 N1 80
AMA: 2014,Jan,11; 2012,Feb,9-10

71130 **sternoclavicular joint or joints, minimum of 3 views**
1.12 1.12 FUD XXX Q1 N1 80
AMA: 2014,Jan,11; 2012,Feb,9-10

71250-71271 Computerized Tomography: Thorax

INCLUDES Imaging using tomographic technique enhanced by computer imaging to create cross-sectional body plane view

EXCLUDES *3D rendering (76376-76377)*
CT breast (0633T-0638T)
CT heart (75571-75574)

71250 **Computed tomography, thorax, diagnostic; without contrast material**
CT thorax with contrast (71260-71270)
EXCLUDES *CT thorax for lung cancer screening (71271)*
4.45 4.45 FUD XXX Q3 Z2 80
AMA: 2020,Sep,11; 2018,Jan,8; 2017,Jan,8; 2016,Jan,13

71260 **with contrast material(s)**
EXCLUDES *CT thorax for lung cancer screening (71271)*
CT thorax without contrast (71250, 71270)
5.52 5.52 FUD XXX Q3 Z2 80
AMA: 2020,Sep,11; 2018,Jan,8; 2017,Jan,8; 2016,Jan,13

71270 **without contrast material, followed by contrast material(s) and further sections**
EXCLUDES *CT thorax for lung cancer screening (71271)*
CT thorax with or without contrast only (71250, 71260)
6.53 6.53 FUD XXX Q3 Z2 80
AMA: 2020,Sep,11; 2018,Jan,8; 2017,Jan,8; 2016,Jan,13

71271 **Computed tomography, thorax, low dose for lung cancer screening, without contrast material(s)**
EXCLUDES *CT thorax not for lung cancer screening (71250, 71260, 71270)*
4.32 4.32 FUD XXX 80

71275 Computerized Tomographic Angiography: Thorax

CMS: 100-04,4,250.16 Multiple Procedure Payment Reduction: Certain Diagnostic Imaging Procedures Rendered by Physicians

INCLUDES Multiple rapid thin section CT scans to create cross-sectional bone, organ, and tissue images

EXCLUDES *CT angiography coronary arteries including calcification score and/or cardiac morphology (75574)*

71275 **Computed tomographic angiography, chest (noncoronary), with contrast material(s), including noncontrast images, if performed, and image postprocessing**
8.53 8.53 FUD XXX Q3 Z2 80
AMA: 2020,Sep,11; 2018,Jan,8; 2017,Jan,8; 2016,Jan,13

71550-71552 Magnetic Resonance Imaging: Thorax

CMS: 100-04,4,250.16 Multiple Procedure Payment Reduction: Certain Diagnostic Imaging Procedures Rendered by Physicians

INCLUDES Three-dimensional imaging that measures response atomic nuclei in soft tissues to high-frequency radio waves when strong magnetic field applied

EXCLUDES *MRI of the breast (77046-77049)*

71550 **Magnetic resonance (eg, proton) imaging, chest (eg, for evaluation of hilar and mediastinal lymphadenopathy); without contrast material(s)**
11.4 11.4 FUD XXX Q3 Z2 80
AMA: 2018,Jan,8; 2017,Jan,8; 2016,Jan,13

71551 **with contrast material(s)**
12.3 12.3 FUD XXX Q3 Z3 80
AMA: 2018,Jan,8; 2017,Jan,8; 2016,Jan,13

71552 **without contrast material(s), followed by contrast material(s) and further sequences**
15.9 15.9 FUD XXX Q3 Z2 80
AMA: 2018,Jan,8; 2017,Jan,8; 2016,Jan,13

71555 Magnetic Resonance Angiography: Thorax

CMS: 100-04,13,40.1.1 Magnetic Resonance Angiography; 100-04,13,40.1.2 HCPCS Coding Requirements; 100-04,4,250.16 Multiple Procedure Payment Reduction: Certain Diagnostic Imaging Procedures Rendered by Physicians

71555 **Magnetic resonance angiography, chest (excluding myocardium), with or without contrast material(s)**
10.8 10.8 FUD XXX B 80
AMA: 2018,Jan,8; 2017,Jan,8; 2016,Jan,13

72020-72120 Radiography: Spine

INCLUDES Minimum number views or more views when needed to adequately complete study
Radiographs repeated during encounter due to substandard quality; only one unit reported

EXCLUDES *Obtaining more films after initial film review, based on the radiologist discretion, an order for the test, and change in patient's condition*

72020 **Radiologic examination, spine, single view, specify level**
EXCLUDES *Single view entire thoracic and lumbar spine (72081)*
0.68 0.68 FUD XXX Q1 N1 80
AMA: 2018,Jan,8; 2017,Jan,8; 2016,Sep,4; 2016,Jan,13

72040 **Radiologic examination, spine, cervical; 2 or 3 views**
1.07 1.07 **FUD** XXX Q1 N1 80
AMA: 2018,Aug,10; 2018,Jan,8; 2017,Jan,8; 2016,Jan,13

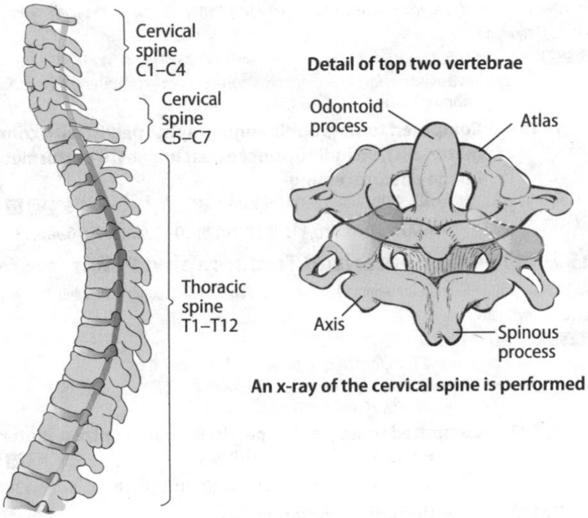

An x-ray of the cervical spine is performed

72050 **4 or 5 views**
1.42 1.42 **FUD** XXX Q1 N1 80
AMA: 2014,Jan,11; 2012,Feb,9-10

72052 **6 or more views**
1.67 1.67 **FUD** XXX Q1 N1 80
AMA: 2014,Jan,11; 2012,Feb,9-10

72070 **Radiologic examination, spine; thoracic, 2 views**
0.96 0.96 **FUD** XXX Q1 N1 80
AMA: 2018,Jan,8; 2017,Jan,8; 2016,Jan,13

72072 **thoracic, 3 views**
1.08 1.08 **FUD** XXX Q1 N1 80
AMA: 2018,Jan,8; 2017,Jan,8; 2016,Jan,13

72074 **thoracic, minimum of 4 views**
1.21 1.21 **FUD** XXX Q1 N1 80
AMA: 2018,Jan,8; 2017,Jan,8; 2016,Jan,13

72080 **thoracolumbar junction, minimum of 2 views**
EXCLUDES *Single view thoracolumbar junction (72020)*
0.96 0.96 **FUD** XXX Q1 N1 80
AMA: 2018,Jan,8; 2017,Jan,8; 2016,Sep,4; 2016,Jan,13

72081 **Radiologic examination, spine, entire thoracic and lumbar, including skull, cervical and sacral spine if performed (eg, scoliosis evaluation); one view**
1.17 1.17 **FUD** XXX Q1 N1 80
AMA: 2018,Jan,8; 2017,Jan,8; 2016,Sep,4

72082 **2 or 3 views**
1.90 1.90 **FUD** XXX Q1 N1 80
AMA: 2018,Jan,8; 2017,Jan,8; 2016,Sep,4

72083 **4 or 5 views**
2.16 2.16 **FUD** XXX S Z2 80
AMA: 2018,Jan,8; 2017,Jan,8; 2016,Sep,4

72084 **minimum of 6 views**
2.52 2.52 **FUD** XXX S Z2 80
AMA: 2018,Jan,8; 2017,Jan,8; 2016,Sep,4

72100 **Radiologic examination, spine, lumbosacral; 2 or 3 views**
1.07 1.07 **FUD** XXX Q1 N1 80
AMA: 2018,Jan,8; 2017,Jan,8; 2016,Jan,13

72110 **minimum of 4 views**
1.36 1.36 **FUD** XXX Q1 N1 80
AMA: 2018,Jan,8; 2017,Jan,8; 2016,Jan,13

72114 **complete, including bending views, minimum of 6 views**
1.64 1.64 **FUD** XXX Q1 N1 80
AMA: 2014,Jan,11; 2012,Feb,9-10

72120 **bending views only, 2 or 3 views**
1.11 1.11 **FUD** XXX Q1 N1 80
AMA: 2018,Jan,8; 2017,Jan,8; 2016,Aug,7

72125-72133 Computerized Tomography: Spine

CMS: 100-04,12,20.4.7 Services Not Meeting National Electrical Manufacturers Association (NEMA) Standard; 100-04,4,20.6.12 Use of HCPCS Modifier – CT; 100-04,4,250.16 Multiple Procedure Payment Reduction: Certain Diagnostic Imaging Procedures Rendered by Physicians

INCLUDES Imaging using tomographic technique enhanced by computer imaging to create cross-sectional body plane view

EXCLUDES *3D rendering (76376-76377)*

Code also intrathecal injection procedure when performed (61055, 62284)

72125 **Computed tomography, cervical spine; without contrast material**
4.38 4.38 **FUD** XXX Q3 Z2 80
AMA: 2020,Sep,11

72126 **with contrast material**
6.40 6.40 **FUD** XXX Q3 Z3 80
AMA: 2020,Sep,11; 2018,Jan,8; 2017,Jan,8; 2016,Jan,13

72127 **without contrast material, followed by contrast material(s) and further sections**
6.48 6.48 **FUD** XXX Q3 Z2 80
AMA: 2020,Sep,11

72128 **Computed tomography, thoracic spine; without contrast material**
5.08 5.08 **FUD** XXX Q3 Z2 80
AMA: 2020,Sep,11

72129 **with contrast material**
5.54 5.54 **FUD** XXX Q3 Z2 80
AMA: 2020,Sep,11; 2019,Jan,14; 2018,Jan,8; 2017,Jan,8; 2016,Jan,13

72130 **without contrast material, followed by contrast material(s) and further sections**
6.49 6.49 **FUD** XXX Q3 Z2 80
AMA: 2020,Sep,11

72131 **Computed tomography, lumbar spine; without contrast material**
4.36 4.36 **FUD** XXX Q3 Z2 80
AMA: 2020,Sep,11

72132 **with contrast material**
5.51 5.51 **FUD** XXX Q3 Z3 80
AMA: 2020,Sep,11; 2019,Jan,14; 2018,Jan,8; 2017,Jan,8; 2016,Jan,13

72133 **without contrast material, followed by contrast material(s) and further sections**
6.45 6.45 **FUD** XXX Q3 Z2 80
AMA: 2020,Sep,11

72141-72158 Magnetic Resonance Imaging: Spine

CMS: 100-04,4,250.16 Multiple Procedure Payment Reduction: Certain Diagnostic Imaging Procedures Rendered by Physicians

INCLUDES Three-dimensional imaging that measures response atomic nuclei in soft tissues to high-frequency radio waves when strong magnetic field applied

EXCLUDES *MR spectroscopy (0609T-0610T)*

Code also intrathecal injection procedure when performed (61055, 62284)

72141 **Magnetic resonance (eg, proton) imaging, spinal canal and contents, cervical; without contrast material**
6.11 6.11 **FUD** XXX Q3 Z2 80
AMA: 2018,Jan,8; 2017,Jan,8; 2016,Jan,13

72142 **with contrast material(s)**
EXCLUDES *MRI cervical spinal canal performed without contrast followed by repeating study with contrast (72156)*
8.88 8.88 **FUD** XXX Q3 Z2 80
AMA: 2018,Jan,8; 2017,Jan,8; 2016,Jan,13

72146 **Magnetic resonance (eg, proton) imaging, spinal canal and contents, thoracic; without contrast material**

6.11 6.11 FUD XXX 03 Z2 80

AMA: 2018,Jan,8; 2017,Jan,8; 2016,Jan,13

72147 **with contrast material(s)**

EXCLUDES *MRI thoracic spinal canal performed without contrast followed by repeating study with contrast (72157)*

8.82 8.82 FUD XXX 03 Z2 80

AMA: 2018,Jan,8; 2017,Jan,8; 2016,Jan,13

72148 **Magnetic resonance (eg, proton) imaging, spinal canal and contents, lumbar; without contrast material**

6.12 6.12 FUD XXX 03 Z2 80

AMA: 2018,Jan,8; 2017,Jan,8; 2016,Jan,13

72149 **with contrast material(s)**

EXCLUDES *MRI lumbar spinal canal performed without contrast followed by repeating study with contrast (72158)*

8.74 8.74 FUD XXX 03 Z2 80

AMA: 2014,Jan,11; 2012,Feb,9-10

72156 **Magnetic resonance (eg, proton) imaging, spinal canal and contents, without contrast material, followed by contrast material(s) and further sequences; cervical**

10.3 10.3 FUD XXX 03 Z2 80

AMA: 2014,Jan,11; 2012,Feb,9-10

72157 **thoracic**

10.5 10.5 FUD XXX 03 Z2 80

AMA: 2014,Jan,11; 2012,Feb,9-10

72158 **lumbar**

10.5 10.5 FUD XXX 03 Z2 80

AMA: 2014,Jan,11; 2012,Feb,9-10

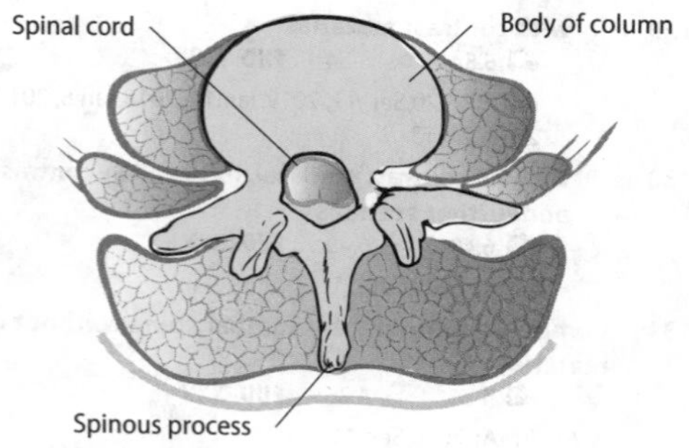

Superior view of thoracic spine and surrounding paraspinal muscles

72159 Magnetic Resonance Angiography: Spine

CMS: 100-04,13,40.1.1 Magnetic Resonance Angiography; 100-04,13,40.1.2 HCPCS Coding Requirements; 100-04,4,250.16 Multiple Procedure Payment Reduction: Certain Diagnostic Imaging Procedures Rendered by Physicians

72159 **Magnetic resonance angiography, spinal canal and contents, with or without contrast material(s)**

11.2 11.2 FUD XXX B 80

AMA: 2018,Jan,8; 2017,Jan,8; 2016,Jan,13

72170-72190 Radiography: Pelvis

INCLUDES Minimum number views or more views when needed to adequately complete study

Radiographs repeated during encounter due to substandard quality; only one unit reported

EXCLUDES *Combined CT or CT angiography abdomen and pelvis (74174, 74176-74178)*

Obtaining more films after initial film review, based on radiologist discretion, order for test, and change in patient's condition

Pelvimetry (74710)

Second interpretation by requesting physician (included in E/M service)

72170 **Radiologic examination, pelvis; 1 or 2 views**

0.80 0.80 FUD XXX 01 N1 80

AMA: 2018,Jan,8; 2017,Jan,8; 2016,Aug,7; 2016,Jun,5; 2016,Jan,13

72190 **complete, minimum of 3 views**

1.14 1.14 FUD XXX 01 N1 80

AMA: 2016,Jun,5

72191 Computerized Tomographic Angiography: Pelvis

CMS: 100-04,4,250.16 Multiple Procedure Payment Reduction: Certain Diagnostic Imaging Procedures Rendered by Physicians

EXCLUDES *Computed tomographic angiography (73706, 74174-74175, 75635)*

Noninvasive arterial plaque analysis non-coronary computerized tomography angiography (0710T-0713T)

72191 **Computed tomographic angiography, pelvis, with contrast material(s), including noncontrast images, if performed, and image postprocessing**

9.08 9.08 FUD XXX 03 Z2 80

AMA: 2020,Sep,11; 2018,Jan,8; 2017,Jan,8; 2016,Jan,13

72192-72194 Computerized Tomography: Pelvis

CMS: 100-04,4,250.16 Multiple Procedure Payment Reduction: Certain Diagnostic Imaging Procedures Rendered by Physicians

EXCLUDES *3D rendering (76376-76377)*

Combined CT abdomen and pelvis (74176-74178)

CT colonography, diagnostic (74261-74262)

CT colonography, screening (74263)

72192 **Computed tomography, pelvis; without contrast material**

4.09 4.09 FUD XXX 03 Z2 80

AMA: 2020,Sep,11; 2018,Jan,8; 2017,Jan,8; 2016,Jan,13

72193 **with contrast material(s)**

6.81 6.81 FUD XXX 03 Z2 80

AMA: 2020,Sep,11; 2018,Jan,8; 2017,Jan,8; 2016,Jan,13

72194 **without contrast material, followed by contrast material(s) and further sections**

7.66 7.66 FUD XXX 03 Z2 80

AMA: 2020,Sep,11; 2018,Jan,8; 2017,Jan,8; 2016,Jan,13

72195-72197 Magnetic Resonance Imaging: Pelvis

CMS: 100-04,4,250.16 Multiple Procedure Payment Reduction: Certain Diagnostic Imaging Procedures Rendered by Physicians

INCLUDES Three-dimensional imaging that measures response atomic nuclei in soft tissues to high-frequency radio waves when strong magnetic field applied

EXCLUDES *MRI fetus(es) (74712-74713)*

72195 **Magnetic resonance (eg, proton) imaging, pelvis; without contrast material(s)**

7.49 7.49 FUD XXX 03 Z2 80

AMA: 2018,Jul,11; 2018,Jan,8; 2017,Jan,8; 2016,Jun,5; 2016,Jan,13

72196 **with contrast material(s)**

8.74 8.74 FUD XXX 03 Z2 80

AMA: 2018,Jul,11; 2018,Jan,8; 2017,Jan,8; 2016,Jun,5; 2016,Jan,13

72197 **without contrast material(s), followed by contrast material(s) and further sequences**

10.9 10.9 FUD XXX 03 Z2 80

AMA: 2018,Jul,11; 2018,Jan,8; 2017,Jan,8; 2016,Jun,5; 2016,Jan,13

72198 Magnetic Resonance Angiography: Pelvis

CMS: 100-04,13,40.1.1 Magnetic Resonance Angiography; 100-04,13,40.1.2 HCPCS Coding Requirements; 100-04,4,250.16 Multiple Procedure Payment Reduction: Certain Diagnostic Imaging Procedures Rendered by Physicians

INCLUDES Magnetic fields and radio waves to produce detailed cross-sectional images arteries and veins

72198 **Magnetic resonance angiography, pelvis, with or without contrast material(s)**

11.0 11.0 FUD XXX B 80

AMA: 2018,Jan,8; 2017,Jan,8; 2016,Jan,13

72200-72220 Radiography: Pelvisacral

INCLUDES Minimum number views or more views when needed to adequately complete study
Radiographs repeated during encounter due to substandard quality; only one unit reported

EXCLUDES *Obtaining more films after initial film review, based on radiologist discretion, order for, and change in patient's condition*
Second interpretation by requesting physician (included in E/M service)

72200 **Radiologic examination, sacroiliac joints; less than 3 views**
0.90 0.90 **FUD** XXX Q1 N1 80
AMA: 2014,Jan,11; 2012,Feb,9-10

72202 **3 or more views**
1.07 1.07 **FUD** XXX Q1 N1 80
AMA: 2014,Jan,11; 2012,Feb,9-10

72220 **Radiologic examination, sacrum and coccyx, minimum of 2 views**
0.88 0.88 **FUD** XXX Q1 N1 80
AMA: 2014,Jan,11; 2012,Feb,9-10

72240-72270 Myelography with Contrast: Spinal Cord

CMS: 100-04,13,30.1.3.1 Payment for Low Osmolar Contrast Material

EXCLUDES *Injection procedure for myelography (62284)*
Myelography (62302-62305)

Code also injection at C1-C2 for complete myelography (61055)

72240 **Myelography, cervical, radiological supervision and interpretation**
3.14 3.14 **FUD** XXX Q2 N1 80
AMA: 2018,Jan,8; 2017,Jan,8; 2016,Jan,13

72255 **Myelography, thoracic, radiological supervision and interpretation**
2.99 2.99 **FUD** XXX Q2 N1 80
AMA: 2018,Jan,8; 2017,Jan,8; 2016,Jan,13

72265 **Myelography, lumbosacral, radiological supervision and interpretation**
2.90 2.90 **FUD** XXX Q2 N1 80
AMA: 2018,Jan,8; 2017,Jan,8; 2016,Jan,13

72270 **Myelography, 2 or more regions (eg, lumbar/thoracic, cervical/thoracic, lumbar/cervical, lumbar/thoracic/cervical), radiological supervision and interpretation**
4.00 4.00 **FUD** XXX Q2 N1 80
AMA: 2018,Jan,8; 2017,Jan,8; 2016,Jan,13

72275 Radiography: Epidural Space

~~**72275**~~ ~~**Epidurography, radiological supervision and interpretation**~~
To report, see (62281-62282, 62321, 62323, 62325, 62327, 64479, 64480, 64483-64484)

72285 Radiography: Intervertebral Disc (Cervical/Thoracic)

CMS: 100-04,13,30.1.3.1 Payment for Low Osmolar Contrast Material

Code also discography injection procedure (62291)

72285 **Discography, cervical or thoracic, radiological supervision and interpretation**
3.45 3.45 **FUD** XXX Q2 N1 80
AMA: 2018,Jan,8; 2017,Jan,8; 2016,Jan,13

72295 Radiography: Intervertebral Disc (Lumbar)

CMS: 100-04,13,30.1.3.1 Payment for Low Osmolar Contrast Material

Code also discography injection procedure (62290)

72295 **Discography, lumbar, radiological supervision and interpretation**
3.02 3.02 **FUD** XXX Q2 N1 80
AMA: 2018,Jan,8; 2017,Feb,12; 2017,Jan,8; 2016,Jan,13

73000-73085 Radiography: Shoulder and Upper Arm

INCLUDES Minimum number views or more views when needed to adequately complete study
Radiographs repeated during encounter due to substandard quality; only one unit reported

EXCLUDES *Obtaining more films after initial film review, based on radiologist discretion, order for test, and change in patient's condition*
Second interpretation by requesting physician (included in E/M service)
Stress views upper body joint(s), when performed (77071)

73000 **Radiologic examination; clavicle, complete**
0.88 0.88 **FUD** XXX Q1 N1 80
AMA: 2014,Jan,11; 2012,Feb,9-10

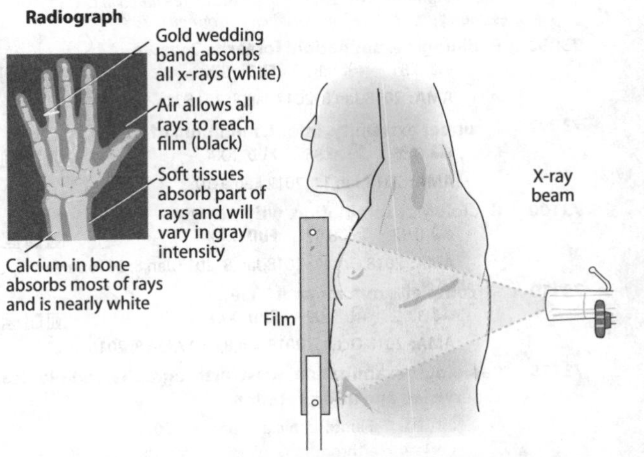
Radiograph
Gold wedding band absorbs all x-rays (white)
Air allows all rays to reach film (black)
Soft tissues absorb part of rays and will vary in gray intensity
Calcium in bone absorbs most of rays and is nearly white
X-ray beam
Film

Posterioranterior (PA) chest study; lateral views also common

73010 **scapula, complete**
0.78 0.78 **FUD** XXX Q1 N1 80
AMA: 2014,Jan,11; 2012,Feb,9-10

73020 **Radiologic examination, shoulder; 1 view**
0.60 0.60 **FUD** XXX Q1 N1 80
AMA: 2014,Jan,11; 2012,Feb,9-10

73030 **complete, minimum of 2 views**
0.93 0.93 **FUD** XXX Q1 N1 80
AMA: 2014,Jan,11; 2012,Feb,9-10

73040 **Radiologic examination, shoulder, arthrography, radiological supervision and interpretation**
INCLUDES Fluoroscopic guidance (77002)
Code also arthrography injection procedure (23350)
3.39 3.39 **FUD** XXX Q2 N1 80
AMA: 2018,Jan,8; 2017,Jan,8; 2016,Jan,13

73050 **Radiologic examination; acromioclavicular joints, bilateral, with or without weighted distraction**
0.88 0.88 **FUD** XXX Q1 N1 80
AMA: 2014,Jan,11; 2012,Feb,9-10

73060 **humerus, minimum of 2 views**
0.88 0.88 **FUD** XXX Q1 N1 80
AMA: 2014,Jan,11; 2012,Feb,9-10

73070 **Radiologic examination, elbow; 2 views**
0.80 0.80 **FUD** XXX Q1 N1 80
AMA: 2018,Jan,8; 2017,Jan,8; 2016,Jan,13

73080 **complete, minimum of 3 views**
0.87 0.87 **FUD** XXX Q1 N1 80
AMA: 2014,Jan,11; 2012,Feb,9-10

73085 **Radiologic examination, elbow, arthrography, radiological supervision and interpretation**

INCLUDES Fluoroscopic guidance (77002)

Code also arthrography injection procedure (24220)

3.18 3.18 FUD XXX Q2 N1 80

AMA: 2018,Jan,8; 2017,Jan,8; 2016,Jan,13

73090-73140 Radiography: Forearm and Hand

INCLUDES Minimum number views or more views when needed to adequately complete study

Radiographs repeated during encounter due to substandard quality; only one unit reported

EXCLUDES *Obtaining more films after initial film review, based on radiologist discretion, order for test, and change in patient's condition*

Second interpretation by requesting physician (included in E/M service)

Stress views upper body joint(s), when performed (77071)

73090 **Radiologic examination; forearm, 2 views**

0.81 0.81 FUD XXX Q1 N1 80

AMA: 2018,Jan,8; 2017,Jan,8; 2016,Jan,13

73092 **upper extremity, infant, minimum of 2 views** A

0.85 0.85 FUD XXX Q1 N1 80

AMA: 2014,Jan,11; 2012,Feb,9-10

73100 **Radiologic examination, wrist; 2 views**

0.92 0.92 FUD XXX Q1 N1 80

AMA: 2018,Oct,11; 2018,Jan,8; 2017,Jan,8; 2016,Jan,13

73110 **complete, minimum of 3 views**

1.09 1.09 FUD XXX Q1 N1 80

AMA: 2018,Oct,11; 2018,Jan,8; 2017,Jan,8; 2016,Jan,13

73115 **Radiologic examination, wrist, arthrography, radiological supervision and interpretation**

INCLUDES Fluoroscopic guidance (77002)

Code also arthrography injection procedure (25246)

3.56 3.56 FUD XXX Q2 N1 80

AMA: 2018,Jan,8; 2017,Jan,8; 2016,Jan,13

73120 **Radiologic examination, hand; 2 views**

0.85 0.85 FUD XXX Q1 N1 80

AMA: 2018,Oct,11

73130 **minimum of 3 views**

0.94 0.94 FUD XXX Q1 N1 80

AMA: 2014,Jan,11; 2012,Feb,9-10

73140 **Radiologic examination, finger(s), minimum of 2 views**

1.00 1.00 FUD XXX Q1 N1 80

AMA: 2018,Jan,8; 2017,Jan,8; 2016,Jan,13

73200-73202 Computerized Tomography: Shoulder, Arm, Hand

CMS: 100-04,4,250.16 Multiple Procedure Payment Reduction: Certain Diagnostic Imaging Procedures Rendered by Physicians

INCLUDES Imaging using tomographic technique enhanced by computer imaging to create cross-sectional body plane view

Intravascular, intrathecal, or intra-articular contrast materials when noted in code descriptor

EXCLUDES *3D rendering (76376-76377)*

73200 **Computed tomography, upper extremity; without contrast material**

5.03 5.03 FUD XXX Q3 Z2 80

AMA: 2018,Jan,8; 2017,Jan,8; 2016,Jan,13

73201 **with contrast material(s)**

6.28 6.28 FUD XXX Q3 Z3 80

AMA: 2018,Jan,8; 2017,Jan,8; 2016,Jan,13

73202 **without contrast material, followed by contrast material(s) and further sections**

7.82 7.82 FUD XXX Q3 Z2 80

AMA: 2014,Jan,11; 2012,Feb,9-10

73206 Computerized Tomographic Angiography: Shoulder, Arm, and Hand

CMS: 100-04,4,250.16 Multiple Procedure Payment Reduction: Certain Diagnostic Imaging Procedures Rendered by Physicians

INCLUDES Intravascular, intrathecal, or intra-articular contrast materials when noted in code descriptor

Multiple rapid thin section CT scans to create cross-sectional images arteries and veins

73206 **Computed tomographic angiography, upper extremity, with contrast material(s), including noncontrast images, if performed, and image postprocessing**

9.24 9.24 FUD XXX Q3 Z2 80

AMA: 2018,Jan,8; 2017,Jan,8; 2016,Jan,13

73218-73223 Magnetic Resonance Imaging: Shoulder, Arm, Hand

CMS: 100-04,4,250.16 Multiple Procedure Payment Reduction: Certain Diagnostic Imaging Procedures Rendered by Physicians

INCLUDES Intravascular, intrathecal, or intra-articular contrast materials when noted in code descriptor

Three-dimensional imaging that measures response atomic nuclei in soft tissues to high-frequency radio waves when strong magnetic field applied

73218 **Magnetic resonance (eg, proton) imaging, upper extremity, other than joint; without contrast material(s)**

10.1 10.1 FUD XXX Q3 Z2 80

AMA: 2018,Jan,8; 2017,Jan,8; 2016,Jan,13

73219 **with contrast material(s)**

10.9 10.9 FUD XXX Q3 Z2 80

AMA: 2018,Jan,8; 2017,Jan,8; 2016,Jan,13

73220 **without contrast material(s), followed by contrast material(s) and further sequences**

13.4 13.4 FUD XXX Q3 Z2 80

AMA: 2018,Jan,8; 2017,Jan,8; 2016,Jan,13

73221 **Magnetic resonance (eg, proton) imaging, any joint of upper extremity; without contrast material(s)**

6.47 6.47 FUD XXX Q3 Z2 80

AMA: 2018,Jan,8; 2017,Jan,8; 2016,Jan,13

73222 **with contrast material(s)**

10.2 10.2 FUD XXX Q3 Z3 80

AMA: 2018,Jan,8; 2017,Jan,8; 2016,Jan,13

73223 **without contrast material(s), followed by contrast material(s) and further sequences**

12.7 12.7 FUD XXX Q3 Z2 80

AMA: 2018,Jan,8; 2017,Jan,8; 2016,Jan,13

73225 Magnetic Resonance Angiography: Shoulder, Arm, Hand

CMS: 100-04,13,40.1.1 Magnetic Resonance Angiography; 100-04,4,250.16 Multiple Procedure Payment Reduction: Certain Diagnostic Imaging Procedures Rendered by Physicians

INCLUDES Intravascular, intrathecal, or intra-articular contrast materials when noted in code descriptor

Magnetic fields and radio waves to produce detailed cross-sectional images arteries and veins

73225 **Magnetic resonance angiography, upper extremity, with or without contrast material(s)**

11.1 11.1 FUD XXX B 80

AMA: 2018,Jan,8; 2017,Jan,8; 2016,Jan,13

73501-73552 Radiography: Pelvic Region and Thigh

EXCLUDES *Stress views lower body joint(s), when performed (77071)*

73501 **Radiologic examination, hip, unilateral, with pelvis when performed; 1 view**

0.89 0.89 FUD XXX Q1 N1 80

AMA: 2018,Jan,8; 2017,Jan,8; 2016,Aug,7; 2016,Jun,8; 2016,Jan,13

73502 **2-3 views**

1.27 1.27 FUD XXX Q1 N1 80

AMA: 2018,Jan,8; 2017,Jan,8; 2016,Aug,7; 2016,Jun,8; 2016,Jan,13

73503 **minimum of 4 views**
1.57 1.57 FUD XXX Q1 N1 80
AMA: 2018,Jan,8; 2017,Jan,8; 2016,Aug,7; 2016,Jun,8; 2016,Jan,13

73521 **Radiologic examination, hips, bilateral, with pelvis when performed; 2 views**
1.12 1.12 FUD XXX Q1 N1 80
AMA: 2018,Jan,8; 2017,Jan,8; 2016,Aug,7; 2016,Jun,8; 2016,Jan,13

73522 **3-4 views**
1.46 1.46 FUD XXX Q1 N1 80
AMA: 2018,Jan,8; 2017,Jan,8; 2016,Aug,7; 2016,Jun,8; 2016,Jan,13

73523 **minimum of 5 views**
1.65 1.65 FUD XXX S N1 80
AMA: 2018,Jan,8; 2017,Jan,8; 2016,Aug,7; 2016,Jun,8; 2016,Jan,13

73525 **Radiologic examination, hip, arthrography, radiological supervision and interpretation**
INCLUDES Fluoroscopic guidance (77002)
3.47 3.47 FUD XXX Q2 N1 80
AMA: 2018,Jan,8; 2017,Jan,8; 2016,Nov,10; 2016,Aug,7; 2016,Jan,13

73551 **Radiologic examination, femur; 1 view**
0.82 0.82 FUD XXX Q1 N1 80
AMA: 2018,Jan,8; 2017,Jan,8; 2016,Aug,7

73552 **minimum 2 views**
0.97 0.97 FUD XXX Q1 N1 80
AMA: 2018,Jan,8; 2017,Nov,10; 2017,Jan,8; 2016,Aug,7

73560-73660 Radiography: Lower Leg, Ankle, and Foot

EXCLUDES *Stress views lower body joint(s), when performed (77071)*

73560 **Radiologic examination, knee; 1 or 2 views**
0.94 0.94 FUD XXX Q1 N1 80
AMA: 2018,Jan,8; 2017,Jan,8; 2016,Jan,13

73562 **3 views**
1.10 1.10 FUD XXX Q1 N1 80
AMA: 2014,Jan,11; 2012,Feb,9-10

73564 **complete, 4 or more views**
1.23 1.23 FUD XXX Q1 N1 80
AMA: 2018,Jan,8; 2017,Jan,8; 2016,Jan,13

73565 **both knees, standing, anteroposterior**
1.09 1.09 FUD XXX Q1 N1 80
AMA: 2018,Jan,8; 2017,Jan,8; 2016,Jan,13

73580 **Radiologic examination, knee, arthrography, radiological supervision and interpretation**
INCLUDES Fluoroscopic guidance (77002)
3.84 3.84 FUD XXX Q2 N1 80
AMA: 2019,Aug,7; 2018,Jan,8; 2017,Jan,8; 2016,Jan,13

73590 **Radiologic examination; tibia and fibula, 2 views**
0.86 0.86 FUD XXX Q1 N1 80
AMA: 2018,Jan,8; 2017,Nov,10; 2017,Jan,8; 2016,Jan,13

73592 **lower extremity, infant, minimum of 2 views** A
0.85 0.85 FUD XXX Q1 N1 80
AMA: 2018,Jan,8; 2017,Nov,10

73600 **Radiologic examination, ankle; 2 views**
0.87 0.87 FUD XXX Q1 N1 80
AMA: 2018,Jan,8; 2017,Jan,8; 2016,Jan,13

73610 **complete, minimum of 3 views**
0.98 0.98 FUD XXX Q1 N1 80
AMA: 2018,Jan,8; 2017,Jan,8; 2016,Jan,13

73615 **Radiologic examination, ankle, arthrography, radiological supervision and interpretation**
INCLUDES Fluoroscopic guidance (77002)
3.61 3.61 FUD XXX Q2 N1 80
AMA: 2018,Jan,8; 2017,Jan,8; 2016,Jan,13

73620 **Radiologic examination, foot; 2 views**
0.78 0.78 FUD XXX Q1 N1 80
AMA: 2018,Jan,8; 2017,Jan,8; 2016,Jan,13

73630 **complete, minimum of 3 views**
0.92 0.92 FUD XXX Q1 N1 80
AMA: 2014,Jan,11; 2012,Feb,9-10

73650 **Radiologic examination; calcaneus, minimum of 2 views**
0.79 0.79 FUD XXX Q1 N1 80
AMA: 2014,Jan,11; 2012,Feb,9-10

73660 **toe(s), minimum of 2 views**
0.79 0.79 FUD XXX Q1 N1 80
AMA: 2014,Jan,11; 2012,Feb,9-10

73700-73702 Computerized Tomography: Leg, Ankle, and Foot

CMS: 100-04,4,250.16 Multiple Procedure Payment Reduction: Certain Diagnostic Imaging Procedures Rendered by Physicians

EXCLUDES *3D rendering (76376-76377)*

73700 **Computed tomography, lower extremity; without contrast material**
5.06 5.06 FUD XXX Q3 Z2 80
AMA: 2018,Jan,8; 2017,Jan,8; 2016,Jan,13

73701 **with contrast material(s)**
5.45 5.45 FUD XXX Q3 Z2 80
AMA: 2019,Aug,7; 2018,Jan,8; 2017,Jan,8; 2016,Jan,13

73702 **without contrast material, followed by contrast material(s) and further sections**
6.56 6.56 FUD XXX Q3 Z2 80
AMA: 2019,Aug,7; 2018,Jan,8; 2017,Jan,8; 2016,Jan,13

73706 Computerized Tomographic Angiography: Leg, Ankle, and Foot

CMS: 100-04,4,250.16 Multiple Procedure Payment Reduction: Certain Diagnostic Imaging Procedures Rendered by Physicians

EXCLUDES *CT angiography for aorto-iliofemoral runoff (75635)*
Noninvasive arterial plaque analysis non-coronary computerized tomography angiography (0710T-0713T)

73706 **Computed tomographic angiography, lower extremity, with contrast material(s), including noncontrast images, if performed, and image postprocessing**
10.0 10.0 FUD XXX Q3 Z2 80
AMA: 2018,Jan,8; 2017,Jan,8; 2016,Jan,13

73718-73723 Magnetic Resonance Imaging: Leg, Ankle, and Foot

CMS: 100-04,4,250.16 Multiple Procedure Payment Reduction: Certain Diagnostic Imaging Procedures Rendered by Physicians

73718 **Magnetic resonance (eg, proton) imaging, lower extremity other than joint; without contrast material(s)**
7.25 7.25 FUD XXX Q3 Z2 80
AMA: 2018,Jan,8; 2017,Jan,8; 2016,Jan,13

73719 **with contrast material(s)**
8.58 8.58 FUD XXX Q3 Z2 80
AMA: 2019,Aug,7; 2018,Jan,8; 2017,Jan,8; 2016,Jan,13

73720 **without contrast material(s), followed by contrast material(s) and further sequences**
10.9 10.9 FUD XXX Q3 Z2 80
AMA: 2019,Aug,7; 2018,Jan,8; 2017,Jan,8; 2016,Jan,13

73721 **Magnetic resonance (eg, proton) imaging, any joint of lower extremity; without contrast material**
6.44 6.44 FUD XXX Q3 Z2 80
AMA: 2018,Jan,8; 2017,Jan,8; 2016,Jan,13

73722 **with contrast material(s)**
10.3 10.3 FUD XXX Q3 Z3 80
AMA: 2019,Aug,7; 2018,Jan,8; 2017,Jan,8; 2016,Jan,13

73723 **without contrast material(s), followed by contrast material(s) and further sequences**
12.7 12.7 **FUD** XXX Q3 Z2 80
AMA: 2019,Aug,7; 2018,Jan,8; 2017,Jan,8; 2016,Jan,13

73725 Magnetic Resonance Angiography: Leg, Ankle, and Foot

CMS: 100-04,13,40.1.2 HCPCS Coding Requirements; 100-04,4,250.16 Multiple Procedure Payment Reduction: Certain Diagnostic Imaging Procedures Rendered by Physicians

73725 **Magnetic resonance angiography, lower extremity, with or without contrast material(s)**
10.8 10.8 **FUD** XXX B 80
AMA: 2018,Jan,8; 2017,Jan,8; 2016,Jan,13

74018-74022 Radiography: Abdomen--General

74018 **Radiologic examination, abdomen; 1 view**
0.80 0.80 **FUD** XXX Q1 N1 80
AMA: 2020,Apr,10; 2019,May,10; 2018,Apr,7

74019 **2 views**
1.01 1.01 **FUD** XXX Q1 N1 80
AMA: 2018,Apr,7

74021 **3 or more views**
1.17 1.17 **FUD** XXX Q1 N1 80
AMA: 2018,Apr,7

74022 **Radiologic examination, complete acute abdomen series, including 2 or more views of the abdomen (eg, supine, erect, decubitus), and a single view chest**
1.36 1.36 **FUD** XXX Q1 N1 80
AMA: 2019,May,10; 2018,Apr,7; 2016,Jun,5

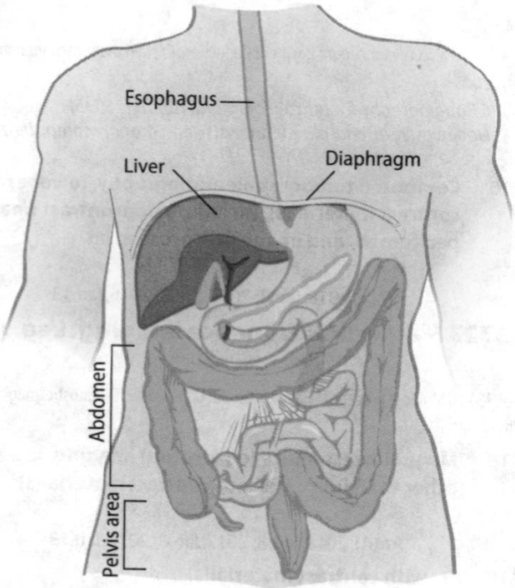

74150-74170 Computerized Tomography: Abdomen–General

CMS: 100-04,4,250.16 Multiple Procedure Payment Reduction: Certain Diagnostic Imaging Procedures Rendered by Physicians

EXCLUDES *3D rendering (76376-76377)*
Combined CT abdomen and pelvis (74176-74178)
CT colonography, diagnostic (74261-74262)
CT colonography, screening (74263)

74150 **Computed tomography, abdomen; without contrast material**
4.20 4.20 **FUD** XXX Q3 Z2 80
AMA: 2020,Sep,11; 2018,Jan,8; 2017,Jan,8; 2016,Jun,5; 2016,Jan,13

74160 **with contrast material(s)**
6.96 6.96 **FUD** XXX Q3 Z2 80
AMA: 2020,Sep,11; 2018,Jan,8; 2017,Jan,8; 2016,Jun,5; 2016,Jan,13

74170 **without contrast material, followed by contrast material(s) and further sections**
7.85 7.85 **FUD** XXX Q3 Z2 80
AMA: 2020,Sep,11; 2018,Jan,8; 2017,Jan,8; 2016,Jun,5; 2016,Jan,13

74174-74175 Computerized Tomographic Angiography: Abdomen and Pelvis

CMS: 100-04,4,250.16 Multiple Procedure Payment Reduction: Certain Diagnostic Imaging Procedures Rendered by Physicians

EXCLUDES *CT angiography for aorto-iliofemoral runoff (75635)*
CT angiography, lower extremity (73706)
CT angiography, pelvis (72191)
Noninvasive arterial plaque analysis non-coronary computerized tomography angiography (0710T-0713T)

74174 **Computed tomographic angiography, abdomen and pelvis, with contrast material(s), including noncontrast images, if performed, and image postprocessing**
EXCLUDES *3D rendering (76376-76377)*
CT angiography abdomen (74175)
11.4 11.4 **FUD** XXX S Z2 80
AMA: 2020,Sep,11

74175 **Computed tomographic angiography, abdomen, with contrast material(s), including noncontrast images, if performed, and image postprocessing**
9.10 9.10 **FUD** XXX Q3 Z2 80
AMA: 2020,Sep,11; 2018,Jan,8; 2017,Jan,8; 2016,Jan,13

74176-74178 Computerized Tomography: Abdomen and Pelvis

CMS: 100-04,4,250.16 Multiple Procedure Payment Reduction: Certain Diagnostic Imaging Procedures Rendered by Physicians

EXCLUDES *CT abdomen or pelvis alone (72192-72194, 74150-74170)*
Procedure performed more than one time for each combined abdomen and pelvis examination

74176 **Computed tomography, abdomen and pelvis; without contrast material**
5.63 5.63 **FUD** XXX Q3 Z3
AMA: 2020,Sep,11; 2018,Jan,8; 2017,Jan,8; 2016,Jan,13

74177 **with contrast material(s)**
9.21 9.21 **FUD** XXX Q3 Z2
AMA: 2020,Sep,11; 2018,Jan,8; 2017,Jan,8; 2016,Jan,13

74178 **without contrast material in one or both body regions, followed by contrast material(s) and further sections in one or both body regions**
10.3 10.3 **FUD** XXX Q3 Z2
AMA: 2020,Sep,11; 2018,Jan,8; 2017,Jan,8; 2016,Jan,13

74181-74183 Magnetic Resonance Imaging: Abdomen–General

CMS: 100-04,4,250.16 Multiple Procedure Payment Reduction: Certain Diagnostic Imaging Procedures Rendered by Physicians

74181 **Magnetic resonance (eg, proton) imaging, abdomen; without contrast material(s)**
6.34 6.34 **FUD** XXX Q3 Z2 80
AMA: 2018,Mar,11; 2018,Jan,8; 2017,Jan,8; 2016,Jan,13

74182 **with contrast material(s)**
9.90 9.90 **FUD** XXX Q3 Z2 80
AMA: 2018,Mar,11; 2018,Jan,8; 2017,Jan,8; 2016,Jan,13

74183 **without contrast material(s), followed by with contrast material(s) and further sequences**
11.0 11.0 **FUD** XXX Q3 Z2 80
AMA: 2018,Mar,11; 2018,Jan,8; 2017,Jan,8; 2016,Jan,13

74185 Magnetic Resonance Angiography: Abdomen–General

CMS: 100-04,13,40.1.1 Magnetic Resonance Angiography; 100-04,13,40.1.2 HCPCS Coding Requirements; 100-04,4,250.16 Multiple Procedure Payment Reduction: Certain Diagnostic Imaging Procedures Rendered by Physicians

74185 **Magnetic resonance angiography, abdomen, with or without contrast material(s)**
10.9 10.9 FUD XXX B 80
AMA: 2018,Jan,8; 2017,Jan,8; 2016,Jan,13

74190 Peritoneography

74190 **Peritoneogram (eg, after injection of air or contrast), radiological supervision and interpretation**
EXCLUDES *CT pelvis or abdomen (72192, 74150)*
Code also injection procedure (49400)
0.00 0.00 FUD XXX Q2 N1 80
AMA: 2018,Jan,8; 2017,Jan,8; 2016,Jan,13

74210-74235 Radiography: Throat and Esophagus

EXCLUDES *Percutaneous placement gastrostomy tube, endoscopic (43246)*
Percutaneous placement gastrostomy tube, fluoroscopic guidance (49440)

74210 **Radiologic examination, pharynx and/or cervical esophagus, including scout neck radiograph(s) and delayed image(s), when performed, contrast (eg, barium) study**
2.66 2.66 FUD XXX Q1 N1 80
AMA: 2020,Aug,9

74220 **Radiologic examination, esophagus, including scout chest radiograph(s) and delayed image(s), when performed; single-contrast (eg, barium) study**
EXCLUDES *Double-contrast study (74221)*
Small bowel follow-through (74248)
Upper GI tract studies (74240-74246)
2.73 2.73 FUD XXX Q1 N1 80
AMA: 2020,Aug,9

74221 **double-contrast (eg, high-density barium and effervescent agent) study**
EXCLUDES *Single-contrast study (74220)*
Small bowel follow-through (74248)
Upper GI tract studies (74240-74246)
3.06 3.06 FUD XXX 80
AMA: 2020,Aug,9

74230 **Radiologic examination, swallowing function, with cineradiography/videoradiography, including scout neck radiograph(s) and delayed image(s), when performed, contrast (eg, barium) study**
EXCLUDES *Swallowing function motion fluoroscopic examination (92611)*
3.64 3.64 FUD XXX Q1 Z2 80
AMA: 2020,Aug,9; 2018,Jan,8; 2017,Jan,8; 2016,Jan,13

74235 **Removal of foreign body(s), esophageal, with use of balloon catheter, radiological supervision and interpretation**
Code also procedure (43499)
0.00 0.00 FUD XXX N N1 80
AMA: 2014,Jan,11; 2012,Feb,9-10

74240-74283 Radiography: Intestines

EXCLUDES *Percutaneous placement gastrostomy tube, endoscopic (43246)*
Percutaneous placement gastrostomy tube, fluoroscopic guidance (49440)

74240 **Radiologic examination, upper gastrointestinal tract, including scout abdominal radiograph(s) and delayed image(s), when performed; single-contrast (eg, barium) study**
INCLUDES Upper GI with KUB
EXCLUDES *Double-contrast study (74246)*
Esophagus studies (74220-74221)
Code also small bowel follow-through when performed (74248)
3.39 3.39 FUD XXX Q1 Z3 80
AMA: 2020,Aug,9; 2018,Jan,8; 2017,Jan,8; 2016,Sep,7

74246 **double-contrast (eg, high-density barium and effervescent agent) study, including glucagon, when administered**
INCLUDES Upper GI with KUB
EXCLUDES *Esophagus studies (74220-74221)*
Single-contrast study (74240)
3.90 3.90 FUD XXX Q1 Z2 80
AMA: 2020,Aug,9; 2018,Jan,8; 2017,Jan,8; 2016,Sep,7

+ **74248** **Radiologic small intestine follow-through study, including multiple serial images (List separately in addition to code for primary procedure for upper GI radiologic examination)**
EXCLUDES *Single- or double-contrast small intestine studies (74250-74251)*
Code first (74240, 74246)
2.32 2.32 FUD ZZZ 80
AMA: 2020,Aug,9

74250 **Radiologic examination, small intestine, including multiple serial images and scout abdominal radiograph(s), when performed; single-contrast (eg, barium) study**
EXCLUDES *Double-contrast study (74251)*
Small bowel follow-through (74248)
3.18 3.18 FUD XXX Q1 Z3 80
AMA: 2020,Aug,9; 2018,Jan,8; 2017,Jan,8; 2016,Sep,7

74251 **double-contrast (eg, high-density barium and air via enteroclysis tube) study, including glucagon, when administered**
EXCLUDES *Single-contrast study (74250)*
Small bowel follow-through (74248)
Code also insertion long gastrointestinal tube (44500, 74340)
11.3 11.3 FUD XXX S Z2 80
AMA: 2020,Aug,9; 2018,Jan,8; 2017,Jan,8; 2016,Sep,7

74261 **Computed tomographic (CT) colonography, diagnostic, including image postprocessing; without contrast material**
EXCLUDES *3D rendering (76376-76377)*
CT abdomen or pelvis alone (72192-72194, 74150-74170)
Screening CT colonography (74263)
13.4 13.4 FUD XXX Q3 Z2 80
AMA: 2020,Sep,11; 2020,Feb,13; 2018,Jan,8; 2017,Jan,8; 2016,Jan,13

74262 **with contrast material(s) including non-contrast images, if performed**
EXCLUDES *3D rendering (76376-76377)*
CT abdomen or pelvis alone (72192-72194, 74150-74170)
Screening CT colonography (74263)
15.1 15.1 FUD XXX Q3 Z2 80
AMA: 2020,Sep,11; 2020,Feb,13; 2018,Jan,8; 2017,Jan,8; 2016,Jan,13

74263 **Computed tomographic (CT) colonography, screening, including image postprocessing**
EXCLUDES *3D rendering (76376-76377)*
CT abdomen or pelvis alone (72192-72194, 74150-74170)
CT colonography (74261-74262)
21.1 21.1 FUD XXX E
AMA: 2020,Sep,11; 2020,Feb,13; 2018,Jan,8; 2017,Jan,8; 2016,Jan,13

74270 **Radiologic examination, colon, including scout abdominal radiograph(s) and delayed image(s), when performed; single-contrast (eg, barium) study**
EXCLUDES *Double-contrast study (74280)*
4.34 4.34 FUD XXX Q1 N1 80
AMA: 2020,Aug,9; 2018,Jan,8; 2017,Jan,8; 2016,Jan,13

74280 **double-contrast (eg, high density barium and air) study, including glucagon, when administered**
EXCLUDES *Single-contrast study (74270)*
6.24 6.24 FUD XXX S N1 80
AMA: 2020,Aug,9

74283   **Therapeutic enema, contrast or air, for reduction of intussusception or other intraluminal obstruction (eg, meconium ileus)**

🔧 7.00   ⚕ 7.00   **FUD** XXX   S Z2 80 💻

AMA: 2014,Jan,11; 2012,Feb,9-10

74290-74330 Radiography: Biliary Tract

74290   **Cholecystography, oral contrast**

🔧 2.15   ⚕ 2.15   **FUD** XXX   Q1 N1 80 💻

AMA: 2014,Jan,11; 2012,Feb,9-10

74300   **Cholangiography and/or pancreatography; intraoperative, radiological supervision and interpretation**

🔧 0.00   ⚕ 0.00   **FUD** XXX   N N1 80 💻

AMA: 2018,Jan,8; 2017,Jan,8; 2016,Jan,13

+   **74301**   **additional set intraoperative, radiological supervision and interpretation (List separately in addition to code for primary procedure)**

Code first (74300)

🔧 0.00   ⚕ 0.00   **FUD** ZZZ   N N1 80 💻

AMA: 2015,Dec,3; 2014,Jan,11

74328   **Endoscopic catheterization of the biliary ductal system, radiological supervision and interpretation**

Code also ERCP (43261-43265, 43274-43278 [43274, 43275, 43276, 43277, 43278])

🔧 0.00   ⚕ 0.00   **FUD** XXX   N N1 80 💻

AMA: 2018,Jan,8; 2017,Jan,8; 2016,Jan,13

74329   **Endoscopic catheterization of the pancreatic ductal system, radiological supervision and interpretation**

Code also ERCP (43261-43265, 43274-43278 [43274, 43275, 43276, 43277, 43278])

🔧 0.00   ⚕ 0.00   **FUD** XXX   N N1 80 💻

AMA: 2014,Jan,11; 2012,Feb,9-10

74330   **Combined endoscopic catheterization of the biliary and pancreatic ductal systems, radiological supervision and interpretation**

Code also ERCP (43261-43265, 43274-43278 [43274, 43275, 43276, 43277, 43278])

🔧 0.00   ⚕ 0.00   **FUD** XXX   N N1 80 💻

AMA: 2014,Jan,11; 2012,Feb,9-10

74340-74363 Radiography: Bilidigestive Intubation

EXCLUDES   *Percutaneous placement gastrostomy tube, endoscopic (43246)*
Percutaneous placement gastrotomy tube, fluoroscopic guidance (49440)

74340   **Introduction of long gastrointestinal tube (eg, Miller-Abbott), including multiple fluoroscopies and images, radiological supervision and interpretation**

Code also placement tube (44500)

🔧 0.00   ⚕ 0.00   **FUD** XXX   N N1 80 💻

AMA: 2020,Aug,9; 2018,Jan,8; 2017,Jan,8; 2016,Sep,9

74355   **Percutaneous placement of enteroclysis tube, radiological supervision and interpretation**

INCLUDES   Fluoroscopic guidance (77002)

🔧 0.00   ⚕ 0.00   **FUD** XXX   N N1 80 💻

AMA: 2018,Jan,8; 2017,Jan,8; 2016,Jan,13

74360   **Intraluminal dilation of strictures and/or obstructions (eg, esophagus), radiological supervision and interpretation**

EXCLUDES   *Esophagogastroduodenoscopy, flexible, transoral; with dilation esophagus (43233)*
Esophagoscopy, flexible, transoral; with dilation esophagus (43213-43214)

🔧 0.00   ⚕ 0.00   **FUD** XXX   N N1 80 💻

AMA: 2018,Jan,8; 2017,Jan,8; 2016,Jan,13

74363   **Percutaneous transhepatic dilation of biliary duct stricture with or without placement of stent, radiological supervision and interpretation**

EXCLUDES   *Surgical procedure (47555-47556)*

🔧 0.00   ⚕ 0.00   **FUD** XXX   N N1 80 💻

AMA: 2014,Jan,11; 2012,Feb,9-10

74400-74775 Radiography: Urogenital

74400   **Urography (pyelography), intravenous, with or without KUB, with or without tomography**

🔧 3.60   ⚕ 3.60   **FUD** XXX   S Z2 80 💻

AMA: 2014,Jan,11; 2012,Feb,9-10

74410   **Urography, infusion, drip technique and/or bolus technique;**

🔧 3.66   ⚕ 3.66   **FUD** XXX   S Z2 80 💻

AMA: 2014,Jan,11; 2012,Feb,9-10

74415   **with nephrotomography**

🔧 4.28   ⚕ 4.28   **FUD** XXX   S Z2 80 💻

AMA: 2014,Jan,11; 2012,Feb,9-10

74420   **Urography, retrograde, with or without KUB**

🔧 2.08   ⚕ 2.08   **FUD** XXX   S Z2 80 💻

AMA: 2018,Jan,8; 2017,Jan,8; 2016,Jan,13

74425   **Urography, antegrade, radiological supervision and interpretation**

EXCLUDES   *Injection for antegrade nephrostogram and/or ureterogram ([50430, 50431, 50432, 50433, 50434, 50435])*
Ureteral stent placement (50693-50695)

Code also aspiration/injection renal cyst or pelvis, percutaneous (50390)

Code also injection procedure:
   ureterography or ureteropyelography (50684)
   visualization ileal conduit/ureteropyelography (50690)

Code also manometric study through nephrostomy or pyelostomy tube (50396)

🔧 3.66   ⚕ 3.66   **FUD** XXX   Q2 N1 80 💻

AMA: 2018,Jan,8; 2017,Jan,8; 2016,Jan,13; 2016,Jan,3

Nephrostomy catheter

Syringe with contrast

Ureter

Bladder

Contrast in urinary system

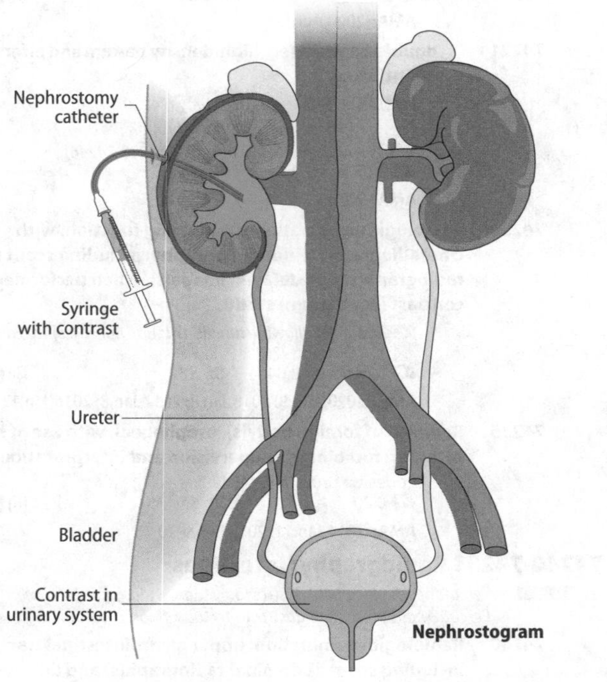

Nephrostogram

74430   **Cystography, minimum of 3 views, radiological supervision and interpretation**

🔧 1.13   ⚕ 1.13   **FUD** XXX   Q2 N1 80 💻

AMA: 2014,Jan,11; 2012,Feb,9-10

74440   **Vasography, vesiculography, or epididymography, radiological supervision and interpretation**   ♂

🔧 2.59   ⚕ 2.59   **FUD** XXX   Q2 N1 80 💻

AMA: 2014,Jan,11; 2012,Feb,9-10

26/TC PC/TC Only   A2-Z3 ASC Payment   50 Bilateral   ♂ Male Only   ♀ Female Only   🔧 Facility RVU   ⚕ Non-Facility RVU   💻 CCI   ✖ CLIA
FUD Follow-up Days   **CMS:** IOM   **AMA:** CPT Asst   A-Y OPPSI   80/80 Surg Assist Allowed / w/Doc   Lab Crosswalk   Radiology Crosswalk

330   CPT © 2021 American Medical Association. All Rights Reserved.   © 2021 Optum360, LLC

74445 Corpora cavernosography, radiological supervision and interpretation ♂

INCLUDES Needle placement with fluoroscopic guidance (77002)

0.00 0.00 FUD XXX Q2 N1 80

AMA: 2018,Jan,8; 2017,Jan,8; 2016,Jan,13

74450 Urethrocystography, retrograde, radiological supervision and interpretation

0.00 0.00 FUD XXX Q2 N1 80

AMA: 2019,Oct,10

74455 Urethrocystography, voiding, radiological supervision and interpretation

2.55 2.55 FUD XXX Q2 N1 80

AMA: 2019,Oct,10

74470 Radiologic examination, renal cyst study, translumbar, contrast visualization, radiological supervision and interpretation

INCLUDES Needle placement with fluoroscopic guidance (77002)

0.00 0.00 FUD XXX Q2 N1 80

AMA: 2018,Jan,8; 2017,Jan,8; 2016,Jan,13

74485 Dilation of ureter(s) or urethra, radiological supervision and interpretation

EXCLUDES *Change pyelostomy/nephrostomy tube ([50435])*
Nephrostomy tract dilation for procedure ([50436, 50437])
Ureter dilation without radiologic guidance (52341, 52344)

3.19 3.19 FUD XXX Q2 N1 80

AMA: 2018,Jan,8; 2017,Jan,8; 2016,Jan,13; 2016,Jan,3

74710 Pelvimetry, with or without placental localization ♀

EXCLUDES *Imaging procedures on abdomen and pelvis (72170-72190, 74018-74019, 74021-74022, 74150-74170)*

1.12 1.12 FUD XXX Q1 N1 80

AMA: 2014,Jan,11; 2012,Feb,9-10

74712 Magnetic resonance (eg, proton) imaging, fetal, including placental and maternal pelvic imaging when performed; single or first gestation ♀

EXCLUDES *Imaging maternal pelvis or placenta without fetal imaging (72195-72197)*

13.3 13.3 FUD XXX S Z2 80

AMA: 2018,Jan,8; 2017,Jan,8; 2016,Jun,5

\+ **74713 each additional gestation (List separately in addition to code for primary procedure)** ♀

EXCLUDES *Imaging maternal pelvis or placenta without fetal imaging (72195-72197)*

Code first (74712)

6.46 6.46 FUD ZZZ N N1 80

AMA: 2018,Jan,8; 2017,Jan,8; 2016,Jun,5

74740 Hysterosalpingography, radiological supervision and interpretation ♀

EXCLUDES *Imaging procedures abdomen and pelvis (72170-72190, 74018-74019, 74021-74022, 74150-74170)*

Code also injection saline/contrast (58340)

2.54 2.54 FUD XXX Q2 N1 80

AMA: 2018,Jan,8; 2017,Jan,8; 2016,Jan,13

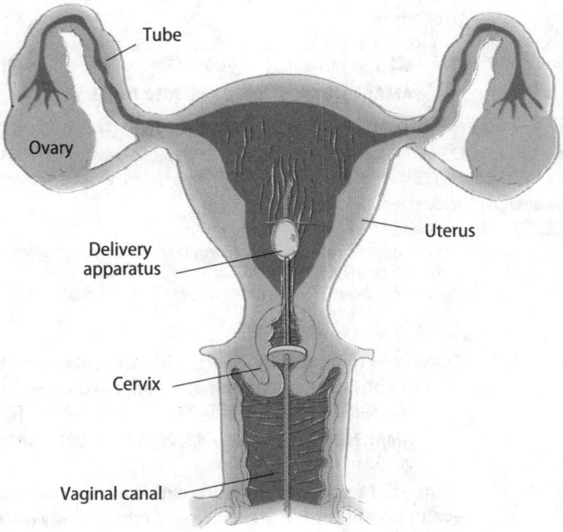

Hysterosalpingography (imaging of the uterus and tubes) is performed. Report for radiological supervision and interpretation

74742 Transcervical catheterization of fallopian tube, radiological supervision and interpretation ♀

EXCLUDES *Imaging procedures abdomen and pelvis (72170-72190, 74018-74019, 74021-74022, 74150-74170)*

Code also transcervical fallopian tube catheter (58345)

0.00 0.00 FUD XXX N N1 80

AMA: 2018,Jan,8; 2017,Jan,8; 2016,Jan,13

74775 Perineogram (eg, vaginogram, for sex determination or extent of anomalies) M ♀

EXCLUDES *Imaging procedures abdomen and pelvis (72170-72190, 74018-74019, 74021-74022, 74150-74170)*

0.00 0.00 FUD XXX S Z2 80

AMA: 2014,Jan,11; 2012,Feb,9-10

75557-75565 Magnetic Resonance Imaging: Heart Structure and Physiology

INCLUDES Physiologic evaluation cardiac function

EXCLUDES *3D rendering (76376-76377)*
Cardiac catheterization procedures (93451-93572)
Reporting more than one code in this group per session

Code also separate vascular injection (36000-36299)

75557 Cardiac magnetic resonance imaging for morphology and function without contrast material;

9.01 9.01 FUD XXX Q3 Z2 80

AMA: 2018,Jan,8; 2017,Jan,8; 2016,Jan,13

75559 with stress imaging

INCLUDES Pharmacologic wall motion stress evaluation without contrast

Code also stress testing when performed (93015-93018)

12.5 12.5 FUD XXX Q3 Z2 80

AMA: 2018,Jan,8; 2017,Jan,8; 2016,Jan,13

75561 Cardiac magnetic resonance imaging for morphology and function without contrast material(s), followed by contrast material(s) and further sequences;

11.8 11.8 FUD XXX Q3 Z2 80

AMA: 2018,Jan,8; 2017,Jan,8; 2016,Jan,13

75563 **with stress imaging**

INCLUDES Pharmacologic perfusion stress evaluation with contrast

Code also stress testing when performed (93015-93018)

14.0 14.0 FUD XXX Q3 Z3 80

AMA: 2018,Jan,8; 2017,Jan,8; 2016,Jan,13

+ **75565** **Cardiac magnetic resonance imaging for velocity flow mapping (List separately in addition to code for primary procedure)**

Code first (75557, 75559, 75561, 75563)

1.51 1.51 FUD ZZZ N N1 80

AMA: 2018,Jan,8; 2017,Jan,8; 2016,Jan,13

75571-75574 Computed Tomographic Imaging: Heart

CMS: 100-04,12,20.4.7 Services Not Meeting National Electrical Manufacturers Association (NEMA) Standard; 100-04,4,20.6.12 Use of HCPCS Modifier – CT; 100-04,4,250.16 Multiple Procedure Payment Reduction: Certain Diagnostic Imaging Procedures Rendered by Physicians

EXCLUDES *3D rendering (76376-76377)*

Automated quantification/characterization coronary atherosclerotic plaque ([0623T, 0624T, 0625T, 0626T])

Fractional flow reserve (FFR) from coronary CT angiography data (0501T-0504T)

Reporting more than one code in this group per session

75571 **Computed tomography, heart, without contrast material, with quantitative evaluation of coronary calcium**

2.95 2.95 FUD XXX Q1 N1 80

AMA: 2020,Sep,11; 2020,Jul,5; 2018,Jan,8; 2017,Jan,8; 2016,Jan,13

75572 **Computed tomography, heart, with contrast material, for evaluation of cardiac structure and morphology (including 3D image postprocessing, assessment of cardiac function, and evaluation of venous structures, if performed)**

INCLUDES Quantitative assessment(s) such as quantification coronary percentage stenosis, ejection fraction, stroke volume, ventricular volume, when performed

7.52 7.52 FUD XXX S Z2 80

AMA: 2020,Sep,11; 2018,Jan,8; 2017,Jan,8; 2016,Jan,13

▲ **75573** **Computed tomography, heart, with contrast material, for evaluation of cardiac structure and morphology in the setting of congenital heart disease (including 3D image postprocessing, assessment of left ventricular [LV] cardiac function, right ventricular [RV] structure and function and evaluation of vascular structures, if performed)**

INCLUDES Quantitative assessment(s) such as quantification coronary percentage stenosis, ejection fraction, stroke volume, ventricular volume, when performed

10.1 10.1 FUD XXX S Z2 80

AMA: 2020,Sep,11; 2018,Jan,8; 2017,Jan,8; 2016,Jan,13

75574 **Computed tomographic angiography, heart, coronary arteries and bypass grafts (when present), with contrast material, including 3D image postprocessing (including evaluation of cardiac structure and morphology, assessment of cardiac function, and evaluation of venous structures, if performed)**

INCLUDES Quantitative assessment(s) such as quantification coronary percentage stenosis, ejection fraction, stroke volume, ventricular volume, when performed

Code also:

Automated data analysis separately from CTA, when performed ([0623T, 0624T, 0625T, 0626T])

Noninvasive estimated coronary fractional flow reserve separately from CTA, when performed (0501T, 0502T, 0503T, 0504T)

10.1 10.1 FUD XXX S Z2 80

AMA: 2020,Sep,11; 2018,Jan,8; 2017,Jan,8; 2016,Jan,13

75600-75774 Radiography: Arterial

INCLUDES Diagnostic angiography specifically included in interventional code description

Diagnostic procedures with interventional supervision and interpretation:

- Angiography
- Contrast injection
- Fluoroscopic guidance for intervention
- Post-angioplasty/atherectomy/stent angiography
- Roadmapping
- Vessel measurement

EXCLUDES *Catheterization codes for diagnostic angiography lower extremity when access site other than site used for therapy required*

Diagnostic angiogram during separate encounter from interventional procedure

Diagnostic angiography with interventional procedure if:

1. No previous catheter-based angiogram accessible and complete diagnostic procedure performed, and decision to proceed with interventional procedure based on diagnostic service, OR

2. Previous diagnostic angiogram accessible but documentation in medical record specifies that:

A. patient's condition has changed

B. insufficient imaging patient's anatomy and/or disease, OR

C. clinical change during procedure that necessitates new examination away from intervention site

3. Modifier 59 appended to code(s) for diagnostic radiological supervision and interpretation service to indicate guidelines were met

Intra-arterial procedures (36100-36248)

Intravenous procedures (36000, 36005-36015)

75600 **Aortography, thoracic, without serialography, radiological supervision and interpretation**

EXCLUDES *Supravalvular aortography (93567)*

5.65 5.65 FUD XXX Q2 N1 80

AMA: 2014,Jan,11; 2012,Feb,9-10

75605 **Aortography, thoracic, by serialography, radiological supervision and interpretation**

EXCLUDES *Supravalvular aortography (93567)*

3.67 3.67 FUD XXX Q2 N1 80

AMA: 2018,Jan,8; 2017,Jan,8; 2016,Jan,13

75625 **Aortography, abdominal, by serialography, radiological supervision and interpretation**

EXCLUDES *Supravalvular aortography (93567)*

3.92 3.92 FUD XXX Q2 N1 80

AMA: 2020,Sep,14; 2018,Jan,8; 2017,Jan,8; 2016,Jan,13

75630 **Aortography, abdominal plus bilateral iliofemoral lower extremity, catheter, by serialography, radiological supervision and interpretation**

EXCLUDES *Supravalvular aortography (93567)*

4.81 4.81 FUD XXX Q2 N1 80

AMA: 2020,Sep,14; 2018,Jan,8; 2017,Jan,8; 2016,Jan,13

75635 **Computed tomographic angiography, abdominal aorta and bilateral iliofemoral lower extremity runoff, with contrast material(s), including noncontrast images, if performed, and image postprocessing**

EXCLUDES *3D rendering (76376-76377)*

CT angiography, abdomen, lower extremity, pelvis (72191, 73706, 74174-74175)

Noninvasive arterial plaque analysis non-coronary computerized tomography angiography (0710T-0713T)

12.4 12.4 FUD XXX Q2 N1 80

AMA: 2020,Sep,11; 2018,Jan,8; 2017,Jan,8; 2016,Jan,13

75705 **Angiography, spinal, selective, radiological supervision and interpretation**

7.13 7.13 FUD XXX Q2 N1 80

AMA: 2014,Jan,11; 2012,Feb,9-10

75710 **Angiography, extremity, unilateral, radiological supervision and interpretation**

4.73 4.73 FUD XXX Q2 N1 80

AMA: 2018,Jan,8; 2017,Mar,3; 2017,Jan,8; 2016,Jan,13

75716 **Angiography, extremity, bilateral, radiological supervision and interpretation**
4.94 4.94 FUD XXX Q2 N1 80
AMA: 2020,Sep,14; 2018,Jan,8; 2017,Jan,8; 2016,Jan,13

75726 **Angiography, visceral, selective or supraselective (with or without flush aortogram), radiological supervision and interpretation**
EXCLUDES *Selective angiography, each additional visceral vessel examined after basic examination (75774)*
4.08 4.08 FUD XXX Q2 N1 80
AMA: 2014,Jan,11; 2012,Feb,9-10

75731 **Angiography, adrenal, unilateral, selective, radiological supervision and interpretation**
4.60 4.60 FUD XXX Q2 Z3 80
AMA: 2014,Jan,11; 2012,Feb,9-10

75733 **Angiography, adrenal, bilateral, selective, radiological supervision and interpretation**
4.97 4.97 FUD XXX Q2 N1 80
AMA: 2014,Jan,11; 2012,Feb,9-10

75736 **Angiography, pelvic, selective or supraselective, radiological supervision and interpretation**
4.25 4.25 FUD XXX Q2 N1 80
AMA: 2014,Jan,11; 2012,Feb,9-10

75741 **Angiography, pulmonary, unilateral, selective, radiological supervision and interpretation**
4.03 4.03 FUD XXX Q2 N1 80
AMA: 2019,Jun,3; 2018,Jan,8; 2017,Jan,8; 2016,Jan,13

75743 **Angiography, pulmonary, bilateral, selective, radiological supervision and interpretation**
4.55 4.55 FUD XXX Q2 N1 80
AMA: 2019,Jun,3; 2018,Jan,8; 2017,Jan,8; 2016,Jan,13

75746 **Angiography, pulmonary, by nonselective catheter or venous injection, radiological supervision and interpretation**
EXCLUDES *Nonselective injection procedure or catheter introduction with cardiac cath (93568)*
4.07 4.07 FUD XXX Q2 Z3 80
AMA: 2019,Jun,3

75756 **Angiography, internal mammary, radiological supervision and interpretation**
EXCLUDES *Internal mammary angiography with cardiac cath (93455, 93457, 93459, 93461, 93564)*
4.62 4.62 FUD XXX Q2 N1 80
AMA: 2018,Jan,8; 2017,Jan,8; 2016,Jan,13

+ **75774** **Angiography, selective, each additional vessel studied after basic examination, radiological supervision and interpretation (List separately in addition to code for primary procedure)**
EXCLUDES *Angiography (75600-75756)*
Cardiac cath procedures (93452-93462, 93563-93568, 93593-93597)
Catheterizations (36215-36248)
Dialysis circuit angiography (current access), report modifier 52 with (36901)
Nonselective catheter placement, thoracic aorta (36221-36228)
Code also diagnostic angiography upper extremities and other vascular beds (except cervicocerebral vessels), when appropriate
Code first initial vessel
3.04 3.04 FUD ZZZ N N1 80
AMA: 2020,Sep,14; 2018,Jan,8; 2017,Jan,8; 2016,Jan,13

75801-75893 Radiography: Lymphatic and Venous

INCLUDES Diagnostic venography specifically included in interventional code description
Diagnostic procedures with interventional supervision and interpretation:
- Contrast injection
- Fluoroscopic guidance for intervention
- Post-angioplasty/venography
- Roadmapping
- Venography
- Vessel measurement

EXCLUDES *Diagnostic venogram during separate encounter from interventional procedure*
Diagnostic venography with interventional procedure if:
1. No previous catheter-based venogram accessible and complete diagnostic procedure performed and decision to proceed with interventional procedure based on diagnostic service, OR
2. Previous diagnostic venogram accessible but documentation in medical record specifies that:
A. patient's condition has changed
B. insufficient imaging patient's anatomy and/or disease, OR
C. clinical change during procedure that necessitates new examination away from intervention site
Intravenous procedures (36000-36015, 36400-36510 [36465, 36466, 36482, 36483])
Lymphatic injection procedures (38790)

75801 **Lymphangiography, extremity only, unilateral, radiological supervision and interpretation**
0.00 0.00 FUD XXX Q2 N1 80
AMA: 2014,Jan,11; 2012,Feb,9-10

75803 **Lymphangiography, extremity only, bilateral, radiological supervision and interpretation**
0.00 0.00 FUD XXX Q2 Z2 80
AMA: 2014,Jan,11; 2012,Feb,9-10

75805 **Lymphangiography, pelvic/abdominal, unilateral, radiological supervision and interpretation**
0.00 0.00 FUD XXX Q2 Z2 80
AMA: 2014,Jan,11; 2012,Feb,9-10

75807 **Lymphangiography, pelvic/abdominal, bilateral, radiological supervision and interpretation**
0.00 0.00 FUD XXX Q2 N1 80
AMA: 2014,Jan,11; 2012,Feb,9-10

75809 **Shuntogram for investigation of previously placed indwelling nonvascular shunt (eg, LeVeen shunt, ventriculoperitoneal shunt, indwelling infusion pump), radiological supervision and interpretation**
Code also surgical procedure (49427, 61070)
2.57 2.57 FUD XXX Q2 N1 80
AMA: 2018,Jan,8; 2017,Jan,8; 2016,Jan,13

75810 **Splenoportography, radiological supervision and interpretation**
0.00 0.00 FUD XXX Q2 Z2 80
AMA: 2018,Jan,8; 2017,Jan,8; 2016,Jan,13

75820 **Venography, extremity, unilateral, radiological supervision and interpretation**
3.04 3.04 FUD XXX Q2 N1 80
AMA: 2019,Mar,6; 2018,Jan,8; 2017,Jan,8; 2016,May,5; 2016,Jan,13

75822 **Venography, extremity, bilateral, radiological supervision and interpretation**
3.56 3.56 FUD XXX Q2 Z3 80
AMA: 2014,Jan,11; 2012,Feb,9-10

75825 **Venography, caval, inferior, with serialography, radiological supervision and interpretation**
3.55 3.55 FUD XXX Q2 N1 80
AMA: 2018,Jan,8; 2017,Feb,14; 2017,Jan,8; 2016,Jan,13

75827 **Venography, caval, superior, with serialography, radiological supervision and interpretation**
3.69 3.69 FUD XXX Q2 N1 80
AMA: 2018,Jan,8; 2017,Jan,8; 2016,Jan,13

75831 **Venography, renal, unilateral, selective, radiological supervision and interpretation**
3.84 3.84 FUD XXX Q2 N1 80
AMA: 2014,Jan,11; 2012,Feb,9-10

75833 **Venography, renal, bilateral, selective, radiological supervision and interpretation**
4.45 4.45 FUD XXX Q2 N1 80
AMA: 2014,Jan,11; 2012,Feb,9-10

75840 **Venography, adrenal, unilateral, selective, radiological supervision and interpretation**
3.97 3.97 FUD XXX Q2 N1 80
AMA: 2014,Jan,11; 2012,Feb,9-10

75842 **Venography, adrenal, bilateral, selective, radiological supervision and interpretation**
4.84 4.84 FUD XXX Q2 N1 80
AMA: 2014,Jan,11; 2012,Feb,9-10

75860 **Venography, venous sinus (eg, petrosal and inferior sagittal) or jugular, catheter, radiological supervision and interpretation**
3.89 3.89 FUD XXX Q2 N1 80
AMA: 2014,Jan,11; 2012,Feb,9-10

75870 **Venography, superior sagittal sinus, radiological supervision and interpretation**
5.30 5.30 FUD XXX Q2 Z3 80
AMA: 2014,Jan,11; 2012,Feb,9-10

75872 **Venography, epidural, radiological supervision and interpretation**
3.97 3.97 FUD XXX Q2 N1 80
AMA: 2014,Jan,11; 2012,Feb,9-10

75880 **Venography, orbital, radiological supervision and interpretation**
3.44 3.44 FUD XXX Q2 N1 80
AMA: 2014,Jan,11; 2012,Feb,9-10

75885 **Percutaneous transhepatic portography with hemodynamic evaluation, radiological supervision and interpretation**
4.29 4.29 FUD XXX Q2 N1 80
AMA: 2018,Jan,8; 2017,Jan,8; 2016,Jan,13

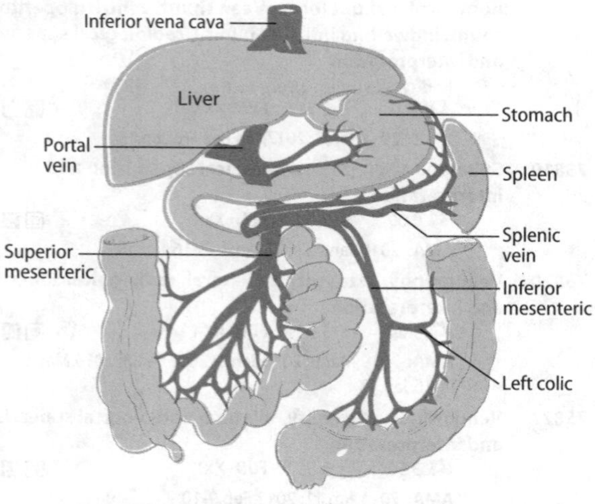

Schematic showing the portal vein

75887 **Percutaneous transhepatic portography without hemodynamic evaluation, radiological supervision and interpretation**
4.24 4.24 FUD XXX Q2 Z3 80
AMA: 2018,Jan,8; 2017,Jan,8; 2016,Jan,13

75889 **Hepatic venography, wedged or free, with hemodynamic evaluation, radiological supervision and interpretation**
3.81 3.81 FUD XXX Q2 N1 80
AMA: 2014,Jan,11; 2012,Feb,9-10

75891 **Hepatic venography, wedged or free, without hemodynamic evaluation, radiological supervision and interpretation**
3.87 3.87 FUD XXX Q2 N1 80
AMA: 2014,Jan,11; 2012,Feb,9-10

75893 **Venous sampling through catheter, with or without angiography (eg, for parathyroid hormone, renin), radiological supervision and interpretation**
Code also surgical procedure (36500)
3.25 3.25 FUD XXX Q2 N1 80
AMA: 2014,Jan,11; 2012,Feb,9-10

75894-75902 Transcatheter Procedures

INCLUDES Diagnostic procedures with interventional supervision and interpretation:
- Angiography/venography
- Completion angiography/venography except for those services allowed by (75898)
- Contrast injection
- Fluoroscopic guidance for intervention
- Roadmapping
- Vessel measurement

EXCLUDES *Diagnostic angiography/venography performed same session as transcatheter therapy unless specifically included in code descriptor or excluded in venography/angiography notes (75600-75893)*

75894 **Transcatheter therapy, embolization, any method, radiological supervision and interpretation**
EXCLUDES *Endovenous ablation therapy incompetent vein (36478-36479)*
Transluminal balloon angioplasty (36475-36476)
Vascular embolization or occlusion (37241-37244)
0.00 0.00 FUD XXX N N1 80
AMA: 2018,Mar,3; 2018,Jan,8; 2017,Jan,8; 2016,Nov,3; 2016,Jan,13

75898 **Angiography through existing catheter for follow-up study for transcatheter therapy, embolization or infusion, other than for thrombolysis**
EXCLUDES *Percutaneous arterial transluminal mechanical thrombectomy (61645)*
Prolonged endovascular intracranial administration pharmacologic agent(s) (61650-61651)
Transcatheter therapy, arterial infusion for thrombolysis (37211-37214)
Vascular embolization or occlusion (37241-37244)
0.00 0.00 FUD XXX Q2 Z2 80
AMA: 2019,Sep,6; 2018,Jan,8; 2017,Jan,8; 2016,Jan,13

75901 **Mechanical removal of pericatheter obstructive material (eg, fibrin sheath) from central venous device via separate venous access, radiologic supervision and interpretation**
EXCLUDES *Venous catheterization (36010-36012)*
Code also surgical procedure (36595)
6.15 6.15 FUD XXX N N1 80
AMA: 2018,Jan,8; 2017,Jan,8; 2016,Jan,13

75902 **Mechanical removal of intraluminal (intracatheter) obstructive material from central venous device through device lumen, radiologic supervision and interpretation**
EXCLUDES *Venous catheterization (36010-36012)*
Code also surgical procedure (36596)
2.40 2.40 FUD XXX N N1 80
AMA: 2018,Jan,8; 2017,Jan,8; 2016,Jan,13

75956-75959 Endovascular Aneurysm Repair

INCLUDES Diagnostic procedures with interventional supervision and interpretation:
- Angiography/venography
- Completion angiography/venography except for those services allowed by (75898)
- Contrast injection
- Fluoroscopic guidance for intervention
- Injection procedure only for transcatheter therapy or biopsy (36100-36299)
- Percutaneous needle biopsy;
  - Pancreas (48102)
  - Retroperitoneal lymph node/mass (49180)
- Roadmapping
- Vessel measurement

EXCLUDES *Diagnostic angiography/venography performed same session as transcatheter therapy unless specifically included in code descriptor (75600-75893)*
Radiological supervision and interpretation for transluminal angioplasty in:
- *Femoral/popliteal arteries (37224-37227)*
- *Iliac artery (37220-37223)*
- *Tibial/peroneal artery (37228-37235)*

75956 Endovascular repair of descending thoracic aorta (eg, aneurysm, pseudoaneurysm, dissection, penetrating ulcer, intramural hematoma, or traumatic disruption); involving coverage of left subclavian artery origin, initial endoprosthesis plus descending thoracic aortic extension(s), if required, to level of celiac artery origin, radiological supervision and interpretation

Code also endovascular graft implantation (33880)
0.00 0.00 FUD XXX C 80
AMA: 2018,Jan,8; 2017,Jan,8; 2016,Jan,13

75957 not involving coverage of left subclavian artery origin, initial endoprosthesis plus descending thoracic aortic extension(s), if required, to level of celiac artery origin, radiological supervision and interpretation

Code also endovascular graft implantation (33881)
0.00 0.00 FUD XXX C 80
AMA: 2018,Jan,8; 2017,Jan,8; 2016,Jan,13

75958 Placement of proximal extension prosthesis for endovascular repair of descending thoracic aorta (eg, aneurysm, pseudoaneurysm, dissection, penetrating ulcer, intramural hematoma, or traumatic disruption), radiological supervision and interpretation

Code also:
- Placement each additional proximal extension(s) (75958)
- Proximal endovascular extension implantation (33883-33884)

0.00 0.00 FUD XXX C 80
AMA: 2018,Jan,8; 2017,Jan,8; 2016,Jan,13

75959 Placement of distal extension prosthesis(s) (delayed) after endovascular repair of descending thoracic aorta, as needed, to level of celiac origin, radiological supervision and interpretation

INCLUDES Corresponding services for placement distal thoracic endovascular extension(s) placed during procedure following principal procedure

EXCLUDES *Endovascular repair descending thoracic aorta (75956-75957)*
Reporting code more than one time no matter how many modules are deployed

Code also placement distal endovascular extension (33886)
0.00 0.00 FUD XXX C 80
AMA: 2018,Jan,8; 2017,Jan,8; 2016,Jan,13

75970 Percutaneous Transluminal Angioplasty

INCLUDES Diagnostic procedures with interventional supervision and interpretation:
- Angiography/venography
- Completion angiography/venography except for those services allowed by (75898)
- Contrast injection
- Fluoroscopic guidance for intervention
- Roadmapping
- Vessel measurement

EXCLUDES *Diagnostic angiography/venography performed same session as transcatheter therapy unless specifically included in code descriptor (75600-75893)*
Injection procedure only for transcatheter therapy or biopsy (36100-36299)
Percutaneous needle biopsy (48102)
Pancreas (48102)
Radiological supervision and interpretation for transluminal balloon angioplasty in:
- *Femoral/popliteal arteries (37224-37227)*
- *Iliac artery (37220-37223)*
- *Tibial/peroneal artery (37228-37235)*

Retroperitoneal lymph node/mass (49180)
Transcatheter renal/ureteral biopsy (52007)

75970 Transcatheter biopsy, radiological supervision and interpretation

0.00 0.00 FUD XXX N N1 80
AMA: 2018,Jan,8

75984-75989 Percutaneous Drainage

75984 Change of percutaneous tube or drainage catheter with contrast monitoring (eg, genitourinary system, abscess), radiological supervision and interpretation

EXCLUDES *Change only nephrostomy/pyelostomy tube ([50435])*
Cholecystostomy, percutaneous (47490)
Introduction procedure only for percutaneous biliary drainage (47531-47544)
Nephrostolithotomy/pyelostolithotomy, percutaneous (50080-50081)
Percutaneous replacement gastrointestinal tube using fluoroscopic guidance (49450-49452)
Removal and/or replacement internal ureteral stent using transurethral approach (50385-50386)

2.79 2.79 FUD XXX N N1 80
AMA: 2014,Jan,11; 2012,Feb,9-10

75989 Radiological guidance (ie, fluoroscopy, ultrasound, or computed tomography), for percutaneous drainage (eg, abscess, specimen collection), with placement of catheter, radiological supervision and interpretation

INCLUDES Imaging guidance

EXCLUDES *Cholecystostomy (47490)*
Image-guided fluid collection drainage by catheter (10030, 49405-49407)
Pericardial drainage (33017-33019)
Thoracentesis (32554-32557)

3.42 3.42 FUD XXX N N1 80
AMA: 2020,Jan,7; 2018,Jan,8; 2017,Jan,8; 2016,Jan,13

76000-76145 Miscellaneous Techniques

EXCLUDES *Arthrography:*
Ankle (73615)
Elbow (73085)
Hip (73525)
Knee (73580)
Shoulder (73040)
Wrist (73115)
CT cerebral perfusion test (0042T)

76000 Fluoroscopy (separate procedure), up to 1 hour physician or other qualified health care professional time

EXCLUDES *Extracorporeal membrane oxygenation (ECMO)/extracorporeal life support (ECLS) (33957-33959, [33962, 33963, 33964])*
Insertion/removal/replacement wireless cardiac stimulator (0515T-0520T)
Insertion/replacement/removal leadless pacemaker ([33274, 33275])

1.18 1.18 **FUD** XXX S Z3 80

AMA: 2019,Sep,10; 2019,Sep,5; 2019,Jun,3; 2019,Mar,6; 2018,Apr,7; 2018,Mar,3; 2018,Jan,8; 2017,Jan,8; 2016,Nov,3; 2016,Aug,5; 2016,May,5; 2016,May,13; 2016,Mar,5; 2016,Jan,11; 2016,Jan,13

76010 Radiologic examination from nose to rectum for foreign body, single view, child A

0.81 0.81 **FUD** XXX Q1 N1 80

AMA: 2018,Jan,8; 2017,Jan,8; 2016,Jan,13

76080 Radiologic examination, abscess, fistula or sinus tract study, radiological supervision and interpretation

EXCLUDES *Contrast injections, radiology evaluation, and guidance via fluoroscopy for gastrostomy, duodenostomy, jejunostomy, gastro-jejunostomy, or cecostomy tube (49465)*

1.67 1.67 **FUD** XXX Q2 N1 80

AMA: 2018,Jan,8; 2017,Jan,8; 2016,Jan,13

76098 Radiological examination, surgical specimen

EXCLUDES *Breast biopsy with placement breast localization device(s) (19081-19086)*
3D volumetric imaging/reconstruction breast or axillary lymph node tissue (0694T)

1.21 1.21 **FUD** XXX Q2 N1 80

AMA: 2012,Feb,9-10; 1997,Nov,1

76100 Radiologic examination, single plane body section (eg, tomography), other than with urography

EXCLUDES *Nephrotomography (74415)*
Panoramic x-ray (70355)

2.75 2.75 **FUD** XXX Q1 N1 80

AMA: 2012,Feb,9-10; 1997,Nov,1

~~**76101 Radiologic examination, complex motion (ie, hypercycloidal) body section (eg, mastoid polytomography), other than with urography; unilateral**~~

~~**76102 bilateral**~~

76120 Cineradiography/videoradiography, except where specifically included

3.06 3.06 **FUD** XXX Q1 N1 80

AMA: 2018,Jan,8; 2017,Jan,8; 2016,Jan,13

\+ **76125 Cineradiography/videoradiography to complement routine examination (List separately in addition to code for primary procedure)**

Code first primary procedure

0.00 0.00 **FUD** ZZZ N N1 80

AMA: 2018,Jan,8; 2017,Jan,8; 2016,Jan,13

76140 Consultation on X-ray examination made elsewhere, written report

0.00 0.00 **FUD** XXX E

AMA: 2018,Jan,8; 2017,Jan,8; 2016,Jan,13

76145 Medical physics dose evaluation for radiation exposure that exceeds institutional review threshold, including report

24.3 24.3 **FUD** XXX Z2 80

76376-76377 Three-dimensional Manipulation

INCLUDES 3D manipulation volumetric data set
Concurrent physician supervision image postprocessing
Rendering image

EXCLUDES *3D echocardiographic imaging/postprocessing during transesophageal echocardiography or transthoracic echocardiography for congenital cardiac anomalies ([93319])*
Anatomic guide 3D-printed and designed from image data set (0561T-0562T)
Anatomic model 3D-printed from image data set (0559T-0560T)
Arthrography:
Ankle (73615)
Elbow (73085)
Hip (73525)
Knee (73580)
Shoulder (73040)
Wrist (73115)
Automated quantification/characterization coronary atherosclerotic plaque ([0623T, 0624T, 0625T, 0626T])
Cardiac MRI (75557, 75559, 75561, 75563, 75565)
Computer-aided detection MRI data for lesion, breast MRI (77046-77049)
CT angiography (70496, 70498, 71275, 72191, 73206, 73706, 74174-74175, 74261-74263, 75571-75574, 75635)
CT breast (0633T-0638T)
CT cerebral perfusion test (0042T)
Digital breast tomosynthesis (77061-77063)
Echocardiography, transesophageal (TEE) for guidance (93355)
Intraprocedural coronary fractional flow reserve (FFR) ([0523T])
Magnetic resonance angiography (70544-70549, 71555, 72159, 72198, 73225, 73725, 74185)
Noninvasive arterial plaque analysis non-coronary computerized tomography angiography (0710T-0713T)
Nuclear radiology procedures (78012-78999 [78429, 78430, 78431, 78432, 78433, 78434, 78804, 78830, 78831, 78832, 78835])
Physician planning patient-specific fenestrated visceral aortic endograft (34839)

Code also base imaging procedure(s)

76376 3D rendering with interpretation and reporting of computed tomography, magnetic resonance imaging, ultrasound, or other tomographic modality with image postprocessing under concurrent supervision; not requiring image postprocessing on an independent workstation

EXCLUDES *3D rendering (76377)*
Bronchoscopy, with computer-assisted, image-guided navigation (31627)

0.65 0.65 **FUD** XXX N N1 80

AMA: 2019,Oct,10; 2019,Sep,10; 2019,Aug,5; 2018,Jul,11; 2018,Jan,8; 2017,Jan,8; 2016,Apr,8; 2016,Jan,13

76377 requiring image postprocessing on an independent workstation

EXCLUDES *3D rendering (76376)*

2.01 2.01 **FUD** XXX N N1 80

AMA: 2019,Oct,10; 2019,Sep,10; 2019,Aug,5; 2018,Jul,11; 2018,Jan,8; 2017,Jan,8; 2016,Apr,8; 2016,Jan,13

76380 Computerized Tomography: Delimited

EXCLUDES *Arthrography:*
Ankle (73615)
Elbow (73085)
Hip (73525)
Knee (73580)
Shoulder (73040)
Wrist (73115)
CT cerebral perfusion test (0042T)

76380 Computed tomography, limited or localized follow-up study

4.07 4.07 **FUD** XXX Q1 N1 80

AMA: 2019,Mar,10; 2018,Jan,8; 2017,Jan,8; 2016,Jan,13

76390-76391 Magnetic Resonance Spectroscopy

EXCLUDES *Arthrography:*
Ankle (73615)
Elbow (73085)
Hip (73525)
Knee (73580)
Shoulder (73040)
Wrist (73115)
CT cerebral perfusion test (0042T)

76390 Magnetic resonance spectroscopy
EXCLUDES *MRI*
MR spectroscopy for discogenic pain (0609T-0610T)
11.9 11.9 FUD XXX E Z2
AMA: 2012,Feb,9-10; 1997,Nov,1

76391 Magnetic resonance (eg, vibration) elastography
6.54 6.54 FUD XXX Z2 80
AMA: 2019,Aug,3

76496-76499 Unlisted Radiology Procedures

76496 Unlisted fluoroscopic procedure (eg, diagnostic, interventional)
0.00 0.00 FUD XXX Q1 N1 80
AMA: 2012,Feb,9-10; 1997,Nov,1

76497 Unlisted computed tomography procedure (eg, diagnostic, interventional)
0.00 0.00 FUD XXX Q1 N1 80
AMA: 2018,Sep,10; 2018,Jan,8; 2017,Jan,8; 2016,Jan,13

76498 Unlisted magnetic resonance procedure (eg, diagnostic, interventional)
0.00 0.00 FUD XXX S Z2 80
AMA: 2019,Aug,5; 2018,Jul,11; 2018,Jan,8; 2017,Jan,8; 2016,Jan,13

76499 Unlisted diagnostic radiographic procedure
0.00 0.00 FUD XXX Q1 N1 80
AMA: 2018,Jan,8; 2017,Jan,8; 2016,Dec,15; 2016,Jul,8; 2016,Jan,13

76506 Ultrasound: Brain

INCLUDES Required permanent documentation ultrasound images except when diagnostic purpose is biometric measurement
Written documentation
EXCLUDES *Noninvasive vascular studies, diagnostic (93880-93990)*
Ultrasound not including thorough assessment organ or site, recorded image, and written report

76506 Echoencephalography, real time with image documentation (gray scale) (for determination of ventricular size, delineation of cerebral contents, and detection of fluid masses or other intracranial abnormalities), including A-mode encephalography as secondary component where indicated
3.25 3.25 FUD XXX Q1 N1 80
AMA: 2018,Jan,8; 2017,Jan,8; 2016,Jan,13

76510-76529 Ultrasound: Eyes

INCLUDES Required permanent documentation ultrasound images except when diagnostic purpose is biometric measurement
Written documentation

76510 Ophthalmic ultrasound, diagnostic; B-scan and quantitative A-scan performed during the same patient encounter
2.56 2.56 FUD XXX Q1 N1 80
AMA: 2018,Jan,8; 2017,Jan,8; 2016,Jan,13

76511 quantitative A-scan only
1.75 1.75 FUD XXX Q1 N1 80
AMA: 2019,Jan,12; 2018,Jan,8; 2017,Jan,8; 2016,Jan,13

76512 B-scan (with or without superimposed non-quantitative A-scan)
1.49 1.49 FUD XXX Q1 N1 80
AMA: 2019,Jan,12; 2018,Jan,8; 2017,Jan,8; 2016,Jan,13

76513 anterior segment ultrasound, immersion (water bath) B-scan or high resolution biomicroscopy, unilateral or bilateral
EXCLUDES *Computerized ophthalmic testing other than by ultrasound (92132-92134)*
2.81 2.81 FUD XXX Q1 N1 80
AMA: 2019,Jan,12; 2018,Jan,8; 2017,Jan,8; 2016,Jan,13

76514 corneal pachymetry, unilateral or bilateral (determination of corneal thickness)
INCLUDES Biometric measurement for which permanent image documentation not required
EXCLUDES *Collagen cross-linking cornea (0402T)*
0.34 0.34 FUD XXX Q1 N1 80
AMA: 2019,Jan,12; 2018,Jan,8; 2017,Jan,8; 2016,Feb,12; 2016,Jan,13

76516 Ophthalmic biometry by ultrasound echography, A-scan;
INCLUDES Biometric measurement for which permanent image documentation not required
1.36 1.36 FUD XXX Q1 N1 80
AMA: 2019,Jan,12; 2018,Jan,8; 2017,Jan,8; 2016,Jan,13

76519 with intraocular lens power calculation
INCLUDES Biometric measurement for which permanent image documentation not required
Written prescription that satisfies requirement for written report
EXCLUDES *Partial coherence interferometry (92136)*
1.88 1.88 FUD XXX Q1 N1 80
AMA: 2019,Jan,12; 2018,Jan,8; 2017,Jan,8; 2016,Jan,13

76529 Ophthalmic ultrasonic foreign body localization
2.35 2.35 FUD XXX Q1 N1 80
AMA: 2019,Jan,12; 2018,Jan,8; 2017,Jan,8; 2016,Jan,13

76536-76800 Ultrasound: Neck, Thorax, Abdomen, and Spine

INCLUDES Required permanent documentation ultrasound images except when diagnostic purpose is biometric measurement
Written documentation
EXCLUDES *Focused ultrasound ablation uterine leiomyomata (0071T-0072T)*
Ultrasound exam not including thorough assessment organ or site, recorded image, and written report

76536 Ultrasound, soft tissues of head and neck (eg, thyroid, parathyroid, parotid), real time with image documentation
3.27 3.27 FUD XXX Q1 N1 80
AMA: 2018,Jan,8; 2017,Oct,9; 2017,Jan,8; 2016,Jan,13

76604 Ultrasound, chest (includes mediastinum), real time with image documentation
2.51 2.51 FUD XXX Q1 N1 80
AMA: 2018,Jan,8; 2017,Oct,9; 2017,Jan,8; 2016,Jan,13

76641 Ultrasound, breast, unilateral, real time with image documentation, including axilla when performed; complete
INCLUDES Complete examination all four quadrants, retroareolar region, and axilla when performed
EXCLUDES *Procedure performed more than one time per breast per session*
3.02 3.02 FUD XXX Q1 N1 80 50
AMA: 2018,Jan,8; 2017,Oct,9; 2017,Jan,8; 2016,Jan,13

76642 limited
INCLUDES Examination not including all complete examination elements
EXCLUDES *Procedure performed more than one time per breast per session*
2.47 2.47 FUD XXX Q1 N1 80 50
AMA: 2018,Jan,8; 2017,Oct,9

Radiology
76390 — 76642

76700 **Ultrasound, abdominal, real time with image documentation; complete**

INCLUDES Real time scans:
- Common bile duct
- Gallbladder
- Inferior vena cava
- Kidneys
- Liver
- Pancreas
- Spleen
- Upper abdominal aorta

3.47 3.47 FUD XXX Q3 Z2 80

AMA: 2018,Jan,8; 2017,Oct,9; 2017,Jan,8; 2016,Jan,13

76705 **limited (eg, single organ, quadrant, follow-up)**

2.57 2.57 FUD XXX Q3 Z2 80

AMA: 2018,Jan,8; 2017,Oct,9; 2017,Jan,8; 2016,Jan,13

76706 **Ultrasound, abdominal aorta, real time with image documentation, screening study for abdominal aortic aneurysm (AAA)**

EXCLUDES *Diagnostic ultrasound aorta (76770-76775)*
Duplex scan aorta (93978-93979)

3.21 3.21 FUD XXX S 80

AMA: 2018,Jan,8; 2017,Sep,11

76770 **Ultrasound, retroperitoneal (eg, renal, aorta, nodes), real time with image documentation; complete**

INCLUDES Complete assessment kidneys and bladder when history indicates urinary pathology
Real time scans:
- Abdominal aorta
- Common iliac artery origins
- Inferior vena cava
- Kidneys

3.19 3.19 FUD XXX Q3 Z2 80

AMA: 2018,Jan,8; 2017,Oct,9; 2017,Jan,8; 2016,Jan,13

76775 **limited**

1.66 1.66 FUD XXX Q1 N1 80

AMA: 2018,Jan,8; 2017,Oct,9; 2017,Jan,8; 2016,Jan,13

76776 **Ultrasound, transplanted kidney, real time and duplex Doppler with image documentation**

EXCLUDES *Abdominal/pelvic/scrotal contents/retroperitoneal duplex scan (93975-93976)*
Transplanted kidney ultrasound without duplex doppler (76775)

4.41 4.41 FUD XXX Q3 Z2 80

AMA: 2018,Jan,8; 2017,Jan,8; 2016,Jan,13

76800 **Ultrasound, spinal canal and contents**

4.04 4.04 FUD XXX Q1 N1 80

AMA: 2018,Jan,8; 2017,Jan,8; 2016,Jan,13

76801-76802 Ultrasound: Pregnancy Less Than 14 Weeks

INCLUDES Determination number gestational sacs and fetuses
Gestational sac/fetal measurement appropriate for gestational age (younger than 14 weeks 0 days)
Inspection maternal uterus and adnexa
Quality analysis amniotic fluid volume/gestational sac shape
Visualization fetal and placental anatomic formation
Written documentation each exam component

EXCLUDES *Focused ultrasound ablation uterine leiomyomata (0071T-0072T)*
Ultrasound exam not including thorough assessment organ or site, recorded image, and written report

76801 **Ultrasound, pregnant uterus, real time with image documentation, fetal and maternal evaluation, first trimester (< 14 weeks 0 days), transabdominal approach; single or first gestation** M ♀

EXCLUDES *Fetal nuchal translucency measurement, first trimester (76813)*

3.45 3.45 FUD XXX S Z2 80

AMA: 2018,Jan,8; 2017,Jan,8; 2016,Jan,13

\+ **76802** **each additional gestation (List separately in addition to code for primary procedure)** M ♀

EXCLUDES *Fetal nuchal translucency measurement, first trimester (76814)*

Code first (76801)

1.78 1.78 FUD ZZZ N N1 80

AMA: 2018,Jan,8; 2017,Jan,8; 2016,Jan,13

76805-76810 Ultrasound: Pregnancy of 14 Weeks or More

INCLUDES Determination number gestational/chorionic sacs and fetuses
Evaluation:
- Amniotic fluid
- Four chambered heart
- Intracranial, spinal, abdominal anatomy
- Placenta location
- Umbilical cord insertion site

Examination maternal adnexa if visible
Gestational sac/fetal measurement appropriate for gestational age (older than or equal to 14 weeks 0 days)
Written documentation each exam component

EXCLUDES *Focused ultrasound ablation uterine leiomyomata (0071T-0072T)*
Ultrasound exam not including thorough assessment organ or site, recorded image, and written report

76805 **Ultrasound, pregnant uterus, real time with image documentation, fetal and maternal evaluation, after first trimester (> or = 14 weeks 0 days), transabdominal approach; single or first gestation** M ♀

3.95 3.95 FUD XXX S Z2 80

AMA: 2018,Jan,8; 2017,Jan,8; 2016,Jan,13

\+ **76810** **each additional gestation (List separately in addition to code for primary procedure)** M ♀

Code first (76805)

2.59 2.59 FUD ZZZ N N1 80

AMA: 2018,Jan,8; 2017,Jan,8; 2016,Jan,13

76811-76812 Ultrasound: Pregnancy, with Additional Studies of Fetus

INCLUDES Determination number gestational/chorionic sacs and fetuses
Evaluation:
- Amniotic fluid
- Examination maternal adnexa if visible
- Focused ultrasound ablation uterine leiomyomata (0071T-0072T)
- Four-chambered heart
- Gestational sac/fetal measurement appropriate for gestational age (older than or equal to 14 weeks 0 days)
- Intracranial, spinal, abdominal anatomy
- Placenta location
- Ultrasound exam not including thorough assessment organ or site, recorded image, and written report
- Umbilical cord insertion site
- Written documentation each exam component

Examination of maternal adnexa if visible
Gestational sac/fetal measurement appropriate for gestational age (older than or equal to 14 weeks 0 days)
Written documentation of each component of exam, including reason for nonvisualization, when applicable

EXCLUDES *Focused ultrasound ablation of uterine leiomyomata (0071T-0072T)*
Ultrasound exam that does not include thorough assessment organ or site, recorded image, and written report

76811 **Ultrasound, pregnant uterus, real time with image documentation, fetal and maternal evaluation plus detailed fetal anatomic examination, transabdominal approach; single or first gestation** M ♀

5.01 5.01 FUD XXX S Z3 80

AMA: 2018,Jan,8; 2017,Jan,8; 2016,Jan,13

\+ **76812** **each additional gestation (List separately in addition to code for primary procedure)** M ♀

Code first (76811)

5.61 5.61 FUD ZZZ N N1 80

AMA: 2018,Jan,8; 2017,Jan,8; 2016,Jan,13

76813-76828 Ultrasound: Other Fetal Evaluations

INCLUDES Required permanent documentation ultrasound images except when diagnostic purpose is biometric measurement
Written documentation

EXCLUDES *Focused ultrasound ablation uterine leiomyomata (0071T-0072T)*
Ultrasound exam not including thorough assessment organ or site, recorded image, and written report

76813 **Ultrasound, pregnant uterus, real time with image documentation, first trimester fetal nuchal translucency measurement, transabdominal or transvaginal approach; single or first gestation** M ♀
3.42 3.42 FUD XXX Q1 N1 80
AMA: 2018,Jan,8; 2017,Jan,8; 2016,Jan,13

\+ **76814** **each additional gestation (List separately in addition to code for primary procedure)** M ♀
Code first (76813)
2.22 2.22 FUD XXX N N1 80
AMA: 2018,Jan,8; 2017,Jan,8; 2016,Jan,13

76815 **Ultrasound, pregnant uterus, real time with image documentation, limited (eg, fetal heart beat, placental location, fetal position and/or qualitative amniotic fluid volume), 1 or more fetuses** M ♀
INCLUDES Exam concentrating on one or more elements
Reporting only one time per exam, not per element
EXCLUDES *Fetal nuchal translucency measurement, first trimester (76813-76814)*
2.37 2.37 FUD XXX Q1 N1 80
AMA: 2018,Jan,8; 2017,Jan,8; 2016,Jan,13

76816 **Ultrasound, pregnant uterus, real time with image documentation, follow-up (eg, re-evaluation of fetal size by measuring standard growth parameters and amniotic fluid volume, re-evaluation of organ system(s) suspected or confirmed to be abnormal on a previous scan), transabdominal approach, per fetus** M ♀
INCLUDES Re-evaluation fetal size, interval growth, or aberrancies noted on prior ultrasound
Code also modifier 59 for examination each additional fetus
3.19 3.19 FUD XXX Q1 N1 80
AMA: 2018,Jan,8; 2017,Jan,8; 2016,Jan,13

76817 **Ultrasound, pregnant uterus, real time with image documentation, transvaginal** M ♀
EXCLUDES *Transvaginal ultrasound, non-obstetrical (76830)*
Code also transabdominal obstetrical ultrasound, when performed
2.73 2.73 FUD XXX Q1 N1 80
AMA: 2018,Jan,8; 2017,Jan,8; 2016,Jan,13

76818 **Fetal biophysical profile; with non-stress testing** M ♀
Code also modifier 59 for each additional fetus
3.44 3.44 FUD XXX S Z2 80
AMA: 2018,Jan,8; 2017,Jan,8; 2016,Jan,13

76819 **without non-stress testing** M ♀
EXCLUDES *Amniotic fluid index without non-stress test (76815)*
Code also modifier 59 for each additional fetus
2.52 2.52 FUD XXX S Z3 80
AMA: 2018,Jan,8; 2017,Jan,8; 2016,Jan,13

76820 **Doppler velocimetry, fetal; umbilical artery** M
1.35 1.35 FUD XXX Q1 N1 80
AMA: 2018,Jan,8; 2017,Jan,8; 2016,Jul,8; 2016,Jan,13

76821 **middle cerebral artery** M
2.61 2.61 FUD XXX Q1 N1 80
AMA: 2018,Jan,8; 2017,Jan,8; 2016,Jan,13

76825 **Echocardiography, fetal, cardiovascular system, real time with image documentation (2D), with or without M-mode recording;** M ♀
7.71 7.71 FUD XXX S Z3 80
AMA: 2018,Jan,8; 2017,Sep,14; 2017,Jan,8; 2016,Jan,13

76826 **follow-up or repeat study** M ♀
4.58 4.58 FUD XXX S Z2 80
AMA: 2018,Jan,8; 2017,Sep,14

76827 **Doppler echocardiography, fetal, pulsed wave and/or continuous wave with spectral display; complete** M ♀
2.07 2.07 FUD XXX Q1 N1 80
AMA: 2018,Jan,8; 2017,Jan,8; 2016,Jan,13

76828 **follow-up or repeat study** M ♀
EXCLUDES *Color mapping (93325)*
1.47 1.47 FUD XXX Q1 N1 80
AMA: 2018,Jan,8; 2017,Jan,8; 2016,Jan,13

76830-76873 Ultrasound: Male and Female Genitalia

INCLUDES Required permanent documentation ultrasound images except when diagnostic purpose is biometric measurement
Written documentation

EXCLUDES *Focused ultrasound ablation uterine leiomyomata (0071T-0072T)*
Ultrasound exam not including thorough assessment organ or site, recorded image, and written report

76830 **Ultrasound, transvaginal** ♀
EXCLUDES *Transvaginal ultrasound, obstetric (76817)*
Code also transabdominal nonobstetrical ultrasound, when performed
3.47 3.47 FUD XXX S Z2 80
AMA: 2018,Jan,8; 2017,Oct,9; 2017,Jan,8; 2016,Jan,13

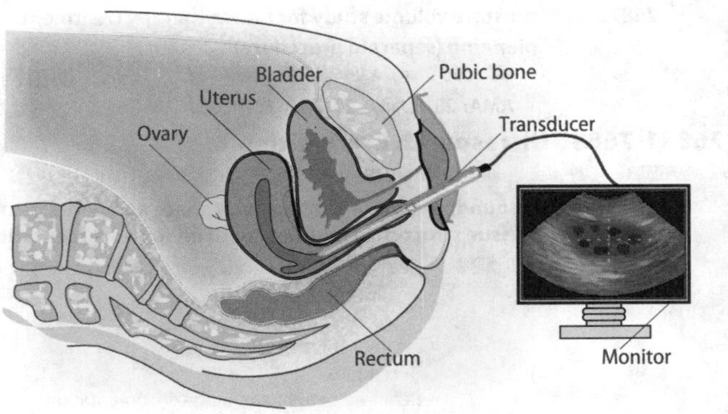

Ultrasound is performed in real time with image documentation by a transvaginal approach

76831 **Saline infusion sonohysterography (SIS), including color flow Doppler, when performed** ♀
Code also saline introduction for saline infusion sonohysterography (58340)
3.36 3.36 FUD XXX Q3 Z3 80
AMA: 2018,Jan,8; 2017,Jan,8; 2016,Jan,13

76856 **Ultrasound, pelvic (nonobstetric), real time with image documentation; complete**
INCLUDES Total examination female pelvic anatomy including:
- Bladder measurement
- Description and measurement uterus and adnexa
- Description any pelvic pathology
- Measurement, endometrium

Total examination male pelvis including:
- Bladder measurement
- Description any pelvic pathology
- Evaluation prostate and seminal vesicles

3.09 3.09 FUD XXX Q3 Z2 80
AMA: 2018,Jan,8; 2017,Oct,9; 2017,Jan,8; 2016,Aug,9; 2016,Jan,13

76857 **limited or follow-up (eg, for follicles)**

INCLUDES Focused evaluation limited to:
- Evaluation one or more elements listed in 76856 and/or
- Re-evaluation one or more pelvic aberrancies noted on prior ultrasound

Urinary bladder alone

EXCLUDES *Bladder volume or post-voided residual measurement without bladder imaging (51798)*
Urinary bladder and kidneys (76770)

1.37 1.37 FUD XXX Q3 Z3 80

AMA: 2018,Jan,8; 2017,Oct,9; 2017,Jan,8; 2016,Jan,13

76870 **Ultrasound, scrotum and contents** ♂

2.96 2.96 FUD XXX Q1 N1 80

AMA: 2018,Jan,8; 2017,Oct,9

76872 **Ultrasound, transrectal;**

EXCLUDES *Colonoscopy (45391-45392)*
Cystourethroscopy with transurethral anterior prostate commissurotomy/drug delivery (0619T)
Hemorrhoidectomy by transanal hemorrhoidal dearterialization ([46948])
Sigmoidoscopy (45341-45342)
Transurethral prostate ablation (0421T)

3.62 3.62 FUD XXX S Z2 80

AMA: 2020,Feb,11; 2018,Nov,10; 2018,Jul,11; 2018,Jan,8; 2017,Oct,9; 2017,Jan,8; 2016,Jan,13

76873 **prostate volume study for brachytherapy treatment planning (separate procedure)** ♂

4.96 4.96 FUD XXX S Z2 80

AMA: 2018,Jan,8; 2017,Jan,8; 2016,Jan,13

76881-76886 Ultrasound: Extremities

EXCLUDES *Doppler studies extremities (93925-93926, 93930-93931, 93970-93971)*

76881 **Ultrasound, complete joint (ie, joint space and peri-articular soft tissue structures) real-time with image documentation**

INCLUDES Real-time scans specific joint including assessment:
- Joint space
- Muscles
- Other soft tissue
- Tendons

Required permanent image documentation
Stress manipulations and dynamic imaging when performed
Written documentation including explanation any joint components not visualized

2.19 2.19 FUD XXX S Z3 80

AMA: 2018,Jan,8; 2017,Oct,9; 2017,Jan,8; 2016,Sep,9

76882 **Ultrasound, limited, joint or other nonvascular extremity structure(s) (eg, joint space, peri-articular tendon[s], muscle[s], nerve[s], other soft tissue structure[s], or soft tissue mass[es]), real-time with image documentation**

INCLUDES Limited joint examination or evaluation due to mass or other abnormality not requiring all complete joint evaluation components (76881)
Real-time scans specific joint including assessment:
- Joint space
- Muscles
- Other soft tissue
- Tendons

Required permanent image documentation
Written documentation including explanation any joint components not visualized

1.62 1.62 FUD XXX Q1 N1 80

AMA: 2018,Jan,8; 2017,Oct,9; 2017,Jan,8; 2016,Sep,9

76885 **Ultrasound, infant hips, real time with imaging documentation; dynamic (requiring physician or other qualified health care professional manipulation)** A

4.05 4.05 FUD XXX Q1 N1 80

AMA: 2012,Feb,9-10; 2002,May,7

76886 **limited, static (not requiring physician or other qualified health care professional manipulation)** A

2.97 2.97 FUD XXX Q1 N1 80

AMA: 2012,Feb,9-10; 2002,May,7

76932-76965 Imaging Guidance: Ultrasound

INCLUDES Required permanent documentation ultrasound images except when diagnostic purpose is biometric measurement
Written documentation

EXCLUDES *Focused ultrasound ablation uterine leiomyomata (0071T-0072T)*
Ultrasound exam not including thorough assessment organ or site, recorded image, and written report

76932 **Ultrasonic guidance for endomyocardial biopsy, imaging supervision and interpretation**

0.00 0.00 FUD YYY N N1 80

AMA: 2012,Feb,9-10; 2001,Sep,4

76936 **Ultrasound guided compression repair of arterial pseudoaneurysm or arteriovenous fistulae (includes diagnostic ultrasound evaluation, compression of lesion and imaging)**

7.60 7.60 FUD XXX S Z2 80

AMA: 2012,Feb,9-10; 2002,May,7

+ **76937** **Ultrasound guidance for vascular access requiring ultrasound evaluation of potential access sites, documentation of selected vessel patency, concurrent realtime ultrasound visualization of vascular needle entry, with permanent recording and reporting (List separately in addition to code for primary procedure)**

INCLUDES Ultrasound guidance, needle placement (76942)

EXCLUDES *Endovascular venous arterialization, tibial or peroneal vein ([0620T])*
Endovenous femoral-popliteal arterial revascularization (0505T)
Extremity venous noninvasive vascular diagnostic study performed separately from venous access guidance (93970-93971)
Insertion or replacement peripherally inserted central venous catheter (36568-36569, [36572, 36573], 36584)
Insertion, removal, or replacement permanent leadless pacemaker ([33274, 33275])
Insertion, removal, or repositioning vena cava filter (37191-37193)
Ligation perforator veins (37760-37761)

Code first primary procedure

1.03 1.03 FUD ZZZ N N1 80

AMA: 2019,May,3; 2019,Mar,6; 2018,Mar,3; 2018,Jan,8; 2017,Dec,3; 2017,Aug,10; 2017,Jul,3; 2017,Mar,3; 2017,Jan,8; 2016,Nov,3; 2016,Jul,6; 2016,Jan,13

76940 **Ultrasound guidance for, and monitoring of, parenchymal tissue ablation**

EXCLUDES *Ablation (20982-20983, [32994], 32998, 47370-47383, 50250, 50542, 50592-50593, 0582T, 0600T-0601T)*
Ultrasound guidance:
- *Intraoperative (76998)*
- *Needle placement (76942)*

0.00 0.00 FUD YYY N N1 80

AMA: 2018,Jan,8; 2017,Nov,8; 2017,Jan,8; 2016,Jan,13

76941 **Ultrasonic guidance for intrauterine fetal transfusion or cordocentesis, imaging supervision and interpretation** M ♀

Code also surgical procedure (36460, 59012)

0.00 0.00 FUD XXX N N1 80

AMA: 2012,Feb,9-10; 2001,Sep,4

76942 **Ultrasonic guidance for needle placement (eg, biopsy, aspiration, injection, localization device), imaging supervision and interpretation**

EXCLUDES *Arthrocentesis (20604, 20606, 20611)*
Autologous WBC injection (0481T)
Breast biopsy with placement localization device(s) (19083)
Core needle biopsy, lung or mediastinum (32408)
Esophagogastroduodenoscopy (43237, 43242)
Esophagoscopy (43232)
Fine needle aspiration biopsy ([10004, 10005, 10006], 10021)
Gastrointestinal endoscopic ultrasound (76975)
Hemorrhoidectomy by transanal hemorrhoidal dearterialization ([46948])
Image-guided fluid collection drainage by catheter (10030)
Injection procedures (27096, 64479-64484, 0232T)
Ligation (37760-37761)
Paravertebral facet joint injections (64490-64491, 64493-64495, 0213T-0218T)
Placement breast localization device(s) (19285)
Sigmoidoscopy (45341-45342)
Thoracentesis (32554-32557)
Transperineal placement, periprostatic biodegradable material (55874)
Transurethral ablation, malignant prostate tissue (0582T)

1.61 1.61 **FUD** XXX N N1 80

AMA: 2020,Jun,10; 2020,Feb,11; 2020,Feb,9; 2020,Jan,7; 2019,Aug,10; 2019,Apr,4; 2019,Feb,8; 2018,Jul,11; 2018,Mar,3; 2018,Jan,8; 2017,Dec,13; 2017,Sep,6; 2017,Jun,10; 2017,Jan,8; 2016,Nov,3; 2016,Jun,3; 2016,Jan,13; 2016,Jan,9

76945 **Ultrasonic guidance for chorionic villus sampling, imaging supervision and interpretation** M ♀

Code also surgical procedure (59015)

0.00 0.00 **FUD** XXX N N1 80

AMA: 2012,Feb,9-10; 2001,Sep,4

76946 **Ultrasonic guidance for amniocentesis, imaging supervision and interpretation** M ♀

0.91 0.91 **FUD** XXX N N1 80

AMA: 2012,Feb,9-10; 2001,Sep,4

76948 **Ultrasonic guidance for aspiration of ova, imaging supervision and interpretation** M ♀

2.15 2.15 **FUD** XXX N N1 80

AMA: 2012,Feb,9-10; 2001,Sep,4

76965 **Ultrasonic guidance for interstitial radioelement application**

2.64 2.64 **FUD** XXX N N1 80

AMA: 2012,Feb,9-10; 1997,Nov,1

76975 Endoscopic Ultrasound

INCLUDES Required permanent documentation ultrasound images except when diagnostic purpose is biometric measurement
Written documentation

EXCLUDES *Focused ultrasound ablation uterine leiomyomata (0071T-0072T)*
Ultrasound exam not including thorough assessment organ or site, recorded image, and written report

76975 **Gastrointestinal endoscopic ultrasound, supervision and interpretation**

INCLUDES Ultrasonic guidance (76942)

EXCLUDES *Colonoscopy (44406-44407, 45391-45392)*
Esophagogastroduodenoscopy (43237-43238, 43240, 43242, 43259)
Esophagoscopy (43231-43232)
Sigmoidoscopy (45341-45342)

0.00 0.00 **FUD** XXX Q2 N1 80

AMA: 2018,Jan,8; 2017,Jan,8; 2016,Jan,13

76977 Bone Density Measurements: Ultrasound

CMS: 100-02,15,80.5.5 Frequency Standards

INCLUDES Required permanent documentation ultrasound images except when diagnostic purpose is biometric measurement
Written documentation

EXCLUDES *Ultrasound exam not including thorough assessment organ or site, recorded image, and written report*

76977 **Ultrasound bone density measurement and interpretation, peripheral site(s), any method**

0.20 0.20 **FUD** XXX S Z3 80

AMA: 2012,Feb,9-10; 1998,Nov,1

76978-76979 Targeted Dynamic Microbubble Sonographic Contrast Characterization: Ultrasound

INCLUDES Intravenous injection (96374)

76978 **Ultrasound, targeted dynamic microbubble sonographic contrast characterization (non-cardiac); initial lesion**

9.21 9.21 **FUD** XXX Z2 80

AMA: 2019,Jun,9

+ **76979** **each additional lesion with separate injection (List separately in addition to code for primary procedure)**

Code first (76978)

6.23 6.23 **FUD** ZZZ N1 80

AMA: 2019,Jun,9

76981-76983 Elastography: Ultrasound

EXCLUDES *Quantitative ultrasound tissue characterization (0689T)*
Shear wave liver elastography (91200)

76981 **Ultrasound, elastography; parenchyma (eg, organ)**

EXCLUDES *Reporting code more than one time each session for same parenchymal organ and/or parenchymal organ and lesion*

3.04 3.04 **FUD** XXX Z2 80

AMA: 2019,Aug,3

76982 **first target lesion**

2.71 2.71 **FUD** XXX Z2 80

AMA: 2019,Aug,3

+ **76983** **each additional target lesion (List separately in addition to code for primary procedure)**

EXCLUDES *Reporting code more than one time each session for same parenchymal organ and/or parenchymal organ and lesion*

Code first (76982)

1.67 1.67 **FUD** ZZZ N1 80

AMA: 2019,Aug,3

76998-76999 Imaging Guidance During Surgery: Ultrasound

INCLUDES Required permanent documentation ultrasound images except when diagnostic purpose is biometric measurement
Written documentation

EXCLUDES *Focused ultrasound ablation uterine leiomyomata (0071T-0072T)*
Ultrasound exam not including thorough assessment organ or site, recorded image, and written report

76998 **Ultrasonic guidance, intraoperative**

EXCLUDES *Ablation (47370-47371, 47380-47382)*
Endovenous ablation therapy incompetent vein (36475, 36479)
Hemorrhoidectomy by transanal hemorrhoidal dearterialization ([46948])
Ligation (37760-37761)
Wireless cardiac stimulator (0515T-0520T)

0.00 0.00 **FUD** XXX N N1 80

AMA: 2020,Feb,11; 2018,Mar,3; 2018,Jan,8; 2017,Apr,7; 2017,Jan,8; 2016,Nov,3; 2016,Jan,13

76999 **Unlisted ultrasound procedure (eg, diagnostic, interventional)**

0.00 0.00 **FUD** XXX Q1 N1 80

AMA: 2019,Dec,8; 2018,Jul,11; 2018,Jan,8; 2017,Jan,8; 2016,Jan,13

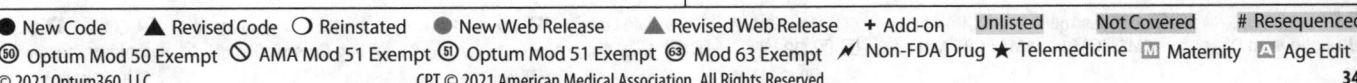

77001-77022 Imaging Guidance Techniques

EXCLUDES *Imaging guidance, breast localization device(s) (19081, 19281, 19283)*

\+ **77001** **Fluoroscopic guidance for central venous access device placement, replacement (catheter only or complete), or removal (includes fluoroscopic guidance for vascular access and catheter manipulation, any necessary contrast injections through access site or catheter with related venography radiologic supervision and interpretation, and radiographic documentation of final catheter position) (List separately in addition to code for primary procedure)**

INCLUDES Fluoroscopic guidance for needle placement (77002)

EXCLUDES *Any procedure codes that include fluoroscopic guidance in code descriptor*
Extracorporeal membrane oxygenation (ECMO)/extracorporeal life support (ECLS) (33957-33959, [33962, 33963, 33964])
Formal extremity venography performed separately from venous access and interpreted separately (36005, 75820, 75822, 75825, 75827)
Insertion peripherally inserted central venous catheter (PICC) (36568-36569, [36572, 36573])
Replacement peripherally inserted central venous catheter (PICC) (36584)

Code first primary procedure

2.71 2.71 **FUD** ZZZ N N1 80

AMA: 2019,May,3; 2018,Jan,8; 2017,Jan,8; 2016,Jan,13

\+ **77002** **Fluoroscopic guidance for needle placement (eg, biopsy, aspiration, injection, localization device) (List separately in addition to code for primary procedure)**

EXCLUDES *Ablation therapy (20982-20983)*
Any procedure codes that include fluoroscopic guidance in code descriptor:
Radiological guidance for percutaneous drainage by catheter (75989)
Transhepatic portography (75885, 75887)
Arthrography procedure(s) (70332, 73040, 73085, 73115, 73525, 73580, 73615)
Biopsy, breast, with placement breast localization device(s) (19081-19086)
Image-guided fluid collection drainage by catheter (10030)
Placement breast localization device(s) (19281-19288)
Platelet rich plasma injection(s) (0232T)
Thoracentesis (32554-32557)

Code first surgical procedure (10160, 20206, 20220, 20225, 20520, 20525-20526, 20550, 20551, 20552, 20553, 20555, 20600, 20605, 20610, 20612, 20615, 21116, 21550, 23350, 24220, 25246, 27093-27095, 27369, 27648, 32400, 32553, 36002, 38220-38222, 38505, 38794, 41019, 42400-42405, 47000-47001, 48102, 49180, 49411, 50200, 50390, 51100-51102, 55700, 55876, 60100, 62268-62269, 64400-64448, 64450, 64455, 64505, 64600-64605)

3.05 3.05 **FUD** ZZZ N N1 80

AMA: 2020,Feb,9; 2020,Jan,7; 2019,Dec,8; 2019,Dec,12; 2019,Aug,7; 2019,Mar,6; 2019,Apr,4; 2019,Feb,8; 2018,Dec,10; 2018,Dec,10; 2018,Jan,8; 2017,Jun,10; 2017,Jan,8; 2016,Sep,9; 2016,Aug,7; 2016,Jun,3; 2016,Jan,9; 2016,Jan,13

\+ **77003** **Fluoroscopic guidance and localization of needle or catheter tip for spine or paraspinous diagnostic or therapeutic injection procedures (epidural or subarachnoid) (List separately in addition to code for primary procedure)**

EXCLUDES *Any procedure codes that include fluoroscopic guidance in code descriptor*
Arthrodesis (22586)
Image-guided fluid collection drainage by catheter (10030)
Injection allogenic cellular and/or tissue-based product, intervertebral disc (0627T-0628T)
Injection medication (subarachnoid/interlaminar epidural) (62320-62327)
Spinal puncture (62270, [62328], 62272, [62329])

Code first (61050-61055, 62267, 62273, 62280-62284, 64449, 64510, 64517, 64520, 64610, 96450)

2.85 2.85 **FUD** ZZZ N N1 80

AMA: 2020,Jun,10; 2019,Dec,8; 2018,Jan,8; 2017,Dec,13; 2017,Sep,6; 2017,Feb,9; 2017,Feb,12; 2017,Jan,8; 2016,Jan,11; 2016,Jan,9; 2016,Jan,13

77011 **Computed tomography guidance for stereotactic localization**

EXCLUDES *Arthrodesis (22586)*

6.57 6.57 **FUD** XXX N N1

AMA: 2018,Jan,8; 2017,Jan,8; 2016,Jan,13

77012 **Computed tomography guidance for needle placement (eg, biopsy, aspiration, injection, localization device), radiological supervision and interpretation**

EXCLUDES *Arthrodesis (22586)*
Autologous white blood cell concentrate (0481T)
Core needle biopsy, lung or mediastinum (32408)
Destruction paravertebral facet joint nerve by neurolysis ([64633, 64634, 64635, 64636])
Fine needle aspiration biopsy using CT guidance ([10009, 10010])
Image-guided fluid collection drainage by catheter (10030)
Injection allogenic cellular and/or tissue-based product, intervertebral disc (0629T-0630T)
Injection, paravertebral facet joint (64490-64495)
Platelet rich plasma injection(s) (0232T)
Sacroiliac joint arthrography (27096)
Spinal puncture (62270, [62328], 62272, [62329])
Thoracentesis (32554-32557)
Transforaminal epidural needle placement/injection (64479-64480, 64483-64484)

4.26 4.26 **FUD** XXX N N1

AMA: 2020,Jun,10; 2020,Jan,7; 2019,Dec,8; 2019,Apr,4; 2019,Feb,8; 2018,Jan,8; 2017,Sep,6; 2017,Feb,12; 2017,Jan,8; 2016,Jun,3; 2016,Jan,13

77013 **Computed tomography guidance for, and monitoring of, parenchymal tissue ablation**

EXCLUDES *Ablation therapy (20982-20983, [32994], 32998, 47382-47383, 50592-50593)*
Ablation, irreversible electroporation (0600T)

0.00 0.00 **FUD** XXX N N1 80

AMA: 2018,Jan,8; 2017,Nov,8; 2017,Jan,8; 2016,Jan,13

77014 **Computed tomography guidance for placement of radiation therapy fields**

Code also placement interstitial device(s) for radiation therapy guidance (31627, 32553, 49411, 55876)

3.45 3.45 **FUD** XXX N N1

AMA: 2018,Jan,8; 2017,Jan,8; 2016,Feb,3; 2016,Jan,13

77021 **Magnetic resonance imaging guidance for needle placement (eg, for biopsy, needle aspiration, injection, or placement of localization device) radiological supervision and interpretation**

EXCLUDES *Autologous white blood cell concentrate (0481T)*
Biopsy, breast, with placement breast localization device(s) (19085)
Core needle biopsy, lung or mediastinum (32408)
Fine needle aspiration biopsy using MR guidance ([10011, 10012])
Image-guided fluid collection drainage by catheter (10030)
Placement breast localization device(s) (19287)
Platelet rich plasma injection(s) (0232T)
Surgical procedure
Thoracentesis (32554-32557)

13.1 13.1 FUD XXX N N1

AMA: 2020,Jun,10; 2020,Feb,9; 2020,Jan,7; 2019,Apr,4; 2019,Feb,8; 2018,Jul,11; 2018,Jan,8; 2017,Jun,10; 2017,Jan,8; 2016,Jun,3; 2016,Jan,13

77022 **Magnetic resonance imaging guidance for, and monitoring of, parenchymal tissue ablation**

EXCLUDES *Ablation:*
Irreversible electroporation (0600T)
Percutaneous radiofrequency ([32994], 32998, 47382-47383, 50592-50593)
Reduction or eradication one or more bone tumors (20982-20983)
Uterine leiomyomata by focused ablation (0071T-0072T)

0.00 0.00 FUD XXX N N1 80

AMA: 2019,Sep,10; 2018,Mar,3; 2018,Jan,8; 2017,Nov,8; 2017,Jan,8; 2016,Nov,3; 2016,Jan,13

77046-77067 Radiography: Breast

77046 **Magnetic resonance imaging, breast, without contrast material; unilateral**

7.02 7.02 FUD XXX Z2 80

AMA: 2019,Aug,5

77047 **bilateral**

7.08 7.08 FUD XXX Z2 80

AMA: 2019,Aug,5

77048 **Magnetic resonance imaging, breast, without and with contrast material(s), including computer-aided detection (CAD real-time lesion detection, characterization and pharmacokinetic analysis), when performed; unilateral**

11.1 11.1 FUD XXX 80

AMA: 2019,Dec,14; 2019,Aug,5

77049 **bilateral**

11.1 11.1 FUD XXX 80

AMA: 2019,Dec,14; 2019,Aug,5

77053 **Mammary ductogram or galactogram, single duct, radiological supervision and interpretation**

Code also injection procedure (19030)

1.60 1.60 FUD XXX Q2 N1

AMA: 2018,Jan,8; 2017,Jan,8; 2016,Jan,13

77054 **Mammary ductogram or galactogram, multiple ducts, radiological supervision and interpretation**

2.07 2.07 FUD XXX Q2 N1

AMA: 2018,Jan,8; 2017,Jan,8; 2016,Jan,13

77061 **Diagnostic digital breast tomosynthesis; unilateral**

EXCLUDES *3D rendering (76376-76377)*
Screening mammography (77067)

0.00 0.00 FUD XXX E

AMA: 2020,Sep,14; 2018,Jan,8

77062 **bilateral**

EXCLUDES *3D rendering (76376-76377)*
Screening mammography (77067)

0.00 0.00 FUD XXX E

AMA: 2020,Sep,14; 2018,Jan,8; 2017,Jan,8; 2016,Dec,15

+ **77063** **Screening digital breast tomosynthesis, bilateral (List separately in addition to code for primary procedure)**

EXCLUDES *3D rendering (76376-76377)*
Diagnostic mammography (77065-77066)

Code first (77067)

1.55 1.55 FUD ZZZ A

AMA: 2020,Sep,14; 2018,Jan,8; 2017,Jan,8; 2016,Dec,15

77065 **Diagnostic mammography, including computer-aided detection (CAD) when performed; unilateral**

3.78 3.78 FUD XXX A 80

AMA: 2020,Sep,14; 2019,Aug,5; 2018,Jan,8; 2017,Jan,8; 2016,Dec,15

77066 **bilateral**

4.76 4.76 FUD XXX A 80

AMA: 2020,Sep,14; 2019,Aug,5; 2018,Jan,8; 2017,Jan,8; 2016,Dec,15

77067 **Screening mammography, bilateral (2-view study of each breast), including computer-aided detection (CAD) when performed**

EXCLUDES *Breast scan, electrical impedance (76499)*

3.86 3.86 FUD XXX A 80

AMA: 2020,Sep,14; 2019,Aug,5; 2018,Jan,8; 2017,Jan,8; 2016,Dec,15

77071-77092 [77085, 77086] Additional Evaluations of Bones and Joints

77071 **Manual application of stress performed by physician or other qualified health care professional for joint radiography, including contralateral joint if indicated**

Code also interpretation stressed images according to anatomical site and number of views

1.50 1.50 FUD XXX Q1 N1 80 26

AMA: 2018,Jan,8; 2017,Jan,8; 2016,Jan,13

77072 **Bone age studies**

0.71 0.71 FUD XXX Q1 N1 80

AMA: 2018,Jan,8; 2017,Jan,8; 2016,Jan,13

77073 **Bone length studies (orthoroentgenogram, scanogram)**

1.24 1.24 FUD XXX Q1 N1 80

AMA: 2018,Jan,8; 2017,Jan,8; 2016,Jan,13

77074 **Radiologic examination, osseous survey; limited (eg, for metastases)**

1.78 1.78 FUD XXX Q1 N1 80

AMA: 2018,Jan,8; 2017,Jan,8; 2016,Jan,13

77075 **complete (axial and appendicular skeleton)**

2.68 2.68 FUD XXX Q1 N1 80

AMA: 2018,Jan,8; 2017,Jan,8; 2016,Jan,13

77076 **Radiologic examination, osseous survey, infant**

2.90 2.90 FUD XXX Q1 N1 80

AMA: 2018,Jan,8; 2017,Jan,8; 2016,Jan,13

77077 **Joint survey, single view, 2 or more joints (specify)**

1.29 1.29 FUD XXX Q1 N1 80

AMA: 2018,Jan,8; 2017,Jan,8; 2016,Jan,13

77078 **Computed tomography, bone mineral density study, 1 or more sites, axial skeleton (eg, hips, pelvis, spine)**

3.22 3.22 FUD XXX S Z2 80

AMA: 2018,Jan,8; 2017,Jan,8; 2016,Jan,13

77080 **Dual-energy X-ray absorptiometry (DXA), bone density study, 1 or more sites; axial skeleton (eg, hips, pelvis, spine)**

EXCLUDES *Dual-energy x-ray absorptiometry (DXA), bone density study ([77085])*
Vertebral fracture assessment via dual-energy x-ray absorptiometry (DXA) ([77086])

1.11 1.11 FUD XXX S Z3 80

AMA: 2018,Jan,8; 2017,Jan,8; 2016,Jan,13

77081 **appendicular skeleton (peripheral) (eg, radius, wrist, heel)**

0.91 0.91 FUD XXX S Z3 80

AMA: 2018,Jan,8; 2017,Jan,8; 2016,Jan,13

\# **77085** **axial skeleton (eg, hips, pelvis, spine), including vertebral fracture assessment**

EXCLUDES *Dual-energy x-ray absorptiometry (DXA), bone density study (77080)*
Vertebral fracture assessment via dual-energy x-ray absorptiometry (DXA) ([77086])

1.50 1.50 FUD XXX Q1 N1 80

\# **77086** **Vertebral fracture assessment via dual-energy X-ray absorptiometry (DXA)**

EXCLUDES *Dual-energy x-ray absorptiometry (DXA), bone density study (77080)*
Therapy performed more than one time for treatment to specific area
Vertebral fracture assessment via dual-energy X-ray absorptiometry (DXA) ([77085])

0.99 0.99 FUD XXX Q1 N1 80

77084 **Magnetic resonance (eg, proton) imaging, bone marrow blood supply**

10.4 10.4 FUD XXX S Z2 80

AMA: 2018,Jan,8; 2017,Jan,8; 2016,Jan,13

77085 **Resequenced code. See code following 77081.**

77086 **Resequenced code. See code before 77084.**

● **77089** **Trabecular bone score (TBS), structural condition of the bone microarchitecture; using dual X-ray absorptiometry (DXA) or other imaging data on gray-scale variogram, calculation, with interpretation and report on fracture-risk**

EXCLUDES *Interpretation and report only by other qualified health care professional (QHCP) (77092)*
Technical calculation only (77091)
Technical preparation and data transmission to be performed elsewhere (77090)

● **77090** **technical preparation and transmission of data for analysis to be performed elsewhere**

EXCLUDES *Trabecular bone score (TBS), complete (77089)*

● **77091** **technical calculation only**

EXCLUDES *Trabecular bone score (TBS), complete (77089)*

● **77092** **interpretation and report on fracture-risk only by other qualified health care professional**

EXCLUDES *Trabecular bone score (TBS), complete (77089)*

77261-77263 Therapeutic Radiology: Treatment Planning

INCLUDES Determination:
- Appropriate treatment devices
- Number and size treatment ports
- Treatment method
- Treatment time/dosage
- Treatment volume

Interpretation special testing
Tumor localization

EXCLUDES *Brachytherapy (0394T-0395T)*
Radiation treatment delivery, superficial (77401)

77261 **Therapeutic radiology treatment planning; simple**

INCLUDES Planning for single treatment area included in single port or simple parallel opposed ports with simple or no blocking

2.03 2.03 FUD XXX B 80 26

AMA: 2018,Jan,8; 2017,Jan,8; 2016,Feb,3; 2016,Jan,13

77262 **intermediate**

INCLUDES Planning for three or more converging ports, two separate treatment sites, multiple blocks, or special time dose constraints

3.06 3.06 FUD XXX B 80 26

AMA: 2018,Jan,8; 2017,Jan,8; 2016,Feb,3; 2016,Jan,13

77263 **complex**

INCLUDES Planning for very complex blocking, custom shielding blocks, tangential ports, special wedges or compensators, three or more separate treatment areas, rotational or special beam considerations, treatment modality combinations

4.78 4.78 FUD XXX B 80 26

AMA: 2018,Jan,8; 2017,Jan,8; 2016,Feb,3; 2016,Jan,13

77280-77299 [77295] Radiation Therapy Simulation

77280 **Therapeutic radiology simulation-aided field setting; simple**

INCLUDES Simulation single treatment site

7.85 7.85 FUD XXX S Z2 80

AMA: 2018,Jan,8; 2017,Jan,8; 2016,Jan,13

77285 **intermediate**

INCLUDES Two different treatment sites

13.1 13.1 FUD XXX S Z2 80

AMA: 2018,Jan,8; 2017,Jan,8; 2016,Jan,13

77290 **complex**

INCLUDES
- Brachytherapy
- Complex blocking
- Contrast material
- Custom shielding blocks
- Hyperthermia probe verification
- Rotation, arc or particle therapy
- Simulation to ≥ 3 treatment sites

14.0 14.0 FUD XXX S Z2 80

AMA: 2018,Jan,8; 2017,Jan,8; 2016,Sep,9; 2016,Jan,13

\+ **77293** **Respiratory motion management simulation (List separately in addition to code for primary procedure)**

Code first (77295, 77301)

12.7 12.7 FUD ZZZ N N1 80

AMA: 2018,Jan,8; 2017,Jan,8; 2016,Jan,13

77295 **Resequenced code. See code before 77300.**

77299 **Unlisted procedure, therapeutic radiology clinical treatment planning**

0.00 0.00 FUD XXX S Z2 80

AMA: 2018,Jan,8; 2017,Jan,8; 2016,Jan,13

77295-77370 [77295] Radiation Physics Services

\# **77295** **3-dimensional radiotherapy plan, including dose-volume histograms**

13.8 13.8 FUD XXX S Z3 80

AMA: 2018,Jan,8; 2017,Jan,8; 2016,Jan,13

77300 **Basic radiation dosimetry calculation, central axis depth dose calculation, TDF, NSD, gap calculation, off axis factor, tissue inhomogeneity factors, calculation of non-ionizing radiation surface and depth dose, as required during course of treatment, only when prescribed by the treating physician**

EXCLUDES *Brachytherapy (77316-77318, 77767-77772, 0394T-0395T)*
Teletherapy plan (77306-77307, 77321)

1.88 1.88 FUD XXX S Z3 80

AMA: 2018,Jan,8; 2017,Jan,8; 2016,Jan,13

77301 **Intensity modulated radiotherapy plan, including dose-volume histograms for target and critical structure partial tolerance specifications**

54.0 54.0 FUD XXX S Z2 80

AMA: 2018,Jan,8; 2017,Jan,8; 2016,Jan,13

77306 **Teletherapy isodose plan; simple (1 or 2 unmodified ports directed to a single area of interest), includes basic dosimetry calculation(s)**

EXCLUDES *Brachytherapy (0394T-0395T)*
Radiation dosimetry calculation (77300)
Radiation treatment delivery (77401)
Therapy performed more than one time for treatment to specific area

4.23 4.23 FUD XXX S Z3 80

AMA: 2018,Jan,8; 2017,Jan,8; 2016,Feb,3

77307 **complex (multiple treatment areas, tangential ports, the use of wedges, blocking, rotational beam, or special beam considerations), includes basic dosimetry calculation(s)**

EXCLUDES *Brachytherapy (0394T-0395T)*
Radiation dosimetry calculation (77300)
Radiation treatment delivery (77401)
Therapy performed more than one time for treatment to specific area

8.20 8.20 **FUD** XXX S Z3 80

AMA: 2018,Jan,8; 2017,Jan,8; 2016,Feb,3

77316 **Brachytherapy isodose plan; simple (calculation[s] made from 1 to 4 sources, or remote afterloading brachytherapy, 1 channel), includes basic dosimetry calculation(s)**

EXCLUDES *Brachytherapy (0394T-0395T)*
Radiation dosimetry calculation (77300)
Radiation treatment delivery (77401)

6.17 6.17 **FUD** XXX S Z3 80

AMA: 2018,Jan,8; 2017,Jan,8; 2016,Feb,3

77317 **intermediate (calculation[s] made from 5 to 10 sources, or remote afterloading brachytherapy, 2-12 channels), includes basic dosimetry calculation(s)**

EXCLUDES *Brachytherapy (0394T-0395T)*
Radiation dosimetry calculation (77300)
Radiation treatment delivery (77401)

8.09 8.09 **FUD** XXX S Z2 80

AMA: 2018,Jan,8; 2017,Jan,8

77318 **complex (calculation[s] made from over 10 sources, or remote afterloading brachytherapy, over 12 channels), includes basic dosimetry calculation(s)**

EXCLUDES *Brachytherapy (0394T-0395T)*
Radiation dosimetry calculation (77300)
Radiation treatment delivery (77401)

11.5 11.5 **FUD** XXX S Z2 80

AMA: 2018,Jan,8; 2017,Jan,8; 2016,Feb,3

77321 **Special teletherapy port plan, particles, hemibody, total body**

2.68 2.68 **FUD** XXX S Z3 80

AMA: 2018,Jan,8; 2017,Jan,8; 2016,Jan,13

77331 **Special dosimetry (eg, TLD, microdosimetry) (specify), only when prescribed by the treating physician**

1.84 1.84 **FUD** XXX S Z3 80

AMA: 2018,Jan,8; 2017,Jan,8; 2016,Jan,13

77332 **Treatment devices, design and construction; simple (simple block, simple bolus)**

EXCLUDES *Brachytherapy (0394T-0395T)*
Radiation treatment delivery (77401)

1.34 1.34 **FUD** XXX S Z3 80

AMA: 2018,Jan,8; 2017,Jan,8; 2016,Feb,3; 2016,Jan,13

77333 **intermediate (multiple blocks, stents, bite blocks, special bolus)**

EXCLUDES *Brachytherapy (0394T-0395T)*
Radiation treatment delivery (77401)

3.41 3.41 **FUD** XXX S Z2 80

AMA: 2018,Jan,8; 2017,Jan,8; 2016,Feb,3; 2016,Jan,13

77334 **complex (irregular blocks, special shields, compensators, wedges, molds or casts)**

EXCLUDES *Brachytherapy (0394T-0395T)*
Radiation treatment delivery (77401)

3.61 3.61 **FUD** XXX S Z3 80

AMA: 2018,Jan,8; 2017,Jan,8; 2016,Sep,9; 2016,Feb,3; 2016,Jan,13

77336 **Continuing medical physics consultation, including assessment of treatment parameters, quality assurance of dose delivery, and review of patient treatment documentation in support of the radiation oncologist, reported per week of therapy**

EXCLUDES *Brachytherapy (0394T-0395T)*
Radiation treatment delivery (77401)

2.26 2.26 **FUD** XXX S Z2 80 TC

AMA: 2018,Jan,8; 2017,Jan,8; 2016,Feb,3; 2016,Jan,13

77338 **Multi-leaf collimator (MLC) device(s) for intensity modulated radiation therapy (IMRT), design and construction per IMRT plan**

EXCLUDES *Immobilization in IMRT treatment (77332-77334)*
Intensity modulated radiation treatment delivery (IMRT) (77385)
Reporting code more than one time per IMRT plan

14.1 14.1 **FUD** XXX S Z2 80

AMA: 2018,Jan,8; 2017,Jan,8; 2016,Jan,13

77370 **Special medical radiation physics consultation**

3.52 3.52 **FUD** XXX S Z2 80 TC

AMA: 2018,Jan,8; 2017,Jan,8; 2016,Feb,3; 2016,Jan,13

77371-77399 [77385, 77386, 77387] Stereotactic Radiosurgery (SRS) Planning and Delivery

77371 **Radiation treatment delivery, stereotactic radiosurgery (SRS), complete course of treatment of cranial lesion(s) consisting of 1 session; multi-source Cobalt 60 based**

EXCLUDES *Guidance with computed tomography for radiation therapy field placement (77014)*

0.00 0.00 **FUD** XXX J 80 TC

AMA: 2018,Jan,8; 2017,Jan,8; 2016,Jan,13

77372 **linear accelerator based**

EXCLUDES *Guidance with computed tomography for radiation therapy field placement (77014)*
Radiation treatment supervision (77432)

30.2 30.2 **FUD** XXX J 80 TC

AMA: 2018,Jan,8; 2017,Jan,8; 2016,Jan,13

77373 **Stereotactic body radiation therapy, treatment delivery, per fraction to 1 or more lesions, including image guidance, entire course not to exceed 5 fractions**

EXCLUDES *Guidance with computed tomography for radiation therapy field placement (77014)*
Intensity modulated radiation treatment delivery (IMRT) (77385-77386)
Radiation treatment delivery (77401-77402, 77407, 77412)
Single fraction cranial lesion(s) (77371-77372)

36.6 36.6 **FUD** XXX S 80 TC

AMA: 2018,Jan,8; 2017,Jan,8; 2016,Jan,13

77385 **Resequenced code. See code following 77417.**

77386 **Resequenced code. See code following 77417.**

77387 **Resequenced code. See code following 77417.**

77399 **Unlisted procedure, medical radiation physics, dosimetry and treatment devices, and special services**

0.00 0.00 **FUD** XXX S Z2 80

AMA: 2018,Jan,8; 2017,Jan,8; 2016,Jan,13

77401-77425 [77385, 77386, 77387, 77424, 77425] Radiation Treatment

INCLUDES Technical component and assorted energy levels

77401 Radiation treatment delivery, superficial and/or ortho voltage, per day

EXCLUDES *Continuing medical physics consultation (77336)*
Isodose plan:
Brachytherapy (77316-77318)
Teletherapy (77306-77307)
Management:
Intraoperative radiation treatment (77469-77470)
Radiation therapy (77431-77432)
Radiation treatment (77427)
Stereotactic body radiation therapy (77435)
Stereotactic body radiation therapy, treatment delivery (77373)
Unlisted procedure, therapeutic radiology treatment management (77499)
Therapeutic radiology treatment planning (77261-77263)
Treatment devices, design and construction (77332-77334)

Code also E/M services when performed alone, as appropriate
0.70 0.70 FUD XXX S Z3 80 TC
AMA: 2018,Jan,8; 2017,Jan,8; 2016,Feb,3; 2016,Jan,13

77402 Radiation treatment delivery, ≥1 MeV; simple

EXCLUDES *Stereotactic body radiation therapy, treatment delivery (77373)*
0.00 0.00 FUD XXX S Z2 80 TC
AMA: 2018,Jan,8; 2017,Jan,8; 2016,Jun,9; 2016,Mar,7; 2016,Feb,3; 2016,Jan,13

77407 intermediate

EXCLUDES *Stereotactic body radiation therapy, treatment delivery (77373)*
0.00 0.00 FUD XXX S Z2 80 TC
AMA: 2018,Jan,8; 2017,Jan,8; 2016,Jun,9; 2016,Mar,7; 2016,Feb,3; 2016,Jan,13

77412 complex

0.00 0.00 FUD XXX S Z2 80 TC
AMA: 2018,Jan,8; 2017,Jan,8; 2016,Jun,9; 2016,Mar,7; 2016,Feb,3; 2016,Jan,13

77417 Therapeutic radiology port image(s)

0.32 0.32 FUD XXX N N1 80 TC
AMA: 2018,Jan,8; 2017,Dec,14; 2017,Jan,8; 2016,Jan,13

\# **77385 Intensity modulated radiation treatment delivery (IMRT), includes guidance and tracking, when performed; simple**

0.00 0.00 FUD XXX S Z2 80 TC
AMA: 2018,Jan,8; 2017,Jan,8; 2016,Feb,3

\# **77386 complex**

0.00 0.00 FUD XXX S Z2 80 TC
AMA: 2018,Jan,8; 2017,Jan,8; 2016,Feb,3

\# **77387 Guidance for localization of target volume for delivery of radiation treatment, includes intrafraction tracking, when performed**

0.00 0.00 FUD XXX N N1 80
AMA: 2018,Jan,8; 2017,Jan,8; 2016,Feb,3; 2016,Jan,13

\# **77424 Intraoperative radiation treatment delivery, x-ray, single treatment session**

0.00 0.00 FUD XXX J Z2
AMA: 2018,Jan,8; 2017,Jan,8; 2016,Jan,13

\# **77425 Intraoperative radiation treatment delivery, electrons, single treatment session**

0.00 0.00 FUD XXX J Z2
AMA: 2018,Jan,8; 2017,Jan,8; 2016,Jan,13

77423-77425 [77424, 77425] Neutron Therapy

77423 High energy neutron radiation treatment delivery, 1 or more isocenter(s) with coplanar or non-coplanar geometry with blocking and/or wedge, and/or compensator(s)

0.00 0.00 FUD XXX S Z3 80 TC
AMA: 2018,Jan,8; 2017,Jan,8; 2016,Jan,13

77424 Resequenced code. See code following 77417.

77425 Resequenced code. See code following 77417.

77427-77499 Radiation Therapy Management

INCLUDES Assessment patient for medical evaluation and management (at least one per treatment management service) including:
Coordination care/treatment
Evaluation patient's response to treatment
Review:
Dose delivery
Dosimetry
Lab tests
Patient treatment set-up
Port film
Treatment parameters
X-rays
Five fractions or treatment sessions regardless of time. Two or more fractions performed same day can be reported separately provided a distinct break in service exists between sessions and fractions are usually furnished on different days

EXCLUDES *High dose rate electronic brachytherapy (0394T-0395T)*
Radiation treatment delivery (77401)

77427 Radiation treatment management, 5 treatments

5.44 5.44 FUD XXX B 26
AMA: 2018,Jan,8; 2017,Jan,8; 2016,Feb,3; 2016,Jan,13

77431 Radiation therapy management with complete course of therapy consisting of 1 or 2 fractions only

2.96 2.96 FUD XXX B 80 26
AMA: 2018,Jan,8; 2017,Jan,8; 2016,Feb,3; 2016,Jan,13

77432 Stereotactic radiation treatment management of cranial lesion(s) (complete course of treatment consisting of 1 session)

12.1 12.1 FUD XXX B 80 26
AMA: 2018,Jan,8; 2017,Jan,8; 2016,Feb,3; 2016,Jan,13

77435 Stereotactic body radiation therapy, treatment management, per treatment course, to 1 or more lesions, including image guidance, entire course not to exceed 5 fractions

18.1 18.1 FUD XXX N N1 80 26
AMA: 2018,Jan,8; 2017,Jan,8; 2016,Feb,3; 2016,Jan,13

77469 Intraoperative radiation treatment management

9.00 9.00 FUD XXX B 80
AMA: 2018,Jan,8; 2017,Jan,8; 2016,Feb,3

77470 Special treatment procedure (eg, total body irradiation, hemibody radiation, per oral or endocavitary irradiation)

3.79 3.79 FUD XXX S Z3 80
AMA: 2018,Jan,8; 2017,Jan,8; 2016,Feb,3; 2016,Jan,13

77499 Unlisted procedure, therapeutic radiology treatment management

0.00 0.00 FUD XXX B 80
AMA: 2018,Jan,8; 2017,Jan,8; 2016,Feb,3; 2016,Jan,13

77520-77525 Proton Therapy

EXCLUDES *High dose rate electronic brachytherapy, per fraction (0394T-0395T)*

77520 Proton treatment delivery; simple, without compensation

0.00 0.00 FUD XXX S Z2 80 TC
AMA: 2018,Jan,8; 2017,Jan,8; 2016,Jan,13

77522 simple, with compensation

0.00 0.00 FUD XXX S Z2 80 TC
AMA: 2012,Feb,9-10; 2010,Oct,3-4

77523 intermediate

0.00 0.00 FUD XXX S Z2 80 TC
AMA: 2018,Jan,8; 2017,Jan,8; 2016,Jan,13

77525 **complex**
0.00 0.00 **FUD** XXX S Z2 80 TC
AMA: 2012,Feb,9-10; 2010,Oct,3-4

77600-77620 Hyperthermia Treatment

CMS: 100-03,110.1 Hyperthermia for Treatment of Cancer

INCLUDES Heat generating devices
Interstitial insertion temperature sensors
Management during course therapy
Normal follow-up care for three months after completion
Physics planning

EXCLUDES *Initial E/M service*
Radiation therapy treatment (77371-77373, 77401-77412, 77423)

77600 **Hyperthermia, externally generated; superficial (ie, heating to a depth of 4 cm or less)**
12.7 12.7 **FUD** XXX S Z2 80
AMA: 2018,Jan,8; 2017,Jan,8; 2016,Jan,13

77605 **deep (ie, heating to depths greater than 4 cm)**
22.0 22.0 **FUD** XXX S Z2 80
AMA: 2018,Jan,8; 2017,Jan,8; 2016,Jan,13

77610 **Hyperthermia generated by interstitial probe(s); 5 or fewer interstitial applicators**
19.2 19.2 **FUD** XXX S Z2 80
AMA: 2018,Jan,8; 2017,Jan,8; 2016,Jan,13

77615 **more than 5 interstitial applicators**
30.1 30.1 **FUD** XXX S Z2 80
AMA: 2018,Jan,8; 2017,Jan,8; 2016,Jan,13

77620 **Hyperthermia generated by intracavitary probe(s)**
17.3 17.3 **FUD** XXX S Z2 80
AMA: 2018,Jan,8; 2017,Jan,8; 2016,Jan,13

77750-77799 Brachytherapy

CMS: 100-04,13,70.4 Clinical Brachytherapy; 100-04,13,70.5 Radiation Physics Services; 100-04,4,61.4.4 Billing for Brachytherapy Source Supervision, Handling and Loading Costs

INCLUDES Hospital admission and daily visits

EXCLUDES *Placement:*
Heyman capsules (58346)
Ovoids and tandems (57155)

77750 **Infusion or instillation of radioelement solution (includes 3-month follow-up care)**
10.9 10.9 **FUD** 090 S Z2 80
AMA: 2018,Jan,8; 2017,Jan,8; 2016,Jan,13

77761 **Intracavitary radiation source application; simple**
11.4 11.4 **FUD** 090 S Z3 80
AMA: 2018,Jan,8; 2017,Jan,8; 2016,Jan,13

77762 **intermediate**
15.1 15.1 **FUD** 090 S Z3 80
AMA: 2018,Jan,8; 2017,Jan,8; 2016,Jan,13

77763 **complex**
21.4 21.4 **FUD** 090 S Z3 80
AMA: 2018,Jan,8; 2017,Jan,8; 2016,Jan,13

77767 **Remote afterloading high dose rate radionuclide skin surface brachytherapy, includes basic dosimetry, when performed; lesion diameter up to 2.0 cm or 1 channel**
6.78 6.78 **FUD** XXX S Z2 80

77768 **lesion diameter over 2.0 cm and 2 or more channels, or multiple lesions**
10.1 10.1 **FUD** XXX S Z2 80

77770 **Remote afterloading high dose rate radionuclide interstitial or intracavitary brachytherapy, includes basic dosimetry, when performed; 1 channel**
9.51 9.51 **FUD** XXX S Z3 80

77771 **2-12 channels**
16.9 16.9 **FUD** XXX S Z2 80

77772 **over 12 channels**
25.5 25.5 **FUD** XXX S Z2 80

77778 **Interstitial radiation source application, complex, includes supervision, handling, loading of radiation source, when performed**
24.5 24.5 **FUD** 000 S Z2 80
AMA: 2018,Jan,8; 2017,Jan,8; 2016,Jan,13

77789 **Surface application of low dose rate radionuclide source**
3.63 3.63 **FUD** 000 S Z2 80
AMA: 2018,Jan,8; 2017,Jan,8; 2016,Jan,13

77790 **Supervision, handling, loading of radiation source**
0.43 0.43 **FUD** XXX N N1 80 TC
AMA: 2018,Jan,8; 2017,Jan,8; 2016,Jan,13

77799 **Unlisted procedure, clinical brachytherapy**
0.00 0.00 **FUD** XXX S Z2 80
AMA: 2018,Jan,8; 2017,Jan,8; 2016,Jan,13

78012-78099 Nuclear Radiology: Thyroid, Parathyroid, Adrenal

EXCLUDES *Diagnostic services (see appropriate sections)*
Follow-up care (see appropriate section)

Code also radiopharmaceutical(s) and/or drug(s) supplied

78012 **Thyroid uptake, single or multiple quantitative measurement(s) (including stimulation, suppression, or discharge, when performed)**
2.34 2.34 **FUD** XXX S Z2 80
AMA: 2018,Jan,8; 2017,Jan,8; 2016,Jan,13

78013 **Thyroid imaging (including vascular flow, when performed);**
5.54 5.54 **FUD** XXX S Z2 80
AMA: 2018,Jan,8; 2017,Jan,8; 2016,Jan,13

78014 **with single or multiple uptake(s) quantitative measurement(s) (including stimulation, suppression, or discharge, when performed)**
6.86 6.86 **FUD** XXX S Z2 80
AMA: 2018,Jan,8; 2017,Jan,8; 2016,Jan,13

78015 **Thyroid carcinoma metastases imaging; limited area (eg, neck and chest only)**
6.43 6.43 **FUD** XXX S Z2 80
AMA: 2018,Jan,8; 2017,Jan,8; 2016,Jan,13

78016 **with additional studies (eg, urinary recovery)**
8.12 8.12 **FUD** XXX S Z2 80
AMA: 2018,Jan,8; 2017,Jan,8; 2016,Jan,13

78018 **whole body**
8.96 8.96 **FUD** XXX S Z2 80
AMA: 2018,Jan,8; 2017,Jan,8; 2016,Jan,13

+ 78020 **Thyroid carcinoma metastases uptake (List separately in addition to code for primary procedure)**
Code first (78018)
2.37 2.37 **FUD** ZZZ N N1 80
AMA: 2018,Jan,8; 2017,Jan,8; 2016,Jan,13

78070 **Parathyroid planar imaging (including subtraction, when performed);**
EXCLUDES *Distribution radiopharmaceutical agents or tumor localization (78800-78802, [78804], 78803)*
Radiopharmaceutical quantification measurements ([78835])
SPECT with concurrently acquired CT transmission scan ([78830, 78831, 78832])
8.48 8.48 **FUD** XXX S Z2 80
AMA: 2020,Oct,3; 2018,Jan,8; 2017,Jan,8; 2016,Dec,9; 2016,Dec,16; 2016,Jan,13

78071 **with tomographic (SPECT)**
EXCLUDES *Distribution radiopharmaceutical agents or tumor localization (78800-78802, [78804], 78803)*
Radiopharmaceutical quantification measurements ([78835])
SPECT with concurrently acquired CT transmission scan ([78830, 78831, 78832])
10.1 10.1 **FUD** XXX S Z2 80
AMA: 2020,Oct,3; 2018,Jan,8; 2017,Jan,8; 2016,Dec,16; 2016,Dec,9

78072 **with tomographic (SPECT), and concurrently acquired computed tomography (CT) for anatomical localization**
EXCLUDES *Distribution radiopharmaceutical agents or tumor localization (78800-78802, [78804], 78803)*
Radiopharmaceutical quantification measurements ([78835])
SPECT with concurrently acquired CT transmission scan ([78830, 78831, 78832])
12.7 12.7 **FUD** XXX S Z2 80
AMA: 2020,Oct,3; 2018,Jan,8; 2017,Jan,8; 2016,Dec,16; 2016,Dec,9

78075 **Adrenal imaging, cortex and/or medulla**
13.0 13.0 **FUD** XXX S Z2 80
AMA: 2018,Jan,8; 2017,Jan,8; 2016,Jan,13

78099 **Unlisted endocrine procedure, diagnostic nuclear medicine**
0.00 0.00 **FUD** XXX S Z2 80
AMA: 2018,Jan,8; 2017,Jan,8; 2016,Dec,9; 2016,Jan,13

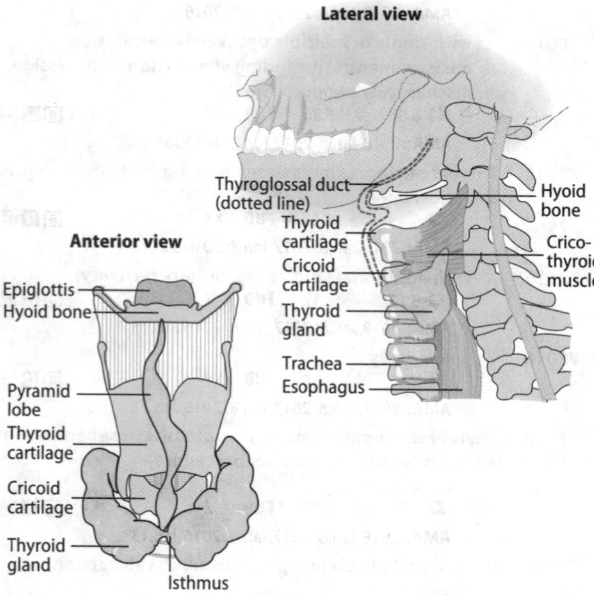

78102-78199 Nuclear Radiology: Blood Forming Organs

EXCLUDES *Diagnostic services (see appropriate sections)*
Follow-up care (see appropriate section)
Radioimmunoassays (82009-84999 [82042, 82652])
Code also radiopharmaceutical(s) and/or drug(s) supplied

78102 **Bone marrow imaging; limited area**
4.89 4.89 **FUD** XXX S Z2 80
AMA: 2018,Jan,8; 2017,Jan,8; 2016,Jan,13

78103 **multiple areas**
6.27 6.27 **FUD** XXX S Z2 80
AMA: 2012,Feb,9-10; 2007,Jan,28-31

78104 **whole body**
7.14 7.14 **FUD** XXX S Z2 80
AMA: 2012,Feb,9-10; 2007,Jan,28-31

78110 **Plasma volume, radiopharmaceutical volume-dilution technique (separate procedure); single sampling**
1.99 1.99 **FUD** XXX S Z2 80
AMA: 2012,Feb,9-10; 2007,Jan,28-31

78111 **multiple samplings**
2.11 2.11 **FUD** XXX S Z2 80
AMA: 2012,Feb,9-10; 2007,Jan,28-31

78120 **Red cell volume determination (separate procedure); single sampling**
2.04 2.04 **FUD** XXX S Z2 80
AMA: 2012,Feb,9-10; 2007,Jan,28-31

78121 **multiple samplings**
2.23 2.23 **FUD** XXX S Z2 80
AMA: 2012,Feb,9-10; 2007,Jan,28-31

78122 **Whole blood volume determination, including separate measurement of plasma volume and red cell volume (radiopharmaceutical volume-dilution technique)**
2.75 2.75 **FUD** XXX S Z2 80
AMA: 2012,Feb,9-10; 2007,Jan,28-31

78130 **Red cell survival study**
3.56 3.56 **FUD** XXX S Z2 80
AMA: 2012,Feb,9-10; 2007,Jan,28-31

78140 **Labeled red cell sequestration, differential organ/tissue (eg, splenic and/or hepatic)**
3.19 3.19 **FUD** XXX S Z2 80
AMA: 2012,Feb,9-10; 2007,Jan,28-31

78185 **Spleen imaging only, with or without vascular flow**
EXCLUDES *Liver imaging (78215-78216)*
4.88 4.88 **FUD** XXX S Z2 80
AMA: 2012,Feb,9-10; 2007,Jan,28-31

78191 **Platelet survival study**
3.59 3.59 **FUD** XXX S Z2 80
AMA: 2012,Feb,9-10; 2007,Jan,28-31

78195 **Lymphatics and lymph nodes imaging**
EXCLUDES *Sentinel node identification without scintigraphy (38792)*
Sentinel node removal (38500-38542)
10.1 10.1 **FUD** XXX S Z2 80
AMA: 2018,Jan,8; 2017,Jan,8; 2016,Jan,13

78199 **Unlisted hematopoietic, reticuloendothelial and lymphatic procedure, diagnostic nuclear medicine**
0.00 0.00 **FUD** XXX S Z2 80
AMA: 2018,Jan,8; 2017,Jan,8; 2016,Jan,13

78201-78299 Nuclear Radiology: Digestive System

EXCLUDES *Diagnostic services (see appropriate sections)*
Follow-up care (see appropriate section)
Code also radiopharmaceutical(s) and/or drug(s) supplied

78201 **Liver imaging; static only**
EXCLUDES *Spleen imaging only (78185)*
5.46 5.46 **FUD** XXX S Z2 80
AMA: 2018,Jan,8; 2017,Jan,8; 2016,Jan,13

78202 **with vascular flow**
EXCLUDES *Spleen imaging only (78185)*
5.88 5.88 **FUD** XXX S Z2 80
AMA: 2012,Feb,9-10; 2007,Jan,28-31

78215 **Liver and spleen imaging; static only**
5.59 5.59 **FUD** XXX S Z2 80
AMA: 2012,Feb,9-10; 2007,Jan,28-31

78216 **with vascular flow**
3.69 3.69 **FUD** XXX S Z2 80
AMA: 2012,Feb,9-10; 2007,Jan,28-31

78226 **Hepatobiliary system imaging, including gallbladder when present;**
9.38 9.38 **FUD** XXX S Z2 80
AMA: 2012,Feb,9-10

78227 **with pharmacologic intervention, including quantitative measurement(s) when performed**
12.6 12.6 FUD XXX
AMA: 2012,Feb,9-10

78230 **Salivary gland imaging;**
5.03 5.03 FUD XXX
AMA: 2012,Feb,9-10; 2007,Jan,28-31

78231 **with serial images**
3.02 3.02 FUD XXX
AMA: 2012,Feb,9-10; 2007,Jan,28-31

78232 **Salivary gland function study**
2.96 2.96 FUD XXX
AMA: 2012,Feb,9-10; 2007,Jan,28-31

78258 **Esophageal motility**
6.19 6.19 FUD XXX
AMA: 2012,Feb,9-10; 2007,Jan,28-31

78261 **Gastric mucosa imaging**
5.84 5.84 FUD XXX
AMA: 2012,Feb,9-10; 2007,Jan,28-31

78262 **Gastroesophageal reflux study**
6.86 6.86 FUD XXX
AMA: 2018,Jan,8; 2017,Jan,8; 2016,Jan,13

78264 **Gastric emptying imaging study (eg, solid, liquid, or both);**
EXCLUDES *Procedure performed more than one time per study*
9.52 9.52 FUD XXX
AMA: 2018,Jan,8; 2017,Jan,8; 2016,Jan,13

78265 **with small bowel transit**
EXCLUDES *Procedure performed more than one time per study*
11.2 11.2 FUD XXX
AMA: 2018,Jan,8; 2017,Jan,8

78266 **with small bowel and colon transit, multiple days**
EXCLUDES *Procedure performed more than one time per study*
12.3 12.3 FUD XXX
AMA: 2018,Jan,8; 2017,Jan,8

78267 **Urea breath test, C-14 (isotopic); acquisition for analysis**
EXCLUDES *Breath hydrogen/methane test (91065)*
0.00 0.00 FUD XXX
AMA: 2020,OctSE,1; 2020,OctSE,1; 2018,Jan,8; 2017,Jan,8; 2016,Jan,13

78268 **analysis**
EXCLUDES *Breath hydrogen/methane test (91065)*
0.00 0.00 FUD XXX
AMA: 2020,OctSE,1; 2020,OctSE,1; 2018,Jan,8; 2017,Jan,8; 2016,Jan,13

78278 **Acute gastrointestinal blood loss imaging**
9.97 9.97 FUD XXX
AMA: 2012,Feb,9-10; 2007,Jan,28-31

78282 **Gastrointestinal protein loss**
0.00 0.00 FUD XXX
AMA: 2018,Jul,14

78290 **Intestine imaging (eg, ectopic gastric mucosa, Meckel's localization, volvulus)**
9.44 9.44 FUD XXX
AMA: 2012,Feb,9-10; 2007,Jan,28-31

78291 **Peritoneal-venous shunt patency test (eg, for LeVeen, Denver shunt)**
Code also (49427)
7.30 7.30 FUD XXX
AMA: 2012,Feb,9-10; 2007,Jan,28-31

78299 **Unlisted gastrointestinal procedure, diagnostic nuclear medicine**
0.00 0.00 FUD XXX
AMA: 2018,Jan,8; 2017,Jan,8; 2016,Jan,13

78300-78399 Nuclear Radiology: Bones and Joints

EXCLUDES *Diagnostic services (see appropriate sections)*
Follow-up care (see appropriate section)
Code also radiopharmaceutical(s) and/or drug(s) supplied

78300 **Bone and/or joint imaging; limited area**
6.56 6.56 FUD XXX
AMA: 2020,Oct,3; 2018,Jan,8; 2017,Jan,8; 2016,Jan,13

78305 **multiple areas**
8.08 8.08 FUD XXX
AMA: 2020,Oct,3; 2018,Jan,8; 2017,Jan,8; 2016,Jan,13

78306 **whole body**
8.71 8.71 FUD XXX
AMA: 2020,Oct,3; 2018,Jan,8; 2017,Jan,8; 2016,Jan,13

78315 **3 phase study**
9.91 9.91 FUD XXX
AMA: 2020,Oct,3; 2018,Jan,8; 2017,Jan,8; 2016,Jan,13

78350 **Bone density (bone mineral content) study, 1 or more sites; single photon absorptiometry**
0.91 0.91 FUD XXX
AMA: 2012,Feb,9-10; 2007,Jan,28-31

78351 **dual photon absorptiometry, 1 or more sites**
0.44 0.44 FUD XXX
AMA: 2012,Feb,9-10; 2007,Jan,28-31

78399 **Unlisted musculoskeletal procedure, diagnostic nuclear medicine**
0.00 0.00 FUD XXX
AMA: 2018,Jan,8; 2017,Jan,8; 2016,Jan,13

78414-78499 [78429, 78430, 78431, 78432, 78433, 78434] Nuclear Radiology: Heart and Vascular

EXCLUDES *Diagnostic services (see appropriate sections)*
Follow-up care (see appropriate section)
Code also radiopharmaceutical(s) and/or drug(s) supplied

78414 **Determination of central c-v hemodynamics (non-imaging) (eg, ejection fraction with probe technique) with or without pharmacologic intervention or exercise, single or multiple determinations**
0.00 0.00 FUD XXX
AMA: 2018,Jan,8; 2017,Jan,8; 2016,Jan,13

78428 **Cardiac shunt detection**
5.30 5.30 FUD XXX
AMA: 2018,Jan,8; 2017,Jan,8; 2016,Jan,13

78429 **Resequenced code. See code following 78459.**

78430 **Resequenced code. See code following 78491.**

78431 **Resequenced code. See code following 78492.**

78432 **Resequenced code. See code following 78492.**

78433 **Resequenced code. See code following 78492.**

78434 **Resequenced code. See code following 78492.**

78445 **Non-cardiac vascular flow imaging (ie, angiography, venography)**
5.60 5.60 FUD XXX
AMA: 2018,Jan,8; 2017,Jan,8; 2016,Jan,13

78451 **Myocardial perfusion imaging, tomographic (SPECT) (including attenuation correction, qualitative or quantitative wall motion, ejection fraction by first pass or gated technique, additional quantification, when performed); single study, at rest or stress (exercise or pharmacologic)**
EXCLUDES *Distribution radiopharmaceutical agents or tumor localization (78800-78802, [78804], 78803)*
Radiopharmaceutical quantification measurements ([78835])
SPECT with concurrently acquired CT transmission scan ([78830, 78831, 78832])
Code also stress testing when performed (93015-93018)
9.63 9.63 FUD XXX
AMA: 2020,Oct,3; 2020,Jul,5; 2018,Jan,8; 2017,Jan,8; 2016,Jan,13

78452 **multiple studies, at rest and/or stress (exercise or pharmacologic) and/or redistribution and/or rest reinjection**

EXCLUDES *Distribution radiopharmaceutical agents or tumor localization (78800-78802, [78804], 78803)*
Radiopharmaceutical quantification measurements ([78835])
SPECT with concurrently acquired CT transmission scan ([78830, 78831, 78832])

Code also stress testing when performed (93015-93018)
13.4 13.4 FUD XXX
AMA: 2020,Oct,3; 2020,Jul,5; 2018,Jan,8; 2017,Jan,8; 2016,Jan,13

78453 **Myocardial perfusion imaging, planar (including qualitative or quantitative wall motion, ejection fraction by first pass or gated technique, additional quantification, when performed); single study, at rest or stress (exercise or pharmacologic)**

Code also stress testing when performed (93015-93018)
8.78 8.78 FUD XXX
AMA: 2020,Jul,5; 2018,Jan,8; 2017,Jan,8; 2016,Jan,13

78454 **multiple studies, at rest and/or stress (exercise or pharmacologic) and/or redistribution and/or rest reinjection**

Code also stress testing when performed (93015-93018)
12.4 12.4 FUD XXX
AMA: 2020,Jul,5; 2018,Jan,8; 2017,Jan,8; 2016,Jan,13

78456 **Acute venous thrombosis imaging, peptide**

8.82 8.82 FUD XXX
AMA: 2018,Jan,8; 2017,Jan,8; 2016,Jan,13

78457 **Venous thrombosis imaging, venogram; unilateral**

5.02 5.02 FUD XXX
AMA: 2018,Jan,8; 2017,Jan,8; 2016,Jan,13

78458 **bilateral**

5.88 5.88 FUD XXX
AMA: 2018,Jan,8; 2017,Jan,8; 2016,Jan,13

78459 **Myocardial imaging, positron emission tomography (PET), metabolic evaluation study (including ventricular wall motion[s] and/or ejection fraction[s], when performed), single study;**

INCLUDES Examination CT transmission images for field of view anatomy review

EXCLUDES *CT coronary calcium scoring (75571)*
CT for other than attenuation correction/anatomical localization; report site-specific CT code with modifier 59
Myocardial perfusion studies (78491-78492)

0.00 0.00 FUD XXX
AMA: 2020,Jul,5; 2018,Jan,8; 2017,Jan,8; 2016,Jan,13

\# **78429** **with concurrently acquired computed tomography transmission scan**

INCLUDES Examination CT transmission images for field of view anatomy review

EXCLUDES *CT coronary calcium scoring (75571)*
CT for other than attenuation correction/anatomical localization; report site-specific CT code with modifier 59

0.00 0.00 FUD XXX
AMA: 2020,Jul,5

78466 **Myocardial imaging, infarct avid, planar; qualitative or quantitative**

5.67 5.67 FUD XXX
AMA: 2012,Feb,9-10; 2010,May,5-6

78468 **with ejection fraction by first pass technique**

5.51 5.51 FUD XXX
AMA: 2018,Jan,8; 2017,Jan,8; 2016,Jan,13

78469 **tomographic SPECT with or without quantification**

EXCLUDES *Distribution radiopharmaceutical agents or tumor localization (78800-78802, [78804], 78803)*
Myocardial sympathetic innervation imaging (0331T-0332T)
Radiopharmaceutical quantification measurements ([78835])
SPECT with concurrently acquired CT transmission scan ([78830, 78831, 78832])

6.39 6.39 FUD XXX
AMA: 2020,Oct,3; 2018,Nov,11; 2018,Jan,8; 2017,Jan,8; 2016,Jan,13

78472 **Cardiac blood pool imaging, gated equilibrium; planar, single study at rest or stress (exercise and/or pharmacologic), wall motion study plus ejection fraction, with or without additional quantitative processing**

EXCLUDES *Cardiac blood pool imaging (78481, 78483, 78494)*
Myocardial perfusion imaging (78451-78454)
Right ventricular ejection fraction by first pass technique (78496)

Code also stress testing when performed (93015-93018)
6.51 6.51 FUD XXX
AMA: 2018,Jan,8; 2017,Jan,8; 2016,Jan,13

78473 **multiple studies, wall motion study plus ejection fraction, at rest and stress (exercise and/or pharmacologic), with or without additional quantification**

EXCLUDES *Cardiac blood pool imaging (78481, 78483, 78494)*
Myocardial perfusion imaging (78451-78454)

Code also stress testing when performed (93015-93018)
8.26 8.26 FUD XXX
AMA: 2018,Jan,8; 2017,Jan,8; 2016,Jan,13

78481 **Cardiac blood pool imaging (planar), first pass technique; single study, at rest or with stress (exercise and/or pharmacologic), wall motion study plus ejection fraction, with or without quantification**

EXCLUDES *Myocardial perfusion imaging (78451-78454)*

Code also stress testing when performed (93015-93018)
5.03 5.03 FUD XXX
AMA: 2018,Jan,8; 2017,Jan,8; 2016,Jan,13

78483 **multiple studies, at rest and with stress (exercise and/or pharmacologic), wall motion study plus ejection fraction, with or without quantification**

EXCLUDES *Blood flow studies brain (78610)*
Myocardial perfusion imaging (78451-78454)

Code also stress testing when performed (93015-93018)
6.89 6.89 FUD XXX
AMA: 2018,Jan,8; 2017,Jan,8; 2016,Jan,13

78491 **Myocardial imaging, positron emission tomography (PET), perfusion study (including ventricular wall motion[s] and/or ejection fraction[s], when performed); single study, at rest or stress (exercise or pharmacologic)**

Code also stress testing when performed (93015-93018)
0.00 0.00 FUD XXX
AMA: 2020,Jul,5; 2018,Jan,8; 2017,Jan,8; 2016,Jan,13

\# **78430** **single study, at rest or stress (exercise or pharmacologic), with concurrently acquired computed tomography transmission scan**

INCLUDES Examination CT transmission images for field of view anatomy review

Code also stress testing when performed (93015-93018)
0.00 0.00 FUD XXX
AMA: 2020,Jul,5

78492 **multiple studies at rest and stress (exercise or pharmacologic)**

Code also stress testing when performed (93015-93018)
0.00 0.00 FUD XXX
AMA: 2020,Jul,5; 2018,Jan,8; 2017,Jan,8; 2016,Jan,13

\# **78431** **multiple studies at rest and stress (exercise or pharmacologic), with concurrently acquired computed tomography transmission scan**

INCLUDES Examination CT transmission images for field of view anatomy review

Code also stress testing when performed (93015-93018)

2.62 2.62 FUD XXX Z2 80

AMA: 2020,Jul,5

\# **78432** **Myocardial imaging, positron emission tomography (PET), combined perfusion with metabolic evaluation study (including ventricular wall motion[s] and/or ejection fraction[s], when performed), dual radiotracer (eg, myocardial viability);**

Code also stress testing when performed (93015-93018)

0.00 0.00 FUD XXX Z2 80

AMA: 2020,Jul,5

\# **78433** **with concurrently acquired computed tomography transmission scan**

INCLUDES Examination CT transmission images for field of view anatomy review

EXCLUDES *CT for other than attenuation correction/anatomical localization; use site-specific CT code with modifier 59*

Code also stress testing when performed (93015-93018)

0.00 0.00 FUD XXX Z2 80

AMA: 2020,Jul,5

\+ # **78434** **Absolute quantitation of myocardial blood flow (AQMBF), positron emission tomography (PET), rest and pharmacologic stress (List separately in addition to code for primary procedure)**

EXCLUDES *CT coronary calcium scoring (75571)*

Myocardial imaging by planar or SPECT (78451-78454)

Code first ([78431], 78492)

0.00 0.00 FUD ZZZ N1 80

AMA: 2020,Jul,5

78494 **Cardiac blood pool imaging, gated equilibrium, SPECT, at rest, wall motion study plus ejection fraction, with or without quantitative processing**

EXCLUDES *Distribution radiopharmaceutical agents or tumor localization (78800-78802, [78804], 78803)*

Radiopharmaceutical quantification measurements ([78835])

SPECT with concurrently acquired CT transmission scan ([78830, 78831, 78832])

6.47 6.47 FUD XXX S Z2 80

AMA: 2020,Oct,3; 2018,Jan,8; 2017,Jan,8; 2016,Jan,13

\+ **78496** **Cardiac blood pool imaging, gated equilibrium, single study, at rest, with right ventricular ejection fraction by first pass technique (List separately in addition to code for primary procedure)**

Code first (78472)

1.23 1.23 FUD ZZZ N N1 80

AMA: 2018,Jan,8; 2017,Jan,8; 2016,Jan,13

78499 **Unlisted cardiovascular procedure, diagnostic nuclear medicine**

0.00 0.00 FUD XXX S Z2 80

AMA: 2018,Jan,8; 2017,Jan,8; 2016,Jan,13

78579-78599 Nuclear Radiology: Lungs

EXCLUDES *Diagnostic services (see appropriate sections)*

Follow-up care (see appropriate sections)

Code also radiopharmaceutical(s) and/or drug(s) supplied

78579 **Pulmonary ventilation imaging (eg, aerosol or gas)**

EXCLUDES *Procedure performed more than one time per imaging session*

5.36 5.36 FUD XXX S Z2 80

AMA: 2012,Feb,9-10

78580 **Pulmonary perfusion imaging (eg, particulate)**

EXCLUDES *Myocardial perfusion imaging (78451-78454)*

Procedure performed more than one time per imaging session

6.77 6.77 FUD XXX S Z2 80

AMA: 2018,Jan,8; 2017,Jan,8; 2016,Jan,13

78582 **Pulmonary ventilation (eg, aerosol or gas) and perfusion imaging**

EXCLUDES *Myocardial perfusion imaging (78451-78454)*

Procedure performed more than one time per imaging session

9.54 9.54 FUD XXX S Z2 80

AMA: 2012,Feb,9-10

78597 **Quantitative differential pulmonary perfusion, including imaging when performed**

EXCLUDES *Myocardial perfusion imaging (78451-78454)*

Procedure performed more than one time per imaging session

5.74 5.74 FUD XXX S Z2 80

AMA: 2012,Feb,9-10

78598 **Quantitative differential pulmonary perfusion and ventilation (eg, aerosol or gas), including imaging when performed**

EXCLUDES *Myocardial perfusion imaging (78451-78454)*

Procedure performed more than one time per imaging session

8.70 8.70 FUD XXX S Z2 80

AMA: 2012,Feb,9-10

78599 **Unlisted respiratory procedure, diagnostic nuclear medicine**

0.00 0.00 FUD XXX S Z2 80

AMA: 2018,Jan,8; 2017,Jan,8; 2016,Jan,13

78600-78650 Nuclear Radiology: Brain/Cerebrospinal Fluid

EXCLUDES *Diagnostic services (see appropriate sections)*

Follow-up care (see appropriate section)

Code also radiopharmaceutical(s) and/or drug(s) supplied

78600 **Brain imaging, less than 4 static views;**

5.26 5.26 FUD XXX S Z2 80

AMA: 2018,Jan,8; 2017,Jan,8; 2016,Jan,13

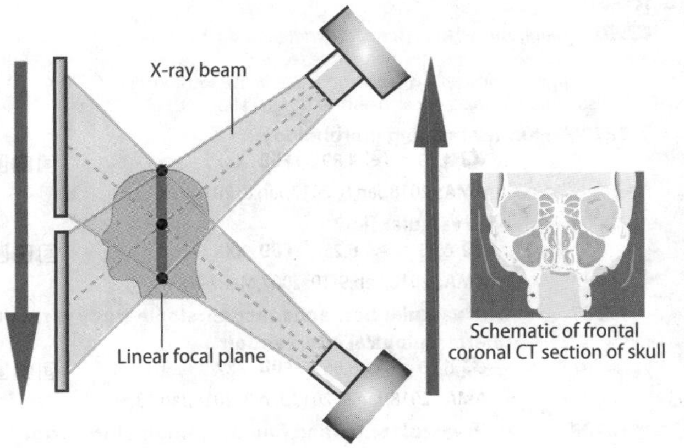

Schematic of frontal coronal CT section of skull

78601 **with vascular flow**

6.20 6.20 FUD XXX S Z2 80

AMA: 2012,Feb,9-10; 2007,Jan,28-31

78605 **Brain imaging, minimum 4 static views;**

5.71 5.71 FUD XXX S Z2 80

AMA: 2012,Feb,9-10; 2007,Jan,28-31

78606 **with vascular flow**

9.50 9.50 FUD XXX S Z2 80

AMA: 2012,Feb,9-10; 2007,Jan,28-31

78608 **Brain imaging, positron emission tomography (PET); metabolic evaluation**
0.00 0.00 FUD XXX S Z2 80
AMA: 2012,Feb,9-10; 2007,Jan,28-31

78609 **perfusion evaluation**
2.16 2.16 FUD XXX E
AMA: 2012,Feb,9-10; 2007,Jan,28-31

78610 **Brain imaging, vascular flow only**
4.97 4.97 FUD XXX S Z2 80
AMA: 2012,Feb,9-10; 2007,Jan,28-31

78630 **Cerebrospinal fluid flow, imaging (not including introduction of material); cisternography**
Code also injection procedure (61000-61070, 62270-62327)
9.66 9.66 FUD XXX S Z2 80
AMA: 2018,Jan,8

78635 **ventriculography**
Code also injection procedure (61000-61070, 62270-62294)
9.77 9.77 FUD XXX S Z2 80
AMA: 2012,Feb,9-10; 2007,Jan,28-31

78645 **shunt evaluation**
Code also injection procedure (61000-61070, 62270-62294)
9.28 9.28 FUD XXX S Z2 80
AMA: 2012,Feb,9-10; 2007,Jan,28-31

78650 **Cerebrospinal fluid leakage detection and localization**
Code also injection procedure (61000-61070, 62270-62294)
7.89 7.89 FUD XXX S Z2 80
AMA: 2012,Feb,9-10; 2007,Jan,28-31

78660-78699 Nuclear Radiology: Lacrimal Duct System

Code also radiopharmaceutical(s) and/or drug(s) supplied

78660 **Radiopharmaceutical dacryocystography**
5.27 5.27 FUD XXX S Z2 80
AMA: 2012,Feb,9-10; 2007,Jan,28-31

78699 **Unlisted nervous system procedure, diagnostic nuclear medicine**
0.00 0.00 FUD XXX S Z2 80
AMA: 2018,Jan,8; 2017,Jan,8; 2016,Jan,13

78700-78725 Nuclear Radiology: Renal Anatomy and Function

EXCLUDES *Diagnostic services (see appropriate sections)*
Follow-up care (see appropriate section)
Renal endoscopy with insertion radioactive substances (77778)
Code also radiopharmaceutical(s) and/or drug(s) supplied

78700 **Kidney imaging morphology;**
4.89 4.89 FUD XXX S Z2 80
AMA: 2018,Jan,8; 2017,Jan,8; 2016,Jan,13

78701 **with vascular flow**
6.25 6.25 FUD XXX S Z2 80
AMA: 2012,Feb,9-10; 2007,Mar,7-8

78707 **with vascular flow and function, single study without pharmacological intervention**
6.66 6.66 FUD XXX S Z2 80
AMA: 2018,Jan,8; 2017,Jan,8; 2016,Jan,13

78708 **with vascular flow and function, single study, with pharmacological intervention (eg, angiotensin converting enzyme inhibitor and/or diuretic)**
5.06 5.06 FUD XXX S Z2 80
AMA: 2018,Jan,8; 2017,Jan,8; 2016,Jan,13

78709 **with vascular flow and function, multiple studies, with and without pharmacological intervention (eg, angiotensin converting enzyme inhibitor and/or diuretic)**
10.5 10.5 FUD XXX S Z2 80
AMA: 2018,Jan,8; 2017,Jan,8; 2016,Jan,13

78725 **Kidney function study, non-imaging radioisotopic study**
3.10 3.10 FUD XXX S Z2 80
AMA: 2012,Feb,9-10; 2007,Jan,28-31

78730-78799 Nuclear Radiology: Urogenital

EXCLUDES *Diagnostic services (see appropriate sections)*
Follow-up care (see appropriate section)
Code also radiopharmaceutical(s) and/or drug(s) supplied

+ **78730** **Urinary bladder residual study (List separately in addition to code for primary procedure)**
EXCLUDES *Measurement postvoid residual urine and /or bladder capacity using ultrasound (51798)*
Ultrasound imaging bladder only with measurement postvoid residual urine (76857)
Code first (78740)
2.17 2.17 FUD ZZZ N N1 80
AMA: 2018,Jan,8; 2017,Jan,8; 2016,Jan,13

78740 **Ureteral reflux study (radiopharmaceutical voiding cystogram)**
EXCLUDES *Catheterization (51701-51703)*
Code also urinary bladder residual study (78730)
6.21 6.21 FUD XXX S Z2 80
AMA: 2012,Feb,9-10; 2007,Jan,28-31

78761 **Testicular imaging with vascular flow** ♂
6.06 6.06 FUD XXX S Z2 80
AMA: 2018,Jan,8; 2017,Jan,8; 2016,Jan,13

78799 **Unlisted genitourinary procedure, diagnostic nuclear medicine**
0.00 0.00 FUD XXX S Z2 80
AMA: 2018,Jan,8; 2017,Jan,8; 2016,Jan,13

78800-78835 [78804, 78830, 78831, 78832, 78835] Nuclear Radiology: Tumor Localization

EXCLUDES *CSF studies requiring injection procedure (61055, 61070, 62320-62323)*
Code also radiopharmaceutical(s) and/or drug(s) supplied

78800 **Radiopharmaceutical localization of tumor, inflammatory process or distribution of radiopharmaceutical agent(s) (includes vascular flow and blood pool imaging, when performed); planar, single area (eg, head, neck, chest, pelvis), single day imaging**
INCLUDES Ocular radiophosphorus tumor identification
EXCLUDES *Specific organ (see appropriate site)*
7.40 7.40 FUD XXX S Z2 80
AMA: 2020,Oct,3; 2018,Nov,11; 2018,Jan,8; 2017,Jan,8; 2016,Jan,13

78801 **planar, 2 or more areas (eg, abdomen and pelvis, head and chest), 1 or more days imaging or single area imaging over 2 or more days**
8.13 8.13 FUD XXX S Z2 80
AMA: 2020,Oct,3; 2018,Jan,8; 2017,Jan,8; 2016,Jan,13

78802 **planar, whole body, single day imaging**
8.93 8.93 FUD XXX S Z2 80
AMA: 2020,Oct,3

\# **78804** **planar, whole body, requiring 2 or more days imaging**
18.8 18.8 FUD XXX S Z2 80
AMA: 2020,Oct,3

78803 **tomographic (SPECT), single area (eg, head, neck, chest, pelvis), single day imaging**
11.1 11.1 FUD XXX S Z2 80
AMA: 2020,Oct,3; 2020,Oct,14; 2018,Nov,11; 2018,Jan,8; 2017,Jan,8; 2016,Dec,9; 2016,Dec,16; 2016,Jan,13

78804 **Resequenced code. See code following 78802.**

\# **78830** **tomographic (SPECT) with concurrently acquired computed tomography (CT) transmission scan for anatomical review, localization and determination/detection of pathology, single area (eg, head, neck, chest, pelvis), single day imaging**
14.0 14.0 FUD XXX Z2 80
AMA: 2020,Oct,3

\# **78831** **tomographic (SPECT), minimum 2 areas (eg, pelvis and knees, abdomen and pelvis), single day imaging, or single area imaging over 2 or more days**
20.3 20.3 FUD XXX Z2 80
AMA: 2020,Oct,3

\# **78832** **tomographic (SPECT) with concurrently acquired computed tomography (CT) transmission scan for anatomical review, localization and determination/detection of pathology, minimum 2 areas (eg, pelvis and knees, abdomen and pelvis), single day imaging, or single area imaging over 2 or more days**
26.4 26.4 FUD XXX Z2 80
AMA: 2020,Oct,3

\+ # **78835** **Radiopharmaceutical quantification measurement(s) single area (List separately in addition to code for primary procedure)**
Code first ([78830], [78832])
2.95 2.95 FUD ZZZ 80
AMA: 2020,Oct,3

78808 Intravenous Injection for Radiopharmaceutical Localization

Code also radiopharmaceutical(s) and/or drug(s) supplied

78808 **Injection procedure for radiopharmaceutical localization by non-imaging probe study, intravenous (eg, parathyroid adenoma)**
1.14 1.14 FUD XXX Q1 N1 80
AMA: 2018,Jan,8; 2017,Jan,8; 2016,Dec,9

78811-78999 [78830, 78831, 78832, 78835] Nuclear Radiology: Diagnosis, Staging, Restaging or Monitoring Cancer

CMS: 100-03,220.6.17 Positron Emission Tomography (FDG) for Oncologic Conditions; 100-03,220.6.19 NaF-18 PET to Identify Bone Metastasis of Cancer; 100-03,220.6.9 FDG PET for Refractory Seizures; 100-04,13,60 Positron Emission Tomography (PET) Scans - General Information; 100-04,13,60.13 Billing for PET Scans for Specific Indications of Cervical Cancer; 100-04,13,60.15 Billing for CMS-Approved Clinical Trials for PET Scans; 100-04,13,60.16 Billing and Coverage for PET Scans; 100-04,13,60.17 Billing and Coverage Changes for PET Scans for Cervical Cancer; 100-04,13,60.2 Use of Gamma Cameras, Full and Partial Ring PET Scanners; 100-04,13,60.3 PET Scan Qualifying Conditions; 100-04,13,60.3.2 Tracer Codes Required for Positron Emission Tomography (PET) Scans

EXCLUDES *CT scan performed for other than attenuation correction and anatomical localization (report with appropriate site-specific CT code and modifier 59)*
Ocular radiophosphorus tumor identification (78800)
PET brain scan (78608-78609)
PET myocardial imaging (78459, 78491-78492)
Procedure performed more than one time per imaging session

Code also radiopharmaceutical(s) and/or drug(s) supplied

78811 **Positron emission tomography (PET) imaging; limited area (eg, chest, head/neck)**
0.00 0.00 FUD XXX S Z2 80
AMA: 2018,Jan,8; 2017,Jan,8; 2016,Jan,13

78812 **skull base to mid-thigh**
0.00 0.00 FUD XXX S Z2 80
AMA: 2018,Jan,8; 2017,Jan,8; 2016,Jan,13

78813 **whole body**
0.00 0.00 FUD XXX S Z2 80
AMA: 2018,Jan,8; 2017,Jan,8; 2016,Jan,13

78814 **Positron emission tomography (PET) with concurrently acquired computed tomography (CT) for attenuation correction and anatomical localization imaging; limited area (eg, chest, head/neck)**
0.00 0.00 FUD XXX S Z2 80
AMA: 2018,Jan,8; 2017,Jan,8; 2016,Jan,13

78815 **skull base to mid-thigh**
0.00 0.00 FUD XXX S Z2 80
AMA: 2018,Jan,8; 2017,Jan,8; 2016,Jan,13

78816 **whole body**
0.00 0.00 FUD XXX S Z2 80
AMA: 2020,Sep,11; 2018,Jan,8; 2017,Jan,8; 2016,Jan,13

78830 **Resequenced code. See code following numeric code 78804.**

78831 **Resequenced code. See code following numeric code 78804.**

78832 **Resequenced code. See code following numeric code 78804.**

78835 **Resequenced code. See code following numeric code 78804.**

78999 **Unlisted miscellaneous procedure, diagnostic nuclear medicine**
0.00 0.00 FUD XXX S Z2 80
AMA: 2018,Jan,8; 2017,Jan,8; 2016,Dec,9; 2016,Dec,16; 2016,Jan,13

79005-79999 Systemic Radiopharmaceutical Therapy

EXCLUDES *Imaging guidance*
Injection into artery, body cavity, or joint (see appropriate injection codes)
Radiological supervision and interpretation

79005 **Radiopharmaceutical therapy, by oral administration**
EXCLUDES *Monoclonal antibody treatment (79403)*
3.92 3.92 FUD XXX S Z3 80
AMA: 2018,Jan,8; 2017,Jan,8; 2016,Jan,13

79101 **Radiopharmaceutical therapy, by intravenous administration**
EXCLUDES *Administration nonantibody radioelement solution including follow-up care (77750)*
Hydration infusion (96360)
Intravenous injection, IV push (96374-96375, 96409)
Radiolabeled monoclonal antibody IV infusion (79403)
Venipuncture (36400, 36410)
4.23 4.23 FUD XXX S Z3 80
AMA: 2018,Jan,8; 2017,Jan,8; 2016,Jan,13

79200 **Radiopharmaceutical therapy, by intracavitary administration**
3.86 3.86 FUD XXX S Z3 80
AMA: 2018,Jan,8; 2017,Jan,8; 2016,Jan,13

79300 **Radiopharmaceutical therapy, by interstitial radioactive colloid administration**
0.00 0.00 FUD XXX S Z2 80
AMA: 2018,Jan,8; 2017,Jan,8; 2016,Jan,13

79403 **Radiopharmaceutical therapy, radiolabeled monoclonal antibody by intravenous infusion**
EXCLUDES *Intravenous radiopharmaceutical therapy (79101)*
5.39 5.39 FUD XXX S Z3 80
AMA: 2018,Jan,8; 2017,Jan,8; 2016,Jan,13

79440 **Radiopharmaceutical therapy, by intra-articular administration**
3.48 3.48 FUD XXX S Z3 80
AMA: 2018,Jan,8; 2017,Jan,8; 2016,Jan,13

79445 **Radiopharmaceutical therapy, by intra-arterial particulate administration**
EXCLUDES *Intra-arterial injections (96373, 96420)*
Procedural and radiological supervision and interpretation for angiographic and interventional procedures before intra-arterial radiopharmaceutical therapy
0.00 0.00 FUD XXX S Z2 80
AMA: 2018,Jan,8; 2017,Jan,8; 2016,Jan,13

79999 **Radiopharmaceutical therapy, unlisted procedure**
0.00 0.00 FUD XXX S Z2 80
AMA: 2018,Jan,8; 2017,Jan,8; 2016,Jan,13

79005–79999 Systemic Radiopharmaceutical Therapy

79005 Radiopharmaceutical therapy, by oral administration

79101 Radiopharmaceutical therapy, by intravenous administration

79200 Radiopharmaceutical therapy, by intracavitary administration

79300 Radiopharmaceutical therapy, by interstitial radioactive colloid administration

79403 Radiopharmaceutical therapy, radiolabeled monoclonal antibody by intravenous infusion

79440 Radiopharmaceutical therapy, by intra-articular administration

79445 Radiopharmaceutical therapy, by intra-arterial particulate administration

78808 Intravenous Injection for Radiopharmaceutical Localization

78811 Positron emission tomography (PET) imaging; limited area (eg, chest, head/neck)

Medical Decision Making Table for Pathology Clinical Consultations

Medical Decision Making

Pathology clinical consultation services may be based on either the total time for consultation services performed on the date of consultation **or** the level of medical decision making as defined for each service.

The Medical Decision Making (MDM) Table for Pathology Clinical Consultations is a guide to assist in selecting the level of MDM for reporting pathology clinical consultation services. The table includes the levels of MDM (i.e., low, limited, moderate, high, extensive) and the three elements of MDM (i.e., number and complexity of problems addressed at the encounter, amount and/or complexity of data reviewed and analyzed, and risk of complications and/or morbidity or mortality of patient management). To qualify for a particular level of MDM, two of the three elements for that level of MDM must be met or exceeded. See Table 1: Medical Decision Making (MDM) Table for Pathology Clinical Consultations below.

Table 1: Medical Decision Making (MDM) Table for Pathology Clinical Consultations

		Elements of Medical Decision Making		
Code	**Level of MDM (based on 2 out of 3 elements of MDM)**	**Number and Complexity of Problems Addressed**	**Amount and/or Complexity of Data to be Reviewed and Analyzed**	**Risk of Complications and/or Morbidity or Mortality of Patient Management**
80503	**Low**	**Low** • **1** to **2** laboratory or pathology findings; **or** • **2** or more self-limited problems	**Limited** *(Must meet the requirements of at least 1 of the 2 categories)* **Category 1: Tests and documents** • **Any combination of 2 from the following:** - Review of prior note(s) from each unique source*; - Review of result(s) of each unique test*; - Ordering or recommending additional or follow-up testing* **or** **Category 2: Assessment requiring an independent historian(s)** (For the categories of independent interpretation of tests and discussion of management or test interpretation, see moderate or high)	**Low risk of morbidity from additional diagnostic testing or treatment**
80504	**Moderate**	**Moderate** • **3** to **4** laboratory or pathology findings; or • **1** or more chronic illnesses with exacerbation, progression, or side effects of treatment; **or** • **2** or more stable chronic illnesses; **or** • **1** undiagnosed new problem with uncertain prognosis; **or** • **1** acute illness with systemic symptoms	**Moderate** *(Must meet the requirements of at least 1 out of 3 categories)* **Category 1: Tests, documents, or independent historian(s)** **Any combination of 3 from the following:** • Review of prior note(s) from each unique source*; • Review of the result(s) of each unique test*; • Ordering or recommending additional or follow-up testing* • Assessment requiring an independent historian(s) **or** **Category 2: Independent interpretation of tests** • Independent interpretation of a test performed by another physician/other qualified health care professional (not separately reported); **or** **Category 3: Discussion of management or test interpretation** • Discussion of management or test interpretation with external physician/other qualified health care professional/appropriate source (not separately reported)	**Moderate risk of morbidity from additional diagnostic testing or treatment** *Examples only:* Prescription drug management • Decision regarding minor surgery with identified patient or procedure risk factors • Decision regarding elective major surgery without identified patient or procedure risk factors • Diagnosis or treatment significantly limited by social determinants of health

**Each unique test, order, or document contributes to the combination of 2 or combination of 3 in Category 1.*

		Elements of Medical Decision Making		
Code	**Level of MDM (based on 2 out of 3 elements of MDM)**	**Number and Complexity of Problems Addressed**	**Amount and/or Complexity of Data to be Reviewed and Analyzed**	**Risk of Complications and/or Morbidity or Mortality of Patient Management**
80505	**High**	**High** • **5** or more laboratory or pathology findings; **or** • **1** or more chronic illnesses with severe exacerbation, progression, or side effects of treatment; **or** • **1** acute or chronic illness or injury that poses a threat to life or bodily function	**Extensive** *(Must meet the requirements of at least 2 out of 3 categories)* **Category 1: Tests, documents, or independent historian(s)** **Any combination of 3 from the following:** • Review of prior note(s) from each unique source*; • Review of the result(s) of each unique test*; • Ordering or recommending additional or follow-up testing* • Assessment requiring an independent historian(s) **or** **Category 2: Independent interpretation of tests** • Independent interpretation of a test performed by another physician/other qualified health care professional (not separately reported); **or** **Category 3: Discussion of management or test interpretation** • Discussion of management or test interpretation with external physician/other qualified health care professional/appropriate source (not separately reported)	**High risk of morbidity from additional diagnostic testing or treatment** *Examples only:* • Drug therapy requiring intensive monitoring for toxicity • Decision regarding elective major surgery with identified patient or procedure risk factors • Decision regarding emergency major surgery • Decision regarding hospitalization

**Each unique test, order, or document contributes to the combination of 2 or combination of 3 in Category 1.*

80047-80081 [80081] Multi-test Laboratory Panels

INCLUDES Specified test groups that may be reported in a panel

EXCLUDES *Reporting two or more panel codes including same tests; report panel with most tests in common to meet panel code definition*

Code also individual tests not part included in panel, when appropriate

80047 Basic metabolic panel (Calcium, ionized)

INCLUDES Calcium, ionized (82330)
Carbon dioxide (bicarbonate) (82374)
Chloride (82435)
Creatinine (82565)
Glucose (82947)
Potassium (84132)
Sodium (84295)
Urea nitrogen (BUN) (84520)

0.00 0.00 **FUD** XXX

AMA: 2020,Dec,3; 2020,Jun,3; 2018,Jan,8; 2017,Jan,8; 2016,Jan,13

80048 Basic metabolic panel (Calcium, total)

INCLUDES Calcium, total (82310)
Carbon dioxide (bicarbonate) (82374)
Chloride (82435)
Creatinine (82565)
Glucose (82947)
Potassium (84132)
Sodium (84295)
Urea nitrogen (BUN) (84520)

0.00 0.00 **FUD** XXX

AMA: 2020,Dec,3; 2018,Jan,8; 2017,Jan,8; 2016,Jan,13

80050 General health panel

INCLUDES Complete blood count (CBC), automated, with:
Manual differential WBC count
Blood smear with manual differential AND complete (CBC), automated (85007, 85027)
Manual differential WBC count, buffy coat AND complete (CBC), automated (85009, 85027)
OR
Automated differential WBC count
Automated differential WBC count AND complete (CBC), automated/automated differential WBC count (85004, 85025)
Automated differential WBC count AND complete (CBC), automated (85004, 85027)
Comprehensive metabolic profile (80053)
Thyroid stimulating hormone (84443)

0.00 0.00 **FUD** XXX

AMA: 2020,Dec,3; 2018,Jan,8; 2017,Jan,8; 2016,Jan,13

80051 Electrolyte panel

INCLUDES Carbon dioxide (bicarbonate) (82374)
Chloride (82435)
Potassium (84132)
Sodium (84295)

0.00 0.00 **FUD** XXX

AMA: 2020,Dec,3; 2018,Jan,8; 2017,Jan,8; 2016,Jan,13

80053 Comprehensive metabolic panel

INCLUDES Albumin (82040)
Bilirubin, total (82247)
Calcium, total (82310)
Carbon dioxide (bicarbonate) (82374)
Chloride (82435)
Creatinine (82565)
Glucose (82947)
Phosphatase, alkaline (84075)
Potassium (84132)
Protein, total (84155)
Sodium (84295)
Transferase, alanine amino (ALT) (SGPT) (84460)
Transferase, aspartate amino (AST) (SGOT) (84450)
Urea nitrogen (BUN) (84520)

0.00 0.00 **FUD** XXX

AMA: 2020,Dec,3; 2018,Jan,8; 2017,Jan,8; 2016,Jan,13

80055 Obstetric panel M ♀

INCLUDES Complete blood count (CBC), automated, with:
Manual differential WBC count
Blood smear with manual differential AND complete (CBC), automated (85007, 85027)
Manual differential WBC count, buffy coat AND complete (CBC), automated (85009, 85027)
OR
Automated differential WBC count
Automated differential WBC count AND complete (CBC), automated/automated differential WBC count (85004, 85025)
Automated differential WBC count AND complete (CBC), automated (85004, 85027)
Blood typing, ABO and Rh (86900-86901)
Hepatitis B surface antigen (HBsAg) (87340)
RBC antibody screen, each serum technique (86850)
Rubella antibody (86762)
Syphilis test, non-treponemal antibody qualitative (86592)

EXCLUDES *Reporting code when syphilis screening provided using treponemal antibody approach. Instead, assign individual codes for tests performed in OB panel (86780)*

0.00 0.00 **FUD** XXX

AMA: 2020,Dec,3; 2018,Jan,8; 2017,Jan,8; 2016,Jan,13

80081 Obstetric panel (includes HIV testing) M ♀

INCLUDES Complete blood count (CBC), automated, with:
Manual differential WBC count
Blood smear with manual differential AND complete (CBC), automated (85007, 85027)
Manual differential WBC count, buffy count AND complete (CBC), automated (85009, 85027)
OR
Automated differential WBC count
Automated differential WBC count AND complete (CBC), automated/automated differential WBC count (85004, 85025)
Automated differential WBC count AND complete (CBC), automated (85004, 85027)
Blood typing, ABO and Rh (86900-86901)
Hepatitis B surface antigen (HBsAg) (87340)
HIV-1 antigens, with HIV-1 and HIV-2 antibodies, single result (87389)
RBC antibody screen, each serum technique (86850)
Rubella antibody (86762)
Syphilis test, non-treponemal antibody qualitative (86592)

EXCLUDES *Reporting code when syphilis screening provided using treponemal antibody approach. Instead, assign individual codes for tests performed in OB panel (86780)*

0.00 0.00 **FUD** XXX

AMA: 2020,Dec,3; 2018,Jan,8; 2017,Jan,8; 2016,Jan,13

80061 Lipid panel

INCLUDES Cholesterol, serum, total (82465)
Lipoprotein, direct measurement, high density cholesterol (HDL cholesterol) (83718)
Triglycerides (84478)

0.00 0.00 **FUD** XXX

AMA: 2020,Dec,3; 2018,Jan,8; 2017,Sep,11; 2017,Jan,8; 2016,Jan,13

80069 Renal function panel

INCLUDES Albumin (82040)
Calcium, total (82310)
Carbon dioxide (bicarbonate) (82374)
Chloride (82435)
Creatinine (82565)
Glucose (82947)
Phosphorus inorganic (phosphate) (84100)
Potassium (84132)
Sodium (84295)
Urea nitrogen (BUN) (84520)

0.00 0.00 **FUD** XXX

AMA: 2020,Dec,3; 2018,Jan,8; 2017,Jan,8; 2016,Jan,13

80074 Acute hepatitis panel

INCLUDES Hepatitis A antibody (HAAb) IgM (86709)
Hepatitis B core antibody (HBcAb), IgM (86705)
Hepatitis B surface antigen (HBsAg) (87340)
Hepatitis C antibody (86803)

0.00 0.00 FUD XXX

AMA: 2020,Dec,3; 2018,Jan,8; 2017,Jan,8; 2016,Jan,13

80076 Hepatic function panel

INCLUDES Albumin (82040)
Bilirubin, direct (82248)
Bilirubin, total (82247)
Phosphatase, alkaline (84075)
Protein, total (84155)
Transferase, alanine amino (ALT) (SGPT) (84460)
Transferase, aspartate amino (AST) (SGOT) (84450)

0.00 0.00 FUD XXX

AMA: 2020,Dec,3; 2018,Jan,8; 2017,Jan,8; 2016,Jan,13

80081 **Resequenced code. See code following 80055.**

80305-80307 [80305, 80306, 80307] Nonspecific Drug Screening

INCLUDES All class testing procedures performed per modality
Validation testing

EXCLUDES *Confirmatory drug testing ([80320, 80321, 80322, 80323, 80324, 80325, 80326, 80327, 80328, 80329, 80330, 80331, 80332, 80333, 80334, 80335, 80336, 80337, 80338, 80339, 80340, 80341, 80342, 80343, 80344, 80345, 80346, 80347, 80348, 80349, 80350, 80351, 80352, 80353, 80354, 80355, 80356, 80357, 80358, 80359, 80360, 80361, 80362, 80363, 80364, 80365, 80366, 80367, 80368, 80369, 80370, 80371, 80372, 80373, 80374, 80375, 80376, 80377, 83992], [83992])*

\# **80305 Drug test(s), presumptive, any number of drug classes, any number of devices or procedures; capable of being read by direct optical observation only (eg, utilizing immunoassay [eg, dipsticks, cups, cards, or cartridges]), includes sample validation when performed, per date of service**

0.00 0.00 FUD XXX

AMA: 2020,Dec,3; 2018,Jul,14; 2018,Jan,8; 2017,Mar,6

\# **80306 read by instrument assisted direct optical observation (eg, utilizing immunoassay [eg, dipsticks, cups, cards, or cartridges]), includes sample validation when performed, per date of service**

0.00 0.00 FUD XXX

AMA: 2020,Dec,3; 2018,Jan,8; 2017,Mar,6

\# **80307 by instrument chemistry analyzers (eg, utilizing immunoassay [eg, EIA, ELISA, EMIT, FPIA, IA, KIMS, RIA]), chromatography (eg, GC, HPLC), and mass spectrometry either with or without chromatography, (eg, DART, DESI, GC-MS, GC-MS/MS, LC-MS, LC-MS/MS, LDTD, MALDI, TOF) includes sample validation when performed, per date of service**

0.00 0.00 FUD XXX

AMA: 2020,Dec,3; 2018,Jan,8; 2017,Mar,6

80320-80377 [80320, 80321, 80322, 80323, 80324, 80325, 80326, 80327, 80328, 80329, 80330, 80331, 80332, 80333, 80334, 80335, 80336, 80337, 80338, 80339, 80340, 80341, 80342, 80343, 80344, 80345, 80346, 80347, 80348, 80349, 80350, 80351, 80352, 80353, 80354, 80355, 80356, 80357, 80358, 80359, 80360, 80361, 80362, 80363, 80364, 80365, 80366, 80367, 80368, 80369, 80370, 80371, 80372, 80373, 80374, 80375, 80376, 80377, 83992] Confirmatory Drug Testing

INCLUDES Antihistamine drug tests ([80375, 80376, 80377])
Detection specific drugs using methods other than immunoassay or enzymatic technique

EXCLUDES *Definitive drug testing for any drug class not specified; report with NOS codes ([80375, 80376, 80377])*
Metabolites separate from code for drug except when distinct code available

\# **80320 Alcohols**

EXCLUDES *Alcohol (ethanol) therapeutic drug assay (82077)*

0.00 0.00 FUD XXX

AMA: 2020,Dec,3; 2018,Jan,8; 2017,Jan,8; 2016,Jan,13

\# **80321 Alcohol biomarkers; 1 or 2**

0.00 0.00 FUD XXX

AMA: 2020,Dec,3

\# **80322 3 or more**

0.00 0.00 FUD XXX

AMA: 2020,Dec,3

\# **80323 Alkaloids, not otherwise specified**

0.00 0.00 FUD XXX

AMA: 2020,Dec,3

\# **80324 Amphetamines; 1 or 2**

0.00 0.00 FUD XXX

AMA: 2020,Dec,3

\# **80325 3 or 4**

0.00 0.00 FUD XXX

AMA: 2020,Dec,3

\# **80326 5 or more**

0.00 0.00 FUD XXX

AMA: 2020,Dec,3

\# **80327 Anabolic steroids; 1 or 2**

0.00 0.00 FUD XXX

AMA: 2020,Dec,3

\# **80328 3 or more**

EXCLUDES *Analysis dihydrotestosterone for monitoring, endogenous levels of hormone (82642)*

0.00 0.00 FUD XXX

AMA: 2020,Dec,3

\# **80329 Analgesics, non-opioid; 1 or 2**

EXCLUDES *Acetaminophen therapeutic drug assay (80143)*
Salicylate therapeutic drug assay ([80179])

0.00 0.00 FUD XXX

AMA: 2020,Dec,3

\# **80330 3-5**

EXCLUDES *Acetaminophen therapeutic drug assay (80143)*
Salicylate therapeutic drug assay ([80179])

0.00 0.00 FUD XXX

AMA: 2020,Dec,3

\# **80331 6 or more**

EXCLUDES *Acetaminophen therapeutic drug assay (80143)*
Salicylate therapeutic drug assay ([80179])

0.00 0.00 FUD XXX

AMA: 2020,Dec,3

\# **80332 Antidepressants, serotonergic class; 1 or 2**

0.00 0.00 FUD XXX

AMA: 2020,Dec,3

80333 3-5
0.00 0.00 FUD XXX
AMA: 2020,Dec,3

80334 6 or more
0.00 0.00 FUD XXX
AMA: 2020,Dec,3

80335 Antidepressants, tricyclic and other cyclicals; 1 or 2
0.00 0.00 FUD XXX
AMA: 2020,Dec,3

80336 3-5
0.00 0.00 FUD XXX
AMA: 2020,Dec,3

80337 6 or more
0.00 0.00 FUD XXX
AMA: 2020,Dec,3

80338 Antidepressants, not otherwise specified
0.00 0.00 FUD XXX
AMA: 2020,Dec,3

80339 Antiepileptics, not otherwise specified; 1-3
0.00 0.00 FUD XXX
AMA: 2020,Dec,3

80340 4-6
0.00 0.00 FUD XXX
AMA: 2020,Dec,3

80341 7 or more
EXCLUDES *Carbamazepine therapeutic drug assay (80156, 80157, [80161])*
Definitive drug testing for antihistamines ([80375, 80376, 80377])
0.00 0.00 FUD XXX
AMA: 2020,Dec,3

80342 Antipsychotics, not otherwise specified; 1-3
0.00 0.00 FUD XXX
AMA: 2020,Dec,3

80343 4-6
0.00 0.00 FUD XXX
AMA: 2020,Dec,3

80344 7 or more
0.00 0.00 FUD XXX
AMA: 2020,Dec,3

80345 Barbiturates
0.00 0.00 FUD XXX
AMA: 2020,Dec,3

80346 Benzodiazepines; 1-12
0.00 0.00 FUD XXX
AMA: 2020,Dec,3

80347 13 or more
0.00 0.00 FUD XXX
AMA: 2020,Dec,3

80348 Buprenorphine
0.00 0.00 FUD XXX
AMA: 2020,Dec,3

80349 Cannabinoids, natural
0.00 0.00 FUD XXX
AMA: 2020,Dec,3

80350 Cannabinoids, synthetic; 1-3
0.00 0.00 FUD XXX
AMA: 2020,Dec,3

80351 4-6
0.00 0.00 FUD XXX
AMA: 2020,Dec,3

80352 7 or more
0.00 0.00 FUD XXX
AMA: 2020,Dec,3

80353 Cocaine
0.00 0.00 FUD XXX
AMA: 2020,Dec,3

80354 Fentanyl
0.00 0.00 FUD XXX
AMA: 2020,Dec,3

80355 Gabapentin, non-blood
EXCLUDES *Therapeutic drug assay ([80171])*
0.00 0.00 FUD XXX
AMA: 2020,Dec,3; 2018,Jan,8; 2017,Jan,8; 2016,Jan,13

80356 Heroin metabolite
0.00 0.00 FUD XXX
AMA: 2020,Dec,3

80357 Ketamine and norketamine
0.00 0.00 FUD XXX
AMA: 2020,Dec,3

80358 Methadone
0.00 0.00 FUD XXX
AMA: 2020,Dec,3

80359 Methylenedioxyamphetamines (MDA, MDEA, MDMA)
0.00 0.00 FUD XXX
AMA: 2020,Dec,3

80360 Methylphenidate
0.00 0.00 FUD XXX
AMA: 2020,Dec,3

80361 Opiates, 1 or more
0.00 0.00 FUD XXX
AMA: 2020,Dec,3

80362 Opioids and opiate analogs; 1 or 2
0.00 0.00 FUD XXX
AMA: 2020,Dec,3

80363 3 or 4
0.00 0.00 FUD XXX
AMA: 2020,Dec,3

80364 5 or more
0.00 0.00 FUD XXX
AMA: 2020,Dec,3

80365 Oxycodone
0.00 0.00 FUD XXX
AMA: 2020,Dec,3

83992 Phencyclidine (PCP)
0.00 0.00 FUD XXX
AMA: 2020,Dec,3; 2018,Jan,8; 2017,Jan,8; 2016,Jan,13

80366 Pregabalin
0.00 0.00 FUD XXX
AMA: 2020,Dec,3

80367 Propoxyphene
0.00 0.00 FUD XXX
AMA: 2020,Dec,3

80368 Sedative hypnotics (non-benzodiazepines)
0.00 0.00 FUD XXX
AMA: 2020,Dec,3

80369 Skeletal muscle relaxants; 1 or 2
0.00 0.00 FUD XXX
AMA: 2020,Dec,3

80370 3 or more
0.00 0.00 FUD XXX
AMA: 2020,Dec,3

80371 Stimulants, synthetic
0.00 0.00 FUD XXX
AMA: 2020,Dec,3

80372 Tapentadol
0.00 0.00 FUD XXX
AMA: 2020,Dec,3

80373 Tramadol
0.00 0.00 FUD XXX
AMA: 2020,Dec,3

80374 Stereoisomer (enantiomer) analysis, single drug class
Code also index drug analysis when appropriate
0.00 0.00 FUD XXX
AMA: 2020,Dec,3

80375 Drug(s) or substance(s), definitive, qualitative or quantitative, not otherwise specified; 1-3
0.00 0.00 FUD XXX
AMA: 2020,Dec,3; 2018,Jan,8; 2017,Jan,8; 2016,Jan,13

80376 4-6
0.00 0.00 FUD XXX
AMA: 2020,Dec,3; 2018,Jan,8; 2017,Jan,8; 2016,Jan,13

80377 7 or more
EXCLUDES *Definitive drug testing for antihistamines ([80375, 80376, 80377])*
0.00 0.00 FUD XXX
AMA: 2020,Dec,3; 2018,Jan,8; 2017,Jan,8; 2016,Jan,13

80143-80377 [80161, 80164, 80165, 80167, 80171, 80176, 80179, 80181, 80189, 80193, 80204, 80210, 80220, 80230, 80235, 80280, 80285, 80305, 80306, 80307, 80320, 80321, 80322, 80323, 80324, 80325, 80326, 80327, 80328, 80329, 80330, 80331, 80332, 80333, 80334, 80335, 80336, 80337, 80338, 80339, 80340, 80341, 80342, 80343, 80344, 80345, 80346, 80347, 80348, 80349, 80350, 80351, 80352, 80353, 80354, 80355, 80356, 80357, 80358, 80359, 80360, 80361, 80362, 80363, 80364, 80365, 80366, 80367, 80368, 80369, 80370, 80371, 80372, 80373, 80374, 80375, 80376, 80377]

Therapeutic Drug Levels

INCLUDES Monitoring known, prescribed or over-the-counter medication levels
Testing drug and metabolite(s) in primary code
Tests on specimens from blood, blood components, and spinal fluid

80143 Acetaminophen
EXCLUDES *Acetaminophen confirmatory drug testing ([80329, 80330, 80331])*
0.00 0.00 FUD XXX
AMA: 2020,Dec,3

80145 Adalimumab
0.00 0.00 FUD XXX
AMA: 2020,Dec,3

80150 Amikacin
0.00 0.00 FUD XXX
AMA: 2020,Dec,3; 2018,Jan,8; 2017,Jan,8; 2016,Jan,13

80151 Amiodarone
0.00 0.00 FUD XXX
AMA: 2020,Dec,3

80155 Caffeine
0.00 0.00 FUD XXX
AMA: 2020,Dec,3

80156 Carbamazepine; total
0.00 0.00 FUD XXX
AMA: 2020,Dec,3; 2018,Jan,8; 2017,Jan,8; 2016,Jan,13

80157 free
0.00 0.00 FUD XXX
AMA: 2020,Dec,3; 2018,Jan,8; 2017,Jan,8; 2016,Jan,13

80161 -10,11-epoxide
0.00 0.00 FUD XXX
AMA: 2020,Dec,3

80158 Cyclosporine
0.00 0.00 FUD XXX
AMA: 2020,Dec,3; 2018,Jan,8; 2017,Jan,8; 2016,Jan,13

80159 Clozapine
0.00 0.00 FUD XXX
AMA: 2020,Dec,3

80161 Resequenced code. See code following 80157.

80162 Digoxin; total
0.00 0.00 FUD XXX
AMA: 2020,Dec,3; 2018,Jan,8; 2017,Jan,8; 2016,Jan,13

80163 free
0.00 0.00 FUD XXX
AMA: 2020,Dec,3; 2018,Jan,8; 2017,Jan,8; 2016,Jan,13

80164 Resequenced code. See code following 80201.

80165 Resequenced code. See code following 80201.

80167 Resequenced code. See code following 80169.

80168 Ethosuximide
0.00 0.00 FUD XXX
AMA: 2020,Dec,3; 2018,Jan,8; 2017,Jan,8; 2016,Jan,13

80169 Everolimus
0.00 0.00 FUD XXX
AMA: 2020,Dec,3

80167 Felbamate
0.00 0.00 FUD XXX
AMA: 2020,Dec,3

80181 Flecainide
0.00 0.00 FUD XXX
AMA: 2020,Dec,3

80171 Gabapentin, whole blood, serum, or plasma
0.00 0.00 FUD XXX
AMA: 2020,Dec,3; 2018,Jan,8; 2017,Jan,8; 2016,Jan,13

80170 Gentamicin
0.00 0.00 FUD XXX
AMA: 2020,Dec,3; 2018,Jan,8; 2017,Jan,8; 2016,Jan,13

80171 Resequenced code. See code before 80170.

80173 Haloperidol
0.00 0.00 FUD XXX
AMA: 2020,Dec,3; 2018,Jan,8; 2017,Jan,8; 2016,Jan,13

● # 80220 Hydroxychloroquine
0.00 0.00 FUD 000

80230 Infliximab
0.00 0.00 FUD XXX
AMA: 2020,Dec,3

80189 Itraconazole
0.00 0.00 FUD XXX
AMA: 2020,Dec,3

80235 Lacosamide
0.00 0.00 FUD XXX
AMA: 2020,Dec,3

80175 Lamotrigine
0.00 0.00 FUD XXX
AMA: 2020,Dec,3

80176 Resequenced code. See code following 80177.

80193 Leflunomide
0.00 0.00 FUD XXX
AMA: 2020,Dec,3

80177 Levetiracetam
0.00 0.00 FUD XXX
AMA: 2020,Dec,3

80176 Lidocaine
0.00 0.00 FUD XXX
AMA: 2020,Dec,3; 2018,Jan,8; 2017,Jan,8; 2016,Jan,13

80178 Lithium
0.00 0.00 FUD XXX
AMA: 2020,Dec,3; 2018,Jan,8; 2017,Jan,8; 2016,Jan,13

80204 Methotrexate
0.00 0.00 FUD XXX
AMA: 2020,Dec,3

80179 **Resequenced code. See code before 80195.**

80180 Mycophenolate (mycophenolic acid)
0.00 0.00 FUD XXX
AMA: 2020,Dec,3

80181 **Resequenced code. See code following resequenced code 80167.**

80183 Oxcarbazepine
0.00 0.00 FUD XXX
AMA: 2020,Dec,3

80184 Phenobarbital
0.00 0.00 FUD XXX
AMA: 2020,Dec,3; 2018,Jan,8; 2017,Jan,8; 2016,Jan,13

80185 Phenytoin; total
0.00 0.00 FUD XXX
AMA: 2020,Dec,3; 2018,Jan,8; 2017,Jan,8; 2016,Jan,13

80186 free
0.00 0.00 FUD XXX
AMA: 2020,Dec,3; 2018,Jan,8; 2017,Jan,8; 2016,Jan,13

80187 Posaconazole
0.00 0.00 FUD XXX
AMA: 2020,Dec,3

80188 Primidone
0.00 0.00 FUD XXX
AMA: 2020,Dec,3; 2018,Jan,8; 2017,Jan,8; 2016,Jan,13

80189 **Resequenced code. See code following resequenced code 80230.**

80190 Procainamide;
0.00 0.00 FUD XXX
AMA: 2020,Dec,3; 2018,Jan,8; 2017,Jan,8; 2016,Jan,13

80192 with metabolites (eg, n-acetyl procainamide)
0.00 0.00 FUD XXX
AMA: 2020,Dec,3; 2018,Jan,8; 2017,Jan,8; 2016,Jan,13

80193 **Resequenced code. See code before 80177.**

80194 Quinidine
0.00 0.00 FUD XXX
AMA: 2020,Dec,3; 2018,Jan,8; 2017,Jan,8; 2016,Jan,13

80210 Rufinamide
0.00 0.00 FUD XXX
AMA: 2020,Dec,3

80179 Salicylate
EXCLUDES *Salicylate confirmatory drug testing ([80329, 80330, 80331])*
0.00 0.00 FUD XXX
AMA: 2020,Dec,3

80195 Sirolimus
0.00 0.00 FUD XXX
AMA: 2020,Dec,3; 2018,Jan,8; 2017,Jan,8; 2016,Jan,13

80197 Tacrolimus
0.00 0.00 FUD XXX
AMA: 2020,Dec,3; 2018,Jan,8; 2017,Jan,8; 2016,Jan,13

80198 Theophylline
0.00 0.00 FUD XXX
AMA: 2020,Dec,3; 2018,Jan,8; 2017,Jan,8; 2016,Jan,13

80199 Tiagabine
0.00 0.00 FUD XXX
AMA: 2020,Dec,3

80200 Tobramycin
0.00 0.00 FUD XXX
AMA: 2020,Dec,3; 2018,Jan,8; 2017,Jan,8; 2016,Jan,13

80201 Topiramate
0.00 0.00 FUD XXX
AMA: 2020,Dec,3; 2018,Jan,8; 2017,Jan,8; 2016,Jan,13

80164 Valproic acid (dipropylacetic acid); total
0.00 0.00 FUD XXX
AMA: 2020,Dec,3; 2018,Jan,8; 2017,Jan,8; 2016,Jan,13

80165 free
0.00 0.00 FUD XXX
AMA: 2020,Dec,3; 2018,Jan,8; 2017,Jan,8; 2016,Jan,13

80202 Vancomycin
0.00 0.00 FUD XXX
AMA: 2020,Dec,3; 2018,Jan,8; 2017,Jan,8; 2016,Jan,13

80280 Vedolizumab
0.00 0.00 FUD XXX
AMA: 2020,Dec,3

80285 Voriconazole
0.00 0.00 FUD XXX
AMA: 2020,Dec,3

80203 Zonisamide
0.00 0.00 FUD XXX
AMA: 2020,Dec,3

80204 **Resequenced code. See code following 80178.**
80210 **Resequenced code. See code following 80194.**
80220 **Resequenced code. See code following 80173.**
80230 **Resequenced code. See code following 80173.**
80235 **Resequenced code. See code before 80175.**
80280 **Resequenced code. See code following 80202.**
80285 **Resequenced code. See code before 80203.**

80299 Quantitation of therapeutic drug, not elsewhere specified
0.00 0.00 FUD XXX
AMA: 2020,Dec,3; 2018,Jan,8; 2017,Jan,8; 2016,Jan,13

80305 **Resequenced code. See code before 80143.**
80306 **Resequenced code. See code before 80143.**
80307 **Resequenced code. See code before 80143.**
80320 **Resequenced code. See code before 80143.**
80321 **Resequenced code. See code before 80143.**
80322 **Resequenced code. See code before 80143.**
80323 **Resequenced code. See code before 80143.**
80324 **Resequenced code. See code before 80143.**
80325 **Resequenced code. See code before 80143.**
80326 **Resequenced code. See code before 80143.**
80327 **Resequenced code. See code before 80143.**
80328 **Resequenced code. See code before 80143.**
80329 **Resequenced code. See code before 80143.**
80330 **Resequenced code. See code before 80143.**
80331 **Resequenced code. See code before 80143.**
80332 **Resequenced code. See code before 80143.**
80333 **Resequenced code. See code before 80143.**
80334 **Resequenced code. See code before 80143.**
80335 **Resequenced code. See code before 80143.**
80336 **Resequenced code. See code before 80143.**
80337 **Resequenced code. See code before 80143.**
80338 **Resequenced code. See code before 80143.**

80339 **Resequenced code. See code before 80143.**

80340 **Resequenced code. See code following resequenced code 80339.**

80341 **Resequenced code. See code before 80143.**

80342 **Resequenced code. See code before 80143.**

80343 **Resequenced code. See code before 80143.**

80344 **Resequenced code. See code before 80143.**

80345 **Resequenced code. See code before 80143.**

80346 **Resequenced code. See code before 80143.**

80347 **Resequenced code. See code before 80143.**

80348 **Resequenced code. See code before 80143.**

80349 **Resequenced code. See code before 80143.**

80350 **Resequenced code. See code before 80143.**

80351 **Resequenced code. See code before 80143.**

80352 **Resequenced code. See code before 80143.**

80353 **Resequenced code. See code before 80143.**

80354 **Resequenced code. See code before 80143.**

80355 **Resequenced code. See code before 80143.**

80356 **Resequenced code. See code before 80143.**

80357 **Resequenced code. See code before 80143.**

80358 **Resequenced code. See code before 80143.**

80359 **Resequenced code. See code before 80143.**

80360 **Resequenced code. See code before 80143.**

80361 **Resequenced code. See code before 80143.**

80362 **Resequenced code. See code before 80143.**

80363 **Resequenced code. See code before 80143.**

80364 **Resequenced code. See code before 80143.**

80365 **Resequenced code. See code before 80143.**

80366 **Resequenced code. See code before 80143.**

80367 **Resequenced code. See code before 80143.**

80368 **Resequenced code. See code before 80143.**

80369 **Resequenced code. See code before 80143.**

80370 **Resequenced code. See code before 80143.**

80371 **Resequenced code. See code before 80143.**

80372 **Resequenced code. See code before 80143.**

80373 **Resequenced code. See code before 80143.**

80374 **Resequenced code. See code before 80143.**

80375 **Resequenced code. See code before 80143.**

80376 **Resequenced code. See code before 80143.**

80377 **Resequenced code. See code before 80143.**

80400-80439 Stimulation and Suppression Test Panels

EXCLUDES *Administration evocative or suppressive material (96365-96368, 96372, 96374-96376, C8957)*
Evocative or suppression test substances, when applicable
Physician monitoring and attendance during test (see E/M services)

80400 **ACTH stimulation panel; for adrenal insufficiency**
INCLUDES Cortisol x 2 (82533)
0.00 0.00 **FUD** XXX
AMA: 2020,Dec,3; 2018,Jan,8; 2017,Jan,8; 2016,Jan,13

80402 **for 21 hydroxylase deficiency**
INCLUDES 17 hydroxyprogesterone X 2 (83498)
Cortisol x 2 (82533)
0.00 0.00 **FUD** XXX
AMA: 2020,Dec,3

80406 **for 3 beta-hydroxydehydrogenase deficiency**
INCLUDES 17 hydroxypregnenolone x 2 (84143)
Cortisol x 2 (82533)
0.00 0.00 **FUD** XXX
AMA: 2020,Dec,3

80408 **Aldosterone suppression evaluation panel (eg, saline infusion)**
INCLUDES Aldosterone x 2 (82088)
Renin x 2 (84244)
0.00 0.00 **FUD** XXX
AMA: 2020,Dec,3

80410 **Calcitonin stimulation panel (eg, calcium, pentagastrin)**
INCLUDES Calcitonin x 3 (82308)
0.00 0.00 **FUD** XXX
AMA: 2020,Dec,3

80412 **Corticotropic releasing hormone (CRH) stimulation panel**
INCLUDES Adrenocorticotropic hormone (ACTH) x 6 (82024)
Cortisol x 6 (82533)
0.00 0.00 **FUD** XXX
AMA: 2020,Dec,3

80414 **Chorionic gonadotropin stimulation panel; testosterone response**
INCLUDES Testosterone x 2 on three pooled blood samples (84403)
0.00 0.00 **FUD** XXX
AMA: 2020,Dec,3

80415 **estradiol response**
INCLUDES Estradiol x 2 on three pooled blood samples (82670)
0.00 0.00 **FUD** XXX
AMA: 2020,Dec,3

80416 **Renal vein renin stimulation panel (eg, captopril)**
INCLUDES Renin x 6 (84244)
0.00 0.00 **FUD** XXX
AMA: 2020,Dec,3

80417 **Peripheral vein renin stimulation panel (eg, captopril)**
INCLUDES Renin x 2 (84244)
0.00 0.00 **FUD** XXX
AMA: 2020,Dec,3

80418 **Combined rapid anterior pituitary evaluation panel**
INCLUDES Adrenocorticotropic hormone (ACTH) x 4 (82024)
Cortisol x 4 (82533)
Follicle stimulating hormone (FSH) x 4 (83001)
Human growth hormone x 4 (83003)
Luteinizing hormone (LH) x 4 (83002)
Prolactin x 4 (84146)
Thyroid stimulating hormone (TSH) x 4 (84443)
0.00 0.00 **FUD** XXX
AMA: 2020,Dec,3

80420 **Dexamethasone suppression panel, 48 hour**
INCLUDES Cortisol x 2 (82533)
Free cortisol, urine x 2 (82530)
Volume measurement for timed collection x 2 (81050)
EXCLUDES *Single dose dexamethasone (82533)*
0.00 0.00 **FUD** XXX
AMA: 2020,Dec,3

80422 **Glucagon tolerance panel; for insulinoma**
INCLUDES Glucose x 3 (82947)
Insulin x 3 (83525)
0.00 0.00 **FUD** XXX
AMA: 2020,Dec,3

80424 **for pheochromocytoma**
INCLUDES Catecholamines, fractionated x 2 (82384)
0.00 0.00 **FUD** XXX
AMA: 2020,Dec,3

80426 Gonadotropin releasing hormone stimulation panel

INCLUDES Follicle stimulating hormone (FSH) x 4 (83001)
Luteinizing hormone (LH) x 4 (83002)

0.00 0.00 FUD XXX

AMA: 2020,Dec,3

80428 Growth hormone stimulation panel (eg, arginine infusion, l-dopa administration)

INCLUDES Human growth hormone (HGH) x 4 (83003)

0.00 0.00 FUD XXX

AMA: 2020,Dec,3

80430 Growth hormone suppression panel (glucose administration)

INCLUDES Glucose x 3 (82947)
Human growth hormone (HGH) x 4 (83003)

0.00 0.00 FUD XXX

AMA: 2020,Dec,3

80432 Insulin-induced C-peptide suppression panel

INCLUDES C-peptide x 5 (84681)
Glucose x 5 (82947)
Insulin (83525)

0.00 0.00 FUD XXX

AMA: 2020,Dec,3

80434 Insulin tolerance panel; for ACTH insufficiency

INCLUDES Cortisol x 5 (82533)
Glucose x 5 (82947)

0.00 0.00 FUD XXX

AMA: 2020,Dec,3

80435 for growth hormone deficiency

INCLUDES Glucose x 5 (82947)
Human growth hormone (HGH) x 5 (83003)

0.00 0.00 FUD XXX

AMA: 2020,Dec,3

80436 Metyrapone panel

INCLUDES 11 deoxycortisol x 2 (82634)
Cortisol x 2 (82533)

0.00 0.00 FUD XXX

AMA: 2020,Dec,3

80438 Thyrotropin releasing hormone (TRH) stimulation panel; 1 hour

INCLUDES Thyroid stimulating hormone (TSH) x 3 (84443)

0.00 0.00 FUD XXX

AMA: 2020,Dec,3

80439 2 hour

INCLUDES Thyroid stimulating hormone (TSH) x 4 (84443)

0.00 0.00 FUD XXX

AMA: 2020,Dec,3

80500-80506 Consultation By Clinical Pathologist

See also: Table 1: Medical Decision Making (MDM) Table for Pathology Clinical Consultations at beginning of Pathology chapter.

INCLUDES Appropriate consultation level selection based on total time for consultation services performed on date of service OR level of medical decision making
Clinical assessment, evaluation pathology/laboratory findings, other relevant clinical/diagnostic information requiring additional medical interpretative judgement
Consult rendered at request of physician, other qualified healt care professional (QHCP), or when mandated by federal or state regulation (i.e., Clinical Laboratory Improvement Amendments [CLIA])
Consultant time includes, when performed:
- Arriving at tentative conclusion/differential diagnosis
- Clinical consultation report documented in electronic or other health record
- Communicating with/referring to other health care professionals
- Ordering/recommending additional or follow up testing
- Reviewing complete medical history
- Reviewing test results, including all relevant past/current laboratory, pathology, radiology reports and images, and clinical testing/findings
- Total time spent on day of consultation personally spent by consultant, not clinical staff

EXCLUDES *Communicating laboratory/pathology results to patient, family, or caregiver (See appropriate E/M service level, if appropriate)*
Consultation, comprehensive, with records/specimen review and report, referred material (88325)
Consultation/report on referred material or slide prepared elsewhere (88321, 88323)
Reporting laboratory/pathology finding or other relevant clinical diagnostic information without medical interpretative judgement

80500 ~~Clinical pathology consultation; limited, without review of patient's history and medical records~~

To report, see (80503-80506)

80502 ~~comprehensive, for a complex diagnostic problem, with review of patient's history and medical records~~

To report, see (80503-80506)

● **80503 Pathology clinical consultation; for a clinical problem, with limited review of patient's history and medical records and straightforward medical decision making**

EXCLUDES *Consultations including patient examination/evaluation (99241-99245, 99251-99255)*

● **80504 for a moderately complex clinical problem, with review of patient's history and medical records and moderate level of medical decision making**

● **80505 for a highly complex clinical problem, with comprehensive review of patient's history and medical records and high level of medical decision making**

● + **80506 prolonged service, each additional 30 minutes (List separately in addition to code for primary procedure)**

EXCLUDES *Prolonged consultation time less than 15 additional minutes*

Code first (80505)

0.00 0.00 FUD 000

81000-81099 Urine Tests

81000 Urinalysis, by dip stick or tablet reagent for bilirubin, glucose, hemoglobin, ketones, leukocytes, nitrite, pH, protein, specific gravity, urobilinogen, any number of these constituents; non-automated, with microscopy

0.00 0.00 FUD XXX

AMA: 2020,Dec,3; 2018,Jul,14; 2018,Jan,8; 2017,Jan,8; 2016,Jan,13

81001 automated, with microscopy

0.00 0.00 FUD XXX

AMA: 2020,Dec,3

81002 non-automated, without microscopy

INCLUDES Mosenthal test

0.00 0.00 FUD XXX

AMA: 2020,Dec,3; 2018,Jan,8; 2017,Jan,8; 2016,Jan,13

81003 **automated, without microscopy**
0.00 0.00 FUD XXX
AMA: 2020,Dec,3; 2018,Jan,8; 2017,Jan,8; 2016,Jan,13

81005 **Urinalysis; qualitative or semiquantitative, except immunoassays**
INCLUDES Benedict test for dextrose
EXCLUDES *Immunoassay, qualitative or semiquantitative (83518)*
Microalbumin (82043-82044)
Nonimmunoassay reagent strip analysis (81000, 81002)
0.00 0.00 FUD XXX
AMA: 2020,Dec,3; 2018,Jan,8; 2017,Jan,8; 2016,Jan,13

81007 **bacteriuria screen, except by culture or dipstick**
EXCLUDES *Culture (87086-87088)*
Dipstick (81000, 81002)
0.00 0.00 FUD XXX
AMA: 2020,Dec,3

81015 **microscopic only**
EXCLUDES *Sperm evaluation for retrograde ejaculation (89331)*
0.00 0.00 FUD XXX
AMA: 2020,Dec,3; 2018,Jan,8; 2017,Nov,10

81020 **2 or 3 glass test**
INCLUDES Valentine's test
0.00 0.00 FUD XXX
AMA: 2020,Dec,3

81025 **Urine pregnancy test, by visual color comparison methods**
M ♀
0.00 0.00 FUD XXX
AMA: 2020,Dec,3; 2018,Jan,8; 2017,Jan,8; 2016,Jan,13

81050 **Volume measurement for timed collection, each**
0.00 0.00 FUD XXX
AMA: 2020,Dec,3

81099 **Unlisted urinalysis procedure**
0.00 0.00 FUD XXX
AMA: 2020,Dec,3; 2018,Jan,8; 2017,Jan,8; 2016,Jan,13

81105-81364 [81105, 81106, 81107, 81108, 81109, 81110, 81111, 81112, 81120, 81121, 81161, 81162, 81163, 81164, 81165, 81166, 81167, 81168, 81173, 81174, 81184, 81185, 81186, 81187, 81188, 81189, 81190, 81191, 81192, 81193, 81194, 81200, 81201, 81202, 81203, 81204, 81205, 81206, 81207, 81208, 81209, 81210, 81219, 81227, 81230, 81231, 81233, 81234, 81238, 81239, 81245, 81246, 81250, 81257, 81258, 81259, 81261, 81262, 81263, 81264, 81265, 81266, 81267, 81268, 81269, 81271, 81274, 81277, 81278, 81279, 81283, 81284, 81285, 81286, 81287, 81288, 81289, 81291, 81292, 81293, 81294, 81295, 81301, 81302, 81303, 81304, 81306, 81307, 81308, 81309, 81312, 81320, 81324, 81325, 81326, 81332, 81334, 81336, 81337, 81338, 81339, 81343, 81344, 81345, 81347, 81348, 81349, 81351, 81352, 81353, 81357, 81361, 81362, 81363, 81364] Gene Analysis: Tier 1 Procedures

INCLUDES All analytical procedures in evaluation:
- Amplification
- Cell lysis
- Detection
- Digestion
- Extraction
- Nucleic acid stabilization

Code selection based on specific gene being reviewed
Evaluation constitutional or somatic gene variations
Evaluation gene variant presence using common gene variant name
Gene specific and genomic testing
Generally, all listed gene variants in code description (lists not all inclusive)
Genes described using Human Genome Organization (HUGO) approved names
Protein or disease examples in code description not all inclusive
Qualitative results unless otherwise stated
Tier 1 molecular pathology codes (81105-81254 [81161, 81162, 81163, 81164, 81165, 81166, 81167, 81173, 81174, 81184, 81185, 81186, 81187, 81188, 81189, 81190, 81200, 81201, 81202, 81203, 81204, 81205, 81206, 81207, 81208, 81209, 81210, 81219, 81227, 81230, 81231, 81233, 81234, 81238, 81239, 81245, 81246, 81250, 81257, 81258, 81259, 81265, 81266, 81267, 81268, 81269, 81284, 81285, 81286, 81289, 81361, 81362, 81363, 81364])

EXCLUDES *Full gene sequencing using separate gene variant assessment codes unless specifically stated in code description*
In situ hybridization analyses (88271-88275, 88365-88368 [88364, 88373, 88374])
Microbial identification (87149-87153, 87471-87801 [87623, 87624, 87625], 87900-87904 [87906, 87910, 87912])
Other related gene variants not listed in code description
Tier 1 molecular pathology codes (81370-81383)
Tier 2 codes (81400-81408)
Unlisted molecular pathology procedures ([81479])

Code also:
Modifier 26 when only interpretation and report performed
Services required before cell lysis

81105 **Resequenced code. See code before 81260.**
81106 **Resequenced code. See code before 81260.**
81107 **Resequenced code. See code before 81260.**
81108 **Resequenced code. See code before 81260.**
81109 **Resequenced code. See code before 81260.**
81110 **Resequenced code. See code before 81260.**
81111 **Resequenced code. See code before 81260.**
81112 **Resequenced code. See code before 81260.**
81120 **Resequenced code. See code before 81260.**
81121 **Resequenced code. See code before 81260.**
81161 **Resequenced code. See code following numeric code 81231.**
81162 **Resequenced code. See code following resequenced code 81210.**
81163 **Resequenced code. See code following resequenced code 81210.**
81164 **Resequenced code. See code before 81212.**

Pathology and Laboratory 81003 — 81164

81165 **Resequenced code. See code following 81212.**

81166 **Resequenced code. See code following 81212.**

81167 **Resequenced code. See code following 81216.**

81168 **Resequenced code. See code before 81218.**

81170 ***ABL1 (ABL proto-oncogene 1, non-receptor tyrosine kinase)* (eg, acquired imatinib tyrosine kinase inhibitor resistance), gene analysis, variants in the kinase domain**
0.00 0.00 **FUD** XXX A
AMA: 2020,Dec,3; 2018,Jan,8; 2017,Jan,8; 2016,Aug,9

81171 ***AFF2 (AF4/FMR2 family, member 2 [FMR2])* (eg, fragile X mental retardation 2 [FRAXE]) gene analysis; evaluation to detect abnormal (eg, expanded) alleles**
0.00 0.00 **FUD** XXX
AMA: 2020,Dec,3

81172 **characterization of alleles (eg, expanded size and methylation status)**
0.00 0.00 **FUD** XXX
AMA: 2020,Dec,3

81173 **Resequenced code. See code following resequenced code 81204.**

81174 **Resequenced code. See code following resequenced code 81204.**

\# **81201** ***APC (adenomatous polyposis coli)* (eg, familial adenomatosis polyposis [FAP], attenuated FAP) gene analysis; full gene sequence**
0.00 0.00 **FUD** XXX A
AMA: 2020,Dec,3; 2020,OctSE,1; 2020,OctSE,1; 2018,Nov,9; 2018,Jan,8; 2017,Jan,8; 2016,Aug,9; 2016,Jan,13

\# **81202** **known familial variants**
0.00 0.00 **FUD** XXX A
AMA: 2020,Dec,3; 2020,OctSE,1; 2020,OctSE,1; 2018,Nov,9; 2018,Jan,8; 2017,Jan,8; 2016,Aug,9; 2016,Jan,13

\# **81203** **duplication/deletion variants**
0.00 0.00 **FUD** XXX A
AMA: 2020,Dec,3; 2020,OctSE,1; 2020,OctSE,1; 2018,Nov,9; 2018,Jan,8; 2017,Jan,8; 2016,Aug,9; 2016,Jan,13

\# **81204** ***AR (androgen receptor)* (eg, spinal and bulbar muscular atrophy, Kennedy disease, X chromosome inactivation) gene analysis; characterization of alleles (eg, expanded size or methylation status)**
0.00 0.00 **FUD** XXX
AMA: 2020,Dec,3; 2020,OctSE,1; 2020,OctSE,1; 2018,Nov,9

\# **81173** **full gene sequence**
0.00 0.00 **FUD** XXX
AMA: 2020,Dec,3

\# **81174** **known familial variant**
0.00 0.00 **FUD** XXX
AMA: 2020,Dec,3

\# **81200** ***ASPA (aspartoacylase)* (eg, Canavan disease) gene analysis, common variants (eg, E285A, Y231X)**
0.00 0.00 **FUD** XXX A
AMA: 2020,Dec,3; 2020,OctSE,1; 2020,OctSE,1; 2018,Nov,9; 2018,Jan,8; 2017,Jan,8; 2016,Aug,9; 2016,Jan,13

81175 ***ASXL1 (additional sex combs like 1, transcriptional regulator)* (eg, myelodysplastic syndrome, myeloproliferative neoplasms, chronic myelomonocytic leukemia), gene analysis; full gene sequence**
0.00 0.00 **FUD** XXX A
AMA: 2020,Dec,3

81176 **targeted sequence analysis (eg, exon 12)**
0.00 0.00 **FUD** XXX A
AMA: 2020,Dec,3

81177 ***ATN1 (atrophin 1)* (eg, dentatorubral-pallidoluysian atrophy) gene analysis, evaluation to detect abnormal (eg, expanded) alleles**
0.00 0.00 **FUD** XXX
AMA: 2020,Dec,3

81178 ***ATXN1 (ataxin 1)* (eg, spinocerebellar ataxia) gene analysis, evaluation to detect abnormal (eg, expanded) alleles**
0.00 0.00 **FUD** XXX
AMA: 2020,Dec,3; 2019,Sep,7

81179 ***ATXN2 (ataxin 2)* (eg, spinocerebellar ataxia) gene analysis, evaluation to detect abnormal (eg, expanded) alleles**
0.00 0.00 **FUD** XXX
AMA: 2020,Dec,3; 2019,Sep,7

81180 ***ATXN3 (ataxin 3)* (eg, spinocerebellar ataxia, Machado-Joseph disease) gene analysis, evaluation to detect abnormal (eg, expanded) alleles**
0.00 0.00 **FUD** XXX
AMA: 2020,Dec,3; 2019,Sep,7

81181 ***ATXN7 (ataxin 7)* (eg, spinocerebellar ataxia) gene analysis, evaluation to detect abnormal (eg, expanded) alleles**
0.00 0.00 **FUD** XXX
AMA: 2020,Dec,3; 2019,Sep,7

81182 ***ATXN8OS (ATXN8 opposite strand [non-protein coding])* (eg, spinocerebellar ataxia) gene analysis, evaluation to detect abnormal (eg, expanded) alleles**
0.00 0.00 **FUD** XXX
AMA: 2020,Dec,3; 2019,Sep,7

81183 ***ATXN10 (ataxin 10)* (eg, spinocerebellar ataxia) gene analysis, evaluation to detect abnormal (eg, expanded) alleles**
0.00 0.00 **FUD** XXX
AMA: 2020,Dec,3; 2019,Sep,7

81184 **Resequenced code. See code following resequenced code 81233.**

81185 **Resequenced code. See code following resequenced code 81233.**

81186 **Resequenced code. See code following resequenced code 81233.**

81187 **Resequenced code. See code following resequenced code 81268.**

81188 **Resequenced code. See code following resequenced code 81266.**

81189 **Resequenced code. See code following resequenced code 81266.**

81190 **Resequenced code. See code following resequenced code 81266.**

81191 **Resequenced code. See code following numeric code 81312.**

81192 **Resequenced code. See code following numeric code 81312.**

81193 **Resequenced code. See code following numeric code 81312.**

81194 **Resequenced code. See code following numeric code 81312.**

81200 **Resequenced code. See code before 81175.**

81201 **Resequenced code. See code following numeric code 81174.**

81202 **Resequenced code. See code following numeric code 81174.**

81203 **Resequenced code. See code following numeric code 81174.**

81204 **Resequenced code. See code following numeric code 81174.**

81205 **Resequenced code. See code following numeric code 81210.**

81206 **Resequenced code. See code following numeric code 81210.**

81207 **Resequenced code. See code following numeric code 81210.**

81208 **Resequenced code. See code following numeric code 81210.**

81209 **Resequenced code. See code following numeric code 81210.**

81210 **Resequenced code. See code following resequenced code 81209.**

\# **81205** ***BCKDHB (branched-chain keto acid dehydrogenase E1, beta polypeptide)* (eg, maple syrup urine disease) gene analysis, common variants (eg, R183P, G278S, E422X)**
0.00 0.00 **FUD** XXX
AMA: 2020,Dec,3; 2020,OctSE,1; 2020,OctSE,1; 2018,Nov,9; 2018,Jan,8; 2017,Jan,8; 2016,Aug,9; 2016,Jan,13

\# **81206** ***BCR/ABL1 (t(9;22))* (eg, chronic myelogenous leukemia) translocation analysis; major breakpoint, qualitative or quantitative**
0.00 0.00 **FUD** XXX
AMA: 2020,Dec,3; 2020,OctSE,1; 2020,OctSE,1; 2018,Nov,9; 2018,Jan,8; 2017,Jan,8; 2016,Aug,9; 2016,Jan,13

\# **81207** **minor breakpoint, qualitative or quantitative**
0.00 0.00 **FUD** XXX
AMA: 2020,Dec,3; 2020,OctSE,1; 2020,OctSE,1; 2018,Nov,9; 2018,Jan,8; 2017,Jan,8; 2016,Aug,9; 2016,Jan,13

\# **81208** **other breakpoint, qualitative or quantitative**
0.00 0.00 **FUD** XXX
AMA: 2020,Dec,3; 2020,OctSE,1; 2020,OctSE,1; 2018,Nov,9; 2018,Jan,8; 2017,Jan,8; 2016,Aug,9; 2016,Jan,13

\# **81209** ***BLM (Bloom syndrome, RecQ helicase-like)* (eg, Bloom syndrome) gene analysis, 2281del6ins7 variant**
0.00 0.00 **FUD** XXX
AMA: 2020,Dec,3; 2020,OctSE,1; 2020,OctSE,1; 2018,Nov,9; 2018,Jan,8; 2017,Jan,8; 2016,Aug,9; 2016,Jan,13

\# **81210** ***BRAF (B-Raf proto-oncogene, serine/threonine kinase)* (eg, colon cancer, melanoma), gene analysis, V600 variant(s)**
0.00 0.00 **FUD** XXX
AMA: 2020,Dec,3; 2020,OctSE,1; 2020,OctSE,1; 2018,Nov,9; 2018,Jan,8; 2017,Jan,8; 2016,Aug,9; 2016,Jan,13

\# **81162** ***BRCA1 (BRCA1, DNA repair associated), BRCA2 (BRCA2, DNA repair associated)* (eg, hereditary breast and ovarian cancer) gene analysis; full sequence analysis and full duplication/deletion analysis (ie, detection of large gene rearrangements)**

EXCLUDES *BRCA1 common duplication/deletion variant ([81479])*
BRCA1, BRCA2 full duplication/deletion analysis only (81164, 81166-81167, 81216)
BRCA1, BRCA2 full sequence analysis only (81163, 81165)
BRCA1, BRCA2 known familial variant only (81215, 81217)
Hereditary breast cancer genomic sequence analysis panel (81432)

0.00 0.00 **FUD** XXX
AMA: 2020,Dec,3; 2019,May,5; 2018,Jan,8; 2017,Jan,8; 2016,Aug,9

\# **81163** **full sequence analysis**

EXCLUDES *BRCA1 common duplication/deletion variant ([81479])*
BRCA1, BRCA2 full duplication/deletion analysis only (81164, 81216)
BRCA1, BRCA2 full sequence analysis and full duplication/deletion analysis (81162)
BRCA1, BRCA2 full sequence analysis only (81165)
Hereditary breast cancer genomic sequence analysis panel (81432)

0.00 0.00 **FUD** XXX
AMA: 2020,Dec,3; 2019,May,5

\# **81164** **full duplication/deletion analysis (ie, detection of large gene rearrangements)**

EXCLUDES *BRCA1 common duplication/deletion variant ([81479])*
BRCA1, BRCA2 full sequence analysis and full duplication/deletion analysis (81162)
BRCA1, BRCA2 full sequence analysis only (81163)
BRCA1, BRCA2 full duplication/deletion analysis only (81166-81167)
BRCA1, BRCA2 known familial variant only (81217)

0.00 0.00 **FUD** XXX
AMA: 2020,Dec,3; 2019,May,5

81212 **185delAG, 5385insC, 6174delT variants**
0.00 0.00 **FUD** XXX
AMA: 2020,Dec,3; 2020,OctSE,1; 2020,OctSE,1; 2019,May,5; 2018,Nov,9; 2018,Jan,8; 2017,Jan,8; 2016,Aug,9; 2016,Jan,13

\# **81165** ***BRCA1 (BRCA1, DNA repair associated)* (eg, hereditary breast and ovarian cancer) gene analysis; full sequence analysis**

EXCLUDES *BRCA1 common duplication/deletion variant ([81479])*
BRCA1, BRCA2 full sequence analysis and full duplication/deletion analysis (81162)
BRCA1, BRCA2 full sequence analysis only (81163)
Hereditary breast cancer genomic sequence analysis panel (81432)

0.00 0.00 **FUD** XXX
AMA: 2020,Dec,3; 2019,May,5

\# **81166** **full duplication/deletion analysis (ie, detection of large gene rearrangements)**

EXCLUDES *BRCA1 common duplication/deletion variant ([81479])*
BRCA1, BRCA2 full duplication/deletion analysis only (81164)
BRCA1, BRCA2 full sequence analysis and full duplication/deletion analysis (81162)

0.00 0.00 **FUD** XXX
AMA: 2020,Dec,3; 2019,May,5

81215 **known familial variant**

EXCLUDES *BRCA1 common duplication/deletion variant ([81479])*

0.00 0.00 **FUD** XXX
AMA: 2020,Dec,3; 2020,OctSE,1; 2020,OctSE,1; 2019,May,5; 2018,Nov,9; 2018,Jan,8; 2017,Jan,8; 2016,Aug,9; 2016,Jan,13

81216 ***BRCA2 (BRCA2, DNA repair associated)* (eg, hereditary breast and ovarian cancer) gene analysis; full sequence analysis**

EXCLUDES *BRCA1, BRCA2 full sequence analysis only (81163)*
BRCA1, BRCA2 full sequence analysis and full duplication/deletion analysis (81162)
Hereditary breast cancer genomic sequence analysis panel (81432)

0.00 0.00 **FUD** XXX
AMA: 2020,Dec,3; 2020,OctSE,1; 2020,OctSE,1; 2019,May,5; 2018,Nov,9; 2018,Jan,8; 2017,Jan,8; 2016,Aug,9; 2016,Jan,13

\# **81167** **full duplication/deletion analysis (ie, detection of large gene rearrangements)**

EXCLUDES *BRCA1, BRCA2 full duplication/deletion analysis only (81164, 81167)*
BRCA1, BRCA2 full sequence analysis and full duplication/deletion analysis (81162)

0.00 0.00 **FUD** XXX
AMA: 2020,Dec,3; 2019,May,5

81217 **known familial variant**

EXCLUDES *BRCA1, BRCA2 full duplication/deletion analysis only (81164, 81167)*
BRCA1, BRCA2 full sequence analysis and full duplication/deletion analysis (81162)

0.00 0.00 **FUD** XXX
AMA: 2020,Dec,3; 2020,OctSE,1; 2020,OctSE,1; 2019,May,5; 2018,Nov,9; 2018,Jan,8; 2017,Jan,8; 2016,Aug,9; 2016,Jan,13

\# **81233** ***BTK (Bruton's tyrosine kinase)* (eg, chronic lymphocytic leukemia) gene analysis, common variants (eg, C481S, C481R, C481F)**
0.00 0.00 **FUD** XXX
AMA: 2020,Dec,3; 2020,OctSE,1; 2020,OctSE,1; 2018,Nov,9

81184 *CACNA1A (calcium voltage-gated channel subunit alpha1 A)* (eg, spinocerebellar ataxia) gene analysis; evaluation to detect abnormal (eg, expanded) alleles
0.00 0.00 FUD XXX
AMA: 2020,Dec,3

81185 full gene sequence
0.00 0.00 FUD XXX
AMA: 2020,Dec,3

81186 known familial variant
0.00 0.00 FUD XXX
AMA: 2020,Dec,3

81219 *CALR (calreticulin)* (eg, myeloproliferative disorders), gene analysis, common variants in exon 9
0.00 0.00 FUD XXX
AMA: 2020,Dec,3; 2020,OctSE,1; 2020,OctSE,1; 2018,Nov,9; 2018,Jan,8; 2017,Jan,8; 2016,Aug,9

81168 *CCND1/IGH (t(11;14))* (eg, mantle cell lymphoma) translocation analysis, major breakpoint, qualitative and quantitative, if performed
0.00 0.00 FUD XXX
AMA: 2020,Dec,3

81218 *CEBPA (CCAAT/enhancer binding protein [C/EBP], alpha)* (eg, acute myeloid leukemia), gene analysis, full gene sequence
0.00 0.00 FUD XXX
AMA: 2020,Dec,3; 2020,OctSE,1; 2020,OctSE,1; 2018,Nov,9; 2018,Jan,8; 2017,Jan,8; 2016,Aug,9

81219 **Resequenced code. See code before 81218.**

81220 *CFTR (cystic fibrosis transmembrane conductance regulator)* (eg, cystic fibrosis) gene analysis; common variants (eg, ACMG/ACOG guidelines)

EXCLUDES *Excludes Intron 8 poly-T analysis performed in conjunction with 81220 in R117H positive patient*

0.00 0.00 FUD XXX
AMA: 2020,Dec,3; 2020,OctSE,1; 2020,OctSE,1; 2018,Nov,9; 2018,Jan,8; 2017,Jan,8; 2016,Aug,9; 2016,Jan,13

81221 known familial variants
0.00 0.00 FUD XXX
AMA: 2020,Dec,3; 2020,OctSE,1; 2020,OctSE,1; 2018,Nov,9; 2018,Jan,8; 2017,Jan,8; 2016,Aug,9; 2016,Jan,13

81222 duplication/deletion variants
0.00 0.00 FUD XXX
AMA: 2020,Dec,3; 2020,OctSE,1; 2020,OctSE,1; 2018,Nov,9; 2018,Jan,8; 2017,Jan,8; 2016,Aug,9; 2016,Jan,13

81223 full gene sequence
0.00 0.00 FUD XXX
AMA: 2020,Dec,3; 2020,OctSE,1; 2020,OctSE,1; 2018,Nov,9; 2018,Jan,8; 2017,Jan,8; 2016,Aug,9; 2016,Jan,13

81224 intron 8 poly-T analysis (eg, male infertility)
0.00 0.00 FUD XXX
AMA: 2020,Dec,3; 2020,OctSE,1; 2020,OctSE,1; 2018,Nov,9; 2018,Jan,8; 2017,Jan,8; 2016,Aug,9; 2016,Jan,13

81267 Chimerism (engraftment) analysis, post transplantation specimen (eg, hematopoietic stem cell), includes comparison to previously performed baseline analyses; without cell selection
0.00 0.00 FUD XXX
AMA: 2020,Dec,3; 2020,OctSE,1; 2020,OctSE,1; 2018,Nov,9; 2018,Jan,8; 2017,Jan,8; 2016,Aug,9; 2016,Jan,13

81268 with cell selection (eg, CD3, CD33), each cell type
0.00 0.00 FUD XXX
AMA: 2020,Dec,3; 2020,OctSE,1; 2020,OctSE,1; 2018,Nov,9; 2018,Jan,8; 2017,Jan,8; 2016,Aug,9; 2016,Jan,13

81187 *CNBP (CCHC-type zinc finger nucleic acid binding protein)* (eg, myotonic dystrophy type 2) gene analysis, evaluation to detect abnormal (eg, expanded) alleles
0.00 0.00 FUD XXX
AMA: 2020,Dec,3

81265 Comparative analysis using Short Tandem Repeat (STR) markers; patient and comparative specimen (eg, pre-transplant recipient and donor germline testing, post-transplant non-hematopoietic recipient germline [eg, buccal swab or other germline tissue sample] and donor testing, twin zygosity testing, or maternal cell contamination of fetal cells)
0.00 0.00 FUD XXX
AMA: 2020,Dec,3; 2020,OctSE,1; 2020,OctSE,1; 2018,Nov,9; 2018,Jan,8; 2017,Jan,8; 2016,Aug,9; 2016,Jan,13

+ # **81266** each additional specimen (eg, additional cord blood donor, additional fetal samples from different cultures, or additional zygosity in multiple birth pregnancies) (List separately in addition to code for primary procedure)
Code first ([81265])
0.00 0.00 FUD XXX
AMA: 2020,Dec,3; 2020,OctSE,1; 2020,OctSE,1; 2018,Nov,9; 2018,Jan,8; 2017,Jan,8; 2016,Aug,9; 2016,Jan,13

81188 *CSTB (cystatin B)* (eg, Unverricht-Lundborg disease) gene analysis; evaluation to detect abnormal (eg, expanded) alleles
0.00 0.00 FUD XXX
AMA: 2020,Dec,3

81189 full gene sequence
0.00 0.00 FUD XXX
AMA: 2020,Dec,3

81190 known familial variant(s)
0.00 0.00 FUD XXX
AMA: 2020,Dec,3

81227 *CYP2C9 (cytochrome P450, family 2, subfamily C, polypeptide 9)* (eg, drug metabolism), gene analysis, common variants (eg, *2, *3, *5, *6)
0.00 0.00 FUD XXX
AMA: 2020,Dec,3; 2020,OctSE,1; 2020,OctSE,1; 2018,Nov,9; 2018,Jan,8; 2017,Jan,8; 2016,Aug,9; 2016,Jan,13

81225 *CYP2C19 (cytochrome P450, family 2, subfamily C, polypeptide 19)* (eg, drug metabolism), gene analysis, common variants (eg, *2, *3, *4, *8, *17)
0.00 0.00 FUD XXX
AMA: 2020,Dec,3; 2020,OctSE,1; 2020,OctSE,1; 2018,Nov,9; 2018,Jan,8; 2017,Jan,8; 2016,Aug,9; 2016,Jan,13

81226 *CYP2D6 (cytochrome P450, family 2, subfamily D, polypeptide 6)* (eg, drug metabolism), gene analysis, common variants (eg, *2, *3, *4, *5, *6, *9, *10, *17, *19, *29, *35, *41, *1XN, *2XN, *4XN)
0.00 0.00 FUD XXX
AMA: 2020,Dec,3; 2020,OctSE,1; 2020,OctSE,1; 2018,Nov,9; 2018,Jan,8; 2017,Jan,8; 2016,Aug,9; 2016,Jan,13

81227 **Resequenced code. See code before 81225.**

81230 *CYP3A4 (cytochrome P450 family 3 subfamily A member 4)* (eg, drug metabolism), gene analysis, common variant(s) (eg, *2, *22)
0.00 0.00 FUD XXX
AMA: 2020,Dec,3; 2020,OctSE,1; 2020,OctSE,1; 2018,Nov,9

81231 *CYP3A5 (cytochrome P450 family 3 subfamily A member 5)* (eg, drug metabolism), gene analysis, common variants (eg, *2, *3, *4, *5, *6, *7)
0.00 0.00 FUD XXX
AMA: 2020,Dec,3; 2020,OctSE,1; 2020,OctSE,1; 2018,Nov,9

▲ **81228 Cytogenomic (genome-wide) analysis for constitutional chromosomal abnormalities; interrogation of genomic regions for copy number variants, comparative genomic hybridization [CGH] microarray analysis**

EXCLUDES *Analyte-specific molecular pathology procedures included in microarray analysis*
When performed in conjunction with:
Cytogenomic (genome-wide) analysis for constitutional chromosomal abnormalities ([81349])
Single nucleotide polymorphism interrogation (81229)

0.00 0.00 FUD XXX

AMA: 2020,Dec,3; 2020,OctSE,1; 2020,OctSE,1; 2018,Nov,9; 2018,Jan,8; 2017,Apr,3; 2017,Jan,8; 2016,Aug,9; 2016,Jan,13

▲ **81229 interrogation of genomic regions for copy number and single nucleotide polymorphism (SNP) variants, comparative genomic hybridization (CGH) microarray analysis**

EXCLUDES *Analyte-specific molecular pathology procedures included in microarray analysis*
Copy number variant detection using oligonucleotide interrogation only (81228)
Cytogenomic (genome-wide) analysis for constitutional chromosomal abnormalities ([81349])
Fetal genomic sequencing or other molecular multianalyte assays using circulating cell-free DNA in maternal blood ([81479], 81420, 81422)
Molecular cytogenetics; DNA probe (88271)

0.00 0.00 FUD XXX

AMA: 2020,Dec,3; 2020,OctSE,1; 2020,OctSE,1; 2018,Nov,9; 2018,Jan,8; 2017,Apr,3; 2017,Jan,8; 2016,Aug,9; 2016,Jan,13

● # **81349 interrogation of genomic regions for copy number and loss-of-heterozygosity variants, low-pass sequencing analysis**

EXCLUDES *Analyte-specific molecular pathology procedures included in microarray analysis*
Chromosomal abnormalities by sequence analysis (81425-81426)
Chromosomal abnormalities not genome-wide, report instead code for targeted analyis or unlisted code ([81479])
Cytogenomic (genome-wide) analysis for constitutional chromosomal abnormalities (81228-81229)

0.00 0.00 FUD 000

81277 Cytogenomic neoplasia (genome-wide) microarray analysis, interrogation of genomic regions for copy number and loss-of-heterozygosity variants for chromosomal abnormalities

EXCLUDES *Analyte-specific molecular pathology procedures included in microarray analysis for neoplasia*
Molecular cytogenetics; DNA probe (88271)

0.00 0.00 FUD XXX

AMA: 2020,Dec,3; 2020,OctSE,1; 2020,OctSE,1; 2020,Feb,10

81230 **Resequenced code. See code following numeric code 81227.**

81231 **Resequenced code. See code following numeric code 81227.**

81161 *DMD (dystrophin)* (eg, Duchenne/Becker muscular dystrophy) deletion analysis, and duplication analysis, if performed

0.00 0.00 FUD XXX

AMA: 2020,Dec,3; 2020,OctSE,1; 2020,OctSE,1; 2018,Nov,9; 2018,Jan,8; 2017,Jan,8; 2016,Aug,9

81234 *DMPK (DM1 protein kinase)* (eg, myotonic dystrophy type 1) gene analysis; evaluation to detect abnormal (expanded) alleles

0.00 0.00 FUD XXX

AMA: 2020,Dec,3; 2020,OctSE,1; 2020,OctSE,1; 2018,Nov,9

81239 characterization of alleles (eg, expanded size)

0.00 0.00 FUD XXX

AMA: 2020,Dec,3; 2020,OctSE,1; 2020,OctSE,1; 2018,Nov,9

81232 *DPYD (dihydropyrimidine dehydrogenase)* (eg, 5-fluorouracil/5-FU and capecitabine drug metabolism), gene analysis, common variant(s) (eg, *2A, *4, *5, *6)

0.00 0.00 FUD XXX

AMA: 2020,Dec,3; 2020,OctSE,1; 2020,OctSE,1; 2018,Nov,9

81233 **Resequenced code. See code following 81217.**

81234 **Resequenced code. See code following numeric code 81231.**

81235 *EGFR (epidermal growth factor receptor)* (eg, non-small cell lung cancer) gene analysis, common variants (eg, exon 19 LREA deletion, L858R, T790M, G719A, G719S, L861Q)

0.00 0.00 FUD XXX

AMA: 2020,Dec,3; 2020,OctSE,1; 2020,OctSE,1; 2018,Nov,9; 2018,Jan,8; 2017,Jan,8; 2016,Aug,9; 2016,Jan,13

81236 *EZH2 (enhancer of zeste 2 polycomb repressive complex 2 subunit)* (eg, myelodysplastic syndrome, myeloproliferative neoplasms) gene analysis, full gene sequence

0.00 0.00 FUD XXX

AMA: 2020,Dec,3; 2020,OctSE,1; 2020,OctSE,1; 2019,Jul,3; 2018,Nov,9

81237 *EZH2 (enhancer of zeste 2 polycomb repressive complex 2 subunit)* (eg, diffuse large B-cell lymphoma) gene analysis, common variant(s) (eg, codon 646)

0.00 0.00 FUD XXX

AMA: 2020,Dec,3; 2020,OctSE,1; 2020,OctSE,1; 2019,Jul,3; 2018,Nov,9

81238 **Resequenced code. See code following 81241.**

81239 **Resequenced code. See code before 81232.**

81240 *F2 (prothrombin, coagulation factor II)* (eg, hereditary hypercoagulability) gene analysis, 20210G>A variant

0.00 0.00 FUD XXX

AMA: 2020,Dec,3; 2020,OctSE,1; 2020,OctSE,1; 2018,Nov,9; 2018,Jan,8; 2017,Jan,8; 2016,Aug,9; 2016,Jan,13

81241 *F5 (coagulation factor V)* (eg, hereditary hypercoagulability) gene analysis, Leiden variant

0.00 0.00 FUD XXX

AMA: 2020,Dec,3; 2020,OctSE,1; 2020,OctSE,1; 2018,Nov,9; 2018,Jan,8; 2017,Jan,8; 2016,Aug,9; 2016,Jan,13

81238 *F9 (coagulation factor IX)* (eg, hemophilia B), full gene sequence

0.00 0.00 FUD XXX

AMA: 2020,Dec,3; 2020,OctSE,1; 2020,OctSE,1; 2018,Nov,9

81242 *FANCC (Fanconi anemia, complementation group C)* (eg, Fanconi anemia, type C) gene analysis, common variant (eg, IVS4+4A>T)

0.00 0.00 FUD XXX

AMA: 2020,Dec,3; 2020,OctSE,1; 2020,OctSE,1; 2018,Nov,9; 2018,Jan,8; 2017,Jan,8; 2016,Aug,9; 2016,Jan,13

81245 *FLT3 (fms-related tyrosine kinase 3)* (eg, acute myeloid leukemia), gene analysis; internal tandem duplication (ITD) variants (ie, exons 14, 15)

0.00 0.00 FUD XXX

AMA: 2020,Dec,3; 2020,OctSE,1; 2020,OctSE,1; 2018,Nov,9; 2018,Jan,8; 2017,Jan,8; 2016,Aug,9; 2016,Jan,13

81246 tyrosine kinase domain (TKD) variants (eg, D835, I836)

0.00 0.00 FUD XXX

AMA: 2020,Dec,3; 2020,OctSE,1; 2020,OctSE,1; 2018,Nov,9; 2018,Jan,8; 2017,Jan,8; 2016,Aug,9; 2016,Jan,13

81243 *FMR1 (fragile X mental retardation 1)* (eg, fragile X mental retardation) gene analysis; evaluation to detect abnormal (eg, expanded) alleles

INCLUDES Evaluation to detect and characterize abnormal alleles using single assay [i.e., PCR]

EXCLUDES *Evaluation to detect and characterize abnormal alleles (81244)*

0.00 0.00 FUD XXX

AMA: 2020,Dec,3; 2020,OctSE,1; 2020,OctSE,1; 2019,Jul,3; 2018,Nov,9; 2018,Jan,8; 2017,Jan,8; 2016,Aug,9; 2016,Jan,13

81244 **characterization of alleles (eg, expanded size and promoter methylation status)**

EXCLUDES *Evaluation to detect and characterize abnormal alleles using single assay [i.e., PCR] (81243)*

0.00 0.00 **FUD** XXX A

AMA: 2020,Dec,3; 2020,OctSE,1; 2020,OctSE,1; 2019,Jul,3; 2018,Nov,9; 2018,Jan,8; 2017,Jan,8; 2016,Aug,9; 2016,Jan,13

81245 **Resequenced code. See code following 81242.**

81246 **Resequenced code. See code following 81242.**

\# 81284 ***FXN (frataxin)* (eg, Friedreich ataxia) gene analysis; evaluation to detect abnormal (expanded) alleles**

0.00 0.00 **FUD** XXX

AMA: 2020,Dec,3; 2020,OctSE,1; 2020,OctSE,1; 2018,Nov,9

\# 81285 **characterization of alleles (eg, expanded size)**

0.00 0.00 **FUD** XXX

AMA: 2020,Dec,3; 2020,OctSE,1; 2020,OctSE,1; 2018,Nov,9

\# 81286 **full gene sequence**

0.00 0.00 **FUD** XXX

AMA: 2020,Dec,3; 2020,OctSE,1; 2020,OctSE,1; 2018,Nov,9

\# 81289 **known familial variant(s)**

0.00 0.00 **FUD** XXX

AMA: 2020,Dec,3; 2020,OctSE,1; 2020,OctSE,1; 2018,Nov,9

\# 81250 ***G6PC (glucose-6-phosphatase, catalytic subunit)* (eg, Glycogen storage disease, type 1a, von Gierke disease) gene analysis, common variants (eg, R83C, Q347X)**

0.00 0.00 **FUD** XXX A

AMA: 2020,Dec,3; 2020,OctSE,1; 2020,OctSE,1; 2018,Nov,9; 2018,Jan,8; 2017,Jan,8; 2016,Aug,9; 2016,Jan,13

81247 ***G6PD (glucose-6-phosphate dehydrogenase)* (eg, hemolytic anemia, jaundice), gene analysis; common variant(s) (eg, A, A-)**

0.00 0.00 **FUD** XXX A

AMA: 2020,Dec,3; 2020,OctSE,1; 2020,OctSE,1; 2018,Nov,9

81248 **known familial variant(s)**

0.00 0.00 **FUD** XXX A

AMA: 2020,Dec,3; 2020,OctSE,1; 2020,OctSE,1; 2018,Nov,9

81249 **full gene sequence**

0.00 0.00 **FUD** XXX A

AMA: 2020,Dec,3; 2020,OctSE,1; 2020,OctSE,1; 2018,Nov,9

81250 **Resequenced code. See code before 81247.**

81251 ***GBA (glucosidase, beta, acid)* (eg, Gaucher disease) gene analysis, common variants (eg, N370S, 84GG, L444P, IVS2+1G>A)**

0.00 0.00 **FUD** XXX A

AMA: 2020,Dec,3; 2020,OctSE,1; 2020,OctSE,1; 2018,Nov,9; 2018,Jan,8; 2017,Jan,8; 2016,Aug,9; 2016,Jan,13

81252 ***GJB2 (gap junction protein, beta 2, 26kDa, connexin 26)* (eg, nonsyndromic hearing loss) gene analysis; full gene sequence**

0.00 0.00 **FUD** XXX A

AMA: 2020,Dec,3; 2020,OctSE,1; 2020,OctSE,1; 2018,Nov,9; 2018,Jan,8; 2017,Jan,8; 2016,Aug,9; 2016,Jan,13

81253 **known familial variants**

0.00 0.00 **FUD** XXX A

AMA: 2020,Dec,3; 2020,OctSE,1; 2020,OctSE,1; 2018,Nov,9; 2018,Jan,8; 2017,Jan,8; 2016,Aug,9; 2016,Jan,13

81254 ***GJB6 (gap junction protein, beta 6, 30kDa, connexin 30)* (eg, nonsyndromic hearing loss) gene analysis, common variants (eg, 309kb [del(GJB6-D13S1830)] and 232kb [del(GJB6-D13S1854)])**

0.00 0.00 **FUD** XXX A

AMA: 2020,Dec,3; 2020,OctSE,1; 2020,OctSE,1; 2018,Nov,9; 2018,Jan,8; 2017,Jan,8; 2016,Aug,9; 2016,Jan,13

\# 81257 ***HBA1/HBA2 (alpha globin 1 and alpha globin 2)* (eg, alpha thalassemia, Hb Bart hydrops fetalis syndrome, HbH disease), gene analysis; common deletions or variant (eg, Southeast Asian, Thai, Filipino, Mediterranean, alpha3.7, alpha4.2, alpha20.5, Constant Spring)**

0.00 0.00 **FUD** XXX A

AMA: 2020,Dec,3; 2020,OctSE,1; 2020,OctSE,1; 2018,Nov,9; 2018,Jan,8; 2017,Jan,8; 2016,Aug,9; 2016,Jan,13

\# 81258 **known familial variant**

0.00 0.00 **FUD** XXX A

AMA: 2020,Dec,3; 2020,OctSE,1; 2020,OctSE,1; 2018,Nov,9

\# 81259 **full gene sequence**

0.00 0.00 **FUD** XXX A

AMA: 2020,Dec,3; 2020,OctSE,1; 2020,OctSE,1; 2018,Nov,9

\# 81269 **duplication/deletion variants**

0.00 0.00 **FUD** XXX A

AMA: 2020,Dec,3; 2020,OctSE,1; 2020,OctSE,1; 2018,Nov,9

\# 81361 ***HBB (hemoglobin, subunit beta)* (eg, sickle cell anemia, beta thalassemia, hemoglobinopathy); common variant(s) (eg, HbS, HbC, HbE)**

0.00 0.00 **FUD** XXX A

AMA: 2020,Dec,3; 2020,OctSE,1; 2020,OctSE,1; 2018,Nov,9

\# 81362 **known familial variant(s)**

0.00 0.00 **FUD** XXX A

AMA: 2020,Dec,3; 2020,OctSE,1; 2020,OctSE,1; 2018,Nov,9

\# 81363 **duplication/deletion variant(s)**

0.00 0.00 **FUD** XXX A

AMA: 2020,Dec,3; 2020,OctSE,1; 2020,OctSE,1; 2018,Nov,9; 2018,Sep,14

\# 81364 **full gene sequence**

0.00 0.00 **FUD** XXX A

AMA: 2020,Dec,3; 2020,OctSE,1; 2020,OctSE,1; 2018,Nov,9; 2018,Sep,14

81255 ***HEXA (hexosaminidase A [alpha polypeptide])* (eg, Tay-Sachs disease) gene analysis, common variants (eg, 1278insTATC, 1421+1G>C, G269S)**

0.00 0.00 **FUD** XXX A

AMA: 2020,Dec,3; 2020,OctSE,1; 2020,OctSE,1; 2018,Nov,9; 2018,Jan,8; 2017,Jan,8; 2016,Aug,9; 2016,Jan,13

81256 ***HFE (hemochromatosis)* (eg, hereditary hemochromatosis) gene analysis, common variants (eg, C282Y, H63D)**

0.00 0.00 **FUD** XXX A

AMA: 2020,Dec,3; 2020,OctSE,1; 2020,OctSE,1; 2018,Nov,9; 2018,Jan,8; 2017,Jan,8; 2016,Aug,9; 2016,Jan,13

81257 **Resequenced code. See code following 81254.**

81258 **Resequenced code. See code following 81254.**

81259 **Resequenced code. See code following 81254.**

\# 81271 ***HTT (huntingtin)* (eg, Huntington disease) gene analysis; evaluation to detect abnormal (eg, expanded) alleles**

0.00 0.00 **FUD** XXX

AMA: 2020,Dec,3; 2020,OctSE,1; 2020,OctSE,1; 2018,Nov,9

\# 81274 **characterization of alleles (eg, expanded size)**

0.00 0.00 **FUD** XXX

AMA: 2020,Dec,3; 2020,OctSE,1; 2020,OctSE,1; 2018,Nov,9

\# 81105 ***Human Platelet Antigen 1 genotyping (HPA-1), ITGB3 (integrin, beta 3 [platelet glycoprotein IIIa], antigen CD61 [GPIIIa])* (eg, neonatal alloimmune thrombocytopenia [NAIT], post-transfusion purpura), gene analysis, common variant, HPA-1a/b (L33P)**

0.00 0.00 **FUD** XXX A

AMA: 2020,Dec,3

\# **81106** ***Human Platelet Antigen 2 genotyping (HPA-2), GP1BA (glycoprotein Ib [platelet], alpha polypeptide [GPIba])*** **(eg, neonatal alloimmune thrombocytopenia [NAIT], post-transfusion purpura), gene analysis, common variant, HPA-2a/b (T145M)**
0.00 0.00 FUD XXX
AMA: 2020,Dec,3

\# **81107** ***Human Platelet Antigen 3 genotyping (HPA-3), ITGA2B (integrin, alpha 2b [platelet glycoprotein IIb of IIb/IIIa complex], antigen CD41 [GPIIb])*** **(eg, neonatal alloimmune thrombocytopenia [NAIT], post-transfusion purpura), gene analysis, common variant, HPA-3a/b (I843S)**
0.00 0.00 FUD XXX
AMA: 2020,Dec,3

\# **81108** ***Human Platelet Antigen 4 genotyping (HPA-4), ITGB3 (integrin, beta 3 [platelet glycoprotein IIIa], antigen CD61 [GPIIIa])*** **(eg, neonatal alloimmune thrombocytopenia [NAIT], post-transfusion purpura), gene analysis, common variant, HPA-4a/b (R143Q)**
0.00 0.00 FUD XXX
AMA: 2020,Dec,3

\# **81109** ***Human Platelet Antigen 5 genotyping (HPA-5), ITGA2 (integrin, alpha 2 [CD49B, alpha 2 subunit of VLA-2 receptor] [GPIa])*** **(eg, neonatal alloimmune thrombocytopenia [NAIT], post-transfusion purpura), gene analysis, common variant (eg, HPA-5a/b (K505E))**
0.00 0.00 FUD XXX
AMA: 2020,Dec,3

\# **81110** ***Human Platelet Antigen 6 genotyping (HPA-6w), ITGB3 (integrin, beta 3 [platelet glycoprotein IIIa, antigen CD61] [GPIIIa])*** **(eg, neonatal alloimmune thrombocytopenia [NAIT], post-transfusion purpura), gene analysis, common variant, HPA-6a/b (R489Q)**
0.00 0.00 FUD XXX
AMA: 2020,Dec,3

\# **81111** ***Human Platelet Antigen 9 genotyping (HPA-9w), ITGA2B (integrin, alpha 2b [platelet glycoprotein IIb of IIb/IIIa complex, antigen CD41] [GPIIb])*** **(eg, neonatal alloimmune thrombocytopenia [NAIT], post-transfusion purpura), gene analysis, common variant, HPA-9a/b (V837M)**
0.00 0.00 FUD XXX
AMA: 2020,Dec,3

\# **81112** ***Human Platelet Antigen 15 genotyping (HPA-15), CD109 (CD109 molecule)*** **(eg, neonatal alloimmune thrombocytopenia [NAIT], post-transfusion purpura), gene analysis, common variant, HPA-15a/b (S682Y)**
0.00 0.00 FUD XXX
AMA: 2020,Dec,3

\# **81120** ***IDH1 (isocitrate dehydrogenase 1 [NADP+], soluble)*** **(eg, glioma), common variants (eg, R132H, R132C)**
0.00 0.00 FUD XXX
AMA: 2020,Dec,3

\# **81121** ***IDH2 (isocitrate dehydrogenase 2 [NADP+], mitochondrial)*** **(eg, glioma), common variants (eg, R140W, R172M)**
0.00 0.00 FUD XXX
AMA: 2020,Dec,3

\# **81283** ***IFNL3 (interferon, lambda 3)*** **(eg, drug response), gene analysis, rs12979860 variant**
0.00 0.00 FUD XXX
AMA: 2020,Dec,3; 2020,OctSE,1; 2020,OctSE,1; 2018,Nov,9

\# **81261** ***IGH@ (Immunoglobulin heavy chain locus)*** **(eg, leukemias and lymphomas, B-cell), gene rearrangement analysis to detect abnormal clonal population(s); amplified methodology (eg, polymerase chain reaction)**
0.00 0.00 FUD XXX
AMA: 2020,Dec,3; 2020,OctSE,1; 2020,OctSE,1; 2018,Nov,9; 2018,Jan,8; 2017,Jan,8; 2016,Aug,9; 2016,Jan,13

\# **81262** **direct probe methodology (eg, Southern blot)**
0.00 0.00 FUD XXX
AMA: 2020,Dec,3; 2020,OctSE,1; 2020,OctSE,1; 2018,Nov,9; 2018,Jan,8; 2017,Jan,8; 2016,Aug,9; 2016,Jan,13

\# **81263** ***IGH@ (Immunoglobulin heavy chain locus)*** **(eg, leukemia and lymphoma, B-cell), variable region somatic mutation analysis**
0.00 0.00 FUD XXX
AMA: 2020,Dec,3; 2020,OctSE,1; 2020,OctSE,1; 2018,Nov,9; 2018,Jan,8; 2017,Jan,8; 2016,Aug,9; 2016,Jan,13

\# **81278** ***IGH@/BCL2 (t(14;18))*** **(eg, follicular lymphoma) translocation analysis, major breakpoint region (MBR) and minor cluster region (mcr) breakpoints, qualitative or quantitative**
0.00 0.00 FUD XXX
AMA: 2020,Dec,3; 2020,OctSE,1

\# **81264** ***IGK@ (Immunoglobulin kappa light chain locus)*** **(eg, leukemia and lymphoma, B-cell), gene rearrangement analysis, evaluation to detect abnormal clonal population(s)**
0.00 0.00 FUD XXX
AMA: 2020,Dec,3; 2020,OctSE,1; 2020,OctSE,1; 2018,Nov,9; 2018,Jan,8; 2017,Jan,8; 2016,Aug,9; 2016,Jan,13

81260 ***IKBKAP (inhibitor of kappa light polypeptide gene enhancer in B-cells, kinase complex-associated protein)*** **(eg, familial dysautonomia) gene analysis, common variants (eg, 2507+6T>C, R696P)**
0.00 0.00 FUD XXX
AMA: 2020,Dec,3; 2020,OctSE,1; 2020,OctSE,1; 2018,Nov,9; 2018,Jan,8; 2017,Jan,8; 2016,Aug,9; 2016,Jan,13

81261 **Resequenced code. See code before 81260.**

81262 **Resequenced code. See code before 81260.**

81263 **Resequenced code. See code before 81260.**

81264 **Resequenced code. See code before 81260.**

81265 **Resequenced code. See code following resequenced code 81187.**

81266 **Resequenced code. See code following resequenced code 81265.**

81267 **Resequenced code. See code following 81224.**

81268 **Resequenced code. See code following 81224.**

81269 **Resequenced code. See code following resequenced code 81259.**

81270 ***JAK2 (Janus kinase 2)*** **(eg, myeloproliferative disorder) gene analysis, p.Val617Phe (V617F) variant**
0.00 0.00 FUD XXX
AMA: 2020,Dec,3; 2020,OctSE,1; 2020,OctSE,1; 2018,Nov,9; 2018,Jan,8; 2017,Jan,8; 2016,Aug,9; 2016,Jan,13

\# **81279** ***JAK2 (Janus kinase 2)*** **(eg, myeloproliferative disorder) targeted sequence analysis (eg, exons 12 and 13)**
0.00 0.00 FUD XXX
AMA: 2020,Dec,3; 2020,OctSE,1

81271 **Resequenced code. See code following numeric code 81259.**

81272 ***KIT (v-kit Hardy-Zuckerman 4 feline sarcoma viral oncogene homolog)*** **(eg, gastrointestinal stromal tumor [GIST], acute myeloid leukemia, melanoma), gene analysis, targeted sequence analysis (eg, exons 8, 11, 13, 17, 18)**
0.00 0.00 FUD XXX
AMA: 2020,Dec,3; 2020,OctSE,1; 2020,OctSE,1; 2018,Nov,9; 2018,Jan,8; 2017,Jan,8; 2016,Aug,9

81273 ***KIT (v-kit Hardy-Zuckerman 4 feline sarcoma viral oncogene homolog)*** **(eg, mastocytosis), gene analysis, D816 variant**
0.00 0.00 FUD XXX
AMA: 2020,Dec,3; 2020,OctSE,1; 2020,OctSE,1; 2018,Nov,9; 2018,Jan,8; 2017,Jan,8; 2016,Aug,9

81274 **Resequenced code. See code following resequenced code 81271.**

81275 ***KRAS (Kirsten rat sarcoma viral oncogene homolog)*** **(eg, carcinoma) gene analysis; variants in exon 2 (eg, codons 12 and 13)**
0.00 0.00 FUD XXX
AMA: 2020,Dec,3; 2020,OctSE,1; 2020,OctSE,1; 2018,Nov,9; 2018,Jan,8; 2017,Jan,8; 2016,Aug,9; 2016,Jan,13

81276 **additional variant(s) (eg, codon 61, codon 146)**
0.00 0.00 FUD XXX
AMA: 2020,Dec,3; 2020,OctSE,1; 2020,OctSE,1; 2018,Nov,9; 2018,Jan,8; 2017,Jan,8; 2016,Aug,9

81277 **Resequenced code. See code following 81229.**

81278 **Resequenced code. See code following resequenced code 81263.**

81279 **Resequenced code. See code following 81270.**

81283 **Resequenced code. See code following resequenced code 81121.**

81284 **Resequenced code. See code following numeric code 81246.**

81285 **Resequenced code. See code following numeric code 81246.**

81286 **Resequenced code. See code following numeric code 81246.**

81287 **Resequenced code. See code following resequenced code 81304.**

81288 **Resequenced code. See code following resequenced code 81292.**

81289 **Resequenced code. See code following numeric code 81246.**

81290 ***MCOLN1 (mucolipin 1)*** **(eg, Mucolipidosis, type IV) gene analysis, common variants (eg, IVS3-2A>G, del6.4kb)**
0.00 0.00 FUD XXX
AMA: 2020,Dec,3; 2020,OctSE,1; 2020,OctSE,1; 2018,Nov,9; 2018,Jan,8; 2017,Jan,8; 2016,Aug,9; 2016,Jan,13

81302 ***MECP2 (methyl CpG binding protein 2)*** **(eg, Rett syndrome) gene analysis; full sequence analysis**
0.00 0.00 FUD XXX
AMA: 2020,Dec,3; 2020,OctSE,1; 2020,OctSE,1; 2018,Nov,9; 2018,Jan,8; 2017,Jan,8; 2016,Aug,9; 2016,Jan,13

81303 **known familial variant**
0.00 0.00 FUD XXX
AMA: 2020,Dec,3; 2020,OctSE,1; 2020,OctSE,1; 2018,Nov,9; 2018,Jan,8; 2017,Jan,8; 2016,Aug,9; 2016,Jan,13

81304 **duplication/deletion variants**
0.00 0.00 FUD XXX
AMA: 2020,Dec,3; 2020,OctSE,1; 2020,OctSE,1; 2018,Nov,9; 2018,Jan,8; 2017,Jan,8; 2016,Aug,9; 2016,Jan,13

81287 ***MGMT (O-6-methylguanine-DNA methyltransferase)*** **(eg, glioblastoma multiforme), promoter methylation analysis**
0.00 0.00 FUD XXX
AMA: 2020,Dec,3; 2020,OctSE,1; 2020,OctSE,1; 2019,Jul,3; 2018,Dec,10; 2018,Dec,10; 2018,Nov,9; 2018,Jan,8; 2017,Jan,8; 2016,Aug,9

81301 **Microsatellite instability analysis (eg, hereditary non-polyposis colorectal cancer, Lynch syndrome) of markers for mismatch repair deficiency (eg, BAT25, BAT26), includes comparison of neoplastic and normal tissue, if performed**
0.00 0.00 FUD XXX
AMA: 2020,Dec,3; 2020,OctSE,1; 2020,OctSE,1; 2018,Nov,9; 2018,Jan,8; 2017,Jan,8; 2016,Aug,9; 2016,Jan,13

81292 ***MLH1 (mutL homolog 1, colon cancer, nonpolyposis type 2)*** **(eg, hereditary non-polyposis colorectal cancer, Lynch syndrome) gene analysis; full sequence analysis**
0.00 0.00 FUD XXX
AMA: 2020,Dec,3; 2020,OctSE,1; 2020,OctSE,1; 2018,Nov,9; 2018,Jan,8; 2017,Jan,8; 2016,Aug,9; 2016,Jan,13

81288 **promoter methylation analysis**
0.00 0.00 FUD XXX
AMA: 2020,Dec,3; 2020,OctSE,1; 2020,OctSE,1; 2018,Nov,9; 2018,Jan,8; 2017,Jan,8; 2016,Aug,9; 2016,Jan,13

81293 **known familial variants**
0.00 0.00 FUD XXX
AMA: 2020,Dec,3; 2020,OctSE,1; 2020,OctSE,1; 2018,Nov,9; 2018,Jan,8; 2017,Jan,8; 2016,Aug,9; 2016,Jan,13

81294 **duplication/deletion variants**
0.00 0.00 FUD XXX
AMA: 2020,Dec,3; 2020,OctSE,1; 2020,OctSE,1; 2018,Nov,9; 2018,Jan,8; 2017,Jan,8; 2016,Aug,9; 2016,Jan,13

81338 ***MPL (MPL proto-oncogene, thrombopoietin receptor)*** **(eg, myeloproliferative disorder) gene analysis; common variants (eg, W515A, W515K, W515L, W515R)**
0.00 0.00 FUD XXX
AMA: 2020,Dec,3; 2020,OctSE,1

81339 **sequence analysis, exon 10**
0.00 0.00 FUD XXX
AMA: 2020,Dec,3; 2020,OctSE,1

81295 ***MSH2 (mutS homolog 2, colon cancer, nonpolyposis type 1)*** **(eg, hereditary non-polyposis colorectal cancer, Lynch syndrome) gene analysis; full sequence analysis**
0.00 0.00 FUD XXX
AMA: 2020,Dec,3; 2020,OctSE,1; 2020,OctSE,1; 2018,Nov,9; 2018,Jan,8; 2017,Jan,8; 2016,Aug,9; 2016,Jan,13

81291 **Resequenced code. See code before 81305.**

81292 **Resequenced code. See code before numeric code 81291.**

81293 **Resequenced code. See code before numeric code 81291.**

81294 **Resequenced code. See code before numeric code 81291.**

81295 **Resequenced code. See code before numeric code 81291.**

81296 **known familial variants**
0.00 0.00 FUD XXX
AMA: 2020,Dec,3; 2020,OctSE,1; 2020,OctSE,1; 2018,Nov,9; 2018,Jan,8; 2017,Jan,8; 2016,Aug,9; 2016,Jan,13

81297 **duplication/deletion variants**
0.00 0.00 FUD XXX
AMA: 2020,Dec,3; 2020,OctSE,1; 2020,OctSE,1; 2018,Nov,9; 2018,Jan,8; 2017,Jan,8; 2016,Aug,9; 2016,Jan,13

81298 ***MSH6 (mutS homolog 6 [E. coli])*** **(eg, hereditary non-polyposis colorectal cancer, Lynch syndrome) gene analysis; full sequence analysis**
0.00 0.00 FUD XXX
AMA: 2020,Dec,3; 2020,OctSE,1; 2020,OctSE,1; 2018,Nov,9; 2018,Jan,8; 2017,Jan,8; 2016,Aug,9; 2016,Jan,13

81299 **known familial variants**
0.00 0.00 FUD XXX
AMA: 2020,Dec,3; 2020,OctSE,1; 2020,OctSE,1; 2018,Nov,9; 2018,Jan,8; 2017,Jan,8; 2016,Aug,9; 2016,Jan,13

81300 **duplication/deletion variants**
0.00 0.00 FUD XXX
AMA: 2020,Dec,3; 2020,OctSE,1; 2020,OctSE,1; 2018,Nov,9; 2018,Jan,8; 2017,Jan,8; 2016,Aug,9; 2016,Jan,13

81301 **Resequenced code. See code following resequenced code 81287.**

81302 **Resequenced code. See code following 81290.**

81303 **Resequenced code. See code following 81290.**

81304 **Resequenced code. See code following 81290.**

81291 ***MTHFR (5,10-methylenetetrahydrofolate reductase)*** **(eg, hereditary hypercoagulability) gene analysis, common variants (eg, 677T, 1298C)**
0.00 0.00 FUD XXX
AMA: 2020,Dec,3; 2020,OctSE,1; 2020,OctSE,1; 2018,Nov,9; 2018,Jan,8; 2017,Jan,8; 2016,Aug,9; 2016,Jan,13

81305 ***MYD88 (myeloid differentiation primary response 88)*** **(eg, Waldenstrom's macroglobulinemia, lymphoplasmacytic leukemia) gene analysis, p.Leu265Pro (L265P) variant**
0.00 0.00 FUD XXX
AMA: 2020,Dec,3; 2020,OctSE,1; 2020,OctSE,1; 2019,Jul,3; 2018,Nov,9

81306 **Resequenced code. See code before resequenced code 81312.**

81307 **Resequenced code. See code before 81313.**

81308 **Resequenced code. See code before 81313.**

81309 **Resequenced code. See code following 81314.**

81310 ***NPM1 (nucleophosmin)*** **(eg, acute myeloid leukemia) gene analysis, exon 12 variants**
0.00 0.00 FUD XXX
AMA: 2020,Dec,3; 2020,OctSE,1; 2020,OctSE,1; 2018,Nov,9; 2018,Jan,8; 2017,Jan,8; 2016,Aug,9; 2016,Jan,13

81311 ***NRAS (neuroblastoma RAS viral [v-ras] oncogene homolog)*** **(eg, colorectal carcinoma), gene analysis, variants in exon 2 (eg, codons 12 and 13) and exon 3 (eg, codon 61)**
0.00 0.00 FUD XXX
AMA: 2020,Dec,3; 2020,OctSE,1; 2020,OctSE,1; 2018,Nov,9; 2018,Jan,8; 2017,Jan,8; 2016,Aug,9

81312 **Resequenced code. See code before resequenced code 81307.**

\# **81191** ***NTRK1 (neurotrophic receptor tyrosine kinase 1)*** **(eg, solid tumors) translocation analysis**
0.00 0.00 FUD XXX
AMA: 2020,Dec,3

\# **81192** ***NTRK2 (neurotrophic receptor tyrosine kinase 2)*** **(eg, solid tumors) translocation analysis**
0.00 0.00 FUD XXX
AMA: 2020,Dec,3

\# **81193** ***NTRK3 (neurotrophic receptor tyrosine kinase 3)*** **(eg, solid tumors) translocation analysis**
0.00 0.00 FUD XXX
AMA: 2020,Dec,3

\# **81194** ***NTRK (neurotrophic receptor tyrosine kinase 1, 2, and 3)*** **(eg, solid tumors) translocation analysis**
INCLUDES Analysis NTRK1, NTRK2, and NTRK3 by single assay
0.00 0.00 FUD XXX
AMA: 2020,Dec,3

\# **81306** ***NUDT15 (nudix hydrolase 15)*** **(eg, drug metabolism) gene analysis, common variant(s) (eg, *2, *3, *4, *5, *6)**
0.00 0.00 FUD XXX
AMA: 2020,Dec,3; 2020,OctSE,1; 2020,OctSE,1; 2019,Jul,3; 2018,Nov,9

\# **81312** ***PABPN1 (poly[A] binding protein nuclear 1)*** **(eg, oculopharyngeal muscular dystrophy) gene analysis, evaluation to detect abnormal (eg, expanded) alleles**
0.00 0.00 FUD XXX
AMA: 2020,Dec,3; 2020,OctSE,1; 2020,OctSE,1; 2018,Nov,9

\# **81307** ***PALB2 (partner and localizer of BRCA2)*** **(eg, breast and pancreatic cancer) gene analysis; full gene sequence**
0.00 0.00 FUD XXX
AMA: 2020,Dec,3; 2020,OctSE,1; 2020,OctSE,1

\# **81308** **known familial variant**
0.00 0.00 FUD XXX
AMA: 2020,Dec,3; 2020,OctSE,1; 2020,OctSE,1

81313 ***PCA3/KLK3 (prostate cancer antigen 3 [non-protein coding]/kallikrein-related peptidase 3 [prostate specific antigen])*** **ratio (eg, prostate cancer)**
0.00 0.00 FUD XXX
AMA: 2020,Dec,3; 2020,OctSE,1; 2020,OctSE,1; 2018,Nov,9; 2018,Jan,8; 2017,Jan,8; 2016,Aug,9; 2016,Jan,13

81314 ***PDGFRA (platelet-derived growth factor receptor, alpha polypeptide)*** **(eg, gastrointestinal stromal tumor [GIST]), gene analysis, targeted sequence analysis (eg, exons 12, 18)**
0.00 0.00 FUD XXX
AMA: 2020,Dec,3; 2020,OctSE,1; 2020,OctSE,1; 2018,Nov,9; 2018,Jan,8; 2017,Jan,8; 2016,Aug,9

\# **81309** ***PIK3CA (phosphatidylinositol-4, 5-biphosphate 3-kinase, catalytic subunit alpha)*** **(eg, colorectal and breast cancer) gene analysis, targeted sequence analysis (eg, exons 7, 9, 20)**
0.00 0.00 FUD XXX
AMA: 2020,Dec,3; 2020,OctSE,1; 2020,OctSE,1; 2020,Apr,10

\# **81320** ***PLCG2 (phospholipase C gamma 2)*** **(eg, chronic lymphocytic leukemia) gene analysis, common variants (eg, R665W, S707F, L845F)**
0.00 0.00 FUD XXX
AMA: 2020,Dec,3; 2020,OctSE,1; 2020,OctSE,1; 2019,Jul,3; 2018,Nov,9

81315 ***PML/RARalpha, (t(15;17)), (promyelocytic leukemia/retinoic acid receptor alpha)*** **(eg, promyelocytic leukemia) translocation analysis; common breakpoints (eg, intron 3 and intron 6), qualitative or quantitative**
0.00 0.00 FUD XXX
AMA: 2020,Dec,3; 2020,OctSE,1; 2020,OctSE,1; 2018,Nov,9; 2018,Jan,8; 2017,Jan,8; 2016,Aug,9; 2016,Jan,13

81316 **single breakpoint (eg, intron 3, intron 6 or exon 6), qualitative or quantitative**
0.00 0.00 FUD XXX
AMA: 2020,Dec,3; 2020,OctSE,1; 2020,OctSE,1; 2018,Nov,9; 2018,Jan,8; 2017,Jan,8; 2016,Aug,9; 2016,Jan,13

\# **81324** ***PMP22 (peripheral myelin protein 22)*** **(eg, Charcot-Marie-Tooth, hereditary neuropathy with liability to pressure palsies) gene analysis; duplication/deletion analysis**
0.00 0.00 FUD XXX
AMA: 2020,Dec,3; 2020,OctSE,1; 2020,OctSE,1; 2018,Nov,9; 2018,Jan,8; 2017,Jan,8; 2016,Aug,9; 2016,Jan,13

\# **81325** **full sequence analysis**
0.00 0.00 FUD XXX
AMA: 2020,Dec,3; 2020,OctSE,1; 2020,OctSE,1; 2018,Nov,9; 2018,May,6; 2018,Jan,8; 2017,Jan,8; 2016,Aug,9; 2016,Jan,13

\# **81326** **known familial variant**
0.00 0.00 FUD XXX
AMA: 2020,Dec,3; 2020,OctSE,1; 2020,OctSE,1; 2018,Nov,9; 2018,Jan,8; 2017,Jan,8; 2016,Aug,9; 2016,Jan,13

81317 ***PMS2 (postmeiotic segregation increased 2 [S. cerevisiae])*** **(eg, hereditary non-polyposis colorectal cancer, Lynch syndrome) gene analysis; full sequence analysis**
0.00 0.00 FUD XXX
AMA: 2020,Dec,3; 2020,OctSE,1; 2020,OctSE,1; 2018,Nov,9; 2018,Jan,8; 2017,Jan,8; 2016,Aug,9; 2016,Jan,13

81318 **known familial variants**
0.00 0.00 FUD XXX
AMA: 2020,Dec,3; 2020,OctSE,1; 2020,OctSE,1; 2018,Nov,9; 2018,Jan,8; 2017,Jan,8; 2016,Aug,9; 2016,Jan,13

81319 **duplication/deletion variants**
0.00 0.00 FUD XXX
AMA: 2020,Dec,3; 2020,OctSE,1; 2020,OctSE,1; 2018,Nov,9; 2018,Jan,8; 2017,Jan,8; 2016,Aug,9; 2016,Jan,13

81320 **Resequenced code. See code before 81315.**

\# **81343** ***PPP2R2B (protein phosphatase 2 regulatory subunit Bbeta)*** **(eg, spinocerebellar ataxia) gene analysis, evaluation to detect abnormal (eg, expanded) alleles**
0.00 0.00 FUD XXX
AMA: 2020,Dec,3; 2020,OctSE,1; 2020,OctSE,1; 2018,Nov,9

81321 *PTEN (phosphatase and tensin homolog)* (eg, Cowden syndrome, PTEN hamartoma tumor syndrome) gene analysis; full sequence analysis
0.00 0.00 FUD XXX
AMA: 2020,Dec,3; 2020,OctSE,1; 2020,OctSE,1; 2018,Nov,9; 2018,Jan,8; 2017,Jan,8; 2016,Aug,9; 2016,Jan,13

81322 known familial variant
0.00 0.00 FUD XXX
AMA: 2020,Dec,3; 2020,OctSE,1; 2020,OctSE,1; 2018,Nov,9; 2018,Jan,8; 2017,Jan,8; 2016,Aug,9; 2016,Jan,13

81323 duplication/deletion variant
0.00 0.00 FUD XXX
AMA: 2020,Dec,3; 2020,OctSE,1; 2020,OctSE,1; 2018,Nov,9; 2018,Jan,8; 2017,Jan,8; 2016,Aug,9; 2016,Jan,13

81324 Resequenced code. See code following 81316.

81325 Resequenced code. See code following 81316.

81326 Resequenced code. See code following 81316.

81334 *RUNX1 (runt related transcription factor 1)* (eg, acute myeloid leukemia, familial platelet disorder with associated myeloid malignancy), gene analysis, targeted sequence analysis (eg, exons 3-8)
0.00 0.00 FUD XXX
AMA: 2020,Dec,3; 2020,OctSE,1; 2020,OctSE,1; 2018,Nov,9

81327 *SEPT9 (Septin9)* (eg, colorectal cancer) promoter methylation analysis
0.00 0.00 FUD XXX
AMA: 2020,Dec,3; 2020,OctSE,1; 2020,OctSE,1; 2019,Jul,3; 2018,Nov,9

81332 *SERPINA1 (serpin peptidase inhibitor, clade A, alpha-1 antiproteinase, antitrypsin, member 1)* (eg, alpha-1-antitrypsin deficiency), gene analysis, common variants (eg, *S and *Z)
0.00 0.00 FUD XXX
AMA: 2020,Dec,3; 2020,OctSE,1; 2020,OctSE,1; 2018,Nov,9; 2018,Jan,8; 2017,Jan,8; 2016,Aug,9; 2016,Jan,13

81347 *SF3B1 (splicing factor [3b] subunit B1)* (eg, myelodysplastic syndrome/acute myeloid leukemia) gene analysis, common variants (eg, A672T, E622D, L833F, R625C, R625L)
0.00 0.00 FUD XXX
AMA: 2020,Dec,3; 2020,OctSE,1

81328 *SLCO1B1 (solute carrier organic anion transporter family, member 1B1)* (eg, adverse drug reaction), gene analysis, common variant(s) (eg, *5)
0.00 0.00 FUD XXX
AMA: 2020,Dec,3; 2020,OctSE,1; 2020,OctSE,1; 2018,Nov,9

81329 *SMN1 (survival of motor neuron 1, telomeric)* (eg, spinal muscular atrophy) gene analysis; dosage/deletion analysis (eg, carrier testing), includes SMN2 (survival of motor neuron 2, centromeric) analysis, if performed
0.00 0.00 FUD XXX
AMA: 2020,Dec,3; 2020,OctSE,1; 2020,OctSE,1; 2019,Jul,3; 2018,Nov,9

81336 full gene sequence
0.00 0.00 FUD XXX
AMA: 2020,Dec,3; 2020,OctSE,1; 2020,OctSE,1; 2019,Jul,3; 2018,Nov,9

81337 known familial sequence variant(s)
0.00 0.00 FUD XXX
AMA: 2020,Dec,3; 2020,OctSE,1; 2020,OctSE,1; 2019,Jul,3; 2018,Nov,9

81330 *SMPD1(sphingomyelin phosphodiesterase 1, acid lysosomal)* (eg, Niemann-Pick disease, Type A) gene analysis, common variants (eg, R496L, L302P, fsP330)
0.00 0.00 FUD XXX
AMA: 2020,Dec,3; 2020,OctSE,1; 2020,OctSE,1; 2018,Nov,9; 2018,Jan,8; 2017,Jan,8; 2016,Aug,9; 2016,Jan,13

81331 *SNRPN/UBE3A (small nuclear ribonucleoprotein polypeptide N and ubiquitin protein ligase E3A)* (eg, Prader-Willi syndrome and/or Angelman syndrome), methylation analysis
0.00 0.00 FUD XXX
AMA: 2020,Dec,3; 2020,OctSE,1; 2020,OctSE,1; 2018,Nov,9; 2018,Jan,8; 2017,Jan,8; 2016,Aug,9; 2016,Jan,13

81332 Resequenced code. See code following 81327.

81348 *SRSF2 (serine and arginine-rich splicing factor 2)* (eg, myelodysplastic syndrome, acute myeloid leukemia) gene analysis, common variants (eg, P95H, P95L)
0.00 0.00 FUD XXX
AMA: 2020,Dec,3; 2020,OctSE,1

81344 *TBP (TATA box binding protein)* (eg, spinocerebellar ataxia) gene analysis, evaluation to detect abnormal (eg, expanded) alleles
0.00 0.00 FUD XXX
AMA: 2020,Dec,3; 2020,OctSE,1; 2020,OctSE,1; 2018,Nov,9

81345 *TERT (telomerase reverse transcriptase)* (eg, thyroid carcinoma, glioblastoma multiforme) gene analysis, targeted sequence analysis (eg, promoter region)
0.00 0.00 FUD XXX
AMA: 2020,Dec,3; 2020,OctSE,1; 2020,OctSE,1; 2019,Jul,3; 2018,Nov,9

81333 *TGFBI (transforming growth factor beta-induced)* (eg, corneal dystrophy) gene analysis, common variants (eg, R124H, R124C, R124L, R555W, R555Q)
0.00 0.00 FUD XXX
AMA: 2020,Dec,3; 2020,OctSE,1; 2020,OctSE,1; 2019,Jul,3; 2018,Nov,9

81334 Resequenced code. See code following numeric code 81326.

81351 *TP53 (tumor protein 53)* (eg, Li-Fraumeni syndrome) gene analysis; full gene sequence
0.00 0.00 FUD XXX
AMA: 2020,Dec,3; 2020,OctSE,1

81352 targeted sequence analysis (eg, 4 oncology)
0.00 0.00 FUD XXX
AMA: 2020,Dec,3; 2020,OctSE,1

81353 known familial variant
0.00 0.00 FUD XXX
AMA: 2020,Dec,3; 2020,OctSE,1

81335 *TPMT (thiopurine S-methyltransferase)* (eg, drug metabolism), gene analysis, common variants (eg, *2, *3)
0.00 0.00 FUD XXX
AMA: 2020,Dec,3; 2020,OctSE,1; 2020,OctSE,1; 2018,Nov,9

81336 Resequenced code. See code following 81329.

81337 Resequenced code. See code following 81329.

81338 Resequenced code. See code following resequenced code 81294.

81339 Resequenced code. See code before resequenced code 81295.

81340 *TRB@ (T cell antigen receptor, beta)* (eg, leukemia and lymphoma), gene rearrangement analysis to detect abnormal clonal population(s); using amplification methodology (eg, polymerase chain reaction)
0.00 0.00 FUD XXX
AMA: 2020,Dec,3; 2020,OctSE,1; 2020,OctSE,1; 2018,Nov,9; 2018,Jan,8; 2017,Jan,8; 2016,Aug,9; 2016,Jan,13

81341 using direct probe methodology (eg, Southern blot)
0.00 0.00 FUD XXX
AMA: 2020,Dec,3; 2020,OctSE,1; 2020,OctSE,1; 2018,Nov,9; 2018,Jan,8; 2017,Jan,8; 2016,Aug,9; 2016,Jan,13

81342 ***TRG@ (T cell antigen receptor, gamma)*** **(eg, leukemia and lymphoma), gene rearrangement analysis, evaluation to detect abnormal clonal population(s)**
0.00 0.00 **FUD** XXX A
AMA: 2020,Dec,3; 2020,OctSE,1; 2020,OctSE,1; 2018,Nov,9; 2018,Jan,8; 2017,Jan,8; 2016,Aug,9; 2016,Jan,13

81343 **Resequenced code. See code following numeric code 81320.**

81344 **Resequenced code. See code following numeric code 81332.**

81345 **Resequenced code. See code following numeric code 81332.**

81346 ***TYMS (thymidylate synthetase)*** **(eg, 5-fluorouracil/5-FU drug metabolism), gene analysis, common variant(s) (eg, tandem repeat variant)**
0.00 0.00 **FUD** XXX A
AMA: 2020,Dec,3; 2020,OctSE,1; 2020,OctSE,1; 2018,Nov,9

81347 **Resequenced code. See code before 81328.**

81348 **Resequenced code. See code following numeric code 81332.**

\# **81357** ***U2AF1 (U2 small nuclear RNA auxiliary factor 1)*** **(eg, myelodysplastic syndrome, acute myeloid leukemia) gene analysis, common variants (eg, S34F, S34Y, Q157R, Q157P)**
0.00 0.00 **FUD** XXX
AMA: 2020,Dec,3; 2020,OctSE,1

81349 **Resequenced code. See code following 81229.**

81350 ***UGT1A1 (UDP glucuronosyltransferase 1 family, polypeptide A1)*** **(eg, drug metabolism, hereditary unconjugated hyperbilirubinemia [Gilbert syndrome]) gene analysis, common variants (eg, *28, *36, *37)**
0.00 0.00 **FUD** XXX A
AMA: 2020,Dec,3; 2020,OctSE,1; 2020,OctSE,1; 2020,Apr,9; 2018,Nov,9; 2018,Jan,8; 2017,Jan,8; 2016,Aug,9; 2016,Jan,13

81351 **Resequenced code. See code following 81333.**

81352 **Resequenced code. See code following 81333.**

81353 **Resequenced code. See code following 81333.**

81355 ***VKORC1 (vitamin K epoxide reductase complex, subunit 1)*** **(eg, warfarin metabolism), gene analysis, common variant(s) (eg, -1639G>A, c.173+1000C>T)**
0.00 0.00 **FUD** XXX A
AMA: 2020,Dec,3; 2020,OctSE,1; 2020,OctSE,1; 2018,Nov,9; 2018,Jan,8; 2017,Jan,8; 2016,Aug,9; 2016,Jan,13

81357 **Resequenced code. See code following 81346.**

81360 ***ZRSR2 (zinc finger CCCH-type, RNA binding motif and serine/arginine-rich 2)*** **(eg, myelodysplastic syndrome, acute myeloid leukemia) gene analysis, common variant(s) (eg, E65fs, E122fs, R448fs)**
0.00 0.00 **FUD** XXX
AMA: 2020,Dec,3; 2020,OctSE,1

81361 **Resequenced code. See code following resequenced code 81269.**

81362 **Resequenced code. See code following resequenced code 81269.**

81363 **Resequenced code. See code following resequenced code 81269.**

81364 **Resequenced code. See code following resequenced code 81269.**

81370-81383 Human Leukocyte Antigen (HLA) Testing

INCLUDES Additional testing performed to resolve ambiguous allele combinations for high-resolution typing
All analytical procedures in evaluation:
- Amplification
- Cell lysis
- Detection
- Digestion
- Extraction
- Nucleic acid stabilization

Analysis to identify human leukocyte antigen (HLA) alleles and allele groups connected to specific diseases and individual response to drug therapy in addition to other clinical uses
Code selection based on specific gene being reviewed
Evaluation gene variant presence using common gene variant name
Generally, all listed gene variants in code description tested (lists not all inclusive)
Genes described using Human Genome Organization (HUGO) approved names
High-resolution typing resolves common well-defined (CWD) alleles usually identified by at least four-digits. Some instances when high-resolution typing may include ambiguities for rare alleles may be reported as string of alleles or National Marrow Donor Program (NMDP) code
Histocompatibility antigen testing
Intermediate resolution HLA testing identified by string of alleles or NMDP code
Low and intermediate resolution considered low resolution for code assignment
Low-resolution HLA type reporting identified by two-digit HLA name
Multiple variant alleles or allele groups identified by typing
One or more HLA genes in specific clinical circumstances
Protein or disease examples in code description not all inclusive
Qualitative results unless otherwise stated
Typing performed to determine recipient compatibility and potential donors undergoing solid organ or hematopoietic stem cell pretransplantation testing

EXCLUDES *Full gene sequencing using separate gene variant assessment codes unless specifically stated in code description*
HLA antigen typing by nonmolecular pathology methods (86812-86821)
In situ hybridization analyses (88271-88275, 88368-88375 [88377])
Microbial identification (87149-87153, 87471-87801 [87623, 87624, 87625], 87900-87904 [87906, 87910, 87912])
Other related gene variants not listed in code description
Tier 1 molecular pathology codes (81105-81254 [81161, 81162, 81163, 81164, 81165, 81166, 81167, 81173, 81174, 81184, 81185, 81186, 81187, 81188, 81189, 81190, 81200, 81201, 81202, 81203, 81204, 81205, 81206, 81207, 81208, 81209, 81210, 81219, 81227, 81230, 81231, 81233, 81234, 81238, 81239, 81245, 81246, 81250, 81257, 81258, 81259, 81265, 81266, 81267, 81268, 81269, 81284, 81285, 81286, 81289, 81361, 81362, 81363, 81364])
Tier 2 and unlisted molecular pathology procedures (81400-81408, [81479])

Code also:
Modifier 26 when only interpretation and report performed
Services required before cell lysis

81370 **HLA Class I and II typing, low resolution (eg, antigen equivalents);** ***HLA-A, -B, -C, -DRB1/3/4/5, and -DQB1***
0.00 0.00 **FUD** XXX A
AMA: 2020,Dec,3; 2020,OctSE,1; 2020,OctSE,1; 2018,Nov,9; 2018,Jan,8; 2017,Jan,8; 2016,Aug,9; 2016,Jan,13

81371 ***HLA-A, -B, and -DRB1*** **(eg, verification typing)**
0.00 0.00 **FUD** XXX A
AMA: 2020,Dec,3; 2020,OctSE,1; 2020,OctSE,1; 2018,Nov,9; 2018,Jan,8; 2017,Jan,8; 2016,Aug,9; 2016,Jan,13

81372 **HLA Class I typing, low resolution (eg, antigen equivalents); complete** ***(ie, HLA-A, -B, and -C)***
EXCLUDES *Class I and II low-resolution HLA typing for HLA-A, -B, -C, -DRB1/3/4/5, and -DQB1 (81370)*
0.00 0.00 **FUD** XXX A
AMA: 2020,Dec,3; 2020,OctSE,1; 2020,OctSE,1; 2018,Nov,9; 2018,Jan,8; 2017,Jan,8; 2016,Aug,9; 2016,Jan,13

81373 **one locus** ***(eg, HLA-A, -B, or -C)*****, each**
EXCLUDES *Complete Class 1 (HLA-A, -B, and -C) low-resolution typing (81372)*
Reporting presence or absence single antigen equivalent using low-resolution methodology (81374)
0.00 0.00 **FUD** XXX A
AMA: 2020,Dec,3; 2020,OctSE,1; 2020,OctSE,1; 2018,Nov,9; 2018,Jan,8; 2017,Jan,8; 2016,Aug,9; 2016,Jan,13

81374 **one antigen equivalent *(eg, B*27)*, each**

EXCLUDES *Testing for presence or absence more than two antigen equivalents at locus, report for each locus test (81373)*

0.00 0.00 FUD XXX A

AMA: 2020,Dec,3; 2020,OctSE,1; 2020,OctSE,1; 2018,Nov,9; 2018,Jan,8; 2017,Jan,8; 2016,Aug,9; 2016,Jan,13

81375 **HLA Class II typing, low resolution (eg, antigen equivalents); *HLA-DRB1/3/4/5 and -DQB1***

EXCLUDES *Class I and II low-resolution HLA typing for HLA-A, -B, -C, -DRB 1/3/4/5, and DQB1 (81370)*

0.00 0.00 FUD XXX A

AMA: 2020,Dec,3; 2020,OctSE,1; 2020,OctSE,1; 2018,Nov,9; 2018,Jan,8; 2017,Jan,8; 2016,Aug,9; 2016,Jan,13

81376 **one locus *(eg, HLA-DRB1, -DRB3/4/5, -DQB1, -DQA1, -DPB1, or -DPA1)*, each**

INCLUDES Low-resolution typing, HLA-DRB1/3/4/5 reported as single locus

EXCLUDES *Low-resolution typing for HLA-DRB1/3/4/5 and -DQB1 (81375)*

0.00 0.00 FUD XXX A

AMA: 2020,Dec,3; 2020,OctSE,1; 2020,OctSE,1; 2018,Nov,9; 2018,Jan,8; 2017,Jan,8; 2016,Aug,9; 2016,Jan,13

81377 **one antigen equivalent, each**

EXCLUDES *Testing for presence or absence more than two antigen equivalents at locus (81376)*

0.00 0.00 FUD XXX A

AMA: 2020,Dec,3; 2020,OctSE,1; 2020,OctSE,1; 2018,Nov,9; 2018,Jan,8; 2017,Jan,8; 2016,Aug,9; 2016,Jan,13

81378 **HLA Class I and II typing, high resolution (ie, alleles or allele groups), *HLA-A, -B, -C, and -DRB1***

0.00 0.00 FUD XXX A

AMA: 2020,Dec,3; 2020,OctSE,1; 2020,OctSE,1; 2018,Nov,9; 2018,Jan,8; 2017,Jan,8; 2016,Aug,9; 2016,Jan,13

81379 **HLA Class I typing, high resolution (ie, alleles or allele groups); complete (ie, *HLA-A, -B, and -C*)**

0.00 0.00 FUD XXX A

AMA: 2020,Dec,3; 2020,OctSE,1; 2020,OctSE,1; 2018,Nov,9; 2018,Jan,8; 2017,Jan,8; 2016,Aug,9; 2016,Jan,13

81380 **one locus (eg, *HLA-A, -B, or -C*), each**

EXCLUDES *Complete Class I high-resolution typing for HLA-A, -B, and -C (81379)*

Testing for presence or absence single allele or allele group using high-resolution methodology (81381)

0.00 0.00 FUD XXX A

AMA: 2020,Dec,3; 2020,OctSE,1; 2020,OctSE,1; 2018,Nov,9; 2018,Jan,8; 2017,Jan,8; 2016,Aug,9; 2016,Jan,13

81381 **one allele or allele group (eg, *B*57:01P*), each**

EXCLUDES *Testing for presence or absence more than two alleles or allele groups at locus, report for each locus (81380)*

0.00 0.00 FUD XXX A

AMA: 2020,Dec,3; 2020,OctSE,1; 2020,OctSE,1; 2018,Nov,9; 2018,Jan,8; 2017,Jan,8; 2016,Aug,9; 2016,Jan,13

81382 **HLA Class II typing, high resolution (ie, alleles or allele groups); one locus (eg, *HLA-DRB1, -DRB3/4/5, -DQB1, -DQA1, -DPB1, or -DPA1*), each**

INCLUDES Typing one or all DRB3/4/5 genes regarded as one locus

EXCLUDES *Testing for just presence or absence single allele or allele group using high-resolution methodology (81383)*

0.00 0.00 FUD XXX A

AMA: 2020,Dec,3; 2020,OctSE,1; 2020,OctSE,1; 2018,Nov,9; 2018,Jan,8; 2017,Jan,8; 2016,Jan,13

81383 **one allele or allele group (eg, *HLA-DQB1*06:02P*), each**

EXCLUDES *Testing for presence or absence more than two alleles or allele groups at locus, report for each locus (81382)*

0.00 0.00 FUD XXX A

AMA: 2020,Dec,3; 2020,OctSE,1; 2020,OctSE,1; 2018,Nov,9; 2018,Jan,8; 2017,Jan,8; 2016,Jan,13

81400-81479 [81479] Molecular Pathology Tier 2 Procedures

INCLUDES All analytical procedures in evaluation:
- Amplification
- Cell lysis
- Detection
- Digestion
- Extraction
- Nucleic acid stabilization

Code selection based on specific gene being reviewed
Codes arranged by technical resource level and work involved
Evaluation gene variant presence using common gene variant name
Generally, all listed gene variants in code description tested (lists not all inclusive)
Genes described using Human Genome Organization (HUGO) approved names
Histocompatibility testing
Protein or disease examples in code description (lists not all inclusive)
Qualitative results unless otherwise stated
Specific analytes listed after code description for selecting appropriate molecular pathology procedure
Targeted genomic testing (81410-81471 [81448])
Testing for more rare diseases

EXCLUDES *Full gene sequencing using separate gene variant assessment codes unless specifically stated in code description*
In situ hybridization analyses (88271-88275, 88365-88368 [88364, 88373, 88374])
Microbial identification (87149-87153, 87471-87801 [87623, 87624, 87625], 87900-87904 [87906, 87910, 87912])
Other related gene variants not listed in code description
Tier 1 molecular pathology (81105-81254 [81161, 81162, 81163, 81164, 81165, 81166, 81167, 81173, 81174, 81184, 81185, 81186, 81187, 81188, 81189, 81190, 81200, 81201, 81202, 81203, 81204, 81205, 81206, 81207, 81208, 81209, 81210, 81219, 81227, 81230, 81231, 81233, 81234, 81238, 81239, 81245, 81246, 81250, 81257, 81258, 81259, 81265, 81266, 81267, 81268, 81269, 81284, 81285, 81286, 81289, 81361, 81362, 81363, 81364])
Unlisted molecular pathology procedures ([81479])

Code also:
Services required before cell lysis
Modifier 26 when only interpretation and report performed

81400 **Molecular pathology procedure, Level 1 (eg, identification of single germline variant [eg, SNP] by techniques such as restriction enzyme digestion or melt curve analysis)**

ACADM (acyl-CoA dehydrogenase, C-4 to C-12 straight chain, MCAD) (eg, medium chain acyl dehydrogenase deficiency), K304E variant

ACE (angiotensin converting enzyme) (eg, hereditary blood pressure regulation), insertion/deletion variant

AGTR1 (angiotensin II receptor, type 1) (eg, essential hypertension), 1166A>C variant

BCKDHA (branched chain keto acid dehydrogenase E1, alpha polypeptide) (eg, maple syrup urine disease, type 1A), Y438N variant

CCR5 (chemokine C-C motif receptor 5) (eg, HIV resistance), 32-bp deletion mutation/794 825del32 deletion

CLRN1 (clarin 1) (eg, Usher syndrome, type 3), N48K variant

F2 (coagulation factor 2) (eg, hereditary hypercoagulability), 1199G>A variant

F5 (coagulation factor V) (eg, hereditary hypercoagulability), HR2 variant

F7 (coagulation factor VII [serum prothrombin conversion accelerator]) (eg, hereditary hypercoagulability), R353Q variant

F13B (coagulation factor XIII, B polypeptide) (eg, hereditary hypercoagulability), V34L variant

FGB (fibrinogen beta chain) (eg, hereditary ischemic heart disease), -455G>A variant

FGFR1 (fibroblast growth factor receptor 1) (eg, Pfeiffer syndrome type 1, craniosynostosis), P252R variant

FGFR3 (fibroblast growth factor receptor 3) (eg, Muenke syndrome), P250R variant

FKTN (fukutin) (eg, Fukuyama congenital muscular dystrophy), retrotransposon insertion variant

GNE (glucosamine [UDP-N-acetyl]-2-epimerase/N-acetylmannosamine kinase) (eg, inclusion body myopathy 2 [IBM2], Nonaka myopathy), M712T variant

IVD (isovaleryl-CoA dehydrogenase) (eg, isovaleric acidemia), A282V variant

LCT (lactase-phlorizin hydrolase) (eg, lactose intolerance), 13910 C>T variant

NEB (nebulin) (eg, nemaline myopathy 2), exon 55 deletion variant

PCDH15 (protocadherin-related 15) (eg, Usher syndrome type 1F), R245X variant

SERPINE1 (serpine peptidase inhibitor clade E, member 1, plasminogen activator inhibitor -1, PAI-1) (eg, thrombophilia), 4G variant

SHOC2 (soc-2 suppressor of clear homolog) (eg, Noonan-like syndrome with loose anagen hair), S2G variant

SRY (sex determining region Y) (eg, 46,XX testicular disorder of sex development, gonadal dysgenesis), gene analysis

TOR1A (torsin family 1, member A [torsin A]) (eg, early-onset primary dystonia [DYT1]), 907_909delGAG (904_906delGAG) variant

0.00 0.00 **FUD** XXX A

AMA: 2020,Dec,3; 2020,OctSE,1; 2020,OctSE,1; 2019,Jul,3; 2018,Nov,9; 2018,Jan,8; 2017,Jan,8; 2016,Aug,9; 2016,Jan,13

81401 **Molecular pathology procedure, Level 2 (eg, 2-10 SNPs, 1 methylated variant, or 1 somatic variant [typically using nonsequencing target variant analysis], or detection of a dynamic mutation disorder/triplet repeat)**

ABCC8 (ATP-binding cassette, sub-family C [CFTR/MRP], member 8) (eg, familial hyperinsulinism), common variants (eg, c.3898-9G>A [c.3992-9G>A], F1388del)

ABL1 (ABL proto oncogene 1, non-receptor tyrosine kinase) (eg, acquired imatinib resistance), T315I variant

ACADM (acyl-CoA dehydrogenase, C-4 to C-12 straight chain, MCAD) (eg, medium chain acyl dehydrogenase deficiency), common variants (eg, K304E, Y42H)

ADRB2 (adrenergic beta-2 receptor surface) (eg, drug metabolism), common variants (eg, G16R, Q27E)

APOB (apolipoprotein B) (eg, familial hypercholesterolemia type B), common variants (eg, R3500Q, R3500W)

*APOE (apolipoprotein E) (eg, hyperlipoproteinemia type III, cardiovascular disease, Alzheimer disease), common variants (eg, *2, *3, *4)*

CBFB/MYH11 (inv(16)) (eg, acute myeloid leukemia), qualitative, and quantitative, if performed

CBS (cystathionine-beta-synthase) (eg, homocystinuria, cystathionine beta-synthase deficiency), common variants (eg, I278T, G307S)

CFH/ARMS2 (complement factor H/age-related maculopathy susceptibility 2) (eg, macular degeneration), common variants (eg, Y402H [CFH], A69S [ARMS2])

DEK/NUP214 (t(6;9))(eg, acute myeloid leukemia), translocation analysis, qualitative, and quantitative, if performed

E2A/PBX1 (t(1;19)) (eg, acute lymphocytic leukemia), translocation analysis, qualitative, and quantitative, if performed

EML4/ALK (inv(2)) (eg, non-small cell lung cancer), translocation or inversion analysis

ETV6/RUNX1 (t(12;21)) (eg, acute lymphocytic leukemia), translocation analysis, qualitative and quantitative, if performed

EWSR1/ATF1 (t(12;22)) (eg, clear cell sarcoma), translocation analysis, qualitative, and quantitative, if performed

EWSR1/ERG (t(21;22)) (eg, Ewing sarcoma/peripheral neuroectodermal tumor), translocation analysis, qualitative and quantitative, if performed

EWSR1/FLI1 (t(11;22)) (eg, Ewing sarcoma/peripheral neuroectodermal tumor), translocation analysis, qualitative and quantitative, if performed

EWSR1/WT1 (t(11;22)) (eg, desmoplastic small round cell tumor), translocation analysis, qualitative and quantitative, if performed

F11 (coagulation factor XI) (eg, coagulation disorder), common variants (eg, E117X [Type II], F283L [Type III], IVS14del14, and IVS14+1G>A [Type I])

FGFR3 (fibroblast growth factor receptor 3) (eg, achondroplasia, hypochondroplasia), common variants (eg, 1138G>A, 1138G>C, 1620C>A, 1620C>G)

FIP1L1/PDGFRA (del[4q12]) (eg, imatinib-sensitive chronic eosinophilic leukemia), qualitative and quantitative, if performed

FLG (filaggrin) (eg, ichthyosis vulgaris), common variants (eg, R501X, 2282del4, R2447X, S3247X, 3702delG)

FOXO1/PAX3 (t(2;13)) (eg, alveolar rhabdomyosarcoma), translocation analysis, qualitative and quantitative, if performed

FOXO1/PAX7 (t(1;13)) (eg, alveolar rhabdomyosarcoma), translocation analysis, qualitative and quantitative, if performed

FUS/DDIT3 (t(12;16)) (eg, myxoid liposarcoma), translocation analysis, qualitative, and quantitative, if performed

GALC (galactosylceramidase) (eg, Krabbe disease), common variants (eg, c.857G>A, 30-kb deletion)

GALT (galactose-1-phosphate uridylyltransferase) (eg, galactosemia), common variants (eg, Q188R, S135L, K285N, T138M, L195P, Y209C, IVS2-2A>G, P171S, del5kb, N314D, L218L/N314D)

H19 (imprinted maternally expressed transcript [non-protein coding]) (eg, Beckwith-Wiedemann syndrome), methylation analysis

IGH@/BCL2 (t(14;18)) (eg, follicular lymphoma), translocation and analysis; single breakpoint (eg) major breakpoint region [MBR] or minor cluster region [mcr]), qualitative or quantitative

(When both MBR and mcr breakpoints are performed, report [81278])

KCNQ1OT1 (KCNQ1 overlapping transcript 1 [non-protein coding]) (e.g, Beckwith-Wiedemann syndrome), methylation analysis

LINC00518 (long intergenic non-protein coding RNA 518) (eg, melanoma), expression analysis

LRRK2 (leucine-rich repeat kinase 2) (eg, Parkinson disease), common variants (eg, R1441G, G2019S, I2020T)

MED12 (mediator complex subunit 12) (eg, FG syndrome type 1, Lujan syndrome), common variants (eg, R961W, N1007S)

MEG3/DLK1 (maternally expressed 3 [non-protein coding]/delta-like 1 homolog [Drosophila]) (eg, intrauterine growth retardation), methylation analysis

MLL/AFF1 (t(4;11)) (eg acute lymphoblastic leukemia), translocation analysis, qualitative and quantitative, if performed

MLL/MLLT3 (t(9;11)) (eg, acute myeloid leukemia) translocation analysis, qualitative and quantitative, if performed

MT-RNR1 (mitochondrially encoded 12S RNA) (eg, nonsyndromic hearing loss), common variants (eg, m.1555>G, m1494C>T)

MUTYH (mutY homolog [E.coli]) (eg, MYH-associated polyposis), common variants (eg, Y165C, G382D)

MT-ATP6 (mitochondrially encoded ATP synthase 6) (eg, neuropathy with ataxia and retinitis pigmentosa [NARP], Leigh syndrome), common variants (eg, m.8993T>G, m.8993T>C)

MT-ND4, MT-ND6 (mitochondrially encoded NADH dehydrogenase 4, mitochondrially encoded NADH dehydrogenase 6) (eg, Leber hereditary optic neuropathy [LHON]), common variants (eg m.11778G>A, m3460G>A, m14484T>C)

MT-ND5 (mitochondrially encoded tRNA leucine 1 [UUA/G], mitochondrially encoded NADH dehydrogenase 5) (eg, mitochondrial encephalopathy with lactic acidosis and stroke-like episodes [MELAS]), common variants (eg, m.3243A>G, m.3271T>C, m.3252A>G, m.13513G>A)

MT-TK (mitochondrially encoded tRNA lysine) (eg, myoclonic epilepsy with ragged-red fibers [MERRF]), common variants (eg, m8344A>G, m.8356T>C)

MT-TL1 (mitochondrially encoded tRNA leucine 1[UUA/G]) (eg, diabetes and hearing loss), common variants (eg, m.3243A>G, m.14709 T>C) MT-TL1

MT-TS1, MT-RNR1 (mitochondrially encoded tRNA serine 1 [UCN], mitochondrially encoded 12S RNA) (eg, nonsyndromic sensorineural deafness [including aminoglycoside-induced nonsyndromic deafness]) common variants (eg, m.7445A>G, m.1555A>G)

NOD2 (nucleotide-binding oligomerization domain containing 2) (eg, Crohn's disease, Blau syndrome), common variants (eg, SNP 8, SNP 12, SNP 13)

NPM/ALK (t(2;5)) (eg, anaplastic large cell lymphoma), translocation analysis

PAX8/PPARG (t(2;3) (q13;p25)) (eg, follicular thyroid carcinoma), translocation analysis

PRAME (preferentially expressed antigen in melanoma)(eg, melanoma), expression analysis

PRSS1 (protease, serine, 1 [trypsin 1]) (eg, hereditary pancreatitis), common variants (eg, N29I, A16V, R122H)

PYGM (phosphorylase, glycogen, muscle) (eg, glycogen storage disease type V, McArdle disease), common variants (eg, R50X, G205S)

RUNX1/RUNX1T1 (t(8;21)) (eg, acute myeloid leukemia) translocation analysis, qualitative and quantitative, if performed

SS18/SSX1 (t(X;18)) (eg, synovial sarcoma), translocation analysis, qualitative and quantitative, if performed

SS18/SSX2 (t(X;18)) (eg, synovial sarcoma), translocation analysis, qualitative and quantitative, if performed

VWF (von Willebrand factor) (eg, von Willebrand disease type 2N), common variants (eg, T791M, R816W, R854Q)

0.00 0.00 **FUD** XXX A

AMA: 2020,Dec,3; 2020,OctSE,1; 2020,OctSE,1; 2019,Sep,7; 2019,Jul,3; 2018,Nov,9; 2018,Jan,8; 2017,Jan,8; 2016,Aug,9; 2016,Jan,13

81402 **Molecular pathology procedure, Level 3 (eg, >10 SNPs, 2-10 methylated variants, or 2-10 somatic variants [typically using non-sequencing target variant analysis], immunoglobulin and T-cell receptor gene rearrangements, duplication/deletion variants of 1 exon, loss of heterozygosity [LOH], uniparental disomy [UPD])**

Chromosome 1p-/19q- (eg, glial tumors), deletion analysis

Chromosome 18q- (eg, D18S55, D18S58, D18S61, D18S64, and D18S69) (eg, colon cancer), allelic imbalance assessment (ie, loss of heterozygosity)

COL1A1/PDGFB (t(17;22)) (eg, dermatofibrosarcoma protuberans), translocation analysis, multiple breakpoints, qualitative, and quantitative, if performed

CYP21A2 (cytochrome P450, family 21, subfamily A, polypeptide 2) (eg, congenital adrenal hyperplasia, 21-hydroxylase deficiency), common variants (eg, IVS2-13G, P30L, I172N, exon 6 mutation cluster [I235N, V236E, M238K], V281L, L307FfsX6, Q318X, R356W, P453S, G110VfsX21, 30-kb deletion variant)

ESR1/PGR (receptor 1/progesterone receptor) ratio (eg, breast cancer)

MEFV (Mediterranean fever) (eg, familial Mediterranean fever), common variants (eg, E148Q, P369S, F479L, M680I, I692del, M694V, M694I, K695R, V726A, A744S, R761H)

TRD@ (T cell antigen receptor, delta) (eg, leukemia and lymphoma), gene rearrangement analysis, evaluation to detect abnormal clonal population

Uniparental disomy (UPD) (eg, Russell-Silver syndrome, Prader-Willi/Angelman syndrome), short tandem repeat (STR) analysis

0.00 0.00 **FUD** XXX A

AMA: 2020,Dec,3; 2020,OctSE,1; 2020,OctSE,1; 2018,Nov,9; 2018,Jan,8; 2017,Jan,8; 2016,Aug,9; 2016,Jan,13

81403 **Molecular pathology procedure, Level 4 (eg, analysis of single exon by DNA sequence analysis, analysis of >10 amplicons using multiplex PCR in 2 or more independent reactions, mutation scanning or duplication/deletion variants of 2-5 exons)**

ANG (angiogenin, ribonuclease, RNase A family, 5) (eg, amyotrophic lateral sclerosis), full gene sequence

ARX (aristaless-related homeobox) (eg, X-linked lissencephaly with ambiguous genitalia, X-linked mental retardation), duplication/deletion analysis

CEL (carboxyl ester lipase [bile salt-stimulated lipase]) (eg, maturity-onset diabetes of the young [MODY]), targeted sequence analysis of exon 11 (eg, c.1785delC, c.1686delT)

CTNNB1 (catenin [cadherin-associated protein], beta 1, 88kDa) (eg, desmoid tumors), targeted sequence analysis (eg, exon 3)

DAZ/SRY (deleted in azoospermia and sex determining region Y) (eg, male infertility), common deletions (eg, AZFa, AZFb, AZFc, AZFd)

DNMT3A (DNA [cytosine-5-]-methyltransferase 3 alpha) (eg, acute myeloid leukemia), targeted sequence analysis (eg, exon 23)

EPCAM (epithelial cell adhesion molecule) (eg, Lynch syndrome), duplication/deletion analysis

F8 (coagulation factor VIII) (eg, hemophilia A), inversion analysis, intron 1 and intron 22A

F12 (coagulation factor XII [Hageman factor]) (eg, angioedema, hereditary, type III; factor XII deficiency), targeted sequence analysis of exon 9

FGFR3 (fibroblast growth factor receptor 3) (eg, isolated craniosynostosis), targeted sequence analysis (eg, exon 7)

(For targeted sequence analysis of multiple FGFR3 exons, use 81404) (81404)

GJB1 (gap junction protein, beta 1) (eg, Charcot-Marie-Tooth X-linked), full gene sequence

GNAQ (guanine nucleotide-binding protein G[q] subunit alpha) (eg, uveal melanoma), common variants (eg, R183, Q209)

HRAS (v-Ha-ras Harvey rat sarcoma viral oncogene homolog) (eg, Costello syndrome), exon 2 sequence

Human erythrocyte antigen gene analyses (eg, SLC14A1 [Kidd blood group], BCAM [Lutheran blood group], ICAM4 [Landsteiner-Wiener blood group], SLC4A1 [Diego blood group], AQP1 [Colton blood group], ERMAP [Scianna blood group], RHCE [Rh blood group, CcEe antigens], KEL [Kell blood group], DARC [Duffy blood group], GYPA, GYPB, GYPE [MNS blood group], ART4 [Dombrock blood group]) (eg, sickle-cell disease, thalassemia, hemolytic transfusion reactions, hemolytic disease of the fetus or newborn), common variants

KCNC3 (potassium voltage-gated channel, Shaw-related subfamily, member 3) (eg, spinocerebellar ataxia), targeted sequence analysis (eg, exon 2)

KCNJ2 (potassium inwardly-rectifying channel, subfamily J, member 2) (eg, Andersen-Tawil syndrome), full gene sequence

KCNJ11 (potassium inwardly-rectifying channel, subfamily J, member 11) (eg, familial hyperinsulinism), full gene sequence

Killer cell immunoglobulin-like receptor (KIR) gene family (eg, hematopoietic stem cell transplantation), genotyping of KIR family genes

Known familial variant, not otherwise specified, for gene listed in Tier 1 or Tier 2, or identified during a genomic sequencing procedure, DNA sequence analysis, each variant exon

(For a known familial variant that is considered a common variant, use specific common variant Tier 1 or Tier 2 code)

MC4R (melanocortin 4 receptor) (eg, obesity), full gene sequence

*MICA (MHC class I polypeptide-related sequence A) (eg, solid organ transplantation), common variants (eg, *001, *002)*

MT-RNR1 (mitochondrially encoded 12S RNA) (eg, nonsyndromic hearing loss), full gene sequence

MT-TS1 (mitochondrially encoded tRNA serine 1) (eg, nonsyndromic hearing loss), full gene sequence

NDP (Norrie disease [pseudoglioma]) (eg, Norrie disease), duplication/deletion analysis

NHLRC1 (NHL repeat containing 1) (eg, progressive myoclonus epilepsy), full gene sequence

PHOX2B (paired-like homeobox 2b) (eg, congenital central hypoventilation syndrome), duplication/deletion analysis

PLN (phospholamban) (eg, dilated cardiomyopathy, hypertrophic cardiomyopathy), full gene sequence

RHD (Rh blood group, D antigen) (eg, hemolytic disease of the fetus and newborn, Rh maternal/fetal compatibility), deletion analysis (eg, exons 4, 5, and 7, pseudogene)

RHD (Rh blood group, D antigen) (eg, hemolytic disease of the fetus and newborn, Rh maternal/fetal compatibility), deletion analysis (eg, exons 4, 5, and 7, pseudogene), performed on cell-free fetal DNA in maternal blood

(For human erythrocyte gene analysis of RHD, use a separate unit of 81403)

SH2D1A (SH2 domain containing 1A) (eg, X-linked lymphoproliferative syndrome), duplication/deletion analysis

TWIST1 (twist homolog 1 [Drosophila]) (eg, Saethre-Chotzen syndrome), duplication/deletion analysis

UBA1 (ubiquitin-like modifier activating enzyme 1) (eg, spinal muscular atrophy, X-linked), targeted sequence analysis (eg, exon 15)

VHL (von Hippel-Lindau tumor suppressor) (eg, von Hippel-Lindau familial cancer syndrome), deletion/duplication analysis

VWF (von Willebrand factor) (eg, von Willebrand disease types 2A, 2B, 2M), targeted sequence analysis (eg, exon 28)

0.00 0.00 **FUD** XXX A

AMA: 2020,Dec,3; 2020,OctSE,1; 2020,OctSE,1; 2019,Jul,3; 2018,Nov,9; 2018,May,6; 2018,Jan,8; 2017,Jan,8; 2016,Aug,9; 2016,Jan,13

81404 **Molecular pathology procedure, Level 5 (eg, analysis of 2-5 exons by DNA sequence analysis, mutation scanning or duplication/deletion variants of 6-10 exons, or characterization of a dynamic mutation disorder/triplet repeat by Southern blot analysis)**

ACADS (acyl-CoA dehydrogenase, C-2 to C-3 short chain) (eg, short chain acyl-CoA dehydrogenase deficiency), targeted sequence analysis (eg, exons 5 and 6)

AQP2 (aquaporin 2 [collecting duct]) (eg, nephrogenic diabetes insipidus), full gene sequence

ARX (aristaless related homeobox) (eg, X-linked lissencephaly with ambiguous genitalia, X-linked mental retardation), full gene sequence

AVPR2 (arginine vasopressin receptor 2) (eg, nephrogenic diabetes insipidus), full gene sequence

BBS10 (Bardet-Biedl syndrome 10) (eg, Bardet-Biedl syndrome), full gene sequence

BTD (biotinidase) (eg, biotinidase deficiency), full gene sequence

C10orf2 (chromosome 10 open reading frame 2) (eg, mitochondrial DNA depletion syndrome), full gene sequence

CAV3 (caveolin 3) (eg, CAV3-related distal myopathy, limb-girdle muscular dystrophy type 1C), full gene sequence

CD40LG (CD40 ligand) (eg, X-linked hyper IgM syndrome), full gene sequence

CDKN2A (cyclin-dependent kinase inhibitor 2A) (eg, CDKN2A-related cutaneous malignant melanoma, familial atypical mole-malignant melanoma syndrome), full gene sequence

CLRN1 (clarin 1) (eg, Usher syndrome, type 3), full gene sequence

COX6B1 (cytochrome c oxidase subunit VIb polypeptide 1) (eg, mitochondrial respiratory chain complex IV deficiency), full gene sequence

CPT2 (carnitine palmitoyltransferase 2) (eg, carnitine palmitoyltransferase II deficiency), full gene sequence

CRX (cone-rod homeobox) (eg, cone-rod dystrophy 2, Leber congenital amaurosis), full gene sequence

CYP1B1 (cytochrome P450, family 1, subfamily B, polypeptide 1) (eg, primary congenital glaucoma), full gene sequence

EGR2 (early growth response 2) (eg, Charcot-Marie-Tooth), full gene sequence

EMD (emerin) (eg, Emery-Dreifuss muscular dystrophy), duplication/deletion analysis

EPM2A (epilepsy, progressive myoclonus type 2A, Lafora disease [laforin]) (eg, progressive myoclonus epilepsy), full gene sequence

FGF23 (fibroblast growth factor 23) (eg, hypophosphatemic rickets), full gene sequence

FGFR2 (fibroblast growth factor receptor 2) (eg, craniosynostosis, Apert syndrome, Crouzon syndrome), targeted sequence analysis (eg, exons 8, 10)

FGFR3 (fibroblast growth factor receptor 3) (eg, achondroplasia, hypochondroplasia), targeted sequence analysis (eg, exons 8, 11, 12, 13)

FHL1 (four and a half LIM domains 1) (eg, Emery-Dreifuss muscular dystrophy), full gene sequence

FKRP (Fukutin related protein) (eg, congenital muscular dystrophy type 1C [MDC1C], limb-girdle muscular dystrophy [LGMD] type 2I), full gene sequence

FOXG1 (forkhead box G1) (eg, Rett syndrome), full gene sequence

FSHMD1A (facioscapulohumeral muscular dystrophy 1A) (eg, facioscapulohumeral muscular dystrophy), evaluation to detect abnormal (eg, deleted) alleles

FSHMD1A (facioscapulohumeral muscular dystrophy 1A) (eg, facioscapulohumeral muscular dystrophy), characterization of haplotype(s) (ie, chromosome 4A and 4B haplotypes)

GH1 (growth hormone 1) (eg, growth hormone deficiency), full gene sequence

GP1BB (glycoprotein Ib [platelet], beta polypeptide) (eg, Bernard-Soulier syndrome type B), full gene sequence

(For common deletion variants of alpha globin 1 and alpha globin 2 genes, use 81257)

HNF1B (HNF1 homeobox B) (eg, maturity-onset diabetes of the young [MODY]), duplication/deletion analysis

HRAS (v-Ha-ras Harvey rat sarcoma viral oncogene homolog) (eg, Costello syndrome), full gene sequence

HSD3B2 (hydroxy-delta-5-steroid dehydrogenase, 3 beta- and steroid delta-isomerase 2) (eg, 3-beta-hydroxysteroid dehydrogenase type II deficiency), full gene sequence

HSD11B2 (hydroxysteroid [11-beta] dehydrogenase 2) (eg, mineralocorticoid excess syndrome), full gene sequence

HSPB1 (heat shock 27kDa protein 1) (eg, Charcot-Marie-Tooth disease), full gene sequence

INS (insulin) (eg, diabetes mellitus), full gene sequence

KCNJ1 (potassium inwardly-rectifying channel, subfamily J, member 1) (eg, Bartter syndrome), full gene sequence

KCNJ10 (potassium inwardly-rectifying channel, subfamily J, member 10) (eg, SeSAME syndrome, EAST syndrome, sensorineural hearing loss), full gene sequence

LITAF (lipopolysaccharide-induced TNF factor) (eg, Charcot-Marie-Tooth), full gene sequence

MEFV (Mediterranean fever) (eg, familial Mediterranean fever), full gene sequence

MEN1 (multiple endocrine neoplasia I) (eg, multiple endocrine neoplasia type 1, Wermer syndrome), duplication/deletion analysis

MMACHC (methylmalonic aciduria [cobalamin deficiency] cblC type, with homocystinuria) (eg, methylmalonic acidemia and homocystinuria), full gene sequence

MPV17 (MpV17 mitochondrial inner membrane protein) (eg, mitochondrial DNA depletion syndrome), duplication/deletion analysis

NDP (Norrie disease [pseudoglioma]) (eg, Norrie disease), full gene sequence

NDUFA1 (NADH dehydrogenase [ubiquinone] 1 alpha subcomplex, 1, 7.5kDa) (eg, Leigh syndrome, mitochondrial complex I deficiency), full gene sequence

NDUFAF2 (NADH dehydrogenase [ubiquinone] 1 alpha subcomplex, assembly factor 2) (eg, Leigh syndrome, mitochondrial complex I deficiency), full gene sequence

NDUFS4 (NADH dehydrogenase [ubiquinone] Fe-S protein 4, 18kDa [NADH-coenzyme Q reductase]) (eg, Leigh syndrome, mitochondrial complex I deficiency), full gene sequence

NIPA1 (non-imprinted in Prader-Willi/Angelman syndrome 1) (eg, spastic paraplegia), full gene sequence

NLGN4X (neuroligin 4, X-linked) (eg, autism spectrum disorders), duplication/deletion analysis

NPC2 (Niemann-Pick disease, type C2 [epididymal secretory protein E1]) (eg, Niemann-Pick disease type C2), full gene sequence

NR0B1 (nuclear receptor subfamily 0, group B, member 1) (eg, congenital adrenal hypoplasia), full gene sequence

PDX1 (pancreatic and duodenal homeobox 1) (eg, maturity-onset diabetes of the young [MODY]), full gene sequence

PHOX2B (paired-like homeobox 2b) (eg, congenital central hypoventilation syndrome), full gene sequence

PIK3CA (phosphatidylinositol-4,5-bisphosphate 3-kinase, catalytic subunit alpha) (eg, colorectal cancer), targeted sequence analysis (eg, exons 9 and 20)

PLP1 (proteolipid protein 1) (eg, Pelizaeus-Merzbacher disease, spastic paraplegia), duplication/deletion analysis

PQBP1 (polyglutamine binding protein 1) (eg, Renpenning syndrome), duplication/deletion analysis

PRNP (prion protein) (eg, genetic prion disease), full gene sequence

PROP1 (PROP paired-like homeobox 1) (eg, combined pituitary hormone deficiency), full gene sequence

PRPH2 (peripherin 2 [retinal degeneration, slow]) (eg, retinitis pigmentosa), full gene sequence

PRSS1 (protease, serine, 1 [trypsin 1]) (eg, hereditary pancreatitis), full gene sequence

RAF1 (v-raf-1 murine leukemia viral oncogene homolog 1) (eg, LEOPARD syndrome), targeted sequence analysis (eg, exons 7, 12, 14, 17)

RET (ret proto-oncogene) (eg, multiple endocrine neoplasia, type 2B and familial medullary thyroid carcinoma), common variants (eg, M918T, 2647_2648delinsTT, A883F)

RHO (rhodopsin) (eg, retinitis pigmentosa), full gene sequence

RP1 (retinitis pigmentosa 1) (eg, retinitis pigmentosa), full gene sequence

SCN1B (sodium channel, voltage-gated, type I, beta) (eg, Brugada syndrome), full gene sequence

SCO2 (SCO cytochrome oxidase deficient homolog 2 [SCO1L]) (eg, mitochondrial respiratory chain complex IV deficiency), full gene sequence

SDHC (succinate dehydrogenase complex, subunit C, integral membrane protein, 15kDa) (eg, hereditary paraganglioma-pheochromocytoma syndrome), duplication/deletion analysis

SDHD (succinate dehydrogenase complex, subunit D, integral membrane protein) (eg, hereditary paraganglioma), full gene sequence

SGCG (sarcoglycan, gamma [35kDa dystrophin-associated glycoprotein]) (eg, limb-girdle muscular dystrophy), duplication/deletion analysis

SH2D1A (SH2 domain containing 1A) (eg, X-linked lymphoproliferative syndrome), full gene sequence

SLC16A2 (solute carrier family 16, member 2 [thyroid hormone transporter]) (eg, specific thyroid hormone cell transporter deficiency, Allan-Herndon-Dudley syndrome), duplication/deletion analysis

SLC25A20 (solute carrier family 25 [carnitine/acylcarnitine translocase], member 20) (eg, carnitine-acylcarnitine translocase deficiency), duplication/deletion analysis

SLC25A4 (solute carrier family 25 [mitochondrial carrier; adenine nucleotide translocation], member 4) (eg, progressive external ophthalmoplegia), full gene sequence

SOD1 (superoxide dismutase 1, soluble) (eg, amyotrophic lateral sclerosis), full gene sequence

SPINK1 (serine peptidase inhibitor, Kazal type 1) (eg, hereditary pancreatitis), full gene sequence

STK11 (serine/threonine kinase 11) (eg, Peutz-Jeghers syndrome), duplication/deletion analysis

TACO1 (translational activator of mitochondrial encoded cytochrome c oxidase I) (eg, mitochondrial respiratory chain complex IV deficiency), full gene sequence

THAP1 (THAP domain containing, apoptosis associated protein 1) (eg, torsion dystonia), full gene sequence

TOR1A (torsin family 1, member A [torsin A]) (eg, torsion dystonia), full gene sequence

TTPA (tocopherol [alpha] transfer protein) (eg, ataxia), full gene sequence

TTR (transthyretin) (eg, familial transthyretin amyloidosis), full gene sequence

TWIST1 (twist homolog 1 [Drosophila]) (eg, Saethre-Chotzen syndrome), full gene sequence

TYR (tyrosinase [oculocutaneous albinism IA]) (eg, oculocutaneous albinism IA), full gene sequence

UGT1A1 (UDP glucuronosyltransferase 1 family, polypeptide A1) (eg, hereditary unconjugated hyperbilirubinemia [Crigler-Najjar syndrome]) full gene sequence

USH1G (Usher syndrome 1G [autosomal recessive]) (eg, Usher syndrome, type 1), full gene sequence

VWF (von Willebrand factor) (eg, von Willebrand disease type 1C), targeted sequence analysis (eg, exons 26, 27, 37)

VHL (von Hippel-Lindau tumor suppressor) (eg, von Hippel-Lindau familial cancer syndrome), full gene sequence

ZEB2 (zinc finger E-box binding homeobox 2) (eg, Mowat-Wilson syndrome), duplication/deletion analysis

ZNF41 (zinc finger protein 41) (eg, X-linked mental retardation 89), full gene sequence

0.00 0.00 **FUD** XXX A

AMA: 2020,Dec,3; 2020,OctSE,1; 2020,OctSE,1; 2020,Apr,9; 2019,Jul,3; 2018,Nov,9; 2018,May,6; 2018,Jan,8; 2017,Jan,8; 2016,Aug,9; 2016,Jan,13

▲ **81405** **Molecular pathology procedure, Level 6 (eg, analysis of 6-10 exons by DNA sequence analysis, mutation scanning or duplication/deletion variants of 11-25 exons, regionally targeted cytogenomic array analysis)**

ABCD1 (ATP-binding cassette, sub-family D [ALD], member 1) (eg, adrenoleukodystrophy), full gene sequence

ACADS (acyl-CoA dehydrogenase, C-2 to C-3 short chain) (eg, short chain acyl-CoA dehydrogenase deficiency), full gene sequence

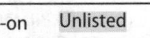

ACTA2 (actin, alpha 2, smooth muscle, aorta) (eg, thoracic aortic aneurysms and aortic dissections), full gene sequence

ACTC1 (actin, alpha, cardiac muscle 1) (eg, familial hypertrophic cardiomyopathy), full gene sequence

ANKRD1 (ankyrin repeat domain 1) (eg, dilated cardiomyopathy), full gene sequence

APTX (aprataxin) (eg, ataxia with oculomotor apraxia 1), full gene sequence

ARSA (arylsulfatase A) (eg, arylsulfatase A deficiency), full gene sequence

BCKDHA (branched chain keto acid dehydrogenase E1, alpha polypeptide) (eg, maple syrup urine disease, type 1A), full gene sequence

BCS1L (BCS1-like [S. cerevisiae]) (eg, Leigh syndrome, mitochondrial complex III deficiency, GRACILE syndrome), full gene sequence

BMPR2 (bone morphogenetic protein receptor, type II [serine/threonine kinase]) (eg, heritable pulmonary arterial hypertension), duplication/deletion analysis

CASQ2 (calsequestrin 2 [cardiac muscle]) (eg, catecholaminergic polymorphic ventricular tachycardia), full gene sequence

CASR (calcium-sensing receptor) (eg, hypocalcemia), full gene sequence

CDKL5 (cyclin-dependent kinase-like 5) (eg, early infantile epileptic encephalopathy), duplication/deletion analysis

CHRNA4 (cholinergic receptor, nicotinic, alpha 4) (eg, nocturnal frontal lobe epilepsy), full gene sequence

CHRNB2 (cholinergic receptor, nicotinic, beta 2 [neuronal]) (eg, nocturnal frontal lobe epilepsy), full gene sequence

COX10 (COX10 homolog, cytochrome c oxidase assembly protein) (eg, mitochondrial respiratory chain complex IV deficiency), full gene sequence

COX15 (COX15 homolog, cytochrome c oxidase assembly protein) (eg, mitochondrial respiratory chain complex IV deficiency), full gene sequence

CPOX (coproporphyrinogen oxidase) (eg, hereditary coproporphyria), full gene sequence

CTRC (chymotrypsin C) (eg, hereditary pancreatitis), full gene sequence

CYP11B1 (cytochrome P450, family 11, subfamily B, polypeptide 1) (eg, congenital adrenal hyperplasia), full gene sequence

CYP17A1 (cytochrome P450, family 17, subfamily A, polypeptide 1) (eg, congenital adrenal hyperplasia), full gene sequence

CYP21A2 (cytochrome P450, family 21, subfamily A, polypeptide2) (eg, steroid 21-hydroxylase isoform, congenital adrenal hyperplasia), full gene sequence

Cytogenomic constitutional targeted microarray analysis of chromosome 22q13 by interrogation of genomic regions for copy number and single nucleotide polymorphism (SNP) variants for chromosomal abnormalities

(When performing cytogenomic [genome-wide] analysis for constitutional chromosomal abnormalities, see 81228, 81229, 81349)

(Do not report analyte-specific molecular pathology procedures separately when the specific analytes are included as part of the microarray analysis of chromosome 22q13)

(Do not report 88271 when performing cytogenomic microarray analysis)

DBT (dihydrolipoamide branched chain transacylase E2) (eg, maple syrup urine disease, type 2), duplication/deletion analysis

DCX (doublecortin) (eg, X-linked lissencephaly), full gene sequence

DES (desmin) (eg, myofibrillar myopathy), full gene sequence

DFNB59 (deafness, autosomal recessive 59) (eg, autosomal recessive nonsyndromic hearing impairment), full gene sequence

DGUOK (deoxyguanosine kinase) (eg, hepatocerebral mitochondrial DNA depletion syndrome), full gene sequence

DHCR7 (7-dehydrocholesterol reductase) (eg, Smith-Lemli-Opitz syndrome), full gene sequence

EIF2B2 (eukaryotic translation initiation factor 2B, subunit 2 beta, 39kDa) (eg, leukoencephalopathy with vanishing white matter), full gene sequence

EMD (emerin) (eg, Emery-Dreifuss muscular dystrophy), full gene sequence

ENG (endoglin) (eg, hereditary hemorrhagic telangiectasia, type 1), duplication/deletion analysis

EYA1 (eyes absent homolog 1 [Drosophila]) (eg, branchio-oto-renal [BOR] spectrum disorders), duplication/deletion analysis

FGFR1 (fibroblast growth factor receptor 1) (eg, Kallmann syndrome 2), full gene sequence

FH (fumarate hydratase) (eg, fumarate hydratase deficiency, hereditary leiomyomatosis with renal cell cancer), full gene sequence

FKTN (fukutin) (eg, limb-girdle muscular dystrophy [LGMD] type 2M or 2L), full gene sequence

FTSJ1 (FtsJ RNA methyltransferase homolog 1 [E. coli]) (eg, X-linked mental retardation 9), duplication/deletion analysis

GABRG2 (gamma-aminobutyric acid [GABA] A receptor, gamma 2) (eg, generalized epilepsy with febrile seizures), full gene sequence

GCH1 (GTP cyclohydrolase 1) (eg, autosomal dominant dopa-responsive dystonia), full gene sequence

GDAP1 (ganglioside-induced differentiation-associated protein 1) (eg, Charcot-Marie-Tooth disease), full gene sequence

GFAP (glial fibrillary acidic protein) (eg, Alexander disease), full gene sequence

GHR (growth hormone receptor) (eg, Laron syndrome), full gene sequence

GHRHR (growth hormone releasing hormone receptor) (eg, growth hormone deficiency), full gene sequence

GLA (galactosidase, alpha) (eg, Fabry disease), full gene sequence

HNF1A (HNF1 homeobox A) (eg, maturity-onset diabetes of the young [MODY]), full gene sequence

HNF1B (HNF1 homeobox B) (eg, maturity-onset diabetes of the young [MODY]), full gene sequence

HTRA1 (HtrA serine peptidase 1) (eg, macular degeneration), full gene sequence

IDS (iduronate 2-sulfatase) (eg, mucopolysaccharidosis, type II), full gene sequence

IL2RG (interleukin 2 receptor, gamma) (eg, X-linked severe combined immunodeficiency), full gene sequence

ISPD (isoprenoid synthase domain containing) (eg, muscle-eye-brain disease, Walker-Warburg syndrome), full gene sequence

KRAS (Kirsten rat sarcoma viral oncogene homolog) (eg, Noonan syndrome), full gene sequence

LAMP2 (lysosomal-associated membrane protein 2) (eg, Danon disease), full gene sequence

LDLR (low density lipoprotein receptor) (eg, familial hypercholesterolemia), duplication/deletion analysis

MEN1 (multiple endocrine neoplasia I) (eg, multiple endocrine neoplasia type 1, Wermer syndrome), full gene sequence

MMAA (methylmalonic aciduria [cobalamine deficiency] type A) (eg, MMAA-related methylmalonic acidemia), full gene sequence

MMAB (methylmalonic aciduria [cobalamine deficiency] type B) (eg, MMAA-related methylmalonic acidemia), full gene sequence

MPI (mannose phosphate isomerase) (eg, congenital disorder of glycosylation 1b), full gene sequence

MPV17 (MpV17 mitochondrial inner membrane protein) (eg, mitochondrial DNA depletion syndrome), full gene sequence

MPZ (myelin protein zero) (eg, Charcot-Marie-Tooth), full gene sequence

MTM1 (myotubularin 1) (eg, X-linked centronuclear myopathy), duplication/deletion analysis

MYL2 (myosin, light chain 2, regulatory, cardiac, slow) (eg, familial hypertrophic cardiomyopathy), full gene sequence

MYL3 (myosin, light chain 3, alkali, ventricular, skeletal, slow) (eg, familial hypertrophic cardiomyopathy), full gene sequence

MYOT (myotilin) (eg, limb-girdle muscular dystrophy), full gene sequence

NDUFS7 (NADH dehydrogenase [ubiquinone] Fe-S protein 7, 20kDa [NADH-coenzyme Q reductase]) (eg, Leigh syndrome, mitochondrial complex I deficiency), full gene sequence

NDUFS8 (NADH dehydrogenase [ubiquinone] Fe-S protein 8, 23kDa [NADH-coenzyme Q reductase]) (eg, Leigh syndrome, mitochondrial complex I deficiency), full gene sequence

NDUFV1 (NADH dehydrogenase [ubiquinone] flavoprotein 1, 51kDa) (eg, Leigh syndrome, mitochondrial complex I deficiency), full gene sequence

NEFL (neurofilament, light polypeptide) (eg, Charcot-Marie-Tooth), full gene sequence

NF2 (neurofibromin 2 [merlin]) (eg, neurofibromatosis, type 2), duplication/deletion analysis

NLGN3 (neuroligin 3) (eg, autism spectrum disorders), full gene sequence

NLGN4X (neuroligin 4, X-linked) (eg, autism spectrum disorders), full gene sequence

NPHP1 (nephronophthisis 1 [juvenile]) (eg, Joubert syndrome), deletion analysis, and duplication analysis, if performed

NPHS2 (nephrosis 2, idiopathic, steroid-resistant [podocin]) (eg, steroid-resistant nephrotic syndrome), full gene sequence

NSD1 (nuclear receptor binding SET domain protein 1) (eg, Sotos syndrome), duplication/deletion analysis

OTC (ornithine carbamoyltransferase) (eg, ornithine transcarbamylase deficiency), full gene sequence

PAFAH1B1 (platelet-activating factor acetylhydrolase 1b, regulatory subunit 1 [45kDa]) (eg, lissencephaly, Miller-Dieker syndrome), duplication/deletion analysis

PARK2 (Parkinson protein 2, E3 ubiquitin protein ligase [parkin]) (eg, Parkinson disease), duplication/deletion analysis

PCCA (propionyl CoA carboxylase, alpha polypeptide) (eg, propionic acidemia, type 1), duplication/deletion analysis

PCDH19 (protocadherin 19) (eg, epileptic encephalopathy), full gene sequence

PDHA1 (pyruvate dehydrogenase [lipoamide] alpha 1) (eg, lactic acidosis), duplication/deletion analysis

PDHB (pyruvate dehydrogenase [lipoamide] beta) (eg, lactic acidosis), full gene sequence

PINK1 (PTEN induced putative kinase 1) (eg, Parkinson disease), full gene sequence

PKLR (pyruvate kinase, liver and RBC) (eg, pyruvate kinase deficiency), full gene sequence

PLP1 (proteolipid protein 1) (eg, Pelizaeus-Merzbacher disease, spastic paraplegia), full gene sequence

POU1F1 (POU class 1 homeobox 1) (eg, combined pituitary hormone deficiency), full gene sequence

PQBP1 (polyglutamine binding protein 1) (eg, Renpenning syndrome), full gene sequence

PRX (periaxin) (eg, Charcot-Marie-Tooth disease), full gene sequence

PSEN1 (presenilin 1) (eg, Alzheimer's disease), full gene sequence

RAB7A (RAB7A, member RAS oncogene family) (eg, Charcot-Marie-Tooth disease), full gene sequence

RAI1 (retinoic acid induced 1) (eg, Smith-Magenis syndrome), full gene sequence

REEP1 (receptor accessory protein 1) (eg, spastic paraplegia), full gene sequence

RET (ret proto-oncogene) (eg, multiple endocrine neoplasia, type 2A and familial medullary thyroid carcinoma), targeted sequence analysis (eg, exons 10, 11, 13-16)

RPS19 (ribosomal protein S19) (eg, Diamond-Blackfan anemia), full gene sequence

RRM2B (ribonucleotide reductase M2 B [TP53 inducible]) (eg, mitochondrial DNA depletion), full gene sequence

SCO1 (SCO cytochrome oxidase deficient homolog 1) (eg, mitochondrial respiratory chain complex IV deficiency), full gene sequence

SDHB (succinate dehydrogenase complex, subunit B, iron sulfur) (eg, hereditary paraganglioma), full gene sequence

SDHC (succinate dehydrogenase complex, subunit C, integral membrane protein, 15kDa) (eg, hereditary paraganglioma-pheochromocytoma syndrome), full gene sequence

SGCA (sarcoglycan, alpha [50kDa dystrophin-associated glycoprotein]) (eg, limb-girdle muscular dystrophy), full gene sequence

SGCB (sarcoglycan, beta [43kDa dystrophin-associated glycoprotein]) (eg, limb-girdle muscular dystrophy), full gene sequence

SGCD (sarcoglycan, delta [35kDa dystrophin-associated glycoprotein]) (eg, limb-girdle muscular dystrophy), full gene sequence

SGCE (sarcoglycan, epsilon) (eg, myoclonic dystonia), duplication/deletion analysis

SGCG (sarcoglycan, gamma [35kDa dystrophin-associated glycoprotein]) (eg, limb-girdle muscular dystrophy), full gene sequence

SHOC2 (soc-2 suppressor of clear homolog) (eg, Noonan-like syndrome with loose anagen hair), full gene sequence

SHOX (short stature homeobox) (eg, Langer mesomelic dysplasia), full gene sequence

SIL1 (SIL1 homolog, endoplasmic reticulum chaperone [S. cerevisiae]) (eg, ataxia), full gene sequence

SLC2A1 (solute carrier family 2 [facilitated glucose transporter], member 1) (eg, glucose transporter type 1 [GLUT 1] deficiency syndrome), full gene sequence

SLC16A2 (solute carrier family 16, member 2 [thyroid hormone transporter]) (eg, specific thyroid hormone cell transporter deficiency, Allan-Herndon-Dudley syndrome), full gene sequence

SLC22A5 (solute carrier family 22 [organic cation/carnitine transporter], member 5) (eg, systemic primary carnitine deficiency), full gene sequence

SLC25A20 (solute carrier family 25 [carnitine/acylcarnitine translocase], member 20) (eg, carnitine-acylcarnitine translocase deficiency), full gene sequence

SMAD4 (SMAD family member 4) (eg, hemorrhagic telangiectasia syndrome, juvenile polyposis), duplication/deletion analysis

SPAST (spastin) (eg, spastic paraplegia), duplication/deletion analysis

SPG7 (spastic paraplegia 7 [pure and complicated autosomal recessive]) (eg, spastic paraplegia), duplication/deletion analysis

SPRED1 (sprouty-related, EVH1 domain containing 1) (eg, Legius syndrome), full gene sequence

STAT3 (signal transducer and activator of transcription 3 [acute-phase response factor]) (eg, autosomal dominant hyper-IgE syndrome), targeted sequence analysis (eg, exons 12, 13, 14, 16, 17, 20, 21)

STK11 (serine/threonine kinase 11) (eg, Peutz-Jeghers syndrome), full gene sequence

SURF1 (surfeit 1) (eg, mitochondrial respiratory chain complex IV deficiency), full gene sequence

TARDBP (TAR DNA binding protein) (eg, amyotrophic lateral sclerosis), full gene sequence

TBX5 (T-box 5) (eg, Holt-Oram syndrome), full gene sequence

TCF4 (transcription factor 4) (eg, Pitt-Hopkins syndrome), duplication/deletion analysis

TGFBR1 (transforming growth factor, beta receptor 1) (eg, Marfan syndrome), full gene sequence

TGFBR2 (transforming growth factor, beta receptor 2) (eg, Marfan syndrome), full gene sequence

THRB (thyroid hormone receptor, beta) (eg, thyroid hormone resistance, thyroid hormone beta receptor deficiency), full gene sequence or targeted sequence analysis of >5 exons

TK2 (thymidine kinase 2, mitochondrial) (eg, mitochondrial DNA depletion syndrome), full gene sequence

TNNC1 (troponin C type 1 [slow]) (eg, hypertrophic cardiomyopathy or dilated cardiomyopathy), full gene sequence

TNNI3 (troponin 1, type 3 [cardiac]) (eg, familial hypertrophic cardiomyopathy), full gene sequence

TPM1 (tropomyosin 1 [alpha]) (eg, familial hypertrophic cardiomyopathy), full gene sequence

TSC1 (tuberous sclerosis 1) (eg, tuberous sclerosis), duplication/deletion analysis

TYMP (thymidine phosphorylase) (eg, mitochondrial DNA depletion syndrome), full gene sequence

VWF (von Willebrand factor) (eg, von Willebrand disease type 2N), targeted sequence analysis (eg, exons 18-20, 23-25)

WT1 (Wilms tumor 1) (eg, Denys-Drash syndrome, familial Wilms tumor), full gene sequence

ZEB2 (zinc finger E-box binding homeobox 2) (eg, Mowat-Wilson syndrome), full gene sequence

0.00 0.00 **FUD** XXX A

AMA: 2020,Dec,3; 2020,OctSE,1; 2020,OctSE,1; 2019,Jul,3; 2018,Nov,9; 2018,Sep,14; 2018,May,6; 2018,Jan,8; 2017,Jan,8; 2016,Aug,9; 2016,Jan,13

81406 **Molecular pathology procedure, Level 7 (eg, analysis of 11-25 exons by DNA sequence analysis, mutation scanning or duplication/deletion variants of 26-50 exons)**

ACADVL (acyl-CoA dehydrogenase, very long chain) (eg, very long chain acyl-coenzyme A dehydrogenase deficiency), full gene sequence

ACTN4 (actinin, alpha 4) (eg, focal segmental glomerulosclerosis), full gene sequence

AFG3L2 (AFG3 ATPase family gene 3-like 2 [S. cerevisiae]) (eg, spinocerebellar ataxia), full gene sequence

AIRE (autoimmune regulator) (eg, autoimmune polyendocrinopathy syndrome type 1), full gene sequence

ALDH7A1 (aldehyde dehydrogenase 7 family, member A1) (eg, pyridoxine-dependent epilepsy), full gene sequence

ANO5 (anoctamin 5) (eg, limb-girdle muscular dystrophy), full gene sequence

ANOS1 (anosim-1) (eg, Kallmann syndrome 1), full gene sequence

APP (amyloid beta [A4] precursor protein) (eg, Alzheimer's disease), full gene sequence

ASS1 (argininosuccinate synthase 1) (eg, citrullinemia type I), full gene sequence

ATL1 (atlastin GTPase 1) (eg, spastic paraplegia), full gene sequence

ATP1A2 (ATPase, Na+/K+ transporting, alpha 2 polypeptide) (eg, familial hemiplegic migraine), full gene sequence

ATP7B (ATPase, Cu++ transporting, beta polypeptide) (eg, Wilson disease), full gene sequence

BBS1 (Bardet-Biedl syndrome 1) (eg, Bardet-Biedl syndrome), full gene sequence

BBS2 (Bardet-Biedl syndrome 2) (eg, Bardet-Biedl syndrome), full gene sequence

BCKDHB (branched-chain keto acid dehydrogenase E1, beta polypeptide) (eg, maple syrup urine disease, type 1B), full gene sequence

BEST1 (bestrophin 1) (eg, vitelliform macular dystrophy), full gene sequence

BMPR2 (bone morphogenetic protein receptor, type II [serine/threonine kinase]) (eg, heritable pulmonary arterial hypertension), full gene sequence

BRAF (B-Raf proto-oncogene, serine/threonine kinase) (eg, Noonan syndrome), full gene sequence

BSCL2 (Berardinelli-Seip congenital lipodystrophy 2 [seipin]) (eg, Berardinelli-Seip congenital lipodystrophy), full gene sequence

BTK (Bruton agammaglobulinemia tyrosine kinase) (eg, X-linked agammaglobulinemia), full gene sequence

CACNB2 (calcium channel, voltage-dependent, beta 2 subunit) (eg, Brugada syndrome), full gene sequence

CAPN3 (calpain 3) (eg, limb-girdle muscular dystrophy [LGMD] type 2A, calpainopathy), full gene sequence

CBS (cystathionine-beta-synthase) (eg, homocystinuria, cystathionine beta-synthase deficiency), full gene sequence

CDH1 (cadherin 1, type 1, E-cadherin [epithelial]) (eg, hereditary diffuse gastric cancer), full gene sequence

CDKL5 (cyclin-dependent kinase-like 5) (eg, early infantile epileptic encephalopathy), full gene sequence

CLCN1 (chloride channel 1, skeletal muscle) (eg, myotonia congenita), full gene sequence

CLCNKB (chloride channel, voltage-sensitive Kb) (eg, Bartter syndrome 3 and 4b), full gene sequence

CNTNAP2 (contactin-associated protein-like 2) (eg, Pitt-Hopkins-like syndrome 1), full gene sequence

COL6A2 (collagen, type VI, alpha 2) (eg, collagen type VI-related disorders), duplication/deletion analysis

CPT1A (carnitine palmitoyltransferase 1A [liver]) (eg, carnitine palmitoyltransferase 1A [CPT1A] deficiency), full gene sequence

CRB1 (crumbs homolog 1 [Drosophila]) (eg, Leber congenital amaurosis), full gene sequence

CREBBP (CREB binding protein) (eg, Rubinstein-Taybi syndrome), duplication/deletion analysis

DBT (dihydrolipoamide branched chain transacylase E2) (eg, maple syrup urine disease, type 2), full gene sequence

DLAT (dihydrolipoamide S-acetyltransferase) (eg, pyruvate dehydrogenase E2 deficiency), full gene sequence

DLD (dihydrolipoamide dehydrogenase) (eg, maple syrup urine disease, type III), full gene sequence

DSC2 (desmocollin) (eg, arrhythmogenic right ventricular dysplasia/cardiomyopathy 11), full gene sequence

DSG2 (desmoglein 2) (eg, arrhythmogenic right ventricular dysplasia/cardiomyopathy 10), full gene sequence

DSP (desmoplakin) (eg, arrhythmogenic right ventricular dysplasia/cardiomyopathy 8), full gene sequence

EFHC1 (EF-hand domain [C-terminal] containing 1) (eg, juvenile myoclonic epilepsy), full gene sequence

EIF2B3 (eukaryotic translation initiation factor 2B, subunit 3 gamma, 58kDa) (eg, leukoencephalopathy with vanishing white matter), full gene sequence

EIF2B4 (eukaryotic translation initiation factor 2B, subunit 4 delta, 67kDa) (eg, leukoencephalopathy with vanishing white matter), full gene sequence

EIF2B5 (eukaryotic translation initiation factor 2B, subunit 5 epsilon, 82kDa) (eg, childhood ataxia with central nervous system hypomyelination/vanishing white matter), full gene sequence

ENG (endoglin) (eg, hereditary hemorrhagic telangiectasia, type 1), full gene sequence

EYA1 (eyes absent homolog 1 [Drosophila]) (eg, branchio-oto-renal [BOR] spectrum disorders), full gene sequence

F8 (coagulation factor VIII) (eg, hemophilia A), duplication/deletion analysis

FAH (fumarylacetoacetate hydrolase [fumarylacetoacetase]) (eg, tyrosinemia, type 1), full gene sequence

FASTKD2 (FAST kinase domains 2) (eg, mitochondrial respiratory chain complex IV deficiency), full gene sequence

FIG4 (FIG4 homolog, SAC1 lipid phosphatase domain containing [S. cerevisiae]) (eg, Charcot-Marie-Tooth disease), full gene sequence

FTSJ1 (FtsJ RNA methyltransferase homolog 1 [E. coli]) (eg, X-linked mental retardation 9), full gene sequence

FUS (fused in sarcoma) (eg, amyotrophic lateral sclerosis), full gene sequence

GAA (glucosidase, alpha; acid) (eg, glycogen storage disease type II [Pompe disease]), full gene sequence

GALC (galactosylceramidase) (eg, Krabbe disease), full gene sequence

GALT (galactose-1-phosphate uridylyltransferase) (eg, galactosemia), full gene sequence

GARS (glycyl-tRNA synthetase) (eg, Charcot-Marie-Tooth disease), full gene sequence

GCDH (glutaryl-CoA dehydrogenase) (eg, glutaricacidemia type 1), full gene sequence

GCK (glucokinase [hexokinase 4]) (eg, maturity-onset diabetes of the young [MODY]), full gene sequence

GLUD1 (glutamate dehydrogenase 1) (eg, familial hyperinsulinism), full gene sequence

GNE (glucosamine [UDP-N-acetyl]-2-epimerase/N-acetylmannosamine kinase) (eg, inclusion body myopathy 2 [IBM2], Nonaka myopathy), full gene sequence

GRN (granulin) (eg, frontotemporal dementia), full gene sequence

HADHA (hydroxyacyl-CoA dehydrogenase/3-ketoacyl-CoA thiolase/enoyl-CoA hydratase [trifunctional protein] alpha subunit) (eg, long chain acyl-coenzyme A dehydrogenase deficiency), full gene sequence

HADHB (hydroxyacyl-CoA dehydrogenase/3-ketoacyl-CoA thiolase/enoyl-CoA hydratase [trifunctional protein], beta subunit) (eg, trifunctional protein deficiency), full gene sequence

HEXA (hexosaminidase A, alpha polypeptide) (eg, Tay-Sachs disease), full gene sequence

HLCS (HLCS holocarboxylase synthetase) (eg, holocarboxylase synthetase deficiency), full gene sequence

HMBS (hydroxymethylbilane synthase) (eg, acute intermittent porphyria), full gene sequence

HNF4A (hepatocyte nuclear factor 4, alpha) (eg, maturity-onset diabetes of the young [MODY]), full gene sequence

IDUA (iduronidase, alpha-L-) (eg, mucopolysaccharidosis type I), full gene sequence

INF2 (inverted formin, FH2 and WH2 domain containing) (eg, focal segmental glomerulosclerosis), full gene sequence

IVD (isovaleryl-CoA dehydrogenase) (eg, isovaleric acidemia), full gene sequence

JAG1 (jagged 1) (eg, Alagille syndrome), duplication/deletion analysis

JUP (junction plakoglobin) (eg, arrhythmogenic right ventricular dysplasia/cardiomyopathy 11), full gene sequence

KCNH2 (potassium voltage-gated channel, subfamily H [eag-related], member 2) (eg, short QT syndrome, long QT syndrome), full gene sequence

KCNQ1 (potassium voltage-gated channel, KQT-like subfamily, member 1) (eg, short QT syndrome, long QT syndrome), full gene sequence

KCNQ2 (potassium voltage-gated channel, KQT-like subfamily, member 2) (eg, epileptic encephalopathy), full gene sequence

LDB3 (LIM domain binding 3) (eg, familial dilated cardiomyopathy, myofibrillar myopathy), full gene sequence

LDLR (low density lipoprotein receptor) (eg, familial hypercholesterolemia), full gene sequence

LEPR (leptin receptor(eg, obesity with hypogonadism), full gene sequence

LHCGR (luteinizing hormone/choriogonadotropin receptor) (eg, precocious male puberty), full gene sequence

LMNA (lamin A/C) (eg, Emery-Dreifuss muscular dystrophy [EDMD1, 2 and 3] limb-girdle muscular dystrophy [LGMD] type 1B, dilated cardiomyopathy [CMD1A], familial partial lipodystrophy [FPLD2]), full gene sequence

LRP5 (low density lipoprotein receptor-related protein 5) (eg, osteopetrosis), full gene sequence

MAP2K1 (mitogen-activated protein kinase 1) (eg, cardiofaciocutaneous syndrome), full gene sequence

MAP2K2 (mitogen-activated protein kinase 2) (eg, cardiofaciocutaneous syndrome), full gene sequence

MAPT (microtubule-associated protein tau) (eg, frontotemporal dementia), full gene sequence

MCCC1 (methylcrotonoyl-CoA carboxylase 1 [alpha]) (eg, 3-methylcrotonyl-CoA carboxylase deficiency), full gene sequence

MCCC2 (methylcrotonoyl-CoA carboxylase 2 [beta]) (eg, 3-methylcrotonyl carboxylase deficiency), full gene sequence

MFN2 (mitofusin 2) (eg, Charcot-Marie-Tooth disease), full gene sequence

MTM1 (myotubularin 1) (eg, X-linked centronuclear myopathy), full gene sequence

MUT (methylmalonyl CoA mutase) (eg, methylmalonic acidemia), full gene sequence

MUTYH (mutY homolog [E. coli]) (eg, MYH-associated polyposis), full gene sequence

NDUFS1 (NADH dehydrogenase [ubiquinone] Fe-S protein 1, 75kDa [NADH-coenzyme Q reductase]) (eg, Leigh syndrome, mitochondrial complex I deficiency), full gene sequence

NF2 (neurofibromin 2 [merlin]) (eg, neurofibromatosis, type 2), full gene sequence

NOTCH3 (notch 3) (eg, cerebral autosomal dominant arteriopathy with subcortical infarcts and leukoencephalopathy [CADASIL]), targeted sequence analysis (eg, exons 1-23)

NPC1 (Niemann-Pick disease, type C1) (eg, Niemann-Pick disease), full gene sequence

NPHP1 (nephronophthisis 1 [juvenile]) (eg, Joubert syndrome), full gene sequence

NSD1 (nuclear receptor binding SET domain protein 1) (eg, Sotos syndrome), full gene sequence

OPA1 (optic atrophy 1) (eg, optic atrophy), duplication/deletion analysis

OPTN (optineurin) (eg, amyotrophic lateral sclerosis), full gene sequence

PAFAH1B1 (platelet-activating factor acetylhydrolase 1b, regulatory subunit 1 [45kDa]) (eg, lissencephaly, Miller-Dieker syndrome), full gene sequence

PAH (phenylalanine hydroxylase) (eg, phenylketonuria), full gene sequence

PALB2 (partner and localizer of BRCA2) (eg, breast and pancreatic cancer), full gene sequence

PARK2 (Parkinson protein 2, E3 ubiquitin protein ligase [parkin]) (eg, Parkinson disease), full gene sequence

PAX2 (paired box 2) (eg, renal coloboma syndrome), full gene sequence

PC (pyruvate carboxylase) (eg, pyruvate carboxylase deficiency), full gene sequence

PCCA (propionyl CoA carboxylase, alpha polypeptide) (eg, propionic acidemia, type 1), full gene sequence

PCCB (propionyl CoA carboxylase, beta polypeptide) (eg, propionic acidemia), full gene sequence

PCDH15 (protocadherin-related 15) (eg, Usher syndrome type 1F), duplication/deletion analysis

PCSK9 (proprotein convertase subtilisin/kexin type 9) (eg familial hypercholesterolemia), full gene sequence

PDHA1 (pyruvate dehydrogenase [lipoamide] alpha 1) (eg, lactic acidosis), full gene sequence

PDHX (pyruvate dehydrogenase complex, component X) (eg, lactic acidosis), full gene sequence

PHEX (phosphate-regulating endopeptidase homolog, X-linked) (eg, hypophosphatemic rickets), full gene sequence

PKD2 (polycystic kidney disease 2 [autosomal dominant]) (eg, polycystic kidney disease), full gene sequence

PKP2 (plakophilin 2) (eg, arrhythmogenic right ventricular dysplasia/cardiomyopathy 9), full gene sequence

PNKD (eg, paroxysmal nonkinesigenic dyskinesia), full gene sequence

POLG (polymerase [DNA directed], gamma) (eg, Alpers-Huttenlocher syndrome, autosomal dominant progressive external ophthalmoplegia), full gene sequence

POMGNT1 (protein O-linked mannose beta1, 2-N acetylglucosaminyltransferase) (eg, muscle-eye-brain disease, Walker-Warburg syndrome), full gene sequence

POMT1 (protein-O-mannosyltransferase 1) (eg, limb-girdle muscular dystrophy [LGMD] type 2K, Walker-Warburg syndrome), full gene sequence

POMT2 (protein-O-mannosyltransferase 2) (eg, limb-girdle muscular dystrophy [LGMD] type 2N, Walker-Warburg syndrome), full gene sequence

PPOX (protoporphyrinogen oxidase) (eg, variegate porphyria), full gene sequence

PRKAG2 (protein kinase, AMP-activated, gamma 2 non-catalytic subunit) (eg, familial hypertrophic cardiomyopathy with Wolff-Parkinson-White syndrome, lethal congenital glycogen storage disease of heart), full gene sequence

PRKCG (protein kinase C, gamma) (eg, spinocerebellar ataxia), full gene sequence

PSEN2 (presenilin 2[Alzheimer's disease 4]) (eg, Alzheimer's disease), full gene sequence

PTPN11 (protein tyrosine phosphatase, non-receptor type 11) (eg, Noonan syndrome, LEOPARD syndrome), full gene sequence

PYGM (phosphorylase, glycogen, muscle) (eg, glycogen storage disease type V, McArdle disease), full gene sequence

RAF1 (v-raf-1 murine leukemia viral oncogene homolog 1) (eg, LEOPARD syndrome), full gene sequence

RET (ret proto-oncogene) (eg, Hirschsprung disease), full gene sequence

RPE65 (retinal pigment epithelium-specific protein 65kDa) (eg, retinitis pigmentosa, Leber congenital amaurosis), full gene sequence

RYR1 (ryanodine receptor 1, skeletal) (eg, malignant hyperthermia), targeted sequence analysis of exons with functionally-confirmed mutations

SCN4A (sodium channel, voltage-gated, type IV, alpha subunit) (eg, hyperkalemic periodic paralysis), full gene sequence

SCNN1A (sodium channel, nonvoltage-gated 1 alpha) (eg, pseudohypoaldosteronism), full gene sequence

SCNN1B (sodium channel, nonvoltage-gated 1, beta) (eg, Liddle syndrome, pseudohypoaldosteronism), full gene sequence

SCNN1G (sodium channel, nonvoltage-gated 1, gamma) (eg, Liddle syndrome, pseudohypoaldosteronism), full gene sequence

SDHA (succinate dehydrogenase complex, subunit A, flavoprotein [Fp]) (eg, Leigh syndrome, mitochondrial complex II deficiency), full gene sequence

SETX (senataxin) (eg, ataxia), full gene sequence

SGCE (sarcoglycan, epsilon) (eg, myoclonic dystonia), full gene sequence

SH3TC2 (SH3 domain and tetratricopeptide repeats 2) (eg, Charcot-Marie-Tooth disease), full gene sequence

SLC9A6 (solute carrier family 9 [sodium/hydrogen exchanger], member 6) (eg, Christianson syndrome), full gene sequence

SLC26A4 (solute carrier family 26, member 4) (eg, Pendred syndrome), full gene sequence

SLC37A4 (solute carrier family 37 [glucose-6-phosphate transporter], member 4) (eg, glycogen storage disease type Ib), full gene sequence

SMAD4 (SMAD family member 4) (eg, hemorrhagic telangiectasia syndrome, juvenile polyposis), full gene sequence

SOS1 (son of sevenless homolog 1) (eg, Noonan syndrome, gingival fibromatosis), full gene sequence

SPAST (spastin) (eg, spastic paraplegia), full gene sequence

SPG7 (spastic paraplegia 7 [pure and complicated autosomal recessive]) (eg, spastic paraplegia), full gene sequence

STXBP1 (syntaxin-binding protein 1) (eg, epileptic encephalopathy), full gene sequence

TAZ (tafazzin) (eg, methylglutaconic aciduria type 2, Barth syndrome), full gene sequence

TCF4 (transcription factor 4) (eg, Pitt-Hopkins syndrome), full gene sequence

TH (tyrosine hydroxylase) (eg, Segawa syndrome), full gene sequence

TMEM43 (transmembrane protein 43) (eg, arrhythmogenic right ventricular cardiomyopathy), full gene sequence

TNNT2 (troponin T, type 2 [cardiac]) (eg, familial hypertrophic cardiomyopathy), full gene sequence

TRPC6 (transient receptor potential cation channel, subfamily C, member 6) (eg, focal segmental glomerulosclerosis), full gene sequence

TSC1 (tuberous sclerosis 1) (eg, tuberous sclerosis), full gene sequence

TSC2 (tuberous sclerosis 2) (eg, tuberous sclerosis), duplication/deletion analysis

UBE3A (ubiquitin protein ligase E3A) (eg, Angelman syndrome) full gene sequence

UMOD (uromodulin) (eg, glomerulocystic kidney disease with hyperuricemia and isosthenuria), full gene sequence

VWF (von Willebrand factor) (von Willebrand disease type 2A), extended targeted sequence analysis (eg, exons 11-16, 24-26, 51, 52)

WAS (Wiskott-Aldrich syndrome [eczema-thrombocytopenia]) (eg, Wiskott-Aldrich syndrome), full gene sequence

0.00 0.00 **FUD** XXX A

AMA: 2020,Dec,3; 2020,OctSE,1; 2020,OctSE,1; 2020,Feb,10; 2018,Nov,9; 2018,May,6; 2018,Jan,8; 2017,Apr,9; 2017,Jan,8; 2016,Aug,9; 2016,Jan,13

81407 Molecular pathology procedure, Level 8 (eg, analysis of 26-50 exons by DNA sequence analysis, mutation scanning or duplication/deletion variants of >50 exons, sequence analysis of multiple genes on one platform)

ABCC8 (ATP-binding cassette, sub-family C [CFTR/MRP], member 8) (eg, familial hyperinsulinism), full gene sequence

AGL (amylo-alpha-1, 6-glucosidase, 4-alpha-glucanotransferase) (eg, glycogen storage disease type III), full gene sequence

AHI1 (Abelson helper integration site 1) (eg, Joubert syndrome), full gene sequence

APOB (apolipoprotein B) (eg, familial hypercholesterolemia type B) full gene sequence

ASPM (asp [abnormal spindle] homolog, microcephaly associated [Drosophila]) (eg, primary microcephaly), full gene sequence

CHD7 (chromodomain helicase DNA binding protein 7) (eg, CHARGE syndrome), full gene sequence

COL4A4 (collagen, type IV, alpha 4) (eg, Alport syndrome), full gene sequence

COL4A5 (collagen, type IV, alpha 5) (eg, Alport syndrome), duplication/deletion analysis

COL6A1 (collagen, type VI, alpha 1) (eg, collagen type VI-related disorders), full gene sequence

COL6A2 (collagen, type VI, alpha 2) (eg, collagen type VI-related disorders), full gene sequence

COL6A3 (collagen, type VI, alpha 3) (eg, collagen type VI-related disorders), full gene sequence

CREBBP (CREB binding protein) (eg, Rubinstein-Taybi syndrome), full gene sequence

F8 (coagulation factor VIII) (eg, hemophilia A), full gene sequence

JAG1 (jagged 1) (eg, Alagille syndrome), full gene sequence

KDM5C (lysine [K]-specific demethylase 5C) (eg, X-linked mental retardation), full gene sequence

KIAA0196 (KIAA0196) (eg, spastic paraplegia), full gene sequence

L1CAM (L1 cell adhesion molecule) (eg, MASA syndrome, X-linked hydrocephaly), full gene sequence

LAMB2 (laminin, beta 2 [laminin S]) (eg, Pierson syndrome), full gene sequence

MYBPC3 (myosin binding protein C, cardiac) (eg, familial hypertrophic cardiomyopathy), full gene sequence

MYH6 (myosin, heavy chain 6, cardiac muscle, alpha) (eg, familial dilated cardiomyopathy), full gene sequence

MYH7 (myosin, heavy chain 7, cardiac muscle, beta) (eg, familial hypertrophic cardiomyopathy, Liang distal myopathy), full gene sequence

MYO7A (myosin VIIA) (eg, Usher syndrome, type 1), full gene sequence

NOTCH1 (notch 1) (eg, aortic valve disease), full gene sequence

NPHS1 (nephrosis 1, congenital, Finnish type [nephrin]) (eg, congenital Finnish nephrosis), full gene sequence

OPA1 (optic atrophy 1) (eg, optic atrophy), full gene sequence

PCDH15 (protocadherin-related 15) (eg, Usher syndrome, type 1), full gene sequence

PKD1 (polycystic kidney disease 1 [autosomal dominant]) (eg, polycystic kidney disease), full gene sequence

PLCE1 (phospholipase C, epsilon 1) (eg, nephrotic syndrome type 3), full gene sequence

SCN1A (sodium channel, voltage-gated, type 1, alpha subunit) (eg, generalized epilepsy with febrile seizures), full gene sequence

SCN5A (sodium channel, voltage-gated, type V, alpha subunit) (eg, familial dilated cardiomyopathy), full gene sequence

SLC12A1 (solute carrier family 12 [sodium/potassium/chloride transporters], member 1) (eg, Bartter syndrome), full gene sequence

SLC12A3 (solute carrier family 12 [sodium/chloride transporters], member 3) (eg, Gitelman syndrome), full gene sequence

SPG11 (spastic paraplegia 11 [autosomal recessive]) (eg, spastic paraplegia), full gene sequence

SPTBN2 (spectrin, beta, non-erythrocytic 2) (eg, spinocerebellar ataxia), full gene sequence

TMEM67 (transmembrane protein 67) (eg, Joubert syndrome), full gene sequence

TSC2 (tuberous sclerosis 2) (eg, tuberous sclerosis), full gene sequence

USH1C (Usher syndrome 1C [autosomal recessive, severe]) (eg, Usher syndrome, type 1), full gene sequence

VPS13B (vacuolar protein sorting 13 homolog B [yeast]) (eg, Cohen syndrome), duplication/deletion analysis

WDR62 (WD repeat domain 62) (eg, primary autosomal recessive microcephaly), full gene sequence

0.00 0.00 **FUD** XXX A

AMA: 2020,Dec,3; 2020,OctSE,1; 2020,OctSE,1; 2019,Jul,3; 2018,Nov,9; 2018,May,6; 2018,Jan,8; 2017,Jan,8; 2016,Aug,9; 2016,Jan,13

81408 Molecular pathology procedure, Level 9 (eg, analysis of >50 exons in a single gene by DNA sequence analysis)

ABCA4 (ATP-binding cassette, sub-family A [ABC1], member 4) (eg, Stargardt disease, age-related macular degeneration), full gene sequence

ATM (ataxia telangiectasia mutated) (eg, ataxia telangiectasia), full gene sequence

CDH23 (cadherin-related 23) (eg, Usher syndrome, type 1), full gene sequence

CEP290 (centrosomal protein 290kDa) (eg, Joubert syndrome), full gene sequence

COL1A1 (collagen, type I, alpha 1) (eg, osteogenesis imperfecta, type I), full gene sequence

COL1A2 (collagen, type I, alpha 2) (eg, osteogenesis imperfecta, type I), full gene sequence

COL4A1 (collagen, type IV, alpha 1) (eg, brain small-vessel disease with hemorrhage), full gene sequence

COL4A3 (collagen, type IV, alpha 3 [Goodpasture antigen]) (eg, Alport syndrome), full gene sequence

COL4A5 (collagen, type IV, alpha 5) (eg, Alport syndrome), full gene sequence

DMD (dystrophin) (eg, Duchenne/Becker muscular dystrophy), full gene sequence

DYSF (dysferlin, limb girdle muscular dystrophy 2B [autosomal recessive]) (eg, limb-girdle muscular dystrophy), full gene sequence

FBN1 (fibrillin 1) (eg, Marfan syndrome), full gene sequence

ITPR1 (inositol 1,4,5-trisphosphate receptor, type 1) (eg, spinocerebellar ataxia), full gene sequence

LAMA2 (laminin, alpha 2) (eg, congenital muscular dystrophy), full gene sequence

LRRK2 (leucine-rich repeat kinase 2) (eg, Parkinson disease), full gene sequence

MYH11 (myosin, heavy chain 11, smooth muscle) (eg, thoracic aortic aneurysms and aortic dissections), full gene sequence

NEB (nebulin) (eg, nemaline myopathy 2), full gene sequence

NF1 (neurofibromin 1) (eg, neurofibromatosis, type 1), full gene sequence

PKHD1 (polycystic kidney and hepatic disease 1) (eg, autosomal recessive polycystic kidney disease), full gene sequence

RYR1 (ryanodine receptor 1, skeletal) (eg, malignant hyperthermia), full gene sequence

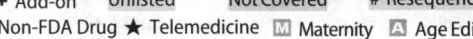

RYR2 (ryanodine receptor 2 [cardiac]) (eg, catecholaminergic polymorphic ventricular tachycardia, arrhythmogenic right ventricular

dysplasia), full gene sequence or targeted sequence analysis of > 50 exons

USH2A (Usher syndrome 2A [autosomal recessive, mild]) (eg, Usher syndrome, type 2), full gene sequence

VPS13B (vacuolar protein sorting 13 homolog B [yeast]) (eg, Cohen syndrome), full gene sequence

VWF (von Willebrand factor) (eg, von Willebrand disease types 1 and 3), full gene sequence

0.00 0.00 FUD XXX A

AMA: 2020,Dec,3; 2020,OctSE,1; 2020,OctSE,1; 2018,Nov,9; 2018,May,6; 2018,Jan,8; 2017,Jan,8; 2016,Aug,9; 2016,Jan,13

\# **81479** **Unlisted molecular pathology procedure**

0.00 0.00 FUD XXX A

AMA: 2020,Dec,13; 2020,Dec,3; 2020,Oct,8; 2019,Jun,11; 2019,May,5; 2018,Dec,10; 2018,Dec,10; 2018,Nov,9; 2018,Sep,14; 2018,Jun,8; 2018,May,6; 2018,Jan,8; 2017,Apr,9; 2017,Jan,8; 2016,Sep,9; 2016,Aug,9; 2016,Apr,4; 2016,Jan,13

81410-81479 [81419, 81443, 81448, 81479] Genomic Sequencing

EXCLUDES *Cytogenomic (genome-wide) analysis for constitutional chromosomal abnormalities (81228-81229, [81349], 81405-81406)*
In situ hybridization analyses (88271-88275, 88365-88368 [88364, 88373, 88374])
Microbial identification (87149-87153, 87471-87801 [87623, 87624, 87625], 87900-87904 [87906, 87910, 87912])

81410 **Aortic dysfunction or dilation (eg, Marfan syndrome, Loeys Dietz syndrome, Ehler Danlos syndrome type IV, arterial tortuosity syndrome); genomic sequence analysis panel, must include sequencing of at least 9 genes, including *FBN1, TGFBR1, TGFBR2, COL3A1, MYH11, ACTA2, SLC2A10, SMAD3,* and *MYLK***

0.00 0.00 FUD XXX A

AMA: 2020,Dec,3; 2018,Jan,8; 2017,Jan,8; 2016,Jan,13

81411 **duplication/deletion analysis panel, must include analyses for *TGFBR1, TGFBR2, MYH11, and COL3A1***

0.00 0.00 FUD XXX A

AMA: 2020,Dec,3; 2018,Jan,8; 2017,Jan,8; 2016,Jan,13

81412 **Ashkenazi Jewish associated disorders (eg, Bloom syndrome, Canavan disease, cystic fibrosis, familial dysautonomia, Fanconi anemia group C, Gaucher disease, Tay-Sachs disease), genomic sequence analysis panel, must include sequencing of at least 9 genes, including *ASPA, BLM, CFTR, FANCC, GBA, HEXA, IKBKAP, MCOLN1,* and *SMPD1***

0.00 0.00 FUD XXX A

AMA: 2020,Dec,3; 2018,Nov,9; 2018,Jan,8; 2017,Jan,8; 2016,Apr,4

81413 **Cardiac ion channelopathies (eg, Brugada syndrome, long QT syndrome, short QT syndrome, catecholaminergic polymorphic ventricular tachycardia); genomic sequence analysis panel, must include sequencing of at least 10 genes, including ANK2, CASQ2, CAV3, KCNE1, KCNE2, KCNH2, KCNJ2, KCNQ1, RYR2, and SCN5A**

EXCLUDES *Evaluation cardiomyopathy (81439)*

0.00 0.00 FUD XXX A

AMA: 2020,Dec,3; 2018,Jan,8; 2017,Apr,3

81414 **duplication/deletion gene analysis panel, must include analysis of at least 2 genes, including KCNH2 and KCNQ1**

EXCLUDES *Evaluation cardiomyopathy (81439)*

0.00 0.00 FUD XXX A

AMA: 2020,Dec,3; 2018,Jan,8; 2017,Apr,3

\# **81419** **Epilepsy genomic sequence analysis panel, must include analyses for *ALDH7A1, CACNA1A, CDKL5, CHD2, GABRG2, GRIN2A, KCNQ2, MECP2, PCDH19, POLG, PRRT2, SCN1A, SCN1B, SCN2A, SCN8A, SLC2A1, SLC9A6, STXBP1, SYNGAP1, TCF4, TPP1, TSC1, TSC2,* and *ZEB2***

0.00 0.00 FUD XXX

AMA: 2020,Dec,3

81415 **Exome (eg, unexplained constitutional or heritable disorder or syndrome); sequence analysis**

INCLUDES Chromosomal abnormality sequence analysis ([81349])

0.00 0.00 FUD XXX A

AMA: 2020,Dec,3; 2018,Jan,8; 2017,Jan,8; 2016,Jan,13

\+ **81416** **sequence analysis, each comparator exome (eg, parents, siblings) (List separately in addition to code for primary procedure)**

INCLUDES Chromosomal abnormality sequence analysis ([81349])

Code first (81415)

0.00 0.00 FUD XXX A

AMA: 2020,Dec,3; 2018,Jan,8; 2017,Jan,8; 2016,Jan,13

81417 **re-evaluation of previously obtained exome sequence (eg, updated knowledge or unrelated condition/syndrome)**

INCLUDES Chromosomal abnormality sequence analysis ([81349])

EXCLUDES *Incidental results*

0.00 0.00 FUD XXX A

AMA: 2020,Dec,3; 2018,Jan,8; 2017,Jan,8; 2016,Jan,13

81419 **Resequenced code. See code following 81414.**

81420 **Fetal chromosomal aneuploidy (eg, trisomy 21, monosomy X) genomic sequence analysis panel, circulating cell-free fetal DNA in maternal blood, must include analysis of chromosomes 13, 18, and 21** M

EXCLUDES *Molecular cytogenetics (88271)*

0.00 0.00 FUD XXX A

AMA: 2020,Dec,3; 2018,Apr,10; 2018,Jan,8; 2017,Jan,8; 2016,Jan,13

81422 **Fetal chromosomal microdeletion(s) genomic sequence analysis (eg, DiGeorge syndrome, Cri-du-chat syndrome), circulating cell-free fetal DNA in maternal blood**

EXCLUDES *Molecular cytogenetics (88271)*

0.00 0.00 FUD XXX A

AMA: 2020,Dec,3; 2018,Jan,8; 2017,Apr,3

\# **81443** **Genetic testing for severe inherited conditions (eg, cystic fibrosis, Ashkenazi Jewish-associated disorders [eg, Bloom syndrome, Canavan disease, Fanconi anemia type C, mucolipidosis type VI, Gaucher disease, Tay-Sachs disease], beta hemoglobinopathies, phenylketonuria, galactosemia), genomic sequence analysis panel, must include sequencing of at least 15 genes (eg, *ACADM, ARSA, ASPA, ATP7B, BCKDHA, BCKDHB, BLM, CFTR, DHCR7, FANCC, G6PC, GAA, GALT, GBA, GBE1, HBB, HEXA, IKBKAP, MCOLN1, PAH*)**

EXCLUDES *When performed separately:*
Ashkenazi Jewish-associated disorder analysis only (81412)
Fragile X mental retardation (FMR1) analysis (81243)
Hemoglobin A testing ([81257])
Spinal muscular atrophy (SMN1) analysis (81329)

0.00 0.00 FUD XXX

AMA: 2020,Dec,3; 2019,Jul,3; 2018,Nov,9

81425 **Genome (eg, unexplained constitutional or heritable disorder or syndrome); sequence analysis**

INCLUDES Chromosomal abnormality sequence analysis ([81349])

0.00 0.00 FUD XXX A

AMA: 2020,Dec,3; 2018,Jan,8; 2017,Jan,8; 2016,Jan,13

\+ **81426** **sequence analysis, each comparator genome (eg, parents, siblings) (List separately in addition to code for primary procedure)**

INCLUDES Chromosomal abnormality sequence analysis ([81349])

Code first (81425)

0.00 0.00 FUD XXX A

AMA: 2020,Dec,3; 2018,Jan,8; 2017,Jan,8; 2016,Jan,13

81427 **re-evaluation of previously obtained genome sequence (eg, updated knowledge or unrelated condition/syndrome)**

EXCLUDES *Incidental results*

0.00 0.00 FUD XXX A

AMA: 2020,Dec,3; 2018,Jan,8; 2017,Jan,8; 2016,Jan,13

81430 **Hearing loss (eg, nonsyndromic hearing loss, Usher syndrome, Pendred syndrome); genomic sequence analysis panel, must include sequencing of at least 60 genes, including *CDH23, CLRN1, GJB2, GPR98, MTRNR1, MYO7A, MYO15A, PCDH15, OTOF, SLC26A4, TMC1, TMPRSS3, USH1C, USH1G, USH2A,* and *WFS1***

0.00 0.00 FUD XXX A

AMA: 2020,Dec,3; 2018,Jan,8; 2017,Jan,8; 2016,Jan,13

81431 **duplication/deletion analysis panel, must include copy number analyses for *STRC* and *DFNB1* deletions in *GJB2* and *GJB6* genes**

0.00 0.00 FUD XXX A

AMA: 2020,Dec,3; 2018,Jan,8; 2017,Jan,8; 2016,Jan,13

81432 **Hereditary breast cancer-related disorders (eg, hereditary breast cancer, hereditary ovarian cancer, hereditary endometrial cancer); genomic sequence analysis panel, must include sequencing of at least 10 genes, always including *BRCA1, BRCA2, CDH1, MLH1, MSH2, MSH6, PALB2, PTEN, STK11, and TP53***

0.00 0.00 FUD XXX A

AMA: 2020,Dec,3; 2019,May,5; 2018,Jan,8; 2017,Jan,8; 2016,Apr,4

81433 **duplication/deletion analysis panel, must include analyses for *BRCA1, BRCA2, MLH1, MSH2,* and *STK11***

0.00 0.00 FUD XXX A

AMA: 2020,Dec,3; 2018,Jan,8; 2017,Jan,8; 2016,Apr,4

81434 **Hereditary retinal disorders (eg, retinitis pigmentosa, Leber congenital amaurosis, cone-rod dystrophy), genomic sequence analysis panel, must include sequencing of at least 15 genes, including *ABCA4, CNGA1, CRB1, EYS, PDE6A, PDE6B, PRPF31, PRPH2, RDH12, RHO, RP1, RP2, RPE65, RPGR,* and *USH2A***

0.00 0.00 FUD XXX A

AMA: 2020,Dec,3; 2018,Jan,8; 2017,Jan,8; 2016,Apr,4

81435 **Hereditary colon cancer disorders (eg, Lynch syndrome, PTEN hamartoma syndrome, Cowden syndrome, familial adenomatosis polyposis); genomic sequence analysis panel, must include sequencing of at least 10 genes, including *APC, BMPR1A, CDH1, MLH1, MSH2, MSH6, MUTYH, PTEN, SMAD4,* and *STK11***

0.00 0.00 FUD XXX A

AMA: 2020,Dec,3; 2018,Jan,8; 2017,Jan,8; 2016,Apr,4; 2016,Jan,13

81436 **duplication/deletion analysis panel, must include analysis of at least 5 genes, including *MLH1, MSH2, EPCAM, SMAD4,* and *STK11***

0.00 0.00 FUD XXX A

AMA: 2020,Dec,3; 2018,Jan,8; 2017,Jan,8; 2016,Apr,4; 2016,Jan,13

81437 **Hereditary neuroendocrine tumor disorders (eg, medullary thyroid carcinoma, parathyroid carcinoma, malignant pheochromocytoma or paraganglioma); genomic sequence analysis panel, must include sequencing of at least 6 genes, including *MAX, SDHB, SDHC, SDHD, TMEM127,* and *VHL***

0.00 0.00 FUD XXX A

AMA: 2020,Dec,3; 2018,Jan,8; 2017,Jan,8; 2016,Apr,4

81438 **duplication/deletion analysis panel, must include analyses for *SDHB, SDHC, SDHD,* and *VHL***

0.00 0.00 FUD XXX A

AMA: 2020,Dec,3; 2018,Jan,8; 2017,Jan,8; 2016,Apr,4

\# **81448** **Hereditary peripheral neuropathies (eg, Charcot-Marie-Tooth, spastic paraplegia), genomic sequence analysis panel, must include sequencing of at least 5 peripheral neuropathy-related genes (eg, *BSCL2, GJB1, MFN2, MPZ, REEP1, SPAST, SPG11, SPTLC1*)**

0.00 0.00 FUD XXX A

AMA: 2020,Dec,3; 2018,May,6

81439 **Hereditary cardiomyopathy (eg, hypertrophic cardiomyopathy, dilated cardiomyopathy, arrhythmogenic right ventricular cardiomyopathy), genomic sequence analysis panel, must include sequencing of at least 5 cardiomyopathy-related genes (eg, *DSG2, MYBPC3, MYH7, PKP2, TTN*)**

EXCLUDES *Genetic sequencing for cardiac ion channelopathies (81413-81414)*

0.00 0.00 FUD XXX A

AMA: 2020,Dec,3; 2020,Dec,13; 2018,Sep,14; 2018,Jan,8; 2017,Apr,3

81440 **Nuclear encoded mitochondrial genes (eg, neurologic or myopathic phenotypes), genomic sequence panel, must include analysis of at least 100 genes, including *BCS1L, C10orf2, COQ2, COX10, DGUOK, MPV17, OPA1, PDSS2, POLG, POLG2, RRM2B, SCO1, SCO2, SLC25A4, SUCLA2, SUCLG1, TAZ, TK2,* and *TYMP***

0.00 0.00 FUD XXX A

AMA: 2020,Dec,3; 2018,Jan,8; 2017,Jan,8; 2016,Jan,13

81442 **Noonan spectrum disorders (eg, Noonan syndrome, cardio-facio-cutaneous syndrome, Costello syndrome, LEOPARD syndrome, Noonan-like syndrome), genomic sequence analysis panel, must include sequencing of at least 12 genes, including *BRAF, CBL, HRAS, KRAS, MAP2K1, MAP2K2, NRAS, PTPN11, RAF1, RIT1, SHOC2,* and *SOS1***

0.00 0.00 FUD XXX A

AMA: 2020,Dec,3; 2018,Jan,8; 2017,Jan,8; 2016,Apr,4

81443 **Resequenced code. See code following 81422.**

81445 **Targeted genomic sequence analysis panel, solid organ neoplasm, DNA analysis, and RNA analysis when performed, 5-50 genes (eg, *ALK, BRAF, CDKN2A, EGFR, ERBB2, KIT, KRAS, NRAS, MET, PDGFRA, PDGFRB, PGR, PIK3CA, PTEN, RET*), interrogation for sequence variants and copy number variants or rearrangements, if performed**

0.00 0.00 FUD XXX A

AMA: 2020,Dec,3; 2018,Jan,8; 2017,Jan,8; 2016,Apr,4; 2016,Jan,13

81448 **Resequenced code. See code following 81438.**

81450 **Targeted genomic sequence analysis panel, hematolymphoid neoplasm or disorder, DNA analysis, and RNA analysis when performed, 5-50 genes (eg, *BRAF, CEBPA, DNMT3A, EZH2, FLT3, IDH1, IDH2, JAK2, KRAS, KIT, MLL, NRAS, NPM1, NOTCH1*), interrogation for sequence variants, and copy number variants or rearrangements, or isoform expression or mRNA expression levels, if performed**

0.00 0.00 FUD XXX A

AMA: 2020,Dec,3; 2018,Jan,8; 2017,Jan,8; 2016,Apr,4; 2016,Jan,13

81455 **Targeted genomic sequence analysis panel, solid organ or hematolymphoid neoplasm, DNA analysis, and RNA analysis when performed, 51 or greater genes (eg, *ALK, BRAF, CDKN2A, CEBPA, DNMT3A, EGFR, ERBB2, EZH2, FLT3, IDH1, IDH2, JAK2, KIT, KRAS, MLL, NPM1, NRAS, MET, NOTCH1, PDGFRA, PDGFRB, PGR, PIK3CA, PTEN, RET*), interrogation for sequence variants and copy number variants or rearrangements, if performed**

0.00 0.00 FUD XXX A

AMA: 2020,Dec,3; 2018,Jan,8; 2017,Jan,8; 2016,Apr,4; 2016,Jan,13

81460 **Whole mitochondrial genome (eg, Leigh syndrome, mitochondrial encephalomyopathy, lactic acidosis, and stroke-like episodes [MELAS], myoclonic epilepsy with ragged-red fibers [MERFF], neuropathy, ataxia, and retinitis pigmentosa [NARP], Leber hereditary optic neuropathy [LHON]), genomic sequence, must include sequence analysis of entire mitochondrial genome with heteroplasmy detection**

0.00 0.00 FUD XXX A

AMA: 2020,Dec,3; 2018,Jan,8; 2017,Jan,8; 2016,Jan,13

81465 **Whole mitochondrial genome large deletion analysis panel (eg, Kearns-Sayre syndrome, chronic progressive external ophthalmoplegia), including heteroplasmy detection, if performed**

0.00 0.00 FUD XXX A

AMA: 2020,Dec,3; 2018,Jan,8; 2017,Jan,8; 2016,Jan,13

81470 **X-linked intellectual disability (XLID) (eg, syndromic and non-syndromic XLID); genomic sequence analysis panel, must include sequencing of at least 60 genes, including *ARX, ATRX, CDKL5, FGD1, FMR1, HUWE1, IL1RAPL, KDM5C, L1CAM, MECP2, MED12, MID1, OCRL, RPS6KA3,* and *SLC16A2***

0.00 0.00 FUD XXX A

AMA: 2020,Dec,3; 2018,Jan,8; 2017,Jan,8; 2016,Jan,13

81471 **duplication/deletion gene analysis, must include analysis of at least 60 genes, including *ARX, ATRX, CDKL5, FGD1, FMR1, HUWE1, IL1RAPL, KDM5C, L1CAM, MECP2, MED12, MID1, OCRL, RPS6KA3,* and *SLC16A2***

0.00 0.00 FUD XXX A

AMA: 2020,Dec,3; 2018,Jan,8; 2017,Jan,8; 2016,Jan,13

81479 **Resequenced code. See code following 81408.**

81490-81599 [81500, 81503, 81504, 81522, 81540, 81546, 81595, 81596] Multianalyte Assays

INCLUDES Procedures using multiple assay panel results (eg, molecular pathology, fluorescent in situ hybridization, non-nucleic acid-based) and other patient information to perform algorithmic analysis
Required analytical services (eg, amplification, cell lysis, detection, digestion, extraction, hybridization, nucleic acid stabilization) and algorithmic analysis

EXCLUDES *Genomic resequencing tests (81410-81471 [81448])*
In situ hybridization analyses (88271-88275, 88365-88368 [88364, 88373, 88374])
Microbial identification (87149-87153, 87471-87801 [87623, 87624, 87625], 87900-87904 [87906, 87910, 87912])
Multianalyte assays with algorithmic analyses without a Category I code (0002M-0007M, 0011M-0013M)

Code also procedures performed prior to cell lysis (eg, microdissection) (88380-88381)

81490 **Autoimmune (rheumatoid arthritis), analysis of 12 biomarkers using immunoassays, utilizing serum, prognostic algorithm reported as a disease activity score**

EXCLUDES *C-reactive protein (86140)*

0.00 0.00 FUD XXX Q

AMA: 2020,Dec,3

\# **81595** **Cardiology (heart transplant), mRNA, gene expression profiling by real-time quantitative PCR of 20 genes (11 content and 9 housekeeping), utilizing subfraction of peripheral blood, algorithm reported as a rejection risk score**

0.00 0.00 FUD XXX A

AMA: 2020,Dec,3; 2019,Jun,11

81493 **Coronary artery disease, mRNA, gene expression profiling by real-time RT-PCR of 23 genes, utilizing whole peripheral blood, algorithm reported as a risk score**

0.00 0.00 FUD XXX A

AMA: 2020,Dec,3

81500 **Resequenced code. See code following 81538.**

81503 **Resequenced code. See code before 81539.**

81504 **Resequenced code. See code following resequenced code 81546.**

81506 **Endocrinology (type 2 diabetes), biochemical assays of seven analytes (glucose, HbA1c, insulin, hs-CRP, adiponectin, ferritin, interleukin 2-receptor alpha), utilizing serum or plasma, algorithm reporting a risk score**

EXCLUDES *C-reactive protein; high sensitivity (hsCRP) (86141)*
Ferritin (82728)
Glucose (82947)
Hemoglobin; glycosylated (A1C) (83036)
Immunoassay for analyte other than infectious agent antibody or infectious agent antigen (83520)
Insulin; total (83525)
Unlisted chemistry procedure (84999)

0.00 0.00 FUD XXX E

AMA: 2020,Dec,3; 2019,Jun,11

81507 **Fetal aneuploidy (trisomy 21, 18, and 13) DNA sequence analysis of selected regions using maternal plasma, algorithm reported as a risk score for each trisomy** ♀

EXCLUDES *Genome-wide microarray analysis (81228-81229)*
Low-pass sequencing analysis ([81349])
Molecular cytogenetics (88271)

0.00 0.00 FUD XXX A

AMA: 2020,Dec,3; 2019,Jun,11; 2018,Apr,10

81508 **Fetal congenital abnormalities, biochemical assays of two proteins (PAPP-A, hCG [any form]), utilizing maternal serum, algorithm reported as a risk score** ♀

EXCLUDES *Gonadotropin, chorionic (hCG) (84702)*
Pregnancy-associated plasma protein-A (PAPP-A) (84163)

0.00 0.00 FUD XXX E

AMA: 2020,Dec,3; 2019,Jun,11

81509 **Fetal congenital abnormalities, biochemical assays of three proteins (PAPP-A, hCG [any form], DIA), utilizing maternal serum, algorithm reported as a risk score** ♀

EXCLUDES *Gonadotropin, chorionic (hCG) (84702)*
Inhibin A (86336)
Pregnancy-associated plasma protein-A (PAPP-A) (84163)

0.00 0.00 FUD XXX E

AMA: 2020,Dec,3; 2019,Jun,11

81510 **Fetal congenital abnormalities, biochemical assays of three analytes (AFP, uE3, hCG [any form]), utilizing maternal serum, algorithm reported as a risk score** ♀

EXCLUDES *Alpha-fetoprotein (AFP) (82105)*
Estriol (82677)
Gonadotropin, chorionic (hCG) (84702)

0.00 0.00 FUD XXX E

AMA: 2020,Dec,3; 2019,Jun,11

81511 **Fetal congenital abnormalities, biochemical assays of four analytes (AFP, uE3, hCG [any form], DIA) utilizing maternal serum, algorithm reported as a risk score (may include additional results from previous biochemical testing)** ♀

EXCLUDES *Alpha-fetoprotein (AFP) (82105)*
Estriol (82677)
Gonadotropin, chorionic (hCG) (84702)
Inhibin A (86336)

0.00 0.00 FUD XXX E

AMA: 2020,Dec,3; 2019,Jun,11

81512 **Fetal congenital abnormalities, biochemical assays of five analytes (AFP, uE3, total hCG, hyperglycosylated hCG, DIA) utilizing maternal serum, algorithm reported as a risk score** ♀

EXCLUDES *Alpha-fetoprotein (AFP) (82105)*
Estriol (82677)
Gonadotropin, chorionic (hCG) (84702)
Inhibin A (86336)

0.00 0.00 FUD XXX E

AMA: 2020,Dec,3; 2019,Jun,11

81513 **Infectious disease, bacterial vaginosis, quantitative real-time amplification of RNA markers for Atopobium vaginae, Gardnerella vaginalis, and Lactobacillus species, utilizing vaginal-fluid specimens, algorithm reported as a positive or negative result for bacterial vaginosis** ♀
0.00 0.00 FUD XXX
AMA: 2020,Dec,3

81514 **Infectious disease, bacterial vaginosis and vaginitis, quantitative real-time amplification of DNA markers for Gardnerella vaginalis, Atopobium vaginae, Megasphaera type 1, Bacterial Vaginosis Associated Bacteria-2 (BVAB-2), and Lactobacillus species (L. crispatus and L. jensenii), utilizing vaginal-fluid specimens, algorithm reported as a positive or negative for high likelihood of bacterial vaginosis, includes separate detection of Trichomonas vaginalis and/or Candida species (C. albicans, C. tropicalis, C. parapsilosis, C. dubliniensis), Candida glabrata, Candida krusei, when reported** ♀
EXCLUDES *Candida (87480-87482)*
Gardnerella vaginalis (87510-87512)
Trichomonas vaginalis (87660-87661)
0.00 0.00 FUD XXX
AMA: 2020,Dec,3

\# **81596** **Infectious disease, chronic hepatitis C virus (HCV) infection, six biochemical assays (ALT, A2-macroglobulin, apolipoprotein A-1, total bilirubin, GGT, and haptoglobin) utilizing serum, prognostic algorithm reported as scores for fibrosis and necroinflammatory activity in liver**
0.00 0.00 FUD XXX
AMA: 2020,Dec,3; 2019,Jun,11; 2019,Jul,3

81518 **Oncology (breast), mRNA, gene expression profiling by real-time RT-PCR of 11 genes (7 content and 4 housekeeping), utilizing formalin-fixed paraffin-embedded tissue, algorithms reported as percentage risk for metastatic recurrence and likelihood of benefit from extended endocrine therapy**
0.00 0.00 FUD XXX
AMA: 2020,Dec,3; 2019,Jun,11; 2019,Jul,3

\# **81522** **Oncology (breast), mRNA, gene expression profiling by RT-PCR of 12 genes (8 content and 4 housekeeping), utilizing formalin-fixed paraffin-embedded tissue, algorithm reported as recurrence risk score**
0.00 0.00 FUD XXX
AMA: 2020,Dec,3

81519 **Oncology (breast), mRNA, gene expression profiling by real-time RT-PCR of 21 genes, utilizing formalin-fixed paraffin embedded tissue, algorithm reported as recurrence score**
0.00 0.00 FUD XXX A
AMA: 2020,Dec,3; 2019,Jun,11; 2018,Jan,8; 2017,Jan,8; 2016,Jan,13

81520 **Oncology (breast), mRNA gene expression profiling by hybrid capture of 58 genes (50 content and 8 housekeeping), utilizing formalin-fixed paraffin-embedded tissue, algorithm reported as a recurrence risk score**
0.00 0.00 FUD XXX A
AMA: 2020,Dec,3; 2019,Jun,11; 2018,Jun,8

81521 **Oncology (breast), mRNA, microarray gene expression profiling of 70 content genes and 465 housekeeping genes, utilizing fresh frozen or formalin-fixed paraffin-embedded tissue, algorithm reported as index related to risk of distant metastasis**
EXCLUDES *Oncology (breast), mRNA, next-generation sequencing gene expression profiling, when performed on same specimen (81523)*
0.00 0.00 FUD XXX A
AMA: 2020,Dec,3; 2019,Jun,11; 2018,Jun,8

81522 **Resequenced code. See code following 81518.**

● **81523** **Oncology (breast), mRNA, next-generation sequencing gene expression profiling of 70 content genes and 31 housekeeping genes, utilizing formalin-fixed paraffin-embedded tissue, algorithm reported as index related to risk to distant metastasis**
EXCLUDES *Oncology (breast), mRNA, microarray gene expression profiling, when performed on same specimen (81521)*

81525 **Oncology (colon), mRNA, gene expression profiling by real-time RT-PCR of 12 genes (7 content and 5 housekeeping), utilizing formalin-fixed paraffin-embedded tissue, algorithm reported as a recurrence score**
0.00 0.00 FUD XXX A
AMA: 2020,Dec,3; 2019,Jun,11

81528 **Oncology (colorectal) screening, quantitative real-time target and signal amplification of 10 DNA markers (*KRAS* mutations, promoter methylation of *NDRG4* and *BMP3*) and fecal hemoglobin, utilizing stool, algorithm reported as a positive or negative result**
EXCLUDES *Blood, occult, by fecal hemoglobin (82274)*
KRAS (Kirsten rat sarcoma viral oncogene homolog) (81275)
0.00 0.00 FUD XXX A
AMA: 2020,Dec,3; 2019,Jun,11

81529 **Oncology (cutaneous melanoma), mRNA, gene expression profiling by real-time RT-PCR of 31 genes (28 content and 3 housekeeping), utilizing formalin-fixed paraffin-embedded tissue, algorithm reported as recurrence risk, including likelihood of sentinel lymph node metastasis**
0.00 0.00 FUD XXX
AMA: 2020,Dec,3

81535 **Oncology (gynecologic), live tumor cell culture and chemotherapeutic response by DAPI stain and morphology, predictive algorithm reported as a drug response score; first single drug or drug combination**
0.00 0.00 FUD XXX Q
AMA: 2020,Dec,3; 2019,Jun,11

\+ **81536** **each additional single drug or drug combination (List separately in addition to code for primary procedure)**
Code first (81535)
0.00 0.00 FUD XXX Q
AMA: 2020,Dec,3; 2019,Jun,11

81538 **Oncology (lung), mass spectrometric 8-protein signature, including amyloid A, utilizing serum, prognostic and predictive algorithm reported as good versus poor overall survival**
0.00 0.00 FUD XXX Q
AMA: 2020,Dec,3; 2019,Jun,11

\# **81500** **Oncology (ovarian), biochemical assays of two proteins (CA-125 and HE4), utilizing serum, with menopausal status, algorithm reported as a risk score** ♀
EXCLUDES *Human epididymis protein 4 (HE4) (86305)*
Immunoassay for tumor antigen, quantitative; CA 125 (86304)
0.00 0.00 FUD XXX E
AMA: 2020,Dec,3; 2019,Jun,11

\# **81503** **Oncology (ovarian), biochemical assays of five proteins (CA-125, apolipoprotein A1, beta-2 microglobulin, transferrin, and pre-albumin), utilizing serum, algorithm reported as a risk score** ♀
EXCLUDES *Apolipoprotein (82172)*
Beta-2 microglobulin (82232)
Immunoassay for tumor antigen, quantitative; CA 125 (86304)
Prealbumin (84134)
Transferrin (84466)
0.00 0.00 FUD XXX Q
AMA: 2020,Dec,3; 2019,Jun,11

81539 **Oncology (high-grade prostate cancer), biochemical assay of four proteins (Total PSA, Free PSA, Intact PSA, and human kallikrein-2 [hK2]), utilizing plasma or serum, prognostic algorithm reported as a probability score** ♂
0.00 0.00 **FUD** XXX Q
AMA: 2020,Dec,3; 2019,Jun,11; 2018,Jan,8; 2017,Apr,3

81540 **Resequenced code. See code before 81552.**

81541 **Oncology (prostate), mRNA gene expression profiling by real-time RT-PCR of 46 genes (31 content and 15 housekeeping), utilizing formalin-fixed paraffin-embedded tissue, algorithm reported as a disease-specific mortality risk score**
0.00 0.00 **FUD** XXX A
AMA: 2020,Dec,3; 2019,Jun,11; 2018,Aug,8

81542 **Oncology (prostate), mRNA, microarray gene expression profiling of 22 content genes, utilizing formalin-fixed paraffin-embedded tissue, algorithm reported as metastasis risk score** ♂
0.00 0.00 **FUD** XXX
AMA: 2020,Dec,3; 2020,Oct,8

81546 **Resequenced code. See code following 81551.**

81551 **Oncology (prostate), promoter methylation profiling by real-time PCR of 3 genes (*GSTP1, APC, RASSF1*), utilizing formalin-fixed paraffin-embedded tissue, algorithm reported as a likelihood of prostate cancer detection on repeat biopsy**
0.00 0.00 **FUD** XXX A
AMA: 2020,Dec,3; 2019,Jun,11; 2018,Aug,8

81546 **Oncology (thyroid), mRNA, gene expression analysis of 10,196 genes, utilizing fine needle aspirate, algorithm reported as a categorical result (eg, benign or suspicious)**
0.00 0.00 **FUD** XXX
AMA: 2020,Dec,3

81504 **Oncology (tissue of origin), microarray gene expression profiling of > 2000 genes, utilizing formalin-fixed paraffin-embedded tissue, algorithm reported as tissue similarity scores**
0.00 0.00 **FUD** XXX A
AMA: 2020,Dec,3; 2019,Jun,11

81540 **Oncology (tumor of unknown origin), mRNA, gene expression profiling by real-time RT-PCR of 92 genes (87 content and 5 housekeeping) to classify tumor into main cancer type and subtype, utilizing formalin-fixed paraffin-embedded tissue, algorithm reported as a probability of a predicted main cancer type and subtype**
0.00 0.00 **FUD** XXX A
AMA: 2020,Dec,3; 2019,Jun,11

81552 **Oncology (uveal melanoma), mRNA, gene expression profiling by real-time RT-PCR of 15 genes (12 content and 3 housekeeping), utilizing fine needle aspirate or formalin-fixed paraffin-embedded tissue, algorithm reported as risk of metastasis**
0.00 0.00 **FUD** XXX
AMA: 2020,Dec,3; 2020,Jan,10

81554 **Pulmonary disease (idiopathic pulmonary fibrosis [IPF]), mRNA, gene expression analysis of 190 genes, utilizing transbronchial biopsies, diagnostic algorithm reported as categorical result (eg, positive or negative for high probability of usual interstitial pneumonia [UIP])**
0.00 0.00 **FUD** XXX
AMA: 2020,Dec,3

● **81560** **Transplantation medicine (allograft rejection, pediatric liver and small bowel), measurement of donor and third-party-induced CD154+T-cytotoxic memory cells, utilizing whole peripheral blood, algorithm reported as a rejection risk score**

EXCLUDES *Blood count (85032)*
Cryopreservation (88240)
Flow cytometry (88184-88185, 88187)
HLA typing (86821)
Lymphocyte transformation, mitogen, antigen induced blastogenesis (86353)
Thawing, expansion frozen cells (88241)
Tissue cultures, non-neoplastic disorders (88230)

81595 **Resequenced code. See code following 81490.**

81596 **Resequenced code. See code following 81514.**

81599 **Unlisted multianalyte assay with algorithmic analysis**
0.00 0.00 **FUD** XXX E
AMA: 2020,Dec,3; 2019,Jun,11; 2018,Jun,8; 2018,Apr,10

82009-82030 Chemistry: Acetaldehyde—Adenosine

INCLUDES Clinical information not requested by ordering physician
Mathematically calculated results
Quantitative analysis unless otherwise specified
Specimens from any source unless otherwise specified

EXCLUDES *Analytes from nonrequested laboratory analysis*
Calculated results representing score or probability derived by algorithm
Drug testing ([80305, 80306, 80307], [80324, 80325, 80326, 80327, 80328, 80329, 80330, 80331, 80332, 80333, 80334, 80335, 80336, 80337, 80338, 80339, 80340, 80341, 80342, 80343, 80344, 80345, 80346, 80347, 80348, 80349, 80350, 80351, 80352, 80353, 80354, 80355, 80356, 80357, 80358, 80359, 80360, 80361, 80362, 80363, 80364, 80365, 80366, 80367, 80368, 80369, 80370, 80371, 80372, 80373, 80374, 80375, 80376, 80377, 83992])
Organ or disease panels (80048-80076 [80081])
Therapeutic drug assays (80150-80299 [80164, 80165, 80171])

82009 **Ketone body(s) (eg, acetone, acetoacetic acid, beta-hydroxybutyrate); qualitative**
0.00 0.00 **FUD** XXX Q
AMA: 2020,Dec,3; 2018,Jan,8; 2017,Jan,8; 2016,Jan,13

82010 **quantitative**
0.00 0.00 **FUD** XXX Q
AMA: 2020,Dec,3; 2018,Jan,8; 2017,Jan,8; 2016,Jan,13

82013 **Acetylcholinesterase**
EXCLUDES *Acid phosphatase (84060-84066)*
Gastric acid analysis (82930)
0.00 0.00 **FUD** XXX Q
AMA: 2020,Dec,3

82016 **Acylcarnitines; qualitative, each specimen**
0.00 0.00 **FUD** XXX Q
AMA: 2020,Dec,3

82017 **quantitative, each specimen**
EXCLUDES *Carnitine (82379)*
0.00 0.00 **FUD** XXX Q
AMA: 2020,Dec,3

82024 **Adrenocorticotropic hormone (ACTH)**
0.00 0.00 **FUD** XXX Q
AMA: 2020,Dec,3

82030 **Adenosine, 5-monophosphate, cyclic (cyclic AMP)**
0.00 0.00 **FUD** XXX Q
AMA: 2020,Dec,3

82040-82042 [82042] Chemistry: Albumin

INCLUDES Clinical information not requested by ordering physician
Mathematically calculated results
Quantitative analysis unless otherwise specified
Specimens from any other sources unless otherwise specified

EXCLUDES *Analytes from nonrequested laboratory analysis*
Calculated results representing score or probability derived by algorithm
Drug testing ([80305, 80306, 80307], [80324, 80325, 80326, 80327, 80328, 80329, 80330, 80331, 80332, 80333, 80334, 80335, 80336, 80337, 80338, 80339, 80340, 80341, 80342, 80343, 80344, 80345, 80346, 80347, 80348, 80349, 80350, 80351, 80352, 80353, 80354, 80355, 80356, 80357, 80358, 80359, 80360, 80361, 80362, 80363, 80364, 80365, 80366, 80367, 80368, 80369, 80370, 80371, 80372, 80373, 80374, 80375, 80376, 80377, 83992])
Organ or disease panels (80048-80076 [80081])
Therapeutic drug assays (80150-80299 [80164, 80165, 80171])

82040 Albumin; serum, plasma or whole blood
0.00 0.00 FUD XXX
AMA: 2020,Dec,3; 2018,Jan,8; 2017,Jan,8; 2016,Jan,13

82042 **Resequenced code. See code following 82045.**

82043 urine (eg, microalbumin), quantitative
0.00 0.00 FUD XXX
AMA: 2020,Dec,3; 2018,Jan,8; 2017,Jan,8; 2016,Jan,13

82044 urine (eg, microalbumin), semiquantitative (eg, reagent strip assay)
EXCLUDES *Prealbumin (84134)*
0.00 0.00 FUD XXX
AMA: 2020,Dec,3; 2018,Jan,8; 2017,Jan,8; 2016,Jan,13

82045 ischemia modified
0.00 0.00 FUD XXX
AMA: 2020,Dec,3

82042 other source, quantitative, each specimen
EXCLUDES *Total protein (84155-84157, 84160)*
0.00 0.00 FUD XXX
AMA: 2020,Dec,3

82075-82107 Chemistry: Alcohol—Alpha-fetoprotein (AFP)

INCLUDES Clinical information not requested by ordering physician
Mathematically calculated results
Quantitative analysis unless otherwise specified
Specimens from any source unless otherwise specified

EXCLUDES *Analytes from nonrequested laboratory analysis*
Calculated results representing score or probability derived by algorithm
Drug testing ([80305, 80306, 80307], [80324, 80325, 80326, 80327, 80328, 80329, 80330, 80331, 80332, 80333, 80334, 80335, 80336, 80337, 80338, 80339, 80340, 80341, 80342, 80343, 80344, 80345, 80346, 80347, 80348, 80349, 80350, 80351, 80352, 80353, 80354, 80355, 80356, 80357, 80358, 80359, 80360, 80361, 80362, 80363, 80364, 80365, 80366, 80367, 80368, 80369, 80370, 80371, 80372, 80373, 80374, 80375, 80376, 80377, 83992])
Organ or disease panels (80048-80076 [80081])
Therapeutic drug assays (80150-80299 [80164, 80165, 80171])

82075 Alcohol (ethanol); breath
0.00 0.00 FUD XXX
AMA: 2020,Dec,3

82077 any specimen except urine and breath, immunoassay (eg, IA, EIA, ELISA, RIA, EMIT, FPIA) and enzymatic methods (eg, alcohol dehydrogenase)
EXCLUDES *Alcohol (ethanol) confirmatory drug testing ([80320])*
0.00 0.00 FUD XXX
AMA: 2020,Dec,3

82085 Aldolase
0.00 0.00 FUD XXX
AMA: 2020,Dec,3

82088 Aldosterone
EXCLUDES *Alkaline phosphatase (84075, 84080)*
Alphaketoglutarate (82009-82010)
Alphatocopherol (VitaminE) (84446)
0.00 0.00 FUD XXX
AMA: 2020,Dec,3

82103 Alpha-1-antitrypsin; total
0.00 0.00 FUD XXX
AMA: 2020,Dec,3

82104 phenotype
0.00 0.00 FUD XXX
AMA: 2020,Dec,3

82105 Alpha-fetoprotein (AFP); serum
0.00 0.00 FUD XXX
AMA: 2020,Dec,3

82106 amniotic fluid M
0.00 0.00 FUD XXX
AMA: 2020,Dec,3

82107 AFP-L3 fraction isoform and total AFP (including ratio)
0.00 0.00 FUD XXX
AMA: 2020,Dec,3

82108 Chemistry: Aluminum

CMS: 100-02,11,20.2 ESRD Laboratory Services

INCLUDES Clinical information not requested by ordering physician
Mathematically calculated results
Quantitative analysis unless otherwise specified
Specimens from any source unless otherwise specified

EXCLUDES *Analytes from nonrequested laboratory analysis*
Calculated results representing score or probability derived by algorithm
Drug testing ([80305, 80306, 80307], [80324, 80325, 80326, 80327, 80328, 80329, 80330, 80331, 80332, 80333, 80334, 80335, 80336, 80337, 80338, 80339, 80340, 80341, 80342, 80343, 80344, 80345, 80346, 80347, 80348, 80349, 80350, 80351, 80352, 80353, 80354, 80355, 80356, 80357, 80358, 80359, 80360, 80361, 80362, 80363, 80364, 80365, 80366, 80367, 80368, 80369, 80370, 80371, 80372, 80373, 80374, 80375, 80376, 80377, 83992])
Organ or disease panels (80048-80076 [80081])
Therapeutic drug assays (80150-80299 [80164, 80165, 80171])

82108 Aluminum
0.00 0.00 FUD XXX
AMA: 2020,Dec,3

82120-82261 Chemistry: Amines—Biotinidase

INCLUDES Clinical information not requested by ordering physician
Mathematically calculated results
Quantitative analysis unless otherwise specified
Specimens from any source unless otherwise specified

EXCLUDES *Analytes from nonrequested laboratory analysis*
Calculated results representing score or probability derived by algorithm
Drug testing ([80305, 80306, 80307], [80324, 80325, 80326, 80327, 80328, 80329, 80330, 80331, 80332, 80333, 80334, 80335, 80336, 80337, 80338, 80339, 80340, 80341, 80342, 80343, 80344, 80345, 80346, 80347, 80348, 80349, 80350, 80351, 80352, 80353, 80354, 80355, 80356, 80357, 80358, 80359, 80360, 80361, 80362, 80363, 80364, 80365, 80366, 80367, 80368, 80369, 80370, 80371, 80372, 80373, 80374, 80375, 80376, 80377, 83992])
Organ or disease panels (80048-80076 [80081])
Therapeutic drug assays (80150-80299 [80164, 80165, 80171])

82120 Amines, vaginal fluid, qualitative ♀
EXCLUDES *Combined pH and amines test for vaginitis (82120, 83986)*
0.00 0.00 FUD XXX
AMA: 2020,Dec,3; 2018,Jan,8; 2017,Jan,8; 2016,Jan,13

82127 Amino acids; single, qualitative, each specimen
0.00 0.00 FUD XXX
AMA: 2020,Dec,3

82128 multiple, qualitative, each specimen
0.00 0.00 FUD XXX
AMA: 2020,Dec,3

82131 single, quantitative, each specimen
INCLUDES Van Slyke method
0.00 0.00 FUD XXX
AMA: 2020,Dec,3; 2018,Jan,8; 2017,Jan,8; 2016,Jan,13

82135 Aminolevulinic acid, delta (ALA)
0.00 0.00 FUD XXX
AMA: 2020,Dec,3

82136 Amino acids, 2 to 5 amino acids, quantitative, each specimen
0.00 0.00 FUD XXX
AMA: 2020,Dec,3

Pathology and Laboratory

82040 — 82136

82139 **Amino acids, 6 or more amino acids, quantitative, each specimen**
0.00 0.00 FUD XXX
AMA: 2020,Dec,3

82140 **Ammonia**
0.00 0.00 FUD XXX
AMA: 2020,Dec,3

82143 **Amniotic fluid scan (spectrophotometric)**
EXCLUDES *Amobarbital ([80345])*
L/S ratio (83661)
0.00 0.00 FUD XXX
AMA: 2020,Dec,3

82150 **Amylase**
0.00 0.00 FUD XXX
AMA: 2020,Dec,3

82154 **Androstanediol glucuronide**
0.00 0.00 FUD XXX
AMA: 2020,Dec,3; 2018,Jan,8; 2017,Jan,8; 2016,Jan,13

82157 **Androstenedione**
0.00 0.00 FUD XXX
AMA: 2020,Dec,3

82160 **Androsterone**
0.00 0.00 FUD XXX
AMA: 2020,Dec,3

82163 **Angiotensin II**
0.00 0.00 FUD XXX
AMA: 2020,Dec,3

82164 **Angiotensin I - converting enzyme (ACE)**
EXCLUDES *Antidiuretic hormone (ADH) (84588)*
Antimony (83015)
Antitrypsin, alpha-1- (82103-82104)
0.00 0.00 FUD XXX
AMA: 2020,Dec,3

82172 **Apolipoprotein, each**
0.00 0.00 FUD XXX
AMA: 2020,Dec,3

82175 **Arsenic**
EXCLUDES *Heavy metal screening (83015)*
0.00 0.00 FUD XXX
AMA: 2020,Dec,3

82180 **Ascorbic acid (Vitamin C), blood**
EXCLUDES *Aspirin (acetylsalicylic acid) ([80329, 80330, 80331])*
Atherogenic index, blood, ultracentrifugation, quantitative (83701)
Salicylate therapeutic drug assay ([80179])
0.00 0.00 FUD XXX
AMA: 2020,Dec,3

82190 **Atomic absorption spectroscopy, each analyte**
0.00 0.00 FUD XXX
AMA: 2020,Dec,3

82232 **Beta-2 microglobulin**
0.00 0.00 FUD XXX
AMA: 2020,Dec,3

82239 **Bile acids; total**
0.00 0.00 FUD XXX
AMA: 2020,Dec,3

82240 **cholylglycine**
EXCLUDES *Bile pigments, urine (81000-81005)*
0.00 0.00 FUD XXX
AMA: 2020,Dec,3

82247 **Bilirubin; total**
INCLUDES Van Den Bergh test
0.00 0.00 FUD XXX
AMA: 2020,Dec,3; 2018,Jan,8; 2017,Jan,8; 2016,Jan,13

82248 **direct**
0.00 0.00 FUD XXX
AMA: 2020,Dec,3; 2018,Jan,8; 2017,Jan,8; 2016,Jan,13

82252 **feces, qualitative**
0.00 0.00 FUD XXX
AMA: 2020,Dec,3

82261 **Biotinidase, each specimen**
0.00 0.00 FUD XXX
AMA: 2020,Dec,3

82270-82274 Chemistry: Occult Blood

CMS: 100-04,16,70.8 CLIA Waived Tests; 100-04,18,60 Colorectal Cancer Screening

INCLUDES Clinical information not requested by ordering physician
Mathematically calculated results
Quantitative analysis unless otherwise specified
Specimens from any source unless otherwise specified

EXCLUDES *Analytes from nonrequested laboratory analysis*
Calculated results representing score or probability derived by algorithm
Drug testing ([80305, 80306, 80307], [80324, 80325, 80326, 80327, 80328, 80329, 80330, 80331, 80332, 80333, 80334, 80335, 80336, 80337, 80338, 80339, 80340, 80341, 80342, 80343, 80344, 80345, 80346, 80347, 80348, 80349, 80350, 80351, 80352, 80353, 80354, 80355, 80356, 80357, 80358, 80359, 80360, 80361, 80362, 80363, 80364, 80365, 80366, 80367, 80368, 80369, 80370, 80371, 80372, 80373, 80374, 80375, 80376, 80377, 83992])
Organ or disease panels (80048-80076 [80081])
Therapeutic drug assays (80150-80299 [80164, 80165, 80171])

82270 **Blood, occult, by peroxidase activity (eg, guaiac), qualitative; feces, consecutive collected specimens with single determination, for colorectal neoplasm screening (ie, patient was provided 3 cards or single triple card for consecutive collection)**
INCLUDES Day test
0.00 0.00 FUD XXX
AMA: 2020,Dec,3; 2018,Jan,8; 2017,Jan,8; 2016,Jan,13

82271 **other sources**
0.00 0.00 FUD XXX
AMA: 2020,Dec,3

82272 **Blood, occult, by peroxidase activity (eg, guaiac), qualitative, feces, 1-3 simultaneous determinations, performed for other than colorectal neoplasm screening**
0.00 0.00 FUD XXX
AMA: 2020,Dec,3; 2018,Jan,8; 2017,Jan,8; 2016,Jan,13

82274 **Blood, occult, by fecal hemoglobin determination by immunoassay, qualitative, feces, 1-3 simultaneous determinations**
0.00 0.00 FUD XXX
AMA: 2020,Dec,3

82286-82308 [82652] Chemistry: Bradykinin—Calcitonin

INCLUDES Clinical information not requested by ordering physician
Mathematically calculated results
Quantitative analysis unless otherwise specified
Specimens from any source unless otherwise specified

EXCLUDES *Analytes from nonrequested laboratory analysis*
Calculated results representing score or probability derived by algorithm
Drug testing ([80305, 80306, 80307], [80324, 80325, 80326, 80327, 80328, 80329, 80330, 80331, 80332, 80333, 80334, 80335, 80336, 80337, 80338, 80339, 80340, 80341, 80342, 80343, 80344, 80345, 80346, 80347, 80348, 80349, 80350, 80351, 80352, 80353, 80354, 80355, 80356, 80357, 80358, 80359, 80360, 80361, 80362, 80363, 80364, 80365, 80366, 80367, 80368, 80369, 80370, 80371, 80372, 80373, 80374, 80375, 80376, 80377, 83992])
Organ or disease panels (80048-80076 [80081])
Therapeutic drug assays (80150-80299 [80164, 80165, 80171])

82286 **Bradykinin**
0.00 0.00 FUD XXX
AMA: 2020,Dec,3

82300 **Cadmium**
0.00 0.00 FUD XXX
AMA: 2020,Dec,3

82306 **Vitamin D; 25 hydroxy, includes fraction(s), if performed**
0.00 0.00 FUD XXX
AMA: 2020,Dec,3

\# **82652** **1, 25 dihydroxy, includes fraction(s), if performed**
0.00 0.00 FUD XXX
AMA: 2020,Dec,3

82308 **Calcitonin**
0.00 0.00 FUD XXX
AMA: 2020,Dec,3

82310-82373 Chemistry: Calcium, total; Carbohydrate Deficient Transferrin

INCLUDES Clinical information not requested by ordering physician
Mathematically calculated results
Quantitative analysis unless otherwise specified
Specimens from any source unless otherwise specified

EXCLUDES *Analytes from nonrequested laboratory analysis*
Calculated results representing score or probability derived by algorithm
Drug testing ([80305, 80306, 80307], [80324, 80325, 80326, 80327, 80328, 80329, 80330, 80331, 80332, 80333, 80334, 80335, 80336, 80337, 80338, 80339, 80340, 80341, 80342, 80343, 80344, 80345, 80346, 80347, 80348, 80349, 80350, 80351, 80352, 80353, 80354, 80355, 80356, 80357, 80358, 80359, 80360, 80361, 80362, 80363, 80364, 80365, 80366, 80367, 80368, 80369, 80370, 80371, 80372, 80373, 80374, 80375, 80376, 80377, 83992])
Organ or disease panels (80048-80076 [80081])
Therapeutic drug assays (80150-80299 [80164, 80165, 80171])

82310 **Calcium; total**
0.00 0.00 FUD XXX
AMA: 2020,Dec,3; 2018,Jan,8; 2017,Jan,8; 2016,Jan,13

82330 **ionized**
0.00 0.00 FUD XXX
AMA: 2020,Dec,3; 2018,Jan,8; 2017,Jan,8; 2016,Jan,13

82331 **after calcium infusion test**
0.00 0.00 FUD XXX
AMA: 2020,Dec,3

82340 **urine quantitative, timed specimen**
0.00 0.00 FUD XXX
AMA: 2020,Dec,3

82355 **Calculus; qualitative analysis**
0.00 0.00 FUD XXX
AMA: 2020,Dec,3

82360 **quantitative analysis, chemical**
0.00 0.00 FUD XXX
AMA: 2020,Dec,3

82365 **infrared spectroscopy**
0.00 0.00 FUD XXX
AMA: 2020,Dec,3

82370 **X-ray diffraction**
0.00 0.00 FUD XXX
AMA: 2020,Dec,3

82373 **Carbohydrate deficient transferrin**
0.00 0.00 FUD XXX
AMA: 2020,Dec,3

82374 Chemistry: Carbon Dioxide

CMS: 100-02,11,20.2 ESRD Laboratory Services; 100-02,11,30.2.2 Automated Multi-Channel Chemistry (AMCC) Tests; 100-04,16,40.6.1 Automated Multi-Channel Chemistry (AMCC) Tests for ESRD Beneficiaries; 100-04,16,70.8 CLIA Waived Tests; 100-04,16,90.2 Organ or Disease Oriented Panels

INCLUDES Clinical information not requested by ordering physician
Mathematically calculated results
Quantitative analysis unless otherwise specified
Specimens from any source unless otherwise specified

EXCLUDES *Analytes from nonrequested laboratory analysis*
Calculated results representing score or probability derived by algorithm
Drug testing ([80305, 80306, 80307], [80324, 80325, 80326, 80327, 80328, 80329, 80330, 80331, 80332, 80333, 80334, 80335, 80336, 80337, 80338, 80339, 80340, 80341, 80342, 80343, 80344, 80345, 80346, 80347, 80348, 80349, 80350, 80351, 80352, 80353, 80354, 80355, 80356, 80357, 80358, 80359, 80360, 80361, 80362, 80363, 80364, 80365, 80366, 80367, 80368, 80369, 80370, 80371, 80372, 80373, 80374, 80375, 80376, 80377, 83992])
Organ or disease panels (80048-80076 [80081])
Therapeutic drug assays (80150-80299 [80164, 80165, 80171])

82374 **Carbon dioxide (bicarbonate)**
EXCLUDES *Blood gases (82803)*
0.00 0.00 FUD XXX
AMA: 2020,Dec,3; 2018,Jan,8; 2017,Jan,8; 2016,Jan,13

82375-82376 Chemistry: Carboxyhemoglobin (Carbon Monoxide)

INCLUDES Clinical information not requested by ordering physician
Mathematically calculated results
Specimens from any source unless otherwise specified

EXCLUDES *Analytes from nonrequested laboratory analysis*
Calculated results representing score or probability derived by algorithm
Drug testing ([80305, 80306, 80307], [80324, 80325, 80326, 80327, 80328, 80329, 80330, 80331, 80332, 80333, 80334, 80335, 80336, 80337, 80338, 80339, 80340, 80341, 80342, 80343, 80344, 80345, 80346, 80347, 80348, 80349, 80350, 80351, 80352, 80353, 80354, 80355, 80356, 80357, 80358, 80359, 80360, 80361, 80362, 80363, 80364, 80365, 80366, 80367, 80368, 80369, 80370, 80371, 80372, 80373, 80374, 80375, 80376, 80377, 83992])
Organ or disease panels (80048-80076 [80081])
Transcutaneous measurement of carboxyhemoglobin (88740)

82375 **Carboxyhemoglobin; quantitative**
0.00 0.00 FUD XXX
AMA: 2020,Dec,3; 2018,Jan,8; 2017,Jan,8; 2016,Jan,13

82376 **qualitative**
0.00 0.00 FUD XXX
AMA: 2020,Dec,3

82378 Chemistry: Carcinoembryonic Antigen (CEA)

CMS: 100-03,190.26 Carcinoembryonic Antigen (CEA)

INCLUDES Clinical information not requested by ordering physician

EXCLUDES *Analytes from nonrequested laboratory analysis*
Calculated results representing score or probability derived by algorithm

82378 **Carcinoembryonic antigen (CEA)**
0.00 0.00 FUD XXX
AMA: 2020,Dec,3; 2018,Jan,8; 2017,Jan,8; 2016,Jan,13

82379-82415 Chemistry: Carnitine—Chloramphenicol

INCLUDES Clinical information not requested by ordering physician
Mathematically calculated results
Quantitative analysis unless otherwise specified
Specimens from any source unless otherwise specified

EXCLUDES *Analytes from nonrequested laboratory analysis*
Calculated results representing score or probability derived by algorithm
Drug testing ([80305, 80306, 80307], [80324, 80325, 80326, 80327, 80328, 80329, 80330, 80331, 80332, 80333, 80334, 80335, 80336, 80337, 80338, 80339, 80340, 80341, 80342, 80343, 80344, 80345, 80346, 80347, 80348, 80349, 80350, 80351, 80352, 80353, 80354, 80355, 80356, 80357, 80358, 80359, 80360, 80361, 80362, 80363, 80364, 80365, 80366, 80367, 80368, 80369, 80370, 80371, 80372, 80373, 80374, 80375, 80376, 80377, 83992])
Organ or disease panels (80048-80076 [80081])
Therapeutic drug assays (80150-80299 [80164, 80165, 80171])

82379 **Carnitine (total and free), quantitative, each specimen**
EXCLUDES *Acylcarnitine (82016-82017)*
0.00 0.00 FUD XXX
AMA: 2020,Dec,3

82380 **Carotene**
0.00 0.00 FUD XXX
AMA: 2020,Dec,3

Pathology and Laboratory 82652 — 82380

82382 **Catecholamines; total urine**
0.00 0.00 FUD XXX
AMA: 2020,Dec,3

82383 **blood**
0.00 0.00 FUD XXX
AMA: 2020,Dec,3

82384 **fractionated**
EXCLUDES *Urine metabolites (83835, 84585)*
0.00 0.00 FUD XXX
AMA: 2020,Dec,3

82387 **Cathepsin-D**
0.00 0.00 FUD XXX
AMA: 2020,Dec,3

82390 **Ceruloplasmin**
0.00 0.00 FUD XXX
AMA: 2020,Dec,3

82397 **Chemiluminescent assay**
0.00 0.00 FUD XXX
AMA: 2020,Dec,3; 2018,Jan,8; 2017,Jan,8; 2016,Jan,13

82415 **Chloramphenicol**
0.00 0.00 FUD XXX
AMA: 2020,Dec,3

82435-82438 Chemistry: Chloride

INCLUDES Clinical information not requested by ordering physician
Mathematically calculated results
Quantitative analysis unless otherwise specified
Specimens from any source unless otherwise specified

EXCLUDES *Analytes from nonrequested laboratory analysis*
Calculated results representing score or probability derived by algorithm
Organ or disease panels (80048-80076 [80081])
Therapeutic drug assays (80150-80299 [80164, 80165, 80171])

82435 **Chloride; blood**
0.00 0.00 FUD XXX
AMA: 2020,Dec,3; 2018,Jan,8; 2017,Jan,8; 2016,Jan,13

82436 **urine**
0.00 0.00 FUD XXX
AMA: 2020,Dec,3

82438 **other source**
EXCLUDES *Sweat collections by iontophoresis (89230)*
0.00 0.00 FUD XXX
AMA: 2020,Dec,3; 2018,Jan,8; 2017,Jan,8; 2016,Jan,13

82441 Chemistry: Chlorinated Hydrocarbons

INCLUDES Clinical information not requested by ordering physician
Mathematically calculated results
Quantitative analysis unless otherwise specified
Specimens from any source unless otherwise specified

EXCLUDES *Analytes from nonrequested laboratory analysis*
Calculated results representing a score or probability derived by algorithm

82441 **Chlorinated hydrocarbons, screen**
EXCLUDES *Cholecalciferol (Vitamin D) (82306)*
0.00 0.00 FUD XXX
AMA: 2020,Dec,3

82465 Chemistry: Cholesterol, Total

CMS: 100-03,190.23 Lipid Testing; 100-04,16,40.6.1 Automated Multi-Channel Chemistry (AMCC) Tests for ESRD Beneficiaries; 100-04,16,70.8 CLIA Waived Tests; 100-04,16,90.2 Organ or Disease Oriented Panels

INCLUDES Clinical information not requested by ordering physician
Mathematically calculated results
Quantitative analysis unless otherwise specified

EXCLUDES *Analytes from nonrequested laboratory analysis*
Calculated results representing score or probability derived by algorithm
Organ or disease panels (80048-80076 [80081])

82465 **Cholesterol, serum or whole blood, total**
EXCLUDES *High density lipoprotein (HDL) (83718)*
0.00 0.00 FUD XXX
AMA: 2020,Dec,3; 2018,Jan,8; 2017,Jan,8; 2016,Jan,13

82480-82507 Chemistry: Cholinesterase—Citrate

INCLUDES Clinical information not requested by ordering physician
Mathematically calculated results
Quantitative analysis unless otherwise specified
Specimens from any source unless otherwise specified

EXCLUDES *Analytes from nonrequested laboratory analysis*
Calculated results representing score or probability derived by algorithm
Drug testing ([80305, 80306, 80307], [80324, 80325, 80326, 80327, 80328, 80329, 80330, 80331, 80332, 80333, 80334, 80335, 80336, 80337, 80338, 80339, 80340, 80341, 80342, 80343, 80344, 80345, 80346, 80347, 80348, 80349, 80350, 80351, 80352, 80353, 80354, 80355, 80356, 80357, 80358, 80359, 80360, 80361, 80362, 80363, 80364, 80365, 80366, 80367, 80368, 80369, 80370, 80371, 80372, 80373, 80374, 80375, 80376, 80377, 83992])
Organ or disease panels (80048-80076 [80081])
Therapeutic drug assays (80150-80299 [80164, 80165, 80171])

82480 **Cholinesterase; serum**
0.00 0.00 FUD XXX
AMA: 2020,Dec,3

82482 **RBC**
0.00 0.00 FUD XXX
AMA: 2020,Dec,3

82485 **Chondroitin B sulfate, quantitative**
EXCLUDES *Chorionic gonadotropin (84702-84703)*
0.00 0.00 FUD XXX
AMA: 2020,Dec,3

82495 **Chromium**
0.00 0.00 FUD XXX
AMA: 2020,Dec,3

82507 **Citrate**
EXCLUDES *Cocaine, qualitative analysis ([80353])*
Codeine, qualitative analysis ([80361])
Complement (86160-86162)
0.00 0.00 FUD XXX
AMA: 2020,Dec,3

82523 Chemistry: Collagen Crosslinks, Any Method

CMS: 100-03,190.19 NCD for Collagen Crosslinks, Any Method; 100-04,16,70.8 CLIA Waived Tests

INCLUDES Clinical information not requested by ordering physician
Mathematically calculated results
Quantitative analysis unless otherwise specified
Specimens from any source unless otherwise specified

EXCLUDES *Analytes from nonrequested laboratory analysis*
Calculated results representing score or probability derived by algorithm
Organ or disease panels (80048-80076 [80081])
Therapeutic drug assays (80150-80299 [80164, 80165, 80171])

82523 **Collagen cross links, any method**
0.00 0.00 FUD XXX
AMA: 2020,Dec,3

82525-82735 [82652, 82653, 82681] Chemistry: Copper—Fluoride

INCLUDES Clinical information not requested by ordering physician
Mathematically calculated results
Quantitative analysis unless otherwise specified
Specimens from any source unless otherwise specified

EXCLUDES *Analytes from nonrequested laboratory analysis*
Calculated results representing score or probability derived by algorithm
Drug testing ([80305, 80306, 80307], [80324, 80325, 80326, 80327, 80328, 80329, 80330, 80331, 80332, 80333, 80334, 80335, 80336, 80337, 80338, 80339, 80340, 80341, 80342, 80343, 80344, 80345, 80346, 80347, 80348, 80349, 80350, 80351, 80352, 80353, 80354, 80355, 80356, 80357, 80358, 80359, 80360, 80361, 80362, 80363, 80364, 80365, 80366, 80367, 80368, 80369, 80370, 80371, 80372, 80373, 80374, 80375, 80376, 80377, 83992])
Organ or disease panels (80048-80076 [80081])
Therapeutic drug assays (80150-80299 [80164, 80165, 80171])

82525 **Copper**
EXCLUDES *Coproporphyrin (84119-84120)*
Corticosteroids (83491)
0.00 0.00 FUD XXX
AMA: 2020,Dec,3

82528 **Corticosterone**
INCLUDES Porter-Silber test
0.00 0.00 FUD XXX
AMA: 2020,Dec,3

82530 **Cortisol; free**
0.00 0.00 FUD XXX
AMA: 2020,Dec,3; 2018,Jan,8; 2017,Jan,8; 2016,Jan,13

82533 **total**
0.00 0.00 FUD XXX
AMA: 2020,Dec,3; 2018,Jan,8; 2017,Jan,8; 2016,Jan,13

82540 **Creatine**
0.00 0.00 FUD XXX
AMA: 2020,Dec,3

82542 **Column chromatography, includes mass spectrometry, if performed (eg, HPLC, LC, LC/MS, LC/MS-MS, GC, GC/MS-MS, GC/MS, HPLC/MS), non-drug analyte(s) not elsewhere specified, qualitative or quantitative, each specimen**
EXCLUDES *Column chromatography/mass spectrometry drugs/substances ([80305, 80306, 80307], [80320, 80321, 80322, 80323, 80324, 80325, 80326, 80327, 80328, 80329, 80330, 80331, 80332, 80333, 80334, 80335, 80336, 80337, 80338, 80339, 80340, 80341, 80342, 80343, 80344, 80345, 80346, 80347, 80348, 80349, 80350, 80351, 80352, 80353, 80354, 80355, 80356, 80357, 80358, 80359, 80360, 80361, 80362, 80363, 80364, 80365, 80366, 80367, 80368, 80369, 80370, 80371, 80372, 80373, 80374, 80375, 80376, 80377, 83992])*
Procedure performed more than one time per specimen
0.00 0.00 FUD XXX
AMA: 2020,Dec,3; 2018,Jan,8; 2017,Jan,8; 2016,Jan,13

82550 **Creatine kinase (CK), (CPK); total**
0.00 0.00 FUD XXX
AMA: 2020,Dec,3; 2018,Jan,8; 2017,Jan,8; 2016,Jan,13

82552 **isoenzymes**
0.00 0.00 FUD XXX
AMA: 2020,Dec,3; 2018,Jan,8; 2017,Jan,8; 2016,Jan,13

82553 **MB fraction only**
0.00 0.00 FUD XXX
AMA: 2020,Dec,3; 2018,Jan,8; 2017,Jan,8; 2016,Jan,13

82554 **isoforms**
0.00 0.00 FUD XXX
AMA: 2020,Dec,3; 2018,Jan,8; 2017,Jan,8; 2016,Jan,13

82565 **Creatinine; blood**
0.00 0.00 FUD XXX
AMA: 2020,Dec,3; 2018,Jan,8; 2017,Jan,8; 2016,Jan,13

82570 **other source**
0.00 0.00 FUD XXX
AMA: 2020,Dec,3

82575 **clearance**
INCLUDES Holten test
0.00 0.00 FUD XXX
AMA: 2020,Dec,3

82585 **Cryofibrinogen**
0.00 0.00 FUD XXX
AMA: 2020,Dec,3

82595 **Cryoglobulin, qualitative or semi-quantitative (eg, cryocrit)**
EXCLUDES *Crystals, pyrophosphate vs urate (89060)*
Quantitative, cryoglobulin (82784-82785)
0.00 0.00 FUD XXX
AMA: 2020,Dec,3

82600 **Cyanide**
0.00 0.00 FUD XXX
AMA: 2020,Dec,3

82607 **Cyanocobalamin (Vitamin B-12);**
EXCLUDES *Cyclic AMP (82030)*
Cyclosporine (80158)
0.00 0.00 FUD XXX
AMA: 2020,Dec,3

82608 **unsaturated binding capacity**
EXCLUDES *Cyclic AMP (82030)*
Cyclosporine (80158)
0.00 0.00 FUD XXX
AMA: 2020,Dec,3

82610 **Cystatin C**
0.00 0.00 FUD XXX
AMA: 2020,Dec,3; 2018,Jan,8; 2017,Jan,8; 2016,Jan,13

82615 **Cystine and homocystine, urine, qualitative**
0.00 0.00 FUD XXX
AMA: 2020,Dec,3

82626 **Dehydroepiandrosterone (DHEA)**
EXCLUDES *Anabolic steroids ([80327, 80328])*
0.00 0.00 FUD XXX
AMA: 2020,Dec,3; 2018,Jan,8; 2017,Jan,8; 2016,Jan,13

82627 **Dehydroepiandrosterone-sulfate (DHEA-S)**
EXCLUDES *Delta-aminolevulinicacid (ALA) (82135)*
0.00 0.00 FUD XXX
AMA: 2020,Dec,3; 2018,Jan,8; 2017,Jan,8; 2016,Jan,13

82633 **Desoxycorticosterone, 11-**
0.00 0.00 FUD XXX
AMA: 2020,Dec,3

82634 **Deoxycortisol, 11-**
EXCLUDES *Dexamethasone suppression test (80420)*
Diastase, urine (82150)
0.00 0.00 FUD XXX
AMA: 2020,Dec,3

82638 **Dibucaine number**
EXCLUDES *Dichloroethane (82441)*
Dichloromethane (82441)
Diethylether (84600)
0.00 0.00 FUD XXX
AMA: 2020,Dec,3

82642 **Dihydrotestosterone (DHT)**
EXCLUDES *Anabolic drug testing analysis dihydrotestosterone ([80327, 80328])*
Dipropylaceticacid ([80164])
Dopamine (82382)
Duodenal contents, individual enzymes for intubation and collection (43756-43757)
0.00 0.00 FUD XXX
AMA: 2020,Dec,3

82652 **Resequenced code. See code following 82306.**

82653 **Resequnced code. See code following 82656.**

▲ **82656** **Elastase, pancreatic (EL-1), fecal; qualitative or semi-quantitative**
0.00 0.00 FUD XXX
AMA: 2020,Dec,3; 2018,Jan,8; 2017,Jan,8; 2016,Jan,13

● # **82653** **quantitative**
0.00 0.00 FUD 000

82657 **Enzyme activity in blood cells, cultured cells, or tissue, not elsewhere specified; nonradioactive substrate, each specimen**
0.00 0.00 FUD XXX
AMA: 2020,Dec,3

82658 **radioactive substrate, each specimen**
0.00 0.00 FUD XXX
AMA: 2020,Dec,3

Pathology and Laboratory

82664 — 82803

82664 Electrophoretic technique, not elsewhere specified
EXCLUDES *Endocrine receptor assays (84233-84235)*
0.00 0.00 FUD XXX
AMA: 2020,Dec,3

82668 Erythropoietin
0.00 0.00 FUD XXX
AMA: 2020,Dec,3

82670 Estradiol; total
0.00 0.00 FUD XXX
AMA: 2020,Dec,3

82681 free, direct measurement (eg, equilibrium dialysis)
0.00 0.00 FUD XXX
AMA: 2020,Dec,3

82671 Estrogens; fractionated
EXCLUDES *Estrogen receptor assay (84233)*
0.00 0.00 FUD XXX
AMA: 2020,Dec,3

82672 total
EXCLUDES *Estrogen receptor assay (84233)*
0.00 0.00 FUD XXX
AMA: 2020,Dec,3

82677 Estriol
0.00 0.00 FUD XXX
AMA: 2020,Dec,3

82679 Estrone
EXCLUDES *Alcohol (ethanol) definitive drug testing ([80320])*
Alcohol (ethanol) therapeutic drug assay (82077)
0.00 0.00 FUD XXX
AMA: 2020,Dec,3

82681 Resequenced code. See code following 82670.

82693 Ethylene glycol
0.00 0.00 FUD XXX
AMA: 2020,Dec,3

82696 Etiocholanolone
EXCLUDES *Fractionation ketosteroids (83593)*
0.00 0.00 FUD XXX
AMA: 2020,Dec,3

82705 Fat or lipids, feces; qualitative
0.00 0.00 FUD XXX
AMA: 2020,Dec,3

82710 quantitative
0.00 0.00 FUD XXX
AMA: 2020,Dec,3

82715 Fat differential, feces, quantitative
0.00 0.00 FUD XXX
AMA: 2020,Dec,3

82725 Fatty acids, nonesterified
0.00 0.00 FUD XXX
AMA: 2020,Dec,3

82726 Very long chain fatty acids
EXCLUDES *Long-chain (C20-22) omega-3 fatty acids in red blood cell (RBC) membranes (84999)*
0.00 0.00 FUD XXX
AMA: 2020,Dec,3

82728 Ferritin
EXCLUDES *Fetal hemoglobin (83030, 83033, 85460)*
Fetoprotein, alpha-1 (82105-82106)
0.00 0.00 FUD XXX
AMA: 2020,Dec,3

82731 Fetal fibronectin, cervicovaginal secretions, semi-quantitative
M ♀
0.00 0.00 FUD XXX
AMA: 2020,Dec,3

82735 Fluoride
EXCLUDES *Foam stability test (83662)*
0.00 0.00 FUD XXX
AMA: 2020,Dec,3

82746-82941 Chemistry: Folic Acid—Gastrin

INCLUDES Clinical information not requested by ordering physician
Mathematically calculated results
Quantitative analysis unless otherwise specified
Specimens from any source unless otherwise specified

EXCLUDES *Analytes from nonrequested laboratory analysis*
Calculated results representing score or probability derived by algorithm
Drug testing ([80305, 80306, 80307], [80324, 80325, 80326, 80327, 80328, 80329, 80330, 80331, 80332, 80333, 80334, 80335, 80336, 80337, 80338, 80339, 80340, 80341, 80342, 80343, 80344, 80345, 80346, 80347, 80348, 80349, 80350, 80351, 80352, 80353, 80354, 80355, 80356, 80357, 80358, 80359, 80360, 80361, 80362, 80363, 80364, 80365, 80366, 80367, 80368, 80369, 80370, 80371, 80372, 80373, 80374, 80375, 80376, 80377, 83992])
Organ or disease panels (80048-80076 [80081])
Therapeutic drug assays (80150-80299 [80164, 80165, 80171])

82746 Folic acid; serum
0.00 0.00 FUD XXX
AMA: 2020,Dec,3

82747 RBC
EXCLUDES *Follicle stimulating hormone (FSH) (83001)*
0.00 0.00 FUD XXX
AMA: 2020,Dec,3

82757 Fructose, semen
EXCLUDES *Fructosamine (82985)*
Fructose, TLC screen (84375)
0.00 0.00 FUD XXX
AMA: 2020,Dec,3

82759 Galactokinase, RBC
0.00 0.00 FUD XXX
AMA: 2020,Dec,3

82760 Galactose
0.00 0.00 FUD XXX
AMA: 2020,Dec,3

82775 Galactose-1-phosphate uridyl transferase; quantitative
0.00 0.00 FUD XXX
AMA: 2020,Dec,3

82776 screen
0.00 0.00 FUD XXX
AMA: 2020,Dec,3

82777 Galectin-3
0.00 0.00 FUD XXX
AMA: 2020,Dec,3

82784 Gammaglobulin (immunoglobulin); IgA, IgD, IgG, IgM, each
INCLUDES Farr test
0.00 0.00 FUD XXX
AMA: 2020,Dec,3; 2018,Jan,8; 2017,Jan,8; 2016,Jan,13

82785 IgE
INCLUDES Farr test
EXCLUDES *Allergen specific, IgE (86003, 86005)*
0.00 0.00 FUD XXX
AMA: 2020,Dec,3; 2018,Jan,8; 2017,Jan,8; 2016,Jan,13

82787 immunoglobulin subclasses (eg, IgG1, 2, 3, or 4), each
EXCLUDES *Gamma-glutamyltransferase (GGT) (82977)*
0.00 0.00 FUD XXX
AMA: 2020,Dec,3

82800 Gases, blood, pH only
0.00 0.00 FUD XXX
AMA: 2020,Dec,3

82803 Gases, blood, any combination of pH, pCO2, pO2, CO2, HCO3 (including calculated O2 saturation);
INCLUDES Two or more listed analytes
0.00 0.00 FUD XXX
AMA: 2020,Dec,3

82805 **with O2 saturation, by direct measurement, except pulse oximetry**
0.00 0.00 FUD XXX
AMA: 2020,Dec,3

82810 **Gases, blood, O2 saturation only, by direct measurement, except pulse oximetry**
EXCLUDES *Pulse oximetry (94760)*
0.00 0.00 FUD XXX
AMA: 2020,Dec,3

82820 **Hemoglobin-oxygen affinity (pO2 for 50% hemoglobin saturation with oxygen)**
EXCLUDES *Gastric acid analysis (82930)*
0.00 0.00 FUD XXX
AMA: 2020,Dec,3

82930 **Gastric acid analysis, includes pH if performed, each specimen**
0.00 0.00 FUD XXX
AMA: 2020,Dec,3; 2018,Jan,8; 2017,Jan,8; 2016,Jan,13

82938 **Gastrin after secretin stimulation**
0.00 0.00 FUD XXX
AMA: 2020,Dec,3

82941 **Gastrin**
EXCLUDES *Gentamicin (80170)*
GGT (82977)
Qualitative column chromatography report specific analyte or (82542)
0.00 0.00 FUD XXX
AMA: 2020,Dec,3

82943-82962 Chemistry: Glucagon—Glucose Testing

CMS: 100-03,190.20 Blood Glucose Testing

INCLUDES Clinical information not requested by ordering physician
Mathematically calculated results
Quantitative analysis unless otherwise specified
Specimens from any source unless otherwise specified

EXCLUDES *Analytes from nonrequested laboratory analysis*
Calculated results representing score or probability derived by algorithm
Organ or disease panels (80048-80076 [80081])
Therapeutic drug assays (80150-80299 [80164, 80165, 80171])

Code also glucose administration injection (96374)

82943 **Glucagon**
0.00 0.00 FUD XXX
AMA: 2020,Dec,3

82945 **Glucose, body fluid, other than blood**
0.00 0.00 FUD XXX
AMA: 2020,Dec,3

82946 **Glucagon tolerance test**
0.00 0.00 FUD XXX
AMA: 2020,Dec,3

82947 **Glucose; quantitative, blood (except reagent strip)**
0.00 0.00 FUD XXX
AMA: 2020,Dec,3; 2018,Jan,8; 2017,Jan,8; 2016,Jan,13

82948 **blood, reagent strip**
0.00 0.00 FUD XXX
AMA: 2020,Dec,3; 2018,Jan,8; 2017,Jan,8; 2016,Jan,13

82950 **post glucose dose (includes glucose)**
0.00 0.00 FUD XXX
AMA: 2020,Dec,3; 2018,Jan,8; 2017,Jan,8; 2016,Jan,13

82951 **tolerance test (GTT), 3 specimens (includes glucose)**
0.00 0.00 FUD XXX
AMA: 2020,Dec,3; 2018,Jan,8; 2017,Jan,8; 2016,Jan,13

+ **82952** **tolerance test, each additional beyond 3 specimens (List separately in addition to code for primary procedure)**
EXCLUDES *Insulin tolerance test (80434-80435)*
Leucine tolerance test (80428)
Semiquantitative urine glucose (81000, 81002, 81005, 81099)
Code first (82951)
0.00 0.00 FUD XXX
AMA: 2020,Dec,3; 2018,Jan,8; 2017,Jan,8; 2016,Jan,13

82955 **Glucose-6-phosphate dehydrogenase (G6PD); quantitative**
Code also glucose tolerance test with medication, when performed (96374)
0.00 0.00 FUD XXX
AMA: 2020,Dec,3

82960 **screen**
Code also glucose tolerance test with medication, when performed (96374)
0.00 0.00 FUD XXX
AMA: 2020,Dec,3

82962 **Glucose, blood by glucose monitoring device(s) cleared by the FDA specifically for home use**
0.00 0.00 FUD XXX
AMA: 2020,Dec,3; 2018,Jan,8; 2017,Jan,8; 2016,Jan,13

82963-83690 [83529] Chemistry: Glucosidase—Lipase

INCLUDES Clinical information not requested by ordering physician
Mathematically calculated results
Quantitative analysis unless otherwise specified
Specimens from any source unless otherwise specified

EXCLUDES *Analytes from nonrequested laboratory analysis*
Calculated results representing score or probability derived by algorithm
Drug testing ([80305, 80306, 80307], [80324, 80325, 80326, 80327, 80328, 80329, 80330, 80331, 80332, 80333, 80334, 80335, 80336, 80337, 80338, 80339, 80340, 80341, 80342, 80343, 80344, 80345, 80346, 80347, 80348, 80349, 80350, 80351, 80352, 80353, 80354, 80355, 80356, 80357, 80358, 80359, 80360, 80361, 80362, 80363, 80364, 80365, 80366, 80367, 80368, 80369, 80370, 80371, 80372, 80373, 80374, 80375, 80376, 80377, 83992])
Organ or disease panels (80048-80076 [80081])
Therapeutic drug assays (80150-80299 [80164, 80165, 80171])

82963 **Glucosidase, beta**
0.00 0.00 FUD XXX
AMA: 2020,Dec,3

82965 **Glutamate dehydrogenase**
0.00 0.00 FUD XXX
AMA: 2020,Dec,3

82977 **Glutamyltransferase, gamma (GGT)**
0.00 0.00 FUD XXX
AMA: 2020,Dec,3; 2018,Jan,8; 2017,Jan,8; 2016,Jan,13

82978 **Glutathione**
0.00 0.00 FUD XXX
AMA: 2020,Dec,3

82979 **Glutathione reductase, RBC**
EXCLUDES *Glycohemoglobin (83036)*
0.00 0.00 FUD XXX
AMA: 2020,Dec,3

82985 **Glycated protein**
EXCLUDES *Gonadotropin chorionic (hCG) (84702-84703)*
0.00 0.00 FUD XXX
AMA: 2020,Dec,3; 2018,Jan,8; 2017,Jan,8; 2016,Jan,13

83001 **Gonadotropin; follicle stimulating hormone (FSH)**
0.00 0.00 FUD XXX
AMA: 2020,Dec,3

83002 **luteinizing hormone (LH)**
EXCLUDES *Luteinizing releasing factor (LRH) (83727)*
0.00 0.00 FUD XXX
AMA: 2020,Dec,3

83003 **Growth hormone, human (HGH) (somatotropin)**
EXCLUDES *Antibody to human growth hormone (86277)*
0.00 0.00 FUD XXX
AMA: 2020,Dec,3

83006 Growth stimulation expressed gene 2 (ST2, Interleukin 1 receptor like-1)
0.00 0.00 FUD XXX
AMA: 2020,Dec,3

83009 Helicobacter pylori, blood test analysis for urease activity, non-radioactive isotope (eg, C-13)
EXCLUDES *H. pylori, breath test analysis for urease activity (83013-83014)*
0.00 0.00 FUD XXX
AMA: 2020,Dec,3

83010 Haptoglobin; quantitative
0.00 0.00 FUD XXX
AMA: 2020,Dec,3

83012 phenotypes
0.00 0.00 FUD XXX
AMA: 2020,Dec,3

83013 Helicobacter pylori; breath test analysis for urease activity, non-radioactive isotope (eg, C-13)
0.00 0.00 FUD XXX
AMA: 2020,Dec,3; 2020,OctSE,1; 2020,OctSE,1; 2018,Jan,8; 2017,Jan,8; 2016,Jan,13

83014 drug administration
EXCLUDES *H. pylori:*
Blood test analysis for urease activity (83009)
Enzyme immunoassay (87339)
Liquid scintillation counter (78267-78268)
Stool (87338)
0.00 0.00 FUD XXX
AMA: 2020,Dec,3; 2020,OctSE,1; 2020,OctSE,1; 2018,Jan,8; 2017,Jan,8; 2016,Jan,13

83015 Heavy metal (eg, arsenic, barium, beryllium, bismuth, antimony, mercury); qualitative, any number of analytes
INCLUDES Reinsch test
0.00 0.00 FUD XXX
AMA: 2020,Dec,3

83018 quantitative, each, not elsewhere specified
EXCLUDES *Evaluation known heavy metal with specific code*
0.00 0.00 FUD XXX
AMA: 2020,Dec,3

83020 Hemoglobin fractionation and quantitation; electrophoresis (eg, A2, S, C, and/or F)
0.00 0.00 FUD XXX
AMA: 2020,Dec,3

83021 chromatography (eg, A2, S, C, and/or F)
EXCLUDES *Analysis glycosylated (A1c) hemoglobin by chromatography or electrophoresis without identified hemoglobin variant (83036)*
0.00 0.00 FUD XXX
AMA: 2020,Dec,3; 2018,Jan,8; 2017,Jan,8; 2016,Jan,13

83026 Hemoglobin; by copper sulfate method, non-automated
0.00 0.00 FUD XXX
AMA: 2020,Dec,3

83030 F (fetal), chemical
0.00 0.00 FUD XXX
AMA: 2020,Dec,3

83033 F (fetal), qualitative
0.00 0.00 FUD XXX
AMA: 2020,Dec,3

83036 glycosylated (A1C)
EXCLUDES *Analysis glycosylated (A1c) hemoglobin by chromatography or electrophoresis without identified hemoglobin variant (83020-83021)*
Detection hemoglobin, fecal, by immunoassay (82274)
0.00 0.00 FUD XXX
AMA: 2020,Dec,3; 2018,Jan,8; 2017,Jan,8; 2016,Jan,13

83037 glycosylated (A1C) by device cleared by FDA for home use
0.00 0.00 FUD XXX
AMA: 2020,Dec,3; 2018,Jan,8; 2017,Jan,8; 2016,Jan,13

83045 methemoglobin, qualitative
0.00 0.00 FUD XXX
AMA: 2020,Dec,3

83050 methemoglobin, quantitative
EXCLUDES *Transcutaneous methemoglobin test (88741)*
0.00 0.00 FUD XXX
AMA: 2020,Dec,3; 2018,Jan,8; 2017,Jan,8; 2016,Jan,13

83051 plasma
0.00 0.00 FUD XXX
AMA: 2020,Dec,3

83060 sulfhemoglobin, quantitative
0.00 0.00 FUD XXX
AMA: 2020,Dec,3

83065 thermolabile
0.00 0.00 FUD XXX
AMA: 2020,Dec,3

83068 unstable, screen
0.00 0.00 FUD XXX
AMA: 2020,Dec,3

83069 urine
0.00 0.00 FUD XXX
AMA: 2020,Dec,3

83070 Hemosiderin, qualitative
EXCLUDES *HIAA (83497)*
Qualitative column chromatography report specific analyte or (82542)
0.00 0.00 FUD XXX
AMA: 2020,Dec,3

83080 b-Hexosaminidase, each assay
0.00 0.00 FUD XXX
AMA: 2020,Dec,3

83088 Histamine
EXCLUDES *Hollander test (43754-43755)*
0.00 0.00 FUD XXX
AMA: 2020,Dec,3

83090 Homocysteine
0.00 0.00 FUD XXX
AMA: 2020,Dec,3; 2018,Jan,8; 2017,Jan,8; 2016,Jan,13

83150 Homovanillic acid (HVA)
EXCLUDES *Hormone testing report from alphabetic list in Chemistry section*
Hydrogen/methane breath test (91065)
0.00 0.00 FUD XXX
AMA: 2020,Dec,3

83491 Hydroxycorticosteroids, 17- (17-OHCS)
EXCLUDES *Cortisol (82530, 82533)*
Deoxycortisol (82634)
0.00 0.00 FUD XXX
AMA: 2020,Dec,3

83497 Hydroxyindolacetic acid, 5-(HIAA)
EXCLUDES *5-Hydroxytryptamine (84260)*
Urine qualitative test (81005)
0.00 0.00 FUD XXX
AMA: 2020,Dec,3

83498 Hydroxyprogesterone, 17-d
0.00 0.00 FUD XXX
AMA: 2020,Dec,3

83500 Hydroxyproline; free
0.00 0.00 FUD XXX
AMA: 2020,Dec,3

83505 **total**
0.00 0.00 FUD XXX
AMA: 2020,Dec,3

83516 **Immunoassay for analyte other than infectious agent antibody or infectious agent antigen; qualitative or semiquantitative, multiple step method**
0.00 0.00 FUD XXX
AMA: 2020,Dec,3; 2020,OctSE,1; 2020,OctSE,1; 2020,AugSE,1; 2020,AugSE,1; 2020,AugSE,1

83518 **qualitative or semiquantitative, single step method (eg, reagent strip)**
0.00 0.00 FUD XXX
AMA: 2020,Dec,3; 2020,OctSE,1; 2020,OctSE,1

83519 **quantitative, by radioimmunoassay (eg, RIA)**
0.00 0.00 FUD XXX
AMA: 2020,Dec,3; 2020,OctSE,1; 2020,OctSE,1; 2018,Jan,8; 2017,Jan,8; 2016,Jan,13

83520 **quantitative, not otherwise specified**
EXCLUDES *Immunoassays for antibodies to infectious agent antigen report specific analyte/method from Immunology*
Immunoassay of tumor antigens not elsewhere specified (86316)
Immunoglobulins (82784, 82785)
0.00 0.00 FUD XXX
AMA: 2020,Dec,3; 2020,OctSE,1; 2020,OctSE,1

● **83521** **Immunoglobulin light chains (ie, kappa, lambda), free, each**

83525 **Insulin; total**
EXCLUDES *Proinsulin (84206)*
0.00 0.00 FUD XXX
AMA: 2020,Dec,3

83527 **free**
0.00 0.00 FUD XXX
AMA: 2020,Dec,3; 2018,Jan,8; 2017,Jan,8; 2016,Jan,13

● # **83529** **Interleukin-6 (IL-6)**
0.00 0.00 FUD 000

83528 **Intrinsic factor**
EXCLUDES *Intrinsic factor antibodies (86340)*
0.00 0.00 FUD XXX
AMA: 2020,Dec,3

83529 **Resequnced code. See code following 83527.**

83540 **Iron**
0.00 0.00 FUD XXX
AMA: 2020,Dec,3; 2018,Jan,8; 2017,Jan,8; 2016,Jan,13

83550 **Iron binding capacity**
0.00 0.00 FUD XXX
AMA: 2020,Dec,3

83570 **Isocitric dehydrogenase (IDH)**
EXCLUDES *Isonicotinic acid hydrazide, INH, report specific method*
Isopropyl alcohol ([80320])
0.00 0.00 FUD XXX
AMA: 2020,Dec,3

83582 **Ketogenic steroids, fractionation**
EXCLUDES *Ketone bodies:*
Serum (82009, 82010)
Urine (81000-81003)
0.00 0.00 FUD XXX
AMA: 2020,Dec,3

83586 **Ketosteroids, 17- (17-KS); total**
0.00 0.00 FUD XXX
AMA: 2020,Dec,3

83593 **fractionation**
0.00 0.00 FUD XXX
AMA: 2020,Dec,3

83605 **Lactate (lactic acid)**
0.00 0.00 FUD XXX
AMA: 2020,Dec,3

83615 **Lactate dehydrogenase (LD), (LDH);**
0.00 0.00 FUD XXX
AMA: 2020,Dec,3; 2018,Jan,8; 2017,Jan,8; 2016,Jan,13

83625 **isoenzymes, separation and quantitation**
0.00 0.00 FUD XXX
AMA: 2020,Dec,3; 2018,Jan,8; 2017,Jan,8; 2016,Jan,13

83630 **Lactoferrin, fecal; qualitative**
0.00 0.00 FUD XXX
AMA: 2020,Dec,3; 2018,Jan,8; 2017,Jan,8; 2016,Jan,13

83631 **quantitative**
0.00 0.00 FUD XXX
AMA: 2020,Dec,3; 2018,Jan,8; 2017,Jan,8; 2016,Jan,13

83632 **Lactogen, human placental (HPL) human chorionic somatomammotropin**
0.00 0.00 FUD XXX
AMA: 2020,Dec,3

83633 **Lactose, urine, qualitative**
EXCLUDES *Lactase deficiency breath hydrogen/methane test (91065)*
Lactose tolerance test (82951, 82952)
0.00 0.00 FUD XXX
AMA: 2020,Dec,3

83655 **Lead**
0.00 0.00 FUD XXX
AMA: 2020,Dec,3

83661 **Fetal lung maturity assessment; lecithin sphingomyelin (L/S) ratio**
0.00 0.00 FUD XXX
AMA: 2020,Dec,3; 2018,Jan,8; 2017,Jan,8; 2016,Jan,13

83662 **foam stability test**
0.00 0.00 FUD XXX
AMA: 2020,Dec,3

83663 **fluorescence polarization**
0.00 0.00 FUD XXX
AMA: 2020,Dec,3

83664 **lamellar body density**
EXCLUDES *Phosphatidylglycerol (84081)*
0.00 0.00 FUD XXX
AMA: 2020,Dec,3

83670 **Leucine aminopeptidase (LAP)**
0.00 0.00 FUD XXX
AMA: 2020,Dec,3

83690 **Lipase**
0.00 0.00 FUD XXX
AMA: 2020,Dec,3

83695-83727 Chemistry: Lipoprotein—Luteinizing Releasing Factor

INCLUDES Clinical information not requested by ordering physician
Mathematically calculated results
Quantitative analysis unless otherwise specified
Specimens from any source unless otherwise specified

EXCLUDES *Analytes from nonrequested laboratory analysis*
Calculated results representing score or probability derived by algorithm
Organ or disease panels (80048-80076 [80081])
Therapeutic drug assays (80150-80299 [80164, 80165, 80171])

83695 **Lipoprotein (a)**
0.00 0.00 FUD XXX
AMA: 2020,Dec,3; 2018,Jan,8; 2017,Jan,8; 2016,Jan,13

83698 **Lipoprotein-associated phospholipase A2 (Lp-PLA2)**
0.00 0.00 FUD XXX
AMA: 2020,Dec,3

Pathology and Laboratory

83505 — 83698

83700 Lipoprotein, blood; electrophoretic separation and quantitation
0.00 0.00 FUD XXX
AMA: 2020,Dec,3; 2018,Jan,8; 2017,Jan,8; 2016,Jan,13

83701 high resolution fractionation and quantitation of lipoproteins including lipoprotein subclasses when performed (eg, electrophoresis, ultracentrifugation)
0.00 0.00 FUD XXX
AMA: 2020,Dec,3; 2018,Jan,8; 2017,Jan,8; 2016,Jan,13

83704 quantitation of lipoprotein particle number(s) (eg, by nuclear magnetic resonance spectroscopy), includes lipoprotein particle subclass(es), when performed
0.00 0.00 FUD XXX
AMA: 2020,Dec,3; 2018,Jan,8; 2017,Jan,8; 2016,Jan,13

83718 Lipoprotein, direct measurement; high density cholesterol (HDL cholesterol)
0.00 0.00 FUD XXX
AMA: 2020,Dec,3; 2018,Jan,8; 2017,Jan,8; 2016,Jan,13

83719 VLDL cholesterol
0.00 0.00 FUD XXX
AMA: 2020,Dec,3; 2018,Jan,8; 2017,Jan,8; 2016,Jan,13

83721 LDL cholesterol
EXCLUDES *Fractionation by high resolution electrophoresis or ultracentrifugation (83701)*
Lipoprotein particle numbers and subclasses analysis by nuclear magnetic resonance spectroscopy (83704)
0.00 0.00 FUD XXX
AMA: 2020,Dec,3; 2018,Jan,8; 2017,Jan,8; 2016,Jan,13

83722 small dense LDL cholesterol
EXCLUDES *Fractionation by high resolution electrophoresis or ultracentrifugation (83701)*
Lipoprotein particle numbers/subclass analysis by nuclear magnetic resonance spectroscopy (83704)
0.00 0.00 FUD XXX
AMA: 2020,Dec,3

83727 Luteinizing releasing factor (LRH)
EXCLUDES *alpha-2-Macroglobulin (86329)*
Luteinizing hormone (LH) (83002)
0.00 0.00 FUD XXX
AMA: 2020,Dec,3

83735-83885 Chemistry: Magnesium—Nickel

INCLUDES Clinical information not requested by the ordering physician
Mathematically calculated results
Quantitative analysis unless otherwise specified
Specimens from any source unless otherwise specified

EXCLUDES *Analytes from nonrequested laboratory analysis*
Calculated results representing a score or probability derived by algorithm
Organ or disease panels (80048-80076 [80081])
Therapeutic drug assays (80150-80299 [80164, 80165, 80171])

83735 Magnesium
0.00 0.00 FUD XXX
AMA: 2020,Dec,3

83775 Malate dehydrogenase
EXCLUDES *Maltose tolerance (82951, 82952)*
Mammotropin (84146)
0.00 0.00 FUD XXX
AMA: 2020,Dec,3

83785 Manganese
0.00 0.00 FUD XXX
AMA: 2020,Dec,3

83789 Mass spectrometry and tandem mass spectrometry (eg, MS, MS/MS, MALDI, MS-TOF, QTOF), non-drug analyte(s) not elsewhere specified, qualitative or quantitative, each specimen
EXCLUDES *Column chromatography/mass spectrometry drugs or substances ([80305], [80306], [80307], [80320, 80321, 80322, 80323, 80324, 80325, 80326, 80327, 80328, 80329, 80330, 80331, 80332, 80333, 80334, 80335, 80336, 80337, 80338, 80339, 80340, 80341, 80342, 80343, 80344, 80345, 80346, 80347, 80348, 80349, 80350, 80351, 80352, 80353, 80354, 80355, 80356, 80357, 80358, 80359, 80360, 80361, 80362, 80363, 80364, 80365, 80366, 80367, 80368, 80369, 80370, 80371, 80372, 80373, 80374, 80375, 80376, 80377, 83992])*
Procedure performed more than one time per specimen
Report specific analyte testing with code(s) from Chemistry section
0.00 0.00 FUD XXX
AMA: 2020,Dec,3

83825 Mercury, quantitative
EXCLUDES *Mercury screen (83015)*
0.00 0.00 FUD XXX
AMA: 2020,Dec,3

83835 Metanephrines
EXCLUDES *Catecholamines (82382-82384)*
Methamphetamine ([80324], [80325], [80326])
Methane breath test (91065)
0.00 0.00 FUD XXX
AMA: 2020,Dec,3

83857 Methemalbumin
EXCLUDES *Methemoglobin (83045, 83050)*
Methyl alcohol ([80320])
Microalbumin
Quantitative (82043)
Semiquantitative (82044)
0.00 0.00 FUD XXX
AMA: 2020,Dec,3

83861 Microfluidic analysis utilizing an integrated collection and analysis device, tear osmolarity
EXCLUDES *beta-2 Microglobulin (82232)*
Code also when performed on both eyes 83861 X 2
0.00 0.00 FUD XXX
AMA: 2020,Dec,3

83864 Mucopolysaccharides, acid, quantitative
0.00 0.00 FUD XXX
AMA: 2020,Dec,3

83872 Mucin, synovial fluid (Ropes test)
0.00 0.00 FUD XXX
AMA: 2020,Dec,3

83873 Myelin basic protein, cerebrospinal fluid
EXCLUDES *Oligoclonal bands (83916)*
0.00 0.00 FUD XXX
AMA: 2020,Dec,3

83874 Myoglobin
0.00 0.00 FUD XXX
AMA: 2020,Dec,3; 2018,Jan,8; 2017,Jan,8; 2016,Jan,13

83876 Myeloperoxidase (MPO)
0.00 0.00 FUD XXX
AMA: 2020,Dec,3

83880 Natriuretic peptide
0.00 0.00 FUD XXX
AMA: 2020,Dec,3; 2018,Jan,8; 2017,Jan,8; 2016,Jan,13

83883 Nephelometry, each analyte not elsewhere specified
0.00 0.00 FUD XXX
AMA: 2020,Dec,3

83885 Nickel
0.00 0.00 FUD XXX
AMA: 2020,Dec,3

83915-84066 [83992] Chemistry: Nucleotidase 5'-—Phosphatase (Acid)

INCLUDES Clinical information not requested by ordering physician
Mathematically calculated results
Quantitative analysis unless otherwise specified
Specimens from any source unless otherwise specified

EXCLUDES *Analytes from nonrequested laboratory analysis*
Calculated results representing score or probability derived by algorithm
Drug testing ([80305, 80306, 80307], [80324, 80325, 80326, 80327, 80328, 80329, 80330, 80331, 80332, 80333, 80334, 80335, 80336, 80337, 80338, 80339, 80340, 80341, 80342, 80343, 80344, 80345, 80346, 80347, 80348, 80349, 80350, 80351, 80352, 80353, 80354, 80355, 80356, 80357, 80358, 80359, 80360, 80361, 80362, 80363, 80364, 80365, 80366, 80367, 80368, 80369, 80370, 80371, 80372, 80373, 80374, 80375, 80376, 80377, 83992])
Organ or disease panels (80048-80076 [80081])
Therapeutic drug assays (80150-80299 [80164, 80165, 80171])

83915 **Nucleotidase 5'-**
0.00 0.00 FUD XXX
AMA: 2020,Dec,3

83916 **Oligoclonal immune (oligoclonal bands)**
0.00 0.00 FUD XXX
AMA: 2020,Dec,3

83918 **Organic acids; total, quantitative, each specimen**
0.00 0.00 FUD XXX
AMA: 2020,Dec,3; 2018,Jan,8; 2017,Jan,8; 2016,Jan,13

83919 **qualitative, each specimen**
0.00 0.00 FUD XXX
AMA: 2020,Dec,3

83921 **Organic acid, single, quantitative**
0.00 0.00 FUD XXX
AMA: 2020,Dec,3

83930 **Osmolality; blood**
EXCLUDES *Tear osmolarity (83861)*
0.00 0.00 FUD XXX
AMA: 2020,Dec,3

83935 **urine**
EXCLUDES *Tear osmolarity (83861)*
0.00 0.00 FUD XXX
AMA: 2020,Dec,3

83937 **Osteocalcin (bone g1a protein)**
0.00 0.00 FUD XXX
AMA: 2020,Dec,3; 2018,Jan,8; 2017,Jan,8; 2016,Jan,13

83945 **Oxalate**
0.00 0.00 FUD XXX
AMA: 2020,Dec,3

83950 **Oncoprotein; HER-2/neu**
EXCLUDES *Tissue (88342, 88365)*
0.00 0.00 FUD XXX
AMA: 2020,Dec,3

83951 **des-gamma-carboxy-prothrombin (DCP)**
0.00 0.00 FUD XXX
AMA: 2020,Dec,3

83970 **Parathormone (parathyroid hormone)**
EXCLUDES *Chlorinated hydrocarbon screen (82441)*
Quantitative pesticide report code for specific method
0.00 0.00 FUD XXX
AMA: 2020,Dec,3

83986 **pH; body fluid, not otherwise specified**
EXCLUDES *Blood pH (82800, 82803)*
0.00 0.00 FUD XXX
AMA: 2020,Dec,3; 2018,Jan,8; 2017,Jan,8; 2016,May,13; 2016,Jan,13

83987 **exhaled breath condensate**
EXCLUDES *Blood pH (82800, 82803)*
Phenobarbital ([80345])
0.00 0.00 FUD XXX
AMA: 2020,Dec,3

83992 **Resequenced code. See code following resequenced code 80365.**

83993 **Calprotectin, fecal**
0.00 0.00 FUD XXX
AMA: 2020,Dec,3; 2018,Jan,8; 2017,Jan,8; 2016,Jan,13

84030 **Phenylalanine (PKU), blood**
INCLUDES Guthrie test
EXCLUDES *Phenylalanine-tyrosine ratio (84030, 84510)*
0.00 0.00 FUD XXX
AMA: 2020,Dec,3

84035 **Phenylketones, qualitative**
0.00 0.00 FUD XXX
AMA: 2020,Dec,3

84060 **Phosphatase, acid; total**
0.00 0.00 FUD XXX
AMA: 2020,Dec,3

84066 **prostatic**
0.00 0.00 FUD XXX
AMA: 2020,Dec,3

84075-84080 Chemistry: Phosphatase (Alkaline)

CMS: 100-03,160.17 Payment for L-Dopa /Associated Inpatient Hospital Services

INCLUDES Clinical information not requested by ordering physician
Mathematically calculated results
Quantitative analysis unless otherwise specified
Specimens from any source unless otherwise specified

EXCLUDES *Analytes from nonrequested laboratory analysis*
Calculated results representing score or probability derived by algorithm
Organ or disease panels (80048-80076 [80081])

84075 **Phosphatase, alkaline;**
0.00 0.00 FUD XXX
AMA: 2020,Dec,3; 2018,Jan,8; 2017,Jan,8; 2016,Jan,13

84078 **heat stable (total not included)**
0.00 0.00 FUD XXX
AMA: 2020,Dec,3

84080 **isoenzymes**
0.00 0.00 FUD XXX
AMA: 2020,Dec,3

84081-84150 Chemistry: Phosphatidylglycerol—Prostaglandin

INCLUDES Clinical information not requested by ordering physician
Mathematically calculated results
Quantitative analysis unless otherwise specified
Specimens from any source unless otherwise specified

EXCLUDES *Analytes from nonrequested laboratory analysis*
Calculated results representing score or probability derived by algorithm
Organ or disease panels (80048-80076 [80081])
Therapeutic drug assays (80150-80299 [80164, 80165, 80171])

84081 **Phosphatidylglycerol**
EXCLUDES *Cholinesterase (82480, 82482)*
Inorganic phosphates (84100)
Organic phosphates, report code for specific method
0.00 0.00 FUD XXX
AMA: 2020,Dec,3

84085 **Phosphogluconate, 6-, dehydrogenase, RBC**
0.00 0.00 FUD XXX
AMA: 2020,Dec,3

84087 **Phosphohexose isomerase**
0.00 0.00 FUD XXX
AMA: 2020,Dec,3

84100 **Phosphorus inorganic (phosphate);**
0.00 0.00 FUD XXX
AMA: 2020,Dec,3; 2018,Jan,8; 2017,Jan,8; 2016,Jan,13

84105 **urine**
EXCLUDES *Pituitary gonadotropins (83001-83002)*
PKU (84030, 84035)
0.00 0.00 FUD XXX
AMA: 2020,Dec,3

84106 **Porphobilinogen, urine; qualitative**
0.00 0.00 FUD XXX
AMA: 2020,Dec,3

84110 **quantitative**
0.00 0.00 FUD XXX
AMA: 2020,Dec,3

84112 **Evaluation of cervicovaginal fluid for specific amniotic fluid protein(s) (eg, placental alpha microglobulin-1 [PAMG-1], placental protein 12 [PP12], alpha-fetoprotein), qualitative, each specimen** ♀
0.00 0.00 FUD XXX
AMA: 2020,Dec,3

84119 **Porphyrins, urine; qualitative**
0.00 0.00 FUD XXX
AMA: 2020,Dec,3

84120 **quantitation and fractionation**
0.00 0.00 FUD XXX
AMA: 2020,Dec,3

84126 **Porphyrins, feces, quantitative**
EXCLUDES *Porphyrin precursors (82135, 84106, 84110)*
Protoporphyrin, RBC (84202, 84203)
0.00 0.00 FUD XXX
AMA: 2020,Dec,3

84132 **Potassium; serum, plasma or whole blood**
0.00 0.00 FUD XXX
AMA: 2020,Dec,3; 2018,Jan,8; 2017,Jan,8; 2016,Jan,13

84133 **urine**
0.00 0.00 FUD XXX
AMA: 2020,Dec,3

84134 **Prealbumin**
EXCLUDES *Microalbumin (82043-82044)*
0.00 0.00 FUD XXX
AMA: 2020,Dec,3

84135 **Pregnanediol** ♀
0.00 0.00 FUD XXX
AMA: 2020,Dec,3

84138 **Pregnanetriol** ♀
0.00 0.00 FUD XXX
AMA: 2020,Dec,3

84140 **Pregnenolone**
0.00 0.00 FUD XXX
AMA: 2020,Dec,3; 2018,Jan,8; 2017,Jan,8;,2016,Jan,13

84143 **17-hydroxypregnenolone**
0.00 0.00 FUD XXX
AMA: 2020,Dec,3; 2018,Jan,8; 2017,Jan,8; 2016,Jan,13

84144 **Progesterone**
EXCLUDES *Progesterone receptor assay (84234)*
Proinsulin (84206)
0.00 0.00 FUD XXX
AMA: 2020,Dec,3

84145 **Procalcitonin (PCT)**
0.00 0.00 FUD XXX
AMA: 2020,Dec,3

84146 **Prolactin**
0.00 0.00 FUD XXX
AMA: 2020,Dec,3

84150 **Prostaglandin, each**
0.00 0.00 FUD XXX
AMA: 2020,Dec,3

84152-84154 Chemistry: Prostate Specific Antigen

CMS: 100-03,190.31 Prostate Specific Antigen (PSA); 100-03,210.1 Prostate Cancer Screening Tests

INCLUDES Clinical information not requested by ordering physician
Mathematically calculated results
Quantitative analysis unless otherwise specified

EXCLUDES *Analytes from nonrequested laboratory analysis*
Calculated results representing score or probability derived by algorithm

84152 **Prostate specific antigen (PSA); complexed (direct measurement)** ♂
0.00 0.00 FUD XXX
AMA: 2020,Dec,3

84153 **total** ♂
0.00 0.00 FUD XXX
AMA: 2020,Dec,3; 2018,Jan,8; 2017,Jan,8; 2016,Jan,13

84154 **free** ♂
0.00 0.00 FUD XXX
AMA: 2020,Dec,3; 2018,Jan,8; 2017,Jan,8; 2016,Jan,13

84155-84157 Chemistry: Protein, Total (Not by Refractometry)

INCLUDES Clinical information not requested by ordering physician
Mathematically calculated results

EXCLUDES *Analytes from nonrequested laboratory analysis*
Calculated results representing score or probability derived by algorithm
Organ or disease panels (80048-80076 [80081])

84155 **Protein, total, except by refractometry; serum, plasma or whole blood**
0.00 0.00 FUD XXX
AMA: 2020,Dec,3; 2018,Jan,8; 2017,Jan,8; 2016,Jan,13

84156 **urine**
0.00 0.00 FUD XXX
AMA: 2020,Dec,3

84157 **other source (eg, synovial fluid, cerebrospinal fluid)**
0.00 0.00 FUD XXX
AMA: 2020,Dec,3

84160-84432 Chemistry: Protein, Total (Refractometry)—Thyroglobulin

INCLUDES Clinical information not requested by ordering physician
Mathematically calculated results
Quantitative analysis unless otherwise specified
Specimens from any source unless otherwise specified

EXCLUDES *Analytes from nonrequested laboratory analysis*
Calculated results representing score or probability derived by algorithm
Drug testing ([80305, 80306, 80307], [80324, 80325, 80326, 80327, 80328, 80329, 80330, 80331, 80332, 80333, 80334, 80335, 80336, 80337, 80338, 80339, 80340, 80341, 80342, 80343, 80344, 80345, 80346, 80347, 80348, 80349, 80350, 80351, 80352, 80353, 80354, 80355, 80356, 80357, 80358, 80359, 80360, 80361, 80362, 80363, 80364, 80365, 80366, 80367, 80368, 80369, 80370, 80371, 80372, 80373, 80374, 80375, 80376, 80377, 83992])
Organ or disease panels (80048-80076 [80081])
Therapeutic drug assays (80150-80299 [80164, 80165, 80171])

84160 **Protein, total, by refractometry, any source**
EXCLUDES *Urine total protein, dipstick method (81000-81003)*
0.00 0.00 FUD XXX
AMA: 2020,Dec,3

84163 **Pregnancy-associated plasma protein-A (PAPP-A)** ♀
0.00 0.00 FUD XXX
AMA: 2020,Dec,3

84165 **Protein; electrophoretic fractionation and quantitation, serum**
0.00 0.00 FUD XXX
AMA: 2020,Dec,3

84166 **electrophoretic fractionation and quantitation, other fluids with concentration (eg, urine, CSF)**
0.00 0.00 FUD XXX
AMA: 2020,Dec,3

84181 **Western Blot, with interpretation and report, blood or other body fluid**
0.00 0.00 FUD XXX
AMA: 2020,Dec,3

84182 **Western Blot, with interpretation and report, blood or other body fluid, immunological probe for band identification, each**
EXCLUDES *Western Blot tissue analysis (88371)*
0.00 0.00 FUD XXX
AMA: 2020,Dec,3

84202 **Protoporphyrin, RBC; quantitative**
0.00 0.00 FUD XXX
AMA: 2020,Dec,3

84203 **screen**
0.00 0.00 FUD XXX
AMA: 2020,Dec,3

84206 **Proinsulin**
EXCLUDES *Pseudocholinesterase (82480)*
0.00 0.00 FUD XXX
AMA: 2020,Dec,3

84207 **Pyridoxal phosphate (Vitamin B-6)**
0.00 0.00 FUD XXX
AMA: 2020,Dec,3

84210 **Pyruvate**
0.00 0.00 FUD XXX
AMA: 2020,Dec,3

84220 **Pyruvate kinase**
0.00 0.00 FUD XXX
AMA: 2020,Dec,3

84228 **Quinine**
0.00 0.00 FUD XXX
AMA: 2020,Dec,3; 2018,Jan,8; 2017,Jan,8; 2016,Jan,13

84233 **Receptor assay; estrogen**
0.00 0.00 FUD XXX
AMA: 2020,Dec,3

84234 **progesterone**
0.00 0.00 FUD XXX
AMA: 2020,Dec,3

84235 **endocrine, other than estrogen or progesterone (specify hormone)**
0.00 0.00 FUD XXX
AMA: 2020,Dec,3

84238 **non-endocrine (specify receptor)**
0.00 0.00 FUD XXX
AMA: 2020,Dec,3; 2018,Jan,8; 2017,Jan,8; 2016,Jan,13

84244 **Renin**
0.00 0.00 FUD XXX
AMA: 2020,Dec,3

84252 **Riboflavin (Vitamin B-2)**
EXCLUDES *Salicylates ([80329], [80330], [80331])*
Salicylate therapeutic drug assay ([80179])
Secretin test reported with appropriate analyses (43756, 43757, 99070)
0.00 0.00 FUD XXX
AMA: 2020,Dec,3

84255 **Selenium**
0.00 0.00 FUD XXX
AMA: 2020,Dec,3

84260 **Serotonin**
EXCLUDES *Urine metabolites (HIAA) (83497)*
0.00 0.00 FUD XXX
AMA: 2020,Dec,3

84270 **Sex hormone binding globulin (SHBG)**
0.00 0.00 FUD XXX
AMA: 2020,Dec,3; 2018,Jan,8; 2017,Jan,8; 2016,Jan,13

84275 **Sialic acid**
EXCLUDES *Sickle hemoglobin (85660)*
0.00 0.00 FUD XXX
AMA: 2020,Dec,3

84285 **Silica**
0.00 0.00 FUD XXX
AMA: 2020,Dec,3

84295 **Sodium; serum, plasma or whole blood**
0.00 0.00 FUD XXX
AMA: 2020,Dec,3; 2018,Jan,8; 2017,Jan,8; 2016,Jan,13

84300 **urine**
0.00 0.00 FUD XXX
AMA: 2020,Dec,3

84302 **other source**
EXCLUDES *Somatomammotropin (83632)*
Somatotropin (83003)
0.00 0.00 FUD XXX
AMA: 2020,Dec,3; 2018,Jan,8; 2017,Jan,8; 2016,Jan,13

84305 **Somatomedin**
0.00 0.00 FUD XXX
AMA: 2020,Dec,3; 2018,Jan,8; 2017,Jan,8; 2016,Jan,13

84307 **Somatostatin**
0.00 0.00 FUD XXX
AMA: 2020,Dec,3; 2018,Jan,8; 2017,Jan,8; 2016,Jan,13

84311 **Spectrophotometry, analyte not elsewhere specified**
0.00 0.00 FUD XXX
AMA: 2020,Dec,3

84315 **Specific gravity (except urine)**
EXCLUDES *Stone analysis (82355-82370)*
Suppression of growth stimulation expressed gene 2 [ST2] testing (83006)
Urine specific gravity (81000-81003)
0.00 0.00 FUD XXX
AMA: 2020,Dec,3

84375 **Sugars, chromatographic, TLC or paper chromatography**
0.00 0.00 FUD XXX
AMA: 2020,Dec,3

84376 **Sugars (mono-, di-, and oligosaccharides); single qualitative, each specimen**
0.00 0.00 FUD XXX
AMA: 2020,Dec,3; 2018,Jan,8; 2017,Jan,8; 2016,Jan,13

84377 **multiple qualitative, each specimen**
0.00 0.00 FUD XXX
AMA: 2020,Dec,3; 2018,Jan,8; 2017,Jan,8; 2016,Jan,13

84378 **single quantitative, each specimen**
0.00 0.00 FUD XXX
AMA: 2020,Dec,3

84379 **multiple quantitative, each specimen**
0.00 0.00 FUD XXX
AMA: 2020,Dec,3; 2018,Jan,8; 2017,Jan,8; 2016,Jan,13

84392 **Sulfate, urine**
EXCLUDES *Sulfhemoglobin (83060)*
T-3 (84479-84481)
T-4 (84436-84439)
0.00 0.00 FUD XXX
AMA: 2020,Dec,3

84402 **Testosterone; free**
EXCLUDES *Anabolic steroids ([80327, 80328])*
0.00 0.00 FUD XXX
AMA: 2020,Dec,3

84403 **total**
EXCLUDES *Anabolic steroids ([80327, 80328])*
0.00 0.00 FUD XXX
AMA: 2020,Dec,3

84410 **bioavailable, direct measurement (eg, differential precipitation)**
0.00 0.00 FUD XXX
AMA: 2020,Dec,3

84425 **Thiamine (Vitamin B-1)**
0.00 0.00 FUD XXX
AMA: 2020,Dec,3

84430 **Thiocyanate**
0.00 0.00 FUD XXX
AMA: 2020,Dec,3

84431 **Thromboxane metabolite(s), including thromboxane if performed, urine**
Code also determination concurrent urine creatinine (82570)
0.00 0.00 FUD XXX
AMA: 2020,Dec,3

84432 **Thyroglobulin**
EXCLUDES *Thyroglobulin antibody (86800)*
Thyrotropin releasing hormone (TRH) (80438, 80439)
0.00 0.00 FUD XXX
AMA: 2020,Dec,3; 2018,Jan,8; 2017,Jan,8; 2016,Jan,13

84436-84445 Chemistry: Thyroid Tests

CMS: 100-03,190.22 Thyroid Testing

INCLUDES Clinical information not requested by the ordering physician
Mathematically calculated results
Quantitative analysis unless otherwise specified
Specimens from any source unless otherwise specified

EXCLUDES *Analytes from nonrequested laboratory analysis*
Calculated results representing a score or probability derived by algorithm
Organ or disease panels (80048-80076 [80081])
Therapeutic drug assays (80150-80299 [80164, 80165, 80171])

84436 **Thyroxine; total**
0.00 0.00 FUD XXX
AMA: 2020,Dec,3; 2018,Jan,8; 2017,Jan,8; 2016,Jan,13

84437 **requiring elution (eg, neonatal)**
0.00 0.00 FUD XXX
AMA: 2020,Dec,3

84439 **free**
0.00 0.00 FUD XXX
AMA: 2020,Dec,3

84442 **Thyroxine binding globulin (TBG)**
0.00 0.00 FUD XXX
AMA: 2020,Dec,3

84443 **Thyroid stimulating hormone (TSH)**
0.00 0.00 FUD XXX
AMA: 2020,Dec,3

84445 **Thyroid stimulating immune globulins (TSI)**
EXCLUDES *Tobramycin (80200)*
0.00 0.00 FUD XXX
AMA: 2020,Dec,3; 2018,Jan,8; 2017,Jan,8; 2016,Jan,13

84446-84449 Chemistry: Tocopherol Alpha—Transcortin

INCLUDES Clinical information not requested by ordering physician
Mathematically calculated results
Quantitative analysis unless otherwise specified
Specimens from any source unless otherwise specified

EXCLUDES *Analytes from nonrequested laboratory analysis*
Calculated results representing score or probability derived by algorithm
Organ or disease panels (80048-80076 [80081])
Therapeutic drug assays (80150-80299 [80164, 80165, 80171])

84446 **Tocopherol alpha (Vitamin E)**
0.00 0.00 FUD XXX
AMA: 2020,Dec,3

84449 **Transcortin (cortisol binding globulin)**
0.00 0.00 FUD XXX
AMA: 2020,Dec,3; 2018,Jan,8; 2017,Jan,8; 2016,Jan,13

84450-84460 Chemistry: Transferase

CMS: 100-02,11,30.2.2 Automated Multi-Channel Chemistry (AMCC) Tests; 100-03,160.17 Payment for L-Dopa /Associated Inpatient Hospital Services; 100-04,16,40.6.1 Automated Multi-Channel Chemistry (AMCC) Tests for ESRD Beneficiaries; 100-04,16,70.8 CLIA Waived Tests

INCLUDES Clinical information not requested by ordering physician
Mathematically calculated results
Quantitative analysis unless otherwise specified

EXCLUDES *Analytes from nonrequested laboratory analysis*
Calculated results representing score or probability derived by algorithm

84450 **Transferase; aspartate amino (AST) (SGOT)**
0.00 0.00 FUD XXX
AMA: 2020,Dec,3; 2018,Jan,8; 2017,Jan,8; 2016,Jan,13

84460 **alanine amino (ALT) (SGPT)**
0.00 0.00 FUD XXX
AMA: 2020,Dec,3; 2018,Jan,8; 2017,Jan,8; 2016,Jan,13

84466 Chemistry: Transferrin

CMS: 100-02,11,20.2 ESRD Laboratory Services; 100-03,190.18 Serum Iron Studies

INCLUDES Clinical information not requested by ordering physician
Mathematically calculated results
Quantitative analysis unless otherwise specified

EXCLUDES *Analytes from nonrequested laboratory analysis*
Calculated results representing score or probability derived by algorithm

84466 **Transferrin**
EXCLUDES *Iron binding capacity (83550)*
0.00 0.00 FUD XXX
AMA: 2020,Dec,3; 2018,Jan,8; 2017,Jan,8; 2016,Jan,13

84478 Chemistry: Triglycerides

CMS: 100-02,11,30.2.2 Automated Multi-Channel Chemistry (AMCC) Tests; 100-03,190.23 Lipid Testing; 100-04,16,70.8 CLIA Waived Tests; 100-04,16,90.2 Organ or Disease Oriented Panels

INCLUDES Clinical information not requested by ordering physician
Mathematically calculated results

EXCLUDES *Analytes from nonrequested laboratory analysis*
Calculated results representing score or probability derived by algorithm
Organ or disease panels (80048-80076 [80081])

84478 **Triglycerides**
0.00 0.00 FUD XXX
AMA: 2020,Dec,3; 2018,Jan,8; 2017,Jan,8; 2016,Jan,13

84479-84482 Chemistry: Thyroid Hormone—Triiodothyronine

CMS: 100-03,190.22 Thyroid Testing

INCLUDES Clinical information not requested by ordering physician
Mathematically calculated results
Quantitative analysis unless otherwise specified
Specimens from any source unless otherwise specified

EXCLUDES *Analytes from nonrequested laboratory analysis*
Calculated results representing score or probability derived by algorithm
Organ or disease panels (80048-80076 [80081])

84479 **Thyroid hormone (T3 or T4) uptake or thyroid hormone binding ratio (THBR)**
0.00 0.00 FUD XXX
AMA: 2020,Dec,3; 2018,Jan,8; 2017,Jan,8; 2016,Jan,13

84480 **Triiodothyronine T3; total (TT-3)**
0.00 0.00 FUD XXX
AMA: 2020,Dec,3

84481 **free**
0.00 0.00 FUD XXX
AMA: 2020,Dec,3

84482 **reverse**
0.00 0.00 FUD XXX
AMA: 2020,Dec,3; 2018,Jan,8; 2017,Jan,8; 2016,Jan,13

Pathology and Laboratory
84410 — 84482

84484-84512 Chemistry: Troponin (Quantitative)—Troponin (Qualitative)

INCLUDES Clinical information not requested by ordering physician
Mathematically calculated results
Specimens from any source unless otherwise specified

EXCLUDES *Analytes from nonrequested laboratory analysis*
Calculated results representing score or probability derived by algorithm
Organ or disease panels

84484 Troponin, quantitative
EXCLUDES *Qualitative troponin assay (84512)*
0.00 0.00 FUD XXX
AMA: 2020,Dec,3; 2018,Jan,8; 2017,Jan,8; 2016,Jan,13

84485 Trypsin; duodenal fluid
0.00 0.00 FUD XXX
AMA: 2020,Dec,3

84488 feces, qualitative
0.00 0.00 FUD XXX
AMA: 2020,Dec,3

84490 feces, quantitative, 24-hour collection
0.00 0.00 FUD XXX
AMA: 2020,Dec,3

84510 Tyrosine
EXCLUDES *Urate crystal identification (89060)*
0.00 0.00 FUD XXX
AMA: 2020,Dec,3

84512 Troponin, qualitative
EXCLUDES *Quantitative troponin assay (84484)*
0.00 0.00 FUD XXX
AMA: 2020,Dec,3; 2018,Jan,8; 2017,Jan,8; 2016,Jan,13

84520-84525 Chemistry: Urea Nitrogen (Blood)

CMS: 100-03,160.17 Payment for L-Dopa /Associated Inpatient Hospital Services

INCLUDES Clinical information not requested by ordering physician
Mathematically calculated results

EXCLUDES *Analytes from nonrequested laboratory analysis*
Calculated results representing score or probability derived by algorithm
Organ or disease panels (80048-80076 [80081])

84520 Urea nitrogen; quantitative
0.00 0.00 FUD XXX
AMA: 2020,Dec,3; 2018,Jan,8; 2017,Jan,8; 2016,Jan,13

84525 semiquantitative (eg, reagent strip test)
INCLUDES Patterson's test
0.00 0.00 FUD XXX
AMA: 2020,Dec,3; 2018,Jan,8; 2017,Jan,8; 2016,Jan,13

84540-84630 Chemistry: Urea Nitrogen (Urine)—Zinc

INCLUDES Clinical information not requested by ordering physician
Mathematically calculated results
Quantitative analysis unless otherwise specified
Specimens from any source unless otherwise specified

EXCLUDES *Analytes from nonrequested laboratory analysis*
Calculated results representing score or probability derived by algorithm
Organ or disease panels (80048-80076 [80081])
Therapeutic drug assays (80150-80299 [80164, 80165, 80171])

84540 Urea nitrogen, urine
0.00 0.00 FUD XXX
AMA: 2020,Dec,3

84545 Urea nitrogen, clearance
0.00 0.00 FUD XXX
AMA: 2020,Dec,3

84550 Uric acid; blood
0.00 0.00 FUD XXX
AMA: 2020,Dec,3; 2018,Jan,8; 2017,Jan,8; 2016,Jan,13

84560 other source
0.00 0.00 FUD XXX
AMA: 2020,Dec,3

84577 Urobilinogen, feces, quantitative
0.00 0.00 FUD XXX
AMA: 2020,Dec,3

84578 Urobilinogen, urine; qualitative
0.00 0.00 FUD XXX
AMA: 2020,Dec,3

84580 quantitative, timed specimen
0.00 0.00 FUD XXX
AMA: 2020,Dec,3

84583 semiquantitative
EXCLUDES *Uroporphyrins (84120)*
Valproic acid (dipropylacetic acid) ([80164])
0.00 0.00 FUD XXX
AMA: 2020,Dec,3

84585 Vanillylmandelic acid (VMA), urine
0.00 0.00 FUD XXX
AMA: 2020,Dec,3

84586 Vasoactive intestinal peptide (VIP)
0.00 0.00 FUD XXX
AMA: 2020,Dec,3; 2018,Jan,8; 2017,Jan,8; 2016,Jan,13

84588 Vasopressin (antidiuretic hormone, ADH)
0.00 0.00 FUD XXX
AMA: 2020,Dec,3; 2018,Jan,7

84590 Vitamin A
EXCLUDES *Vitamin B-1 (84425)*
Vitamin B-2 (84252)
Vitamin B-6 (84207)
Vitamin B-12 (82607)
Vitamin C (82180)
Vitamin D (82306, [82652])
Vitamin E (84446)
0.00 0.00 FUD XXX
AMA: 2020,Dec,3

84591 Vitamin, not otherwise specified
0.00 0.00 FUD XXX
AMA: 2020,Dec,3

84597 Vitamin K
EXCLUDES *Vanillylmandelic acid (VMA) (84585)*
0.00 0.00 FUD XXX
AMA: 2020,Dec,3

84600 Volatiles (eg, acetic anhydride, diethylether)
EXCLUDES *Carbon tetrachloride, dichloroethane, dichloromethane (82441)*
Isopropyl alcohol and methanol ([80320])
Volume, blood, RISA, or Cr-51 (78110, 78111)
0.00 0.00 FUD XXX
AMA: 2020,Dec,3

84620 Xylose absorption test, blood and/or urine
EXCLUDES *Administration (99070)*
0.00 0.00 FUD XXX
AMA: 2020,Dec,3

84630 Zinc
0.00 0.00 FUD XXX
AMA: 2020,Dec,3

84681-84999 Other and Unlisted Chemistry Tests

INCLUDES Clinical information not requested by ordering physician
Mathematically calculated results
Quantitative analysis unless otherwise specified
Specimens from any source unless otherwise specified

EXCLUDES *Analytes from nonrequested laboratory analysis*
Calculated results representing score or probability derived by algorithm
Confirmational testing, not otherwise specified drug ([80375, 80376, 80377], 80299)
Organ or disease panels (80048-80076 [80081])

84681 C-peptide
0.00 0.00 FUD XXX
AMA: 2020,Dec,3

84702 Gonadotropin, chorionic (hCG); quantitative
0.00 0.00 FUD XXX
AMA: 2020,Dec,3

84703 **qualitative**
EXCLUDES *Urine pregnancy test by visual color comparison (81025)*
0.00 0.00 FUD XXX
AMA: 2020,Dec,3

84704 **free beta chain**
0.00 0.00 FUD XXX
AMA: 2020,Dec,3; 2018,Jan,8; 2017,Jan,8; 2016,Jan,13

84830 **Ovulation tests, by visual color comparison methods for human luteinizing hormone** ♀
0.00 0.00 FUD XXX
AMA: 2020,Dec,3; 2018,Jan,8; 2017,Jan,8; 2016,Jan,13

84999 **Unlisted chemistry procedure**
EXCLUDES *Definitive drug testing, not otherwise specified ([80375], [80376], [80377], 80299)*
0.00 0.00 FUD XXX
AMA: 2020,Dec,3; 2018,Jan,8; 2017,Jan,8; 2016,Jan,13

85002 Bleeding Time Test

EXCLUDES *Agglutinins (86000, 86156, 86157)*
Antiplasmin (85410)
Antithrombin III (85300, 85301)
Blood banking procedures (86077-86079)

85002 **Bleeding time**
0.00 0.00 FUD XXX
AMA: 2020,Dec,3; 2018,Jan,8; 2017,Jan,8; 2016,Jan,13

85004-85049 Blood Counts

CMS: 100-03,190.15 Blood Counts
EXCLUDES *Agglutinins (86000, 86156-86157)*
Antiplasmin (85410)
Antithrombin III (85300-85301)
Blood banking procedures (86850-86999)

85004 **Blood count; automated differential WBC count**
0.00 0.00 FUD XXX
AMA: 2020,Dec,3; 2018,Jan,8; 2017,Jan,8; 2016,Jan,13

85007 **blood smear, microscopic examination with manual differential WBC count**
0.00 0.00 FUD XXX
AMA: 2020,Dec,3; 2018,Jan,8; 2017,Jan,8; 2016,Jan,13

85008 **blood smear, microscopic examination without manual differential WBC count**
EXCLUDES *Cell count other fluids (eg, CSF) (89050-89051)*
0.00 0.00 FUD XXX
AMA: 2020,Dec,3; 2018,Jan,8; 2017,Jan,8; 2016,Jan,13

85009 **manual differential WBC count, buffy coat**
EXCLUDES *Eosinophils, nasal smear (89190)*
0.00 0.00 FUD XXX
AMA: 2020,Dec,3; 2018,Jan,8; 2017,Jan,8; 2016,Jan,13

85013 **spun microhematocrit**
0.00 0.00 FUD XXX
AMA: 2020,Dec,3

85014 **hematocrit (Hct)**
0.00 0.00 FUD XXX
AMA: 2020,Dec,3; 2018,Jan,8; 2017,Jan,8; 2016,Jan,13

85018 **hemoglobin (Hgb)**
EXCLUDES *Immunoassay, hemoglobin, fecal (82274)*
Other hemoglobin determination (83020-83069)
Transcutaneous hemoglobin measurement (88738)
0.00 0.00 FUD XXX
AMA: 2020,Dec,3; 2018,Jan,8; 2017,Jan,8; 2016,Jan,13

85025 **complete (CBC), automated (Hgb, Hct, RBC, WBC and platelet count) and automated differential WBC count**
0.00 0.00 FUD XXX
AMA: 2020,Dec,3; 2018,Jan,8; 2017,Jan,8; 2016,Jan,13

85027 **complete (CBC), automated (Hgb, Hct, RBC, WBC and platelet count)**
0.00 0.00 FUD XXX
AMA: 2020,Dec,3; 2018,Jan,8; 2017,Jan,8; 2016,Jan,13

85032 **manual cell count (erythrocyte, leukocyte, or platelet) each**
0.00 0.00 FUD XXX
AMA: 2020,Dec,3; 2018,Jan,8; 2017,Jan,8; 2016,Jan,13

85041 **red blood cell (RBC), automated**
EXCLUDES *Complete blood count (85025, 85027)*
0.00 0.00 FUD XXX
AMA: 2020,Dec,3; 2018,Jan,8; 2017,Jan,8; 2016,Jan,13

85044 **reticulocyte, manual**
0.00 0.00 FUD XXX
AMA: 2020,Dec,3; 2018,Jan,8; 2017,Jan,8; 2016,Jan,13

85045 **reticulocyte, automated**
0.00 0.00 FUD XXX
AMA: 2020,Dec,3; 2018,Jan,8; 2017,Jan,8; 2016,Jan,13

85046 **reticulocytes, automated, including 1 or more cellular parameters (eg, reticulocyte hemoglobin content [CHr], immature reticulocyte fraction [IRF], reticulocyte volume [MRV], RNA content), direct measurement**
0.00 0.00 FUD XXX
AMA: 2020,Dec,3

85048 **leukocyte (WBC), automated**
0.00 0.00 FUD XXX
AMA: 2020,Dec,3; 2018,Jan,8; 2017,Jan,8; 2016,Jan,13

85049 **platelet, automated**
0.00 0.00 FUD XXX
AMA: 2020,Dec,3

85055-85705 Coagulopathy Testing

EXCLUDES *Agglutinins (86000, 86156-86157)*
Antiplasmin (85410)
Antithrombin III (85300-85301)
Blood banking procedures (86850-86999)

85055 **Reticulated platelet assay**
0.00 0.00 FUD XXX
AMA: 2020,Dec,3

85060 **Blood smear, peripheral, interpretation by physician with written report**
0.70 0.70 FUD XXX
AMA: 2020,Dec,3

85097 **Bone marrow, smear interpretation**
EXCLUDES *Bone biopsy (20220, 20225, 20240, 20245, 20250-20251)*
Special stains (88312-88313)
1.42 2.11 FUD XXX
AMA: 2020,Dec,3; 2018,Jan,8; 2017,Jan,8; 2016,Jan,13

85130 **Chromogenic substrate assay**
EXCLUDES *Circulating anticoagulant screen (mixing studies) (85611, 85732)*
0.00 0.00 FUD XXX
AMA: 2020,Dec,3

85170 **Clot retraction**
0.00 0.00 FUD XXX
AMA: 2020,Dec,3

85175 **Clot lysis time, whole blood dilution**
EXCLUDES *Clotting factor I (fibrinogen) (85384, 85385)*
0.00 0.00 FUD XXX
AMA: 2020,Dec,3

85210 **Clotting; factor II, prothrombin, specific**
EXCLUDES *Prothrombin time (85610-85611)*
Russell viper venom time (85612-85613)
0.00 0.00 FUD XXX
AMA: 2020,Dec,3

85220 **factor V (AcG or proaccelerin), labile factor**
0.00 0.00 FUD XXX
AMA: 2020,Dec,3

85230 **factor VII (proconvertin, stable factor)**
0.00 0.00 FUD XXX
AMA: 2020,Dec,3

85240 **factor VIII (AHG), 1-stage**
0.00 0.00 FUD XXX
AMA: 2020,Dec,3

85244 **factor VIII related antigen**
0.00 0.00 FUD XXX
AMA: 2020,Dec,3

85245 **factor VIII, VW factor, ristocetin cofactor**
0.00 0.00 FUD XXX
AMA: 2020,Dec,3

85246 **factor VIII, VW factor antigen**
0.00 0.00 FUD XXX
AMA: 2020,Dec,3

85247 **factor VIII, von Willebrand factor, multimetric analysis**
0.00 0.00 FUD XXX
AMA: 2020,Dec,3

85250 **factor IX (PTC or Christmas)**
0.00 0.00 FUD XXX
AMA: 2020,Dec,3

85260 **factor X (Stuart-Prower)**
0.00 0.00 FUD XXX
AMA: 2020,Dec,3

85270 **factor XI (PTA)**
0.00 0.00 FUD XXX
AMA: 2020,Dec,3

85280 **factor XII (Hageman)**
0.00 0.00 FUD XXX
AMA: 2020,Dec,3

85290 **factor XIII (fibrin stabilizing)**
0.00 0.00 FUD XXX
AMA: 2020,Dec,3

85291 **factor XIII (fibrin stabilizing), screen solubility**
0.00 0.00 FUD XXX
AMA: 2020,Dec,3

85292 **prekallikrein assay (Fletcher factor assay)**
0.00 0.00 FUD XXX
AMA: 2020,Dec,3

85293 **high molecular weight kininogen assay (Fitzgerald factor assay)**
0.00 0.00 FUD XXX
AMA: 2020,Dec,3

85300 **Clotting inhibitors or anticoagulants; antithrombin III, activity**
0.00 0.00 FUD XXX
AMA: 2020,Dec,3

85301 **antithrombin III, antigen assay**
0.00 0.00 FUD XXX
AMA: 2020,Dec,3

85302 **protein C, antigen**
0.00 0.00 FUD XXX
AMA: 2020,Dec,3

85303 **protein C, activity**
0.00 0.00 FUD XXX
AMA: 2020,Dec,3

85305 **protein S, total**
0.00 0.00 FUD XXX
AMA: 2020,Dec,3

85306 **protein S, free**
0.00 0.00 FUD XXX
AMA: 2020,Dec,3

85307 **Activated Protein C (APC) resistance assay**
0.00 0.00 FUD XXX
AMA: 2020,Dec,3

85335 **Factor inhibitor test**
0.00 0.00 FUD XXX
AMA: 2020,Dec,3

85337 **Thrombomodulin**
EXCLUDES *Mixing studies for inhibitors (85732)*
0.00 0.00 FUD XXX
AMA: 2020,Dec,3

85345 **Coagulation time; Lee and White**
0.00 0.00 FUD XXX
AMA: 2020,Dec,3

85347 **activated**
0.00 0.00 FUD XXX
AMA: 2020,Dec,3; 2019,Apr,10

85348 **other methods**
EXCLUDES *Differential count (85007-85009, 85025)*
Duke bleeding time (85002)
Eosinophils, nasal smear (89190)
0.00 0.00 FUD XXX
AMA: 2020,Dec,3

85360 **Euglobulin lysis**
EXCLUDES *Fetal hemoglobin (83030, 83033, 85460)*
0.00 0.00 FUD XXX
AMA: 2020,Dec,3

85362 **Fibrin(ogen) degradation (split) products (FDP) (FSP); agglutination slide, semiquantitative**
EXCLUDES *Immunoelectrophoresis (86320)*
0.00 0.00 FUD XXX
AMA: 2020,Dec,3

85366 **paracoagulation**
0.00 0.00 FUD XXX
AMA: 2020,Dec,3

85370 **quantitative**
0.00 0.00 FUD XXX
AMA: 2020,Dec,3

85378 **Fibrin degradation products, D-dimer; qualitative or semiquantitative**
0.00 0.00 FUD XXX
AMA: 2020,Dec,3; 2018,Jan,8; 2017,Jan,8; 2016,Jan,13

85379 **quantitative**
INCLUDES Ultrasensitive and standard sensitivity quantitative D-dimer (85379)
0.00 0.00 FUD XXX
AMA: 2020,Dec,3

85380 **ultrasensitive (eg, for evaluation for venous thromboembolism), qualitative or semiquantitative**
0.00 0.00 FUD XXX
AMA: 2020,Dec,3; 2018,Jan,8; 2017,Jan,8; 2016,Jan,13

85384 **Fibrinogen; activity**
0.00 0.00 FUD XXX
AMA: 2020,Dec,3; 2019,Apr,10

85385 **antigen**
0.00 0.00 FUD XXX
AMA: 2020,Dec,3

85390 **Fibrinolysins or coagulopathy screen, interpretation and report**
0.00 0.00 FUD XXX
AMA: 2020,Dec,3; 2019,Apr,10

85396 **Coagulation/fibrinolysis assay, whole blood (eg, viscoelastic clot assessment), including use of any pharmacologic additive(s), as indicated, including interpretation and written report, per day**
0.58 0.58 FUD XXX
AMA: 2020,Dec,3; 2019,Apr,10

85397 **Coagulation and fibrinolysis, functional activity, not otherwise specified (eg, ADAMTS-13), each analyte**
0.00 0.00 FUD XXX
AMA: 2020,Dec,3

Pathology and Laboratory

85400 — 85705

85400 Fibrinolytic factors and inhibitors; plasmin
0.00 0.00 FUD XXX
AMA: 2020,Dec,3

85410 alpha-2 antiplasmin
0.00 0.00 FUD XXX
AMA: 2020,Dec,3

85415 plasminogen activator
0.00 0.00 FUD XXX
AMA: 2020,Dec,3

85420 plasminogen, except antigenic assay
0.00 0.00 FUD XXX
AMA: 2020,Dec,3

85421 plasminogen, antigenic assay
EXCLUDES *Fragility, red blood cell (85547, 85555-85557)*
0.00 0.00 FUD XXX
AMA: 2020,Dec,3

85441 Heinz bodies; direct
0.00 0.00 FUD XXX
AMA: 2020,Dec,3

85445 induced, acetyl phenylhydrazine
EXCLUDES *Hematocrit (PCV) (85014, 85025, 85027)*
Hemoglobin (83020-83068, 85018, 85025, 85027)
0.00 0.00 FUD XXX
AMA: 2020,Dec,3

85460 Hemoglobin or RBCs, fetal, for fetomaternal hemorrhage; differential lysis (Kleihauer-Betke) M ♀
EXCLUDES *Hemoglobin F (83030, 83033)*
Hemolysins (86940-86941)
0.00 0.00 FUD XXX
AMA: 2020,Dec,3; 2018,Jan,8; 2017,Jan,8; 2016,Jan,13

85461 rosette M ♀
0.00 0.00 FUD XXX
AMA: 2020,Dec,3

85475 Hemolysin, acid
INCLUDES Ham test
EXCLUDES *Hemolysins and agglutinins (86940-86941)*
0.00 0.00 FUD XXX
AMA: 2020,Dec,3

85520 Heparin assay
0.00 0.00 FUD XXX
AMA: 2020,Dec,3

85525 Heparin neutralization
0.00 0.00 FUD XXX
AMA: 2020,Dec,3; 2018,Jan,8; 2017,Aug,9

85530 Heparin-protamine tolerance test
0.00 0.00 FUD XXX
AMA: 2020,Dec,3

85536 Iron stain, peripheral blood
EXCLUDES *Iron stains on bone marrow or other tissues with physician evaluation (88313)*
0.00 0.00 FUD XXX
AMA: 2020,Dec,3

85540 Leukocyte alkaline phosphatase with count
0.00 0.00 FUD XXX
AMA: 2020,Dec,3

85547 Mechanical fragility, RBC
0.00 0.00 FUD XXX
AMA: 2020,Dec,3

85549 Muramidase
EXCLUDES *Nitroblue tetrazolium dye test (86384)*
0.00 0.00 FUD XXX
AMA: 2020,Dec,3

85555 Osmotic fragility, RBC; unincubated
0.00 0.00 FUD XXX
AMA: 2020,Dec,3

85557 incubated
EXCLUDES *Packed cell volume (85013)*
Parasites, blood (eg, malaria smears) (87207)
Partial thromboplastin time (85730, 85732)
Plasmin (85400)
Plasminogen (85420)
Plasminogen activator (85415)
0.00 0.00 FUD XXX
AMA: 2020,Dec,3

85576 Platelet, aggregation (in vitro), each agent
EXCLUDES *Thromboxane metabolite(s), including thromboxane, when performed, in urine (84431)*
0.00 0.00 FUD XXX
AMA: 2020,Dec,3; 2019,Apr,10; 2018,Jan,8; 2017,Jan,8; 2016,Jan,13

85597 Phospholipid neutralization; platelet
0.00 0.00 FUD XXX
AMA: 2020,Dec,3; 2018,Jan,8; 2017,Jan,8; 2016,Jan,13

85598 hexagonal phospholipid
0.00 0.00 FUD XXX
AMA: 2020,Dec,3; 2018,Jan,8; 2017,Jan,8; 2016,Jan,13

85610 Prothrombin time;
0.00 0.00 FUD XXX
AMA: 2020,Dec,3

85611 substitution, plasma fractions, each
0.00 0.00 FUD XXX
AMA: 2020,Dec,3

85612 Russell viper venom time (includes venom); undiluted
0.00 0.00 FUD XXX
AMA: 2020,Dec,3

85613 diluted
EXCLUDES *Red blood cell count (85025, 85027, 85041)*
0.00 0.00 FUD XXX
AMA: 2020,Dec,3

85635 Reptilase test
EXCLUDES *Reticulocyte count (85044-85045)*
0.00 0.00 FUD XXX
AMA: 2020,Dec,3

85651 Sedimentation rate, erythrocyte; non-automated
0.00 0.00 FUD XXX
AMA: 2020,Dec,3

85652 automated
INCLUDES Westergren test
0.00 0.00 FUD XXX
AMA: 2020,Dec,3

85660 Sickling of RBC, reduction
EXCLUDES *Hemoglobin electrophoresis (83020)*
Smears (87207)
0.00 0.00 FUD XXX
AMA: 2020,Dec,3

85670 Thrombin time; plasma
0.00 0.00 FUD XXX
AMA: 2020,Dec,3

85675 titer
0.00 0.00 FUD XXX
AMA: 2020,Dec,3

85705 Thromboplastin inhibition, tissue
EXCLUDES *Individual clotting factors (85245-85247)*
0.00 0.00 FUD XXX
AMA: 2020,Dec,3

85730-85732 Partial Thromboplastin Time (PTT)

EXCLUDES *Agglutinins (86000, 86156-86157)*
Antiplasmin (85410)
Antithrombin III (85300-85301)
Blood banking procedures (86850-86999)

85730 **Thromboplastin time, partial (PTT); plasma or whole blood**
INCLUDES Hicks-Pitney test
0.00 0.00 FUD XXX
AMA: 2020,Dec,3

85732 **substitution, plasma fractions, each**
0.00 0.00 FUD XXX
AMA: 2020,Dec,3; 2018,Jan,8; 2017,Jan,8; 2016,Jan,13

85810-85999 Blood Viscosity and Unlisted Hematology Procedures

85810 **Viscosity**
EXCLUDES *von Willebrand factor assay (85245-85247)*
WBC count (85025, 85027, 85048, 89050)
0.00 0.00 FUD XXX
AMA: 2020,Dec,3; 2018,Jan,8; 2017,Jan,8; 2016,Jan,13

85999 **Unlisted hematology and coagulation procedure**
0.00 0.00 FUD XXX
AMA: 2020,Dec,3; 2018,Jan,8; 2017,Aug,9; 2017,Jan,8; 2016,Jan,13

86015-86053 [86015, 86051, 86052, 86053] Antibody Testing

● # **86015** **Actin (smooth muscle) antibody (ASMA), each**
EXCLUDES *Antibodies:*
Actinomyces (86602)
Adrenal cortex (86255-86256)
0.00 0.00 FUD 000

86000 **Agglutinins, febrile (eg, Brucella, Francisella, Murine typhus, Q fever, Rocky Mountain spotted fever, scrub typhus), each antigen**
EXCLUDES *Infectious agent antibodies (86602-86804)*
0.00 0.00 FUD XXX
AMA: 2020,Dec,3; 2018,Jan,8; 2017,Jan,8; 2016,Jan,13

86001 **Allergen specific IgG quantitative or semiquantitative, each allergen**
EXCLUDES *Agglutinins and autohemolysins (86940-86941)*
0.00 0.00 FUD XXX
AMA: 2020,Dec,3

86003 **Allergen specific IgE; quantitative or semiquantitative, crude allergen extract, each**
EXCLUDES *Total quantitative IgE (82785)*
0.00 0.00 FUD XXX
AMA: 2020,Dec,3; 2018,Jan,8; 2017,Jan,8; 2016,Jan,13

86005 **qualitative, multiallergen screen (eg, disk, sponge, card)**
EXCLUDES *Total qualitative IgE (83518)*
0.00 0.00 FUD XXX
AMA: 2020,Dec,3; 2018,Jan,8; 2017,Jan,8; 2016,Jan,13

86008 **quantitative or semiquantitative, recombinant or purified component, each**
EXCLUDES *Alpha-1 antitrypsin (82103, 82104)*
Alpha-1 feto-protein (82105, 82106)
Anti-AChR (acetylcholine receptor) antibody titer (86255, 86256)
Anticardiolipin antibody (86147)
Anti-deoxyribonuclease titer (86215)
Anti-DNA (86225)
0.00 0.00 FUD XXX
AMA: 2020,Dec,3

86015 **Resequenced code. See code before 86000.**

86021 **Antibody identification; leukocyte antibodies**
0.00 0.00 FUD XXX
AMA: 2020,Dec,3; 2020,AugSE,1; 2020,AugSE,1; 2020,AugSE,1

86022 **platelet antibodies**
0.00 0.00 FUD XXX
AMA: 2020,Dec,3; 2020,AugSE,1; 2020,AugSE,1; 2020,AugSE,1

86023 **platelet associated immunoglobulin assay**
0.00 0.00 FUD XXX
AMA: 2020,Dec,3; 2020,AugSE,1; 2020,AugSE,1; 2020,AugSE,1

● **86036** **Antineutrophil cytoplasmic antibody (ANCA); screen, each antibody**

● **86037** **titer, each antibody**

86038 **Antinuclear antibodies (ANA);**
0.00 0.00 FUD XXX
AMA: 2020,Dec,3

86039 **titer**
EXCLUDES *Antistreptococcal antibody, ie, anti-DNAse (86215)*
Antistreptokinase titer (86590)
0.00 0.00 FUD XXX
AMA: 2020,Dec,3

86051 **Resequenced code. See code following 86063.**

86052 **Resequenced code. See code following 86063.**

86053 **Resequenced code. See code following 86063.**

86060 **Antistreptolysin 0; titer**
EXCLUDES *Antibodies, infectious agents (86602-86804)*
0.00 0.00 FUD XXX
AMA: 2020,Dec,3

86063 **screen**
EXCLUDES *Antibodies to blastomyces (86612)*
Antibodies, infectious agents (86602-86804)
0.00 0.00 FUD XXX
AMA: 2020,Dec,3

● # **86051** **Aquaporin-4 (neuromyelitis optica [NMO]) antibody; enzyme-linked immunosorbent immunoassay (ELISA)**
0.00 0.00 FUD 000

● # **86052** **cell-based immunofluorescence assay (CBA), each**
0.00 0.00 FUD 000

● # **86053** **flow cytometry (ie, fluorescence-activated cell sorting [FACS]), each**
0.00 0.00 FUD 000

86077-86079 Blood Bank Services

86077 **Blood bank physician services; difficult cross match and/or evaluation of irregular antibody(s), interpretation and written report**
1.46 1.57 FUD XXX
AMA: 2020,Dec,3

86078 **investigation of transfusion reaction including suspicion of transmissible disease, interpretation and written report**
1.46 1.57 FUD XXX
AMA: 2020,Dec,3

86079 **authorization for deviation from standard blood banking procedures (eg, use of outdated blood, transfusion of Rh incompatible units), with written report**
EXCLUDES *Brucella antibodies (86622)*
Candida antibodies (86628)
Candida skin test (86485)
1.46 1.56 FUD XXX
AMA: 2020,Dec,3

86140-86344 [86152, 86153, 86328] Diagnostic Immunology Testing

86140 **C-reactive protein;**
EXCLUDES *Candidiasis (86628)*
0.00 0.00 FUD XXX
AMA: 2020,Dec,3

86141 **high sensitivity (hsCRP)**
0.00 0.00 FUD XXX
AMA: 2020,Dec,3

86146 **Beta 2 Glycoprotein I antibody, each**
0.00 0.00 FUD XXX
AMA: 2020,Dec,3

86147 **Cardiolipin (phospholipid) antibody, each Ig class**
0.00 0.00 FUD XXX
AMA: 2020,Dec,3

86152 **Cell enumeration using immunologic selection and identification in fluid specimen (eg, circulating tumor cells in blood);**
EXCLUDES *Flow cytometric immunophenotyping (88184-88189)*
Flow cytometric quantitation (86355-86357, 86359-86361, 86367)
Code also physician interpretation/report when performed ([86153])
0.00 0.00 FUD XXX
AMA: 2020,Dec,3

86153 **physician interpretation and report, when required**
EXCLUDES *Flow cytometric immunophenotyping (88184-88189)*
Flow cytometric quantitation (86355-86357, 86359-86361, 86367)
Code first cell enumeration, when performed ([86152])
0.00 0.00 FUD 000
AMA: 2020,Dec,3

86148 **Anti-phosphatidylserine (phospholipid) antibody**
EXCLUDES *Antiprothrombin (phospholipid cofactor) antibody (86849)*
0.00 0.00 FUD XXX
AMA: 2020,Dec,3; 2018,Jan,8; 2017,Jan,8; 2016,Jan,13

86152 **Resequenced code. See code following 86147.**

86153 **Resequenced code. See code before 86148.**

86155 **Chemotaxis assay, specify method**
EXCLUDES *Antibodies, coccidioides (86635)*
Clostridium difficile toxin (87230)
Skin test, coccidioides (86490)
0.00 0.00 FUD XXX
AMA: 2020,Dec,3

86156 **Cold agglutinin; screen**
0.00 0.00 FUD XXX
AMA: 2020,Dec,3

86157 **titer**
0.00 0.00 FUD XXX
AMA: 2020,Dec,3

86160 **Complement; antigen, each component**
0.00 0.00 FUD XXX
AMA: 2020,Dec,3

86161 **functional activity, each component**
0.00 0.00 FUD XXX
AMA: 2020,Dec,3

86162 **total hemolytic (CH50)**
0.00 0.00 FUD XXX
AMA: 2020,Dec,3

86171 **Complement fixation tests, each antigen**
EXCLUDES *Coombs test*
0.00 0.00 FUD XXX
AMA: 2020,Dec,3

86200 **Cyclic citrullinated peptide (CCP), antibody**
0.00 0.00 FUD XXX
AMA: 2020,Dec,3; 2018,Jan,8; 2017,Jan,8; 2016,Jan,13

86215 **Deoxyribonuclease, antibody**
0.00 0.00 FUD XXX
AMA: 2020,Dec,3

86225 **Deoxyribonucleic acid (DNA) antibody; native or double stranded**
EXCLUDES *Echinococcus antibodies, report code for specific method*
HIV antibody tests (86701-86703)
0.00 0.00 FUD XXX
AMA: 2020,Dec,3

86226 **single stranded**
EXCLUDES *Anti D.S, DNA, IFA, eg, using C. Lucilae (86255-86256)*
0.00 0.00 FUD XXX
AMA: 2020,Dec,3

● **86231** **Endomysial antibody (EMA), each immunoglobulin (Ig) class**

86235 **Extractable nuclear antigen, antibody to, any method (eg, nRNP, SS-A, SS-B, Sm, RNP, Sc170, J01), each antibody**
0.00 0.00 FUD XXX
AMA: 2020,Dec,3

86255 **Fluorescent noninfectious agent antibody; screen, each antibody**
0.00 0.00 FUD XXX
AMA: 2020,Dec,3; 2020,AugSE,1; 2020,AugSE,1; 2020,AugSE,1

86256 **titer, each antibody**
EXCLUDES *Fluorescent technique for antigen identification in tissue (88346, [88350])*
FTA (86780)
Gel (agar) diffusion tests (86331)
Indirect fluorescence (88346, [88350])
0.00 0.00 FUD XXX
AMA: 2020,Dec,3; 2020,AugSE,1; 2020,AugSE,1; 2020,AugSE,1

● **86258** **Gliadin (deamidated) (DGP) antibody, each immunoglobulin (Ig) class**

86277 **Growth hormone, human (HGH), antibody**
0.00 0.00 FUD XXX
AMA: 2020,Dec,3

86280 **Hemagglutination inhibition test (HAI)**
EXCLUDES *Antibodies to infectious agents (86602-86804)*
Rubella (86762)
0.00 0.00 FUD XXX
AMA: 2020,Dec,3

86294 **Immunoassay for tumor antigen, qualitative or semiquantitative (eg, bladder tumor antigen)**
EXCLUDES *Qualitative NMP22 protein (86386)*
0.00 0.00 FUD XXX
AMA: 2020,Dec,3

86300 **Immunoassay for tumor antigen, quantitative; CA 15-3 (27.29)**
0.00 0.00 FUD XXX
AMA: 2020,Dec,3

86301 **CA 19-9**
0.00 0.00 FUD XXX
AMA: 2020,Dec,3

86304 **CA 125**
EXCLUDES *Antibody, hepatitis delta agent (86692)*
Measurement serum HER-2/neu oncoprotein (83950)
0.00 0.00 FUD XXX
AMA: 2020,Dec,3

86305 **Human epididymis protein 4 (HE4)**
0.00 0.00 FUD XXX
AMA: 2020,Dec,3

86308 **Heterophile antibodies; screening**
EXCLUDES *Antibodies, infectious agents (86602-86804)*
0.00 0.00 FUD XXX
AMA: 2020,Dec,3

86309 **titer**
EXCLUDES *Antibodies, infectious agents (86602-86804)*
0.00 0.00 FUD XXX
AMA: 2020,Dec,3

86310 **titers after absorption with beef cells and guinea pig kidney**

EXCLUDES *Antibodies, infectious agents (86602-86804)*
Histoplasma antibodies (86698)
Histoplasmosis skin test (86510)
Human growth hormone antibody (86277)

0.00 0.00 FUD XXX

AMA: 2020,Dec,3

86316 **Immunoassay for tumor antigen, other antigen, quantitative (eg, CA 50, 72-4, 549), each**

0.00 0.00 FUD XXX

AMA: 2020,Dec,3; 2018,Jan,8; 2017,Jan,8; 2016,Jan,13

86317 **Immunoassay for infectious agent antibody, quantitative, not otherwise specified**

EXCLUDES *Immunoassay techniques for infectious antigens (87301-87451)*
Immunoassay techniques for noninfectious antigens (83516, 83518-83520)
Immunoassay techniques with direct/visual observation for infectious antigens (87802-87899 [87806, 87811])
Particle agglutination test (86403)

0.00 0.00 FUD XXX

AMA: 2020,Dec,3; 2020,OctSE,1; 2020,OctSE,1

86318 **Immunoassay for infectious agent antibody(ies), qualitative or semiquantitative, single-step method (eg, reagent strip);**

0.00 0.00 FUD XXX

AMA: 2020,Dec,3; 2020,AugSE,1; 2020,AugSE,1; 2020,AugSE,1; 2018,Jan,8; 2017,Jan,8; 2016,Jan,13

\# **86328** **severe acute respiratory syndrome coronavirus 2 (SARS-CoV-2) (Coronavirus disease [COVID-19])**

INCLUDES Testing for antibodies only

EXCLUDES *Severe acute respiratory syndrome coronavirus 2 [SARS-CoV-2] [coronavirus disease {COVID-19}] testing via multiple-step method (86769)*
Testing for presence neutralizing antibodies that block cell infection ([86408, 86409])

0.00 0.00 FUD XXX

AMA: 2020,Dec,3; 2020,SepSE,1; 2020,AugSE,1; 2020,SepSE,1; 2020,AugSE,1; 2020,AugSE,1

86320 **Immunoelectrophoresis; serum**

0.00 0.00 FUD XXX

AMA: 2020,Dec,3

86325 **other fluids (eg, urine, cerebrospinal fluid) with concentration**

0.00 0.00 FUD XXX

AMA: 2020,Dec,3

86327 **crossed (2-dimensional assay)**

0.00 0.00 FUD XXX

AMA: 2020,Dec,3

86328 **Resequenced code. See code following 86318.**

86329 **Immunodiffusion; not elsewhere specified**

0.00 0.00 FUD XXX

AMA: 2020,Dec,3; 2018,Jan,8; 2017,Jan,8; 2016,Jan,13

86331 **gel diffusion, qualitative (Ouchterlony), each antigen or antibody**

0.00 0.00 FUD XXX

AMA: 2020,Dec,3

86332 **Immune complex assay**

0.00 0.00 FUD XXX

AMA: 2020,Dec,3

86334 **Immunofixation electrophoresis; serum**

0.00 0.00 FUD XXX

AMA: 2020,Dec,3

86335 **other fluids with concentration (eg, urine, CSF)**

0.00 0.00 FUD XXX

AMA: 2020,Dec,3

86336 **Inhibin A**

0.00 0.00 FUD XXX

AMA: 2020,Dec,3

86337 **Insulin antibodies**

0.00 0.00 FUD XXX

AMA: 2020,Dec,3

86340 **Intrinsic factor antibodies**

EXCLUDES *Antibodies, leptospira (86720)*
Leukoagglutinins (86021)

0.00 0.00 FUD XXX

AMA: 2020,Dec,3

86341 **Islet cell antibody**

0.00 0.00 FUD XXX

AMA: 2020,Dec,3; 2018,Jan,8; 2017,Jan,8; 2016,Jan,13

86343 **Leukocyte histamine release test (LHR)**

0.00 0.00 FUD XXX

AMA: 2020,Dec,3

86344 **Leukocyte phagocytosis**

0.00 0.00 FUD XXX

AMA: 2020,Dec,3

86352 Assay Cellular Function

86352 **Cellular function assay involving stimulation (eg, mitogen or antigen) and detection of biomarker (eg, ATP)**

0.00 0.00 FUD XXX

AMA: 2020,Dec,3

86353 Lymphocyte Mitogen Response Assay

CMS: 100-03,190.8 Lymphocyte Mitogen Response Assays

86353 **Lymphocyte transformation, mitogen (phytomitogen) or antigen induced blastogenesis**

EXCLUDES *Cellular function assay with stimulation and biomarker detection (86352)*
Malaria antibodies (86750)

0.00 0.00 FUD XXX

AMA: 2020,Dec,3

86355-86596 [86362, 86363, 86364, 86408, 86409, 86413] Additional Diagnostic Immunology Testing

86355 **B cells, total count**

EXCLUDES *Flow cytometry interpretation (88187-88189)*

0.00 0.00 FUD XXX

AMA: 2020,Dec,3; 2018,Jan,8; 2017,Jan,8; 2016,Jan,13

86356 **Mononuclear cell antigen, quantitative (eg, flow cytometry), not otherwise specified, each antigen**

EXCLUDES *Flow cytometry interpretation (88187-88189)*

0.00 0.00 FUD XXX

AMA: 2020,Dec,3; 2018,Jan,8; 2017,Jan,8; 2016,Jan,13

● # **86362** **Myelin oligodendrocyte glycoprotein (MOG-IgG1) antibody; cell-based immunofluorescence assay (CBA), each**

0.00 0.00 FUD 000

● # **86363** **flow cytometry (ie, fluorescence-activated cell sorting [FACS]), each**

0.00 0.00 FUD 000

86357 **Natural killer (NK) cells, total count**

EXCLUDES *Flow cytometry interpretation (88187-88189)*

0.00 0.00 FUD XXX

AMA: 2020,Dec,3; 2018,Jan,8; 2017,Jan,8; 2016,Jan,13

● # **86364** **Tissue transglutaminase, each immunoglobulin (Ig) class**

0.00 0.00 FUD 000

86359 **T cells; total count**

EXCLUDES *Flow cytometry interpretation (88187-88189)*

0.00 0.00 FUD XXX

AMA: 2020,Dec,3; 2018,Jan,8; 2017,Jan,8; 2016,Jan,13

86360 **absolute CD4 and CD8 count, including ratio**

EXCLUDES *Flow cytometry interpretation (88187-88189)*

0.00 0.00 FUD XXX

AMA: 2020,Dec,3; 2018,Jan,8; 2017,Jan,8; 2016,Jan,13

86361 **absolute CD4 count**

EXCLUDES *Flow cytometry interpretation (88187-88189)*

0.00 0.00 FUD XXX

AMA: 2020,Dec,3; 2018,Jan,8; 2017,Jan,8; 2016,Jan,13

86362 **Resequenced code. See code following 86356.**

86363 **Resequenced code. See code following 86356.**

86364 **Resequenced code. See code following 86357.**

86367 **Stem cells (ie, CD34), total count**

EXCLUDES *Flow cytometric immunophenotyping, potential hematolymphoid neoplasia assessment (88184-88189)*

Flow cytometry interpretation (88187-88189)

0.00 0.00 FUD XXX

AMA: 2020,Dec,3; 2018,Jan,8; 2017,Jan,8; 2016,Jan,13

86376 **Microsomal antibodies (eg, thyroid or liver-kidney), each**

0.00 0.00 FUD XXX

AMA: 2020,Dec,3; 2020,AugSE,1; 2020,AugSE,1; 2020,AugSE,1

● **86381** **Mitochondrial antibody (eg, M2), each**

86382 **Neutralization test, viral**

0.00 0.00 FUD XXX

AMA: 2020,Dec,3

● # **86408** **Neutralizing antibody, severe acute respiratory syndrome coronavirus 2 (SARS-CoV-2) (Coronavirus disease [COVID-19]); screen**

INCLUDES Testing for presence neutralizing antibodies that block cell infection

EXCLUDES *Testing for presence antibodies only ([86328])*

0.00 0.00 FUD XXX

AMA: 2020,Dec,3; 2020,AugSE,1

● # **86409** **titer**

INCLUDES Testing for presence neutralizing antibodies that block cell infection

EXCLUDES *Testing for presence antibodies only ([86328])*

0.00 0.00 FUD XXX

AMA: 2020,Dec,3; 2020,AugSE,1

● # **86413** **Severe acute respiratory syndrome coronavirus 2 (SARS-CoV-2) (Coronavirus disease [COVID-19]) antibody, quantitative**

INCLUDES Testing for presence and adaptive immune response to SARS-CoV-2

0.00 0.00 FUD XXX

AMA: 2020,Dec,3; 2020,SepSE,1

86384 **Nitroblue tetrazolium dye test (NTD)**

0.00 0.00 FUD XXX

AMA: 2020,Dec,3

86386 **Nuclear Matrix Protein 22 (NMP22), qualitative**

EXCLUDES *Ouchterlony diffusion (86331)*

Platelet antibodies (86022, 86023)

0.00 0.00 FUD XXX

AMA: 2020,Dec,3

86403 **Particle agglutination; screen, each antibody**

0.00 0.00 FUD XXX

AMA: 2020,Dec,3; 2020,OctSE,1; 2020,OctSE,1

86406 **titer, each antibody**

EXCLUDES *Pregnancy test (84702, 84703)*

Rapid plasma reagin test (RPR) (86592, 86593)

0.00 0.00 FUD XXX

AMA: 2020,Dec,3

86408 **Resequenced code. See code following 86382.**

86409 **Resequenced code. See code following 86382.**

86413 **Resequenced code. See code following resequenced code 86409.**

86430 **Rheumatoid factor; qualitative**

0.00 0.00 FUD XXX

AMA: 2020,Dec,3

86431 **quantitative**

EXCLUDES *Serologic syphilis testing (86592, 86593)*

0.00 0.00 FUD XXX

AMA: 2020,Dec,3

86480 **Tuberculosis test, cell mediated immunity antigen response measurement; gamma interferon**

0.00 0.00 FUD XXX

AMA: 2020,Dec,3; 2019,Dec,12; 2018,Jan,8; 2017,Jan,8; 2016,Jan,13

86481 **enumeration of gamma interferon-producing T-cells in cell suspension**

0.00 0.00 FUD XXX

AMA: 2020,Dec,3; 2019,Dec,12

86485 **Skin test; candida**

EXCLUDES *Candida antibody (86628)*

0.00 0.00 FUD XXX

AMA: 2020,Dec,3

86486 **unlisted antigen, each**

0.15 0.15 FUD XXX

AMA: 2020,Dec,3

86490 **coccidioidomycosis**

2.49 2.49 FUD XXX

AMA: 2020,Dec,3

86510 **histoplasmosis**

EXCLUDES *Histoplasma antibody (86698)*

0.19 0.19 FUD XXX

AMA: 2020,Dec,3

86580 **tuberculosis, intradermal**

INCLUDES Heaf test

Intradermal Mantoux test

EXCLUDES *Antibodies to sporothrix, report code for specific method*

Skin test for allergy (95012-95199)

Smooth muscle antibody ([86015])

Tuberculosis test, cell mediated immunity measurement gamma interferon antigen response (86480)

0.26 0.26 FUD XXX

AMA: 2020,Dec,3

86590 **Streptokinase, antibody**

EXCLUDES *Antibodies, infectious agents (86602-86804)*

Streptolysin O antibody, antistreptolysin O (86060, 86063)

0.00 0.00 FUD XXX

AMA: 2020,Dec,3

86592 **Syphilis test, non-treponemal antibody; qualitative (eg, VDRL, RPR, ART)**

INCLUDES Wasserman test

EXCLUDES *Antibodies to infectious agents (86602-86804)*

0.00 0.00 FUD XXX

AMA: 2020,Dec,3

86593 **quantitative**

EXCLUDES *Antibodies, infectious agents (86602-86804)*

Tetanus antibody (86774)

Thyroglobulin (84432)

Thyroglobulin antibody (86800)

Thyroid microsomal antibody (86376)

Toxoplasma antibody (86777-86778)

0.00 0.00 FUD XXX

AMA: 2020,Dec,3

● **86596** **Voltage-gated calcium channel antibody, each**

86602-86698 Testing for Antibodies to Infectious Agents: Actinomyces—Histoplasma

INCLUDES Qualitative or semiquantitative immunoassays performed by multiple-step methods for detection, antibodies to infectious agents

EXCLUDES *Detection:*
Antibodies other than those to infectious agents, see specific antibody or method
Infectious agent/antigen (87260-87899 [87623, 87624, 87625, 87806])
Immunoassays by single-step method (86318, [86328])

86602 Antibody; actinomyces
0.00 0.00 FUD XXX
AMA: 2020,Dec,3; 2020,OctSE,1; 2020,OctSE,1; 2020,AugSE,1; 2020,AugSE,1; 2020,AugSE,1; 2018,Jan,8; 2017,Jan,8; 2016,Jan,13

86603 adenovirus
0.00 0.00 FUD XXX
AMA: 2020,Dec,3; 2020,OctSE,1; 2020,OctSE,1; 2020,AugSE,1; 2020,AugSE,1; 2020,AugSE,1

86606 Aspergillus
0.00 0.00 FUD XXX
AMA: 2020,Dec,3; 2020,OctSE,1; 2020,OctSE,1; 2020,AugSE,1; 2020,AugSE,1; 2020,AugSE,1

86609 bacterium, not elsewhere specified
0.00 0.00 FUD XXX
AMA: 2020,Dec,3; 2020,OctSE,1; 2020,OctSE,1; 2020,AugSE,1; 2020,AugSE,1; 2020,AugSE,1

86611 Bartonella
0.00 0.00 FUD XXX
AMA: 2020,Dec,3; 2020,OctSE,1; 2020,OctSE,1; 2020,AugSE,1; 2020,AugSE,1; 2020,AugSE,1

86612 Blastomyces
0.00 0.00 FUD XXX
AMA: 2020,Dec,3; 2020,OctSE,1; 2020,OctSE,1; 2020,AugSE,1; 2020,AugSE,1; 2020,AugSE,1

86615 Bordetella
0.00 0.00 FUD XXX
AMA: 2020,Dec,3; 2020,OctSE,1; 2020,OctSE,1; 2020,AugSE,1; 2020,AugSE,1; 2020,AugSE,1

86617 Borrelia burgdorferi (Lyme disease) confirmatory test (eg, Western Blot or immunoblot)
0.00 0.00 FUD XXX
AMA: 2020,Dec,3; 2020,OctSE,1; 2020,OctSE,1; 2020,AugSE,1; 2020,AugSE,1; 2020,AugSE,1

86618 Borrelia burgdorferi (Lyme disease)
0.00 0.00 FUD XXX
AMA: 2020,Dec,3; 2020,OctSE,1; 2020,OctSE,1; 2020,AugSE,1; 2020,AugSE,1; 2020,AugSE,1

86619 Borrelia (relapsing fever)
0.00 0.00 FUD XXX
AMA: 2020,Dec,3; 2020,OctSE,1; 2020,OctSE,1; 2020,AugSE,1; 2020,AugSE,1; 2020,AugSE,1

86622 Brucella
0.00 0.00 FUD XXX
AMA: 2020,Dec,3; 2020,OctSE,1; 2020,OctSE,1; 2020,AugSE,1; 2020,AugSE,1; 2020,AugSE,1

86625 Campylobacter
0.00 0.00 FUD XXX
AMA: 2020,Dec,3; 2020,OctSE,1; 2020,OctSE,1; 2020,AugSE,1; 2020,AugSE,1; 2020,AugSE,1

86628 Candida
EXCLUDES *Candida skin test (86485)*
0.00 0.00 FUD XXX
AMA: 2020,Dec,3; 2020,OctSE,1; 2020,OctSE,1; 2020,AugSE,1; 2020,AugSE,1; 2020,AugSE,1

86631 Chlamydia
0.00 0.00 FUD XXX
AMA: 2020,Dec,3; 2020,OctSE,1; 2020,OctSE,1; 2020,AugSE,1; 2020,AugSE,1; 2020,AugSE,1

86632 Chlamydia, IgM
EXCLUDES *Chlamydia antigen (87270, 87320)*
Fluorescent antibody technique (86255-86256)
0.00 0.00 FUD XXX
AMA: 2020,Dec,3; 2020,OctSE,1; 2020,OctSE,1; 2020,AugSE,1; 2020,AugSE,1; 2020,AugSE,1

86635 Coccidioides
EXCLUDES *Severe Acute Respiratory Syndrome Coronavirus 2 [SARS-CoV-2] [Coronavirus disease {COVID-19}] antibody testing ([86328], 86769)*
0.00 0.00 FUD XXX
AMA: 2020,Dec,3; 2020,OctSE,1; 2020,OctSE,1; 2020,AugSE,1; 2020,AugSE,1; 2020,AugSE,1

86638 Coxiella burnetii (Q fever)
0.00 0.00 FUD XXX
AMA: 2020,Dec,3; 2020,OctSE,1; 2020,OctSE,1; 2020,AugSE,1; 2020,AugSE,1; 2020,AugSE,1

86641 Cryptococcus
0.00 0.00 FUD XXX
AMA: 2020,Dec,3; 2020,OctSE,1; 2020,OctSE,1; 2020,AugSE,1; 2020,AugSE,1; 2020,AugSE,1

86644 cytomegalovirus (CMV)
0.00 0.00 FUD XXX
AMA: 2020,Dec,3; 2020,OctSE,1; 2020,OctSE,1; 2020,AugSE,1; 2020,AugSE,1; 2020,AugSE,1

86645 cytomegalovirus (CMV), IgM
0.00 0.00 FUD XXX
AMA: 2020,Dec,3; 2020,OctSE,1; 2020,OctSE,1; 2020,AugSE,1; 2020,AugSE,1; 2020,AugSE,1; 2018,Jan,8; 2017,Jan,8; 2016,Jan,13

86648 Diphtheria
0.00 0.00 FUD XXX
AMA: 2020,Dec,3; 2020,OctSE,1; 2020,OctSE,1; 2020,AugSE,1; 2020,AugSE,1; 2020,AugSE,1

86651 encephalitis, California (La Crosse)
0.00 0.00 FUD XXX
AMA: 2020,Dec,3; 2020,OctSE,1; 2020,OctSE,1; 2020,AugSE,1; 2020,AugSE,1; 2020,AugSE,1

86652 encephalitis, Eastern equine
0.00 0.00 FUD XXX
AMA: 2020,Dec,3; 2020,OctSE,1; 2020,OctSE,1; 2020,AugSE,1; 2020,AugSE,1; 2020,AugSE,1

86653 encephalitis, St. Louis
0.00 0.00 FUD XXX
AMA: 2020,Dec,3; 2020,OctSE,1; 2020,OctSE,1; 2020,AugSE,1; 2020,AugSE,1; 2020,AugSE,1

86654 encephalitis, Western equine
0.00 0.00 FUD XXX
AMA: 2020,Dec,3; 2020,OctSE,1; 2020,OctSE,1; 2020,AugSE,1; 2020,AugSE,1; 2020,AugSE,1

86658 enterovirus (eg, coxsackie, echo, polio)
EXCLUDES *Antibodies to:*
Trichinella (86784)
Trypanosoma—see code for specific methodology
Tuberculosis (86580)
Viral—see code for specific methodology
0.00 0.00 FUD XXX
AMA: 2020,Dec,3; 2020,OctSE,1; 2020,OctSE,1; 2020,AugSE,1; 2020,AugSE,1; 2020,AugSE,1

86663 Epstein-Barr (EB) virus, early antigen (EA)
0.00 0.00 FUD XXX
AMA: 2020,Dec,3; 2020,OctSE,1; 2020,OctSE,1; 2020,AugSE,1; 2020,AugSE,1; 2020,AugSE,1

86664 Epstein-Barr (EB) virus, nuclear antigen (EBNA)
0.00 0.00 FUD XXX
AMA: 2020,Dec,3; 2020,OctSE,1; 2020,OctSE,1; 2020,AugSE,1; 2020,AugSE,1; 2020,AugSE,1

86665 **Epstein-Barr (EB) virus, viral capsid (VCA)**
0.00 0.00 **FUD** XXX
AMA: 2020,Dec,3; 2020,OctSE,1; 2020,OctSE,1; 2020,AugSE,1; 2020,AugSE,1; 2020,AugSE,1

86666 **Ehrlichia**
0.00 0.00 **FUD** XXX
AMA: 2020,Dec,3; 2020,OctSE,1; 2020,OctSE,1; 2020,AugSE,1; 2020,AugSE,1; 2020,AugSE,1

86668 **Francisella tularensis**
0.00 0.00 **FUD** XXX
AMA: 2020,Dec,3; 2020,OctSE,1; 2020,OctSE,1; 2020,AugSE,1; 2020,AugSE,1; 2020,AugSE,1

86671 **fungus, not elsewhere specified**
0.00 0.00 **FUD** XXX
AMA: 2020,Dec,3; 2020,OctSE,1; 2020,OctSE,1; 2020,AugSE,1; 2020,AugSE,1; 2020,AugSE,1

86674 **Giardia lamblia**
0.00 0.00 **FUD** XXX
AMA: 2020,Dec,3; 2020,OctSE,1; 2020,OctSE,1; 2020,AugSE,1; 2020,AugSE,1; 2020,AugSE,1

86677 **Helicobacter pylori**
0.00 0.00 **FUD** XXX
AMA: 2020,Dec,3; 2020,OctSE,1; 2020,OctSE,1; 2020,AugSE,1; 2020,AugSE,1; 2020,AugSE,1; 2018,Jan,8; 2017,Jan,8; 2016,Jan,13

86682 **helminth, not elsewhere specified**
0.00 0.00 **FUD** XXX
AMA: 2020,Dec,3; 2020,OctSE,1; 2020,OctSE,1; 2020,AugSE,1; 2020,AugSE,1; 2020,AugSE,1

86684 **Haemophilus influenza**
0.00 0.00 **FUD** XXX
AMA: 2020,Dec,3; 2020,OctSE,1; 2020,OctSE,1; 2020,AugSE,1; 2020,AugSE,1; 2020,AugSE,1

86687 **HTLV-I**
0.00 0.00 **FUD** XXX
AMA: 2020,Dec,3; 2020,OctSE,1; 2020,OctSE,1; 2020,AugSE,1; 2020,AugSE,1; 2020,AugSE,1

86688 **HTLV-II**
0.00 0.00 **FUD** XXX
AMA: 2020,Dec,3; 2020,OctSE,1; 2020,OctSE,1; 2020,AugSE,1; 2020,AugSE,1; 2020,AugSE,1

86689 **HTLV or HIV antibody, confirmatory test (eg, Western Blot)**
0.00 0.00 **FUD** XXX
AMA: 2020,Dec,3; 2020,OctSE,1; 2020,OctSE,1; 2020,AugSE,1; 2020,AugSE,1; 2020,AugSE,1; 2018,Jan,8; 2017,Jan,8; 2016,Jan,13

86692 **hepatitis, delta agent**
EXCLUDES *Hepatitis delta agent, antigen (87380)*
0.00 0.00 **FUD** XXX
AMA: 2020,Dec,3; 2020,OctSE,1; 2020,OctSE,1; 2020,AugSE,1; 2020,AugSE,1; 2020,AugSE,1

86694 **herpes simplex, non-specific type test**
0.00 0.00 **FUD** XXX
AMA: 2020,Dec,3; 2020,OctSE,1; 2020,OctSE,1; 2020,AugSE,1; 2020,AugSE,1; 2020,AugSE,1

86695 **herpes simplex, type 1**
0.00 0.00 **FUD** XXX
AMA: 2020,Dec,3; 2020,OctSE,1; 2020,OctSE,1; 2020,AugSE,1; 2020,AugSE,1; 2020,AugSE,1; 2018,Jan,8; 2017,Jan,8; 2016,Jan,13

86696 **herpes simplex, type 2**
0.00 0.00 **FUD** XXX
AMA: 2020,Dec,3; 2020,OctSE,1; 2020,OctSE,1; 2020,AugSE,1; 2020,AugSE,1; 2020,AugSE,1

86698 **histoplasma**
0.00 0.00 **FUD** XXX
AMA: 2020,Dec,3; 2020,OctSE,1; 2020,OctSE,1; 2020,AugSE,1; 2020,AugSE,1; 2020,AugSE,1

86701-86703 Testing for HIV Antibodies

CMS: 100-03,190.14 Human Immunodeficiency Virus Testing (Diagnosis); 100-03,190.9 Serologic Testing for Acquired Immunodeficiency Syndrome (AIDS)

INCLUDES Qualitative or semiquantitative immunoassays performed by multiple-step methods for detection, antibodies to infectious agents

EXCLUDES *Confirmatory test for HIV antibody (86689)*
HIV-1 antigen (87390)
HIV-1 antigen(s) with HIV 1 and 2 antibodies, single result (87389)
HIV-2 antigen (87391)
Immunoassays by single-step method (86318)

Code also modifier 92 for test performed using kit or transportable instrument comprising (all or part) single-use, disposable analytical chamber

86701 **Antibody; HIV-1**
0.00 0.00 **FUD** XXX
AMA: 2020,Dec,3; 2020,OctSE,1; 2020,OctSE,1; 2020,AugSE,1; 2020,AugSE,1; 2020,AugSE,1; 2018,Jan,8; 2017,Jan,8; 2016,Jan,13

86702 **HIV-2**
0.00 0.00 **FUD** XXX
AMA: 2020,Dec,3; 2020,OctSE,1; 2020,OctSE,1; 2020,AugSE,1; 2020,AugSE,1; 2020,AugSE,1; 2018,Jan,8; 2017,Jan,8; 2016,Jan,13

86703 **HIV-1 and HIV-2, single result**
0.00 0.00 **FUD** XXX
AMA: 2020,Dec,3; 2020,OctSE,1; 2020,OctSE,1; 2020,AugSE,1; 2020,AugSE,1; 2020,AugSE,1; 2018,Jan,8; 2017,Jan,8; 2016,Jan,13

86704-86804 Testing for Infectious Disease Antibodies: Hepatitis—Yersinia

INCLUDES Qualitative or semiquantitative immunoassays performed by multiple-step methods for detection, antibodies to infectious agents

EXCLUDES *Detection of:*
Antibodies other than those to infectious agents, see specific antibody or method
Infectious agent/antigen (87260-87899 [87623, 87624, 87625, 87806])
Immunoassays by single-step method (86318)

86704 **Hepatitis B core antibody (HBcAb); total**
0.00 0.00 **FUD** XXX
AMA: 2020,Dec,3; 2020,OctSE,1; 2020,OctSE,1; 2020,AugSE,1; 2020,AugSE,1; 2020,AugSE,1; 2018,Jan,8; 2017,Jan,8; 2016,Jan,13

86705 **IgM antibody**
0.00 0.00 **FUD** XXX
AMA: 2020,Dec,3; 2020,OctSE,1; 2020,OctSE,1; 2020,AugSE,1; 2020,AugSE,1; 2020,AugSE,1; 2018,Jan,8; 2017,Jan,8; 2016,Jan,13

86706 **Hepatitis B surface antibody (HBsAb)**
0.00 0.00 **FUD** XXX
AMA: 2020,Dec,3; 2020,OctSE,1; 2020,OctSE,1; 2020,AugSE,1; 2020,AugSE,1; 2020,AugSE,1

86707 **Hepatitis Be antibody (HBeAb)**
0.00 0.00 **FUD** XXX
AMA: 2020,Dec,3; 2020,OctSE,1; 2020,OctSE,1; 2020,AugSE,1; 2020,AugSE,1; 2020,AugSE,1

86708 **Hepatitis A antibody (HAAb)**
0.00 0.00 **FUD** XXX
AMA: 2020,Dec,3; 2020,OctSE,1; 2020,OctSE,1; 2020,AugSE,1; 2020,AugSE,1; 2020,AugSE,1; 2018,Jan,8; 2017,Jan,8; 2016,Jan,13

86709 **Hepatitis A antibody (HAAb), IgM antibody**
0.00 0.00 **FUD** XXX
AMA: 2020,Dec,3; 2020,OctSE,1; 2020,OctSE,1; 2020,AugSE,1; 2020,AugSE,1; 2020,AugSE,1; 2018,Jan,8; 2017,Jan,8; 2016,Jan,13

86710 **Antibody; influenza virus**
0.00 0.00 **FUD** XXX
AMA: 2020,Dec,3; 2020,OctSE,1; 2020,OctSE,1; 2020,AugSE,1; 2020,AugSE,1; 2020,AugSE,1; 2018,Jan,8; 2017,Jan,8; 2016,Jan,13

86711 **JC (John Cunningham) virus**
0.00 0.00 **FUD** XXX
AMA: 2020,Dec,3; 2020,OctSE,1; 2020,OctSE,1; 2020,AugSE,1; 2020,AugSE,1; 2020,AugSE,1

86713 **Legionella**
0.00 0.00 **FUD** XXX
AMA: 2020,Dec,3; 2020,OctSE,1; 2020,OctSE,1; 2020,AugSE,1; 2020,AugSE,1; 2020,AugSE,1

86717 **Leishmania**
0.00 0.00 FUD XXX
AMA: 2020,Dec,3; 2020,OctSE,1; 2020,OctSE,1; 2020,AugSE,1; 2020,AugSE,1; 2020,AugSE,1

86720 **Leptospira**
0.00 0.00 FUD XXX
AMA: 2020,Dec,3; 2020,OctSE,1; 2020,OctSE,1; 2020,AugSE,1; 2020,AugSE,1; 2020,AugSE,1

86723 **Listeria monocytogenes**
0.00 0.00 FUD XXX
AMA: 2020,Dec,3; 2020,OctSE,1; 2020,OctSE,1; 2020,AugSE,1; 2020,AugSE,1; 2020,AugSE,1

86727 **lymphocytic choriomeningitis**
0.00 0.00 FUD XXX
AMA: 2020,Dec,3; 2020,OctSE,1; 2020,OctSE,1; 2020,AugSE,1; 2020,AugSE,1; 2020,AugSE,1

86732 **mucormycosis**
0.00 0.00 FUD XXX
AMA: 2020,Dec,3; 2020,OctSE,1; 2020,OctSE,1; 2020,AugSE,1; 2020,AugSE,1; 2020,AugSE,1

86735 **mumps**
0.00 0.00 FUD XXX
AMA: 2020,Dec,3; 2020,OctSE,1; 2020,OctSE,1; 2020,AugSE,1; 2020,AugSE,1; 2020,AugSE,1; 2018,Jan,8; 2017,Jan,8; 2016,Jan,13

86738 **mycoplasma**
0.00 0.00 FUD XXX
AMA: 2020,Dec,3; 2020,OctSE,1; 2020,OctSE,1; 2020,AugSE,1; 2020,AugSE,1; 2020,AugSE,1

86741 **Neisseria meningitidis**
0.00 0.00 FUD XXX
AMA: 2020,Dec,3; 2020,OctSE,1; 2020,OctSE,1; 2020,AugSE,1; 2020,AugSE,1; 2020,AugSE,1

86744 **Nocardia**
0.00 0.00 FUD XXX
AMA: 2020,Dec,3; 2020,OctSE,1; 2020,OctSE,1; 2020,AugSE,1; 2020,AugSE,1; 2020,AugSE,1

86747 **parvovirus**
0.00 0.00 FUD XXX
AMA: 2020,Dec,3; 2020,OctSE,1; 2020,OctSE,1; 2020,AugSE,1; 2020,AugSE,1; 2020,AugSE,1

86750 **Plasmodium (malaria)**
0.00 0.00 FUD XXX
AMA: 2020,Dec,3; 2020,OctSE,1; 2020,OctSE,1; 2020,AugSE,1; 2020,AugSE,1; 2020,AugSE,1

86753 **protozoa, not elsewhere specified**
0.00 0.00 FUD XXX
AMA: 2020,Dec,3; 2020,OctSE,1; 2020,OctSE,1; 2020,AugSE,1; 2020,AugSE,1; 2020,AugSE,1

86756 **respiratory syncytial virus**
0.00 0.00 FUD XXX
AMA: 2020,Dec,3; 2020,OctSE,1; 2020,OctSE,1; 2020,AugSE,1; 2020,AugSE,1; 2020,AugSE,1

86757 **Rickettsia**
0.00 0.00 FUD XXX
AMA: 2020,Dec,3; 2020,OctSE,1; 2020,OctSE,1; 2020,AugSE,1; 2020,AugSE,1; 2020,AugSE,1

86759 **rotavirus**
0.00 0.00 FUD XXX
AMA: 2020,Dec,3; 2020,OctSE,1; 2020,OctSE,1; 2020,AugSE,1; 2020,AugSE,1; 2020,AugSE,1

86762 **rubella**
0.00 0.00 FUD XXX
AMA: 2020,Dec,3; 2020,OctSE,1; 2020,OctSE,1; 2020,AugSE,1; 2020,AugSE,1; 2020,AugSE,1

86765 **rubeola**
0.00 0.00 FUD XXX
AMA: 2020,Dec,3; 2020,OctSE,1; 2020,OctSE,1; 2020,AugSE,1; 2020,AugSE,1; 2020,AugSE,1

86768 **Salmonella**
0.00 0.00 FUD XXX
AMA: 2020,Dec,3; 2020,OctSE,1; 2020,OctSE,1; 2020,AugSE,1; 2020,AugSE,1; 2020,AugSE,1

86769 **severe acute respiratory syndrome coronavirus 2 (SARS-CoV-2) (Coronavirus disease [COVID-19])**
EXCLUDES *Antibody, severe acute respiratory syndrome coronavirus 2 (SARS-CoV-2) (coronavirus disease [COVID-19]), includes titer(s) (0224U)*
Severe acute respiratory syndrome coronavirus 2 (SARS-CoV-2) (coronavirus disease [COVID-19]) antibody testing via single-step method ([86328])
0.00 0.00 FUD XXX
AMA: 2020,Dec,3; 2020,OctSE,1; 2020,SepSE,1; 2020,OctSE,1; 2020,AugSE,1; 2020,SepSE,1; 2020,AugSE,1; 2020,AugSE,1; 2020,May,3; 2020,JuneSE,1

86771 **Shigella**
0.00 0.00 FUD XXX
AMA: 2020,Dec,3; 2020,OctSE,1; 2020,OctSE,1; 2020,AugSE,1; 2020,AugSE,1; 2020,AugSE,1

86774 **tetanus**
0.00 0.00 FUD XXX
AMA: 2020,Dec,3; 2020,OctSE,1; 2020,OctSE,1; 2020,AugSE,1; 2020,AugSE,1; 2020,AugSE,1

86777 **Toxoplasma**
0.00 0.00 FUD XXX
AMA: 2020,Dec,3; 2020,OctSE,1; 2020,OctSE,1; 2020,AugSE,1; 2020,AugSE,1; 2020,AugSE,1

86778 **Toxoplasma, IgM**
0.00 0.00 FUD XXX
AMA: 2020,Dec,3; 2020,OctSE,1; 2020,OctSE,1; 2020,AugSE,1; 2020,AugSE,1; 2020,AugSE,1

86780 **Treponema pallidum**
EXCLUDES *Nontreponemal antibody analysis syphilis testing (86592-86593)*
0.00 0.00 FUD XXX
AMA: 2020,Dec,3; 2020,OctSE,1; 2020,OctSE,1; 2020,AugSE,1; 2020,AugSE,1; 2020,AugSE,1

86784 **Trichinella**
0.00 0.00 FUD XXX
AMA: 2020,Dec,3; 2020,OctSE,1; 2020,OctSE,1; 2020,AugSE,1; 2020,AugSE,1; 2020,AugSE,1

86787 **varicella-zoster**
0.00 0.00 FUD XXX
AMA: 2020,Dec,3; 2020,OctSE,1; 2020,OctSE,1; 2020,AugSE,1; 2020,AugSE,1; 2020,AugSE,1

86788 **West Nile virus, IgM**
0.00 0.00 FUD XXX
AMA: 2020,Dec,3; 2020,OctSE,1; 2020,OctSE,1; 2020,AugSE,1; 2020,AugSE,1; 2020,AugSE,1

86789 **West Nile virus**
0.00 0.00 FUD XXX
AMA: 2020,Dec,3; 2020,OctSE,1; 2020,OctSE,1; 2020,AugSE,1; 2020,AugSE,1; 2020,AugSE,1

86790 **virus, not elsewhere specified**
0.00 0.00 FUD XXX
AMA: 2020,Dec,3; 2020,OctSE,1; 2020,OctSE,1; 2020,AugSE,1; 2020,AugSE,1; 2020,AugSE,1

86793 **Yersinia**
0.00 0.00 FUD XXX
AMA: 2020,Dec,3; 2020,OctSE,1; 2020,OctSE,1; 2020,AugSE,1; 2020,AugSE,1; 2020,AugSE,1

86794 **Zika virus, IgM**
0.00 0.00 FUD XXX
AMA: 2020,Dec,3; 2020,OctSE,1; 2020,OctSE,1; 2020,AugSE,1; 2020,AugSE,1; 2020,AugSE,1

86800 **Thyroglobulin antibody**
EXCLUDES *Thyroglobulin (84432)*
0.00 0.00 FUD XXX
AMA: 2020,Dec,3; 2020,OctSE,1; 2020,OctSE,1; 2020,AugSE,1; 2020,AugSE,1; 2020,AugSE,1

86803 **Hepatitis C antibody;**
0.00 0.00 FUD XXX
AMA: 2020,Dec,3; 2020,OctSE,1; 2020,OctSE,1; 2020,AugSE,1; 2020,AugSE,1; 2020,AugSE,1

86804 **confirmatory test (eg, immunoblot)**
0.00 0.00 FUD XXX
AMA: 2020,Dec,3; 2020,OctSE,1; 2020,OctSE,1; 2020,AugSE,1; 2020,AugSE,1; 2020,AugSE,1; 2018,Jan,8; 2017,Jan,8; 2016,Jan,13

86805-86808 Pre-Transplant Antibody Cross Matching

86805 **Lymphocytotoxicity assay, visual crossmatch; with titration**
0.00 0.00 FUD XXX
AMA: 2020,Dec,3; 2018,Jan,8; 2017,Jan,8; 2016,Jan,13

86806 **without titration**
0.00 0.00 FUD XXX
AMA: 2020,Dec,3

86807 **Serum screening for cytotoxic percent reactive antibody (PRA); standard method**
0.00 0.00 FUD XXX
AMA: 2020,Dec,3; 2018,Jan,8; 2017,Jan,8; 2016,Jan,13

86808 **quick method**
0.00 0.00 FUD XXX
AMA: 2020,Dec,3; 2018,Jan,8; 2017,Jan,8; 2016,Jan,13

86812-86826 Histocompatibility Testing

CMS: 100-03,110.23 Stem Cell Transplantation; 100-03,190.1 Histocompatibility Testing; 100-04,3,90.3 Stem Cell Transplantation; 100-04,3,90.3.1 Allogeneic Stem Cell Transplantation; 100-04,3,90.3.3 Billing for Allogeneic Stem Cell Transplants; 100-04,32,90 Billing for Stem Cell Transplantation; 100-04,4,231.11 Billing for Allogeneic Stem Cell Transplants

EXCLUDES *HLA typing by molecular pathology techniques (81370-81383)*

86812 **HLA typing; A, B, or C (eg, A10, B7, B27), single antigen**
0.00 0.00 FUD XXX
AMA: 2020,Dec,3; 2018,Jan,8; 2017,Jan,8; 2016,Jan,13

86813 **A, B, or C, multiple antigens**
0.00 0.00 FUD XXX
AMA: 2020,Dec,3; 2018,Jan,8; 2017,Jan,8; 2016,Jan,13

86816 **DR/DQ, single antigen**
0.00 0.00 FUD XXX
AMA: 2020,Dec,3; 2018,Jan,8; 2017,Jan,8; 2016,Jan,13

86817 **DR/DQ, multiple antigens**
0.00 0.00 FUD XXX
AMA: 2020,Dec,3; 2018,Jan,8; 2017,Jan,8; 2016,Jan,13

86821 **lymphocyte culture, mixed (MLC)**
0.00 0.00 FUD XXX
AMA: 2020,Dec,3; 2018,Jan,8; 2017,Jan,8; 2016,Jan,13

86825 **Human leukocyte antigen (HLA) crossmatch, non-cytotoxic (eg, using flow cytometry); first serum sample or dilution**
INCLUDES Autologous HLA crossmatch
EXCLUDES *B cells (86355)*
Flow cytometry (88184-88189)
Lymphocytotoxicity visual crossmatch (86805-86806)
T cells (86359)
0.00 0.00 FUD XXX
AMA: 2020,Dec,3; 2020,Aug,14

\+ **86826** **each additional serum sample or sample dilution (List separately in addition to primary procedure)**
INCLUDES Autologous HLA crossmatch
EXCLUDES *B cells (86355)*
Flow cytometry (88184-88189)
Lymphocytotoxicity visual crossmatch (86805-86806)
T cells (86359)
Code first (86825)
0.00 0.00 FUD XXX
AMA: 2020,Dec,3; 2020,Aug,14

86828-86849 HLA Antibodies

86828 **Antibody to human leukocyte antigens (HLA), solid phase assays (eg, microspheres or beads, ELISA, flow cytometry); qualitative assessment of the presence or absence of antibody(ies) to HLA Class I and Class II HLA antigens**
Code also solid phase testing, untreated and treated specimens, either class of HLA after treatment (86828-86833)
0.00 0.00 FUD XXX
AMA: 2020,Dec,3

86829 **qualitative assessment of the presence or absence of antibody(ies) to HLA Class I or Class II HLA antigens**
Code also solid phase testing, untreated and treated specimens, either class of HLA after treatment (86828-86833)
0.00 0.00 FUD XXX
AMA: 2020,Dec,3

86830 **antibody identification by qualitative panel using complete HLA phenotypes, HLA Class I**
Code also solid phase testing, untreated and treated specimens, either class of HLA after treatment (86828-86833)
0.00 0.00 FUD XXX
AMA: 2020,Dec,3

86831 **antibody identification by qualitative panel using complete HLA phenotypes, HLA Class II**
Code also solid phase testing, untreated and treated specimens, either class of HLA after treatment (86828-86833)
0.00 0.00 FUD XXX
AMA: 2020,Dec,3

86832 **high definition qualitative panel for identification of antibody specificities (eg, individual antigen per bead methodology), HLA Class I**
Code also solid phase testing, untreated and treated specimens, either class of HLA after treatment (86828-86833)
0.00 0.00 FUD XXX
AMA: 2020,Dec,3

86833 **high definition qualitative panel for identification of antibody specificities (eg, individual antigen per bead methodology), HLA Class II**
Code also solid phase testing, untreated and treated specimens, either class of HLA after treatment (86828-86833)
0.00 0.00 FUD XXX
AMA: 2020,Dec,3

86834 **semi-quantitative panel (eg, titer), HLA Class I**
0.00 0.00 FUD XXX
AMA: 2020,Dec,3

86835 **semi-quantitative panel (eg, titer), HLA Class II**
0.00 0.00 FUD XXX
AMA: 2020,Dec,3

86849 **Unlisted immunology procedure**
0.00 0.00 FUD XXX
AMA: 2020,Dec,3; 2019,Dec,12; 2018,Jan,8; 2017,Jan,8; 2016,Jan,13

86850-86999 Transfusion Services

EXCLUDES *Apheresis (36511-36512)*
Therapeutic phlebotomy (99195)

86850 **Antibody screen, RBC, each serum technique**
0.00 0.00 FUD XXX
AMA: 2020,Dec,3; 2020,AugSE,1; 2020,AugSE,1; 2020,AugSE,1; 2018,Jan,8; 2017,Jan,8; 2016,Jan,13

86860 Antibody elution (RBC), each elution
0.00 0.00 FUD XXX Q1
AMA: 2020,Dec,3; 2020,AugSE,1; 2020,AugSE,1; 2020,AugSE,1

86870 Antibody identification, RBC antibodies, each panel for each serum technique
0.00 0.00 FUD XXX Q2
AMA: 2020,Dec,3; 2020,AugSE,1; 2020,AugSE,1; 2020,AugSE,1; 2018,Jan,8; 2017,Jan,8; 2016,Jan,13

86880 Antihuman globulin test (Coombs test); direct, each antiserum
0.00 0.00 FUD XXX Q1
AMA: 2020,Dec,3

86885 indirect, qualitative, each reagent red cell
0.00 0.00 FUD XXX Q1
AMA: 2020,Dec,3; 2018,Jan,8; 2017,Jan,8; 2016,Jan,13

86886 indirect, each antibody titer
EXCLUDES *Indirect antihuman globulin (Coombs) test for RBC antibody identification using reagent red cell panels (86870)*
Indirect antihuman globulin (Coombs) test for RBC antibody screening (86850)
0.00 0.00 FUD XXX Q1
AMA: 2020,Dec,3; 2018,Jan,8; 2017,Jan,8; 2016,Jan,13

86890 Autologous blood or component, collection processing and storage; predeposited
0.00 0.00 FUD XXX Q1
AMA: 2020,Dec,3; 2018,Jan,8; 2017,Jan,8; 2016,Jan,13

86891 intra- or postoperative salvage
0.00 0.00 FUD XXX Q1
AMA: 2020,Dec,3

86900 Blood typing, serologic; ABO
0.00 0.00 FUD XXX Q1
AMA: 2020,Dec,3

86901 Rh (D)
0.00 0.00 FUD XXX Q1
AMA: 2020,Dec,3; 2018,Jan,8; 2017,Jan,8; 2016,Jan,13

86902 antigen testing of donor blood using reagent serum, each antigen test
Code also one time for each antigen, each unit blood, when multiple units tested for same antigen
0.00 0.00 FUD XXX Q1
AMA: 2020,Dec,3

86904 antigen screening for compatible unit using patient serum, per unit screened
0.00 0.00 FUD XXX Q1
AMA: 2020,Dec,3

86905 RBC antigens, other than ABO or Rh (D), each
0.00 0.00 FUD XXX Q1
AMA: 2020,Dec,3

86906 Rh phenotyping, complete
EXCLUDES *Reporting molecular pathology procedures for human erythrocyte antigen typing (81403)*
0.00 0.00 FUD XXX Q1
AMA: 2020,Dec,3

86910 Blood typing, for paternity testing, per individual; ABO, Rh and MN
0.00 0.00 FUD XXX E
AMA: 2020,Dec,3

86911 each additional antigen system
0.00 0.00 FUD XXX E
AMA: 2020,Dec,3

86920 Compatibility test each unit; immediate spin technique
0.00 0.00 FUD XXX Q1
AMA: 2020,Dec,3; 2018,Jan,8; 2017,Jan,8; 2016,Jan,13

86921 incubation technique
0.00 0.00 FUD XXX Q1
AMA: 2020,Dec,3; 2018,Jan,8; 2017,Jan,8; 2016,Jan,13

86922 antiglobulin technique
0.00 0.00 FUD XXX Q1
AMA: 2020,Dec,3; 2018,Jan,8; 2017,Jan,8; 2016,Jan,13

86923 electronic
EXCLUDES *Other compatibility test techniques (86920-86922)*
0.00 0.00 FUD XXX Q1
AMA: 2020,Dec,3; 2018,Jan,8; 2017,Jan,8; 2016,Jan,13

86927 Fresh frozen plasma, thawing, each unit
0.00 0.00 FUD XXX S
AMA: 2020,Dec,3

86930 Frozen blood, each unit; freezing (includes preparation)
0.00 0.00 FUD XXX Q1
AMA: 2020,Dec,3; 2018,Jan,8; 2017,Jan,8; 2016,Jan,13

86931 thawing
0.00 0.00 FUD XXX Q1
AMA: 2020,Dec,3; 2018,Jan,8; 2017,Jan,8; 2016,Jan,13

86932 freezing (includes preparation) and thawing
0.00 0.00 FUD XXX Q1
AMA: 2020,Dec,3; 2018,Jan,8; 2017,Jan,8; 2016,Jan,13

86940 Hemolysins and agglutinins; auto, screen, each
0.00 0.00 FUD XXX Q
AMA: 2020,Dec,3

86941 incubated
0.00 0.00 FUD XXX Q
AMA: 2020,Dec,3

86945 Irradiation of blood product, each unit
0.00 0.00 FUD XXX Q1
AMA: 2020,Dec,3; 2018,Jan,8; 2017,Jan,8; 2016,Jan,13

86950 Leukocyte transfusion
EXCLUDES *Infusion allogeneic lymphocytes (38242)*
Leukapheresis (36511)
0.00 0.00 FUD XXX Q1
AMA: 2020,Dec,3; 2018,Jan,8; 2017,Jan,8; 2016,Jan,13

86960 Volume reduction of blood or blood product (eg, red blood cells or platelets), each unit
0.00 0.00 FUD XXX Q1
AMA: 2020,Dec,3; 2018,Jan,8; 2017,Jan,8; 2016,Jan,13

86965 Pooling of platelets or other blood products
EXCLUDES *Autologous WBC injection (0481T)*
Injection platelet rich plasma (0232T)
0.00 0.00 FUD XXX Q1
AMA: 2020,Dec,3; 2018,Jan,8; 2017,Jan,8; 2016,Jan,13

86970 Pretreatment of RBCs for use in RBC antibody detection, identification, and/or compatibility testing; incubation with chemical agents or drugs, each
0.00 0.00 FUD XXX Q1
AMA: 2020,Dec,3

86971 incubation with enzymes, each
0.00 0.00 FUD XXX Q1
AMA: 2020,Dec,3

86972 by density gradient separation
0.00 0.00 FUD XXX Q1
AMA: 2020,Dec,3

86975 Pretreatment of serum for use in RBC antibody identification; incubation with drugs, each
0.00 0.00 FUD XXX Q1
AMA: 2020,Dec,3

86976 by dilution
0.00 0.00 FUD XXX Q1
AMA: 2020,Dec,3

86977 incubation with inhibitors, each
0.00 0.00 FUD XXX Q1
AMA: 2020,Dec,3

Pathology and Laboratory 86860 — 86977

86978 **by differential red cell absorption using patient RBCs or RBCs of known phenotype, each absorption**
0.00 0.00 FUD XXX
AMA: 2020,Dec,3

86985 **Splitting of blood or blood products, each unit**
0.00 0.00 FUD XXX
AMA: 2020,Dec,3; 2018,Jan,8; 2017,Jan,8; 2016,Jan,13

86999 **Unlisted transfusion medicine procedure**
0.00 0.00 FUD XXX
AMA: 2020,Dec,3; 2018,Jan,8; 2017,Jan,8; 2016,Jan,13

87003-87118 Identification of Microorganisms

INCLUDES Bacteriology, mycology, parasitology, and virology

EXCLUDES *Additional tests using molecular probes, chromatography, nucleic acid resequencing, or immunologic techniques (87140-87158)*

Code also:
Modifier 59 for multiple specimens or sites
Modifier 91 for repeat procedures performed on same day

87003 **Animal inoculation, small animal, with observation and dissection**
0.00 0.00 FUD XXX
AMA: 2020,Dec,3

87015 **Concentration (any type), for infectious agents**
EXCLUDES *Direct smear for ova and parasites (87177)*
0.00 0.00 FUD XXX
AMA: 2020,Dec,3

87040 **Culture, bacterial; blood, aerobic, with isolation and presumptive identification of isolates (includes anaerobic culture, if appropriate)**
0.00 0.00 FUD XXX
AMA: 2020,Dec,3; 2018,Jan,8; 2017,Jan,8; 2016,Jan,13

87045 **stool, aerobic, with isolation and preliminary examination (eg, KIA, LIA), Salmonella and Shigella species**
0.00 0.00 FUD XXX
AMA: 2020,Dec,3

87046 **stool, aerobic, additional pathogens, isolation and presumptive identification of isolates, each plate**
0.00 0.00 FUD XXX
AMA: 2020,Dec,3; 2018,Jan,8; 2017,Jan,8; 2016,Jan,13

87070 **any other source except urine, blood or stool, aerobic, with isolation and presumptive identification of isolates**
EXCLUDES *Urine (87088)*
0.00 0.00 FUD XXX
AMA: 2020,Dec,3; 2018,Jan,8; 2017,Jan,8; 2016,Jan,13

87071 **quantitative, aerobic with isolation and presumptive identification of isolates, any source except urine, blood or stool**
EXCLUDES *Urine (87088)*
0.00 0.00 FUD XXX
AMA: 2020,Dec,3; 2018,Jan,8; 2017,Jan,8; 2016,Jan,13

87073 **quantitative, anaerobic with isolation and presumptive identification of isolates, any source except urine, blood or stool**
EXCLUDES *Definitive identification isolates (87076, 87077)*
Typing isolates (87140-87158)
0.00 0.00 FUD XXX
AMA: 2020,Dec,3; 2018,Jan,8; 2017,Jan,8; 2016,Jan,13

87075 **any source, except blood, anaerobic with isolation and presumptive identification of isolates**
0.00 0.00 FUD XXX
AMA: 2020,Dec,3

87076 **anaerobic isolate, additional methods required for definitive identification, each isolate**
0.00 0.00 FUD XXX
AMA: 2020,Dec,3; 2018,Jan,8; 2017,Jan,8; 2016,Jan,13

87077 **aerobic isolate, additional methods required for definitive identification, each isolate**
0.00 0.00 FUD XXX
AMA: 2020,Dec,3; 2018,Jan,8; 2017,Jan,8; 2016,Jan,13

87081 **Culture, presumptive, pathogenic organisms, screening only;**
0.00 0.00 FUD XXX
AMA: 2020,Dec,3; 2018,Jan,8; 2017,Jan,8; 2016,Jan,13

87084 **with colony estimation from density chart**
0.00 0.00 FUD XXX
AMA: 2020,Dec,3

87086 **Culture, bacterial; quantitative colony count, urine**
0.00 0.00 FUD XXX
AMA: 2020,Dec,3; 2018,Jan,8; 2017,Jan,8; 2016,Jan,13

87088 **with isolation and presumptive identification of each isolate, urine**
0.00 0.00 FUD XXX
AMA: 2020,Dec,3; 2018,Jan,8; 2017,Jan,8; 2016,Jan,13

87101 **Culture, fungi (mold or yeast) isolation, with presumptive identification of isolates; skin, hair, or nail**
0.00 0.00 FUD XXX
AMA: 2020,Dec,3; 2018,Jan,8; 2017,Jan,8; 2016,Jan,13

87102 **other source (except blood)**
0.00 0.00 FUD XXX
AMA: 2020,Dec,3

87103 **blood**
0.00 0.00 FUD XXX
AMA: 2020,Dec,3

87106 **Culture, fungi, definitive identification, each organism; yeast**
0.00 0.00 FUD XXX
AMA: 2020,Dec,3

87107 **mold**
0.00 0.00 FUD XXX
AMA: 2020,Dec,3

87109 **Culture, mycoplasma, any source**
0.00 0.00 FUD XXX
AMA: 2020,Dec,3

87110 **Culture, chlamydia, any source**
EXCLUDES *Immunofluorescence staining shell vials (87140)*
0.00 0.00 FUD XXX
AMA: 2020,Dec,3

87116 **Culture, tubercle or other acid-fast bacilli (eg, TB, AFB, mycobacteria) any source, with isolation and presumptive identification of isolates**
EXCLUDES *Concentration (87015)*
0.00 0.00 FUD XXX
AMA: 2020,Dec,3

87118 **Culture, mycobacterial, definitive identification, each isolate**
0.00 0.00 FUD XXX
AMA: 2020,Dec,3

87140-87158 [87154] Additional Culture Typing Techniques

INCLUDES Bacteriology, mycology, parasitology, and virology

EXCLUDES *Reporting molecular procedure codes as substitute for codes in this range (81105-81183 [81173, 81174, 81200, 81201, 81202, 81203, 81204], 81400-81408, [81479])*

Code also:
Definitive identification
Modifier 59 for multiple specimens or sites
Modifier 91 for repeat procedures performed on same day

87140 **Culture, typing; immunofluorescent method, each antiserum**
0.00 0.00 FUD XXX
AMA: 2020,Dec,3; 2020,OctSE,1; 2020,OctSE,1; 2018,Jan,8; 2017,Jan,8; 2016,Jan,13

87143 **gas liquid chromatography (GLC) or high pressure liquid chromatography (HPLC) method**
0.00 0.00 FUD XXX
AMA: 2020,Dec,3; 2020,OctSE,1; 2020,OctSE,1

87147 **immunologic method, other than immunofluorescence (eg, agglutination grouping), per antiserum**
0.00 0.00 FUD XXX
AMA: 2020,Dec,3; 2020,OctSE,1; 2020,OctSE,1; 2018,Jan,8; 2017,Jan,8; 2016,Jan,13

87149 **identification by nucleic acid (DNA or RNA) probe, direct probe technique, per culture or isolate, each organism probed**
0.00 0.00 FUD XXX
AMA: 2020,Dec,3; 2020,OctSE,1; 2020,OctSE,1; 2018,Jan,8; 2017,Jan,8; 2016,Jan,13

87150 **identification by nucleic acid (DNA or RNA) probe, amplified probe technique, per culture or isolate, each organism probed**
0.00 0.00 FUD XXX
AMA: 2020,Dec,3; 2020,OctSE,1; 2020,OctSE,1; 2018,Jan,8; 2017,Jan,8; 2016,Jan,13

● # 87154 **identification of blood pathogen and resistance typing, when performed, by nucleic acid (DNA or RNA) probe, multiplexed amplified probe technique including multiplex reverse transcription, when performed, per culture or isolate, 6 or more targets**
0.00 0.00 FUD 000

87152 **identification by pulse field gel typing**
0.00 0.00 FUD XXX
AMA: 2020,Dec,3; 2020,OctSE,1; 2020,OctSE,1; 2018,Jan,8; 2017,Jan,8; 2016,Jan,13

87153 **identification by nucleic acid sequencing method, each isolate (eg, sequencing of the 16S rRNA gene)**
0.00 0.00 FUD XXX
AMA: 2020,Dec,3; 2020,OctSE,1; 2020,OctSE,1; 2018,Jan,8; 2017,Jan,8; 2016,Jan,13

87154 **Resequenced code. See code following 87150.**

87158 **other methods**
0.00 0.00 FUD XXX
AMA: 2020,Dec,3; 2020,OctSE,1; 2020,OctSE,1; 2018,Jan,8; 2017,Jan,8; 2016,Jan,13

87164-87255 Identification of Organism from Primary Source and Sensitivity Studies

INCLUDES Bacteriology, mycology, parasitology, and virology

EXCLUDES *Additional tests using molecular probes, chromatography, or immunologic techniques (87140-87158)*

Code also:
Modifier 59 for multiple specimens or sites
Modifier 91 for repeat procedures performed on same day

87164 **Dark field examination, any source (eg, penile, vaginal, oral, skin); includes specimen collection**
0.00 0.00 FUD XXX
AMA: 2020,Dec,3

87166 **without collection**
0.00 0.00 FUD XXX
AMA: 2020,Dec,3

87168 **Macroscopic examination; arthropod**
0.00 0.00 FUD XXX
AMA: 2020,Dec,3

87169 **parasite**
0.00 0.00 FUD XXX
AMA: 2020,Dec,3

87172 **Pinworm exam (eg, cellophane tape prep)**
0.00 0.00 FUD XXX
AMA: 2020,Dec,3

87176 **Homogenization, tissue, for culture**
0.00 0.00 FUD XXX
AMA: 2020,Dec,3

87177 **Ova and parasites, direct smears, concentration and identification**

EXCLUDES *Coccidia or microsporidia exam (87207)*
Complex special stain (trichrome, iron hematoxylin) (87209)
Concentration for infectious agents (87015)
Direct smears from primary source (87207)
Nucleic acid probes in cytologic material (88365)

0.00 0.00 FUD XXX
AMA: 2020,Dec,3; 2018,Jan,8; 2017,Jan,8; 2016,Jan,13

87181 **Susceptibility studies, antimicrobial agent; agar dilution method, per agent (eg, antibiotic gradient strip)**
0.00 0.00 FUD XXX
AMA: 2020,Dec,3; 2018,Jan,8; 2017,Jan,8; 2016,Jan,13

87184 **disk method, per plate (12 or fewer agents)**
0.00 0.00 FUD XXX
AMA: 2020,Dec,3; 2018,Jan,8; 2017,Jan,8; 2016,Jan,13

87185 **enzyme detection (eg, beta lactamase), per enzyme**
0.00 0.00 FUD XXX
AMA: 2020,Dec,3; 2018,Jan,8; 2017,Jan,8; 2016,Jan,13

87186 **microdilution or agar dilution (minimum inhibitory concentration [MIC] or breakpoint), each multi-antimicrobial, per plate**
0.00 0.00 FUD XXX
AMA: 2020,Dec,3; 2018,Jan,8; 2017,Jan,8; 2016,Jan,13

\+ 87187 **microdilution or agar dilution, minimum lethal concentration (MLC), each plate (List separately in addition to code for primary procedure)**
Code first (87186, 87188)
0.00 0.00 FUD XXX
AMA: 2020,Dec,3; 2018,Jan,8; 2017,Jan,8; 2016,Jan,13

87188 **macrobroth dilution method, each agent**
0.00 0.00 FUD XXX
AMA: 2020,Dec,3; 2018,Jan,8; 2017,Jan,8; 2016,Jan,13

87190 **mycobacteria, proportion method, each agent**

EXCLUDES *Other mycobacterial susceptibility studies (87181, 87184, 87186, 87188)*

0.00 0.00 FUD XXX
AMA: 2020,Dec,3

87197 **Serum bactericidal titer (Schlichter test)**
0.00 0.00 FUD XXX
AMA: 2020,Dec,3

87205 **Smear, primary source with interpretation; Gram or Giemsa stain for bacteria, fungi, or cell types**
0.00 0.00 FUD XXX
AMA: 2020,Dec,3; 2018,Jan,8; 2017,Jan,8; 2016,Jan,13

87206 **fluorescent and/or acid fast stain for bacteria, fungi, parasites, viruses or cell types**
0.00 0.00 FUD XXX
AMA: 2020,Dec,3

87207 **special stain for inclusion bodies or parasites (eg, malaria, coccidia, microsporidia, trypanosomes, herpes viruses)**

EXCLUDES *Direct smears with concentration and identification (87177)*
Fat, fibers, meat, nasal eosinophils, starch (89049-89240)
Thick smear preparation (87015)

0.00 0.00 FUD XXX
AMA: 2020,Dec,3; 2018,Jan,8; 2017,Jan,8; 2016,Jan,13

87209 **complex special stain (eg, trichrome, iron hemotoxylin) for ova and parasites**
0.00 0.00 FUD XXX
AMA: 2020,Dec,3; 2018,Jan,8; 2017,Jan,8; 2016,Jan,13

87210 **wet mount for infectious agents (eg, saline, India ink, KOH preps)**

EXCLUDES *KOH evaluation skin, hair, or nails (87220)*

0.00 0.00 FUD XXX

AMA: 2020,Dec,3; 2018,Jan,8; 2017,Jan,8; 2016,May,13

87220 **Tissue examination by KOH slide of samples from skin, hair, or nails for fungi or ectoparasite ova or mites (eg, scabies)**

0.00 0.00 FUD XXX

AMA: 2020,Dec,3

87230 **Toxin or antitoxin assay, tissue culture (eg, Clostridium difficile toxin)**

0.00 0.00 FUD XXX

AMA: 2020,Dec,3

87250 **Virus isolation; inoculation of embryonated eggs, or small animal, includes observation and dissection**

0.00 0.00 FUD XXX

AMA: 2020,Dec,3; 2020,OctSE,1; 2020,OctSE,1

87252 **tissue culture inoculation, observation, and presumptive identification by cytopathic effect**

0.00 0.00 FUD XXX

AMA: 2020,Dec,3

87253 **tissue culture, additional studies or definitive identification (eg, hemabsorption, neutralization, immunofluorescence stain), each isolate**

EXCLUDES *Electron microscopy (88348)*
Inclusion bodies in:
Fluids (88106)
Smears (87207-87210)
Tissue sections (88304-88309)

0.00 0.00 FUD XXX

AMA: 2020,Dec,3

87254 **centrifuge enhanced (shell vial) technique, includes identification with immunofluorescence stain, each virus**

Code also (87252)

0.00 0.00 FUD XXX

AMA: 2020,Dec,3; 2018,Jan,8; 2017,Jan,8; 2016,Jan,13

87255 **including identification by non-immunologic method, other than by cytopathic effect (eg, virus specific enzymatic activity)**

0.00 0.00 FUD XXX

AMA: 2020,Dec,3; 2020,OctSE,1; 2020,OctSE,1; 2018,Jan,8; 2017,Jan,8; 2016,Jan,13

87260-87300 Fluorescence Microscopy by Organism

INCLUDES Primary source only

EXCLUDES *Comparable tests on culture material (87140-87158)*
Identification antibodies (86602-86804)
Immunoassay techniques with direct/visual observation for infectious antigens (87260-87300)
Microscopic identification infectious agents via direct/indirect immunofluorescent assay (IFA) techniques (87301-87451, 87802-87899 [87806, 87811])
Nonspecific agent detection (87299, 87449, 87797-87799, 87899)

Code also modifier 59 for different species or strains reported by same code

87260 **Infectious agent antigen detection by immunofluorescent technique; adenovirus**

0.00 0.00 FUD XXX

AMA: 2020,Dec,3; 2020,OctSE,1; 2020,OctSE,1; 2020,AugSE,1; 2020,AugSE,1; 2020,AugSE,1

87265 **Bordetella pertussis/parapertussis**

0.00 0.00 FUD XXX

AMA: 2020,Dec,3; 2020,OctSE,1; 2020,OctSE,1; 2020,AugSE,1; 2020,AugSE,1; 2020,AugSE,1

87267 **Enterovirus, direct fluorescent antibody (DFA)**

0.00 0.00 FUD XXX

AMA: 2020,Dec,3; 2020,OctSE,1; 2020,OctSE,1; 2020,AugSE,1; 2020,AugSE,1; 2020,AugSE,1; 2018,Jan,8; 2017,Jan,8; 2016,Jan,13

87269 **giardia**

0.00 0.00 FUD XXX

AMA: 2020,Dec,3; 2020,OctSE,1; 2020,OctSE,1; 2020,AugSE,1; 2020,AugSE,1; 2020,AugSE,1

87270 **Chlamydia trachomatis**

0.00 0.00 FUD XXX

AMA: 2020,Dec,3; 2020,OctSE,1; 2020,OctSE,1; 2020,AugSE,1; 2020,AugSE,1; 2020,AugSE,1

87271 **Cytomegalovirus, direct fluorescent antibody (DFA)**

0.00 0.00 FUD XXX

AMA: 2020,Dec,3; 2020,OctSE,1; 2020,OctSE,1; 2020,AugSE,1; 2020,AugSE,1; 2020,AugSE,1; 2018,Jan,8; 2017,Jan,8; 2016,Jan,13

87272 **cryptosporidium**

0.00 0.00 FUD XXX

AMA: 2020,Dec,3; 2020,OctSE,1; 2020,OctSE,1; 2020,AugSE,1; 2020,AugSE,1; 2020,AugSE,1

87273 **Herpes simplex virus type 2**

0.00 0.00 FUD XXX

AMA: 2020,Dec,3; 2020,OctSE,1; 2020,OctSE,1; 2020,AugSE,1; 2020,AugSE,1; 2020,AugSE,1

87274 **Herpes simplex virus type 1**

0.00 0.00 FUD XXX

AMA: 2020,Dec,3; 2020,OctSE,1; 2020,OctSE,1; 2020,AugSE,1; 2020,AugSE,1; 2020,AugSE,1

87275 **influenza B virus**

0.00 0.00 FUD XXX

AMA: 2020,Dec,3; 2020,OctSE,1; 2020,OctSE,1; 2020,AugSE,1; 2020,AugSE,1; 2020,AugSE,1; 2018,Jan,8; 2017,Jan,8; 2016,Jan,13

87276 **influenza A virus**

0.00 0.00 FUD XXX

AMA: 2020,Dec,3; 2020,OctSE,1; 2020,OctSE,1; 2020,AugSE,1; 2020,AugSE,1; 2020,AugSE,1; 2018,Jan,8; 2017,Jan,8; 2016,Jan,13

87278 **Legionella pneumophila**

0.00 0.00 FUD XXX

AMA: 2020,Dec,3; 2020,OctSE,1; 2020,OctSE,1; 2020,AugSE,1; 2020,AugSE,1; 2020,AugSE,1

87279 **Parainfluenza virus, each type**

0.00 0.00 FUD XXX

AMA: 2020,Dec,3; 2020,OctSE,1; 2020,OctSE,1; 2020,AugSE,1; 2020,AugSE,1; 2020,AugSE,1

87280 **respiratory syncytial virus**

0.00 0.00 FUD XXX

AMA: 2020,Dec,3; 2020,OctSE,1; 2020,OctSE,1; 2020,AugSE,1; 2020,AugSE,1; 2020,AugSE,1

87281 **Pneumocystis carinii**

0.00 0.00 FUD XXX

AMA: 2020,Dec,3; 2020,OctSE,1; 2020,OctSE,1; 2020,AugSE,1; 2020,AugSE,1; 2020,AugSE,1

87283 **Rubeola**

0.00 0.00 FUD XXX

AMA: 2020,Dec,3; 2020,OctSE,1; 2020,OctSE,1; 2020,AugSE,1; 2020,AugSE,1; 2020,AugSE,1

87285 **Treponema pallidum**

0.00 0.00 FUD XXX

AMA: 2020,Dec,3; 2020,OctSE,1; 2020,OctSE,1; 2020,AugSE,1; 2020,AugSE,1; 2020,AugSE,1

87290 **Varicella zoster virus**

0.00 0.00 FUD XXX

AMA: 2020,Dec,3; 2020,OctSE,1; 2020,OctSE,1; 2020,AugSE,1; 2020,AugSE,1; 2020,AugSE,1

87299 **not otherwise specified, each organism**

0.00 0.00 FUD XXX

AMA: 2020,Dec,3; 2020,OctSE,1; 2020,OctSE,1; 2020,AugSE,1; 2020,AugSE,1; 2020,AugSE,1; 2018,Jan,8; 2017,Jan,8; 2016,Jan,13

87300 **Infectious agent antigen detection by immunofluorescent technique, polyvalent for multiple organisms, each polyvalent antiserum**

EXCLUDES *Physician evaluation infectious disease agents by immunofluorescence (88346)*

0.00 0.00 FUD XXX

AMA: 2020,Dec,3; 2020,OctSE,1; 2020,OctSE,1; 2020,AugSE,1; 2020,AugSE,1; 2020,AugSE,1

87301-87451 [87428] Enzyme Immunoassay Technique by Organism

INCLUDES Primary source only

EXCLUDES *Comparable tests on culture material (87140-87158)*
Identification antibodies (86602-86804)
Nonspecific agent detection (87449, 87797-87799, 87899)

Code also modifier 59 for different species or strains reported by same code

▲ 87301 **Infectious agent antigen detection by immunoassay technique, (eg, enzyme immunoassay [EIA], enzyme-linked immunosorbent assay [ELISA], fluorescence immunoassay [FIA], immunochemiluminometric assay [IMCA]) qualitative or semiquantitative; adenovirus enteric types 40/41**

0.00 0.00 FUD XXX

AMA: 2020,Dec,3; 2020,OctSE,1; 2020,NovSE,1; 2020,OctSE,1; 2020,AugSE,1; 2020,AugSE,1; 2020,AugSE,1; 2020,May,3; 2020,JuneSE,1; 2018,Jan,8; 2017,Jan,8; 2016,Jan,13

▲ 87305 **Aspergillus**

0.00 0.00 FUD XXX

AMA: 2020,Dec,3; 2020,OctSE,1; 2020,OctSE,1; 2020,AugSE,1; 2020,AugSE,1; 2020,AugSE,1

▲ 87320 **Chlamydia trachomatis**

0.00 0.00 FUD XXX

AMA: 2020,Dec,3; 2020,OctSE,1; 2020,OctSE,1; 2020,AugSE,1; 2020,AugSE,1; 2020,AugSE,1

▲ 87324 **Clostridium difficile toxin(s)**

0.00 0.00 FUD XXX

AMA: 2020,Dec,3; 2020,OctSE,1; 2020,OctSE,1; 2020,AugSE,1; 2020,AugSE,1; 2020,AugSE,1

▲ 87327 **Cryptococcus neoformans**

EXCLUDES *Cryptococcus latex agglutination (86403)*

0.00 0.00 FUD XXX

AMA: 2020,Dec,3; 2020,OctSE,1; 2020,OctSE,1; 2020,AugSE,1; 2020,AugSE,1; 2020,AugSE,1

▲ 87328 **cryptosporidium**

0.00 0.00 FUD XXX

AMA: 2020,Dec,3; 2020,OctSE,1; 2020,OctSE,1; 2020,AugSE,1; 2020,AugSE,1; 2020,AugSE,1

▲ 87329 **giardia**

0.00 0.00 FUD XXX

AMA: 2020,Dec,3; 2020,OctSE,1; 2020,OctSE,1; 2020,AugSE,1; 2020,AugSE,1; 2020,AugSE,1

▲ 87332 **cytomegalovirus**

0.00 0.00 FUD XXX

AMA: 2020,Dec,3; 2020,OctSE,1; 2020,OctSE,1; 2020,AugSE,1; 2020,AugSE,1; 2020,AugSE,1

▲ 87335 **Escherichia coli 0157**

EXCLUDES *Giardia antigen (87329)*

0.00 0.00 FUD XXX

AMA: 2020,Dec,3; 2020,OctSE,1; 2020,OctSE,1; 2020,AugSE,1; 2020,AugSE,1; 2020,AugSE,1

▲ 87336 **Entamoeba histolytica dispar group**

0.00 0.00 FUD XXX

AMA: 2020,Dec,3; 2020,OctSE,1; 2020,OctSE,1; 2020,AugSE,1; 2020,AugSE,1; 2020,AugSE,1

▲ 87337 **Entamoeba histolytica group**

0.00 0.00 FUD XXX

AMA: 2020,Dec,3; 2020,OctSE,1; 2020,OctSE,1; 2020,AugSE,1; 2020,AugSE,1; 2020,AugSE,1

▲ 87338 **Helicobacter pylori, stool**

0.00 0.00 FUD XXX

AMA: 2020,Dec,3; 2020,OctSE,1; 2020,OctSE,1; 2020,AugSE,1; 2020,AugSE,1; 2020,AugSE,1; 2018,Jan,8; 2017,Jan,8; 2016,Jan,13

▲ 87339 **Helicobacter pylori**

EXCLUDES *H. pylori:*
Breath and blood by mass spectrometry (83013-83014)
Liquid scintillation counter (78267-78268)
Stool (87338)

0.00 0.00 FUD XXX

AMA: 2020,Dec,3; 2020,OctSE,1; 2020,OctSE,1; 2020,AugSE,1; 2020,AugSE,1; 2020,AugSE,1

▲ 87340 **hepatitis B surface antigen (HBsAg)**

0.00 0.00 FUD XXX

AMA: 2020,Dec,3; 2020,OctSE,1; 2020,OctSE,1; 2020,AugSE,1; 2020,AugSE,1; 2020,AugSE,1; 2018,Jan,8; 2017,Jan,8; 2016,Jan,13

▲ 87341 **hepatitis B surface antigen (HBsAg) neutralization**

0.00 0.00 FUD XXX

AMA: 2020,Dec,3; 2020,OctSE,1; 2020,OctSE,1; 2020,AugSE,1; 2020,AugSE,1; 2020,AugSE,1

▲ 87350 **hepatitis Be antigen (HBeAg)**

0.00 0.00 FUD XXX

AMA: 2020,Dec,3; 2020,OctSE,1; 2020,OctSE,1; 2020,AugSE,1; 2020,AugSE,1; 2020,AugSE,1

▲ 87380 **hepatitis, delta agent**

0.00 0.00 FUD XXX

AMA: 2020,Dec,3; 2020,OctSE,1; 2020,OctSE,1; 2020,AugSE,1; 2020,AugSE,1; 2020,AugSE,1

▲ 87385 **Histoplasma capsulatum**

0.00 0.00 FUD XXX

AMA: 2020,Dec,3; 2020,OctSE,1; 2020,OctSE,1; 2020,AugSE,1; 2020,AugSE,1; 2020,AugSE,1

▲ 87389 **HIV-1 antigen(s), with HIV-1 and HIV-2 antibodies, single result**

Code also modifier 92 for test performed using kit or transportable instrument comprising (all or part) single-use, disposable analytical chamber

0.00 0.00 FUD XXX

AMA: 2020,Dec,3; 2020,OctSE,1; 2020,OctSE,1; 2020,AugSE,1; 2020,AugSE,1; 2020,AugSE,1

▲ 87390 **HIV-1**

0.00 0.00 FUD XXX

AMA: 2020,Dec,3; 2020,OctSE,1; 2020,OctSE,1; 2020,AugSE,1; 2020,AugSE,1; 2020,AugSE,1

▲ 87391 **HIV-2**

0.00 0.00 FUD XXX

AMA: 2020,Dec,3; 2020,OctSE,1; 2020,OctSE,1; 2020,AugSE,1; 2020,AugSE,1; 2020,AugSE,1

▲ 87400 **Influenza, A or B, each**

0.00 0.00 FUD XXX

AMA: 2020,Dec,3; 2020,OctSE,1; 2020,NovSE,1; 2020,OctSE,1; 2020,AugSE,1; 2020,AugSE,1; 2020,AugSE,1; 2018,Jan,8; 2017,Jan,8; 2016,Jan,13

▲ 87420 **respiratory syncytial virus**

0.00 0.00 FUD XXX

AMA: 2020,Dec,3; 2020,OctSE,1; 2020,OctSE,1; 2020,AugSE,1; 2020,AugSE,1; 2020,AugSE,1

▲ 87425 **rotavirus**

0.00 0.00 FUD XXX

AMA: 2020,Dec,3; 2020,OctSE,1; 2020,OctSE,1; 2020,AugSE,1; 2020,AugSE,1; 2020,AugSE,1

▲ 87426 **severe acute respiratory syndrome coronavirus (eg, SARS-CoV, SARS-CoV-2 [COVID-19])**

AMA: 2020,Dec,3; 2020,OctSE,1; 2020,NovSE,1; 2020,OctSE,1; 2020,AugSE,1; 2020,AugSE,1; 2020,AugSE,1

● # **87428** **severe acute respiratory syndrome coronavirus (eg, SARS-CoV, SARS-CoV-2 [COVID-19]) and influenza virus types A and B**
0.00 0.00 FUD XXX
AMA: 2020,Dec,3; 2020,OctSE,1

▲ **87427** **Shiga-like toxin**
0.00 0.00 FUD XXX
AMA: 2020,Dec,3; 2020,OctSE,1; 2020,OctSE,1; 2020,AugSE,1; 2020,AugSE,1; 2020,AugSE,1

87428 **Resequenced code. See code following 87426.**

▲ **87430** **Streptococcus, group A**
0.00 0.00 FUD XXX
AMA: 2020,Dec,3; 2020,OctSE,1; 2020,OctSE,1; 2020,AugSE,1; 2020,AugSE,1; 2020,AugSE,1; 2018,Jan,8; 2017,Jan,8; 2016,Jan,13

▲ **87449** **not otherwise specified, each organism**
0.00 0.00 FUD XXX
AMA: 2020,Dec,3; 2020,OctSE,1; 2020,OctSE,1; 2020,AugSE,1; 2020,AugSE,1; 2020,AugSE,1; 2018,Jan,8; 2017,Jan,8; 2016,Jan,13

87450 ~~**single step method, not otherwise specified, each organism**~~
To report, see (87301-87451 [87428], 87802-87899 [87806, 87811])

▲ **87451** **polyvalent for multiple organisms, each polyvalent antiserum**
0.00 0.00 FUD XXX
AMA: 2020,Dec,3; 2020,OctSE,1; 2020,OctSE,1; 2020,AugSE,1; 2020,AugSE,1; 2020,AugSE,1

87471-87801 [87623, 87624, 87625] Detection Infectious Agent by Probe Techniques

INCLUDES Primary source only

EXCLUDES *Comparable tests on culture material (87140-87158)*
Identification antibodies (86602-86804)
Nonspecific agent detection (87299, 87449, 87797-87799, 87899)
Reporting molecular procedure codes as substitute for codes in this range (81161-81408 [81105, 81106, 81107, 81108, 81109, 81110, 81111, 81112, 81120, 81121, 81161, 81162, 81230, 81231, 81238, 81269, 81283, 81287, 81288, 81334])

Code also modifier 59 for different species or strains reported by same code

87471 **Infectious agent detection by nucleic acid (DNA or RNA); Bartonella henselae and Bartonella quintana, amplified probe technique**
0.00 0.00 FUD XXX
AMA: 2020,Dec,3; 2020,OctSE,1; 2020,Oct,11; 2020,OctSE,1; 2020,AugSE,1; 2020,AugSE,1; 2020,AugSE,1; 2018,Jan,8; 2017,Jan,8; 2016,Jan,13

87472 **Bartonella henselae and Bartonella quintana, quantification**
0.00 0.00 FUD XXX
AMA: 2020,Dec,3; 2020,OctSE,1; 2020,OctSE,1; 2020,AugSE,1; 2020,AugSE,1; 2020,AugSE,1; 2020,AugSE,1; 2018,Jan,8; 2017,Jan,8; 2016,Jan,13

87475 **Borrelia burgdorferi, direct probe technique**
0.00 0.00 FUD XXX
AMA: 2020,Dec,3; 2020,OctSE,1; 2020,OctSE,1; 2020,AugSE,1; 2020,AugSE,1; 2020,AugSE,1; 2018,Jan,8; 2017,Jan,8; 2016,Jan,13

87476 **Borrelia burgdorferi, amplified probe technique**
0.00 0.00 FUD XXX
AMA: 2020,Dec,3; 2020,OctSE,1; 2020,OctSE,1; 2020,AugSE,1; 2020,AugSE,1; 2020,AugSE,1; 2018,Jan,8; 2017,Jan,8; 2016,Jan,13

87480 **Candida species, direct probe technique**
0.00 0.00 FUD XXX
AMA: 2020,Dec,3; 2020,OctSE,1; 2020,OctSE,1; 2020,AugSE,1; 2020,AugSE,1; 2020,AugSE,1; 2018,Jan,8; 2017,Jan,8; 2016,Jan,13

87481 **Candida species, amplified probe technique**
0.00 0.00 FUD XXX
AMA: 2020,Dec,3; 2020,OctSE,1; 2020,OctSE,1; 2020,AugSE,1; 2020,AugSE,1; 2020,AugSE,1; 2018,Jan,8; 2017,Jan,8; 2016,Jan,13

87482 **Candida species, quantification**
0.00 0.00 FUD XXX
AMA: 2020,Dec,3; 2020,OctSE,1; 2020,OctSE,1; 2020,AugSE,1; 2020,AugSE,1; 2020,AugSE,1; 2018,Jan,8; 2017,Jan,8; 2016,Jan,13

87483 **central nervous system pathogen (eg, Neisseria meningitidis, Streptococcus pneumoniae, Listeria, Haemophilus influenzae, E. coli, Streptococcus agalactiae, enterovirus, human parechovirus, herpes simplex virus type 1 and 2, human herpesvirus 6, cytomegalovirus, varicella zoster virus, Cryptococcus), includes multiplex reverse transcription, when performed, and multiplex amplified probe technique, multiple types or subtypes, 12-25 targets**
0.00 0.00 FUD XXX
AMA: 2020,Dec,3; 2020,OctSE,1; 2020,OctSE,1; 2020,AugSE,1; 2020,AugSE,1; 2020,AugSE,1

87485 **Chlamydia pneumoniae, direct probe technique**
0.00 0.00 FUD XXX
AMA: 2020,Dec,3; 2020,OctSE,1; 2020,OctSE,1; 2020,AugSE,1; 2020,AugSE,1; 2020,AugSE,1; 2018,Jan,8; 2017,Jan,8; 2016,Jan,13

87486 **Chlamydia pneumoniae, amplified probe technique**
0.00 0.00 FUD XXX
AMA: 2020,Dec,3; 2020,OctSE,1; 2020,OctSE,1; 2020,AugSE,1; 2020,AugSE,1; 2020,AugSE,1; 2018,Jan,8; 2017,Jan,8; 2016,Jan,13

87487 **Chlamydia pneumoniae, quantification**
0.00 0.00 FUD XXX
AMA: 2020,Dec,3; 2020,OctSE,1; 2020,OctSE,1; 2020,AugSE,1; 2020,AugSE,1; 2020,AugSE,1; 2018,Jan,8; 2017,Jan,8; 2016,Jan,13

87490 **Chlamydia trachomatis, direct probe technique**
0.00 0.00 FUD XXX
AMA: 2020,Dec,3; 2020,OctSE,1; 2020,OctSE,1; 2020,AugSE,1; 2020,AugSE,1; 2020,AugSE,1; 2018,Jan,8; 2017,Jan,8; 2016,Jan,13

87491 **Chlamydia trachomatis, amplified probe technique**
0.00 0.00 FUD XXX
AMA: 2020,Dec,3; 2020,OctSE,1; 2020,OctSE,1; 2020,AugSE,1; 2020,AugSE,1; 2020,AugSE,1; 2018,Jan,8; 2017,Jan,8; 2016,Jan,13

87492 **Chlamydia trachomatis, quantification**
0.00 0.00 FUD XXX
AMA: 2020,Dec,3; 2020,OctSE,1; 2020,OctSE,1; 2020,AugSE,1; 2020,AugSE,1; 2020,AugSE,1; 2018,Jan,8; 2017,Jan,8; 2016,Jan,13

87493 **Clostridium difficile, toxin gene(s), amplified probe technique**
0.00 0.00 FUD XXX
AMA: 2020,Dec,3; 2020,OctSE,1; 2020,OctSE,1; 2020,AugSE,1; 2020,AugSE,1; 2020,AugSE,1; 2018,Jan,8; 2017,Jan,8; 2016,Jan,13

87495 **cytomegalovirus, direct probe technique**
0.00 0.00 FUD XXX
AMA: 2020,Dec,3; 2020,OctSE,1; 2020,OctSE,1; 2020,AugSE,1; 2020,AugSE,1; 2020,AugSE,1; 2018,Jan,8; 2017,Jan,8; 2016,Jan,13

87496 **cytomegalovirus, amplified probe technique**
0.00 0.00 FUD XXX
AMA: 2020,Dec,3; 2020,OctSE,1; 2020,OctSE,1; 2020,AugSE,1; 2020,AugSE,1; 2020,AugSE,1; 2018,Jan,8; 2017,Jan,8; 2016,Jan,13

87497 **cytomegalovirus, quantification**
0.00 0.00 FUD XXX
AMA: 2020,Dec,3; 2020,OctSE,1; 2020,OctSE,1; 2020,AugSE,1; 2020,AugSE,1; 2020,AugSE,1; 2018,Jan,8; 2017,Jan,8; 2016,Jan,13

87498 **enterovirus, amplified probe technique, includes reverse transcription when performed**
0.00 0.00 FUD XXX
AMA: 2020,Dec,3; 2020,OctSE,1; 2020,OctSE,1; 2020,AugSE,1; 2020,AugSE,1; 2020,AugSE,1; 2018,Jan,8; 2017,Jan,8; 2016,Jan,13

87500 **vancomycin resistance (eg, enterococcus species van A, van B), amplified probe technique**
0.00 0.00 FUD XXX
AMA: 2020,Dec,3; 2020,OctSE,1; 2020,OctSE,1; 2020,AugSE,1; 2020,AugSE,1; 2020,AugSE,1; 2018,Jan,8; 2017,Jan,8; 2016,Jan,13

87501 **influenza virus, includes reverse transcription, when performed, and amplified probe technique, each type or subtype**
0.00 0.00 FUD XXX
AMA: 2020,Dec,3; 2020,OctSE,1; 2020,OctSE,1; 2020,AugSE,1; 2020,AugSE,1; 2020,AugSE,1; 2018,Jan,8; 2017,Jan,8; 2016,Jan,13

87502 **influenza virus, for multiple types or sub-types, includes multiplex reverse transcription, when performed, and multiplex amplified probe technique, first 2 types or sub-types**
0.00 0.00 FUD XXX
AMA: 2020,Dec,3; 2020,OctSE,1; 2020,OctSE,1; 2020,AugSE,1; 2020,AugSE,1; 2020,AugSE,1; 2018,Jan,8; 2017,Jan,8; 2016,Jan,13

\+ **87503** **influenza virus, for multiple types or sub-types, includes multiplex reverse transcription, when performed, and multiplex amplified probe technique, each additional influenza virus type or sub-type beyond 2 (List separately in addition to code for primary procedure)**
Code first (87502)
0.00 0.00 FUD XXX
AMA: 2020,Dec,3; 2020,OctSE,1; 2020,OctSE,1; 2020,AugSE,1; 2020,AugSE,1; 2020,AugSE,1; 2018,Jan,8; 2017,Jan,8; 2016,Jan,13

87505 **gastrointestinal pathogen (eg, Clostridium difficile, E. coli, Salmonella, Shigella, norovirus, Giardia), includes multiplex reverse transcription, when performed, and multiplex amplified probe technique, multiple types or subtypes, 3-5 targets**
0.00 0.00 FUD XXX
AMA: 2020,Dec,3; 2020,OctSE,1; 2020,OctSE,1; 2020,AugSE,1; 2020,AugSE,1; 2020,AugSE,1

87506 **gastrointestinal pathogen (eg, Clostridium difficile, E. coli, Salmonella, Shigella, norovirus, Giardia), includes multiplex reverse transcription, when performed, and multiplex amplified probe technique, multiple types or subtypes, 6-11 targets**
0.00 0.00 FUD XXX
AMA: 2020,Dec,3; 2020,OctSE,1; 2020,OctSE,1; 2020,AugSE,1; 2020,AugSE,1; 2020,AugSE,1

87507 **gastrointestinal pathogen (eg, Clostridium difficile, E. coli, Salmonella, Shigella, norovirus, Giardia), includes multiplex reverse transcription, when performed, and multiplex amplified probe technique, multiple types or subtypes, 12-25 targets**
0.00 0.00 FUD XXX
AMA: 2020,Dec,3; 2020,OctSE,1; 2020,OctSE,1; 2020,AugSE,1; 2020,AugSE,1; 2020,AugSE,1

87510 **Gardnerella vaginalis, direct probe technique**
0.00 0.00 FUD XXX
AMA: 2020,Dec,3; 2020,OctSE,1; 2020,OctSE,1; 2020,AugSE,1; 2020,AugSE,1; 2020,AugSE,1; 2018,Jan,8; 2017,Jan,8; 2016,Jan,13

87511 **Gardnerella vaginalis, amplified probe technique**
0.00 0.00 FUD XXX
AMA: 2020,Dec,3; 2020,OctSE,1; 2020,OctSE,1; 2020,AugSE,1; 2020,AugSE,1; 2020,AugSE,1; 2018,Jan,8; 2017,Jan,8; 2016,Jan,13

87512 **Gardnerella vaginalis, quantification**
0.00 0.00 FUD XXX
AMA: 2020,Dec,3; 2020,OctSE,1; 2020,OctSE,1; 2020,AugSE,1; 2020,AugSE,1; 2020,AugSE,1; 2018,Jan,8; 2017,Jan,8; 2016,Jan,13

87516 **hepatitis B virus, amplified probe technique**
0.00 0.00 FUD XXX
AMA: 2020,Dec,3; 2020,OctSE,1; 2020,OctSE,1; 2020,AugSE,1; 2020,AugSE,1; 2020,AugSE,1; 2018,Jan,8; 2017,Jan,8; 2016,Jan,13

87517 **hepatitis B virus, quantification**
0.00 0.00 FUD XXX
AMA: 2020,Dec,3; 2020,OctSE,1; 2020,OctSE,1; 2020,AugSE,1; 2020,AugSE,1; 2020,AugSE,1; 2018,Jan,8; 2017,Jan,8; 2016,Jan,13

87520 **hepatitis C, direct probe technique**
0.00 0.00 FUD XXX
AMA: 2020,Dec,3; 2020,OctSE,1; 2020,OctSE,1; 2020,AugSE,1; 2020,AugSE,1; 2020,AugSE,1; 2018,Jan,8; 2017,Jan,8; 2016,Jan,13

87521 **hepatitis C, amplified probe technique, includes reverse transcription when performed**
0.00 0.00 FUD XXX
AMA: 2020,Dec,3; 2020,OctSE,1; 2020,OctSE,1; 2020,AugSE,1; 2020,AugSE,1; 2020,AugSE,1; 2018,Jan,8; 2017,Jan,8; 2016,Jan,13

87522 **hepatitis C, quantification, includes reverse transcription when performed**
0.00 0.00 FUD XXX
AMA: 2020,Dec,3; 2020,OctSE,1; 2020,OctSE,1; 2020,AugSE,1; 2020,AugSE,1; 2020,AugSE,1; 2018,Jan,8; 2017,Jan,8; 2016,Jan,13

87525 **hepatitis G, direct probe technique**
0.00 0.00 FUD XXX
AMA: 2020,Dec,3; 2020,OctSE,1; 2020,OctSE,1; 2020,AugSE,1; 2020,AugSE,1; 2020,AugSE,1; 2018,Jan,8; 2017,Jan,8; 2016,Jan,13

87526 **hepatitis G, amplified probe technique**
0.00 0.00 FUD XXX
AMA: 2020,Dec,3; 2020,OctSE,1; 2020,OctSE,1; 2020,AugSE,1; 2020,AugSE,1; 2020,AugSE,1; 2018,Jan,8; 2017,Jan,8; 2016,Jan,13

87527 **hepatitis G, quantification**
0.00 0.00 FUD XXX
AMA: 2020,Dec,3; 2020,OctSE,1; 2020,OctSE,1; 2020,AugSE,1; 2020,AugSE,1; 2020,AugSE,1; 2018,Jan,8; 2017,Jan,8; 2016,Jan,13

87528 **Herpes simplex virus, direct probe technique**
0.00 0.00 FUD XXX
AMA: 2020,Dec,3; 2020,OctSE,1; 2020,OctSE,1; 2020,AugSE,1; 2020,AugSE,1; 2020,AugSE,1; 2018,Jan,8; 2017,Jan,8; 2016,Jan,13

87529 **Herpes simplex virus, amplified probe technique**
0.00 0.00 FUD XXX
AMA: 2020,Dec,3; 2020,OctSE,1; 2020,OctSE,1; 2020,AugSE,1; 2020,AugSE,1; 2020,AugSE,1; 2018,Jan,8; 2017,Jan,8; 2016,Jan,13

87530 **Herpes simplex virus, quantification**
0.00 0.00 FUD XXX
AMA: 2020,Dec,3; 2020,OctSE,1; 2020,OctSE,1; 2020,AugSE,1; 2020,AugSE,1; 2020,AugSE,1; 2018,Jan,8; 2017,Jan,8; 2016,Jan,13

87531 **Herpes virus-6, direct probe technique**
0.00 0.00 FUD XXX
AMA: 2020,Dec,3; 2020,OctSE,1; 2020,OctSE,1; 2020,AugSE,1; 2020,AugSE,1; 2020,AugSE,1; 2018,Jan,8; 2017,Jan,8; 2016,Jan,13

87532 **Herpes virus-6, amplified probe technique**
0.00 0.00 FUD XXX
AMA: 2020,Dec,3; 2020,OctSE,1; 2020,OctSE,1; 2020,AugSE,1; 2020,AugSE,1; 2020,AugSE,1; 2018,Jan,8; 2017,Jan,8; 2016,Jan,13

87533 **Herpes virus-6, quantification**
0.00 0.00 FUD XXX
AMA: 2020,Dec,3; 2020,OctSE,1; 2020,OctSE,1; 2020,AugSE,1; 2020,AugSE,1; 2020,AugSE,1; 2018,Jan,8; 2017,Jan,8; 2016,Jan,13

87534 **HIV-1, direct probe technique**
0.00 0.00 FUD XXX
AMA: 2020,Dec,3; 2020,OctSE,1; 2020,OctSE,1; 2020,AugSE,1; 2020,AugSE,1; 2020,AugSE,1; 2018,Jan,8; 2017,Jan,8; 2016,Jan,13

87535 **HIV-1, amplified probe technique, includes reverse transcription when performed**
0.00 0.00 FUD XXX
AMA: 2020,Dec,3; 2020,OctSE,1; 2020,OctSE,1; 2020,AugSE,1; 2020,AugSE,1; 2020,AugSE,1; 2018,Jan,8; 2017,Jan,8; 2016,Jan,13

87536 **HIV-1, quantification, includes reverse transcription when performed**
0.00 0.00 FUD XXX
AMA: 2020,Dec,3; 2020,OctSE,1; 2020,OctSE,1; 2020,AugSE,1; 2020,AugSE,1; 2020,AugSE,1; 2018,Jan,8; 2017,Jan,8; 2016,Jan,13

87537 **HIV-2, direct probe technique**
0.00 0.00 FUD XXX
AMA: 2020,Dec,3; 2020,OctSE,1; 2020,OctSE,1; 2020,AugSE,1; 2020,AugSE,1; 2020,AugSE,1; 2018,Jan,8; 2017,Jan,8; 2016,Jan,13

87538 **HIV-2, amplified probe technique, includes reverse transcription when performed**
0.00 0.00 FUD XXX
AMA: 2020,Dec,3; 2020,OctSE,1; 2020,OctSE,1; 2020,AugSE,1; 2020,AugSE,1; 2020,AugSE,1; 2018,Jan,8; 2017,Jan,8; 2016,Jan,13

87539 **HIV-2, quantification, includes reverse transcription when performed**
0.00 0.00 FUD XXX
AMA: 2020,Dec,3; 2020,OctSE,1; 2020,OctSE,1; 2020,AugSE,1; 2020,AugSE,1; 2020,AugSE,1; 2018,Jan,8; 2017,Jan,8; 2016,Jan,13

87623 **Human Papillomavirus (HPV), low-risk types (eg, 6, 11, 42, 43, 44)**
0.00 0.00 FUD XXX
AMA: 2020,Dec,3; 2020,OctSE,1; 2020,OctSE,1; 2020,AugSE,1; 2020,AugSE,1; 2020,AugSE,1

87624 **Human Papillomavirus (HPV), high-risk types (eg, 16, 18, 31, 33, 35, 39, 45, 51, 52, 56, 58, 59, 68)**
INCLUDES Low- and high-risk types in one assay
0.00 0.00 FUD XXX
AMA: 2020,Dec,3; 2020,OctSE,1; 2020,OctSE,1; 2020,AugSE,1; 2020,AugSE,1; 2020,AugSE,1; 2018,Jan,8; 2017,Jan,8; 2016,Jan,13

87625 **Human Papillomavirus (HPV), types 16 and 18 only, includes type 45, if performed**
EXCLUDES *HPV detection (genotyping) (0500T)*
0.00 0.00 FUD XXX
AMA: 2020,Dec,3; 2020,OctSE,1; 2020,OctSE,1; 2020,AugSE,1; 2020,AugSE,1; 2020,AugSE,1; 2018,Jan,8; 2017,Jan,8; 2016,Jan,13

87540 **Legionella pneumophila, direct probe technique**
0.00 0.00 FUD XXX
AMA: 2020,Dec,3; 2020,OctSE,1; 2020,OctSE,1; 2020,AugSE,1; 2020,AugSE,1; 2020,AugSE,1; 2018,Jan,8; 2017,Jan,8; 2016,Jan,13

87541 **Legionella pneumophila, amplified probe technique**
0.00 0.00 FUD XXX
AMA: 2020,Dec,3; 2020,OctSE,1; 2020,OctSE,1; 2020,AugSE,1; 2020,AugSE,1; 2020,AugSE,1; 2018,Jan,8; 2017,Jan,8; 2016,Jan,13

87542 **Legionella pneumophila, quantification**
0.00 0.00 FUD XXX
AMA: 2020,Dec,3; 2020,OctSE,1; 2020,OctSE,1; 2020,AugSE,1; 2020,AugSE,1; 2020,AugSE,1; 2018,Jan,8; 2017,Jan,8; 2016,Jan,13

87550 **Mycobacteria species, direct probe technique**
0.00 0.00 FUD XXX
AMA: 2020,Dec,3; 2020,OctSE,1; 2020,OctSE,1; 2020,AugSE,1; 2020,AugSE,1; 2020,AugSE,1; 2018,Jan,8; 2017,Jan,8; 2016,Jan,13

87551 **Mycobacteria species, amplified probe technique**
0.00 0.00 FUD XXX
AMA: 2020,Dec,3; 2020,OctSE,1; 2020,OctSE,1; 2020,AugSE,1; 2020,AugSE,1; 2020,AugSE,1; 2018,Jan,8; 2017,Jan,8; 2016,Jan,13

87552 **Mycobacteria species, quantification**
0.00 0.00 FUD XXX
AMA: 2020,Dec,3; 2020,OctSE,1; 2020,OctSE,1; 2020,AugSE,1; 2020,AugSE,1; 2020,AugSE,1; 2018,Jan,8; 2017,Jan,8; 2016,Jan,13

87555 **Mycobacteria tuberculosis, direct probe technique**
0.00 0.00 FUD XXX
AMA: 2020,Dec,3; 2020,OctSE,1; 2020,OctSE,1; 2020,AugSE,1; 2020,AugSE,1; 2020,AugSE,1; 2018,Jan,8; 2017,Jan,8; 2016,Jan,13

87556 **Mycobacteria tuberculosis, amplified probe technique**
0.00 0.00 FUD XXX
AMA: 2020,Dec,3; 2020,OctSE,1; 2020,OctSE,1; 2020,AugSE,1; 2020,AugSE,1; 2020,AugSE,1; 2018,Jan,8; 2017,Jan,8; 2016,Jan,13

87557 **Mycobacteria tuberculosis, quantification**
0.00 0.00 FUD XXX
AMA: 2020,Dec,3; 2020,OctSE,1; 2020,OctSE,1; 2020,AugSE,1; 2020,AugSE,1; 2020,AugSE,1; 2018,Jan,8; 2017,Jan,8; 2016,Jan,13

87560 **Mycobacteria avium-intracellulare, direct probe technique**
0.00 0.00 FUD XXX
AMA: 2020,Dec,3; 2020,OctSE,1; 2020,OctSE,1; 2020,AugSE,1; 2020,AugSE,1; 2020,AugSE,1; 2018,Jan,8; 2017,Jan,8; 2016,Jan,13

87561 **Mycobacteria avium-intracellulare, amplified probe technique**
0.00 0.00 FUD XXX
AMA: 2020,Dec,3; 2020,OctSE,1; 2020,OctSE,1; 2020,AugSE,1; 2020,AugSE,1; 2020,AugSE,1; 2018,Jan,8; 2017,Jan,8; 2016,Jan,13

87562 **Mycobacteria avium-intracellulare, quantification**
0.00 0.00 FUD XXX
AMA: 2020,Dec,3; 2020,OctSE,1; 2020,OctSE,1; 2020,AugSE,1; 2020,AugSE,1; 2020,AugSE,1; 2018,Jan,8; 2017,Jan,8; 2016,Jan,13

87563 **Mycoplasma genitalium, amplified probe technique**
0.00 0.00 FUD XXX
AMA: 2020,Dec,3; 2020,OctSE,1; 2020,Oct,11; 2020,OctSE,1; 2020,AugSE,1; 2020,AugSE,1; 2020,AugSE,1

87580 **Mycoplasma pneumoniae, direct probe technique**
0.00 0.00 FUD XXX
AMA: 2020,Dec,3; 2020,OctSE,1; 2020,OctSE,1; 2020,AugSE,1; 2020,AugSE,1; 2020,AugSE,1; 2018,Jan,8; 2017,Jan,8; 2016,Jan,13

87581 **Mycoplasma pneumoniae, amplified probe technique**
0.00 0.00 FUD XXX
AMA: 2020,Dec,3; 2020,OctSE,1; 2020,OctSE,1; 2020,AugSE,1; 2020,AugSE,1; 2020,AugSE,1; 2018,Jan,8; 2017,Jan,8; 2016,Jan,13

87582 **Mycoplasma pneumoniae, quantification**
0.00 0.00 FUD XXX
AMA: 2020,Dec,3; 2020,OctSE,1; 2020,OctSE,1; 2020,AugSE,1; 2020,AugSE,1; 2020,AugSE,1; 2018,Jan,8; 2017,Jan,8; 2016,Jan,13

87590 **Neisseria gonorrhoeae, direct probe technique**
0.00 0.00 FUD XXX
AMA: 2020,Dec,3; 2020,OctSE,1; 2020,OctSE,1; 2020,AugSE,1; 2020,AugSE,1; 2020,AugSE,1; 2018,Jan,8; 2017,Jan,8; 2016,Jan,13

87591 **Neisseria gonorrhoeae, amplified probe technique**
0.00 0.00 FUD XXX
AMA: 2020,Dec,3; 2020,OctSE,1; 2020,OctSE,1; 2020,AugSE,1; 2020,AugSE,1; 2020,AugSE,1; 2018,Jan,8; 2017,Jan,8; 2016,Jan,13

87592 **Neisseria gonorrhoeae, quantification**
0.00 0.00 FUD XXX
AMA: 2020,Dec,3; 2020,OctSE,1; 2020,OctSE,1; 2020,AugSE,1; 2020,AugSE,1; 2020,AugSE,1; 2018,Jan,8; 2017,Jan,8; 2016,Jan,13

87623 **Resequenced code. See code following 87539.**

87624 **Resequenced code. See code following 87539.**

87625 **Resequenced code. See code before 87540.**

87631 **respiratory virus (eg, adenovirus, influenza virus, coronavirus, metapneumovirus, parainfluenza virus, respiratory syncytial virus, rhinovirus), includes multiplex reverse transcription, when performed, and multiplex amplified probe technique, multiple types or subtypes, 3-5 targets**
INCLUDES Detection multiple respiratory viruses with one test
EXCLUDES *Assay for severe acute respiratory syndrome coronavirus 2 (SARS-CoV-2) (Coronavirus disease) (COVID-19) (87635)*
Assays for typing or subtyping influenza viruses only (87501-87503)
Single test for detection multiple infectious organisms (87800-87801)
0.00 0.00 FUD XXX
AMA: 2020,Dec,3; 2020,OctSE,1; 2020,OctSE,1; 2020,AugSE,1; 2020,AugSE,1; 2020,AugSE,1; 2020,Apr,3; 2020,Mar,3; 2018,Jan,8; 2017,Jan,8; 2016,Jan,13

87632 **respiratory virus (eg, adenovirus, influenza virus, coronavirus, metapneumovirus, parainfluenza virus, respiratory syncytial virus, rhinovirus), includes multiplex reverse transcription, when performed, and multiplex amplified probe technique, multiple types or subtypes, 6-11 targets**

INCLUDES Detection multiple respiratory viruses with one test

EXCLUDES *Assay for severe acute respiratory syndrome coronavirus 2 (SARS-CoV-2) (Coronavirus disease) (COVID-19) (87635)*

Assays for typing or subtyping influenza viruses only (87501-87503)

Single test to detect multiple infectious organisms (87800-87801)

0.00 0.00 **FUD** XXX

AMA: 2020,Dec,3; 2020,OctSE,1; 2020,OctSE,1; 2020,AugSE,1; 2020,AugSE,1; 2020,AugSE,1; 2020,Apr,3; 2020,Mar,3; 2018,Jan,8; 2017,Jan,8; 2016,Jan,13

87633 **respiratory virus (eg, adenovirus, influenza virus, coronavirus, metapneumovirus, parainfluenza virus, respiratory syncytial virus, rhinovirus), includes multiplex reverse transcription, when performed, and multiplex amplified probe technique, multiple types or subtypes, 12-25 targets**

INCLUDES Detection multiple respiratory viruses with one test

EXCLUDES *Assay for severe acute respiratory syndrome coronavirus 2 (SARS-CoV-2) (Coronavirus disease) (COVID-19) (87635)*

Assays for typing or subtyping influenza viruses only (87501-87503)

Single test to detect multiple infectious organisms (87800-87801)

0.00 0.00 **FUD** XXX

AMA: 2020,Dec,3; 2020,OctSE,1; 2020,OctSE,1; 2020,AugSE,1; 2020,AugSE,1; 2020,AugSE,1; 2020,Apr,3; 2020,Mar,3; 2018,Jan,8; 2017,Jan,8; 2016,Jan,13

87634 **respiratory syncytial virus, amplified probe technique**

EXCLUDES *Assays for RSV with other respiratory viruses (87631-87633)*

0.00 0.00 **FUD** XXX

AMA: 2020,Dec,3; 2020,OctSE,1; 2020,OctSE,1; 2020,AugSE,1; 2020,AugSE,1; 2020,AugSE,1

87635 **severe acute respiratory syndrome coronavirus 2 (SARS-CoV-2) (Coronavirus disease [COVID-19]), amplified probe technique**

EXCLUDES *HCPCS codes for reporting coronavirus testing (U0001-U0002)*

Single procedure nucleic acid assays to detect multiple respiratory viruses by multiplex reaction (87631-87633)

Code also code 87635, with modifier 59, for assays performed on specimens from different anatomic locations, when performed

0.00 0.00 **FUD** XXX

AMA: 2020,Dec,3; 2020,OctSE,1; 2020,OctSE,1; 2020,AugSE,1; 2020,AugSE,1; 2020,AugSE,1; 2020,Apr,3; 2020,Mar,3

● **87636** **severe acute respiratory syndrome coronavirus 2 (SARS-CoV-2) (Coronavirus disease [COVID-19]) and influenza virus types A and B, multiplex amplified probe technique**

EXCLUDES *Nucleic acid detection multiple respiratory infectious agents (87631-87633):*

Including severe acute respiratory syndrome coronavirus 2 (SARS-CoV-2) (Coronavirus disease) (COVID-19) with additional agents beyond influenza A and B and respiratory syncytial virus

Not including severe acute respiratory syndrome coronavirus 2 (SARS-CoV-2) (Coronavirus disease) (COVID-19)

0.00 0.00 **FUD** XXX

AMA: 2020,Dec,3; 2020,OctSE,1; 2020,NovSE,1

● **87637** **severe acute respiratory syndrome coronavirus 2 (SARS-CoV-2) (Coronavirus disease [COVID-19]), influenza virus types A and B, and respiratory syncytial virus, multiplex amplified probe technique**

EXCLUDES *Nucleic acid detection multiple respiratory infectious agents (87631-87633):*

Including severe acute respiratory syndrome coronavirus 2 (SARS-CoV-2) (coronavirus disease) (COVID-19) with additional agents beyond influenza A and B and respiratory syncytial virus

Not including severe acute respiratory syndrome coronavirus 2 (SARS-CoV-2) (coronavirus disease) (COVID-19)

0.00 0.00 **FUD** XXX

AMA: 2020,Dec,3; 2020,OctSE,1; 2020,NovSE,1

87640 **Staphylococcus aureus, amplified probe technique**

0.00 0.00 **FUD** XXX

AMA: 2020,Dec,3; 2020,OctSE,1; 2020,OctSE,1; 2020,AugSE,1; 2020,AugSE,1; 2020,AugSE,1; 2018,Jan,8; 2017,Jan,8; 2016,Jan,13

87641 **Staphylococcus aureus, methicillin resistant, amplified probe technique**

EXCLUDES *Assays that detect methicillin resistance and identify Staphylococcus aureus using single nucleic acid sequence (87641)*

0.00 0.00 **FUD** XXX

AMA: 2020,Dec,3; 2020,OctSE,1; 2020,OctSE,1; 2020,AugSE,1; 2020,AugSE,1; 2020,AugSE,1; 2018,Jan,8; 2017,Jan,8; 2016,Jan,13

87650 **Streptococcus, group A, direct probe technique**

0.00 0.00 **FUD** XXX

AMA: 2020,Dec,3; 2020,OctSE,1; 2020,OctSE,1; 2020,AugSE,1; 2020,AugSE,1; 2020,AugSE,1; 2018,Jan,8; 2017,Jan,8; 2016,Jan,13

87651 **Streptococcus, group A, amplified probe technique**

0.00 0.00 **FUD** XXX

AMA: 2020,Dec,3; 2020,OctSE,1; 2020,OctSE,1; 2020,AugSE,1; 2020,AugSE,1; 2020,AugSE,1; 2018,Jan,8; 2017,Jan,8; 2016,Jan,13

87652 **Streptococcus, group A, quantification**

0.00 0.00 **FUD** XXX

AMA: 2020,Dec,3; 2020,OctSE,1; 2020,OctSE,1; 2020,AugSE,1; 2020,AugSE,1; 2020,AugSE,1; 2018,Jan,8; 2017,Jan,8; 2016,Jan,13

87653 **Streptococcus, group B, amplified probe technique**

0.00 0.00 **FUD** XXX

AMA: 2020,Dec,3; 2020,OctSE,1; 2020,OctSE,1; 2020,AugSE,1; 2020,AugSE,1; 2020,AugSE,1; 2018,Jan,8; 2017,Jan,8; 2016,Jan,13

87660 **Trichomonas vaginalis, direct probe technique**

0.00 0.00 **FUD** XXX

AMA: 2020,Dec,3; 2020,OctSE,1; 2020,OctSE,1; 2020,AugSE,1; 2020,AugSE,1; 2020,AugSE,1; 2018,Jan,8; 2017,Jan,8; 2016,Jan,13

87661 **Trichomonas vaginalis, amplified probe technique**

0.00 0.00 **FUD** XXX

AMA: 2020,Dec,3; 2020,OctSE,1; 2020,OctSE,1; 2020,AugSE,1; 2020,AugSE,1; 2020,AugSE,1

87662 **Zika virus, amplified probe technique**

0.00 0.00 **FUD** XXX

AMA: 2020,Dec,3; 2020,OctSE,1; 2020,OctSE,1; 2020,AugSE,1; 2020,AugSE,1; 2020,AugSE,1

87797 **Infectious agent detection by nucleic acid (DNA or RNA), not otherwise specified; direct probe technique, each organism**

0.00 0.00 **FUD** XXX

AMA: 2020,Dec,3; 2020,OctSE,1; 2020,OctSE,1; 2020,AugSE,1; 2020,AugSE,1; 2020,AugSE,1; 2018,Jan,8; 2017,Jan,8; 2016,Aug,9; 2016,Jan,13

87798 **amplified probe technique, each organism**

0.00 0.00 **FUD** XXX

AMA: 2020,Dec,3; 2020,Oct,11; 2020,OctSE,1; 2020,OctSE,1; 2020,AugSE,1; 2020,AugSE,1; 2020,AugSE,1; 2018,Jan,8; 2017,Jan,8; 2016,Jan,13

87799 **quantification, each organism**
0.00 0.00 **FUD** XXX
AMA: 2020,Dec,3; 2020,OctSE,1; 2020,OctSE,1; 2020,AugSE,1; 2020,AugSE,1; 2020,AugSE,1; 2018,Jan,8; 2017,Jan,8; 2016,Jan,13

87800 **Infectious agent detection by nucleic acid (DNA or RNA), multiple organisms; direct probe(s) technique**
INCLUDES Single test to detect multiple infectious organisms
EXCLUDES *Detection specific infectious agents not otherwise specified (87797-87799)*
Each specific organism nucleic acid detection from primary source (87471-87660 [87623, 87624, 87625])
0.00 0.00 **FUD** XXX
AMA: 2020,Dec,3; 2020,OctSE,1; 2020,OctSE,1; 2020,AugSE,1; 2020,AugSE,1; 2020,AugSE,1; 2018,Jan,8; 2017,Jan,8; 2016,Aug,9; 2016,Jan,13

87801 **amplified probe(s) technique**
INCLUDES Single test to detect multiple infectious organisms
EXCLUDES *Detection multiple respiratory viruses with one test (87631-87633)*
Detection specific infectious agents not otherwise specified (87797-87799)
Each specific organism nucleic acid detection from primary source (87471-87660 [87623, 87624, 87625])
0.00 0.00 **FUD** XXX
AMA: 2020,Dec,3; 2020,OctSE,1; 2020,OctSE,1; 2020,AugSE,1; 2020,AugSE,1; 2020,AugSE,1; 2018,Jan,8; 2017,Jan,8; 2016,Jan,13

87802-87899 [87806, 87811] Detection Infectious Agent by Immunoassay with Direct Optical Observation

▲ **87802** **Infectious agent antigen detection by immunoassay with direct optical (ie, visual) observation; Streptococcus, group B**
0.00 0.00 **FUD** XXX
AMA: 2020,Dec,3; 2020,OctSE,1; 2020,OctSE,1; 2020,AugSE,1; 2020,AugSE,1; 2020,AugSE,1

▲ **87803** **Clostridium difficile toxin A**
0.00 0.00 **FUD** XXX
AMA: 2020,Dec,3; 2020,OctSE,1; 2020,OctSE,1; 2020,AugSE,1; 2020,AugSE,1; 2020,AugSE,1

▲ # **87806** **HIV-1 antigen(s), with HIV-1 and HIV-2 antibodies**
0.00 0.00 **FUD** XXX
AMA: 2020,Dec,3; 2020,OctSE,1; 2020,OctSE,1; 2020,AugSE,1; 2020,AugSE,1; 2020,AugSE,1

▲ **87804** **Influenza**
0.00 0.00 **FUD** XXX
AMA: 2020,Dec,3; 2020,OctSE,1; 2020,OctSE,1; 2020,AugSE,1; 2020,AugSE,1; 2020,AugSE,1; 2018,Jan,8; 2017,Jan,8; 2016,Jan,13

87806 **Resequenced code. See code following 87803.**

▲ **87807** **respiratory syncytial virus**
0.00 0.00 **FUD** XXX
AMA: 2020,Dec,3; 2020,OctSE,1; 2020,OctSE,1; 2020,AugSE,1; 2020,AugSE,1; 2020,AugSE,1

● # **87811** **severe acute respiratory syndrome coronavirus 2 (SARS-CoV-2) (Coronavirus disease [COVID-19])**
0.00 0.00 **FUD** XXX
AMA: 2020,Dec,3; 2020,OctSE,1

▲ **87808** **Trichomonas vaginalis**
0.00 0.00 **FUD** XXX
AMA: 2020,Dec,3; 2020,OctSE,1; 2020,OctSE,1; 2020,AugSE,1; 2020,AugSE,1; 2020,AugSE,1

▲ **87809** **adenovirus**
0.00 0.00 **FUD** XXX
AMA: 2020,Dec,3; 2020,OctSE,1; 2020,OctSE,1; 2020,AugSE,1; 2020,AugSE,1; 2020,AugSE,1; 2018,Jan,8; 2017,Jan,8; 2016,Jan,13

▲ **87810** **Chlamydia trachomatis**
0.00 0.00 **FUD** XXX
AMA: 2020,Dec,3; 2020,OctSE,1; 2020,OctSE,1; 2020,AugSE,1; 2020,AugSE,1; 2020,AugSE,1; 2018,Jan,8; 2017,Jan,8; 2016,Jan,13

87811 **Resequenced code. See code following 87807.**

▲ **87850** **Neisseria gonorrhoeae**
0.00 0.00 **FUD** XXX
AMA: 2020,Dec,3; 2020,OctSE,1; 2020,OctSE,1; 2020,AugSE,1; 2020,AugSE,1; 2020,AugSE,1; 2018,Jan,8; 2017,Jan,8; 2016,Jan,13

▲ **87880** **Streptococcus, group A**
0.00 0.00 **FUD** XXX
AMA: 2020,Dec,3; 2020,OctSE,1; 2020,OctSE,1; 2020,AugSE,1; 2020,AugSE,1; 2020,AugSE,1; 2018,Jan,8; 2017,Jan,8; 2016,Jan,13

▲ **87899** **not otherwise specified**
0.00 0.00 **FUD** XXX
AMA: 2020,Dec,3; 2020,OctSE,1; 2020,OctSE,1; 2020,AugSE,1; 2020,AugSE,1; 2020,AugSE,1; 2018,Jan,8; 2017,Jan,8; 2016,Jan,13

87900-87999 [87906, 87910, 87912] Drug Sensitivity Genotype/Phenotype

87900 **Infectious agent drug susceptibility phenotype prediction using regularly updated genotypic bioinformatics**
0.00 0.00 **FUD** XXX
AMA: 2020,Dec,3; 2020,OctSE,1; 2020,OctSE,1; 2018,Jan,8; 2017,Jan,8; 2016,Jan,13

87910 **Infectious agent genotype analysis by nucleic acid (DNA or RNA); cytomegalovirus**
EXCLUDES *HPV detection (genotyping) (0500T)*
HIV-1 infectious agent phenotype prediction (87900)
0.00 0.00 **FUD** XXX
AMA: 2020,Dec,3; 2018,Jan,8; 2017,Jan,8; 2016,Jan,13

87901 **HIV-1, reverse transcriptase and protease regions**
EXCLUDES *Infectious agent drug susceptibility phenotype prediction for HIV-1 (87900)*
0.00 0.00 **FUD** XXX
AMA: 2020,Dec,3; 2020,OctSE,1; 2020,OctSE,1; 2018,Jan,8; 2017,Jan,8; 2016,Jan,13

87906 **HIV-1, other region (eg, integrase, fusion)**
EXCLUDES *HIV-1 infectious agent phenotype prediction (87900)*
0.00 0.00 **FUD** XXX
AMA: 2020,Dec,3; 2018,Jan,8; 2017,Jan,8; 2016,Jan,13

87912 **Hepatitis B virus**
0.00 0.00 **FUD** XXX
AMA: 2020,Dec,3; 2018,Jan,8; 2017,Jan,8; 2016,Jan,13

87902 **Hepatitis C virus**
0.00 0.00 **FUD** XXX
AMA: 2020,Dec,3; 2020,OctSE,1; 2020,OctSE,1; 2018,Jan,8; 2017,Jan,8; 2016,Jan,13

87903 **Infectious agent phenotype analysis by nucleic acid (DNA or RNA) with drug resistance tissue culture analysis, HIV 1; first through 10 drugs tested**
0.00 0.00 **FUD** XXX
AMA: 2020,Dec,3; 2020,OctSE,1; 2020,OctSE,1; 2018,Jan,8; 2017,Jan,8; 2016,Jan,13

\+ **87904** **each additional drug tested (List separately in addition to code for primary procedure)**
Code first (87903)
0.00 0.00 **FUD** XXX
AMA: 2020,Dec,3; 2018,Jan,8; 2017,Jan,8; 2016,Jan,13

87905 **Infectious agent enzymatic activity other than virus (eg, sialidase activity in vaginal fluid)**
EXCLUDES *Virus isolation identified by nonimmunologic method, and by noncytopathic effect (87255)*
0.00 0.00 **FUD** XXX
AMA: 2020,Dec,3

87906 **Resequenced code. See code following 87901.**

87910 **Resequenced code. See code following 87900.**

#87912 **Resequenced code. See code before 87902.**

87999 **Unlisted microbiology procedure**
0.00 0.00 FUD XXX N
AMA: 2020,Dec,3; 2018,Jan,8; 2017,Jan,8; 2016,Jan,13

88000-88099 Autopsy Services

CMS: 100-02,15,80.1 Payment for Clinical Laboratory Services

INCLUDES Services for physicians only

88000 **Necropsy (autopsy), gross examination only; without CNS**
0.00 0.00 FUD XXX E
AMA: 2020,Dec,3; 2018,Jan,8; 2017,Jan,8; 2016,Jan,13

88005 **with brain**
0.00 0.00 FUD XXX E
AMA: 2020,Dec,3

88007 **with brain and spinal cord**
0.00 0.00 FUD XXX E
AMA: 2020,Dec,3

88012 **infant with brain** A
0.00 0.00 FUD XXX E
AMA: 2020,Dec,3

88014 **stillborn or newborn with brain** A
0.00 0.00 FUD XXX E
AMA: 2020,Dec,3

88016 **macerated stillborn** A
0.00 0.00 FUD XXX E
AMA: 2020,Dec,3

88020 **Necropsy (autopsy), gross and microscopic; without CNS**
0.00 0.00 FUD XXX E
AMA: 2020,Dec,3

88025 **with brain**
0.00 0.00 FUD XXX E
AMA: 2020,Dec,3

88027 **with brain and spinal cord**
0.00 0.00 FUD XXX E
AMA: 2020,Dec,3

88028 **infant with brain** A
0.00 0.00 FUD XXX E
AMA: 2020,Dec,3

88029 **stillborn or newborn with brain** A
0.00 0.00 FUD XXX E
AMA: 2020,Dec,3

88036 **Necropsy (autopsy), limited, gross and/or microscopic; regional**
0.00 0.00 FUD XXX E
AMA: 2020,Dec,3

88037 **single organ**
0.00 0.00 FUD XXX E
AMA: 2020,Dec,3

88040 **Necropsy (autopsy); forensic examination**
0.00 0.00 FUD XXX E
AMA: 2020,Dec,3

88045 **coroner's call**
0.00 0.00 FUD XXX E
AMA: 2020,Dec,3

88099 **Unlisted necropsy (autopsy) procedure**
0.00 0.00 FUD XXX E
AMA: 2020,Dec,3; 2018,Jan,8; 2017,Jan,8; 2016,Jan,13

88104-88140 Cytopathology: Other Than Cervical/Vaginal

88104 **Cytopathology, fluids, washings or brushings, except cervical or vaginal; smears with interpretation**
1.93 1.93 FUD XXX Q1 80
AMA: 2020,Dec,3; 2018,Jan,8; 2017,Jan,8; 2016,Jan,13

88106 **simple filter method with interpretation**
EXCLUDES *Cytopathology smears with interpretation (88104)*
Selective cellular enhancement (nongynecological) including filter transfer techniques (88112)
1.81 1.81 FUD XXX Q1 80
AMA: 2020,Dec,3; 2018,Jan,8; 2017,Jan,8; 2016,Jan,13

88108 **Cytopathology, concentration technique, smears and interpretation (eg, Saccomanno technique)**
EXCLUDES *Cervical or vaginal smears (88150-88155)*
Gastric intubation with lavage (43754-43755)
(74340)
1.75 1.75 FUD XXX Q1 80
AMA: 2020,Dec,3; 2018,Jan,8; 2017,Jan,8; 2016,Jan,13

88112 **Cytopathology, selective cellular enhancement technique with interpretation (eg, liquid based slide preparation method), except cervical or vaginal**
EXCLUDES *Cytopathology cellular enhancement technique (88108)*
1.90 1.90 FUD XXX Q1 80
AMA: 2020,Dec,3

88120 **Cytopathology, in situ hybridization (eg, FISH), urinary tract specimen with morphometric analysis, 3-5 molecular probes, each specimen; manual**
EXCLUDES *More than five probes (88399)*
Morphometric in situ hybridization on specimens other than urinary tract (88367-88368 [88373, 88374])
16.3 16.3 FUD XXX Q2 80
AMA: 2020,Dec,3

88121 **using computer-assisted technology**
EXCLUDES *More than five probes (88399)*
Morphometric in situ hybridization on specimens other than urinary tract (88367-88368 [88373, 88374])
12.4 12.4 FUD XXX Q1 80
AMA: 2020,Dec,3

88125 **Cytopathology, forensic (eg, sperm)**
0.75 0.75 FUD XXX Q1 80
AMA: 2020,Dec,3

88130 **Sex chromatin identification; Barr bodies**
0.00 0.00 FUD XXX Q
AMA: 2020,Dec,3

88140 **peripheral blood smear, polymorphonuclear drumsticks**
EXCLUDES *Guard stain (88313)*
0.00 0.00 FUD XXX Q
AMA: 2020,Dec,3; 2018,Jan,8; 2017,Jan,8; 2016,Jan,13

88141-88155 Pap Smears

CMS: 100-03,210.2 Screening Pap Smears/Pelvic Examinations for Early Cancer Detection

EXCLUDES *Non-Bethesda method (88150-88153)*

88141 **Cytopathology, cervical or vaginal (any reporting system), requiring interpretation by physician** ♀
Code also (88142-88153, 88164-88167, 88174-88175)
0.90 0.90 FUD XXX N 80 26
AMA: 2020,Dec,3; 2018,Jan,8; 2017,Jan,8; 2016,Jan,13

88142 **Cytopathology, cervical or vaginal (any reporting system), collected in preservative fluid, automated thin layer preparation; manual screening under physician supervision** ♀
INCLUDES Bethesda or non-Bethesda method
0.00 0.00 FUD XXX Q
AMA: 2020,Dec,3; 2018,Jan,8; 2017,Jan,8; 2016,Jan,13

88143 **with manual screening and rescreening under physician supervision** ♀
INCLUDES Bethesda or non-Bethesda method
EXCLUDES *Automated screening automated thin layer preparation (88174-88175)*
0.00 0.00 FUD XXX Q
AMA: 2020,Dec,3; 2018,Jan,8; 2017,Jan,8; 2016,Jan,13

88147 **Cytopathology smears, cervical or vaginal; screening by automated system under physician supervision** ♀
0.00 0.00 FUD XXX
AMA: 2020,Dec,3; 2018,Jan,8; 2017,Jan,8; 2016,Jan,13

88148 **screening by automated system with manual rescreening under physician supervision** ♀
0.00 0.00 FUD XXX
AMA: 2020,Dec,3; 2018,Jan,8; 2017,Jan,8; 2016,Jan,13

88150 **Cytopathology, slides, cervical or vaginal; manual screening under physician supervision** ♀
EXCLUDES *Bethesda method Pap smears (88164-88167)*
0.00 0.00 FUD XXX
AMA: 2020,Dec,3; 2018,Jan,8; 2017,Jan,8; 2016,Jan,13

88152 **with manual screening and computer-assisted rescreening under physician supervision**
EXCLUDES *Bethesda method Pap smears (88164-88167)*
0.00 0.00 FUD XXX
AMA: 2020,Dec,3; 2018,Jan,8; 2017,Jan,8; 2016,Jan,13

88153 **with manual screening and rescreening under physician supervision** ♀
EXCLUDES *Bethesda method Pap smears (88164-88167)*
0.00 0.00 FUD XXX
AMA: 2020,Dec,3; 2018,Jan,8; 2017,Jan,8; 2016,Jan,13

+ **88155** **Cytopathology, slides, cervical or vaginal, definitive hormonal evaluation (eg, maturation index, karyopyknotic index, estrogenic index) (List separately in addition to code[s] for other technical and interpretation services)** ♀
Code first (88142-88153, 88164-88167, 88174-88175)
0.00 0.00 FUD XXX
AMA: 2020,Dec,3; 2018,Jan,8; 2017,Jan,8; 2016,Jan,13

88160-88162 Cytopathology Smears (Other Than Pap)

88160 **Cytopathology, smears, any other source; screening and interpretation**
2.01 2.01 FUD XXX
AMA: 2020,Dec,3

88161 **preparation, screening and interpretation**
1.93 1.93 FUD XXX
AMA: 2020,Dec,3; 2018,Jan,8; 2017,Jan,8; 2016,Jan,13

88162 **extended study involving over 5 slides and/or multiple stains**
EXCLUDES *Aerosol collection sputum (89220)*
Special stains (88312-88314)
2.80 2.80 FUD XXX
AMA: 2020,Dec,3

88164-88167 Pap Smears: Bethesda System

CMS: 100-03,210.2 Screening Pap Smears/Pelvic Examinations for Early Cancer Detection
EXCLUDES *Non-Bethesda method (88150-88153)*

88164 **Cytopathology, slides, cervical or vaginal (the Bethesda System); manual screening under physician supervision** ♀
0.00 0.00 FUD XXX
AMA: 2020,Dec,3; 2018,Jan,8; 2017,Jan,8; 2016,Jan,13

88165 **with manual screening and rescreening under physician supervision** ♀
0.00 0.00 FUD XXX
AMA: 2020,Dec,3; 2018,Jan,8; 2017,Jan,8; 2016,Jan,13

88166 **with manual screening and computer-assisted rescreening under physician supervision** ♀
0.00 0.00 FUD XXX
AMA: 2020,Dec,3; 2018,Jan,8; 2017,Jan,8; 2016,Jan,13

88167 **with manual screening and computer-assisted rescreening using cell selection and review under physician supervision** ♀
EXCLUDES *Fine needle aspiration ([10004, 10005, 10006, 10007, 10008, 10009, 10010, 10011, 10012])*
0.00 0.00 FUD XXX
AMA: 2020,Dec,3; 2018,Jan,8; 2017,Jan,8; 2016,Jan,13

88172-88177 [88177] Cytopathology of Needle Biopsy

EXCLUDES *Fine needle aspiration (10021, [10004, 10005, 10006, 10007, 10008, 10009, 10010, 10011, 10012])*

88172 **Cytopathology, evaluation of fine needle aspirate; immediate cytohistologic study to determine adequacy for diagnosis, first evaluation episode, each site**
INCLUDES Submission complete set cytologic material for evaluation no matter how many needle passes performed or slides prepared from each site
EXCLUDES *Cytologic examination during intraoperative pathology consultation (88333-88334)*
1.58 1.58 FUD XXX
AMA: 2020,Dec,3; 2019,Feb,8; 2019,Apr,4; 2018,Jan,8; 2017,Jan,8; 2016,Jan,13; 2016,Jan,11

88173 **interpretation and report**
INCLUDES Interpretation and report from each anatomical site no matter how many passes or evaluation episodes performed during aspiration
EXCLUDES *Cytologic examination during intraoperative pathology consultation (88333-88334)*
4.36 4.36 FUD XXX
AMA: 2020,Dec,3; 2019,Apr,4; 2019,Feb,8; 2018,Jan,8; 2017,Jan,8; 2016,Jan,13

+ # **88177** **immediate cytohistologic study to determine adequacy for diagnosis, each separate additional evaluation episode, same site (List separately in addition to code for primary procedure)**
Code also each additional immediate repeat evaluation episode(s) required from same site (i.e., previous sample inadequate)
Code first (88172)
0.84 0.84 FUD ZZZ
AMA: 2020,Dec,3; 2019,Apr,4; 2018,Jan,8; 2017,Jan,8; 2016,Jan,11

88174-88177 [88177] Pap Smears: Automated Screening

EXCLUDES *Non-Bethesda method (88150-88153)*

88174 **Cytopathology, cervical or vaginal (any reporting system), collected in preservative fluid, automated thin layer preparation; screening by automated system, under physician supervision** ♀
INCLUDES Bethesda or non-Bethesda method
0.00 0.00 FUD XXX
AMA: 2020,Dec,3; 2018,Jan,8; 2017,Jan,8; 2016,Jan,13

88175 **with screening by automated system and manual rescreening or review, under physician supervision** ♀
INCLUDES Bethesda or non-Bethesda method
EXCLUDES *Manual screening (88142-88143)*
0.00 0.00 FUD XXX
AMA: 2020,Dec,3; 2018,Jan,8; 2017,Jan,8; 2016,Jan,13

88177 **Resequenced code. See code following 88173.**

88182-88199 Cytopathology Using the Fluorescence-Activated Cell Sorter

88182 **Flow cytometry, cell cycle or DNA analysis**
EXCLUDES *DNA ploidy analysis by morphometric technique (88358)*
3.89 3.89 FUD XXX
AMA: 2020,Dec,3; 2018,Jan,8; 2017,Jan,8; 2016,Jan,13

88184 **Flow cytometry, cell surface, cytoplasmic, or nuclear marker, technical component only; first marker**
1.88 1.88 FUD XXX
AMA: 2020,Dec,3; 2018,Jan,8; 2017,Jan,8; 2016,Jan,13

+ **88185** **each additional marker (List separately in addition to code for first marker)**
Code first (88184)
0.69 0.69 FUD ZZZ N 80 TC
AMA: 2020,Dec,3; 2018,Jan,8; 2017,Jan,8; 2016,Jan,13

88187 **Flow cytometry, interpretation; 2 to 8 markers**
EXCLUDES *Antibody assessment by flow cytometry (83516-83520, 86000-86849 [86152, 86153])*
Cell enumeration by immunologic selection and identification ([86152, 86153])
Interpretation (86355-86357, 86359-86361, 86367)
1.08 1.08 FUD XXX B 80 26
AMA: 2020,Dec,3; 2018,Jan,8; 2017,Jan,8; 2016,Jan,13

88188 **9 to 15 markers**
EXCLUDES *Antibody assessment by flow cytometry (83516-83520, 86000-86849 [86152, 86153])*
Cell enumeration by immunologic selection and identification ([86152, 86153])
Interpretation (86355-86357, 86359-86361, 86367)
1.83 1.83 FUD XXX B 80 26
AMA: 2020,Dec,3; 2018,Jan,8; 2017,Jan,8; 2016,Jan,13

88189 **16 or more markers**
EXCLUDES *Antibody assessment by flow cytometry (83516-83520, 86000-86849 [86152, 86153])*
Cell enumeration using immunologic selection and identification in fluid sample ([86152, 86153])
Interpretation (86355-86357, 86359-86361, 86367)
2.45 2.45 FUD XXX B 80 26
AMA: 2020,Dec,3; 2018,Jan,8; 2017,Jan,8; 2016,Jan,13

88199 **Unlisted cytopathology procedure**
EXCLUDES *Electron microscopy (88348)*
0.00 0.00 FUD XXX Q1 80
AMA: 2020,Dec,3; 2018,Jan,8; 2017,Jan,8; 2016,Jan,13

88230-88299 Cytogenic Studies

CMS: 100-03,190.3 Cytogenic Studies
EXCLUDES *Acetylcholinesterase (82013)*
Alpha-fetoprotein (amniotic fluid or serum) (82105-82106)
Microdissection (88380)
Molecular pathology codes (81105-81383 [81105, 81106, 81107, 81108, 81109, 81110, 81111, 81112, 81120, 81121, 81161, 81162, 81163, 81164, 81165, 81166, 81167, 81173, 81174, 81184, 81185, 81186, 81187, 81188, 81189, 81190, 81200, 81201, 81202, 81203, 81204, 81205, 81206, 81207, 81208, 81209, 81210, 81219, 81227, 81230, 81231, 81233, 81234, 81238, 81239, 81245, 81246, 81250, 81257, 81258, 81259, 81261, 81262, 81263, 81264, 81265, 81266, 81267, 81268, 81269, 81271, 81274, 81283, 81284, 81285, 81286, 81287, 81288, 81289, 81291, 81292, 81293, 81294, 81295, 81301, 81302, 81303, 81304, 81306, 81312, 81320, 81324, 81325, 81326, 81332, 81334, 81336, 81337, 81343, 81344, 81345, 81361, 81362, 81363, 81364], 81400-81408, [81479], 81410-81471 [81448], 81500-81512, 81599)

88230 **Tissue culture for non-neoplastic disorders; lymphocyte**
0.00 0.00 FUD XXX Q
AMA: 2020,Dec,3; 2018,Jan,8; 2017,Jan,8; 2016,Jan,13

88233 **skin or other solid tissue biopsy**
0.00 0.00 FUD XXX Q
AMA: 2020,Dec,3; 2018,Jan,8; 2017,Jan,8; 2016,Jan,13

88235 **amniotic fluid or chorionic villus cells** M
0.00 0.00 FUD XXX Q
AMA: 2020,Dec,3; 2018,Jan,8; 2017,Jan,8; 2016,Jan,13

88237 **Tissue culture for neoplastic disorders; bone marrow, blood cells**
0.00 0.00 FUD XXX Q
AMA: 2020,Dec,3; 2018,Jan,8; 2017,Jan,8; 2016,Jan,13

88239 **solid tumor**
0.00 0.00 FUD XXX Q
AMA: 2020,Dec,3; 2018,Jan,8; 2017,Jan,8; 2016,Jan,13

88240 **Cryopreservation, freezing and storage of cells, each cell line**
EXCLUDES *Therapeutic cryopreservation and storage (38207)*
0.00 0.00 FUD XXX Q
AMA: 2020,Dec,3; 2018,Jan,8; 2017,Jan,8; 2016,Jan,13

88241 **Thawing and expansion of frozen cells, each aliquot**
EXCLUDES *Therapeutic thawing of prior harvest (38208)*
0.00 0.00 FUD XXX Q
AMA: 2020,Dec,3; 2018,Jan,8; 2017,Jan,8; 2016,Jan,13

88245 **Chromosome analysis for breakage syndromes; baseline Sister Chromatid Exchange (SCE), 20-25 cells**
0.00 0.00 FUD XXX Q
AMA: 2020,Dec,3; 2018,Jan,8; 2017,Jan,8; 2016,Jan,13

88248 **baseline breakage, score 50-100 cells, count 20 cells, 2 karyotypes (eg, for ataxia telangiectasia, Fanconi anemia, fragile X)**
0.00 0.00 FUD XXX Q
AMA: 2020,Dec,3; 2018,Jan,8; 2017,Jan,8; 2016,Jan,13

88249 **score 100 cells, clastogen stress (eg, diepoxybutane, mitomycin C, ionizing radiation, UV radiation)**
0.00 0.00 FUD XXX Q
AMA: 2020,Dec,3; 2018,Jan,8; 2017,Jan,8; 2016,Jan,13

88261 **Chromosome analysis; count 5 cells, 1 karyotype, with banding**
0.00 0.00 FUD XXX Q
AMA: 2020,Dec,3; 2018,Jan,8; 2017,Jan,8; 2016,Jan,13

88262 **count 15-20 cells, 2 karyotypes, with banding**
0.00 0.00 FUD XXX Q
AMA: 2020,Dec,3; 2019,Aug,10; 2018,Jan,8; 2017,Jan,8; 2016,Jan,13

88263 **count 45 cells for mosaicism, 2 karyotypes, with banding**
0.00 0.00 FUD XXX Q
AMA: 2020,Dec,3; 2018,Jan,8; 2017,Jan,8; 2016,Jan,13

88264 **analyze 20-25 cells**
0.00 0.00 FUD XXX Q
AMA: 2020,Dec,3; 2019,Aug,10; 2018,Jan,8; 2017,Jan,8; 2016,Jan,13

88267 **Chromosome analysis, amniotic fluid or chorionic villus, count 15 cells, 1 karyotype, with banding** M ♀
0.00 0.00 FUD XXX Q
AMA: 2020,Dec,3; 2018,Jan,8; 2017,Jan,8; 2016,Jan,13

88269 **Chromosome analysis, in situ for amniotic fluid cells, count cells from 6-12 colonies, 1 karyotype, with banding** M ♀
0.00 0.00 FUD XXX Q
AMA: 2020,Dec,3; 2018,Jan,8; 2017,Jan,8; 2016,Jan,13

88271 **Molecular cytogenetics; DNA probe, each (eg, FISH)**
EXCLUDES *Cytogenomic microarray analysis (81228-81229, [81349], 81405-81406, [81479])*
Fetal chromosome analysis using maternal blood (81420-81422)
0.00 0.00 FUD XXX Q
AMA: 2020,Dec,3; 2020,Feb,10; 2018,Jan,8; 2017,Apr,3; 2017,Jan,8; 2016,Jan,13

88272 **chromosomal in situ hybridization, analyze 3-5 cells (eg, for derivatives and markers)**
0.00 0.00 FUD XXX Q
AMA: 2020,Dec,3; 2018,Jan,8; 2017,Jan,8; 2016,Jan,13

88273 **chromosomal in situ hybridization, analyze 10-30 cells (eg, for microdeletions)**
0.00 0.00 FUD XXX Q
AMA: 2020,Dec,3; 2018,Jan,8; 2017,Jan,8; 2016,Jan,13

88274 **interphase in situ hybridization, analyze 25-99 cells**
0.00 0.00 FUD XXX Q
AMA: 2020,Dec,3; 2018,Jan,8; 2017,Jan,8; 2016,Jan,13

88275 **interphase in situ hybridization, analyze 100-300 cells**
0.00 0.00 FUD XXX Q
AMA: 2020,Dec,3; 2018,Jan,8; 2017,Jan,8; 2016,Jan,13

88280 **Chromosome analysis; additional karyotypes, each study**
0.00 0.00 FUD XXX Q
AMA: 2020,Dec,3; 2018,Jan,8; 2017,Jan,8; 2016,Jan,13

88283 **additional specialized banding technique (eg, NOR, C-banding)**
0.00 0.00 FUD XXX
AMA: 2020,Dec,3; 2018,Jan,8; 2017,Jan,8; 2016,Jan,13

88285 **additional cells counted, each study**
0.00 0.00 FUD XXX
AMA: 2020,Dec,3; 2018,Jan,8; 2017,Jan,8; 2016,Jan,13

88289 **additional high resolution study**
0.00 0.00 FUD XXX
AMA: 2020,Dec,3; 2018,Jan,8; 2017,Jan,8; 2016,Jan,13

88291 **Cytogenetics and molecular cytogenetics, interpretation and report**
0.94 0.94 FUD XXX
AMA: 2020,Dec,3; 2018,Jan,8; 2017,Jan,8; 2016,Jan,13

88299 **Unlisted cytogenetic study**
0.00 0.00 FUD XXX
AMA: 2020,Dec,3; 2018,Jan,8; 2017,Jan,8; 2016,Jan,13

88300 Evaluation of Surgical Specimen: Gross Anatomy

CMS: 100-02,15,80.1 Payment for Clinical Laboratory Services

INCLUDES Attainment, examination, and reporting
Unit of service is the specimen

EXCLUDES *Additional procedures (88311-88365 [88341, 88350], 88399)*
Microscopic exam (88302-88309)

88300 **Level I - Surgical pathology, gross examination only**
0.44 0.44 FUD XXX
AMA: 2020,Dec,3; 2018,Jan,8; 2017,Jan,8; 2016,Jan,13

88302-88309 Evaluation of Surgical Specimens: Gross and Microscopic Anatomy

CMS: 100-02,15,80.1 Payment for Clinical Laboratory Services

INCLUDES Attainment, examination, and reporting
Unit of service is the specimen

EXCLUDES *Additional procedures (88311-88365 [88341, 88350], 88399)*
Mohs surgery (17311-17315)

88302 **Level II - Surgical pathology, gross and microscopic examination**

INCLUDES Confirming identification and disease absence:
- Appendix, incidental
- Fallopian tube, sterilization
- Fingers or toes traumatic amputation
- Foreskin, newborn
- Hernia sac, any site
- Hydrocele sac
- Nerve
- Skin, plastic repair
- Sympathetic ganglion
- Testis, castration
- Vaginal mucosa, incidental
- Vas deferens, sterilization

0.87 0.87 FUD XXX
AMA: 2020,Dec,3; 2018,Jan,8; 2017,Jan,8; 2016,Jan,13

88304 **Level III - Surgical pathology, gross and microscopic examination**

INCLUDES
- Abortion, induced
- Abscess
- Anal tag
- Aneurysm-atrial/ventricular
- Appendix, other than incidental
- Artery, atheromatous plaque
- Bartholin's gland cyst
- Bone fragment(s), other than pathologic fracture
- Bursa/ synovial cyst
- Carpal tunnel tissue
- Cartilage, shavings
- Cholesteatoma
- Colon, colostomy stoma
- Conjunctiva-biopsy/pterygium
- Cornea
- Diverticulum-esophagus/small intestine
- Dupuytren's contracture tissue
- Femoral head, other than fracture
- Fissure/fistula
- Foreskin, other than newborn
- Gallbladder
- Ganglion cyst
- Hematoma
- Hemorrhoids
- Hydatid of Morgagni
- Intervertebral disc
- Joint, loose body
- Meniscus
- Mucocele, salivary
- Neuroma-Morton's/traumatic
- Pilonidal cyst/sinus
- Polyps, inflammatory-nasal/sinusoidal
- Skin-cyst/tag/debridement
- Soft tissue, debridement
- Soft tissue, lipoma
- Spermatocele
- Tendon/tendon sheath
- Testicular appendage
- Thrombus or embolus
- Tonsil and/or adenoids
- Varicocele
- Vas deferens, other than sterilization
- Vein, varicosity

1.16 1.16 FUD XXX
AMA: 2020,Dec,3; 2018,Jan,8; 2017,Jan,8; 2016,Jan,13

88305 **Level IV - Surgical pathology, gross and microscopic examination**

INCLUDES
- Abortion, spontaneous/missed
- Artery, biopsy
- Bone exostosis
- Bone marrow, biopsy
- Brain/meninges, other than for tumor resection
- Breast biopsy without microscopic assessment of surgical margin
- Breast reduction mammoplasty
- Bronchus, biopsy
- Cell block, any source
- Cervix, biopsy
- Colon, biopsy
- Duodenum, biopsy
- Endocervix, curettings/biopsy
- Endometrium, curettings/biopsy
- Esophagus, biopsy
- Extremity, amputation, traumatic
- Fallopian tube, biopsy
- Fallopian tube, ectopic pregnancy
- Femoral head, fracture
- Finger/toes, amputation, nontraumatic
- Gingiva/oral mucosa, biopsy
- Heart valve
- Joint resection
- Kidney biopsy
- Larynx biopsy

Leiomyoma(s), uterine myomectomy-without uterus
Lip, biopsy/wedge resection
Lung, transbronchial biopsy
Lymph node, biopsy
Muscle, biopsy
Nasal mucosa, biopsy
Nasopharynx/oropharynx, biopsy
Nerve biopsy
Odontogenic/dental cyst
Omentum, biopsy
Ovary, biopsy/wedge resection
Ovary with or without tube, nonneoplastic
Parathyroid gland
Peritoneum, biopsy
Pituitary tumor
Placenta, other than third trimester
Pleura/pericardium-biopsy/tissue
Polyp:
- Cervical/endometrial
- Colorectal
- Stomach/small intestine

Prostate:
- Needle biopsy
- TUR

Salivary gland, biopsy
Sinus, paranasal biopsy
Skin, other than cyst/tag/debridement/plastic repair
Small intestine, biopsy
Soft tissue, other than tumor/mas/lipoma/debridement
Spleen
Stomach biopsy
Synovium
Testis, other than tumor/biopsy, castration
Thyroglossal duct/brachial cleft cyst
Tongue, biopsy
Tonsil, biopsy
Trachea biopsy
Ureter, biopsy
Urethra, biopsy
Urinary bladder, biopsy
Uterus, with or without tubes and ovaries, for prolapse
Vagina biopsy
Vulva/labial biopsy

1.95 1.95 FUD XXX Q1 80

AMA: 2020,Dec,3; 2018,May,3; 2018,Jan,8; 2017,Jan,8; 2016,Jan,13

88307 Level V - Surgical pathology, gross and microscopic examination

INCLUDES
Adrenal resection
Bone, biopsy/curettings
Bone fragment(s), pathologic fractures
Brain, biopsy
Brain meninges, tumor resection
Breast, excision of lesion, requiring microscopic evaluation of surgical margins
Breast, mastectomy-partial/simple
Cervix, conization
Colon, segmental resection, other than for tumor
Extremity, amputation, nontraumatic
Eye, enucleation
Kidney, partial/total nephrectomy
Larynx, partial/total resection
Liver
- Biopsy, needle/wedge
- Partial resection

Lung, wedge biopsy
Lymph nodes, regional resection
Mediastinum, mass
Myocardium, biopsy
Odontogenic tumor
Ovary with or without tube, neoplastic
Pancreas, biopsy
Placenta, third trimester
Prostate, except radical resection
Salivary gland
Sentinel lymph node
Small intestine, resection, other than for tumor
Soft tissue mass (except lipoma)-biopsy/simple excision
Stomach-subtotal/total resection, other than for tumor
Testis, biopsy
Thymus, tumor
Thyroid, total/lobe
Ureter, resection
Urinary bladder, TUR
Uterus, with or without tubes and ovaries, other than neoplastic/prolapse

7.80 7.80 FUD XXX Q2 80

AMA: 2020,Dec,3; 2018,Jan,8; 2017,Jan,8; 2016,Jan,13

88309 Level VI - Surgical pathology, gross and microscopic examination

INCLUDES
Bone resection
Breast, mastectomy-with regional lymph nodes
Colon:
- Segmental resection for tumor
- Total resection

Esophagus, partial/total resection
Extremity, disarticulation
Fetus, with dissection
Larynx, partial/total resection-with regional lymph nodes
Lung-total/lobe/segment resection
Pancreas, total/subtotal resection
Prostate, radical resection
Small intestine, resection for tumor
Soft tissue tumor, extensive resection
Stomach, subtotal/total resection for tumor
Testis, tumor
Tongue/tonsil, resection for tumor
Urinary bladder, partial/total resection
Uterus, with or without tubes and ovaries, neoplastic
Vulva, total/subtotal resection

EXCLUDES
Evaluation fine needle aspirate (88172-88173)
Fine needle aspiration (10021, [10004, 10005, 10006, 10007, 10008, 10009, 10010, 10011, 10012])

11.8 11.8 FUD XXX Q2 80

AMA: 2020,Dec,3; 2018,Jan,8; 2017,Jan,8; 2016,Jan,13

Pathology and Laboratory

88305 — 88309

88311-88399 [88341, 88350, 88364, 88373, 88374, 88377] Additional Surgical Pathology Services

CMS: 100-02,15,80.1 Payment for Clinical Laboratory Services

\+ **88311** **Decalcification procedure (List separately in addition to code for surgical pathology examination)**

Code first surgical pathology exam (88302-88309)

0.61 0.61 **FUD** XXX N 80

AMA: 2020,Dec,3; 2018,Jan,8; 2017,Jan,8; 2016,Jan,13

88312 **Special stain including interpretation and report; Group I for microorganisms (eg, acid fast, methenamine silver)**

INCLUDES Reporting one unit for each special stain performed on surgical pathology block, cytologic sample, or hematologic smear

2.97 2.97 **FUD** XXX Q1 80

AMA: 2020,Dec,3; 2018,Jan,8; 2017,Jan,8; 2016,Jan,13

88313 **Group II, all other (eg, iron, trichrome), except stain for microorganisms, stains for enzyme constituents, or immunocytochemistry and immunohistochemistry**

INCLUDES Reporting one unit for each special stain performed on surgical pathology block, cytologic sample, or hematologic smear

EXCLUDES *Immunocytochemistry and immunohistochemistry (88342)*

2.14 2.14 **FUD** XXX Q1 80

AMA: 2020,Dec,3; 2018,Jan,8; 2017,Jan,8; 2016,Jan,13

\+ **88314** **histochemical stain on frozen tissue block (List separately in addition to code for primary procedure)**

INCLUDES Reporting one unit for each special stain on each frozen surgical pathology block

EXCLUDES *Routine frozen section stain during Mohs surgery (17311-17315)*

Special stain performed on frozen tissue section specimen to identify enzyme constituents (88319)

Code also modifier 59 for nonroutine histochemical stain on frozen section during Mohs surgery

Code first (17311-17315, 88302-88309, 88331-88332)

2.60 2.60 **FUD** XXX N 80

AMA: 2020,Dec,3; 2018,Jan,8; 2017,Jan,8; 2016,Jan,13

88319 **Group III, for enzyme constituents**

INCLUDES Reporting one unit for each special stain on each frozen surgical pathology block

EXCLUDES *Detection of enzyme constituents by immunohistochemical or immunocytochemical methodology (88342)*

3.15 3.15 **FUD** XXX Q2 80

AMA: 2020,Dec,3; 2018,Jan,8; 2017,Jan,8; 2016,Jan,13

88321 **Consultation and report on referred slides prepared elsewhere**

2.42 2.85 **FUD** XXX Q1 80

AMA: 2020,Dec,3; 2018,Jan,8; 2017,Jan,8; 2016,Jan,13

88323 **Consultation and report on referred material requiring preparation of slides**

3.26 3.26 **FUD** XXX Q1 80

AMA: 2020,Dec,3; 2018,Jan,8; 2017,Jan,8; 2016,Jan,13

88325 **Consultation, comprehensive, with review of records and specimens, with report on referred material**

4.18 4.96 **FUD** XXX Q1 80

AMA: 2020,Dec,3; 2018,Jan,8; 2017,Jan,8; 2016,Jan,13

88329 **Pathology consultation during surgery;**

1.04 1.47 **FUD** XXX Q1 80

AMA: 2020,Dec,3; 2018,Jan,8; 2017,Jan,8; 2016,Jan,13

88331 **first tissue block, with frozen section(s), single specimen**

Code also cytologic evaluation performed at same time (88334)

2.78 2.78 **FUD** XXX Q1 80

AMA: 2020,Dec,3; 2018,Jan,8; 2017,Jan,8; 2016,Jan,13

\+ **88332** **each additional tissue block with frozen section(s) (List separately in addition to code for primary procedure)**

Code first (88331)

1.51 1.51 **FUD** XXX N 80

AMA: 2020,Dec,3; 2018,Jan,8; 2017,Jan,8; 2016,Jan,13

88333 **cytologic examination (eg, touch prep, squash prep), initial site**

EXCLUDES *Intraprocedural cytologic evaluation fine needle aspirate (88172)*

Nonintraoperative cytologic examination (88160-88162)

2.55 2.55 **FUD** XXX Q2 80

AMA: 2020,Dec,3; 2018,Jan,8; 2017,Jan,8; 2016,Jan,13

\+ **88334** **cytologic examination (eg, touch prep, squash prep), each additional site (List separately in addition to code for primary procedure)**

EXCLUDES *Intraprocedural cytologic evaluation fine needle aspirate (88172)*

Nonintraoperative cytologic examination (88160-88162)

Percutaneous needle biopsy requiring intraprocedural cytologic examination (88333)

Code first (88331, 88333)

1.60 1.60 **FUD** ZZZ N 80

AMA: 2020,Dec,3; 2018,Jan,8; 2017,Jan,8; 2016,Jan,13

88341 **Resequenced code. See code following 88342.**

88342 **Immunohistochemistry or immunocytochemistry, per specimen; initial single antibody stain procedure**

EXCLUDES *Morphometric analysis, tumor immunohistochemistry, on same antibody (88360-88361)*

Multiplex antibody stain (88344)

Reporting code more than one time for each specific antibody

2.97 2.97 **FUD** XXX Q2 80

AMA: 2020,Dec,3; 2018,Jan,8; 2017,Jan,8; 2016,Jan,13

\+ # **88341** **each additional single antibody stain procedure (List separately in addition to code for primary procedure)**

EXCLUDES *Morphometric analysis (88360-88361)*

Multiplex antibody stain (88344)

Reporting code more than one time for each specific antibody

Code first (88342)

2.61 2.61 **FUD** ZZZ N 80

AMA: 2020,Dec,3; 2018,Jan,8; 2017,Jan,8; 2016,Jan,13

88344 **each multiplex antibody stain procedure**

INCLUDES Staining with multiple antibodies on same slide

EXCLUDES *Morphometric analysis, tumor immunohistochemistry, on same antibody (88360-88361)*

Reporting code more than one time for each specific antibody

4.86 4.86 **FUD** XXX Q1 80

AMA: 2020,Dec,3; 2018,Jan,8; 2017,Jan,8; 2016,Jan,13

88346 **Immunofluorescence, per specimen; initial single antibody stain procedure**

EXCLUDES *Fluorescent in situ hybridization studies (88364-88369 [88364, 88373, 88374, 88377])*

Multiple immunofluorescence analysis (88399)

3.56 3.56 **FUD** XXX Q2 80

AMA: 2020,Dec,3; 2018,Jan,8; 2017,Jan,8; 2016,Jan,13

\+ # **88350** **each additional single antibody stain procedure (List separately in addition to code for primary procedure)**

EXCLUDES *Fluorescent in situ hybridization studies (88364-88369 [88364, 88373, 88374, 88377])*

Multiple immunofluorescence analysis (88399)

Code first (88346)

2.18 2.18 **FUD** ZZZ N 80

AMA: 2020,Dec,3

88348 **Electron microscopy, diagnostic**

10.1 10.1 **FUD** XXX Q2 80

AMA: 2020,Dec,3

88350 **Resequenced code. See code following 88346.**

88355 **Morphometric analysis; skeletal muscle**
3.88 3.88 FUD XXX Q1 80
AMA: 2020,Dec,3; 2018,Jan,8; 2017,Jan,8; 2016,Jan,13

88356 **nerve**
6.66 6.66 FUD XXX Q1 80
AMA: 2020,Dec,3; 2018,Jan,8; 2017,Jan,8; 2016,Jan,13

88358 **tumor (eg, DNA ploidy)**
EXCLUDES *Special stain, Group II (88313)*
3.77 3.77 FUD XXX Q2 80
AMA: 2020,Dec,3; 2018,Jan,8; 2017,Jan,8; 2016,Jan,13

88360 **Morphometric analysis, tumor immunohistochemistry (eg, Her-2/neu, estrogen receptor/progesterone receptor), quantitative or semiquantitative, per specimen, each single antibody stain procedure; manual**
EXCLUDES *Additional stain procedures unless each test for different antibody (88341, 88342, 88344)*
Morphometric analysis using in situ hybridization techniques (88367-88368 [88373, 88374])
3.53 3.53 FUD XXX Q2 80
AMA: 2020,Dec,3; 2018,Jan,8; 2017,Jan,8; 2016,Jan,13

88361 **using computer-assisted technology**
EXCLUDES *Additional stain procedures unless each test for different antibody (88341, 88342, 88344)*
Morphometric analysis using in situ hybridization techniques (88367-88368 [88373, 88374])
3.58 3.58 FUD XXX Q2 80
AMA: 2020,Dec,3; 2018,Jan,8; 2017,Jan,8; 2016,Jan,13

88362 **Nerve teasing preparations**
6.44 6.44 FUD XXX Q2 80
AMA: 2020,Dec,3; 2018,Jan,8; 2017,Jan,8; 2016,Jan,13

88363 **Examination and selection of retrieved archival (ie, previously diagnosed) tissue(s) for molecular analysis (eg, KRAS mutational analysis)**
INCLUDES Archival retrieval only
0.57 0.67 FUD XXX Q1 80
AMA: 2020,Dec,3; 2018,Jan,8; 2017,Jan,8; 2016,Jan,13

88364 **Resequenced code. See code following 88365.**

88365 **In situ hybridization (eg, FISH), per specimen; initial single probe stain procedure**
EXCLUDES *Morphometric analysis probe stain procedures with same probe (88367, [88374], 88368, [88377])*
4.99 4.99 FUD XXX Q1 80
AMA: 2020,Dec,3; 2018,Nov,11; 2018,Jan,8; 2017,Jan,8; 2016,Jan,13

\+ # **88364** **each additional single probe stain procedure (List separately in addition to code for primary procedure)**
Code first (88365)
3.89 3.89 FUD ZZZ N 80
AMA: 2020,Dec,3

88366 **each multiplex probe stain procedure**
EXCLUDES *Morphometric analysis probe stain procedures (88367, [88374], 88368, [88377])*
7.80 7.80 FUD XXX Q1 80
AMA: 2020,Dec,3

88367 **Morphometric analysis, in situ hybridization (quantitative or semi-quantitative), using computer-assisted technology, per specimen; initial single probe stain procedure**
EXCLUDES *In situ hybridization probe stain procedures for same probe (88365, 88366, 88368, [88377])*
Morphometric in situ hybridization evaluation urinary tract cytologic specimens (88120-88121)
3.19 3.19 FUD XXX Q2 80
AMA: 2020,Dec,3; 2018,Jan,8; 2017,Jan,8; 2016,Jan,13

\+ # **88373** **each additional single probe stain procedure (List separately in addition to code for primary procedure)**
Code first (88367)
2.08 2.08 FUD ZZZ N 80
AMA: 2020,Dec,3

\# **88374** **each multiplex probe stain procedure**
EXCLUDES *In situ hybridization probe stain procedures for same probe (88365, 88366, 88368, [88377])*
9.65 9.65 FUD XXX Q1 80
AMA: 2020,Dec,3

88368 **Morphometric analysis, in situ hybridization (quantitative or semi-quantitative), manual, per specimen; initial single probe stain procedure**
EXCLUDES *In situ hybridization probe stain procedures for same probe (88365, 88366-88367, [88374])*
Morphometric in situ hybridization evaluation urinary tract cytologic specimens (88120-88121)
3.71 3.71 FUD XXX Q2 80
AMA: 2020,Dec,3; 2018,Jan,8; 2017,Jan,8; 2016,Jan,13

\+ **88369** **each additional single probe stain procedure (List separately in addition to code for primary procedure)**
Code first (88368)
3.23 3.23 FUD ZZZ N 80
AMA: 2020,Dec,3

\# **88377** **each multiplex probe stain procedure**
EXCLUDES *In situ hybridization probe stain procedures for same probe (88365, 88366-88367, [88374])*
Morphometric in situ hybridization evaluation, urinary tract cytologic specimens (88120-88121)
11.4 11.4 FUD XXX Q1 80
AMA: 2020,Dec,3

88371 **Protein analysis of tissue by Western Blot, with interpretation and report;**
0.00 0.00 FUD XXX N 80
AMA: 2020,Dec,3; 2018,Jan,8; 2017,Jan,8; 2016,Jan,13

88372 **immunological probe for band identification, each**
0.00 0.00 FUD XXX N 80
AMA: 2020,Dec,3; 2018,Jan,8; 2017,Jan,8; 2016,Jan,13

88373 **Resequenced code. See code following 88367.**

88374 **Resequenced code. See code following 88367.**

88375 **Optical endomicroscopic image(s), interpretation and report, real-time or referred, each endoscopic session**
EXCLUDES *Endoscopic procedures that include optical endomicroscopy (43206, 43252, 0397T)*
1.42 1.42 FUD XXX B 80 26
AMA: 2020,Dec,3; 2018,Jan,8; 2017,Jan,8; 2016,Jan,13

88377 **Resequenced code. See code following 88369.**

88380 **Microdissection (ie, sample preparation of microscopically identified target); laser capture**
EXCLUDES *Microdissection, manual procedure (88381)*
3.82 3.82 FUD XXX N 80
AMA: 2020,Dec,3; 2018,Aug,3; 2018,Jan,8; 2017,Jan,8; 2016,Jan,13

88381 **manual**
EXCLUDES *Microdissection, laser capture procedure (88380)*
5.07 5.07 FUD XXX N 80
AMA: 2020,Dec,3; 2018,Aug,3; 2018,Jan,8; 2017,Jan,8; 2016,Jan,13

88387 **Macroscopic examination, dissection, and preparation of tissue for non-microscopic analytical studies (eg, nucleic acid-based molecular studies); each tissue preparation (eg, a single lymph node)**
EXCLUDES *Pathology consultation during surgery (88329-88334, 88388)*
Tissue preparation for microbiologic cultures or flow cytometric studies
1.00 1.00 FUD XXX N 80
AMA: 2020,Dec,3; 2018,Jan,8; 2017,Jan,8; 2016,Jan,13

+ **88388** **in conjunction with a touch imprint, intraoperative consultation, or frozen section, each tissue preparation (eg, a single lymph node) (List separately in addition to code for primary procedure)**

EXCLUDES *Tissue preparation for microbiologic cultures or flow cytometric studies*

Code first (88329-88334)

1.04 1.04 FUD XXX N 80

AMA: 2020,Dec,3; 2018,Jan,8; 2017,Jan,8; 2016,Jan,13

88399 **Unlisted surgical pathology procedure**

0.00 0.00 FUD XXX Q1 80

AMA: 2020,Dec,3; 2018,Jan,8; 2017,Jan,8; 2016,Jan,13

88720-88749 Transcutaneous Procedures

EXCLUDES *Transcutaneous oxyhemoglobin measurement (0493T)*

Wavelength fluorescent spectroscopy advanced glycation end products (skin) (88749)

88720 **Bilirubin, total, transcutaneous**

EXCLUDES *Transdermal oxygen saturation testing (94760-94762)*

0.00 0.00 FUD XXX Q

AMA: 2020,Dec,3; 2020,May,13; 2018,Jan,8; 2017,Jan,8; 2016,Jan,13

88738 **Hemoglobin (Hgb), quantitative, transcutaneous**

EXCLUDES *In vitro hemoglobin measurement (85018)*

0.00 0.00 FUD XXX Q

AMA: 2020,Dec,3; 2018,Jan,8; 2017,Jan,8; 2016,Jan,13

88740 **Hemoglobin, quantitative, transcutaneous, per day; carboxyhemoglobin**

EXCLUDES *In vitro carboxyhemoglobin measurement (82375)*

0.00 0.00 FUD XXX Q

AMA: 2020,Dec,3; 2018,Jan,8; 2017,Jan,8; 2016,Jan,13

88741 **methemoglobin**

EXCLUDES *In vitro quantitative methemoglobin measurement (83050)*

0.00 0.00 FUD XXX Q

AMA: 2020,Dec,3; 2018,Jan,8; 2017,Jan,8; 2016,Jan,13

88749 **Unlisted in vivo (eg, transcutaneous) laboratory service**

INCLUDES All in vivo measurements not specifically listed

0.00 0.00 FUD XXX Q

AMA: 2020,Dec,3

89049-89240 Other Pathology Services

89049 **Caffeine halothane contracture test (CHCT) for malignant hyperthermia susceptibility, including interpretation and report**

1.75 7.13 FUD XXX Q1 80

AMA: 2020,Dec,3; 2018,Jan,8; 2017,Jan,8; 2016,Jan,13

89050 **Cell count, miscellaneous body fluids (eg, cerebrospinal fluid, joint fluid), except blood;**

0.00 0.00 FUD XXX Q

AMA: 2020,Dec,3; 2018,Jan,8; 2017,Jan,8; 2016,Jan,13

89051 **with differential count**

0.00 0.00 FUD XXX Q

AMA: 2020,Dec,3; 2018,Jan,8; 2017,Jan,8; 2016,Jan,13

89055 **Leukocyte assessment, fecal, qualitative or semiquantitative**

0.00 0.00 FUD XXX Q

AMA: 2020,Dec,3; 2018,Jan,8; 2017,Jan,8; 2016,Jan,13

89060 **Crystal identification by light microscopy with or without polarizing lens analysis, tissue or any body fluid (except urine)**

EXCLUDES *Crystal identification on paraffin embedded tissue*

0.00 0.00 FUD XXX Q 80

AMA: 2020,Dec,3; 2018,Jan,8; 2017,Jan,8; 2016,Jan,13

89125 **Fat stain, feces, urine, or respiratory secretions**

0.00 0.00 FUD XXX Q

AMA: 2020,Dec,3; 2018,Jan,8; 2017,Jan,8; 2016,Jan,13

89160 **Meat fibers, feces**

0.00 0.00 FUD XXX Q

AMA: 2020,Dec,3; 2018,Jan,8; 2017,Jan,8; 2016,Jan,13

89190 **Nasal smear for eosinophils**

EXCLUDES *Occult blood feces (82270)*

Paternity tests (86910)

0.00 0.00 FUD XXX Q

AMA: 2020,Dec,3; 2018,Jan,8; 2017,Jan,8; 2016,Jan,13

89220 **Sputum, obtaining specimen, aerosol induced technique (separate procedure)**

0.46 0.46 FUD XXX Q1 80 TC

AMA: 2020,Dec,3; 2018,Jan,8; 2017,Jan,8; 2016,Jan,13

89230 **Sweat collection by iontophoresis**

0.08 0.08 FUD XXX Q1 80 TC

AMA: 2020,Dec,3; 2018,Jan,8; 2017,Jan,8; 2016,Jan,13

89240 **Unlisted miscellaneous pathology test**

0.00 0.00 FUD XXX Q1 80

AMA: 2020,Dec,3; 2018,Jan,8; 2017,Jan,8; 2016,Jan,13

89250-89398 Infertility Treatment Services

CMS: 100-02,1,100 Treatment for Infertility

89250 **Culture of oocyte(s)/embryo(s), less than 4 days;**

0.00 0.00 FUD XXX Q1

AMA: 2020,Dec,3; 2018,Jan,8; 2017,Jan,8; 2016,Jan,13

89251 **with co-culture of oocyte(s)/embryos**

EXCLUDES *Extended culture oocyte(s)/embryo(s) (89272)*

0.00 0.00 FUD XXX Q2

AMA: 2020,Dec,3; 2018,Jan,8; 2017,Jan,8; 2016,Jan,13

89253 **Assisted embryo hatching, microtechniques (any method)**

0.00 0.00 FUD XXX Q1

AMA: 2020,Dec,3; 2018,Jan,8; 2017,Jan,8; 2016,Jan,13

89254 **Oocyte identification from follicular fluid**

0.00 0.00 FUD XXX Q1

AMA: 2020,Dec,3; 2018,Jan,8; 2017,Jan,8; 2016,Jan,13

89255 **Preparation of embryo for transfer (any method)**

0.00 0.00 FUD XXX Q1

AMA: 2020,Dec,3; 2018,Jan,8; 2017,Jan,8; 2016,Jan,13

89257 **Sperm identification from aspiration (other than seminal fluid)**

EXCLUDES *Semen analysis (89300-89320)*

Sperm identification from testis tissue (89264)

0.00 0.00 FUD XXX Q1

AMA: 2020,Dec,3; 2018,Jan,8; 2017,Jan,8; 2016,Jan,13

89258 **Cryopreservation; embryo(s)**

0.00 0.00 FUD XXX Q2

AMA: 2020,Dec,3; 2018,Jan,8; 2017,Jan,8; 2016,Jan,13

89259 **sperm**

EXCLUDES *Cryopreservation testicular reproductive tissue (89335)*

0.00 0.00 FUD XXX Q1

AMA: 2020,Dec,3; 2018,Jan,8; 2017,Jan,8; 2016,Jan,13

89260 **Sperm isolation; simple prep (eg, sperm wash and swim-up) for insemination or diagnosis with semen analysis**

0.00 0.00 FUD XXX Q1

AMA: 2020,Dec,3; 2018,Jan,8; 2017,Jan,8; 2016,Jan,13

89261 **complex prep (eg, Percoll gradient, albumin gradient) for insemination or diagnosis with semen analysis**

EXCLUDES *Semen analysis without sperm wash or swim-up (89320)*

0.00 0.00 FUD XXX Q1

AMA: 2020,Dec,3; 2018,Jan,8; 2017,Jan,8; 2016,Jan,13

89264 **Sperm identification from testis tissue, fresh or cryopreserved** ♂

EXCLUDES *Biopsy testis (54500, 54505)*

Semen analysis (89300-89320)

Sperm identification from aspiration (89257)

0.00 0.00 FUD XXX Q1

AMA: 2020,Dec,3; 2018,Jan,8; 2017,Jan,8; 2016,Jan,13

89268 **Insemination of oocytes**
0.00 0.00 FUD XXX Q1
AMA: 2020,Dec,3; 2018,Jan,8; 2017,Jan,8; 2016,Jan,13

89272 **Extended culture of oocyte(s)/embryo(s), 4-7 days**
0.00 0.00 FUD XXX Q2
AMA: 2020,Dec,3; 2018,Jan,8; 2017,Jan,8; 2016,Jan,13

89280 **Assisted oocyte fertilization, microtechnique; less than or equal to 10 oocytes**
0.00 0.00 FUD XXX Q2
AMA: 2020,Dec,3; 2018,Jan,8; 2017,Jan,8; 2016,Jan,13

89281 **greater than 10 oocytes**
0.00 0.00 FUD XXX Q1
AMA: 2020,Dec,3; 2018,Jan,8; 2017,Jan,8; 2016,Jan,13

89290 **Biopsy, oocyte polar body or embryo blastomere, microtechnique (for pre-implantation genetic diagnosis); less than or equal to 5 embryos**
0.00 0.00 FUD XXX Q1
AMA: 2020,Dec,3; 2018,Jan,8; 2017,Jan,8; 2016,Jan,13

89291 **greater than 5 embryos**
0.00 0.00 FUD XXX Q1
AMA: 2020,Dec,3; 2018,Jan,8; 2017,Jan,8; 2016,Jan,13

89300 **Semen analysis; presence and/or motility of sperm including Huhner test (post coital)**
0.00 0.00 FUD XXX ☒ Q
AMA: 2020,Dec,3; 2018,Jan,8; 2017,Jan,8; 2016,Jan,13

89310 **motility and count (not including Huhner test)** ♂
0.00 0.00 FUD XXX Q
AMA: 2020,Dec,3; 2018,Jan,8; 2017,Jan,8; 2016,Jan,13

89320 **volume, count, motility, and differential** ♂
EXCLUDES *Skin testing (86485-86580, 95012-95199)*
0.00 0.00 FUD XXX Q
AMA: 2020,Dec,3; 2018,Jan,8; 2017,Jan,8; 2016,Jan,13

89321 **sperm presence and motility of sperm, if performed** ♂
EXCLUDES *Hyaluronan binding assay (HBA) (89398)*
0.00 0.00 FUD XXX ☒ Q
AMA: 2020,Dec,3; 2018,Jan,8; 2017,Jan,8; 2016,Jan,13

89322 **volume, count, motility, and differential using strict morphologic criteria (eg, Kruger)** ♂
0.00 0.00 FUD XXX Q
AMA: 2020,Dec,3; 2018,Jan,8; 2017,Jan,8; 2016,Jan,13

89325 **Sperm antibodies** ♂
EXCLUDES *Medicolegal identification sperm (88125)*
0.00 0.00 FUD XXX Q
AMA: 2020,Dec,3; 2018,Jan,8; 2017,Jan,8; 2016,Jan,13

89329 **Sperm evaluation; hamster penetration test** ♂
0.00 0.00 FUD XXX Q
AMA: 2020,Dec,3; 2018,Jan,8; 2017,Jan,8; 2016,Jan,13

89330 **cervical mucus penetration test, with or without spinnbarkeit test** ♂
0.00 0.00 FUD XXX Q
AMA: 2020,Dec,3; 2018,Jan,8; 2017,Jan,8; 2016,Jan,13

89331 **Sperm evaluation, for retrograde ejaculation, urine (sperm concentration, motility, and morphology, as indicated)** ♂
EXCLUDES *Detection sperm in urine (81015)*
Code also semen analysis on concurrent sperm specimen (89300-89322)
0.00 0.00 FUD XXX Q
AMA: 2020,Dec,3; 2018,Jan,8; 2017,Jan,8; 2016,Jan,13

89335 **Cryopreservation, reproductive tissue, testicular**
EXCLUDES *Cryopreservation:*
Embryo(s) (89258)
Immature oocyte(s) (89398)
Mature oocytes (89337)
Ovarian reproductive tissue (89398)
Sperm (89259)
0.00 0.00 FUD XXX Q1
AMA: 2020,Dec,3; 2018,Jan,8; 2017,Jan,8; 2016,Jan,13

89337 **Cryopreservation, mature oocyte(s)** ♀
EXCLUDES *Cryopreservation immature oocyte[s] (89398)*
0.00 0.00 FUD XXX Q1
AMA: 2020,Dec,3; 2018,Jan,8; 2017,Jan,8; 2016,Jan,13

89342 **Storage (per year); embryo(s)**
0.00 0.00 FUD XXX Q1
AMA: 2020,Dec,3; 2018,Jan,8; 2017,Jan,8; 2016,Jan,13

89343 **sperm/semen**
0.00 0.00 FUD XXX Q1
AMA: 2020,Dec,3; 2018,Jan,8; 2017,Jan,8; 2016,Jan,13

89344 **reproductive tissue, testicular/ovarian**
0.00 0.00 FUD XXX Q1
AMA: 2020,Dec,3; 2018,Jan,8; 2017,Jan,8; 2016,Jan,13

89346 **oocyte(s)**
0.00 0.00 FUD XXX Q2
AMA: 2020,Dec,3; 2018,Jan,8; 2017,Jan,8; 2016,Jan,13

89352 **Thawing of cryopreserved; embryo(s)**
0.00 0.00 FUD XXX Q1
AMA: 2020,Dec,3; 2018,Jan,8; 2017,Jan,8; 2016,Jan,13

89353 **sperm/semen, each aliquot**
0.00 0.00 FUD XXX Q1
AMA: 2020,Dec,3; 2018,Jan,8; 2017,Jan,8; 2016,Jan,13

89354 **reproductive tissue, testicular/ovarian**
0.00 0.00 FUD XXX Q1
AMA: 2020,Dec,3; 2018,Jan,8; 2017,Jan,8; 2016,Jan,13

89356 **oocytes, each aliquot**
0.00 0.00 FUD XXX Q1
AMA: 2020,Dec,3; 2018,Jan,8; 2017,Jan,8; 2016,Jan,13

89398 **Unlisted reproductive medicine laboratory procedure**
INCLUDES Cryopreservation:
Immature oocytes
Ovarian reproductive tissue
Hyaluronan binding assay (HBA)
0.00 0.00 FUD XXX Q1
AMA: 2020,Dec,3

0001U-0305U Proprietary Laboratory Analysis (PLA)

In response to the Protecting Access to Medicare Act of 2014 (PAMA), which focuses on payment and coding of clinical laboratory studies paid for under the Medicare Clinical Laboratory Fee Schedule (CLFS), the AMA has developed a new category of CPT codes known as Proprietary Laboratory Analyses (PLA), which are released on a quarterly basis. These alphanumeric codes appear at the end of the Pathology and Laboratory chapter of the CPT book and include a wide range of tests. Codes in this section can also be found in Appendix L along with the procedure's proprietary name and clinical laboratory or manufacturer. When multiple codes have identical code descriptors and can only be distinguished by a proprietary test name, instructional notes are provided to help ensure accurate code assignment.

INCLUDES All necessary investigative services
PLA codes take priority over other CPT codes

EXCLUDES *Additional procedures necessary before cell lysis (88380-88381)*

0001U **Red blood cell antigen typing, DNA, human erythrocyte antigen gene analysis of 35 antigens from 11 blood groups, utilizing whole blood, common RBC alleles reported**
INCLUDES PreciseType® HEA Test, Immucor, Inc
0.00 0.00 FUD 000 A
AMA: 2019,Jun,11

0002U Oncology (colorectal), quantitative assessment of three urine metabolites (ascorbic acid, succinic acid and carnitine) by liquid chromatography with tandem mass spectrometry (LC-MS/MS) using multiple reaction monitoring acquisition, algorithm reported as likelihood of adenomatous polyps

INCLUDES PolypDX™, Atlantic Diagnostic Laboratories, LLC, Metabolomic Technologies Inc

0.00 0.00 FUD 000 Q

AMA: 2018,Aug,3

0003U Oncology (ovarian) biochemical assays of five proteins (apolipoprotein A-1, CA 125 II, follicle stimulating hormone, human epididymis protein 4, transferrin), utilizing serum, algorithm reported as a likelihood score

INCLUDES Overa (OVA1 Next Generation), Aspira Labs, Inc, Vermillion, Inc

0.00 0.00 FUD 000 Q

0005U Oncology (prostate) gene expression profile by real-time RT-PCR of 3 genes (*ERG, PCA3,* and *SPDEF*), urine, algorithm reported as risk score

INCLUDES ExosomeDx® Prostate (IntelliScore), Exosome Diagnostics, Inc, Exosome Diagnostics, Inc

0.00 0.00 FUD 000 Q

0007U Drug test(s), presumptive, with definitive confirmation of positive results, any number of drug classes, urine, includes specimen verification including DNA authentication in comparison to buccal DNA, per date of service

INCLUDES ToxProtect, Genotox Laboratories LTD

0.00 0.00 FUD 000 Q

AMA: 2018,Jan,6

0008U Helicobacter pylori detection and antibiotic resistance, DNA, 16S and 23S rRNA, gyrA, pbp1, rdxA and rpoB, next-generation sequencing, formalin-fixed paraffin-embedded or fresh tissue or fecal sample, predictive, reported as positive or negative for resistance to clarithromycin, fluoroquinolones, metronidazole, amoxicillin, tetracycline, and rifabutin

INCLUDES AmHPR® H. pylori Antibiotic Resistance Panel, American Molecular Laboratories, Inc

0.00 0.00 FUD 000 A

0009U Oncology (breast cancer), ERBB2 (HER2) copy number by FISH, tumor cells from formalin fixed paraffin embedded tissue isolated using image-based dielectrophoresis (DEP) sorting, reported as ERBB2 gene amplified or non-amplified

INCLUDES DEPArray™ HER2, PacificDx

0.00 0.00 FUD 000 Q

0010U Infectious disease (bacterial), strain typing by whole genome sequencing, phylogenetic-based report of strain relatedness, per submitted isolate

INCLUDES Bacterial Typing by Whole Genome Sequencing, Mayo Clinic

0.00 0.00 FUD 000 A

0011U Prescription drug monitoring, evaluation of drugs present by LC-MS/MS, using oral fluid, reported as a comparison to an estimated steady-state range, per date of service including all drug compounds and metabolites

INCLUDES Cordant CORE™, Cordant Health Solutions

0.00 0.00 FUD 000 Q

0012U Germline disorders, gene rearrangement detection by whole genome next-generation sequencing, DNA, whole blood, report of specific gene rearrangement(s)

INCLUDES MatePair Targeted Rearrangements, Congenital, Mayo Clinic

0.00 0.00 FUD 000 A

0013U Oncology (solid organ neoplasia), gene rearrangement detection by whole genome next-generation sequencing, DNA, fresh or frozen tissue or cells, report of specific gene rearrangement(s)

INCLUDES MatePair Targeted Rearrangements, Oncology, Mayo Clinic

0.00 0.00 FUD 000 A

0014U Hematology (hematolymphoid neoplasia), gene rearrangement detection by whole genome next-generation sequencing, DNA, whole blood or bone marrow, report of specific gene rearrangement(s)

INCLUDES MatePair Targeted Rearrangements, Hematologic, Mayo Clinic

0.00 0.00 FUD 000 A

0016U Oncology (hematolymphoid neoplasia), RNA, *BCR/ABL1* major and minor breakpoint fusion transcripts, quantitative PCR amplification, blood or bone marrow, report of fusion not detected or detected with quantitation

INCLUDES BCR-ABL1 major and minor breakpoint fusion transcripts, University of Iowa, Department of Pathology, Asuragen

0.00 0.00 FUD 000 A

0017U Oncology (hematolymphoid neoplasia), *JAK2* mutation, DNA, PCR amplification of exons 12-14 and sequence analysis, blood or bone marrow, report of *JAK2* mutation not detected or detected

INCLUDES *JAK2* Mutation, University of Iowa, Department of Pathology

0.00 0.00 FUD 000 A

0018U Oncology (thyroid), microRNA profiling by RT-PCR of 10 microRNA sequences, utilizing fine needle aspirate, algorithm reported as a positive or negative result for moderate to high risk of malignancy

INCLUDES ThyraMIR™, Interpace Diagnostics

0.00 0.00 FUD 000 A

0019U Oncology, RNA, gene expression by whole transcriptome sequencing, formalin-fixed paraffin embedded tissue or fresh frozen tissue, predictive algorithm reported as potential targets for therapeutic agents

INCLUDES OncoTarget/OncoTreat, Columbia University Department of Pathology and Cell Biology, Darwin Health

0.00 0.00 FUD 000 A

0021U Oncology (prostate), detection of 8 autoantibodies (ARF 6, NKX3-1, 5'-UTR-BMI1, CEP 164, 3'-UTR-Ropporin, Desmocollin, AURKAIP-1, CSNK2A2), multiplexed immunoassay and flow cytometry serum, algorithm reported as risk score

INCLUDES Apifiny®, Armune BioScience, Inc

0.00 0.00 FUD 000 Q

0022U Targeted genomic sequence analysis panel, non-small cell lung neoplasia, DNA and RNA analysis, 23 genes, interrogation for sequence variants and rearrangements, reported as presence/absence of variants and associated therapy(ies) to consider

INCLUDES Oncomine™ Dx Target Test, Thermo Fisher Scientific

0.00 0.00 FUD 000 A

0023U Oncology (acute myelogenous leukemia), DNA, genotyping of internal tandem duplication, p.D835, p.I836, using mononuclear cells, reported as detection or non-detection of *FLT3* mutation and indication for or against the use of midostaurin

INCLUDES LeukoStrat® CDx *FLT3* Mutation Assay, LabPMM LLC, an Invivoscribe Technologies, Inc Company, Invivoscribe Technologies, Inc

0.00 0.00 FUD 000 A

0024U Glycosylated acute phase proteins (GlycA), nuclear magnetic resonance spectroscopy, quantitative

INCLUDES GlycA, Laboratory Corporation of America, Laboratory Corporation of America

0.00 0.00 FUD 000 Q

0025U Tenofovir, by liquid chromatography with tandem mass spectrometry (LC-MS/MS), urine, quantitative

INCLUDES UrSure Tenofovir Quantification Test, Synergy Medical Laboratories, UrSure Inc

0.00 0.00 FUD 000 Q

0026U Oncology (thyroid), DNA and mRNA of 112 genes, next-generation sequencing, fine needle aspirate of thyroid nodule, algorithmic analysis reported as a categorical result ("Positive, high probability of malignancy" or "Negative, low probability of malignancy")

INCLUDES Thyroseq Genomic Classifier, CBLPath, Inc, University of Pittsburgh Medical Center

0.00 0.00 FUD 000

0027U *JAK2 (Janus kinase 2)* (eg, myeloproliferative disorder) gene analysis, targeted sequence analysis exons 12-15

INCLUDES *JAK2* Exons 12 to 15 Sequencing, Mayo Clinic, Mayo Clinic

0.00 0.00 FUD 000

0029U Drug metabolism (adverse drug reactions and drug response), targeted sequence analysis (ie, *CYP1A2, CYP2C19, CYP2C9, CYP2D6, CYP3A4, CYP3A5, CYP4F2, SLCO1B1, VKORC1* and rs12777823)

INCLUDES Focused Pharmacogenomics Panel, Mayo Clinic, Mayo Clinic

0.00 0.00 FUD 000

0030U Drug metabolism (warfarin drug response), targeted sequence analysis (ie, *CYP2C9, CYP4F2, VKORC1*, rs12777823)

INCLUDES Warfarin Response Genotype, Mayo Clinic, Mayo Clinic

0.00 0.00 FUD 000

0031U *CYP1A2 (cytochrome P450 family 1, subfamily A, member 2)*(eg, drug metabolism) gene analysis, common variants (ie, *1F, *1K, *6, *7)

INCLUDES Cytochrome P450 1A2 Genotype, Mayo Clinic, Mayo Clinic

0.00 0.00 FUD 000

0032U *COMT (catechol-O-methyltransferase)(drug metabolism)* gene analysis, c.472G>A (rs4680) variant

INCLUDES Catechol-O-Methyltransferase (*COMT*) Genotype, Mayo Clinic, Mayo Clinic

0.00 0.00 FUD 000

0033U *HTR2A (5-hydroxytryptamine receptor 2A), HTR2C (5-hydroxytryptamine receptor 2C)* (eg, citalopram metabolism) gene analysis, common variants (ie, *HTR2A* rs7997012 [c.614-2211T>C], *HTR2C* rs3813929 [c.-759C>T] and rs1414334 [c.551-3008C>G])

INCLUDES Serotonin Receptor Genotype (*HTR2A* and *HTR2C*), Mayo Clinic, Mayo Clinic

0.00 0.00 FUD 000

0034U *TPMT (thiopurine S-methyltransferase), NUDT15 (nudix hydroxylase 15)(eg, thiopurine metabolism)*, gene analysis, common variants (ie, *TPMT* *2, *3A, *3B, *3C, *4, *5, *6, *8, *12; *NUDT15* *3, *4, *5)

INCLUDES Thiopurine Methyltransferase (*TPMT*) and Nudix Hydrolase (*NUDT15*) Genotyping, Mayo Clinic, Mayo Clinic

0.00 0.00 FUD 000

0035U Neurology (prion disease), cerebrospinal fluid, detection of prion protein by quaking-induced conformational conversion, qualitative

INCLUDES Real-time quaking-induced conversion for prion detection (RT-QuIC), National Prion Disease Pathology Surveillance Center

0.00 0.00 FUD 000

0036U Exome (ie, somatic mutations), paired formalin-fixed paraffin-embedded tumor tissue and normal specimen, sequence analyses

INCLUDES EXaCT-1 Whole Exome Testing, Lab of Oncology-Molecular Detection, Weill Cornell Medicine-Clinical Genomics Laboratory

0.00 0.00 FUD 000

0037U Targeted genomic sequence analysis, solid organ neoplasm, DNA analysis of 324 genes, interrogation for sequence variants, gene copy number amplifications, gene rearrangements, microsatellite instability and tumor mutational burden

INCLUDES FoundationOne CDx™ (F1CDx), Foundation Medicine, Inc, Foundation Medicine, Inc

0.00 0.00 FUD 000

0038U Vitamin D, 25 hydroxy D2 and D3, by LC-MS/MS, serum microsample, quantitative

INCLUDES Sensieva™ Droplet 25OH Vitamin D2/D3 Microvolume LC/MS Assay, InSource Diagnostics, InSource Diagnostics

0.00 0.00 FUD 000

0039U Deoxyribonucleic acid (DNA) antibody, double stranded, high avidity

INCLUDES Anti-dsDNA, High Salt/Avidity, University of Washington, Department of Laboratory Medicine, Bio-Rad

0.00 0.00 FUD 000

0040U *BCR/ABL1 (t(9;22))* (eg, chronic myelogenous leukemia) translocation analysis, major breakpoint, quantitative

INCLUDES MRDx BCR-ABL Test, MolecularMD, MolecularMD

0.00 0.00 FUD 000

0041U Borrelia burgdorferi, antibody detection of 5 recombinant protein groups, by immunoblot, IgM

INCLUDES Lyme ImmunoBlot IgM, IGeneX Inc, ID-FISH Technology Inc. (ASR) (Lyme ImmunoBlot IgM Strips Only)

0.00 0.00 FUD 000

0042U Borrelia burgdorferi, antibody detection of 12 recombinant protein groups, by immunoblot, IgG

INCLUDES Lyme ImmunoBlot IgG, IGeneX Inc, ID-FISH Technology Inc (ASR) (Lyme ImmunoBlot IgG Strips Only)

0.00 0.00 FUD 000

0043U Tick-borne relapsing fever Borrelia group, antibody detection to 4 recombinant protein groups, by immunoblot, IgM

INCLUDES Tick-Borne Relapsing Fever (TBRF) Borrelia ImmunoBlots IgM Test, IGeneX Inc, ID-FISH Technology Inc (Provides TBRF ImmunoBlot IgM Strips)

0.00 0.00 FUD 000

0044U Tick-borne relapsing fever Borrelia group, antibody detection to 4 recombinant protein groups, by immunoblot, IgG

INCLUDES Tick-Borne Relapsing Fever (TBRF) Borrelia ImmunoBlots IgG Test, IGeneX Inc, ID-FISH Technology Inc (Provides TBRF ImmunoBlot IgG Strips)

0.00 0.00 FUD 000

0045U Oncology (breast ductal carcinoma in situ), mRNA, gene expression profiling by real-time RT-PCR of 12 genes (7 content and 5 housekeeping), utilizing formalin-fixed paraffin-embedded tissue, algorithm reported as recurrence score

INCLUDES The Oncotype DX® Breast DCIS Score™ Test, Genomic Health, Inc, Genomic Health, Inc

0.00 0.00 FUD 000

0046U *FLT3* (fms-related tyrosine kinase 3) (eg, acute myeloid leukemia) internal tandem duplication (ITD) variants, quantitative

INCLUDES FLT3 ITD MRD by NGS, LabPMM LLC, an Invivoscribe Technologies, Inc Company

0.00 0.00 FUD 000

0047U Oncology (prostate), mRNA, gene expression profiling by real-time RT-PCR of 17 genes (12 content and 5 housekeeping), utilizing formalin-fixed paraffin-embedded tissue, algorithm reported as a risk score

INCLUDES Oncotype DX Genomic Prostate Score, Genomic Health, Inc, Genomic Health, Inc

0.00 0.00 FUD 000

0048U Oncology (solid organ neoplasia), DNA, targeted sequencing of protein-coding exons of 468 cancer-associated genes, including interrogation for somatic mutations and microsatellite instability, matched with normal specimens, utilizing formalin-fixed paraffin-embedded tumor tissue, report of clinically significant mutation(s)

INCLUDES MSK-IMPACT (Integrated Mutation Profiling of Actionable Cancer Targets), Memorial Sloan Kettering Cancer Center

0.00 0.00 FUD 000

0049U NPM1 (nucleophosmin) (eg, acute myeloid leukemia) gene analysis, quantitative

INCLUDES *NPM1* MRD by NGS, LabPMM LLC, an Invivoscribe Technologies, Inc Company

0.00 0.00 FUD 000

0050U Targeted genomic sequence analysis panel, acute myelogenous leukemia, DNA analysis, 194 genes, interrogation for sequence variants, copy number variants or rearrangements

INCLUDES MyAML NGS Panel, LabPMM LLC, an Invivoscribe Technologies, Inc Company

0.00 0.00 FUD 000

▲ **0051U Prescription drug monitoring, evaluation of drugs present by liquid chromatography tandem mass spectrommetry (LC-MS/MS), urine or blood, 31 drug panel, reported as quantitative results, detected or not detected, per date of service**

INCLUDES UCompliDx, Elite Medical Laboratory Solutions, LLC, Elite Medical Laboratory Solutions, LLC (LDT)

0.00 0.00 FUD 000

0052U Lipoprotein, blood, high resolution fractionation and quantitation of lipoproteins, including all five major lipoprotein classes and subclasses of HDL, LDL, and VLDL by vertical auto profile ultracentrifugation

INCLUDES VAP Cholesterol Test, VAP Diagnostics Laboratory, Inc, VAP Diagnostics Laboratory, Inc

0.00 0.00 FUD 000

0053U Oncology (prostate cancer), FISH analysis of 4 genes (*ASAP1, HDAC9, CHD1* and *PTEN*), needle biopsy specimen, algorithm reported as probability of higher tumor grade

INCLUDES Prostate Cancer Risk Panel, Mayo Clinic, Laboratory Developed Test

0.00 0.00 FUD 000

0054U Prescription drug monitoring, 14 or more classes of drugs and substances, definitive tandem mass spectrometry with chromatography, capillary blood, quantitative report with therapeutic and toxic ranges, including steady-state range for the prescribed dose when detected, per date of service

INCLUDES AssuranceRx Micro Serum, Firstox Laboratories, LLC, Firstox Laboratories, LLC

0.00 0.00 FUD 000

0055U Cardiology (heart transplant), cell-free DNA, PCR assay of 96 DNA target sequences (94 single nucleotide polymorphism targets and two control targets), plasma

INCLUDES myTAIHEART, TAI Diagnostics, Inc, TAI Diagnostics, Inc

0.00 0.00 FUD 000

0056U Hematology (acute myelogenous leukemia), DNA, whole genome next-generation sequencing to detect gene rearrangement(s), blood or bone marrow, report of specific gene rearrangement(s)

INCLUDES MatePair Acute Myeloid Leukemia Panel, Mayo Clinic, Laboratory Developed Test

0.00 0.00 FUD 000

0058U Oncology (Merkel cell carcinoma), detection of antibodies to the Merkel cell polyoma virus oncoprotein (small T antigen), serum, quantitative

INCLUDES Merkel SmT Oncoprotein Antibody Titer, University of Washington, Department of Laboratory Medicine

0.00 0.00 FUD 000

0059U Oncology (Merkel cell carcinoma), detection of antibodies to the Merkel cell polyoma virus capsid protein (VP1), serum, reported as positive or negative

INCLUDES Merkel Virus VP1 Capsid Antibody, University of Washington, Department of Laboratory Medicine

0.00 0.00 FUD 000

0060U Twin zygosity, genomic targeted sequence analysis of chromosome 2, using circulating cell-free fetal DNA in maternal blood

INCLUDES Twins Zygosity PLA, Natera, Inc, Natera, Inc

0.00 0.00 FUD 000

0061U Transcutaneous measurement of five biomarkers (tissue oxygenation [StO2], oxyhemoglobin [ctHbO2], deoxyhemoglobin [ctHbR], papillary and reticular dermal hemoglobin concentrations [ctHb1 and ctHb2]), using spatial frequency domain imaging (SFDI) and multi-spectral analysis

INCLUDES Transcutaneous multispectral measurement of tissue oxygenation and hemoglobin using spatial frequency domain imaging (SFDI), Modulated Imaging, Inc, Modulated Imaging, Inc

0.00 0.00 FUD 000

0062U Autoimmune (systemic lupus erythematosus), IgG and IgM analysis of 80 biomarkers, utilizing serum, algorithm reported with a risk score

INCLUDES SLE-key® Rule Out, Veracis Inc, Veracis Inc

0.00 0.00 FUD 000

0063U Neurology (autism), 32 amines by LC-MS/MS, using plasma, algorithm reported as metabolic signature associated with autism spectrum disorder

INCLUDES NPDX ASD ADM Panel I, Stemina Biomarker Discovery, Inc, Stemina Biomarker Discovery, Inc d/b/a NeuroPointDX

0.00 0.00 FUD 000

0064U Antibody, Treponema pallidum, total and rapid plasma reagin (RPR), immunoassay, qualitative

INCLUDES BioPlex 2200 Syphilis Total & RPR Assay, Bio-Rad Laboratories, Bio-Rad Laboratories

0.00 0.00 FUD 000

0065U Syphilis test, non-treponemal antibody, immunoassay, qualitative (RPR)

INCLUDES BioPlex 2200 RPR Assay, Bio-Rad Laboratories, Bio-Rad Laboratories

0.00 0.00 FUD 000

0066U Placental alpha-micro globulin-1 (PAMG-1), immunoassay with direct optical observation, cervico-vaginal fluid, each specimen

INCLUDES PartoSure™ Test, Parsagen Diagnostics, Inc, Parsagen Diagnostics, Inc, a QIAGEN Company

0.00 0.00 FUD 000

0067U **Oncology (breast), immunohistochemistry, protein expression profiling of 4 biomarkers (matrix metalloproteinase-1 [MMP-1], carcinoembryonic antigen-related cell adhesion molecule 6 [CEACAM6], hyaluronoglucosaminidase [HYAL1], highly expressed in cancer protein [HEC1]), formalin-fixed paraffin-embedded precancerous breast tissue, algorithm reported as carcinoma risk score**

INCLUDES BBDRisk Dx™, Silbiotech, Inc, Silbiotech, Inc

0.00 0.00 FUD 000

0068U **Candida species panel *(C. albicans, C. glabrata, C. parapsilosis, C. kruseii, C tropicalis, and C. auris)*, amplified probe technique with qualitative report of the presence or absence of each species**

INCLUDES MYCODART-PCR™ Dual Amplification Real Time PCR Panel for 6 Candida species, RealTime Laboratories, Inc/MycoDART, Inc, RealTime Laboratories, Inc

0.00 0.00 FUD 000

0069U **Oncology (colorectal), microRNA, RT-PCR expression profiling of miR-31-3p, formalin-fixed paraffin-embedded tissue, algorithm reported as an expression score**

INCLUDES miR-31now™, GoPath Laboratories, GoPath Laboratories

0.00 0.00 FUD 000

0070U ***CYP2D6 (cytochrome P450, family 2, subfamily D, polypeptide 6)* (eg, drug metabolism) gene analysis, common and select rare variants (ie, *2, *3, *4, *4N, *5, *6, *7, *8, *9, *10, *11, *12, *13, *14A, *14B, *15, *17, *29, *35, *36, *41, *57, *61, *63, *68, *83, *xN)**

INCLUDES *CYP2D6* Common Variants and Copy Number, Mayo Clinic, Laboratory Developed Test

0.00 0.00 FUD 000

+ **0071U** ***CYP2D6 (cytochrome P450, family 2, subfamily D, polypeptide 6)* (eg, drug metabolism) gene analysis, full gene sequence (List separately in addition to code for primary procedure)**

INCLUDES *CYP2D6* Full Gene Sequencing, Mayo Clinic, Laboratory Developed Test

Code first (0070U)

0.00 0.00 FUD 000

+ **0072U** ***CYP2D6 (cytochrome P450, family 2, subfamily D, polypeptide 6)* (eg, drug metabolism) gene analysis, targeted sequence analysis (ie, CYP2D6-2D7 hybrid gene) (List separately in addition to code for primary procedure)**

INCLUDES *CYP2D6-2D7* Hybrid Gene Targeted Sequence Analysis, Mayo Clinic, Laboratory Developed Test

Code first (0070U)

0.00 0.00 FUD 000

+ **0073U** ***CYP2D6 (cytochrome P450, family 2, subfamily D, polypeptide 6)* (eg, drug metabolism) gene analysis, targeted sequence analysis (ie, CYP2D7-2D6 hybrid gene) (List separately in addition to code for primary procedure)**

INCLUDES *CYP2D7-2D6* Hybrid Gene Targeted Sequence Analysis, Mayo Clinic, Laboratory Developed Test

Code first (0070U)

0.00 0.00 FUD 000

+ **0074U** ***CYP2D6 (cytochrome P450, family 2, subfamily D, polypeptide 6)* (eg, drug metabolism) gene analysis, targeted sequence analysis (ie, non-duplicated gene when duplication/multiplication is trans) (List separately in addition to code for primary procedure)**

INCLUDES *CYP2D6* trans-duplication/multiplication non-duplicated gene targeted sequence analysis, Mayo Clinic, Laboratory Developed Test

Code first (0070U)

0.00 0.00 FUD 000

+ **0075U** ***CYP2D6 (cytochrome P450, family 2, subfamily D, polypeptide 6)* (eg, drug metabolism) gene analysis, targeted sequence analysis (ie, 5' gene duplication/multiplication) (List separately in addition to code for primary procedure)**

INCLUDES *CYP2D6* 5' gene duplication/multiplication targeted sequence analysis, Mayo Clinic, Laboratory Developed Test

Code first (0070U)

0.00 0.00 FUD 000

+ **0076U** ***CYP2D6 (cytochrome P450, family 2, subfamily D, polypeptide 6)* (eg, drug metabolism) gene analysis, targeted sequence analysis (ie, 3' gene duplication/ multiplication) (List separately in addition to code for primary procedure)**

INCLUDES *CYP2D6* 3' gene duplication/multiplication targeted sequence analysis, Mayo Clinic, Laboratory Developed Test

Code first (0070U)

0.00 0.00 FUD 000

0077U **Immunoglobulin paraprotein (M-protein), qualitative, immunoprecipitation and mass spectrometry, blood or urine, including isotype**

INCLUDES M-Protein Detection and Isotyping by MALDI-TOF Mass Spectrometry, Mayo Clinic, Laboratory Developed Test

0.00 0.00 FUD 000

0078U **Pain management (opioid-use disorder) genotyping panel, 16 common variants (ie, *ABCB1, COMT, DAT1, DBH, DOR, DRD1, DRD2, DRD4, GABA, GAL, HTR2A, HTTLPR, MTHFR, MUOR, OPRK1, OPRM1*), buccal swab or other germline tissue sample, algorithm reported as positive or negative risk of opioid-use disorder**

INCLUDES INFINITI® Neural Response Panel, PersonalizeDx Labs, AutoGenomics Inc

0.00 0.00 FUD 000

0079U **Comparative DNA analysis using multiple selected single-nucleotide polymorphisms (SNPs), urine and buccal DNA, for specimen identity verification**

INCLUDES ToxLok™, InSource Diagnostics, InSource Diagnostics

0.00 0.00 FUD 000

0080U **Oncology (lung), mass spectrometric analysis of galectin-3-binding protein and scavenger receptor cysteine-rich type 1 protein M130, with five clinical risk factors (age, smoking status, nodule diameter, nodule-spiculation status and nodule location), utilizing plasma, algorithm reported as a categorical probability of malignancy**

INCLUDES BDX-XL2, Biodesix®, Inc, Biodesix®, Inc

0.00 0.00 FUD 000

0082U **Drug test(s), definitive, 90 or more drugs or substances, definitive chromatography with mass spectrometry, and presumptive, any number of drug classes, by instrument chemistry analyzer (utilizing immunoassay), urine, report of presence or absence of each drug, drug metabolite or substance with description and severity of significant interactions per date of service**

INCLUDES NextGen Precision™ Testing, Precision Diagnostics, Precision Diagnostics LBN Precision Toxicology, LLC

0.00 0.00 FUD 000

0083U **Oncology, response to chemotherapy drugs using motility contrast tomography, fresh or frozen tissue, reported as likelihood of sensitivity or resistance to drugs or drug combinations**

INCLUDES Onco4D™, Animated Dynamics, Inc, Animated Dynamics, Inc

0.00 0.00 FUD 000

Pathology and Laboratory

0084U — 0097U

0084U Red blood cell antigen typing, DNA, genotyping of 10 blood groups with phenotype prediction of 37 red blood cell antigens

INCLUDES BLOODchip® ID CORE XT™, Grifols Diagnostic Solutions Inc

0.00 0.00 FUD 000

0086U Infectious disease (bacterial and fungal), organism identification, blood culture, using rRNA FISH, 6 or more organism targets, reported as positive or negative with phenotypic minimum inhibitory concentration (MIC)-based antimicrobial susceptibility

INCLUDES Accelerate PhenoTest™ BC kit, Accelerate Diagnostics, Inc

0.00 0.00 FUD 000

0087U Cardiology (heart transplant), mRNA gene expression profiling by microarray of 1283 genes, transplant biopsy tissue, allograft rejection and injury algorithm reported as a probability score

INCLUDES Molecular Microscope® MMDx—Heart, Kashi Clinical Laboratories

0.00 0.00 FUD 000

0088U Transplantation medicine (kidney allograft rejection), microarray gene expression profiling of 1494 genes, utilizing transplant biopsy tissue, algorithm reported as a probability score for rejection

INCLUDES Molecular Microscope® MMDx—Kidney, Kashi Clinical Laboratories

0.00 0.00 FUD 000

0089U Oncology (melanoma), gene expression profiling by RTqPCR, *PRAME* and *LINC00518*, superficial collection using adhesive patch(es)

INCLUDES Pigmented Lesion Assay (PLA), DermTech

0.00 0.00 FUD 000

▲ **0090U Oncology (cutaneous melanoma), mRNA gene expression profiling by RT-PCR of 23 genes (14 content and 9 housekeeping), utilizing formalin-fixed paraffin-embedded (FFPE) tissue, algorithm reported as a categorical result (ie, benign, intermediate, malignant)**

INCLUDES myPath® Melanoma, Castle Biosciences, Inc

0.00 0.00 FUD 000

0091U Oncology (colorectal) screening, cell enumeration of circulating tumor cells, utilizing whole blood, algorithm, for the presence of adenoma or cancer, reported as a positive or negative result

INCLUDES FirstSightCRC™, CellMax Life

0.00 0.00 FUD 000

0092U Oncology (lung), three protein biomarkers, immunoassay using magnetic nanosensor technology, plasma, algorithm reported as risk score for likelihood of malignancy

INCLUDES REVEAL Lung Nodule Characterization, MagArray, Inc

0.00 0.00 FUD 000

0093U Prescription drug monitoring, evaluation of 65 common drugs by LC-MS/MS, urine, each drug reported detected or not detected

INCLUDES ComplyRX, Claro Labs

0.00 0.00 FUD 000

0094U Genome (eg, unexplained constitutional or heritable disorder or syndrome), rapid sequence analysis

INCLUDES RCIGM Rapid Whole Genome Sequencing, Rady Children's Institute for Genomic Medicine (RCIGM)

0.00 0.00 FUD 000

0095U Inflammation (eosinophilic esophagitis), ELISA analysis of eotaxin-3 *(CCL26 [C-C motif chemokine ligand 26])* and major basic protein *(PRG2 [proteoglycan 2, pro eosinophil major basic protein])*, specimen obtained by swallowed nylon string, algorithm reported as predictive probability index for active eosinophilic esophagitis

INCLUDES Esophageal String Test™ (EST), Cambridge Biomedical, Inc

0.00 0.00 FUD 000

0096U Human papillomavirus (HPV), high-risk types (ie, 16, 18, 31, 33, 35, 39, 45, 51, 52, 56, 58, 59, 66, 68), male urine

INCLUDES HPV, High-Risk, Male Urine, Molecular Testing Labs

0.00 0.00 FUD 000

0097U Gastrointestinal pathogen, multiplex reverse transcription and multiplex amplified probe technique, multiple types or subtypes, 22 targets (Campylobacter [C. jejuni/C. coli/C. upsaliensis], Clostridium difficile [C. difficile] toxin A/B, Plesiomonas shigelloides, Salmonella, Vibrio [V. parahaemolyticus/V. vulnificus/V. cholerae], including specific identification of Vibrio cholerae, Yersinia enterocolitica, Enteroaggregative Escherichia coli [EAEC], Enteropathogenic Escherichia coli [EPEC], Enterotoxigenic Escherichia coli [ETEC] lt/st, Shiga-like toxin-producing Escherichia coli [STEC] stx1/stx2 [including specific identification of the E. coli O157 serogroup within STEC], Shigella/Enteroinvasive Escherichia coli [EIEC], Cryptosporidium, Cyclospora cayetanensis, Entamoeba histolytica, Giardia lamblia [also known as G. intestinalis and G. duodenalis], adenovirus F 40/41, astrovirus, norovirus GI/GII, rotavirus A, sapovirus [Genogroups I, II, IV, and V])

INCLUDES BioFire® FilmArray® Gastrointestinal (GI) Panel, BioFire® Diagnostics

0.00 0.00 FUD 000

~~**0098U Respiratory pathogen, multiplex reverse transcription and multiplex amplified probe technique, multiple types or subtypes, 14 targets (adenovirus, coronavirus, human metapneumovirus, influenza A, influenza A subtype H1, influenza A subtype H3, influenza A subtype H1-2009, influenza B, parainfluenza virus, human rhinovirus/enterovirus, respiratory syncytial virus, Bordetella pertussis, Chlamydophila pneumoniae, Mycoplasma pneumoniae)**~~

~~**0099U Respiratory pathogen, multiplex reverse transcription and multiplex amplified probe technique, multiple types or subtypes, 20 targets (adenovirus, coronavirus 229E, coronavirus HKU1, coronavirus, coronavirus OC43, human metapneumovirus, influenza A, influenza A subtype, influenza A subtype H3, influenza A subtype H1-2009, influenza, parainfluenza virus, parainfluenza virus 2, parainfluenza virus 3, parainfluenza virus 4, human rhinovirus/enterovirus, respiratory syncytial virus, Bordetella pertussis, Chlamydophila pneumonia, Mycoplasma pneumoniae)**~~

~~**0100U Respiratory pathogen, multiplex reverse transcription and multiplex amplified probe technique, multiple types or subtypes, 21 targets (adenovirus, coronavirus 229E, coronavirus HKU1, coronavirus NL63, coronavirus OC43, human metapneumovirus, human rhinovirus/enterovirus, influenza A, including subtypes H1, H1-2009, and H3, influenza B, parainfluenza virus 1, parainfluenza virus 2, parainfluenza virus 3, parainfluenza virus 4, respiratory syncytial virus, Bordetella parapertussis [IS1001], Bordetella pertussis [ptxP], Chlamydia pneumoniae, Mycoplasma pneumoniae)**~~

0101U **Hereditary colon cancer disorders (eg, Lynch syndrome, *PTEN* hamartoma syndrome, Cowden syndrome, familial adenomatosis polyposis), genomic sequence analysis panel utilizing a combination of NGS, Sanger, MLPA, and array CGH, with MRNA analytics to resolve variants of unknown significance when indicated (15 genes [sequencing and deletion/duplication], *EPCAM* and *GREM1* [deletion/duplication only])**

INCLUDES ColoNext®, Ambry Genetics®, Ambry Genetics®

0.00 0.00 FUD 000

0102U **Hereditary breast cancer-related disorders (eg, hereditary breast cancer, hereditary ovarian cancer, hereditary endometrial cancer), genomic sequence analysis panel utilizing a combination of NGS, Sanger, MLPA, and array CGH, with mRNA analytics to resolve variants of unknown significance when indicated (17 genes [sequencing and deletion/duplication])**

INCLUDES BreastNext®, Ambry Genetics®, Ambry Genetics®

0.00 0.00 FUD 000

0103U **Hereditary ovarian cancer (eg, hereditary ovarian cancer, hereditary endometrial cancer), genomic sequence analysis panel utilizing a combination of NGS, Sanger, MLPA, and array CGH, with MRNA analytics to resolve variants of unknown significance when indicated (24 genes [sequencing and deletion/duplication], *EPCAM* [deletion/duplication only])**

INCLUDES OvaNext®, Ambry Genetics®, Ambry Genetics®

0.00 0.00 FUD 000

0105U **Nephrology (chronic kidney disease), multiplex electrochemiluminescent immunoassay (ECLIA) of tumor necrosis factor receptor 1A, receptor superfamily 2 *(TNFR1, TNFR2)*, and kidney injury molecule-1 (KIM-1) combined with longitudinal clinical data, including *APOL1* genotype if available, and plasma (isolated fresh or frozen), algorithm reported as probability score for rapid kidney function decline (RKFD)**

INCLUDES KidneyIntelX™, RenalytixAI, RenalytixAI

0.00 0.00 FUD 000

0106U **Gastric emptying, serial collection of 7 timed breath specimens, non-radioisotope carbon-13 (^{13}C) spirulina substrate, analysis of each specimen by gas isotope ratio mass spectrometry, reported as rate of $^{13}CO_2$ excretion**

INCLUDES 13C-Spirulina Gastric Emptying Breath Test (GEBT), Cairn Diagnostics d/b/a Advanced Breath Diagnostics, LLC, Cairn Diagnostics d/b/a Advanced Breath Diagnostics, LLC

0.00 0.00 FUD 000

0107U **Clostridium difficile toxin(s) antigen detection by immunoassay technique, stool, qualitative, multiple-step method**

INCLUDES Singulex Clarity C. diff toxins A/B assay, Singulex

0.00 0.00 FUD 000

0108U **Gastroenterology (Barrett's esophagus), whole slide-digital imaging, including morphometric analysis, computer-assisted quantitative immunolabeling of 9 protein biomarkers (p16, AMACR, p53, CD68, COX-2, CD45RO, HIF1a, HER-2, K20) and morphology, formalin-fixed paraffin-embedded tissue, algorithm reported as risk of progression to high-grade dysplasia or cancer**

INCLUDES TissueCypher® Barrett's Esophagus Assay, Cernostics, Cernostics

0.00 0.00 FUD 000

0109U **Infectious disease (Aspergillus species), real-time PCR for detection of DNA from 4 species *(A. fumigatus, A. terreus, A. niger,* and *A. flavus)*, blood, lavage fluid, or tissue, qualitative reporting of presence or absence of each species**

INCLUDES MYCODART-PCR™ Dual Amplification Real Time PCR Panel for 4 Aspergillus species, RealTime Laboratories, Inc/MycoDART, Inc

0.00 0.00 FUD 000

0110U **Prescription drug monitoring, one or more oral oncology drug(s) and substances, definitive tandem mass spectrometry with chromatography, serum or plasma from capillary blood or venous blood, quantitative report with steady-state range for the prescribed drug(s) when detected**

INCLUDES Oral OncolyticAssuranceRX, Firstox Laboratories, LLC, Firstox Laboratories, LLC

0.00 0.00 FUD 000

0111U **Oncology (colon cancer), targeted *KRAS* (codons 12, 13, and 61) and *NRAS* (codons 12, 13, and 61) gene analysis utilizing formalin-fixed paraffin-embedded tissue**

INCLUDES Praxis(™) Extended RAS Panel, Illumina, Illumina

0.00 0.00 FUD 000

0112U **Infectious agent detection and identification, targeted sequence analysis (16S and 18S rRNA genes) with drug-resistance gene**

INCLUDES MicroGenDX qPCR & NGS For Infection, MicroGenDX, MicroGenDX

0.00 0.00 FUD 000

0113U **Oncology (prostate), measurement of *PCA3* and *TMPRSS2-ERG* in urine and PSA in serum following prostatic massage, by RNA amplification and fluorescence-based detection, algorithm reported as risk score**

INCLUDES MiPS (Mi-Prostate Score), MLabs, Mlabs

0.00 0.00 FUD 000

0114U **Gastroenterology (Barrett's esophagus), *VIM* and *CCNA1* methylation analysis, esophageal cells, algorithm reported as likelihood for Barrett's esophagus**

INCLUDES EsoGuard™, Lucid Diagnostics, Lucid Diagnostics

0.00 0.00 FUD 000

0115U **Respiratory infectious agent detection by nucleic acid (DNA and RNA), 18 viral types and subtypes and 2 bacterial targets, amplified probe technique, including multiplex reverse transcription for RNA targets, each analyte reported as detected or not detected**

INCLUDES ePlex Respiratory Pathogen (RP) Panel, GenMark Diagnostics, Inc, GenMark Diagnostics, Inc

0.00 0.00 FUD 000

AMA: 2020,Apr,3

0116U **Prescription drug monitoring, enzyme immunoassay of 35 or more drugs confirmed with LC-MS/MS, oral fluid, algorithm results reported as a patient-compliance measurement with risk of drug to drug interactions for prescribed medications**

INCLUDES Snapshot Oral Fluid Compliance, Ethos Laboratories

0.00 0.00 FUD 000

0117U **Pain management, analysis of 11 endogenous analytes (methylmalonic acid, xanthurenic acid, homocysteine, pyroglutamic acid, vanilmandelate, 5-hydroxyindoleacetic acid, hydroxymethylglutarate, ethylmalonate, 3-hydroxypropyl mercapturic acid (3-HPMA), quinolinic acid, kynurenic acid), LC-MS/MS, urine, algorithm reported as a pain-index score with likelihood of atypical biochemical function associated with pain**

INCLUDES Foundation PI[SM], Ethos Laboratories

0.00 0.00 FUD 000

0118U Transplantation medicine, quantification of donor-derived cell-free DNA using whole genome next-generation sequencing, plasma, reported as percentage of donor-derived cell-free DNA in the total cell-free DNA

INCLUDES Viracor TRAC™ dd-cfDNA, Viracor Eurofins, Viracor Eurofins

0.00 0.00 **FUD** 000

0119U Cardiology, ceramides by liquid chromatography-tandem mass spectrometry, plasma, quantitative report with risk score for major cardiovascular events

INCLUDES MI-HEART Ceramides, Plasma, Mayo Clinic, Laboratory Developed Test

0.00 0.00 **FUD** 000

0120U Oncology (B-cell lymphoma classification), mRNA, gene expression profiling by fluorescent probe hybridization of 58 genes (45 content and 13 housekeeping genes), formalin-fixed paraffin-embedded tissue, algorithm reported as likelihood for primary mediastinal B-cell lymphoma (PMBCL) and diffuse large B-cell lymphoma (DLBCL) with cell of origin subtyping in the latter

INCLUDES Lymph3Cx Lymphoma Molecular Subtyping Assay, Mayo Clinic, Laboratory Developed Test

EXCLUDES *Oncology (diffuse large B-cell lymphoma [DLBCL]), mRNA, gene expression profiling by fluorescent probe hybridization of 20 genes (0017M)*

0.00 0.00 **FUD** 000

0121U Sickle cell disease, microfluidic flow adhesion (VCAM-1), whole blood

INCLUDES Flow Adhesion of Whole Blood on VCAM-1 (FAB-V), Functional Fluidics, Functional Fluidics

0.00 0.00 **FUD** 000

0122U Sickle cell disease, microfluidic flow adhesion (P-Selectin), whole blood

INCLUDES Flow Adhesion of Whole Blood to P-SELECTIN (WB-PSEL), Functional Fluidics, Functional Fluidics

0.00 0.00 **FUD** 000

0123U Mechanical fragility, RBC, shear stress and spectral analysis profiling

INCLUDES Mechanical Fragility, RBC by shear stress profiling and spectral analysis, Functional Fluidics, Functional Fluidics

0.00 0.00 **FUD** 000

0129U Hereditary breast cancer-related disorders (eg, hereditary breast cancer, hereditary ovarian cancer, hereditary endometrial cancer), genomic sequence analysis and deletion/duplication analysis panel *(ATM, BRCA1, BRCA2, CDH1, CHEK2, PALB2, PTEN,* and *TP53)*

INCLUDES BRCAplus, Ambry Genetics

0.00 0.00 **FUD** 000

\+ **0130U Hereditary colon cancer disorders (eg, Lynch syndrome, PTEN hamartoma syndrome, Cowden syndrome, familial adenomatosis polyposis), targeted mRNA sequence analysis panel *(APC, CDH1, CHEK2, MLH1, MSH2, MSH6, MUTYH, PMS2, PTEN,* and *TP53)* (List separately in addition to code for primary procedure)**

INCLUDES +RNAinsight™ for ColoNext®, Ambry Genetics

Code first (81435, 0101U)

0.00 0.00 **FUD** 000

\+ **0131U Hereditary breast cancer-related disorders (eg, hereditary breast cancer, hereditary ovarian cancer, hereditary endometrial cancer), targeted mRNA sequence analysis panel (13 genes) (List separately in addition to code for primary procedure)**

INCLUDES +RNAinsight™ for BreastNext®, Ambry Genetics

Code first ([81162], 81432, 0102U)

0.00 0.00 **FUD** 000

\+ **0132U Hereditary ovarian cancer-related disorders (eg, hereditary breast cancer, hereditary ovarian cancer, hereditary endometrial cancer), targeted mRNA sequence analysis panel (17 genes) (List separately in addition to code for primary procedure)**

INCLUDES +RNAinsight™ for OvaNext®, Ambry Genetics

Code first ([81162], 81432, 0103U)

0.00 0.00 **FUD** 000

\+ **0133U Hereditary prostate cancer-related disorders, targeted mRNA sequence analysis panel (11 genes) (List separately in addition to code for primary procedure)**

INCLUDES +RNAinsight™ for ProstateNext®, Ambry Genetics

Code first ([81162])

0.00 0.00 **FUD** 000

\+ **0134U Hereditary pan cancer (eg, hereditary breast and ovarian cancer, hereditary endometrial cancer, hereditary colorectal cancer), targeted mRNA sequence analysis panel (18 genes) (List separately in addition to code for primary procedure)**

INCLUDES +RNAinsight™ for CancerNext®, Ambry Genetics

Code first ([81162], 81432, 81435)

0.00 0.00 **FUD** 000

\+ **0135U Hereditary gynecological cancer (eg, hereditary breast and ovarian cancer, hereditary endometrial cancer, hereditary colorectal cancer), targeted mRNA sequence analysis panel (12 genes) (List separately in addition to code for primary procedure)**

INCLUDES +RNAinsight™ for GYNPlus®, Ambry Genetics

Code first ([81162])

0.00 0.00 **FUD** 000

\+ **0136U *ATM (ataxia telangiectasia mutated)* (eg, ataxia telangiectasia) mRNA sequence analysis (List separately in addition to code for primary procedure)**

INCLUDES +RNAinsight™ for *ATM*, Ambry Genetics

Code first (81408)

0.00 0.00 **FUD** 000

\+ **0137U *PALB2 (partner and localizer of BRCA2)* (eg, breast and pancreatic cancer) mRNA sequence analysis (List separately in addition to code for ...**

INCLUDES +RNAinsight™ for *PALB2*, Ambry Genetics

Code first (81406)

0.00 0.00 **FUD** 000

\+ **0138U *BRCA1 (BRCA1, DNA repair associated), BRCA2 (BRCA2, DNA repair associated)* (eg, hereditary breast and ovarian cancer) mRNA sequence analysis (List separately in addition to code for primary procedure)**

INCLUDES +RNAinsight™ for *BRCA1/2*, Ambry Genetics

Code first ([81162])

0.00 0.00 **FUD** 000

~~**0139U Neurology (autism spectrum disorder [ASD]), quantitative measurements of 6 central carbon metabolites (ie, a-ketoglutarate, alanine, lactate, phenylalanine, pyruvate, and succinate), LC-MS/MS, plasma, algorithmic analysis with result reported as negative or positive (with metabolic subtypes of ASD)**~~

0140U Infectious disease (fungi), fungal pathogen identification, DNA (15 fungal targets), blood culture, amplified probe technique, each target reported as detected or not detected

INCLUDES ePlex® BCID Fungal Pathogens Panel, GenMark Diagnostics, Inc, GenMark Diagnostics, Inc

0.00 0.00 **FUD** 000

0141U **Infectious disease (bacteria and fungi), gram-positive organism identification and drug resistance element detection, DNA (20 gram-positive bacterial targets, 4 resistance genes, 1 pan gram-negative bacterial target, 1 pan Candida target), blood culture, amplified probe technique, each target reported as detected or not detected**

INCLUDES ePlex® BCID Gram-Positive Panel, GenMark Diagnostics, Inc, GenMark Diagnostics, Inc

0.00 0.00 **FUD** 000

0142U **Infectious disease (bacteria and fungi), gram-negative bacterial identification and drug resistance element detection, DNA (21 gram-negative bacterial targets, 6 resistance genes, 1 pan gram-positive bacterial target, 1 pan Candida target), amplified probe technique, each target reported as detected or not detected**

INCLUDES ePlex® BCID Gram-Negative Panel, GenMark Diagnostics, Inc, GenMark Diagnostics, Inc

0.00 0.00 **FUD** 000

0143U **Drug assay, definitive, 120 or more drugs or metabolites, urine, quantitative liquid chromatography with tandem mass spectrometry (LC-MS/MS) using multiple reaction monitoring (MRM), with drug or metabolite description, comments including sample validation, per date of service**

INCLUDES CareViewRx, Newstar Medical Laboratories, LLC, Newstar Medical Laboratories, LLC

EXCLUDES *PsychViewRx Plus analysis by Newstar Medical Laboratories, LLC. To report, see (0150U)*

0.00 0.00 **FUD** 000

0144U **Drug assay, definitive, 160 or more drugs or metabolites, urine, quantitative liquid chromatography with tandem mass spectrometry (LC-MS/MS) using multiple reaction monitoring (MRM), with drug or metabolite description, comments including sample validation, per date of service**

INCLUDES CareViewRx Plus, Newstar Medical Laboratories, LLC, Newstar Medical Laboratories, LLC

0.00 0.00 **FUD** 000

0145U **Drug assay, definitive, 65 or more drugs or metabolites, urine, quantitative liquid chromatography with tandem mass spectrometry (LC-MS/MS) using multiple reaction monitoring (MRM), with drug or metabolite description, comments including sample validation, per date of service**

INCLUDES PainViewRx, Newstar Medical Laboratories, LLC, Newstar Medical Laboratories, LLC

0.00 0.00 **FUD** 000

0146U **Drug assay, definitive, 80 or more drugs or metabolites, urine, by quantitative liquid chromatography with tandem mass spectrometry (LC-MS/MS) using multiple reaction monitoring (MRM), with drug or metabolite description, comments including sample validation, per date of service**

INCLUDES PainViewRx Plus, Newstar Medical Laboratories, LLC, Newstar Medical Laboratories, LLC

0.00 0.00 **FUD** 000

0147U **Drug assay, definitive, 85 or more drugs or metabolites, urine, quantitative liquid chromatography with tandem mass spectrometry (LC-MS/MS) using multiple reaction monitoring (MRM), with drug or metabolite description, comments including sample validation, per date of service**

INCLUDES RiskViewRx, Newstar Medical Laboratories, LLC, Newstar Medical Laboratories, LLC

0.00 0.00 **FUD** 000

0148U **Drug assay, definitive, 100 or more drugs or metabolites, urine, quantitative liquid chromatography with tandem mass spectrometry (LC-MS/MS) using multiple reaction monitoring (MRM), with drug or metabolite description, comments including sample validation, per date of service**

INCLUDES RiskViewRx Plus, Newstar Medical Laboratories, LLC, Newstar Medical Laboratories, LLC

0.00 0.00 **FUD** 000

0149U **Drug assay, definitive, 60 or more drugs or metabolites, urine, quantitative liquid chromatography with tandem mass spectrometry (LC-MS/MS) using multiple reaction monitoring (MRM), with drug or metabolite description, comments including sample validation, per date of service**

INCLUDES PsychViewRx, Newstar Medical Laboratories, LLC, Newstar Medical Laboratories, LLC

0.00 0.00 **FUD** 000

0150U **Drug assay, definitive, 120 or more drugs or metabolites, urine, quantitative liquid chromatography with tandem mass spectrometry (LC-MS/MS) using multiple reaction monitoring (MRM), with drug or metabolite description, comments including sample validation, per date of service**

INCLUDES PsychViewRx Plus, Newstar Medical Laboratories, LLC, Newstar Medical Laboratories, LLC

EXCLUDES *CareViewRx analysis by Newstar Medical Laboratories, LLC. To report, see (0143U)*

0.00 0.00 **FUD** 000

0151U **Infectious disease (bacterial or viral respiratory tract infection), pathogen specific nucleic acid (DNA or RNA), 33 targets, real-time semi-quantitative PCR, bronchoalveolar lavage, sputum, or endotracheal aspirate, detection of 33 organismal and antibiotic resistance genes with limited semi-quantitative results**

INCLUDES BioFire® FilmArray® Pneumonia Panel, BioFire® Diagnostics, BioFire® Diagnostics

0.00 0.00 **FUD** 000

AMA: 2020,Apr,3

▲ **0152U** **Infectious disease (bacteria, fungi, parasites, and DNA viruses), microbial cell-free DNA, plasma, untargeted next-generation sequencing, report for significant positive pathogens**

INCLUDES Karius® Test, Karius Inc, Karius Inc

0153U **Oncology (breast), mRNA, gene expression profiling by next-generation sequencing of 101 genes, utilizing formalin-fixed paraffin-embedded tissue, algorithm reported as a triple negative breast cancer clinical subtype(s) with information on immune cell involvement**

INCLUDES Insight TNBCtype™, Insight Molecular Labs

0.00 0.00 **FUD** 000

0154U **Oncology (urothelial cancer), RNA, analysis by real-time RT-PCR of the *FGFR3 (fibroblast growth factor receptor3)* gene analysis (ie, p.R248C [c.742C>T], p.S249C [c.746C>G], p.G370C [c.1108G>T], p.Y373C [c.1118A>G], FGFR3-TACC3v1, and FGFR3-TACC3v3) utilizing formalin-fixed paraffin-embedded urothelial cancer tumor tissue, reported as *FGFR* gene alteration status**

INCLUDES therascreen® *FGFR* RGQ RT-PCR Kit, QIAGEN, QIAGEN GmbH

0.00 0.00 **FUD** 000

AMA: 2020,Jun,11

0155U **Oncology (breast cancer), DNA, *PIK3CA (phosphatidylinositol-4,5-bisphosphate 3-kinase, catalytic subunit alpha)* (eg, breast cancer) gene analysis (ie, p.C420R, p.E542K, p.E545A, p.E545D [g.1635G>T only], p.E545G, p.E545K, p.Q546E, p.Q546R, p.H1047L, p.H1047R, p.H1047Y), utilizing formalin-fixed paraffin-embedded breast tumor tissue, reported as *PIK3CA* gene mutation status**

INCLUDES therascreen® *PIK3CA* RGQ PCR Kit, QIAGEN, QIAGEN GmbH

0.00 0.00 **FUD** 000

AMA: 2020,Jun,11

0156U **Copy number (eg, intellectual disability, dysmorphology), sequence analysis**

INCLUDES SMASH™, New York Genome Center, Marvel Genomics™

0.00 0.00 **FUD** 000

\+ **0157U** ***APC (APC regulator of WNT signaling pathway)*** **(eg, familial adenomatous polyposis [FAP]) mRNA sequence analysis (List separately in addition to code for primary procedure)**

INCLUDES CustomNext + RNA: APC, Ambry Genetics®, Ambry Genetics®

Code first ([81201])

0.00 0.00 FUD 000

\+ **0158U** ***MLH1 (mutL homolog 1)*** **(eg, hereditary non-polyposis colorectal cancer, Lynch syndrome) mRNA sequence analysis (List separately in addition to code for primary procedure)**

INCLUDES CustomNext + RNA: *MLH1*, Ambry Genetics®, Ambry Genetics®

Code first ([81292])

0.00 0.00 FUD 000

\+ **0159U** ***MSH2 (mutS homolog 2)*** **(eg, hereditary colon cancer, Lynch syndrome) mRNA sequence analysis (List separately in addition to code for primary procedure)**

INCLUDES CustomNext + RNA: *MSH2*, Ambry Genetics®, Ambry Genetics®

Code first ([81295])

0.00 0.00 FUD 000

\+ **0160U** ***MSH6 (mutS homolog 6)*** **(eg, hereditary colon cancer, Lynch syndrome) mRNA sequence analysis (List separately in addition to code for primary procedure)**

INCLUDES CustomNext + RNA: *MSH6*, Ambry Genetics®, Ambry Genetics®

Code first (81298)

0.00 0.00 FUD 000

\+ **0161U** ***PMS2 (PMS1 homolog 2, mismatch repair system component)*** **(eg, hereditary non-polyposis colorectal cancer, Lynch syndrome) mRNA sequence analysis (List separately in addition to code for primary procedure)**

INCLUDES CustomNext + RNA: *PMS2*, Ambry Genetics®, Ambry Genetics®

Code first (81317)

0.00 0.00 FUD 000

\+ **0162U Hereditary colon cancer (Lynch syndrome), targeted mRNA sequence analysis panel *(MLH1, MSH2, MSH6, PMS2)* (List separately in addition to code for primary procedure)**

INCLUDES CustomNext + RNA: Lynch *(MLH1, MSH2, MSH6, PMS2)*, Ambry Genetics®, Ambry Genetics®

Code first ([81292], [81295], 81298, 81317, 81435)

0.00 0.00 FUD 000

0163U Oncology (colorectal) screening, biochemical enzyme-linked immunosorbent assay (ELISA) of 3 plasma or serum proteins (teratocarcinoma derived growth factor-1 [TDGF-1, Cripto-1], carcinoembryonic antigen [CEA], extracellular matrix protein [ECM]), with demographic data (age, gender, CRC-screening compliance) using a proprietary algorithm and reported as likelihood of CRC or advanced adenomas

INCLUDES BeScreened™-CRC, Beacon Biomedical Inc, Beacon Biomedical Inc

0.00 0.00 FUD 000

AMA: 2020,Jun,11

0164U Gastroenterology (irritable bowel syndrome [IBS]), immunoassay for anti-CdtB and anti-vinculin antibodies, utilizing plasma, algorithm for elevated or not elevated qualitative results

INCLUDES ibs-smart™, Gemelli Biotech, Gemelli Biotech

0.00 0.00 FUD 000

AMA: 2020,Jun,11

0165U Peanut allergen-specific quantitative assessment of multiple epitopes using enzyme-linked immunosorbent assay (ELISA), blood, individual epitope results and probability of peanut allergy

INCLUDES VeriMAP™ Peanut Dx – Bead-based Epitope Assay, AllerGenis™ Clinical Laboratory, AllerGenis™ LLC

0.00 0.00 FUD 000

AMA: 2020,Jun,11

0166U Liver disease, 10 biochemical assays (α2-macroglobulin, haptoglobin, apolipoprotein A1, bilirubin, GGT, ALT, AST, triglycerides, cholesterol, fasting glucose) and biometric and demographic data, utilizing serum, algorithm reported as scores for fibrosis, necroinflammatory activity, and steatosis with a summary interpretation

INCLUDES LiverFASt™, Fibronostics, Fibronostics

0.00 0.00 FUD 000

AMA: 2020,Jun,11

0167U Gonadotropin, chorionic (hCG), immunoassay with direct optical observation, blood

INCLUDES ADEXUSDx hCG Test, NOWDiagnostics, NOWDiagnostics

0.00 0.00 FUD 000

AMA: 2020,Jun,11

~~**0168U Fetal aneuploidy (trisomy 21, 18, and 13) DNA sequence analysis of selected regions using maternal plasma without fetal fraction cutoff, algorithm reported as a risk score for each trisomy**~~

0169U *NUDT15 (nudix hydrolase 15)* and *TPMT (thiopurine S-methyltransferase)* (eg, drug metabolism) gene analysis, common variants

INCLUDES NT *(NUDT15* and *TPMT)* genotyping panel, RPRD Diagnostics

0.00 0.00 FUD 000

AMA: 2020,Jun,11

0170U Neurology (autism spectrum disorder [ASD]), RNA, next-generation sequencing, saliva, algorithmic analysis, and results reported as predictive probability of ASD diagnosis

INCLUDES Clarifi™, Quadrant Biosciences, Inc, Quadrant Biosciences, Inc

0.00 0.00 FUD 000

AMA: 2020,Jun,11

0171U Targeted genomic sequence analysis panel, acute myeloid leukemia, myelodysplastic syndrome, and myeloproliferative neoplasms, DNA analysis, 23 genes, interrogation for sequence variants, rearrangements and minimal residual disease, reported as presence/absence

INCLUDES MyMRD® NGS Panel, Laboratory for Personalized Molecular Medicine, Laboratory for Personalized Molecular Medicine

0.00 0.00 FUD 000

AMA: 2020,Jun,11

0172U Oncology (solid tumor as indicated by the label), somatic mutation analysis of *BRCA1 (BRCA1, DNA repair associated), BRCA2 (BRCA2, DNA repair associated)* and analysis of homologous recombination deficiency pathways, DNA, formalin-fixed paraffin-embedded tissue, algorithm quantifying tumor genomic instability score

INCLUDES myChoice® CDx, Myriad Genetics Laboratories, Inc, Myriad Genetics Laboratories, Inc

0.00 0.00 FUD 000

0173U Psychiatry (ie, depression, anxiety), genomic analysis panel, includes variant analysis of 14 genes

INCLUDES Psych HealthPGx Panel, RPRD Diagnostics, RPRD Diagnostics

0.00 0.00 FUD 000

0174U Oncology (solid tumor), mass spectrometric 30 protein targets, formalin-fixed paraffin-embedded tissue, prognostic and predictive algorithm reported as likely, unlikely, or uncertain benefit of 39 chemotherapy and targeted therapeutic oncology agents

INCLUDES LC-MS/MS Targeted Proteomic Assay, OncoOmicDx Laboratory, LDT

0.00 0.00 FUD 000

0175U Psychiatry (eg, depression, anxiety), genomic analysis panel, variant analysis of 15 genes

INCLUDES Genomind® Professional PGx Express™ CORE, Genomind, Inc, Genomind, Inc

0.00 0.00 FUD 000

0176U Cytolethal distending toxin B (CdtB) and vinculin IgG antibodies by immunoassay (ie, ELISA)

INCLUDES IBSSchek®, Commonwealth Diagnostics International, Inc, Commonwealth Diagnostics International, Inc

0.00 0.00 FUD 000

0177U Oncology (breast cancer), DNA, *PIK3CA (phosphatidylinositol-4,5-bisphosphate 3-kinase catalytic subunit alpha)* gene analysis of 11 gene variants utilizing plasma, reported as *PIK3CA* gene mutation status

INCLUDES therascreen® *PIK3CA* RGQ PCR Kit, QIAGEN, QIAGEN GmbH

0.00 0.00 FUD 000

0178U Peanut allergen-specific quantitative assessment of multiple epitopes using enzyme-linked immunosorbent assay (ELISA), blood, report of minimum eliciting exposure for a clinical reaction

INCLUDES VeriMAP™ Peanut Reactivity Threshold - Bead Based Epitope Assay, AllerGenis™ Clinical Laboratory, AllerGenis™ LLC

0.00 0.00 FUD 000

0179U Oncology (non-small cell lung cancer), cell-free DNA, targeted sequence analysis of 23 genes (single nucleotide variations, insertions and deletions, fusions without prior knowledge of partner/breakpoint, copy number variations), with report of significant mutation(s)

INCLUDES Resolution ctDx Lung™, Resolution Bioscience, Resolution Bioscience, Inc

0.00 0.00 FUD 000

0180U Red cell antigen (ABO blood group) genotyping (ABO), gene analysis Sanger/chain termination/conventional sequencing, *ABO (ABO, alpha 1-3-N-acetylgalactosaminyltransferase and alpha 1-3-galactosyltransferase)* gene, including subtyping, 7 exons

INCLUDES Navigator ABO Sequencing, Grifols Immunohematology Center, Grifols Immunohematology Center

0.00 0.00 FUD 000

0181U Red cell antigen (Colton blood group) genotyping (CO), gene analysis, *AQP1 (aquaporin 1 [Colton blood group])* exon 1

INCLUDES Navigator CO Sequencing, Grifols Immunohematology Center, Grifols Immunohematology Center

0.00 0.00 FUD 000

0182U Red cell antigen (Cromer blood group) genotyping (CROM), gene analysis, *CD55 (CD55 molecule [Cromer blood group])* exons 1-10

INCLUDES Navigator CROM Sequencing, Grifols Immunohematology Center, Grifols Immunohematology Center

0.00 0.00 FUD 000

0183U Red cell antigen (Diego blood group) genotyping (DI), gene analysis, *SLC4A1 (solute carrier family 4 member 1 [Diego blood group])* exon 19

INCLUDES Navigator DI Sequencing, Grifols Immunohematology Center, Grifols Immunohematology Center

0.00 0.00 FUD 000

0184U Red cell antigen (Dombrock blood group) genotyping (DO), gene analysis, *ART4 (ADP-ribosyltransferase 4 [Dombrock blood group])* exon 2

INCLUDES Navigator DO Sequencing, Grifols Immunohematology Center, Grifols Immunohematology Center

0.00 0.00 FUD 000

0185U Red cell antigen (H blood group) genotyping (FUT1), gene analysis, *FUT1 (fucosyltransferase 1 [H blood group])* exon 4

INCLUDES Navigator FUT1 Sequencing, Grifols Immunohematology Center, Grifols Immunohematology Center

0.00 0.00 FUD 000

0186U Red cell antigen (H blood group) genotyping (FUT2), gene analysis, *FUT2 (fucosyltransferase 2)* exon 2

INCLUDES Navigator FUT2 Sequencing, Grifols Immunohematology Center, Grifols Immunohematology Center

0.00 0.00 FUD 000

0187U Red cell antigen (Duffy blood group) genotyping (FY), gene analysis, *ACKR1 (atypical chemokine receptor 1 [Duffy blood group])* exons 1-2

INCLUDES Navigator FY Sequencing, Grifols Immunohematology Center, Grifols Immunohematology Center

0.00 0.00 FUD 000

0188U Red cell antigen (Gerbich blood group) genotyping (GE), gene analysis, *GYPC (glycophorin C [Gerbich blood group])* exons 1-4

INCLUDES Navigator GE Sequencing, Grifols Immunohematology Center, Grifols Immunohematology Center

0.00 0.00 FUD 000

0189U Red cell antigen (MNS blood group) genotyping (GYPA), gene analysis, *GYPA (glycophorin A [MNS blood group])* introns 1, 5, exon 2

INCLUDES Navigator GYPA Sequencing, Grifols Immunohematology Center, Grifols Immunohematology Center

0.00 0.00 FUD 000

0190U Red cell antigen (MNS blood group) genotyping (GYPB), gene analysis, *GYPB (glycophorin B [MNS blood group])* introns 1, 5, pseudoexon 3

INCLUDES Navigator GYPB Sequencing, Grifols Immunohematology Center, Grifols Immunohematology Center

0.00 0.00 FUD 000

0191U Red cell antigen (Indian blood group) genotyping (IN), gene analysis, *CD44 (CD44 molecule [Indian blood group])* exons 2, 3, 6

INCLUDES Navigator IN Sequencing, Grifols Immunohematology Center, Grifols Immunohematology Center

0.00 0.00 FUD 000

0192U Red cell antigen (Kidd blood group) genotyping (JK), gene analysis, *SLC14A1 (solute carrier family 14 member 1 [Kidd blood group])* gene promoter, exon 9

INCLUDES Navigator JK Sequencing, Grifols Immunohematology Center, Grifols Immunohematology Center

0.00 0.00 FUD 000

0193U Red cell antigen (JR blood group) genotyping (JR), gene analysis, *ABCG2 (ATP binding cassette subfamily G member 2 [Junior blood group])* exons 2-26

INCLUDES Navigator JR Sequencing, Grifols Immunohematology Center, Grifols Immunohematology Center

0.00 0.00 FUD 000

0194U Red cell antigen (Kell blood group) genotyping (KEL), gene analysis, *KEL (Kell metallo-endopeptidase [Kell blood group])* exon 8

INCLUDES Navigator KEL Sequencing, Grifols Immunohematology Center, Grifols Immunohematology Center

0.00 0.00 FUD 000

0195U *KLF1 (Kruppel-like factor 1)*, targeted sequencing (ie, exon 13)

INCLUDES Navigator *KLF1* Sequencing, Grifols Immunohematology Center, Grifols Immunohematology Center

0.00 0.00 FUD 000

0196U **Red cell antigen (Lutheran blood group) genotyping (LU), gene analysis, *BCAM (basal cell adhesion molecule [Lutheran blood group])* exon 3**

INCLUDES Navigator LU Sequencing, Grifols Immunohematology Center, Grifols Immunohematology Center

0.00 0.00 **FUD** 000

0197U **Red cell antigen (Landsteiner-Wiener blood group) genotyping (LW), gene analysis, *ICAM4 (intercellular adhesion molecule 4 [Landsteiner-Wiener blood group])* exon 1**

INCLUDES Navigator LW Sequencing, Grifols Immunohematology Center, Grifols Immunohematology Center

0.00 0.00 **FUD** 000

0198U **Red cell antigen (RH blood group) genotyping (RHD and RHCE), gene analysis Sanger/chain termination/conventional sequencing, *RHD (Rh blood group D antigen) exons 1-10 and RHCE (Rh blood group CcEe antigens)* exon 5**

INCLUDES Navigator RHD/CE Sequencing, Grifols Immunohematology Center, Grifols Immunohematology Center

0.00 0.00 **FUD** 000

0199U **Red cell antigen (Scianna blood group) genotyping (SC), gene analysis, *ERMAP (erythroblast membrane associated protein [Scianna blood group])* exons 4, 12**

INCLUDES Navigator SC Sequencing, Grifols Immunohematology Center, Grifols Immunohematology Center

0.00 0.00 **FUD** 000

0200U **Red cell antigen (Kx blood group) genotyping (XK), gene analysis, *XK (X-linked Kx blood group)* exons 1-3**

INCLUDES Navigator XK Sequencing, Grifols Immunohematology Center, Grifols Immunohematology Center

0.00 0.00 **FUD** 000

0201U **Red cell antigen (Yt blood group) genotyping (YT), gene analysis, *ACHE (acetylcholinesterase [Cartwright blood group])* exon 2**

INCLUDES Navigator YT Sequencing, Grifols Immunohematology Center, Grifols Immunohematology Center

0.00 0.00 **FUD** 000

0202U **Infectious disease (bacterial or viral respiratory tract infection), pathogen-specific nucleic acid (DNA or RNA), 22 targets including severe acute respiratory syndrome coronavirus 2 (SARS-CoV-2), qualitative RT-PCR, nasopharyngeal swab, each pathogen reported as detected or not detected**

INCLUDES BioFire® Respiratory Panel 2.1 (RP2.1), BioFire® Diagnostics, BioFire® Diagnostics, LLC

EXCLUDES *QIAstat-Dx Respiratory SARS CoV-2 Panel, QIAGEN Sciences, QIAGEN GmbH. To report, see (0223U)*

0.00 0.00 **FUD** 000

AMA: 2020,AugSE,1; 2020,AugSE,1; 2020,AugSE,1; 2020,MaySE,1; 2020,May,3; 2020,JuneSE,1

0203U **Autoimmune (inflammatory bowel disease), mRNA, gene expression profiling by quantitative RT-PCR, 17 genes (15 target and 2 reference genes), whole blood, reported as a continuous risk score and classification of inflammatory bowel disease aggressiveness**

INCLUDES PredictSURE IBD™ Test, KSL Diagnostics, PredictImmune Ltd

0.00 0.00 **FUD** 000

0204U **Oncology (thyroid), mRNA, gene expression analysis of 593 genes (including *BRAF, RAS, RET, PAX8,* and *NTRK*) for sequence variants and rearrangements, utilizing fine needle aspirate, reported as detected or not detected**

INCLUDES Afirma Xpression Atlas, Veracyte, Inc, Veracyte, Inc

0.00 0.00 **FUD** 000

0205U **Ophthalmology (age-related macular degeneration), analysis of 3 gene variants (2 *CFH* gene, 1 *ARMS2* gene), using PCR and MALDI-TOF, buccal swab, reported as positive or negative for neovascular age-related macular-degeneration risk associated with zinc supplements**

INCLUDES Vita Risk®, Arctic Medical Laboratories, Arctic Medical Laboratories

0.00 0.00 **FUD** 000

0206U **Neurology (Alzheimer disease); cell aggregation using morphometric imaging and protein kinase C-epsilon (PKCe) concentration in response to amylospheroid treatment by ELISA, cultured skin fibroblasts, each reported as positive or negative for Alzheimer disease**

INCLUDES DISCERN™, NeuroDiagnostics, NeuroDiagnostics

0.00 0.00 **FUD** 000

+ **0207U** **quantitative imaging of phosphorylated *ERK1* and *ERK2* in response to bradykinin treatment by in situ immunofluorescence, using cultured skin fibroblasts, reported as a probability index for Alzheimer disease (List separately in addition to code for primary procedure)**

INCLUDES DISCERN™, NeuroDiagnostics, NeuroDiagnostics

Code first (0206U)

0.00 0.00 **FUD** 000

~~**0208U** **Oncology (medullary thyroid carcinoma), mRNA, gene expression analysis of 108 genes, utilizing fine needle aspirate, algorithm reported as positive or negative for medullary thyroid carcinoma**~~

0209U **Cytogenomic constitutional (genome-wide) analysis, interrogation of genomic regions for copy number, structural changes and areas of homozygosity for chromosomal abnormalities**

INCLUDES CNGnome™, PerkinElmer Genomics, PerkinElmer Genomics

0.00 0.00 **FUD** 000

0210U **Syphilis test, non-treponemal antibody, immunoassay, quantitative (RPR)**

INCLUDES BioPlex 2200 RPR Assay - Quantitative, Bio-Rad Laboratories, Bio-Rad Laboratories

0.00 0.00 **FUD** 000

0211U **Oncology (pan-tumor), DNA and RNA by next-generation sequencing, utilizing formalin-fixed paraffin-embedded tissue, interpretative report for single nucleotide variants, copy number alterations, tumor mutational burden, and microsatellite instability, with therapy association**

INCLUDES MI Cancer Seek™ - NGS Analysis, Caris MPI d/b/a Caris Life Sciences, Caris MPI d/b/a Caris Life Sciences

0.00 0.00 **FUD** 000

0212U **Rare diseases (constitutional/heritable disorders), whole genome and mitochondrial DNA sequence analysis, including small sequence changes, deletions, duplications, short tandem repeat gene expansions, and variants in non-uniquely mappable regions, blood or saliva, identification and categorization of genetic variants, proband**

INCLUDES Genomic Unity® Whole Genome Analysis – Proband, Variantyx Inc, Variantyx Inc

EXCLUDES *Genome (e.g., unexplained constitutional or heritable disorder or syndrome); sequence analysis (81425)*

0.00 0.00 **FUD** 000

0213U Rare diseases (constitutional/heritable disorders), whole genome and mitochondrial DNA sequence analysis, including small sequence changes, deletions, duplications, short tandem repeat gene expansions, and variants in non-uniquely mappable regions, blood or saliva, identification and categorization of genetic variants, each comparator genome (eg, parent, sibling)

INCLUDES Genomic Unity® Whole Genome Analysis - Comparator, Variantyx Inc, Variantyx Inc

EXCLUDES *Genome (e.g., unexplained constitutional or heritable disorder or syndrome); sequence analysis, each comparator genome (e.g., parents, siblings) (81426)*

0.00 0.00 FUD 000

0214U Rare diseases (constitutional/heritable disorders), whole exome and mitochondrial DNA sequence analysis, including small sequence changes, deletions, duplications, short tandem repeat gene expansions, and variants in non-uniquely mappable regions, blood or saliva, identification and categorization of genetic variants, proband

INCLUDES Genomic Unity® Exome Plus Analysis - Proband, Variantyx Inc, Variantyx Inc

EXCLUDES *Exome (e.g., unexplained constitutional or heritable disorder or syndrome); sequence analysis (81415)*

0.00 0.00 FUD 000

0215U Rare diseases (constitutional/heritable disorders), whole exome and mitochondrial DNA sequence analysis, including small sequence changes, deletions, duplications, short tandem repeat gene expansions, and variants in non-uniquely mappable regions, blood or saliva, identification and categorization of genetic variants, each comparator exome (eg, parent, sibling)

INCLUDES Genomic Unity® Exome Plus Analysis - Comparator, Variantyx Inc, Variantyx Inc

EXCLUDES *Exome (e.g., unexplained constitutional or heritable disorder or syndrome); sequence analysis, each comparator exome (e.g., parents, siblings) (81416)*

0.00 0.00 FUD 000

0216U Neurology (inherited ataxias), genomic DNA sequence analysis of 12 common genes including small sequence changes, deletions, duplications, short tandem repeat gene expansions, and variants in non-uniquely mappable regions, blood or saliva, identification and categorization of genetic variants

INCLUDES Genomic Unity® Ataxia Repeat Expansion and Sequence Analysis, Variantyx Inc, Variantyx Inc

0.00 0.00 FUD 000

0217U Neurology (inherited ataxias), genomic DNA sequence analysis of 51 genes including small sequence changes, deletions, duplications, short tandem repeat gene expansions, and variants in non-uniquely mappable regions, blood or saliva, identification and categorization of genetic variants

INCLUDES Genomic Unity® Comprehensive Ataxia Repeat Expansion and Sequence Analysis, Variantyx Inc, Variantyx Inc

0.00 0.00 FUD 000

0218U Neurology (muscular dystrophy), *DMD* gene sequence analysis, including small sequence changes, deletions, duplications, and variants in non-uniquely mappable regions, blood or saliva, identification and characterization of genetic variants

INCLUDES Genomic Unity® DMD Analysis, Variantyx Inc, Variantyx Inc

0.00 0.00 FUD 000

0219U Infectious agent (human immunodeficiency virus), targeted viral next-generation sequence analysis (ie, protease [PR], reverse transcriptase [RT], integrase [INT]), algorithm reported as prediction of antiviral drug susceptibility

INCLUDES *Sentosa®* SQ HIV-1 Genotyping Assay, Vela Diagnostics USA, Inc, Vela Operations Singapore Pte Ltd

0.00 0.00 FUD 000

0220U Oncology (breast cancer), image analysis with artificial intelligence assessment of 12 histologic and immunohistochemical features, reported as a recurrence score

INCLUDES PreciseDx™ Breast Cancer Test, PreciseDx, PreciseDx

0.00 0.00 FUD 000

0221U Red cell antigen (ABO blood group) genotyping (ABO), gene analysis, next-generation sequencing, *ABO (ABO, alpha 1-3-N-acetylgalactosaminyltransferase and alpha 1-3-galactosyltransferase)* gene

INCLUDES Navigator ABO Blood Group NGS, Grifols Immunohematology Center, Grifols Immunohematology Center

0.00 0.00 FUD 000

0222U Red cell antigen (RH blood group) genotyping (RHD and RHCE), gene analysis, next-generation sequencing, RH proximal promoter, exons 1-10, portions of introns 2-3

INCLUDES Navigator Rh Blood Group NGS, Grifols Immunohematology Center, Grifols Immunohematology Center

0.00 0.00 FUD 000

● **0223U Infectious disease (bacterial or viral respiratory tract infection), pathogen-specific nucleic acid (DNA or RNA), 22 targets including severe acute respiratory syndrome coronavirus 2 (SARS-CoV-2), qualitative RT-PCR, nasopharyngeal swab, each pathogen reported as detected or not detected**

INCLUDES QIAstat-Dx Respiratory SARS CoV-2 Panel, QIAGEN Sciences, QIAGEN GmbH

EXCLUDES *BioFire® Respiratory Panel 2.1 (RP2.1), BioFire® Diagnostics, BioFire® Diagnostics, LLC. To report, see (0202U)*

AMA: 2020,AugSE,1; 2020,AugSE,1; 2020,AugSE,1

● **0224U Antibody, severe acute respiratory syndrome coronavirus 2 (SARS-CoV-2) (coronavirus disease [COVID-19]), includes titer(s), when performed**

INCLUDES COVID-19 Antibody Test, Mt Sinai, Mount Sinai Laboratory

EXCLUDES *Antibody; severe acute respiratory syndrome coronavirus 2 (SARS-CoV-2) (coronavirus disease [COVID-19]) (86769)*

AMA: 2020,AugSE,1; 2020,AugSE,1; 2020,AugSE,1

● **0225U Infectious disease (bacterial or viral respiratory tract infection) pathogen-specific DNA and RNA, 21 targets, including severe acute respiratory syndrome coronavirus 2 (SARS-CoV-2), amplified probe technique, including multiplex reverse transcription for RNA targets, each analyte reported as detected or not detected**

INCLUDES ePlex® Respiratory Pathogen Panel 2, GenMark Dx, GenMark Diagnostics, Inc

AMA: 2020,AugSE,1

● **0226U Surrogate viral neutralization test (sVNT), severe acute respiratory syndrome coronavirus 2 (SARS-CoV-2) (coronavirus disease [COVID-19]), ELISA, plasma, serum**

INCLUDES Tru-Immune™, Ethos Laboratories, GenScript® USA Inc

AMA: 2020,AugSE,1

● **0227U Drug assay, presumptive, 30 or more drugs or metabolites, urine, liquid chromatography with tandem mass spectrometry (LC-MS/MS) using multiple reaction monitoring (MRM), with drug or metabolite description, includes sample validation**

INCLUDES Comprehensive Screen, Aspenti Health

0.00 0.00 FUD 000

● **0228U** **Oncology (prostate), multianalyte molecular profile by photometric detection of macromolecules adsorbed on nanosponge array slides with machine learning, utilizing first morning voided urine, algorithm reported as likelihood of prostate cancer**

INCLUDES PanGIA Prostate, Genetics Institute of America, Entopsis, LLC

● **0229U** ***BCAT1 (Branched chain amino acid transaminase 1)* or *IKZF1 (IKAROS family zinc finger 1)* (eg, colorectal cancer) promoter methylation analysis**

INCLUDES Colvera®, Clinical Genomics Pathology Inc

● **0230U** ***AR (androgen receptor)* (eg, spinal and bulbar muscular atrophy, Kennedy disease, X chromosome inactivation), full sequence analysis, including small sequence changes in exonic and intronic regions, deletions, duplications, short tandem repeat (STR) expansions, mobile element insertions, and variants in non-uniquely mappable regions**

INCLUDES Genomic Unity® AR Analysis, Variantyx Inc, Variantyx Inc

● **0231U** ***CACNA1A (calcium voltage-gated channel subunit alpha 1A)* (eg, spinocerebellar ataxia), full gene analysis, including small sequence changes in exonic and intronic regions, deletions, duplications, short tandem repeat (STR) gene expansions, mobile element insertions, and variants in non-uniquely mappable regions**

INCLUDES Genomic Unity® CACNA1A Analysis, Variantyx Inc, Variantyx Inc

● **0232U** ***CSTB (cystatin B)* (eg, progressive myoclonic epilepsy type 1A, Unverricht-Lundborg disease), full gene analysis, including small sequence changes in exonic and intronic regions, deletions, duplications, short tandem repeat (STR) expansions, mobile element insertions, and variants in non-uniquely mappable regions**

INCLUDES Genomic Unity® CSTB Analysis, Variantyx Inc, Variantyx Inc

● **0233U** ***FXN (frataxin)* (eg, Friedreich ataxia), gene analysis, including small sequence changes in exonic and intronic regions, deletions, duplications, short tandem repeat (STR) expansions, mobile element insertions, and variants in non-uniquely mappable regions**

INCLUDES Genomic Unity® FXN Analysis, Variantyx Inc, Variantyx Inc

● **0234U** ***MECP2 (methyl CpG binding protein 2)* (eg, Rett syndrome), full gene analysis, including small sequence changes in exonic and intronic regions, deletions, duplications, mobile element insertions, and variants in non-uniquely mappable regions**

INCLUDES Genomic Unity® MECP2 Analysis, Variantyx Inc, Variantyx Inc

● **0235U** ***PTEN (phosphatase and tensin homolog)* (eg, Cowden syndrome, PTEN hamartoma tumor syndrome), full gene analysis, including small sequence changes in exonic and intronic regions, deletions, duplications, mobile element insertions, and variants in non-uniquely mappable regions**

INCLUDES Genomic Unity® PTEN Analysis, Variantyx Inc, Variantyx Inc

● **0236U** ***SMN1 (survival of motor neuron 1, telomeric)* and *SMN2 (survival of motor neuron 2, centromeric)* (eg, spinal muscular atrophy) full gene analysis, including small sequence changes in exonic and intronic regions, duplications, deletions, and mobile element insertions**

INCLUDES Genomic Unity® SMN1/2 Analysis, Variantyx Inc, Variantyx Inc

● **0237U** **Cardiac ion channelopathies (eg, Brugada syndrome, long QT syndrome, short QT syndrome, catecholaminergic polymorphic ventricular tachycardia), genomic sequence analysis panel including *ANK2, CASQ2, CAV3, KCNE1, KCNE2, KCNH2, KCNJ2, KCNQ1, RYR2,* and *SCN5A*, including small sequence changes in exonic and intronic regions, deletions, duplications, mobile element insertions, and variants in non-uniquely mappable regions**

INCLUDES Genomic Unity® Cardiac Ion Channelopathies Analysis, Variantyx Inc, Variantyx Inc

● **0238U** **Oncology (Lynch syndrome), genomic DNA sequence analysis of *MLH1, MSH2, MSH6, PMS2,* and *EPCAM*, including small sequence changes in exonic and intronic regions, deletions, duplications, mobile element insertions, and variants in non-uniquely mappable regions**

INCLUDES Genomic Unity® Lynch Syndrome Analysis, Variantyx Inc, Variantyx Inc

● **0239U** **Targeted genomic sequence analysis panel, solid organ neoplasm, cell-free DNA, analysis of 311 or more genes, interrogation for sequence variants, including substitutions, insertions, deletions, select rearrangements, and copy number variations**

INCLUDES FoundationOne® Liquid CDx, Foundation Medicine, Inc, Foundation Medicine, Inc

● **0240U** **Infectious disease (viral respiratory tract infection), pathogen-specific RNA, 3 targets (severe acute respiratory syndrome coronavirus 2 [SARS-CoV-2], influenza A, influenza B), upper respiratory specimen, each pathogen reported as detected or not detected**

INCLUDES Xpert® Xpress SARS-CoV-2/Flu/RSV (SARS-CoV-2 & Flu targets only), Cepheid

0.00   0.00   **FUD** 000

AMA: 2020,OctSE,1

● **0241U** **Infectious disease (viral respiratory tract infection), pathogen-specific RNA, 4 targets (severe acute respiratory syndrome coronavirus 2 [SARS-CoV-2], influenza A, influenza B, respiratory syncytial virus [RSV]), upper respiratory specimen, each pathogen reported as detected or not detected**

INCLUDES Xpert® Xpress SARS-CoV-2/Flu/RSV (all targets), Cepheid

0.00   0.00   **FUD** 000

AMA: 2020,OctSE,1

● **0242U** **Targeted genomic sequence analysis panel, solid organ neoplasm, cell-free circulating DNA analysis of 55-74 genes, interrogation for sequence variants, gene copy number amplifications, and gene rearrangements**

INCLUDES Guardant360® CDx, Guardant Health Inc, Guardant Health Inc

● **0243U** **Obstetrics (preeclampsia), biochemical assay of placental-growth factor, time-resolved fluorescence immunoassay, maternal serum, predictive algorithm reported as a risk score for preeclampsia** ♀

INCLUDES PIGF Preeclampsia Screen, PerkinElmer Genetics, PerkinElmer Genetics, Inc

0.00   0.00   **FUD** 000

● **0244U** **Oncology (solid organ), DNA, comprehensive genomic profiling, 257 genes, interrogation for single-nucleotide variants, insertions/deletions, copy number alterations, gene rearrangements, tumor-mutational burden and microsatellite instability, utilizing formalin-fixed paraffin-embedded tumor tissue**

INCLUDES Oncotype MAP™ Pan-Cancer Tissue Test, Paradigm Diagnostics, Inc, Paradigm Diagnostics, Inc

● **0245U** **Oncology (thyroid), mutation analysis of 10 genes and 37 RNA fusions and expression of 4 mRNA markers using next-generation sequencing, fine needle aspirate, report includes associated risk of malignancy expressed as a percentage**

INCLUDES ThyGeNEXT® Thyroid Oncogene Panel, Interpace Diagnostics, Interpace Diagnostics

● **0246U** **Red blood cell antigen typing, DNA, genotyping of at least 16 blood groups with phenotype prediction of at least 51 red blood cell antigens**

INCLUDES PrecisionBlood™, San Diego Blood Bank, San Diego Blood Bank

● **0247U** **Obstetrics (preterm birth), insulin-like growth factor-binding protein 4 (IBP4), sex hormone-binding globulin (SHBG), quantitative measurement by LC-MS/MS, utilizing maternal serum, combined with clinical data, reported as predictive-risk stratification for spontaneous preterm birth**

INCLUDES PreTRM®, Sera Prognostics, Sera Prognostics, Inc®

● **0248U** **Oncology (brain), spheroid cell culture in a 3D microenvironment, 12 drug panel, tumor-response prediction for each drug**

INCLUDES 3D Predict Glioma, KIYATEC®, Inc

● **0249U** **Oncology (breast), semiquantitative analysis of 32 phosphoproteins and protein analytes, includes laser capture microdissection, with algorithmic analysis and interpretative report**

INCLUDES Theralink® Reverse Phase Protein Array (RPPA), Theralink® Technologies, Inc, Theralink® Technologies, Inc

● **0250U** **Oncology (solid organ neoplasm), targeted genomic sequence DNA analysis of 505 genes, interrogation for somatic alterations (SNVs [single nucleotide variant], small insertions and deletions, one amplification, and four translocations), microsatellite instability and tumor-mutation burden**

INCLUDES PGDx elio™ tissue complete, Personal Genome Diagnostics, Inc, Personal Genome Diagnostics, Inc

● **0251U** **Hepcidin-25, enzyme-linked immunosorbent assay (ELISA), serum or plasma**

INCLUDES Intrinsic Hepcidin IDx™ Test, IntrinsicDx, Intrinsic LifeSciences™ LLC

● **0252U** **Fetal aneuploidy short tandem–repeat comparative analysis, fetal DNA from products of conception, reported as normal (euploidy), monosomy, trisomy, or partial deletion/duplication, mosaicism, and segmental aneuploidy**

INCLUDES POC (Products of Conception), Igenomix®, Igenomix® USA

● **0253U** **Reproductive medicine (endometrial receptivity analysis), RNA gene expression profile, 238 genes by next-generation sequencing, endometrial tissue, predictive algorithm reported as endometrial window of implantation (eg, pre-receptive, receptive, post-receptive)** ♀

INCLUDES ERA® (Endometrial Receptivity Analysis), Igenomix®, Igenomix® USA

0.00 0.00 FUD 000

● **0254U** **Reproductive medicine (preimplantation genetic assessment), analysis of 24 chromosomes using embryonic DNA genomic sequence analysis for aneuploidy, and a mitochondrial DNA score in euploid embryos, results reported as normal (euploidy), monosomy, trisomy, or partial deletion/duplication, mosaicism, and segmental aneuploidy, per embryo tested**

INCLUDES SMART PGT-A (Pre-implantation Genetic Testing - Aneuploidy), Igenomix®, Igenomix® USA

● **0255U** **Andrology (infertility), sperm-capacitation assessment of ganglioside GM1 distribution patterns, fluorescence microscopy, fresh or frozen specimen, reported as percentage of capacitated sperm and probability of generating a pregnancy score**

INCLUDES Cap-Score™ Test, Androvia LifeSciences, Avantor Clinical Services (previously known as Therapak)

● **0256U** **Trimethylamine/trimethylamine N-oxide (TMA/TMAO) profile, tandem mass spectrometry (MS/MS), urine, with algorithmic analysis and interpretive report**

INCLUDES Trimethylamine (TMA) and TMA N-Oxide, Children's Hospital Colorado Laboratory

● **0257U** **Very long chain acyl-coenzyme A (CoA) dehydrogenase (VLCAD), leukocyte enzyme activity, whole blood**

INCLUDES Very-Long Chain Acyl-CoA Dehydrogenase (VLCAD) Enzyme Activity, Children's Hospital Colorado Laboratory

● **0258U** **Autoimmune (psoriasis), mRNA, next-generation sequencing, gene expression profiling of 50-100 genes, skin-surface collection using adhesive patch, algorithm reported as likelihood of response to psoriasis biologics**

INCLUDES Mind.Px, Mindera, Mindera Corporation

● **0259U** **Nephrology (chronic kidney disease), nuclear magnetic resonance spectroscopy measurement of myo-inositol, valine, and creatinine, algorithmically combined with cystatin C (by immunoassay) and demographic data to determine estimated glomerular filtration rate (GFR), serum, quantitative**

INCLUDES GFR by NMR, Labtech™ Diagnostics

● **0260U** **Rare diseases (constitutional/heritable disorders), identification of copy number variations, inversions, insertions, translocations, and other structural variants by optical genome mapping**

INCLUDES Augusta Optical Genome Mapping, Georgia Esoteric and Molecular (GEM) Laboratory, LLC, Bionano Genomics Inc

EXCLUDES *Praxis Optical Genome Mapping, Praxis Genomics LLC (0264U)*

● **0261U** **Oncology (colorectal cancer), image analysis with artificial intelligence assessment of 4 histologic and immunohistochemical features (CD3 and CD8 within tumor-stroma border and tumor core), tissue, reported as immune response and recurrence-risk score**

INCLUDES Immunoscore®, HalioDx, HalioDx

● **0262U** **Oncology (solid tumor), gene expression profiling by real-time RT-PCR of 7 gene pathways *(ER, AR, PI3K, MAPK, HH, TGFB,* Notch), formalin-fixed paraffin-embedded (FFPE), algorithm reported as gene pathway activity score**

INCLUDES OncoSignal 7 Pathway Signal, Protean BioDiagnostics, Philips Electronics Nederland BV

● **0263U** **Neurology (autism spectrum disorder [ASD]), quantitative measurements of 16 central carbon metabolites (ie, α-ketoglutarate, alanine, lactate, phenylalanine, pyruvate, succinate, carnitine, citrate, fumarate, hypoxanthine, inosine, malate, S-sulfocysteine, taurine, urate, and xanthine), liquid chromatography tandem mass spectrometry (LC-MS/MS), plasma, algorithmic analysis with result reported as negative or positive (with metabolic subtypes of ASD)**

INCLUDES NPDX ASD and Central Carbon Energy Metabolism, Stemina Biomarker Discovery, Inc, Stemina Biomarker Discovery, Inc

● **0264U** **Rare diseases (constitutional/heritable disorders), identification of copy number variations, inversions, insertions, translocations, and other structural variants by optical genome mapping**

INCLUDES Praxis Optical Genome Mapping, Praxis Genomics LLC

EXCLUDES *Augusta Optical Genome Mapping, Georgia Esoteric and Molecular (GEM) Laboratory, LLC, Bionano Genomics Inc (0260U)*

● **0265U Rare constitutional and other heritable disorders, whole genome and mitochondrial DNA sequence analysis, blood, frozen and formalin-fixed paraffin-embedded (FFPE) tissue, saliva, buccal swabs or cell lines, identification of single nucleotide and copy number variants**

INCLUDES Praxis Whole Genome Sequencing, Praxis Genomics LLC

● **0266U Unexplained constitutional or other heritable disorders or syndromes, tissue-specific gene expression by whole-transcriptome and next-generation sequencing, blood, formalin-fixed paraffin-embedded (FFPE) tissue or fresh frozen tissue, reported as presence or absence of splicing or expression changes**

INCLUDES Praxis Transcriptome, Praxis Genomics LLC

● **0267U Rare constitutional and other heritable disorders, identification of copy number variations, inversions, insertions, translocations, and other structural variants by optical genome mapping and whole genome sequencing**

INCLUDES Praxis Combined Whole Genome Sequencing and Optical Genome Mapping, Praxis Genomics LLC

● **0268U Hematology (atypical hemolytic uremic syndrome [aHUS]), genomic sequence analysis of 15 genes, blood, buccal swab, or amniotic fluid**

INCLUDES Versiti™ aHUS Genetic Evaluation, Versiti™ Diagnostic Laboratories, Versiti™

● **0269U Hematology (autosomal dominant congenital thrombocytopenia), genomic sequence analysis of 14 genes, blood, buccal swab, or amniotic fluid**

INCLUDES Versiti™ Autosomal Dominant Thrombocytopenia Panel, Versiti™ Diagnostic Laboratories, Versiti™

● **0270U Hematology (congenital coagulation disorders), genomic sequence analysis of 20 genes, blood, buccal swab, or amniotic fluid**

INCLUDES Versiti™ Coagulation Disorder Panel, Versiti™ Diagnostic Laboratories, Versiti™

● **0271U Hematology (congenital neutropenia), genomic sequence analysis of 23 genes, blood, buccal swab, or amniotic fluid**

INCLUDES Versiti™ Congenital Neutropenia Panel, Versiti™ Diagnostic Laboratories, Versiti™

● **0272U Hematology (genetic bleeding disorders), genomic sequence analysis of 51 genes, blood, buccal swab, or amniotic fluid, comprehensive**

INCLUDES Versiti™ Comprehensive Bleeding Disorder Panel, Versiti™ Diagnostic Laboratories, Versiti™

● **0273U Hematology (genetic hyperfibrinolysis, delayed bleeding), genomic sequence analysis of 8 genes *(F13A1, F13B, FGA, FGB, FGG, SERPINA1, SERPINE1, SERPINF2, PLAU)*, blood, buccal swab, or amniotic fluid**

INCLUDES Versiti™ Fibrinolytic Disorder Panel, Versiti™ Diagnostic Laboratories, Versiti™

● **0274U Hematology (genetic platelet disorders), genomic sequence analysis of 43 genes, blood, buccal swab, or amniotic fluid**

INCLUDES Versiti™ Comprehensive Platelet Disorder Panel, Versiti™ Diagnostic Laboratories, Versiti™

● **0275U Hematology (heparin-induced thrombocytopenia), platelet antibody reactivity by flow cytometry, serum**

INCLUDES Versiti™ Heparin-Induced Thrombocytopenia Evaluation – PEA, Versiti™ Diagnostic Laboratories, Versiti™

● **0276U Hematology (inherited thrombocytopenia), genomic sequence analysis of 23 genes, blood, buccal swab, or amniotic fluid**

INCLUDES Versiti™ Inherited Thrombocytopenia Panel, Versiti™ Diagnostic Laboratories, Versiti™

● **0277U Hematology (genetic platelet function disorder), genomic sequence analysis of 31 genes, blood, buccal swab, or amniotic fluid**

INCLUDES Versiti™ Platelet Function Disorder Panel, Versiti™ Diagnostic Laboratories, Versiti™

● **0278U Hematology (genetic thrombosis), genomic sequence analysis of 12 genes, blood, buccal swab, or amniotic fluid**

INCLUDES Versiti™ Thrombosis Panel, Versiti™ Diagnostic Laboratories, Versiti™

● **0279U Hematology (von Willebrand disease [VWD]), von Willebrand factor (VWF) and collagen III binding by enzyme-linked immunosorbent assays (ELISA), plasma, report of collagen III binding**

INCLUDES Versiti™ VWF Collagen III Binding, Versiti™ Diagnostic Laboratories, Versiti™

● **0280U Hematology (von Willebrand disease [VWD]), von Willebrand factor (VWF) and collagen IV binding by enzyme-linked immunosorbent assays (ELISA), plasma, report of collagen IV binding**

INCLUDES Versiti™ VWF Collagen IV Binding, Versiti™ Diagnostic Laboratories, Versiti™

● **0281U Hematology (von Willebrand disease [VWD]), von Willebrand propeptide, enzyme-linked immunosorbent assays (ELISA), plasma, diagnostic report of von Willebrand factor (VWF) propeptide antigen level**

INCLUDES Versiti™ VWF Propeptide Antigen, Versiti™ Diagnostic Laboratories, Versiti™

● **0282U Red blood cell antigen typing, DNA, genotyping of 12 blood group system genes to predict 44 red blood cell antigen phenotypes**

INCLUDES Versiti™ Red Cell Genotyping Panel, Versiti™ Diagnostic Laboratories, Versiti™

● **0283U von Willebrand factor (VWF), type 2B, platelet-binding evaluation, radioimmunoassay, plasma**

INCLUDES Versiti™ VWD Type 2B Evaluation, Versiti™ Diagnostic Laboratories, Versiti™

● **0284U von Willebrand factor (VWF), type 2N, factor VIII and VWF binding evaluation, enzyme-linked immunosorbent assays (ELISA), plasma**

INCLUDES Versiti™ VWD Type 2N Binding, Versiti™ Diagnostic Laboratories, Versiti™

● **0285U Oncology, response to radiation, cell-free DNA, quantitative branched chain DNA amplification, plasma, reported as a radiation toxicity score**

INCLUDES RadTox™ cfDNA test, DiaCarta Clinical Lab, DiaCarta Inc

● **0286U *CEP72 (centrosomal protein, 72-KDa), NUDT15 (nudix hydrolase 15)* and *TPMT (thiopurine S-methyltransferase)* (eg, drug metabolism) gene analysis, common variants**

INCLUDES CNT *(CEP72, TPMT and NUDT15)* genotyping panel, RPRD Diagnostics

● **0287U Oncology (thyroid), DNA and mRNA, next-generation sequencing analysis of 112 genes, fine needle aspirate or formalin-fixed paraffin-embedded (FFPE) tissue, algorithmic prediction of cancer recurrence, reported as a categorical risk result (low, intermediate, high)**

INCLUDES ThyroSeq® CRC, CBLPath, Inc, University of Pittsburgh Medical Center

● **0288U Oncology (lung), mRNA, quantitative PCR analysis of 11 genes *(BAG1, BRCA1, CDC6, CDK2AP1, ERBB3, FUT3, IL11, LCK, RND3, SH3BGR, WNT3A)* and 3 reference genes *(ESD, TBP, YAP1)*, formalin-fixed paraffin-embedded (FFPE) tumor tissue, algorithmic interpretation reported as a recurrence risk score**

INCLUDES DetermaRx™, Oncocyte Corporation

● **0289U** **Neurology (Alzheimer disease), mRNA, gene expression profiling by RNA sequencing of 24 genes, whole blood, algorithm reported as predictive risk score**

INCLUDES MindX Blood Test™ - Memory/Alzheimer's, MindX Sciences™ Laboratory, MindX Sciences™ Inc

● **0290U** **Pain management, mRNA, gene expression profiling by RNA sequencing of 36 genes, whole blood, algorithm reported as predictive risk score**

INCLUDES MindX Blood Test™ - Pain, MindX Sciences™ Laboratory, MindX Sciences™ Inc

● **0291U** **Psychiatry (mood disorders), mRNA, gene expression profiling by RNA sequencing of 144 genes, whole blood, algorithm reported as predictive risk score**

INCLUDES MindX Blood Test™ - Mood, MindX Sciences™ Laboratory, MindX Sciences™ Inc

● **0292U** **Psychiatry (stress disorders), mRNA, gene expression profiling by RNA sequencing of 72 genes, whole blood, algorithm reported as predictive risk score**

INCLUDES MindX Blood Test™ - Stress, MindX Sciences™ Laboratory, MindX Sciences™ Inc

● **0293U** **Psychiatry (suicidal ideation), mRNA, gene expression profiling by RNA sequencing of 54 genes, whole blood, algorithm reported as predictive risk score**

INCLUDES MindX Blood Test™ - Suicidality, MindX Sciences™ Laboratory, MindX Sciences™ Inc

● **0294U** **Longevity and mortality risk, mRNA, gene expression profiling by RNA sequencing of 18 genes, whole blood, algorithm reported as predictive risk score**

INCLUDES MindX Blood Test™ - Longevity, MindX Sciences™ Laboratory, MindX Sciences™ Inc

● **0295U** **Oncology (breast ductal carcinoma in situ), protein expression profiling by immunohistochemistry of 7 proteins (COX2, FOXA1, HER2, Ki-67, p16, PR, SIAH2), with 4 clinicopathologic factors (size, age, margin status, palpability), utilizing formalin-fixed paraffin-embedded (FFPE) tissue, algorithm reported as a recurrence risk score**

INCLUDES DCISionRT®, PreludeDx™, Prelude Corporation

● **0296U** **Oncology (oral and/or oropharyngeal cancer), gene expression profiling by RNA sequencing at least 20 molecular features (eg, human and/or microbial mRNA), saliva, algorithm reported as positive or negative for signature associated with malignancy**

INCLUDES mRNA CancerDetect™, Viome Life Sciences, Inc, Viome Life Sciences, Inc

● **0297U** **Oncology (pan tumor), whole genome sequencing of paired malignant and normal DNA specimens, fresh or formalin-fixed paraffin-embedded (FFPE) tissue, blood or bone marrow, comparative sequence analyses and variant identification**

INCLUDES Praxis Somatic Whole Genome Sequencing, Praxis Genomics LLC

● **0298U** **Oncology (pan tumor), whole transcriptome sequencing of paired malignant and normal RNA specimens, fresh or formalin-fixed paraffin-embedded (FFPE) tissue, blood or bone marrow, comparative sequence analyses and expression level and chimeric transcript identification**

INCLUDES Praxis Somatic Transcriptome, Praxis Genomics LLC

● **0299U** **Oncology (pan tumor), whole genome optical genome mapping of paired malignant and normal DNA specimens, fresh frozen tissue, blood, or bone marrow, comparative structural variant identification**

INCLUDES Praxis Somatic Optical Genome Mapping, Praxis Genomics LLC

● **0300U** **Oncology (pan tumor), whole genome sequencing and optical genome mapping of paired malignant and normal DNA specimens, fresh tissue, blood, or bone marrow, comparative sequence analyses and variant identification**

INCLUDES Praxis Somatic Combined Whole Genome Sequencing and Optical Genome Mapping, Praxis Genomics LLC

● **0301U** **Infectious agent detection by nucleic acid (DNA or RNA), Bartonella henselae and Bartonella quintana, droplet digital PCR (ddPCR);**

INCLUDES Bartonella ddPCR, Galaxy Diagnostics Inc

● **0302U** **following liquid enhancement**

INCLUDES Bartonella Digital ePCR™, Galaxy Diagnostics Inc

● **0303U** **Hematology, red blood cell (RBC) adhesion to endothelial/subendothelial adhesion molecules, functional assessment, whole blood, with algorithmic analysis and result reported as an RBC adhesion index; hypoxic**

INCLUDES Hypoxic BioChip Adhesion, BioChip Labs™, BioChip Labs™

● **0304U** **normoxic**

INCLUDES Normoxic BioChip Adhesion, BioChip Labs™, BioChip Labs™

● **0305U** **Hematology, red blood cell (RBC) functionality and deformity as a function of shear stress, whole blood, reported as a maximum elongation index**

INCLUDES Ektacytometry, BioChip Labs™, BioChip Labs™

90281-90399 Immunoglobulin Products

INCLUDES Immune globulin product only
Anti-infectives
Antitoxins
Isoantibodies
Monoclonal antibodies

Code also (96365-96372, 96374-96375)

90281 Immune globulin (Ig), human, for intramuscular use
INCLUDES Gamastan
0.00 0.00 FUD XXX
AMA: 2020,NovSE,1; 2020,Jan,11; 2018,Jan,8; 2017,Jan,8; 2016,Jan,13

90283 Immune globulin (IgIV), human, for intravenous use
0.00 0.00 FUD XXX
AMA: 2020,NovSE,1; 2020,Jan,11; 2018,Jan,8; 2017,Jan,8; 2016,Jan,13

90284 Immune globulin (SCIg), human, for use in subcutaneous infusions, 100 mg, each
0.00 0.00 FUD XXX
AMA: 2020,NovSE,1; 2020,Jan,11; 2018,Jan,8; 2017,Jan,8; 2016,Jan,13

90287 Botulinum antitoxin, equine, any route
0.00 0.00 FUD XXX
AMA: 2020,NovSE,1; 2020,Jan,11; 2018,Jan,8; 2017,Jan,8; 2016,Jan,13

90288 Botulism immune globulin, human, for intravenous use
0.00 0.00 FUD XXX
AMA: 2020,NovSE,1; 2020,Jan,11; 2018,Jan,8; 2017,Jan,8; 2016,Jan,13

90291 Cytomegalovirus immune globulin (CMV-IgIV), human, for intravenous use
INCLUDES Cytogram
0.00 0.00 FUD XXX
AMA: 2020,NovSE,1; 2020,Jan,11; 2018,Jan,8; 2017,Jan,8; 2016,Jan,13

90296 Diphtheria antitoxin, equine, any route
0.00 0.00 FUD XXX
AMA: 2020,NovSE,1; 2020,Jan,11; 2018,Jan,8; 2017,Jan,8; 2016,Jan,13

90371 Hepatitis B immune globulin (HBIg), human, for intramuscular use
INCLUDES HBIG
0.00 0.00 FUD XXX
AMA: 2020,NovSE,1; 2020,Jan,11; 2018,Jan,8; 2017,Jan,8; 2016,Jan,13

90375 Rabies immune globulin (RIg), human, for intramuscular and/or subcutaneous use
INCLUDES HyperRAB
0.00 0.00 FUD XXX
AMA: 2020,NovSE,1; 2020,Jan,11; 2018,Jan,8; 2017,Jan,8; 2016,Jan,13

90376 Rabies immune globulin, heat-treated (RIg-HT), human, for intramuscular and/or subcutaneous use
0.00 0.00 FUD XXX
AMA: 2020,NovSE,1; 2020,Jan,11; 2018,Jan,8; 2017,Jan,8; 2016,Jan,13

90377 Rabies immune globulin, heat- and solvent/detergent-treated (RIg-HT S/D), human, for intramuscular and/or subcutaneous use
0.00 0.00 FUD XXX

90378 Respiratory syncytial virus, monoclonal antibody, recombinant, for intramuscular use, 50 mg, each
INCLUDES Synagis
0.00 0.00 FUD XXX
AMA: 2020,NovSE,1; 2020,Jan,11; 2018,Jan,8; 2017,Jan,8; 2016,Jan,13

90384 Rho(D) immune globulin (RhIg), human, full-dose, for intramuscular use
0.00 0.00 FUD XXX
AMA: 2020,NovSE,1; 2020,Jan,11; 2018,Jan,8; 2017,Jan,8; 2016,Jan,13

90385 Rho(D) immune globulin (RhIg), human, mini-dose, for intramuscular use
0.00 0.00 FUD XXX
AMA: 2020,NovSE,1; 2020,Jan,11; 2018,Jan,8; 2017,Jan,8; 2016,Jan,13

90386 Rho(D) immune globulin (RhIgIV), human, for intravenous use
0.00 0.00 FUD XXX
AMA: 2020,NovSE,1; 2020,Jan,11; 2018,Jan,8; 2017,Jan,8; 2016,Jan,13

90389 Tetanus immune globulin (TIg), human, for intramuscular use
INCLUDES HyperTET S/D (Tetanus Immune Globulin)
0.00 0.00 FUD XXX
AMA: 2020,NovSE,1; 2020,Jan,11; 2018,Jan,8; 2017,Jan,8; 2016,Jan,13

90393 Vaccinia immune globulin, human, for intramuscular use
0.00 0.00 FUD XXX
AMA: 2020,NovSE,1; 2020,Jan,11; 2018,Jan,8; 2017,Jan,8; 2016,Jan,13

90396 Varicella-zoster immune globulin, human, for intramuscular use
INCLUDES VariZIG
0.00 0.00 FUD XXX
AMA: 2020,NovSE,1; 2020,Jan,11; 2018,Jan,8; 2017,Jan,8; 2016,Jan,13

90399 Unlisted immune globulin
0.00 0.00 FUD XXX
AMA: 2020,NovSE,1; 2020,Jan,11; 2018,Jan,8; 2017,Jan,8; 2016,Jan,13

90460-90461 Injections Provided with Counseling

INCLUDES All components influenza vaccine, report one time only
Combination vaccines which comprise multiple vaccine components
Components (all antigens) in vaccines to prevent disease due to specific organisms
Counseling by physician or other qualified health care professional
Multivalent antigens or multiple antigen serotypes against single organisms considered one component
Patient/family face-to-face counseling by doctor or qualified health care professional for patients age 18 years and younger

EXCLUDES *Administration influenza and pneumococcal vaccine for Medicare patients (G0008-G0009)*
Allergy testing (95004-95028)
Bacterial/viral/fungal skin tests (86485-86580)
Diagnostic or therapeutic injections (96365-96371, 96372-96379)
Reporting with severe acute respiratory syndrome coronavirus 2 (SARS-CoV-2) (coronavirus disease [COVID-19]) vaccine when not administered with separately identifiable vaccine/toxoid ([91300, 91301, 91302, 91303, 91304, 91305, 91306, 91307])
Vaccines provided without face-to-face counseling from physician or qualified health care professional or to patients age 18 years and older (90471-90474)

Code also:
Significant, separately identifiable E/M service when appropriate
Toxoid/vaccine (90476-90749 [90619, 90620, 90621, 90625, 90630, 90644, 90672, 90673, 90674, 90750, 90756])

90460 Immunization administration through 18 years of age via any route of administration, with counseling by physician or other qualified health care professional; first or only component of each vaccine or toxoid administered
Code also each additional component in vaccine (e.g., 5-year-old receives DtaP-IPV IM administration, and MMR/Varicella vaccines SQ administration. Report initial component two times, and additional components six times)
0.47 0.47 FUD XXX
AMA: 2020,DecSE,1; 2020,DecSE,1; 2020,NovBULL,2; 2020,NovSE,1; 2020,Jul,11; 2020,Jan,11; 2018,Nov,7; 2018,Jan,8; 2017,Jan,8; 2016,Oct,6; 2016,Jan,13

+ **90461** **each additional vaccine or toxoid component administered (List separately in addition to code for primary procedure)** A

Code also each additional component in vaccine (e.g., 5-year-old receives DtaP-IPV IM administration, and MMR/Varicella vaccines SQ administration. Report initial component two times, and additional components six times)

Code first initial component in each vaccine provided (90460)

0.36 0.36 FUD ZZZ B 80

AMA: 2020,DecSE,1; 2020,DecSE,1; 2020,NovSE,1; 2020,Jul,11; 2020,Jan,11; 2018,Nov,7; 2018,Jan,8; 2017,Jan,8; 2016,Oct,6; 2016,Jan,13

90471-0104A [0001A, 0002A, 0003A, 0004A, 0011A, 0012A, 0013A, 0014A, 0021A, 0022A, 0023A, 0024A, 0031A, 0032A, 0033A, 0034A, 0041A, 0042A, 0043A, 0044A, 0051A, 0052A, 0053A, 0054A, 0061A, 0062A, 0063A, 0064A, 0071A, 0072A, 0073A, 0074A, 0081A, 0082A, 0083A, 0084A, 0091A, 0092A, 0093A, 0094A, 0101A, 0102A, 0103A, 0104A] Injections and Other Routes of Administration Without Physician Counseling

EXCLUDES *Administration influenza and pneumococcal vaccine for Medicare patients (G0008-G0009)*
Administration vaccine with counseling (90460-90461)
Allergy testing (95004-95028)
Bacterial/viral/fungal skin tests (86485-86580)
Diagnostic or therapeutic injections (96365-96371, 96374)
Patient/family face-to-face counseling
Reporting with severe acute respiratory syndrome coronavirus 2 (SARS-CoV-2) (Coronavirus disease [COVID-19]) vaccine when not administered with separately identifiable vaccine/toxoid ([91300, 91301, 91302, 91303, 91304, 91305, 91306, 91307])

Code also:
Significant, separately identifiable E/M service when appropriate
Toxoid/vaccine (90476-90749 [90619, 90620, 90621, 90625, 90630, 90644, 90672, 90673, 90674, 90750, 90756])

90471 **Immunization administration (includes percutaneous, intradermal, subcutaneous, or intramuscular injections); 1 vaccine (single or combination vaccine/toxoid)**

EXCLUDES *Intranasal/oral administration (90473)*

0.47 0.47 FUD XXX Q1 80

AMA: 2020,NovSE,1; 2020,Jul,11; 2020,Jan,11; 2019,Jun,11; 2018,Nov,7; 2018,Jan,8; 2017,Jan,8; 2016,Oct,6; 2016,Jan,13

+ **90472** **each additional vaccine (single or combination vaccine/toxoid) (List separately in addition to code for primary procedure)**

EXCLUDES *BCG vaccine, intravesical administration (51720, 90586)*
Immune globulin administration (96365-96371, 96374)
Immune globulin product (90281-90399)

Code first initial vaccine (90460, 90471, 90473)

0.36 0.36 FUD ZZZ N 80

AMA: 2020,NovSE,1; 2020,Jul,11; 2020,Jan,11; 2018,Nov,7; 2018,Jan,8; 2017,Jan,8; 2016,Oct,6; 2016,Jan,13

90473 **Immunization administration by intranasal or oral route; 1 vaccine (single or combination vaccine/toxoid)**

EXCLUDES *Administration by injection (90471)*

0.47 0.47 FUD XXX Q1 80

AMA: 2020,NovSE,1; 2020,Jan,11; 2018,Nov,7; 2018,Jan,8; 2017,Jan,8; 2016,Jan,13

+ **90474** **each additional vaccine (single or combination vaccine/toxoid) (List separately in addition to code for primary procedure)**

Code first initial vaccine (90460, 90471, 90473)

0.36 0.36 FUD ZZZ N 80

AMA: 2020,NovSE,1; 2018,Nov,7; 2018,Jan,8; 2017,Jan,8; 2016,Jan,13

● **0001A** **Immunization administration by intramuscular injection of severe acute respiratory syndrome coronavirus 2 (SARS-CoV-2) (coronavirus disease [COVID-19]) vaccine, mRNA-LNP, spike protein, preservative free, 30 mcg/0.3mL dosage, diluent reconstituted; first dose**

INCLUDES Pfizer-BioNTech COVID-19 vaccine, Comirnaty

Code also vaccine ([91300])

0.00 0.00 FUD XXX

● **0002A** **second dose**

INCLUDES Pfizer-BioNTech COVID-19 vaccine, Comirnaty

Code also vaccine ([91300])

0.00 0.00 FUD XXX

● **0003A** **third dose**

INCLUDES Pfizer-BioNTech COVID-19 vaccine, Comirnaty

Code also vaccine ([91300])

0.00 0.00 FUD 000

● **0004A** **booster dose**

INCLUDES Pfizer-BioNTech COVID-19 vaccine, Comirnaty

Code also vaccine ([91300])

0.00 0.00 FUD 000

● # **0051A** **Immunization administration by intramuscular injection of severe acute respiratory syndrome coronavirus 2 (SARS-CoV-2) (coronavirus disease [COVID-19]) vaccine, mRNA-LNP, spike protein, preservative free, 30 mcg/0.3 mL dosage, tris-sucrose formulation; first dose**

INCLUDES Pfizer-BioNTech COVID-19 vaccine

Code also vaccine ([91305])

0.00 0.00 FUD 000

● # **0052A** **second dose**

INCLUDES Pfizer-BioNTech COVID-19 vaccine

Code also vaccine ([91305])

0.00 0.00 FUD 000

● # **0053A** **third dose**

INCLUDES Pfizer-BioNTech COVID-19 vaccine

Code also vaccine ([91305])

0.00 0.00 FUD 000

● # **0054A** **booster dose**

INCLUDES Pfizer-BioNTech COVID-19 vaccine

Code also vaccine ([91305])

0.00 0.00 FUD 000

● # **0071A** **Immunization administration by intramuscular injection of severe acute respiratory syndrome coronavirus 2 (SARS-CoV-2) (coronavirus disease [COVID-19]) vaccine, mRNA-LNP, spike protein, preservative free, 10 mcg/0.2 mL dosage, diluent reconstituted, tris-sucrose formulation; first dose**

INCLUDES Pfizer-BioNTech COVID-19 vaccine

Code also vaccine ([91307])

0.00 0.00 FUD 000

● # **0072A** **second dose**

INCLUDES Pfizer-BioNTech COVID-19 vaccine

Code also vaccine ([91307])

0.00 0.00 FUD 000

● **0011A** **Immunization administration by intramuscular injection of severe acute respiratory syndrome coronavirus 2 (SARS-CoV-2) (coronavirus disease [COVID-19]) vaccine, mRNA-LNP, spike protein, preservative free, 100 mcg/0.5mL dosage; first dose**

INCLUDES Moderna COVID-19 vaccine

Code also vaccine ([91301])

0.00 0.00 FUD XXX

● **0012A** **second dose**

INCLUDES Moderna COVID-19 vaccine

Code also vaccine ([91301])

0.00 0.00 FUD XXX

● 0013A **third dose**

INCLUDES Moderna COVID-19 vaccine

Code also vaccine ([91301])

0.00 0.00 FUD 000

● # 0064A **Immunization administration by intramuscular injection of severe acute respiratory syndrome coronavirus 2 (SARS-CoV-2) (coronavirus disease [COVID-19]) vaccine, mRNA-LNP, spike protein, preservative free, 50 mcg/0.25 mL dosage, booster dose**

INCLUDES Moderna COVID-19 vaccine

Code also vaccine ([91306])

0.00 0.00 FUD 000

● 0014A **PLACEHOLDER ONLY**

0.00 0.00 FUD 000

● 0021A **Immunization administration by intramuscular injection of severe acute respiratory syndrome coronavirus 2 (SARS-CoV-2) (coronavirus disease [COVID-19]) vaccine, DNA, spike protein, chimpanzee adenovirus Oxford 1 (ChAdOx1) vector, preservative free, $5x10^{10}$ viral particles/0.5mL dosage; first dose**

INCLUDES AstraZeneca COVID-19 vaccine

Code also vaccine [91302]

0.00 0.00 FUD 000

● 0022A **second dose**

INCLUDES AstraZeneca COVID-19 vaccine

Code also vaccine [91302]

0.00 0.00 FUD 000

● 0023A **PLACEHOLDER ONLY**

0.00 0.00 FUD 000

● 0024A **PLACEHOLDER ONLY**

0.00 0.00 FUD 000

● 0031A **Immunization administration by intramuscular injection of severe acute respiratory syndrome coronavirus 2 (SARS-CoV-2) (coronavirus disease [COVID-19]) vaccine, DNA, spike protein, adenovirus type 26 (Ad26) vector, preservative free, $5x10^{10}$ viral particles/0.5mL dosage; single dose**

INCLUDES Janssen COVID-19 vaccine

Code also vaccine ([91303])

0.00 0.00 FUD XXX

● 0034A **booster dose**

INCLUDES Janssen COVID-19 vaccine

Code also vaccine ([91303])

0.00 0.00 FUD 000

● 0032A **PLACEHOLDER ONLY**

0.00 0.00 FUD 000

● 0033A **PLACEHOLDER ONLY**

0.00 0.00 FUD 000

● 0041A **Immunization administration by intramuscular injection of severe acute respiratory syndrome coronavirus 2 (SARS-CoV-2) (coronavirus disease [COVID-19]) vaccine, recombinant spike protein nanoparticle, saponin-based adjuvant, preservative free, 5 mcg/0.5mL dosage; first dose**

INCLUDES Novavax COVID-19 vaccine

Code also vaccine ([91304])

0.00 0.00 FUD 000

● 0042A **second dose**

INCLUDES Novavax COVID-19 vaccine

Code also vaccine ([91304])

0.00 0.00 FUD 000

● 0043A **PLACEHOLDER ONLY**

0.00 0.00 FUD 000

● 0044A **PLACEHOLDER ONLY**

0.00 0.00 FUD 000

● 0061A **PLACEHOLDER ONLY**

0.00 0.00 FUD 000

● 0062A **PLACEHOLDER ONLY**

0.00 0.00 FUD 000

● 0063A **PLACEHOLDER ONLY**

0.00 0.00 FUD 000

● 0073A **PLACEHOLDER ONLY**

0.00 0.00 FUD 000

● 0074A **PLACEHOLDER ONLY**

0.00 0.00 FUD 000

● 0081A **PLACEHOLDER ONLY**

0.00 0.00 FUD 000

● 0082A **PLACEHOLDER ONLY**

0.00 0.00 FUD 000

● 0083A **PLACEHOLDER ONLY**

0.00 0.00 FUD 000

● 0084A **PLACEHOLDER ONLY**

0.00 0.00 FUD 000

● 0091A **PLACEHOLDER ONLY**

0.00 0.00 FUD 000

● 0092A **PLACEHOLDER ONLY**

0.00 0.00 FUD 000

● 0093A **PLACEHOLDER ONLY**

0.00 0.00 FUD 000

● 0094A **PLACEHOLDER ONLY**

0.00 0.00 FUD 000

● 0101A **PLACEHOLDER ONLY**

0.00 0.00 FUD 000

● 0102A **PLACEHOLDER ONLY**

0.00 0.00 FUD 000

● 0103A **PLACEHOLDER ONLY**

0.00 0.00 FUD 000

● 0104A **PLACEHOLDER ONLY**

0.00 0.00 FUD 000

91300-90759 [90619, 90620, 90621, 90625, 90626, 90627, 90630, 90644, 90672, 90673, 90674, 90677, 90694, 90750, 90756, 90758, 90759, 91300, 91301, 91302, 91303, 91304, 91305, 91306, 91307, 91308, 91309, 91310] Vaccination Products

INCLUDES Patient's age for reporting purposes, not for product license
Vaccine product only

EXCLUDES *Immune globulins and administration (90281-90399, 96365-96375)*
Reporting each combination vaccine component individually

Code also:
Administration vaccine (90460-90461, 90471-90474, [0001A, 0002A, 0003A, 0004A], [0011A, 0012A], [0013A], [0021A, 0022A], [0031A], [0034A], [0041A, 0042A], [0051A, 0052A, 0053A, 0054A], [0064A], [0071A, 0072A]
Significant separately identifiable E/M service when appropriate

● # 91300 **Severe acute respiratory syndrome coronavirus 2 (SARS-CoV-2) (coronavirus disease [COVID-19]) vaccine, mRNA-LNP, spike protein, preservative free, 30 mcg/0.3mL dosage, diluent reconstituted, for intramuscular use**

INCLUDES Pfizer-BioNTech COVID-19 vaccine, Comirnaty

Code also vaccine administration ([0001A], [0002A], [0003A], [0004A])

0.00 0.00 FUD XXX

AMA: 2020,DecSE,1; 2020,DecSE,1

● New Code ▲ Revised Code ○ Reinstated ● New Web Release ▲ Revised Web Release + Add-on Unlisted Not Covered # Resequenced
⑸ Optum Mod 50 Exempt ⊘ AMA Mod 51 Exempt ⑸ Optum Mod 51 Exempt ⑹ Mod 63 Exempt ✓ Non-FDA Drug ★ Telemedicine M Maternity A Age Edit

● # **91305** **Severe acute respiratory syndrome coronavirus 2 (SARS-CoV-2) (coronavirus disease [COVID-19]) vaccine, mRNA-LNP, spike protein, preservative free, 30 mcg/0.3 mL dosage, tris-sucrose formulation, for intramuscular use**

INCLUDES Pfizer-BioNTech COVID-19 vaccine

Code also vaccine administration ([0051A], [0052A], [0053A], [0054A])

0.00 0.00 **FUD** 000

● # **91307** **Severe acute respiratory syndrome coronavirus 2 (SARS-CoV-2) (coronavirus disease [COVID-19]) vaccine, mRNA-LNP, spike protein, preservative free, 10 mcg/0.2 mL dosage, diluent reconstituted, tris-sucrose formulation, for intramuscular use**

INCLUDES Pfizer-BioNTech COVID-19 vaccine

Code also vaccine administration ([0071A, 0072A])

0.00 0.00 **FUD** 000

● # **91301** **Severe acute respiratory syndrome coronavirus 2 (SARS-CoV2) (coronavirus disease [COVID-19]) vaccine, mRNA-LNP, spike protein, preservative free, 100 mcg/0.5mL dosage, for intramuscular use**

INCLUDES Moderna COVID-19 vaccine

Code also vaccine administration ([0011A], [0012A], [0013A])

0.00 0.00 **FUD** XXX

AMA: 2020,DecSE,1; 2020,DecSE,1

● # **91306** **Severe acute respiratory syndrome coronavirus 2 (SARS-CoV-2) (coronavirus disease [COVID-19]) vaccine, mRNA-LNP, spike protein, preservative free, 50 mcg/0.25 mL dosage, for intramuscular use**

INCLUDES Moderna COVID-19 vaccine

Code also vaccine administration ([0064A])

0.00 0.00 **FUD** 000

● # **91302** **Severe acute respiratory syndrome coronavirus 2 (SARS-CoV-2) (coronavirus disease [COVID-19]) vaccine, DNA, spike protein, chimpanzee adenovirus Oxford 1 (ChAdOx1) vector, preservative free, $5x10^{10}$ viral particles/0.5mL dosage, for intramuscular use**

INCLUDES AstraZeneca COVID-19 vaccine

Code also vaccine administration ([0021A], [0022A])

0.00 0.00 **FUD** 000

AMA: 2020,DecSE,1; 2020,DecSE,1

● # **91303** **Severe acute respiratory syndrome coronavirus 2 (SARSCoV-2) (coronavirus disease [COVID-19]) vaccine, DNA, spike protein, adenovirus type 26 (Ad26) vector, preservative free, $5x10^{10}$ viral particles/0.5mL dosage, for intramuscular use**

INCLUDES Janssen COVID-19 vaccine

Code also vaccine administration ([0031A], [0034A])

0.00 0.00 **FUD** XXX

● # **91304** **Severe acute respiratory syndrome coronavirus 2 (SARS-CoV-2) (coronavirus disease [COVID-19]) vaccine, recombinant spike protein nanoparticle, saponin-based adjuvant, preservative free, 5 mcg/0.5mL dosage, for intramuscular use**

INCLUDES Novavax COVID-19 vaccine

Code also vaccine administration ([0041A, 0042A])

0.00 0.00 **FUD** 000

● # **91308** **PLACEHOLDER ONLY**

0.00 0.00 **FUD** 000

● # **91309** **PLACEHOLDER ONLY**

0.00 0.00 **FUD** 000

● # **91310** **PLACEHOLDER ONLY**

0.00 0.00 **FUD** 000

90476 **Adenovirus vaccine, type 4, live, for oral use**

INCLUDES Adeno-4

0.00 0.00 **FUD** XXX

AMA: 2020,DecSE,1; 2020,DecSE,1; 2020,NovSE,1; 2018,Jan,8; 2017,Jan,8; 2016,Jan,13

90477 **Adenovirus vaccine, type 7, live, for oral use**

INCLUDES Adeno-7

0.00 0.00 **FUD** XXX

AMA: 2020,DecSE,1; 2020,DecSE,1; 2020,NovSE,1; 2018,Jan,8; 2017,Jan,8; 2016,Jan,13

90581 **Anthrax vaccine, for subcutaneous or intramuscular use**

INCLUDES BioThrax

0.00 0.00 **FUD** XXX

AMA: 2020,DecSE,1; 2020,DecSE,1; 2020,NovSE,1; 2018,Jan,8; 2017,Jan,8; 2016,Jan,13

90585 **Bacillus Calmette-Guerin vaccine (BCG) for tuberculosis, live, for percutaneous use**

INCLUDES Mycobax

0.00 0.00 **FUD** XXX

AMA: 2020,DecSE,1; 2020,DecSE,1; 2020,NovSE,1; 2018,Jan,8; 2017,Jan,8; 2016,Jan,13

90586 **Bacillus Calmette-Guerin vaccine (BCG) for bladder cancer, live, for intravesical use**

INCLUDES TheraCys
TICE BCG

0.00 0.00 **FUD** XXX

AMA: 2020,DecSE,1; 2020,DecSE,1; 2020,NovSE,1; 2020,Jan,11; 2018,Jan,8; 2017,Jan,8; 2016,Jan,13

90587 **Dengue vaccine, quadrivalent, live, 3 dose schedule, for subcutaneous use**

0.00 0.00 **FUD** XXX

AMA: 2020,DecSE,1; 2020,DecSE,1; 2020,NovSE,1; 2018,Nov,7; 2018,Jan,8

90619 **Resequenced code. See code following 90734.**

90620 **Resequenced code. See code following 90734.**

90621 **Resequenced code. See code following 90734.**

90625 **Resequenced code. See code following 90723.**

90626 **Resequenced code. See code following 90715.**

90627 **Resequenced code. See code following 90715.**

90630 **Resequenced code. See code following 90654.**

90632 **Hepatitis A vaccine (HepA), adult dosage, for intramuscular use**

INCLUDES Havrix
Vaqta

0.00 0.00 **FUD** XXX

AMA: 2020,DecSE,1; 2020,DecSE,1; 2020,NovSE,1; 2018,Jan,8; 2017,Jan,8; 2016,Jan,13

90633 **Hepatitis A vaccine (HepA), pediatric/adolescent dosage-2 dose schedule, for intramuscular use**

INCLUDES Havrix
Vaqta

0.00 0.00 **FUD** XXX

AMA: 2020,DecSE,1; 2020,DecSE,1; 2020,NovSE,1; 2018,Jan,8; 2017,Jan,8; 2016,Jan,13

90634 **Hepatitis A vaccine (HepA), pediatric/adolescent dosage-3 dose schedule, for intramuscular use**

INCLUDES Havrix

0.00 0.00 **FUD** XXX

AMA: 2020,DecSE,1; 2020,DecSE,1; 2020,NovSE,1; 2018,Jan,8; 2017,Jan,8; 2016,Jan,13

90636 **Hepatitis A and hepatitis B vaccine (HepA-HepB), adult dosage, for intramuscular use**

INCLUDES Twinrix

0.00 0.00 **FUD** XXX

AMA: 2020,DecSE,1; 2020,DecSE,1; 2020,NovSE,1; 2018,Jan,8; 2017,Jan,8; 2016,Jan,13

90644 **Resequenced code. See code following 90732.**

90647 Haemophilus influenzae type b vaccine (Hib), PRP-OMP conjugate, 3 dose schedule, for intramuscular use

INCLUDES PedvaxHIB
0.00 0.00 FUD XXX
AMA: 2020,DecSE,1; 2020,DecSE,1; 2020,NovSE,1; 2018,Jan,8; 2017,Jan,8; 2016,Jan,13

90648 Haemophilus influenzae type b vaccine (Hib), PRP-T conjugate, 4 dose schedule, for intramuscular use

INCLUDES ActHIB
Hiberix
OmniHIB
0.00 0.00 FUD XXX
AMA: 2020,DecSE,1; 2020,DecSE,1; 2020,NovSE,1; 2018,Jan,8; 2017,Jan,8; 2016,Jan,13

90649 Human Papillomavirus vaccine, types 6, 11, 16, 18, quadrivalent (4vHPV), 3 dose schedule, for intramuscular use

INCLUDES Gardasil
0.00 0.00 FUD XXX
AMA: 2020,DecSE,1; 2020,DecSE,1; 2020,NovSE,1; 2018,Jan,8; 2017,Jan,8; 2016,Jan,13

90650 Human Papillomavirus vaccine, types 16, 18, bivalent (2vHPV), 3 dose schedule, for intramuscular use

INCLUDES Cervarix
0.00 0.00 FUD XXX
AMA: 2020,DecSE,1; 2020,DecSE,1; 2020,NovSE,1; 2018,Jan,8; 2017,Jan,8; 2016,Jan,13

90651 Human Papillomavirus vaccine types 6, 11, 16, 18, 31, 33, 45, 52, 58, nonavalent (9vHPV), 2 or 3 dose schedule, for intramuscular use

INCLUDES GARDASIL 9
0.00 0.00 FUD XXX
AMA: 2020,DecSE,1; 2020,DecSE,1; 2020,NovSE,1; 2018,Nov,7; 2018,Jan,8; 2017,Jan,8; 2016,Jan,13

90653 Influenza vaccine, inactivated (IIV), subunit, adjuvanted, for intramuscular use

INCLUDES Fluad
0.00 0.00 FUD XXX
AMA: 2020,DecSE,1; 2020,DecSE,1; 2020,NovSE,1; 2019,Jun,11; 2018,Jan,8; 2017,Jan,8; 2016,Oct,6; 2016,Jan,13

90654 Influenza virus vaccine, trivalent (IIV3), split virus, preservative-free, for intradermal use

INCLUDES Fluzone intradermal
0.00 0.00 FUD XXX
AMA: 2020,DecSE,1; 2020,DecSE,1; 2020,NovSE,1; 2018,Jan,8; 2017,Jan,8; 2016,Jan,13

90630 Influenza virus vaccine, quadrivalent (IIV4), split virus, preservative free, for intradermal use

INCLUDES Fluzone Intradermal Quadrivalent
0.00 0.00 FUD XXX
AMA: 2020,DecSE,1; 2020,DecSE,1; 2020,NovSE,1; 2018,Jan,8; 2017,Jan,8; 2016,Jan,13

90655 Influenza virus vaccine, trivalent (IIV3), split virus, preservative free, 0.25 mL dosage, for intramuscular use

INCLUDES Afluria
Fluzone, no preservative, pediatric dose
0.00 0.00 FUD XXX
AMA: 2020,DecSE,1; 2020,DecSE,1; 2020,NovSE,1; 2018,Jan,8; 2017,Jan,8; 2016,Oct,6; 2016,May,9; 2016,Jan,13

90656 Influenza virus vaccine, trivalent (IIV3), split virus, preservative free, 0.5 mL dosage, for intramuscular use

INCLUDES Afluria
0.00 0.00 FUD XXX
AMA: 2020,DecSE,1; 2020,DecSE,1; 2020,NovSE,1; 2018,Jan,8; 2017,Jan,8; 2016,Oct,6; 2016,May,9; 2016,Jan,13

90657 Influenza virus vaccine, trivalent (IIV3), split virus, 0.25 mL dosage, for intramuscular use

INCLUDES Afluria
Flulaval
Fluvirin
Fluzone (5 ml vial [0.25ml dose])
0.00 0.00 FUD XXX
AMA: 2020,DecSE,1; 2020,DecSE,1; 2020,NovSE,1; 2018,Jan,8; 2017,Jan,8; 2016,Oct,6; 2016,May,9; 2016,Jan,13

90658 Influenza virus vaccine, trivalent (IIV3), split virus, 0.5 mL dosage, for intramuscular use

INCLUDES Afluria
Flulaval
Fluvirin
Fluzone
0.00 0.00 FUD XXX
AMA: 2020,DecSE,1; 2020,DecSE,1; 2020,NovSE,1; 2018,Jan,8; 2017,Jan,8; 2016,Oct,6; 2016,May,9; 2016,Jan,13

90660 Influenza virus vaccine, trivalent, live (LAIV3), for intranasal use

INCLUDES FluMist
0.00 0.00 FUD XXX
AMA: 2020,DecSE,1; 2020,DecSE,1; 2020,NovSE,1; 2018,Jan,8; 2017,Jan,8; 2016,Jan,13

90672 Influenza virus vaccine, quadrivalent, live (LAIV4), for intranasal use

INCLUDES FluMist Quadrivalent
0.00 0.00 FUD XXX
AMA: 2020,DecSE,1; 2020,DecSE,1; 2020,NovSE,1; 2018,Jan,8; 2017,Jan,8; 2016,Jan,13

90661 Influenza virus vaccine (ccIIV3), derived from cell cultures, subunit, preservative and antibiotic free, for intramuscular use

INCLUDES Flucelvax
0.00 0.00 FUD XXX
AMA: 2020,DecSE,1; 2020,DecSE,1; 2020,NovSE,1; 2018,Jan,8; 2017,Jan,8; 2016,Oct,6; 2016,Jan,13

90674 Influenza virus vaccine, quadrivalent (ccIIV4), derived from cell cultures, subunit, preservative and antibiotic free, 0.5 mL dosage, for intramuscular use

INCLUDES Flucelvax Quadrivalent
0.00 0.00 FUD XXX
AMA: 2020,DecSE,1; 2020,DecSE,1; 2020,NovSE,1; 2018,Jan,8; 2017,Jan,8; 2016,Oct,6

90756 Influenza virus vaccine, quadrivalent (ccIIV4), derived from cell cultures, subunit, antibiotic free, 0.5mL dosage, for intramuscular use

INCLUDES Flucelvax Quadrivalent
0.00 0.00 FUD XXX
AMA: 2018,Nov,7

90673 Influenza virus vaccine, trivalent (RIV3), derived from recombinant DNA, hemagglutinin (HA) protein only, preservative and antibiotic free, for intramuscular use

0.00 0.00 FUD XXX
AMA: 2020,DecSE,1; 2020,DecSE,1; 2020,NovSE,1; 2018,Jan,8; 2017,Jan,8; 2016,Jan,13

90662 Influenza virus vaccine (IIV), split virus, preservative free, enhanced immunogenicity via increased antigen content, for intramuscular use

INCLUDES Fluzone high-dose Quadrivalent
0.00 0.00 FUD XXX
AMA: 2020,DecSE,1; 2020,DecSE,1; 2020,NovSE,1; 2018,Jan,8; 2017,Jan,8; 2016,Jan,13

90664 Influenza virus vaccine, live (LAIV), pandemic formulation, for intranasal use

0.00 0.00 FUD XXX
AMA: 2020,DecSE,1; 2020,DecSE,1; 2020,NovSE,1; 2018,Jan,8; 2017,Jan,8; 2016,Jan,13

90666 **Influenza virus vaccine (IIV), pandemic formulation, split virus, preservative free, for intramuscular use**

0.00 0.00 FUD XXX

AMA: 2020,DecSE,1; 2020,DecSE,1; 2020,NovSE,1; 2018,Jan,8; 2017,Jan,8; 2016,Jan,13

90667 **Influenza virus vaccine (IIV), pandemic formulation, split virus, adjuvanted, for intramuscular use**

0.00 0.00 FUD XXX

AMA: 2020,DecSE,1; 2020,DecSE,1; 2020,NovSE,1; 2018,Jan,8; 2017,Jan,8; 2016,Jan,13

90668 **Influenza virus vaccine (IIV), pandemic formulation, split virus, for intramuscular use**

0.00 0.00 FUD XXX

AMA: 2020,DecSE,1; 2020,DecSE,1; 2020,NovSE,1; 2018,Jan,8; 2017,Jan,8; 2016,Jan,13

90670 **Pneumococcal conjugate vaccine, 13 valent (PCV13), for intramuscular use**

INCLUDES Prevnar 13

0.00 0.00 FUD XXX

AMA: 2020,DecSE,1; 2020,DecSE,1; 2020,NovSE,1; 2018,Jan,8; 2017,Jan,8; 2016,Jan,13

● **90671** **Pneumococcal conjugate vaccine, 15 valent (PCV15), for intramuscular use**

0.00 0.00 FUD XXX

● # **90677** **Pneumococcal conjugate vaccine, 20 valent (PCV20), for intramuscular use**

0.00 0.00 FUD XXX

90672 **Resequenced code. See code following 90660.**

90673 **Resequenced code. See code before 90662.**

90674 **Resequenced code. See code following 90661.**

90675 **Rabies vaccine, for intramuscular use**

INCLUDES Imovax

RabAvert

0.00 0.00 FUD XXX

AMA: 2020,DecSE,1; 2020,DecSE,1; 2020,NovSE,1; 2018,Jan,8; 2017,Jan,8; 2016,Jan,13

90676 **Rabies vaccine, for intradermal use**

0.00 0.00 FUD XXX

AMA: 2020,DecSE,1; 2020,DecSE,1; 2020,NovSE,1; 2018,Jan,8; 2017,Jan,8; 2016,Jan,13

90677 **Resequenced code. See code following 90671.**

90680 **Rotavirus vaccine, pentavalent (RV5), 3 dose schedule, live, for oral use**

INCLUDES RotaTeq

0.00 0.00 FUD XXX

AMA: 2020,DecSE,1; 2020,DecSE,1; 2020,NovSE,1; 2018,Jan,8; 2017,Jan,8; 2016,Jan,13

90681 **Rotavirus vaccine, human, attenuated (RV1), 2 dose schedule, live, for oral use**

INCLUDES Rotarix

0.00 0.00 FUD XXX

AMA: 2020,DecSE,1; 2020,DecSE,1; 2020,NovSE,1; 2018,Jan,8; 2017,Jan,8; 2016,Jan,13

90682 **Influenza virus vaccine, quadrivalent (RIV4), derived from recombinant DNA, hemagglutinin (HA) protein only, preservative and antibiotic free, for intramuscular use**

INCLUDES Flublok Quadrivalent

0.00 0.00 FUD XXX

AMA: 2020,DecSE,1; 2020,DecSE,1; 2020,NovSE,1; 2018,Nov,7; 2018,Jan,8; 2017,Jan,8

90685 **Influenza virus vaccine, quadrivalent (IIV4), split virus, preservative free, 0.25 mL, for intramuscular use** A

INCLUDES Afluria Quadrivalent

0.00 0.00 FUD XXX

AMA: 2020,DecSE,1; 2020,DecSE,1; 2020,NovSE,1; 2018,Jan,8; 2017,Jan,8; 2016,Oct,6; 2016,May,9; 2016,Jan,13

90686 **Influenza virus vaccine, quadrivalent (IIV4), split virus, preservative free, 0.5 mL dosage, for intramuscular use** A

INCLUDES Afluria Quadrivalent

Fluarix Quadrivalent

Flulaval Quadrivalent

Fluzone Quadrivalent

0.00 0.00 FUD XXX

AMA: 2020,DecSE,1; 2020,DecSE,1; 2020,NovSE,1; 2018,Jan,8; 2017,Jan,8; 2016,Oct,6; 2016,May,9; 2016,Jan,13

90687 **Influenza virus vaccine, quadrivalent (IIV4), split virus, 0.25 mL dosage, for intramuscular use** A

INCLUDES Afluria Quadrivalent

Fluzone Quadrivalent

0.00 0.00 FUD XXX

AMA: 2020,DecSE,1; 2020,DecSE,1; 2020,NovSE,1; 2018,Jan,8; 2017,Jan,8; 2016,Oct,6; 2016,May,9; 2016,Jan,13

90688 **Influenza virus vaccine, quadrivalent (IIV4), split virus, 0.5 mL dosage, for intramuscular use** A

INCLUDES Afluria Quadrivalent

Fluzone Quadrivalent

0.00 0.00 FUD XXX

AMA: 2020,DecSE,1; 2020,DecSE,1; 2020,NovSE,1; 2020,Jul,11; 2018,Jan,8; 2017,Jan,8; 2016,Oct,6; 2016,May,9; 2016,Jan,13

90689 **Influenza virus vaccine quadrivalent (IIV4), inactivated, adjuvanted, preservative free, 0.25 mL dosage, for intramuscular use**

0.00 0.00 FUD XXX

AMA: 2020,DecSE,1; 2020,DecSE,1; 2020,NovSE,1; 2020,Jul,11; 2019,Jul,10; 2018,Nov,7

90694 **Influenza virus vaccine, quadrivalent (aIIV4), inactivated, adjuvanted, preservative free, 0.5 mL dosage, for intramuscular use**

INCLUDES Fluad Quadrivalent

0.00 0.00 FUD XXX

AMA: 2020,DecSE,1; 2020,DecSE,1; 2020,NovSE,1; 2020,Jul,11

90690 **Typhoid vaccine, live, oral**

INCLUDES Vivotif

0.00 0.00 FUD XXX

AMA: 2020,DecSE,1; 2020,DecSE,1; 2020,NovSE,1; 2020,Jul,11; 2018,Jan,8; 2017,Jan,8; 2016,Jan,13

90691 **Typhoid vaccine, Vi capsular polysaccharide (ViCPs), for intramuscular use**

INCLUDES Typhim Vi

0.00 0.00 FUD XXX

AMA: 2020,DecSE,1; 2020,DecSE,1; 2020,NovSE,1; 2020,Jul,11; 2018,Jan,8; 2017,Jan,8; 2016,Jan,13

90694 **Resequenced code. See code following 90689.**

90696 **Diphtheria, tetanus toxoids, acellular pertussis vaccine and inactivated poliovirus vaccine (DTaP-IPV), when administered to children 4 through 6 years of age, for intramuscular use** A

INCLUDES KINRIX

Quadracel

0.00 0.00 FUD XXX

AMA: 2020,DecSE,1; 2020,DecSE,1; 2020,NovSE,1; 2018,Jan,8; 2017,Jan,8; 2016,Jan,13

90697 **Diphtheria, tetanus toxoids, acellular pertussis vaccine, inactivated poliovirus vaccine, Haemophilus influenzae type b PRP-OMP conjugate vaccine, and hepatitis B vaccine (DTaP-IPV-Hib-HepB), for intramuscular use**

0.00 0.00 FUD XXX

AMA: 2020,DecSE,1; 2020,DecSE,1; 2020,NovSE,1; 2018,Jan,8; 2017,Jan,8; 2016,Jan,13

90698 Diphtheria, tetanus toxoids, acellular pertussis vaccine, Haemophilus influenzae type b, and inactivated poliovirus vaccine, (DTaP-IPV/Hib), for intramuscular use

INCLUDES Pentacel

0.00 0.00 FUD XXX

AMA: 2020,DecSE,1; 2020,DecSE,1; 2020,NovSE,1; 2018,Jan,8; 2017,Jan,8; 2016,Jan,13

90700 Diphtheria, tetanus toxoids, and acellular pertussis vaccine (DTaP), when administered to individuals younger than 7 years, for intramuscular use

INCLUDES Daptacel
Infanrix

0.00 0.00 FUD XXX

AMA: 2020,DecSE,1; 2020,DecSE,1; 2020,NovSE,1; 2018,Jan,8; 2017,Jan,8; 2016,Jan,13

90702 Diphtheria and tetanus toxoids adsorbed (DT) when administered to individuals younger than 7 years, for intramuscular use

INCLUDES Diphtheria and Tetanus Toxoids Adsorbed USP (For Pediatric Use)

0.00 0.00 FUD XXX

AMA: 2020,DecSE,1; 2020,DecSE,1; 2020,NovSE,1; 2018,Jan,8; 2017,Jan,8; 2016,Jan,13

90707 Measles, mumps and rubella virus vaccine (MMR), live, for subcutaneous use

INCLUDES M-M-R II

0.00 0.00 FUD XXX

AMA: 2020,DecSE,1; 2020,DecSE,1; 2020,NovSE,1; 2018,Jan,8; 2017,Jan,8; 2016,Jan,13

90710 Measles, mumps, rubella, and varicella vaccine (MMRV), live, for subcutaneous use

INCLUDES ProQuad

0.00 0.00 FUD XXX

AMA: 2020,DecSE,1; 2020,DecSE,1; 2020,NovSE,1; 2018,Jan,8; 2017,Jan,8; 2016,Jan,13

90713 Poliovirus vaccine, inactivated (IPV), for subcutaneous or intramuscular use

INCLUDES IPOL

0.00 0.00 FUD XXX

AMA: 2020,DecSE,1; 2020,DecSE,1; 2020,NovSE,1; 2018,Jan,8; 2017,Jan,8; 2016,Jan,13

90714 Tetanus and diphtheria toxoids adsorbed (Td), preservative free, when administered to individuals 7 years or older, for intramuscular use

INCLUDES Tenivac
Tetanus-diphtheria toxoids absorbed

0.00 0.00 FUD XXX

AMA: 2020,DecSE,1; 2020,DecSE,1; 2020,NovSE,1; 2018,Jan,8; 2017,Jan,8; 2016,Jan,13

90715 Tetanus, diphtheria toxoids and acellular pertussis vaccine (Tdap), when administered to individuals 7 years or older, for intramuscular use

INCLUDES Adacel
Boostrix

0.00 0.00 FUD XXX

AMA: 2020,DecSE,1; 2020,DecSE,1; 2020,NovSE,1; 2018,Jan,8; 2017,Jan,8; 2016,Jan,13

● # **90626 Tick-borne encephalitis virus vaccine, inactivated; 0.25 mL dosage, for intramuscular use**

INCLUDES TicoVac Junior®

0.00 0.00 FUD XXX

● # **90627 0.5 mL dosage, for intramuscular use**

INCLUDES TicoVac®

0.00 0.00 FUD XXX

90716 Varicella virus vaccine (VAR), live, for subcutaneous use

INCLUDES Varivax

0.00 0.00 FUD XXX

AMA: 2020,DecSE,1; 2020,DecSE,1; 2020,NovSE,1; 2018,Jan,8; 2017,Jan,8; 2016,Jan,13

90717 Yellow fever vaccine, live, for subcutaneous use

INCLUDES YF-VAX

0.00 0.00 FUD XXX

AMA: 2020,DecSE,1; 2020,DecSE,1; 2020,NovSE,1; 2018,Jan,8; 2017,Jan,8; 2016,Jan,13

90723 Diphtheria, tetanus toxoids, acellular pertussis vaccine, hepatitis B, and inactivated poliovirus vaccine (DTaP-HepB-IPV), for intramuscular use

INCLUDES PEDIARIX

0.00 0.00 FUD XXX

AMA: 2020,DecSE,1; 2020,DecSE,1; 2020,NovSE,1; 2018,Jan,8; 2017,Jan,8; 2016,Jan,13

90625 Cholera vaccine, live, adult dosage, 1 dose schedule, for oral use

0.00 0.00 FUD XXX

AMA: 2020,DecSE,1; 2020,DecSE,1; 2020,NovSE,1; 2018,Jan,8; 2017,Jan,8; 2016,Oct,6; 2016,Jan,13

90732 Pneumococcal polysaccharide vaccine, 23-valent (PPSV23), adult or immunosuppressed patient dosage, when administered to individuals 2 years or older, for subcutaneous or intramuscular use

INCLUDES Pneumovax 23

0.00 0.00 FUD XXX

AMA: 2020,DecSE,1; 2020,DecSE,1; 2020,NovSE,1; 2018,Jan,8; 2017,Jan,8; 2016,Jan,13

90644 Meningococcal conjugate vaccine, serogroups C & Y and Haemophilus influenzae type b vaccine (Hib-MenCY), 4 dose schedule, when administered to children 6 weeks-18 months of age, for intramuscular use

INCLUDES MenHibrix

0.00 0.00 FUD XXX

AMA: 2020,DecSE,1; 2020,DecSE,1; 2020,NovSE,1; 2018,Jan,8; 2017,Jan,8; 2016,Jan,13

90733 Meningococcal polysaccharide vaccine, serogroups A, C, Y, W-135, quadrivalent (MPSV4), for subcutaneous use

INCLUDES Menomune-A/C/Y/W-135

0.00 0.00 FUD XXX

AMA: 2020,DecSE,1; 2020,DecSE,1; 2020,NovSE,1; 2018,Jan,8; 2017,Jan,8; 2016,Jan,13

90734 Meningococcal conjugate vaccine, serogroups A, C, W, Y, quadrivalent, diphtheria toxoid carrier (MenACWY-D) or CRM197 carrier (MenACWY-CRM), for intramuscular use

INCLUDES Menactra
Menveo

0.00 0.00 FUD XXX

AMA: 2020,DecSE,1; 2020,DecSE,1; 2020,NovSE,1; 2020,Jan,11; 2018,Jan,8; 2017,Jan,8; 2016,Oct,6; 2016,Jan,13

90619 Meningococcal conjugate vaccine, serogroups A, C, W, Y, quadrivalent, tetanus toxoid carrier (MenACWY-TT), for intramuscular use

0.00 0.00 FUD XXX

AMA: 2020,DecSE,1; 2020,DecSE,1; 2020,NovSE,1; 2020,Jan,11

90620 Meningococcal recombinant protein and outer membrane vesicle vaccine, serogroup B (MenB-4C), 2 dose schedule, for intramuscular use

INCLUDES Bexsero

0.00 0.00 FUD XXX

AMA: 2020,DecSE,1; 2020,DecSE,1; 2020,NovSE,1; 2018,Nov,7; 2018,Jan,8; 2017,Jan,8; 2016,Jan,13

\# **90621 Meningococcal recombinant lipoprotein vaccine, serogroup B (MenB-FHbp), 2 or 3 dose schedule, for intramuscular use**

INCLUDES Trumenba

0.00 0.00 FUD XXX

AMA: 2020,DecSE,1; 2020,DecSE,1; 2020,NovSE,1; 2018,Nov,7; 2018,Jan,8; 2017,Jan,8; 2016,Jan,13

90736 Zoster (shingles) vaccine (HZV), live, for subcutaneous injection

INCLUDES Zostavax

0.00 0.00 FUD XXX

AMA: 2020,DecSE,1; 2020,DecSE,1; 2020,NovSE,1; 2018,Nov,7; 2018,Jan,8; 2017,Jan,8; 2016,Jan,13

\# **90750 Zoster (shingles) vaccine (HZV), recombinant, subunit, adjuvanted, for intramuscular use**

0.00 0.00 FUD XXX

AMA: 2018,Nov,7

90738 Japanese encephalitis virus vaccine, inactivated, for intramuscular use

INCLUDES Ixiaro

0.00 0.00 FUD XXX

AMA: 2020,DecSE,1; 2020,DecSE,1; 2020,NovSE,1; 2018,Jan,8; 2017,Jan,8; 2016,Jan,13

90739 Hepatitis B vaccine (HepB), adult dosage, 2 dose schedule, for intramuscular use

0.00 0.00 FUD XXX

AMA: 2020,DecSE,1; 2020,DecSE,1; 2020,NovSE,1; 2018,Nov,7; 2018,Jan,8; 2017,Jan,8; 2016,Jan,13

90740 Hepatitis B vaccine (HepB), dialysis or immunosuppressed patient dosage, 3 dose schedule, for intramuscular use

INCLUDES Recombivax HB

0.00 0.00 FUD XXX

AMA: 2020,DecSE,1; 2020,DecSE,1; 2020,NovSE,1; 2018,Jan,8; 2017,Jan,8; 2016,Jan,13

90743 Hepatitis B vaccine (HepB), adolescent, 2 dose schedule, for intramuscular use

INCLUDES Energix-B
Recombivax HB

0.00 0.00 FUD XXX

AMA: 2020,DecSE,1; 2020,DecSE,1; 2020,NovSE,1; 2018,Jan,8; 2017,Jan,8; 2016,Jan,13

90744 Hepatitis B vaccine (HepB), pediatric/adolescent dosage, 3 dose schedule, for intramuscular use

INCLUDES Energix-B
Flucelvax Quadrivalent
Recombivax HB

0.00 0.00 FUD XXX

AMA: 2020,DecSE,1; 2020,DecSE,1; 2020,NovSE,1; 2018,Jan,8; 2017,Jan,8; 2016,Jan,13

90746 Hepatitis B vaccine (HepB), adult dosage, 3 dose schedule, for intramuscular use

INCLUDES Energix-B
Recombivax HB

0.00 0.00 FUD XXX

AMA: 2020,DecSE,1; 2020,DecSE,1; 2020,NovSE,1; 2018,Jan,8; 2017,Jan,8; 2016,Jan,13

● # **90759 Hepatitis B vaccine (HepB), 3-antigen (S, Pre-S1, Pre-S2), 10 mcg dosage, 3 dose schedule, for intramuscular use**

0.00 0.00 FUD 000

90747 Hepatitis B vaccine (HepB), dialysis or immunosuppressed patient dosage, 4 dose schedule, for intramuscular use

INCLUDES Energix-B
RECOMBIVAX dialysis

0.00 0.00 FUD XXX

AMA: 2020,DecSE,1; 2020,DecSE,1; 2020,NovSE,1; 2018,Jan,8; 2017,Jan,8; 2016,Jan,13

90748 Hepatitis B and Haemophilus influenzae type b vaccine (Hib-HepB), for intramuscular use

INCLUDES COMVAX

0.00 0.00 FUD XXX

AMA: 2020,DecSE,1; 2020,DecSE,1; 2020,NovSE,1; 2018,Jan,8; 2017,Jan,8; 2016,Jan,13

● # **90758 Zaire ebolavirus vaccine, live, for intramuscular use**

INCLUDES Ervebo®

0.00 0.00 FUD XXX

90749 Unlisted vaccine/toxoid

0.00 0.00 FUD XXX

AMA: 2020,DecSE,1; 2020,DecSE,1; 2020,NovSE,1; 2018,Jan,8; 2017,Jan,8; 2016,Jan,13

***90750* Resequenced code. See code following 90736.**

***90756* Resequenced code. See code following 90661.**

***90758* Resequenced code. See code following 90748.**

***90759* Resequenced code. See code following 90746.**

90785 Complex Interactive Encounter

CMS: 100-02,15,160 Clinical Psychologist Services; 100-02,15,170 Clinical Social Worker (CSW) Services; 100-03,10.3 Inpatient Pain Rehabilitation Programs; 100-03,10.4 Outpatient Hospital Pain Rehabilitation Programs; 100-03,130.1 Inpatient Stays for Alcoholism Treatment; 100-04,12,100 Teaching Physician Services; 100-04,4,260.1 Special Partial Hospitalization Billing Requirements forHospitals, Community Mental Health Centers, and Critical Access Hospitals; 100-04,4,260.1.1 Bill Review for Partial Hospitalization Services Provided in Community Mental Health Centers (CMHC)

INCLUDES Complicated communication issues affecting psychiatric service
Involved communication with:
- Emotionally charged or dissonant family members
- Patients wanting others present during visit (e.g., family member, translator)
- Patients with impaired or undeveloped verbal skills
- Patients with third parties responsible for their care (e.g., parents, guardians)
- Third-party involvement (e.g., schools, probation and parole officers, child protective agencies)

One or more following activity:
- Discussion sentinel event demanding third-party involvement (i.e., abuse or neglect reported to state agency)
- Interference by caregiver's behavior or emotional state to understand and assist in treatment plan
- Managing discordant communication complicating care among participating members (e.g., arguing, reactivity)
- Nonverbal communication methods (e.g., toys, other devices, or translator) to eliminate communication barriers

EXCLUDES *Adaptive behavior assessment/treatment ([97151, 97152, 97153, 97154, 97155, 97156, 97157, 97158], 0362T, 0373T)*
Crisis psychotherapy (90839-90840)
Psychological or neuropsychological test administration (96136-96139, 96146)
Psychological testing evaluation services (96130-96133)

\+ **90785 Interactive complexity (List separately in addition to the code for primary procedure)**

Code first, when performed (90791-90792, 90832-90834, 90836-90838, 90853)

0.39 0.42 FUD ZZZ ★

AMA: 2020,Aug,3; 2018,Nov,3; 2018,Jul,12; 2018,Apr,9; 2018,Jan,8; 2017,Jan,8; 2016,Dec,11; 2016,Jan,13

90791-90792 Psychiatric Evaluations

CMS: 100-02,15,170 Clinical Social Worker (CSW) Services; 100-03,10.3 Inpatient Pain Rehabilitation Programs; 100-03,130.1 Inpatient Stays for Alcoholism Treatment; 100-03,130.2 Outpatient Hospital Services for Alcoholism; 100-04,12,100 Teaching Physician Services; 100-04,12,190.3 List of Telehealth Services; 100-04,12,190.6 Payment Methodology for Physician/Practitioner at the Distant Site ; 100-04,12,190.6.1 Submission of Telehealth Claims for Distant Site Practitioners; 100-04,12,190.7 Contractor Editing of Telehealth Claims; 100-04,4,260.1 Special Partial Hospitalization Billing Requirements forHospitals, Community Mental Health Centers, and Critical Access Hospitals; 100-04,4,260.1.1 Bill Review for Partial Hospitalization Services Provided in Community Mental Health Centers (CMHC)

INCLUDES Diagnostic assessment or reassessment without psychotherapy services

EXCLUDES *Adaptive behavior assessment/treatment ([97151, 97152, 97153, 97154, 97155, 97156, 97157, 97158], 0362T, 0373T)*
Crisis psychotherapy (90839-90840)
E/M services (99202-99337 [99224, 99225, 99226], 99341-99350, 99366-99368, 99401-99443 [99415, 99416, 99417, 99421, 99422, 99423, 99439])

Code also interactive complexity services when applicable (90785)

90791 Psychiatric diagnostic evaluation
3.54 3.89 FUD XXX ★ 03
AMA: 2020,Oct,14; 2020,Aug,3; 2018,Nov,3; 2018,Jul,12; 2018,Apr,9; 2018,Jan,8; 2017,Nov,3; 2017,Jan,8; 2016,Jan,13

90792 Psychiatric diagnostic evaluation with medical services
4.01 4.37 FUD XXX ★ 03
AMA: 2020,Oct,14; 2020,Aug,3; 2019,Dec,14; 2018,Nov,3; 2018,Jul,12; 2018,Apr,9; 2018,Jan,8; 2017,Nov,3; 2017,Jan,8; 2016,Jan,13

90832-90838 Psychotherapy Services

CMS: 100-02,15,160 Clinical Psychologist Services; 100-02,15,170 Clinical Social Worker (CSW) Services; 100-03,130.1 Inpatient Stays for Alcoholism Treatment; 100-03,130.2 Outpatient Hospital Services for Alcoholism; 100-03,130.3 Chemical Aversion Therapy for Treatment of Alcoholism; 100-04,12,100 Teaching Physician Services; 100-04,12,160 Independent Psychologist Services; 100-04,12,170 Clinical Psychologist Services; 100-04,12,190.3 List of Telehealth Services; 100-04,12,190.6 Payment Methodology for Physician/Practitioner at the Distant Site ; 100-04,12,190.6.1 Submission of Telehealth Claims for Distant Site Practitioners; 100-04,12,190.7 Contractor Editing of Telehealth Claims

INCLUDES Face-to-face time with patient (family, other informers may also be present)
Pharmacologic management in time allocated to psychotherapy service codes
Psychotherapy only (90832, 90834, 90837)
Psychotherapy with separately identifiable medical E/M services includes add-on codes (90833, 90836, 90838)
Service times no less than 16 minutes
Services provided in all settings
Therapeutic communication to:
- Ameliorate patient's mental and behavioral symptoms
- Modify behavior
- Support and encourage personality growth and development

Treatment for:
- Behavior disturbances
- Mental illness

EXCLUDES *Adaptive behavior assessment/treatment ([97151, 97152, 97153, 97154, 97155, 97156, 97157, 97158], 0362T, 0373T)*
Crisis psychotherapy (90839-90840)
Family psychotherapy (90846-90847)

Code also interactive complexity services with time provider spends performing service reflected in time for appropriate psychotherapy code (90785)

90832 Psychotherapy, 30 minutes with patient
1.76 1.90 FUD XXX ★ 03
AMA: 2020,Dec,13; 2020,Aug,3; 2018,Nov,3; 2018,Jul,12; 2018,Jan,8; 2017,Nov,3; 2017,Sep,11; 2017,Jan,8; 2016,Dec,11; 2016,Jan,13

\+ **90833 Psychotherapy, 30 minutes with patient when performed with an evaluation and management service (List separately in addition to the code for primary procedure)**
Code first (99202-99255 [99224, 99225, 99226], 99304-99337, 99341-99350)
1.84 1.97 FUD ZZZ ★ N
AMA: 2020,Dec,13; 2020,Aug,3; 2018,Nov,3; 2018,Jul,12; 2018,Jan,8; 2017,Nov,3; 2017,Jan,8; 2016,Dec,11; 2016,Jan,13

90834 Psychotherapy, 45 minutes with patient
2.35 2.53 FUD XXX ★ 03
AMA: 2020,Dec,13; 2020,Aug,3; 2018,Nov,3; 2018,Jul,12; 2018,Jan,8; 2017,Nov,3; 2017,Jan,8; 2016,Dec,11; 2016,Jan,13

\+ **90836 Psychotherapy, 45 minutes with patient when performed with an evaluation and management service (List separately in addition to the code for primary procedure)**
Code first (99202-99255 [99224, 99225, 99226], 99304-99337, 99341-99350)
2.33 2.49 FUD ZZZ ★ N
AMA: 2020,Dec,13; 2020,Aug,3; 2018,Nov,3; 2018,Jul,12; 2018,Jan,8; 2017,Nov,3; 2017,Jan,8; 2016,Dec,11; 2016,Jan,13

90837 Psychotherapy, 60 minutes with patient
Code also prolonged service for psychotherapy performed without E/M service face-to-face with patient lasting 90 minutes or longer (99354-99357)
3.53 3.80 FUD XXX ★ 03
AMA: 2020,Dec,13; 2020,Sep,3; 2020,Aug,3; 2018,Nov,3; 2018,Jul,12; 2018,Jan,8; 2017,Nov,3; 2017,Jan,8; 2016,Dec,11; 2016,Jan,13

\+ **90838 Psychotherapy, 60 minutes with patient when performed with an evaluation and management service (List separately in addition to the code for primary procedure)**
Code first (99202-99255 [99224, 99225, 99226], 99304-99337, 99341-99350)
3.08 3.29 FUD ZZZ ★ N
AMA: 2020,Dec,13; 2020,Aug,3; 2018,Nov,3; 2018,Jul,12; 2018,Jan,8; 2017,Nov,3; 2017,Jan,8; 2016,Dec,11; 2016,Jan,13

90839-90840 Services for Patients in Crisis

CMS: 100-02,15,170 Clinical Social Worker (CSW) Services; 100-03,130.1 Inpatient Stays for Alcoholism Treatment; 100-03,130.3 Chemical Aversion Therapy for Treatment of Alcoholism; 100-04,12,100 Teaching Physician Services; 100-04,12,160 Independent Psychologist Services; 100-04,12,160.1 Payment of Independent Psychologist Services; 100-04,12,170 Clinical Psychologist Services

INCLUDES 30 minutes or more face-to-face time with patient (for all or part service) and/or family providing crisis psychotherapy
All time spent exclusively with patient (for all or part service) and/or family, even if time not continuous
Emergent care to patient in severe distress (e.g., life threatening or complex)
Institute interventions to minimize psychological trauma
Measures to ease crisis and reestablish safety
Psychotherapy

EXCLUDES *Adaptive behavior assessment/treatment ([97151, 97152, 97153, 97154, 97155, 97156, 97157, 97158], 0362T, 0373T)*
Other psychiatric services (90785-90899)

90839 Psychotherapy for crisis; first 60 minutes
INCLUDES First 30-74 minutes crisis psychotherapy per day
EXCLUDES *Reporting code more than one time per day, even when service not continuous on that date*
3.69 3.96 FUD XXX ★ 03 80
AMA: 2020,Aug,3; 2018,Nov,3; 2018,Jul,12; 2018,Jan,8; 2017,Nov,3; 2017,Jan,8; 2016,Jan,13

\+ **90840 each additional 30 minutes (List separately in addition to code for primary service)**
INCLUDES Up to 30 minutes time beyond initial 74 minutes
Code first (90839)
1.76 1.90 FUD ZZZ ★ N 80
AMA: 2020,Aug,3; 2018,Nov,3; 2018,Jul,12; 2018,Jan,8; 2017,Nov,3; 2017,Jan,8; 2016,Jan,13

90845-90863 Additional Psychotherapy Services

CMS: 100-02,15,170 Clinical Social Worker (CSW) Services; 100-03,10.3 Inpatient Pain Rehabilitation Programs; 100-03,10.4 Outpatient Hospital Pain Rehabilitation Programs

EXCLUDES *Adaptive behavior assessment/treatment ([97151, 97152, 97153, 97154, 97155, 97156, 97157, 97158], 0362T, 0373T)*
Analysis/programming neurostimulators for vagus nerve stimulation therapy (95970, 95976-95977)
Crisis psychotherapy (90839-90840)

90845 Psychoanalysis
2.52 2.70 FUD XXX ★ 03 80
AMA: 2020,Aug,3; 2018,Nov,3; 2018,Jul,12; 2018,Jan,8; 2017,Jan,8; 2016,Jan,13

90846 **Family psychotherapy (without the patient present), 50 minutes**

EXCLUDES *Service times less than 26 minutes*

2.85 3.06 FUD XXX ★ Q3 80

AMA: 2020,Aug,3; 2018,Nov,3; 2018,Jul,12; 2018,Jan,8; 2017,Nov,3; 2017,Mar,10; 2017,Jan,8; 2016,Dec,11; 2016,Jan,13

90847 **Family psychotherapy (conjoint psychotherapy) (with patient present), 50 minutes**

EXCLUDES *Service times less than 26 minutes*

Service times more than 80 minutes, see prolonged services (99354-99357)

2.96 3.18 FUD XXX ★ Q3 80

AMA: 2020,Sep,3; 2020,Aug,3; 2018,Nov,3; 2018,Jul,12; 2018,Jan,8; 2017,Nov,3; 2017,Jan,8; 2016,Dec,11; 2016,Jan,13

90849 **Multiple-family group psychotherapy**

0.87 1.17 FUD XXX Q3 80

AMA: 2020,Aug,3; 2018,Nov,3; 2018,Jul,12; 2018,Jan,8; 2017,Nov,3; 2017,Jan,8; 2016,Jan,13

90853 **Group psychotherapy (other than of a multiple-family group)**

Code also group psychotherapy with interactive complexity (90785)

0.70 0.76 FUD XXX Q3 80

AMA: 2020,Aug,3; 2018,Nov,3; 2018,Jul,12; 2018,Jan,8; 2017,Nov,3; 2017,Mar,10; 2017,Jan,8; 2016,Jan,13

+ **90863** **Pharmacologic management, including prescription and review of medication, when performed with psychotherapy services (List separately in addition to the code for primary procedure)**

INCLUDES Pharmacologic management in time allocated to psychotherapy service codes

Code first (90832, 90834, 90837)

0.70 0.74 FUD XXX ★ E

AMA: 2020,Aug,3; 2018,Nov,3; 2018,Jul,12; 2018,Jan,8; 2017,Jan,8; 2016,Jan,13

90865-90870 Other Psychiatric Treatment

EXCLUDES *Adaptive behavior assessment/treatment ([97151, 97152, 97153, 97154, 97155, 97156, 97157, 97158], 0362T, 0373T)*

Analysis/programming neurostimulators for vagus nerve stimulation therapy (95970, 95976-95977)

Crisis psychotherapy (90839-90840)

90865 **Narcosynthesis for psychiatric diagnostic and therapeutic purposes (eg, sodium amobarbital (Amytal) interview)**

3.61 4.80 FUD XXX Q3 80

AMA: 2020,Aug,3; 2018,Nov,3; 2018,Jul,12; 2018,Jan,8; 2017,Jan,8; 2016,Jan,13

90867 **Therapeutic repetitive transcranial magnetic stimulation (TMS) treatment; initial, including cortical mapping, motor threshold determination, delivery and management**

INCLUDES E/M services related directly to:
- Cortical mapping
- Delivery and management TMS services
- Motor threshold determination

EXCLUDES *Electromyography (95860, 95870)*

Evoked potential studies (95928, 95929, [95939])

Medication management

Reporting code more than one time for each treatment course

Significant, separately identifiable E/M service

Significant, separately identifiable psychotherapy service

Subsequent transcranial magnetic stimulation (TMS) treatment:
- *Delivery and management (90868)*
- *Motor threshold redetermination (90869)*

0.00 0.00 FUD 000 S

AMA: 2020,Aug,3; 2018,Nov,3; 2018,Jul,12

90868 **subsequent delivery and management, per session**

INCLUDES E/M services related directly to:
- Cortical mapping
- Delivery and management TMS services
- Motor threshold determination

EXCLUDES *Medication management*

Significant, separately identifiable E/M service

Significant, separately identifiable psychotherapy service

0.00 0.00 FUD 000 S

AMA: 2020,Aug,3; 2018,Nov,3; 2018,Jul,12

90869 **subsequent motor threshold re-determination with delivery and management**

INCLUDES E/M services related directly to:
- Cortical mapping
- Delivery and management TMS services
- Motor threshold determination

EXCLUDES *Electromyography (95860, 95870)*

Evoked potential studies (95928-95929, [95939])

Medication management

Significant, separately identifiable E/M service

Significant, separately identifiable psychotherapy service

Transcranial magnetic stimulation (TMS) treatment:
- *Initial (90867)*
- *Subsequent delivery and managment (90868)*

0.00 0.00 FUD 000 S

AMA: 2020,Aug,3; 2018,Nov,3; 2018,Jul,12

90870 **Electroconvulsive therapy (includes necessary monitoring)**

3.11 4.99 FUD 000 S 80

AMA: 2020,Aug,3; 2018,Nov,3; 2018,Jul,12; 2018,Jan,8; 2017,Jan,8; 2016,Jan,13

90875-90880 Psychiatric Therapy with Biofeedback or Hypnosis

CMS: 100-02,15,170 Clinical Social Worker (CSW) Services; 100-04,12,160 Independent Psychologist Services; 100-04,12,160.1 Payment of Independent Psychologist Services; 100-04,12,170 Clinical Psychologist Services

EXCLUDES *Adaptive behavior assessment/treatment ([97151, 97152, 97153, 97154, 97155, 97156, 97157, 97158], 0362T, 0373T)*

Analysis/programming neurostimulators for vagus nerve stimulation therapy (95970, 95976-95977)

Crisis psychotherapy (90839-90840)

90875 **Individual psychophysiological therapy incorporating biofeedback training by any modality (face-to-face with the patient), with psychotherapy (eg, insight oriented, behavior modifying or supportive psychotherapy); 30 minutes**

1.73 1.80 FUD XXX E

AMA: 2020,Aug,3; 2018,Nov,3; 2018,Jul,12; 2018,Jan,8; 2017,Jan,8; 2016,Jan,13

90876 **45 minutes**

2.74 3.05 FUD XXX E

AMA: 2020,Aug,3; 2018,Nov,3; 2018,Jul,12; 2018,Jan,8; 2017,Jan,8; 2016,Jan,13

90880 **Hypnotherapy**

2.58 2.98 FUD XXX Q3 80

AMA: 2020,Aug,3; 2018,Nov,3; 2018,Jul,12; 2018,Jan,8; 2017,Jan,8; 2016,Jan,13

90882-90899 Psychiatric Services without Patient Face-to-Face Contact

CMS: 100-04,12,160 Independent Psychologist Services; 100-04,12,160.1 Payment of Independent Psychologist Services

EXCLUDES *Analysis/programming neurostimulators for vagus nerve stimulation therapy (95970, 95976-95977)*

Crisis psychotherapy (90839-90840)

90882 **Environmental intervention for medical management purposes on a psychiatric patient's behalf with agencies, employers, or institutions**

0.00 0.00 FUD XXX E

AMA: 2020,Aug,3; 2018,Nov,3; 2018,Jul,12; 2018,Jan,8; 2017,Jan,8; 2016,Jan,13

90885 Psychiatric evaluation of hospital records, other psychiatric reports, psychometric and/or projective tests, and other accumulated data for medical diagnostic purposes

1.41 1.41 FUD XXX N

AMA: 2020,Dec,13; 2020,Aug,3; 2018,Nov,3; 2018,Jul,12; 2018,Jan,8; 2017,Jan,8; 2016,Jan,13

90887 Interpretation or explanation of results of psychiatric, other medical examinations and procedures, or other accumulated data to family or other responsible persons, or advising them how to assist patient

EXCLUDES *Adaptive behavior assessment/treatment ([97151, 97152, 97153, 97154, 97155, 97156, 97157, 97158], 0362T, 0373T)*

2.14 2.48 FUD XXX N

AMA: 2020,Aug,3; 2018,Nov,3; 2018,Jul,12; 2018,Jan,8; 2017,Jan,8; 2016,Jan,13

90889 Preparation of report of patient's psychiatric status, history, treatment, or progress (other than for legal or consultative purposes) for other individuals, agencies, or insurance carriers

0.00 0.00 FUD XXX N

AMA: 2020,Aug,3; 2018,Nov,3; 2018,Jul,12; 2018,Jan,8; 2017,Jan,8; 2016,Jan,13

90899 Unlisted psychiatric service or procedure

0.00 0.00 FUD XXX 03 80

AMA: 2020,Aug,3; 2018,Nov,3; 2018,Jul,12; 2018,Jan,8; 2017,Jan,8; 2016,Jan,13

90901-90913 Biofeedback Therapy

EXCLUDES *Psychophysiological therapy utilizing biofeedback training (90875-90876)*

90901 Biofeedback training by any modality

0.57 1.15 FUD 000 A 80

AMA: 2020,Jun,13; 2018,Jan,8; 2017,Jan,8; 2016,Jan,13

90912 Biofeedback training, perineal muscles, anorectal or urethral sphincter, including EMG and/or manometry, when performed; initial 15 minutes of one-on-one physician or other qualified health care professional contact with the patient

EXCLUDES *Incontinence treatment using pulsed magnetic neuromodulation (53899)*

Testing rectal sensation, tone, and compliance (91120)

1.26 2.27 FUD 000 80

AMA: 2020,Jun,13

+ **90913 each additional 15 minutes of one-on-one physician or other qualified health care professional contact with the patient (List separately in addition to code for primary procedure)**

EXCLUDES *Incontinence treatment using pulsed magnetic neuromodulation (53899)*

Testing rectal sensation, tone, and compliance (91120)

Code first (90912)

0.70 0.92 FUD ZZZ 80

AMA: 2020,Jun,13

90935-90940 Hemodialysis Services: Inpatient ESRD and Outpatient Non-ESRD

CMS: 100-02,11,20 Renal Dialysis Items and Services ; 100-04,3,100.6 Inpatient Renal Services

EXCLUDES *Attendance by physician or other qualified health care provider for prolonged period of time (99354-99360 [99415, 99416])*

Blood specimen collection from partial/complete implantable venous access device (36591)

Declotting cannula (36831, 36833, 36860-36861)

Hemodialysis home visit by non-physician health care professional (99512)

Therapeutic apheresis procedures (36511-36516)

Therapeutic ultrafiltration (0692T)

Thrombolytic agent declotting implanted vascular access device/catheter (36593)

Code also significant separately identifiable E/M service not related to dialysis procedure or renal failure with modifier 25 (99202-99215, 99217-99223 [99224, 99225, 99226], 99231-99239, 99241-99245, 99281-99285, 99291-99292, 99304-99318, 99324-99337, 99341-99350, 99466-99467, 99468-99472, 99475-99480)

90935 Hemodialysis procedure with single evaluation by a physician or other qualified health care professional

INCLUDES All E/M services related to patient's renal disease rendered on day dialysis performed

Inpatient ESRD and non-ESRD procedures

Only one patient evaluation related to hemodialysis procedure

Outpatient non-ESRD dialysis

2.07 2.07 FUD 000 S 80

AMA: 2018,Jan,8; 2017,Jan,8; 2016,Jan,13

90937 Hemodialysis procedure requiring repeated evaluation(s) with or without substantial revision of dialysis prescription

INCLUDES All E/M services related to patient's renal disease rendered on day dialysis performed

Inpatient ESRD and non-ESRD procedures

Outpatient non-ESRD dialysis

Re-evaluation patient during hemodialysis procedure

2.95 2.95 FUD 000 B 80

AMA: 2018,Jan,8; 2017,Jan,8; 2016,Jan,13

90940 Hemodialysis access flow study to determine blood flow in grafts and arteriovenous fistulae by an indicator method

EXCLUDES *Hemodialysis access duplex scan (93990)*

0.00 0.00 FUD XXX N

AMA: 2018,Jan,8; 2017,Jan,8; 2016,Jan,13

90945-90947 Dialysis Techniques Other Than Hemodialysis

CMS: 100-04,12,40.3 Global Surgery Review; 100-04,3,100.6 Inpatient Renal Services

INCLUDES All E/M services related to patient's renal disease rendered on day dialysis performed

Procedures other than hemodialysis:

- Continuous renal replacement therapies
- Hemofiltration
- Peritoneal dialysis

EXCLUDES *Attendance by physician or other qualified health care provider for prolonged time period (99354-99360 [99415, 99416])*

Hemodialysis

Therapeutic ultrafiltration (0692T)

Tunneled intraperitoneal catheter insertion

Open (49421)

Percutaneous (49418)

Code also significant, separately identifiable E/M service not related to dialysis procedure or renal failure with modifier 25 (99202-99215, 99217-99223 [99224, 99225, 99226], 99231-99239, 99241-99245, 99281-99285, 99291-99292, 99304-99318, 99324-99337, 99341-99350, 99466-99467, 99468-99472, 99475-99480)

90945 Dialysis procedure other than hemodialysis (eg, peritoneal dialysis, hemofiltration, or other continuous renal replacement therapies), with single evaluation by a physician or other qualified health care professional

INCLUDES Only one patient evaluation related to procedure

EXCLUDES *Peritoneal dialysis home infusion (99601, 99602)*

2.42 2.42 FUD 000 V 80

AMA: 2018,Jan,8; 2017,Jan,8; 2016,Jan,13

90947 **Dialysis procedure other than hemodialysis (eg, peritoneal dialysis, hemofiltration, or other continuous renal replacement therapies) requiring repeated evaluations by a physician or other qualified health care professional, with or without substantial revision of dialysis prescription**

EXCLUDES *Re-evaluation during procedure*

3.51 3.51 **FUD** 000

AMA: 2018,Jan,8; 2017,Jan,8; 2016,Jan,13

90951-90962 End-stage Renal Disease Monthly Outpatient Services

CMS: 100-02,11,20 Renal Dialysis Items and Services ; 100-04,12,190.3 List of Telehealth Services; 100-04,12,190.3.4 ESRD-Related Services as a Telehealth Service; 100-04,8,140.1 ESRD-Related Services Under the Monthly Capitation Payment

INCLUDES Establishing dialyzing cycle
Management dialysis visits
Outpatient E/M dialysis visits
Patient management during dialysis for month
Telephone calls

EXCLUDES *ESRD/non-ESRD dialysis services performed in inpatient setting (90935-90937, 90945-90947)*
Non-ESRD dialysis services performed in outpatient setting (90935-90937, 90945-90947)
Non-ESRD related E/M services that cannot be performed during dialysis session
Services provided in same month with:
Chronic care management ([99437], [99439, 99490, 99491])
Complex chronic care management (99487-99489)
Principal care management services ([99424, 99425, 99426, 99427])
Therapeutic ultrafiltration (0692T)

90951 **End-stage renal disease (ESRD) related services monthly, for patients younger than 2 years of age to include monitoring for the adequacy of nutrition, assessment of growth and development, and counseling of parents; with 4 or more face-to-face visits by a physician or other qualified health care professional per month**

26.6 26.6 **FUD** XXX

AMA: 2018,Feb,11; 2018,Jan,8; 2017,Jan,8; 2016,Jan,13

90952 **with 2-3 face-to-face visits by a physician or other qualified health care professional per month**

0.00 0.00 **FUD** XXX

AMA: 2018,Feb,11; 2018,Jan,8; 2017,Jan,8; 2016,Jan,13

90953 **with 1 face-to-face visit by a physician or other qualified health care professional per month**

0.00 0.00 **FUD** XXX

AMA: 2018,Feb,11; 2018,Jan,8; 2017,Jan,8; 2016,Jan,13

90954 **End-stage renal disease (ESRD) related services monthly, for patients 2-11 years of age to include monitoring for the adequacy of nutrition, assessment of growth and development, and counseling of parents; with 4 or more face-to-face visits by a physician or other qualified health care professional per month**

23.0 23.0 **FUD** XXX

AMA: 2018,Feb,11; 2018,Jan,8; 2017,Jan,8; 2016,Jan,13

90955 **with 2-3 face-to-face visits by a physician or other qualified health care professional per month**

13.0 13.0 **FUD** XXX

AMA: 2018,Feb,11; 2018,Jan,8; 2017,Jan,8; 2016,Jan,13

90956 **with 1 face-to-face visit by a physician or other qualified health care professional per month**

9.05 9.05 **FUD** XXX

AMA: 2018,Feb,11; 2018,Jan,8; 2017,Jan,8; 2016,Jan,13

90957 **End-stage renal disease (ESRD) related services monthly, for patients 12-19 years of age to include monitoring for the adequacy of nutrition, assessment of growth and development, and counseling of parents; with 4 or more face-to-face visits by a physician or other qualified health care professional per month**

18.3 18.3 **FUD** XXX

AMA: 2018,Feb,11; 2018,Jan,8; 2017,Jan,8; 2016,Jan,13

90958 **with 2-3 face-to-face visits by a physician or other qualified health care professional per month**

12.3 12.3 **FUD** XXX

AMA: 2018,Feb,11; 2018,Jan,8; 2017,Jan,8; 2016,Jan,13

90959 **with 1 face-to-face visit by a physician or other qualified health care professional per month**

8.40 8.40 **FUD** XXX

AMA: 2018,Feb,11; 2018,Jan,8; 2017,Jan,8; 2016,Jan,13

90960 **End-stage renal disease (ESRD) related services monthly, for patients 20 years of age and older; with 4 or more face-to-face visits by a physician or other qualified health care professional per month**

8.02 8.02 **FUD** XXX

AMA: 2018,Feb,11; 2018,Jan,8; 2017,Jan,8; 2016,Jan,13

90961 **with 2-3 face-to-face visits by a physician or other qualified health care professional per month**

6.78 6.78 **FUD** XXX

AMA: 2018,Feb,11; 2018,Jan,8; 2017,Jan,8; 2016,Jan,13

90962 **with 1 face-to-face visit by a physician or other qualified health care professional per month**

5.23 5.23 **FUD** XXX

AMA: 2018,Feb,11; 2018,Jan,8; 2017,Jan,8; 2016,Jan,13

90963-90966 End-stage Renal Disease Monthly Home Dialysis Services

CMS: 100-02,11,20 Renal Dialysis Items and Services ; 100-04,12,190.3.4 ESRD-Related Services as a Telehealth Service; 100-04,8,140.1 ESRD-Related Services Under the Monthly Capitation Payment; 100-04,8,140.1.1 Payment for Managing Patients on Home Dialysis

INCLUDES ESRD services for home dialysis patients
Services provided for full month

EXCLUDES *Services provided in same month with:*
Chronic care management ([99437], [99439, 99490, 99491])
Complex chronic care management (99487-99489)
Principal care management services ([99424, 99425, 99426, 99427])
Therapeutic ultrafiltration (0692T)

90963 **End-stage renal disease (ESRD) related services for home dialysis per full month, for patients younger than 2 years of age to include monitoring for the adequacy of nutrition, assessment of growth and development, and counseling of parents**

15.4 15.4 **FUD** XXX

AMA: 2018,Feb,11; 2018,Jan,8; 2017,Jan,8; 2016,Jan,13

90964 **End-stage renal disease (ESRD) related services for home dialysis per full month, for patients 2-11 years of age to include monitoring for the adequacy of nutrition, assessment of growth and development, and counseling of parents**

13.4 13.4 **FUD** XXX

AMA: 2018,Feb,11; 2018,Jan,8; 2017,Jan,8; 2016,Jan,13

90965 **End-stage renal disease (ESRD) related services for home dialysis per full month, for patients 12-19 years of age to include monitoring for the adequacy of nutrition, assessment of growth and development, and counseling of parents**

12.8 12.8 **FUD** XXX

AMA: 2018,Feb,11; 2018,Jan,8; 2017,Jan,8; 2016,Jan,13

90966 **End-stage renal disease (ESRD) related services for home dialysis per full month, for patients 20 years of age and older**

6.77 6.77 **FUD** XXX

AMA: 2018,Feb,11; 2018,Jan,8; 2017,Jan,8; 2016,Jan,13

90967-90970 End-stage Renal Disease Services: Partial Month

CMS: 100-02,11,20 Renal Dialysis Items and Services

INCLUDES ESRD services for less than full month, such as:
- Outpatient ESRD-related services initiated prior to assessment completion
- Patient spending partial month as hospital inpatient
- Patient who is transient, dies, recovers, or undergoes kidney transplant

Services reported on daily basis, less hospitalization days

EXCLUDES *Services provided in same month with:*
- *Chronic care management ([99437], [99439, 99490, 99491])*
- *Complex chronic care management (99487-99489)*
- *Principal care management services ([99424, 99425, 99426, 99427])*

Therapeutic ultrafiltration (0692T)

90967 **End-stage renal disease (ESRD) related services for dialysis less than a full month of service, per day; for patients younger than 2 years of age** A
0.51 0.51 FUD XXX ★ M 80
AMA: 2018,Feb,11; 2018,Jan,8; 2017,Jan,8; 2016,Jan,13

90968 **for patients 2-11 years of age** A
0.45 0.45 FUD XXX ★ M 80
AMA: 2018,Feb,11; 2018,Jan,8; 2017,Jan,8; 2016,Jan,13

90969 **for patients 12-19 years of age** A
0.43 0.43 FUD XXX ★ M 80
AMA: 2018,Feb,11; 2018,Jan,8; 2017,Jan,8; 2016,Jan,13

90970 **for patients 20 years of age and older** A
0.22 0.22 FUD XXX ★ M 80
AMA: 2018,Feb,11; 2018,Jan,8; 2017,Jan,8; 2016,Jan,13

90989-90993 Dialysis Training Services

CMS: 100-04,3,100.6 Inpatient Renal Services

EXCLUDES *Therapeutic ultrafiltration (0692T)*

90989 **Dialysis training, patient, including helper where applicable, any mode, completed course**
0.00 0.00 FUD XXX B
AMA: 2018,Feb,11; 2018,Jan,8; 2017,Jan,8; 2016,Jan,13

90993 **Dialysis training, patient, including helper where applicable, any mode, course not completed, per training session**
0.00 0.00 FUD XXX B
AMA: 2018,Feb,11; 2018,Jan,8; 2017,Jan,8; 2016,Jan,13

90997-90999 Hemoperfusion and Unlisted Dialysis Procedures

CMS: 100-04,3,100.6 Inpatient Renal Services

EXCLUDES *Therapeutic ultrafiltration (0692T)*

90997 **Hemoperfusion (eg, with activated charcoal or resin)**
2.56 2.56 FUD 000 B 80
AMA: 2018,Feb,11

90999 **Unlisted dialysis procedure, inpatient or outpatient**
0.00 0.00 FUD XXX B 80
AMA: 2018,Feb,11

91010-91022 Esophageal Manometry

91010 **Esophageal motility (manometric study of the esophagus and/or gastroesophageal junction) study with interpretation and report;**

EXCLUDES *Esophageal motility studies with high-resolution esophageal pressure topography (91299)*

Code also for esophageal motility studies with stimulant or perfusion (91013)
5.70 5.70 FUD 000 S 80
AMA: 2018,Feb,11

\+ **91013** **with stimulation or perfusion (eg, stimulant, acid or alkali perfusion) (List separately in addition to code for primary procedure)**

EXCLUDES *Esophageal motility studies with high-resolution esophageal pressure topography (91299)*
Reporting code more than one time for each session

Code first (91010)
0.73 0.73 FUD ZZZ N 80
AMA: 2018,Feb,11

91020 **Gastric motility (manometric) studies**

EXCLUDES *Gastrointestinal imaging by wireless capsule (91112)*
7.35 7.35 FUD 000 S 80
AMA: 2018,Feb,11; 2018,Jan,8; 2017,Jan,8; 2016,Jan,13

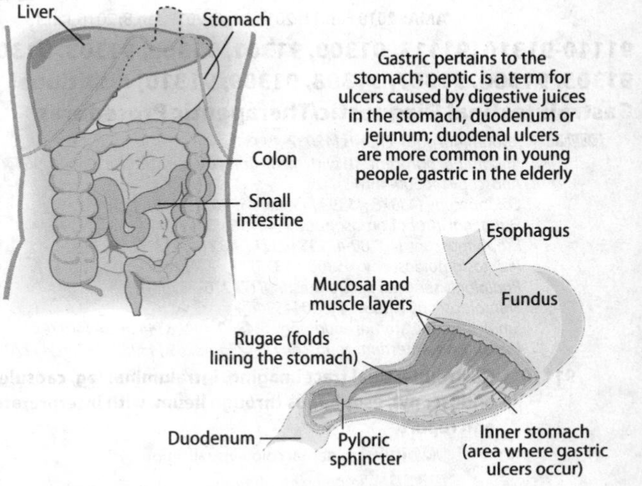

91022 **Duodenal motility (manometric) study**

EXCLUDES *Fluoroscopy (76000)*
Gastric motility study (91020)
Gastrointestinal imaging by wireless capsule (91112)
4.79 4.79 FUD 000 S 80
AMA: 2018,Feb,11; 2018,Jan,8; 2017,Jan,8; 2016,Jan,13

91030-91040 Esophageal Reflux Tests

EXCLUDES *Duodenal intubation/aspiration (43756-43757)*
Esophagoscopy (43180-43233 [43211, 43212, 43213, 43214])
Insertion:
- *Esophageal tamponade tube (43460)*
- *Insertion long gastrointestinal tube (44500)*

Radiologic services, gastrointestinal (74210-74363)
Upper gastrointestinal endoscopy (43235-43259 [43233, 43266, 43270])

91030 **Esophagus, acid perfusion (Bernstein) test for esophagitis**
3.94 3.94 FUD 000 S 80
AMA: 2018,Feb,11

91034 **Esophagus, gastroesophageal reflux test; with nasal catheter pH electrode(s) placement, recording, analysis and interpretation**
5.41 5.41 FUD 000 S 80
AMA: 2018,Feb,11; 2018,Jan,8; 2017,Jan,8; 2016,Jan,13

91035 **with mucosal attached telemetry pH electrode placement, recording, analysis and interpretation**

INCLUDES Endoscopy only to place device
13.7 13.7 FUD 000 S Z2 80
AMA: 2018,Feb,11; 2018,Jan,8; 2017,Jan,8; 2016,Jan,13

91037 **Esophageal function test, gastroesophageal reflux test with nasal catheter intraluminal impedance electrode(s) placement, recording, analysis and interpretation;**
4.71 4.71 FUD 000 S 80
AMA: 2018,Feb,11

91038 **prolonged (greater than 1 hour, up to 24 hours)**
12.4 12.4 FUD 000 S 80
AMA: 2018,Feb,11; 2018,Jan,8; 2017,Jan,8; 2016,Jan,13

91040 **Esophageal balloon distension study, diagnostic, with provocation when performed**

EXCLUDES *Reporting code more than one time for each session*

14.4 14.4 **FUD** 000 S 80

AMA: 2018,Feb,11; 2018,Jan,8; 2017,Jan,6

91065 Breath Analysis

CMS: 100-03,100.5 Diagnostic Breath Analysis

EXCLUDES *H. pylori breath test analysis, radioactive (C-14) or nonradioactive (C-13) (78268, 83013)*

Code also each challenge administered

91065 **Breath hydrogen or methane test (eg, for detection of lactase deficiency, fructose intolerance, bacterial overgrowth, or oro-cecal gastrointestinal transit)**

2.26 2.26 **FUD** 000 S 80

AMA: 2018,Feb,11; 2018,Jan,8; 2017,Jan,8; 2016,Jan,13

91110-91310 [91113, 91300, 91301, 91302, 91303, 91304, 91305, 91306, 91307, 91308, 91309, 91310] Additional Gastrointestinal Diagnostic/Therapeutic Procedures

EXCLUDES *Abdominal paracentesis (49082-49084)*
Abdominal paracentesis with medication administration (96440, 96446)
Anoscopy (46600-46615)
Colonoscopy (45378-45393 [45388, 45390, 45398])
Duodenal intubation/aspiration (43756-43757)
Esophagoscopy (43180-43233 [43211, 43212, 43213, 43214])
Proctosigmoidoscopy (45300-45327)
Radiologic services, gastrointestinal (74210-74363)
Sigmoidoscopy (45330-45350 [45346])
Small intestine/stomal endoscopy (44360-44408 [44381, 44401])
Upper gastrointestinal endoscopy (43235-43259 [43233, 43266, 43270])

91110 **Gastrointestinal tract imaging, intraluminal (eg, capsule endoscopy), esophagus through ileum, with interpretation and report**

INCLUDES Incidental colon visualization

EXCLUDES *Imaging esophagus (91111)*
Intraluminal capsule endoscopy GI tract ([91113])
Magnetically controlled capsule endoscopy (0651T)

Code also modifier 52 when ileum not visualized

24.3 24.3 **FUD** XXX T 80

AMA: 2018,Feb,11; 2018,Jan,8; 2017,Jan,8; 2016,Jan,13

91111 **Gastrointestinal tract imaging, intraluminal (eg, capsule endoscopy), esophagus with interpretation and report**

INCLUDES Incidental colon, duodenum, esophagus, ileum, or stomach visualization

EXCLUDES *Imaging esophagus through ileum (91110)*
Intraluminal capsule endoscopy GI tract ([91113])
Magnetically controlled capsule endoscopy (0651T)
Wireless capsule to measure transit times or pressure in gastrointestinal tract (91112)

22.8 22.8 **FUD** XXX T 80

AMA: 2018,Feb,11; 2018,Jan,8; 2017,Jan,8; 2016,Jan,13

● # **91113** **Gastrointestinal tract imaging, intraluminal (eg, capsule endoscopy), colon, with interpretation and report**

INCLUDES Incidental duodenum, esophagus, ileum, or stomach visualization

EXCLUDES *Imaging esophagus or esophagus through ileum (91110, 91111)*

0.00 0.00 **FUD** 000

91112 **Gastrointestinal transit and pressure measurement, stomach through colon, wireless capsule, with interpretation and report**

EXCLUDES *Colon motility study (91117)*
Duodenal motility study (91022)
Gastric motility studies (91020)
pH body fluid (83986)

40.9 40.9 **FUD** XXX T 80

AMA: 2018,Feb,11; 2018,Jan,8; 2017,Jan,8; 2016,Jan,13

91113 **Resequenced code. See code following 91111.**

91117 **Colon motility (manometric) study, minimum 6 hours continuous recording (including provocation tests, eg, meal, intracolonic balloon distension, pharmacologic agents, if performed), with interpretation and report**

EXCLUDES *Anal manometry (91122)*
Rectal sensation, tone and compliance testing (91120)
Reporting code more than one time no matter how many provocations
Wireless capsule to measure transit times or pressure in gastrointestinal tract (91112)

3.96 3.96 **FUD** 000 T 80

AMA: 2018,Feb,11; 2018,Jan,8; 2017,Jan,8; 2016,Jan,13

91120 **Rectal sensation, tone, and compliance test (ie, response to graded balloon distention)**

EXCLUDES *Anorectal manometry (91122)*
Biofeedback training (90912, 90913)
Colon motility study (91117)

13.7 13.7 **FUD** XXX S 80

AMA: 2020,Jun,13; 2018,Feb,11; 2018,Jan,8; 2017,Jan,8; 2016,Jan,13

91122 **Anorectal manometry**

EXCLUDES *Colon motility study (91117)*

7.13 7.13 **FUD** 000 T 80

AMA: 2018,Feb,11

91132 **Electrogastrography, diagnostic, transcutaneous;**

9.16 9.16 **FUD** XXX S 80

AMA: 2018,Feb,11

91133 **with provocative testing**

7.44 7.44 **FUD** XXX Q1 80

AMA: 2018,Feb,11

91200 **Liver elastography, mechanically induced shear wave (eg, vibration), without imaging, with interpretation and report**

EXCLUDES *Ultrasound elastography parenchyma (76981-76983)*

1.05 1.05 **FUD** XXX Q1 80

AMA: 2019,Aug,3; 2018,Feb,11; 2018,Jan,8; 2017,Oct,9

91299 **Unlisted diagnostic gastroenterology procedure**

0.00 0.00 **FUD** XXX S 80

AMA: 2018,Feb,11; 2018,Jan,8; 2017,Jan,8; 2016,Jan,13

91300 **Resequenced code. See code before 90476.**

91301 **Resequenced code. See code before 90476.**

91302 **Resequenced code. See code before 90476.**

91303 **Resequenced code. See code before 90476.**

91304 **Resequenced code. See code before 90476.**

91305 **Resequenced code. See code following resequenced code 91300.**

91306 **Resequenced code. See code following resequenced code 91301.**

91307 **Resequenced code. See code following resequenced code 91305.**

91308 **Resequenced code. See code before 90476.**

91309 **Resequenced code. See code before 90476.**

91310 **Resequenced code. See code before 90476.**

92002-92014 Ophthalmic Medical Services

CMS: 100-02,15,30.4 Optometrist's Services

INCLUDES Routine ophthalmoscopy
Services provided to established patients who have received professional services from physician or other qualified health care provider or another physician or other qualified health care professional within same group practice/exact same specialty and subspecialty within past three years
Services provided to new patients who have received no professional services from physician or other qualified health care provider or another physician or other qualified health care professional within same group practice/exact same specialty and subspecialty within past three years

EXCLUDES *Retinal polarization scan (0469T)*
Surgical procedures on eye/ocular adnexa (65091-68899 [66987, 66988, 67810])
Visual screening tests (99173-99174 [99177])

92002 **Ophthalmological services: medical examination and evaluation with initiation of diagnostic and treatment program; intermediate, new patient**

INCLUDES Evaluation new/existing condition complicated by new diagnostic or management problem
Integrated services where medical decision making cannot be separated from examination methods
Intermediate services:
External ocular/adnexal examination
General medical observation
History
Other diagnostic procedures:
Biomicroscopy
Mydriasis
Ophthalmoscopy
Tonometry
Problems not related to primary diagnosis

1.34 2.37 **FUD** XXX V 80

AMA: 2018,Feb,11; 2018,Feb,3; 2018,Jan,8; 2017,Sep,14; 2017,Jan,8; 2016,Jan,13

92004 **comprehensive, new patient, 1 or more visits**

INCLUDES Comprehensive services:
Basic sensorimotor examination
Biomicroscopy
Dilation (cycloplegia)
External examinations
General medical observation
Gross visual fields
History
Initiation diagnostic/treatment programs
Mydriasis
Ophthalmoscopic examinations
Other diagnostic procedures
Prescription medication
Special diagnostic/treatment services
Tonometry
General evaluation complete visual system
Integrated services where medical decision making cannot be separated from examination methods
Single service that need not be performed at one session

2.81 4.26 **FUD** XXX V 80

AMA: 2018,Feb,11; 2018,Feb,3; 2018,Jan,8; 2017,Sep,14; 2017,Jan,8; 2016,Nov,9; 2016,Jan,13

92012 **Ophthalmological services: medical examination and evaluation, with initiation or continuation of diagnostic and treatment program; intermediate, established patient**

INCLUDES Evaluation new/existing condition complicated by new diagnostic or management problem
Integrated services where medical decision making cannot be separated from examination methods
Problems not related to primary diagnosis
Intermediate services:
External ocular/adnexal examination
General medical observation
History
Other diagnostic procedures:
Biomicroscopy
Mydriasis
Ophthalmoscopy
Tonometry

1.49 2.49 **FUD** XXX V 80

AMA: 2018,Feb,11; 2018,Feb,3; 2018,Jan,8; 2017,Sep,14; 2017,Jan,8; 2016,Jan,13

92014 **comprehensive, established patient, 1 or more visits**

INCLUDES General evaluation complete visual system
Integrated services where medical decision making cannot be separated from examination methods
Single service that need not be performed at one session
Comprehensive services:
Basic sensorimotor examination
Biomicroscopy
Dilation (cycloplegia)
External examinations
General medical observation
Gross visual fields
History
Initiation diagnostic/treatment programs
Mydriasis
Ophthalmoscopic examinations
Other diagnostic procedures
Prescription medication
Special diagnostic/treatment services
Tonometry

2.25 3.57 **FUD** XXX V 80

AMA: 2018,Feb,11; 2018,Feb,3; 2018,Jan,8; 2017,Sep,14; 2017,Jan,8; 2016,Nov,9; 2016,Jan,13

92015-92145 Ophthalmic Special Services

INCLUDES Routine ophthalmoscopy

EXCLUDES *Surgical procedures on eye/ocular adnexa (65091-68899 [66987, 66988, 67810])*

Code also:
E/M services, when performed
General ophthalmological services, when performed (92002-92014)

92015 **Determination of refractive state**

INCLUDES Lens prescription:
Absorptive factor
Axis
Impact resistance
Lens power
Prism
Specification lens type:
Bifocal
Monofocal

EXCLUDES *Ocular screening, instrument based (99173-99174 [99177])*

0.55 0.56 **FUD** XXX E

AMA: 2020,Dec,13; 2018,Feb,11; 2018,Jan,8; 2017,Jan,8; 2016,Mar,10; 2016,Jan,13

92018 **Ophthalmological examination and evaluation, under general anesthesia, with or without manipulation of globe for passive range of motion or other manipulation to facilitate diagnostic examination; complete**

4.06 4.06 **FUD** XXX J 80

AMA: 2018,Feb,11; 2018,Jan,8; 2017,Jan,8; 2016,Jan,13

92019 **limited**
2.05 2.05 FUD XXX J 80
AMA: 2018,Feb,11; 2018,Jan,8; 2017,Jan,8; 2016,Jan,13

92020 **Gonioscopy (separate procedure)**
EXCLUDES *Gonioscopy under general anesthesia (92018)*
Laser trabeculostomy ab interno (0621T-0622T)
0.60 0.78 FUD XXX Q1 80
AMA: 2018,Feb,11; 2018,Jan,8; 2017,Jan,8; 2016,Jan,13

92025 **Computerized corneal topography, unilateral or bilateral, with interpretation and report**
EXCLUDES *Corneal transplant procedures (65710-65771)*
Manual keratoscopy
1.04 1.04 FUD XXX Q1 80
AMA: 2018,Feb,11; 2018,Jan,8; 2017,Jan,8; 2016,Jan,13

92060 **Sensorimotor examination with multiple measurements of ocular deviation (eg, restrictive or paretic muscle with diplopia) with interpretation and report (separate procedure)**
1.79 1.79 FUD XXX Q1 80
AMA: 2018,Feb,11; 2018,Jan,8; 2017,Jan,8; 2016,Jan,13

▲ **92065** **Orthoptic training**
1.49 1.49 FUD XXX Q1 80
AMA: 2018,Feb,11; 2018,Jan,8; 2017,Jan,8; 2016,Jan,13

92071 **Fitting of contact lens for treatment of ocular surface disease**
EXCLUDES *Contact lens service for keratoconus (92072)*
Code also lens supply with appropriate supply code or (99070)
0.95 1.07 FUD XXX N 80 50
AMA: 2018,Feb,11

92072 **Fitting of contact lens for management of keratoconus, initial fitting**
EXCLUDES *Contact lens service for disease ocular surface (92071)*
Subsequent fittings (99211-99215, 92012-92014)
Code also lens supply with appropriate supply code or (99070)
2.84 3.72 FUD XXX N 80
AMA: 2018,Feb,11; 2018,Jan,8; 2017,Sep,14; 2017,Jan,8; 2016,Jan,13

92081 **Visual field examination, unilateral or bilateral, with interpretation and report; limited examination (eg, tangent screen, Autoplot, arc perimeter, or single stimulus level automated test, such as Octopus 3 or 7 equivalent)**
INCLUDES Gross visual testing/confrontation testing
0.95 0.95 FUD XXX Q1 80
AMA: 2018,Feb,11; 2018,Jan,8; 2017,Jan,8; 2016,Jan,13

92082 **intermediate examination (eg, at least 2 isopters on Goldmann perimeter, or semiquantitative, automated suprathreshold screening program, Humphrey suprathreshold automatic diagnostic test, Octopus program 33)**
INCLUDES Gross visual testing/confrontation testing
1.34 1.34 FUD XXX Q1 80
AMA: 2018,Feb,11; 2018,Jan,8; 2017,Jan,8; 2016,Jan,13

92083 **extended examination (eg, Goldmann visual fields with at least 3 isopters plotted and static determination within the central 30°, or quantitative, automated threshold perimetry, Octopus program G-1, 32 or 42, Humphrey visual field analyzer full threshold programs 30-2, 24-2, or 30/60-2)**
INCLUDES Gross visual field testing/confrontation testing
EXCLUDES *Assessment visual field, by data transmission, by patient to surveillance center (0378T-0379T)*
1.78 1.78 FUD XXX Q1 80
AMA: 2018,Feb,11; 2018,Jan,8; 2017,Jan,8; 2016,Jan,13

92100 **Serial tonometry (separate procedure) with multiple measurements of intraocular pressure over an extended time period with interpretation and report, same day (eg, diurnal curve or medical treatment of acute elevation of intraocular pressure)**
EXCLUDES *Intraocular pressure monitoring for 24 hours or more (0329T)*
Ocular blood flow measurements (0198T)
Single-episode tonometry (99202-99215, 92002-92004)
0.96 2.32 FUD XXX N 80
AMA: 2018,Feb,11; 2018,Jan,8; 2017,Jan,8; 2016,Jan,13

92132 **Scanning computerized ophthalmic diagnostic imaging, anterior segment, with interpretation and report, unilateral or bilateral**
EXCLUDES *Imaging anterior segment with specular microscopy and endothelial cell analysis (92286)*
Scanning computerized ophthalmic diagnostic imaging optic nerve and retina (92133-92134)
Tear film imaging (0330T)
0.89 0.89 FUD XXX Q1 80
AMA: 2018,Feb,11; 2018,Jan,8; 2017,Jan,8; 2016,Jan,13

92133 **Scanning computerized ophthalmic diagnostic imaging, posterior segment, with interpretation and report, unilateral or bilateral; optic nerve**
EXCLUDES *Remote imaging for retinal disease (92227-92228)*
Scanning computerized ophthalmic imaging retina same visit (92134)
1.05 1.05 FUD XXX Q1 80
AMA: 2018,Feb,11; 2018,Jan,8; 2017,Jan,8; 2016,Jan,13

92134 **retina**
EXCLUDES *Remote imaging for retinal disease (92227-92228)*
Scanning computerized ophthalmic imaging retina same visit (92134)
1.15 1.15 FUD XXX Q1 80
AMA: 2018,Feb,11; 2018,Jan,8; 2017,Jan,8; 2016,Jan,13

92136 **Ophthalmic biometry by partial coherence interferometry with intraocular lens power calculation**
EXCLUDES *Tear film imaging (0330T)*
1.76 1.76 FUD XXX Q1 80
AMA: 2018,Feb,11; 2018,Jan,8; 2017,Jan,8; 2016,Jan,13

92145 **Corneal hysteresis determination, by air impulse stimulation, unilateral or bilateral, with interpretation and report**
0.42 0.42 FUD XXX Q1 80
AMA: 2018,Feb,11

92201-92287 Other Ophthalmology Services

EXCLUDES *Ophthalmological exam under anesthesia (92018)*
Prescription, fitting, and/or medical supervision ocular prosthesis adaptation by physician (99202-99215, 99241-99245, 92002-92014)
Surgical procedures on eye/ocular adnexa (65091-68899 [66987, 66988, 67810])

92201 **Ophthalmoscopy, extended; with retinal drawing and scleral depression of peripheral retinal disease (eg, for retinal tear, retinal detachment, retinal tumor) with interpretation and report, unilateral or bilateral**
EXCLUDES *Fundus photography with interpretation and report (92250)*
0.65 0.71 FUD XXX 80
AMA: 2019,Dec,3

92202 **with drawing of optic nerve or macula (eg, for glaucoma, macular pathology, tumor) with interpretation and report, unilateral or bilateral**
EXCLUDES *Fundus photography with interpretation and report (92250)*
0.42 0.45 FUD XXX 80
AMA: 2019,Dec,3

92227 **Imaging of retina for detection or monitoring of disease; with remote clinical staff review and report, unilateral or bilateral**

EXCLUDES *Fundus photography with interpretation and report (92250)*
Imaging for retinal disease:
Point of care automated analysis and report (92229)
Remote interpretation and report (92228)
Scanning computerized ophthalmic imaging:
Optic nerve (92133)
Retina (92134)

0.40 0.40 FUD XXX ★ Q1 80 TC

AMA: 2019,Aug,10; 2018,Feb,11; 2018,Jan,8; 2017,Jan,8; 2016,Jul,8; 2016,Jan,13

92228 **with remote physician or other qualified health care professional interpretation and report, unilateral or bilateral**

EXCLUDES *Fundus photography with interpretation and report (92250)*
Imaging for retinal disease:
Point of care automated analysis and report (92229)
Remote clinical staff review and report (92227)
Scanning computerized ophthalmic imaging:
Optic nerve (92133)
Retina (92134)

0.97 0.97 FUD XXX ★ Q1 80

AMA: 2018,Feb,11; 2018,Jan,8; 2017,Jan,8; 2016,Jan,13

92229 **point-of-care automated analysis and report, unilateral or bilateral**

EXCLUDES *Fundus photography with interpretation and report (92250)*
Remote imaging for retinal disease (92227-92228)
Scanning computerized ophthalmic imaging:
Optic nerve (92133)
Retina (92134)

0.00 0.00 FUD XXX 80 TC

92230 **Fluorescein angioscopy with interpretation and report**

0.95 1.83 FUD XXX Q1 80

AMA: 2018,Feb,11; 2018,Jan,8; 2017,Jan,8; 2016,Jan,13

92235 **Fluorescein angiography (includes multiframe imaging) with interpretation and report, unilateral or bilateral**

EXCLUDES *Fluorescein and indocyanine-green angiography (92242)*

2.93 2.93 FUD XXX S 80

AMA: 2018,Feb,11; 2018,Jan,8; 2017,Jun,8; 2017,Jan,8; 2016,Jan,13

92240 **Indocyanine-green angiography (includes multiframe imaging) with interpretation and report, unilateral or bilateral**

EXCLUDES *Fluorescein and indocyanine-green angiography (92242)*

5.69 5.69 FUD XXX S 80

AMA: 2018,Feb,11; 2018,Jan,8; 2017,Jun,8; 2017,Jan,8; 2016,Jan,13

92242 **Fluorescein angiography and indocyanine-green angiography (includes multiframe imaging) performed at the same patient encounter with interpretation and report, unilateral or bilateral**

6.71 6.71 FUD XXX S 80

AMA: 2018,Feb,11; 2018,Jan,8; 2017,Jun,8

92250 **Fundus photography with interpretation and report**

1.27 1.27 FUD XXX Q1 80

AMA: 2019,Dec,3; 2018,Feb,11; 2018,Jan,8; 2017,Jan,8; 2016,Jul,8; 2016,Jan,13

92260 **Ophthalmodynamometry**

0.31 0.55 FUD XXX Q1 80

AMA: 2018,Feb,11; 2018,Jan,8; 2017,Jan,8; 2016,Jan,13

92265 **Needle oculoelectromyography, 1 or more extraocular muscles, 1 or both eyes, with interpretation and report**

2.45 2.45 FUD XXX Q1 80

AMA: 2018,Feb,11; 2018,Jan,8; 2017,Jan,8; 2016,Jan,13

92270 **Electro-oculography with interpretation and report**

EXCLUDES *Recording saccadic eye movement (92700)*
Vestibular function testing (92537-92538, 92540-92542, 92544-92549)

2.73 2.73 FUD XXX Q1 80

AMA: 2020,Apr,7; 2018,Feb,11; 2018,Jan,8; 2017,Jan,8; 2016,Jan,13

92273 **Electroretinography (ERG), with interpretation and report; full field (ie, ffERG, flash ERG, Ganzfeld ERG)**

EXCLUDES *Pattern electroretinography (PERG) (0509T)*

3.78 3.78 FUD XXX 80

AMA: 2019,Jan,12

92274 **multifocal (mfERG)**

EXCLUDES *Pattern electroretinography (PERG) (0509T)*

2.56 2.56 FUD XXX 80

AMA: 2019,Jan,12

92283 **Color vision examination, extended, eg, anomaloscope or equivalent**

1.49 1.49 FUD XXX Q1 80

AMA: 2018,Feb,11; 2018,Jan,8; 2017,Jan,8; 2016,Jan,13

92284 **Dark adaptation examination with interpretation and report**

1.68 1.68 FUD XXX Q1 80

AMA: 2018,Feb,11; 2018,Jan,8; 2017,Jan,8; 2016,Jan,13

92285 **External ocular photography with interpretation and report for documentation of medical progress (eg, close-up photography, slit lamp photography, goniophotography, stereo-photography)**

0.62 0.62 FUD XXX Q1 80

AMA: 2018,Feb,11; 2018,Jan,8; 2017,Jan,8; 2016,Jan,13

92286 **Anterior segment imaging with interpretation and report; with specular microscopy and endothelial cell analysis**

1.10 1.10 FUD XXX Q1 80

AMA: 2018,Feb,11; 2018,Jan,8; 2017,Jan,8; 2016,Jan,13

92287 **with fluorescein angiography**

4.46 4.46 FUD XXX Q1 80

AMA: 2018,Feb,11; 2018,Jan,8; 2017,Jan,8; 2016,Jan,13

92310-92326 Services Related to Contact Lenses

CMS: 100-02,15,30.4 Optometrist's Services

INCLUDES Incidental revision lens during training period
Patient training/instruction
Specification optical/physical characteristics:
Curvature
Flexibility
Gas-permeability
Power
Size

EXCLUDES *Extended wear lenses follow up (92012-92014)*
General ophthalmological services
Therapeutic/surgical use contact lens (68340, 92071-92072)

92310 **Prescription of optical and physical characteristics of and fitting of contact lens, with medical supervision of adaptation; corneal lens, both eyes, except for aphakia**

Code also modifier 52 for prescription and fitting only one eye

1.69 2.80 FUD XXX E

AMA: 2018,Feb,11; 2018,Jan,8; 2017,Jan,8; 2016,Jan,13

92311 **corneal lens for aphakia, 1 eye**

1.57 2.94 FUD XXX Q1 80

AMA: 2018,Feb,11; 2018,Jan,8; 2017,Jan,8; 2016,Jan,13

92312 **corneal lens for aphakia, both eyes**

1.81 3.40 FUD XXX Q1 80

AMA: 2018,Feb,11; 2018,Jan,8; 2017,Jan,8; 2016,Jan,13

92313 **corneoscleral lens**
Facility RVU 1.31 Non-Facility RVU 2.78 **FUD** XXX Q1 80
AMA: 2018,Feb,11; 2018,Jan,8; 2017,Jan,8; 2016,Jan,13

92314 **Prescription of optical and physical characteristics of contact lens, with medical supervision of adaptation and direction of fitting by independent technician; corneal lens, both eyes except for aphakia**
Code also modifier 52 for prescription and fitting only one eye
Facility RVU 1.00 Non-Facility RVU 2.36 **FUD** XXX E
AMA: 2018,Feb,11; 2018,Jan,8; 2017,Jan,8; 2016,Jan,13

92315 **corneal lens for aphakia, 1 eye**
Facility RVU 0.62 Non-Facility RVU 2.19 **FUD** XXX Q1 80
AMA: 2018,Feb,11; 2018,Jan,8; 2017,Jan,8; 2016,Jan,13

92316 **corneal lens for aphakia, both eyes**
Facility RVU 0.92 Non-Facility RVU 2.76 **FUD** XXX Q1 80
AMA: 2018,Feb,11; 2018,Jan,8; 2017,Jan,8; 2016,Jan,13

92317 **corneoscleral lens**
Facility RVU 0.61 Non-Facility RVU 2.32 **FUD** XXX Q1 80
AMA: 2018,Feb,11; 2018,Jan,8; 2017,Jan,8; 2016,Jan,13

92325 **Modification of contact lens (separate procedure), with medical supervision of adaptation**
Facility RVU 1.24 Non-Facility RVU 1.24 **FUD** XXX Q1 80
AMA: 2018,Feb,11; 2018,Jan,8; 2017,Jan,8; 2016,Jan,13

92326 **Replacement of contact lens**
Facility RVU 1.06 Non-Facility RVU 1.06 **FUD** XXX Q1 80
AMA: 2018,Feb,11; 2018,Jan,8; 2017,Jan,8; 2016,Jan,13

92340-92499 Services Related to Eyeglasses

CMS: 100-02,15,30.4 Optometrist's Services

INCLUDES Anatomical facial characteristics measurement
Final adjustment of spectacles to visual axes/anatomical topography
Written laboratory specifications

EXCLUDES *Materials supply*

92340 **Fitting of spectacles, except for aphakia; monofocal**
Facility RVU 0.53 Non-Facility RVU 0.99 **FUD** XXX E
AMA: 2018,Feb,11; 2018,Jan,8; 2017,Jan,8; 2016,Jan,13

92341 **bifocal**
Facility RVU 0.68 Non-Facility RVU 1.14 **FUD** XXX E
AMA: 2018,Feb,11; 2018,Jan,8; 2017,Jan,8; 2016,Jan,13

92342 **multifocal, other than bifocal**
Facility RVU 0.78 Non-Facility RVU 1.23 **FUD** XXX E
AMA: 2018,Feb,11; 2018,Jan,8; 2017,Jan,8; 2016,Jan,13

92352 **Fitting of spectacle prosthesis for aphakia; monofocal**
Facility RVU 0.53 Non-Facility RVU 1.17 **FUD** XXX Q1
AMA: 2018,Feb,11; 2018,Jan,8; 2017,Jan,8; 2016,Jan,13

92353 **multifocal**
Facility RVU 0.72 Non-Facility RVU 1.36 **FUD** XXX Q1
AMA: 2018,Feb,11; 2018,Jan,8; 2017,Jan,8; 2016,Jan,13

92354 **Fitting of spectacle mounted low vision aid; single element system**
Facility RVU 0.37 Non-Facility RVU 0.37 **FUD** XXX Q1
AMA: 2018,Feb,11; 2018,Jan,8; 2017,Jan,8; 2016,Jan,13

92355 **telescopic or other compound lens system**
Facility RVU 0.59 Non-Facility RVU 0.59 **FUD** XXX Q1
AMA: 2018,Feb,11; 2018,Jan,8; 2017,Jan,8; 2016,Jan,13

92358 **Prosthesis service for aphakia, temporary (disposable or loan, including materials)**
Facility RVU 0.31 Non-Facility RVU 0.31 **FUD** XXX Q1
AMA: 2018,Feb,11; 2018,Jan,8; 2017,Jan,8; 2016,Jan,13

92370 **Repair and refitting spectacles; except for aphakia**
Facility RVU 0.46 Non-Facility RVU 0.88 **FUD** XXX E
AMA: 2018,Feb,11; 2018,Jan,8; 2017,Jan,8; 2016,Jan,13

92371 **spectacle prosthesis for aphakia**
Facility RVU 0.33 Non-Facility RVU 0.33 **FUD** XXX Q1
AMA: 2018,Feb,11; 2018,Jan,8; 2017,Jan,8; 2016,Jan,13

92499 **Unlisted ophthalmological service or procedure**
Facility RVU 0.00 Non-Facility RVU 0.00 **FUD** XXX Q1 80
AMA: 2020,Dec,13; 2020,Aug,14; 2019,Jan,12; 2018,Jul,3; 2018,Feb,11; 2018,Jan,8; 2017,Jan,8; 2016,Jan,13

92502-92526 [92517, 92518, 92519] Special Procedures of the Ears/Nose/Throat

INCLUDES Anterior rhinoscopy, tuning fork testing, otoscopy, or removal non-impacted cerumen
Diagnostic/treatment services not generally included in E/M service

EXCLUDES *Laryngoscopy with stroboscopy (31579)*

92502 **Otolaryngologic examination under general anesthesia**
Facility RVU 2.73 Non-Facility RVU 2.73 **FUD** 000 T 80
AMA: 2018,Feb,11; 2018,Jan,8; 2017,Jan,8; 2016,Sep,6

92504 **Binocular microscopy (separate diagnostic procedure)**
Facility RVU 0.27 Non-Facility RVU 0.83 **FUD** XXX N 80
AMA: 2018,Feb,11; 2018,Jan,8; 2017,Jan,8; 2016,Sep,6; 2016,Jan,13

92507 **Treatment of speech, language, voice, communication, and/or auditory processing disorder; individual**
EXCLUDES *Adaptive behavior treatment ([97153], [97155])*
Auditory rehabilitation:
Postlingual hearing loss (92633)
Prelingual hearing loss (92630)
Programming cochlear implant (92601-92604)
Facility RVU 2.23 Non-Facility RVU 2.23 **FUD** XXX A 80
AMA: 2018,Dec,7; 2018,Dec,7; 2018,Nov,3; 2018,Feb,11; 2018,Jan,8; 2017,Jan,8; 2016,Sep,6; 2016,Jan,13

92508 **group, 2 or more individuals**
EXCLUDES *Adaptive behavior treatment ([97154], [97158])*
Auditory rehabilitation:
Postlingual hearing loss (92633)
Prelingual hearing loss (92630)
Programming cochlear implant (92601-92604)
Facility RVU 0.68 Non-Facility RVU 0.68 **FUD** XXX A 80
AMA: 2018,Nov,3; 2018,Feb,11; 2018,Jan,8; 2017,Jan,8; 2016,Sep,6; 2016,Jan,13

92511 **Nasopharyngoscopy with endoscope (separate procedure)**
EXCLUDES *Diagnostic flexible laryngoscopy (31575)*
Drug-induced sleep endoscopy (42975)
Nasopharyngoscopic dilation eustachian tube (69705-69706)
Transnasal esophagoscopy (43197-43198)
Facility RVU 1.08 Non-Facility RVU 3.15 **FUD** 000 T 80
AMA: 2018,Feb,11; 2018,Jan,8; 2017,Jul,7; 2017,Jan,8; 2016,Dec,13; 2016,Sep,6

92512 **Nasal function studies (eg, rhinomanometry)**
Facility RVU 0.80 Non-Facility RVU 1.68 **FUD** XXX S 80
AMA: 2018,Feb,11; 2018,Jan,8; 2017,Jan,8; 2016,Sep,6

92516 **Facial nerve function studies (eg, electroneuronography)**
Facility RVU 0.65 Non-Facility RVU 1.94 **FUD** XXX S 80
AMA: 2018,Feb,11; 2018,Jan,8; 2017,Jan,8; 2016,Sep,6

92517 **Resequenced code. See code following 92549.**

92518 **Resequenced code. See code following 92549.**

92519 **Resequenced code. See code following 92549.**

92520 **Laryngeal function studies (ie, aerodynamic testing and acoustic testing)**
EXCLUDES *Other laryngeal function testing (92700)*
Swallowing/laryngeal sensory testing with flexible fiberoptic endoscope (92611-92617)
Code also modifier 52 for single test
Facility RVU 1.15 Non-Facility RVU 2.23 **FUD** XXX Q1 80
AMA: 2018,Feb,11; 2018,Jan,8; 2017,Jan,8; 2016,Sep,6; 2016,Jan,13

92521 **Evaluation of speech fluency (eg, stuttering, cluttering)**

INCLUDES Ability to execute motor movements needed for speech
Comprehension written and verbal expression
Determination patient's ability to create and communicate expressive thought
Evaluation ability to produce speech sound

3.21 3.21 FUD XXX A 80

AMA: 2018,Feb,11; 2018,Jan,8; 2017,Jan,8; 2016,Sep,6; 2016,Jan,13

92522 **Evaluation of speech sound production (eg, articulation, phonological process, apraxia, dysarthria);**

INCLUDES Ability to execute motor movements needed for speech
Comprehension written and verbal expression
Determination patient's ability to create and communicate expressive thought
Evaluation ability to produce speech sound

2.60 2.60 FUD XXX A 80

AMA: 2018,Feb,11; 2018,Jan,8; 2017,Jan,8; 2016,Sep,6; 2016,Jan,13

92523 **with evaluation of language comprehension and expression (eg, receptive and expressive language)**

INCLUDES Ability to execute motor movements needed for speech
Comprehension written and verbal expression
Determination patient's ability to create and communicate expressive thought
Evaluation ability to produce speech sound

5.54 5.54 FUD XXX A 80

AMA: 2018,Feb,11; 2018,Jan,8; 2017,Jan,8; 2016,Sep,6; 2016,Jan,13

92524 **Behavioral and qualitative analysis of voice and resonance**

INCLUDES Ability to execute motor movements needed for speech
Comprehension written and verbal expression
Determination patient's ability to create and communicate expressive thought
Evaluation ability to produce speech sound

2.51 2.51 FUD XXX A 80

AMA: 2018,Feb,11; 2018,Jan,8; 2017,Jan,8; 2016,Sep,6; 2016,Jan,13

92526 **Treatment of swallowing dysfunction and/or oral function for feeding**

2.44 2.44 FUD XXX A 80

AMA: 2018,Feb,11; 2018,Jan,8; 2017,Jan,8; 2016,Sep,6

92531-92519 [92517, 92518, 92519] Vestibular Function Tests

92531 **Spontaneous nystagmus, including gaze**

EXCLUDES *When performed with E/M services (99202-99215, 99218-99223 [99224, 99225, 99226], 99231-99236, 99241-99245, 99304-99318, 99324-99337)*

0.00 0.00 FUD XXX N

AMA: 2020,Aug,14; 2018,Feb,11

92532 **Positional nystagmus test**

EXCLUDES *When performed with E/M services (99202-99215, 99218-99223 [99224, 99225, 99226], 99231-99236, 99241-99245, 99304-99318, 99324-99337)*

0.00 0.00 FUD XXX N

AMA: 2020,Aug,14; 2018,Feb,11

92533 **Caloric vestibular test, each irrigation (binaural, bithermal stimulation constitutes 4 tests)**

INCLUDES Barany caloric test

0.00 0.00 FUD XXX N

AMA: 2020,Aug,14; 2018,Feb,11; 2018,Jan,8; 2017,Jan,8; 2016,Jan,13

92534 **Optokinetic nystagmus test**

0.00 0.00 FUD XXX N

AMA: 2020,Aug,14; 2018,Feb,11

92537 **Caloric vestibular test with recording, bilateral; bithermal (ie, one warm and one cool irrigation in each ear for a total of four irrigations)**

EXCLUDES *Electro-oculography (92270)*
Monothermal caloric vestibular test (92538)

Code also modifier 52 when only three irrigations performed

1.18 1.18 FUD XXX S 80

AMA: 2020,Aug,14; 2018,Feb,11

92538 **monothermal (ie, one irrigation in each ear for a total of two irrigations)**

EXCLUDES *Bithermal caloric vestibular test (92537)*
Electro-oculography (92270)

Code also modifier 52 only one irrigation performed

0.64 0.64 FUD XXX S 80

AMA: 2020,Aug,14; 2018,Feb,11

92540 **Basic vestibular evaluation, includes spontaneous nystagmus test with eccentric gaze fixation nystagmus, with recording, positional nystagmus test, minimum of 4 positions, with recording, optokinetic nystagmus test, bidirectional foveal and peripheral stimulation, with recording, and oscillating tracking test, with recording**

EXCLUDES *Vestibular function tests (92270, 92541-92542, 92544-92545)*

3.04 3.04 FUD XXX S 80

AMA: 2020,Aug,14; 2018,Feb,11; 2018,Jan,8; 2017,Jan,8; 2016,Jan,13

92541 **Spontaneous nystagmus test, including gaze and fixation nystagmus, with recording**

EXCLUDES *Vestibular function tests (92270, 92540, 92542, 92544-92545)*

0.72 0.72 FUD XXX Q1 80

AMA: 2020,Aug,14; 2019,Jan,12; 2018,Feb,11; 2018,Jan,8; 2017,Jan,8; 2016,Jan,13

92542 **Positional nystagmus test, minimum of 4 positions, with recording**

EXCLUDES *Vestibular function tests (92270, 92540-92541, 92544-92545)*

0.84 0.84 FUD XXX Q1 80

AMA: 2020,Aug,14; 2018,Feb,11; 2018,Jan,8; 2017,Jan,8; 2016,Jan,13

92544 **Optokinetic nystagmus test, bidirectional, foveal or peripheral stimulation, with recording**

EXCLUDES *Vestibular function tests (92270, 92540-92542, 92545)*

0.50 0.50 FUD XXX S 80

AMA: 2020,Aug,14; 2018,Feb,11; 2018,Jan,8; 2017,Jan,8; 2016,Jan,13

92545 **Oscillating tracking test, with recording**

EXCLUDES *Vestibular function tests (92270, 92540-92542, 92544)*

0.47 0.47 FUD XXX S 80

AMA: 2020,Aug,14; 2018,Feb,11; 2018,Jan,8; 2017,Jan,8; 2016,Jan,13

92546 **Sinusoidal vertical axis rotational testing**

EXCLUDES *Electro-oculography (92270)*

3.15 3.15 FUD XXX S 80

AMA: 2020,Aug,14; 2018,Feb,11; 2018,Jan,8; 2017,Jan,8; 2016,Jan,13

+ **92547** **Use of vertical electrodes (List separately in addition to code for primary procedure)**

EXCLUDES *Electro-oculography (92270)*
Unlisted vestibular tests (92700)

Code first (92540-92546)

0.21 0.21 FUD ZZZ N 80 TC

AMA: 2020,Aug,14; 2018,Feb,11; 2018,Jan,8; 2017,Jan,8; 2016,Jan,13

92548 **Computerized dynamic posturography sensory organization test (CDP-SOT), 6 conditions (ie, eyes open, eyes closed, visual sway, platform sway, eyes closed platform sway, platform and visual sway), including interpretation and report;**

EXCLUDES *Electro-oculography (92270)*

1.41 1.41 FUD XXX Q1 80

AMA: 2020,Aug,14; 2020,Apr,7; 2018,Feb,11; 2018,Jan,8; 2017,Jan,8; 2016,Jan,13

92549 **with motor control test (MCT) and adaptation test (ADT)**

EXCLUDES *Electro-oculography (92270)*

1.80 1.80 FUD XXX 80

AMA: 2020,Aug,14; 2020,Apr,7

\# **92517** **Vestibular evoked myogenic potential (VEMP) testing, with interpretation and report; cervical (cVEMP)**

EXCLUDES *Electro-oculography (92270)*
Vestibular evoked myogenic potential testing:
Cervical and ocular ([92519])
Ocular ([92518])

1.26 2.50 FUD XXX 80

\# **92518** **ocular (oVEMP)**

EXCLUDES *Electro-oculography (92270)*
Vestibular evoked myogenic potential testing:
Cervical ([92517])
Cervical and ocular ([92519])

1.26 2.33 FUD XXX 80

\# **92519** **cervical (cVEMP) and ocular (oVEMP)**

EXCLUDES *Electro-oculography (92270)*
Vestibular evoked myogenic potential testing:
Cervical only ([92517])
Ocular only ([92518])

1.89 3.88 FUD XXX 80

92550-92597 [92558, 92597, 92650, 92651, 92652, 92653] Hearing and Speech Tests

INCLUDES Calibrated electronic equipment, recording results, and report with interpretation
Diagnostic/treatment services not generally included in comprehensive otorhinolaryngologic evaluation or office visit
Testing both ears
Tuning fork and whisper tests

EXCLUDES *Evaluation speech/language/hearing problems using performance observation/assessment (92521-92524)*

Code also modifier 52 for unilateral testing

92550 **Tympanometry and reflex threshold measurements**

INCLUDES Tympanometry, acoustic reflex testing individual codes (92567-92568)

0.62 0.62 FUD XXX Q1 80

AMA: 2018,Feb,11; 2018,Jan,8; 2017,Jan,8; 2016,Jan,13

92551 **Screening test, pure tone, air only**

0.33 0.33 FUD XXX E

AMA: 2018,Feb,11; 2018,Jan,8; 2017,Jan,8; 2016,Jan,13

92552 **Pure tone audiometry (threshold); air only**

EXCLUDES *Automated test (0208T)*

0.89 0.89 FUD XXX Q1 80 TC

AMA: 2018,Feb,11; 2018,Jan,8; 2017,Jan,8; 2016,Jan,13

92553 **air and bone**

EXCLUDES *Automated test (0209T)*

1.08 1.08 FUD XXX Q1 80 TC

AMA: 2018,Feb,11; 2018,Jan,8; 2017,Jan,8; 2016,Jan,13

92555 **Speech audiometry threshold;**

EXCLUDES *Automated test (0210T)*

0.68 0.68 FUD XXX Q1 80 TC

AMA: 2018,Feb,11; 2018,Jan,8; 2017,Jan,8; 2016,Jan,13

92556 **with speech recognition**

EXCLUDES *Automated test (0211T)*

1.07 1.07 FUD XXX Q1 80 TC

AMA: 2018,Feb,11; 2018,Jan,8; 2017,Jan,8; 2016,Jan,13

92557 **Comprehensive audiometry threshold evaluation and speech recognition (92553 and 92556 combined)**

EXCLUDES *Automated test (0208T-0212T)*
Evaluation/selection hearing aid (92590-92595)

0.93 1.08 FUD XXX Q1 80

AMA: 2018,Feb,11; 2018,Jan,8; 2017,Jan,8; 2016,Jan,13

92558 **Resequenced code. See code before 92587.**

92559 **~~Audiometric testing of groups~~**

To report, see (92700)

92560 **~~Bekesy audiometry; screening~~**

To report, see (92700)

92561 **~~diagnostic~~**

To report, see (92700)

92562 **Loudness balance test, alternate binaural or monaural**

INCLUDES ABLB test

1.25 1.25 FUD XXX Q1 80 TC

AMA: 2018,Feb,11; 2018,Jan,8; 2017,Jan,8; 2016,Jan,13

92563 **Tone decay test**

0.86 0.86 FUD XXX Q1 80 TC

AMA: 2018,Feb,11; 2018,Jan,8; 2017,Jan,8; 2016,Jan,13

92564 **~~Short increment sensitivity index (SISI)~~**

To report, see (92700)

92565 **Stenger test, pure tone**

0.44 0.44 FUD XXX Q1 80 TC

AMA: 2018,Feb,11; 2018,Jan,8; 2017,Jan,8; 2016,Jan,13

92567 **Tympanometry (impedance testing)**

0.31 0.45 FUD XXX Q1 80

AMA: 2018,Feb,11; 2018,Jan,8; 2017,Jan,8; 2016,Jan,13

92568 **Acoustic reflex testing, threshold**

0.44 0.45 FUD XXX Q1 80

AMA: 2018,Feb,11; 2018,Jan,8; 2017,Jan,8; 2016,Jan,13

92570 **Acoustic immittance testing, includes tympanometry (impedance testing), acoustic reflex threshold testing, and acoustic reflex decay testing**

INCLUDES Tympanometry, acoustic reflex testing individual codes (92567-92568)

0.85 0.92 FUD XXX Q1 80

AMA: 2018,Feb,11; 2018,Jan,8; 2017,Jan,8; 2016,Jan,13

92571 **Filtered speech test**

0.76 0.76 FUD XXX Q1 80 TC

AMA: 2018,Feb,11; 2018,Jan,8; 2017,Jan,8; 2016,Jan,13

92572 **Staggered spondaic word test**

1.21 1.21 FUD XXX Q1 80 TC

AMA: 2018,Feb,11; 2018,Jan,8; 2017,Jan,8; 2016,Jan,13

92575 **Sensorineural acuity level test**

1.79 1.79 FUD XXX Q1 80 TC

AMA: 2018,Feb,11; 2018,Jan,8; 2017,Jan,8; 2016,Jan,13

92576 **Synthetic sentence identification test**

1.03 1.03 FUD XXX Q1 80 TC

AMA: 2018,Feb,11; 2018,Jan,8; 2017,Jan,8; 2016,Jan,13

92577 **Stenger test, speech**

0.39 0.39 FUD XXX Q1 80 TC

AMA: 2018,Feb,11; 2018,Jan,8; 2017,Jan,8; 2016,Jan,13

92579 **Visual reinforcement audiometry (VRA)**

1.09 1.32 FUD XXX Q1 80

AMA: 2018,Feb,11; 2018,Jan,8; 2017,Jan,8; 2016,Jan,13

92582 **Conditioning play audiometry**

2.06 2.06 FUD XXX Q1 80 TC

AMA: 2018,Feb,11; 2018,Jan,8; 2017,Jan,8; 2016,Jan,13

92583 **Select picture audiometry**

1.35 1.35 FUD XXX Q1 80 TC

AMA: 2018,Feb,11; 2018,Jan,8; 2017,Jan,8; 2016,Jan,13

92584 **Electrocochleography**

2.09 2.09 FUD XXX S 80

AMA: 2018,Feb,11; 2018,Jan,8; 2017,Jan,8; 2016,Jan,13

\# **92650** **Auditory evoked potentials; screening of auditory potential with broadband stimuli, automated analysis**
0.83 0.83 FUD XXX
AMA: 2020,Oct,9

\# **92651** **for hearing status determination, broadband stimuli, with interpretation and report**
EXCLUDES *Auditory evoked potentials, neurodiagnostic ([92653])*
Threshold estimation ([92652])
2.62 2.62 FUD XXX
AMA: 2020,Oct,9

\# **92652** **for threshold estimation at multiple frequencies, with interpretation and report**
EXCLUDES *Hearing status determination ([92651])*
Auditory evoked potentials, neurodiagnostic ([92653])
3.43 3.43 FUD XXX
AMA: 2020,Oct,9

\# **92653** **neurodiagnostic, with interpretation and report**
EXCLUDES *Hearing status determination ([92651])*
Threshold estimation ([92652])
2.51 2.51 FUD XXX
AMA: 2020,Oct,9

\# **92558** **Evoked otoacoustic emissions, screening (qualitative measurement of distortion product or transient evoked otoacoustic emissions), automated analysis**
0.25 0.28 FUD XXX
AMA: 2018,Feb,11; 2018,Jan,8; 2017,Jan,8; 2016,Jan,13

92587 **Distortion product evoked otoacoustic emissions; limited evaluation (to confirm the presence or absence of hearing disorder, 3-6 frequencies) or transient evoked otoacoustic emissions, with interpretation and report**
0.63 0.63 FUD XXX
AMA: 2018,Feb,11; 2018,Jan,8; 2017,Jan,8; 2016,Jan,13

92588 **comprehensive diagnostic evaluation (quantitative analysis of outer hair cell function by cochlear mapping, minimum of 12 frequencies), with interpretation and report**
EXCLUDES *Evaluation central auditory function (92620-92621)*
0.96 0.96 FUD XXX
AMA: 2018,Feb,11; 2018,Jan,8; 2017,Jan,8; 2016,Jan,13

92590 **Hearing aid examination and selection; monaural**
0.00 0.00 FUD XXX
AMA: 2020,Jul,3; 2018,Feb,11; 2018,Jan,8; 2017,Jan,8; 2016,Jan,13

92591 **binaural**
0.00 0.00 FUD XXX
AMA: 2020,Jul,3; 2018,Feb,11; 2018,Jan,8; 2017,Jan,8; 2016,Jan,13

92592 **Hearing aid check; monaural**
0.00 0.00 FUD XXX
AMA: 2020,Jul,3; 2018,Feb,11; 2018,Jan,8; 2017,Jan,8; 2016,Jan,13

92593 **binaural**
0.00 0.00 FUD XXX
AMA: 2020,Jul,3; 2018,Feb,11; 2018,Jan,8; 2017,Jan,8; 2016,Jan,13

92594 **Electroacoustic evaluation for hearing aid; monaural**
0.00 0.00 FUD XXX
AMA: 2020,Jul,3; 2018,Feb,11; 2018,Jan,8; 2017,Jan,8; 2016,Jan,13

92595 **binaural**
0.00 0.00 FUD XXX
AMA: 2020,Jul,3; 2018,Feb,11; 2018,Jan,8; 2017,Jan,8; 2016,Jan,13

92596 **Ear protector attenuation measurements**
1.84 1.84 FUD XXX
AMA: 2018,Feb,11; 2018,Jan,8; 2017,Jan,8; 2016,Jan,13

92597 **Resequenced code. See code following 92604.**

92601-92609 [92597, 92618] Services Related to Hearing and Speech Devices

INCLUDES Diagnostic/treatment services not generally included in comprehensive otorhinolaryngologic evaluation or office visit

92601 **Diagnostic analysis of cochlear implant, patient younger than 7 years of age; with programming**
INCLUDES Connection to cochlear implant
Postoperative analysis/fitting previously placed external devices
Stimulator programming
EXCLUDES *Cochlear implant placement (69930)*
3.57 4.68 FUD XXX
AMA: 2020,Jul,3; 2018,Feb,11; 2018,Jan,8; 2017,Jan,8; 2016,Sep,6; 2016,Jan,13

92602 **subsequent reprogramming**
INCLUDES Internal stimulator re-programming
Subsequent sessions for external transmitter measurements/adjustment
EXCLUDES *Analysis with programming (92601)*
Aural rehabilitation services after cochlear implant (92626-92627, 92630-92633)
Cochlear implant placement (69930)
2.03 2.96 FUD XXX
AMA: 2020,Jul,3; 2018,Feb,11; 2018,Jan,8; 2017,Jan,8; 2016,Sep,6; 2016,Jan,13

92603 **Diagnostic analysis of cochlear implant, age 7 years or older; with programming**
INCLUDES Connection to cochlear implant
Postoperative analysis/fitting previously placed external devices
Stimulator programming
EXCLUDES *Cochlear implant placement (69930)*
3.47 4.37 FUD XXX
AMA: 2020,Jul,3; 2018,Feb,11; 2018,Jan,8; 2017,Jan,8; 2016,Sep,6; 2016,Jan,13

92604 **subsequent reprogramming**
INCLUDES Internal stimulator reprogramming
Subsequent sessions for external transmitter measurements/adjustment
EXCLUDES *Analysis with programming (92603)*
Cochlear implant placement (69930)
1.94 2.64 FUD XXX
AMA: 2020,Jul,3; 2018,Feb,11; 2018,Jan,8; 2017,Jan,8; 2016,Sep,6; 2016,Jan,13

\# **92597** **Evaluation for use and/or fitting of voice prosthetic device to supplement oral speech**
EXCLUDES *Augmentative or alternative communication device services (92605, [92618], 92607-92608)*
2.06 2.06 FUD XXX
AMA: 2018,Feb,11; 2018,Jan,8; 2017,Jan,8; 2016,Jan,13

92605 **Evaluation for prescription of non-speech-generating augmentative and alternative communication device, face-to-face with the patient; first hour**
EXCLUDES *Prosthetic voice device fitting or use evaluation (92597)*
2.53 2.65 FUD XXX
AMA: 2018,Feb,11; 2018,Jan,8; 2017,Jan,8; 2016,Jan,13

\+ # **92618** **each additional 30 minutes (List separately in addition to code for primary procedure)**
Code first (92605)
0.94 0.96 FUD ZZZ
AMA: 2018,Feb,11

92606 **Therapeutic service(s) for the use of non-speech-generating device, including programming and modification**
2.05 2.39 FUD XXX
AMA: 2018,Feb,11; 2018,Jan,8; 2017,Jan,8; 2016,Jan,13

92607 **Evaluation for prescription for speech-generating augmentative and alternative communication device, face-to-face with the patient; first hour**

EXCLUDES *Evaluation for prescription non-speech generating device (92605)*

Evaluation for use/fitting voice prosthetic (92597)

3.66 3.66 FUD XXX A 80

AMA: 2018,Feb,11; 2018,Jan,8; 2017,Jan,8; 2016,Jan,13

+ **92608** **each additional 30 minutes (List separately in addition to code for primary procedure)**

Code first initial hour (92607)

1.47 1.47 FUD ZZZ A 80

AMA: 2018,Feb,11; 2018,Jan,8; 2017,Jan,8; 2016,Jan,13

92609 **Therapeutic services for the use of speech-generating device, including programming and modification**

EXCLUDES *Therapeutic services for use non-speech generating device (92606)*

3.08 3.08 FUD XXX A 80

AMA: 2018,Feb,11; 2018,Jan,8; 2017,Jan,8; 2016,Jan,13

92610-92618 [92618] Swallowing Evaluations

92610 **Evaluation of oral and pharyngeal swallowing function**

EXCLUDES *Evaluation with flexible endoscope (92612-92617)*

Motion fluoroscopic evaluation swallowing function (92611)

2.07 2.47 FUD XXX A 80

AMA: 2018,Feb,11; 2018,Jan,8; 2017,Apr,8; 2017,Jan,8; 2016,Jan,13

92611 **Motion fluoroscopic evaluation of swallowing function by cine or video recording**

EXCLUDES *Diagnostic flexible laryngoscopy (31575)*

Evaluation oral/pharyngeal swallowing function (92610)

(74230)

2.55 2.55 FUD XXX A 80

AMA: 2020,Aug,9; 2018,Feb,11; 2018,Jan,8; 2017,Apr,8; 2017,Jan,8; 2016,Sep,6; 2016,Jan,13

92612 **Flexible endoscopic evaluation of swallowing by cine or video recording;**

EXCLUDES *Diagnostic flexible fiberoptic laryngoscopy (31575)*

Flexible endoscopic examination/testing without cine or video recording (92700)

1.94 5.42 FUD XXX A 80

AMA: 2018,Feb,11; 2018,Jan,8; 2017,Jul,7; 2017,Apr,8; 2017,Jan,8; 2016,Dec,13; 2016,Sep,6; 2016,Jan,13

92613 **interpretation and report only**

EXCLUDES *Diagnostic flexible laryngoscopy (31575)*

Oral/pharyngeal swallowing function examination (92610)

Swallowing function motion fluoroscopic examination (92611)

1.07 1.07 FUD XXX B 80

AMA: 2018,Feb,11; 2018,Jan,8; 2017,Jul,7; 2017,Apr,8; 2017,Jan,8; 2016,Dec,13; 2016,Sep,6; 2016,Jan,13

92614 **Flexible endoscopic evaluation, laryngeal sensory testing by cine or video recording;**

EXCLUDES *Diagnostic flexible laryngoscopy (31575)*

Flexible endoscopic examination/testing without cine or video recording (92700)

1.90 4.03 FUD XXX A 80

AMA: 2018,Feb,11; 2018,Jan,8; 2017,Jul,7; 2017,Apr,8; 2017,Jan,8; 2016,Dec,13; 2016,Sep,6; 2016,Jan,13

92615 **interpretation and report only**

EXCLUDES *Diagnostic flexible laryngoscopy (31575)*

0.95 0.95 FUD XXX E 80

AMA: 2018,Feb,11; 2018,Jan,8; 2017,Jul,7; 2017,Apr,8; 2017,Jan,8; 2016,Dec,13; 2016,Sep,6; 2016,Jan,13

92616 **Flexible endoscopic evaluation of swallowing and laryngeal sensory testing by cine or video recording;**

EXCLUDES *Diagnostic flexible fiberoptic laryngoscopy (31575)*

Flexible endoscopic examination/testing without cine or video recording (92700)

2.84 5.85 FUD XXX A 80

AMA: 2018,Feb,11; 2018,Jan,8; 2017,Jul,7; 2017,Apr,8; 2017,Jan,8; 2016,Dec,13; 2016,Sep,6; 2016,Jan,13

92617 **interpretation and report only**

EXCLUDES *Diagnostic flexible laryngoscopy (31575)*

1.18 1.18 FUD XXX E 80

AMA: 2018,Feb,11; 2018,Jan,8; 2017,Jul,7; 2017,Apr,8; 2017,Jan,8; 2016,Dec,13; 2016,Sep,6; 2016,Jan,13

92618 **Resequenced code. See code following 92605.**

92620-92700 [92650, 92651, 92652, 92653] Diagnostic Hearing Evaluations and Rehabilitation

INCLUDES Diagnostic/treatment services not generally included in comprehensive otorhinolaryngologic evaluation or office visit

92620 **Evaluation of central auditory function, with report; initial 60 minutes**

EXCLUDES *Voice analysis (92521-92524)*

2.33 2.67 FUD XXX Q1 80

AMA: 2018,Feb,11; 2018,Jan,8; 2017,Jan,8; 2016,Jan,13

+ **92621** **each additional 15 minutes (List separately in addition to code for primary procedure)**

EXCLUDES *Voice analysis (92521-92524)*

Code first (92620)

0.54 0.64 FUD ZZZ N 80

AMA: 2018,Feb,11; 2018,Jan,8; 2017,Jan,8; 2016,Jan,13

92625 **Assessment of tinnitus (includes pitch, loudness matching, and masking)**

EXCLUDES *Loudness test (92562)*

Code also modifier 52 for unilateral procedure

1.78 1.99 FUD XXX Q1 80

AMA: 2018,Feb,11; 2018,Jan,8; 2017,Jan,8; 2016,Jan,13

92626 **Evaluation of auditory function for surgically implanted device(s) candidacy or postoperative status of a surgically implanted device(s); first hour**

INCLUDES Assessment to determine patient's proficiency in remaining hearing to identify speech

Face-to-face time spent with patient or family

EXCLUDES *Hearing aid evaluation, fitting, follow-up, or selection (92590-92591, 92592-92593, 92594-92595)*

2.16 2.55 FUD XXX Q1 80

AMA: 2020,Jul,3; 2018,Feb,11; 2018,Jan,8; 2017,Jan,8; 2016,Sep,6; 2016,Jan,13

+ **92627** **each additional 15 minutes (List separately in addition to code for primary procedure)**

INCLUDES Assessment to determine patient's proficiency in remaining hearing to identify speech

Face-to-face time spent with patient or family

EXCLUDES *Hearing aid evaluation, fitting, follow-up, or selection (92590-92591, 92592-92593, 92594-92595)*

Code first initial hour (92626)

0.51 0.64 FUD ZZZ N 80

AMA: 2020,Jul,3; 2018,Feb,11; 2018,Jan,8; 2017,Jan,8; 2016,Sep,6; 2016,Jan,13

92630 **Auditory rehabilitation; prelingual hearing loss**

0.00 0.00 FUD XXX E

AMA: 2018,Feb,11; 2018,Jan,8; 2017,Jan,8; 2016,Sep,6; 2016,Jan,13

92633 **postlingual hearing loss**

0.00 0.00 FUD XXX E

AMA: 2018,Feb,11; 2018,Jan,8; 2017,Jan,8; 2016,Sep,6; 2016,Jan,13

92640 **Diagnostic analysis with programming of auditory brainstem implant, per hour**

EXCLUDES *Nonprogramming services (cardiac monitoring)*

2.74 3.24 FUD XXX S 80

AMA: 2018,Feb,11

92650 **Resequenced code. See code following 92584.**

92651 **Resequenced code. See code following 92584.**

92652 **Resequenced code. See code following 92584.**

92653 **Resequenced code. See code following 92584.**

92700 **Unlisted otorhinolaryngological service or procedure**

INCLUDES Lombard test

0.00 0.00 FUD XXX Q1 80

AMA: 2018,Feb,11; 2018,Jan,8; 2017,Apr,8; 2017,Jan,8; 2016,Sep,6; 2016,Jan,13

92920-92953 [92920, 92921, 92924, 92925, 92928, 92929, 92933, 92934, 92937, 92938, 92941, 92943, 92944] Emergency Cardiac Procedures

92920 **Resequenced code. See code following 92998.**

92921 **Resequenced code. See code following 92998.**

92924 **Resequenced code. See code following 92998.**

92925 **Resequenced code. See code following 92998.**

92928 **Resequenced code. See code following 92998.**

92929 **Resequenced code. See code following 92998.**

92933 **Resequenced code. See code following 92998.**

92934 **Resequenced code. See code following 92998.**

92937 **Resequenced code. See code following 92998.**

92938 **Resequenced code. See code following 92998.**

92941 **Resequenced code. See code following 92998.**

92943 **Resequenced code. See code following 92998.**

92944 **Resequenced code. See code following 92998.**

92950 **Cardiopulmonary resuscitation (eg, in cardiac arrest)**

INCLUDES Cardiac defibrillation

EXCLUDES *Critical care services (99291-99292)*

5.36 9.16 FUD 000 S 80

AMA: 2018,Feb,11; 2018,Jan,8; 2017,Jan,8; 2016,Jan,13

92953 **Temporary transcutaneous pacing**

EXCLUDES *Direction ambulance/rescue personnel by physician or other qualified health care professional (99288)*

0.03 0.03 FUD 000 Q3 80

AMA: 2019,Aug,8; 2018,Feb,11; 2018,Jan,8; 2017,Jan,8; 2016,Jan,13

92960-92961 Cardioversion

92960 **Cardioversion, elective, electrical conversion of arrhythmia; external**

3.13 4.51 FUD 000 S 80

AMA: 2018,Feb,11; 2018,Jan,8; 2017,Jan,8; 2016,Jan,13

92961 **internal (separate procedure)**

EXCLUDES *Device evaluation for implantable defibrillator/multi-lead pacemaker system (93282-93284, 93287, 93289, 93295-93296)*

Electrophysiological studies (93618-93624, 93631, 93640-93642)

Intracardiac ablation (93650-93657, 93662)

7.17 7.17 FUD 000 S

AMA: 2018,Feb,11; 2018,Jan,8; 2017,Jan,8; 2016,Jan,13

92970-92979 [92973, 92974, 92975, 92977, 92978, 92979] Circulatory Assist: External/Internal

EXCLUDES *Atrial septostomy, any method (33741)*

Catheter placement for use in circulatory assist devices (intra-aortic balloon pump) (33970)

92970 **Cardioassist-method of circulatory assist; internal**

5.49 5.49 FUD 000 C 80

AMA: 2018,Feb,11

92971 **external**

2.91 2.91 FUD 000 C 80

AMA: 2018,Feb,11

92973 **Resequenced code. See code following 92998.**

92974 **Resequenced code. See code following 92998.**

92975 **Resequenced code. See code following 92998.**

92977 **Resequenced code. See code following 92998.**

92978 **Resequenced code. See code following 92998.**

92979 **Resequenced code. See code following 92998.**

92986-92990 Percutaneous Procedures of Heart Valves and Septum

EXCLUDES *Atrial septostomy, any method (33741)*

92986 **Percutaneous balloon valvuloplasty; aortic valve**

38.1 38.1 FUD 090 J 80

AMA: 2018,Feb,11; 2018,Jan,8; 2017,Jan,8; 2016,Jan,13

92987 **mitral valve**

39.5 39.5 FUD 090 J 80

AMA: 2018,Feb,11; 2018,Jan,8; 2017,Jan,8; 2016,Jan,13

92990 **pulmonary valve**

31.6 31.6 FUD 090 J 80

AMA: 2018,Feb,11; 2018,Jan,8; 2017,Jan,8; 2016,Jan,13

92997-92998 Percutaneous Angioplasty: Pulmonary Artery

92997 **Percutaneous transluminal pulmonary artery balloon angioplasty; single vessel**

19.0 19.0 FUD 000 J 80

AMA: 2018,Feb,11; 2018,Jan,8; 2017,Jul,3; 2017,Jan,8; 2016,Mar,5; 2016,Jan,13

\+ **92998** **each additional vessel (List separately in addition to code for primary procedure)**

Code first single vessel (92997)

9.44 9.44 FUD ZZZ N 80

AMA: 2018,Feb,11; 2018,Jan,8; 2017,Jul,3; 2017,Jan,8; 2016,Mar,5; 2016,Jan,13

92920-92944 [92920, 92921, 92924, 92925, 92928, 92929, 92933, 92934, 92937, 92938, 92941, 92943, 92944]
Intravascular Coronary Procedures

INCLUDES Accessing vessel
- Additional procedures performed in third branch, major coronary artery
- All procedures performed in all branch segments, coronary arteries
  - Branches left anterior descending (diagonals), left circumflex (marginals), and right (posterior descending, posterolaterals)
  - Distal, proximal, and mid segments
- All procedures performed in all segments, major coronary arteries through native vessels:
  - Distal, proximal, and mid segments
  - Left main, left anterior descending, left circumflex, right, and ramus intermedius arteries
- All procedures performed in major coronary arteries or recognized coronary artery branches through coronary artery bypass graft
  - Sequential bypass graft with more than single distal anastomosis as one graft
  - Branching bypass grafts (e.g., "Y" grafts) include coronary vessel for primary graft, with each branch off primary graft making up an additional coronary vessel
  - Each coronary artery bypass graft denotes single coronary vessel
  - Embolic protection devices when used
- Arteriotomy closure through access sheath
- Atherectomy (e.g., directional, laser, rotational)
- Balloon angioplasty (e.g., cryoplasty, cutting balloon, wired balloons)
- Cardiac catheterization and related procedures when included in coronary revascularization service (93454-93461, 93563-93564)
- Imaging once procedure complete
- Percutaneous coronary interventions (PCI) for coronary vessel disease, native and bypass grafts
- Procedures in left main and ramus intermedius coronary artery branches as they are unrecognized for individual code assignment
- Radiological supervision and interpretation intervention(s)
- Reporting most comprehensive treatment in given vessel according to intensity hierarchy for base and add-on codes:
  - Add-on codes: 92944 = 92938 > 92934 > 92925 > 92929 > 92921
  - Base codes (report only one): 92943 = 92941 = 92933 > 92924 > 92937 = 92928 > 92920
- Revascularization achieved with single procedure when single lesion continues from one target vessel (major artery, branch, or bypass graft) to another target vessel
- Selective vessel catheterization
- Stenting (e.g., balloon expandable, bare metal, covered, drug eluting, self-expanding)
- Traversing lesion

EXCLUDES *Application intravascular radioelements (77770-77772)*
- *Insertion device for coronary intravascular brachytherapy (92974)*
- *Reduction septum (e.g., alcohol ablation) (93799)*

Code also add-on codes for procedures performed during same session in additional recognized target vessel branches

Code also diagnostic angiography during interventional procedure when:
- No previous catheter-based coronary angiography study available, and full diagnostic study performed, with decision to perform intervention based on that study
- Previous study available, but documentation states patient's condition changed since previous study or target area visualization inadequate, or change occurs during procedure warranting additional evaluation outside current target area

Code also diagnostic angiography performed at session separate from interventional procedure

Code also individual base codes for treatment major native coronary artery segment and another segment same artery requiring treatment through bypass graft when performed at same time

Code also procedures for both vessels for bifurcation lesion

Code also procedures performed in second branch major coronary artery

Code also treatment arterial segment requiring access through bypass graft

\# **92920** **Percutaneous transluminal coronary angioplasty; single major coronary artery or branch**

15.4 15.4 FUD 000 J J8 80

AMA: 2018,Feb,11; 2018,Jan,8; 2017,Jul,3; 2017,Jan,8; 2016,Jan,13

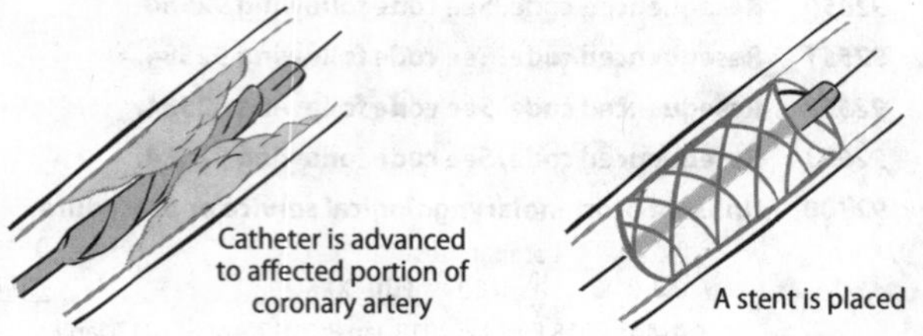
Catheter is advanced to affected portion of coronary artery
A stent is placed

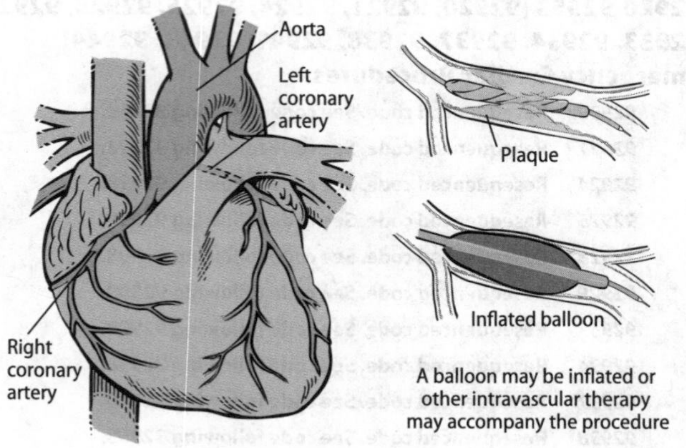
Aorta
Left coronary artery
Plaque
Inflated balloon
Right coronary artery
A balloon may be inflated or other intravascular therapy may accompany the procedure

\+ # **92921** **each additional branch of a major coronary artery (List separately in addition to code for primary procedure)**

Code first (92920, 92924, 92928, 92933, 92937, 92941, 92943)

0.00 0.00 FUD ZZZ N N1

AMA: 2018,Feb,11; 2018,Jan,8; 2017,Jul,3; 2017,Jan,8; 2016,Jan,13

\# **92924** **Percutaneous transluminal coronary atherectomy, with coronary angioplasty when performed; single major coronary artery or branch**

18.4 18.4 FUD 000 J 80

AMA: 2018,Feb,11; 2018,Jan,8; 2017,Jul,3; 2017,Jan,8; 2016,Jan,13

\+ # **92925** **each additional branch of a major coronary artery (List separately in addition to code for primary procedure)**

Code first (92924, 92928, 92933, 92937, 92941, 92943)

0.00 0.00 FUD ZZZ N

AMA: 2018,Feb,11; 2018,Jan,8; 2017,Jul,3; 2017,Jan,8; 2016,Jan,13

\# **92928** **Percutaneous transcatheter placement of intracoronary stent(s), with coronary angioplasty when performed; single major coronary artery or branch**

17.2 17.2 FUD 000 J J8 80

AMA: 2018,Feb,11; 2018,Jan,8; 2017,Jul,3; 2017,Feb,14; 2017,Jan,8; 2017,Jan,6; 2016,Jan,13

\+ # **92929** **each additional branch of a major coronary artery (List separately in addition to code for primary procedure)**

Code first (92928, 92933, 92937, 92941, 92943)

0.00 0.00 FUD ZZZ N N1

AMA: 2018,Feb,11; 2018,Jan,8; 2017,Jul,3; 2017,Jan,8; 2017,Jan,6; 2016,Jan,13

\# **92933** **Percutaneous transluminal coronary atherectomy, with intracoronary stent, with coronary angioplasty when performed; single major coronary artery or branch**

19.3 19.3 FUD 000 J 80

AMA: 2018,Feb,11; 2018,Jan,8; 2017,Jul,3; 2017,Jan,8; 2016,Jan,13

+ # **92934** **each additional branch of a major coronary artery (List separately in addition to code for primary procedure)**
Code first (92933, 92937, 92941, 92943)
0.00 0.00 FUD ZZZ N
AMA: 2018,Feb,11; 2018,Jan,8; 2017,Jul,3; 2017,Jan,8; 2016,Jan,13

92937 **Percutaneous transluminal revascularization of or through coronary artery bypass graft (internal mammary, free arterial, venous), any combination of intracoronary stent, atherectomy and angioplasty, including distal protection when performed; single vessel**
17.2 17.2 FUD 000 J 80
AMA: 2018,Feb,11; 2018,Jan,8; 2017,Jul,3; 2017,Feb,14; 2017,Jan,8; 2016,Jan,13

+ # **92938** **each additional branch subtended by the bypass graft (List separately in addition to code for primary procedure)**
Code first (92937)
0.00 0.00 FUD ZZZ N
AMA: 2018,Feb,11; 2018,Jan,8; 2017,Jul,3; 2017,Jan,8; 2016,Jan,13

92941 **Percutaneous transluminal revascularization of acute total/subtotal occlusion during acute myocardial infarction, coronary artery or coronary artery bypass graft, any combination of intracoronary stent, atherectomy and angioplasty, including aspiration thrombectomy when performed, single vessel**
INCLUDES Aspiration thrombectomy, when performed
Embolic protection
Rheolytic thrombectomy
EXCLUDES *Transcatheter intracoronary infusion supersaturated oxygen therapy [SSO2] (0659T)*
Code also treatment additional vessels, when appropriate (92920-92938, 92943-92944)
19.3 19.3 FUD 000 C 80
AMA: 2020,Jul,13; 2018,Feb,11; 2018,Jan,8; 2017,Jul,3; 2017,Feb,14; 2017,Jan,8; 2016,Jan,13

92943 **Percutaneous transluminal revascularization of chronic total occlusion, coronary artery, coronary artery branch, or coronary artery bypass graft, any combination of intracoronary stent, atherectomy and angioplasty; single vessel**
INCLUDES Antegrade flow deficiency with angiography and clinical criteria indicating chronic total occlusion
19.3 19.3 FUD 000 J 80
AMA: 2018,Feb,11; 2018,Jan,8; 2017,Jul,3; 2017,Jan,8; 2016,Jan,13

+ # **92944** **each additional coronary artery, coronary artery branch, or bypass graft (List separately in addition to code for primary procedure)**
EXCLUDES *Application intravascular radioelements (77770-77772)*
Code first (92924, 92928, 92933, 92937, 92941, 92943)
0.00 0.00 FUD ZZZ N
AMA: 2018,Feb,11; 2018,Jan,8; 2017,Jul,3; 2017,Jan,8; 2016,Jan,13

92973-92979 [92973, 92974, 92975, 92977, 92978, 92979] Additional Coronary Artery Procedures

+ # **92973** **Percutaneous transluminal coronary thrombectomy mechanical (List separately in addition to code for primary procedure)**
EXCLUDES *Aspiration thrombectomy*
Code first (92920, 92924, 92928, 92933, 92937, 92941, 92943, 92975, 93454-93461, 93563-93564)
5.12 5.12 FUD ZZZ N 80
AMA: 2020,Jul,13; 2018,Feb,11; 2018,Jan,8; 2017,Feb,14; 2017,Jan,8; 2016,Jan,13

+ # **92974** **Transcatheter placement of radiation delivery device for subsequent coronary intravascular brachytherapy (List separately in addition to code for primary procedure)**
EXCLUDES *Application intravascular radioelements (77770-77772)*
Code first (92920, 92924, 92928, 92933, 92937, 92941, 92943, 93454-93461)
4.72 4.72 FUD ZZZ N 80
AMA: 2018,Feb,11; 2018,Jan,8; 2017,Feb,14; 2017,Jan,8; 2016,Jan,13

92975 **Thrombolysis, coronary; by intracoronary infusion, including selective coronary angiography**
EXCLUDES *Thrombolysis, cerebral (37195)*
Thrombolysis other than coronary ([37211, 37212, 37213, 37214])
10.9 10.9 FUD 000 C 80
AMA: 2018,Feb,11

92977 **by intravenous infusion**
EXCLUDES *Thrombolysis, cerebral (37195)*
Thrombolysis other than coronary ([37211, 37212, 37213, 37214])
1.51 1.51 FUD XXX T 80
AMA: 2018,Feb,11

+ # **92978** **Endoluminal imaging of coronary vessel or graft using intravascular ultrasound (IVUS) or optical coherence tomography (OCT) during diagnostic evaluation and/or therapeutic intervention including imaging supervision, interpretation and report; initial vessel (List separately in addition to code for primary procedure)**
Code first primary procedure (92920, 92924, 92928, 92933, 92937, 92941, 92943, 92975, 93454-93461, 93563-93564)
0.00 0.00 FUD ZZZ N 80
AMA: 2018,Feb,11; 2018,Jan,8; 2017,Jan,8; 2016,Jan,13

+ # **92979** **each additional vessel (List separately in addition to code for primary procedure)**
INCLUDES Transducer manipulations/repositioning in vessel examined, before and after therapeutic intervention
EXCLUDES *Intravascular spectroscopy (93799)*
Code first initial vessel (92978)
0.00 0.00 FUD ZZZ N 80
AMA: 2018,Feb,11; 2018,Jan,8; 2017,Jan,8; 2016,Jan,13

93000-93010 Electrocardiographic Services

INCLUDES Specific order for service, separate written and signed report, and documentation medical necessity
EXCLUDES *Acoustic cardiography (93799)*
Echocardiography (93303-93350)
Intracardiac ischemia monitoring system (0525T-0532T)
Reporting codes for telemetry monitoring strip review

93000 **Electrocardiogram, routine ECG with at least 12 leads; with interpretation and report**
0.48 0.48 FUD XXX M 80
AMA: 2020,Dec,3; 2018,Feb,11; 2018,Jan,8; 2017,Oct,3; 2017,Jan,8; 2016,Jan,13

93005 **tracing only, without interpretation and report**
0.24 0.24 FUD XXX 01 80 TC
AMA: 2020,Dec,3; 2018,Feb,11; 2018,Jan,8; 2017,Oct,3; 2017,Jan,8; 2016,Apr,8; 2016,Jan,13

93010 **interpretation and report only**
0.24 0.24 **FUD** XXX B 80 26
AMA: 2020,Dec,3; 2018,Feb,11; 2018,Jan,8; 2017,Oct,3; 2017,Jan,8; 2016,Apr,8; 2016,Jan,13

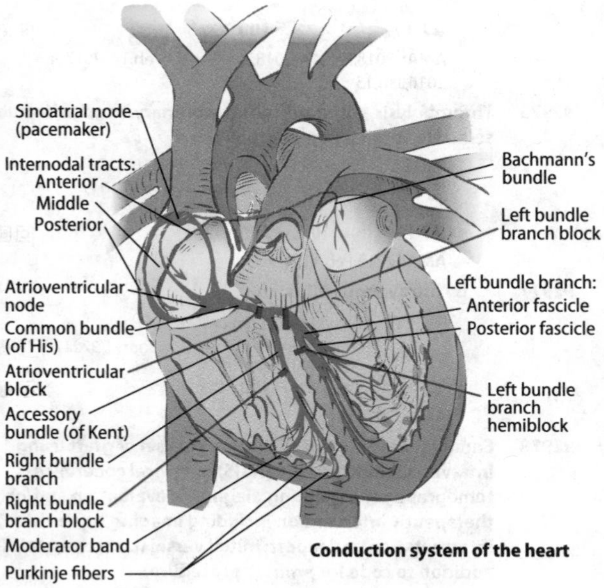

Conduction system of the heart

93015-93018 Stress Test

93015 **Cardiovascular stress test using maximal or submaximal treadmill or bicycle exercise, continuous electrocardiographic monitoring, and/or pharmacological stress; with supervision, interpretation and report**
2.01 2.01 **FUD** XXX B 80
AMA: 2020,Dec,3; 2020,Jul,5; 2018,Feb,11; 2018,Jan,8; 2017,Oct,3; 2017,Jan,8; 2016,Jan,13

93016 **supervision only, without interpretation and report**
0.63 0.63 **FUD** XXX B 80 26
AMA: 2020,Dec,3; 2020,Jul,5; 2018,Feb,11; 2018,Jan,8; 2017,Oct,3; 2017,Jan,8; 2016,Jan,13

93017 **tracing only, without interpretation and report**
0.96 0.96 **FUD** XXX Q1 80 TC
AMA: 2020,Dec,3; 2020,Jul,5; 2018,Feb,11; 2018,Jan,8; 2017,Oct,3; 2017,Jan,8; 2016,Jan,13

93018 **interpretation and report only**
0.42 0.42 **FUD** XXX B 80 26
AMA: 2020,Dec,3; 2020,Jul,5; 2018,Feb,11; 2018,Jan,8; 2017,Oct,3; 2017,Jan,8; 2016,Jan,13

93024 Provocation Test for Coronary Vasospasm

93024 **Ergonovine provocation test**
3.12 3.12 **FUD** XXX Q1 80
AMA: 2018,Feb,11

93025 Microvolt T-Wave Alternans

CMS: 100-03,20.30 Microvolt T-Wave Alternans (MTWA); 100-04,32,370 Microvolt T-wave Alternans; 100-04,32,370.1 Coding and Claims Processing for MTWA; 100-04,32,370.2 Messaging for MTWA

INCLUDES Specific order for service, separate written and signed report, and documentation medical necessity

EXCLUDES *Echocardiography (93303-93350)*
Reporting codes for telemetry monitoring strip review

93025 **Microvolt T-wave alternans for assessment of ventricular arrhythmias**
4.23 4.23 **FUD** XXX S 80
AMA: 2018,Feb,11; 2018,Jan,8; 2017,Jan,8; 2016,Jan,13

93040-93042 Rhythm Strips

INCLUDES Specific order for service, separate written and signed report, and documentation medical necessity

EXCLUDES *Device evaluation ([93261], 93279-93289 [93260], 93291-93296, 93298)*
Echocardiography (93303-93350)
Reporting codes for telemetry monitoring strip review

93040 **Rhythm ECG, 1-3 leads; with interpretation and report**
0.36 0.36 **FUD** XXX B 80
AMA: 2020,Dec,3; 2020,Sep,7; 2018,Feb,11; 2018,Jan,8; 2017,Oct,3; 2017,Jan,8; 2016,Jan,13

93041 **tracing only without interpretation and report**
0.16 0.16 **FUD** XXX Q1 80 TC
AMA: 2020,Dec,3; 2018,Feb,11; 2018,Jan,8; 2017,Oct,3; 2017,Jan,8; 2016,Jan,13

93042 **interpretation and report only**
0.20 0.20 **FUD** XXX B 80 26
AMA: 2020,Dec,3; 2018,Feb,11; 2018,Jan,8; 2017,Oct,3; 2017,Jan,8; 2016,Jan,13

93050 Arterial Waveform Analysis

EXCLUDES *Reporting code with any intra-arterial diagnostic or interventional procedure*

93050 **Arterial pressure waveform analysis for assessment of central arterial pressures, includes obtaining waveform(s), digitization and application of nonlinear mathematical transformations to determine central arterial pressures and augmentation index, with interpretation and report, upper extremity artery, non-invasive**
0.46 0.46 **FUD** XXX Q1 80
AMA: 2018,Feb,11

93224-93227 Holter Monitor

INCLUDES Cardiac monitoring using in-person as well as remote technology for electrocardiographic data assessment
Up to 48 hours recording on continuous basis

EXCLUDES *Echocardiography (93303-93355 [93356])*
Implantable patient activated cardiac event recorders (93285, 93291, 93297-93298)
More than 48 hours monitoring ([93241, 93242, 93243, 93244, 93245, 93246, 93247, 93248])

Code also modifier 52 when less than 12 hours continuous recording provided

93224 **External electrocardiographic recording up to 48 hours by continuous rhythm recording and storage; includes recording, scanning analysis with report, review and interpretation by a physician or other qualified health care professional**
2.51 2.51 **FUD** XXX M 80
AMA: 2020,Nov,10; 2018,Feb,11; 2018,Jan,8; 2017,Jan,8; 2016,Jan,13

93225 **recording (includes connection, recording, and disconnection)**
0.73 0.73 **FUD** XXX Q1 80 TC
AMA: 2020,Nov,10; 2018,Feb,11; 2018,Jan,8; 2017,Jan,8; 2016,Jan,13

93226 **scanning analysis with report**
1.03 1.03 **FUD** XXX Q1 80 TC
AMA: 2020,Nov,10; 2018,Feb,11; 2018,Jan,8; 2017,Jan,8; 2016,Jan,13

93227 **review and interpretation by a physician or other qualified health care professional**
0.75 0.75 **FUD** XXX M 80 26
AMA: 2020,Nov,10; 2018,Mar,5; 2018,Feb,11; 2018,Jan,8; 2017,Jan,8; 2016,Jan,13

93241-93248 [93241, 93242, 93243, 93244, 93245, 93246, 93247, 93248] External Electrocardiographic Recording

INCLUDES Cardiac monitoring using in-person as well as remote technology for electrocardiographic data assessment

EXCLUDES *During same monitoring period:*
External ECG event recording up to 30 days (93268-93272)
External ECG event recording without 24 hour attended monitoring (0497T-0498T)
Remote physiological monitoring, collection and interpretation ([99453, 99454], [99091])
Echocardiography (93303-93355 [93356])
Implantable patient activated cardiac event recorders (93285, 93291, 93297-93298)
Less than 48 hours monitoring (93224-93227)

93241 **External electrocardiographic recording for more than 48 hours up to 7 days by continuous rhythm recording and storage; includes recording, scanning analysis with report, review and interpretation**
EXCLUDES *More than 7 days and up to 15 days monitoring ([93245, 93246, 93247, 93248])*
0.00 0.00 FUD XXX 80

93242 **recording (includes connection and initial recording)**
EXCLUDES *More than 7 days and up to 15 days monitoring ([93245, 93246, 93247, 93248])*
0.44 0.44 FUD XXX 80 TC

93243 **scanning analysis with report**
EXCLUDES *More than 7 days and up to 15 days monitoring ([93245, 93246, 93247, 93248])*
0.00 0.00 FUD XXX 80 TC

93244 **review and interpretation**
EXCLUDES *More than 7 days and up to 15 days monitoring ([93245, 93246, 93247, 93248])*
0.71 0.71 FUD XXX 80 26

93245 **External electrocardiographic recording for more than 7 days up to 15 days by continuous rhythm recording and storage; includes recording, scanning analysis with report, review and interpretation**
EXCLUDES *More than 48 hours up to 7 days monitoring ([93241, 93242, 93243, 93244])*
0.00 0.00 FUD XXX 80

93246 **recording (includes connection and initial recording)**
EXCLUDES *More than 48 hours up to 7 days monitoring ([93241, 93242, 93243, 93244])*
0.44 0.44 FUD XXX 80 TC

93247 **scanning analysis with report**
EXCLUDES *More than 48 hours up to 7 days monitoring ([93241, 93242, 93243, 93244])*
0.00 0.00 FUD XXX 80 TC

93248 **review and interpretation**
EXCLUDES *More than 48 hours up to 7 days monitoring ([93241, 93242, 93243, 93244])*
0.78 0.78 FUD XXX 80 26

93228-93248 [93241, 93242, 93243, 93244, 93245, 93246, 93247, 93248] Remote Cardiovascular Telemetry

INCLUDES Cardiac monitoring using in-person as well as remote technology for electrocardiographic data assessment
Mobile telemetry monitors with capacity to:
Detect arrhythmias
Real-time data analysis for signal quality evaluation quality
Records ECG rhythm on continuous basis using external electrodes on patient
Transmit tracing at any time
Transmit data to attended surveillance center where technician available to respond to device or rhythm alerts and contact physician or qualified health care professional when needed

EXCLUDES *Reporting code more than one time in 30-day period*

93228 **External mobile cardiovascular telemetry with electrocardiographic recording, concurrent computerized real time data analysis and greater than 24 hours of accessible ECG data storage (retrievable with query) with ECG triggered and patient selected events transmitted to a remote attended surveillance center for up to 30 days; review and interpretation with report by a physician or other qualified health care professional**
EXCLUDES *Cardiovascular monitors that do not perform automatic ECG triggered transmissions to attended surveillance center (93224-93227, 93268-93272)*
0.74 0.74 FUD XXX ★ M 80 26
AMA: 2020,Nov,10; 2018,Feb,11; 2018,Jan,8; 2017,Jan,8; 2016,Jan,13

93229 **technical support for connection and patient instructions for use, attended surveillance, analysis and transmission of daily and emergent data reports as prescribed by a physician or other qualified health care professional**
19.9 19.9 FUD XXX ★ S 80 TC
AMA: 2020,Nov,10; 2018,Feb,11; 2018,Jan,8; 2017,Jan,8; 2016,Jan,13

93241 **Resequenced code. See code following 93227.**
93242 **Resequenced code. See code following 93227.**
93243 **Resequenced code. See code following 93227.**
93244 **Resequenced code. See code following 93227.**
93245 **Resequenced code. See code following 93227.**
93246 **Resequenced code. See code following 93227.**
93247 **Resequenced code. See code following 93227.**
93248 **Resequenced code. See code following 93227.**

93260-93272 [93260, 93261, 93264] Event Monitors

INCLUDES ECG rhythm derived elements, which differ from physiologic data and include heart rhythm, rate, ST analysis, heart rate variability, T-wave alternans, among others
Event monitors that:
Record ECGs in response to patient activation or automatic detection algorithm (or both)
Require attended surveillance
Transmit data upon request (although not immediately when activated)

EXCLUDES *Monitoring cardiovascular devices (93279-93289 [93260], 93291-93296, 93298)*

93260 **Resequenced code. See code following 93284.**
93261 **Resequenced code. See code following 93289.**
93264 **Resequenced code. See code before 93279.**

93268 **External patient and, when performed, auto activated electrocardiographic rhythm derived event recording with symptom-related memory loop with remote download capability up to 30 days, 24-hour attended monitoring; includes transmission, review and interpretation by a physician or other qualified health care professional**
EXCLUDES *Implantable patient activated cardiac event recorders (93285, 93291, 93298)*
Subcutaneous cardiac rhythm monitor (33285)
5.70 5.70 FUD XXX ★ M 80
AMA: 2020,Nov,10; 2018,Feb,11; 2018,Jan,8; 2017,Jan,8; 2016,Jan,13

93270 **recording (includes connection, recording, and disconnection)**

0.26 0.26 FUD XXX ★ Q1 80 TC

AMA: 2020,Nov,10; 2018,Feb,11; 2018,Jan,8; 2017,Jan,8; 2016,Jan,13

93271 **transmission and analysis**

4.72 4.72 FUD XXX ★ S 80 TC

AMA: 2020,Nov,10; 2018,Feb,11; 2018,Jan,8; 2017,Jan,8; 2016,Jan,13

93272 **review and interpretation by a physician or other qualified health care professional**

EXCLUDES *Implantable patient activated cardiac event recorders (93285, 93291, 93298)*
Subcutaneous cardiac rhythm monitor (33285)

0.72 0.72 FUD XXX ★ M 80 26

AMA: 2020,Nov,10; 2018,Mar,5; 2018,Feb,11; 2018,Jan,8; 2017,Jan,8; 2016,Jan,13

93278 Signal-averaged Electrocardiography

EXCLUDES *Echocardiography (93303-93355)*

Code also modifier 26 for interpretation and report only

93278 **Signal-averaged electrocardiography (SAECG), with or without ECG**

0.85 0.85 FUD XXX Q1 80

AMA: 2018,Feb,11; 2018,Jan,8; 2017,Jan,8; 2016,Jan,13

93264 [93264] Wireless Pulmonary Artery Pressure Sensor Monitoring

INCLUDES Data collection from internal sensor in pulmonary artery
Downloads, interpretation, analysis, and report that must occur at least one time per week
Transmission and storage of data

EXCLUDES *Reporting code wehn monitoring for less than 30-day period*
Reporting code more than one time in 30 days

93264 **Remote monitoring of a wireless pulmonary artery pressure sensor for up to 30 days, including at least weekly downloads of pulmonary artery pressure recordings, interpretation(s), trend analysis, and report(s) by a physician or other qualified health care professional**

1.03 1.43 FUD XXX 80

AMA: 2020,Feb,7; 2019,Oct,3; 2019,Jun,3

93279-93298 [93260, 93261] Monitoring of Cardiovascular Devices

INCLUDES Implantable cardiovascular monitor (ICM) interrogation:
- Analysis at least one recorded physiologic cardiovascular data element from either internal or external sensors
- Programmed parameters

Implantable defibrillator interrogation:
- Battery
- Capture and sensing functions
- Leads
- Presence or absence therapy for ventricular tachyarrhythmias
- Programmed parameters
- Underlying heart rhythm

Implantable loop recorder (ILR) interrogation:
- Heart rate and rhythm during recorded episodes from both patient-initiated and device detected events
- Programmed parameters

In-person interrogation/device evaluation (93288)
In-person periprocedural device evaluation/programming device system parameters (93286)
Interrogation evaluation device
Pacemaker interrogation:
- Battery
- Capture and sensing functions
- Heart rhythm
- Leads
- Programmed parameters

Time period established by initiation remote monitoring or 91st day implantable defibrillator/pacemaker monitoring or 31st day ILR monitoring and extending for succeeding 30- or 90-day period

EXCLUDES *Wearable device monitoring (93224-93272)*

93279 **Programming device evaluation (in person) with iterative adjustment of the implantable device to test the function of the device and select optimal permanent programmed values with analysis, review and report by a physician or other qualified health care professional; single lead pacemaker system or leadless pacemaker system in one cardiac chamber**

EXCLUDES *External ECG event recording up to 30 days (93268-93272)*
Peri-procedural and interrogation device evaluation (93286, 93288)
Rhythm strips (93040-93042)

Code also body surface-activation mapping, pacemaker or pacing cardioverter-defibrillator lead(s), for electrical synchrony optimization, when performed during same session (0696T)

1.72 1.72 FUD XXX Q1 80

AMA: 2019,Oct,3; 2019,Mar,6; 2018,Feb,11; 2018,Jan,8; 2017,Jan,8; 2016,Aug,5; 2016,May,5; 2016,Jan,13

93280 **dual lead pacemaker system**

EXCLUDES *External ECG event recording up to 30 days (93268-93272)*
Peri-procedural and interrogation device evaluation (93286, 93288)
Rhythm strips (93040-93042)

2.03 2.03 FUD XXX Q1 80

AMA: 2019,Oct,3; 2018,Feb,11; 2018,Jan,8; 2017,Jan,8; 2016,Aug,5; 2016,May,5; 2016,Jan,13

93281 **multiple lead pacemaker system**

EXCLUDES *External ECG event recording up to 30 days (93268-93272)*
Peri-procedural and interrogation device evaluation (93286, 93288)
Rhythm strips (93040-93042)

Code also body surface-activation mapping, pacemaker or pacing cardioverter-defibrillator lead(s), for electrical synchrony optimization, when performed during same session (0696T)

2.17 2.17 FUD XXX Q1 80

AMA: 2019,Oct,3; 2018,Feb,11; 2018,Jan,8; 2017,Jan,8; 2016,Aug,5; 2016,May,5; 2016,Jan,13

93282 single lead transvenous implantable defibrillator system

EXCLUDES *Device evaluation subcutaneous lead defibrillator system (93260)*
External ECG event recording up to 30 days (93268-93272)
Peri-procedural and interrogation device evaluation (93287, 93289)
Rhythm strips (93040-93042)
Wearable cardio-defibrillator system services (93745)

2.08 2.08 FUD XXX Q1 80

AMA: 2019,Oct,3; 2018,Feb,11; 2018,Jan,8; 2017,Jan,8; 2016,Aug,5; 2016,Jan,13

93283 dual lead transvenous implantable defibrillator system

EXCLUDES *External ECG event recording up to 30 days (93268-93272)*
Peri-procedural and interrogation device evaluation (93287, 93289)
Rhythm strips (93040-93042)

2.60 2.60 FUD XXX Q1 80

AMA: 2019,Oct,3; 2018,Feb,11; 2018,Jan,8; 2017,Jan,8; 2016,Aug,5; 2016,Jan,13

93284 multiple lead transvenous implantable defibrillator system

EXCLUDES *External ECG event recording up to 30 days (93268-93272)*
Peri-procedural and interrogation device evaluation (93287, 93289)
Rhythm strips (93040-93042)

Code also body surface-activation mapping, pacemaker or pacing cardioverter-defibrillator lead(s), for electrical synchrony optimization, when performed during same session (0696T)

2.81 2.81 FUD XXX Q1 80

AMA: 2019,Oct,3; 2018,Feb,11; 2018,Jan,8; 2017,Jan,8; 2016,Aug,5; 2016,Jan,13

93260 implantable subcutaneous lead defibrillator system

EXCLUDES *Device evaluation (93261, 93282, 93287)*
External ECG event recording up to 30 days (93268-93272)
Insertion/removal/replacement implantable defibrillator (33240, 33241, [33262], [33270, 33271, 33272, 33273])
Rhythm strips (93040-93042)

2.04 2.04 FUD XXX Q1 80

AMA: 2019,Oct,3; 2018,Feb,11; 2018,Jan,8; 2017,Jan,8; 2016,Aug,5; 2016,Jan,13

93285 subcutaneous cardiac rhythm monitor system

EXCLUDES *Device evaluation (93279-93284, 93291)*
External ECG event recording up to 30 days (93268-93272)
Insertion subcutaneous cardiac rhythm monitor (33285)
Remote programming device evaluation (0650T)
Rhythm strips (93040-93042)

1.52 1.52 FUD XXX Q1 80

AMA: 2019,Oct,3; 2019,Apr,3; 2018,Feb,11; 2018,Jan,8; 2017,Jan,8; 2016,Aug,5; 2016,Jan,13

93286 Peri-procedural device evaluation (in person) and programming of device system parameters before or after a surgery, procedure, or test with analysis, review and report by a physician or other qualified health care professional; single, dual, or multiple lead pacemaker system, or leadless pacemaker system

INCLUDES One evaluation and programming (if performed once before and once after, report as two units)

EXCLUDES *Device evaluation (93279-93281, 93288)*
External ECG event recording up to 30 days (93268-93272)
Rhythm strips (93040-93042)
Services related to cardiac contractility modulation systems (0408T-0411T, 0414T-0415T)
Subcutaneous implantable defibrillator peri-procedural device evaluation and programming (93260, 93261)

Code also body surface-activation mapping, pacemaker or pacing cardioverter-defibrillator lead(s), for electrical synchrony optimization, when performed during same session (0696T)

1.14 1.14 FUD XXX N 80

AMA: 2019,Oct,3; 2019,Mar,6; 2018,Feb,11; 2018,Jan,8; 2017,Jan,8; 2016,Aug,5; 2016,May,5; 2016,Jan,13

93287 single, dual, or multiple lead implantable defibrillator system

INCLUDES One evaluation and programming (if performed once before and once after, report as two units)

EXCLUDES *Device evaluation (93282-93284, 93289)*
External ECG event recording up to 30 days (93268-93272)
Rhythm strips (93040-93042)
Services related to cardiac contractility modulation systems (0408T-0411T, 0414T-0415T)
Subcutaneous implantable defibrillator peri-procedural device evaluation and programming (93260, 93261)

Code also body surface-activation mapping, pacemaker or pacing cardioverter-defibrillator lead(s), for electrical synchrony optimization, when performed during same session (0696T)

1.36 1.36 FUD XXX N 80

AMA: 2019,Oct,3; 2018,Feb,11; 2018,Jan,8; 2017,Jan,8; 2016,Aug,5; 2016,May,5; 2016,Jan,13

93288 Interrogation device evaluation (in person) with analysis, review and report by a physician or other qualified health care professional, includes connection, recording and disconnection per patient encounter; single, dual, or multiple lead pacemaker system, or leadless pacemaker system

EXCLUDES *Device evaluation (93279-93281, 93286, 93294-93295)*
External ECG event recording up to 30 days (93268-93272)
Rhythm strips (93040-93042)

Code also body surface-activation mapping, pacemaker or pacing cardioverter-defibrillator lead(s), for electrical synchrony optimization, when performed during same session (0696T)

1.39 1.39 FUD XXX Q1 80

AMA: 2019,Oct,3; 2019,Mar,6; 2018,Feb,11; 2018,Jan,8; 2017,Jan,8; 2016,Aug,5; 2016,May,5; 2016,Jan,13

93289 single, dual, or multiple lead transvenous implantable defibrillator system, including analysis of heart rhythm derived data elements

EXCLUDES *Monitoring physiologic cardiovascular data elements derived from implantable defibrillator (93290)*
Device evaluation (93261, 93282-93284, 93287, 93295-93296)
External ECG event recording up to 30 days (93268-93272)
Rhythm strips (93040-93042)

Code also body surface-activation mapping, pacemaker or pacing cardioverter-defibrillator lead(s), for electrical synchrony optimization, when performed during same session (0696T)

1.87 1.87 FUD XXX Q1 80

AMA: 2019,Oct,3; 2018,Feb,11; 2018,Jan,8; 2017,Jan,8; 2016,Aug,5; 2016,May,5; 2016,Jan,13

\# **93261** **implantable subcutaneous lead defibrillator system**

EXCLUDES *Device evaluation (93260, 93287, 93289)*
External ECG event recording up to 30 days (93268-93272)
Insertion/removal/replacement implantable defibrillator (33240, 33241, [33262], [33270, 33271, 33272, 33273])
Rhythm strips (93040-93042)

1.87 1.87 FUD XXX

AMA: 2019,Oct,3; 2018,Feb,11; 2018,Jan,8; 2017,Jan,8; 2016,Aug,5; 2016,Jan,13

93290 **implantable cardiovascular physiologic monitor system, including analysis of 1 or more recorded physiologic cardiovascular data elements from all internal and external sensors**

EXCLUDES *Device evaluation (93297)*
Heart rhythm derived data (93289)

1.34 1.34 FUD XXX

AMA: 2020,Feb,7; 2019,Oct,3; 2018,Feb,11; 2018,Jan,8; 2017,Jan,8; 2016,Aug,5; 2016,Jan,13

93291 **subcutaneous cardiac rhythm monitor system, including heart rhythm derived data analysis**

EXCLUDES *Device evaluation (93288-93290 [93261], 93298)*
External ECG event recording up to 30 days (93268-93272)
Insertion subcutaneous cardiac rhythm monitor (33285)
Remote programming device evaluation subcutaneous cardiac rhythm monitor system (0650T)
Rhythm strips (93040-93042)

1.22 1.22 FUD XXX

AMA: 2019,Oct,3; 2019,Apr,3; 2018,Feb,11; 2018,Jan,8; 2017,Jan,8; 2016,Aug,5; 2016,Jan,13

93292 **wearable defibrillator system**

EXCLUDES *External ECG event recording up to 30 days (93268-93272)*
Rhythm strips (93040-93042)
Wearable cardioverter-defibrillator system (93745)

1.14 1.14 FUD XXX

AMA: 2019,Oct,3; 2018,Feb,11; 2018,Jan,8; 2017,Jan,8; 2016,Aug,5; 2016,Jan,13

93293 **Transtelephonic rhythm strip pacemaker evaluation(s) single, dual, or multiple lead pacemaker system, includes recording with and without magnet application with analysis, review and report(s) by a physician or other qualified health care professional, up to 90 days**

EXCLUDES *Device evaluation (93294)*
External ECG event recording up to 30 days (93268-93272)
Rhythm strips (93040-93042)
Reporting code more than one time in 90-day period
Reporting code when monitoring period less than 30 days

1.46 1.46 FUD XXX

AMA: 2019,Oct,3; 2018,Feb,11; 2018,Jan,8; 2017,Jan,8; 2016,Aug,5; 2016,Jan,13

93294 **Interrogation device evaluation(s) (remote), up to 90 days; single, dual, or multiple lead pacemaker system, or leadless pacemaker system with interim analysis, review(s) and report(s) by a physician or other qualified health care professional**

EXCLUDES *Device evaluation (93288, 93293)*
External ECG event recording up to 30 days (93268-93272)
Rhythm strips (93040-93042)
Reporting code more than one time in 90-day period
Reporting code when monitoring period less than 30 days

0.87 0.87 FUD XXX M 80 26

AMA: 2019,Oct,3; 2019,Mar,6; 2018,Feb,11; 2018,Jan,8; 2017,Jan,8; 2016,Aug,5; 2016,Jan,13

93295 **single, dual, or multiple lead implantable defibrillator system with interim analysis, review(s) and report(s) by a physician or other qualified health care professional**

EXCLUDES *Device evaluation (93289)*
External ECG event recording up to 30 days (93268-93272)
Remote interrogation device evaluation implantable cardioverter-defibrillator with substernal lead (0578T, 0579T)
Remote monitoring physiological cardiovascular data (93297)
Rhythm strips (93040-93042)
Reporting code more than one time in 90-day period
Reporting code when monitoring period less than 30 days

1.26 1.26 FUD XXX M 80 26

AMA: 2019,Oct,3; 2018,Feb,11; 2018,Jan,8; 2017,Jan,8; 2016,Aug,5; 2016,Jan,13

93296 **single, dual, or multiple lead pacemaker system, leadless pacemaker system, or implantable defibrillator system, remote data acquisition(s), receipt of transmissions and technician review, technical support and distribution of results**

EXCLUDES *Device evaluation (93288-93289)*
External ECG event recording up to 30 days (93268-93272)
Remote interrogation device evaluation implantable cardioverter-defibrillator with substernal lead (0578T, 0579T)
Rhythm strips (93040-93042)
Reporting code more than one time in 90-day period
Reporting code when monitoring period less than 30 days

0.72 0.72 FUD XXX 01 80 TC

AMA: 2019,Oct,3; 2019,Mar,6; 2019,Jan,6; 2018,Feb,11; 2018,Jan,8; 2017,Jan,8; 2016,Aug,5; 2016,Jan,13

93297 **Interrogation device evaluation(s), (remote) up to 30 days; implantable cardiovascular physiologic monitor system, including analysis of 1 or more recorded physiologic cardiovascular data elements from all internal and external sensors, analysis, review(s) and report(s) by a physician or other qualified health care professional**

EXCLUDES *Collection and interpretation physiologic data digitally stored and/or transmitted ([99091])*
Device evaluation (93290, 93298)
Heart rhythm derived data (93295)
Remote monitoring physiologic parameter(s) with daily recording(s) or programmed alert(s) ([99454])
Remote monitoring wireless pulmonary artery pressure sensor (93264)
Reporting code more than one time in 30-day period
Reporting code when monitoring period less than 10 days

Code also for technical component (G2066)

0.75 0.75 FUD XXX M 80 26

AMA: 2020,Feb,12; 2019,Oct,3; 2018,Feb,11; 2018,Jan,8; 2017,Jan,8; 2016,Aug,5; 2016,Jan,13

93298 **subcutaneous cardiac rhythm monitor system, including analysis of recorded heart rhythm data, analysis, review(s) and report(s) by a physician or other qualified health care professional**

EXCLUDES *Collection and interpretation physiologic data digitally stored and/or transmitted ([99091])*
Device evaluation (93291, 93297)
External ECG event recording up to 30 days (93268-93272)
Implantation patient-activated cardiac event recorder (33285)
Remote monitoring physiologic parameter(s) with daily recording(s) or programmed alert(s) ([99454])

Code also for technical component (G2066)
Reporting code more than one time in 30-day period
Reporting code when monitoring period less than 10 days
Rhythm strips (93040-93042)

0.75 0.75 **FUD** XXX M 80 26

AMA: 2020,Feb,12; 2019,Oct,3; 2019,Apr,3; 2018,Feb,11; 2018,Jan,8; 2017,Jan,8; 2016,Aug,5; 2016,Jan,13

93303-93356 [93319, 93356] Echocardiography

INCLUDES Interpretation and report
Obtaining ultrasonic signals from heart/great arteries
Report study including:
Description recognized abnormalities
Documentation all clinically relevant findings including obtained quantitative measurements
Interpretation all information obtained
Two-dimensional image/doppler ultrasonic signal documentation
Ultrasound exam:
Adjacent great vessels
Cardiac chambers/valves
Pericardium

EXCLUDES *Contrast agents and/or drugs used for pharmacological stress*
Echocardiography, fetal (76825-76828)
Ultrasound with thorough examination organ(s) or anatomic region/documentation image/final written report

93303 **Transthoracic echocardiography for congenital cardiac anomalies; complete**

6.58 6.58 **FUD** XXX S 80

AMA: 2020,Jul,12; 2020,Apr,10; 2020,Jan,7; 2018,Feb,11; 2018,Jan,8; 2017,Jan,8; 2016,Jan,13

93304 **follow-up or limited study**

4.52 4.52 **FUD** XXX S 80

AMA: 2020,Jul,12; 2020,Jan,7; 2018,Feb,11; 2018,Jan,8; 2017,Jan,8; 2016,Jan,13

93306 **Echocardiography, transthoracic, real-time with image documentation (2D), includes M-mode recording, when performed, complete, with spectral Doppler echocardiography, and with color flow Doppler echocardiography**

INCLUDES Doppler and color flow
Two-dimensional and M-mode

EXCLUDES *Transthoracic without spectral and color doppler (93307)*

5.86 5.86 **FUD** XXX S 80

AMA: 2020,Jul,12; 2020,May,12; 2020,Jan,7; 2018,Dec,10; 2018,Dec,10; 2018,Feb,11; 2018,Jan,8; 2017,Jan,8; 2016,Apr,8; 2016,Jan,13

93307 **Echocardiography, transthoracic, real-time with image documentation (2D), includes M-mode recording, when performed, complete, without spectral or color Doppler echocardiography**

INCLUDES Additional structures that may be viewed such as pulmonary vein or artery, pulmonic valve, inferior vena cava
Obtaining/recording appropriate measurements
Two-dimensional/selected M-mode exam:
Adjacent portions aorta
Aortic/mitral/tricuspid valves
Left/right atria
Left/right ventricles
Pericardium
Using multiple views as required to obtain complete functional/anatomic evaluation

EXCLUDES *Doppler echocardiography (93320-93321, 93325)*

3.97 3.97 **FUD** XXX S 80

AMA: 2020,Jul,12; 2020,May,12; 2020,Jan,7; 2018,Feb,11; 2018,Jan,8; 2017,Jan,8; 2016,Apr,8; 2016,Jan,13

93308 **Echocardiography, transthoracic, real-time with image documentation (2D), includes M-mode recording, when performed, follow-up or limited study**

INCLUDES Exam that does not evaluate/document attempt to evaluate all structures comprising complete echocardiographic exam

2.79 2.79 **FUD** XXX S 80

AMA: 2020,Jul,12; 2020,May,12; 2020,Jan,7; 2018,Dec,10; 2018,Dec,10; 2018,Feb,11; 2018,Jan,8; 2017,Jan,8; 2016,Apr,8; 2016,Jan,13

93312 **Echocardiography, transesophageal, real-time with image documentation (2D) (with or without M-mode recording); including probe placement, image acquisition, interpretation and report**

EXCLUDES *Transesophageal echocardiography (93355)*

6.96 6.96 **FUD** XXX S 80

AMA: 2020,Jan,7; 2018,Feb,11; 2018,Jan,8; 2017,Jan,8; 2016,Jan,13

93313 **placement of transesophageal probe only**

EXCLUDES *Procedure when performed by same person performing transesophageal echocardiography (93355)*

0.33 0.33 **FUD** XXX S 80

AMA: 2020,Jan,7; 2018,Feb,11; 2018,Jan,8; 2017,Jan,8; 2016,Jan,13

93314 **image acquisition, interpretation and report only**

EXCLUDES *Transesophageal echocardiography (93355)*

6.68 6.68 **FUD** XXX N 80

AMA: 2020,Jan,7; 2018,Feb,11; 2018,Jan,8; 2017,Jan,8; 2016,Jan,13

93315 **Transesophageal echocardiography for congenital cardiac anomalies; including probe placement, image acquisition, interpretation and report**

EXCLUDES *Transesophageal echocardiography (93355)*

0.00 0.00 **FUD** XXX S 80

AMA: 2020,Jan,7; 2018,Feb,11; 2018,Jan,8; 2017,Jan,8; 2016,Jan,13

93316 **placement of transesophageal probe only**

EXCLUDES *Transesophageal echocardiography (93355)*

0.79 0.79 **FUD** XXX S 80

AMA: 2020,Jan,7; 2018,Feb,11; 2018,Jan,8; 2017,Jan,8; 2016,Jan,13

93317 **image acquisition, interpretation and report only**

EXCLUDES *Transesophageal echocardiography (93355)*

0.00 0.00 **FUD** XXX N 80

AMA: 2020,Jan,7; 2018,Feb,11; 2018,Jan,8; 2017,Jan,8; 2016,Jan,13

● + # **93319** **3D echocardiographic imaging and postprocessing during transesophageal echocardiography, or during transthoracic echocardiography for congenital cardiac anomalies, for the assessment of cardiac structure(s) (eg, cardiac chambers and valves, left atrial appendage, interatrial septum, interventricular septum) and function, when performed (List separately in addition to code for echocardiographic imaging)**

EXCLUDES *3D rendering (76376, 76377)*

Doppler echocardiography color flow velocity mapping (93325)

Echocardiography, transesophageal (TEE) for guidance (93355)

Code first (93303-93304, 93312, 93314-93315, 93317)

0.00 0.00 **FUD** 000

93318 **Echocardiography, transesophageal (TEE) for monitoring purposes, including probe placement, real time 2-dimensional image acquisition and interpretation leading to ongoing (continuous) assessment of (dynamically changing) cardiac pumping function and to therapeutic measures on an immediate time basis**

EXCLUDES *Transesophageal echocardiography (93355)*

0.00 0.00 **FUD** XXX S 80

AMA: 2020,Jan,7; 2018,Feb,11; 2018,Jan,8; 2017,Jan,8; 2016,Jan,13

93319 **Resequenced code. See code following 93317.**

\+ **93320** **Doppler echocardiography, pulsed wave and/or continuous wave with spectral display (List separately in addition to codes for echocardiographic imaging); complete**

EXCLUDES *Transesophageal echocardiography (93355)*

Code first (93303-93304, 93312, 93314-93315, 93317, 93350-93351)

1.51 1.51 **FUD** ZZZ N 80

AMA: 2020,May,12; 2020,Jan,7; 2018,Feb,11; 2018,Jan,8; 2017,Jan,8; 2016,Jan,13

\+ **93321** **follow-up or limited study (List separately in addition to codes for echocardiographic imaging)**

EXCLUDES *Transesophageal echocardiography (93355)*

Code first (93303-93304, 93308, 93312, 93314-93315, 93317, 93350-93351)

0.75 0.75 **FUD** ZZZ N 80

AMA: 2020,Jan,7; 2018,Feb,11; 2018,Jan,8; 2017,Jan,8; 2016,Jan,13

\+ **93325** **Doppler echocardiography color flow velocity mapping (List separately in addition to codes for echocardiography)**

EXCLUDES *Transesophageal echocardiography (93355)*

Code first (76825-76828, 93303-93304, 93308, 93312, 93314-93315, 93317, 93350-93351)

0.70 0.70 **FUD** ZZZ N 80

AMA: 2020,May,12; 2020,Jan,7; 2018,Feb,11; 2018,Jan,8; 2017,Jan,8; 2016,Jul,8; 2016,Jan,13

93350 **Echocardiography, transthoracic, real-time with image documentation (2D), includes M-mode recording, when performed, during rest and cardiovascular stress test using treadmill, bicycle exercise and/or pharmacologically induced stress, with interpretation and report;**

EXCLUDES *Cardiovascular stress test, complete procedure (93015)*

Code also exercise stress testing (93016-93018)

5.31 5.31 **FUD** XXX S 80

AMA: 2020,Jul,12; 2018,Feb,11; 2018,Jan,8; 2017,Jan,8; 2016,Apr,8; 2016,Jan,13

93351 **including performance of continuous electrocardiographic monitoring, with supervision by a physician or other qualified health care professional**

INCLUDES Stress echocardiogram performed with complete cardiovascular stress test

EXCLUDES *Cardiovascular stress test (93015-93018)*

Echocardiography (93350)

Professional only components complete stress test and stress echocardiogram performed in facility by same physician, append modifier 26

Reporting code for professional component (modifier 26 appended) with (93016, 93018, 93350)

Code also components cardiovascular stress test when professional services not performed by same physician performing stress echocardiogram (93016-93018)

6.57 6.57 **FUD** XXX S

AMA: 2020,Jul,12; 2018,Feb,11; 2018,Jan,8; 2017,Jan,8; 2016,Apr,8; 2016,Jan,13

\+ # **93356** **Myocardial strain imaging using speckle tracking-derived assessment of myocardial mechanics (List separately in addition to codes for echocardiography imaging)**

EXCLUDES *Reporting code more than one time for each session*

Code first (93303-93304, 93306, 93307, 93308, 93350-93351)

0.34 1.13 **FUD** ZZZ 80

AMA: 2020,Jul,12; 2020,Apr,10

\+ **93352** **Use of echocardiographic contrast agent during stress echocardiography (List separately in addition to code for primary procedure)**

EXCLUDES *Reporting code more than one time for each stress echocardiogram*

Code first (93350, 93351)

0.95 0.95 **FUD** ZZZ M 80

AMA: 2018,Feb,11; 2018,Jan,8; 2017,Jan,8; 2016,Jan,13

93355 **Echocardiography, transesophageal (TEE) for guidance of a transcatheter intracardiac or great vessel(s) structural intervention(s) (eg,TAVR, transcatheter pulmonary valve replacement, mitral valve repair, paravalvular regurgitation repair, left atrial appendage occlusion/closure, ventricular septal defect closure) (peri-and intra-procedural), real-time image acquisition and documentation, guidance with quantitative measurements, probe manipulation, interpretation, and report, including diagnostic transesophageal echocardiography and, when performed, administration of ultrasound contrast, Doppler, color flow, and 3D**

EXCLUDES *3D rendering (76376-76377)*

Doppler echocardiography (93320-93321, 93325)

Transesophageal echocardiography (93312-93318)

Transesophageal probe positioning by different provider (93313)

6.49 6.49 **FUD** XXX N 80

AMA: 2018,Feb,11

93356 **Resequenced code. See code following 93351.**

93451-93505 Heart Catheterization

INCLUDES Access site imaging and placement closure device
Catheter insertion and positioning
Contrast injection (except as listed below)
Imaging and insertion closure device
Radiology supervision and interpretation
Roadmapping angiography

EXCLUDES *Congenital cardiac catheterization procedures (93593-93597)*

Code also separately identifiable:
Aortography (93567)
Noncardiac angiography (see radiology and vascular codes)
Pulmonary angiography (93568)
Right ventricular or atrial injection (93566)

93451 Right heart catheterization including measurement(s) of oxygen saturation and cardiac output, when performed

INCLUDES Cardiac output review
Insertion catheter into one or more right cardiac chambers or areas
Obtaining samples for blood gas

EXCLUDES *Catheterization procedures including right side heart (93453, 93456-93457, 93460-93461)*
Implantation wireless pulmonary artery pressure sensor (33289)
Indicator dilution studies (93598)
Percutaneous repair congenital interatrial defect (93580)
Swan-Ganz catheter insertion (93503)
Transcatheter implantation interatrial septal shunt device, percutaneous approach (0613T)
Transcatheter left ventricular restoration device implantation ([0643T])
Transcatheter ultrasound ablation nerves innervating pulmonary arteries, percutaneous approach (0632T)
Valve repair or annulus reconstruction (33418, 0345T, 0483T, 0484T, 0544T, 0545T)

Code also administration medication or exercise to repeat assessment hemodynamic measurement (93463-93464)

23.9 23.9 **FUD** 000 J G2 80

AMA: 2019,Jun,3; 2019,Mar,6; 2018,Dec,10; 2018,Dec,10; 2018,Feb,11; 2018,Jan,8; 2017,Dec,13; 2017,Jul,3; 2017,Jan,8; 2016,Mar,5; 2016,Jan,13

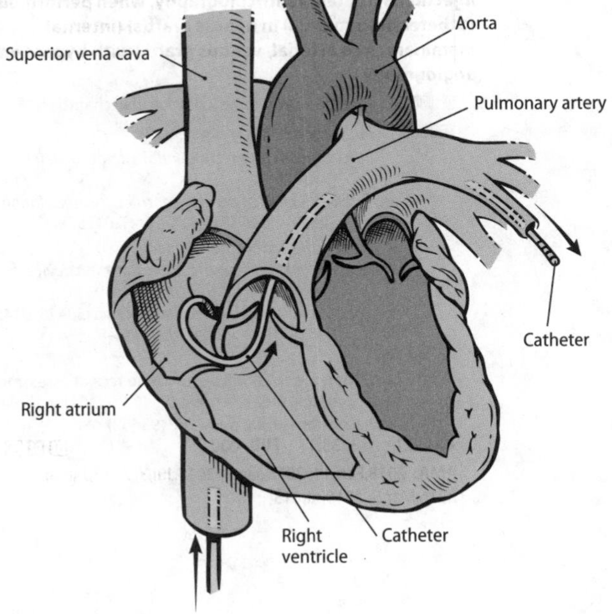

93452 Left heart catheterization including intraprocedural injection(s) for left ventriculography, imaging supervision and interpretation, when performed

INCLUDES Insertion catheter into left cardiac chambers

EXCLUDES *Catheterization procedures including injections for left ventriculography (93453, 93458-93461)*
Indicator dilution studies (93598)
Percutaneous repair congenital interatrial defect (93580)
Services related to cardiac contractility modulation systems (0408T-0411T, 0414T-0415T)
Swan-Ganz catheter insertion (93503)
Transcatheter left ventricular restoration device implantation ([0643T])
Valve repair or annulus reconstruction (33418, 0345T, 0483T, 0484T, 0544T, 0545T)

Code also:
Administration medication or exercise to repeat assessment hemodynamic measurement (93463-93464)
Transapical or transseptal puncture (93462)

25.9 25.9 **FUD** 000 J G2 80

AMA: 2018,Feb,11; 2018,Jan,8; 2017,Jul,3; 2017,Jan,8; 2016,Jan,13

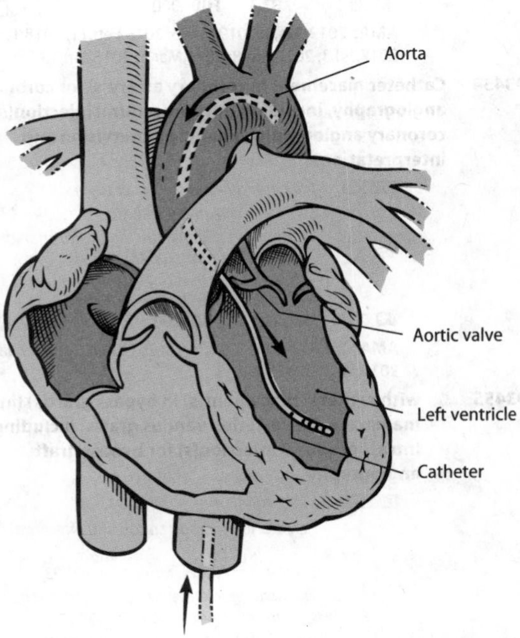

93453 **Combined right and left heart catheterization including intraprocedural injection(s) for left ventriculography, imaging supervision and interpretation, when performed**

INCLUDES Cardiac output review
Insertion catheter into left cardiac chambers
Insertion catheter into one or more right cardiac chambers or areas
Obtaining samples for blood gas

EXCLUDES *Catheterization procedures (93451-93452, 93456-93461)*
Indicator dilution studies (93598)
Percutaneous repair congenital interatrial defect (93580)
Services related to cardiac contractility modulation systems (0408T-0411T, 0414T-0415T)
Swan-Ganz catheter insertion (93503)
Transcatheter left ventricular restoration device implantation ([0643T])
Valve repair or annulus reconstruction (33418, 0345T, 0483T, 0484T, 0544T, 0545T)

Code also:
Administration medication or exercise to repeat assessment hemodynamic measurement (93463-93464)
Transapical or transseptal puncture (93462)

Facility RVU 33.3 Non-Facility RVU 33.3 FUD 000 J G2 80

AMA: 2019,Jun,3; 2019,Mar,6; 2018,Feb,11; 2018,Jan,8; 2017,Jul,3; 2017,Jan,8; 2016,Mar,5; 2016,Jan,13

93454 **Catheter placement in coronary artery(s) for coronary angiography, including intraprocedural injection(s) for coronary angiography, imaging supervision and interpretation;**

EXCLUDES *Indicator dilution studies (93598)*
Swan-Ganz catheter insertion (93503)
Transcatheter left ventricular restoration device implantation ([0643T])
Valve repair or annulus reconstruction (33418, 0345T, 0483T, 0484T, 0544T, 0545T)

Facility RVU 25.9 Non-Facility RVU 25.9 FUD 000 J G2 80

AMA: 2018,Feb,11; 2018,Jan,8; 2017,Feb,14; 2017,Jan,8; 2016,Mar,5; 2016,Jan,13

93455 **with catheter placement(s) in bypass graft(s) (internal mammary, free arterial, venous grafts) including intraprocedural injection(s) for bypass graft angiography**

EXCLUDES *Indicator dilution studies (93598)*
Percutaneous repair congenital interatrial defect (93580)
Swan-Ganz catheter insertion (93503)
Transcatheter left ventricular restoration device implantation ([0643T])
Valve repair or annulus reconstruction (33418, 0345T, 0483T, 0484T, 0544T, 0545T)

Facility RVU 28.6 Non-Facility RVU 28.6 FUD 000 J G2 80

AMA: 2018,Feb,11; 2018,Jan,8; 2017,Jan,8; 2016,Mar,5; 2016,Jan,13

93456 **with right heart catheterization**

INCLUDES Cardiac output review
Insertion catheter into one or more right cardiac chambers or areas
Obtaining samples for blood gas

EXCLUDES *Indicator dilution studies (93598)*
Percutaneous repair congenital interatrial defect (93580)
Swan-Ganz catheter insertion (93503)
Transcatheter left ventricular restoration device implantation ([0643T])
Valve repair or annulus reconstruction (33418, 0345T, 0483T, 0484T, 0544T, 0545T)

Code also administration medication or exercise to repeat assessment hemodynamic measurement (93463-93464)

Facility RVU 32.8 Non-Facility RVU 32.8 FUD 000 J G2 80

AMA: 2019,Jun,3; 2019,Mar,6; 2018,Feb,11; 2018,Jan,8; 2017,Jul,3; 2017,Jan,8; 2016,Mar,5; 2016,Jan,13

93457 **with catheter placement(s) in bypass graft(s) (internal mammary, free arterial, venous grafts) including intraprocedural injection(s) for bypass graft angiography and right heart catheterization**

INCLUDES Cardiac output review
Insertion catheter into one more right cardiac chambers or areas
Obtaining samples for blood gas

EXCLUDES *Indicator dilution studies (93598)*
Percutaneous repair congenital interatrial defect (93580)
Swan-Ganz catheter insertion (93503)
Transcatheter left ventricular restoration device implantation ([0643T])
Valve repair or annulus reconstruction (33418, 0345T, 0483T, 0484T, 0544T, 0545T)

Code also administration medication or exercise to repeat assessment hemodynamic measurement (93463-93464)

Facility RVU 36.4 Non-Facility RVU 36.4 FUD 000 J G2 80

AMA: 2019,Jun,3; 2019,Mar,6; 2018,Feb,11; 2018,Jan,8; 2017,Jan,8; 2016,Mar,5; 2016,Jan,13

93458 **with left heart catheterization including intraprocedural injection(s) for left ventriculography, when performed**

INCLUDES Insertion catheter into left cardiac chambers

EXCLUDES *Indicator dilution studies (93598)*
Percutaneous repair congenital interatrial defect (93580)
Services related to cardiac contractility modulation systems (0408T-0411T, 0414T-0415T)
Swan-Ganz catheter insertion (93503)
Transcatheter left ventricular restoration device implantation ([0643T])
Valve repair or annulus reconstruction (33418, 0345T, 0483T, 0484T, 0544T, 0545T)

Code also:
Administration medication or exercise to repeat assessment hemodynamic measurement (93463-93464)
Transapical or transseptal puncture (93462)

Facility RVU 30.4 Non-Facility RVU 30.4 FUD 000 J G2 80

AMA: 2018,Feb,11; 2018,Jan,8; 2017,Jul,3; 2017,Jan,8; 2016,Mar,5; 2016,Jan,13

93459 **with left heart catheterization including intraprocedural injection(s) for left ventriculography, when performed, catheter placement(s) in bypass graft(s) (internal mammary, free arterial, venous grafts) with bypass graft angiography**

INCLUDES Insertion catheter into left cardiac chambers

EXCLUDES *Indicator dilution studies (93598)*
Percutaneous repair congenital interatrial defect (93580)
Services related to cardiac contractility modulation systems (0408T-0411T, 0414T-0415T)
Swan-Ganz catheter insertion (93503)
Transcatheter left ventricular restoration device implantation ([0643T])
Valve repair or annulus reconstruction (33418, 0345T, 0483T, 0484T, 0544T, 0545T)

Code also:
Administration medication or exercise to repeat assessment hemodynamic measurement (93463-93464)
Transapical or transseptal puncture (93462)

Facility RVU 33.1 Non-Facility RVU 33.1 FUD 000 J G2 80

AMA: 2018,Feb,11; 2018,Jan,8; 2017,Jul,3; 2017,Jan,8; 2016,Mar,5; 2016,Jan,13

93460 **with right and left heart catheterization including intraprocedural injection(s) for left ventriculography, when performed**

INCLUDES Cardiac output review
Insertion catheter into left cardiac chambers
Insertion catheter into one or more right cardiac chambers or areas
Obtaining samples for blood gas

EXCLUDES *Indicator dilution studies (93598)*
Percutaneous repair congenital interatrial defect (93580)
Services related to cardiac contractility modulation systems (0408T-0411T, 0414T-0415T)
Swan-Ganz catheter insertion (93503)
Transcatheter left ventricular restoration device implantation ([0643T])
Valve repair or annulus reconstruction (33418, 0345T, 0483T, 0484T, 0544T, 0545T)

Code also:
Administration medication or exercise to repeat assessment hemodynamic measurement (93463-93464)
Transapical or transseptal puncture (93462)

36.6 36.6 FUD 000 J G2 80

AMA: 2019,Jun,3; 2019,Mar,6; 2018,Feb,11; 2018,Jan,8; 2017,Jul,3; 2017,Jan,8; 2016,Mar,5; 2016,Jan,13

93461 **with right and left heart catheterization including intraprocedural injection(s) for left ventriculography, when performed, catheter placement(s) in bypass graft(s) (internal mammary, free arterial, venous grafts) with bypass graft angiography**

INCLUDES Cardiac output review
Insertion catheter into left cardiac chambers
Insertion catheter into one or more right cardiac chambers or areas
Obtaining samples for blood gas

EXCLUDES *Indicator dilution studies (93598)*
Percutaneous repair congenital interatrial defect (93580)
Services related to cardiac contractility modulation systems (0408T-0411T, 0414T-0415T)
Swan-Ganz catheter insertion (93503)
Transcatheter left ventricular restoration device implantation ([0643T])
Valve repair or annulus reconstruction (33418, 0345T, 0483T, 0484T, 0544T, 0545T)

Code also:
Administration medication or exercise to repeat assessment hemodynamic measurement (93463-93464)
Transapical or transseptal puncture (93462)

41.0 41.0 FUD 000 J G2 80

AMA: 2019,Jun,3; 2019,Mar,6; 2018,Feb,11; 2018,Jan,8; 2017,Jul,3; 2017,Jan,8; 2016,Mar,5; 2016,Jan,13

\+ **93462** **Left heart catheterization by transseptal puncture through intact septum or by transapical puncture (List separately in addition to code for primary procedure)**

INCLUDES Insertion catheter into left cardiac chambers

EXCLUDES *Comprehensive electrophysiologic evaluation (93656)*
Transseptal approach for percutaneous closure paravalvular leak (93590)
Valve repair or annulus reconstruction unless performed with transapical puncture (33418, 0345T, 0544T)

Code also, when performed:
Percutaneous closure paravalvular leak when transapical puncture (93590-93591)
Percutaneous closure ventricular septal defect (93581)

Code first (33477, 33741, 33745, 93452-93453, 93458-93461, 93582, 93595-93597, 93653-93654)

6.11 6.11 FUD ZZZ N N1 80

AMA: 2020,Nov,7; 2018,Feb,11; 2018,Jan,8; 2017,Sep,3; 2017,Jul,3; 2017,Jan,8; 2016,Jan,13

\+ **93463** **Pharmacologic agent administration (eg, inhaled nitric oxide, intravenous infusion of nitroprusside, dobutamine, milrinone, or other agent) including assessing hemodynamic measurements before, during, after and repeat pharmacologic agent administration, when performed (List separately in addition to code for primary procedure)**

EXCLUDES *Coronary interventional procedures (92920-92944, 92975, 92977)*
Reporting code more than one time per catheterization

Code first (33477, 93451-93453, 93456-93461, 93580-93582, 93593-93597)

2.82 2.82 FUD ZZZ N 80

AMA: 2018,Feb,11; 2018,Jan,8; 2017,Jan,8; 2016,Jan,13

\+ **93464** **Physiologic exercise study (eg, bicycle or arm ergometry) including assessing hemodynamic measurements before and after (List separately in addition to code for primary procedure)**

EXCLUDES *Administration of pharmacologic agent (93463)*
Reporting code more than one time per catheterization

Code first (33477, 93451-93453, 93456-93461, 93593-93597)

6.89 6.89 FUD ZZZ N 80

AMA: 2018,Feb,11; 2018,Jan,8; 2017,Jan,8; 2016,Jan,13

93503 **Insertion and placement of flow directed catheter (eg, Swan-Ganz) for monitoring purposes**

EXCLUDES *Diagnostic cardiac catheterization (93451-93461, 93593-93594)*
Subsequent monitoring (99356-99357)
Transcatheter ultrasound ablation nerves innervating pulmonary arteries, percutaneous approach (0632T)

2.55 2.55 FUD 000 T 80

AMA: 2018,Feb,11; 2018,Jan,8; 2017,Jan,8; 2016,Jan,13

93505 **Endomyocardial biopsy**

EXCLUDES *Cardiac blood pool imaging (78472-78473, 78481)*
Transcatheter insertion brachytherapy delivery device (92974)

20.1 20.1 FUD 000 T 80

AMA: 2018,Feb,11; 2018,Jan,8; 2017,Dec,13; 2017,Jan,8; 2016,Jan,13

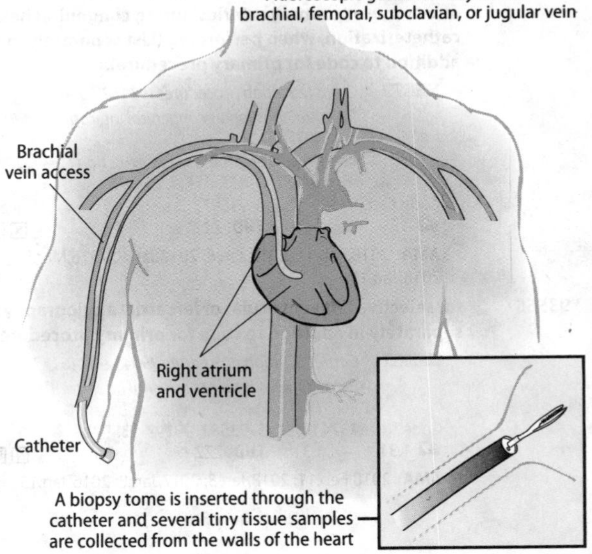
Fluoroscopic guidance may be via brachial, femoral, subclavian, or jugular vein
Brachial vein access
Right atrium and ventricle
Catheter
A biopsy tome is inserted through the catheter and several tiny tissue samples are collected from the walls of the heart

93530-93533 Congenital Heart Defect Catheterization

93530 ~~**Right heart catheterization, for congenital cardiac anomalies**~~

To report, see (93593-93594)

~~93531 Combined right heart catheterization and retrograde left heart catheterization, for congenital cardiac anomalies~~

To report, see (93462, 93596-93597)

~~93532 Combined right heart catheterization and transseptal left heart catheterization through intact septum with or without retrograde left heart catheterization, for congenital cardiac anomalies~~

To report, see (93462, 93596-93597)

~~93533 Combined right heart catheterization and transseptal left heart catheterization through existing septal opening, with or without retrograde left heart catheterization, for congenital cardiac anomalies~~

To report, see (93462, 93596-93597)

93561-93568 Injection Procedures

INCLUDES Automatic power injector
Catheter repositioning
Radiology supervision and interpretation

~~93561 Indicator dilution studies such as dye or thermodilution, including arterial and/or venous catheterization; with cardiac output measurement (separate procedure)~~

To report, see (93598)

~~93562 subsequent measurement of cardiac output~~

To report, see (93598)

\+ **93563 Injection procedure during cardiac catheterization including imaging supervision, interpretation, and report; for selective coronary angiography during congenital heart catheterization (List separately in addition to code for primary procedure)**

EXCLUDES *Catheterization procedures (93452-93461)*
Valve repair or annulus reconstruction (33418, 0345T, 0483T, 0484T, 0544T, 0545T)

Code first (33741, 33745, 93582, 93593-93597)

Facility RVU 1.69 Non-Facility RVU 1.69 FUD ZZZ N 80

AMA: 2018,Feb,11; 2018,Jan,8; 2017,Jan,8; 2016,Mar,5; 2016,Jan,13

\+ **93564 for selective opacification of aortocoronary venous or arterial bypass graft(s) (eg, aortocoronary saphenous vein, free radial artery, or free mammary artery graft) to one or more coronary arteries and in situ arterial conduits (eg, internal mammary), whether native or used for bypass to one or more coronary arteries during congenital heart catheterization, when performed (List separately in addition to code for primary procedure)**

EXCLUDES *Catheterization procedures (93452-93461)*
Percutaneous repair congenital interatrial defect (93580)
Valve repair or annulus reconstruction (33418, 0345T, 0483T, 0484T, 0544T, 0545T)

Code first (93582, 93593-93597)

Facility RVU 1.79 Non-Facility RVU 1.79 FUD ZZZ N 80

AMA: 2018,Feb,11; 2018,Jan,8; 2017,Jan,8; 2016,Mar,5; 2016,Jan,13

\+ **93565 for selective left ventricular or left atrial angiography (List separately in addition to code for primary procedure)**

EXCLUDES *Catheterization procedures (93452-93461)*
Percutaneous repair congenital interatrial defect (93580)

Code first (33741, 33745, 93582, 93593-93597)

Facility RVU 1.31 Non-Facility RVU 1.31 FUD ZZZ N 80

AMA: 2018,Feb,11; 2018,Jan,8; 2017,Jan,8; 2016,Jan,13

\+ **93566 for selective right ventricular or right atrial angiography (List separately in addition to code for primary procedure)**

EXCLUDES *Annulus reconstruction (0545T)*
Percutaneous repair congenital interatrial defect (93580)
Right ventriculography when performed during insertion leadless pacemaker ([33274])

Code first (33741, 33745, 93451, 93453, 93456-93457, 93460-93461, 93582, 93593-93597)

Facility RVU 1.35 Non-Facility RVU 4.38 FUD ZZZ N N1 80

AMA: 2019,Mar,6; 2018,Feb,11; 2018,Jan,8; 2017,Jan,8; 2016,Aug,5; 2016,May,5; 2016,Mar,5; 2016,Jan,13

\+ **93567 for supravalvular aortography (List separately in addition to code for primary procedure)**

EXCLUDES *Abdominal aortography or non-supravalvular thoracic aortography at same time as cardiac catheterization (36221, 75600-75630)*

Code first (33741, 33745, 93451-93461, 93593-93597)

Facility RVU 1.53 Non-Facility RVU 3.71 FUD ZZZ N N1 80

AMA: 2018,Feb,11; 2018,Jan,8; 2017,Jan,8; 2016,Mar,5; 2016,Jan,13

\+ **93568 for pulmonary angiography (List separately in addition to code for primary procedure)**

EXCLUDES *Transcatheter ultrasound ablation nerves innervating pulmonary arteries, percutaneous approach (0632T)*

Code first (33741, 33745, 93451, 93453, 93456-93457, 93460-93461, 93580-93583, 93593-93597)

Facility RVU 1.38 Non-Facility RVU 3.97 FUD ZZZ N N1 80

AMA: 2019,Jun,3; 2019,Apr,10; 2018,Feb,11; 2018,Jan,8; 2017,Jan,8; 2016,Mar,5; 2016,Jan,13

93571-93572 Coronary Artery Doppler Studies

INCLUDES Doppler transducer manipulations/repositioning within vessel examined, during coronary angiography/therapeutic intervention (angioplasty)

EXCLUDES *Intraprocedural coronary fractional flow reserve (FFR) ([0523T])*

\+ **93571 Intravascular Doppler velocity and/or pressure derived coronary flow reserve measurement (coronary vessel or graft) during coronary angiography including pharmacologically induced stress; initial vessel (List separately in addition to code for primary procedure)**

Code first ([92920], [92924], [92928], [92933], [92937], [92941], [92943], [92975], 93454-93461, 93563-93564, 93593-93597)

Facility RVU 0.00 Non-Facility RVU 0.00 FUD ZZZ N N1 80

AMA: 2018,Feb,11; 2018,Jan,8; 2017,Jan,8; 2016,Jan,13

\+ **93572 each additional vessel (List separately in addition to code for primary procedure)**

Code first initial vessel (93571)

Facility RVU 0.00 Non-Facility RVU 0.00 FUD ZZZ N N1 80

AMA: 2018,Feb,11; 2018,Jan,8; 2017,Jan,8; 2016,Jan,13

93580-93583 Percutaneous Repair of Congenital Heart Defects

93580 Percutaneous transcatheter closure of congenital interatrial communication (ie, Fontan fenestration, atrial septal defect) with implant

INCLUDES Injection contrast for atrial/ventricular angiograms (93565-93566)
Right heart catheterization (93451, 93456-93457, 93593-93594)

EXCLUDES *Left heart catheterization (93452, 93458-93459, 93595)*
Measurement cardiac output (93598)
Other contrast injections (93563-93564, 93567-93568)
Right and left heart catheterization (93453, 93460-93461, 93596-93597)

Code also echocardiography, when performed (93303-93317, 93662)

Facility RVU 28.4 Non-Facility RVU 28.4 FUD 000 J 80

AMA: 2018,Feb,11; 2018,Jan,8; 2017,Jan,8; 2016,Jan,13

93581 **Percutaneous transcatheter closure of a congenital ventricular septal defect with implant**

INCLUDES Injection contrast for atrial/ventricular angiograms (93565-93566)
Right heart catheterization (93451, 93456-93457, 93593-93594)

EXCLUDES *Left heart catheterization (93452, 93458-93459, 93595)*
Measurement cardiac output (93598)
Other contrast injections (93563-93564, 93567-93568)
Right and left heart catheterization (93453, 93460-93461, 93596-93597)

Code also echocardiography, when performed (93303-93317, 93662)

38.7 38.7 FUD 000 J 80

AMA: 2018,Feb,11; 2018,Jan,8; 2017,Jan,8; 2016,Jan,13

93582 **Percutaneous transcatheter closure of patent ductus arteriosus**

INCLUDES Aorta catheter placement (36200)
Aortography (75600-75605, 93567)
Heart catheterization (93451, 93453, 93456-93461, 93593-93598)

EXCLUDES *Catheterization pulmonary artery (36013-36014)*
Intracardiac echocardiographic services (93662)
Ligation repair (33820, 33822, 33824)
Other cardiac angiographic procedures (93563-93566, 93568)
Other echocardiographic services by different provider (93315-93317)

19.4 19.4 FUD 000 J 80

AMA: 2019,Apr,10; 2018,Feb,11; 2018,Jan,8; 2017,Jan,8; 2016,Jan,13

93583 **Percutaneous transcatheter septal reduction therapy (eg, alcohol septal ablation) including temporary pacemaker insertion when performed**

INCLUDES Alcohol injection (93463)
Coronary angiography during procedure to roadmap, guide intervention, measure vessel, and complete angiography (93454-93461, 93563, 93563, 93565)
Left heart catheterization (93452-93453, 93458-93461, 93595-93597)
Temporary pacemaker insertion (33210-33211)

EXCLUDES *Intracardiac echocardiographic services when performed (93662)*
Myectomy (surgical ventriculomyotomy) to treat idiopathic hypertrophic subaortic stenosis (33416)
Other echocardiographic services rendered by different provider (93312-93317)

Code also diagnostic cardiac catheterization procedures if patient's condition (clinical indication) changed since intervention or prior study, no available prior catheter-based diagnostic study in treatment zone, or prior study not adequate (93451, 93454-93457, 93563-93564, 93566-93568, 93593-93594, 93598)

21.6 21.6 FUD 000 C 80

AMA: 2018,Feb,11

93590-93592 Percutaneous Repair Paravalvular Leak

INCLUDES Access with insertion and positioning of device
Angiography
Fluoroscopy (76000)
Imaging guidance
Left heart catheterization (93452-93453, 93458-93461, 93565, 93595-93597)

Code also diagnostic cardiac catheterization procedures if patient's condition (clinical indication) changed since intervention or prior study, no available prior catheter-based diagnostic study in treatment zone, or prior study not adequate; append modifier 59 (93451, 93454-93457, 93563-93564, 93593-93594, 93598)

93590 **Percutaneous transcatheter closure of paravalvular leak; initial occlusion device, mitral valve**

INCLUDES Transseptal puncture (93462)

Code also for transapical puncture/left heart catheterization, when performed (93462)

31.2 31.2 FUD 000 J 80

AMA: 2018,Feb,11; 2018,Jan,8; 2017,Sep,3

93591 **initial occlusion device, aortic valve**

Code also for transapical puncture/left heart catheterization, when performed (93462)

25.7 25.7 FUD 000 J 80

AMA: 2018,Feb,11; 2018,Jan,8; 2017,Sep,3

+ **93592** **each additional occlusion device (List separately in addition to code for primary procedure)**

Code first (93590-93591)

11.3 11.3 FUD ZZZ N 80

AMA: 2018,Feb,11; 2018,Jan,8; 2017,Sep,3

93593-93598 Cardiac Catheterization for Congenital Heart Defects

INCLUDES Access site imaging and placement closure device
Cardiac output review
Evaluation anomalous coronary arteries arising from pulmonary arterial system
Insertion catheter into one or more right cardiac chambers or areas
Obtaining samples for blood gas
Radiologic supervision and interpretation
Roadmapping angiography

EXCLUDES *Angiography/ventriculography (93565-93566)*
Angiography native coronary arteries/bypass arteries during same operative session (93563-93564)
Cardiac cath on noncongenital heart (93451-93453, 93456-93461)
Contrast injections (93563-93568)
Percutaneous repair congenital interarterial defect (93580)
Swan-Ganz catheter insertion (93503)

Code also, when performed:
Pharmacologic agent administration (93463)
Physiologic exercise study during procedure (93464)
Transapical or transseptal access (93462)

● **93593** **Right heart catheterization for congenital heart defect(s) including imaging guidance by the proceduralist to advance the catheter to the target zone; normal native connections**

● **93594** **abnormal native connections**

● **93595** **Left heart catheterization for congenital heart defect(s) including imaging guidance by the proceduralist to advance the catheter to the target zone, normal or abnormal native connections**

● **93596** **Right and left heart catheterization for congenital heart defect(s) including imaging guidance by the proceduralist to advance the catheter to the target zone(s); normal native connections**

● **93597** **abnormal native connections**

● + **93598** **Cardiac output measurement(s), thermodilution or other indicator dilution method, performed during cardiac catheterization for the evaluation of congenital heart defects (List separately in addition to code for primary procedure)**

Code first (93593-93597)

0.00 0.00 FUD 000

93600-93603 Recording of Intracardiac Electrograms

INCLUDES Unusual situations in which there may be recording/pacing/attempt at arrhythmia induction from only one side heart

EXCLUDES *Comprehensive electrophysiological studies (93619-93620, 93653-93654, 93656)*

93600 **Bundle of His recording**

0.00 0.00 FUD 000 ⊘ J 80

AMA: 2018,Feb,11; 2018,Jan,8; 2017,Jan,8; 2016,Jan,13

93602 **Intra-atrial recording**

0.00 0.00 FUD 000 ⊘ J 80

AMA: 2018,Feb,11; 2018,Jan,8; 2017,Jan,8; 2016,Jan,13

93603 **Right ventricular recording**

0.00 0.00 FUD 000 ⊘ J 80

AMA: 2018,Feb,11; 2018,Jan,8; 2017,Jan,8; 2016,Jan,13

93609-93613 Intracardiac Mapping and Pacing

\+ **93609** **Intraventricular and/or intra-atrial mapping of tachycardia site(s) with catheter manipulation to record from multiple sites to identify origin of tachycardia (List separately in addition to code for primary procedure)**

EXCLUDES *Intracardiac 3D mapping (93613)*
Intracardiac ablation with 3D mapping (93654)

Code first (93620, 93653, 93656)

0.00   0.00   **FUD** ZZZ   N 80

AMA: 2018,Feb,11; 2018,Jan,8; 2017,Jan,8; 2016,Jan,13

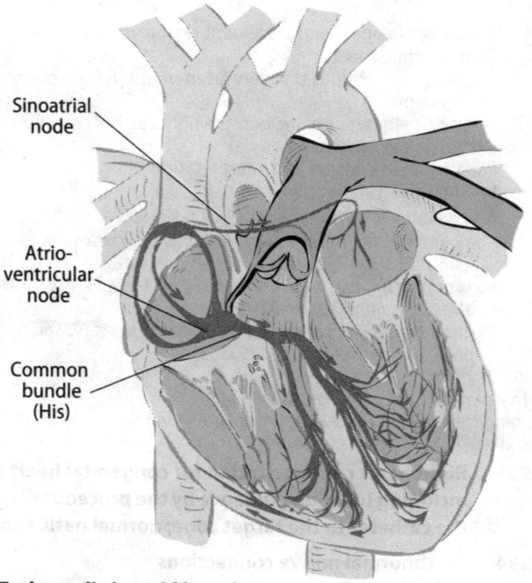

Tachycardia is rapid heartbeat

93610 **Intra-atrial pacing**

INCLUDES Unusual situations in which there may be recording/pacing/attempt at arrhythmia induction from only one side heart

EXCLUDES *Comprehensive electrophysiological studies (93619-93620)*
Intracardiac ablation (93653-93654, 93656)

0.00   0.00   **FUD** 000   J 80

AMA: 2018,Feb,11; 2018,Jan,8; 2017,Jan,8; 2016,Jan,13

93612 **Intraventricular pacing**

INCLUDES Unusual situations in which there may be recording/pacing/attempt at arrhythmia induction from only one side heart

EXCLUDES *Comprehensive electrophysiological studies (93619-93622)*
Intracardiac ablation (93653-93654, 93656)

0.00   0.00   **FUD** 000   J 80

AMA: 2018,Feb,11; 2018,Jan,8; 2017,Jan,8; 2016,Jan,13

\+ **93613** **Intracardiac electrophysiologic 3-dimensional mapping (List separately in addition to code for primary procedure)**

EXCLUDES *Intracardiac ablation with 3D mapping (93654)*
Mapping tachycardia site (93609)

Code first (93620)

8.63   8.63   **FUD** ZZZ   N 80

AMA: 2018,Feb,11; 2018,Jan,8; 2017,Jan,8; 2016,Jan,13

93615-93616 Recording and Pacing via Esophagus

93615 **Esophageal recording of atrial electrogram with or without ventricular electrogram(s);**

0.00   0.00   **FUD** 000   J 80

AMA: 2018,Feb,11; 2018,Jan,8; 2017,Jan,8; 2016,Jan,13

93616 **with pacing**

0.00   0.00   **FUD** 000   J 80

AMA: 2018,Feb,11; 2018,Jan,8; 2017,Jan,8; 2016,Jan,13

93618 Pacing to Produce an Arrhythmia

CMS: 100-03,20.12 Diagnostic Endocardial Electrical Stimulation (Pacing)

INCLUDES Unusual situations in which there may be recording/pacing/attempt at arrhythmia induction from only one side heart

EXCLUDES *Comprehensive electrophysiological studies (93619-93622)*
Intracardiac ablation (93653-93654, 93656)
Intracardiac phonocardiogram (93799)

93618 **Induction of arrhythmia by electrical pacing**

0.00   0.00   **FUD** 000   J 80

AMA: 2018,Feb,11; 2018,Jan,8; 2017,Jan,8; 2016,Jan,13

93619-93623 Comprehensive Electrophysiological Studies

CMS: 100-03,20.12 Diagnostic Endocardial Electrical Stimulation (Pacing)

93619 **Comprehensive electrophysiologic evaluation with right atrial pacing and recording, right ventricular pacing and recording, His bundle recording, including insertion and repositioning of multiple electrode catheters, without induction or attempted induction of arrhythmia**

INCLUDES Evaluation sinus node/atrioventricular node/His-Purkinje conduction system without arrhythmia induction

EXCLUDES *Comprehensive electrophysiological studies (93620-93622)*
Intracardiac ablation (93653-93657)
Intracardiac pacing (93610, 93612, 93618)
Recording intracardiac electrograms (93600-93603)

0.00   0.00   **FUD** 000   J 80

AMA: 2018,Feb,11; 2018,Jan,8; 2017,Jan,8; 2016,Jan,13

93620 **Comprehensive electrophysiologic evaluation including insertion and repositioning of multiple electrode catheters with induction or attempted induction of arrhythmia; with right atrial pacing and recording, right ventricular pacing and recording, His bundle recording**

INCLUDES Recording/pacing/attempted arrhythmia induction from one or more site(s) in heart

EXCLUDES *Comprehensive electrophysiological study without induction/attempted induction arrhythmia (93619)*
Intracardiac ablation (93653-93657)
Intracardiac pacing (93610, 93612, 93618)
Recording intracardiac electrograms (93600-93603)

0.00   0.00   **FUD** 000   J 80

AMA: 2018,Feb,11; 2018,Jan,8; 2017,Jan,8; 2016,Jan,13

\+ **93621** **with left atrial pacing and recording from coronary sinus or left atrium (List separately in addition to code for primary procedure)**

INCLUDES Recording/pacing/attempted arrhythmia induction from one or more site(s) in heart

EXCLUDES *Intracardiac ablation (93656)*

Code first (93620)

0.00   0.00   **FUD** ZZZ   N 80

AMA: 2018,Feb,11; 2018,Jan,8; 2017,Jan,8; 2016,Jan,13

\+ **93622** **with left ventricular pacing and recording (List separately in addition to code for primary procedure)**

EXCLUDES *Intracardiac ablation (93654)*

Code first (93620, 93653, 93656)

0.00   0.00   **FUD** ZZZ   N 80

AMA: 2018,Feb,11; 2018,Jan,8; 2017,Jan,8; 2016,Jan,13

\+ **93623** **Programmed stimulation and pacing after intravenous drug infusion (List separately in addition to code for primary procedure)**

INCLUDES Recording/pacing/attempted arrhythmia induction from one or more site(s) in heart

EXCLUDES *Reporting code more than one time per day*

Code first comprehensive electrophysiologic evaluation (93610, 93612, 93619-93620, 93653-93654, 93656)

0.00   0.00   **FUD** ZZZ   N 80

AMA: 2018,Feb,11; 2018,Jan,8; 2017,Jan,8; 2016,Jan,13

93624-93631 Followup and Intraoperative Electrophysiologic Studies

CMS: 100-03,20.12 Diagnostic Endocardial Electrical Stimulation (Pacing)

93624 **Electrophysiologic follow-up study with pacing and recording to test effectiveness of therapy, including induction or attempted induction of arrhythmia**

INCLUDES Recording/pacing/attempted arrhythmia induction from one or more site(s) in heart

0.00 0.00 **FUD** 000 J 80

AMA: 2018,Feb,11; 2018,Jan,8; 2017,Jan,8; 2016,Jan,13

93631 **Intra-operative epicardial and endocardial pacing and mapping to localize the site of tachycardia or zone of slow conduction for surgical correction**

EXCLUDES *Operative ablation arrhythmogenic focus or pathway by separate provider (33250-33261)*

0.00 0.00 **FUD** 000 N 80

AMA: 2018,Feb,11; 2018,Jan,8; 2017,Jan,8; 2016,Jan,13

93640-93644 Electrophysiologic Studies of Cardioverter-Defibrillators

INCLUDES Recording/pacing/attempted arrhythmia induction from one or more site(s) in heart

93640 **Electrophysiologic evaluation of single or dual chamber pacing cardioverter-defibrillator leads including defibrillation threshold evaluation (induction of arrhythmia, evaluation of sensing and pacing for arrhythmia termination) at time of initial implantation or replacement;**

0.00 0.00 **FUD** 000 N 80

AMA: 2018,Feb,11; 2018,Jan,8; 2017,Jan,8; 2016,Jan,13

93641 **with testing of single or dual chamber pacing cardioverter-defibrillator pulse generator**

EXCLUDES *Single/dual chamber pacing cardioverter-defibrillators reprogramming/electronic analysis, subsequent/periodic (93282-93283, 93289, 93292, 93295, 93642)*

0.00 0.00 **FUD** 000 N 80

AMA: 2018,Feb,11; 2018,Jan,8; 2017,Jan,8; 2016,Jan,13

93642 **Electrophysiologic evaluation of single or dual chamber transvenous pacing cardioverter-defibrillator (includes defibrillation threshold evaluation, induction of arrhythmia, evaluation of sensing and pacing for arrhythmia termination, and programming or reprogramming of sensing or therapeutic parameters)**

9.78 9.78 **FUD** 000 J 80

AMA: 2018,Feb,11; 2018,Jan,8; 2017,Jan,8; 2016,Jan,13

93644 **Electrophysiologic evaluation of subcutaneous implantable defibrillator (includes defibrillation threshold evaluation, induction of arrhythmia, evaluation of sensing for arrhythmia termination, and programming or reprogramming of sensing or therapeutic parameters)**

EXCLUDES *Electrophysiological evaluation subcutaneous implantable defibrillator system with substernal electrode (0577T)*

Insertion/replacement subcutaneous implantable defibrillator ([33270])

Subcutaneous cardioverter-defibrillator electrophysiologic evaluation, subsequent/periodic (93260-93261)

5.63 5.63 **FUD** 000 N 80

AMA: 2018,Feb,11

93650-93657 Intracardiac Ablation

INCLUDES Ablation services include selective delivery cryo-energy or radiofrequency to targeted tissue

Electrophysiologic studies performed in same session with ablation

93650 **Intracardiac catheter ablation of atrioventricular node function, atrioventricular conduction for creation of complete heart block, with or without temporary pacemaker placement**

17.2 17.2 **FUD** 000 J 80

AMA: 2018,Feb,11; 2018,Jan,8; 2017,Jan,8; 2016,Jan,13

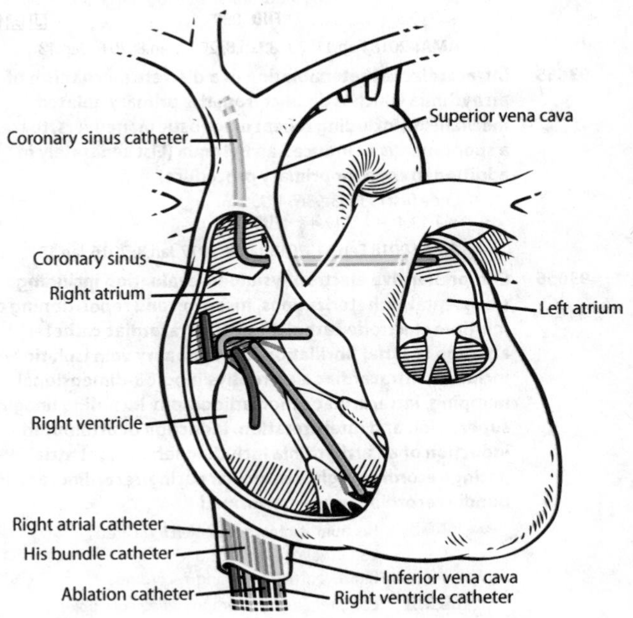

▲ **93653** **Comprehensive electrophysiologic evaluation with insertion and repositioning of multiple electrode catheters, induction or attempted induction of an arrhythmia with right atrial pacing and recording and catheter ablation of arrhythmogenic focus, including intracardiac electrophysiologic 3-dimensional mapping, right ventricular pacing and recording, left atrial pacing and recording from coronary sinus or left atrium, and His bundle recording, when performed; with treatment of supraventricular tachycardia by ablation of fast or slow atrioventricular pathway, accessory atrioventricular connection, cavo-tricuspid isthmus or other single atrial focus or source of atrial re-entry**

EXCLUDES *Comprehensive electrophysiological studies (93619-93621)*

Electrophysiologic evaluation pacing cardioverter defibrillator (93642)

Intracardiac ablation with transseptal catheterization (93656)

Intracardiac ablation with treatment ventricular arrhythmia (93654)

Intracardiac electrophysiologic 3D mapping (93613)

Intracardiac pacing (93610, 93612, 93618)

Recording intracardiac electrograms (93600-93603)

24.3 24.3 **FUD** 000 J 80

AMA: 2018,Feb,11; 2018,Jan,8; 2017,Jan,8; 2016,Jan,13

▲ **93654 with treatment of ventricular tachycardia or focus of ventricular ectopy including left ventricular pacing and recording, when performed**

EXCLUDES *Comprehensive electrophysiological studies (93619-93620, 93622)*
Device evaluation (93279-93284, 93286-93289)
Intracardiac ablation with transseptal catheterization (93656)
Intracardiac ablation with treatment supraventricular tachycardia (93653)
Intracardiac pacing (93609-93613, 93618)
Recording intracardiac electrograms (93600-93603)

32.6 32.6 FUD 000 J 80

AMA: 2018,Feb,11; 2018,Jan,8; 2017,Jan,8; 2016,Jan,13

+ **93655 Intracardiac catheter ablation of a discrete mechanism of arrhythmia which is distinct from the primary ablated mechanism, including repeat diagnostic maneuvers, to treat a spontaneous or induced arrhythmia (List separately in addition to code for primary procedure)**

Code first (93653-93654, 93656)

12.4 12.4 FUD ZZZ N 80

AMA: 2018,Feb,11; 2018,Jan,8; 2017,Jan,8; 2016,Jan,13

▲ **93656 Comprehensive electrophysiologic evaluation including transseptal catheterizations, insertion and repositioning of multiple electrode catheters with intracardiac catheter ablation of atrial fibrillation by pulmonary vein isolation, including intracardiac electrophysiologic 3-dimensional mapping, intracardiac echocardiography including imaging supervision and interpretation, induction or attempted induction of an arrhythmia including left or right atrial pacing/recording, right ventricular pacing/recording, and His bundle recording, when performed**

INCLUDES His bundle recording when indicated
Left atrial pacing/recording
Right ventricular pacing/recording

EXCLUDES *Comprehensive electrophysiological studies (93619-93621)*
Device evaluation (93279-93284, 93286-93289)
Electrophysiologic evaluation with treatment ventricular tachycardia (93654)
Intracardiac ablation with treatment supraventricular tachycardia (93653)
Intracardiac echocardiography during diagnostic/therapeutic intervention (93662)
Intracardiac electrophysiologic 3D mapping (93613)
Intracardiac pacing (93610, 93612, 93618)
Left heart catheterization by transseptal puncture (93462)
Recording intracardiac electrograms (93600-93603)

32.7 32.7 FUD 000 J 80

AMA: 2020,Nov,12; 2019,Sep,10; 2018,Feb,11; 2018,Jan,8; 2017,Jan,8; 2016,Jan,13

+ **93657 Additional linear or focal intracardiac catheter ablation of the left or right atrium for treatment of atrial fibrillation remaining after completion of pulmonary vein isolation (List separately in addition to code for primary procedure)**

Code first (93656)

12.3 12.3 FUD ZZZ N 80

AMA: 2020,Nov,12; 2019,Sep,10; 2018,Feb,11; 2018,Jan,8; 2017,Jan,8; 2016,Jan,13

93660-93662 Other Tests for Cardiac Function

93660 Evaluation of cardiovascular function with tilt table evaluation, with continuous ECG monitoring and intermittent blood pressure monitoring, with or without pharmacological intervention

EXCLUDES *Autonomic nervous system function testing (95921, 95924)*

4.51 4.51 FUD 000 S 80

AMA: 2018,Feb,11; 2018,Jan,8; 2017,Jan,8; 2016,Jan,13

+ **93662 Intracardiac echocardiography during therapeutic/diagnostic intervention, including imaging supervision and interpretation (List separately in addition to code for primary procedure)**

EXCLUDES *Internal cardioversion (92961)*
Transcatheter implantation interatrial septal shunt device, percutaneous approach (0613T)
Transcatheter tricuspid valve repair with prosthesis, percutaneous approach (0569T-0570T)

Code first (as appropriate) ([33274, 33275], 33340, 33361-33366, 33418, 33477, 33741, 33745, 92986-92987, 92990, 92997, 93451-93461, 93505, 93580-93583, 93590-93591, 93593-93597, 93620, 93653-93654, 93656, 0345T, 0483T-0484T, 0543T, 0544T, 0545T)

0.00 0.00 FUD ZZZ N 80

AMA: 2018,Feb,11; 2018,Jan,8; 2017,Jan,8; 2016,Jan,13

93668 Rehabilitation Services: Peripheral Arterial Disease

CMS: 100-03,1,20.35 Supervised Exercise Therapy (SET) for Symptomatic Peripheral Artery Disease (PAD)(Effective May 25, 2017; 100-04,32,390 Supervised exercise therapy (SET) Symptomatic Peripheral Artery Disease; 100-04,32,390.1 General Billing Requirements for Supervised exercise therapy (SET) for PAD; 100-04,32,390.2 Coding Requirements for SET for PAD; 100-04,32,390.3 Special Billing Requirements for Professional Claims; 100-04,32,390.4 Special Billing Requirements for Institutional Claims; 100-04,32,390.5 Common Working File (CWF) Requirements; 100-04,32,390.6 Applicable Medicare Summary Notice (MSN), Remittance Advice Remark Codes (RARCs), and Claim Adjustment Reason Code (CARC) Messaging

INCLUDES Monitoring:
Other cardiovascular limitations for workload adjustment
Patient's claudication threshold
Motorized treadmill or track
Sessions lasting 45-60 minutes
Supervision by exercise physiologist/nurse

Code also appropriate E/M service, when performed

93668 Peripheral arterial disease (PAD) rehabilitation, per session

0.50 0.50 FUD XXX S 80 TC

AMA: 2018,Feb,11

93701-93702 Thoracic Electrical Bioimpedance

EXCLUDES *Bioelectrical impedance analysis whole body (0358T)*
Indirect measurement left ventricular filling pressure by computerized calibration arterial waveform response to Valsalva (93799)

93701 Bioimpedance-derived physiologic cardiovascular analysis

0.71 0.71 FUD XXX Q1 80 TC

AMA: 2018,Feb,11; 2018,Jan,8; 2017,Jan,8; 2016,Jan,13

93702 Bioimpedance spectroscopy (BIS), extracellular fluid analysis for lymphedema assessment(s)

3.50 3.50 FUD XXX S 80 TC

AMA: 2018,Feb,11

93724 Electronic Analysis of Pacemaker Function

93724 Electronic analysis of antitachycardia pacemaker system (includes electrocardiographic recording, programming of device, induction and termination of tachycardia via implanted pacemaker, and interpretation of recordings)

8.04 8.04 FUD 000 S 80

AMA: 2018,Feb,11; 2018,Jan,8; 2017,Jan,8; 2016,Jan,13

93740 Temperature Gradient Assessment

93740 Temperature gradient studies

0.23 0.23 FUD XXX Q1

AMA: 2018,Feb,11

93745 Wearable Cardioverter-Defibrillator System Services

EXCLUDES *Device evaluation (93282, 93292)*

93745 Initial set-up and programming by a physician or other qualified health care professional of wearable cardioverter-defibrillator includes initial programming of system, establishing baseline electronic ECG, transmission of data to data repository, patient instruction in wearing system and patient reporting of problems or events

0.00 0.00 FUD XXX S 80

AMA: 2018,Feb,11

93750 Ventricular Assist Device (VAD) Interrogation

CMS: 100-03,20.9 Artificial Hearts and Related Devices; 100-03,20.9.1 Ventricular Assist Devices; 100-04,32,320.1 Artificial Hearts Prior to May 1, 2008; 100-04,32,320.2 Coding for Artificial Hearts After May 1, 2008; 100-04,32,320.3 Ventricular Assist Devices; 100-04,32,320.3.1 Post-cardiotomy; 100-04,32,320.3.2 Bridge-to-Transplantation; 100-04,32,320.3.3 Other

EXCLUDES *Insertion ventricular assist device (33975-33976, 33979)*
Removal/replacement ventricular assist device (33981-33983)

93750 **Interrogation of ventricular assist device (VAD), in person, with physician or other qualified health care professional analysis of device parameters (eg, drivelines, alarms, power surges), review of device function (eg, flow and volume status, septum status, recovery), with programming, if performed, and report**
1.32 1.58 **FUD** XXX S 80
AMA: 2018,Dec,10; 2018,Dec,10; 2018,Feb,11; 2018,Jan,8; 2017,Jan,8; 2016,Jan,13

93770 Peripheral Venous Blood Pressure Assessment

CMS: 100-03,20.19 Ambulatory Blood Pressure Monitoring (20.19)

EXCLUDES *Cannulization, central venous (36500, 36555-36556)*

93770 **Determination of venous pressure**
0.23 0.23 **FUD** XXX N
AMA: 2018,Feb,11

93784-93790 Ambulatory Blood Pressure Monitoring

CMS: 100-03,20.19 Ambulatory Blood Pressure Monitoring (20.19); 100-04,32,10.1 Ambulatory Blood Pressure Monitoring Billing Requirements

EXCLUDES *Self-measured blood pressure monitoring ([99473, 99474])*

93784 **Ambulatory blood pressure monitoring, utilizing report-generating software, automated, worn continuously for 24 hours or longer; including recording, scanning analysis, interpretation and report**
1.51 1.51 **FUD** XXX B 80
AMA: 2020,Apr,5; 2018,Feb,11

93786 **recording only**
0.83 0.83 **FUD** XXX 01 80 TC
AMA: 2020,Apr,5; 2018,Feb,11

93788 **scanning analysis with report**
0.15 0.15 **FUD** XXX 01 80 TC
AMA: 2020,Apr,5; 2018,Feb,11

93790 **review with interpretation and report**
0.53 0.53 **FUD** XXX M 80 26
AMA: 2020,Apr,5; 2018,Feb,11

93792-93793 INR Monitoring

CMS: 100-03,190.11 Home PT/INR Monitoring for Anticoagulation Management

EXCLUDES *Chronic care management services provided during same month ([99439, 99490, 99491])*
Complex chronic care management services provided during same month (99487-99489)
Online digital assessment and management services by nonphysician healthcare professional (98970-98972)
Online digital evaluation and management services by physician or other qualified health care professional ([99421, 99422, 99423])
Telephone assessment and management service by nonphysician healthcare professional (98966-98968)
Telephone evaluation and management service by physician or other qualified healthcare professional (99441-99443)

93792 **Patient/caregiver training for initiation of home international normalized ratio (INR) monitoring under the direction of a physician or other qualified health care professional, face-to-face, including use and care of the INR monitor, obtaining blood sample, instructions for reporting home INR test results, and documentation of patient's/caregiver's ability to perform testing and report results**
Code also:
INR home monitoring equipment with appropriate supply code or (99070)
Significantly separately identifiable E/M service on same date service; append modifier 25
1.84 1.84 **FUD** XXX B 80 TC
AMA: 2018,Mar,7; 2018,Feb,11

93793 **Anticoagulant management for a patient taking warfarin, must include review and interpretation of a new home, office, or lab international normalized ratio (INR) test result, patient instructions, dosage adjustment (as needed), and scheduling of additional test(s), when performed**
EXCLUDES *E/M services performed same date (99202-99215, 99241-99245)*
Reporting code more than one time per day
0.33 0.33 **FUD** XXX B 80 26
AMA: 2020,Feb,7; 2018,Mar,7; 2018,Feb,11; 2018,Jan,8; 2017,Nov,10

93797-93799 Cardiac Rehabilitation

CMS: 100-02,15,232 Cardiac Rehabilitation (CR) and Intensive Cardiac Rehabilitation (ICR) Services Furnished On or After January 1, 2010; 100-04,32,140.2 Cardiac Rehabilitation On or After January 1, 2010; 100-04,32,140.2.1 Coding Cardiac Rehabilitation Services On or After January 1, 2010; 100-04,32,140.2.2.2 Institutional Claims for CR and ICR Services; 100-04,32,140.2.2.4 CR Services Exceeding 36 Sessions; 100-04,32,140.3 Intensive Cardiac Rehabilitation On or After January 1, 2010; 100-08,15,4.2.8 Cardiac Rehabilitation (CR) and Intensive Cardiac Rehabilitation (ICR)

93797 **Physician or other qualified health care professional services for outpatient cardiac rehabilitation; without continuous ECG monitoring (per session)**
0.25 0.46 **FUD** 000 S 80
AMA: 2018,Feb,11

93798 **with continuous ECG monitoring (per session)**
0.40 0.72 **FUD** 000 S 80
AMA: 2018,Feb,11

93799 **Unlisted cardiovascular service or procedure**
0.00 0.00 **FUD** XXX S 80
AMA: 2020,Nov,7; 2018,Dec,10; 2018,Dec,10; 2018,Sep,10; 2018,Aug,10; 2018,Feb,11; 2018,Jan,8; 2017,Jan,8; 2016,May,5; 2016,Jan,13

93880-93895 Noninvasive Tests Extracranial/Intracranial Arteries

INCLUDES Patient care required to perform/supervise studies and interpret results
EXCLUDES *Hand-held Dopplers that do not provide hard copy or vascular flow bidirectional analysis (see E/M codes)*

93880 **Duplex scan of extracranial arteries; complete bilateral study**
EXCLUDES *Common carotid intima-media thickness (IMT) studies (93895)*
5.70 5.70 **FUD** XXX S 80
AMA: 2018,Feb,11; 2018,Jan,8; 2017,Jan,8; 2016,Jan,13

93882 **unilateral or limited study**
EXCLUDES *Common carotid intima-media thickness (IMT) studies (93895)*
3.64 3.64 **FUD** XXX S 80
AMA: 2018,Feb,11; 2018,Jan,8; 2017,Jan,8; 2016,Jan,13

93886 **Transcranial Doppler study of the intracranial arteries; complete study**
INCLUDES Complete transcranial doppler (TCD) study
Ultrasound evaluation right/left anterior circulation territories and posterior circulation territory
7.67 7.67 **FUD** XXX S 80
AMA: 2018,Feb,11; 2018,Jan,8; 2017,Jan,8; 2016,Jan,13

93888 **limited study**
INCLUDES Limited TCD study
Ultrasound examination two or fewer territories (right/left anterior circulation, posterior circulation)
4.47 4.47 **FUD** XXX S 80
AMA: 2018,Feb,11; 2018,Jan,8; 2017,Jan,8; 2016,Jan,13

93890 **vasoreactivity study**
EXCLUDES *Limited TCD study (93888)*
7.82 7.82 **FUD** XXX 01 80
AMA: 2018,Feb,11; 2018,Jan,8; 2017,Jan,8; 2016,Jan,13

93892 **emboli detection without intravenous microbubble injection**

EXCLUDES *Limited TCD study (93888)*

8.81 8.81 **FUD** XXX Q1 80

AMA: 2018,Feb,11; 2018,Jan,8; 2017,Jan,8; 2016,Jan,13

93893 **emboli detection with intravenous microbubble injection**

EXCLUDES *Limited TCD study (93888)*

10.1 10.1 **FUD** XXX Q1 80

AMA: 2018,Feb,11; 2018,Jan,8; 2017,Jan,8; 2016,Jan,13

93895 **Quantitative carotid intima media thickness and carotid atheroma evaluation, bilateral**

EXCLUDES *Complete and limited duplex studies (93880, 93882)*

0.00 0.00 **FUD** XXX E 80

AMA: 2018,Feb,11

93922-93971 Noninvasive Vascular Studies: Extremities

CMS: 100-04,8,180 Noninvasive Studies for ESRD Patients

INCLUDES Patient care required to perform/supervise studies and interpret results

EXCLUDES *Hand-held Dopplers that do not provide hard copy or vascular flow bidirectional analysis (see E/M codes)*

93922 **Limited bilateral noninvasive physiologic studies of upper or lower extremity arteries, (eg, for lower extremity: ankle/brachial indices at distal posterior tibial and anterior tibial/dorsalis pedis arteries plus bidirectional, Doppler waveform recording and analysis at 1-2 levels, or ankle/brachial indices at distal posterior tibial and anterior tibial/dorsalis pedis arteries plus volume plethysmography at 1-2 levels, or ankle/brachial indices at distal posterior tibial and anterior tibial/dorsalis pedis arteries with, transcutaneous oxygen tension measurement at 1-2 levels)**

INCLUDES Evaluation:
- Doppler analysis bidirectional blood flow
- Nonimaging physiologic recordings pressure
- Oxygen tension measurements and/or plethysmography

Lower extremity (potential levels include high thigh, low thigh, calf, ankle, metatarsal and toes) limited study includes either:
- Ankle/brachial indices distal posterior tibial and anterior tibial/dorsalis pedis arteries plus bidirectional Doppler waveform recording and analysis 1-2 levels; OR
- Ankle/brachial indices distal posterior tibial and anterior tibial/dorsalis pedis arteries plus volume plethysmography 1-2 levels; OR
- Ankle/brachial indices distal posterior tibial and anterior tibial/dorsalis pedis arteries with transcutaneous oxygen tension measurements 1-2 levels

Unilateral provocative functional measurement

Unilateral study 3 or move levels

Upper extremity (potential levels include arm, forearm, wrist, and digits) limited study includes:
- Doppler-determined systolic pressures and bidirectional waveform recording with analysis 1-2 levels; OR
- Doppler-determined systolic pressures and transcutaneous oxygen tension measurements 1-2 levels; OR
- Doppler-determined systolic pressures and volume plethysmography 1-2 levels

EXCLUDES *Reporting code more than one time for lower extremity(ies)*

Reporting code more than one time for upper extremity(ies)

Transcutaneous oxyhemoglobin, deoxyhemoglobin and tissue oxygenation measurement (0631T)

Transcutaneous oxyhemoglobin measurement (0493T)

Code also:
- Modifier 52 for unilateral study 1-2 levels
- Twice for upper and lower extremity study; append modifier 59 on second code

2.40 2.40 **FUD** XXX Q1 80

AMA: 2019,Oct,8; 2018,Feb,11; 2018,Jan,8; 2017,Jan,8; 2016,Jan,13

93923 Complete bilateral noninvasive physiologic studies of upper or lower extremity arteries, 3 or more levels (eg, for lower extremity: ankle/brachial indices at distal posterior tibial and anterior tibial/dorsalis pedis arteries plus segmental blood pressure measurements with bidirectional Doppler waveform recording and analysis, at 3 or more levels, or ankle/brachial indices at distal posterior tibial and anterior tibial/dorsalis pedis arteries plus segmental volume plethysmography at 3 or more levels, or ankle/brachial indices at distal posterior tibial and anterior tibial/dorsalis pedis arteries plus segmental transcutaneous oxygen tension measurements at 3 or more levels), or single level study with provocative functional maneuvers (eg, measurements with postural provocative tests, or measurements with reactive hyperemia)

INCLUDES Evaluation:
- Doppler analysis bidirectional blood flow
- Nonimaging physiologic recordings pressures
- Oxygen tension measurements

Lower extremity:
- Ankle/brachial indices distal posterior tibial and anterior tibial/dorsalis pedis arteries plus bidirectional Doppler waveform recording and analysis 3 or more levels; OR
- Ankle/brachial indices distal posterior tibial and anterior tibial/dorsalis pedis arteries with transcutaneous oxygen tension measurements 3 or more levels; OR
- Ankle/brachial indices distal posterior tibial and anterior tibial/dorsalis pedis arteries plus volume plethysmography 3 or more levels; OR

Provocative functional maneuvers and measurement single level

Upper extremity complete study:
- Doppler-determined systolic pressures and bidirectional waveform recording with analysis 3 or more levels; OR
- Doppler-determined systolic pressures and transcutaneous oxygen tension measurements 3 or more levels; OR
- Doppler-determined systolic pressures and volume plethysmography 3 or more levels; OR

EXCLUDES *Reporting code more than one time for lower extremity(ies)*
Reporting coe more than one time for upper extremity(ies)
Transcutaneous oxyhemoglobin, deoxyhemoglobin and tissue oxygenation measurement (0631T)
Unilateral study 3 or more levels (93922)

Code also twice for upper and lower extremity study and append modifier 59

3.74 3.74 **FUD** XXX S 80

AMA: 2020,Sep,14; 2019,Oct,8; 2018,Feb,11; 2018,Jan,8; 2017,Jan,8; 2016,Jan,13

93924 Noninvasive physiologic studies of lower extremity arteries, at rest and following treadmill stress testing, (ie, bidirectional Doppler waveform or volume plethysmography recording and analysis at rest with ankle/brachial indices immediately after and at timed intervals following performance of a standardized protocol on a motorized treadmill plus recording of time of onset of claudication or other symptoms, maximal walking time, and time to recovery) complete bilateral study

INCLUDES Evaluation:
- Doppler analysis bidirectional blood flow
- Nonimaging physiologic recordings pressures
- Oxygen tension measurements
- Plethysmography

EXCLUDES *Noninvasive vascular studies extremities (93922-93923)*
Other types exercise

4.67 4.67 **FUD** XXX S 80

AMA: 2019,Oct,8; 2018,Feb,11; 2018,Jan,8; 2017,Jan,8; 2016,Jan,13

93925 Duplex scan of lower extremity arteries or arterial bypass grafts; complete bilateral study

EXCLUDES *Preoperative arterial inflow and venous outflow duplex scan for creation hemodialysis access, same extremities (93985)*

7.17 7.17 **FUD** XXX S 80

AMA: 2019,Oct,8; 2018,Feb,11; 2018,Jan,8; 2017,Jan,8; 2016,Sep,9; 2016,Jan,13

93926 unilateral or limited study

EXCLUDES *Preoperative arterial inflow and venous outflow duplex scan for creation hemodialysis access, same extremity (93986)*

4.24 4.24 **FUD** XXX S 80

AMA: 2019,Oct,8; 2018,Feb,11; 2018,Jan,8; 2017,Jan,8; 2016,Sep,9; 2016,Jan,13

93930 Duplex scan of upper extremity arteries or arterial bypass grafts; complete bilateral study

EXCLUDES *Preoperative arterial inflow and venous outflow duplex scan for creation hemodialysis access, same extremity(ies) (93985-93986)*

5.83 5.83 **FUD** XXX S 80

AMA: 2019,Oct,8; 2018,Feb,11; 2018,Jan,8; 2017,Jan,8; 2016,Sep,9; 2016,Jan,13

93931 unilateral or limited study

EXCLUDES *Preoperative arterial inflow and venous outflow duplex scan for creation hemodialysis access, same extremity (93985-93986)*

3.64 3.64 **FUD** XXX S 80

AMA: 2019,Oct,8; 2018,Feb,11; 2018,Jan,8; 2017,Jan,8; 2016,Sep,9; 2016,Jan,13

93970 Duplex scan of extremity veins including responses to compression and other maneuvers; complete bilateral study

EXCLUDES *Endovenous ablation (36475-36476, 36478-36479)*
Preoperative arterial inflow and venous outflow duplex scan for creation hemodialysis access, same extremity(ies) (93985-93986)

5.51 5.51 **FUD** XXX S 80

AMA: 2019,Oct,8; 2018,Mar,3; 2018,Feb,11; 2018,Jan,8; 2017,Jan,8; 2016,Nov,3; 2016,Sep,9; 2016,Jan,13

93971 unilateral or limited study

EXCLUDES *Endovenous ablation (36475-36476, 36478-36479)*
Preoperative arterial inflow and venous outflow duplex scan for creation hemodialysis access, same extremity (93985-93986)

3.44 3.44 **FUD** XXX S 80

AMA: 2019,Oct,8; 2018,Mar,3; 2018,Feb,11; 2018,Jan,8; 2017,Jan,8; 2016,Nov,3; 2016,Sep,9; 2016,Jan,13

93975-93981 Noninvasive Vascular Studies: Abdomen/Chest/Pelvis

93975 Duplex scan of arterial inflow and venous outflow of abdominal, pelvic, scrotal contents and/or retroperitoneal organs; complete study

7.88 7.88 **FUD** XXX S 80

AMA: 2018,Feb,11; 2018,Jan,8; 2017,Jan,8; 2016,Aug,9; 2016,Jan,13

93976 limited study

4.64 4.64 **FUD** XXX S 80

AMA: 2018,Feb,11; 2018,Jan,8; 2017,Jan,8; 2016,Aug,9; 2016,Jan,13

93978 Duplex scan of aorta, inferior vena cava, iliac vasculature, or bypass grafts; complete study

EXCLUDES *Ultrasound screening for abdominal aortic aneurysm (76706)*

5.32 5.32 **FUD** XXX S 80

AMA: 2018,Feb,11; 2018,Jan,8; 2017,Jan,8; 2016,Jan,13

93979 **unilateral or limited study**

EXCLUDES *Ultrasound screening for abdominal aortic aneurysm (76706)*

3.42 3.42 FUD XXX Q1 80

AMA: 2018,Feb,11; 2018,Jan,8; 2017,Jan,8; 2016,Jan,13

93980 **Duplex scan of arterial inflow and venous outflow of penile vessels; complete study**

3.46 3.46 FUD XXX S 80

AMA: 2018,Feb,11; 2018,Jan,8; 2017,Jan,8; 2016,Jan,13

93981 **follow-up or limited study**

2.08 2.08 FUD XXX S 80

AMA: 2018,Feb,11; 2018,Jan,8; 2017,Jan,8; 2016,Jan,13

93985-93998 Noninvasive Vascular Studies: Hemodialysis Access

93985 **Duplex scan of arterial inflow and venous outflow for preoperative vessel assessment prior to creation of hemodialysis access; complete bilateral study**

EXCLUDES *Duplex scan extremity arteries only, same extremity(ies) (93925, 93930)*

Duplex scan extremity veins only, same extremity(ies) (93970)

Duplex scan hemodialysis access, arterial inflow, and venous outflow, same extremity(ies) (93990)

Physiologic arterial evaluation extremities (93922-93924)

7.53 7.53 FUD XXX P2 80

93986 **complete unilateral study**

EXCLUDES *Duplex scan extremity arteries only, same extremity (93926, 93931)*

Duplex scan extremity veins only, same extremity (93971)

Duplex scan hemodialysis access, arterial inflow and venous outflow, same extremity (93990)

Physiologic arterial evaluation extremities (93922-93924)

4.37 4.37 FUD XXX P2 80

93990 **Duplex scan of hemodialysis access (including arterial inflow, body of access and venous outflow)**

EXCLUDES *Hemodialysis access flow measurement by indicator method (90940)*

4.39 4.39 FUD XXX Q1 80

AMA: 2019,Oct,8; 2018,Feb,11; 2018,Jan,8; 2017,Jan,8; 2016,Jan,13

93998 **Unlisted noninvasive vascular diagnostic study**

0.00 0.00 FUD XXX Q1 80

AMA: 2018,Feb,11; 2018,Jan,8; 2017,Jan,8; 2016,Jan,13

94002-94005 Ventilator Management Services

94002 **Ventilation assist and management, initiation of pressure or volume preset ventilators for assisted or controlled breathing; hospital inpatient/observation, initial day**

EXCLUDES *E/M services*

2.64 2.64 FUD XXX Q3 80

AMA: 2019,Aug,8; 2018,Feb,11; 2018,Jan,8; 2017,Jan,8; 2016,Jan,13

94003 **hospital inpatient/observation, each subsequent day**

EXCLUDES *E/M services*

1.89 1.89 FUD XXX Q3 80

AMA: 2019,Aug,8; 2018,Feb,11; 2018,Jan,8; 2017,Jan,8; 2016,Jan,13

94004 **nursing facility, per day**

EXCLUDES *E/M services*

1.40 1.40 FUD XXX B 80

AMA: 2019,Aug,8; 2018,Feb,11; 2018,Jan,8; 2017,Jan,8; 2016,Jan,13

94005 **Home ventilator management care plan oversight of a patient (patient not present) in home, domiciliary or rest home (eg, assisted living) requiring review of status, review of laboratories and other studies and revision of orders and respiratory care plan (as appropriate), within a calendar month, 30 minutes or more**

Code also when different provider reports care plan oversight in same 30 days (99339-99340, 99374-99378)

2.61 2.61 FUD XXX M

AMA: 2018,Feb,11; 2018,Jan,8; 2017,Jan,8; 2016,Jan,13

94010-94799 [94619] Respiratory Services: Diagnostic and Therapeutic

INCLUDES Laboratory procedure(s)

Test results interpretation

EXCLUDES *Separately identifiable E/M service*

94010 **Spirometry, including graphic record, total and timed vital capacity, expiratory flow rate measurement(s), with or without maximal voluntary ventilation**

INCLUDES Measurement expiratory airflow and volumes

EXCLUDES *Diffusing capacity (94729)*

Other respiratory function services (94150, 94200, 94375, 94728)

1.00 1.00 FUD XXX Q1 80

AMA: 2020,Dec,3; 2019,May,10; 2019,Mar,10; 2019,Apr,10; 2018,Feb,11; 2018,Jan,8; 2017,Jan,8; 2016,Jan,13

94011 **Measurement of spirometric forced expiratory flows in an infant or child through 2 years of age**

2.48 2.48 FUD XXX Q1 80

AMA: 2020,Dec,3; 2019,Mar,10; 2018,Feb,11; 2018,Jan,8; 2017,Jan,8; 2016,Jan,13

94012 **Measurement of spirometric forced expiratory flows, before and after bronchodilator, in an infant or child through 2 years of age**

4.01 4.01 FUD XXX Q1 80

AMA: 2020,Dec,3; 2019,Mar,10; 2018,Feb,11; 2018,Jan,8; 2017,Jan,8; 2016,Jan,13

94013 **Measurement of lung volumes (ie, functional residual capacity [FRC], forced vital capacity [FVC], and expiratory reserve volume [ERV]) in an infant or child through 2 years of age**

0.55 0.55 FUD XXX S 80

AMA: 2020,Dec,3; 2019,Mar,10; 2018,Feb,11; 2018,Jan,8; 2017,Jan,8; 2016,Jan,13

94014 **Patient-initiated spirometric recording per 30-day period of time; includes reinforced education, transmission of spirometric tracing, data capture, analysis of transmitted data, periodic recalibration and review and interpretation by a physician or other qualified health care professional**

1.58 1.58 FUD XXX Q1 80

AMA: 2020,Dec,3; 2019,Mar,10; 2018,Feb,11; 2018,Jan,8; 2017,Jan,8; 2016,Jan,13

94015 **recording (includes hook-up, reinforced education, data transmission, data capture, trend analysis, and periodic recalibration)**

0.86 0.86 FUD XXX Q1 80 TC

AMA: 2020,Dec,3; 2019,Mar,10; 2018,Feb,11; 2018,Jan,8; 2017,Jan,8; 2016,Jan,13

94016 **review and interpretation only by a physician or other qualified health care professional**

0.72 0.72 FUD XXX A 80 26

AMA: 2020,Dec,3; 2019,Mar,10; 2018,Feb,11; 2018,Jan,8; 2017,Jan,8; 2016,Jan,13

94060 Bronchodilation responsiveness, spirometry as in 94010, pre- and post-bronchodilator administration

INCLUDES Spirometry performed prior to and after bronchodilator has been administered

EXCLUDES *Bronchospasm prolonged exercise test with pre- and post-spirometry (94617, [94619])*
Diffusing capacity (94729)
Other respiratory function services (94150, 94200, 94375, 94640, 94728)

Code also bronchodilator supply with appropriate supply code or (99070)

1.67 1.67 FUD XXX S 80

AMA: 2020,Dec,3; 2019,Mar,10; 2019,Apr,10; 2018,Feb,11; 2018,Jan,8; 2017,Jan,8; 2016,Jan,13

94070 Bronchospasm provocation evaluation, multiple spirometric determinations as in 94010, with administered agents (eg, antigen[s], cold air, methacholine)

EXCLUDES *Diffusing capacity (94729)*
Inhalation treatment (diagnostic or therapeutic) (94640)

Code also antigen(s) administration with appropriate supply code or (99070)

1.69 1.69 FUD XXX S 80

AMA: 2020,Dec,3; 2019,Mar,10; 2018,Feb,11; 2018,Jan,8; 2017,Jan,8; 2016,Jan,13

94150 Vital capacity, total (separate procedure)

EXCLUDES *Other respiratory function services (94010, 94060, 94728)*
Thoracic gas volumes (94726-94727)

0.71 0.71 FUD XXX Q1

AMA: 2020,Dec,3; 2019,Mar,10; 2018,Sep,14; 2018,Feb,11; 2018,Jan,8; 2017,Jan,8; 2016,Jan,13

94200 Maximum breathing capacity, maximal voluntary ventilation

EXCLUDES *Other respiratory function services (94010, 94060)*

0.63 0.63 FUD XXX Q1 80

AMA: 2020,Dec,3; 2019,Mar,10; 2018,Feb,11; 2018,Jan,8; 2017,Jan,8; 2016,Jan,13

94375 Respiratory flow volume loop

INCLUDES Obstruction pattern identification in central or peripheral airways (inspiratory and/or expiratory)

EXCLUDES *Diffusing capacity (94729)*
Other respiratory function services (94010, 94060, 94728)

1.10 1.10 FUD XXX Q1 80

AMA: 2020,Dec,3; 2019,Mar,10; 2018,Feb,11; 2018,Jan,8; 2017,Jan,8; 2016,Jan,13

94450 Breathing response to hypoxia (hypoxia response curve)

EXCLUDES *HAST - high altitude simulation test (94452, 94453)*

1.88 1.88 FUD XXX Q1 80

AMA: 2020,Dec,3; 2019,Mar,10; 2018,Feb,11; 2018,Jan,8; 2017,Jan,8; 2016,Jan,13

94452 High altitude simulation test (HAST), with interpretation and report by a physician or other qualified health care professional;

EXCLUDES *HAST test with supplemental oxygen titration (94453)*
Noninvasive pulse oximetry (94760-94761)
Obtaining arterial blood gases (36600)

1.48 1.48 FUD XXX Q1 80

AMA: 2020,Dec,3; 2019,Mar,10; 2018,Feb,11; 2018,Jan,8; 2017,Jan,8; 2016,Jan,13

94453 with supplemental oxygen titration

EXCLUDES *HAST test without supplemental oxygen titration (94452)*
Noninvasive pulse oximetry (94760-94761)
Obtaining arterial blood gases (36600)

2.03 2.03 FUD XXX Q1 80

AMA: 2020,Dec,3; 2019,Mar,10; 2018,Feb,11; 2018,Jan,8; 2017,Jan,8; 2016,Jan,13

94610 Intrapulmonary surfactant administration by a physician or other qualified health care professional through endotracheal tube

INCLUDES Reporting once per dosing episode

EXCLUDES *Intubation, endotracheal (31500)*
Neonatal critical care (99468-99472)

1.59 1.59 FUD XXX ⊘ Q1 80

AMA: 2020,Dec,3; 2019,Mar,10; 2018,Feb,11; 2018,Jan,8; 2017,Jan,8; 2016,Jan,13

94617 Exercise test for bronchospasm, including pre- and post-spirometry and pulse oximetry; with electrocardiographic recording(s)

EXCLUDES *Cardiovascular stress test (93015-93018)*
ECG monitoring (93000-93010, 93040-93042)
Pulse oximetry (94760-94761)

2.58 2.58 FUD XXX Q1 80

AMA: 2020,Dec,3; 2019,May,10; 2019,Mar,10; 2018,Feb,11; 2018,Jan,8; 2017,Oct,3

\# **94619 without electrocardiographic recording(s)**

EXCLUDES *Cardiovascular stress test (93015-93018)*
ECG monitoring (93000-93010, 93040-93042)
Pulse oximetry (94760-94761)

2.16 2.16 FUD XXX 80

AMA: 2020,Dec,3

94618 Pulmonary stress testing (eg, 6-minute walk test), including measurement of heart rate, oximetry, and oxygen titration, when performed

EXCLUDES *Pulse oximetry (94760-94761)*

0.95 0.95 FUD XXX Q1 80

AMA: 2020,Dec,3; 2019,May,10; 2019,Mar,10; 2018,Feb,11; 2018,Jan,8; 2017,Oct,3

94619 **Resequenced code. See code following 94617.**

94621 Cardiopulmonary exercise testing, including measurements of minute ventilation, CO2 production, O2 uptake, and electrocardiographic recordings

EXCLUDES *Cardiovascular stress test (93015-93018)*
ECG monitoring (93000-93010, 93040-93042)
Oxygen uptake expired gas analysis (94680-94690)
Pulse oximetry (94760-94761)

4.50 4.50 FUD XXX S 80

AMA: 2020,Dec,3; 2019,May,10; 2019,Mar,10; 2018,Feb,11; 2018,Jan,8; 2017,Oct,3; 2017,Jan,8; 2016,Jan,13

● **94625 Physician or other qualified health care professional services for outpatient pulmonary rehabilitation; without continuous oximetry monitoring (per session)**

EXCLUDES *Pulse oximetry, noninvasive (94760-94761)*

● **94626 with continuous oximetry monitoring (per session)**

EXCLUDES *Pulse oximetry, noninvasive (94760-94761)*

94640 Pressurized or nonpressurized inhalation treatment for acute airway obstruction for therapeutic purposes and/or for diagnostic purposes such as sputum induction with an aerosol generator, nebulizer, metered dose inhaler or intermittent positive pressure breathing (IPPB) device

EXCLUDES *One hour or more continuous inhalation treatment (94644, 94645)*
Other respiratory function services (94060, 94070)

Code also modifier 76 when more than one inhalation treatment performed on same date

0.51 0.51 FUD XXX Q1 80

AMA: 2020,Dec,3; 2019,Mar,10; 2018,Feb,11; 2018,Jan,8; 2017,Jan,8; 2016,Jan,13

94642 Aerosol inhalation of pentamidine for pneumocystis carinii pneumonia treatment or prophylaxis

0.00 0.00 FUD XXX Q1 80

AMA: 2020,Dec,3; 2019,Mar,10; 2018,Feb,11; 2018,Jan,8; 2017,Jan,8; 2016,Jan,13

94644 Continuous inhalation treatment with aerosol medication for acute airway obstruction; first hour

EXCLUDES *Services less than one hour (94640)*

1.40 1.40 FUD XXX Q1 80

AMA: 2020,Dec,3; 2019,Mar,10; 2018,Feb,11; 2018,Jan,8; 2017,Jan,8; 2016,Jan,13

+ **94645 each additional hour (List separately in addition to code for primary procedure)**

Code first initial hour (94644)

0.47 0.47 FUD XXX N 80

AMA: 2020,Dec,3; 2019,Mar,10; 2018,Feb,11; 2018,Jan,8; 2017,Jan,8; 2016,Jan,13

94660 Continuous positive airway pressure ventilation (CPAP), initiation and management

1.09 1.81 FUD XXX Q1 80

AMA: 2020,Dec,3; 2019,Aug,8; 2019,Mar,10; 2018,Feb,11; 2018,Jan,8; 2017,Jan,8; 2016,Jan,13

94662 Continuous negative pressure ventilation (CNP), initiation and management

1.03 1.03 FUD XXX Q3 80

AMA: 2020,Dec,3; 2019,Aug,8; 2019,Mar,10; 2018,Feb,11; 2018,Jan,8; 2017,Jan,8; 2016,Jan,13

94664 Demonstration and/or evaluation of patient utilization of an aerosol generator, nebulizer, metered dose inhaler or IPPB device

INCLUDES Reporting only one time per day

0.48 0.48 FUD XXX Q1 80

AMA: 2020,Dec,3; 2019,Mar,10; 2018,Feb,11; 2018,Jan,8; 2017,Jan,8; 2016,Jan,13

94667 Manipulation chest wall, such as cupping, percussing, and vibration to facilitate lung function; initial demonstration and/or evaluation

0.70 0.70 FUD XXX Q1 80

AMA: 2020,Dec,3; 2019,Mar,10; 2018,Feb,11; 2018,Jan,8; 2017,Jan,8; 2016,Jan,13

94668 subsequent

0.92 0.92 FUD XXX Q1 80

AMA: 2020,Dec,3; 2019,Mar,10; 2018,Feb,11; 2018,Jan,8; 2017,Jan,8; 2016,Jan,13

94669 Mechanical chest wall oscillation to facilitate lung function, per session

INCLUDES Application external wrap or vest to provide mechanical oscillation

0.90 0.90 FUD XXX Q1 80

AMA: 2020,Dec,3; 2019,Mar,10; 2018,Feb,11; 2018,Jan,8; 2017,Jan,8; 2016,Jan,13

94680 Oxygen uptake, expired gas analysis; rest and exercise, direct, simple

EXCLUDES *Cardiopulmonary stress testing (94621)*

1.51 1.51 FUD XXX Q1 80

AMA: 2020,Dec,3; 2019,Mar,10; 2018,Feb,11; 2018,Jan,8; 2017,Oct,3; 2017,Jan,8; 2016,Jan,13

94681 including CO2 output, percentage oxygen extracted

EXCLUDES *Cardiopulmonary stress testing (94621)*

1.49 1.49 FUD XXX Q1 80

AMA: 2020,Dec,3; 2019,Mar,10; 2018,Feb,11; 2018,Jan,8; 2017,Oct,3; 2017,Jan,8; 2016,Jan,13

94690 rest, indirect (separate procedure)

EXCLUDES *Arterial puncture (36600)*
Cardiopulmonary stress testing (94621)

1.43 1.43 FUD XXX Q1 80

AMA: 2020,Dec,3; 2019,Mar,10; 2018,Feb,11; 2018,Jan,8; 2017,Oct,3; 2017,Jan,8; 2016,Jan,13

94726 Plethysmography for determination of lung volumes and, when performed, airway resistance

INCLUDES Airway resistance
Determination:
Functional residual capacity
Residual volume
Total lung capacity

EXCLUDES *Airway resistance by oscillometry (94728)*
Bronchial provocation (94070)
Diffusing capacity (94729)
Gas dilution or washout (94727)
Spirometry (94010, 94060)

1.51 1.51 FUD XXX Q1 80

AMA: 2020,Dec,3; 2019,Mar,10; 2018,Feb,11; 2018,Jan,8; 2017,Jan,8; 2016,Jan,13

94727 Gas dilution or washout for determination of lung volumes and, when performed, distribution of ventilation and closing volumes

INCLUDES Closing volume
Lung volume measurement
Ventilation distribution

EXCLUDES *Bronchial provocation (94070)*
Diffusing capacity (94729)
Plethysmography for lung volume/airway resistance (94726)
Spirometry (94010, 94060)

1.23 1.23 FUD XXX Q1 80

AMA: 2020,Dec,3; 2019,Mar,10; 2018,Feb,11; 2018,Jan,8; 2017,Jan,8; 2016,Jan,13

94728 Airway resistance by oscillometry

EXCLUDES *Diffusing capacity (94729)*
Gas dilution techniques
Other respiratory function services (94010, 94060, 94070, 94375, 94726)

1.15 1.15 FUD XXX Q1 80

AMA: 2020,Dec,3; 2019,Mar,10; 2018,Feb,11; 2018,Jan,8; 2017,Jan,8; 2016,Jan,13

+ **94729 Diffusing capacity (eg, carbon monoxide, membrane) (List separately in addition to code for primary procedure)**

Code first (94010, 94060, 94070, 94375, 94726-94728)

1.59 1.59 FUD ZZZ N 80

AMA: 2020,Dec,3; 2019,Mar,10; 2018,Feb,11; 2018,Jan,8; 2017,Jan,8; 2016,Jan,13

94760 Noninvasive ear or pulse oximetry for oxygen saturation; single determination

EXCLUDES *Blood gases (82803-82810)*
Cardiopulmonary stress testing (94621)
Exercise test for bronchospasm (94617)
Pulmonary stress testing (94618)

0.07 0.07 FUD XXX N 80 TC

AMA: 2020,Dec,3; 2019,Aug,8; 2019,Mar,10; 2019,Jan,6; 2018,Feb,11; 2018,Jan,8; 2017,Oct,3; 2017,Jan,8; 2016,Jan,13

94761 multiple determinations (eg, during exercise)

EXCLUDES *Cardiopulmonary stress testing (94621)*
Exercise test for bronchospasm (94617, [94619])
Pulmonary stress testing (94618)

0.12 0.12 FUD XXX N 80 TC

AMA: 2020,Dec,3; 2019,Aug,8; 2019,Mar,10; 2018,Feb,11; 2018,Jan,8; 2017,Oct,3; 2017,Jan,8; 2016,Jan,13

94762 by continuous overnight monitoring (separate procedure)

0.71 0.71 FUD XXX Q3 80 TC

AMA: 2020,Dec,3; 2019,Aug,8; 2019,Mar,10; 2018,Feb,11; 2018,Jan,8; 2017,Jan,8; 2016,Jan,13

94772 Circadian respiratory pattern recording (pediatric pneumogram), 12-24 hour continuous recording, infant A

EXCLUDES *Electromyograms/EEG/ECG/respiration recordings*

0.00 0.00 FUD XXX S 80

AMA: 2020,Dec,3; 2019,Mar,10; 2018,Feb,11; 2018,Jan,8; 2017,Jan,8; 2016,Jan,13

94774 Pediatric home apnea monitoring event recording including respiratory rate, pattern and heart rate per 30-day period of time; includes monitor attachment, download of data, review, interpretation, and preparation of a report by a physician or other qualified health care professional A

INCLUDES Oxygen saturation monitoring

EXCLUDES *Event monitors (93268-93272)*
Holter monitor (93224-93227)
Pediatric home apnea services (94775-94777)
Remote cardiovascular telemetry (93228-93229)
Sleep testing (95805-95811 [95800, 95801])

0.00 0.00 FUD YYY B 80

AMA: 2020,Dec,3; 2019,Mar,10; 2018,Feb,11; 2018,Jan,8; 2017,Jan,8; 2016,Jan,13

94775 monitor attachment only (includes hook-up, initiation of recording and disconnection) A

INCLUDES Oxygen saturation monitoring

EXCLUDES *Event monitors (93268-93272)*
Holter monitor (93224-93227)
Remote cardiovascular telemetry (93228-93229)
Sleep testing (95805-95811 [95800, 95801])

0.00 0.00 FUD YYY S 80 TC

AMA: 2020,Dec,3; 2019,Mar,10; 2018,Feb,11; 2018,Jan,8; 2017,Jan,8; 2016,Jan,13

94776 monitoring, download of information, receipt of transmission(s) and analyses by computer only A

INCLUDES Oxygen saturation monitoring

EXCLUDES *Event monitors (93268-93272)*
Holter monitor (93224-93227)
Remote cardiovascular telemetry (93228-93229)
Sleep testing (95805-95811 [95800, 95801])

0.00 0.00 FUD YYY S 80 TC

AMA: 2020,Dec,3; 2019,Mar,10; 2018,Feb,11; 2018,Jan,8; 2017,Jan,8; 2016,Jan,13

94777 review, interpretation and preparation of report only by a physician or other qualified health care professional A

INCLUDES Oxygen saturation monitoring

EXCLUDES *Event monitors (93268-93272)*
Holter monitor (93224-93227)
Remote cardiovascular telemetry (93228-93229)
Sleep testing (95805-95811 [95800, 95801])

0.00 0.00 FUD YYY B 80 26

AMA: 2020,Dec,3; 2019,Mar,10; 2018,Feb,11; 2018,Jan,8; 2017,Jan,8; 2016,Jan,13

94780 Car seat/bed testing for airway integrity, for infants through 12 months of age, with continual clinical staff observation and continuous recording of pulse oximetry, heart rate and respiratory rate, with interpretation and report; 60 minutes A

EXCLUDES *Pediatric and neonatal critical care services (99468-99476, 99477-99480)*
Pulse oximetry (94760-94761)
Reporting code for service less than 60 minutes
Rhythm strips (93040-93042)

0.68 1.45 FUD XXX Q1

AMA: 2020,Dec,3; 2019,Mar,10; 2018,Feb,11; 2018,Jan,8; 2017,Jan,8; 2016,Jan,13

\+ **94781 each additional full 30 minutes (List separately in addition to code for primary procedure)** A

Code first (94780)

0.24 0.57 FUD ZZZ N

AMA: 2020,Dec,3; 2019,Mar,10; 2018,Feb,11; 2018,Jan,8; 2017,Jan,8; 2016,Jan,13

94799 Unlisted pulmonary service or procedure

0.00 0.00 FUD XXX Q1 80

AMA: 2020,Dec,3; 2019,Mar,10; 2018,Sep,14; 2018,Feb,11; 2018,Jan,8; 2017,Jan,8; 2016,Jan,13

95004-95070 Allergy Tests

EXCLUDES *Drugs administered for intractable/severe allergic reaction (eg, antihistamines, epinephrine, steroids) (96372)*
E/M services when reporting test interpretation/report
Laboratory tests for allergies (86000-86999 [86152, 86153])

Code also:
Medical conferences regarding equipment use (e.g., air filters, humidifiers, dehumidifiers), climate therapy, physical, occupational, and recreation therapy using appropriate E/M codes
Significant, separately identifiable E/M services appending modifier 25, when performed (99202-99215, 99217-99223 [99224, 99225, 99226], 99231-99233, 99241-99255, 99281-99285, 99304-99318, 99324-99337, 99341-99350, 99381-99429 [99415, 99416, 99417, 99421, 99422, 99423])

95004 Percutaneous tests (scratch, puncture, prick) with allergenic extracts, immediate type reaction, including test interpretation and report, specify number of tests

0.12 0.12 FUD XXX Q1 80

AMA: 2018,Feb,11; 2018,Jan,8; 2017,Jan,8; 2016,Jan,13

95012 Nitric oxide expired gas determination

0.57 0.57 FUD XXX Q1 80

AMA: 2018,Feb,11; 2018,Jan,8; 2017,Jan,8; 2016,Jan,13

95017 Allergy testing, any combination of percutaneous (scratch, puncture, prick) and intracutaneous (intradermal), sequential and incremental, with venoms, immediate type reaction, including test interpretation and report, specify number of tests

0.11 0.23 FUD XXX Q1 80

AMA: 2018,Feb,11; 2018,Jan,8; 2017,Jan,8; 2016,Jan,13

95018 Allergy testing, any combination of percutaneous (scratch, puncture, prick) and intracutaneous (intradermal), sequential and incremental, with drugs or biologicals, immediate type reaction, including test interpretation and report, specify number of tests

0.21 0.61 FUD XXX Q1 80

AMA: 2018,Feb,11; 2018,Jan,8; 2017,Jan,8; 2016,Jan,13

95024 Intracutaneous (intradermal) tests with allergenic extracts, immediate type reaction, including test interpretation and report, specify number of tests

0.03 0.23 FUD XXX Q1 80

AMA: 2018,Feb,11; 2018,Jan,8; 2017,Jan,8; 2016,Jan,13

95027 Intracutaneous (intradermal) tests, sequential and incremental, with allergenic extracts for airborne allergens, immediate type reaction, including test interpretation and report, specify number of tests

0.13 0.13 FUD XXX Q1 80

AMA: 2018,Feb,11; 2018,Jan,8; 2017,Jan,8; 2016,Jan,13

95028 Intracutaneous (intradermal) tests with allergenic extracts, delayed type reaction, including reading, specify number of tests

0.37 0.37 FUD XXX Q1 80 TC

AMA: 2018,Feb,11; 2018,Jan,8; 2017,Jan,8; 2016,Jan,13

95044 Patch or application test(s) (specify number of tests)

0.16 0.16 FUD XXX Q1 80

AMA: 2018,Feb,11; 2018,Jan,8; 2017,Jan,8; 2016,Jan,13

95052 Photo patch test(s) (specify number of tests)

0.19 0.19 FUD XXX Q1 80

AMA: 2018,Feb,11; 2018,Jan,8; 2017,Jan,8; 2016,Jan,13

95056 Photo tests

1.31 1.31 FUD XXX Q1 80

AMA: 2018,Feb,11; 2018,Jan,8; 2017,Jan,8; 2016,Jan,13

95060 Ophthalmic mucous membrane tests

0.99 0.99 FUD XXX Q1 80 TC

AMA: 2018,Feb,11; 2018,Jan,8; 2017,Jan,8; 2016,Jan,13

95065 Direct nasal mucous membrane test

0.74 0.74 FUD XXX Q1 80 TC

AMA: 2018,Feb,11; 2018,Jan,8; 2017,Jan,8; 2016,Jan,13

95070 **Inhalation bronchial challenge testing (not including necessary pulmonary function tests), with histamine, methacholine, or similar compounds**

EXCLUDES *Pulmonary function tests (94060, 94070)*

0.90 0.90 FUD XXX S 80 TC

AMA: 2018,Feb,11; 2018,Jan,8; 2017,Jan,8; 2016,Jan,13

95076-95079 Challenge Ingestion Testing

CMS: 100-03,110.12 Challenge Ingestion Food Testing

INCLUDES Assessment and monitoring for allergic reactions (eg, blood pressure, peak flow meter)

Testing time until test ends or to point E/M service needed

EXCLUDES *Reporting code for testing time less than 61 minutes, such as positive challenge resulting in ending test (report E/M codes as appropriate)*

Code also interventions when appropriate (eg, injection of epinephrine or steroid)

95076 **Ingestion challenge test (sequential and incremental ingestion of test items, eg, food, drug or other substance); initial 120 minutes of testing**

INCLUDES First 120 minutes testing time (not face-to-face time with physician)

2.15 3.43 FUD XXX S 80

AMA: 2018,Feb,11; 2018,Jan,8; 2017,Jan,8; 2016,Jan,13

+ **95079** **each additional 60 minutes of testing (List separately in addition to code for primary procedure)**

INCLUDES Includes each 60 minutes additional testing time (not face-to-face time with physician)

Code first (95076)

1.97 2.42 FUD ZZZ N 80

AMA: 2018,Feb,11; 2018,Jan,8; 2017,Jan,8; 2016,Jan,13

95115-95199 Allergy Immunotherapy

CMS: 100-03,110.9 Antigens Prepared for Sublingual Administration

INCLUDES Allergen immunotherapy professional services

EXCLUDES *Bacterial/viral/fungal extracts skin testing (86485-86580, 95028)*

Procedures for testing: (see Pathology/Immunology section or code:) (95199)

Leukocyte histamine release (LHR)

Lymphocytic transformation test (LTT)

Mast cell degranulation test (MCDT)

Migration inhibitory factor test (MIF)

Nitroblue tetrazolium dye test (NTD)

Radioallergosorbent testing (RAST)

Rat mast cell technique (RMCT)

Transfer factor test (TFT)

Special reports for allergy patients (99080)

Code also significant separately identifiable E/M services, when performed

95115 **Professional services for allergen immunotherapy not including provision of allergenic extracts; single injection**

0.26 0.26 FUD XXX Q1 80

AMA: 2020,Sep,14; 2019,Jun,14; 2018,Feb,11; 2018,Jan,8; 2017,Jan,8; 2016,Jan,13

95117 **2 or more injections**

0.30 0.30 FUD XXX Q1 80

AMA: 2020,Sep,14; 2019,Jun,14; 2018,Feb,11; 2018,Jan,8; 2017,Jan,8; 2016,Jan,13

95120 **Professional services for allergen immunotherapy in the office or institution of the prescribing physician or other qualified health care professional, including provision of allergenic extract; single injection**

0.00 0.00 FUD XXX E

AMA: 2018,Feb,11; 2018,Jan,8; 2017,Jan,8; 2016,Jan,13

95125 **2 or more injections**

0.00 0.00 FUD XXX E

AMA: 2018,Feb,11; 2018,Jan,8; 2017,Jan,8; 2016,Jan,13

95130 **single stinging insect venom**

0.00 0.00 FUD XXX E

AMA: 2018,Feb,11; 2018,Jan,8; 2017,Jan,8; 2016,Jan,13

95131 **2 stinging insect venoms**

0.00 0.00 FUD XXX E

AMA: 2018,Feb,11; 2018,Jan,8; 2017,Jan,8; 2016,Jan,13

95132 **3 stinging insect venoms**

0.00 0.00 FUD XXX E

AMA: 2018,Feb,11; 2018,Jan,8; 2017,Jan,8; 2016,Jan,13

95133 **4 stinging insect venoms**

0.00 0.00 FUD XXX E

AMA: 2018,Feb,11; 2018,Jan,8; 2017,Jan,8; 2016,Jan,13

95134 **5 stinging insect venoms**

0.00 0.00 FUD XXX E

AMA: 2018,Feb,11; 2018,Jan,8; 2017,Jan,8; 2016,Jan,13

95144 **Professional services for the supervision of preparation and provision of antigens for allergen immunotherapy, single dose vial(s) (specify number of vials)**

INCLUDES Single dose vial/single dose of antigen administered in one injection

0.09 0.41 FUD XXX Q1 80

AMA: 2018,Feb,11; 2018,Jan,8; 2017,Jan,8; 2016,Jan,13

95145 **Professional services for the supervision of preparation and provision of antigens for allergen immunotherapy (specify number of doses); single stinging insect venom**

0.09 0.81 FUD XXX Q1 80

AMA: 2018,Feb,11; 2018,Jan,8; 2017,Jan,8; 2016,Jan,13

95146 **2 single stinging insect venoms**

0.09 1.50 FUD XXX Q1 80

AMA: 2018,Feb,11; 2018,Jan,8; 2017,Jan,8; 2016,Jan,13

95147 **3 single stinging insect venoms**

0.09 1.55 FUD XXX Q1 80

AMA: 2018,Feb,11; 2018,Jan,8; 2017,Jan,8; 2016,Jan,13

95148 **4 single stinging insect venoms**

0.09 2.23 FUD XXX Q1 80

AMA: 2018,Feb,11; 2018,Jan,8; 2017,Jan,8; 2016,Jan,13

95149 **5 single stinging insect venoms**

0.09 2.97 FUD XXX Q1 80

AMA: 2018,Feb,11; 2018,Jan,8; 2017,Jan,8; 2016,Jan,13

95165 **Professional services for the supervision of preparation and provision of antigens for allergen immunotherapy; single or multiple antigens (specify number of doses)**

0.09 0.40 FUD XXX Q1 80

AMA: 2018,Feb,11; 2018,Jan,8; 2017,Jan,8; 2016,Jan,13

95170 **whole body extract of biting insect or other arthropod (specify number of doses)**

INCLUDES Dose which is amount of antigen(s) administered in single injection from multiple dose vial

0.09 0.30 FUD XXX Q1 80

AMA: 2018,Feb,11; 2018,Jan,8; 2017,Jan,8; 2016,Jan,13

95180 **Rapid desensitization procedure, each hour (eg, insulin, penicillin, equine serum)**

2.96 3.92 FUD XXX Q1 80

AMA: 2019,Jun,14; 2018,Feb,11; 2018,Jan,8; 2017,Jan,8; 2016,Jan,13

95199 **Unlisted allergy/clinical immunologic service or procedure**

0.00 0.00 FUD XXX Q1 80

AMA: 2018,Feb,11; 2018,Jan,8; 2017,Jan,8; 2016,Jan,13

95249-95251 [95249] Glucose Monitoring By Subcutaneous Device

EXCLUDES *Physiologic data collection/interpretation (99091)*

Code also when data receiver owned by patient for sensor placement, hook-up, monitor calibration, training, and printout (95999)

95249 **Resequenced code. See code following 95250.**

95250 **Ambulatory continuous glucose monitoring of interstitial tissue fluid via a subcutaneous sensor for a minimum of 72 hours; physician or other qualified health care professional (office) provided equipment, sensor placement, hook-up, calibration of monitor, patient training, removal of sensor, and printout of recording**

EXCLUDES *Reporting code more than one time per month*

Subcutaneous pocket with insertion interstitial glucose monitor (0446T)

4.26 4.26 FUD XXX V 80 TC

AMA: 2019,Jan,6; 2018,Jun,6; 2018,Mar,5; 2018,Feb,11; 2018,Jan,8; 2017,Jan,8; 2016,Jan,13

95249 **patient-provided equipment, sensor placement, hook-up, calibration of monitor, patient training, and printout of recording**

INCLUDES Performing complete collection initial data in provider's office

EXCLUDES *Reporting code more than one time during period patient owns data receiver*

Subcutaneous pocket with insertion interstitial glucose monitor (0446T)

1.54 1.54 FUD XXX S 80 TC

AMA: 2018,Jun,6; 2018,Feb,11

95251 **analysis, interpretation and report**

EXCLUDES *Reporting code more than one time per month*

1.02 1.02 FUD XXX B 80 26

AMA: 2018,Jun,6; 2018,Mar,5; 2018,Feb,11; 2018,Jan,8; 2017,Jan,8; 2016,Jan,13

95700-95783 [95700, 95705, 95706, 95707, 95708, 95709, 95710, 95711, 95712, 95713, 95714, 95715, 95716, 95717, 95718, 95719, 95720, 95721, 95722, 95723, 95724, 95725, 95726, 95782, 95783, 95800, 95801] Sleep Studies

INCLUDES Assessment sleep disorders in adults and children
Continuous and simultaneous monitoring and recording physiological sleep parameters six hours or more
Evaluation patient's response to therapies
Physician:
- Interpretation
- Recording
- Report

Portable and in-laboratory technology
Recording sessions may be:
- Attended studies that include technologist or qualified health care professional presence to respond to patient needs or technical issues at bedside
- Remote without technologist or qualified health professional presence
- Unattended without technologist or qualified health care professional presence

Testing parameters include:
- Actigraphy: Noninvasive portable device to record gross motor movements to approximate sleep and wakeful periods
- Electrooculogram (EOG): Records electrical activity associated with eye movements
- Maintenance of wakefulness test (MWT): Attended study to determine patient's ability to stay awake
- Multiple sleep latency test (MSLT): Attended study to determine patient tendency to fall asleep
- Peripheral arterial tonometry (PAT): Pulsatile volume changes in digit measured to determine activity in sympathetic nervous system for respiratory analysis
- Polysomnography: Attended continuous, simultaneous recording physiological sleep parameters for at least six hours in sleep laboratory setting that also includes four or more:
  1. Airflow-oral and/or nasal
  2. Bilateral anterior tibialis EMG
  3. Electrocardiogram (ECG)
  4. Oxyhemoglobin saturation, SpO2
  5. Respiratory effort
- Positive airway pressure (PAP): Noninvasive devices to treat sleep-related disorders
- Respiratory airflow (ventilation): Assessment air movement during inhalation and exhalation as measured by nasal pressure sensors and thermistor
- Respiratory analysis: Assessment respiration components obtained by other methods such as airflow or peripheral arterial tone
- Respiratory effort: Diaphragm and/or intercostal muscle contraction for airflow measured using transducers to estimate thoracic and abdominal motion
- Respiratory movement: Measures chest and abdomen movement during respiration
- Sleep latency: Pertains to time it takes to get to sleep
- Sleep staging: Determining separate sleep levels according to physiological measurements
- Total sleep time: Determined by actigraphy and other methods

EXCLUDES *E/M services*

95700 **Resequenced code. See code following 95967.**
95705 **Resequenced code. See code following 95967.**
95706 **Resequenced code. See code following 95967.**
95707 **Resequenced code. See code following 95967.**
95708 **Resequenced code. See code following 95967.**
95709 **Resequenced code. See code following 95967.**
95710 **Resequenced code. See code following 95967.**
95711 **Resequenced code. See code following 95967.**
95712 **Resequenced code. See code following 95967.**
95713 **Resequenced code. See code following 95967.**
95714 **Resequenced code. See code following 95967.**
95715 **Resequenced code. See code following 95967.**
95716 **Resequenced code. See code following 95967.**
95717 **Resequenced code. See code following 95967.**
95718 **Resequenced code. See code following 95967.**
95719 **Resequenced code. See code following 95967.**
95720 **Resequenced code. See code following 95967.**
95721 **Resequenced code. See code following 95967.**
95722 **Resequenced code. See code following 95967.**
95723 **Resequenced code. See code following 95967.**
95724 **Resequenced code. See code following 95967.**
95725 **Resequenced code. See code following 95967.**
95726 **Resequenced code. See code following 95967.**
95782 **Resequenced code. See code following 95811.**
95783 **Resequenced code. See code following 95811.**
95800 **Resequenced code. See code following 95806.**
95801 **Resequenced code. See code following 95806.**

95803 **Actigraphy testing, recording, analysis, interpretation, and report (minimum of 72 hours to 14 consecutive days of recording)**

EXCLUDES *Reporting code more than one time in 14-day period*

Sleep studies (95806-95811 [95800, 95801])

4.22 4.22 FUD XXX Q1 80

AMA: 2018,Feb,11; 2018,Jan,8; 2017,Jan,8; 2016,Jan,13

95805 **Multiple sleep latency or maintenance of wakefulness testing, recording, analysis and interpretation of physiological measurements of sleep during multiple trials to assess sleepiness**

INCLUDES Physiological sleep parameters as measured by:
- Frontal, central, and occipital EEG leads (three leads)
- Left and right EOG
- Submental EMG lead

EXCLUDES *Polysomnography (95808-95811)*

Sleep study, not attended (95806)

Code also modifier 52 when less than four nap opportunities recorded

11.7 11.7 FUD XXX S 80

AMA: 2018,Feb,11; 2018,Jan,8; 2017,Jan,8; 2016,Jan,13

95806 **Sleep study, unattended, simultaneous recording of, heart rate, oxygen saturation, respiratory airflow, and respiratory effort (eg, thoracoabdominal movement)**

EXCLUDES *Arterial waveform analysis (93050)*

Event monitors (93268-93272)

Holter monitor (93224-93227)

Remote cardiovascular telemetry (93228-93229)

Rhythm strips (93041-93042)

Unattended sleep study with minimum heart rate, oxygen saturation, and respiratory analysis measurement ([95801])

Unattended sleep study with heart rate, oxygen saturation, respiratory analysis, and sleep time measurement ([95800])

Code also modifier 52 for fewer than six hours recording

3.30 3.30 FUD XXX S 80

AMA: 2018,Feb,11; 2018,Jan,8; 2017,Jan,8; 2016,Jan,13

\# **95800 Sleep study, unattended, simultaneous recording; heart rate, oxygen saturation, respiratory analysis (eg, by airflow or peripheral arterial tone), and sleep time**

EXCLUDES *Actigraphy testing (95803)*
Arterial waveform analysis (93050)
Event monitors (93268-93272)
Holter monitor (93224-93227)
Remote cardiovascular telemetry (93228-93229)
Rhythm strips (93041-93042)
Unattended sleep study with heart rate, oxygen saturation, respiratory airflow and respiratory effort measurement (95806)
Unattended sleep study with minimum heart rate, oxygen saturation, and respiratory analysis measurement ([95801])

Code also modifier 52 for fewer than 6 hours recording
4.68 | 4.68 | FUD XXX | S 80
AMA: 2018,Feb,11; 2018,Jan,8; 2017,Jan,8; 2016,Jan,13

\# **95801 minimum of heart rate, oxygen saturation, and respiratory analysis (eg, by airflow or peripheral arterial tone)**

EXCLUDES *Arterial waveform analysis (93050)*
Event monitors (93268-93272)
Holter monitor (93224-93227)
Remote cardiovascular telemetry (93228-93229)
Rhythm strips (93041-93042)
Unattended sleep study with heart rate, oxygen saturation, respiratory airflow and respiratory effort measurement (95806)
Unattended sleep study with heart rate, oxygen saturation, respiratory analysis, and sleep time measurement ([95800])

Code also modifier 52 for fewer than 6 hours recording
2.52 | 2.52 | FUD XXX | Q1 80
AMA: 2018,Feb,11; 2018,Jan,8; 2017,Jan,8; 2016,Jan,13

95807 Sleep study, simultaneous recording of ventilation, respiratory effort, ECG or heart rate, and oxygen saturation, attended by a technologist

EXCLUDES *Polysomnography (95808-95811)*
Sleep study, not attended (95806)

Code also modifier 52 for fewer than six hours recording
11.4 | 11.4 | FUD XXX | S 80
AMA: 2018,Feb,11; 2018,Jan,8; 2017,Jan,8; 2016,Jan,13

95808 Polysomnography; any age, sleep staging with 1-3 additional parameters of sleep, attended by a technologist

EXCLUDES *Sleep study, not attended (95806)*

18.4 | 18.4 | FUD XXX | S 80
AMA: 2018,Feb,11; 2018,Jan,8; 2017,Jan,8; 2016,Jan,13

95810 age 6 years or older, sleep staging with 4 or more additional parameters of sleep, attended by a technologist A

EXCLUDES *Sleep study, not attended (95806)*

Code also modifier 52 for fewer than six hours recording
17.2 | 17.2 | FUD XXX | S 80
AMA: 2018,Feb,11; 2018,Jan,8; 2017,Jan,8; 2016,Jan,13

95811 age 6 years or older, sleep staging with 4 or more additional parameters of sleep, with initiation of continuous positive airway pressure therapy or bilevel ventilation, attended by a technologist A

EXCLUDES *Sleep study, not attended (95806)*

Code also modifier 52 for fewer than six hours recording
18.1 | 18.1 | FUD XXX | S 80
AMA: 2018,Feb,11; 2018,Jan,8; 2017,Jan,8; 2016,Jan,13

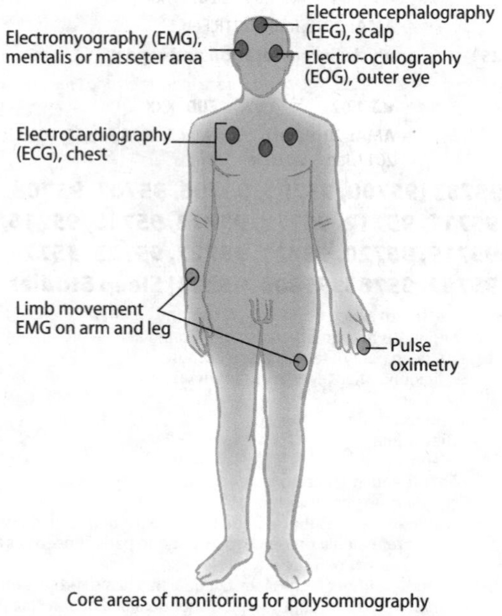

Core areas of monitoring for polysomnography

\# **95782 younger than 6 years, sleep staging with 4 or more additional parameters of sleep, attended by a technologist** A

Code also modifier 52 for fewer than 7 hours recording
25.4 | 25.4 | FUD XXX | S 80
AMA: 2018,Feb,11; 2018,Jan,8; 2017,Jan,8; 2016,Jan,13

\# **95783 younger than 6 years, sleep staging with 4 or more additional parameters of sleep, with initiation of continuous positive airway pressure therapy or bi-level ventilation, attended by a technologist** A

Code also modifier 52 for fewer than seven hours recording
27.1 | 27.1 | FUD XXX | S 80
AMA: 2018,Feb,11; 2018,Jan,8; 2017,Jan,8; 2016,Jan,13

95812-95830 [95829] Evaluation of Brain Activity by Electroencephalogram

INCLUDES Only time when time is recorded, data collected, and does not include set-up and take-down

EXCLUDES *E/M services*

95812 Electroencephalogram (EEG) extended monitoring; 41-60 minutes

INCLUDES Hyperventilation
Photic stimulation
Physician interpretation
Recording 41-60 minutes
Report

EXCLUDES *EEG digital analysis (95957)*
EEG during nonintracranial surgery (95955)
Long-term EEG (two hours or more) ([95700, 95705, 95706, 95707, 95708, 95709, 95710, 95711, 95712, 95713, 95714, 95715, 95716, 95717, 95718, 95719, 95720, 95721, 95722, 95723, 95724, 95725, 95726])
Wada test (95958)

Code also modifier 26 for physician interpretation only

9.19 9.19 **FUD** XXX S 80

AMA: 2018,Dec,3; 2018,Dec,3; 2018,Feb,11; 2018,Jan,8; 2017,Jan,8; 2016,Jan,13

95813 61-119 minutes

INCLUDES Hyperventilation
Photic stimulation
Physician interpretation
Recording 61 minutes or more
Report

EXCLUDES *EEG digital analysis (95957)*
EEG during nonintracranial surgery (95955)
Long-term EEG (two hours or more) ([95700, 95705, 95706, 95707, 95708, 95709, 95710, 95711, 95712, 95713, 95714, 95715, 95716, 95717, 95718, 95719, 95720, 95721, 95722, 95723, 95724, 95725, 95726])
Wada test (95958)

Code also modifier 26 for physician interpretation only

11.5 11.5 **FUD** XXX S 80

AMA: 2018,Dec,3; 2018,Dec,3; 2018,Feb,11; 2018,Jan,8; 2017,Jan,8; 2016,Jan,13

95816 Electroencephalogram (EEG); including recording awake and drowsy

INCLUDES Photic stimulation
Physician interpretation
Recording 20-40 minutes
Report

EXCLUDES *EEG digital analysis (95957)*
EEG during nonintracranial surgery (95955)
Long-term EEG (two hours or more) ([95700, 95705, 95706, 95707, 95708, 95709, 95710, 95711, 95712, 95713, 95714, 95715, 95716, 95717, 95718, 95719, 95720, 95721, 95722, 95723, 95724, 95725, 95726])
Wada test (95958)

Code also modifier 26 for physician interpretation only

10.3 10.3 **FUD** XXX S 80

AMA: 2018,Dec,3; 2018,Dec,3; 2018,Feb,11; 2018,Jan,8; 2017,Jan,8; 2016,Jan,13

95819 including recording awake and asleep

INCLUDES Hyperventilation
Photic stimulation
Physician interpretation
Recording 20-40 minutes
Report

EXCLUDES *EEG digital analysis (95957)*
EEG during nonintracranial surgery (95955)
Long-term EEG (two hours or more) ([95700, 95705, 95706, 95707, 95708, 95709, 95710, 95711, 95712, 95713, 95714, 95715, 95716, 95717, 95718, 95719, 95720, 95721, 95722, 95723, 95724, 95725, 95726])
Wada test (95958)

Code also modifier 26 for interpretation only

12.2 12.2 **FUD** XXX S 80

AMA: 2018,Dec,3; 2018,Dec,3; 2018,Feb,11; 2018,Jan,8; 2017,Jan,8; 2016,Jan,13

95822 recording in coma or sleep only

INCLUDES Hyperventilation
Photic stimulation
Physician interpretation
Recording 20-40 minutes
Report

EXCLUDES *EEG digital analysis (95957)*
EEG during nonintracranial surgery (95955)
Long-term EEG (two hours or more) ([95700, 95705, 95706, 95707, 95708, 95709, 95710, 95711, 95712, 95713, 95714, 95715, 95716, 95717, 95718, 95719, 95720, 95721, 95722, 95723, 95724, 95725, 95726])
Wada test (95958)

Code also modifier 26 for interpretation only

11.0 11.0 **FUD** XXX S 80

AMA: 2018,Dec,3; 2018,Dec,3; 2018,Feb,11; 2018,Jan,8; 2017,Jan,8; 2016,Jan,13

95824 cerebral death evaluation only

INCLUDES Physician interpretation
Recording
Report

EXCLUDES *EEG digital analysis (95957)*
EEG during nonintracranial surgery (95955)
Long-term EEG (two hours or more) ([95700, 95705, 95706, 95707, 95708, 95709, 95710, 95711, 95712, 95713, 95714, 95715, 95716, 95717, 95718, 95719, 95720, 95721, 95722, 95723, 95724, 95725, 95726])
Wada test (95958)

Code also modifier 26 for physician interpretation only

0.00 0.00 **FUD** XXX S 80

AMA: 2018,Feb,11

95829 **Resequenced code. See code following 95830.**

95830 Insertion by physician or other qualified health care professional of sphenoidal electrodes for electroencephalographic (EEG) recording

2.64 10.9 **FUD** XXX B 80

AMA: 2018,Feb,11

95829-95836 [95829, 95836] Evaluation of Brain Activity by Electrocorticography

\# **95829 Electrocorticogram at surgery (separate procedure)**

INCLUDES EEG recording from electrodes placed in or on brain
Interpretation and review during surgical procedure

Code also modifier 26 for interpretation only

53.6 53.6 **FUD** XXX N 80

AMA: 2018,Dec,3; 2018,Dec,3; 2018,Feb,11

\# **95836** **Electrocorticogram from an implanted brain neurostimulator pulse generator/transmitter, including recording, with interpretation and written report, up to 30 days**

INCLUDES Intracranial recordings up to 30 days (unattended) with storage for later review

EXCLUDES *EEG digital analysis (95957)*

Programming neurostimulator during 30-day period ([95983, 95984])

Reporting code more than one time for documented 30-day period

3.19 3.19 FUD XXX 80

AMA: 2018,Dec,3; 2018,Dec,3

95836-95857 [95836] Evaluation of Muscles and Range of Motion

95836 **Resequenced code. See code following 95830.**

95851 **Range of motion measurements and report (separate procedure); each extremity (excluding hand) or each trunk section (spine)**

0.22 0.59 FUD XXX A 80

AMA: 2018,Feb,11; 2018,Jan,8; 2017,Jan,8; 2016,Dec,16; 2016,Jan,13

95852 **hand, with or without comparison with normal side**

0.17 0.53 FUD XXX A 80

AMA: 2018,Feb,11; 2018,Jan,8; 2017,Jan,8; 2016,Jan,13

95857 **Cholinesterase inhibitor challenge test for myasthenia gravis**

0.85 1.54 FUD XXX S 80

AMA: 2018,Feb,11; 2018,Jan,8; 2017,Jan,8; 2016,Jan,13

95860-95887 [95885, 95886, 95887] Evaluation of Nerve and Muscle Function: EMGs with/without Nerve Conduction Studies

INCLUDES Physician interpretation
Recording
Report

EXCLUDES *E/M services*

95860 **Needle electromyography; 1 extremity with or without related paraspinal areas**

INCLUDES Testing five or more muscles per extremity

EXCLUDES *Dynamic electromyography during motion analysis studies (96002-96003)*

Guidance for chemodenervation (95873-95874)

3.40 3.40 FUD XXX Q1 80

AMA: 2018,Feb,11; 2018,Jan,8; 2017,Jan,8; 2016,Jan,13

95861 **2 extremities with or without related paraspinal areas**

INCLUDES Testing five or more muscles per extremity

EXCLUDES *Dynamic electromyography during motion analysis studies (96002-96003)*

Guidance for chemodenervation (95873-95874)

4.87 4.87 FUD XXX Q1 80

AMA: 2018,Feb,11; 2018,Jan,8; 2017,Jan,8; 2016,Jan,13

95863 **3 extremities with or without related paraspinal areas**

INCLUDES Testing five or more muscles per extremity

EXCLUDES *Dynamic electromyography during motion analysis studies (96002-96003)*

Guidance for chemodenervation (95873-95874)

6.02 6.02 FUD XXX S 80

AMA: 2018,Feb,11; 2018,Jan,8; 2017,Jan,8; 2016,Jan,13

95864 **4 extremities with or without related paraspinal areas**

INCLUDES Testing five or more muscles per extremity

EXCLUDES *Dynamic electromyography during motion analysis studies (96002-96003)*

Guidance for chemodenervation (95873-95874)

7.07 7.07 FUD XXX S 80

AMA: 2018,Feb,11; 2018,Jan,8; 2017,Jan,8; 2016,Jan,13

95865 **larynx**

EXCLUDES *Dynamic electromyography during motion analysis studies (96002-96003)*

Guidance for chemodenervation (95873-95874)

Code also modifier 52 for unilateral procedure

4.34 4.34 FUD XXX Q1 80

AMA: 2018,Feb,11; 2018,Jan,8; 2017,Jan,8; 2016,Jan,13

95866 **hemidiaphragm**

EXCLUDES *Dynamic electromyography during motion analysis studies (96002-96003)*

Guidance for chemodenervation (95873-95874)

3.83 3.83 FUD XXX Q1 80

AMA: 2018,Feb,11; 2018,Jan,8; 2017,Jan,8; 2016,Jan,13

95867 **cranial nerve supplied muscle(s), unilateral**

EXCLUDES *Guidance for chemodenervation (95873-95874)*

3.05 3.05 FUD XXX S 80

AMA: 2018,Feb,11; 2018,Jan,8; 2017,Jan,8; 2016,Jan,13

95868 **cranial nerve supplied muscles, bilateral**

EXCLUDES *Guidance for chemodenervation (95873-95874)*

4.00 4.00 FUD XXX S 80

AMA: 2018,Feb,11; 2018,Jan,8; 2017,Jan,8; 2016,Jan,13

95869 **thoracic paraspinal muscles (excluding T1 or T12)**

EXCLUDES *Dynamic electromyography during motion analysis studies (96002-96003)*

Guidance for chemodenervation (95873-95874)

2.71 2.71 FUD XXX Q1 80

AMA: 2018,Feb,11; 2018,Jan,8; 2017,Jan,8; 2016,Jan,13

95870 **limited study of muscles in 1 extremity or non-limb (axial) muscles (unilateral or bilateral), other than thoracic paraspinal, cranial nerve supplied muscles, or sphincters**

INCLUDES Adson test

Testing four or less muscles per extremity

EXCLUDES *Anal/urethral sphincter/detrusor/urethra/perineum musculature (51785-51792)*

Complete study extremities (95860-95864)

Dynamic electromyography during motion analysis studies (96002-96003)

Eye muscles (92265)

Guidance for chemodenervation (95873-95874)

2.56 2.56 FUD XXX Q1 80

AMA: 2018,Feb,11; 2018,Jan,8; 2017,Jan,8; 2016,Jan,13

95872 **Needle electromyography using single fiber electrode, with quantitative measurement of jitter, blocking and/or fiber density, any/all sites of each muscle studied**

EXCLUDES *Dynamic electromyography during motion analysis studies (96002-96003)*

5.66 5.66 FUD XXX S 80

AMA: 2018,Feb,11; 2018,Jan,8; 2017,Jan,8; 2016,Jan,13

\+ # **95885** **Needle electromyography, each extremity, with related paraspinal areas, when performed, done with nerve conduction, amplitude and latency/velocity study; limited (List separately in addition to code for primary procedure)**

INCLUDES Testing four or less muscles per extremity

EXCLUDES *Dynamic electromyography during motion analysis studies (96002-96003)*

Motor and sensory nerve conduction (95905)

Needle electromyography extremities (95860-95864, 95870)

Reporting code more than one time per extremity

Code also, when applicable, for combined maximum total four units per patient when all four extremities tested ([95886])

Code first nerve conduction tests (95907-95913)

1.77 1.77 FUD ZZZ N 80

AMA: 2020,Nov,12; 2018,Feb,11; 2018,Jan,8; 2017,Jul,10; 2017,Jan,8; 2016,Jan,13

+ # **95886** **complete, five or more muscles studied, innervated by three or more nerves or four or more spinal levels (List separately in addition to code for primary procedure)**

INCLUDES Testing five or more muscles per extremity

EXCLUDES *Dynamic electromyography during motion analysis studies (96002-96003)*

Motor and sensory nerve conduction (95905)

Needle electromyography extremities (95860-95864, 95870)

Reporting code more than one time per extremity

Code also, when applicable, for combined maximum total four units per patient when all four extremities tested ([95885])

Code first nerve conduction tests (95907-95913)

2.75 2.75 **FUD** ZZZ N 80

AMA: 2020,Nov,12; 2018,Feb,11; 2018,Jan,8; 2017,Jul,10; 2017,Jan,8; 2016,Jan,13

+ # **95887** **Needle electromyography, non-extremity (cranial nerve supplied or axial) muscle(s) done with nerve conduction, amplitude and latency/velocity study (List separately in addition to code for primary procedure)**

INCLUDES Nerve study unilateral cranial nerve innervated muscles

EXCLUDES *Dynamic electromyography during motion analysis studies (96002-96003)*

Guidance for chemodenervation (95874)

Motor and sensory nerve conduction (95905)

Needle electromyography cranial nerve supplied muscles (95867-95868)

Needle electromyography except for thoracic paraspinal, cranial nerve supplied muscles, or sphincters (95870)

Nerve study extra-ocular or laryngeal nerves

Reporting code more than once per anatomic site

Code also twice when performed bilaterally

Code first nerve conduction tests (95907-95913)

2.40 2.40 **FUD** ZZZ N 80

AMA: 2018,Feb,11; 2018,Jan,8; 2017,Jul,10; 2017,Jan,8; 2016,Jan,13

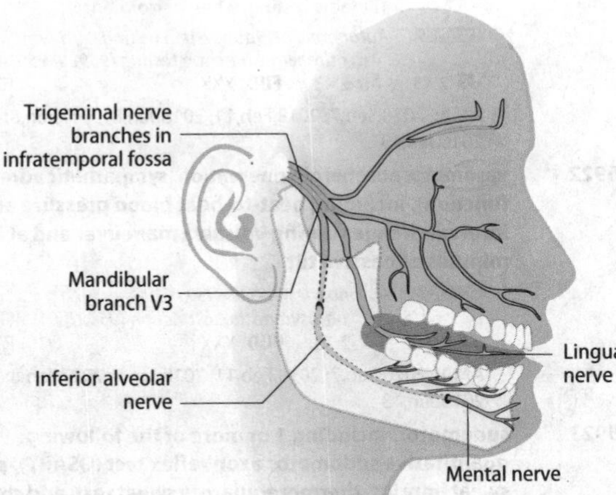

Cranial nerves: trigeminal branches of lower face and select facial nerves

Needle EMG is performed to determine conduction, amplitude, and latency/velocity

+ **95873** **Electrical stimulation for guidance in conjunction with chemodenervation (List separately in addition to code for primary procedure)**

EXCLUDES *Chemodenervation larynx (64617)*

Injection anesthetic or steroid, sacroiliac joint (64451)

Needle electromyography (95860-95870)

Needle electromyography guidance for chemodenervation (95874)

Radiofrequency ablation, sacroiliac joint ([64625])

Reporting more than one guidance code for each chemodenervation code

Code first chemodenervation (64612, 64615-64616, 64642-64647)

2.17 2.17 **FUD** ZZZ N 80

AMA: 2019,Dec,8; 2019,Apr,9; 2018,Feb,11; 2018,Jan,8; 2017,Jan,8; 2016,Jan,13

+ **95874** **Needle electromyography for guidance in conjunction with chemodenervation (List separately in addition to code for primary procedure)**

EXCLUDES *Chemodenervation larynx (64617)*

Injection anesthetic or steroid, sacroiliac joint (64451)

Needle electromyography (95860-95870)

Needle electromyography guidance for chemodenervation (95873)

Radiofrequency ablation, sacroiliac joint ([64625])

Reporting more than one guidance code for each chemodenervation code

Code first chemodenervation (64612, 64615-64616, 64642-64647)

2.23 2.23 **FUD** ZZZ N 80

AMA: 2020,Dec,13; 2019,Dec,8; 2019,Apr,9; 2018,Feb,11; 2018,Jan,8; 2017,Jan,8; 2016,Jan,13

95875 **Ischemic limb exercise test with serial specimen(s) acquisition for muscle(s) metabolite(s)**

3.78 3.78 **FUD** XXX S 80

AMA: 2018,Feb,11; 2018,Jan,8; 2017,Jan,8; 2016,Jan,13

95885 **Resequenced code. See code following 95872.**

95886 **Resequenced code. See code following 95872.**

95887 **Resequenced code. See code before 95873.**

95905-95913 Evaluation of Nerve Function: Nerve Conduction Studies

INCLUDES Conduction studies motor and sensory nerves

Reports from on-site examiner including interpretation results using established methodologies, calculations, comparisons to normal studies, and interpretation by physician or other qualified health care professional

Single conduction study comprising sensory and motor conduction test with/without F or H wave testing, and all orthodromic and antidromic impulses

Total number tests performed indicate appropriate code

EXCLUDES *Reporting code for more than one study when multiple sites on same nerve tested*

Code also electromyography performed with nerve conduction studies, as appropriate ([95885, 95886, 95887])

95905 **Motor and/or sensory nerve conduction, using preconfigured electrode array(s), amplitude and latency/velocity study, each limb, includes F-wave study when performed, with interpretation and report**

INCLUDES Study with preconfigured electrodes that are customized to a specific body location

EXCLUDES *Needle electromyography ([95885, 95886])*

Nerve conduction studies (95907-95913)

Reporting code more than one time for each limb studied

1.53 1.53 **FUD** XXX ⊘ 80

AMA: 2018,Feb,11; 2018,Jan,8; 2017,Jan,8; 2016,Jan,13

95907 **Nerve conduction studies; 1-2 studies**

2.71 2.71 **FUD** XXX S 80

AMA: 2018,Aug,10; 2018,Feb,11; 2018,Jan,8; 2017,Dec,14; 2017,Jan,8; 2016,Jan,13

95908 3-4 studies
3.44 3.44 FUD XXX
AMA: 2018,Aug,10; 2018,Feb,11; 2018,Jan,8; 2017,Jan,8; 2016,Jan,13

95909 5-6 studies
4.12 4.12 FUD XXX
AMA: 2018,Aug,10; 2018,Feb,11; 2018,Jan,8; 2017,Jan,8; 2016,Jan,13

95910 7-8 studies
5.42 5.42 FUD XXX
AMA: 2018,Aug,10; 2018,Feb,11; 2018,Jan,8; 2017,Jan,8; 2016,Jan,13

95911 9-10 studies
6.49 6.49 FUD XXX
AMA: 2018,Aug,10; 2018,Feb,11; 2018,Jan,8; 2017,Jan,8; 2016,Jan,13

95912 11-12 studies
7.43 7.43 FUD XXX
AMA: 2018,Aug,10; 2018,Feb,11; 2018,Jan,8; 2017,Jan,8; 2016,Jan,13

95913 13 or more studies
8.60 8.60 FUD XXX
AMA: 2018,Aug,10; 2018,Feb,11; 2018,Jan,8; 2017,Jan,8; 2016,Jan,13

95940-95941 [95940, 95941] Intraoperative Neurophysiological Monitoring

INCLUDES Monitoring, testing, and data evaluation during surgical procedures by monitoring professional dedicated only to performing necessary testing and monitoring
Monitoring services provided by anesthesiologist or surgeon separately

EXCLUDES *Baseline neurophysiologic monitoring*
EEG during nonintracranial surgery (95955)
Electrocorticography ([95829])
Intraoperative cortical and subcortical mapping (95961-95962)
Neurostimulator programming/analysis (95971-95972, 95976-95977, [95983, 95984])
Time required for set-up, recording, interpretation, and electrode removal

Code also:
Baseline studies (eg, EMGs, NCVs), no more than one time per operative session
Services provided after midnight using date when monitoring started and total monitoring time
Standby time prior to procedure (99360)
Code first ([92653], 95822, 95860-95870, 95907-95913, 95925-95937 [95938, 95939])

\+ # **95940 Continuous intraoperative neurophysiology monitoring in the operating room, one on one monitoring requiring personal attendance, each 15 minutes (List separately in addition to code for primary procedure)**

INCLUDES 15 minute increments monitoring service
Based on time spent monitoring, despite number tests or parameters monitored
Continuous intraoperative neurophysiologic monitoring by dedicated monitoring professional in operating room providing one-on-one patient care
Monitoring time distinct from baseline neurophysiologic study time(s) or other services (e.g., mapping)
Monitoring time may begin prior to incision
Total all monitoring time for procedures overlapping midnight

EXCLUDES *Time spent in executing or interpreting baseline neurophysiologic study or studies*

Code also monitoring from outside operative room, when applicable ([95941])
0.93 0.93 FUD XXX
AMA: 2020,Oct,9; 2020,Oct,14; 2018,Feb,11; 2018,Jan,8; 2017,Aug,8; 2017,Jan,8; 2016,Jan,13

\+ # **95941 Continuous intraoperative neurophysiology monitoring, from outside the operating room (remote or nearby) or for monitoring of more than one case while in the operating room, per hour (List separately in addition to code for primary procedure)**

INCLUDES Based on time spent monitoring, despite number tests or parameters monitored
Monitoring time distinct from baseline neurophysiologic study time(s) or other services (e.g., mapping)
One hour increments monitoring service

0.00 0.00 FUD XXX
AMA: 2020,Oct,9; 2020,Oct,14; 2018,Feb,11; 2018,Jan,8; 2017,Aug,8; 2017,Jan,8; 2016,Jan,13

95921-95924 Evaluation of Autonomic Nervous System

INCLUDES Physician interpretation
Recording
Report
Testing for autonomic dysfunction including site and autonomic subsystems

95921 Testing of autonomic nervous system function; cardiovagal innervation (parasympathetic function), including 2 or more of the following: heart rate response to deep breathing with recorded R-R interval, Valsalva ratio, and 30:15 ratio

INCLUDES Data storage for waveform analysis
Display on monitor
Minimum two elements performed:
Cardiovascular function indicated by 30:15 ration (R/R interval at beat 30)/(R-R interval at beat 15)
Heart rate response to deep breathing obtained by visual quantitative recording analysis with patient taking five to six breaths per minute
Valsalva ratio (at least two) obtained by dividing highest heart rate by lowest
Monitoring heart rate by electrocardiography; rate obtained from time between two successive R waves (R-R interval)
Testing most usually in prone position
Tilt table testing, when performed

EXCLUDES *Autonomic nervous system testing with sympathetic adrenergic function testing (95922, 95924)*

2.43 2.43 FUD XXX
AMA: 2020,Sep,7; 2018,Feb,11; 2018,Jan,8; 2017,Jan,8; 2016,Jan,13

95922 vasomotor adrenergic innervation (sympathetic adrenergic function), including beat-to-beat blood pressure and R-R interval changes during Valsalva maneuver and at least 5 minutes of passive tilt

EXCLUDES *Autonomic nervous system testing with parasympathetic function (95921, 95924)*

2.70 2.70 FUD XXX
AMA: 2020,Sep,7; 2018,Feb,11; 2018,Jan,8; 2017,Jan,8; 2016,Jan,13

95923 sudomotor, including 1 or more of the following: quantitative sudomotor axon reflex test (QSART), silastic sweat imprint, thermoregulatory sweat test, and changes in sympathetic skin potential

3.64 3.64 FUD XXX
AMA: 2020,Sep,7; 2018,Feb,11; 2018,Jan,8; 2017,Jan,8; 2016,Jan,13

95924 combined parasympathetic and sympathetic adrenergic function testing with at least 5 minutes of passive tilt

INCLUDES Tilt table testing adrenergic and parasympathetic function

EXCLUDES *Autonomic nervous system testing with parasympathetic function (95921-95922)*

4.25 4.25 FUD XXX
AMA: 2020,Sep,7; 2018,Feb,11; 2018,Jan,8; 2017,Jan,8; 2016,Jan,13

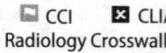

95925-95943 [95938, 95939, 95940, 95941] Neurotransmission Studies

95925 Short-latency somatosensory evoked potential study, stimulation of any/all peripheral nerves or skin sites, recording from the central nervous system; in upper limbs

EXCLUDES *Auditory evoked potentials ([92653])*
Evoked potential study both upper and lower limbs ([95938])
Evoked potential study lower limbs (95926)

3.73 3.73 FUD XXX S 80

AMA: 2018,Feb,11; 2018,Jan,8; 2017,Jan,8; 2016,Jan,13

95926 in lower limbs

EXCLUDES *Auditory evoked potentials ([92653])*
Evoked potential study both upper and lower limbs ([95938])
Evoked potential study upper limbs (95925)

3.76 3.76 FUD XXX S 80

AMA: 2018,Feb,11; 2018,Jan,8; 2017,Jan,8; 2016,Jan,13

95938 in upper and lower limbs

9.88 9.88 FUD XXX S 80

AMA: 2018,Feb,11; 2018,Jan,8; 2017,Jan,8; 2016,Jan,13

95927 in the trunk or head

EXCLUDES *Auditory evoked potentials ([92653])*

Code also modifier 52 for unilateral test

3.75 3.75 FUD XXX S 80

AMA: 2020,Oct,9; 2018,Feb,11; 2018,Jan,8; 2017,Jan,8; 2016,Jan,13

95928 Central motor evoked potential study (transcranial motor stimulation); upper limbs

EXCLUDES *Central motor evoked potential study lower limbs (95929)*

6.20 6.20 FUD XXX S 80

AMA: 2018,Feb,11; 2018,Jan,8; 2017,Jan,8; 2016,Jan,13

95929 lower limbs

EXCLUDES *Central motor evoked potential study upper limbs (95928)*

6.57 6.57 FUD XXX S 80

AMA: 2018,Feb,11; 2018,Jan,8; 2017,Jan,8; 2016,Jan,13

95939 in upper and lower limbs

EXCLUDES *Central motor evoked potential study either lower or upper limbs (95928-95929)*

14.8 14.8 FUD XXX S 80

AMA: 2018,Feb,11; 2018,Jan,8; 2017,Jan,8; 2016,Jan,13

95930 Visual evoked potential (VEP) checkerboard or flash testing, central nervous system except glaucoma, with interpretation and report

EXCLUDES *Visual acuity screening using automated visual evoked potential devices (0333T)*
Visual evoked glaucoma testing ([0464T])

1.88 1.88 FUD XXX S 80

AMA: 2018,Feb,11; 2018,Feb,3; 2018,Jan,8; 2017,Jan,8; 2016,Jan,13

95933 Orbicularis oculi (blink) reflex, by electrodiagnostic testing

2.33 2.33 FUD XXX Q1 80

AMA: 2018,Feb,11; 2018,Jan,8; 2017,Jul,10; 2017,Jan,8; 2016,Jan,13

95937 Neuromuscular junction testing (repetitive stimulation, paired stimuli), each nerve, any 1 method

2.48 2.48 FUD XXX S 80

AMA: 2020,Aug,14; 2018,Feb,11; 2018,Jan,8; 2017,Jan,8; 2016,Feb,13; 2016,Jan,13

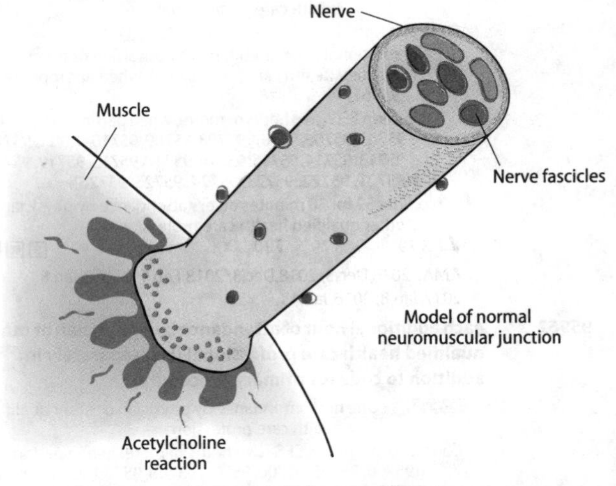

A selected neuromuscular junction is repeatedly stimulated. The test is useful to demonstrate reduced muscle action potential from fatigue

95938 **Resequenced code. See code following 95926.**
95939 **Resequenced code. See code following 95929.**
95940 **Resequenced code. See code following 95913.**
95941 **Resequenced code. See code following 95913.**

95943 ~~**Simultaneous, independent, quantitative measures of both parasympathetic function and sympathetic function, based on time-frequency analysis of heart rate variability concurrent with time-frequency analysis of continuous respiratory activity, with mean heart rate and blood pressure measures, during rest, paced (deep) breathing, Valsalva maneuvers, and head-up postural change**~~

To report, see (95999)

95954-95962 Electroencephalography For Seizure Monitoring/Intraoperative Use

EXCLUDES *E/M services*

95954 Pharmacological or physical activation requiring physician or other qualified health care professional attendance during EEG recording of activation phase (eg, thiopental activation test)

11.0 11.0 FUD XXX S 80

AMA: 2018,Feb,11; 2018,Jan,8; 2017,Jan,8; 2016,Jan,13

95955 Electroencephalogram (EEG) during nonintracranial surgery (eg, carotid surgery)

5.94 5.94 FUD XXX N 80

AMA: 2018,Feb,11; 2018,Jan,8; 2017,Jan,8; 2016,Jan,13

95957 Digital analysis of electroencephalogram (EEG) (eg, for epileptic spike analysis)

EXCLUDES *Use of automated spike and seizure detection/trending software, when performed ([95700, 95705, 95706, 95707, 95708, 95709, 95710, 95711, 95712, 95713, 95714, 95715, 95716, 95717, 95718, 95719, 95720, 95721, 95722, 95723, 95724, 95725, 95726])*

7.24 7.24 FUD XXX N 80

AMA: 2018,Dec,3; 2018,Dec,3; 2018,Feb,11; 2018,Jan,8; 2017,Jan,8; 2016,Jan,13

95958 Wada activation test for hemispheric function, including electroencephalographic (EEG) monitoring

16.4 16.4 FUD XXX S 80

AMA: 2018,Feb,11

95961 **Functional cortical and subcortical mapping by stimulation and/or recording of electrodes on brain surface, or of depth electrodes, to provoke seizures or identify vital brain structures; initial hour of attendance by a physician or other qualified health care professional**

INCLUDES One hour attendance by physician or other qualified health care professional

Code also:

Each additional hour attendance by physician or other qualified health care professional, when appropriate (95962)

Long-term EEG (two hours or more), when performed ([95700, 95705, 95706, 95707, 95708, 95709, 95710, 95711, 95712, 95713, 95714, 95715, 95716, 95717, 95718, 95719, 95720, 95721, 95722, 95723, 95724, 95725, 95726])

Modifier 52 for 30 minutes or less attendance by physician or other qualified health care professional

8.79 8.79 **FUD** XXX S 80

AMA: 2018,Dec,3; 2018,Dec,3; 2018,Feb,11; 2018,Jan,8; 2017,Jan,8; 2016,Jan,13

+ **95962** **each additional hour of attendance by a physician or other qualified health care professional (List separately in addition to code for primary procedure)**

INCLUDES One hour attendance by physician or other qualified health care professional

Code also long-term EEG (two hours or more), when performed ([95700, 95705, 95706, 95707, 95708, 95709, 95710, 95711, 95712, 95713, 95714, 95715, 95716, 95717, 95718, 95719, 95720, 95721, 95722, 95723, 95724, 95725, 95726])

Code first initial hour (95961)

7.44 7.44 **FUD** ZZZ N 80

AMA: 2018,Feb,11; 2018,Jan,8; 2017,Jan,8; 2016,Jan,13

95965-95967 Magnetoencephalography

INCLUDES Physician interpretation
Recording
Report

EXCLUDES *CT provided with magnetoencephalography (70450-70470, 70496)*
Electroencephalography provided with magnetoencephalography (95812-95824)
E/M services
MRI provided with magnetoencephalography (70551-70553)
Somatosensory evoked potentials/auditory evoked potentials/visual evoked potentials provided with magnetic evoked field responses ([92653], 95925, 95926, 95930)

95965 **Magnetoencephalography (MEG), recording and analysis; for spontaneous brain magnetic activity (eg, epileptic cerebral cortex localization)**

0.00 0.00 **FUD** XXX S 80

AMA: 2018,Feb,11

95966 **for evoked magnetic fields, single modality (eg, sensory, motor, language, or visual cortex localization)**

0.00 0.00 **FUD** XXX S 80

AMA: 2018,Feb,11

+ **95967** **for evoked magnetic fields, each additional modality (eg, sensory, motor, language, or visual cortex localization) (List separately in addition to code for primary procedure)**

Code first single modality (95966)

0.00 0.00 **FUD** ZZZ N 80

AMA: 2020,Oct,9; 2018,Feb,11

95700-95726 [95700, 95705, 95706, 95707, 95708, 95709, 95710, 95711, 95712, 95713, 95714, 95715, 95716, 95717, 95718, 95719, 95720, 95721, 95722, 95723, 95724, 95725, 95726] Electroencephalogram (EEG)

INCLUDES Automated spike and seizure detection/trending software, when performed
Determination:
Eligibility for epilepsy surgery
Location and type seizures
Differentiation seizures from other conditions
Monitoring:
Seizure treatment
Status epilepticus

EXCLUDES *Diagnostic EEG recording time less than two hours*
Routine EEG (95812-95813, 95816, 95819, 95822)

Code also cortical or subcortical mapping, when performed (95961-95962)

95700 **Electroencephalogram (EEG) continuous recording, with video when performed, setup, patient education, and takedown when performed, administered in person by EEG technologist, minimum of 8 channels**

INCLUDES Technical component

EXCLUDES *EEG performed using patient-placed electrodes, performed by non-EEG technologist, or remote supervision by EEG technologist (95999)*
Reporting code more than one time each session

0.00 0.00 **FUD** XXX 80

95705 **Electroencephalogram (EEG), without video, review of data, technical description by EEG technologist, 2-12 hours; unmonitored**

INCLUDES Technical component

EXCLUDES *Reporting code more than one time to capture complete long-term EEG session or final 2-12 hour segment past 26 hours*

0.00 0.00 **FUD** XXX 80

95706 **with intermittent monitoring and maintenance**

INCLUDES Technical component

EXCLUDES *Reporting code more than one time to capture complete long-term EEG session or final 2-12 hour segment past 26 hours*

0.00 0.00 **FUD** XXX 80

95707 **with continuous, real-time monitoring and maintenance**

INCLUDES Technical component

EXCLUDES *Reporting code more than one time to capture complete long-term EEG session or final 2-12 hour segment past 26 hours*

0.00 0.00 **FUD** XXX 80

95708 **Electroencephalogram (EEG), without video, review of data, technical description by EEG technologist, each increment of 12-26 hours; unmonitored**

INCLUDES Technical component

0.00 0.00 **FUD** XXX 80

95709 **with intermittent monitoring and maintenance**

INCLUDES Technical component

0.00 0.00 **FUD** XXX 80

95710 **with continuous, real-time monitoring and maintenance**

INCLUDES Technical component

0.00 0.00 **FUD** XXX 80

95711 **Electroencephalogram with video (VEEG), review of data, technical description by EEG technologist, 2-12 hours; unmonitored**

INCLUDES Technical component

EXCLUDES *Reporting code more than one time to capture complete long-term EEG session or final 2-12 hour segment past 26 hours*

0.00 0.00 **FUD** XXX 80

 # 95712 with intermittent monitoring and maintenance

INCLUDES Technical component

EXCLUDES *Reporting code more than one time to capture complete long-term EEG session or final 2-12 hour segment past 26 hours*

0.00 0.00 **FUD** XXX 80

 # 95713 with continuous, real-time monitoring and maintenance

INCLUDES Technical component

EXCLUDES *Reporting code more than one time to capture complete long-term EEG session or final 2-12 hour segment past 26 hours*

0.00 0.00 **FUD** XXX 80

 # 95714 Electroencephalogram with video (VEEG), review of data, technical description by EEG technologist, each increment of 12-26 hours; unmonitored

INCLUDES Technical component

0.00 0.00 **FUD** XXX 80

 # 95715 with intermittent monitoring and maintenance

INCLUDES Technical component

0.00 0.00 **FUD** XXX 80

 # 95716 with continuous, real-time monitoring and maintenance

INCLUDES Technical component

0.00 0.00 **FUD** XXX 80

 # 95717 Electroencephalogram (EEG), continuous recording, physician or other qualified health care professional review of recorded events, analysis of spike and seizure detection, interpretation and report, 2-12 hours of EEG recording; without video

INCLUDES Professional component

EXCLUDES *Professional interpretation for recordings greater than 36 hours and for which entire professional report generated retroactively ([95721, 95722, 95723, 95724, 95725, 95726])*

Reporting code more than one time to capture complete long-term EEG session or final 2-12 hour segment past 24 hours

2.90 2.94 **FUD** XXX 80

 # 95718 with video (VEEG)

INCLUDES Professional component

EXCLUDES *Professional interpretation for recordings greater than 36 hours and for which entire professional report generated retroactively ([95721, 95722, 95723, 95724, 95725, 95726])*

Reporting code more than one time to capture complete long-term EEG session or final 2-12 hour segment past 24 hours

3.81 3.87 **FUD** XXX 80

 # 95719 Electroencephalogram (EEG), continuous recording, physician or other qualified health care professional review of recorded events, analysis of spike and seizure detection, each increment of greater than 12 hours, up to 26 hours of EEG recording, interpretation and report after each 24-hour period; without video

INCLUDES Professional component

Single report or multiple reports during 26-hour reporting period

EXCLUDES *Professional interpretation for recordings greater than 36 hours and for which entire professional report generated retroactively ([95721, 95722, 95723, 95724, 95725, 95726])*

Reporting code more than once for multiple day studies after each 24-hour period during extended EEG recording time ([95719, 95720])

Reporting code more than one time to capture between 12-26 hours

Code also EEG, 2-12 hours for studies longer than 26 hours ([95717, 95718])

4.50 4.55 **FUD** XXX 80

 # 95720 with video (VEEG)

INCLUDES Professional component

Single report or multiple reports during 26-hour reporting period

EXCLUDES *Professional interpretation for recordings greater than 36 hours and for which entire professional report generated retroactively ([95721, 95722, 95723, 95724, 95725, 95726])*

Reporting code more than one time to capture between 12-26 hours

Reporting code more than once for multiple day studies after each 24-hour period during extended EEG recording time ([95719, 95720])

Code also EEG, 2-12 hours for studies longer than 26 hours ([95717, 95718])

5.90 5.99 **FUD** XXX 80

 # 95721 Electroencephalogram (EEG), continuous recording, physician or other qualified health care professional review of recorded events, analysis of spike and seizure detection, interpretation, and summary report, complete study; greater than 36 hours, up to 60 hours of EEG recording, without video

INCLUDES Professional interpretation for recordings greater than 36 hours and for which entire professional report generated retroactively

EXCLUDES *EEG, continuous recording, less than 36 hours ([95717, 95718, 95719, 95720])*

5.92 6.04 **FUD** XXX 80

 # 95722 greater than 36 hours, up to 60 hours of EEG recording, with video (VEEG)

INCLUDES Professional interpretation for recordings greater than 36 hours and for which entire professional report generated retroactively

EXCLUDES *EEG, continuous recording, less than 36 hours ([95717, 95718, 95719, 95720])*

7.20 7.33 **FUD** XXX 80

 # 95723 greater than 60 hours, up to 84 hours of EEG recording, without video

INCLUDES Professional interpretation for recordings greater than 36 hours and for which entire professional report generated retroactively

EXCLUDES *EEG, continuous recording, less than 36 hours ([95717, 95718, 95719, 95720])*

7.33 7.49 **FUD** XXX 80

 # 95724 greater than 60 hours, up to 84 hours of EEG recording, with video (VEEG)

INCLUDES Professional interpretation for recordings greater than 36 hours and for which entire professional report generated retroactively

EXCLUDES *EEG, continuous recording, less than 36 hours ([95717, 95718, 95719, 95720])*

9.18 9.36 **FUD** XXX 80

 # 95725 greater than 84 hours of EEG recording, without video

INCLUDES Professional interpretation for recordings greater than 36 hours and for which entire professional report generated retroactively

EXCLUDES *EEG, continuous recording, less than 36 hours ([95717, 95718, 95719, 95720])*

8.34 8.55 **FUD** XXX 80

AMA: 2011,Jan,11; 2009,Jan,11-31

 # 95726 greater than 84 hours of EEG recording, with video (VEEG)

INCLUDES Professional interpretation for recordings greater than 36 hours and for which entire professional report generated retroactively

EXCLUDES *EEG, continuous recording, less than 36 hours ([95717, 95718, 95719, 95720])*

11.6 11.8 **FUD** XXX 80

95970-95984 [95983, 95984] Evaluation of Implanted Neurostimulator with/without Programming

INCLUDES Documentation settings, electrode impedances system parameters before programming
Insertion electrode array(s) into target area (permanent or trial)
Multiple adjustments to parameters necessary during programming session
Neurostimulators distinguished by nervous system area stimulated:
Brain: Deep brain stimulation or cortical stimulation (brain surface)
Cranial nerves: Includes12 pairs cranial nerves, branches, divisions, intracranial and extracranial segments
Spinal cord and peripheral nerves: Nerves originating in spinal cord and nerves and ganglia outside spinal cord
Parameters (vary by system) include:
Amplitude
Burst
Cycling on/off
Detection algorithms
Dose lockout
Frequency
Pulse width
Responsive neurostimulation

EXCLUDES *Implantation/replacement neurostimulator electrodes (43647, 43881, 61850-61868, 63650-63655, 64553-64581)*
Neurostimulation system, posterior tibial nerve (0587T-0590T)
Neurostimulator pulse generator/receiver:
Insertion (61885-61886, 63685, 64568, 64582, 64590)
Revision/removal (61888, 63688, 64569, 64570, 64583-64584, 64595)
Revision/removal neurostimulator electrodes (43648, 43882, 61880, 63661-63664, 64569-64570, 64583-64585)

95970 **Electronic analysis of implanted neurostimulator pulse generator/transmitter (eg, contact group[s], interleaving, amplitude, pulse width, frequency [Hz], on/off cycling, burst, magnet mode, dose lockout, patient selectable parameters, responsive neurostimulation, detection algorithms, closed loop parameters, and passive parameters) by physician or other qualified health care professional; with brain, cranial nerve, spinal cord, peripheral nerve, or sacral nerve, neurostimulator pulse generator/transmitter, without programming**

INCLUDES Analysis implanted neurostimulator without programming

EXCLUDES *Programming with analysis (95971-95972, 95976-95977, [95983, 95984])*

0.53 | 0.54 | FUD XXX | Q1 80

AMA: 2019,Feb,6; 2018,Oct,8; 2018,Feb,11; 2018,Jan,8; 2017,Jan,8; 2016,Jul,7; 2016,Jan,13

95971 **with simple spinal cord or peripheral nerve (eg, sacral nerve) neurostimulator pulse generator/transmitter programming by physician or other qualified health care professional**

EXCLUDES *Programming neurostimulator for complex spinal cord or peripheral nerve (95972)*

1.17 | 1.44 | FUD XXX | S 80

AMA: 2019,Feb,6; 2018,Oct,8; 2018,Feb,11; 2018,Jan,8; 2017,Jan,8; 2016,Jul,7; 2016,Jan,13

95972 **with complex spinal cord or peripheral nerve (eg, sacral nerve) neurostimulator pulse generator/transmitter programming by physician or other qualified health care professional**

1.19 | 1.62 | FUD XXX | S 80

AMA: 2019,Feb,6; 2018,Oct,8; 2018,Feb,11; 2018,Jan,8; 2017,Jan,8; 2016,Jul,7; 2016,Jan,13

95976 **with simple cranial nerve neurostimulator pulse generator/transmitter programming by physician or other qualified health care professional**

EXCLUDES *Programming neurostimulator for complex cranial nerve (95977)*

1.16 | 1.18 | FUD XXX | 80

AMA: 2019,Feb,6

95977 **with complex cranial nerve neurostimulator pulse generator/transmitter programming by physician or other qualified health care professional**

1.52 | 1.54 | FUD XXX | 80

AMA: 2019,Feb,6

\# **95983** **with brain neurostimulator pulse generator/transmitter programming, first 15 minutes face-to-face time with physician or other qualified health care professional**

1.44 | 1.46 | FUD XXX | 80

AMA: 2019,Feb,6; 2018,Dec,3; 2018,Dec,3

\+ # **95984** **with brain neurostimulator pulse generator/transmitter programming, each additional 15 minutes face-to-face time with physician or other qualified health care professional (List separately in addition to code for primary procedure)**

Code first ([95983])

1.26 | 1.27 | FUD ZZZ | 80

AMA: 2019,Feb,6; 2018,Dec,3; 2018,Dec,3

95980 **Electronic analysis of implanted neurostimulator pulse generator system (eg, rate, pulse amplitude and duration, configuration of wave form, battery status, electrode selectability, output modulation, cycling, impedance and patient measurements) gastric neurostimulator pulse generator/transmitter; intraoperative, with programming**

INCLUDES Gastric neurostimulator lesser curvature

EXCLUDES *Analysis, with programming when performed, vagus nerve trunk stimulator for morbid obesity (0312T, 0317T)*

1.32 | 1.32 | FUD XXX | N 80

AMA: 2018,Feb,11; 2018,Jan,8; 2017,Jan,8; 2016,Jul,7; 2016,Jan,13

95981 **subsequent, without reprogramming**

EXCLUDES *Analysis, with programming when performed, vagus nerve trunk stimulator for morbid obesity (0312T, 0317T)*

0.51 | 0.97 | FUD XXX | Q1 80

AMA: 2018,Feb,11; 2018,Jan,8; 2017,Jan,8; 2016,Jul,7; 2016,Jan,13

95982 **subsequent, with reprogramming**

EXCLUDES *Analysis, with programming when performed, vagus nerve trunk stimulator for morbid obesity (0312T, 0317T)*

1.04 | 1.55 | FUD XXX | Q1 80

AMA: 2018,Feb,11; 2018,Jan,8; 2017,Jan,8; 2016,Jul,7; 2016,Jan,13

95983 **Resequenced code. See code following 95977.**

95984 **Resequenced code. See code following 95977.**

95990-95991 Refill/Upkeep of Implanted Drug Delivery Pump to Central Nervous System

EXCLUDES *Analysis/reprogramming implanted pump for infusion (62367-62370)*
E/M services

95990 **Refilling and maintenance of implantable pump or reservoir for drug delivery, spinal (intrathecal, epidural) or brain (intraventricular), includes electronic analysis of pump, when performed;**

2.62 | 2.62 | FUD XXX | S 80

AMA: 2018,Feb,11; 2018,Jan,8; 2017,Jan,8; 2016,Jan,13

95991 **requiring skill of a physician or other qualified health care professional**

1.14 | 3.30 | FUD XXX | T 80

AMA: 2018,Feb,11; 2018,Jan,8; 2017,Jan,8; 2016,Jan,13

95992-95999 Other and Unlisted Neurological Procedures

95992 **Canalith repositioning procedure(s) (eg, Epley maneuver, Semont maneuver), per day**

EXCLUDES *Nystagmus testing (92531-92532)*

1.07 | 1.25 | FUD XXX | A 80

AMA: 2018,Feb,11; 2018,Jan,8; 2017,Jan,8; 2016,Jan,13

95999 **Unlisted neurological or neuromuscular diagnostic procedure**
0.00 0.00 **FUD** XXX
AMA: 2018,Aug,10; 2018,Feb,11; 2018,Jan,8; 2017,Jan,8; 2016,Jan,13

96000-96004 Motion Analysis Studies

CMS: 100-02,15,230.4 Services By a Physical/Occupational Therapist in Private Practice

INCLUDES Services provided as part major therapeutic/diagnostic decision making
Services provided in dedicated motion analysis department with these capabilities:
3D kinetics/dynamic electromyography
Computerized 3D kinematics
Videotaping from front/back/both sides

EXCLUDES *E/M services*
Gait training (97116)
Needle electromyography (95860-95872 [95885, 95886, 95887])

96000 **Comprehensive computer-based motion analysis by video-taping and 3D kinematics;**
2.72 2.72 **FUD** XXX
AMA: 2018,Feb,11; 2018,Jan,8; 2017,Jan,8; 2016,Jan,13

96001 **with dynamic plantar pressure measurements during walking**
3.65 3.65 **FUD** XXX
AMA: 2018,Feb,11; 2018,Jan,8; 2017,Jan,8; 2016,Jan,13

96002 **Dynamic surface electromyography, during walking or other functional activities, 1-12 muscles**
0.63 0.63 **FUD** XXX
AMA: 2018,Feb,11; 2018,Jan,8; 2017,Jan,8; 2016,Jan,13

96003 **Dynamic fine wire electromyography, during walking or other functional activities, 1 muscle**
0.49 0.49 **FUD** XXX
AMA: 2018,Feb,11; 2018,Jan,8; 2017,Jan,8; 2016,Jan,13

96004 **Review and interpretation by physician or other qualified health care professional of comprehensive computer-based motion analysis, dynamic plantar pressure measurements, dynamic surface electromyography during walking or other functional activities, and dynamic fine wire electromyography, with written report**
3.27 3.27 **FUD** XXX
AMA: 2018,Feb,11; 2018,Jan,8; 2017,Jan,8; 2016,Jan,13

96020 Neurofunctional Brain Testing

INCLUDES Selection/administration, testing:
Cognition
Determining validity neurofunctional testing relative to separately interpreted functional magnetic resonance images
Functional neuroimaging
Language
Memory
Monitoring performance of testing
Movement
Other neurological functions
Sensation

EXCLUDES *Clinical depression treatment by repetitive transcranial magnetic stimulation (90867-90868)*
Developmental test administration (96112-96113)
E/M services on same date
MRI brain (70554-70555)
Neurobehavioral status examination (96116, 96121)
Neuropsychological testing (96132-96133)
Psychological testing (96130-96131)

96020 **Neurofunctional testing selection and administration during noninvasive imaging functional brain mapping, with test administered entirely by a physician or other qualified health care professional (ie, psychologist), with review of test results and report**
0.00 0.00 **FUD** XXX
AMA: 2018,Feb,11; 2018,Jan,8; 2017,Jan,8; 2016,Jan,13

96040 Genetic Counseling Services

INCLUDES Analysis for genetic risk assessment
Counseling patient/family
Counseling services
Face-to-face interviews
Obtaining structured family genetic history
Pedigree construction
Review medical data/family information
Services provided by trained genetic counselor
Services provided during one or more sessions
Thirty minutes face-to-face time, reported one time for each 16-30 minutes service

EXCLUDES *Education/genetic counseling by physician or other qualified health care provider to group (99078)*
Education/genetic counseling by physician or other qualified health care provider to individual; report appropriate E/M code
Education regarding genetic risks by nonphysician to group (98961, 98962)
Genetic counseling and/or risk factor reduction intervention from physician or other qualified health care provider provided to patients without symptoms/diagnosis (99401-99412)
Reporting code when 15 minutes or less face-to-face time provided

96040 **Medical genetics and genetic counseling services, each 30 minutes face-to-face with patient/family**
1.30 1.30 **FUD** XXX ★
AMA: 2018,Feb,11; 2018,Jan,8; 2017,Jan,8; 2016,Jan,13

97151-97158 [97151, 97152, 97153, 97154, 97155, 97156, 97157, 97158] Adaptive Behavior Assessments and Treatments

INCLUDES Adaptive behavior deficits (e.g., impairment in social, communication, self care skills)
Assessment and treatment that focuses on:
Maladaptive behaviors (e.g., repetitive movements, risk harm to self, others, property)
Secondary functional impairment due to consequences deficient adaptive and maladaptive behaviors (e.g., communication, play, leisure, social interactions)
Treatment determined based on goals and targets identified in assessments

97151 **Behavior identification assessment, administered by a physician or other qualified health care professional, each 15 minutes of the physician's or other qualified health care professional's time face-to-face with patient and/or guardian(s)/caregiver(s) administering assessments and discussing findings and recommendations, and non-face-to-face analyzing past data, scoring/interpreting the assessment, and preparing the report/treatment plan**

EXCLUDES *Health and behavior assessment and intervention (96156, 96158-96159, [96164, 96165], [96167, 96168], [96170, 96171])*
Medical team conference (99366-99368)
Neurobehavioral status examination (96116, 96121)
Neuropsychological testing (96132-96133, 96136-96139, 96146)
Psychiatric diagnostic evaluation (90791-90792)
Speech evaluations (92521-92524)

Code also:
More than one time on same or different days until assessment complete
Supporting assessment depending on time patient spends face-to-face with one or more technicians (counting only time spent by one technician) ([97152], 0362T)

0.00 0.00 **FUD** XXX
AMA: 2018,Nov,3

97152 **Behavior identification-supporting assessment, administered by one technician under the direction of a physician or other qualified health care professional, face-to-face with the patient, each 15 minutes**

EXCLUDES *Health and behavior assessment and intervention (96156, 96158-96159, [96164, 96165], [96167, 96168], [96170, 96171])*
Medical team conference (99366-99368)
Neurobehavioral status examination (96116, 96121)
Neuropsychological testing (96132-96133, 96136-96139, 96146)
Psychiatric diagnostic evaluation (90791-90792)
Speech evaluations (92521-92524)

Code also:
More than one time on same or different days until assessment complete
Supporting assessment depending on time patient spends face-to-face with one or more technicians (counting only time spent by one technician) ([97152], 0362T)

0.00 0.00 FUD XXX 80

AMA: 2018,Nov,3

97153 **Adaptive behavior treatment by protocol, administered by technician under the direction of a physician or other qualified health care professional, face-to-face with one patient, each 15 minutes**

INCLUDES Face-to-face service with one patient only
Provided by technician under physician/other qualified healthcare professional direction

EXCLUDES *Aphasia and cognitive performance testing (96105, [96125])*
Behavioral/developmental screening/testing (96110-96113 [96127])
Health and behavior assessment and intervention (96156, 96158-96159, [96164, 96165], [96167, 96168], [96170, 96171])
Health risk assessment (96160-96161)
Neurobehavioral status examination (96116, 96121)
Psychiatric services (90785-90899)
Testing administration with scoring (96136-96139, 96146)
Testing evaluation (96130-96133)
Therapeutic procedure(s), individual patient (97129)
Treatment speech disorders (individual) (92507)

0.00 0.00 FUD XXX 80

AMA: 2020,Jul,10; 2018,Nov,3

97154 **Group adaptive behavior treatment by protocol, administered by technician under the direction of a physician or other qualified health care professional, face-to-face with two or more patients, each 15 minutes**

INCLUDES Face-to-face service with one patient only
Provided by technician under physician/other qualified healthcare professional direction

EXCLUDES *Aphasia and cognitive performance testing (96105, [96125])*
Behavioral/developmental screening/testing (96110-96113, [96127])
Health and behavior assessment and intervention (96156, 96158-96159, [96164, 96165], [96167, 96168], [96170, 96171])
Neurobehavioral status examination (96116, 96121)
Psychiatric services (90785-90899)
Testing administration with scoring (96136-96139, 96146)
Testing evaluation (96130-96133)
Therapeutic procedure(s) group, two or more patients (97150)
Treatment speech disorders (group) (92508)

0.00 0.00 FUD XXX 80

AMA: 2018,Nov,3

97155 **Adaptive behavior treatment with protocol modification, administered by physician or other qualified health care professional, which may include simultaneous direction of technician, face-to-face with one patient, each 15 minutes**

INCLUDES Face-to-face service with one patient only
Provided by technician under physician/other qualified healthcare professional direction

EXCLUDES *Aphasia and cognitive performance testing (96105, [96125])*
Behavioral/developmental screening/testing (96110-96113, [96127])
Health and behavior assessment and intervention (96156, 96158-96159, [96164, 96165], [96167, 96168], [96170, 96171])
Neurobehavioral status examination (96116, 96121)
Psychiatric services (90785-90899)
Testing administration with scoring (96136-96139, 96146)
Testing evaluation (96130-96133)
Therapeutic procedure(s), individual patient (97129)
Treatment speech disorders (individual) (92507)

0.00 0.00 FUD XXX 80

AMA: 2020,Jul,10; 2018,Nov,3

97156 **Family adaptive behavior treatment guidance, administered by physician or other qualified health care professional (with or without the patient present), face-to-face with guardian(s)/caregiver(s), each 15 minutes**

INCLUDES Provided by physician/other qualified healthcare professional
Without patient presence

EXCLUDES *Aphasia and cognitive performance testing (96105, [96125])*
Behavioral/developmental screening/testing (96110-96113 [96127])
Health and behavior assessment and intervention (96156, 96158-96159, [96164, 96165], [96167, 96168], [96170, 96171])
Neurobehavioral status examination (96116, 96121)
Psychiatric services (90785-90899)
Testing administration with scoring (96136-96139, 96146)
Testing evaluation (96130-96133)

0.00 0.00 FUD XXX 80

AMA: 2018,Nov,3

97157 **Multiple-family group adaptive behavior treatment guidance, administered by physician or other qualified health care professional (without the patient present), face-to-face with multiple sets of guardians/caregivers, each 15 minutes**

INCLUDES Provided by physician/other qualified healthcare professional
Without patient presence

EXCLUDES *Aphasia and cognitive performance testing (96105, [96125])*
Behavioral/developmental screening/testing (96110-96113 [96127])
Groups more than eight families
Health and behavior assessment and intervention (96156, 96158-96159, [96164, 96165], [96167, 96168], [96170, 96171])
Neurobehavioral status examination (96116, 96121)
Psychiatric services (90785-90899)
Testing administration with scoring (96136-96139, 96146)
Testing evaluation (96130-96133)

0.00 0.00 FUD XXX 80

AMA: 2018,Nov,3

97158 **Group adaptive behavior treatment with protocol modification, administered by physician or other qualified health care professional, face-to-face with multiple patients, each 15 minutes**

INCLUDES Face-to-face service with one patient only
Provided by technician under physician/other qualified healthcare professional direction

EXCLUDES *Aphasia and cognitive performance testing (96105, [96125])*
Behavioral/developmental screening/testing (96110-96113 [96127])
Groups more than eight families
Health and behavior assessment and intervention (96156, 96158-96159, [96164, 96165], [96167, 96168], [96170, 96171])
Neurobehavioral status examination (96116, 96121)
Psychiatric services (90785-90899)
Testing administration with scoring (96136-96139, 96146)
Testing evaluation (96130-96133)
Therapeutic procedure(s) group of two or more patients (97150)
Treatment speech disorders (group) (92508)

0.00 0.00 FUD XXX 80

AMA: 2018,Nov,3

96105-96146 [96125, 96127] Testing Services

INCLUDES Interpretation and report when performed by qualified healthcare professional
Results when automatically generated

EXCLUDES *Adaptive behavior assessments and treatments ([97151, 97152, 97153, 97154, 97155, 97156, 97157, 97158], 0362T, 0373T)*
Cognitive skills development (97129, 97533)

96105 **Assessment of aphasia (includes assessment of expressive and receptive speech and language function, language comprehension, speech production ability, reading, spelling, writing, eg, by Boston Diagnostic Aphasia Examination) with interpretation and report, per hour**

EXCLUDES *Reporting code for less than 31 minutes*

2.96 2.96 FUD XXX A 80

AMA: 2018,Nov,3; 2018,Oct,5; 2018,Feb,11; 2018,Jan,8; 2017,Jan,8; 2016,Jan,13

96125 **Standardized cognitive performance testing (eg, Ross Information Processing Assessment) per hour of a qualified health care professional's time, both face-to-face time administering tests to the patient and time interpreting these test results and preparing the report**

EXCLUDES *Neuropsychological testing (96132-96139, 96146)*

3.12 3.12 FUD XXX A 80

AMA: 2018,Nov,3; 2018,Oct,5; 2018,Feb,11; 2018,Jan,8; 2017,Jan,8; 2016,Jan,13

96110 **Developmental screening (eg, developmental milestone survey, speech and language delay screen), with scoring and documentation, per standardized instrument**

EXCLUDES *Emotional/behavioral assessment ([96127])*

0.28 0.28 FUD XXX E

AMA: 2018,Nov,3; 2018,Feb,11; 2018,Jan,8; 2017,Feb,14; 2017,Jan,8; 2016,Jan,13

96112 **Developmental test administration (including assessment of fine and/or gross motor, language, cognitive level, social, memory and/or executive functions by standardized developmental instruments when performed), by physician or other qualified health care professional, with interpretation and report; first hour**

EXCLUDES *Reporting code for less than 31 minutes*

3.61 3.83 FUD XXX 80

AMA: 2018,Nov,3

+ **96113** **each additional 30 minutes (List separately in addition to code for primary procedure)**

EXCLUDES *Reporting code for less than 16 minutes*

1.65 1.74 FUD ZZZ 80

AMA: 2018,Nov,3

96127 **Brief emotional/behavioral assessment (eg, depression inventory, attention-deficit/hyperactivity disorder [ADHD] scale), with scoring and documentation, per standardized instrument**

0.15 0.15 FUD XXX Q1 80 TC

AMA: 2018,Nov,3; 2018,Oct,5; 2018,Apr,9; 2018,Feb,11; 2018,Jan,8; 2017,Feb,14; 2017,Jan,8; 2016,Jan,13

96116 **Neurobehavioral status exam (clinical assessment of thinking, reasoning and judgment, [eg, acquired knowledge, attention, language, memory, planning and problem solving, and visual spatial abilities]), by physician or other qualified health care professional, both face-to-face time with the patient and time interpreting test results and preparing the report; first hour**

EXCLUDES *Neuropsychological testing (96132-96139, 96146)*
Reporting code for less than 31 minutes

2.41 2.70 FUD XXX ★ 03 80

AMA: 2018,Nov,3; 2018,Oct,5; 2018,Feb,11; 2018,Jan,8; 2017,Jan,8; 2016,Jan,13

+ **96121** **each additional hour (List separately in addition to code for primary procedure)**

EXCLUDES *Reporting code for less than 31 minutes*
Code first (96116)

2.22 2.39 FUD ZZZ 80

AMA: 2018,Nov,3

96125 **Resequenced code. See code following 96105.**

96127 **Resequenced code. See code following 96113.**

96130 **Psychological testing evaluation services by physician or other qualified health care professional, including integration of patient data, interpretation of standardized test results and clinical data, clinical decision making, treatment planning and report, and interactive feedback to the patient, family member(s) or caregiver(s), when performed; first hour**

EXCLUDES *Reporting code for less than 31 minutes*

3.08 3.38 FUD XXX 80

AMA: 2019,Dec,14; 2019,Sep,10; 2018,Nov,3

+ **96131** **each additional hour (List separately in addition to code for primary procedure)**

EXCLUDES *Reporting code for less than 31 minutes*

2.37 2.60 FUD ZZZ 80

AMA: 2019,Dec,14; 2019,Sep,10; 2018,Nov,3

96132 **Neuropsychological testing evaluation services by physician or other qualified health care professional, including integration of patient data, interpretation of standardized test results and clinical data, clinical decision making, treatment planning and report, and interactive feedback to the patient, family member(s) or caregiver(s), when performed; first hour**

EXCLUDES *Reporting code for less than 31 minutes*

3.04 3.78 FUD XXX 80

AMA: 2019,Dec,14; 2019,Sep,10; 2018,Nov,3

+ **96133** **each additional hour (List separately in addition to code for primary procedure)**

EXCLUDES *Reporting code for less than 31 minutes*

2.34 2.84 FUD ZZZ 80

AMA: 2019,Dec,14; 2019,Sep,10; 2018,Nov,3

96136 **Psychological or neuropsychological test administration and scoring by physician or other qualified health care professional, two or more tests, any method; first 30 minutes**

EXCLUDES *Reporting code for less than 16 minutes*
Code also testing evaluation on same or different days (96130-96133)

0.70 1.33 FUD XXX 80

AMA: 2020,Aug,3; 2019,Dec,14; 2019,Sep,10; 2018,Nov,3

+ **96137** **each additional 30 minutes (List separately in addition to code for primary procedure)**

EXCLUDES *Reporting code for less than 16 minutes*

Code also testing evaluation on same or different days (96130-96133)

0.55 | 1.22 | FUD ZZZ

AMA: 2020,Aug,3; 2019,Dec,14; 2019,Sep,10; 2018,Nov,3

96138 **Psychological or neuropsychological test administration and scoring by technician, two or more tests, any method; first 30 minutes**

EXCLUDES *Reporting code for less than 16 minutes*

Code also testing evaluation on same or different days (96130-96133)

1.07 | 1.07 | FUD XXX

AMA: 2018,Nov,3

+ **96139** **each additional 30 minutes (List separately in addition to code for primary procedure)**

EXCLUDES *Reporting code for less than 16 minutes*

Code also testing evaluation on same or different days (96130-96133)

1.07 | 1.07 | FUD ZZZ

AMA: 2018,Nov,3

96146 **Psychological or neuropsychological test administration, with single automated, standardized instrument via electronic platform, with automated result only**

EXCLUDES *Testing provided by physician, other qualified healthcare professional, or technician ([96127], 96136-96139)*

0.06 | 0.06 | FUD XXX

AMA: 2018,Nov,3

96156-96171 [96164, 96165, 96167, 96168, 96170, 96171] Biopsychosocial Assessment/Intervention

INCLUDES Services for patients that have primary physical illnesses/diagnoses/symptoms who may benefit from assessments/interventions that focus on biopsychosocial factors related to patient's health status

Services used to identify factors important to prevention/treatment/management physical health problems:

- Behavioral
- Cognitive
- Emotional
- Psychological
- Social

EXCLUDES *Adaptive behavior services ([97151, 97152, 97153, 97154, 97155, 97156, 97157, 97158], 0362T, 0373T)*

E/M services same date

Health and behavior assessment and intervention (96156, 96158-96159)

Preventive medicine counseling services (99401-99412)

96156 **Health behavior assessment, or re-assessment (ie, health-focused clinical interview, behavioral observations, clinical decision making)**

EXCLUDES *Psychotherapy services (90785-90899)*

2.51 | 2.77 | FUD XXX

AMA: 2020,Aug,3; 2020,Jul,7

96158 **Health behavior intervention, individual, face-to-face; initial 30 minutes**

EXCLUDES *Psychotherapy services (90785-90899)*

1.71 | 1.89 | FUD XXX

AMA: 2020,Aug,3; 2020,Jul,7

+ **96159** **each additional 15 minutes (List separately in addition to code for primary service)**

EXCLUDES *Psychotherapy services (90785-90899)*

Code first (96158)

0.59 | 0.66 | FUD ZZZ

AMA: 2020,Aug,3; 2020,Jul,7

\# **96164** **Health behavior intervention, group (2 or more patients), face-to-face; initial 30 minutes**

EXCLUDES *Psychotherapy services (90785-90899)*

0.25 | 0.28 | FUD XXX

AMA: 2020,Aug,3; 2020,Jul,7

+ # **96165** **each additional 15 minutes (List separately in addition to code for primary service)**

EXCLUDES *Psychotherapy services (90785-90899)*

Code first ([96164])

0.11 | 0.13 | FUD ZZZ

AMA: 2020,Aug,3; 2020,Jul,7

\# **96167** **Health behavior intervention, family (with the patient present), face-to-face; initial 30 minutes**

EXCLUDES *Psychotherapy services (90785-90899)*

1.83 | 2.03 | FUD XXX

AMA: 2020,Aug,3

+ # **96168** **each additional 15 minutes (List separately in addition to code for primary service)**

EXCLUDES *Psychotherapy services (90785-90899)*

Code first ([96167])

0.65 | 0.72 | FUD ZZZ

AMA: 2020,Aug,3

\# **96170** **Health behavior intervention, family (without the patient present), face-to-face; initial 30 minutes**

EXCLUDES *Psychotherapy services (90785-90899)*

2.19 | 2.30 | FUD XXX

AMA: 2020,Aug,3

+ # **96171** **each additional 15 minutes (List separately in addition to code for primary service)**

EXCLUDES *Psychotherapy services (90785-90899)*

Code first ([96170])

0.80 | 0.84 | FUD ZZZ

AMA: 2020,Aug,3

96160-96171 [96164, 96165, 96167, 96168, 96170, 96171] Health Risk Assessments

96160 **Administration of patient-focused health risk assessment instrument (eg, health hazard appraisal) with scoring and documentation, per standardized instrument**

0.09 | 0.09 | FUD ZZZ ★ S

AMA: 2020,Aug,3; 2018,Feb,11; 2018,Jan,8; 2017,Feb,14; 2017,Jan,8; 2016,Nov,5

96161 **Administration of caregiver-focused health risk assessment instrument (eg, depression inventory) for the benefit of the patient, with scoring and documentation, per standardized instrument**

0.07 | 0.07 | FUD ZZZ ★ S

AMA: 2020,Aug,3; 2018,Feb,11; 2018,Jan,8; 2017,Feb,14; 2017,Jan,8; 2016,Nov,5

96164 **Resequenced code. See code following 96159.**

96165 **Resequenced code. See code following 96159.**

96167 **Resequenced code. See code following 96159.**

96168 **Resequenced code. See code following 96159.**

96170 **Resequenced code. See code following 96159.**

96171 **Resequenced code. See code following 96159.**

96360-96361 Intravenous Fluid Infusion for Hydration (Nonchemotherapy)

CMS: 100-04,4,230.2 OPPS Drug Administration

INCLUDES Administration prepackaged fluids and electrolytes
Coding hierarchy rules for facility reporting only:
Chemotherapy services primary to diagnostic, prophylactic, and therapeutic services
Diagnostic, prophylactic, and therapeutic services primary to hydration services
Infusions primary to pushes
Pushes primary to injections
Constant observance/attendance by person administering drug or substance
Infusion 15 minutes or less
Direct supervision by physician or other qualified health care provider:
Direction personnel
Minimal supervision for:
Consent
Safety oversight
Supervision personnel
If done to facilitate injection/infusion:
Flush at infusion end
Indwelling IV, subcutaneous catheter/port access
Local anesthesia
Start IV
Supplies/tubing/syringes
Report initial code for primary reason for visit despite order infusions or injections given
Treatment plan verification

EXCLUDES *Catheter/port declotting (36593)*
Drugs/other substances
Minimal infusion to keep vein open or during other therapeutic infusions
Reporting code for hydration infusion 31 minutes or less
Reporting code for second initial service on same date for accessing multilumen catheter, restarting IV, or when two IV lines are needed to meet infusion rate
Services provided by physicians or other qualified health care providers in facility settings
Significant separately identifiable E/M service, when performed

96360 **Intravenous infusion, hydration; initial, 31 minutes to 1 hour**

EXCLUDES *Reporting code when service performed as concurrent infusion*

1.07 1.07 **FUD** XXX S 80

AMA: 2019,Jun,5; 2018,Feb,11; 2018,Jan,8; 2017,Jan,8; 2016,Jan,13

\+ **96361** **each additional hour (List separately in addition to code for primary procedure)**

INCLUDES Hydration infusion of more than 30 minutes beyond 1 hour
Hydration provided as secondary or subsequent service after different initial service via same IV access site

Code first (96360)

0.38 0.38 **FUD** ZZZ S 80

AMA: 2019,Jun,5; 2018,Feb,11; 2018,Jan,8; 2017,Jan,8; 2016,Jan,13

96365-96371 Infusions: Diagnostic/Preventive/Therapeutic

CMS: 100-04,4,230.2 OPPS Drug Administration

INCLUDES Administration fluid
Administration substances/drugs
Coding hierarchy rules for facility reporting:
Chemotherapy services primary to diagnostic, prophylactic, and therapeutic services
Diagnostic, prophylactic, and therapeutic services primary to hydration services
Infusions primary to pushes
Pushes primary to injections
Constant presence by health care professional administering substance/drug
Direct supervision by physician or other qualified health care provider:
Consent
Direction personnel
Patient assessment
Safety oversight
Supervision personnel
If done to facilitate injection/infusion:
Flush at infusion end
Indwelling IV, subcutaneous catheter/port access
Local anesthesia
Start IV
Supplies/tubing/syringes
Infusion 16 minutes or more
Training to assess patient and monitor vital signs
Training to prepare/dose/dispose
Treatment plan verification

EXCLUDES *Catheter/port declotting (36593)*
Mechanical scalp cooling (0662T-0663T)
Services provided by physicians or other qualified health care providers in facility settings
Significant separately identifiable E/M service, when performed
Reporting code for second initial service on same date for accessing multilumen catheter, restarting IV, or when two IV lines needed to meet infusion rate
Reporting code with other procedures where IV push or infusion is integral to procedure

Code also drugs/materials

96365 **Intravenous infusion, for therapy, prophylaxis, or diagnosis (specify substance or drug); initial, up to 1 hour**

Code also second initial service with modifier 59 when patient's condition or drug protocol mandates use of two IV lines

2.02 2.02 **FUD** XXX S 80

AMA: 2020,NovSE,1; 2020,Jan,11; 2018,Dec,8; 2018,Dec,8; 2018,Sep,14; 2018,May,10; 2018,Feb,11; 2018,Jan,8; 2017,Jan,8; 2016,Jan,13

\+ **96366** **each additional hour (List separately in addition to code for primary procedure)**

INCLUDES Additional hours sequential infusion
Infusion intervals more than 30 minutes beyond one hour
Second and subsequent infusions same drug or substance

Code also additional infusion, when appropriate (96367)
Code first (96365)

0.61 0.61 **FUD** ZZZ S 80

AMA: 2020,NovSE,1; 2020,Jan,11; 2018,Sep,14; 2018,Feb,11; 2018,Jan,8; 2017,Jan,8; 2016,Jan,13

\+ **96367** **additional sequential infusion of a new drug/substance, up to 1 hour (List separately in addition to code for primary procedure)**

INCLUDES Secondary or subsequent service with new drug or substance after different initial service via same IV access

EXCLUDES *Reporting code more than one time per sequential infusion same mix*

Code first (96365, 96374, 96409, 96413)

0.88 0.88 **FUD** ZZZ S 80

AMA: 2020,NovSE,1; 2020,Jan,11; 2018,Feb,11; 2018,Jan,8; 2017,Jan,8; 2016,Jan,13

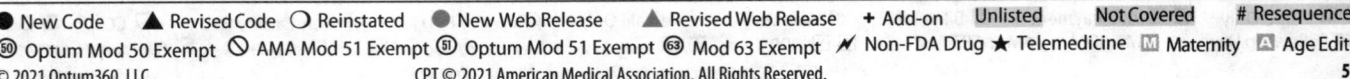

+ 96368 concurrent infusion (List separately in addition to code for primary procedure)

EXCLUDES *Reporting code more than one time per service date*

Code first (96365, 96366, 96413, 96415, 96416)

0.59 0.59 FUD ZZZ N 80

AMA: 2020,NovSE,1; 2020,Jan,11; 2018,Feb,11; 2018,Jan,8; 2017,Jan,8; 2016,Jan,13

96369 Subcutaneous infusion for therapy or prophylaxis (specify substance or drug); initial, up to 1 hour, including pump set-up and establishment of subcutaneous infusion site(s)

EXCLUDES *Infusions 15 minutes or less (96372)*
Reporting code more than one time per encounter

4.69 4.69 FUD XXX S 80

AMA: 2020,NovSE,1; 2020,Jan,11; 2018,Feb,11; 2018,Jan,8; 2017,Jan,8; 2016,Jan,13

+ 96370 each additional hour (List separately in addition to code for primary procedure)

INCLUDES Infusions more than 30 minutes beyond one hour

Code first (96369)

0.44 0.44 FUD ZZZ S 80

AMA: 2020,NovSE,1; 2020,Jan,11; 2018,Feb,11; 2018,Jan,8; 2017,Jan,8; 2016,Jan,13

+ 96371 additional pump set-up with establishment of new subcutaneous infusion site(s) (List separately in addition to code for primary procedure)

EXCLUDES *Reporting code more than one time per encounter*

Code first (96369)

1.84 1.84 FUD ZZZ Q1 80

AMA: 2020,NovSE,1; 2020,Jan,11; 2018,Feb,11; 2018,Jan,8; 2017,Jan,8; 2016,Jan,13

96372-96379 Injections: Diagnostic/Preventive/Therapeutic

CMS: 100-04,4,230.2 OPPS Drug Administration

INCLUDES
- Administration fluid
- Administration substances/drugs
- Coding hierarchy rules for facility reporting:
  - Chemotherapy services primary to diagnostic, prophylactic, and therapeutic services
  - Diagnostic, prophylactic, and therapeutic services primary to hydration services
  - Infusions primary to pushes
  - Pushes primary to injections
- Constant presence by health care professional administering substance/drug
- Direct supervision by physician or other qualified health care provider:
  - Consent
  - Direction personnel
  - Patient assessment
  - Safety oversight
  - Supervision personnel
- If done to facilitate injection/infusion:
  - Flush at infusion end
  - Indwelling IV, subcutaneous catheter/port access
  - Local anesthesia
  - Start IV
  - Supplies/tubing/syringes
- Infusion 15 minutes or less
- Training to assess patient and monitor vital signs
- Training to prepare/dose/dispose
- Treatment plan verification

EXCLUDES
- *Catheter/port declotting (36593)*
- *Mechanical scalp cooling (0662T-0663T)*
- *Reporting code for second initial service on same date for accessing multilumen catheter, restarting IV, or when two IV lines needed to meet infusion rate*
- *Reporting code with other procedures where IV push or infusion is integral to procedure*
- *Services provided by physicians or other qualified health care providers in facility settings*
- *Significant separately identifiable E/M service, when performed*

Code also drugs/materials

96372 Therapeutic, prophylactic, or diagnostic injection (specify substance or drug); subcutaneous or intramuscular

INCLUDES Direct supervision by physician or other qualified health care provider when reported by physician/other qualified health care provider. When reported by hospital, physician/other qualified health care provider need not be present
Hormonal therapy injections (non-antineoplastic) (96372)

EXCLUDES *Administration vaccines/toxoids (90460-90461, 90471-90472, [0001A, 0002A, 0003A, 0004A], [0051A, 0052A, 0053A, 0054A], [0071A, 0072A], [0011A, 0012A, 0013A], [0064A], [0021A, 0022A], [0031A], [0034A], [0041A, 0042A])*
Allergen immunotherapy injections (95115-95117)
Antineoplastic hormonal injections (96402)
Antineoplastic nonhormonal injections (96401)
Injections administered without direct supervision by physician or other qualified health care provider (99211)
Intradermal cancer immunotherapy (0708T-0709T)

0.47 0.47 FUD XXX Q1 80

AMA: 2018,Dec,10; 2018,Dec,10; 2018,Feb,11; 2018,Jan,8; 2017,Jan,8; 2016,Oct,9; 2016,Jan,13

96373 intra-arterial

0.53 0.53 FUD XXX S 80

AMA: 2018,Feb,11; 2018,Jan,8; 2017,Jan,8; 2016,Jan,13

96374 intravenous push, single or initial substance/drug

1.10 1.10 FUD XXX S 80

AMA: 2020,NovSE,1; 2020,Jan,11; 2019,Sep,5; 2019,Jun,9; 2018,Feb,11; 2018,Jan,8; 2017,Jan,8; 2016,Jan,13

+ **96375 each additional sequential intravenous push of a new substance/drug (List separately in addition to code for primary procedure)**

INCLUDES IV push new substance/drug provided as secondary or subsequent service after different initial service via same IV access site

Code first (96365, 96374, 96409, 96413)

0.47 0.47 FUD ZZZ S 80

AMA: 2019,Sep,5; 2018,Feb,11; 2018,Jan,8; 2017,Jan,8; 2016,Jan,13

+ **96376 each additional sequential intravenous push of the same substance/drug provided in a facility (List separately in addition to code for primary procedure)**

INCLUDES Facilities only

EXCLUDES *IV push performed within 30 minutes push same substance or drug*

Services performed by any nonfacilty provider

Code first (96365, 96374, 96409, 96413)

0.00 0.00 FUD ZZZ N

AMA: 2018,Dec,8; 2018,Dec,8; 2018,Feb,11; 2018,Jan,8; 2017,Jan,8; 2016,Jan,13

96377 Application of on-body injector (includes cannula insertion) for timed subcutaneous injection

0.56 0.56 FUD XXX Q1 80

AMA: 2018,Feb,11; 2018,Jan,8; 2017,Jan,8; 2016,Oct,9

96379 Unlisted therapeutic, prophylactic, or diagnostic intravenous or intra-arterial injection or infusion

0.00 0.00 FUD XXX Q1 80

AMA: 2018,Feb,11; 2018,Jan,8; 2017,Jan,8; 2016,Jan,13

96401-96411 Chemotherapy and Other Complex Drugs, Biologicals: Injection and IV Push

CMS: 100-03,110.2 Certain Drugs Distributed by the National Cancer Institute; 100-03,110.6 Scalp Hypothermia During Chemotherapy, to Prevent Hair Loss; 100-04,4,230.2 OPPS Drug Administration

INCLUDES Highly complex services that require direct supervision for:
- Consent
- Patient assessment
- Safety oversight
- Supervision

More intense work and monitoring clinical staff by physician or other qualified health care provider due to greater risk severe patient reactions

Parenteral administration:
- Anti-neoplastic agents for noncancer diagnoses
- Monoclonal antibody agents
- Nonradionuclide antineoplastic drugs
- Other biologic response modifiers

EXCLUDES *Reporting code for second initial service on same date for accessing multilumen catheter, restarting IV, or when two IV lines needed to meet infusion rate*

96401 Chemotherapy administration, subcutaneous or intramuscular; non-hormonal anti-neoplastic

EXCLUDES *Intradermal cancer immunotherapy (0708T-0709T)*

Services performed by physicians or other qualified health care providers in facility settings

2.24 2.24 FUD XXX Q1 80

AMA: 2018,Feb,11; 2018,Jan,8; 2017,Jan,8; 2016,Jan,13

96402 hormonal anti-neoplastic

EXCLUDES *Services performed by physicians or other qualified health care providers in facility settings*

0.87 0.87 FUD XXX Q1 80

AMA: 2018,Feb,11; 2018,Jan,8; 2017,Jan,8; 2016,Jan,13

96405 Chemotherapy administration; intralesional, up to and including 7 lesions

0.84 2.31 FUD 000 Q1

AMA: 2018,Feb,11; 2018,Jan,8; 2017,Jan,8; 2016,Jan,13

96406 intralesional, more than 7 lesions

1.31 3.46 FUD 000 S

AMA: 2018,Feb,11; 2018,Jan,8; 2017,Jan,8; 2016,Jan,13

96409 intravenous, push technique, single or initial substance/drug

INCLUDES Push technique includes:

Administration injection directly into vessel or access line by health care professional; or

Infusion less than or equal to 15 minutes

EXCLUDES *Insertion arterial and venous cannula(s) for extracorpororeal circulation (36823)*

Services performed by physicians or other qualified health care providers in facility settings

3.05 3.05 FUD XXX S 80

AMA: 2018,Feb,11; 2018,Jan,8; 2017,Jan,8; 2016,Jan,13

+ **96411 intravenous, push technique, each additional substance/drug (List separately in addition to code for primary procedure)**

INCLUDES Push technique includes:

Administration injection directly into vessel or access line by health care professional; or

Infusion less than or equal to 15 minutes

EXCLUDES *Insertion arterial and venous cannula(s) for extracorpororeal circulation (36823)*

Services performed by physicians or other qualified health care providers in facility settings

Code first initial substance/drug (96409, 96413)

1.65 1.65 FUD ZZZ S 80

AMA: 2018,Feb,11; 2018,Jan,8; 2017,Jan,8; 2016,Jan,13

96413-96417 Chemotherapy and Complex Drugs, Biologicals: Intravenous Infusion

CMS: 100-03,110.2 Certain Drugs Distributed by the National Cancer Institute; 100-03,110.6 Scalp Hypothermia During Chemotherapy, to Prevent Hair Loss; 100-04,4,230.2 OPPS Drug Administration

INCLUDES Administration:
- Access to IV/catheter/port
- Drug preparation
- Flushing at infusion completion
- Hydration fluid
- Local anesthesia
- Routine tubing/syringe/supplies
- Starting IV

Highly complex services that require direct supervision for:
- Consent
- Patient assessment
- Safety oversight
- Supervision

More intense work and monitoring clinical staff by physician or other qualified health care provider due to greater risk severe patient reactions

Parenteral administration:
- Antineoplastic agents for noncancer diagnoses
- Monoclonal antibody agents
- Nonradionuclide antineoplastic drugs
- Other biologic response modifiers

EXCLUDES *Administration nonchemotherapy agents such as antibiotics/steroids/analgesics*
Declotting catheter/port (36593)
Home infusion (99601-99602)
Insertion arterial and venous cannula(s) for extracorpororeal circulation (36823)
Reporting code for second initial service on same date for accessing multilumen catheter, restarting IV, or when two IV lines needed to meet infusion rate
Services provided by physicians or other qualified health care providers in facility settings

Code also:
- Drug or substance
- Significant separately identifiable E/M service, when performed

96413 Chemotherapy administration, intravenous infusion technique; up to 1 hour, single or initial substance/drug

INCLUDES Push technique includes:
- Administration injection directly into vessel or access line by health care professional; or
- Infusion less than or equal to 15 minutes

EXCLUDES *Hydration administered as secondary or subsequent service via same IV access site (96361)*
Therapeutic/prophylactic/diagnostic drug infusion/injection through the same intravenous access (96366, 96367, 96375)

Code also second initial service with modifier 59 when patient's condition or drug protocol mandates use of two IV lines

Facility RVU 3.97 Non-Facility RVU 3.97 **FUD** XXX S 80

AMA: 2018,Feb,11; 2018,Jan,8; 2017,Jan,8; 2016,Jan,13

\+ **96415 each additional hour (List separately in addition to code for primary procedure)**

INCLUDES Infusion intervals more than 30 minutes past 1-hour increments

Code first initial hour (96413)

Facility RVU 0.86 Non-Facility RVU 0.86 **FUD** ZZZ S 80

AMA: 2018,Feb,11; 2018,Jan,8; 2017,Jan,8; 2016,Jan,13

96416 initiation of prolonged chemotherapy infusion (more than 8 hours), requiring use of a portable or implantable pump

EXCLUDES *Portable or implantable infusion pump/reservoir refilling/maintenance for drug delivery (96521-96523)*

Facility RVU 3.98 Non-Facility RVU 3.98 **FUD** XXX S 80

AMA: 2018,Feb,11; 2018,Jan,8; 2017,Jan,8; 2016,Jan,13

\+ **96417 each additional sequential infusion (different substance/drug), up to 1 hour (List separately in addition to code for primary procedure)**

INCLUDES Push technique includes:
- Administration injection directly into vessel or access line by health care professional; or
- Infusion less than or equal to 15 minutes

EXCLUDES *Additional hour(s) sequential infusion (96415)*
Reporting code more than one time per sequential infusion

Code first initial substance/drug (96413)

Facility RVU 1.92 Non-Facility RVU 1.92 **FUD** ZZZ S 80

AMA: 2018,Feb,11; 2018,Jan,8; 2017,Jan,8; 2016,Jan,13

96420-96425 Chemotherapy and Complex Drugs, Biologicals: Intra-arterial

CMS: 100-03,110.2 Certain Drugs Distributed by the National Cancer Institute; 100-03,110.6 Scalp Hypothermia During Chemotherapy, to Prevent Hair Loss; 100-04,4,230.2 OPPS Drug Administration

INCLUDES Administration:
- Access to IV/catheter/port
- Drug preparation
- Flushing at infusion completion
- Hydration fluid
- Local anesthesia
- Routine tubing/syringe/supplies
- Starting IV

Highly complex services that require direct supervision for:
- Consent
- Patient assessment
- Safety oversight
- Supervision

More intense work and monitoring clinical staff by physician or other qualified health care provider due to greater risk severe patient reactions

Parenteral administration:
- Antineoplastic agents for noncancer diagnoses
- Monoclonal antibody agents
- Nonradionuclide antineoplastic drugs
- Other biologic response modifiers

EXCLUDES *Administration nonchemotherapy agents such as antibiotics/steroids/analgesics*
Declotting catheter/port (36593)
Home infusion (99601-99602)
Reporting code for second initial service on same date for accessing multilumen catheter, restarting IV, or when two IV lines needed to meet an infusion rate
Services provided by physicians or other qualified health care providers in facility settings

Code also:
- Significant separately identifiable E/M service, when performed
- Drug or substance

96420 Chemotherapy administration, intra-arterial; push technique

INCLUDES Push technique includes:
- Administration injection directly into vessel or access line by health care professional; or
- Infusion less than or equal to 15 minutes

Regional chemotherapy perfusion

EXCLUDES *Insertion arterial and venous cannula(s) for extracorpororeal circulation (36823)*
Placement intra-arterial catheter

Facility RVU 2.95 Non-Facility RVU 2.95 **FUD** XXX S 80

AMA: 2018,Feb,11; 2018,Jan,8; 2017,Jan,8; 2016,Mar,3; 2016,Jan,13

96422 infusion technique, up to 1 hour

INCLUDES Push technique includes:
- Administration injection directly into vessel or access line by health care professional; or
- Infusion less than or equal to 15 minutes

Regional chemotherapy perfusion

EXCLUDES *Insertion arterial and venous cannula(s) for extracorpororeal circulation (36823)*
Placement intra-arterial catheter

Facility RVU 4.85 Non-Facility RVU 4.85 **FUD** XXX S 80

AMA: 2018,Feb,11; 2018,Jan,8; 2017,Jan,8; 2016,Mar,3; 2016,Jan,13

+ **96423** **infusion technique, each additional hour (List separately in addition to code for primary procedure)**

INCLUDES Infusion intervals more than 30 minutes past 1-hour increments
Regional chemotherapy perfusion

EXCLUDES *Insertion arterial and venous cannula(s) for extracorpororeal circulation (36823)*
Placement intra-arterial catheter

Code first initial hour (96422)

2.24 2.24 FUD ZZZ S 80

AMA: 2018,Feb,11; 2018,Jan,8; 2017,Jan,8; 2016,Mar,3; 2016,Jan,13

96425 **infusion technique, initiation of prolonged infusion (more than 8 hours), requiring the use of a portable or implantable pump**

INCLUDES Regional chemotherapy perfusion

EXCLUDES *Insertion arterial and venous cannula(s) for extracorpororeal circulation (36823)*
Placement intra-arterial catheter
Portable or implantable infusion pump/reservoir refilling/maintenance for drug delivery (96521-96523)

5.14 5.14 FUD XXX S 80

AMA: 2018,Feb,11; 2018,Jan,8; 2017,Jan,8; 2016,Mar,3; 2016,Jan,13

96440-96450 Chemotherapy Administration: Intrathecal/Peritoneal Cavity/Pleural Cavity

CMS: 100-03,110.2 Certain Drugs Distributed by the National Cancer Institute; 100-04,4,230.2 OPPS Drug Administration

96440 **Chemotherapy administration into pleural cavity, requiring and including thoracentesis**

3.57 23.6 FUD 000 S 80

AMA: 2018,Feb,11; 2018,Jan,8; 2017,Jan,8; 2016,Jan,13

96446 **Chemotherapy administration into the peritoneal cavity via indwelling port or catheter**

0.79 5.78 FUD XXX S 80

AMA: 2018,Feb,11; 2018,Jan,8; 2017,Jan,8; 2016,Jan,13

96450 **Chemotherapy administration, into CNS (eg, intrathecal), requiring and including spinal puncture**

EXCLUDES *Chemotherapy administration, intravesical/bladder (51720)*
Fluoroscopy (77003)
Insertion catheter/reservoir:
Intraventricular (61210, 61215)
Subarachnoid (62350-62351, 62360-62362)

2.27 5.13 FUD 000 S 80

AMA: 2018,Feb,11; 2018,Jan,8; 2017,Jan,8; 2016,Jan,13

96521-96523 Refill/Upkeep of Drug Delivery Device

CMS: 100-04,4,230.2 OPPS Drug Administration

INCLUDES Administration:
- Access to IV/catheter/port
- Drug preparation
- Flushing at infusion completion
- Hydration fluid
- Local anesthesia
- Routine tubing/syringe/supplies
- Starting IV

Highly complex services that require direct supervision for:
- Consent
- Patient assessment
- Safety oversight
- Supervision

Parenteral administration:
- Antineoplastic agents for noncancer diagnoses
- Monoclonal antibody agents
- Nonradionuclide antineoplastic drugs
- Other biologic response modifiers

Therapeutic drugs other than chemotherapy

EXCLUDES *Administration nonchemotherapy agents such as antibiotics/steroids/analgesics*
Blood specimen collection from completely implantable venous access device (36591)
Declotting catheter/port (36593)
Home infusion (99601-99602)
Services provided by physicians or other qualified health care providers in facility settings

Code also:
Drug or substance
Significant separately identifiable E/M service, when performed

96521 **Refilling and maintenance of portable pump**

4.13 4.13 FUD XXX S 80

AMA: 2018,Feb,11; 2018,Jan,8; 2017,Jan,8; 2016,Jan,13

96522 **Refilling and maintenance of implantable pump or reservoir for drug delivery, systemic (eg, intravenous, intra-arterial)**

EXCLUDES *Implantable infusion pump refilling/maintenance for spinal/brain drug delivery (95990-95991)*

3.39 3.39 FUD XXX S 80

AMA: 2018,Feb,11; 2018,Jan,8; 2017,Jan,8; 2016,Jan,13

96523 **Irrigation of implanted venous access device for drug delivery systems**

EXCLUDES *Direct supervision by physician or other qualified health care provider in facility settings*
Reporting code with any other services on same service date

0.77 0.77 FUD XXX 01 80

AMA: 2018,Feb,11; 2018,Jan,8; 2017,Jan,8; 2016,Jan,13

96542-96549 Chemotherapy Injection Into Brain

CMS: 100-04,4,230.2 OPPS Drug Administration

INCLUDES Administration:
- Access to IV/catheter/port
- Drug preparation
- Flushing at infusion completion
- Hydration fluid
- Local anesthesia
- Routine tubing/syringe/supplies
- Starting IV

Highly complex services that require direct supervision for:
- Consent
- Patient assessment
- Safety oversight
- Supervision

Parenteral administration:
- Antineoplastic agents for noncancer diagnoses
- Monoclonal antibody agents
- Nonradionuclide antineoplastic drugs
- Other biologic response modifiers

EXCLUDES *Administration nonchemotherapy agents such as antibiotics/steroids/analgesics*
Blood specimen collection from completely implantable venous access device (36591)
Declotting catheter/port (36593)
Home infusion (99601-99602)

Code also:
- Drug or substance
- Significant separately identifiable E/M service, when performed

96542 Chemotherapy injection, subarachnoid or intraventricular via subcutaneous reservoir, single or multiple agents

EXCLUDES *Oral radioactive isotope therapy (79005)*

1.19 3.77 **FUD** XXX S 80

AMA: 2018,Feb,11; 2018,Jan,8; 2017,Jan,8; 2016,Jan,13

96549 Unlisted chemotherapy procedure

0.00 0.00 **FUD** XXX Q1 80

AMA: 2018,Feb,11; 2018,Jan,8; 2017,Jan,8; 2016,Jan,13

96567-96574 Destruction of Lesions: Photodynamic Therapy

EXCLUDES *Ocular photodynamic therapy (67221)*

96567 Photodynamic therapy by external application of light to destroy premalignant lesions of the skin and adjacent mucosa with application and illumination/activation of photosensitive drug(s), per day

INCLUDES Services provided without direct participation by physician or other qualified healthcare professional

3.50 3.50 **FUD** XXX Q1 80

AMA: 2018,Jul,14; 2018,Feb,10; 2018,Feb,11; 2018,Jan,8; 2017,Jan,8; 2016,Jan,13

\+ **96570 Photodynamic therapy by endoscopic application of light to ablate abnormal tissue via activation of photosensitive drug(s); first 30 minutes (List separately in addition to code for endoscopy or bronchoscopy procedures of lung and gastrointestinal tract)**

Code also:
- For 38-52 minutes (96571)
- Modifier 52 when services with report less than 23 minutes

Code first (31641, 43229)

1.48 1.48 **FUD** ZZZ N

AMA: 2018,Feb,11; 2018,Jan,8; 2017,Jan,8; 2016,Jan,13

\+ **96571 each additional 15 minutes (List separately in addition to code for endoscopy or bronchoscopy procedures of lung and gastrointestinal tract)**

EXCLUDES *23-37 minutes service (96570)*

Code first (96570)

Code first when appropriate (31641, 43229)

0.83 0.83 **FUD** ZZZ N

AMA: 2018,Feb,11; 2018,Jan,8; 2017,Jan,8; 2016,Jan,13

96573 Photodynamic therapy by external application of light to destroy premalignant lesions of the skin and adjacent mucosa with application and illumination/activation of photosensitizing drug(s) provided by a physician or other qualified health care professional, per day

INCLUDES Application photosensitizer to lesions at anatomical site
Debridement, when performed
Light to activate photosensitizer for destruction premalignant lesions

EXCLUDES *Debridement lesion with photodynamic therapy provided by physician or other qualified healthcare professional (96574)*
Photodynamic therapy by external application light to same anatomical site (96567)
Services provided to same area on same date as photodynamic therapy:
- *Biopsy (11102-11107)*
- *Debridement (11000-11001, 11004-11005)*
- *Excision lesion (11400-11471)*
- *Shaving lesion (11300-11313)*

6.03 6.03 **FUD** 000 Q1 80

AMA: 2018,Jul,14; 2018,Feb,11; 2018,Feb,10

96574 Debridement of premalignant hyperkeratotic lesion(s) (ie, targeted curettage, abrasion) followed with photodynamic therapy by external application of light to destroy premalignant lesions of the skin and adjacent mucosa with application and illumination/activation of photosensitizing drug(s) provided by a physician or other qualified health care professional, per day

INCLUDES Application photosensitizer to lesions at anatomical site
Debridement, when performed
Light to activate photosensitizer for destruction premalignant lesions

EXCLUDES *Photodynamic therapy by external application light for destruction premalignant lesions (96573)*
Photodynamic therapy by external application light to same anatomical site (96567)
Services provided to same area on same as photodynamic therapy:
- *Biopsy (11102-11107)*
- *Debridement (11000-11001, 11004-11005)*
- *Excision lesion (11400-11471)*
- *Shaving lesion (11300-11313)*

7.25 7.25 **FUD** 000 Q1 80

AMA: 2018,Feb,10; 2018,Feb,11

96900-96999 Diagnostic/Therapeutic Skin Procedures

EXCLUDES *E/M services*
Injection, intralesional (11900-11901)

96900 Actinotherapy (ultraviolet light)

EXCLUDES *Rhinophototherapy (30999)*

(88160-88161)

0.61 0.61 **FUD** XXX Q1 80

AMA: 2018,Feb,11; 2018,Jan,8; 2017,Jan,8; 2016,Nov,9; 2016,Sep,3; 2016,Jan,13

96902 Microscopic examination of hairs plucked or clipped by the examiner (excluding hair collected by the patient) to determine telogen and anagen counts, or structural hair shaft abnormality

(88160-88161)

0.59 0.62 **FUD** XXX N

AMA: 2018,Feb,11

96904 Whole body integumentary photography, for monitoring of high risk patients with dysplastic nevus syndrome or a history of dysplastic nevi, or patients with a personal or familial history of melanoma

(88160-88161)

1.82 1.82 **FUD** XXX N 80

AMA: 2018,Feb,11

96910 **Photochemotherapy; tar and ultraviolet B (Goeckerman treatment) or petrolatum and ultraviolet B**

(88160-88161)

3.24 3.24 FUD XXX

AMA: 2018,Feb,11; 2018,Jan,8; 2017,Jan,8; 2016,Sep,3; 2016,Jan,13

96912 **psoralens and ultraviolet A (PUVA)**

(88160-88161)

2.75 2.75 FUD XXX

AMA: 2018,Feb,11; 2018,Jan,8; 2017,Jan,8; 2016,Sep,3; 2016,Jan,13

96913 **Photochemotherapy (Goeckerman and/or PUVA) for severe photoresponsive dermatoses requiring at least 4-8 hours of care under direct supervision of the physician (includes application of medication and dressings)**

(88160-88161)

3.91 3.91 FUD XXX

AMA: 2018,Feb,11; 2018,Jan,8; 2017,Jan,8; 2016,Sep,3

96920 **Laser treatment for inflammatory skin disease (psoriasis); total area less than 250 sq cm**

EXCLUDES *Destruction by laser:*
Benign lesions (17110-17111)
Cutaneous vascular proliferative lesions (17106-17108)
Malignant lesions (17260-17286)
Premalignant lesions (17000-17004)

(88160-88161)

1.90 4.64 FUD 000

AMA: 2020,Jul,13; 2018,Feb,11; 2018,Jan,8; 2017,Jan,8; 2016,Sep,3; 2016,Jan,13

96921 **250 sq cm to 500 sq cm**

EXCLUDES *Destruction by laser:*
Benign lesions (17110-17111)
Cutaneous vascular proliferative lesions (17106-17108)
Malignant lesions (17260-17286)
Premalignant lesions (17000-17004)

(88160-88161)

2.14 5.09 FUD 000

AMA: 2020,Jul,13; 2018,Feb,11; 2018,Jan,8; 2017,Jan,8; 2016,Sep,3; 2016,Jan,13

96922 **over 500 sq cm**

EXCLUDES *Destruction by laser:*
Benign lesions (17110-17111)
Cutaneous vascular proliferative lesions (17106-17108)
Malignant lesions (17260-17286)
Premalignant lesions (17000-17004)

(88160-88161)

3.43 6.91 FUD 000

AMA: 2020,Jul,13; 2018,Feb,11; 2018,Jan,8; 2017,Jan,8; 2016,Sep,3; 2016,Jan,13

96931 **Reflectance confocal microscopy (RCM) for cellular and sub-cellular imaging of skin; image acquisition and interpretation and report, first lesion**

EXCLUDES *Optical coherence tomography for skin imaging (0470T-0471T)*
Reflectance confocal microscopy examination without generated mosaic images (96999)

4.83 4.83 FUD XXX

AMA: 2018,Feb,11; 2018,Jan,8; 2017,Sep,9

96932 **image acquisition only, first lesion**

EXCLUDES *Optical coherence tomography for skin imaging (0470T-0471T)*
Reflectance confocal microscopy examination without generated mosaic images (96999)

3.51 3.51 FUD XXX

AMA: 2018,Feb,11; 2018,Jan,8; 2017,Sep,9

96933 **interpretation and report only, first lesion**

EXCLUDES *Optical coherence tomography for skin imaging (0470T-0471T)*
Reflectance confocal microscopy examination without generated mosaic images (96999)

1.16 1.16 FUD XXX

AMA: 2018,Feb,11; 2018,Jan,8; 2017,Sep,9

+ 96934 **image acquisition and interpretation and report, each additional lesion (List separately in addition to code for primary procedure)**

EXCLUDES *Optical coherence tomography for skin imaging (0470T-0471T)*
Reflectance confocal microscopy examination without generated mosaic images (96999)

Code first (96931)

2.74 2.74 FUD ZZZ

AMA: 2018,Feb,11; 2018,Jan,8; 2017,Sep,9

+ 96935 **image acquisition only, each additional lesion (List separately in addition to code for primary procedure)**

EXCLUDES *Optical coherence tomography for skin imaging (0470T-0471T)*
Reflectance confocal microscopy examination without generated mosaic images (96999)

Code first (96932)

1.26 1.26 FUD ZZZ

AMA: 2018,Feb,11; 2018,Jan,8; 2017,Sep,9

+ 96936 **interpretation and report only, each additional lesion (List separately in addition to code for primary procedure)**

EXCLUDES *Optical coherence tomography for skin imaging (0470T-0471T)*
Reflectance confocal microscopy examination without generated mosaic images (96999)

Code first (96933)

1.26 1.26 FUD ZZZ

AMA: 2018,Feb,11; 2018,Jan,8; 2017,Sep,9

96999 **Unlisted special dermatological service or procedure**

0.00 0.00 FUD XXX

AMA: 2020,Jul,13; 2018,Feb,11; 2018,Jan,8; 2017,Sep,9; 2017,Jan,8; 2016,Sep,3; 2016,Jan,13

97161-97164 [97161, 97162, 97163, 97164] Assessment: Physical Therapy

CMS: 100-02,15,220 Coverage of Outpatient Rehabilitation Therapy Services; 100-02,15,220.4 Functional Reporting; 100-02,15,230 Practice of Physical Therapy, Occupational Therapy, and Speech-Language Pathology; 100-02,15,230.1 Practice of Physical Therapy; 100-02,15,230.4 Services By a Physical/Occupational Therapist in Private Practice; 100-04,5,10.3.2 Therapy Cap Exceptions; 100-04,5,10.3.3 Use of the KX Modifier; 100-04,5,10.6 Functional Reporting; 100-04,5,20.2 Reporting Units of Service

INCLUDES Care plan creation
Evaluation body systems as defined in 1997 E/M documentation guidelines:
Cardiovascular system: Vital signs, edema extremities
Integumentary system: Inspection for skin abnormalities
Mental status: Orientation, judgment, thought processes
Musculoskeletal system: Evaluation gait and station, motion range, muscle strength, height, and weight
Neuromuscular evaluation: Balance, abnormal movements

EXCLUDES *Biofeedback traning via EMG (90901)*
Joint motion range (95851-95852)
Transcutaneous nerve stimulation (TENS) (97014, 97032)

97161 **Physical therapy evaluation: low complexity, requiring these components: A history with no personal factors and/or comorbidities that impact the plan of care; An examination of body system(s) using standardized tests and measures addressing 1-2 elements from any of the following: body structures and functions, activity limitations, and/or participation restrictions; A clinical presentation with stable and/or uncomplicated characteristics; and Clinical decision making of low complexity using standardized patient assessment instrument and/or measurable assessment of functional outcome. Typically, 20 minutes are spent face-to-face with the patient and/or family.**

2.40 2.40 FUD XXX ★

AMA: 2018,May,5; 2018,Feb,11; 2018,Jan,8; 2017,Aug,3; 2017,Jun,6; 2017,Jan,8

Medicine 96910 — 97161

● New Code ▲ Revised Code ○ Reinstated ● New Web Release ▲ Revised Web Release + Add-on Unlisted Not Covered # Resequenced
50 Optum Mod 50 Exempt ⊘ AMA Mod 51 Exempt 51 Optum Mod 51 Exempt 63 Mod 63 Exempt Non-FDA Drug ★ Telemedicine M Maternity A Age Edit

\# **97162** **Physical therapy evaluation: moderate complexity, requiring these components: A history of present problem with 1-2 personal factors and/or comorbidities that impact the plan of care; An examination of body systems using standardized tests and measures in addressing a total of 3 or more elements from any of the following: body structures and functions, activity limitations, and/or participation restrictions; An evolving clinical presentation with changing characteristics; and Clinical decision making of moderate complexity using standardized patient assessment instrument and/or measurable assessment of functional outcome. Typically, 30 minutes are spent face-to-face with the patient and/or family.**

2.40 2.40 **FUD** XXX ★ (51) A 80

AMA: 2018,May,5; 2018,Feb,11; 2018,Jan,8; 2017,Aug,3; 2017,Jun,6; 2017,Jan,8

\# **97163** **Physical therapy evaluation: high complexity, requiring these components: A history of present problem with 3 or more personal factors and/or comorbidities that impact the plan of care; An examination of body systems using standardized tests and measures addressing a total of 4 or more elements from any of the following: body structures and functions, activity limitations, and/or participation restrictions; A clinical presentation with unstable and unpredictable characteristics; and Clinical decision making of high complexity using standardized patient assessment instrument and/or measurable assessment of functional outcome. Typically, 45 minutes are spent face-to-face with the patient and/or family.**

2.40 2.40 **FUD** XXX (51) A 80

AMA: 2018,May,5; 2018,Feb,11; 2018,Jan,8; 2017,Aug,3; 2017,Jun,6; 2017,Jan,8

\# **97164** **Re-evaluation of physical therapy established plan of care, requiring these components: An examination including a review of history and use of standardized tests and measures is required; and Revised plan of care using a standardized patient assessment instrument and/or measurable assessment of functional outcome Typically, 20 minutes are spent face-to-face with the patient and/or family.**

1.63 1.63 **FUD** XXX (51) A 80

AMA: 2018,May,5; 2018,Feb,11; 2018,Jan,8; 2017,Aug,3; 2017,Jun,6; 2017,Jan,8

97165-97168 [97165, 97166, 97167, 97168] Assessment: Occupational Therapy

CMS: 100-02,15,220 Coverage of Outpatient Rehabilitation Therapy Services; 100-02,15,220.4 Functional Reporting; 100-02,15,230 Practice of Physical Therapy, Occupational Therapy, and Speech-Language Pathology; 100-02,15,230.1 Practice of Physical Therapy; 100-02,15,230.2 Practice of Occupational Therapy; 100-02,15,230.4 Services By a Physical/Occupational Therapist in Private Practice; 100-04,5,10.3.2 Therapy Cap Exceptions; 100-04,5,10.3.3 Use of the KX Modifier; 100-04,5,10.6 Functional Reporting; 100-04,5,20.2 Reporting Units of Service

INCLUDES Care plan creation
Evaluations as appropriate
Medical history
Occupational status
Past therapy history

\# **97165** **Occupational therapy evaluation, low complexity, requiring these components: An occupational profile and medical and therapy history, which includes a brief history including review of medical and/or therapy records relating to the presenting problem; An assessment(s) that identifies 1-3 performance deficits (ie, relating to physical, cognitive, or psychosocial skills) that result in activity limitations and/or participation restrictions; and Clinical decision making of low complexity, which includes an analysis of the occupational profile, analysis of data from problem-focused assessment(s), and consideration of a limited number of treatment options. Patient presents with no comorbidities that affect occupational performance. Modification of tasks or assistance (eg, physical or verbal) with assessment(s) is not necessary to enable completion of evaluation component. Typically, 30 minutes are spent face-to-face with the patient and/or family.**

2.58 2.58 **FUD** XXX ★ (51) A 80

AMA: 2018,May,5; 2018,Feb,11; 2018,Jan,8; 2017,Jun,6; 2017,Feb,3; 2017,Jan,8

\# **97166** **Occupational therapy evaluation, moderate complexity, requiring these components: An occupational profile and medical and therapy history, which includes an expanded review of medical and/or therapy records and additional review of physical, cognitive, or psychosocial history related to current functional performance; An assessment(s) that identifies 3-5 performance deficits (ie, relating to physical, cognitive, or psychosocial skills) that result in activity limitations and/or participation restrictions; and Clinical decision making of moderate analytic complexity, which includes an analysis of the occupational profile, analysis of data from detailed assessment(s), and consideration of several treatment options. Patient may present with comorbidities that affect occupational performance. Minimal to moderate modification of tasks or assistance (eg, physical or verbal) with assessment(s) is necessary to enable patient to complete evaluation component. Typically, 45 minutes are spent face-to-face with the patient and/or family.**

2.58 2.58 **FUD** XXX ★ (51) A 80

AMA: 2018,May,5; 2018,Feb,11; 2018,Jan,8; 2017,Jun,6; 2017,Feb,3; 2017,Jan,8

97167 Occupational therapy evaluation, high complexity, requiring these components: An occupational profile and medical and therapy history, which includes review of medical and/or therapy records and extensive additional review of physical, cognitive, or psychosocial history related to current functional performance; An assessment(s) that identifies 5 or more performance deficits (ie, relating to physical, cognitive, or psychosocial skills) that result in activity limitations and/or participation restrictions; and Clinical decision making of high analytic complexity, which includes an analysis of the patient profile, analysis of data from comprehensive assessment(s), and consideration of multiple treatment options. Patient presents with comorbidities that affect occupational performance. Significant modification of tasks or assistance (eg, physical or verbal) with assessment(s) is necessary to enable patient to complete evaluation component. Typically, 60 minutes are spent face-to-face with the patient and/or family.

2.58 2.58 **FUD** XXX

AMA: 2018,May,5; 2018,Feb,11; 2018,Jan,8; 2017,Jun,6; 2017,Feb,3; 2017,Jan,8

97168 Re-evaluation of occupational therapy established plan of care, requiring these components: An assessment of changes in patient functional or medical status with revised plan of care; An update to the initial occupational profile to reflect changes in condition or environment that affect future interventions and/or goals; and A revised plan of care. A formal reevaluation is performed when there is a documented change in functional status or a significant change to the plan of care is required. Typically, 30 minutes are spent face-to-face with the patient and/or family.

1.77 1.77 **FUD** XXX

AMA: 2018,May,5; 2018,Feb,11; 2018,Jan,8; 2017,Jun,6; 2017,Feb,3; 2017,Jan,8

97169-97172 [97169, 97170, 97171, 97172] Assessment: Athletic Training

CMS: 100-02,15,220 Coverage of Outpatient Rehabilitation Therapy Services; 100-02,15,230 Practice of Physical Therapy, Occupational Therapy, and Speech-Language Pathology; 100-02,15,230.1 Practice of Physical Therapy

INCLUDES Care plan creation
Evaluation body systems as defined in 1997 E/M documentation guidelines:
- Cardiovascular system: Vital signs, edema extremities
- Integumentary system: Inspection for skin abnormalities
- Musculoskeletal system: Evaluation gait and station, motion range, muscle strength, height, and weight
- Neuromuscular evaluation: Balance, abnormal movements

97169 Athletic training evaluation, low complexity, requiring these components: A history and physical activity profile with no comorbidities that affect physical activity; An examination of affected body area and other symptomatic or related systems addressing 1-2 elements from any of the following: body structures, physical activity, and/or participation deficiencies; and Clinical decision making of low complexity using standardized patient assessment instrument and/or measurable assessment of functional outcome. Typically, 15 minutes are spent face-to-face with the patient and/or family.

0.00 0.00 **FUD** XXX

AMA: 2018,May,5; 2018,Feb,11; 2018,Jan,8; 2017,Jun,6; 2017,Jan,8

97170 Athletic training evaluation, moderate complexity, requiring these components: A medical history and physical activity profile with 1-2 comorbidities that affect physical activity; An examination of affected body area and other symptomatic or related systems addressing a total of 3 or more elements from any of the following: body structures, physical activity, and/or participation deficiencies; and Clinical decision making of moderate complexity using standardized patient assessment instrument and/or measurable assessment of functional outcome. Typically, 30 minutes are spent face-to-face with the patient and/or family.

0.00 0.00 **FUD** XXX

AMA: 2018,May,5; 2018,Feb,11; 2018,Jan,8; 2017,Jun,6; 2017,Jan,8

97171 Athletic training evaluation, high complexity, requiring these components: A medical history and physical activity profile, with 3 or more comorbidities that affect physical activity; A comprehensive examination of body systems using standardized tests and measures addressing a total of 4 or more elements from any of the following: body structures, physical activity, and/or participation deficiencies; Clinical presentation with unstable and unpredictable characteristics; and Clinical decision making of high complexity using standardized patient assessment instrument and/or measurable assessment of functional outcome. Typically, 45 minutes are spent face-to-face with the patient and/or family.

0.00 0.00 **FUD** XXX

AMA: 2018,May,5; 2018,Feb,11; 2018,Jan,8; 2017,Jun,6; 2017,Jan,8

97172 Re-evaluation of athletic training established plan of care requiring these components: An assessment of patient's current functional status when there is a documented change; and A revised plan of care using a standardized patient assessment instrument and/or measurable assessment of functional outcome with an update in management options, goals, and interventions. Typically, 20 minutes are spent face-to-face with the patient and/or family.

0.00 0.00 **FUD** XXX

AMA: 2018,May,5; 2018,Feb,11; 2018,Jan,8; 2017,Jun,6; 2017,Jan,8

97010-97028 Physical Therapy Treatment Modalities: Supervised

CMS: 100-02,15,220 Coverage of Outpatient Rehabilitation Therapy Services; 100-02,15,220.4 Functional Reporting; 100-02,15,230 Practice of Physical Therapy, Occupational Therapy, and Speech-Language Pathology; 100-02,15,230.1 Practice of Physical Therapy; 100-02,15,230.2 Practice of Occupational Therapy; 100-02,15,230.4 Services By a Physical/Occupational Therapist in Private Practice; 100-03,10.3 Inpatient Pain Rehabilitation Programs; 100-03,10.4 Outpatient Hospital Pain Rehabilitation Programs; 100-03,160.17 Payment for L-Dopa /Associated Inpatient Hospital Services; 100-04,5,10 Part B Outpatient Rehabilitation and Comprehensive Outpatient Rehabilitation Facility (CORF) Services - General; 100-04,5,10.3.2 Therapy Cap Exceptions; 100-04,5,10.3.3 Use of the KX Modifier; 100-04,5,20.2 Reporting Units of Service

INCLUDES Adding incremental treatment time intervals for same visit to calculate total service time

EXCLUDES *Direct patient contact by provider*
Electromyography (95860-95872 [95885, 95886, 95887])
EMG biofeedback training (90901)
Muscle and motion range tests ([97161, 97162, 97163, 97164, 97165, 97166, 97167, 97168, 97169, 97170, 97171, 97172])
Nerve conduction studies (95905-95913)

97010 Application of a modality to 1 or more areas; hot or cold packs

0.18 0.18 **FUD** XXX

AMA: 2018,May,5; 2018,Feb,11; 2018,Jan,8; 2017,Jan,8; 2016,Jun,8; 2016,Jan,13

97012 traction, mechanical

0.42 0.42 **FUD** XXX

AMA: 2020,Jul,13; 2018,May,5; 2018,Feb,11; 2018,Jan,8; 2017,Jan,8; 2016,Jun,8; 2016,Jan,13

97014 **electrical stimulation (unattended)**

EXCLUDES *Acupuncture with electrical stimulation (97813, 97814)*

0.42 0.42 FUD XXX

AMA: 2019,Jul,10; 2018,Oct,11; 2018,Oct,8; 2018,May,5; 2018,Feb,11; 2018,Jan,8; 2017,Jan,8; 2016,Jan,13

97016 **vasopneumatic devices**

0.36 0.36 FUD XXX

AMA: 2018,May,5; 2018,Feb,11; 2018,Jan,8; 2017,Jan,8; 2016,Jan,13

97018 **paraffin bath**

0.20 0.20 FUD XXX

AMA: 2018,May,5; 2018,Feb,11; 2018,Jan,8; 2017,Jan,8; 2016,Jan,13

97022 **whirlpool**

0.51 0.51 FUD XXX

AMA: 2018,May,5; 2018,Feb,11; 2018,Jan,8; 2017,Jan,8; 2016,Jan,13

97024 **diathermy (eg, microwave)**

0.20 0.20 FUD XXX

AMA: 2018,May,5; 2018,Feb,11; 2018,Jan,8; 2017,Jan,8; 2016,Jan,13

97026 **infrared**

0.18 0.18 FUD XXX

AMA: 2018,May,5; 2018,Feb,11; 2018,Jan,8; 2017,Jan,8; 2016,Jan,13

97028 **ultraviolet**

0.23 0.23 FUD XXX

AMA: 2018,May,5; 2018,Feb,11; 2018,Jan,8; 2017,Jan,8; 2016,Jan,13

97032-97039 Physical Therapy Treatment Modalities: Constant Attendance

CMS: 100-02,15,220 Coverage of Outpatient Rehabilitation Therapy Services; 100-02,15,220.4 Functional Reporting; 100-02,15,230 Practice of Physical Therapy, Occupational Therapy, and Speech-Language Pathology; 100-02,15,230.1 Practice of Physical Therapy; 100-02,15,230.2 Practice of Occupational Therapy; 100-02,15,230.4 Services By a Physical/Occupational Therapist in Private Practice; 100-03,10.3 Inpatient Pain Rehabilitation Programs; 100-03,10.4 Outpatient Hospital Pain Rehabilitation Programs; 100-03,160.17 Payment for L-Dopa /Associated Inpatient Hospital Services; 100-04,5,10 Part B Outpatient Rehabilitation and Comprehensive Outpatient Rehabilitation Facility (CORF) Services - General; 100-04,5,10.3.2 Therapy Cap Exceptions; 100-04,5,10.3.3 Use of the KX Modifier; 100-04,5,20.2 Reporting Units of Service

INCLUDES Adding incremental treatment time intervals for same visit to calculate total service time
Direct patient contact by provider

EXCLUDES *Electromyography (95860-95872 [95885, 95886, 95887])*
EMG biofeedback training (90901)
Muscle and motion range tests ([97161, 97162, 97163, 97164, 97165, 97166, 97167, 97168, 97169, 97170, 97171, 97172])
Nerve conduction studies (95905-95913)

97032 **Application of a modality to 1 or more areas; electrical stimulation (manual), each 15 minutes**

EXCLUDES *Transcutaneous electrical modulation pain reprocessing (TEMPR) (scrambler therapy) (0278T)*

0.42 0.42 FUD XXX

AMA: 2019,Jul,10; 2018,Oct,11; 2018,Oct,8; 2018,May,5; 2018,Feb,11; 2018,Jan,8; 2017,Jan,8; 2016,Jan,13

97033 **iontophoresis, each 15 minutes**

0.59 0.59 FUD XXX

AMA: 2018,May,5; 2018,Feb,11; 2018,Jan,8; 2017,Jan,8; 2016,Jan,13

97034 **contrast baths, each 15 minutes**

0.43 0.43 FUD XXX

AMA: 2018,May,5; 2018,Feb,11; 2018,Jan,8; 2017,Jan,8; 2016,Jan,13

97035 **ultrasound, each 15 minutes**

0.39 0.39 FUD XXX

AMA: 2018,May,5; 2018,Feb,11; 2018,Jan,8; 2017,Jan,8; 2016,Jan,13

97036 **Hubbard tank, each 15 minutes**

0.99 0.99 FUD XXX

AMA: 2018,May,5; 2018,Feb,11; 2018,Jan,8; 2017,Jan,8; 2016,Jan,13

97039 **Unlisted modality (specify type and time if constant attendance)**

0.00 0.00 FUD XXX

AMA: 2020,Jul,13; 2018,May,5; 2018,Feb,11; 2018,Jan,8; 2017,Jan,8; 2016,Nov,9; 2016,Jun,8; 2016,Jan,13

97110-97546 [97151, 97152, 97153, 97154, 97155, 97156, 97157, 97158, 97161, 97162, 97163, 97164, 97165, 97166, 97167, 97168, 97169, 97170, 97171, 97172] Other Therapeutic Techniques With Direct Patient Contact

CMS: 100-02,15,220 Coverage of Outpatient Rehabilitation Therapy Services; 100-02,15,230 Practice of Physical Therapy, Occupational Therapy, and Speech-Language Pathology; 100-02,15,230.1 Practice of Physical Therapy; 100-02,15,230.2 Practice of Occupational Therapy; 100-02,15,230.4 Services By a Physical/Occupational Therapist in Private Practice; 100-03,10.3 Inpatient Pain Rehabilitation Programs; 100-03,10.4 Outpatient Hospital Pain Rehabilitation Programs; 100-04,5,10 Part B Outpatient Rehabilitation and Comprehensive Outpatient Rehabilitation Facility (CORF) Services - General; 100-04,5,20.2 Reporting Units of Service

INCLUDES Application clinical skills/services to improve function
Direct patient contact by provider

EXCLUDES *Electromyography (95860-95872 [95885, 95886, 95887])*
EMG biofeedback training (90901)
Muscle and motion range tests ([97161, 97162, 97163, 97164, 97165, 97166, 97167, 97168, 97169, 97170, 97171, 97172])
Nerve conduction studies (95905-95913)

97110 **Therapeutic procedure, 1 or more areas, each 15 minutes; therapeutic exercises to develop strength and endurance, range of motion and flexibility**

0.87 0.87 FUD XXX ★

AMA: 2019,Jun,14; 2018,Dec,7; 2018,Dec,7; 2018,May,5; 2018,Feb,11; 2018,Jan,8; 2017,Dec,14; 2017,Jan,8; 2016,Jun,8; 2016,Jan,13

97112 **neuromuscular reeducation of movement, balance, coordination, kinesthetic sense, posture, and/or proprioception for sitting and/or standing activities**

0.99 0.99 FUD XXX ★

AMA: 2018,May,5; 2018,Feb,11; 2018,Jan,8; 2017,Jan,8; 2016,Jan,13

97113 **aquatic therapy with therapeutic exercises**

1.10 1.10 FUD XXX

AMA: 2018,May,5; 2018,Feb,11; 2018,Jan,8; 2017,Jan,8; 2016,Jan,13

97116 **gait training (includes stair climbing)**

EXCLUDES *Comprehensive gait/motion analysis (96000-96003)*

0.86 0.86 FUD XXX ★

AMA: 2018,May,5; 2018,Feb,11; 2018,Jan,8; 2017,Jan,8; 2016,Jan,13

97124 **massage, including effleurage, petrissage and/or tapotement (stroking, compression, percussion)**

EXCLUDES *Myofascial release (97140)*

0.81 0.81 FUD XXX

AMA: 2020,Jul,10; 2019,Jun,14; 2018,May,5; 2018,Feb,11; 2018,Jan,8; 2017,Jan,8; 2016,Jun,8; 2016,Jan,13

97129 **Therapeutic interventions that focus on cognitive function (eg, attention, memory, reasoning, executive function, problem solving, and/or pragmatic functioning) and compensatory strategies to manage the performance of an activity (eg, managing time or schedules, initiating, organizing, and sequencing tasks), direct (one-on-one) patient contact; initial 15 minutes**

EXCLUDES *Adaptive behavior treatment ([97153], [97155])*
Reporting code more than one time per day

0.67 0.68 FUD XXX

AMA: 2020,Jul,10

\+ **97130** **each additional 15 minutes (List separately in addition to code for primary procedure)**
EXCLUDES *Adaptive behavior treatment ([97153], [97155])*
Code first (97129)
0.65 0.65 FUD ZZZ
AMA: 2020,Jul,10

97139 **Unlisted therapeutic procedure (specify)**
0.00 0.00 FUD XXX
AMA: 2018,May,5; 2018,Feb,11; 2018,Jan,8; 2017,Jan,8; 2016,Jan,13

97140 **Manual therapy techniques (eg, mobilization/ manipulation, manual lymphatic drainage, manual traction), 1 or more regions, each 15 minutes**
EXCLUDES *Insertion needle without injection ([20560, 20561])*
0.79 0.79 FUD XXX
AMA: 2020,Jul,10; 2020,Feb,9; 2019,Jun,14; 2018,May,5; 2018,Feb,11; 2018,Jan,8; 2017,Jan,8; 2016,Nov,9; 2016,Sep,9; 2016,Aug,3; 2016,Jan,13

97150 **Therapeutic procedure(s), group (2 or more individuals)**
INCLUDES Constant attendance by physician/therapist
Reporting this procedure for each group member
EXCLUDES *Adaptive behavior services ([97154], [97158])*
Osteopathic manipulative treatment (98925-98929)
0.52 0.52 FUD XXX
AMA: 2020,Jul,7; 2018,Nov,3; 2018,May,5; 2018,Feb,11; 2018,Jan,8; 2017,Jan,8; 2016,Jan,13

97151 **Resequenced code. See code following 96040.**
97152 **Resequenced code. See code following 96040.**
97153 **Resequenced code. See code following 96040.**
97154 **Resequenced code. See code following 96040.**
97155 **Resequenced code. See code following 96040.**
97156 **Resequenced code. See code following 96040.**
97157 **Resequenced code. See code following 96040.**
97158 **Resequenced code. See code following 96040.**
97161 **Resequenced code. See code before 97010.**
97162 **Resequenced code. See code before 97010.**
97163 **Resequenced code. See code before 97010.**
97164 **Resequenced code. See code before 97010.**
97165 **Resequenced code. See code before 97010.**
97166 **Resequenced code. See code before 97010.**
97167 **Resequenced code. See code before 97010.**
97168 **Resequenced code. See code before 97010.**
97169 **Resequenced code. See code before 97010.**
97170 **Resequenced code. See code before 97010.**
97171 **Resequenced code. See code before 97010.**
97172 **Resequenced code. See code before 97010.**

97530 **Therapeutic activities, direct (one-on-one) patient contact (use of dynamic activities to improve functional performance), each 15 minutes**
1.13 1.13 FUD XXX ★
AMA: 2018,Dec,7; 2018,Dec,7; 2018,May,5; 2018,Feb,11; 2018,Jan,8; 2017,Jan,8; 2016,Jan,13

97533 **Sensory integrative techniques to enhance sensory processing and promote adaptive responses to environmental demands, direct (one-on-one) patient contact, each 15 minutes**
1.21 1.21 FUD XXX
AMA: 2018,May,5; 2018,Feb,11; 2018,Jan,8; 2017,Jan,8; 2016,Jan,13

97535 **Self-care/home management training (eg, activities of daily living (ADL) and compensatory training, meal preparation, safety procedures, and instructions in use of assistive technology devices/adaptive equipment) direct one-on-one contact, each 15 minutes**
0.97 0.97 FUD XXX ★
AMA: 2018,May,5; 2018,Feb,11; 2018,Jan,8; 2017,Jan,8; 2016,Aug,3; 2016,Jan,13

97537 **Community/work reintegration training (eg, shopping, transportation, money management, avocational activities and/or work environment/modification analysis, work task analysis, use of assistive technology device/adaptive equipment), direct one-on-one contact, each 15 minutes**
EXCLUDES *Wheelchair management/propulsion training (97542)*
0.93 0.93 FUD XXX
AMA: 2018,May,5; 2018,Feb,11; 2018,Jan,8; 2017,Jan,8; 2016,Jan,13

97542 **Wheelchair management (eg, assessment, fitting, training), each 15 minutes**
0.94 0.94 FUD XXX
AMA: 2018,May,5; 2018,Feb,11; 2018,Jan,8; 2017,Jan,8; 2016,Jan,13

97545 **Work hardening/conditioning; initial 2 hours**
0.00 0.00 FUD XXX
AMA: 2018,May,5; 2018,Feb,11; 2018,Jan,8; 2017,Jan,8; 2016,Jan,13

\+ **97546** **each additional hour (List separately in addition to code for primary procedure)**
Code first initial two hours (97545)
0.00 0.00 FUD ZZZ
AMA: 2018,May,5; 2018,Feb,11; 2018,Jan,8; 2017,Jan,8; 2016,Jan,13

97597-97610 Treatment of Wounds

CMS: 100-02,15,220.4 Functional Reporting; 100-02,15,230.4 Services By a Physical/Occupational Therapist in Private Practice; 100-03,270.3 Blood-derived Products for Chronic Nonhealing Wounds; 100-04,4,200.9 Billing for "Sometimes Therapy" Services that May be Paid as Non-Therapy Services; 100-04,5,10 Part B Outpatient Rehabilitation and Comprehensive Outpatient Rehabilitation Facility (CORF) Services - General; 100-04,5,10.3.2 Therapy Cap Exceptions; 100-04,5,10.3.3 Use of the KX Modifier

INCLUDES Direct patient contact
Removing devitalized/necrotic tissue and promoting healing

EXCLUDES *Burn wound debridement (16020-16030)*

97597 Debridement (eg, high pressure waterjet with/without suction, sharp selective debridement with scissors, scalpel and forceps), open wound, (eg, fibrin, devitalized epidermis and/or dermis, exudate, debris, biofilm), including topical application(s), wound assessment, use of a whirlpool, when performed and instruction(s) for ongoing care, per session, total wound(s) surface area; first 20 sq cm or less

INCLUDES Chemical cauterization (17250)

0.68 2.52 **FUD** 000 (51) T 80

AMA: 2018,May,5; 2018,Feb,11; 2018,Jan,8; 2017,Jan,8; 2016,Oct,3; 2016,Aug,9; 2016,Jan,13

Wound may be washed, addressed with scissors, and/or tweezers and scalpel

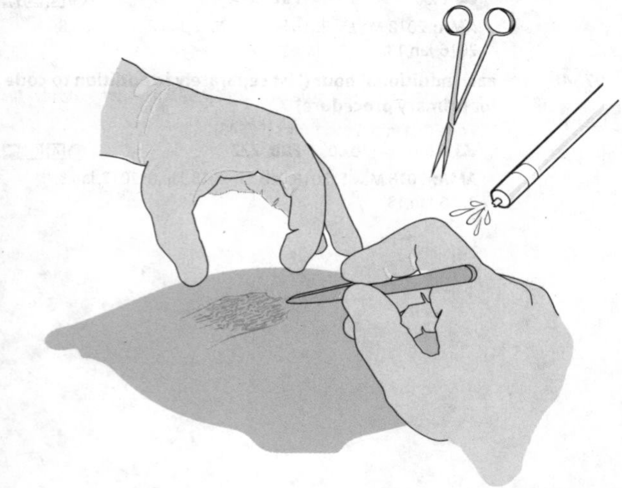

\+ **97598 each additional 20 sq cm, or part thereof (List separately in addition to code for primary procedure)**

INCLUDES Chemical cauterization (17250)

Code first (97597)

0.32 0.79 **FUD** ZZZ (51) N 80

AMA: 2018,May,5; 2018,Feb,11; 2018,Jan,8; 2017,Jan,8; 2016,Oct,3; 2016,Aug,9; 2016,Jan,13

97602 Removal of devitalized tissue from wound(s), non-selective debridement, without anesthesia (eg, wet-to-moist dressings, enzymatic, abrasion, larval therapy), including topical application(s), wound assessment, and instruction(s) for ongoing care, per session

INCLUDES Chemical cauterization (17250)

0.00 0.00 **FUD** XXX (51) Q1

AMA: 2018,May,5; 2018,Feb,11; 2018,Jan,8; 2017,Jan,8; 2016,Oct,3; 2016,Jan,13

97605 Negative pressure wound therapy (eg, vacuum assisted drainage collection), utilizing durable medical equipment (DME), including topical application(s), wound assessment, and instruction(s) for ongoing care, per session; total wound(s) surface area less than or equal to 50 square centimeters

EXCLUDES *Negative pressure wound therapy using disposable medical equipment (97607-97608)*

0.74 1.24 **FUD** XXX (51) Q1 80

AMA: 2018,May,5; 2018,Feb,11; 2018,Jan,8; 2017,Jan,8; 2016,Feb,13; 2016,Jan,13

97606 total wound(s) surface area greater than 50 square centimeters

EXCLUDES *Negative pressure wound therapy using disposable medical equipment (97607-97608)*

0.80 1.46 **FUD** XXX (51) Q1 80

AMA: 2018,May,5; 2018,Feb,11; 2018,Jan,8; 2017,Jan,8; 2016,Feb,13; 2016,Jan,13

97607 Negative pressure wound therapy, (eg, vacuum assisted drainage collection), utilizing disposable, non-durable medical equipment including provision of exudate management collection system, topical application(s), wound assessment, and instructions for ongoing care, per session; total wound(s) surface area less than or equal to 50 square centimeters

EXCLUDES *Negative pressure wound therapy using durable medical equipment (97605-97606)*

0.00 0.00 **FUD** XXX (51) T 80

AMA: 2018,May,5; 2018,Feb,11; 2018,Jan,8; 2017,Jan,8; 2016,Jan,13

97608 total wound(s) surface area greater than 50 square centimeters

EXCLUDES *Negative pressure wound therapy using durable medical equipment (97605-97606)*

0.00 0.00 **FUD** XXX (51) T 80

AMA: 2018,May,5; 2018,Feb,11; 2018,Jan,8; 2017,Jan,8; 2016,Jan,13

97610 Low frequency, non-contact, non-thermal ultrasound, including topical application(s), when performed, wound assessment, and instruction(s) for ongoing care, per day

0.48 6.39 **FUD** XXX (51) Q1 80

AMA: 2018,May,5; 2018,Feb,11; 2018,Jan,8; 2017,Jan,8; 2016,Jan,13

97750-97799 Assessments and Training

CMS: 100-02,15,220 Coverage of Outpatient Rehabilitation Therapy Services; 100-02,15,220.4 Functional Reporting; 100-02,15,230 Practice of Physical Therapy, Occupational Therapy, and Speech-Language Pathology; 100-02,15,230.1 Practice of Physical Therapy; 100-02,15,230.2 Practice of Occupational Therapy; 100-02,15,230.4 Services By a Physical/Occupational Therapist in Private Practice; 100-04,5,10 Part B Outpatient Rehabilitation and Comprehensive Outpatient Rehabilitation Facility (CORF) Services - General; 100-04,5,10.3.2 Exceptions Process; 100-04,5,10.3.3 Use of the KX Modifier

97750 Physical performance test or measurement (eg, musculoskeletal, functional capacity), with written report, each 15 minutes

INCLUDES Direct patient contact

EXCLUDES *Electromyography (95860-95872, [95885, 95886, 95887])*
Joint motion range (95851-95852)
Nerve velocity determination (95905, 95907-95913)

0.99 0.99 **FUD** XXX ★ (51) A 80

AMA: 2018,May,5; 2018,Feb,11; 2018,Jan,8; 2017,Jan,8; 2016,Jan,13

97755 **Assistive technology assessment (eg, to restore, augment or compensate for existing function, optimize functional tasks and/or maximize environmental accessibility), direct one-on-one contact, with written report, each 15 minutes**

INCLUDES Direct patient contact

EXCLUDES *Augmentative/alternative communication device (92605, 92607)*
Electromyography (95860-95872, [95885, 95886, 95887])
Joint motion range (95851-95852)
Nerve velocity determination (95905, 95907-95913)

1.08 1.08 FUD XXX ★ 51 A 80

AMA: 2018,May,5; 2018,Feb,11

97760 **Orthotic(s) management and training (including assessment and fitting when not otherwise reported), upper extremity(ies), lower extremity(ies) and/or trunk, initial orthotic(s) encounter, each 15 minutes**

EXCLUDES *Gait training, when performed on same extremity (97116)*

1.35 1.35 FUD XXX ★ 51 A 80

AMA: 2018,May,5; 2018,Feb,11; 2018,Jan,8; 2017,Jan,8; 2016,Jan,13

97761 **Prosthetic(s) training, upper and/or lower extremity(ies), initial prosthetic(s) encounter, each 15 minutes**

1.16 1.16 FUD XXX ★ 51 A 80

AMA: 2018,May,5; 2018,Feb,11; 2018,Jan,8; 2017,Jan,8; 2016,Jan,13

97763 **Orthotic(s)/prosthetic(s) management and/or training, upper extremity(ies), lower extremity(ies), and/or trunk, subsequent orthotic(s)/prosthetic(s) encounter, each 15 minutes**

EXCLUDES *Initial encounter for orthotics and prosthetics management and training (97760-97761)*

1.50 1.50 FUD XXX 51 A 80

AMA: 2018,May,5; 2018,Feb,11

97799 **Unlisted physical medicine/rehabilitation service or procedure**

0.00 0.00 FUD XXX A 80

AMA: 2018,May,5; 2018,Feb,11; 2018,Jan,8; 2017,Jan,8; 2016,Nov,9; 2016,Jan,13

97802-97804 Medical Nutrition Therapy Services

CMS: 100-02,13,220 Preventive Health Services; 100-03,180.1 Medical Nutrition Therapy; 100-04,12,190.3 List of Telehealth Services; 100-04,12,190.6 Payment Methodology for Physician/Practitioner at the Distant Site ; 100-04,12,190.6.1 Submission of Telehealth Claims for Distant Site Practitioners; 100-04,12,190.7 Contractor Editing of Telehealth Claims; 100-04,4,300 Medical Nutrition Therapy Services; 100-04,4,300.6 CWF Edits for MNT/DSMT

EXCLUDES *Medical nutrition therapy assessment/intervention provided by physician or other qualified health care provider; report appropriate E/M codes*

97802 **Medical nutrition therapy; initial assessment and intervention, individual, face-to-face with the patient, each 15 minutes**

0.96 1.05 FUD XXX ★ A 80

AMA: 2020,Jul,7; 2018,Feb,11; 2018,Jan,8; 2017,Jan,8; 2016,Jan,13

97803 **re-assessment and intervention, individual, face-to-face with the patient, each 15 minutes**

0.82 0.91 FUD XXX ★ A 80

AMA: 2020,Jul,7; 2018,Feb,11; 2018,Jan,8; 2017,Jan,8; 2016,Jan,13

97804 **group (2 or more individual(s)), each 30 minutes**

0.45 0.48 FUD XXX ★ A 80

AMA: 2020,Jul,7; 2018,Feb,11; 2018,Jan,8; 2017,Jan,8; 2016,Jan,13

97810-97814 Acupuncture

CMS: 100-03,10.3 Inpatient Pain Rehabilitation Programs; 100-03,10.4 Outpatient Hospital Pain Rehabilitation Programs; 100-03,30.3 Acupuncture; 100-03,30.3.1 Acupuncture for Fibromyalgia; 100-03,30.3.2 Acupuncture for Osteoarthritis; 100-04,32,410 Acupuncture for Chronic Low Back Pain (cLBP); 100-04,32,410.1 Coverage Requirements; 100-04,32,410.3 Institutional Claims Bill Type and Revenue Coding Information; 100-04,32,410.4 Messaging

INCLUDES 15 minute increments face-to-face contact with patient
Reporting only one code for each 15 minute increment

EXCLUDES *Insertion needle without injection ([20560, 20561])*

Code also significant separately identifiable E/M service with modifier 25, when performed

97810 **Acupuncture, 1 or more needles; without electrical stimulation, initial 15 minutes of personal one-on-one contact with the patient**

EXCLUDES *Treatment with electrical stimulation (97813-97814)*

0.87 1.03 FUD XXX E

AMA: 2020,Feb,9; 2018,Feb,11; 2018,Jan,8; 2017,Jan,8; 2016,Jan,13

+ **97811** **without electrical stimulation, each additional 15 minutes of personal one-on-one contact with the patient, with re-insertion of needle(s) (List separately in addition to code for primary procedure)**

EXCLUDES *Treatment with electrical stimulation (97813-97814)*

Code first initial 15 minutes (97810)

0.72 0.78 FUD ZZZ E

AMA: 2020,Feb,9; 2018,Feb,11; 2018,Jan,8; 2017,Jan,8; 2016,Jan,13

97813 **with electrical stimulation, initial 15 minutes of personal one-on-one contact with the patient**

EXCLUDES *Treatment without electrical stimulation (97813-97814)*

0.94 1.13 FUD XXX E

AMA: 2020,Feb,9; 2018,Feb,11; 2018,Jan,8; 2017,Jan,8; 2016,Jan,13

+ **97814** **with electrical stimulation, each additional 15 minutes of personal one-on-one contact with the patient, with re-insertion of needle(s) (List separately in addition to code for primary procedure)**

EXCLUDES *Treatment without electrical stimulation (97813-97814)*

Code first initial 15 minutes (97813)

0.79 0.91 FUD ZZZ E

AMA: 2020,Feb,9; 2018,Feb,11; 2018,Jan,8; 2017,Jan,8; 2016,Jan,13

98925-98929 Osteopathic Manipulation

CMS: 100-03,150.1 Manipulation

INCLUDES Body regions:
- Abdomen/visceral region
- Cervical region
- Head region
- Lower extremities
- Lumbar region
- Pelvic region
- Rib cage region
- Sacral region
- Thoracic region
- Upper extremities

Physician applied manual treatment done to eliminate/alleviate somatic dysfunction and related disorders with multiple techniques

Code also significant separately identifiable E/M service with modifier 25, when performed

98925 **Osteopathic manipulative treatment (OMT); 1-2 body regions involved**

0.68 0.89 FUD 000 Q1 80

AMA: 2018,Aug,9; 2018,Feb,11; 2018,Jan,8; 2017,Dec,14; 2017,Jan,8; 2016,Jan,13

98926 **3-4 body regions involved**

1.02 1.28 FUD 000 Q1 80

AMA: 2018,Aug,9; 2018,Feb,11; 2018,Jan,8; 2017,Jan,8; 2016,Jan,13

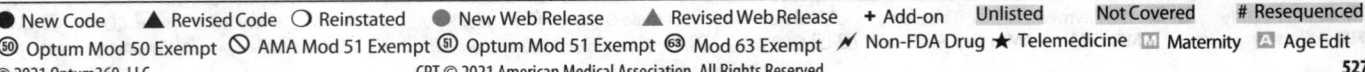

98927 **5-6 body regions involved**
Facility RVU 1.35 Non-Facility RVU 1.68 FUD 000
AMA: 2018,Aug,9; 2018,Feb,11; 2018,Jan,8; 2017,Jan,8; 2016,Jan,13

98928 **7-8 body regions involved**
Facility RVU 1.69 Non-Facility RVU 2.04 FUD 000
AMA: 2018,Aug,9; 2018,Feb,11; 2018,Jan,8; 2017,Jan,8; 2016,Jan,13

98929 **9-10 body regions involved**
Facility RVU 2.05 Non-Facility RVU 2.44 FUD 000
AMA: 2018,Aug,9; 2018,Feb,11; 2018,Jan,8; 2017,Jan,8; 2016,Jan,13

98940-98943 Chiropractic Manipulation

CMS: 100-01,5,70.6 Chiropractors; 100-02,15,240 Chiropractic Services - General; 100-02,15,240.1.3 Necessity for Treatment; 100-02,15,30.5 Chiropractor's Services; 100-03,150.1 Manipulation

INCLUDES Five extraspinal regions:
- Abdomen
- Head, including temporomandibular joint, excluding atlanto-occipital region
- Lower extremities
- Rib cage, not including costotransverse/costovertebral joints
- Upper extremities

Five spinal regions:
- Cervical region (atlanto-occipital joint)
- Lumbar region
- Pelvic region (sacro-iliac joint)
- Sacral region
- Thoracic region (costovertebral/costotransverse joints)

Manual treatment performed to influence joint/neurophysical function

Code also significant separately identifiable E/M service with modifier 25, when performed

98940 **Chiropractic manipulative treatment (CMT); spinal, 1-2 regions**
Facility RVU 0.64 Non-Facility RVU 0.80 FUD 000
AMA: 2018,Nov,11; 2018,Feb,11; 2018,Jan,8; 2017,Jan,8; 2016,Jan,13

98941 **spinal, 3-4 regions**
Facility RVU 0.98 Non-Facility RVU 1.16 FUD 000
AMA: 2018,Nov,11; 2018,Feb,11; 2018,Jan,8; 2017,Jan,8; 2016,Jan,13

98942 **spinal, 5 regions**
Facility RVU 1.33 Non-Facility RVU 1.50 FUD 000
AMA: 2018,Nov,11; 2018,Feb,11; 2018,Jan,8; 2017,Jan,8; 2016,Jan,13

98943 **extraspinal, 1 or more regions**
Facility RVU 0.67 Non-Facility RVU 0.77 FUD XXX
AMA: 2018,Nov,11; 2018,Feb,11; 2018,Jan,8; 2017,Jan,8; 2016,Jan,13

98960-98962 Self-Management Training

INCLUDES Education/training services:
- Prescribed by physician or other qualified health care professional
- Provided by qualified nonphysician health care provider

Standardized curriculum that may be modified as necessary for:
- Clinical needs
- Cultural norms
- Health literacy

Teaching patient how to manage illness/delay comorbidity(s)

EXCLUDES *Collection/interpretation physiologic data ([99091])*
Complex chronic care management (99487, 99489)
Counseling/education to group (99078)
Counseling/risk factor reduction without symptoms/established disease (99401-99412)
Genetic counseling education services (96040, 98961-98962)
Health and behavior assessment and intervention (96156, 96158-96159, [96164, 96165], [96167, 96168], [96170, 96171])
Medical nutrition therapy (97802-97804)
Physician supervision in home, domiciliary, or rest home (99339, 99340, 99374-99375, 99379-99380)
Services provided in which time would be reported with other services
Services provided with cumulative time of less than 5 minutes
Supervision hospice patient (99377-99378)
Transitional care management (99495, 99496)

98960 **Education and training for patient self-management by a qualified, nonphysician health care professional using a standardized curriculum, face-to-face with the patient (could include caregiver/family) each 30 minutes; individual patient**
Facility RVU 0.77 Non-Facility RVU 0.77 FUD XXX ★
AMA: 2020,Jul,7; 2018,Aug,6; 2018,Feb,11; 2018,Jan,8; 2017,Jan,8; 2016,Jan,13

98961 **2-4 patients**
INCLUDES Group education regarding genetic risks
Facility RVU 0.38 Non-Facility RVU 0.38 FUD XXX ★
AMA: 2020,Jul,7; 2018,Aug,6; 2018,Feb,11; 2018,Jan,8; 2017,Jan,8; 2016,Jan,13

98962 **5-8 patients**
INCLUDES Group education regarding genetic risks
Facility RVU 0.28 Non-Facility RVU 0.28 FUD XXX ★
AMA: 2020,Jul,7; 2018,Aug,6; 2018,Feb,11; 2018,Jan,8; 2017,Jan,8; 2016,Jan,13

98966-98968 Nonphysician Telephone Services

INCLUDES Assessment and management services provided by telephone by qualified health care professional
Care episodes initiated by established patient or his/her guardian

EXCLUDES *Call initiated by qualified health care professional*
Calls during postoperative period
Decision to see patient at next available urgent care appointment
Decision to see patient within 24 hours from patient call
Monitoring INR (93792-93793)
Patient management services during same time frame as ([99439, 99490, 99491], 99487-99489)
Principal care management services during same time frame as ([99426], [99427])
Reporting codes when same codes billed within past seven days
Telephone services considered previous or subsequent service component
Telephone services provided by physician (99441-99443)

98966 **Telephone assessment and management service provided by a qualified nonphysician health care professional to an established patient, parent, or guardian not originating from a related assessment and management service provided within the previous 7 days nor leading to an assessment and management service or procedure within the next 24 hours or soonest available appointment; 5-10 minutes of medical discussion**
Facility RVU 0.36 Non-Facility RVU 0.39 FUD XXX
AMA: 2018,Mar,7; 2018,Feb,11; 2018,Jan,8; 2017,Jan,8; 2016,Jan,13

98967 **11-20 minutes of medical discussion**
Facility RVU 0.72 Non-Facility RVU 0.76 FUD XXX
AMA: 2018,Mar,7; 2018,Feb,11; 2018,Jan,8; 2017,Jan,8; 2016,Jan,13

98968 **21-30 minutes of medical discussion**
1.08 1.12 FUD XXX
AMA: 2018,Mar,7; 2018,Feb,11; 2018,Jan,8; 2017,Jan,8; 2016,Jan,13

98970-98972 Nonphysician Online Service

INCLUDES Timely reply to patient as well as:
Ordering laboratory services
Permanent service record; either hard copy or electronic
Providing prescription
Related telephone calls

EXCLUDES *Monitoring INR (93792-93793)*
Online digital assessment and management service provided by qualified health care professional ([99421, 99422, 99423])
Online evaluation service:
Provided during postoperative period
Provided more than once in seven day period
Related to service provided in previous seven days
Provided with cumulative time less than 5 minutes
Where time would be reported as another service
Patient management services during same time frame as:
Chronic care management ([99437], [99439, 99490, 99491])
Collection/interpretation physiologic data ([99091])
Complex chronic care management (99487-99489)
Physician supervision in home, domiciliary, or rest home (99339-99340, 99374-99375, 99379-99380)
Principal care management services ([99426, 99427])
Supervision hospice patient (99377-99378)

98970 **Qualified nonphysician health care professional online digital assessment and management, for an established patient, for up to 7 days, cumulative time during the 7 days; 5-10 minutes**
0.00 0.00 FUD XXX
AMA: 2020,Jan,3

98971 **11-20 minutes**
0.00 0.00 FUD XXX
AMA: 2020,Jan,3

98972 **21 or more minutes**
0.00 0.00 FUD XXX
AMA: 2020,Jan,3

98975-98977 Remote Therapeutic Monitoring Services

INCLUDES Device:
Set-up and patient education
Supply

EXCLUDES *Physiological monitoring services ([99453], [99454])*
Pulse oximetry, noninvasive (94760)
Remote device interrogation (93296)
Remote physiologic monitoring treatment management services ([99457])
Reporting when monitoring less than 16 days
Self-measured blood pressure monitoring ([99473, 99474])
Therapeutic monitoring treatment management services (98980)

● 98975 **Remote therapeutic monitoring (eg, respiratory system status, musculoskeletal system status, therapy adherence, therapy response); initial set-up and patient education on use of equipment**
EXCLUDES *Reporting more than once per episode of care*

● 98976 **device(s) supply with scheduled (eg, daily) recording(s) and/or programmed alert(s) transmission to monitor respiratory system, each 30 days**

● 98977 **device(s) supply with scheduled (eg, daily) recording(s) and/or programmed alert(s) transmission to monitor musculoskeletal system, each 30 days**

98980-98981 Remote Therapeutic Monitoring Treatment Management Services

INCLUDES Patient management via remote therapeutic monitoring for specific treatment plan

EXCLUDES *Time counted during month of reporting for:*
E/M service(s) (99202-99205, 99211-99215, 99221-99223, 99231-99233, 99251-99255, 99324-99328, 99334-99337, 99341-99345, 99347-99350)
Other reported services

● 98980 **Remote therapeutic monitoring treatment management services, physician or other qualified health care professional time in a calendar month requiring at least one interactive communication with the patient or caregiver during the calendar month; first 20 minutes**
INCLUDES Reporting once each 30 days
EXCLUDES *Collection/interpretation physiologic data (99091)*
Remote monitoring wireless pulmonary artery sensor (93264)
Remote physiologic monitoring treatment management services (99457-99458)
Reporting services less than 20 minutes
Self-measured blood pressure monitoring ([99473, 99474])

● + 98981 **each additional 20 minutes (List separately in addition to code for primary procedure)**
EXCLUDES *Reporting services less than additional 20 minutes*
Code first (98980)
0.00 0.00 FUD 000

99000-99091 [99091] Supplemental Services and Supplies

INCLUDES Supplemental reporting for services adjunct to basic service provided

99000 **Handling and/or conveyance of specimen for transfer from the office to a laboratory**
0.00 0.00 FUD XXX
AMA: 2018,Dec,10; 2018,Dec,10; 2018,Feb,11; 2018,Jan,8; 2017,Jan,8; 2016,Jan,13

99001 **Handling and/or conveyance of specimen for transfer from the patient in other than an office to a laboratory (distance may be indicated)**
0.00 0.00 FUD XXX
AMA: 2018,Dec,10; 2018,Dec,10; 2018,Feb,11; 2018,Jan,8; 2017,Jan,8; 2016,Jan,13

99002 **Handling, conveyance, and/or any other service in connection with the implementation of an order involving devices (eg, designing, fitting, packaging, handling, delivery or mailing) when devices such as orthotics, protectives, prosthetics are fabricated by an outside laboratory or shop but which items have been designed, and are to be fitted and adjusted by the attending physician or other qualified health care professional**
EXCLUDES *Venous blood routine collection (36415)*
0.00 0.00 FUD XXX
AMA: 2018,Dec,10; 2018,Dec,10; 2018,Feb,11; 2018,Jan,8; 2017,Jan,8; 2016,Jan,13

99024 **Postoperative follow-up visit, normally included in the surgical package, to indicate that an evaluation and management service was performed during a postoperative period for a reason(s) related to the original procedure**
0.00 0.00 FUD XXX
AMA: 2018,Dec,10; 2018,Dec,10; 2018,Feb,11; 2018,Jan,8; 2017,Jul,9; 2017,Jan,3; 2017,Jan,8; 2016,Jan,13

99026 **Hospital mandated on call service; in-hospital, each hour**
EXCLUDES *Physician stand-by services with prolonged physician attendance (99360)*
Time spent providing procedures or services that may be separately reported
0.00 0.00 FUD XXX
AMA: 2018,Dec,10; 2018,Dec,10; 2018,Feb,11; 2018,Jan,8; 2017,Jan,8; 2016,Jan,13

99027 **out-of-hospital, each hour**

EXCLUDES *Physician stand-by services with prolonged physician attendance (99360)*

Time spent providing procedures or services that may be separately reported

0.00 0.00 FUD XXX E

AMA: 2018,Dec,10; 2018,Dec,10; 2018,Feb,11; 2018,Jan,8; 2017,Jan,8; 2016,Jan,13

99050 **Services provided in the office at times other than regularly scheduled office hours, or days when the office is normally closed (eg, holidays, Saturday or Sunday), in addition to basic service**

Code also more than one adjunct code per encounter when appropriate

Code first basic service provided

0.00 0.00 FUD XXX 51 B

AMA: 2018,Dec,10; 2018,Dec,10; 2018,Feb,11; 2018,Jan,8; 2017,Jan,8; 2016,Jan,13

99051 **Service(s) provided in the office during regularly scheduled evening, weekend, or holiday office hours, in addition to basic service**

Code also more than one adjunct code per encounter when appropriate

Code first basic service provided

0.00 0.00 FUD XXX 51 B

AMA: 2018,Dec,10; 2018,Dec,10; 2018,Feb,11; 2018,Jan,8; 2017,Jan,8; 2016,Jan,13

99053 **Service(s) provided between 10:00 PM and 8:00 AM at 24-hour facility, in addition to basic service**

Code also more than one adjunct code per encounter when appropriate

Code first basic service provided

0.00 0.00 FUD XXX 51 B

AMA: 2018,Dec,10; 2018,Dec,10; 2018,Feb,11; 2018,Jan,8; 2017,Jan,8; 2016,Jan,13

99056 **Service(s) typically provided in the office, provided out of the office at request of patient, in addition to basic service**

Code also more than one adjunct code per encounter when appropriate

Code first basic service provided

0.00 0.00 FUD XXX 51 B

AMA: 2018,Dec,10; 2018,Dec,10; 2018,Feb,11; 2018,Jan,8; 2017,Jan,8; 2016,Jan,13

99058 **Service(s) provided on an emergency basis in the office, which disrupts other scheduled office services, in addition to basic service**

Code also more than one adjunct code per encounter when appropriate

Code first basic service provided

0.00 0.00 FUD XXX 51 B

AMA: 2018,Dec,10; 2018,Dec,10; 2018,Feb,11; 2018,Jan,8; 2017,Jan,8; 2016,Jan,13

99060 **Service(s) provided on an emergency basis, out of the office, which disrupts other scheduled office services, in addition to basic service**

Code also more than one adjunct code per encounter when appropriate

Code first basic service provided

0.00 0.00 FUD XXX 51 B

AMA: 2018,Dec,10; 2018,Dec,10; 2018,Feb,11; 2018,Jan,8; 2017,Jan,8; 2016,Jan,13

99070 **Supplies and materials (except spectacles), provided by the physician or other qualified health care professional over and above those usually included with the office visit or other services rendered (list drugs, trays, supplies, or materials provided)**

EXCLUDES *Additional supplies, materials, and clinical staff time required for patient symptom review, personal protective equipment (PPE) use, and heightened cleaning processes due to respiratory-transmitted infectious disease during a declared public health emergency (PHE), as defined by law (99072)*

Spectacles supply

0.00 0.00 FUD XXX B

AMA: 2020,SepSE,1; 2020,SepSE,1; 2019,Apr,10; 2019,Feb,10; 2018,Dec,10; 2018,Dec,10; 2018,Jun,11; 2018,Mar,7; 2018,Jan,3; 2018,Jan,8; 2017,Sep,14; 2017,Jan,8; 2017,Jan,6; 2016,Jan,13

99071 **Educational supplies, such as books, tapes, and pamphlets, for the patient's education at cost to physician or other qualified health care professional**

0.00 0.00 FUD XXX B

AMA: 2018,Dec,10; 2018,Dec,10; 2018,Jan,8; 2017,Jan,8; 2016,Jan,13

● **99072** **Additional supplies, materials, and clinical staff time over and above those usually included in an office visit or other nonfacility service(s), when performed during a Public Health Emergency, as defined by law, due to respiratory-transmitted infectious disease**

INCLUDES Additional supplies, materials, and clinical staff time required for patient symptom review, personal protective equipment (PPE) use, and heightened cleaning processes due to respiratory-transmitted infectious disease during a declared public health emergency (PHE), as defined by law

EXCLUDES *Reporting more than one time per encounter, despite number services provided during encounter*

Supplies and materials provided, above those normally included in the encounter, unrelated to a declared PHE (99070)

AMA: 2020,SepSE,1

99075 **Medical testimony**

0.00 0.00 FUD XXX E

AMA: 2018,Dec,10; 2018,Dec,10; 2018,Jan,8; 2017,Jan,8; 2016,Jan,13

99078 **Physician or other qualified health care professional qualified by education, training, licensure/regulation (when applicable) educational services rendered to patients in a group setting (eg, prenatal, obesity, or diabetic instructions)**

0.00 0.00 FUD XXX N

AMA: 2018,Dec,10; 2018,Dec,10; 2018,Jan,8; 2017,Jan,8; 2016,Jan,13

99080 **Special reports such as insurance forms, more than the information conveyed in the usual medical communications or standard reporting form**

EXCLUDES *Completion workmen's compensation forms (99455-99456)*

0.00 0.00 FUD XXX B

AMA: 2018,Dec,10; 2018,Dec,10; 2018,Jan,8; 2017,Jan,8; 2016,Jan,13

99082 **Unusual travel (eg, transportation and escort of patient)**

0.00 0.00 FUD XXX B 80

AMA: 2018,Dec,10; 2018,Dec,10; 2018,Jan,8; 2017,Jan,8; 2016,Jan,13

99091 **Resequenced code. See code following resequenced code 99454.**

99100-99140 Modifying Factors for Anesthesia Services

CMS: 100-04,12,140.3 Payment for Qualified Nonphysician Anesthetists; 100-04,12,140.3.3 Billing Modifiers; 100-04,12,140.3.4 General Billing Instructions; 100-04,12,140.4.1 An Anesthesiologist and Qualified Nonphysician Anesthetist Work Together; 100-04,12,140.4.2 Anesthetist and Anesthesiologist in a Single Procedure; 100-04,12,140.4.4 Conversion Factors for Anesthesia Services; 100-04,4,250.3.2 Anesthesia in a Hospital Outpatient Setting

Code first primary anesthesia procedure

\+ **99100 Anesthesia for patient of extreme age, younger than 1 year and older than 70 (List separately in addition to code for primary anesthesia procedure)** A

EXCLUDES *Anesthesia services for infants one year old or less (00326, 00561, 00834, 00836)*

0.00 0.00 **FUD** ZZZ B

AMA: 2019,Oct,10; 2018,Jan,8; 2017,Dec,8; 2017,Jan,8; 2016,Jan,13

\+ **99116 Anesthesia complicated by utilization of total body hypothermia (List separately in addition to code for primary anesthesia procedure)**

EXCLUDES *Anesthesia for procedures on heart/pericardial sac/great vessels chest with pump oxygenator (00561)*

0.00 0.00 **FUD** ZZZ B

AMA: 2019,Oct,10; 2018,Jan,8; 2017,Dec,8; 2017,Jan,8; 2016,Jan,13

\+ **99135 Anesthesia complicated by utilization of controlled hypotension (List separately in addition to code for primary anesthesia procedure)**

EXCLUDES *Anesthesia for procedures on heart/pericardial sac/great vessels chest with pump oxygenator (00561)*

0.00 0.00 **FUD** ZZZ B

AMA: 2019,Oct,10; 2018,Jan,8; 2017,Dec,8; 2017,Jan,8; 2016,Jan,13

\+ **99140 Anesthesia complicated by emergency conditions (specify) (List separately in addition to code for primary anesthesia procedure)**

INCLUDES Conditions where treatment delay could be dangerous to life or health

0.00 0.00 **FUD** ZZZ B

AMA: 2019,Oct,10; 2018,Jan,8; 2017,Dec,8; 2017,Jan,8; 2016,Jan,13

99151-99157 Moderate Sedation Services

INCLUDES Intraservice work that begins with sedation administration and ends when procedure complete
Monitoring:
Patient response to drugs
Vital signs
Ordering and providing drug to patient (first and subsequent)
Pre- and postservice procedures

99151 Moderate sedation services provided by the same physician or other qualified health care professional performing the diagnostic or therapeutic service that the sedation supports, requiring the presence of an independent trained observer to assist in the monitoring of the patient's level of consciousness and physiological status; initial 15 minutes of intraservice time, patient younger than 5 years of age

INCLUDES First 15 minutes intraservice time for patients under age 5
Services provided to patients by same service provider for which moderate sedation necessary with monitoring by trained observer

0.72 2.12 **FUD** XXX ⊘ N

AMA: 2020,Nov,12; 2019,Feb,10; 2018,Jan,8; 2017,Sep,11; 2017,Jun,3; 2017,Jan,3

99152 initial 15 minutes of intraservice time, patient age 5 years or older

INCLUDES First 15 minutes intraservice time for patients age 5 and over
Services provided to patients by same service provider for which moderate sedation necessary with monitoring by trained observer

0.35 1.44 **FUD** XXX ⊘ N

AMA: 2020,Nov,12; 2019,May,10; 2019,Feb,10; 2018,Jan,8; 2017,Sep,11; 2017,Jun,3; 2017,Jan,3

\+ **99153 each additional 15 minutes intraservice time (List separately in addition to code for primary service)**

INCLUDES Services provided to patients by same service provider for which moderate sedation necessary with monitoring by trained observer (99155-99157)

EXCLUDES *Services provided to patients by physician/other qualified health care professional other than provider rendering service*

Code first (99151-99152)

0.30 0.30 **FUD** ZZZ N TC

AMA: 2020,Nov,12; 2019,May,10; 2019,Feb,10; 2018,Jan,8; 2017,Sep,11; 2017,Jun,3; 2017,Jan,3

99155 Moderate sedation services provided by a physician or other qualified health care professional other than the physician or other qualified health care professional performing the diagnostic or therapeutic service that the sedation supports; initial 15 minutes of intraservice time, patient younger than 5 years of age

INCLUDES First 15 minutes intraservice time for patients under age 5
Services provided to patients by physician/other qualified health care professional other than provider rendering service for which moderate sedation necessary

2.54 2.54 **FUD** XXX N

AMA: 2020,Nov,12; 2019,Feb,10; 2018,Jan,8; 2017,Sep,11; 2017,Jun,3; 2017,Jan,3

99156 initial 15 minutes of intraservice time, patient age 5 years or older

INCLUDES First 15 minutes intraservice time for patients age 5 and over
Services provided to patients by physician/other qualified health care professional other than provider rendering service for which moderate sedation necessary

2.24 2.24 **FUD** XXX N

AMA: 2020,Nov,12; 2019,Feb,10; 2018,Jan,8; 2017,Sep,11; 2017,Jun,3; 2017,Jan,3

\+ **99157 each additional 15 minutes intraservice time (List separately in addition to code for primary service)**

INCLUDES Each subsequent 15 minutes services
Services provided to patients by physician/other qualified health care professional other than provider rendering service for which moderate sedation necessary (99151-99152)

EXCLUDES *Services provided to patients by same service provider for which moderate sedation necessary with monitoring by trained observer (99151-99152)*

Code first (99155-99156)

1.82 1.82 **FUD** ZZZ N

AMA: 2020,Nov,12; 2019,Feb,10; 2018,Jan,8; 2017,Sep,11; 2017,Jun,3; 2017,Jan,3

99170 Specialized Examination of Child

EXCLUDES *Moderate sedation (99151-99157)*

99170 Anogenital examination, magnified, in childhood for suspected trauma, including image recording when performed A

2.47 4.48 **FUD** 000 T

AMA: 2018,Jan,8; 2017,Jan,8; 2016,Jan,13

99172-99173 Visual Acuity Screening Tests

INCLUDES Graduated visual acuity stimuli that allow quantitative determination/estimation visual acuity

EXCLUDES *General ophthalmological or E/M services*

99172 **Visual function screening, automated or semi-automated bilateral quantitative determination of visual acuity, ocular alignment, color vision by pseudoisochromatic plates, and field of vision (may include all or some screening of the determination[s] for contrast sensitivity, vision under glare)**

EXCLUDES *Screening for visual acuity, amblyogenic factors, retinal polarization scan (99173, 99174 [99177], 0469T)*

0.00 0.00 FUD XXX E

AMA: 2018,Jan,8; 2017,Jan,8; 2016,Jan,13

99173 **Screening test of visual acuity, quantitative, bilateral**

EXCLUDES *Screening for visual function, amblyogenic factors (99172, 99174, [99177])*

0.08 0.08 FUD XXX E

AMA: 2018,Jan,8; 2017,Jan,8; 2016,Jan,13

99174-99177 [99177] Screening For Amblyogenic Factors

EXCLUDES *General ophthalmological services (92002-92014)*
Screening for visual acuity (99172-99173, [99177])

99174 **Instrument-based ocular screening (eg, photoscreening, automated-refraction), bilateral; with remote analysis and report**

EXCLUDES *Ocular screening on-site analysis ([99177])*

0.16 0.16 FUD XXX E

AMA: 2018,Feb,3; 2018,Jan,8; 2017,Jan,8; 2016,Mar,10; 2016,Jan,13

99177 **with on-site analysis**

EXCLUDES *Remote ocular screening (99174)*
Retinal polarization scan (0469T)

0.13 0.13 FUD XXX E

AMA: 2018,Feb,3; 2018,Jan,8; 2017,Jan,8; 2016,Mar,10

99175-99177 [99177] Drug Administration to Induce Vomiting

EXCLUDES *Diagnostic gastric lavage (43754-43755)*
Diagnostic gastric intubation (43754-43755)

99175 **Ipecac or similar administration for individual emesis and continued observation until stomach adequately emptied of poison**

0.73 0.73 FUD XXX N 80

AMA: 1997,Nov,1

99177 **Resequenced code. See code following 99174.**

99183-99184 Hyperbaric Oxygen Therapy

CMS: 100-03,20.29 Hyperbaric Oxygen Therapy; 100-04,32,30.1 HBO Therapy for Lower Extremity Diabetic Wounds

EXCLUDES *E/M services, when performed*
Other procedures such as wound debridement, when performed

99183 **Physician or other qualified health care professional attendance and supervision of hyperbaric oxygen therapy, per session**

3.12 3.12 FUD XXX B 80 26

AMA: 2018,Jan,8; 2017,Jan,8; 2016,Jan,13

99184 **Initiation of selective head or total body hypothermia in the critically ill neonate, includes appropriate patient selection by review of clinical, imaging and laboratory data, confirmation of esophageal temperature probe location, evaluation of amplitude EEG, supervision of controlled hypothermia, and assessment of patient tolerance of cooling** A

EXCLUDES *Reporting code more than one time per hospitalization*

6.33 6.33 FUD XXX C 80

AMA: 2018,Jan,8; 2017,Jan,8; 2016,Jan,13

99188 Topical Fluoride Application

99188 **Application of topical fluoride varnish by a physician or other qualified health care professional**

0.29 0.35 FUD XXX E 80

99190-99192 Assemble and Manage Pump with Oxygenator/Heat Exchange

99190 **Assembly and operation of pump with oxygenator or heat exchanger (with or without ECG and/or pressure monitoring); each hour**

0.00 0.00 FUD XXX C

AMA: 1997,Nov,1

99191 **45 minutes**

0.00 0.00 FUD XXX C

AMA: 1997,Nov,1

99192 **30 minutes**

0.00 0.00 FUD XXX C

AMA: 1997,Nov,1

99195-99199 Therapeutic Phlebotomy and Unlisted Procedures

99195 **Phlebotomy, therapeutic (separate procedure)**

2.86 2.86 FUD XXX Q1 80

AMA: 2018,Jan,8; 2017,Jan,8; 2016,Jan,13

99199 **Unlisted special service, procedure or report**

0.00 0.00 FUD XXX B 80

AMA: 2018,Jan,8; 2017,Jan,8; 2016,Jan,13

99500-99602 Home Visit By Non-Physician Professionals

INCLUDES Services performed by non-physician providers
Services provided in patient's:
- Assisted living apartment
- Custodial care facility
- Group home
- Nontraditional private home
- Residence
- School

EXCLUDES *Home visits performed by physicians (99341-99350)*
Other services/procedures provided by physicians to patients at home

Code also:
Home visit E/M codes when health care provider authorized to report (99341-99350)
Significant separately identifiable E/M service, when performed

99500 **Home visit for prenatal monitoring and assessment to include fetal heart rate, non-stress test, uterine monitoring, and gestational diabetes monitoring** M ♀

0.00 0.00 FUD XXX E

AMA: 2018,Jan,8; 2017,Jan,8; 2016,Jan,13

99501 **Home visit for postnatal assessment and follow-up care** M ♀

0.00 0.00 FUD XXX E

AMA: 2018,Jan,8; 2017,Jan,8; 2016,Jan,13

99502 **Home visit for newborn care and assessment** A

0.00 0.00 FUD XXX E

AMA: 2018,Jan,8; 2017,Jan,8; 2016,Jan,13

99503 **Home visit for respiratory therapy care (eg, bronchodilator, oxygen therapy, respiratory assessment, apnea evaluation)**

0.00 0.00 FUD XXX E

AMA: 2018,Jan,8; 2017,Jan,8; 2016,Jan,13

99504 **Home visit for mechanical ventilation care**

0.00 0.00 FUD XXX E

AMA: 2018,Jan,8; 2017,Jan,8; 2016,Jan,13

99505 **Home visit for stoma care and maintenance including colostomy and cystostomy**

0.00 0.00 FUD XXX E

AMA: 2018,Jan,8; 2017,Jan,8; 2016,Jan,13

99506 **Home visit for intramuscular injections**

0.00 0.00 FUD XXX E

AMA: 2018,Jan,8; 2017,Jan,8; 2016,Jan,13

99507 Home visit for care and maintenance of catheter(s) (eg, urinary, drainage, and enteral)

0.00 0.00 FUD XXX E

AMA: 2018,Jan,8; 2017,Jan,8; 2016,Jan,13

99509 Home visit for assistance with activities of daily living and personal care

EXCLUDES *Medical nutrition therapy/assessment home services (97802-97804)*
Self-care/home management training (97535)
Speech therapy home services (92507-92508)

0.00 0.00 FUD XXX E

AMA: 2018,Jan,8; 2017,Jan,8; 2016,Jan,13

99510 Home visit for individual, family, or marriage counseling

0.00 0.00 FUD XXX E

AMA: 2018,Jan,8; 2017,Jan,8; 2016,Jan,13

99511 Home visit for fecal impaction management and enema administration

0.00 0.00 FUD XXX E

AMA: 2018,Jan,8; 2017,Jan,8; 2016,Jan,13

99512 Home visit for hemodialysis

EXCLUDES *Peritoneal dialysis home infusion (99601-99602)*

0.00 0.00 FUD XXX E

AMA: 2018,Jan,8; 2017,Jan,8; 2016,Jan,13

99600 Unlisted home visit service or procedure

0.00 0.00 FUD XXX E

AMA: 2018,Jan,8; 2017,Jan,8; 2016,Jan,13

99601 Home infusion/specialty drug administration, per visit (up to 2 hours);

0.00 0.00 FUD XXX E

AMA: 2005,Nov,1-9; 2003,Oct,7

+ **99602 each additional hour (List separately in addition to code for primary procedure)**

Code first (99601)

0.00 0.00 FUD XXX E

AMA: 2005,Nov,1-9; 2003,Oct,7

99605-96607 Medication Management By Pharmacist

INCLUDES Direct (face-to-face) assessment and intervention by pharmacist:
- Managing medication complications and/or interactions
- Maximizing patient's response to drug therapy

Documenting required elements:
- Advice given regarding improvement treatment compliance and outcomes
- Medication profile (prescription and nonprescription)
- Review applicable patient history

EXCLUDES *Routine tasks associated with dispensing and related activities (e.g., providing product information)*

99605 Medication therapy management service(s) provided by a pharmacist, individual, face-to-face with patient, with assessment and intervention if provided; initial 15 minutes, new patient

0.00 0.00 FUD XXX E

AMA: 2018,Apr,9; 2018,Jan,8; 2017,Jan,8; 2016,Jan,13

99606 initial 15 minutes, established patient

0.00 0.00 FUD XXX E

AMA: 2018,Apr,9; 2018,Jan,8; 2017,Jan,8; 2016,Jan,13

+ **99607 each additional 15 minutes (List separately in addition to code for primary service)**

Code first (99605, 99606)

0.00 0.00 FUD XXX E

AMA: 2018,Apr,9; 2018,Jan,8; 2017,Jan,8; 2016,Jan,13

Home visit for ... and/or maintenance of ... attention, drainage, and ...

Home visit for ... of newborn ...

Evaluation and Management Guidelines Common to All E/M Services

Information unique to this section is defined or identified below.

For additional information about evaluation and management services, see Appendix C: Evaluation and Management Extended Guidelines. This appendix includes comprehensive explanations and instructions for the correct selection of an E/M service code based on federal documentation standards.

Classification of Evaluation and Management (E/M) Services

The E/M section is divided into broad categories such as office visits, hospital visits, and consultations. Most of the categories are further divided into two or more subcategories of E/M services. For example, there are two subcategories of office visits (new patient and established patient) and there are two subcategories of hospital visits (initial and subsequent). The subcategories of E/M services are further classified into levels of E/M services that are identified by specific codes.

The basic format of the levels of E/M services is the same for most categories. First, a unique code number is listed. Second, the place and/or type of service is specified, eg, office consultation. Third, the content of the service is defined. Fourth, time is specified. (A detailed discussion of time is provided following the Decision Tree for New vs Established Patients.)

Definitions of Commonly Used Terms

Certain key words and phrases are used throughout the E/M section. The following definitions are intended to reduce the potential for differing interpretations and to increase the consistency of reporting by physicians and other qualified health care professionals. The definitions in the E/M section are provided solely for the basis of code selection.

Some definitions are common to all categories of services, and others are specific to one or more categories only.

New and Established Patient

Solely for the purposes of distinguishing between new and established patients, **professional services** are those face-to-face services rendered by physicians and other qualified health care professionals who may report E/M services with a specific CPT® code or codes. A new patient is one who has not received any professional services from the physician/qualified health care professional or another physician/qualified health care professional of the **exact** same specialty **and subspecialty** who belongs to the same group practice, within the past three years.

An established patient is one who has received professional services from the physician/qualified health care professional or another physician/qualified health care professional of the **exact** same specialty **and subspecialty** who belongs to the same group practice, within the past three years. See the decision tree on the following page.

When a physician/qualified health care professional is on call or covering for another physician/qualified health care professional, the patient's encounter is classified as it would have been by the physician/qualified health care professional who is not available. When advanced practice nurses and physician assistants are working with physicians, they are considered as working in the exact same specialty and exact same subspecialties as the physician.

No distinction is made between new and established patients in the emergency department. E/M services in the emergency department category may be reported for any new or established patient who presents for treatment in the emergency department.

The decision tree on the following page is provided to aid in determining whether to report the E/M service provided as a new or an established patient encounter.

Time

The inclusion of time in the definitions of levels of E/M services has been implicit in prior editions of the CPT codebook. The inclusion of time as an explicit factor beginning in CPT 1992 was done to assist in selecting the most appropriate level of E/M services. Beginning with CPT 2021, except for 99211, time alone may be used to select the appropriate code level for the office or other outpatient E/M services codes (99202, 99203, 99204, 99205, 99212, 99213, 99214, 99215). Different categories of services use time differently. It is important to review the instructions for each category.

Time is **not** a descriptive component for the emergency department levels of E/M services because emergency department services are typically provided on a variable intensity basis, often involving multiple encounters with several patients over an extended period of time. Therefore, it is often difficult to provide accurate estimates of the time spent face-to-face with the patient.

Time may be used to select a code level in office or other outpatient services whether or not counseling and/or coordination of care dominates the service. Time may only be used for selecting the level of the ***other*** E/M services when counseling and/or coordination of care dominates the service.

When time is used for reporting E/M services codes, the time defined in the service descriptors is used for selecting the appropriate level of services. The E/M services for which these guidelines apply require a face-to-face encounter with the physician or other qualified health care professional. For office or other outpatient services, if the physician's or other qualified health care professional's time is spent in the supervision of clinical staff who perform the face-to-face services of the encounter, use 99211.

A shared or split visit is defined as a visit in which a physician and other qualified health care professional(s) jointly provide the face-to-face and non-face-to-face work related to the visit. When time is being used to select the appropriate level of services for which time-based reporting of shared or split visits is allowed, the time personally spent by the physician and other qualified health care professional(s) assessing and managing the patient on the date of the encounter is summed to define total time. Only distinct time should be summed for shared or split visits (ie, when two or more individuals jointly meet with or discuss the patient, only the time of one individual should be counted).

When prolonged time occurs, the appropriate prolonged services code may be reported. The appropriate time should be documented in the medical record when it is used as the basis for code selection.

Face-to-face time (outpatient consultations [99241, 99242, 99243, 99244, 99245], domiciliary, rest home, or custodial services [99324, 99325, 99326, 99327, 99328, 99334, 99335, 99336, 99337], home services [99341, 99342, 99343, 99344, 99345, 99347, 99348, 99349, 99350], cognitive assessment and care plan services [99483]): For coding purposes, face-to-face time for these services is defined as only that time spent face-to-face with the patient and/or family. This includes the time spent performing such tasks as obtaining a history, examination, and counseling the patient.

Unit/floor time (hospital observation services [99218, 99219, 99220, 99224, 99225, 99226, 99234, 99235, 99236], hospital inpatient services [99221, 99222, 99223, 99231, 99232, 99233], inpatient consultations [99251, 99252, 99253, 99254, 99255], nursing facility services [99304, 99305, 99306, 99307, 99308, 99309, 99310, 99315, 99316, 99318]): For coding purposes, time for these services is defined as unit/floor time, which includes the time present on the patient's hospital unit and at the bedside rendering services for that patient. This includes the time to establish and/or review the patient's chart, examine the patient, write notes, and communicate with other professionals and the patient's family.

Total time on the date of the encounter (office or other outpatient services [99202, 99203, 99204, 99205, 99212, 99213, 99214, 99215]): For coding purposes, time for these services is the total time on the date of the encounter. It includes both the face-to-face and non-face-to-face time personally spent by the physician and/or other qualified health care professional(s) on the day of the encounter (includes time in activities that require the physician or other qualified health care professional and does not include time in activities normally performed by clinical staff).

Physician/other qualified health care professional time includes the following activities, when performed:

- Preparing to see the patient (eg, review of tests)
- Obtaining and/or reviewing separately obtained history
- Performing a medically appropriate examination and/or evaluation
- Counseling and educating the patient/family/caregiver
- Ordering medications, tests, or procedures
- Referring and communicating with other health care professionals (when not separately reported)
- Documenting clinical information in the electronic or other health record
- Independently interpreting results (not separately reported) and communicating results to the patient/family/caregiver
- Care coordination (not separately reported)

Do not count time spent on the following:

- The performance of other services that are reported separately
- Travel
- Teaching that is general and not limited to discussion that is required for the management of a specific patient

Concurrent Care and Transfer of Care

Concurrent care is the provision of similar services (eg, hospital visits) to the same patient by more than one physician or other qualified health care professional on the same day. When concurrent care is provided, no special reporting is required. Transfer of care is the process whereby a physician or other qualified health care professional who is managing some or all of a patient's problems relinquishes this responsibility to another physician or other qualified health care professional who explicitly agrees to accept this responsibility and who, from the initial encounter, is not providing consultative services. The physician or other qualified health care professional transferring care is then no longer providing care for these problems though he or she may continue providing care for other conditions when appropriate. Consultation codes should not be reported by the physician or other qualified health care professional who has agreed to accept transfer of care before an initial evaluation, but they are appropriate to report if the decision to accept transfer of care cannot be made until after the initial consultation evaluation, regardless of site of service.

Decision Tree for New vs Established Patients

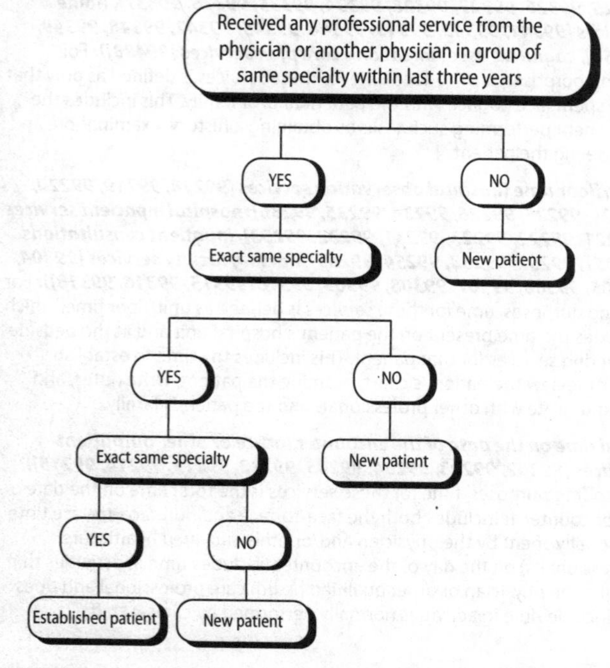

Counseling

Counseling is a discussion with a patient and/or family concerning one or more of the following areas:

- Diagnostic results, impressions, and/or recommended diagnostic studies
- Prognosis
- Risks and benefits of management (treatment) options
- Instructions for management (treatment) and/or follow-up
- Importance of compliance with chosen management (treatment) options
- Risk factor reduction
- Patient and family education
  (For psychotherapy, see 90832–90834, 90836–90840)

Services Reported Separately

Any specifically identifiable procedure or service (ie, identified with a specific CPT code) performed on the date of E/M services may be reported separately.

The ordering and actual performance and/or interpretation of diagnostic tests/studies during a patient encounter are not included in determining the levels of E/M services when the professional interpretation of those tests/studies is reported separately by the physician or other qualified health care professional reporting the E/M service. Tests that do not require separate interpretation (eg, tests that are results only) and are analyzed as part of MDM do not count as an independent interpretation, but may be counted as ordered or reviewed for selecting an MDM level. Physician performance of diagnostic tests/studies for which specific CPT codes are available may be reported separately, in addition to the appropriate E/M code. The physician's interpretation of the results of diagnostic tests/studies (ie, professional component) with preparation of a separation distinctly identifiable signed written report may also be reported separately, using the appropriate CPT code and, if required, with modifier 26 appended. If a test/study is independently interpreted in order to manage the patient as part of the E/M service, but is not separately reported, it is part of MDM.

The physician or other qualified health care professional may need to indicate that on the day a procedure or service identified by a CPT code was performed, the patient's condition required a significant separately identifiable E/M service. The E/M service may be caused or prompted by the symptoms or condition for which the procedure and/or service was provided. This circumstance may be reported by adding modifier 25 to the appropriate level of E/M service. As such, different diagnoses are not required for reporting of the procedure and the E/M services on the same date.

Levels of E/M Services

Within each category or subcategory of E/M service, there are three to five levels of E/M services available for reporting purposes. Levels of E/M services are **not** interchangeable among the different categories or subcategories of service. For example, the first level of E/M services in the subcategory of office visit, new patient, does not have the same definition as the first level of E/M services in the subcategory of office visit, established patient. Each level of E/M services may be used by all physicians or other qualified health care professionals.

The levels of E/M services include examinations, evaluations, treatments, conferences with or concerning patients, preventive pediatric and adult health supervision, and similar medical services, such as the determination of the need and/or location for appropriate care. Medical screening includes the history, examination, and medical decision-making required to determine the need and/or location for appropriate care and treatment of the patient (eg, office and other outpatient setting, emergency department, nursing facility). The levels of E/M services encompass the wide variations in skill, effort, time, responsibility, and medical knowledge required for the prevention or diagnosis and treatment of illness or injury and the promotion of optimal health. Each level of E/M services may be used by all physicians or other qualified health care professionals.

The descriptors for the levels of E/M services recognize seven components, six of which are used in defining the levels of E/M services. These components are:

- History
- Examination
- Medical decision making
- Counseling
- Coordination of care
- Nature of presenting problem
- Time

The first three of these components (history, examination, and medical decision making) are considered the **key** components in selecting a level of E/M services. (See "Determine the Extent of History Obtained.")

The next three components (counseling, coordination of care, and the nature of the presenting problem) are considered **contributory** factors in the majority of encounters. Although the first two of these contributory factors are important E/M services, it is not required that these services be provided at every patient encounter.

Coordination of care with other physicians, other qualified health care professionals, or agencies without a patient encounter on that day is reported using the case management codes.

The final component, time, is discussed in detail before the Decision Tree for New vs Established Patients.

Chief Complaint

A chief complaint is a concise statement describing the symptom, problem, condition, diagnosis, or other factor that is the reason for the encounter, usually stated in the patient's words.

History of Present Illness

A chronological description of the development of the patient's present illness from the first sign and/or symptom to the present. This includes a description of location, quality, severity, timing, context, modifying factors, and associated signs and symptoms significantly related to the presenting problem.

Nature of Presenting Problem

A presenting problem is a disease, condition, illness, injury, symptom, sign, finding, complaint, or other reason for encounter, with or without a diagnosis being established at the time of the encounter. The E/M codes recognize five types of presenting problems that are defined as follows:

Minimal: A problem that may not require the presence of the physician or other qualified health care professional, but service is provided under the physician's or other qualified health care professional's supervision.

Self-limited or minor: A problem that runs a definite and prescribed course, is transient in nature, and is not likely to permanently alter health status.

Low severity: A problem where the risk of morbidity without treatment is low; there is little to no risk of mortality without treatment; full recovery without functional impairment is expected.

Moderate severity: A problem where the risk of morbidity without treatment is moderate; there is moderate risk of mortality without treatment; uncertain prognosis OR increased probability of prolonged functional impairment.

High severity: A problem where the risk of morbidity without treatment is high to extreme; there is a moderate to high risk of mortality without treatment OR high probability of severe, prolonged functional impairment.

Past History

A review of the patient's past experiences with illnesses, injuries, and treatments that includes significant information about:

- Prior major illnesses and injuries
- Prior operations
- Prior hospitalizations
- Current medications
- Allergies (eg, drug, food)
- Age appropriate immunization status
- Age appropriate feeding/dietary status

Family History

A review of medical events in the patient's family that includes significant information about:

- The health status of cause of death of parents, siblings, and children
- Specific diseases related to problems identified in the Chief Complaint or History of the Present Illness, and/or System Review
- Diseases of family members that may be hereditary or place the patient at risk

Social History

An age appropriate review of past and current activities that includes significant information about:

- Marital status and/or living arrangements
- Current employment
- Occupational history
- Military history
- Use of drugs, alcohol, and tobacco
- Level of education
- Sexual history
- Other relevant social factors

System Review (Review of Systems)

An inventory of body systems obtained through a series of questions seeking to identify signs and/or symptoms that the patient may be experiencing or has experienced. For the purposes of the CPT codebook the following elements of a system review have been identified:

- Constitutional symptoms (fever, weight loss, etc)
- Eyes
- Ears, nose, mouth, throat
- Cardiovascular
- Respiratory
- Gastrointestinal
- Genitourinary
- Musculoskeletal
- Integumentary (skin and/or breast)
- Neurological
- Psychiatric
- Endocrine
- Hematologic/lymphatic
- Allergic/immunologic

The review of systems helps define the problem, clarify the differential diagnosis, identify needed testing, or serves as baseline data on other systems that might be affected by any possible management options.

Instructions for Selecting a Level of E/M Service

Review the Reporting Instructions for the Selected Category or Subcategory

Most of the categories and many of the subcategories of service have special guidelines or instructions unique to that category or subcategory. Where these are indicated, eg, "Inpatient Hospital Care," special instructions will be presented preceding the levels of E/M services.

Review the Level of E/M Service Descriptors and Examples in the Selected Category or Subcategory

The descriptors for the levels of E/M services recognize seven components, six of which are used in defining the levels of E/M services. These components are:

- History
- Examination
- Medical decision making
- Counseling
- Coordination of care
- Nature of presenting problem
- Time

The first three of these components (ie, history, examination, and medical decision making) should be considered the **key** components in selecting the level of E/M services. An exception to this rule is in the case of visits that consist predominantly of counseling or coordination of care.

The nature of the presenting problem and time are provided in some levels to assist the physician in determining the appropriate level of E/M service.

Determine the Extent of History Obtained

The extent of the history is dependent upon clinical judgment and on the nature of the presenting problem(s). The levels of E/M services recognize four types of history that are defined as follows:

Problem focused: Chief complaint; brief history of present illness or problem.

Expanded problem focused: Chief complaint; brief history of present illness; problem pertinent system review.

Detailed: Chief complaint; extended history of present illness; problem pertinent system review extended to include a review of a limited number of additional systems; pertinent past, family, and/or social history directly related to the patient's problems.

Comprehensive: Chief complaint; extended history of present illness; review of systems that is directly related to the problem(s) identified in the history of the present illness plus a review of all additional body systems; **complete** past, family, and social history.

The comprehensive history obtained as part of the preventive medicine E/M service is not problem-oriented and does not involve a chief complaint or present illness. It does, however, include a comprehensive system review and comprehensive or interval past, family, and social history as well as a comprehensive assessment/history of pertinent risk factors.

Determine the Extent of Examination Performed

The extent of the examination performed is dependent on clinical judgment and on the nature of the presenting problem(s). The levels of E/M services recognize four types of examination that are defined as follows:

Problem focused: A limited examination of the affected body area or organ system.

Expanded problem focused: A limited examination of the affected body area or organ system and other symptomatic or related organ system(s).

Detailed: An extended examination of the affected body area(s) and other symptomatic or related organ system(s).

Comprehensive: A general multisystem examination or a complete examination of a single organ system. **Note:** The comprehensive examination performed as part of the preventive medicine E/M service is multisystem, but its extent is based on age and risk factors identified.

For the purposes of these CPT definitions, the following body areas are recognized:

- Head, including the face
- Neck
- Chest, including breasts and axilla
- Abdomen
- Genitalia, groin, buttocks
- Back
- Each extremity

For the purposes of these CPT definitions, the following organ systems are recognized:

- Eyes
- Ears, nose, mouth, and throat
- Cardiovascular
- Respiratory
- Gastrointestinal
- Genitourinary
- Musculoskeletal
- Skin
- Neurologic
- Psychiatric
- Hematologic/lymphatic/immunologic

Determine the Complexity of Medical Decision Making

Medical decision making refers to the complexity of establishing a diagnosis and/or selecting a management option as measured by:

- The number of possible diagnoses and/or the number of management options that must be considered
- The amount and/or complexity of medical records, diagnostic tests, and/or other information that must be obtained, reviewed, and analyzed
- The risk of significant complications, morbidity, and/or mortality, as well as comorbidities associated with the patient's presenting problem(s), the diagnostic procedure(s), and/or the possible management options

Four types of medical decision making are recognized: straightforward, low complexity, moderate complexity, and high complexity. To qualify for a given type of decision making, two of the three elements in Table 1 must be met or exceeded.

Comorbidities and underlying diseases, in and of themselves, are not considered in selecting a level of E/M services unless their presence significantly increases the complexity of the medical decision making.

Select the Appropriate Level of E/M Services Based on the Following

For the following categories/subcategories, **all of the key components**, ie, history, examination, and medical decision making, must meet or exceed the stated requirements to qualify for a particular level of E/M service: initial observation care; initial hospital care; observation or inpatient hospital care (including admission and discharge services); office or other outpatient consultations; inpatient consultations; emergency department services; initial nursing facility care; other nursing facility services; domiciliary care, new patient; and home services, new patient.

For the following categories/subcategories, **two of the three key components** (ie, history, examination, and medical decision making) must meet or exceed the stated requirements to qualify for a particular level of E/M services: subsequent observation care; subsequent hospital care; subsequent nursing facility care; domiciliary care, established patient; and home services, established patient.

When counseling and/or coordination of care dominates (more than 50 percent) the encounter with the patient and/or family (face-to-face time in the office or other outpatient setting or floor/unit time in the hospital or nursing facility), then **time** shall be considered the key or controlling factor to qualify for a particular level of E/M services. This includes time spent with parties who have assumed responsibility for the care of the patient or decision making whether or not they are family members (eg, foster parents, person acting in loco parentis, legal guardian). The extent of counseling and/or coordination of care must be documented in the medical record.

CONSULTATION CODES AND MEDICARE REIMBURSEMENT

The Centers for Medicare and Medicaid Services (CMS) no longer provides benefits for CPT consultation codes. CMS has, however, redistributed the value of the consultation codes across the other E/M codes for services which are covered by Medicare. CMS has retained codes 99241 - 99251 in the Medicare Physician Fee Schedule for those private payers that use this data for reimbursement. Note that private payers may choose to follow CMS or CPT guidelines, and the use of consultation codes should be verified with individual payers.

Table 1

Complexity of Medical Decision Making

Number of Diagnoses or Management Options	*Amount and/or Complexity of Data to Be Reviewed*	*Risk of Complications and/or Morbidity or Mortality*	*Type of Decision Making*
minimal	minimal or none	minimal	**straightforward**
limited	limited	low	**low complexity**
multiple	moderate	moderate	**moderate complexity**
extensive	extensive	high	**high complexity**

Guidelines for Office or Other Outpatient E/M Services

History and/or Examination

Office or other outpatient services include a medically appropriate history and/or physical examination, when performed. The nature and extent of the history and/or physical examination are determined by the treating physician or other qualified health care professional reporting the service. The care team may collect information and the patient or caregiver may supply information directly (eg, by electronic health record [EHR] portal or questionnaire) that is reviewed by the reporting physician or other qualified health care professional. The extent of history and physical examination is not an element in selection of the level of office or other outpatient code.

Number and Complexity of Problems Addressed at the Encounter

One element used in selecting the level of office or other outpatient services is the number and complexity of the problems that are addressed at an encounter. Multiple new or established conditions may be addressed at the same time and may affect MDM. Symptoms may cluster around a specific diagnosis and each symptom is not necessarily a unique condition. Comorbidities/underlying diseases, in and of themselves, are not considered in selecting a level of E/M services **unless** they are addressed, and their presence increases the amount and/or complexity of data to be reviewed and analyzed or the risk of complications and/or morbidity or mortality of patient management. The final diagnosis for a condition does not, in and of itself, determine the complexity or risk, as extensive evaluation may be required to reach the conclusion that the signs or symptoms do not represent a highly morbid condition. Therefore, presenting symptoms that are likely to represent a highly morbid condition may "drive" MDM even when the ultimate diagnosis is not highly morbid. The evaluation and/or treatment should be consistent with the likely nature of the condition. Multiple problems of a lower severity may, in the aggregate, create higher risk due to interaction. The term "risk" as used in these definitions relates to risk from the condition. While condition risk and management risk may often correlate, the risk from the condition is distinct from the risk of the management.

Definitions for the elements of MDM (see Table 2, Levels of Medical Decision Making) for other office or other outpatient services are:

Problem: A problem is a disease, condition, illness, injury, symptom, sign, finding, complaint, or other matter addressed at the encounter, with or without a diagnosis being established at the time of the encounter.

Problem addressed: A problem is addressed or managed when it is evaluated or treated at the encounter by the physician or other qualified health care professional reporting the service. This includes consideration of further testing or treatment that may not be elected by virtue of risk/benefit analysis or patient/parent/guardian/surrogate choice. Notation in the patient's medical record that another professional is managing the problem without additional assessment or care coordination documented does not qualify as being addressed or managed by the physician or other qualified health care professional reporting the service. Referral without evaluation (by history, examination, or diagnostic study[ies]) or consideration of treatment does not qualify as being addressed or managed by the physician or other qualified health care professional reporting the service.

Minimal problem: A problem that may not require the presence of the physician or other qualified health care professional, but the service is provided under the physician's or other qualified health care professional's supervision (see 99211).

Self-limited or minor problem: A problem that runs a definite and prescribed course, is transient in nature, and is not likely to permanently alter health status.

Stable, chronic illness: A problem with an expected duration of at least one year or until the death of the patient. For the purpose of defining chronicity, conditions are treated as chronic whether or not stage or severity changes (eg, uncontrolled diabetes and controlled diabetes are a single chronic condition). "Stable" for the purposes of categorizing MDM is defined by the specific treatment goals for an individual patient. A patient who is not at his or her treatment goal is not stable, even if the condition has not changed and there is no short\term threat to life or function. For example, in a patient with persistently poorly controlled blood pressure for whom better control is a goal is not stable, even if the pressures are not changing and the patient is asymptomatic, the risk of morbidity **without** treatment is significant. Examples may include well-controlled hypertension, non-insulin dependent diabetes, cataract, or benign prostatic hyperplasia.

Acute, uncomplicated illness or injury: A recent or new short-term problem with low risk of morbidity for which treatment is considered. There is little to no risk of mortality with treatment, and full recovery without functional impairment is expected. A problem that is normally self-limited or minor but is not resolving consistent with a definite and prescribed course is an acute, uncomplicated illness. Examples may include cystitis, allergic rhinitis, or a simple sprain.

Chronic illness with exacerbation, progression, or side effects of treatment: A chronic illness that is acutely worsening, poorly controlled, or progressing with an intent to control progression and requiring additional supportive care or requiring attention to treatment for side effects but that does not require consideration of hospital level of care.

Undiagnosed new problem with uncertain prognosis: A problem in the differential diagnosis that represents a condition likely to result in a high risk of morbidity without treatment. An example may be a lump in the breast.

Acute illness with systemic symptoms: An illness that causes systemic symptoms and has a high risk of morbidity without treatment. For systemic general symptoms, such as fever, body aches, or fatigue in a minor illness that may be treated to alleviate symptoms, shorten the course of illness, or to prevent complications, see the definitions for **self-limited or minor problem** or **acute, uncomplicated illness or injury**. Systemic symptoms may not be general but may be single system. Examples may include pyelonephritis, pneumonitis, or colitis.

Acute, complicated injury: An injury which requires treatment that includes evaluation of body systems that are not directly part of the injured organ, the injury is extensive, or the treatment options are multiple and/or associated with risk of morbidity. An example may be a head injury with brief loss of consciousness.

Chronic illness with severe exacerbation, progression, or side effects of treatment: The severe exacerbation or progression of a chronic illness or severe side effects of treatment that have significant risk of morbidity and may require hospital level of care.

Acute or chronic illness or injury that poses a threat to life or bodily function: An acute illness with systemic symptoms, an acute complicated injury, or a chronic illness or injury with exacerbation and/or progression or side effects of treatment, that poses a threat to life or bodily function in the near term without treatment. Examples may include acute myocardial infarction, pulmonary embolus, severe respiratory distress, progressive severe rheumatoid arthritis, psychiatric illness with potential threat to self or others, peritonitis, acute renal failure, or an abrupt change in neurologic status.

Analyzed: The process of using the data as part of the MDM. The data element itself may not be subject to analysis (eg, glucose), but it is instead included in the thought processes for diagnosis, evaluation, or treatment. Tests ordered are presumed to be analyzed when the results are reported. Therefore, when they are ordered during an encounter, they are counted in that encounter. Tests that are ordered outside of an encounter may be counted in the encounter in which they are analyzed. In the case of a recurring order, each new result may be counted in the encounter in which it is analyzed. For example, an encounter that includes an order for monthly prothrombin times would count for one prothrombin time ordered and reviewed. Additional future results, if analyzed in a subsequent encounter, may be counted as a single test in that subsequent encounter. Any service for which the professional component is separately reported by the physician or other qualified health care professional reporting the E/M services is not counted as a data element ordered, reviewed, analyzed, or independently interpreted for the purposes of determining the level of MDM.

Test: Tests are imaging, laboratory, psychometric, or physiologic data. A clinical laboratory panel (eg, basic metabolic panel [80047]) is a single test. The differentiation between single or multiple tests is defined in accordance with the CPT code set. For the purposes of data reviewed and analyzed, pulse oximetry is not a test.

Unique: A unique test is defined by the CPT code set. When multiple results of the same unique test (eg, serial blood glucose values) are compared during an E/M service, count it as one unique test. Tests that have overlapping elements are not unique, even if they are identified with distinct CPT codes. For example, a CBC with differential would incorporate the set of hemoglobin, CBC without differential, and platelet count. A unique source is defined as a physician or qualified heath care professional in a distinct group or different specialty or subspecialty, or a unique entity. Review of all materials from any unique source counts as one element toward MDM.

Combination of Data Elements: A combination of different data elements, for example, a combination of notes reviewed, tests ordered, tests reviewed, or independent historian, allows these elements to be summed. It does not require each item type or category to be represented. A unique test ordered, plus a note reviewed and an independent historian would be a combination of three elements.

External: External records, communications and/or test results are from an external physician, other qualified health care professional, facility, or health care organization.

External physician or other qualified health care professional: An external physician or other qualified health care professional who is not in the same group practice or is of a different specialty or subspecialty. This includes licensed professionals who are practicing independently. The individual may also be a facility or organizational provider such as from a hospital, nursing facility, or home health care agency.

Discussion: Discussion requires an interactive exchange. The exchange must be direct and not through intermediaries (eg, clinical staff or trainees). Sending chart notes or written exchanges that are within progress notes does not qualify as an interactive exchange. The discussion does not need to be on the date of the encounter, but it is counted only once and only when it is used in the decision making of the encounter. It may be asynchronous (ie, does not need to be in person), but it must be initiated and completed within a short time period (eg, within a day or two).

Independent historian(s): An individual (eg, parent, guardian, surrogate, spouse, witness) who provides a history in addition to a history provided by the patient who is unable to provide a complete or reliable history (eg, due to developmental stage, dementia, or psychosis) or because a confirmatory history is judged to be necessary. In the case where there may be conflict or poor communication between multiple historians and more than one historian is needed, the independent historian requirement is met. The independent history does not need to be obtained in person but does need to be obtained directly from the historian providing the independent information.

Independent interpretation: The interpretation of a test for which there is a CPT code and an interpretation or report is customary. This does not apply when the physician or other qualified health care professional is reporting the service or has previously report the service for the patient. A form of interpretation should be documented but need not conform to the usual standards of a complete report for the test.

Appropriate source: For the purpose of the discussion of management data element (see Table 2, Levels of Medical Decision Making), an appropriate source includes professionals who are not health care professionals but may be involved in the management of the patient (eg, lawyer, parole officer, case manager, teacher). It does not include discussion with family or informal caregivers.

One element used in selecting the level of service is the risk of complications and/or morbidity or mortality of patient management at an encounter. This is distinct from the risk of the condition itself.

Risk: The probability and/or consequences of an event. The assessment of the level of risk is affected by the nature of the event under consideration. For example, a low probability of death may be high risk, whereas a high chance of a minor, self-limited adverse effect of treatment may be low risk. Definitions of risk are based upon the usual behavior and thought processes of a physician or other qualified health care professional in the same specialty. Trained clinicians apply common language usage meanings to terms such as high, medium, low, or minimal risk and do not require quantification for these definitions (though quantification may be provided when evidence-based medicine has established probabilities). For the purposes of MDM, level of risk is based upon consequences of the problem(s) addressed at the encounter when appropriately treated. Risk also includes MDM related to the need to initiate or forego further testing, treatment, and/or hospitalization. The risk of patient management criteria applies to the patient management decisions made by the reporting physician or other qualified health care professional as part of the reported encounter.

Morbidity: A state of illness or functional impairment that is expected to be of substantial duration during which function is limited, quality of life is impaired, or there is organ damage that may not be transient despite treatment.

Social determinants of health: Economic and social conditions that influence the health of people and communities. Examples may include food and housing insecurity.

Surgery (minor or major, elective, emergency, procedure or patient risk):

- **Surgery—Minor or Major:** The classification of surgery into minor or major is based on the common meaning of such terms when used by trained clinicians, similar to the use of the term "risk." These terms are not defined by a surgical package classification.

- **Surgery—Elective or Emergency:** Elective procedures and emergent or urgent procedures describe the timing of a procedure when the timing is related to the patient's condition. An elective procedure is typically planned in advance (eg, scheduled for weeks later), while an emergent procedure is typically performed immediately or with minimal delay to allow for patient stabilization. Both elective and emergent procedures may be minor or major procedures.
- **Surgery—Risk Factors, Patient or Procedure:** Risk factors are those that are relevant to the patient and procedure. Evidence-based risk calculators may be used, but are not required, in assessing patient and procedure risk.

Drug therapy requiring intensive monitoring for toxicity: A drug that requires intensive monitoring is a therapeutic agent that has the potential to cause serious morbidity or death. The monitoring is performed for assessment of these adverse effects and not primarily for assessment of therapeutic efficacy. The monitoring should be that which is generally accepted practice for the agent but may be patient-specific in some cases. Intensive monitoring may be long-term or short-term. Long-term intensive monitoring is not performed less than quarterly. The monitoring may be performed with a laboratory test, a physiologic test, or imaging. Monitoring by history or examination does not qualify. The monitoring affects the level of MDM in an encounter in which it is considered in the management of the patient. Examples may include monitoring for cytopenia in the use of an antineoplastic agent between dose cycles or the short-term intensive monitoring of electrolytes and renal function in a patient who is undergoing diuresis. Examples of monitoring that do not qualify include monitoring glucose levels during insulin therapy, as the primary reason is the therapeutic effect (unless severe hypoglycemia is a current, significant concern); or annual electrolytes and renal function for a patient on a diuretic, as the frequency does not meet the threshold.

Instructions for Selecting a Level of Office or Other Outpatient E/M Services

Select the appropriate level of E/M services based on the following:

1. The level of the MDM as defined for each service, or
2. The total time for E/M services performed on the date of the encounter.

Medical Decision Making

MDM includes establishing diagnoses, assessing the status of a condition, and/or selecting a management option. MDM in the office or other outpatient services codes is defined by three elements:

- The number and complexity of problem(s) that are addressed during the encounter.
- The amount and/or complexity of data to be reviewed and analyzed. These data include medical records, tests, and/or other information that must be obtained, ordered, reviewed, and analyzed for the encounter. This includes information obtained from multiple sources or interprofessional communications that are not reported separately and interpretation of tests that are not reported separately. Ordering a test is included in the category of test result(s) and the review of the test result is part of the encounter and not a subsequent encounter. Ordering a test may include those considered, but not selected after shared decision making. For example, a patient may request diagnostic imaging that is not necessary for their condition and discussion of the lack of benefit may be required. Alternatively, a test may normally be performed, but due to the risk for a specific patient it is not ordered. These considerations must be documented.
- Data are divided into three categories:
  - — Tests, documents, orders, or independent historian(s). (Each unique test, order, or document is counted to meet a threshold number.)
  - — Independent interpretation of tests.
  - — Discussion of management or test interpretation with external physician or other qualified health care professional or appropriate source.
- The risk of complications and/or morbidity or mortality of patient management decisions made at the visit, associated with the patient's problem(s), the diagnostic procedure(s), treatment(s). This includes the possible management options selected and those considered but not selected, after shared MDM with the patient and/or family. For example, a decision about hospitalization includes consideration of alternative levels of care. Examples may include a psychiatric patient with a sufficient degree of support in the outpatient setting or the decision to not hospitalize a patient with advanced dementia with an acute condition that would generally warrant in patient care, but for whom the goal is palliative treatment.

Four types of MDM are recognized: straightforward, low, moderate, and high. The concept of the level of MDM does not apply to 99211. Shared MDM involves eliciting patient and/or family preferences, patient and/or family education, and explaining risks and benefits of management options. MDM may be impacted by role and management responsibility.

When the physician or other qualified health care professional is reporting a separate CPT code that includes interpretation and/or report, the interpretation and/or report should not count toward the MDM when selecting a level of office or other outpatient services. When the physician or other qualified health care professional is reporting a separate service for discussion of management with a physician or another qualified health care professional, the discussion is not counted toward the MDM when selecting a level of office or other outpatient services.

The Levels of Medical Decision Making (MDM) table (Table2) is a guide to assist in selecting the level of MDM for reporting an office or other outpatient E/M services code. The table includes the four levels of MDM (ie, straightforward, low, moderate, high) and the three elements of MDM (ie, number and complexity of problems addressed at the encounter, amount and/or complexity of data reviewed and analyzed, and risk of complications and/or morbidity or mortality of patient management). To qualify for a particular level of MDM, two of the three elements for that level of MDM must be met or exceeded. See Table 2: Levels of Medical Decision Making (MDM) below.

Table 2: Levels of Medical Decision Making (MDM)

		Elements of Medical Decision Making		
Code	**Level of MDM (Based on 2 out of 3 Elements of MDM)**	**Number and Complexity of Problems Addressed**	**Amount and/or Complexity of Data to be Reviewed and Analyzed**	**Risk of Complications and/or Morbidity or Mortality of Patient Management**
99211	N/A	N/A	N/A	N/A
99202 **99212**	**Straightforward**	**Minimal** • **1** self-limited or minor problem	**Minimal or none**	**Minimal risk of morbidity from additional diagnostic testing or treatment**
99203 **99213**	**Low**	**Low** • **2** or more self-limited or minor problems; **or** • stable chronic illness; **or** • **1** acute, uncomplicated illness or injury	**Limited** *(Must meet the requirements of at least 1 of the 2 categories)* **Category 1: Tests and documents** • Any combination of 2 from the following: - Review of prior external note(s) from each unique source*; - review of the result(s) of each unique test*; - ordering of each unique test* **or** **Category 2: Assessment requiring an independent historian(s)** *(For the categories of independent interpretation of tests and discussion of management or test interpretation, see moderate or high)*	**Low risk of morbidity from additional diagnostic testing or treatment**
99204 **99214**	**Moderate**	**Moderate** • **1** or more chronic illnesses with exacerbation, progression, or side effects of treatment; **or** • **2** or more stable chronic illnesses; **or** • **1** undiagnosed new problem with uncertain prognosis; **or** • **1** acute illness with systemic symptoms; **or** • **1** acute complicated injury	**Moderate** *(Must meet the requirements of at least 1 out of 3 categories)* **Category 1: Tests, documents, or independent historian(s)** • Any combination of 3 from the following: - Review of prior external note(s) from each unique source*; - Review of the result(s) of each unique test*; - Ordering of each unique test*; - Assessment requiring an independent historian(s) **or** **Category 2: Independent interpretation of tests** • Independent interpretation of a test performed by another physician/other qualified health care professional (not separately reported); **or** **Category 3: Discussion of management or test interpretation** Discussion of management or test interpretation with external physician/other qualified health care professional\appropriate source (not separately reported)	**Moderate risk of morbidity from additional diagnostic testing or treatment** *Examples only:* • Prescription drug management • Decision regarding minor surgery with identified patient or procedure risk factors • Decision regarding elective major surgery without identified patient or procedure risk factors Diagnosis or treatment significantly limited by social determinants of health

Each unique test, order, or document contributes to the combination of 2 or combination of 3 in Category 1 below.

		Elements of Medical Decision Making		
Code	**Level of MDM (Based on 2 out of 3 Elements of MDM)**	**Number and Complexity of Problems Addressed**	**Amount and/or Complexity of Data to be Reviewed and Analyzed**	**Risk of Complications and/or Morbidity or Mortality of Patient Management**
99205 **99215**	**High**	**High** • **1** or more chronic illnesses with severe exacerbation, progression, or side effects of treatment; **or** • **1** acute or chronic illness or injury that poses a threat to life or bodily function	**Extensive** *(Must meet the requirements of at least 2 out of 3 categories)* **Category 1: Tests, documents, or independent historian(s)** • **Any combination of 3 from the following:** - Review of prior external note(s) from each unique source*; - Review of the result(s) of each unique test*; - Ordering of each unique test*; - Assessment requiring an independent historian(s) **or** **Category 2: Independent interpretation of tests** • **Independent interpretation of a test performed by another physician/other qualified health care professional (not separately reported);** **or** **Category 3: Discussion of management or test interpretation** • Discussion of management or test interpretation with external physician/other qualified health care professional/appropriate source (not separately reported)	**High risk of morbidity from additional diagnostic testing or treatment** *Examples only:* • Drug therapy requiring intensive monitoring for toxicity • Decision regarding elective major surgery with identified patient or procedure risk factors • Decision regarding emergency major surgery • Decision regarding hospitalization • Decision not to resuscitate or to de-escalate care because of poor prognosis

**Each unique test, order, or document contributes to the combination of 2 or combination of 3 in Category 1 below.*

Time

For instructions on using time to select the level of office or other outpatient E/M services code, see the ***Time*** subsection in the ***Guidelines Common to All E/M Services.***

Unlisted Service

An E/M service may be provided that is not listed in this section of the CPT codebook. When reporting such a service, the appropriate unlisted code may be used to indicate the service, identifying it by "Special Report," as discussed in the following paragraph. The "Unlisted Services" and accompanying codes for the E/M section are as follows:

99429 **Unlisted preventive** medicine service

99499 **Unlisted evaluation and management** service

Special Report

An unlisted service or one that is unusual, variable, or new may require a special report demonstrating the medical appropriateness of the service. Pertinent information should include an adequate definition or description of the nature, extent, and need for the procedure and the time, effort, and equipment necessary to provide the service. Additional items that may be included are complexity of symptoms, final diagnosis, pertinent physical findings, diagnostic and therapeutic procedures, concurrent problems, and follow-up care.

Clinical Examples

Clinical examples of the codes for E/M services are provided to assist in understanding the meaning of the descriptors and selecting the correct code. The clinical examples are listed in Appendix C. Each example was developed by the specialties shown. The same problem, when seen by different specialties, may involve different amounts of work. Therefore, the appropriate level of encounter should be reported using the descriptors rather than the examples.

Evaluation and Management

99202 — 99215

99202-99215 Outpatient and Other Visits

INCLUDES Established patients: received prior professional services from physician or qualified health care professional or another physician or qualified health care professional in exact same specialty practice and subspecialty in previous three years (99211-99215)
New patients: have not received professional services from physician or qualified health care professional or any other physician or qualified health care professional in same practice in exact same specialty and subspecialty in previous three years (99202-99205)
Office visits
Outpatient services (including services prior to formal admission to facility)

EXCLUDES *Services provided in:*
Emergency department (99281-99285)
Hospital observation (99217-99220 [99224, 99225, 99226])
Hospital observation or inpatient with same day admission and discharge (99234-99236)

99202 **Office or other outpatient visit for the evaluation and management of a new patient, which requires a medically appropriate history and/or examination and straightforward medical decision making. When using time for code selection, 15-29 minutes of total time is spent on the date of the encounter.**

1.43 2.15 **FUD** XXX ★ B 80

AMA: 2020,Dec,11; 2020,Oct,14; 2020,Nov,3; 2020,Sep,3; 2020,Sep,14; 2020,Jun,3; 2020,May,3; 2020,Feb,3; 2020,Jan,3; 2019,Oct,10; 2019,Feb,3; 2019,Jan,3; 2018,Sep,14; 2018,Apr,10; 2018,Apr,9; 2018,Mar,7; 2018,Jan,8; 2017,Aug,3; 2017,Jun,6; 2017,Jan,8; 2016,Dec,11; 2016,Sep,6; 2016,Mar,10; 2016,Jan,13; 2016,Jan,7

99203 **Office or other outpatient visit for the evaluation and management of a new patient, which requires a medically appropriate history and/or examination and low level of medical decision making. When using time for code selection, 30-44 minutes of total time is spent on the date of the encounter.**

2.15 3.05 **FUD** XXX ★ B 80

AMA: 2020,Oct,14; 2020,Nov,3; 2020,Sep,14; 2020,Sep,3; 2020,Jun,3; 2020,May,3; 2020,Feb,3; 2020,Jan,3; 2019,Oct,10; 2019,Feb,3; 2019,Jan,3; 2018,Sep,14; 2018,Apr,9; 2018,Apr,10; 2018,Mar,7; 2018,Jan,8; 2017,Aug,3; 2017,Jun,6; 2017,Jan,8; 2016,Dec,11; 2016,Sep,6; 2016,Mar,10; 2016,Jan,13; 2016,Jan,7

99204 **Office or other outpatient visit for the evaluation and management of a new patient, which requires a medically appropriate history and/or examination and moderate level of medical decision making. When using time for code selection, 45-59 minutes of total time is spent on the date of the encounter.**

3.64 4.63 **FUD** XXX ★ B 80

AMA: 2020,Oct,14; 2020,Nov,3; 2020,Nov,12; 2020,Sep,3; 2020,Sep,14; 2020,Jun,3; 2020,May,3; 2020,Feb,3; 2020,Jan,3; 2019,Oct,10; 2019,Feb,3; 2019,Jan,3; 2018,Sep,14; 2018,Apr,10; 2018,Apr,9; 2018,Mar,7; 2018,Jan,8; 2017,Aug,3; 2017,Jun,6; 2017,Jan,8; 2016,Dec,11; 2016,Sep,6; 2016,Mar,10; 2016,Jan,7; 2016,Jan,13

99205 **Office or other outpatient visit for the evaluation and management of a new patient, which requires a medically appropriate history and/or examination and high level of medical decision making. When using time for code selection, 60-74 minutes of total time is spent on the date of the encounter.**

EXCLUDES *Prolonged services (lasting 75 minutes or more) ([99417])*

4.75 5.82 **FUD** XXX ★ B 80

AMA: 2020,Oct,14; 2020,Nov,3; 2020,Nov,12; 2020,Sep,3; 2020,Sep,14; 2020,Jun,3; 2020,May,3; 2020,Feb,3; 2020,Jan,3; 2019,Oct,10; 2019,Feb,3; 2019,Jan,3; 2018,Sep,14; 2018,Apr,10; 2018,Apr,9; 2018,Mar,7; 2018,Jan,8; 2017,Aug,3; 2017,Jun,6; 2017,Jan,8; 2016,Dec,11; 2016,Sep,6; 2016,Mar,10; 2016,Jan,7; 2016,Jan,13

▲ **99211** **Office or other outpatient visit for the evaluation and management of an established patient that may not require the presence of a physician or other qualified health care professional**

0.26 0.64 **FUD** XXX ★ B 80

AMA: 2020,Oct,14; 2020,Nov,12; 2020,Nov,3; 2020,Sep,14; 2020,Sep,3; 2020,Jun,3; 2020,May,3; 2020,Feb,3; 2020,Jan,3; 2019,Oct,10; 2019,Feb,3; 2019,Jan,3; 2018,Sep,14; 2018,Apr,9; 2018,Apr,10; 2018,Mar,7; 2018,Jan,8; 2017,Aug,3; 2017,Jun,6; 2017,Mar,10; 2017,Jan,8; 2016,Dec,11; 2016,Sep,6; 2016,Mar,10; 2016,Jan,7; 2016,Jan,13

99212 **Office or other outpatient visit for the evaluation and management of an established patient, which requires a medically appropriate history and/or examination and straightforward medical decision making. When using time for code selection, 10-19 minutes of total time is spent on the date of the encounter.**

0.72 1.27 **FUD** XXX ★ B 80

AMA: 2020,Oct,14; 2020,Nov,3; 2020,Sep,14; 2020,Sep,3; 2020,Jun,3; 2020,May,3; 2020,Feb,3; 2020,Jan,3; 2019,Oct,10; 2019,Feb,3; 2019,Jan,3; 2018,Sep,14; 2018,Apr,9; 2018,Apr,10; 2018,Mar,7; 2018,Jan,8; 2017,Oct,5; 2017,Aug,3; 2017,Jun,6; 2017,Jan,8; 2016,Dec,11; 2016,Sep,6; 2016,Mar,10; 2016,Jan,13; 2016,Jan,7

99213 **Office or other outpatient visit for the evaluation and management of an established patient, which requires a medically appropriate history and/or examination and low level of medical decision making. When using time for code selection, 20-29 minutes of total time is spent on the date of the encounter.**

1.44 2.09 **FUD** XXX ★ B 80

AMA: 2020,Oct,14; 2020,Nov,3; 2020,Sep,3; 2020,Sep,14; 2020,Jun,3; 2020,May,3; 2020,Feb,3; 2020,Jan,3; 2019,Oct,10; 2019,Feb,3; 2019,Jan,3; 2018,Sep,14; 2018,Apr,10; 2018,Apr,9; 2018,Mar,7; 2018,Jan,8; 2017,Aug,3; 2017,Jun,6; 2017,Jan,8; 2016,Dec,11; 2016,Sep,6; 2016,Mar,10; 2016,Jan,13; 2016,Jan,7

99214 **Office or other outpatient visit for the evaluation and management of an established patient, which requires a medically appropriate history and/or examination and moderate level of medical decision making. When using time for code selection, 30-39 minutes of total time is spent on the date of the encounter.**

2.22 3.06 **FUD** XXX ★ B 80

AMA: 2020,Oct,14; 2020,Nov,3; 2020,Nov,12; 2020,Sep,14; 2020,Sep,3; 2020,Jun,3; 2020,May,3; 2020,Feb,3; 2020,Jan,3; 2019,Oct,10; 2019,Feb,3; 2019,Jan,3; 2018,Sep,14; 2018,Apr,9; 2018,Apr,10; 2018,Mar,7; 2018,Jan,8; 2017,Aug,3; 2017,Jun,6; 2017,Jan,8; 2016,Dec,11; 2016,Sep,6; 2016,Mar,10; 2016,Jan,7; 2016,Jan,13

99215 **Office or other outpatient visit for the evaluation and management of an established patient, which requires a medically appropriate history and/or examination and high level of medical decision making. When using time for code selection, 40-54 minutes of total time is spent on the date of the encounter.**

EXCLUDES *Prolonged services (lasting 55 minutes or more) ([99417])*

3.13 4.10 **FUD** XXX ★ B 80

AMA: 2020,Oct,14; 2020,Nov,12; 2020,Nov,3; 2020,Sep,14; 2020,Sep,3; 2020,Jun,3; 2020,May,3; 2020,Feb,3; 2020,Jan,3; 2019,Oct,10; 2019,Feb,3; 2019,Jan,3; 2018,Sep,14; 2018,Apr,9; 2018,Apr,10; 2018,Mar,7; 2018,Jan,8; 2017,Aug,3; 2017,Jun,6; 2017,Jan,8; 2016,Dec,11; 2016,Sep,6; 2016,Mar,10; 2016,Jan,7; 2016,Jan,13

99217-99220 Facility Observation Visits: Initial and Discharge

CMS: 100-04,11,40.1.3 Independent Attending Physician Services; 100-04,12,30.6.4 Services Furnished Incident to Physician's Service; 100-04,12,30.6.8 Payment for Hospital Observation Services; 100-04,12,40.3 Global Surgery Review; 100-04,32,130.1 Billing and Payment of External counterpulsation (ECP)

INCLUDES Services provided on same date in other settings or departments associated with observation status admission (99202-99215, 99281-99285, 99304-99318, 99324-99337, 99341-99350, 99381-99429 [99415, 99416, 99417, 99421, 99422, 99423])
Services provided to new and established patients admitted to hospital specifically for observation (not required to be designated hospital area)

EXCLUDES *Services provided by physicians or another qualified health care professional other than admitting physician ([99224, 99225, 99226], 99241-99245)*
Services provided to patient admitted and discharged from observation status on same date (99234-99236)
Services provided to patient admitted to hospital following observation status (99221-99223)
Services provided to patient discharged from inpatient care (99238-99239)

99217 **Observation care discharge day management (This code is to be utilized to report all services provided to a patient on discharge from outpatient hospital "observation status" if the discharge is on other than the initial date of "observation status." To report services to a patient designated as "observation status" or "inpatient status" and discharged on the same date, use the codes for Observation or Inpatient Care Services [including Admission and Discharge Services, 99234-99236 as appropriate.])**

INCLUDES Discussing observation admission with patient
Final patient evaluation:
Discharge instructions
Sign off on discharge medical records

2.06 2.06 **FUD** XXX B 80

AMA: 2019,Jul,10; 2018,Jan,8; 2017,Aug,3; 2017,Jun,6; 2017,Jan,8; 2016,Dec,11; 2016,Jan,13; 2016,Jan,7

99218 **Initial observation care, per day, for the evaluation and management of a patient which requires these 3 key components: A detailed or comprehensive history; A detailed or comprehensive examination; and Medical decision making that is straightforward or of low complexity. Counseling and/or coordination of care with other physicians, other qualified health care professionals, or agencies are provided consistent with the nature of the problem(s) and the patient's and/or family's needs. Usually, the problem(s) requiring admission to outpatient hospital "observation status" are of low severity. Typically, 30 minutes are spent at the bedside and on the patient's hospital floor or unit.**

2.81 2.81 **FUD** XXX B 80

AMA: 2020,Sep,3; 2019,Jul,10; 2018,Dec,8; 2018,Dec,8; 2018,Jan,8; 2017,Aug,3; 2017,Jun,6; 2017,Jan,8; 2016,Dec,11; 2016,Jan,7; 2016,Jan,13

99219 **Initial observation care, per day, for the evaluation and management of a patient, which requires these 3 key components: A comprehensive history; A comprehensive examination; and Medical decision making of moderate complexity. Counseling and/or coordination of care with other physicians, other qualified health care professionals, or agencies are provided consistent with the nature of the problem(s) and the patient's and/or family's needs. Usually, the problem(s) requiring admission to outpatient hospital "observation status" are of moderate severity. Typically, 50 minutes are spent at the bedside and on the patient's hospital floor or unit.**

3.83 3.83 **FUD** XXX B 80

AMA: 2020,Sep,3; 2019,Jul,10; 2018,Dec,8; 2018,Dec,8; 2018,Jan,8; 2017,Aug,3; 2017,Jun,6; 2017,Jan,8; 2016,Dec,11; 2016,Jan,13; 2016,Jan,7

99220 **Initial observation care, per day, for the evaluation and management of a patient, which requires these 3 key components: A comprehensive history; A comprehensive examination; and Medical decision making of high complexity. Counseling and/or coordination of care with other physicians, other qualified health care professionals, or agencies are provided consistent with the nature of the problem(s) and the patient's and/or family's needs. Usually, the problem(s) requiring admission to outpatient hospital "observation status" are of high severity. Typically, 70 minutes are spent at the bedside and on the patient's hospital floor or unit.**

5.23 5.23 **FUD** XXX B 80

AMA: 2020,Sep,3; 2019,Jul,10; 2018,Dec,8; 2018,Dec,8; 2018,Jan,8; 2017,Aug,3; 2017,Jun,6; 2017,Jan,8; 2016,Dec,11; 2016,Jan,13; 2016,Jan,7

99224-99226 [99224, 99225, 99226] Facility Observation Visits: Subsequent

CMS: 100-04,11,40.1.3 Independent Attending Physician Services; 100-04,12,30.6.4 Services Furnished Incident to Physician's Service; 100-04,12,30.6.8 Payment for Hospital Observation Services; 100-04,12,30.6.9.1 Initial Hospital Care and Observation or Inpatient Care Services

INCLUDES Changes in patient's status (e.g., physical condition, history; response to medical management)
Medical record review
Review diagnostic test results
Services provided on same date in other settings or departments associated with observation status admission (99202-99215, 99281-99285, 99304-99318, 99324-99337, 99341-99350, 99381-99429 [99415, 99416, 99417, 99421, 99422, 99423])

EXCLUDES *Observation admission and discharge on same day (99234-99236)*

99224 **Subsequent observation care, per day, for the evaluation and management of a patient, which requires at least 2 of these 3 key components: Problem focused interval history; Problem focused examination; Medical decision making that is straightforward or of low complexity. Counseling and/or coordination of care with other physicians, other qualified health care professionals, or agencies are provided consistent with the nature of the problem(s) and the patient's and/or family's needs. Usually, the patient is stable, recovering, or improving. Typically, 15 minutes are spent at the bedside and on the patient's hospital floor or unit.**

1.12 1.12 **FUD** XXX B 80

AMA: 2020,Sep,3; 2019,Jul,10; 2018,Jan,8; 2017,Aug,3; 2017,Jun,6; 2017,Jan,8; 2016,Dec,11; 2016,Jan,7; 2016,Jan,13

99225 **Subsequent observation care, per day, for the evaluation and management of a patient, which requires at least 2 of these 3 key components: An expanded problem focused interval history; An expanded problem focused examination; Medical decision making of moderate complexity. Counseling and/or coordination of care with other physicians, other qualified health care professionals, or agencies are provided consistent with the nature of the problem(s) and the patient's and/or family's needs. Usually, the patient is responding inadequately to therapy or has developed a minor complication. Typically, 25 minutes are spent at the bedside and on the patient's hospital floor or unit.**

2.06 2.06 **FUD** XXX B 80

AMA: 2020,Sep,3; 2019,Jul,10; 2018,Jan,8; 2017,Aug,3; 2017,Jun,6; 2017,Jan,8; 2016,Dec,11; 2016,Jan,7; 2016,Jan,13

\# **99226** **Subsequent observation care, per day, for the evaluation and management of a patient, which requires at least 2 of these 3 key components: A detailed interval history; A detailed examination; Medical decision making of high complexity. Counseling and/or coordination of care with other physicians, other qualified health care professionals, or agencies are provided consistent with the nature of the problem(s) and the patient's and/or family's needs. Usually, the patient is unstable or has developed a significant complication or a significant new problem. Typically, 35 minutes are spent at the bedside and on the patient's hospital floor or unit.**

2.95 2.95 FUD XXX B 80

AMA: 2020,Sep,3; 2019,Jul,10; 2018,Jan,8; 2017,Aug,3; 2017,Jun,6; 2017,Jan,8; 2016,Dec,11; 2016,Jan,7; 2016,Jan,13

99221-99233 [99224, 99225, 99226] Inpatient Hospital Visits: Initial and Subsequent

CMS: 100-04,11,40.1.3 Independent Attending Physician Services; 100-04,12,30.6.10 Consultation Services; 100-04,12,30.6.15.1 Prolonged Services With Direct Face-to-Face Patient Contact; 100-04,12,30.6.4 Services Furnished Incident to Physician's Service; 100-04,12,30.6.9 Hospital Visit and Critical Care on Same Day

INCLUDES Initial physician services provided to patient in hospital or "partial" hospital settings (99221-99223)

Services provided on admission date in other settings or departments associated with observation status admission (99202-99215, 99281-99285, 99304-99318, 99324-99337, 99341-99350, 99381-99397)

Services provided to new or established patient

EXCLUDES *Inpatient admission and discharge on same date (99234-99236)*

Inpatient E/M services provided by other than admitting physician

99221 **Initial hospital care, per day, for the evaluation and management of a patient, which requires these 3 key components: A detailed or comprehensive history; A detailed or comprehensive examination; and Medical decision making that is straightforward or of low complexity. Counseling and/or coordination of care with other physicians, other qualified health care professionals, or agencies are provided consistent with the nature of the problem(s) and the patient's and/or family's needs. Usually, the problem(s) requiring admission are of low severity. Typically, 30 minutes are spent at the bedside and on the patient's hospital floor or unit.**

2.86 2.86 FUD XXX B 80

AMA: 2020,Oct,14; 2020,Sep,3; 2018,Dec,8; 2018,Dec,8; 2018,Jan,8; 2017,Aug,3; 2017,Jun,6; 2017,Jan,8; 2016,Dec,11; 2016,Mar,10; 2016,Jan,13; 2016,Jan,7

99222 **Initial hospital care, per day, for the evaluation and management of a patient, which requires these 3 key components: A comprehensive history; A comprehensive examination; and Medical decision making of moderate complexity. Counseling and/or coordination of care with other physicians, other qualified health care professionals, or agencies are provided consistent with the nature of the problem(s) and the patient's and/or family's needs. Usually, the problem(s) requiring admission are of moderate severity. Typically, 50 minutes are spent at the bedside and on the patient's hospital floor or unit.**

3.86 3.86 FUD XXX B 80

AMA: 2020,Oct,14; 2020,Sep,3; 2018,Dec,8; 2018,Dec,8; 2018,Jan,8; 2017,Aug,3; 2017,Jun,6; 2017,Jan,8; 2016,Dec,11; 2016,Mar,10; 2016,Jan,13; 2016,Jan,7

99223 **Initial hospital care, per day, for the evaluation and management of a patient, which requires these 3 key components: A comprehensive history; A comprehensive examination; and Medical decision making of high complexity. Counseling and/or coordination of care with other physicians, other qualified health care professionals, or agencies are provided consistent with the nature of the problem(s) and the patient's and/or family's needs. Usually, the problem(s) requiring admission are of high severity. Typically, 70 minutes are spent at the bedside and on the patient's hospital floor or unit.**

5.71 5.71 FUD XXX B 80

AMA: 2020,Oct,14; 2020,Sep,3; 2018,Dec,8; 2018,Dec,8; 2018,Jan,8; 2017,Aug,3; 2017,Jun,6; 2017,Jan,8; 2016,Dec,11; 2016,Mar,10; 2016,Jan,13; 2016,Jan,7

99224 **Resequenced code. See code following 99220.**

99225 **Resequenced code. See code following 99220.**

99226 **Resequenced code. See code following 99220.**

99231 **Subsequent hospital care, per day, for the evaluation and management of a patient, which requires at least 2 of these 3 key components: A problem focused interval history; A problem focused examination; Medical decision making that is straightforward or of low complexity. Counseling and/or coordination of care with other physicians, other qualified health care professionals, or agencies are provided consistent with the nature of the problem(s) and the patient's and/or family's needs. Usually, the patient is stable, recovering or improving. Typically, 15 minutes are spent at the bedside and on the patient's hospital floor or unit.**

1.11 1.11 FUD XXX ★ B 80

AMA: 2020,Sep,3; 2018,Dec,8; 2018,Dec,8; 2018,Jan,8; 2017,Aug,3; 2017,Jun,6; 2017,Jan,8; 2016,Dec,11; 2016,Jan,13; 2016,Jan,7

99232 **Subsequent hospital care, per day, for the evaluation and management of a patient, which requires at least 2 of these 3 key components: An expanded problem focused interval history; An expanded problem focused examination; Medical decision making of moderate complexity. Counseling and/or coordination of care with other physicians, other qualified health care professionals, or agencies are provided consistent with the nature of the problem(s) and the patient's and/or family's needs. Usually, the patient is responding inadequately to therapy or has developed a minor complication. Typically, 25 minutes are spent at the bedside and on the patient's hospital floor or unit.**

2.05 2.05 FUD XXX ★ B 80

AMA: 2020,Sep,3; 2018,Dec,8; 2018,Dec,8; 2018,Jan,8; 2017,Aug,3; 2017,Jun,6; 2017,Jan,8; 2016,Dec,11; 2016,Oct,8; 2016,Jan,13; 2016,Jan,7

99233 **Subsequent hospital care, per day, for the evaluation and management of a patient, which requires at least 2 of these 3 key components: A detailed interval history; A detailed examination; Medical decision making of high complexity. Counseling and/or coordination of care with other physicians, other qualified health care professionals, or agencies are provided consistent with the nature of the problem(s) and the patient's and/or family's needs. Usually, the patient is unstable or has developed a significant complication or a significant new problem. Typically, 35 minutes are spent at the bedside and on the patient's hospital floor or unit.**

2.93 2.93 FUD XXX ★ B 80

AMA: 2020,Sep,3; 2018,Dec,8; 2018,Dec,8; 2018,Jan,8; 2017,Aug,3; 2017,Jun,6; 2017,Jan,8; 2016,Dec,11; 2016,Oct,8; 2016,Jan,13; 2016,Jan,7

99234-99236 Observation/Inpatient Visits: Admitted/Discharged on Same Date

CMS: 100-04,11,40.1.3 Independent Attending Physician Services; 100-04,12,30.6.4 Services Furnished Incident to Physician's Service; 100-04,12,30.6.8 Payment for Hospital Observation Services; 100-04,12,30.6.9 Swing Bed Visits; 100-04,12,30.6.9.1 Initial Hospital Care and Observation or Inpatient Care Services; 100-04,12,30.6.9.2 Hospital Discharge Management; 100-04,12,40.3 Global Surgery Review

INCLUDES Admission and discharge services on same date in observation or inpatient setting
All services provided by admitting physician or other qualified health care professional on same date, even when initiated in another setting (e.g., emergency department, nursing facility, office)

EXCLUDES *Services provided to patients admitted to observation and discharged on different date (99217-99220, [99224, 99225, 99226])*

99234 Observation or inpatient hospital care, for the evaluation and management of a patient including admission and discharge on the same date, which requires these 3 key components: A detailed or comprehensive history; A detailed or comprehensive examination; and Medical decision making that is straightforward or of low complexity. Counseling and/or coordination of care with other physicians, other qualified health care professionals, or agencies are provided consistent with the nature of the problem(s) and the patient's and/or family's needs. Usually the presenting problem(s) requiring admission are of low severity. Typically, 40 minutes are spent at the bedside and on the patient's hospital floor or unit.

3.75 3.75 FUD XXX B 80

AMA: 2020,Sep,3; 2018,Dec,8; 2018,Dec,8; 2018,Apr,10; 2018,Jan,8; 2017,Aug,3; 2017,Jun,6; 2017,Jan,8; 2016,Dec,11; 2016,Jan,13

99235 Observation or inpatient hospital care, for the evaluation and management of a patient including admission and discharge on the same date, which requires these 3 key components: A comprehensive history; A comprehensive examination; and Medical decision making of moderate complexity. Counseling and/or coordination of care with other physicians, other qualified health care professionals, or agencies are provided consistent with the nature of the problem(s) and the patient's and/or family's needs. Usually the presenting problem(s) requiring admission are of moderate severity. Typically, 50 minutes are spent at the bedside and on the patient's hospital floor or unit.

4.77 4.77 FUD XXX B 80

AMA: 2020,Sep,3; 2018,Dec,8; 2018,Dec,8; 2018,Apr,10; 2018,Jan,8; 2017,Aug,3; 2017,Jun,6; 2017,Jan,8; 2016,Dec,11; 2016,Jan,13

99236 Observation or inpatient hospital care, for the evaluation and management of a patient including admission and discharge on the same date, which requires these 3 key components: A comprehensive history; A comprehensive examination; and Medical decision making of high complexity. Counseling and/or coordination of care with other physicians, other qualified health care professionals, or agencies are provided consistent with the nature of the problem(s) and the patient's and/or family's needs. Usually the presenting problem(s) requiring admission are of high severity. Typically, 55 minutes are spent at the bedside and on the patient's hospital floor or unit.

6.13 6.13 FUD XXX B 80

AMA: 2020,Sep,3; 2018,Dec,8; 2018,Dec,8; 2018,Apr,10; 2018,Jan,8; 2017,Aug,3; 2017,Jun,6; 2017,Jan,8; 2016,Dec,11; 2016,Jan,13

99238-99239 Inpatient Hospital Discharge Services

CMS: 100-04,11,40.1.3 Independent Attending Physician Services; 100-04,12,30.6.4 Services Furnished Incident to Physician's Service; 100-04,12,30.6.9 Swing Bed Visits; 100-04,12,30.6.9.1 Initial Hospital Care and Observation or Inpatient Care Services; 100-04,12,30.6.9.2 Hospital Discharge Management; 100-04,12,40.3 Global Surgery Review

INCLUDES All services on discharge day when discharge and admission are not on same day
Discharge instructions
Final patient evaluation
Final preparation patient's medical records
Provision prescriptions/referrals, as needed
Review inpatient admission

EXCLUDES *Admission/discharge on same date (99234-99236)*
Discharge from observation (99217)
Discharge from nursing facility (99315-99316)
Healthy newborn evaluated and discharged on same date (99463)
Services provided by other than attending physician or other qualified health care professional on discharge date (99231-99233)

99238 Hospital discharge day management; 30 minutes or less

2.06 2.06 FUD XXX B 80

AMA: 2018,Dec,8; 2018,Dec,8; 2018,Jan,8; 2017,Aug,3; 2017,Jun,6; 2017,Jan,8; 2016,Dec,11; 2016,Jan,13

99239 more than 30 minutes

3.02 3.02 FUD XXX B 80

AMA: 2018,Dec,8; 2018,Dec,8; 2018,Jan,8; 2017,Aug,3; 2017,Jun,6; 2017,Jan,8; 2016,Dec,11; 2016,Jan,13

99241-99245 Consultations: Office and Outpatient

CMS: 100-04,11,40.1.3 Independent Attending Physician Services; 100-04,12,190.6 Payment Methodology for Physician/Practitioner at the Distant Site ; 100-04,12,190.6.1 Submission of Telehealth Claims for Distant Site Practitioners; 100-04,12,190.7 Contractor Editing of Telehealth Claims; 100-04,12,30.6.10 Consultation Services; 100-04,12,30.6.15.1 Prolonged Services With Direct Face-to-Face Patient Contact; 100-04,12,30.6.4 Services Furnished Incident to Physician's Service; 100-04,12,30.6.9.1 Initial Hospital Care and Observation or Inpatient Care Services; 100-04,12,40.3 Global Surgery Review; 100-04,32,130.1 Billing and Payment of External counterpulsation (ECP); 100-04,4,160 Clinic and Emergency Visits Under OPPS

INCLUDES All outpatient consultations provided in office, outpatient or other ambulatory facility, domiciliary/rest home, emergency department, patient's home, and hospital observation
Documentation consultation request from appropriate source
Documentation need for consultation in patient's medical record
One consultation per consultant
Provision by physician or qualified nonphysician practitioner whose advice, opinion, recommendation, suggestion, direction, or counsel, etc., requested for evaluating/treating patient since that individual's specific medical expertise beyond requesting physician knowledge
Provision written report, findings/recommendations from consultant to referring physician
Third-party mandated consultation; append modifier 32

EXCLUDES *Another appropriately requested and documented consultation pertaining to same/new problem; repeat consultation code reporting*
Any distinctly recognizable procedure/service provided on or following consultation
Care assumption (all or partial); report subsequent codes as appropriate for place of service (99211-99215, 99334-99337, 99347-99350)
Consultation prompted by patient/family; report codes for office, domiciliary/rest home, or home visits instead (99202-99215, 99324-99337, 99341-99350)
Services provided to Medicare patients; E/M code as appropriate for place of service or HCPCS code (99202-99215, 99221-99223, 99231-99233, G0406-G0408, G0425-G0427)

99241 Office consultation for a new or established patient, which requires these 3 key components: A problem focused history; A problem focused examination; and Straightforward medical decision making. Counseling and/or coordination of care with other physicians, other qualified health care professionals, or agencies are provided consistent with the nature of the problem(s) and the patient's and/or family's needs. Usually, the presenting problem(s) are self limited or minor. Typically, 15 minutes are spent face-to-face with the patient and/or family.

0.92 1.34 FUD XXX ★ E

AMA: 2020,Oct,14; 2020,Nov,3; 2020,Sep,3; 2018,Apr,9; 2018,Apr,10; 2018,Mar,7; 2018,Jan,8; 2017,Aug,3; 2017,Jun,6; 2017,Jan,8; 2016,Dec,11; 2016,Sep,6; 2016,Jan,13; 2016,Jan,7

99242 **Office consultation for a new or established patient, which requires these 3 key components: An expanded problem focused history; An expanded problem focused examination; and Straightforward medical decision making. Counseling and/or coordination of care with other physicians, other qualified health care professionals, or agencies are provided consistent with the nature of the problem(s) and the patient's and/or family's needs. Usually, the presenting problem(s) are of low severity. Typically, 30 minutes are spent face-to-face with the patient and/or family.**

1.93 2.52 **FUD** XXX ★ E

AMA: 2020,Oct,14; 2020,Nov,3; 2020,Sep,3; 2018,Apr,9; 2018,Apr,10; 2018,Mar,7; 2018,Jan,8; 2017,Aug,3; 2017,Jun,8; 2017,Jun,6; 2017,Jan,8; 2016,Dec,11; 2016,Sep,6; 2016,Jan,13; 2016,Jan,7

99243 **Office consultation for a new or established patient, which requires these 3 key components: A detailed history; A detailed examination; and Medical decision making of low complexity. Counseling and/or coordination of care with other physicians, other qualified health care professionals, or agencies are provided consistent with the nature of the problem(s) and the patient's and/or family's needs. Usually, the presenting problem(s) are of moderate severity. Typically, 40 minutes are spent face-to-face with the patient and/or family.**

2.70 3.45 **FUD** XXX ★ E

AMA: 2020,Oct,14; 2020,Nov,3; 2020,Sep,3; 2018,Apr,9; 2018,Apr,10; 2018,Mar,7; 2018,Jan,8; 2017,Aug,3; 2017,Jun,6; 2017,Jan,8; 2016,Dec,11; 2016,Sep,6; 2016,Jan,13; 2016,Jan,7

99244 **Office consultation for a new or established patient, which requires these 3 key components: A comprehensive history; A comprehensive examination; and Medical decision making of moderate complexity. Counseling and/or coordination of care with other physicians, other qualified health care professionals, or agencies are provided consistent with the nature of the problem(s) and the patient's and/or family's needs. Usually, the presenting problem(s) are of moderate to high severity. Typically, 60 minutes are spent face-to-face with the patient and/or family.**

4.34 5.16 **FUD** XXX ★ E

AMA: 2020,Oct,14; 2020,Nov,3; 2020,Sep,3; 2018,Apr,9; 2018,Apr,10; 2018,Mar,7; 2018,Jan,8; 2017,Aug,3; 2017,Jun,6; 2017,Jan,8; 2016,Dec,11; 2016,Sep,6; 2016,Jan,13; 2016,Jan,7

99245 **Office consultation for a new or established patient, which requires these 3 key components: A comprehensive history; A comprehensive examination; and Medical decision making of high complexity. Counseling and/or coordination of care with other physicians, other qualified health care professionals, or agencies are provided consistent with the nature of the problem(s) and the patient's and/or family's needs. Usually, the presenting problem(s) are of moderate to high severity. Typically, 80 minutes are spent face-to-face with the patient and/or family.**

5.37 6.29 **FUD** XXX ★ E

AMA: 2020,Oct,14; 2020,Nov,3; 2020,Sep,3; 2018,Apr,9; 2018,Apr,10; 2018,Mar,7; 2018,Jan,8; 2017,Aug,3; 2017,Jun,6; 2017,Jan,8; 2016,Dec,11; 2016,Sep,6; 2016,Jan,13; 2016,Jan,7

99251-99255 Consultations: Inpatient

CMS: 100-04,11,40.1.3 Independent Attending Physician Services; 100-04,12,190.6 Payment Methodology for Physician/Practitioner at the Distant Site ; 100-04,12,190.6.1 Submission of Telehealth Claims for Distant Site Practitioners; 100-04,12,190.7 Contractor Editing of Telehealth Claims; 100-04,12,30.6.10 Consultation Services; 100-04,12,30.6.15.1 Prolonged Services With Direct Face-to-Face Patient Contact; 100-04,12,30.6.4 Services Furnished Incident to Physician's Service; 100-04,12,30.6.9.1 Initial Hospital Care and Observation or Inpatient Care Services; 100-04,12,40.3 Global Surgery Review

INCLUDES All outpatient consultations provided in office, outpatient or other ambulatory facility, domiciliary/rest home, emergency department, patient's home, and hospital observation
Documentation consultation request from appropriate source
Documentation need for consultation in patient's medical record
One consultation per consultant
Provision by physician or qualified nonphysician practitioner whose advice, opinion, recommendation, suggestion, direction, or counsel, etc., requested for evaluating/treating patient since that individual's specific medical expertise beyond requesting physician knowledge
Provision written report, findings/recommendations from consultant to referring physician
Third-party mandated consultation; append modifier 32

EXCLUDES *Another appropriately requested and documented consultation pertaining to same/new problem; repeat consultation code reporting*
Any distinctly recognizable procedure/service provided on or following consultation
Care assumption (all or partial); report subsequent codes as appropriate for place of service (99231-99233, 99307-99310)
Consultation prompted by patient/family; report codes for office, domiciliary/rest home, or home visits instead (99202-99215, 99234-99337, 99341-99350)
Services provided to Medicare patients; E/M code as appropriate for place of service or HCPCS code (99202-99215, 99324-99337, 99341-99350)

99251 **Inpatient consultation for a new or established patient, which requires these 3 key components: A problem focused history; A problem focused examination; and Straightforward medical decision making. Counseling and/or coordination of care with other physicians, other qualified health care professionals, or agencies are provided consistent with the nature of the problem(s) and the patient's and/or family's needs. Usually, the presenting problem(s) are self limited or minor. Typically, 20 minutes are spent at the bedside and on the patient's hospital floor or unit.**

1.38 1.38 **FUD** XXX ★ E

AMA: 2020,Sep,3; 2018,Jan,8; 2017,Aug,3; 2017,Jun,6; 2017,Jan,8; 2016,Dec,11; 2016,Jan,7; 2016,Jan,13

99252 **Inpatient consultation for a new or established patient, which requires these 3 key components: An expanded problem focused history; An expanded problem focused examination; and Straightforward medical decision making. Counseling and/or coordination of care with other physicians, other qualified health care professionals, or agencies are provided consistent with the nature of the problem(s) and the patient's and/or family's needs. Usually, the presenting problem(s) are of low severity. Typically, 40 minutes are spent at the bedside and on the patient's hospital floor or unit.**

2.11 2.11 **FUD** XXX ★ E

AMA: 2020,Sep,3; 2018,Jan,8; 2017,Aug,3; 2017,Jun,6; 2017,Jan,8; 2016,Dec,11; 2016,Jan,13; 2016,Jan,7

99253 **Inpatient consultation for a new or established patient, which requires these 3 key components: A detailed history; A detailed examination; and Medical decision making of low complexity. Counseling and/or coordination of care with other physicians, other qualified health care professionals, or agencies are provided consistent with the nature of the problem(s) and the patient's and/or family's needs. Usually, the presenting problem(s) are of moderate severity. Typically, 55 minutes are spent at the bedside and on the patient's hospital floor or unit.**

3.25 3.25 **FUD** XXX ★ E

AMA: 2020,Sep,3; 2018,Jan,8; 2017,Aug,3; 2017,Jun,6; 2017,Jan,8; 2016,Dec,11; 2016,Jan,13; 2016,Jan,7

99254 **Inpatient consultation for a new or established patient, which requires these 3 key components: A comprehensive history; A comprehensive examination; and Medical decision making of moderate complexity. Counseling and/or coordination of care with other physicians, other qualified health care professionals, or agencies are provided consistent with the nature of the problem(s) and the patient's and/or family's needs. Usually, the presenting problem(s) are of moderate to high severity. Typically, 80 minutes are spent at the bedside and on the patient's hospital floor or unit.**

4.72 4.72 **FUD** XXX ★ E

AMA: 2020,Sep,3; 2018,Jan,8; 2017,Aug,3; 2017,Jun,6; 2017,Jan,8; 2016,Dec,11; 2016,Jan,7; 2016,Jan,13

99255 **Inpatient consultation for a new or established patient, which requires these 3 key components: A comprehensive history; A comprehensive examination; and Medical decision making of high complexity. Counseling and/or coordination of care with other physicians, other qualified health care professionals, or agencies are provided consistent with the nature of the problem(s) and the patient's and/or family's needs. Usually, the presenting problem(s) are of moderate to high severity. Typically, 110 minutes are spent at the bedside and on the patient's hospital floor or unit.**

5.76 5.76 **FUD** XXX ★ E

AMA: 2020,Sep,3; 2018,Jan,8; 2017,Aug,3; 2017,Jun,6; 2017,Jan,8; 2016,Dec,11; 2016,Jan,7; 2016,Jan,13

99281-99288 Emergency Department Visits

CMS: 100-04,11,40.1.3 Independent Attending Physician Services; 100-04,12,30.6.11 Emergency Department Visits; 100-04,4,160 Clinic and Emergency Visits Under OPPS

INCLUDES Any time spent with patient, which usually involves multiple encounters while patient in emergency department

Care provided to new and established patients

EXCLUDES *Critical care services (99291-99292)*

Observation services (99217-99220, 99234-99236)

99281 **Emergency department visit for the evaluation and management of a patient, which requires these 3 key components: A problem focused history; A problem focused examination; and Straightforward medical decision making. Counseling and/or coordination of care with other physicians, other qualified health care professionals, or agencies are provided consistent with the nature of the problem(s) and the patient's and/or family's needs. Usually, the presenting problem(s) are self limited or minor.**

0.60 0.60 **FUD** XXX J 80

AMA: 2020,Oct,13; 2020,Jul,13; 2019,Jul,10; 2018,Jan,8; 2017,Aug,3; 2017,Jun,6; 2017,Jan,8; 2016,Jan,13; 2016,Jan,7

99282 **Emergency department visit for the evaluation and management of a patient, which requires these 3 key components: An expanded problem focused history; An expanded problem focused examination; and Medical decision making of low complexity. Counseling and/or coordination of care with other physicians, other qualified health care professionals, or agencies are provided consistent with the nature of the problem(s) and the patient's and/or family's needs. Usually, the presenting problem(s) are of low to moderate severity.**

1.17 1.17 **FUD** XXX J 80

AMA: 2020,Oct,13; 2020,Jul,13; 2019,Jul,10; 2018,Jan,8; 2017,Aug,3; 2017,Jun,6; 2017,Jan,8; 2016,Jan,13; 2016,Jan,7

99283 **Emergency department visit for the evaluation and management of a patient, which requires these 3 key components: An expanded problem focused history; An expanded problem focused examination; and Medical decision making of moderate complexity. Counseling and/or coordination of care with other physicians, other qualified health care professionals, or agencies are provided consistent with the nature of the problem(s) and the patient's and/or family's needs. Usually, the presenting problem(s) are of moderate severity.**

1.75 1.75 **FUD** XXX J 80

AMA: 2020,Oct,13; 2020,Jul,13; 2019,Jul,10; 2018,Jan,8; 2017,Aug,3; 2017,Jun,6; 2017,Jan,8; 2016,Jan,7; 2016,Jan,13

99284 **Emergency department visit for the evaluation and management of a patient, which requires these 3 key components: A detailed history; A detailed examination; and Medical decision making of moderate complexity. Counseling and/or coordination of care with other physicians, other qualified health care professionals, or agencies are provided consistent with the nature of the problem(s) and the patient's and/or family's needs. Usually, the presenting problem(s) are of high severity, and require urgent evaluation by the physician, or other qualified health care professionals but do not pose an immediate significant threat to life or physiologic function.**

3.32 3.32 **FUD** XXX J 80

AMA: 2020,Oct,13; 2020,Jul,13; 2019,Jul,10; 2018,Jan,8; 2017,Aug,3; 2017,Jun,6; 2017,Jan,8; 2016,Jan,13; 2016,Jan,7

99285 **Emergency department visit for the evaluation and management of a patient, which requires these 3 key components within the constraints imposed by the urgency of the patient's clinical condition and/or mental status: A comprehensive history; A comprehensive examination; and Medical decision making of high complexity. Counseling and/or coordination of care with other physicians, other qualified health care professionals, or agencies are provided consistent with the nature of the problem(s) and the patient's and/or family's needs. Usually, the presenting problem(s) are of high severity and pose an immediate significant threat to life or physiologic function.**

4.89 4.89 **FUD** XXX J 80

AMA: 2020,Oct,13; 2020,Jul,13; 2020,Jan,12; 2019,Jul,10; 2018,Jan,8; 2017,Aug,3; 2017,Jun,6; 2017,Jan,8; 2016,Jan,13; 2016,Jan,7

99288 **Physician or other qualified health care professional direction of emergency medical systems (EMS) emergency care, advanced life support**

INCLUDES Management provided by emergency/intensive care based physician or other qualified health care professional via voice contact to ambulance/rescue staff for services such as heart monitoring and drug administration

0.00 0.00 **FUD** XXX B

AMA: 2018,Jan,8; 2017,Aug,3; 2017,Jun,6; 2017,Jan,8; 2016,Jan,13

Evaluation and Management

99254 — 99288

99291-99292 Critical Care Visits: Patients 72 Months of Age and Older

CMS: 100-04,11,40.1.3 Independent Attending Physician Services; 100-04,12,30.6.4 Services Furnished Incident to Physician's Service; 100-04,12,30.6.9 Payment for Inpatient Hospital Visits - General; 100-04,12,40.3 Global Surgery Review; 100-04,4,160 Clinic and Emergency Visits Under OPPS; 100-04,4,160.1 Critical Care Services

INCLUDES 30 minutes or more direct care provided by physician or other qualified health care professional to critically ill or injured patient, any location
All activities performed outside unit or off floor
All time spent exclusively with patient/family/caregivers on nursing unit or elsewhere
Outpatient critical care provided to neonates and pediatric patients age 71 months or younger
Physician or other qualified health care professional presence during interfacility transfer for critically ill/injured patients age 24 months or older
Professional services for interpretation:
Blood gases
Chest films (71045-71046)
Measurement cardiac output (93598)
Other computer stored information
Pulse oximetry (94760-94762)
Professional services:
Gastric intubation (43752-43753)
Transcutaneous pacing, temporary (92953)
Venous access, arterial puncture (36000, 36410, 36415, 36591, 36600)
Ventilation assistance and management, includes CPAP, CNP (94002-94004, 94660, 94662)

EXCLUDES *All services less than 30 minutes; report appropriate E/M code*
Inpatient critical care services provided to child age 2 through 5 years old (99475-99476)
Inpatient critical care services provided to infants age 29 days through 24 months old (99471-99472)
Inpatient critical care services provided to neonates age 28 days or younger (99468-99469)
Other procedures not listed as included performed by physician or other qualified health care professional rendering critical care
Patients not critically ill but in critical care department (report appropriate E/M code)
Physician or other qualified health care professional presence during interfacility transfer for critically ill/injured patients age 24 months or younger (99466-99467)
Supervisory services control physician during interfacility transfer for critically ill/injured patients age 24 months or younger ([99485, 99486])

99291 **Critical care, evaluation and management of the critically ill or critically injured patient; first 30-74 minutes**
6.28 7.82 FUD XXX J 80
AMA: 2020,Feb,7; 2020,Jan,12; 2019,Dec,14; 2019,Aug,8; 2019,Jul,10; 2018,Dec,8; 2018,Dec,8; 2018,Jun,9; 2018,Jan,8; 2017,Aug,3; 2017,Jun,6; 2017,Jan,8; 2016,Oct,8; 2016,Aug,9; 2016,May,3; 2016,Jan,13

+ **99292** **each additional 30 minutes (List separately in addition to code for primary service)**
Code first (99291)
3.15 3.46 FUD ZZZ N 80
AMA: 2020,Feb,7; 2019,Dec,14; 2019,Aug,8; 2019,Jul,10; 2018,Dec,8; 2018,Dec,8; 2018,Jun,9; 2018,Jan,8; 2017,Aug,3; 2017,Jun,6; 2017,Jan,8; 2016,Aug,9; 2016,May,3; 2016,Jan,13

99304-99310 Nursing Facility Visits

CMS: 100-04,11,40.1.3 Independent Attending Physician Services; 100-04,12,230 Primary Care Incentive Payment Program; 100-04,12,230.1 Definition of Primary Care Practitioners and Services; 100-04,12,230.2 Coordination with Other Payments; 100-04,12,230.3 Claims Processing and Payment; 100-04,12,30.6.10 Consultation Services; 100-04,12,30.6.13 Nursing Facility Visits; 100-04,12,30.6.15.1 Prolonged Services With Direct Face-to-Face Patient Contact; 100-04,12,30.6.4 Services Furnished Incident to Physician's Service; 100-04,12,30.6.9 Payment for Inpatient Hospital Visits - General

INCLUDES All E/M services provided by admitting physician on nursing facility admission date in other locations (e.g., office, emergency department)
Initial care, subsequent care, discharge, and yearly assessments
Initial services include patient assessment and physician participation in developing plan of care (99304-99306)
Services provided in psychiatric residential treatment center
Services provided to new and established patients in nursing facility (skilled, intermediate, and long-term care facilities)
Subsequent services include physician review medical records, reassessment, and review test results (99307-99310)

EXCLUDES *Care plan oversight services (99379-99380)*

Code also hospital discharge services on same admission or readmission date to nursing home (99217, 99234-99236, 99238-99239)

99304 **Initial nursing facility care, per day, for the evaluation and management of a patient, which requires these 3 key components: A detailed or comprehensive history; A detailed or comprehensive examination; and Medical decision making that is straightforward or of low complexity. Counseling and/or coordination of care with other physicians, other qualified health care professionals, or agencies are provided consistent with the nature of the problem(s) and the patient's and/or family's needs. Usually, the problem(s) requiring admission are of low severity. Typically, 25 minutes are spent at the bedside and on the patient's facility floor or unit.**
2.54 2.54 FUD XXX B 80
AMA: 2020,Nov,3; 2020,Sep,3; 2018,Jan,8; 2017,Aug,3; 2017,Jun,6; 2017,Jan,8; 2016,Dec,11; 2016,Jan,7; 2016,Jan,13

99305 **Initial nursing facility care, per day, for the evaluation and management of a patient, which requires these 3 key components: A comprehensive history; A comprehensive examination; and Medical decision making of moderate complexity. Counseling and/or coordination of care with other physicians, other qualified health care professionals, or agencies are provided consistent with the nature of the problem(s) and the patient's and/or family's needs. Usually, the problem(s) requiring admission are of moderate severity. Typically, 35 minutes are spent at the bedside and on the patient's facility floor or unit.**
3.67 3.67 FUD XXX B 80
AMA: 2020,Nov,3; 2020,Sep,3; 2018,Jan,8; 2017,Aug,3; 2017,Jun,6; 2017,Jan,8; 2016,Dec,11; 2016,Jan,7; 2016,Jan,13

99306 **Initial nursing facility care, per day, for the evaluation and management of a patient, which requires these 3 key components: A comprehensive history; A comprehensive examination; and Medical decision making of high complexity. Counseling and/or coordination of care with other physicians, other qualified health care professionals, or agencies are provided consistent with the nature of the problem(s) and the patient's and/or family's needs. Usually, the problem(s) requiring admission are of high severity. Typically, 45 minutes are spent at the bedside and on the patient's facility floor or unit.**
4.71 4.71 FUD XXX B 80
AMA: 2020,Nov,3; 2020,Sep,3; 2018,Jan,8; 2017,Aug,3; 2017,Jun,6; 2017,Jan,8; 2016,Dec,11; 2016,Jan,7; 2016,Jan,13

99307 **Subsequent nursing facility care, per day, for the evaluation and management of a patient, which requires at least 2 of these 3 key components: A problem focused interval history; A problem focused examination; Straightforward medical decision making. Counseling and/or coordination of care with other physicians, other qualified health care professionals, or agencies are provided consistent with the nature of the problem(s) and the patient's and/or family's needs. Usually, the patient is stable, recovering, or improving. Typically, 10 minutes are spent at the bedside and on the patient's facility floor or unit.**

1.24 1.24 FUD XXX ★ B 80

AMA: 2020,Nov,3; 2020,Sep,3; 2018,Jan,8; 2017,Aug,3; 2017,Jun,6; 2017,Jan,8; 2016,Dec,11; 2016,Jan,13; 2016,Jan,7

99308 **Subsequent nursing facility care, per day, for the evaluation and management of a patient, which requires at least 2 of these 3 key components: An expanded problem focused interval history; An expanded problem focused examination; Medical decision making of low complexity. Counseling and/or coordination of care with other physicians, other qualified health care professionals, or agencies are provided consistent with the nature of the problem(s) and the patient's and/or family's needs. Usually, the patient is responding inadequately to therapy or has developed a minor complication. Typically, 15 minutes are spent at the bedside and on the patient's facility floor or unit.**

1.94 1.94 FUD XXX ★ B 80

AMA: 2020,Nov,3; 2020,Sep,3; 2018,Jan,8; 2017,Aug,3; 2017,Jun,6; 2017,Jan,8; 2016,Dec,11; 2016,Jan,13; 2016,Jan,7

99309 **Subsequent nursing facility care, per day, for the evaluation and management of a patient, which requires at least 2 of these 3 key components: A detailed interval history; A detailed examination; Medical decision making of moderate complexity. Counseling and/or coordination of care with other physicians, other qualified health care professionals, or agencies are provided consistent with the nature of the problem(s) and the patient's and/or family's needs. Usually, the patient has developed a significant complication or a significant new problem. Typically, 25 minutes are spent at the bedside and on the patient's facility floor or unit.**

2.58 2.58 FUD XXX ★ B 80

AMA: 2020,Nov,3; 2020,Sep,3; 2018,Jan,8; 2017,Aug,3; 2017,Jun,6; 2017,Jan,8; 2016,Dec,11; 2016,Jan,13; 2016,Jan,7

99310 **Subsequent nursing facility care, per day, for the evaluation and management of a patient, which requires at least 2 of these 3 key components: A comprehensive interval history; A comprehensive examination; Medical decision making of high complexity. Counseling and/or coordination of care with other physicians, other qualified health care professionals, or agencies are provided consistent with the nature of the problem(s) and the patient's and/or family's needs. The patient may be unstable or may have developed a significant new problem requiring immediate physician attention. Typically, 35 minutes are spent at the bedside and on the patient's facility floor or unit.**

3.82 3.82 FUD XXX ★ B 80

AMA: 2020,Nov,3; 2020,Sep,3; 2018,Jan,8; 2017,Aug,3; 2017,Jun,6; 2017,Jan,8; 2016,Dec,11; 2016,Jan,13; 2016,Jan,7

99315-99316 Nursing Home Discharge

CMS: 100-04,11,40.1.3 Independent Attending Physician Services; 100-04,12,230 Primary Care Incentive Payment Program; 100-04,12,230.1 Definition of Primary Care Practitioners and Services; 100-04,12,230.2 Coordination with Other Payments; 100-04,12,230.3 Claims Processing and Payment; 100-04,12,30.6.13 Nursing Facility Visits; 100-04,12,30.6.4 Services Furnished Incident to Physician's Service; 100-04,12,40.3 Global Surgery Review

INCLUDES Discharge services include all time spent by physician or other qualified health care professional:
- Completion discharge records
- Discharge instructions for patient and caregivers
- Discussion regarding stay in facility
- Final patient examination
- Provide prescriptions and referrals as appropriate

99315 **Nursing facility discharge day management; 30 minutes or less**

2.07 2.07 FUD XXX B 80

AMA: 2020,Nov,3; 2018,Jan,8; 2017,Aug,3; 2017,Jun,6; 2017,Jan,8; 2016,Dec,11; 2016,Jan,7; 2016,Jan,13

99316 **more than 30 minutes**

2.98 2.98 FUD XXX B 80

AMA: 2020,Nov,3; 2018,Jan,8; 2017,Aug,3; 2017,Jun,6; 2017,Jan,8; 2016,Dec,11; 2016,Jan,7; 2016,Jan,13

99318 Annual Nursing Home Assessment

CMS: 100-04,11,40.1.3 Independent Attending Physician Services; 100-04,12,230 Primary Care Incentive Payment Program; 100-04,12,230.1 Definition of Primary Care Practitioners and Services; 100-04,12,230.2 Coordination with Other Payments; 100-04,12,230.3 Claims Processing and Payment; 100-04,12,30.6.13 Nursing Facility Visits; 100-04,12,30.6.15.1 Prolonged Services With Direct Face-to-Face Patient Contact; 100-04,12,30.6.4 Services Furnished Incident to Physician's Service; 100-04,12,30.6.9 Payment for Inpatient Hospital Visits - General

INCLUDES Includes nursing facility visits on same date as (99304-99316)

99318 **Evaluation and management of a patient involving an annual nursing facility assessment, which requires these 3 key components: A detailed interval history; A comprehensive examination; and Medical decision making that is of low to moderate complexity. Counseling and/or coordination of care with other physicians, other qualified health care professionals, or agencies are provided consistent with the nature of the problem(s) and the patient's and/or family's needs. Usually, the patient is stable, recovering, or improving. Typically, 30 minutes are spent at the bedside and on the patient's facility floor or unit.**

2.70 2.70 FUD XXX B 80

AMA: 2020,Nov,3; 2018,Jan,8; 2017,Aug,3; 2017,Jun,6; 2017,Jan,8; 2016,Dec,11; 2016,Jan,7; 2016,Jan,13

99324-99337 Domiciliary Care, Rest Home, Assisted Living Visits

CMS: 100-04,12,230 Primary Care Incentive Payment Program; 100-04,12,230.1 Definition of Primary Care Practitioners and Services; 100-04,12,230.2 Coordination with Other Payments; 100-04,12,230.3 Claims Processing and Payment; 100-04,12,30.6.14 Domiciliary Care, Rest Home, Assisted Living Visits; 100-04,12,30.6.15.1 Prolonged Services With Direct Face-to-Face Patient Contact; 100-04,12,30.6.4 Services Furnished Incident to Physician's Service

INCLUDES E/M services for patients residing in assisted living, domiciliary care, and rest homes where medical care not included
Services provided to new patients or established patients (99324-99328, 99334-99337)

EXCLUDES *Care plan oversight services provided to patient in rest home under home health agency care (99374-99375)*
Care plan oversight services provided to patient under hospice agency care (99377-99378)

99324 **Domiciliary or rest home visit for the evaluation and management of a new patient, which requires these 3 key components: A problem focused history; A problem focused examination; and Straightforward medical decision making. Counseling and/or coordination of care with other physicians, other qualified health care professionals, or agencies are provided consistent with the nature of the problem(s) and the patient's and/or family's needs. Usually, the presenting problem(s) are of low severity. Typically, 20 minutes are spent with the patient and/or family or caregiver.**

1.56 1.56 **FUD** XXX B 80

AMA: 2020,Sep,3; 2018,Apr,9; 2018,Jan,8; 2017,Aug,3; 2017,Jun,6; 2017,Jan,8; 2016,Dec,11; 2016,Jan,7; 2016,Jan,13

99325 **Domiciliary or rest home visit for the evaluation and management of a new patient, which requires these 3 key components: An expanded problem focused history; An expanded problem focused examination; and Medical decision making of low complexity. Counseling and/or coordination of care with other physicians, other qualified health care professionals, or agencies are provided consistent with the nature of the problem(s) and the patient's and/or family's needs. Usually, the presenting problem(s) are of moderate severity. Typically, 30 minutes are spent with the patient and/or family or caregiver.**

2.26 2.26 **FUD** XXX B 80

AMA: 2020,Sep,3; 2018,Apr,9; 2018,Jan,8; 2017,Aug,3; 2017,Jun,6; 2017,Jan,8; 2016,Dec,11; 2016,Jan,7; 2016,Jan,13

99326 **Domiciliary or rest home visit for the evaluation and management of a new patient, which requires these 3 key components: A detailed history; A detailed examination; and Medical decision making of moderate complexity. Counseling and/or coordination of care with other physicians, other qualified health care professionals, or agencies are provided consistent with the nature of the problem(s) and the patient's and/or family's needs. Usually, the presenting problem(s) are of moderate to high severity. Typically, 45 minutes are spent with the patient and/or family or caregiver.**

3.92 3.92 **FUD** XXX B 80

AMA: 2020,Sep,3; 2018,Apr,9; 2018,Jan,8; 2017,Aug,3; 2017,Jun,6; 2017,Jan,8; 2016,Dec,11; 2016,Jan,7; 2016,Jan,13

99327 **Domiciliary or rest home visit for the evaluation and management of a new patient, which requires these 3 key components: A comprehensive history; A comprehensive examination; and Medical decision making of moderate complexity. Counseling and/or coordination of care with other physicians, other qualified health care professionals, or agencies are provided consistent with the nature of the problem(s) and the patient's and/or family's needs. Usually, the presenting problem(s) are of high severity. Typically, 60 minutes are spent with the patient and/or family or caregiver.**

5.26 5.26 **FUD** XXX B 80

AMA: 2020,Sep,3; 2018,Apr,9; 2018,Jan,8; 2017,Aug,3; 2017,Jun,6; 2017,Jan,8; 2016,Dec,11; 2016,Jan,7; 2016,Jan,13

99328 **Domiciliary or rest home visit for the evaluation and management of a new patient, which requires these 3 key components: A comprehensive history; A comprehensive examination; and Medical decision making of high complexity. Counseling and/or coordination of care with other physicians, other qualified health care professionals, or agencies are provided consistent with the nature of the problem(s) and the patient's and/or family's needs. Usually, the patient is unstable or has developed a significant new problem requiring immediate physician attention. Typically, 75 minutes are spent with the patient and/or family or caregiver.**

6.19 6.19 **FUD** XXX B 80

AMA: 2020,Sep,3; 2018,Apr,9; 2018,Jan,8; 2017,Aug,3; 2017,Jun,6; 2017,Jan,8; 2016,Dec,11; 2016,Jan,7; 2016,Jan,13

99334 **Domiciliary or rest home visit for the evaluation and management of an established patient, which requires at least 2 of these 3 key components: A problem focused interval history; A problem focused examination; Straightforward medical decision making. Counseling and/or coordination of care with other physicians, other qualified health care professionals, or agencies are provided consistent with the nature of the problem(s) and the patient's and/or family's needs. Usually, the presenting problem(s) are self-limited or minor. Typically, 15 minutes are spent with the patient and/or family or caregiver.**

1.70 1.70 **FUD** XXX B 80

AMA: 2020,Sep,3; 2018,Apr,9; 2018,Jan,8; 2017,Aug,3; 2017,Jun,6; 2017,Jan,8; 2016,Dec,11; 2016,Jan,7; 2016,Jan,13

99335 **Domiciliary or rest home visit for the evaluation and management of an established patient, which requires at least 2 of these 3 key components: An expanded problem focused interval history; An expanded problem focused examination; Medical decision making of low complexity. Counseling and/or coordination of care with other physicians, other qualified health care professionals, or agencies are provided consistent with the nature of the problem(s) and the patient's and/or family's needs. Usually, the presenting problem(s) are of low to moderate severity. Typically, 25 minutes are spent with the patient and/or family or caregiver.**

2.68 2.68 **FUD** XXX B 80

AMA: 2020,Sep,3; 2018,Apr,9; 2018,Jan,8; 2017,Aug,3; 2017,Jun,6; 2017,Jan,8; 2016,Dec,11; 2016,Jan,7; 2016,Jan,13

99336 **Domiciliary or rest home visit for the evaluation and management of an established patient, which requires at least 2 of these 3 key components: A detailed interval history; A detailed examination; Medical decision making of moderate complexity. Counseling and/or coordination of care with other physicians, other qualified health care professionals, or agencies are provided consistent with the nature of the problem(s) and the patient's and/or family's needs. Usually, the presenting problem(s) are of moderate to high severity. Typically, 40 minutes are spent with the patient and/or family or caregiver.**

3.82 3.82 **FUD** XXX B 80

AMA: 2020,Sep,3; 2018,Apr,9; 2018,Jan,8; 2017,Aug,3; 2017,Jun,6; 2017,Jan,8; 2016,Dec,11; 2016,Jan,7; 2016,Jan,13

99337 Domiciliary or rest home visit for the evaluation and management of an established patient, which requires at least 2 of these 3 key components: A comprehensive interval history; A comprehensive examination; Medical decision making of moderate to high complexity. Counseling and/or coordination of care with other physicians, other qualified health care professionals, or agencies are provided consistent with the nature of the problem(s) and the patient's and/or family's needs. Usually, the presenting problem(s) are of moderate to high severity. The patient may be unstable or may have developed a significant new problem requiring immediate physician attention. Typically, 60 minutes are spent with the patient and/or family or caregiver.

5.47 5.47 FUD XXX

AMA: 2020,Sep,3; 2018,Apr,9; 2018,Jan,8; 2017,Aug,3; 2017,Jun,6; 2017,Jan,8; 2016,Dec,11; 2016,Jan,7; 2016,Jan,13

99339-99340 Care Plan Oversight: Rest Home, Domiciliary Care, Assisted Living, and Home

CMS: 100-04,12,180 Payment of Care Plan Oversight (CPO); 100-04,12,180.1 Billing for Care Plan Oversight (CPO); 100-04,12,230 Primary Care Incentive Payment Program; 100-04,12,230.1 Definition of Primary Care Practitioners and Services; 100-04,12,230.2 Coordination with Other Payments; 100-04,12,230.3 Claims Processing and Payment; 100-04,12,30.6.14 Domiciliary Care, Rest Home, Assisted Living Visits; 100-04,12,30.6.4 Services Furnished Incident to Physician's Service

INCLUDES Care plan oversight for patients residing in assisted living, domiciliary care, private residences, and rest homes

Online or telephone services during same time frame ([99421, 99422, 99423], 99441-99443, 98966-98968)

EXCLUDES *Care plan oversight services furnished under home health agency, nursing facility, or hospice (99374-99380)*

Services during the same time frame:

Chronic/complex chronic care management ([99437], [99439], [99490], [99491], 99487, 99489)

Principal care management ([99424, 99425, 99426, 99427])

99339 Individual physician supervision of a patient (patient not present) in home, domiciliary or rest home (eg, assisted living facility) requiring complex and multidisciplinary care modalities involving regular physician development and/or revision of care plans, review of subsequent reports of patient status, review of related laboratory and other studies, communication (including telephone calls) for purposes of assessment or care decisions with health care professional(s), family member(s), surrogate decision maker(s) (eg, legal guardian) and/or key caregiver(s) involved in patient's care, integration of new information into the medical treatment plan and/or adjustment of medical therapy, within a calendar month; 15-29 minutes

2.17 2.17 FUD XXX

AMA: 2019,Jan,6; 2018,Oct,9; 2018,Jan,8; 2017,Aug,3; 2017,Jun,6; 2017,Jan,8; 2016,Jan,13

99340 30 minutes or more

3.05 3.05 FUD XXX

AMA: 2019,Jan,6; 2018,Oct,9; 2018,Jan,8; 2017,Aug,3; 2017,Jun,6; 2017,Jan,8; 2016,Jan,13

99341-99350 Home Visits

CMS: 100-04,11,40.1.3 Independent Attending Physician Services; 100-04,12,230 Primary Care Incentive Payment Program; 100-04,12,230.1 Definition of Primary Care Practitioners and Services; 100-04,12,230.2 Coordination with Other Payments; 100-04,12,230.3 Claims Processing and Payment; 100-04,12,30.6.14 Domiciliary Care, Rest Home, Assisted Living Visits; 100-04,12,30.6.14.1 Home Visits; 100-04,12,30.6.15.1 Prolonged Services With Direct Face-to-Face Patient Contact; 100-04,12,30.6.4 Services Furnished Incident to Physician's Service; 100-04,12,40.3 Global Surgery Review; 100-04,30.6.14.1 Home Services (Codes 99341 - 99350)

INCLUDES Services for new or established patient (99341-99345, 99347-99350)

Services provided to patient in private home (e.g., private residence, temporary or short-term housing such as campground, cruise ship, hostel, or hotel)

EXCLUDES *Services provided to patients under home health agency or hospice care (99374-99378)*

99341 Home visit for the evaluation and management of a new patient, which requires these 3 key components: A problem focused history; A problem focused examination; and Straightforward medical decision making. Counseling and/or coordination of care with other physicians, other qualified health care professionals, or agencies are provided consistent with the nature of the problem(s) and the patient's and/or family's needs. Usually, the presenting problem(s) are of low severity. Typically, 20 minutes are spent face-to-face with the patient and/or family.

1.56 1.56 FUD XXX

AMA: 2020,Nov,3; 2020,Sep,3; 2018,Apr,9; 2018,Jan,8; 2017,Aug,3; 2017,Jun,6; 2017,Jan,8; 2016,Dec,11; 2016,Jan,13; 2016,Jan,7

99342 Home visit for the evaluation and management of a new patient, which requires these 3 key components: An expanded problem focused history; An expanded problem focused examination; and Medical decision making of low complexity. Counseling and/or coordination of care with other physicians, other qualified health care professionals, or agencies are provided consistent with the nature of the problem(s) and the patient's and/or family's needs. Usually, the presenting problem(s) are of moderate severity. Typically, 30 minutes are spent face-to-face with the patient and/or family.

2.25 2.25 FUD XXX

AMA: 2020,Nov,3; 2020,Sep,3; 2018,Apr,9; 2018,Jan,8; 2017,Aug,3; 2017,Jun,6; 2017,Jan,8; 2016,Dec,11; 2016,Jan,7; 2016,Jan,13

99343 Home visit for the evaluation and management of a new patient, which requires these 3 key components: A detailed history; A detailed examination; and Medical decision making of moderate complexity. Counseling and/or coordination of care with other physicians, other qualified health care professionals, or agencies are provided consistent with the nature of the problem(s) and the patient's and/or family's needs. Usually, the presenting problem(s) are of moderate to high severity. Typically, 45 minutes are spent face-to-face with the patient and/or family.

3.67 3.67 FUD XXX

AMA: 2020,Nov,3; 2020,Sep,3; 2018,Apr,9; 2018,Jan,8; 2017,Aug,3; 2017,Jun,6; 2017,Jan,8; 2016,Dec,11; 2016,Jan,13; 2016,Jan,7

99344 Home visit for the evaluation and management of a new patient, which requires these 3 key components: A comprehensive history; A comprehensive examination; and Medical decision making of moderate complexity. Counseling and/or coordination of care with other physicians, other qualified health care professionals, or agencies are provided consistent with the nature of the problem(s) and the patient's and/or family's needs. Usually, the presenting problem(s) are of high severity. Typically, 60 minutes are spent face-to-face with the patient and/or family.

5.14 5.14 FUD XXX

AMA: 2020,Nov,3; 2020,Sep,3; 2018,Apr,9; 2018,Jan,8; 2017,Aug,3; 2017,Jun,6; 2017,Jan,8; 2016,Dec,11; 2016,Jan,13; 2016,Jan,7

99345 **Home visit for the evaluation and management of a new patient, which requires these 3 key components: A comprehensive history; A comprehensive examination; and Medical decision making of high complexity. Counseling and/or coordination of care with other physicians, other qualified health care professionals, or agencies are provided consistent with the nature of the problem(s) and the patient's and/or family's needs. Usually, the patient is unstable or has developed a significant new problem requiring immediate physician attention. Typically, 75 minutes are spent face-to-face with the patient and/or family.**

6.25 6.25 FUD XXX B 80

AMA: 2020,Nov,3; 2020,Sep,3; 2018,Apr,9; 2018,Jan,8; 2017,Aug,3; 2017,Jun,6; 2017,Jan,8; 2016,Dec,11; 2016,Jan,13; 2016,Jan,7

99347 **Home visit for the evaluation and management of an established patient, which requires at least 2 of these 3 key components: A problem focused interval history; A problem focused examination; Straightforward medical decision making. Counseling and/or coordination of care with other physicians, other qualified health care professionals, or agencies are provided consistent with the nature of the problem(s) and the patient's and/or family's needs. Usually, the presenting problem(s) are self limited or minor. Typically, 15 minutes are spent face-to-face with the patient and/or family.**

1.56 1.56 FUD XXX B 80

AMA: 2020,Nov,3; 2020,Sep,3; 2018,Apr,9; 2018,Jan,8; 2017,Aug,3; 2017,Jun,6; 2017,Jan,8; 2016,Dec,11; 2016,Jan,13; 2016,Jan,7

99348 **Home visit for the evaluation and management of an established patient, which requires at least 2 of these 3 key components: An expanded problem focused interval history; An expanded problem focused examination; Medical decision making of low complexity. Counseling and/or coordination of care with other physicians, other qualified health care professionals, or agencies are provided consistent with the nature of the problem(s) and the patient's and/or family's needs. Usually, the presenting problem(s) are of low to moderate severity. Typically, 25 minutes are spent face-to-face with the patient and/or family.**

2.37 2.37 FUD XXX B 80

AMA: 2020,Nov,3; 2020,Sep,3; 2018,Apr,9; 2018,Jan,8; 2017,Aug,3; 2017,Jun,6; 2017,Jan,8; 2016,Dec,11; 2016,Jan,13; 2016,Jan,7

99349 **Home visit for the evaluation and management of an established patient, which requires at least 2 of these 3 key components: A detailed interval history; A detailed examination; Medical decision making of moderate complexity. Counseling and/or coordination of care with other physicians, other qualified health care professionals, or agencies are provided consistent with the nature of the problem(s) and the patient's and/or family's needs. Usually, the presenting problem(s) are moderate to high severity. Typically, 40 minutes are spent face-to-face with the patient and/or family.**

3.64 3.64 FUD XXX B 80

AMA: 2020,Nov,3; 2020,Sep,3; 2018,Apr,9; 2018,Jan,8; 2017,Aug,3; 2017,Jun,6; 2017,Jan,8; 2016,Dec,11; 2016,Jan,13; 2016,Jan,7

99350 **Home visit for the evaluation and management of an established patient, which requires at least 2 of these 3 key components: A comprehensive interval history; A comprehensive examination; Medical decision making of moderate to high complexity. Counseling and/or coordination of care with other physicians, other qualified health care professionals, or agencies are provided consistent with the nature of the problem(s) and the patient's and/or family's needs. Usually, the presenting problem(s) are of moderate to high severity. The patient may be unstable or may have developed a significant new problem requiring immediate physician attention. Typically, 60 minutes are spent face-to-face with the patient and/or family.**

5.05 5.05 FUD XXX B 80

AMA: 2020,Nov,3; 2020,Sep,3; 2018,Apr,9; 2018,Jan,8; 2017,Aug,3; 2017,Jun,6; 2017,Jan,8; 2016,Dec,11; 2016,Jan,13; 2016,Jan,7

99354-99357 Prolonged Services Direct Contact

CMS: 100-04,11,40.1.3 Independent Attending Physician Services; 100-04,12,30.6.15.1 Prolonged Services With Direct Face-to-Face Patient Contact; 100-04,12,30.6.4 Services Furnished Incident to Physician's Service

INCLUDES Personal contact with patient by physician or other qualified health professional
Services extending beyond customary service provided in inpatient, observation, or outpatient setting
Time spent providing additional indirect contact services on floor, hospital unit, or nursing facility during same session as direct contact
Time spent providing prolonged services on service date, even when time not continuous

EXCLUDES *Services less than 30 minutes, less than 15 minutes after first hour, or after final 30 minutes*
Services provided independent from personal contact date with patient (99358-99359)

Code first E/M service code, as appropriate

\+ **99354** **Prolonged service(s) in the outpatient setting requiring direct patient contact beyond the time of the usual service; first hour (List separately in addition to code for outpatient Evaluation and Management or psychotherapy service, except with office or other outpatient services [99202, 99203, 99204, 99205, 99212, 99213, 99214, 99215])**

EXCLUDES *Office or other outpatient visit (99202-99205, 99212-99215)*
Prolonged office/outpatient services ([99417])
Prolonged service provided by clinical staff under supervision ([99415, 99416])
Reporting code more than one time per service date

Code first (99241-99245, 99324-99337, 99341-99350, 90837, 90847)

3.44 3.67 FUD ZZZ ★ N 80

AMA: 2020,Dec,11; 2020,Sep,3; 2020,Feb,3; 2019,Oct,10; 2019,Jun,7; 2018,Jan,8; 2017,Jan,8; 2016,Dec,11; 2016,Jan,13

\+ **99355** **each additional 30 minutes (List separately in addition to code for prolonged service)**

EXCLUDES *Office or other outpatient visit (99202-99205, 99212-99215)*
Prolonged office/outpatient services ([99417])
Prolonged service provided by clinical staff under supervision ([99415, 99416])

Code first (99354)

2.60 2.80 FUD ZZZ ★ N 80

AMA: 2020,Dec,11; 2020,Sep,3; 2020,Feb,3; 2019,Oct,10; 2019,Jun,7; 2018,Jan,8; 2017,Jan,8; 2016,Dec,11; 2016,Jan,13

\+ **99356** **Prolonged service in the inpatient or observation setting, requiring unit/floor time beyond the usual service; first hour (List separately in addition to code for inpatient or observation Evaluation and Management service)**

EXCLUDES *Reporting code more than one time per service date*

Code first (99218-99223 [99224, 99225, 99226], 99231-99236, 99251-99255, 99304-99310, 90837, 90847)

2.60 2.60 FUD ZZZ ★ C 80

AMA: 2020,Dec,11; 2020,Sep,3; 2019,Jun,7; 2018,Jan,8; 2017,Jan,8; 2016,Dec,11; 2016,Jan,13

+ **99357** **each additional 30 minutes (List separately in addition to code for prolonged service)**

Code first (99356)

2.61 2.61 FUD ZZZ ★ C 80

AMA: 2020,Dec,11; 2020,Sep,3; 2019,Jun,7; 2018,Jan,8; 2017,Jan,8; 2016,Dec,11; 2016,Jan,13

99358-99359 Prolonged Services Indirect Contact

CMS: 100-04,11,40.1.3 Independent Attending Physician Services; 100-04,12,30.6.15.2 Prolonged Services Without Face to Face Service; 100-04,12,30.6.4 Services Furnished Incident to Physician's Service

INCLUDES Services extending beyond customary service

Time spent providing indirect contact services by physician or other qualified health care professional in relation to patient management where face-to-face services have or will occur on different date

Time spent providing prolonged services on service date, even when time not continuous

EXCLUDES *Any additional unit or floor time in hospital or nursing facility during same evaluation and management session*

Behavioral health integration care management services (99484)

Patient management services during same time frame as (99487-99489, 99495-99496)

Psychiatric collaborative care management services during same month (99492-99494)

Reporting code more than one time per service date

Services less than 30 minutes, less than15 minutes after first hour, or after final 30 minutes

Time without direct patient contact for other services:

Care plan oversight (99339-99340, 99374-99380)

Chronic care management services provided during same month ([99491])

INR monitoring services (93792-93793)

Medical team conference (99366-99368)

Online and telephone consultative services (99446-99452 [99451, 99452])

Online medical services ([99421, 99422, 99423])

Principal care management services ([99424])

Code also E/M or other services provided, excluding (99202-99205, 99212-99215, 99217)

99358 **Prolonged evaluation and management service before and/or after direct patient care; first hour**

EXCLUDES *Use of code more than one time per date of service*

3.15 3.15 FUD XXX N 80

AMA: 2020,Sep,3; 2020,Feb,3; 2019,Jun,7; 2019,Jan,13; 2018,Oct,9; 2018,Jan,8; 2017,Jan,8; 2016,Jan,13

+ **99359** **each additional 30 minutes (List separately in addition to code for prolonged service)**

Code first (99358)

1.52 1.52 FUD ZZZ N 80

AMA: 2020,Sep,3; 2020,Feb,3; 2019,Jun,7; 2019,Jan,13; 2018,Oct,9; 2018,Jan,8; 2017,Jan,8; 2016,Jan,13

99415-99417 [99415, 99416, 99417] Prolonged Clinical Staff Services Under Supervision

INCLUDES Time spent by clinical staff providing prolonged face-to-face services extending beyond customary service under physician or other qualified health professional supervision

Time spent by clinical staff providing prolonged services on service date, even when time not continuous

EXCLUDES *Prolonged service provided by physician or other qualified health care professional (99354-99355, [99417])*

+ # **99415** **Prolonged clinical staff service (the service beyond the highest time in the range of total time of the service) during an evaluation and management service in the office or outpatient setting, direct patient contact with physician supervision; first hour (List separately in addition to code for outpatient Evaluation and Management service)**

EXCLUDES *Reporting code more than one time per service date*

Reporting code with ([99417])

Services less than 30 minutes

Services provided to more than two patients at same time

Code first (99202-99205, 99212-99215)

0.28 0.28 FUD ZZZ N 80 TC

AMA: 2020,Nov,12; 2020,Sep,3; 2020,Feb,3; 2019,Oct,10; 2018,Jan,8; 2017,Jan,8; 2016,Mar,8; 2016,Feb,13; 2016,Jan,13

+ # **99416** **each additional 30 minutes (List separately in addition to code for prolonged service)**

EXCLUDES *Reporting code with ([99417])*

Services less than 30 minutes, less than15 minutes after first hour, or after final 30 minutes

Services provided to more than two patients at same time

Code first ([99415])

0.12 0.12 FUD ZZZ N 80 TC

AMA: 2020,Nov,12; 2020,Sep,3; 2020,Feb,3; 2019,Oct,10; 2018,Jan,8; 2017,Jan,8; 2016,Mar,8; 2016,Feb,13; 2016,Jan,13

+ # **99417** **Prolonged office or other outpatient evaluation and management service(s) beyond the minimum required time of the primary procedure which has been selected using total time, requiring total time with or without direct patient contact beyond the usual service, on the date of the primary service, each 15 minutes of total time (List separately in addition to codes 99205, 99215 for office or other outpatient Evaluation and Management services)**

INCLUDES Total time prolonged services provided same date with both direct and indirect patient contact by physician or QHCP

EXCLUDES *Services less than 15 minutes*

Code first (99205 or 99215)

0.93 0.96 FUD XXX ★

99360 Standby Services

CMS: 100-04,11,40.1.3 Independent Attending Physician Services; 100-04,12,30.6.15.3 Standby Services; 100-04,12,30.6.4 Services Furnished Incident to Physician's Service

INCLUDES Services requested by physician or qualified health care professional that involve no direct patient contact

Total standby time for day

EXCLUDES *Delivery attendance (99464)*

Less than 30 minutes standby time

On-call services mandated by hospital (99026-99027)

Code also as appropriate (99460, 99465)

99360 **Standby service, requiring prolonged attendance, each 30 minutes (eg, operative standby, standby for frozen section, for cesarean/high risk delivery, for monitoring EEG)**

1.73 1.73 FUD XXX B

AMA: 2018,Jan,8; 2017,Jan,8; 2016,Jan,13

99366-99368 Interdisciplinary Conferences

CMS: 100-04,11,40.1.3 Independent Attending Physician Services

INCLUDES Documentation conference participation, contribution, and recommendations

Face-to-face participation by minimum of three qualified people from different specialties or disciplines

Individual patient review from start to conclusion

Only participants who have performed face-to-face evaluations or direct treatment to patient within previous 60 days

Team conferences 30 minutes or more

EXCLUDES *Conferences less than 30 minutes (not reportable)*

More than one individual from same specialty at same encounter

Patient management services during same month as ([99424, 99425, 99426, 99427], [99437], [99439, 99490, 99491], 99487-99489)

Time spent record keeping or writing report

99366 **Medical team conference with interdisciplinary team of health care professionals, face-to-face with patient and/or family, 30 minutes or more, participation by nonphysician qualified health care professional**

EXCLUDES *Team conferences by physician with patient or family present, see appropriate E/M service code*

1.19 1.21 FUD XXX N

AMA: 2018,Apr,9; 2018,Jan,8; 2017,Jan,8; 2016,Jan,13

99367 **Medical team conference with interdisciplinary team of health care professionals, patient and/or family not present, 30 minutes or more; participation by physician**

1.60 1.60 FUD XXX N

AMA: 2019,Dec,14; 2018,Apr,9; 2018,Jan,8; 2017,Jan,8; 2016,Jan,13

99368 **participation by nonphysician qualified health care professional**
1.04 1.04 FUD XXX N
AMA: 2018,Apr,9; 2018,Jan,8; 2017,Jan,8; 2016,Jan,13

99374-99380 Care Plan Oversight: Patient Under Care of HHA, Hospice, or Nursing Facility

CMS: 100-04,11,40.1.3 Independent Attending Physician Services; 100-04,12,180 Payment of Care Plan Oversight (CPO); 100-04,12,180.1 Billing for Care Plan Oversight (CPO); 100-04,12,30.6.4 Services Furnished Incident to Physician's Service

INCLUDES Analysis reports, diagnostic tests, treatment plans
Discussions with other health care providers, outside practice, involved in patient's care
Establishment and revisions to care plans within 30-day period
Payment to one physician per month for covered care plan oversight services (must be same one who signed plan of care)

EXCLUDES *Care plan oversight services provided in hospice agency (99377-99378)*
Care plan oversight services provided in assisted living, domiciliary care, or private residence, not under home health agency or hospice care (99339-99340)
Patient management services during same time frame as ([99421, 99422, 99423], 99441-99443, 98966-98968)
Routine postoperative care provided during global surgery period
Time discussing treatment with patient and/or caregivers

Code also office/outpatient visits, hospital, home, nursing facility, domiciliary, or non-face-to-face services

99374 **Supervision of a patient under care of home health agency (patient not present) in home, domiciliary or equivalent environment (eg, Alzheimer's facility) requiring complex and multidisciplinary care modalities involving regular development and/or revision of care plans by that individual, review of subsequent reports of patient status, review of related laboratory and other studies, communication (including telephone calls) for purposes of assessment or care decisions with health care professional(s), family member(s), surrogate decision maker(s) (eg, legal guardian) and/or key caregiver(s) involved in patient's care, integration of new information into the medical treatment plan and/or adjustment of medical therapy, within a calendar month; 15-29 minutes**
EXCLUDES *Complex chronic care management services during same time frame as (99487, 99489)*
1.60 1.96 FUD XXX B
AMA: 2019,Jan,6; 2018,Jan,8; 2017,Jan,8; 2016,Jan,13

99375 **30 minutes or more**
EXCLUDES *Complex chronic care management services during same time frame as (99487, 99489)*
2.50 2.94 FUD XXX E
AMA: 2019,Jan,6; 2018,Jan,8; 2017,Jan,8; 2016,Jan,13

99377 **Supervision of a hospice patient (patient not present) requiring complex and multidisciplinary care modalities involving regular development and/or revision of care plans by that individual, review of subsequent reports of patient status, review of related laboratory and other studies, communication (including telephone calls) for purposes of assessment or care decisions with health care professional(s), family member(s), surrogate decision maker(s) (eg, legal guardian) and/or key caregiver(s) involved in patient's care, integration of new information into the medical treatment plan and/or adjustment of medical therapy, within a calendar month; 15-29 minutes**
EXCLUDES *Complex chronic care management services during same time frame as (99487, 99489)*
1.60 1.96 FUD XXX B
AMA: 2019,Jan,6; 2018,Jan,8; 2017,Jan,8; 2016,Jan,13

99378 **30 minutes or more**
EXCLUDES *Complex chronic care management services during same time frame as (99487, 99489)*
2.50 2.94 FUD XXX E
AMA: 2019,Jan,6; 2018,Jan,8; 2017,Jan,8; 2016,Jan,13

99379 **Supervision of a nursing facility patient (patient not present) requiring complex and multidisciplinary care modalities involving regular development and/or revision of care plans by that individual, review of subsequent reports of patient status, review of related laboratory and other studies, communication (including telephone calls) for purposes of assessment or care decisions with health care professional(s), family member(s), surrogate decision maker(s) (eg, legal guardian) and/or key caregiver(s) involved in patient's care, integration of new information into the medical treatment plan and/or adjustment of medical therapy, within a calendar month; 15-29 minutes**
1.60 1.96 FUD XXX B
AMA: 2019,Jan,6; 2018,Jan,8; 2017,Jan,8; 2016,Jan,13

99380 **30 minutes or more**
2.50 2.94 FUD XXX B
AMA: 2019,Jan,6; 2018,Jan,8; 2017,Jan,8; 2016,Jan,13

99381-99397 Preventive Medicine Visits

CMS: 100-04,11,40.1.3 Independent Attending Physician Services; 100-04,12,30.6.2 Medically Necessary and Preventive Medicine Service on Same Date; 100-04,12,30.6.4 Services Furnished Incident to Physician's Service

INCLUDES Care for small problem or pre-existing condition that requires no extra work
New patients or established patients (99381-99387, 99391-99397)
Regular preventive care (e.g., well-child exams) for all age groups

EXCLUDES *Behavioral change interventions (99406-99409)*
Counseling/risk factor reduction interventions not provided with preventive medical examination (99401-99412)
Diagnostic tests and other procedures

Code also:
Immunization counseling, administration, and product (90460-90461, 90471-90474, [0001A, 0002A], [0051A, 0052A, 0053A, 0054A], [0071A, 0072A], [0011A, 0012A], [0064A], [0021A, 0022A], [0031A], [0034A], [0041A, 0042A], [91300], [91305], [91307], [91301], [91306], [91302], [91303], [91304], [90619, 90620, 90621, 90625, 90626, 90627, 90630, 90644, 90672, 90673, 90674, 90677, 90694, 90750, 90756, 90758, 90759])
Significant, separately identifiable E/M service on same date for substantial problems requiring additional work append modifier 25 to (99202-99215)

99381 **Initial comprehensive preventive medicine evaluation and management of an individual including an age and gender appropriate history, examination, counseling/anticipatory guidance/risk factor reduction interventions, and the ordering of laboratory/diagnostic procedures, new patient; infant (age younger than 1 year)** A
2.17 3.13 FUD XXX E
AMA: 2018,Jan,8; 2017,Jan,8; 2016,Mar,8; 2016,Jan,13

99382 **early childhood (age 1 through 4 years)** A
2.32 3.28 FUD XXX E
AMA: 2018,Jan,8; 2017,Jan,8; 2016,Mar,8; 2016,Jan,13

99383 **late childhood (age 5 through 11 years)** A
2.46 3.41 FUD XXX E
AMA: 2018,Jan,8; 2017,Jan,8; 2016,Mar,8; 2016,Jan,13

99384 **adolescent (age 12 through 17 years)** A
2.88 3.85 FUD XXX E
AMA: 2018,Jan,8; 2017,Jan,8; 2016,Mar,8; 2016,Jan,13

99385 **18-39 years** A
2.76 3.72 FUD XXX E
AMA: 2018,Jan,8; 2017,Jan,8; 2016,Mar,8; 2016,Jan,13

99386 **40-64 years** A
3.36 4.32 FUD XXX E
AMA: 2018,Jan,8; 2017,Jan,8; 2016,Mar,8; 2016,Jan,13

99387 **65 years and older** A
3.61 4.68 FUD XXX E
AMA: 2018,Jan,8; 2017,Jan,8; 2016,Mar,8; 2016,Jan,13

99391 **Periodic comprehensive preventive medicine reevaluation and management of an individual including an age and gender appropriate history, examination, counseling/anticipatory guidance/risk factor reduction interventions, and the ordering of laboratory/diagnostic procedures, established patient; infant (age younger than 1 year)**
1.98 2.82 FUD XXX
AMA: 2018,Jan,8; 2017,Jan,8; 2016,Mar,8; 2016,Jan,13

99392 **early childhood (age 1 through 4 years)**
2.17 3.01 FUD XXX
AMA: 2018,Jan,8; 2017,Jan,8; 2016,Mar,8; 2016,Jan,13

99393 **late childhood (age 5 through 11 years)**
2.17 3.00 FUD XXX
AMA: 2018,Jan,8; 2017,Jan,8; 2016,Mar,8; 2016,Jan,13

99394 **adolescent (age 12 through 17 years)**
2.46 3.29 FUD XXX
AMA: 2018,Jan,8; 2017,Jan,8; 2016,Mar,8; 2016,Jan,13

99395 **18-39 years**
2.53 3.36 FUD XXX
AMA: 2018,Jan,8; 2017,Jan,8; 2016,Mar,8; 2016,Jan,13

99396 **40-64 years**
2.74 3.58 FUD XXX
AMA: 2018,Jan,8; 2017,Sep,11; 2017,Jan,8; 2016,Mar,8; 2016,Jan,13

99397 **65 years and older**
2.88 3.85 FUD XXX
AMA: 2018,Jan,8; 2017,Jan,8; 2016,Mar,8; 2016,Jan,13

99401-99423 [99415, 99416, 99417, 99421, 99422, 99423] Counseling Services: Risk Factor and Behavioral Change Modification

INCLUDES Face-to-face services for new and established patients based on 15- to 60-minute time increments
Health and behavioral services provided on same day (96156-96159 [96164, 96165, 96167, 96168, 96170, 96171])
Issues such as healthy diet, exercise, alcohol, and drug abuse
Services provided by physician or other qualified healthcare professional for promoting health and reducing illness and injury

EXCLUDES *Counseling and risk factor reduction interventions included in preventive medicine services (99381-99397)*
Counseling services provided to patient groups with existing symptoms or illness (99078)

Code also:
Immunization counseling, administration, and product (90460-90461, 90471-90474, [0001A, 0002A], [0051A, 0052A, 0053A, 0054A], [0071A, 0072A], [0011A, 0012A], [0064A], [0021A, 0022A], [0031A], [0034A], [0041A, 0042A], [91300], [91305], [91307], [91301], [91306], [91302], [91303], [91304], [90619, 90620, 90621, 90625, 90626, 90627, 90630, 90644, 90672, 90673, 90674, 90677, 90694, 90750, 90756, 90758, 90759])
Significant, separately identifiable E/M services when performed and append modifier 25 to service

99401 **Preventive medicine counseling and/or risk factor reduction intervention(s) provided to an individual (separate procedure); approximately 15 minutes**
0.70 1.10 FUD XXX
AMA: 2020,Aug,3; 2018,Jan,8; 2017,Jan,8; 2016,Mar,8; 2016,Jan,13

99402 **approximately 30 minutes**
1.42 1.81 FUD XXX
AMA: 2020,Aug,3; 2018,Jan,8; 2017,Jan,8; 2016,Mar,8; 2016,Jan,13

99403 **approximately 45 minutes**
2.12 2.51 FUD XXX
AMA: 2020,Aug,3; 2018,Jan,8; 2017,Jan,8; 2016,Mar,8; 2016,Jan,13

99404 **approximately 60 minutes**
2.81 3.21 FUD XXX
AMA: 2020,Aug,3; 2018,Jan,8; 2017,Jan,8; 2016,Mar,8; 2016,Jan,13

99406 **Smoking and tobacco use cessation counseling visit; intermediate, greater than 3 minutes up to 10 minutes**
0.35 0.42 FUD XXX ★
AMA: 2020,Sep,14; 2020,Aug,3; 2018,Jan,8; 2017,Nov,3; 2017,Jan,8; 2016,Mar,8; 2016,Jan,13

99407 **intensive, greater than 10 minutes**
INCLUDES Services 11-14 minutes
0.73 0.80 FUD XXX ★
AMA: 2020,Aug,3; 2018,Jan,8; 2017,Nov,3; 2017,Jan,8; 2016,Mar,8; 2016,Jan,13

99408 **Alcohol and/or substance (other than tobacco) abuse structured screening (eg, AUDIT, DAST), and brief intervention (SBI) services; 15 to 30 minutes**
INCLUDES Health risk assessment (96160-96161)
Services 15 minutes or more
Only initial screening and brief intervention
0.94 1.01 FUD XXX ★
AMA: 2020,Aug,3; 2018,Jan,8; 2017,Nov,3; 2017,Jan,8; 2016,Nov,5; 2016,Mar,8; 2016,Jan,13

99409 **greater than 30 minutes**
INCLUDES Health risk assessment (96160-96161)
Only initial screening and brief intervention
Services 31 minutes or more
1.88 1.95 FUD XXX ★
AMA: 2020,Aug,3; 2018,Jan,8; 2017,Nov,3; 2017,Jan,8; 2016,Nov,5; 2016,Mar,8; 2016,Jan,13

99411 **Preventive medicine counseling and/or risk factor reduction intervention(s) provided to individuals in a group setting (separate procedure); approximately 30 minutes**
0.22 0.55 FUD XXX
AMA: 2020,Aug,3; 2018,Jan,8; 2017,Jan,8; 2016,Mar,8; 2016,Jan,13

99412 **approximately 60 minutes**
0.36 0.69 FUD XXX
AMA: 2020,Aug,3; 2018,Jan,8; 2017,Jan,8; 2016,Mar,8; 2016,Jan,13

99415 **Resequenced code. See code following 99359.**

99416 **Resequenced code. See code following 99359.**

99417 **Resequenced code. See code following 99416.**

99421 **Resequenced code. See code following 99443.**

99422 **Resequenced code. See code following 99443.**

99423 **Resequenced code. See code following 99443.**

99424-99439 [99424, 99425, 99426, 99427, 99437, 99439] Other Preventive Medicine

Code also immunization counseling, administration, and product (90460-90461, 90471-90474, [0001A, 0002A], [0051A, 0052A, 0053A, 0054A], [0071A, 0072A], [0011A, 0012A], [0064A], [0021A, 0022A], [0031A], [0034A], [0041A, 0042A], [91300], [91305], [91307], [91301], [91306], [91302], [91303], [91304], [90619, 90620, 90621, 90625, 90626, 90627, 90630, 90644, 90672, 90673, 90674, 90677, 90694, 90750, 90756, 90758, 90759])

99424 **Resequenced code. See code following 99489.**

99425 **Resequenced code. See code following 99489.**

99426 **Resequenced code. See code following 99489.**

99427 **Resequenced code. See code following 99489.**

99429 **Unlisted preventive medicine service**
0.00 0.00 FUD XXX
AMA: 2018,Jan,8; 2017,Jan,8; 2016,Mar,8; 2016,Jan,13

99437 **Resequenced code. See code following resequenced code 99491.**

99439 **Resequenced code. See code following resequenced code 99490.**

Evaluation and Management
99441 — 99451

99441-99443 Telephone Calls for Patient Management

CMS: 100-04,11,40.1.3 Independent Attending Physician Services

INCLUDES Care initiated by established patient or patient's guardian
Non-face-to-face E/M services provided by physician or other health care provider qualified to report E/M services
Related E/M services provided within:
Postoperative period
Seven days prior to service

EXCLUDES *Patient management services during same time frame as (99339-99340, 99374-99380, 99487-99489, 99495-99496, 93792-93793)*
Reporting codes more than one time for telephone and online services when reported within 7-day time period by same provider
Services provided by qualified nonphysician health care professional unable to report E/M codes (98966-98968)

99441 Telephone evaluation and management service by a physician or other qualified health care professional who may report evaluation and management services provided to an established patient, parent, or guardian not originating from a related E/M service provided within the previous 7 days nor leading to an E/M service or procedure within the next 24 hours or soonest available appointment; 5-10 minutes of medical discussion

0.36 0.39 **FUD** XXX E 80
AMA: 2020,JulBULL,1; 2019,Mar,8; 2018,Mar,7; 2018,Jan,8; 2017,Jan,8; 2016,Jan,13

99442 11-20 minutes of medical discussion

0.72 0.76 **FUD** XXX E 80
AMA: 2020,JulBULL,1; 2019,Mar,8; 2018,Mar,7; 2018,Jan,8; 2017,Jan,8; 2016,Jan,13

99443 21-30 minutes of medical discussion

1.08 1.12 **FUD** XXX E 80
AMA: 2020,JulBULL,1; 2019,Mar,8; 2018,Mar,7; 2018,Jan,8; 2017,Jan,8; 2016,Jan,13

99421-99423 [99421, 99422, 99423] Digital Evaluation and Management Services

CMS: 100-04,11,40.1.3 Independent Attending Physician Services

INCLUDES Cumulative service time within seven-day time frame needed to evaluate, assess, and manage the patient:
Ordering tests
Prescription generation
Separate digital inquiry for new and unrelated problem
Subsequent communication digitally supported (i.e., email, online, telephone)
Digital service initiated by established patient

EXCLUDES *Clinical staff time*
Digital evaluation by qualified nonphysician health care professional (98970-98972)
Digital evaluation peformed with separately reportable E/M services during same time frame for new or established patient:
Inquiries related to previously completed procedure and within postoperative period
INR monitoring (93792-93793)
Office consultation (99241-99245)
Office or other outpatient visit (99202-99205, 99212-99215)
Patient management services (99339-99340, 99374-99380, [99424, 99425, 99426, 99427], [99437], [99091], [99491], 99487-99489, 99495-99496)
Digital service less than 5 minutes
Reporting code more than one time in 7 days

\# **99421 Online digital evaluation and management service, for an established patient, for up to 7 days, cumulative time during the 7 days; 5-10 minutes**

0.37 0.43 **FUD** XXX 80
AMA: 2020,Jan,3

\# **99422 11-20 minutes**

0.76 0.86 **FUD** XXX 80
AMA: 2020,Jan,3

\# **99423 21 or more minutes**

1.21 1.39 **FUD** XXX 80
AMA: 2020,Jan,3

99446-99452 [99451, 99452] Online and Telephone Consultative Services

INCLUDES Multiple telephone and/or internet contact needed to complete consultation (e.g., test result(s) follow-up)
New or established patient with new problem or exacerbation existing problem and not seen within last 14 days
Review pertinent lab, imaging and/or pathology studies, medical records, medications

EXCLUDES *Any service less than 5 minutes*
Communication with family with or without patient present ([99421, 99422, 99423], 99441-99443, 98966-98967)
Transfer care only

99446 Interprofessional telephone/Internet/electronic health record assessment and management service provided by a consultative physician, including a verbal and written report to the patient's treating/requesting physician or other qualified health care professional; 5-10 minutes of medical consultative discussion and review

INCLUDES Verbal and written reports from consultant to requesting provider

EXCLUDES *Prolonged services without direct patient contact (99358-99359)*
Reporting code more than one time in 7 days

0.51 0.51 **FUD** XXX E 80
AMA: 2019,Jun,7; 2019,Jan,3; 2018,Jan,8; 2017,Jan,8; 2016,Jan,13

99447 11-20 minutes of medical consultative discussion and review

INCLUDES Verbal and written reports from consultant to requesting provider

EXCLUDES *Prolonged services without direct patient contact (99358-99359)*
Reporting code more than one time in 7 days

1.01 1.01 **FUD** XXX E 80
AMA: 2019,Jun,7; 2019,Jan,3; 2018,Jan,8; 2017,Jan,8; 2016,Jan,13

99448 21-30 minutes of medical consultative discussion and review

INCLUDES Verbal and written reports from consultant to requesting provider

EXCLUDES *Prolonged services without direct patient contact (99358-99359)*
Reporting code more than one time in 7 days

1.52 1.52 **FUD** XXX E 80
AMA: 2019,Jun,7; 2019,Jan,3; 2018,Jan,8; 2017,Jan,8; 2016,Jan,13

99449 31 minutes or more of medical consultative discussion and review

INCLUDES Verbal and written reports from consultant to requesting provider

EXCLUDES *Prolonged services without direct patient contact (99358-99359)*
Reporting code more than one time in 7 days

2.02 2.02 **FUD** XXX E 80
AMA: 2019,Jun,7; 2019,Jan,3; 2018,Jan,8; 2017,Jan,8; 2016,Jan,13

\# **99451 Interprofessional telephone/Internet/electronic health record assessment and management service provided by a consultative physician, including a written report to the patient's treating/requesting physician or other qualified health care professional, 5 minutes or more of medical consultative time**

INCLUDES Verbal and written reports from consultant to requesting provider

EXCLUDES *Prolonged services without direct patient contact (99358-99359)*
Reporting code more than one time in 7 days

1.04 1.04 **FUD** XXX 80
AMA: 2019,Jun,7; 2019,Jan,3

99452 **Interprofessional telephone/Internet/electronic health record referral service(s) provided by a treating/requesting physician or other qualified health care professional, 30 minutes**

INCLUDES Time preparing for referral, 16 to 30 minutes

EXCLUDES *Requesting physician's time 30 minutes over typical E/M service, patient not on site (99358-99359)*

Requesting physician's time 30 minutes over typical E/M service, patient on site (99354-99357)

Reporting code more than one time every 14 days

1.04 1.04 FUD XXX 80

AMA: 2020,Jun,3; 2019,Jun,7; 2019,Jan,3

99453-99474 [99091, 99453, 99454, 99473, 99474] Remote Monitoring/Collection Biological Data

99453 **Remote monitoring of physiologic parameter(s) (eg, weight, blood pressure, pulse oximetry, respiratory flow rate), initial; set-up and patient education on use of equipment**

INCLUDES 30-day period physiologic monitoring parameters such as weight, blood pressure, pulse oximetry

Services ordered by physician or other qualified healthcare professional

Services provided for each care episode (starts when monitoring begins and ends when treatment goals achieved)

Set-up and instructions for use

Treatment with device approved by FDA

EXCLUDES *Monitoring less than 16 days*

Reporting codes when services included in other monitoring services (e.g., 93296, 94760, 95250)

0.52 0.52 FUD XXX 80

AMA: 2020,Nov,10; 2020,Apr,5; 2019,Mar,10; 2019,Jan,3; 2019,Jan,6

99454 **device(s) supply with daily recording(s) or programmed alert(s) transmission, each 30 days**

INCLUDES 30-day period physiologic monitoring parameters such as weight, blood pressure, pulse oximetry

Service ordered by physician or other qualified healthcare professional

Supplying device

Treatment with device approved by FDA

EXCLUDES *Monitoring less than 16 days*

Remote monitoring treatment management ([99457])

Remote therapeutic monitoring (98975-98977)

Reporting codes when services included in other monitoring services (e.g., 93296, 94760, 95250)

Self-measured blood pressure monitoring ([99473, 99474])

1.73 1.73 FUD XXX 80

AMA: 2020,Nov,10; 2020,Apr,5; 2019,Oct,3; 2019,Mar,10; 2019,Jan,3; 2019,Jan,6

99091 **Collection and interpretation of physiologic data (eg, ECG, blood pressure, glucose monitoring) digitally stored and/or transmitted by the patient and/or caregiver to the physician or other qualified health care professional, qualified by education, training, licensure/regulation (when applicable) requiring a minimum of 30 minutes of time, each 30 days**

INCLUDES E/M services provided on same service date

EXCLUDES *Care plan oversight services within same calendar month (99339-99340, 99374-99380)*

Chronic care management services within same calendar month ([99437], [99491], 99487)

Data transfer/interpretation from clinical lab or hospital computers

Principal care management services within same calendar month ([99424, 99425, 99426, 99427])

Remote physiologic monitoring treatment management within same calendar month ([99457, 99458])

Reporting code more than one time in 30 days

Reporting codes when services included in other monitoring services such as (93227, 93272, 95250)

Services for which more specific codes exist, such as:

Ambulatory continuous glucose monitoring (95250)

Electrocardiographic services (93227, 93272)

1.62 1.62 FUD XXX N 80

AMA: 2020,Nov,10; 2020,Apr,5; 2020,Feb,7; 2019,Oct,3; 2019,Jun,3; 2019,Jan,6; 2018,Dec,10; 2018,Dec,10; 2018,Jun,6; 2018,Mar,5; 2018,Feb,7; 2018,Jan,8; 2017,Jan,8; 2016,Jan,13

99473 **Self-measured blood pressure using a device validated for clinical accuracy; patient education/training and device calibration**

EXCLUDES *Reporting code more than once per device*

Reporting codes when services included in same calendar month as:

Ambulatory blood pressure monitoring (93784-93790)

Chronic care management services ([99437], [99439, 99490, 99491], 99487-99489)

Principal care management services ([99424, 99425, 99426, 99427])

Remote physiologic monitoring, collection and interpretation ([99453, 99454], [99091], [99457])

0.31 0.31 FUD XXX 80

AMA: 2020,Apr,5; 2020,Feb,7; 2020,Jan,3

99474 **separate self-measurements of two readings one minute apart, twice daily over a 30-day period (minimum of 12 readings), collection of data reported by the patient and/or caregiver to the physician or other qualified health care professional, with report of average systolic and diastolic pressures and subsequent communication of a treatment plan to the patient**

EXCLUDES *Reporting code more than once per device*

Reporting codes when services included in same calendar month as:

Ambulatory blood pressure monitoring (93784-93790)

Chronic care management services ([99437], [99439, 99490, 99491], 99487-99489)

Principal care management services within same calendar month ([99424, 99425, 99426, 99427])

Remote physiologic monitoring, collection and interpretation services ([99453, 99454], [99091], [99457])

0.25 0.42 FUD XXX 80

AMA: 2020,Apr,5; 2020,Feb,7; 2020,Jan,3

99457-99458 [99457, 99458] Remote Monitoring Management

CMS: 100-04,11,40.1.3 Independent Attending Physician Services

INCLUDES Interactive live communication with patient at least 20 minutes per month
Remote monitoring results used for patient management
Reporting code each 30 days no matter number parameters monitored
Service ordered by physician or other qualified healthcare professional
Time managing care when more specific service codes not available
Treatment with device approved by FDA

EXCLUDES *Remote therapeutic monitoring (98980-98981)*
Reporting code for services lasting less than 20 minutes
Reporting code on same service date as E/M services (99202-99215, 99221-99223, 99231-99233, 99251-99255, 99324-99328, 99334-99337, 99341-99350)

Code also, when appropriate:
Behavioral health integration services ([99484], 99492-99494)
Chronic care management services ([99437], [99439, 99490, 99491], 99487-99489)
Principal care management services ([99424, 99425, 99426, 99427])
Transitional care management services (99495-99496)

99457 **Remote physiologic monitoring treatment management services, clinical staff/physician/other qualified health care professional time in a calendar month requiring interactive communication with the patient/caregiver during the month; first 20 minutes**

EXCLUDES *Collection and interpretation physiologic data ([99091])*
0.90 1.43 FUD XXX 80
AMA: 2020,Apr,5; 2020,Feb,7; 2019,Jun,3; 2019,Jan,3; 2019,Jan,6

+ # **99458** **each additional 20 minutes (List separately in addition to code for primary procedure)**

EXCLUDES *Reporting code when 20 minutes additional treatment time not obtained ([99457])*
Code first ([99457])
0.91 1.17 FUD ZZZ 80
AMA: 2020,Feb,7

99450-99458 [99451, 99452, 99453, 99454, 99457, 99458] Life/Disability Insurance Eligibility Visits

INCLUDES Assessment services for insurance eligibility and work-related disability without medical management of the patient's illness/injury
Services provided to new/established patients at any site of service

EXCLUDES *Any additional E&M services or procedures performed on the same date of service: report with appropriate code*

99450 **Basic life and/or disability examination that includes: Measurement of height, weight, and blood pressure; Completion of a medical history following a life insurance pro forma; Collection of blood sample and/or urinalysis complying with "chain of custody" protocols; and Completion of necessary documentation/certificates.**
0.00 0.00 FUD XXX E
AMA: 2019,Jun,7; 2018,Jan,8; 2017,Jan,8; 2016,Jan,13

99451 **Resequenced code. See code following 99449.**

99452 **Resequenced code. See code following 99449.**

99453 **Resequenced code. See code following 99449.**

99454 **Resequenced code. See code following 99449.**

99455 **Work related or medical disability examination by the treating physician that includes: Completion of a medical history commensurate with the patient's condition; Performance of an examination commensurate with the patient's condition; Formulation of a diagnosis, assessment of capabilities and stability, and calculation of impairment; Development of future medical treatment plan; and Completion of necessary documentation/certificates and report.**

INCLUDES Special reports (99080)
0.00 0.00 FUD XXX B 80
AMA: 2018,Jan,8; 2017,Jan,8; 2016,Jan,13

99456 **Work related or medical disability examination by other than the treating physician that includes: Completion of a medical history commensurate with the patient's condition; Performance of an examination commensurate with the patient's condition; Formulation of a diagnosis, assessment of capabilities and stability, and calculation of impairment; Development of future medical treatment plan; and Completion of necessary documentation/certificates and report.**

INCLUDES Special reports (99080)
0.00 0.00 FUD XXX B 80
AMA: 2018,Jan,8; 2017,Jan,8; 2016,Jan,13

99457 **Resequenced code. See code before 99450.**

99458 **Resequenced code. See code before 99450.**

99460-99463 Evaluation and Management Services for Age 28 Days or Less

CMS: 100-04,12,30.6.4 Services Furnished Incident to Physician's Service

INCLUDES Family consultation
Healthy newborn history and physical
Medical record documentation
Ordering diagnostic test and treatments
Services provided to healthy newborns age 28 days or younger

EXCLUDES *Neonatal intensive and critical care services (99466-99469 [99485, 99486], 99477-99480)*
Newborn follow-up services in office or outpatient setting (99202-99215, 99381, 99391)
Newborn hospital discharge services when provided on date subsequent to admission (99238-99239)
Nonroutine neonatal inpatient evaluation and management services (99221-99233)

Code also:
Attendance at delivery (99464)
Circumcision (54150)
Emergency resuscitation services (99465)

99460 **Initial hospital or birthing center care, per day, for evaluation and management of normal newborn infant** A
2.71 2.71 FUD XXX V 80
AMA: 2018,Jan,8; 2017,Jan,8; 2016,Jan,13

99461 **Initial care, per day, for evaluation and management of normal newborn infant seen in other than hospital or birthing center** A
1.78 2.58 FUD XXX M 80
AMA: 2018,Jan,8; 2017,Jan,8; 2016,Jan,13

99462 **Subsequent hospital care, per day, for evaluation and management of normal newborn** A
1.19 1.19 FUD XXX C 80
AMA: 2018,Jan,8; 2017,Jan,8; 2016,Jan,13

99463 **Initial hospital or birthing center care, per day, for evaluation and management of normal newborn infant admitted and discharged on the same date** A
3.13 3.13 FUD XXX V 80
AMA: 2018,Jan,8; 2017,Jan,8; 2016,Jan,13

99464-99465 Newborn Delivery Attendance/Resuscitation

CMS: 100-04,12,30.6.4 Services Furnished Incident to Physician's Service

99464 **Attendance at delivery (when requested by the delivering physician or other qualified health care professional) and initial stabilization of newborn** A

EXCLUDES *Resuscitation at delivery (99465)*
2.12 2.12 FUD XXX N 80
AMA: 2018,Jan,8; 2017,Jan,8; 2016,Jan,13

99465 Delivery/birthing room resuscitation, provision of positive pressure ventilation and/or chest compressions in the presence of acute inadequate ventilation and/or cardiac output A

EXCLUDES *Attendance at delivery (99464)*

Code also any necessary procedures performed as resuscitation component

4.13 4.13 **FUD** XXX S 80

AMA: 2018,Jan,8; 2017,Jan,8; 2016,Jan,13

99466-99467 Critical Care Transport Age 24 Months or Younger

CMS: 100-04,12,30.6.4 Services Furnished Incident to Physician's Service

INCLUDES Face-to-face care starting when physician assumes patient responsibility at referring facility until receiving facility accepts patient
Physician presence during interfacility transfer critically ill/injured patient age 24 months or younger
Services provided by physician during transport:
- Blood gases
- Chest x-rays (71045-71046)
- Data stored in computers (e.g., ECGs, blood pressures, hematologic data)
- Gastric intubation (43752-43753)
- Interpretation cardiac output measurements (93598)
- Pulse oximetry (94760-94762)
- Routine monitoring:
  - Heart rate
  - Respiratory rate
- Temporary transcutaneous pacing (92953)
- Vascular access procedures (36000, 36400, 36405-36406, 36415, 36591, 36600)
- Ventilatory management (94002-94003, 94660, 94662)

EXCLUDES *Neonatal hypothermia (99184)*
Patient critical care transport services with personal patient contact less than 30 minutes
Physician directed emergency care via two-way voice communication with transporting staff (99288, [99485, 99486])
Physician services directing transport (control physician) ([99485, 99486])
Services less than 30 minutes in duration (see E/M codes)

Code also any services not designated as included in critical care transport service

99466 Critical care face-to-face services, during an interfacility transport of critically ill or critically injured pediatric patient, 24 months of age or younger; first 30-74 minutes of hands-on care during transport A

6.75 6.75 **FUD** XXX N 80

AMA: 2018,Jun,9; 2018,Jan,8; 2017,Jan,8; 2016,Jan,13

\+ **99467 each additional 30 minutes (List separately in addition to code for primary service)** A

Code first (99466)

3.37 3.37 **FUD** ZZZ N 80

AMA: 2018,Jun,9; 2018,Jan,8; 2017,Jan,8; 2016,Jan,13

99485-99486 [99485, 99486] Critical Care Transport Supervision Age 24 Months or Younger

INCLUDES Advice for treatment to transport team from control physician
Non face-to-face care starts with first contact by control physician with transport team and ends when patient responsibility assumed by receiving facility

EXCLUDES *Emergency systems physician direction for pediatric patient older than 24 months (99288)*
Services less than 15 minutes
Services performed by control physician for same time period
Services performed by same physician providing critical care transport (99466-99467)
Services provided by transport team

\# **99485 Supervision by a control physician of interfacility transport care of the critically ill or critically injured pediatric patient, 24 months of age or younger, includes two-way communication with transport team before transport, at the referring facility and during the transport, including data interpretation and report; first 30 minutes** A

2.17 2.17 **FUD** XXX B

AMA: 2018,Jun,9; 2018,Jan,8; 2017,Jan,8; 2016,Jan,13

\+ # **99486 each additional 30 minutes (List separately in addition to code for primary procedure)** A

Code first ([99485])

1.88 1.88 **FUD** XXX B

AMA: 2018,Jun,9; 2018,Jan,8; 2017,Jan,8; 2016,Jan,13

99468-99476 [99473, 99474] Critical Care Age 5 Years or Younger

CMS: 100-04,12,30.6.4 Services Furnished Incident to Physician's Service

INCLUDES All services included in codes 99291-99292 as well as (which may be reported by facilities only):
- Administration blood/blood components (36430, 36440)
- Administration intravenous fluids (96360-96361)
- Administration surfactant (94610)
- Bladder aspiration, suprapubic (51100)
- Bladder catheterization (51701, 51702)
- Car seat evaluation (94780-94781)
- Catheterization umbilical artery (36660)
- Catheterization umbilical vein (36510)
- Central venous catheter, centrally inserted (36555)
- Endotracheal intubation (31500)
- Lumbar puncture (62270)
- Oral or nasogastric tube placement (43752)
- Pulmonary function testing, performed at bedside (94375)
- Pulse or ear oximetry (94760-94762)
- Vascular access, arteries (36140, 36620)
- Vascular access, venous (36400-36406, 36420, 36600)
- Ventilatory management (94002-94004, 94660)

Initial and subsequent care provided to critically ill infant or child
Other hospital care or intensive care services by same group or individual done on same day patient transferred to initial neonatal/pediatric critical care
Readmission to critical unit on same day or during same stay (subsequent care)

EXCLUDES *Critical care services for patients age six years or older (99291-99292)*
Critical care services provided by second physician or different physician specialty (99291-99292)
Interfacility transport services by same or different individual, same or different specialty or group, on same service date (99466-99467, [99485, 99486])
Neonatal hypothermia (99184)
Services performed by individual in another group receiving patient transferred to lower care level (99231-99233, 99478-99480)
Services performed by individual transferring patient to lower care level (99231-99233, 99291-99292)
Services performed by same or different individual in same group on same day (99291-99292)
Services performed by transferring individual prior to patient transfer to individual in different group (99221-99233, 99291-99292, 99460-99462, 99477-99480)

Code also normal newborn care when done on same day by same group or individual providing critical care. Report modifier 25 with initial critical care code (99460-99462)

99468 Initial inpatient neonatal critical care, per day, for the evaluation and management of a critically ill neonate, 28 days of age or younger A

26.0 26.0 **FUD** XXX C 80

AMA: 2018,Dec,8; 2018,Dec,8; 2018,Jun,9; 2018,Jan,8; 2017,Jan,8; 2016,May,3; 2016,Jan,13

99469 Subsequent inpatient neonatal critical care, per day, for the evaluation and management of a critically ill neonate, 28 days of age or younger A

11.2 11.2 **FUD** XXX C 80

AMA: 2018,Dec,8; 2018,Dec,8; 2018,Jun,9; 2018,Jan,8; 2017,Jan,8; 2016,May,3; 2016,Jan,13

99471 Initial inpatient pediatric critical care, per day, for the evaluation and management of a critically ill infant or young child, 29 days through 24 months of age A

22.5 22.5 **FUD** XXX C 80

AMA: 2018,Dec,8; 2018,Dec,8; 2018,Jun,9; 2018,Jan,8; 2017,Jan,8; 2016,May,3; 2016,Jan,13

99472 Subsequent inpatient pediatric critical care, per day, for the evaluation and management of a critically ill infant or young child, 29 days through 24 months of age A

11.5 11.5 **FUD** XXX C 80

AMA: 2018,Dec,8; 2018,Dec,8; 2018,Jun,9; 2018,Jan,8; 2017,Jan,8; 2016,May,3; 2016,Jan,13

99473 Resequenced code. See code before 99450.

99474 Resequenced code. See code before 99450.

99475 **Initial inpatient pediatric critical care, per day, for the evaluation and management of a critically ill infant or young child, 2 through 5 years of age** A
15.8 15.8 FUD XXX C 80
AMA: 2018,Dec,8; 2018,Dec,8; 2018,Jun,9; 2018,Jan,8; 2017,Jan,8; 2016,May,3; 2016,Jan,13

99476 **Subsequent inpatient pediatric critical care, per day, for the evaluation and management of a critically ill infant or young child, 2 through 5 years of age** A
9.86 9.86 FUD XXX C 80
AMA: 2018,Dec,8; 2018,Dec,8; 2018,Jun,9; 2018,Jan,8; 2017,Jan,8; 2016,May,3; 2016,Jan,13

99477-99480 Initial Inpatient Neonatal Intensive Care and Other Services

CMS: 100-04,12,30.6.4 Services Furnished Incident to Physician's Service

INCLUDES <insert title here>

INCLUDES All services included in codes 99291-99292 as well as (which may be reported by facilities only):
- Adjustments to enteral and/or parenteral nutrition
- Airway and ventilator management (31500, 94002-94004, 94375, 94610, 94660)
- Bladder catheterization (51701-51702)
- Blood transfusion (36430, 36440)
- Car seat evaluation (94780-94781)
- Constant and/or frequent monitoring vital signs
- Continuous observation by the healthcare team
- Heat maintenance
- Intensive cardiac or respiratory monitoring
- Oral or nasogastric tube insertion (43752)
- Oxygen saturation (94760-94762)
- Spinal puncture (62270)
- Suprapubic catheterization (51100)
- Vascular access procedures (36000, 36140, 36400, 36405-36406, 36420, 36510, 36555, 36600, 36620, 36660)

EXCLUDES *Critical care services for patient transferred after initial or subsequent intensive care provided (99291-99292)*
Initial day intensive care provided by transferring individual same day neonate/infant transferred to lower care level (99477)
Inpatient neonatal/pediatric critical care services received on same day (99468-99476)
Necessary resuscitation services done as delivery care component prior to admission
Neonatal hypothermia (99184)
Services provided by receiving individual when patient transferred for critical care (99468-99476)
Services for receiving provider when patient improves after initial day and transferred to lower care level (99231-99233, 99478-99480)
Subsequent care sick neonate, under age 28 days, more than 5000 grams, not requiring critical or intensive care services (99231-99233)

Code also:
Care provided by receiving individual when patient transferred to individual in different group (99231-99233, 99462)
Initial neonatal intensive care service when physician or other qualified health care professional present for delivery and/or neonate requires resuscitation (99464-99465); append modifier 25 to (99477)

99477 **Initial hospital care, per day, for the evaluation and management of the neonate, 28 days of age or younger, who requires intensive observation, frequent interventions, and other intensive care services** A
EXCLUDES *Initiation care critically ill neonate (99468)*
Initiation inpatient care normal newborn (99460)
9.85 9.85 FUD XXX C 80
AMA: 2018,Dec,8; 2018,Dec,8; 2018,Jan,8; 2017,Jan,8; 2016,Jan,13

99478 **Subsequent intensive care, per day, for the evaluation and management of the recovering very low birth weight infant (present body weight less than 1500 grams)** A
3.87 3.87 FUD XXX C 80
AMA: 2018,Dec,8; 2018,Dec,8; 2018,Jun,11; 2018,Jan,8; 2017,Jan,8; 2016,Jan,13

99479 **Subsequent intensive care, per day, for the evaluation and management of the recovering low birth weight infant (present body weight of 1500-2500 grams)** A
3.52 3.52 FUD XXX C 80
AMA: 2018,Dec,8; 2018,Dec,8; 2018,Jun,11; 2018,Jan,8; 2017,Jan,8; 2016,Jan,13

99480 **Subsequent intensive care, per day, for the evaluation and management of the recovering infant (present body weight of 2501-5000 grams)** A
3.37 3.37 FUD XXX C 80
AMA: 2018,Dec,8; 2018,Dec,8; 2018,Jun,11; 2018,Jan,8; 2017,Jan,8; 2016,Jan,13

99483-99486 [99484, 99485, 99486] Cognitive Impairment Services

INCLUDES Assessment and care plan services during same time frame as:
- E/M services (99202-99215, 99241-99245, 99324-99337, 99341-99350, 99366-99368, 99497-99498)
- Medication management (99605-99607)
- Need for services evaluation (e.g., legal, financial, meals, personal care)
- Patient and caregiver focused risk assessment (96160-96161)
- Psychiatric and psychological services (90785, 90791-90792, [96127])
- Psychological or neuropsychological tests (96146)

Consideration other conditions that may cause cognitive impairment (e.g., infection, hydrocephalus, stroke, medications)
Evaluation and care plans for new or existing patients with cognitive impairment symptoms

EXCLUDES *Reporting code more than one time per 180-day period*

▲ **99483** **Assessment of and care planning for a patient with cognitive impairment, requiring an independent historian, in the office or other outpatient, home or domiciliary or rest home, with all of the following required elements: Cognition-focused evaluation including a pertinent history and examination, Medical decision making of moderate or high complexity, Functional assessment (eg, basic and instrumental activities of daily living), including decision-making capacity, Use of standardized instruments for staging of dementia (eg, functional assessment staging test [FAST], clinical dementia rating [CDR]), Medication reconciliation and review for high-risk medications, Evaluation for neuropsychiatric and behavioral symptoms, including depression, including use of standardized screening instrument(s), Evaluation of safety (eg, home), including motor vehicle operation, Identification of caregiver(s), caregiver knowledge, caregiver needs, social supports, and the willingness of caregiver to take on caregiving tasks, Development, updating or revision, or review of an Advance Care Plan, Creation of a written care plan, including initial plans to address any neuropsychiatric symptoms, neuro-cognitive symptoms, functional limitations, and referral to community resources as needed (eg, rehabilitation services, adult day programs, support groups) shared with the patient and/or caregiver with initial education and support. Typically, 50 minutes are spent face-to-face with the patient and/or family or caregiver.**
5.12 7.35 FUD XXX S 80
AMA: 2020,Sep,3; 2018,Jul,12; 2018,Apr,9; 2018,Jan,8

99484 Resequenced code. See code following 99498.

99485 Resequenced code. See code following 99467.

99486 Resequenced code. See code following 99467.

99490-99437 [99437, 99439, 99490, 99491] Chronic Care Management Services

INCLUDES Case management services provided to patients that:
- Have two or more conditions anticipated to endure more than 12 months or until patient's death
- High risk that conditions will result in decompensation, deterioration, or death

Only services given by physician or other qualified health caregiver who has care coordination role for patient for month

EXCLUDES *Patient management services during same time frame as (99339-99340, 99374-99380, [99424, 99425, 99426, 99427], [99437], [99491], 99487-99489, 90951-90970, 99605-99607)*

Service time reported with (99358-99359, 99366-99368, [99421, 99422, 99423], 99441-99443, [99091], [99484], 99492-99494, 93792-93793, 98960-98962, 98966-98968, 99071, 99078, 99080)

▲ # 99490 **Chronic care management services with the following required elements: multiple (two or more) chronic conditions expected to last at least 12 months, or until the death of the patient, chronic conditions that place the patient at significant risk of death, acute exacerbation/decompensation, or functional decline, comprehensive care plan established, implemented, revised, or monitored; first 20 minutes of clinical staff time directed by a physician or other qualified health care professional, per calendar month.**

EXCLUDES *Chronic care management provided personally by physician or other qualified health care professional ([99437], [99491])*

Less than 20 minutes staff time monthly

Qualified nonphysician health care professional online digital assessment and management (98970-98972)

Reporting code more than once per calendar month

0.90 1.17 FUD XXX S 80

AMA: 2020,Apr,5; 2020,Feb,7; 2019,Jan,6; 2018,Oct,9; 2018,Jul,12; 2018,Apr,9; 2018,Mar,7; 2018,Mar,5; 2018,Feb,7; 2018,Jan,8; 2017,Jan,8; 2016,Jan,13

▲ + # 99439 **each additional 20 minutes of clinical staff time directed by a physician or other qualified health care professional, per calendar month (List separately in addition to code for primary procedure)**

EXCLUDES *Qualified nonphysician health care professional online digital assessment and management (98970-98972)*

Reporting code more than twice per calendar month

Code first ([99490])

0.81 1.08 FUD ZZZ 80

▲ # 99491 **Chronic care management services with the following required elements: multiple (two or more) chronic conditions expected to last at least 12 months, or until the death of the patient, chronic conditions that place the patient at significant risk of death, acute exacerbation/decompensation, or functional decline, comprehensive care plan established, implemented, revised, or monitored; first 30 minutes provided personally by a physician or other qualified health care professional, per calendar month.**

EXCLUDES *Chronic care management provided by medically directed clinical staff only ([99439], [99490])*

Less than 30 minutes staff time monthly

Reporting code more than once per calendar month

Service time reported for transitional care management services (99495-99496)

2.33 2.33 FUD XXX 80

AMA: 2020,Apr,5

● + # 99437 **each additional 30 minutes by a physician or other qualified health care professional, per calendar month (List separately in addition to code for primary procedure)**

Code first ([99491])

0.00 0.00 FUD 000

99487-99489 Complex Chronic Care Management Services

CMS: 100-04,11,40.1.3 Independent Attending Physician Services

INCLUDES All clinical non-face-to-face time with patient, family, and caregivers

Patient management services during same time frame as (99339-99340, 99374-99380, [99437], [99439, 99490, 99491], 90951-90970, 99605-99607)

Service time reported with (99358-99359, 99366-99368, [99421, 99422, 99423], 99441-99443, [99091], 93792-93793, 98960-98962, 98966-98972, 99071, 99078, 99080, 99605-99607)

Services provided to patients in rest home, domiciliary, assisted living facility, or at home including:
- Caregiver education to family or patient, addressing independent living and self-management
- Communication with patient and all caregivers and professionals regarding care
- Determining which community and health resources benefit patient
- Developing and maintaining care plan
- Facilitation services and care
- Health outcomes data and registry documentation
- Providing communication with home health and other patient utilized services
- Support for treatment and medication adherence

Services that address activities daily living, psychosocial, and medical needs

EXCLUDES *E/M services by same/different individual during care management services time frame*

Psychiatric collaborative care management (99484, 99492-99494)

▲ 99487 **Complex chronic care management services with the following required elements: multiple (two or more) chronic conditions expected to last at least 12 months, or until the death of the patient, chronic conditions that place the patient at significant risk of death, acute exacerbation/decompensation, or functional decline, comprehensive care plan established, implemented, revised, or monitored, moderate or high complexity medical decision making; first 60 minutes of clinical staff time directed by a physician or other qualified health care professional, per calendar month.**

INCLUDES Clinical services, 60 to 74 minutes, during calendar month

Only services given by physician or other qualified health caregiver who has care coordination role for patient for month

EXCLUDES *Clinical staff time focusing on only one of multiple chronic conditions ([99424, 99425, 99426, 99427])*

Reporting code more than once per calendar month

1.47 2.58 FUD XXX S 80

AMA: 2020,Apr,5; 2020,Feb,7; 2019,Jan,6; 2018,Oct,9; 2018,Jul,12; 2018,Apr,9; 2018,Mar,7; 2018,Mar,5; 2018,Feb,7; 2018,Jan,8; 2017,Apr,9; 2017,Jan,8; 2016,Jan,13

▲ + 99489 **each additional 30 minutes of clinical staff time directed by a physician or other qualified health care professional, per calendar month (List separately in addition to code for primary procedure)**

INCLUDES Only services given by physician or other qualified health caregiver who has care coordination role for patient for month

EXCLUDES *Clinical services less than 30 minutes beyond initial 60 minutes, per calendar month*

Code first (99487)

0.74 1.29 FUD ZZZ N 80

AMA: 2020,Apr,5; 2020,Feb,7; 2019,Jan,6; 2018,Oct,9; 2018,Jul,12; 2018,Apr,9; 2018,Mar,7; 2018,Mar,5; 2018,Feb,7; 2018,Jan,8; 2017,Apr,9; 2017,Jan,8; 2016,Jan,13

99424-99491 [99424, 99425, 99426, 99427, 99490, 99491] Principal Care Management Services

INCLUDES Establishing, implementing, revising, and monitoring care plan specific to single disease
Medical/psychological need management single, complex chronic condition 3 months duration or longer

● # **99424** **Principal care management services, for a single high-risk disease, with the following required elements: one complex chronic condition expected to last at least 3 months, and that places the patient at significant risk of hospitalization, acute exacerbation/decompensation, functional decline, or death, the condition requires development, monitoring, or revision of disease-specific care plan, the condition requires frequent adjustments in the medication regimen and/or the management of the condition is unusually complex due to comorbidities, ongoing communication and care coordination between relevant practitioners furnishing care; first 30 minutes provided personally by a physician or other qualified health care professional, per calendar month.**

EXCLUDES *Clinical staff time focused on multiple chronic conditions (99487-99489)*
Less than 30 minutes staff time monthly
Principal care management provided by medically directed clinical staff only ([99426, 99427])
Reporting code more than once per calendar month

0.00 0.00 FUD 000

● + # **99425** **each additional 30 minutes provided personally by a physician or other qualified health care professional, per calendar month (List separately in addition to code for primary procedure)**

Code first ([99424])

0.00 0.00 FUD 000

● # **99426** **Principal care management services, for a single high-risk disease, with the following required elements: one complex chronic condition expected to last at least 3 months, and that places the patient at significant risk of hospitalization, acute exacerbation/decompensation, functional decline, or death, the condition requires development, monitoring, or revision of disease-specific care plan, the condition requires frequent adjustments in the medication regimen and/or the management of the condition is unusually complex due to comorbidities, ongoing communication and care coordination between relevant practitioners furnishing care; first 30 minutes of clinical staff time directed by physician or other qualified health care professional, per calendar month.**

EXCLUDES *Clinical staff time focused on multiple chronic conditions (99487-99489)*
Less than 30 minutes staff time monthly
Principal care management provided personally by physician or other qualified health care professional ([99424, 99425])
Reporting code more than once per calendar month

0.00 0.00 FUD 000

● + # **99427** **each additional 30 minutes of clinical staff time directed by a physician or other qualified health care professional, per calendar month (List separately in addition to code for primary procedure)**

EXCLUDES *Reporting code more than twice per calendar month*

Code first ([99426])

0.00 0.00 FUD 000

99490 **Resequenced code. See code before 99487.**

99491 **Resequenced code. See code before 99487.**

99492-99494 Psychiatric Collaborative Care

CMS: 100-02,13,230.2 Chronic Care Management and General Behavioral Health Integration Services

INCLUDES Services provided during calendar month by physician or other qualified healthcare profession for patients with psychiatric diagnosis
Assessment behavioral health status
Creation and care plan revision
Treatment provided during care episode during which goals may be met, not achieved, or lack of services during six-month period

EXCLUDES *Additional services provided by behavioral health care manager during same calendar month period (do not count as time for 99492-99494):*
Psychiatric evaluation (90791-90792)
Psychotherapy (99406-99407, 99408-99409, 90832-90834, 90836-90838, 90839-90840, 90846-90847, 90849, 90853)
Services provided by psychiatric consultant (do not count as time for 99492-99494): (E/M services) and psychiatric evaluation (90791-90792)

▲ **99492** **Initial psychiatric collaborative care management, first 70 minutes in the first calendar month of behavioral health care manager activities, in consultation with a psychiatric consultant, and directed by the treating physician or other qualified health care professional, with the following required elements: outreach to and engagement in treatment of a patient directed by the treating physician or other qualified health care professional, initial assessment of the patient, including administration of validated rating scales, with the development of an individualized treatment plan, review by the psychiatric consultant with modifications of the plan if recommended, entering patient in a registry and tracking patient follow-up and progress using the registry, with appropriate documentation, and participation in weekly caseload consultation with the psychiatric consultant, and provision of brief interventions using evidence-based techniques such as behavioral activation, motivational interviewing, and other focused treatment strategies.**

EXCLUDES *Services less than 36 minutes*
Subsequent collaborative care managment in same calendar month (99493)

2.50 4.35 FUD XXX S 80

AMA: 2020,Feb,7; 2019,Jan,6; 2018,Jul,12; 2018,Mar,5; 2018,Feb,7; 2018,Jan,8; 2017,Nov,3

▲ **99493** **Subsequent psychiatric collaborative care management, first 60 minutes in a subsequent month of behavioral health care manager activities, in consultation with a psychiatric consultant, and directed by the treating physician or other qualified health care professional, with the following required elements: tracking patient follow-up and progress using the registry, with appropriate documentation, participation in weekly caseload consultation with the psychiatric consultant, ongoing collaboration with and coordination of the patient's mental health care with the treating physician or other qualified health care professional and any other treating mental health providers, additional review of progress and recommendations for changes in treatment, as indicated, including medications, based on recommendations provided by the psychiatric consultant, provision of brief interventions using evidence-based techniques such as behavioral activation, motivational interviewing, and other focused treatment strategies, monitoring of patient outcomes using validated rating scales, and relapse prevention planning with patients as they achieve remission of symptoms and/or other treatment goals and are prepared for discharge from active treatment.**

EXCLUDES *Initial collaborative care managment in same calendar month (99492)*

2.25 3.50 FUD XXX S 80

AMA: 2020,Feb,7; 2019,Jan,6; 2018,Jul,12; 2018,Mar,5; 2018,Feb,7; 2018,Jan,8; 2017,Nov,3

\+ **99494** **Initial or subsequent psychiatric collaborative care management, each additional 30 minutes in a calendar month of behavioral health care manager activities, in consultation with a psychiatric consultant, and directed by the treating physician or other qualified health care professional (List separately in addition to code for primary procedure)**

INCLUDES Coordination care with emergency department staff

Code first (99492, 99493)

1.20 1.77 FUD ZZZ N 80

AMA: 2020,Feb,7; 2019,Jan,6; 2018,Jul,12; 2018,Mar,5; 2018,Feb,7; 2018,Jan,8; 2017,Nov,3

99495-99496 Management of Transitional Care Services

CMS: 100-02,13,230.1 Transitional Care Management Services; 100-04,11,40.1.3 Independent Attending Physician Services; 100-04,12,190.3 List of Telehealth Services

INCLUDES First interaction (face-to-face, by telephone, or electronic) with patient or his/her caregiver and must be done within two working days from discharge

Initial face-to-face; must be done within code time frame and include medication management

New or established patient with moderate to high complexity medical decision making needs during care transitions

Patient management services during same time frame as (99339-99340, 99358-99359, 99366-99368, 99374-99380, 99441-99443, [99091], 99487-99489, 90951-90970, 93792-93793, 98960-98962, 98966-98968, 99071, 99078, 99080, 99605-99607)

Services from discharge day up to 29 days post discharge

Subsequent discharge within 30 days

Without face-to-face patient care given by physician or other qualified health care professional includes:

- Contacting qualified health care professionals for specific patient problems
- Discharge information review
- Follow-up and referral arrangements with community resources and providers
- Need for follow-up care review based on tests and treatments
- Patient, family, and caregiver education

Without face-to-face patient care given by staff under physician guidance or other qualified health care professional includes:

- Caregiver education to family or patient, addressing independent living and self-management
- Communication with patient and all caregivers and professionals regarding care
- Determining which community and health resources benefit patient
- Facilitation services and care
- Providing communication with home health and other patient utilized services
- Support for treatment and medication adherence

EXCLUDES *E/M services after first face-to-face visit*

99495 **Transitional Care Management Services with the following required elements: Communication (direct contact, telephone, electronic) with the patient and/or caregiver within 2 business days of discharge Medical decision making of at least moderate complexity during the service period Face-to-face visit, within 14 calendar days of discharge**

3.11 4.62 FUD XXX ★ V 80

AMA: 2020,Feb,7; 2020,Jan,3; 2019,Jan,6; 2018,Jul,12; 2018,Apr,9; 2018,Mar,5; 2018,Mar,7; 2018,Feb,7; 2018,Jan,8; 2017,Jan,8; 2016,Jan,13

99496 **Transitional Care Management Services with the following required elements: Communication (direct contact, telephone, electronic) with the patient and/or caregiver within 2 business days of discharge Medical decision making of high complexity during the service period Face-to-face visit, within 7 calendar days of discharge**

4.51 6.52 FUD XXX ★ V 80

AMA: 2020,Feb,7; 2020,Jan,3; 2019,Jan,6; 2018,Jul,12; 2018,Apr,9; 2018,Mar,5; 2018,Mar,7; 2018,Feb,7; 2018,Jan,8; 2017,Jan,8; 2016,Jan,13

99497-99498 Advance Directive Guidance

CMS: 100-02,15,280.5.1 Advance Care Planning with an Annual Wellness Visit; 100-04,11,40.1.3 Independent Attending Physician Services; 100-04,18,140.8 Advance Care Planning with an Annual Wellness Visit (AWV); 100-04,4,200.11 Advance Care Planning as an Optional Element of an Annual Wellness Visit

EXCLUDES *Critical care services (99291-99292, 99468-99469, 99471-99472, 99475-99476, 99477-99480)*

Services for cognitive care (99483)

Treatment/management for active problem (see appropriate E/M service)

99497 **Advance care planning including the explanation and discussion of advance directives such as standard forms (with completion of such forms, when performed), by the physician or other qualified health care professional; first 30 minutes, face-to-face with the patient, family member(s), and/or surrogate**

2.23 2.40 FUD XXX ★ Q1 80

AMA: 2018,Apr,9; 2018,Jan,8; 2017,Jan,8; 2016,Feb,7; 2016,Jan,13

\+ **99498** **each additional 30 minutes (List separately in addition to code for primary procedure)**

Code first (99497)

2.10 2.11 FUD ZZZ ★ N 80

AMA: 2018,Apr,9; 2018,Jan,8; 2017,Jan,8; 2016,Feb,7; 2016,Jan,13

99484 [99484] Behavioral Health Integration Care

CMS: 100-02,13,230.2 Chronic Care Management and General Behavioral Health Integration Services

INCLUDES Care management services requiring 20 minutes or more per calendar month

Coordination of care with emergency department staff

Face to face services when necessary

Provided as outpatient service

Provision services by clinical staff and reported by supervising physician or other qualified healthcare professional

Provision services to patients with ongoing relationship

Treatment plan and specific service components

EXCLUDES *Other services for which time or activities associated with service not used to meet requirements for 99484:*

- *Behavioral health integration care in same month ([99484])*
- *Chronic care management ([99437], [99439], [99490], 99487-99489)*
- *Principal care management ([99424, 99425, 99426, 99427])*
- *Psychiatric collaborative care in same calendar month (99492-99494)*
- *Psychotherapy services (90785-90899)*
- *Transitional care management (99495-99496)*

▲ # **99484** **Care management services for behavioral health conditions, at least 20 minutes of clinical staff time, directed by a physician or other qualified health care professional, per calendar month, with the following required elements: initial assessment or follow-up monitoring, including the use of applicable validated rating scales, behavioral health care planning in relation to behavioral/psychiatric health problems, including revision for patients who are not progressing or whose status changes, facilitating and coordinating treatment such as psychotherapy, pharmacotherapy, counseling and/or psychiatric consultation, and continuity of care with a designated member of the care team.**

0.91 1.33 FUD XXX S 80

AMA: 2020,Feb,7; 2019,Jan,6; 2018,Jul,12; 2018,Mar,5; 2018,Feb,7; 2018,Jan,8

99499 Unlisted Evaluation and Management Services

CMS: 100-04,12,30.6.10 Consultation Services; 100-04,12,30.6.4 Services Furnished Incident to Physician's Service; 100-04,12,30.6.9.1 Initial Hospital Care and Observation or Inpatient Care Services

99499 **Unlisted evaluation and management service**

0.00 0.00 FUD XXX B 80

AMA: 2019,Aug,8; 2018,Jan,8; 2017,Jan,8; 2016,Jan,13

[illegible]

[illegible]

[illegible]

[illegible]

[illegible]

AMA: [illegible]

[illegible]

[illegible]

AMA: [illegible]

[illegible]

[illegible] Management Services

[illegible]

0001F-0015F Quality Measures with Multiple Components

INCLUDES Several measures grouped within single code descriptor to make possible reporting for clinical conditions when all components have been met

0001F **Heart failure assessed (includes assessment of all the following components) (CAD): Blood pressure measured (2000F) Level of activity assessed (1003F) Clinical symptoms of volume overload (excess) assessed (1004F) Weight, recorded (2001F) Clinical signs of volume overload (excess) assessed (2002F)**

INCLUDES Blood pressure measured (2000F)
Clinical signs volume overload (excess) assessed (2002F)
Clinical symptoms volume overload (excess) assessed (1004F)
Level activity assessed (1003F)
Weight recorded (2001F)

0.00 0.00 FUD XXX E

AMA: 2018,Jan,8; 2017,Jan,8; 2016,Jan,13

0005F **Osteoarthritis assessed (OA) Includes assessment of all the following components: Osteoarthritis symptoms and functional status assessed (1006F) Use of anti-inflammatory or over-the-counter (OTC) analgesic medications assessed (1007F) Initial examination of the involved joint(s) (includes visual inspection, palpation, range of motion) (2004F)**

INCLUDES Anti-inflammatory or over-the-counter (OTC) analgesic medication usage assessed (1007F)
Initial examination involved joint(s) (includes visual inspection/palpation/range) (2004F)
Osteoarthritis symptoms and functional status assessed (1006F)

0.00 0.00 FUD XXX E

AMA: 2005,Oct,1-5

0012F **Community-acquired bacterial pneumonia assessment (includes all of the following components) (CAP): Co-morbid conditions assessed (1026F) Vital signs recorded (2010F) Mental status assessed (2014F) Hydration status assessed (2018F)**

INCLUDES Co-morbid conditions assessed (1026F)
Hydration status assessed (2018F)
Mental status assessed (2014F)
Vital signs recorded (2010F)

0.00 0.00 FUD XXX E

0014F **Comprehensive preoperative assessment performed for cataract surgery with intraocular lens (IOL) placement (includes assessment of all of the following components) (EC): Dilated fundus evaluation performed within 12 months prior to cataract surgery (2020F) Pre-surgical (cataract) axial length, corneal power measurement and method of intraocular lens power calculation documented (must be performed within 12 months prior to surgery) (3073F) Preoperative assessment of functional or medical indication(s) for surgery prior to the cataract surgery with intraocular lens placement (must be performed within 12 months prior to cataract surgery) (3325F)**

INCLUDES Evaluation dilated fundus done within 12 months prior to surgery (2020F)
Preoperative assessment functional or medical indications done within 12 months prior to surgery (3325F)
Presurgical measurement axial length, corneal power, and IOL power calculation performed within 12 months prior to surgery (3073F)

0.00 0.00 FUD XXX E

AMA: 2008,Mar,8-12

0015F **Melanoma follow up completed (includes assessment of all of the following components) (ML): History obtained regarding new or changing moles (1050F) Complete physical skin exam performed (2029F) Patient counseled to perform a monthly self skin examination (5005F)**

INCLUDES Complete physical skin exam (2029F)
Counseling to perform monthly skin self-examination (5005F)
History obtained new or changing moles (1050F)

0.00 0.00 FUD XXX E

AMA: 2008,Mar,8-12

0500F-0584F Care Provided According to Prevailing Guidelines

INCLUDES Utilization measures or patient care provided for certain clinical purposes

0500F **Initial prenatal care visit (report at first prenatal encounter with health care professional providing obstetrical care. Report also date of visit and, in a separate field, the date of the last menstrual period [LMP]) (Prenatal)** M ♀

0.00 0.00 FUD XXX E

AMA: 2018,Jan,8; 2017,Jan,8; 2016,Jan,13

0501F **Prenatal flow sheet documented in medical record by first prenatal visit (documentation includes at minimum blood pressure, weight, urine protein, uterine size, fetal heart tones, and estimated date of delivery). Report also: date of visit and, in a separate field, the date of the last menstrual period [LMP] (Note: If reporting 0501F Prenatal flow sheet, it is not necessary to report 0500F Initial prenatal care visit) (Prenatal)** M ♀

0.00 0.00 FUD XXX E

AMA: 2004,Nov,1

0502F **Subsequent prenatal care visit (Prenatal) [Excludes: patients who are seen for a condition unrelated to pregnancy or prenatal care (eg, an upper respiratory infection; patients seen for consultation only, not for continuing care)]** M ♀

EXCLUDES *Patients seen for unrelated pregnancy/prenatal care condition (e.g., upper respiratory infection; patients seen for consultation only, not for continuing care)*

0.00 0.00 FUD XXX E

AMA: 2004,Nov,1

0503F **Postpartum care visit (Prenatal)** M ♀

0.00 0.00 FUD XXX E

AMA: 2004,Nov,1

0505F **Hemodialysis plan of care documented (ESRD, P-ESRD)**

0.00 0.00 FUD XXX E

AMA: 2008,Mar,8-12

0507F **Peritoneal dialysis plan of care documented (ESRD)**

0.00 0.00 FUD XXX E

AMA: 2008,Mar,8-12

0509F **Urinary incontinence plan of care documented (GER)**

0.00 0.00 FUD XXX M

0513F **Elevated blood pressure plan of care documented (CKD)**

0.00 0.00 FUD XXX M

AMA: 2008,Mar,8-12

0514F **Plan of care for elevated hemoglobin level documented for patient receiving Erythropoiesis-Stimulating Agent therapy (ESA) (CKD)**

0.00 0.00 FUD XXX E

AMA: 2008,Mar,8-12

0516F **Anemia plan of care documented (ESRD)**

0.00 0.00 FUD XXX E

AMA: 2008,Mar,8-12

0517F **Glaucoma plan of care documented (EC)**

0.00 0.00 FUD XXX M

AMA: 2008,Mar,8-12

0518F **Falls plan of care documented (GER)**
0.00 0.00 **FUD** XXX M
AMA: 2008,Mar,8-12

0519F **Planned chemotherapy regimen, including at a minimum: drug(s) prescribed, dose, and duration, documented prior to initiation of a new treatment regimen (ONC)**
0.00 0.00 **FUD** XXX E
AMA: 2008,Mar,8-12

0520F **Radiation dose limits to normal tissues established prior to the initiation of a course of 3D conformal radiation for a minimum of 2 tissue/organ (ONC)**
0.00 0.00 **FUD** XXX M
AMA: 2008,Mar,8-12

0521F **Plan of care to address pain documented (COA) (ONC)**
0.00 0.00 **FUD** XXX M
AMA: 2008,Mar,8-12

0525F **Initial visit for episode (BkP)**
0.00 0.00 **FUD** XXX E
AMA: 2008,Mar,8-12

0526F **Subsequent visit for episode (BkP)**
0.00 0.00 **FUD** XXX M
AMA: 2008,Mar,8-12

0528F **Recommended follow-up interval for repeat colonoscopy of at least 10 years documented in colonoscopy report (End/Polyp)**
0.00 0.00 **FUD** XXX M

0529F **Interval of 3 or more years since patient's last colonoscopy, documented (End/Polyp)**
0.00 0.00 **FUD** XXX M

0535F **Dyspnea management plan of care, documented (Pall Cr)**
0.00 0.00 **FUD** XXX E

0540F **Glucorticoid Management Plan Documented (RA)**
0.00 0.00 **FUD** XXX M

0545F **Plan for follow-up care for major depressive disorder, documented (MDD ADOL)**
0.00 0.00 **FUD** XXX E

0550F **Cytopathology report on routine nongynecologic specimen finalized within two working days of accession date (PATH)**
0.00 0.00 **FUD** XXX E

0551F **Cytopathology report on nongynecologic specimen with documentation that the specimen was non-routine (PATH)**
0.00 0.00 **FUD** XXX E

0555F **Symptom management plan of care documented (HF)**
0.00 0.00 **FUD** XXX E

0556F **Plan of care to achieve lipid control documented (CAD)**
0.00 0.00 **FUD** XXX E

0557F **Plan of care to manage anginal symptoms documented (CAD)**
0.00 0.00 **FUD** XXX E

0575F **HIV RNA control plan of care, documented (HIV)**
0.00 0.00 **FUD** XXX E

0580F **Multidisciplinary care plan developed or updated (ALS)**
0.00 0.00 **FUD** XXX E

0581F **Patient transferred directly from anesthetizing location to critical care unit (Peri2)**
0.00 0.00 **FUD** XXX M

0582F **Patient not transferred directly from anesthetizing location to critical care unit (Peri2)**
0.00 0.00 **FUD** XXX E

0583F **Transfer of care checklist used (Peri2)**
0.00 0.00 **FUD** XXX M

0584F **Transfer of care checklist not used (Peri2)**
0.00 0.00 **FUD** XXX E

1000F-1505F Elements of History/Review of Systems

INCLUDES Measures for specific aspects patient history or systems review

1000F **Tobacco use assessed (CAD, CAP, COPD, PV) (DM)**
0.00 0.00 **FUD** XXX E
AMA: 2018,Jan,8; 2017,Jan,8; 2016,Jan,13

1002F **Anginal symptoms and level of activity assessed (NMA-No Measure Associated)**
0.00 0.00 **FUD** XXX E
AMA: 2004,Nov,1

1003F **Level of activity assessed (NMA-No Measure Associated)**
0.00 0.00 **FUD** XXX E
AMA: 2006,Dec,10-12

1004F **Clinical symptoms of volume overload (excess) assessed (NMA-No Measure Associated)**
0.00 0.00 **FUD** XXX E
AMA: 2006,Dec,10-12

1005F **Asthma symptoms evaluated (includes documentation of numeric frequency of symptoms or patient completion of an asthma assessment tool/survey/questionnaire) (NMA-No Measure Associated)**
0.00 0.00 **FUD** XXX E

1006F **Osteoarthritis symptoms and functional status assessed (may include the use of a standardized scale or the completion of an assessment questionnaire, such as the SF-36, AAOS Hip & Knee Questionnaire) (OA) [Instructions: Report when osteoarthritis is addressed during the patient encounter]**
INCLUDES Osteoarthritis when addressed during patient encounter
0.00 0.00 **FUD** XXX M

1007F **Use of anti-inflammatory or analgesic over-the-counter (OTC) medications for symptom relief assessed (OA)**
0.00 0.00 **FUD** XXX E

1008F **Gastrointestinal and renal risk factors assessed for patients on prescribed or OTC non-steroidal anti-inflammatory drug (NSAID) (OA)**
0.00 0.00 **FUD** XXX E

1010F **Severity of angina assessed by level of activity (CAD)**
0.00 0.00 **FUD** XXX E

1011F **Angina present (CAD)**
0.00 0.00 **FUD** XXX E

1012F **Angina absent (CAD)**
0.00 0.00 **FUD** XXX E

1015F **Chronic obstructive pulmonary disease (COPD) symptoms assessed (Includes assessment of at least 1 of the following: dyspnea, cough/sputum, wheezing), or respiratory symptom assessment tool completed (COPD)**
0.00 0.00 **FUD** XXX E

1018F **Dyspnea assessed, not present (COPD)**
0.00 0.00 **FUD** XXX E

1019F **Dyspnea assessed, present (COPD)**
0.00 0.00 **FUD** XXX E

1022F **Pneumococcus immunization status assessed (CAP, COPD)**
0.00 0.00 **FUD** XXX E
AMA: 2010,Jul,3-5; 2008,Mar,8-12

1026F **Co-morbid conditions assessed (eg, includes assessment for presence or absence of: malignancy, liver disease, congestive heart failure, cerebrovascular disease, renal disease, chronic obstructive pulmonary disease, asthma, diabetes, other co-morbid conditions) (CAP)**
0.00 0.00 **FUD** XXX E

1030F **Influenza immunization status assessed (CAP)**
0.00 0.00 **FUD** XXX E
AMA: 2008,Mar,8-12

1031F **Smoking status and exposure to second hand smoke in the home assessed (Asthma)**
0.00 0.00 FUD XXX E

1032F **Current tobacco smoker or currently exposed to secondhand smoke (Asthma)**
0.00 0.00 FUD XXX E

1033F **Current tobacco non-smoker and not currently exposed to secondhand smoke (Asthma)**
0.00 0.00 FUD XXX E

1034F **Current tobacco smoker (CAD, CAP, COPD, PV) (DM)**
0.00 0.00 FUD XXX E
AMA: 2008,Mar,8-12

1035F **Current smokeless tobacco user (eg, chew, snuff) (PV)**
0.00 0.00 FUD XXX E
AMA: 2008,Mar,8-12

1036F **Current tobacco non-user (CAD, CAP, COPD, PV) (DM) (IBD)**
0.00 0.00 FUD XXX M
AMA: 2008,Mar,8-12

1038F **Persistent asthma (mild, moderate or severe) (Asthma)**
0.00 0.00 FUD XXX M
AMA: 2018,Jan,8; 2017,Jan,8; 2016,Jan,13

1039F **Intermittent asthma (Asthma)**
0.00 0.00 FUD XXX M
AMA: 2018,Jan,8; 2017,Jan,8; 2016,Jan,13

1040F **DSM-5 criteria for major depressive disorder documented at the initial evaluation (MDD, MDD ADOL)**
0.00 0.00 FUD XXX E
AMA: 2008,Mar,8-12

1050F **History obtained regarding new or changing moles (ML)**
0.00 0.00 FUD XXX E
AMA: 2008,Mar,8-12

1052F **Type, anatomic location, and activity all assessed (IBD)**
0.00 0.00 FUD XXX E

1055F **Visual functional status assessed (EC)**
0.00 0.00 FUD XXX E

1060F **Documentation of permanent or persistent or paroxysmal atrial fibrillation (STR)**
0.00 0.00 FUD XXX E

1061F **Documentation of absence of permanent and persistent and paroxysmal atrial fibrillation (STR)**
0.00 0.00 FUD XXX E

1065F **Ischemic stroke symptom onset of less than 3 hours prior to arrival (STR)**
0.00 0.00 FUD XXX E

1066F **Ischemic stroke symptom onset greater than or equal to 3 hours prior to arrival (STR)**
0.00 0.00 FUD XXX E

1070F **Alarm symptoms (involuntary weight loss, dysphagia, or gastrointestinal bleeding) assessed; none present (GERD)**
0.00 0.00 FUD XXX E

1071F **1 or more present (GERD)**
0.00 0.00 FUD XXX E

1090F **Presence or absence of urinary incontinence assessed (GER)**
0.00 0.00 FUD XXX M

1091F **Urinary incontinence characterized (eg, frequency, volume, timing, type of symptoms, how bothersome) (GER)**
0.00 0.00 FUD XXX E

1100F **Patient screened for future fall risk; documentation of 2 or more falls in the past year or any fall with injury in the past year (GER)**
0.00 0.00 FUD XXX M
AMA: 2008,Mar,8-12

1101F **documentation of no falls in the past year or only 1 fall without injury in the past year (GER)**
0.00 0.00 FUD XXX M
AMA: 2008,Mar,8-12

1110F **Patient discharged from an inpatient facility (eg, hospital, skilled nursing facility, or rehabilitation facility) within the last 60 days (GER)**
0.00 0.00 FUD XXX E

1111F **Discharge medications reconciled with the current medication list in outpatient medical record (COA) (GER)**
0.00 0.00 FUD XXX M

1116F **Auricular or periauricular pain assessed (AOE)**
0.00 0.00 FUD XXX E
AMA: 2008,Mar,8-12

1118F **GERD symptoms assessed after 12 months of therapy (GERD)**
0.00 0.00 FUD XXX E
AMA: 2008,Mar,8-12

1119F **Initial evaluation for condition (HEP C)(EPI, DSP)**
0.00 0.00 FUD XXX E
AMA: 2008,Mar,8-12

1121F **Subsequent evaluation for condition (HEP C)(EPI)**
0.00 0.00 FUD XXX E
AMA: 2008,Mar,8-12

1123F **Advance Care Planning discussed and documented advance care plan or surrogate decision maker documented in the medical record (DEM) (GER, Pall Cr)**
0.00 0.00 FUD XXX M
AMA: 2008,Mar,8-12

1124F **Advance Care Planning discussed and documented in the medical record, patient did not wish or was not able to name a surrogate decision maker or provide an advance care plan (DEM) (GER, Pall Cr)**
0.00 0.00 FUD XXX M
AMA: 2008,Mar,8-12

1125F **Pain severity quantified; pain present (COA) (ONC)**
0.00 0.00 FUD XXX M
AMA: 2008,Mar,8-12

1126F **no pain present (COA) (ONC)**
0.00 0.00 FUD XXX M
AMA: 2008,Mar,8-12

1127F **New episode for condition (NMA-No Measure Associated)**
0.00 0.00 FUD XXX E
AMA: 2008,Mar,8-12

1128F **Subsequent episode for condition (NMA-No Measure Associated)**
0.00 0.00 FUD XXX E
AMA: 2008,Mar,8-12

1130F **Back pain and function assessed, including all of the following: Pain assessment and functional status and patient history, including notation of presence or absence of "red flags" (warning signs) and assessment of prior treatment and response, and employment status (BkP)**
0.00 0.00 FUD XXX E
AMA: 2008,Mar,8-12

1134F **Episode of back pain lasting 6 weeks or less (BkP)**
0.00 0.00 FUD XXX E
AMA: 2008,Mar,8-12

1135F **Episode of back pain lasting longer than 6 weeks (BkP)**
0.00 0.00 FUD XXX E
AMA: 2008,Mar,8-12

1136F **Episode of back pain lasting 12 weeks or less (BkP)**
0.00 0.00 FUD XXX E
AMA: 2008,Mar,8-12

1137F **Episode of back pain lasting longer than 12 weeks (BkP)**
0.00 0.00 FUD XXX E
AMA: 2008,Mar,8-12

1150F **Documentation that a patient has a substantial risk of death within 1 year (Pall Cr)**
0.00 0.00 FUD XXX E

1151F **Documentation that a patient does not have a substantial risk of death within one year (Pall Cr)**
0.00 0.00 FUD XXX E

1152F **Documentation of advanced disease diagnosis, goals of care prioritize comfort (Pall Cr)**
0.00 0.00 FUD XXX E

1153F **Documentation of advanced disease diagnosis, goals of care do not prioritize comfort (Pall Cr)**
0.00 0.00 FUD XXX E

1157F **Advance care plan or similar legal document present in the medical record (COA)**
0.00 0.00 FUD XXX E

1158F **Advance care planning discussion documented in the medical record (COA)**
0.00 0.00 FUD XXX M

1159F **Medication list documented in medical record (COA)**
0.00 0.00 FUD XXX E

1160F **Review of all medications by a prescribing practitioner or clinical pharmacist (such as, prescriptions, OTCs, herbal therapies and supplements) documented in the medical record (COA)**
0.00 0.00 FUD XXX E

1170F **Functional status assessed (COA) (RA)**
0.00 0.00 FUD XXX M

1175F **Functional status for dementia assessed and results reviewed (DEM)**
0.00 0.00 FUD XXX E

1180F **All specified thromboembolic risk factors assessed (AFIB)**
0.00 0.00 FUD XXX E

1181F **Neuropsychiatric symptoms assessed and results reviewed (DEM)**
0.00 0.00 FUD XXX E

1182F **Neuropsychiatric symptoms, one or more present (DEM)**
0.00 0.00 FUD XXX E

1183F **Neuropsychiatric symptoms, absent (DEM)**
0.00 0.00 FUD XXX E

1200F **Seizure type(s) and current seizure frequency(ies) documented (EPI)**
0.00 0.00 FUD XXX E

1205F **Etiology of epilepsy or epilepsy syndrome(s) reviewed and documented (EPI)**
0.00 0.00 FUD XXX E

1220F **Patient screened for depression (SUD)**
0.00 0.00 FUD XXX E

1400F **Parkinson's disease diagnosis reviewed (Prkns)**
0.00 0.00 FUD XXX E

1450F **Symptoms improved or remained consistent with treatment goals since last assessment (HF)**
0.00 0.00 FUD XXX E

1451F **Symptoms demonstrated clinically important deterioration since last assessment (HF)**
0.00 0.00 FUD XXX E

1460F **Qualifying cardiac event/diagnosis in previous 12 months (CAD)**
0.00 0.00 FUD XXX M

1461F **No qualifying cardiac event/diagnosis in previous 12 months (CAD)**
0.00 0.00 FUD XXX M

1490F **Dementia severity classified, mild (DEM)**
0.00 0.00 FUD XXX E

1491F **Dementia severity classified, moderate (DEM)**
0.00 0.00 FUD XXX E

1493F **Dementia severity classified, severe (DEM)**
0.00 0.00 FUD XXX E

1494F **Cognition assessed and reviewed (DEM)**
0.00 0.00 FUD XXX E

1500F **Symptoms and signs of distal symmetric polyneuropathy reviewed and documented (DSP)**
0.00 0.00 FUD XXX E

1501F **Not initial evaluation for condition (DSP)**
0.00 0.00 FUD XXX E

1502F **Patient queried about pain and pain interference with function using a valid and reliable instrument (DSP)**
0.00 0.00 FUD XXX E

1503F **Patient queried about symptoms of respiratory insufficiency (ALS)**
0.00 0.00 FUD XXX E

1504F **Patient has respiratory insufficiency (ALS)**
0.00 0.00 FUD XXX E

1505F **Patient does not have respiratory insufficiency (ALS)**
0.00 0.00 FUD XXX E

2000F-2060F [2033F] Elements of Examination

INCLUDES Components clinical assessment or physical exam

2000F **Blood pressure measured (CKD)(DM)**
0.00 0.00 FUD XXX M
AMA: 2018,Jan,8; 2017,Jan,8; 2016,Jan,13

2001F **Weight recorded (PAG)**
0.00 0.00 FUD XXX E
AMA: 2006,Dec,10-12

2002F **Clinical signs of volume overload (excess) assessed (NMA-No Measure Associated)**
0.00 0.00 FUD XXX E
AMA: 2006,Dec,10-12

2004F **Initial examination of the involved joint(s) (includes visual inspection, palpation, range of motion) (OA) [Instructions: Report only for initial osteoarthritis visit or for visits for new joint involvement]**
INCLUDES Visits for initial osteoarthritis examination or new joint involvement
0.00 0.00 FUD XXX E
AMA: 2004,Feb,3; 2003,Aug,1

2010F **Vital signs (temperature, pulse, respiratory rate, and blood pressure) documented and reviewed (CAP) (EM)**
0.00 0.00 FUD XXX E

2014F **Mental status assessed (CAP) (EM)**
0.00 0.00 FUD XXX E

2015F **Asthma impairment assessed (Asthma)**
0.00 0.00 FUD XXX E

2016F **Asthma risk assessed (Asthma)**
0.00 0.00 FUD XXX E

2018F **Hydration status assessed (normal/mildly dehydrated/severely dehydrated) (CAP)**
0.00 0.00 FUD XXX E

2019F **Dilated macular exam performed, including documentation of the presence or absence of macular thickening or hemorrhage and the level of macular degeneration severity (EC)**
0.00 0.00 FUD XXX E

2020F **Dilated fundus evaluation performed within 12 months prior to cataract surgery (EC)**
0.00 0.00 FUD XXX E
AMA: 2008,Mar,8-12

2021F **Dilated macular or fundus exam performed, including documentation of the presence or absence of macular edema and level of severity of retinopathy (EC)**
0.00 0.00 FUD XXX E

2022F **Dilated retinal eye exam with interpretation by an ophthalmologist or optometrist documented and reviewed; with evidence of retinopathy (DM)**
0.00 0.00 FUD XXX M
AMA: 2008,Mar,8-12

2023F **without evidence of retinopathy (DM)**
0.00 0.00 FUD XXX

2024F **7 standard field stereoscopic retinal photos with interpretation by an ophthalmologist or optometrist documented and reviewed; with evidence of retinopathy (DM)**
0.00 0.00 FUD XXX M
AMA: 2008,Mar,8-12

2025F **without evidence of retinopathy (DM)**
0.00 0.00 FUD XXX

2026F **Eye imaging validated to match diagnosis from 7 standard field stereoscopic retinal photos results documented and reviewed; with evidence of retinopathy (DM)**
0.00 0.00 FUD XXX M
AMA: 2008,Mar,8-12

2033F **without evidence of retinopathy (DM)**
0.00 0.00 FUD XXX

2027F **Optic nerve head evaluation performed (EC)**
0.00 0.00 FUD XXX M

2028F **Foot examination performed (includes examination through visual inspection, sensory exam with monofilament, and pulse exam - report when any of the 3 components are completed) (DM)**
0.00 0.00 FUD XXX E

2029F **Complete physical skin exam performed (ML)**
0.00 0.00 FUD XXX E
AMA: 2008,Mar,8-12

2030F **Hydration status documented, normally hydrated (PAG)**
0.00 0.00 FUD XXX E

2031F **Hydration status documented, dehydrated (PAG)**
0.00 0.00 FUD XXX E

2033F **Resequenced code. See code following 2026F.**

2035F **Tympanic membrane mobility assessed with pneumatic otoscopy or tympanometry (OME)**
0.00 0.00 FUD XXX E
AMA: 2008,Mar,8-12

2040F **Physical examination on the date of the initial visit for low back pain performed, in accordance with specifications (BkP)**
0.00 0.00 FUD XXX E
AMA: 2008,Mar,8-12

2044F **Documentation of mental health assessment prior to intervention (back surgery or epidural steroid injection) or for back pain episode lasting longer than 6 weeks (BkP)**
0.00 0.00 FUD XXX E
AMA: 2008,Mar,8-12

2050F **Wound characteristics including size and nature of wound base tissue and amount of drainage prior to debridement documented (CWC)**
0.00 0.00 FUD XXX E

2060F **Patient interviewed directly on or before date of diagnosis of major depressive disorder (MDD ADOL)**
0.00 0.00 FUD XXX E

3006F-3776F [3051F, 3052F] Findings from Diagnostic or Screening Tests

INCLUDES Results and medical decision making with regards to ordered tests:
- Clinical laboratory tests
- Other examination procedures
- Radiological examinations

3006F **Chest X-ray results documented and reviewed (CAP)**
0.00 0.00 FUD XXX E
AMA: 2018,Jan,8; 2017,Jan,8; 2016,Jan,13

3008F **Body Mass Index (BMI), documented (PV)**
0.00 0.00 FUD XXX E

3011F **Lipid panel results documented and reviewed (must include total cholesterol, HDL-C, triglycerides and calculated LDL-C) (CAD)**
0.00 0.00 FUD XXX E

3014F **Screening mammography results documented and reviewed (PV)**
0.00 0.00 FUD XXX E
AMA: 2008,Mar,8-12

3015F **Cervical cancer screening results documented and reviewed (PV)** ♀
0.00 0.00 FUD XXX E

3016F **Patient screened for unhealthy alcohol use using a systematic screening method (PV) (DSP)**
0.00 0.00 FUD XXX E

3017F **Colorectal cancer screening results documented and reviewed (PV)**
0.00 0.00 FUD XXX M
AMA: 2008,Mar,8-12

3018F **Pre-procedure risk assessment and depth of insertion and quality of the bowel prep and complete description of polyp(s) found, including location of each polyp, size, number and gross morphology and recommendations for follow-up in final colonoscopy report documented (End/Polyp)**
0.00 0.00 FUD XXX E

3019F **Left ventricular ejection fraction (LVEF) assessment planned post discharge (HF)**
0.00 0.00 FUD XXX E

3020F **Left ventricular function (LVF) assessment (eg, echocardiography, nuclear test, or ventriculography) documented in the medical record (Includes quantitative or qualitative assessment results) (NMA-No Measure Associated)**
0.00 0.00 FUD XXX E
AMA: 2006,Dec,10-12

3021F **Left ventricular ejection fraction (LVEF) less than 40% or documentation of moderately or severely depressed left ventricular systolic function (CAD, HF)**
0.00 0.00 FUD XXX M

3022F **Left ventricular ejection fraction (LVEF) greater than or equal to 40% or documentation as normal or mildly depressed left ventricular systolic function (CAD, HF)**
0.00 0.00 FUD XXX M

3023F **Spirometry results documented and reviewed (COPD)**
0.00 0.00 FUD XXX M

3025F **Spirometry test results demonstrate FEV1/FVC less than 70% with COPD symptoms (eg, dyspnea, cough/sputum, wheezing) (CAP, COPD)**
0.00 0.00 FUD XXX E

3027F **Spirometry test results demonstrate FEV1/FVC greater than or equal to 70% or patient does not have COPD symptoms (COPD)**
0.00 0.00 FUD XXX E

3028F **Oxygen saturation results documented and reviewed (includes assessment through pulse oximetry or arterial blood gas measurement) (CAP, COPD) (EM)**
0.00 0.00 FUD XXX E

3035F **Oxygen saturation less than or equal to 88% or a PaO2 less than or equal to 55 mm Hg (COPD)**
0.00 0.00 FUD XXX E

3037F **Oxygen saturation greater than 88% or PaO2 greater than 55 mm Hg (COPD)**
0.00 0.00 FUD XXX E

3038F **Pulmonary function test performed within 12 months prior to surgery (Lung/Esop Cx)**
0.00 0.00 FUD XXX E

3040F **Functional expiratory volume (FEV1) less than 40% of predicted value (COPD)**
0.00 0.00 FUD XXX E

3042F **Functional expiratory volume (FEV1) greater than or equal to 40% of predicted value (COPD)**
0.00 0.00 FUD XXX E

3044F **Most recent hemoglobin A1c (HbA1c) level less than 7.0% (DM)**
0.00 0.00 FUD XXX M

3051F **Most recent hemoglobin A1c (HbA1c) level greater than or equal to 7.0% and less than 8.0% (DM)**
0.00 0.00 FUD XXX

3052F **Most recent hemoglobin A1c (HbA1c) level greater than or equal to 8.0% and less than or equal to 9.0% (DM)**
0.00 0.00 FUD XXX

3046F **Most recent hemoglobin A1c level greater than 9.0% (DM)**
EXCLUDES *Hemoglobin A1c less than or equal to 9.0% (3044F, [3051F], [3052F])*
0.00 0.00 FUD XXX M

3048F **Most recent LDL-C less than 100 mg/dL (CAD) (DM)**
0.00 0.00 FUD XXX E

3049F **Most recent LDL-C 100-129 mg/dL (CAD) (DM)**
0.00 0.00 FUD XXX E

3050F **Most recent LDL-C greater than or equal to 130 mg/dL (CAD) (DM)**
0.00 0.00 FUD XXX E

3051F **Resequenced code. See code following 3044F.**

3052F **Resequenced code. See code before 3046F.**

3055F **Left ventricular ejection fraction (LVEF) less than or equal to 35% (HF)**
0.00 0.00 FUD XXX E

3056F **Left ventricular ejection fraction (LVEF) greater than 35% or no LVEF result available (HF)**
0.00 0.00 FUD XXX E

3060F **Positive microalbuminuria test result documented and reviewed (DM)**
0.00 0.00 FUD XXX M

3061F **Negative microalbuminuria test result documented and reviewed (DM)**
0.00 0.00 FUD XXX M

3062F **Positive macroalbuminuria test result documented and reviewed (DM)**
0.00 0.00 FUD XXX M

3066F **Documentation of treatment for nephropathy (eg, patient receiving dialysis, patient being treated for ESRD, CRF, ARF, or renal insufficiency, any visit to a nephrologist) (DM)**
0.00 0.00 FUD XXX M

3072F **Low risk for retinopathy (no evidence of retinopathy in the prior year) (DM)**
0.00 0.00 FUD XXX M
AMA: 2008,Mar,8-12

3073F **Pre-surgical (cataract) axial length, corneal power measurement and method of intraocular lens power calculation documented within 12 months prior to surgery (EC)**
0.00 0.00 FUD XXX E
AMA: 2008,Mar,8-12

3074F **Most recent systolic blood pressure less than 130 mm Hg (DM), (HTN, CKD, CAD)**
0.00 0.00 FUD XXX E
AMA: 2008,Mar,8-12

3075F **Most recent systolic blood pressure 130-139 mm Hg (DM) (HTN, CKD, CAD)**
0.00 0.00 FUD XXX E
AMA: 2008,Mar,8-12

3077F **Most recent systolic blood pressure greater than or equal to 140 mm Hg (HTN, CKD, CAD) (DM)**
0.00 0.00 FUD XXX E
AMA: 2008,Mar,8-12

3078F **Most recent diastolic blood pressure less than 80 mm Hg (HTN, CKD, CAD) (DM)**
0.00 0.00 FUD XXX E
AMA: 2008,Mar,8-12

3079F **Most recent diastolic blood pressure 80-89 mm Hg (HTN, CKD, CAD) (DM)**
0.00 0.00 FUD XXX E
AMA: 2008,Mar,8-12

3080F **Most recent diastolic blood pressure greater than or equal to 90 mm Hg (HTN, CKD, CAD) (DM)**
0.00 0.00 FUD XXX E
AMA: 2008,Mar,8-12

3082F **Kt/V less than 1.2 (Clearance of urea [Kt]/volume [V]) (ESRD, P-ESRD)**
0.00 0.00 FUD XXX E
AMA: 2008,Mar,8-12

3083F **Kt/V equal to or greater than 1.2 and less than 1.7 (Clearance of urea [Kt]/volume [V]) (ESRD, P-ESRD)**
0.00 0.00 FUD XXX E
AMA: 2008,Mar,8-12

3084F **Kt/V greater than or equal to 1.7 (Clearance of urea [Kt]/volume [V]) (ESRD, P-ESRD)**
0.00 0.00 FUD XXX E
AMA: 2008,Mar,8-12

3085F **Suicide risk assessed (MDD, MDD ADOL)**
0.00 0.00 FUD XXX E

3088F **Major depressive disorder, mild (MDD)**
0.00 0.00 FUD XXX E

3089F **Major depressive disorder, moderate (MDD)**
0.00 0.00 FUD XXX E

3090F **Major depressive disorder, severe without psychotic features (MDD)**
0.00 0.00 FUD XXX E

3091F **Major depressive disorder, severe with psychotic features (MDD)**
0.00 0.00 FUD XXX E

3092F **Major depressive disorder, in remission (MDD)**
0.00 0.00 FUD XXX E

3093F **Documentation of new diagnosis of initial or recurrent episode of major depressive disorder (MDD)**
0.00 0.00 FUD XXX E
AMA: 2008,Mar,8-12

3095F **Central dual-energy X-ray absorptiometry (DXA) results documented (OP)(IBD)**
0.00 0.00 FUD XXX M

3096F **Central dual-energy X-ray absorptiometry (DXA) ordered (OP)(IBD)**
0.00 0.00 FUD XXX E

3100F **Carotid imaging study report (includes direct or indirect reference to measurements of distal internal carotid diameter as the denominator for stenosis measurement) (STR, RAD)**
0.00 0.00 FUD XXX M
AMA: 2008,Mar,8-12

3110F **Documentation in final CT or MRI report of presence or absence of hemorrhage and mass lesion and acute infarction (STR)**
0.00 0.00 FUD XXX E

3111F **CT or MRI of the brain performed in the hospital within 24 hours of arrival or performed in an outpatient imaging center, to confirm initial diagnosis of stroke, TIA or intracranial hemorrhage (STR)**
0.00 0.00 FUD XXX E

3112F **CT or MRI of the brain performed greater than 24 hours after arrival to the hospital or performed in an outpatient imaging center for purpose other than confirmation of initial diagnosis of stroke, TIA, or intracranial hemorrhage (STR)**
0.00 0.00 FUD XXX E

3115F **Quantitative results of an evaluation of current level of activity and clinical symptoms (HF)**
0.00 0.00 FUD XXX E

3117F **Heart failure disease specific structured assessment tool completed (HF)**
0.00 0.00 FUD XXX E

3118F **New York Heart Association (NYHA) Class documented (HF)**
0.00 0.00 FUD XXX E

3119F **No evaluation of level of activity or clinical symptoms (HF)**
0.00 0.00 FUD XXX E

3120F **12-Lead ECG Performed (EM)**
0.00 0.00 FUD XXX E

3126F **Esophageal biopsy report with a statement about dysplasia (present, absent, or indefinite, and if present, contains appropriate grading) (PATH)**
0.00 0.00 FUD XXX M

3130F **Upper gastrointestinal endoscopy performed (GERD)**
0.00 0.00 FUD XXX E

3132F **Documentation of referral for upper gastrointestinal endoscopy (GERD)**
0.00 0.00 FUD XXX E

3140F **Upper gastrointestinal endoscopy report indicates suspicion of Barrett's esophagus (GERD)**
0.00 0.00 FUD XXX E

3141F **Upper gastrointestinal endoscopy report indicates no suspicion of Barrett's esophagus (GERD)**
0.00 0.00 FUD XXX E

3142F **Barium swallow test ordered (GERD)**
INCLUDES Documentation barium swallow test
0.00 0.00 FUD XXX E

3150F **Forceps esophageal biopsy performed (GERD)**
0.00 0.00 FUD XXX E

3155F **Cytogenetic testing performed on bone marrow at time of diagnosis or prior to initiating treatment (HEM)**
0.00 0.00 FUD XXX M
AMA: 2008,Mar,8-12

3160F **Documentation of iron stores prior to initiating erythropoietin therapy (HEM)**
0.00 0.00 FUD XXX M
AMA: 2008,Mar,8-12

3170F **Baseline flow cytometry studies performed at time of diagnosis or prior to initiating treatment (HEM)**
0.00 0.00 FUD XXX M
AMA: 2008,Mar,8-12

3200F **Barium swallow test not ordered (GERD)**
0.00 0.00 FUD XXX E

3210F **Group A Strep Test Performed (PHAR)**
0.00 0.00 FUD XXX M
AMA: 2008,Mar,8-12

3215F **Patient has documented immunity to Hepatitis A (HEP-C)**
0.00 0.00 FUD XXX E
AMA: 2008,Mar,8-12

3216F **Patient has documented immunity to Hepatitis B (HEP-C)(IBD)**
0.00 0.00 FUD XXX E
AMA: 2008,Mar,8-12

3218F **RNA testing for Hepatitis C documented as performed within 6 months prior to initiation of antiviral treatment for Hepatitis C (HEP-C)**
0.00 0.00 FUD XXX E
AMA: 2008,Mar,8-12

3220F **Hepatitis C quantitative RNA testing documented as performed at 12 weeks from initiation of antiviral treatment (HEP-C)**
0.00 0.00 FUD XXX E
AMA: 2008,Mar,8-12

3230F **Documentation that hearing test was performed within 6 months prior to tympanostomy tube insertion (OME)**
0.00 0.00 FUD XXX E
AMA: 2008,Mar,8-12

3250F **Specimen site other than anatomic location of primary tumor (PATH)**
0.00 0.00 FUD XXX M

3260F **pT category (primary tumor), pN category (regional lymph nodes), and histologic grade documented in pathology report (PATH)**
0.00 0.00 FUD XXX M
AMA: 2008,Mar,8-12

3265F **Ribonucleic acid (RNA) testing for Hepatitis C viremia ordered or results documented (HEP C)**
0.00 0.00 FUD XXX E
AMA: 2008,Mar,8-12

3266F **Hepatitis C genotype testing documented as performed prior to initiation of antiviral treatment for Hepatitis C (HEP C)**
0.00 0.00 FUD XXX E
AMA: 2008,Mar,8-12

3267F **Pathology report includes pT category, pN category, Gleason score, and statement about margin status (PATH)**
0.00 0.00 FUD XXX M

3268F **Prostate-specific antigen (PSA), and primary tumor (T) stage, and Gleason score documented prior to initiation of treatment (PRCA)**
0.00 0.00 FUD XXX E
AMA: 2008,Mar,8-12

Category II Codes

3093F — 3268F

Category II Codes

3269F **Bone scan performed prior to initiation of treatment or at any time since diagnosis of prostate cancer (PRCA)**
0.00 0.00 FUD XXX M
AMA: 2008,Mar,8-12

3270F **Bone scan not performed prior to initiation of treatment nor at any time since diagnosis of prostate cancer (PRCA)**
0.00 0.00 FUD XXX M
AMA: 2008,Mar,8-12

3271F **Low risk of recurrence, prostate cancer (PRCA)**
0.00 0.00 FUD XXX E
AMA: 2008,Mar,8-12

3272F **Intermediate risk of recurrence, prostate cancer (PRCA)**
0.00 0.00 FUD XXX E
AMA: 2008,Mar,8-12

3273F **High risk of recurrence, prostate cancer (PRCA)**
0.00 0.00 FUD XXX E
AMA: 2008,Mar,8-12

3274F **Prostate cancer risk of recurrence not determined or neither low, intermediate nor high (PRCA)**
0.00 0.00 FUD XXX E
AMA: 2008,Mar,8-12

3278F **Serum levels of calcium, phosphorus, intact Parathyroid Hormone (PTH) and lipid profile ordered (CKD)**
0.00 0.00 FUD XXX E
AMA: 2008,Mar,8-12

3279F **Hemoglobin level greater than or equal to 13 g/dL (CKD, ESRD)**
0.00 0.00 FUD XXX E
AMA: 2008,Mar,8-12

3280F **Hemoglobin level 11 g/dL to 12.9 g/dL (CKD, ESRD)**
0.00 0.00 FUD XXX E
AMA: 2008,Mar,8-12

3281F **Hemoglobin level less than 11 g/dL (CKD, ESRD)**
0.00 0.00 FUD XXX E
AMA: 2008,Mar,8-12

3284F **Intraocular pressure (IOP) reduced by a value of greater than or equal to 15% from the pre-intervention level (EC)**
0.00 0.00 FUD XXX M
AMA: 2008,Mar,8-12

3285F **Intraocular pressure (IOP) reduced by a value less than 15% from the pre-intervention level (EC)**
0.00 0.00 FUD XXX M
AMA: 2008,Mar,8-12

3288F **Falls risk assessment documented (GER)**
0.00 0.00 FUD XXX M
AMA: 2008,Mar,8-12

3290F **Patient is D (Rh) negative and unsensitized (Pre-Cr)**
0.00 0.00 FUD XXX E
AMA: 2008,Mar,8-12

3291F **Patient is D (Rh) positive or sensitized (Pre-Cr)**
0.00 0.00 FUD XXX E
AMA: 2008,Mar,8-12

3292F **HIV testing ordered or documented and reviewed during the first or second prenatal visit (Pre-Cr)**
0.00 0.00 FUD XXX E

3293F **ABO and Rh blood typing documented as performed (Pre-Cr)**
0.00 0.00 FUD XXX E

3294F **Group B Streptococcus (GBS) screening documented as performed during week 35-37 gestation (Pre-Cr)**
0.00 0.00 FUD XXX E

3300F **American Joint Committee on Cancer (AJCC) stage documented and reviewed (ONC)**
0.00 0.00 FUD XXX M
AMA: 2008,Mar,8-12

3301F **Cancer stage documented in medical record as metastatic and reviewed (ONC)**
EXCLUDES *Cancer staging measures (3321F-3390F)*
0.00 0.00 FUD XXX M
AMA: 2008,Mar,8-12

3315F **Estrogen receptor (ER) or progesterone receptor (PR) positive breast cancer (ONC)**
0.00 0.00 FUD XXX E
AMA: 2008,Mar,8-12

3316F **Estrogen receptor (ER) and progesterone receptor (PR) negative breast cancer (ONC)**
0.00 0.00 FUD XXX E
AMA: 2008,Mar,8-12

3317F **Pathology report confirming malignancy documented in the medical record and reviewed prior to the initiation of chemotherapy (ONC)**
0.00 0.00 FUD XXX E
AMA: 2008,Mar,8-12

3318F **Pathology report confirming malignancy documented in the medical record and reviewed prior to the initiation of radiation therapy (ONC)**
0.00 0.00 FUD XXX E
AMA: 2008,Mar,8-12

3319F **1 of the following diagnostic imaging studies ordered: chest x-ray, CT, Ultrasound, MRI, PET, or nuclear medicine scans (ML)**
0.00 0.00 FUD XXX M
AMA: 2008,Mar,8-12

3320F **None of the following diagnostic imaging studies ordered: chest X-ray, CT, Ultrasound, MRI, PET, or nuclear medicine scans (ML)**
0.00 0.00 FUD XXX M
AMA: 2008,Mar,8-12

3321F **AJCC Cancer Stage 0 or IA Melanoma, documented (ML)**
0.00 0.00 FUD XXX M

3322F **Melanoma greater than AJCC Stage 0 or IA (ML)**
0.00 0.00 FUD XXX M

3323F **Clinical tumor, node and metastases (TNM) staging documented and reviewed prior to surgery (Lung/Esop Cx)**
0.00 0.00 FUD XXX E

3324F **MRI or CT scan ordered, reviewed or requested (EPI)**
0.00 0.00 FUD XXX E

3325F **Preoperative assessment of functional or medical indication(s) for surgery prior to the cataract surgery with intraocular lens placement (must be performed within 12 months prior to cataract surgery) (EC)**
0.00 0.00 FUD XXX E
AMA: 2008,Mar,8-12

3328F **Performance status documented and reviewed within 2 weeks prior to surgery (Lung/Esop Cx)**
0.00 0.00 FUD XXX E

3330F **Imaging study ordered (BkP)**
0.00 0.00 FUD XXX E
AMA: 2008,Mar,8-12

3331F **Imaging study not ordered (BkP)**
0.00 0.00 FUD XXX E
AMA: 2008,Mar,8-12

3340F **Mammogram assessment category of "incomplete: need additional imaging evaluation" documented (RAD)**
0.00 0.00 FUD XXX M
AMA: 2008,Mar,8-12

3341F **Mammogram assessment category of "negative," documented (RAD)**
0.00 0.00 FUD XXX M
AMA: 2008,Mar,8-12

3269F — 3341F

3342F **Mammogram assessment category of "benign," documented (RAD)**
0.00 0.00 FUD XXX M
AMA: 2008,Mar,8-12

3343F **Mammogram assessment category of "probably benign," documented (RAD)**
0.00 0.00 FUD XXX M
AMA: 2008,Mar,8-12

3344F **Mammogram assessment category of "suspicious," documented (RAD)**
0.00 0.00 FUD XXX M
AMA: 2008,Mar,8-12

3345F **Mammogram assessment category of "highly suggestive of malignancy," documented (RAD)**
0.00 0.00 FUD XXX M
AMA: 2008,Mar,8-12

3350F **Mammogram assessment category of "known biopsy proven malignancy," documented (RAD)**
0.00 0.00 FUD XXX M
AMA: 2008,Mar,8-12

3351F **Negative screen for depressive symptoms as categorized by using a standardized depression screening/assessment tool (MDD)**
0.00 0.00 FUD XXX E

3352F **No significant depressive symptoms as categorized by using a standardized depression assessment tool (MDD)**
0.00 0.00 FUD XXX E

3353F **Mild to moderate depressive symptoms as categorized by using a standardized depression screening/assessment tool (MDD)**
0.00 0.00 FUD XXX E

3354F **Clinically significant depressive symptoms as categorized by using a standardized depression screening/assessment tool (MDD)**
0.00 0.00 FUD XXX E

3370F **AJCC Breast Cancer Stage 0 documented (ONC)**
0.00 0.00 FUD XXX E

3372F **AJCC Breast Cancer Stage I: T1mic, T1a or T1b (tumor size ≤ 1 cm) documented (ONC)**
0.00 0.00 FUD XXX E

3374F **AJCC Breast Cancer Stage I: T1c (tumor size > 1 cm to 2 cm) documented (ONC)**
0.00 0.00 FUD XXX E

3376F **AJCC Breast Cancer Stage II documented (ONC)**
0.00 0.00 FUD XXX E

3378F **AJCC Breast Cancer Stage III documented (ONC)**
0.00 0.00 FUD XXX E

3380F **AJCC Breast Cancer Stage IV documented (ONC)**
0.00 0.00 FUD XXX E

3382F **AJCC colon cancer, Stage 0 documented (ONC)**
0.00 0.00 FUD XXX E

3384F **AJCC colon cancer, Stage I documented (ONC)**
0.00 0.00 FUD XXX E

3386F **AJCC colon cancer, Stage II documented (ONC)**
0.00 0.00 FUD XXX E

3388F **AJCC colon cancer, Stage III documented (ONC)**
0.00 0.00 FUD XXX E

3390F **AJCC colon cancer, Stage IV documented (ONC)**
0.00 0.00 FUD XXX E

3394F **Quantitative HER2 immunohistochemistry (IHC) evaluation of breast cancer consistent with the scoring system defined in the ASCO/CAP guidelines (PATH)**
0.00 0.00 FUD XXX M

3395F **Quantitative non-HER2 immunohistochemistry (IHC) evaluation of breast cancer (eg, testing for estrogen or progesterone receptors [ER/PR]) performed (PATH)**
0.00 0.00 FUD XXX M

3450F **Dyspnea screened, no dyspnea or mild dyspnea (Pall Cr)**
0.00 0.00 FUD XXX E

3451F **Dyspnea screened, moderate or severe dyspnea (Pall Cr)**
0.00 0.00 FUD XXX E

3452F **Dyspnea not screened (Pall Cr)**
0.00 0.00 FUD XXX E

3455F **TB screening performed and results interpreted within six months prior to initiation of first-time biologic disease modifying anti-rheumatic drug therapy for RA (RA)**
0.00 0.00 FUD XXX M

3470F **Rheumatoid arthritis (RA) disease activity, low (RA)**
0.00 0.00 FUD XXX M

3471F **Rheumatoid arthritis (RA) disease activity, moderate (RA)**
0.00 0.00 FUD XXX M

3472F **Rheumatoid arthritis (RA) disease activity, high (RA)**
0.00 0.00 FUD XXX M

3475F **Disease prognosis for rheumatoid arthritis assessed, poor prognosis documented (RA)**
0.00 0.00 FUD XXX M

3476F **Disease prognosis for rheumatoid arthritis assessed, good prognosis documented (RA)**
0.00 0.00 FUD XXX M

3490F **History of AIDS-defining condition (HIV)**
0.00 0.00 FUD XXX E

3491F **HIV indeterminate (infants of undetermined HIV status born of HIV-infected mothers) (HIV)**
0.00 0.00 FUD XXX E

3492F **History of nadir CD4+ cell count <350 cells/mm3 (HIV)**
0.00 0.00 FUD XXX E

3493F **No history of nadir CD4+ cell count <350 cells/mm3 and no history of AIDS-defining condition (HIV)**
0.00 0.00 FUD XXX E

3494F **CD4+ cell count <200 cells/mm3 (HIV)**
0.00 0.00 FUD XXX E

3495F **CD4+ cell count 200 - 499 cells/mm3 (HIV)**
0.00 0.00 FUD XXX E

3496F **CD4+ cell count ≥ 500 cells/mm3 (HIV)**
0.00 0.00 FUD XXX E

3497F **CD4+ cell percentage <15% (HIV)**
0.00 0.00 FUD XXX E

3498F **CD4+ cell percentage ≥ 15% (HIV)**
0.00 0.00 FUD XXX E

3500F **CD4+ cell count or CD4+ cell percentage documented as performed (HIV)**
0.00 0.00 FUD XXX E

3502F **HIV RNA viral load below limits of quantification (HIV)**
0.00 0.00 FUD XXX E

3503F **HIV RNA viral load not below limits of quantification (HIV)**
0.00 0.00 FUD XXX E

3510F **Documentation that tuberculosis (TB) screening test performed and results interpreted (HIV) (IBD)**
0.00 0.00 FUD XXX E

3511F **Chlamydia and gonorrhea screenings documented as performed (HIV)**
0.00 0.00 FUD XXX E

3512F **Syphilis screening documented as performed (HIV)**
0.00 0.00 FUD XXX E

3513F **Hepatitis B screening documented as performed (HIV)**
0.00 0.00 FUD XXX E

3514F **Hepatitis C screening documented as performed (HIV)**
0.00 0.00 FUD XXX E

3515F **Patient has documented immunity to Hepatitis C (HIV)**
0.00 0.00 FUD XXX E

3517F **Hepatitis B Virus (HBV) status assessed and results interpreted within one year prior to receiving a first course of anti-TNF (tumor necrosis factor) therapy (IBD)**
0.00 0.00 FUD XXX E

3520F **Clostridium difficile testing performed (IBD)**
0.00 0.00 FUD XXX E

3550F **Low risk for thromboembolism (AFIB)**
0.00 0.00 FUD XXX E

3551F **Intermediate risk for thromboembolism (AFIB)**
0.00 0.00 FUD XXX E

3552F **High risk for thromboembolism (AFIB)**
0.00 0.00 FUD XXX E

3555F **Patient had International Normalized Ratio (INR) measurement performed (AFIB)**
0.00 0.00 FUD XXX E
AMA: 2010,Jul,3-5

3570F **Final report for bone scintigraphy study includes correlation with existing relevant imaging studies (eg, X-ray, MRI, CT) corresponding to the same anatomical region in question (NUC_MED)**
0.00 0.00 FUD XXX M

3572F **Patient considered to be potentially at risk for fracture in a weight-bearing site (NUC_MED)**
0.00 0.00 FUD XXX E

3573F **Patient not considered to be potentially at risk for fracture in a weight-bearing site (NUC_MED)**
0.00 0.00 FUD XXX E

3650F **Electroencephalogram (EEG) ordered, reviewed or requested (EPI)**
0.00 0.00 FUD XXX E

3700F **Psychiatric disorders or disturbances assessed (Prkns)**
0.00 0.00 FUD XXX E

3720F **Cognitive impairment or dysfunction assessed (Prkns)**
0.00 0.00 FUD XXX M

3725F **Screening for depression performed (DEM)**
0.00 0.00 FUD XXX M

3750F **Patient not receiving dose of corticosteroids greater than or equal to 10mg/day for 60 or greater consecutive days (IBD)**
0.00 0.00 FUD XXX E

3751F **Electrodiagnostic studies for distal symmetric polyneuropathy conducted (or requested), documented, and reviewed within 6 months of initial evaluation for condition (DSP)**
0.00 0.00 FUD XXX E

3752F **Electrodiagnostic studies for distal symmetric polyneuropathy not conducted (or requested), documented, or reviewed within 6 months of initial evaluation for condition (DSP)**
0.00 0.00 FUD XXX E

3753F **Patient has clear clinical symptoms and signs that are highly suggestive of neuropathy AND cannot be attributed to another condition, AND has an obvious cause for the neuropathy (DSP)**
0.00 0.00 FUD XXX E

3754F **Screening tests for diabetes mellitus reviewed, requested, or ordered (DSP)**
0.00 0.00 FUD XXX E

3755F **Cognitive and behavioral impairment screening performed (ALS)**
0.00 0.00 FUD XXX E

3756F **Patient has pseudobulbar affect, sialorrhea, or ALS-related symptoms (ALS)**
0.00 0.00 FUD XXX E

3757F **Patient does not have pseudobulbar affect, sialorrhea, or ALS-related symptoms (ALS)**
0.00 0.00 FUD XXX E

3758F **Patient referred for pulmonary function testing or peak cough expiratory flow (ALS)**
0.00 0.00 FUD XXX E

3759F **Patient screened for dysphagia, weight loss, and impaired nutrition, and results documented (ALS)**
0.00 0.00 FUD XXX E

3760F **Patient exhibits dysphagia, weight loss, or impaired nutrition (ALS)**
0.00 0.00 FUD XXX E

3761F **Patient does not exhibit dysphagia, weight loss, or impaired nutrition (ALS)**
0.00 0.00 FUD XXX E

3762F **Patient is dysarthric (ALS)**
0.00 0.00 FUD XXX E

3763F **Patient is not dysarthric (ALS)**
0.00 0.00 FUD XXX E

3775F **Adenoma(s) or other neoplasm detected during screening colonoscopy (SCADR)**
0.00 0.00 FUD XXX E

3776F **Adenoma(s) or other neoplasm not detected during screening colonoscopy (SCADR)**
0.00 0.00 FUD XXX E

4000F-4563F Therapies Provided (Includes Preventive Services)

INCLUDES Behavioral/pharmacologic/procedural therapies
Preventive services including patient education/counseling

4000F **Tobacco use cessation intervention, counseling (COPD, CAP, CAD, Asthma) (DM) (PV)**
0.00 0.00 FUD XXX E
AMA: 2018,Jan,8; 2017,Jan,8; 2016,Jan,13

4001F **Tobacco use cessation intervention, pharmacologic therapy (COPD, CAD, CAP, PV, Asthma) (DM) (PV)**
0.00 0.00 FUD XXX E
AMA: 2008,Mar,8-12; 2004,Nov,1

4003F **Patient education, written/oral, appropriate for patients with heart failure, performed (NMA-No Measure Associated)**
0.00 0.00 FUD XXX E
AMA: 2004,Nov,1

4004F **Patient screened for tobacco use and received tobacco cessation intervention (counseling, pharmacotherapy, or both), if identified as a tobacco user (PV, CAD)**
0.00 0.00 FUD XXX M

4005F **Pharmacologic therapy (other than minerals/vitamins) for osteoporosis prescribed (OP) (IBD)**
0.00 0.00 FUD XXX E

4008F **Beta-blocker therapy prescribed or currently being taken (CAD,HF)**
0.00 0.00 FUD XXX M

4010F **Angiotensin Converting Enzyme (ACE) Inhibitor or Angiotensin Receptor Blocker (ARB) therapy prescribed or currently being taken (CAD, CKD, HF) (DM)**
0.00 0.00 FUD XXX M

4011F Oral antiplatelet therapy prescribed (CAD)
0.00 0.00 FUD XXX E
AMA: 2004,Nov,1

4012F Warfarin therapy prescribed (NMA-No Measure Associated)
0.00 0.00 FUD XXX E

4013F Statin therapy prescribed or currently being taken (CAD)
0.00 0.00 FUD XXX E

4014F Written discharge instructions provided to heart failure patients discharged home (Instructions include all of the following components: activity level, diet, discharge medications, follow-up appointment, weight monitoring, what to do if symptoms worsen) (NMA-No Measure Associated)
0.00 0.00 FUD XXX E

4015F Persistent asthma, preferred long term control medication or an acceptable alternative treatment, prescribed (NMA-No Measure Associated)
EXCLUDES *Reporting code with modifier 1P*
Code also modifier 2P for patient reasons for not prescribing
0.00 0.00 FUD XXX E

4016F Anti-inflammatory/analgesic agent prescribed (OA) (Use for prescribed or continued medication[s], including over-the-counter medication[s])
INCLUDES Over-the-counter medication(s)
Prescribed/continued medication(s)
0.00 0.00 FUD XXX E

4017F Gastrointestinal prophylaxis for NSAID use prescribed (OA)
0.00 0.00 FUD XXX E

4018F Therapeutic exercise for the involved joint(s) instructed or physical or occupational therapy prescribed (OA)
0.00 0.00 FUD XXX E

4019F Documentation of receipt of counseling on exercise and either both calcium and vitamin D use or counseling regarding both calcium and vitamin D use (OP)
0.00 0.00 FUD XXX E

4025F Inhaled bronchodilator prescribed (COPD)
0.00 0.00 FUD XXX E

4030F Long-term oxygen therapy prescribed (more than 15 hours per day) (COPD)
0.00 0.00 FUD XXX E

4033F Pulmonary rehabilitation exercise training recommended (COPD)
Code also dyspnea assessed, present (1019F)
0.00 0.00 FUD XXX E

4035F Influenza immunization recommended (COPD) (IBD)
0.00 0.00 FUD XXX E
AMA: 2008,Mar,8-12

4037F Influenza immunization ordered or administered (COPD, PV, CKD, ESRD)(IBD)
0.00 0.00 FUD XXX E
AMA: 2008,Mar,8-12

4040F Pneumococcal vaccine administered or previously received (COPD) (PV), (IBD)
0.00 0.00 FUD XXX M
AMA: 2008,Mar,8-12

4041F Documentation of order for cefazolin OR cefuroxime for antimicrobial prophylaxis (PERI 2)
0.00 0.00 FUD XXX E

4042F Documentation that prophylactic antibiotics were neither given within 4 hours prior to surgical incision nor given intraoperatively (PERI 2)
0.00 0.00 FUD XXX E

4043F Documentation that an order was given to discontinue prophylactic antibiotics within 48 hours of surgical end time, cardiac procedures (PERI 2)
0.00 0.00 FUD XXX E

4044F Documentation that an order was given for venous thromboembolism (VTE) prophylaxis to be given within 24 hours prior to incision time or 24 hours after surgery end time (PERI 2)
0.00 0.00 FUD XXX M

4045F Appropriate empiric antibiotic prescribed (CAP), (EM)
0.00 0.00 FUD XXX E

4046F Documentation that prophylactic antibiotics were given within 4 hours prior to surgical incision or given intraoperatively (PERI 2)
0.00 0.00 FUD XXX E

4047F Documentation of order for prophylactic parenteral antibiotics to be given within 1 hour (if fluoroquinolone or vancomycin, 2 hours) prior to surgical incision (or start of procedure when no incision is required) (PERI 2)
0.00 0.00 FUD XXX E

4048F Documentation that administration of prophylactic parenteral antibiotic was initiated within 1 hour (if fluoroquinolone or vancomycin, 2 hours) prior to surgical incision (or start of procedure when no incision is required) as ordered (PERI 2)
0.00 0.00 FUD XXX E

4049F Documentation that order was given to discontinue prophylactic antibiotics within 24 hours of surgical end time, non-cardiac procedure (PERI 2)
0.00 0.00 FUD XXX E

4050F Hypertension plan of care documented as appropriate (NMA-No Measure Associated)
0.00 0.00 FUD XXX E

4051F Referred for an arteriovenous (AV) fistula (ESRD, CKD)
0.00 0.00 FUD XXX E
AMA: 2008,Mar,8-12

4052F Hemodialysis via functioning arteriovenous (AV) fistula (ESRD)
0.00 0.00 FUD XXX E
AMA: 2008,Mar,8-12

4053F Hemodialysis via functioning arteriovenous (AV) graft (ESRD)
0.00 0.00 FUD XXX E
AMA: 2008,Mar,8-12

4054F Hemodialysis via catheter (ESRD)
0.00 0.00 FUD XXX E
AMA: 2008,Mar,8-12

4055F Patient receiving peritoneal dialysis (ESRD)
0.00 0.00 FUD XXX E
AMA: 2008,Mar,8-12

4056F Appropriate oral rehydration solution recommended (PAG)
0.00 0.00 FUD XXX E

4058F Pediatric gastroenteritis education provided to caregiver (PAG)
0.00 0.00 FUD XXX E

4060F Psychotherapy services provided (MDD, MDD ADOL)
0.00 0.00 FUD XXX E

4062F Patient referral for psychotherapy documented (MDD, MDD ADOL)
0.00 0.00 FUD XXX E

4063F Antidepressant pharmacotherapy considered and not prescribed (MDD ADOL)
0.00 0.00 FUD XXX E

4064F **Antidepressant pharmacotherapy prescribed (MDD, MDD ADOL)**
0.00 0.00 FUD XXX E

4065F **Antipsychotic pharmacotherapy prescribed (MDD)**
0.00 0.00 FUD XXX E

4066F **Electroconvulsive therapy (ECT) provided (MDD)**
0.00 0.00 FUD XXX E

4067F **Patient referral for electroconvulsive therapy (ECT) documented (MDD)**
0.00 0.00 FUD XXX E

4069F **Venous thromboembolism (VTE) prophylaxis received (IBD)**
0.00 0.00 FUD XXX E

4070F **Deep vein thrombosis (DVT) prophylaxis received by end of hospital day 2 (STR)**
0.00 0.00 FUD XXX E

4073F **Oral antiplatelet therapy prescribed at discharge (STR)**
0.00 0.00 FUD XXX E

4075F **Anticoagulant therapy prescribed at discharge (STR)**
0.00 0.00 FUD XXX E

4077F **Documentation that tissue plasminogen activator (t-PA) administration was considered (STR)**
0.00 0.00 FUD XXX E

4079F **Documentation that rehabilitation services were considered (STR)**
0.00 0.00 FUD XXX E

4084F **Aspirin received within 24 hours before emergency department arrival or during emergency department stay (EM)**
0.00 0.00 FUD XXX E

4086F **Aspirin or clopidogrel prescribed or currently being taken (CAD)**
0.00 0.00 FUD XXX M

4090F **Patient receiving erythropoietin therapy (HEM)**
0.00 0.00 FUD XXX M
AMA: 2008,Mar,8-12

4095F **Patient not receiving erythropoietin therapy (HEM)**
0.00 0.00 FUD XXX E
AMA: 2008,Mar,8-12

4100F **Bisphosphonate therapy, intravenous, ordered or received (HEM)**
0.00 0.00 FUD XXX M
AMA: 2008,Mar,8-12

4110F **Internal mammary artery graft performed for primary, isolated coronary artery bypass graft procedure (CABG)**
0.00 0.00 FUD XXX M

4115F **Beta blocker administered within 24 hours prior to surgical incision (CABG)**
0.00 0.00 FUD XXX M

4120F **Antibiotic prescribed or dispensed (URI, PHAR), (A-BRONCH)**
0.00 0.00 FUD XXX M
AMA: 2008,Mar,8-12

4124F **Antibiotic neither prescribed nor dispensed (URI, PHAR), (A-BRONCH)**
0.00 0.00 FUD XXX M
AMA: 2008,Mar,8-12

4130F **Topical preparations (including OTC) prescribed for acute otitis externa (AOE)**
0.00 0.00 FUD XXX M
AMA: 2010,Jan,6-7; 2008,Mar,8-12

4131F **Systemic antimicrobial therapy prescribed (AOE)**
0.00 0.00 FUD XXX M
AMA: 2008,Mar,8-12

4132F **Systemic antimicrobial therapy not prescribed (AOE)**
0.00 0.00 FUD XXX M
AMA: 2008,Mar,8-12

4133F **Antihistamines or decongestants prescribed or recommended (OME)**
0.00 0.00 FUD XXX E
AMA: 2008,Mar,8-12

4134F **Antihistamines or decongestants neither prescribed nor recommended (OME)**
0.00 0.00 FUD XXX E
AMA: 2008,Mar,8-12

4135F **Systemic corticosteroids prescribed (OME)**
0.00 0.00 FUD XXX E
AMA: 2008,Mar,8-12

4136F **Systemic corticosteroids not prescribed (OME)**
0.00 0.00 FUD XXX E
AMA: 2008,Mar,8-12

4140F **Inhaled corticosteroids prescribed (Asthma)**
0.00 0.00 FUD XXX E

4142F **Corticosteroid sparing therapy prescribed (IBD)**
0.00 0.00 FUD XXX E

4144F **Alternative long-term control medication prescribed (Asthma)**
0.00 0.00 FUD XXX E

4145F **Two or more anti-hypertensive agents prescribed or currently being taken (CAD, HTN)**
0.00 0.00 FUD XXX E

4148F **Hepatitis A vaccine injection administered or previously received (HEP-C)**
0.00 0.00 FUD XXX E

4149F **Hepatitis B vaccine injection administered or previously received (HEP-C, HIV) (IBD)**
0.00 0.00 FUD XXX E

4150F **Patient receiving antiviral treatment for Hepatitis C (HEP-C)**
0.00 0.00 FUD XXX E
AMA: 2008,Mar,8-12

4151F **Patient did not start or is not receiving antiviral treatment for Hepatitis C during the measurement period (HEP-C)**
0.00 0.00 FUD XXX E
AMA: 2008,Mar,8-12

4153F **Combination peginterferon and ribavirin therapy prescribed (HEP-C)**
0.00 0.00 FUD XXX E
AMA: 2008,Mar,8-12

4155F **Hepatitis A vaccine series previously received (HEP-C)**
0.00 0.00 FUD XXX E
AMA: 2008,Mar,8-12

4157F **Hepatitis B vaccine series previously received (HEP-C)**
0.00 0.00 FUD XXX E
AMA: 2008,Mar,8-12

4158F **Patient counseled about risks of alcohol use (HEP-C)**
0.00 0.00 FUD XXX E
AMA: 2008,Mar,8-12

4159F **Counseling regarding contraception received prior to initiation of antiviral treatment (HEP-C)**
0.00 0.00 FUD XXX E
AMA: 2008,Mar,8-12

4163F **Patient counseling at a minimum on all of the following treatment options for clinically localized prostate cancer: active surveillance, and interstitial prostate brachytherapy, and external beam radiotherapy, and radical prostatectomy, provided prior to initiation of treatment (PRCA)**
0.00 0.00 FUD XXX E
AMA: 2008,Mar,8-12

4164F **Adjuvant (ie, in combination with external beam radiotherapy to the prostate for prostate cancer) hormonal therapy (gonadotropin-releasing hormone [GnRH] agonist or antagonist) prescribed/administered (PRCA)**
0.00 0.00 FUD XXX E
AMA: 2008,Mar,8-12

4165F **3-dimensional conformal radiotherapy (3D-CRT) or intensity modulated radiation therapy (IMRT) received (PRCA)**
0.00 0.00 FUD XXX E
AMA: 2008,Mar,8-12

4167F **Head of bed elevation (30-45 degrees) on first ventilator day ordered (CRIT)**
0.00 0.00 FUD XXX E
AMA: 2008,Mar,8-12

4168F **Patient receiving care in the intensive care unit (ICU) and receiving mechanical ventilation, 24 hours or less (CRIT)**
0.00 0.00 FUD XXX E
AMA: 2008,Mar,8-12

4169F **Patient either not receiving care in the intensive care unit (ICU) OR not receiving mechanical ventilation OR receiving mechanical ventilation greater than 24 hours (CRIT)**
0.00 0.00 FUD XXX E
AMA: 2008,Mar,8-12

4171F **Patient receiving erythropoiesis-stimulating agents (ESA) therapy (CKD)**
0.00 0.00 FUD XXX E
AMA: 2008,Mar,8-12

4172F **Patient not receiving erythropoiesis-stimulating agents (ESA) therapy (CKD)**
0.00 0.00 FUD XXX E
AMA: 2008,Mar,8-12

4174F **Counseling about the potential impact of glaucoma on visual functioning and quality of life, and importance of treatment adherence provided to patient and/or caregiver(s) (EC)**
0.00 0.00 FUD XXX E
AMA: 2008,Mar,8-12

4175F **Best-corrected visual acuity of 20/40 or better (distance or near) achieved within the 90 days following cataract surgery (EC)**
0.00 0.00 FUD XXX M
AMA: 2008,Mar,8-12

4176F **Counseling about value of protection from UV light and lack of proven efficacy of nutritional supplements in prevention or progression of cataract development provided to patient and/or caregiver(s) (NMA-No Measure Associated)**
0.00 0.00 FUD XXX E

4177F **Counseling about the benefits and/or risks of the Age-Related Eye Disease Study (AREDS) formulation for preventing progression of age-related macular degeneration (AMD) provided to patient and/or caregiver(s) (EC)**
0.00 0.00 FUD XXX M
AMA: 2008,Mar,8-12

4178F **Anti-D immune globulin received between 26 and 30 weeks gestation (Pre-Cr)**
0.00 0.00 FUD XXX M E
AMA: 2008,Mar,8-12

4179F **Tamoxifen or aromatase inhibitor (AI) prescribed (ONC)**
0.00 0.00 FUD XXX E
AMA: 2008,Mar,8-12

4180F **Adjuvant chemotherapy referred, prescribed, or previously received for Stage III colon cancer (ONC)**
0.00 0.00 FUD XXX E
AMA: 2008,Mar,8-12

4181F **Conformal radiation therapy received (NMA-No Measure Associated)**
0.00 0.00 FUD XXX E

4182F **Conformal radiation therapy not received (NMA-No Measure Associated)**
0.00 0.00 FUD XXX E

4185F **Continuous (12-months) therapy with proton pump inhibitor (PPI) or histamine H2 receptor antagonist (H2RA) received (GERD)**
0.00 0.00 FUD XXX E
AMA: 2008,Mar,8-12

4186F **No continuous (12-months) therapy with either proton pump inhibitor (PPI) or histamine H2 receptor antagonist (H2RA) received (GERD)**
0.00 0.00 FUD XXX E
AMA: 2008,Mar,8-12

4187F **Disease modifying anti-rheumatic drug therapy prescribed or dispensed (RA)**
0.00 0.00 FUD XXX E

4188F **Appropriate angiotensin converting enzyme (ACE)/angiotensin receptor blockers (ARB) therapeutic monitoring test ordered or performed (AM)**
0.00 0.00 FUD XXX E
AMA: 2008,Mar,8-12

4189F **Appropriate digoxin therapeutic monitoring test ordered or performed (AM)**
0.00 0.00 FUD XXX E
AMA: 2008,Mar,8-12

4190F **Appropriate diuretic therapeutic monitoring test ordered or performed (AM)**
0.00 0.00 FUD XXX E
AMA: 2008,Mar,8-12

4191F **Appropriate anticonvulsant therapeutic monitoring test ordered or performed (AM)**
0.00 0.00 FUD XXX E
AMA: 2008,Mar,8-12

4192F **Patient not receiving glucocorticoid therapy (RA)**
0.00 0.00 FUD XXX M

4193F **Patient receiving <10 mg daily prednisone (or equivalent), or RA activity is worsening, or glucocorticoid use is for less than 6 months (RA)**
0.00 0.00 FUD XXX M

4194F **Patient receiving ≥10 mg daily prednisone (or equivalent) for longer than 6 months, and improvement or no change in disease activity (RA)**
0.00 0.00 FUD XXX M

4195F **Patient receiving first-time biologic disease modifying anti-rheumatic drug therapy for rheumatoid arthritis (RA)**
0.00 0.00 FUD XXX M

4196F **Patient not receiving first-time biologic disease modifying anti-rheumatic drug therapy for rheumatoid arthritis (RA)**
0.00 0.00 FUD XXX M

4200F **External beam radiotherapy as primary therapy to prostate with or without nodal irradiation (PRCA)**
0.00 0.00 FUD XXX E
AMA: 2008,Mar,8-12

4201F **External beam radiotherapy with or without nodal irradiation as adjuvant or salvage therapy for prostate cancer patient (PRCA)**
0.00 0.00 FUD XXX E
AMA: 2008,Mar,8-12

4210F **Angiotensin converting enzyme (ACE) or angiotensin receptor blockers (ARB) medication therapy for 6 months or more (MM)**
0.00 0.00 FUD XXX E
AMA: 2008,Mar,8-12

4220F **Digoxin medication therapy for 6 months or more (MM)**
0.00 0.00 FUD XXX E
AMA: 2008,Mar,8-12

4221F **Diuretic medication therapy for 6 months or more (MM)**
0.00 0.00 FUD XXX E
AMA: 2008,Mar,8-12

4230F **Anticonvulsant medication therapy for 6 months or more (MM)**
0.00 0.00 FUD XXX E
AMA: 2008,Mar,8-12

4240F **Instruction in therapeutic exercise with follow-up provided to patients during episode of back pain lasting longer than 12 weeks (BkP)**
0.00 0.00 FUD XXX E
AMA: 2008,Mar,8-12

4242F **Counseling for supervised exercise program provided to patients during episode of back pain lasting longer than 12 weeks (BkP)**
0.00 0.00 FUD XXX E
AMA: 2008,Mar,8-12

4245F **Patient counseled during the initial visit to maintain or resume normal activities (BkP)**
0.00 0.00 FUD XXX E
AMA: 2008,Mar,8-12

4248F **Patient counseled during the initial visit for an episode of back pain against bed rest lasting 4 days or longer (BkP)**
0.00 0.00 FUD XXX E
AMA: 2008,Mar,8-12

4250F **Active warming used intraoperatively for the purpose of maintaining normothermia, or at least 1 body temperature equal to or greater than 36 degrees Centigrade (or 96.8 degrees Fahrenheit) recorded within the 30 minutes immediately before or the 15 minutes immediately after anesthesia end time (CRIT)**
0.00 0.00 FUD XXX E
AMA: 2008,Mar,8-12

4255F **Duration of general or neuraxial anesthesia 60 minutes or longer, as documented in the anesthesia record (CRIT) (Peri2)**
0.00 0.00 FUD XXX M

4256F **Duration of general or neuraxial anesthesia less than 60 minutes, as documented in the anesthesia record (CRIT) (Peri2)**
0.00 0.00 FUD XXX E

4260F **Wound surface culture technique used (CWC)**
0.00 0.00 FUD XXX E

4261F **Technique other than surface culture of the wound exudate used (eg, Levine/deep swab technique, semi-quantitative or quantitative swab technique) or wound surface culture technique not used (CWC)**
0.00 0.00 FUD XXX E

4265F **Use of wet to dry dressings prescribed or recommended (CWC)**
0.00 0.00 FUD XXX E

4266F **Use of wet to dry dressings neither prescribed nor recommended (CWC)**
0.00 0.00 FUD XXX E

4267F **Compression therapy prescribed (CWC)**
0.00 0.00 FUD XXX E

4268F **Patient education regarding the need for long term compression therapy including interval replacement of compression stockings received (CWC)**
0.00 0.00 FUD XXX E

4269F **Appropriate method of offloading (pressure relief) prescribed (CWC)**
0.00 0.00 FUD XXX E

4270F **Patient receiving potent antiretroviral therapy for 6 months or longer (HIV)**
0.00 0.00 FUD XXX E

4271F **Patient receiving potent antiretroviral therapy for less than 6 months or not receiving potent antiretroviral therapy (HIV)**
0.00 0.00 FUD XXX E

4274F **Influenza immunization administered or previously received (HIV) (P-ESRD)**
0.00 0.00 FUD XXX E

4276F **Potent antiretroviral therapy prescribed (HIV)**
0.00 0.00 FUD XXX E

4279F **Pneumocystis jiroveci pneumonia prophylaxis prescribed (HIV)**
0.00 0.00 FUD XXX E

4280F **Pneumocystis jiroveci pneumonia prophylaxis prescribed within 3 months of low CD4+ cell count or percentage (HIV)**
0.00 0.00 FUD XXX E

4290F **Patient screened for injection drug use (HIV)**
0.00 0.00 FUD XXX E

4293F **Patient screened for high-risk sexual behavior (HIV)**
0.00 0.00 FUD XXX E

4300F **Patient receiving warfarin therapy for nonvalvular atrial fibrillation or atrial flutter (AFIB)**
0.00 0.00 FUD XXX E

4301F **Patient not receiving warfarin therapy for nonvalvular atrial fibrillation or atrial flutter (AFIB)**
0.00 0.00 FUD XXX E

4305F **Patient education regarding appropriate foot care and daily inspection of the feet received (CWC)**
0.00 0.00 FUD XXX E

4306F **Patient counseled regarding psychosocial and pharmacologic treatment options for opioid addiction (SUD)**
0.00 0.00 FUD XXX E

4320F **Patient counseled regarding psychosocial and pharmacologic treatment options for alcohol dependence (SUD)**
0.00 0.00 FUD XXX E

4322F **Caregiver provided with education and referred to additional resources for support (DEM)**
0.00 0.00 FUD XXX M

4324F **Patient (or caregiver) queried about Parkinson's disease medication related motor complications (Prkns)**
0.00 0.00 FUD XXX E

4325F **Medical and surgical treatment options reviewed with patient (or caregiver) (Prkns)**
0.00 0.00 FUD XXX M

4326F **Patient (or caregiver) queried about symptoms of autonomic dysfunction (Prkns)**
0.00 0.00 FUD XXX E

4328F **Patient (or caregiver) queried about sleep disturbances (Prkns)**
0.00 0.00 FUD XXX E

4330F **Counseling about epilepsy specific safety issues provided to patient (or caregiver(s)) (EPI)**
0.00 0.00 FUD XXX E

4340F **Counseling for women of childbearing potential with epilepsy (EPI)**
0.00 0.00 FUD XXX M

4350F **Counseling provided on symptom management, end of life decisions, and palliation (DEM)**
0.00 0.00 FUD XXX E

4400F **Rehabilitative therapy options discussed with patient (or caregiver) (Prkns)**
0.00 0.00 FUD XXX M

4450F **Self-care education provided to patient (HF)**
0.00 0.00 FUD XXX E

4470F **Implantable cardioverter-defibrillator (ICD) counseling provided (HF)**
0.00 0.00 FUD XXX E

4480F **Patient receiving ACE inhibitor/ARB therapy and beta-blocker therapy for 3 months or longer (HF)**
0.00 0.00 FUD XXX E

4481F **Patient receiving ACE inhibitor/ARB therapy and beta-blocker therapy for less than 3 months or patient not receiving ACE inhibitor/ARB therapy and beta-blocker therapy (HF)**
0.00 0.00 FUD XXX E

4500F **Referred to an outpatient cardiac rehabilitation program (CAD)**
0.00 0.00 FUD XXX M

4510F **Previous cardiac rehabilitation for qualifying cardiac event completed (CAD)**
0.00 0.00 FUD XXX M

4525F **Neuropsychiatric intervention ordered (DEM)**
0.00 0.00 FUD XXX E

4526F **Neuropsychiatric intervention received (DEM)**
0.00 0.00 FUD XXX E

4540F **Disease modifying pharmacotherapy discussed (ALS)**
0.00 0.00 FUD XXX E

4541F **Patient offered treatment for pseudobulbar affect, sialorrhea, or ALS-related symptoms (ALS)**
0.00 0.00 FUD XXX E

4550F **Options for noninvasive respiratory support discussed with patient (ALS)**
0.00 0.00 FUD XXX E

4551F **Nutritional support offered (ALS)**
0.00 0.00 FUD XXX E

4552F **Patient offered referral to a speech language pathologist (ALS)**
0.00 0.00 FUD XXX E

4553F **Patient offered assistance in planning for end of life issues (ALS)**
0.00 0.00 FUD XXX E

4554F **Patient received inhalational anesthetic agent (Peri2)**
0.00 0.00 FUD XXX M

4555F **Patient did not receive inhalational anesthetic agent (Peri2)**
0.00 0.00 FUD XXX E

4556F **Patient exhibits 3 or more risk factors for post-operative nausea and vomiting (Peri2)**
0.00 0.00 FUD XXX M

4557F **Patient does not exhibit 3 or more risk factors for post-operative nausea and vomiting (Peri2)**
0.00 0.00 FUD XXX E

4558F **Patient received at least 2 prophylactic pharmacologic anti-emetic agents of different classes preoperatively and intraoperatively (Peri2)**
0.00 0.00 FUD XXX E

4559F **At least 1 body temperature measurement equal to or greater than 35.5 degrees Celsius (or 95.9 degrees Fahrenheit) recorded within the 30 minutes immediately before or the 15 minutes immediately after anesthesia end time (Peri2)**
0.00 0.00 FUD XXX E

4560F **Anesthesia technique did not involve general or neuraxial anesthesia (Peri2)**
0.00 0.00 FUD XXX E

4561F **Patient has a coronary artery stent (Peri2)**
0.00 0.00 FUD XXX E

4562F **Patient does not have a coronary artery stent (Peri2)**
0.00 0.00 FUD XXX E

4563F **Patient received aspirin within 24 hours prior to anesthesia start time (Peri2)**
0.00 0.00 FUD XXX E

5005F-5250F Results Conveyed and Documented

INCLUDES Patient's:
- Functional status
- Morbidity/mortality
- Satisfaction/experience with care

Review/communication test results to patients

5005F **Patient counseled on self-examination for new or changing moles (ML)**
0.00 0.00 FUD XXX E
AMA: 2008,Mar,8-12

5010F **Findings of dilated macular or fundus exam communicated to the physician or other qualified health care professional managing the diabetes care (EC)**
0.00 0.00 FUD XXX M

5015F **Documentation of communication that a fracture occurred and that the patient was or should be tested or treated for osteoporosis (OP)**
0.00 0.00 FUD XXX M

5020F **Treatment summary report communicated to physician(s) or other qualified health care professional(s) managing continuing care and to the patient within 1 month of completing treatment (ONC)**
0.00 0.00 FUD XXX E
AMA: 2008,Mar,8-12

5050F **Treatment plan communicated to provider(s) managing continuing care within 1 month of diagnosis (ML)**
0.00 0.00 FUD XXX M
AMA: 2008,Mar,8-12

5060F **Findings from diagnostic mammogram communicated to practice managing patient's on-going care within 3 business days of exam interpretation (RAD)**
0.00 0.00 FUD XXX E
AMA: 2008,Mar,8-12

5062F **Findings from diagnostic mammogram communicated to the patient within 5 days of exam interpretation (RAD)**
0.00 0.00 FUD XXX E
AMA: 2008,Mar,8-12

5100F **Potential risk for fracture communicated to the referring physician or other qualified health care professional within 24 hours of completion of the imaging study (NUC_MED)**
0.00 0.00 FUD XXX E

5200F **Consideration of referral for a neurological evaluation of appropriateness for surgical therapy for intractable epilepsy within the past 3 years (EPI)**
0.00 0.00 FUD XXX E

5250F **Asthma discharge plan provided to patient (Asthma)**
0.00 0.00 FUD XXX E

6005F-6150F Elements Related to Patient Safety Processes

INCLUDES Patient safety practices

6005F **Rationale (eg, severity of illness and safety) for level of care (eg, home, hospital) documented (CAP)**
0.00 0.00 **FUD** XXX E
AMA: 2018,Jan,8; 2017,Jan,8; 2016,Jan,13

6010F **Dysphagia screening conducted prior to order for or receipt of any foods, fluids, or medication by mouth (STR)**
0.00 0.00 **FUD** XXX E

6015F **Patient receiving or eligible to receive foods, fluids, or medication by mouth (STR)**
0.00 0.00 **FUD** XXX E

6020F **NPO (nothing by mouth) ordered (STR)**
0.00 0.00 **FUD** XXX E

6030F **All elements of maximal sterile barrier technique, hand hygiene, skin preparation and, if ultrasound is used, sterile ultrasound techniques followed (CRIT)**
0.00 0.00 **FUD** XXX M
AMA: 2008,Mar,8-12

6040F **Use of appropriate radiation dose reduction devices OR manual techniques for appropriate moderation of exposure, documented (RAD)**
0.00 0.00 **FUD** XXX E

6045F **Radiation exposure or exposure time in final report for procedure using fluoroscopy, documented (RAD)**
0.00 0.00 **FUD** XXX E
AMA: 2008,Mar,8-12

6070F **Patient queried and counseled about anti-epileptic drug (AED) side effects (EPI)**
0.00 0.00 **FUD** XXX E

6080F **Patient (or caregiver) queried about falls (Prkns, DSP)**
0.00 0.00 **FUD** XXX E

6090F **Patient (or caregiver) counseled about safety issues appropriate to patient's stage of disease (Prkns)**
0.00 0.00 **FUD** XXX E

6100F **Timeout to verify correct patient, correct site, and correct procedure, documented (PATH)**
0.00 0.00 **FUD** XXX E

6101F **Safety counseling for dementia provided (DEM)**
0.00 0.00 **FUD** XXX E

6102F **Safety counseling for dementia ordered (DEM)**
0.00 0.00 **FUD** XXX E

6110F **Counseling provided regarding risks of driving and the alternatives to driving (DEM)**
0.00 0.00 **FUD** XXX E

6150F **Patient not receiving a first course of anti-TNF (tumor necrosis factor) therapy (IBD)**
0.00 0.00 **FUD** XXX E

7010F-7025F Recall/Reminder System in Place

INCLUDES Measures that address setting or care system provided
Provider capabilities

7010F **Patient information entered into a recall system that includes: target date for the next exam specified and a process to follow up with patients regarding missed or unscheduled appointments (ML)**
0.00 0.00 **FUD** XXX M
AMA: 2008,Mar,8-12

7020F **Mammogram assessment category (eg, Mammography Quality Standards Act [MQSA], Breast Imaging Reporting and Data System [BI-RADS], or FDA approved equivalent categories) entered into an internal database to allow for analysis of abnormal interpretation (recall) rate (RAD)**
0.00 0.00 **FUD** XXX E
AMA: 2008,Mar,8-12

7025F **Patient information entered into a reminder system with a target due date for the next mammogram (RAD)**
0.00 0.00 **FUD** XXX M
AMA: 2008,Mar,8-12

9001F-9007F No Measure Associated

INCLUDES Care aspects not associated with measures at current time

9001F **Aortic aneurysm less than 5.0 cm maximum diameter on centerline formatted CT or minor diameter on axial formatted CT (NMA-No Measure Associated)**
0.00 0.00 **FUD** XXX E

9002F **Aortic aneurysm 5.0 - 5.4 cm maximum diameter on centerline formatted CT or minor diameter on axial formatted CT (NMA-No Measure Associated)**
0.00 0.00 **FUD** XXX E

9003F **Aortic aneurysm 5.5 - 5.9 cm maximum diameter on centerline formatted CT or minor diameter on axial formatted CT (NMA-No Measure Associated)**
0.00 0.00 **FUD** XXX M

9004F **Aortic aneurysm 6.0 cm or greater maximum diameter on centerline formatted CT or minor diameter on axial formatted CT (NMA-No Measure Associated)**
0.00 0.00 **FUD** XXX M

9005F **Asymptomatic carotid stenosis: No history of any transient ischemic attack or stroke in any carotid or vertebrobasilar territory (NMA-No Measure Associated)**
0.00 0.00 **FUD** XXX E

9006F **Symptomatic carotid stenosis: Ipsilateral carotid territory TIA or stroke less than 120 days prior to procedure (NMA-No Measure Associated)**
0.00 0.00 **FUD** XXX M

9007F **Other carotid stenosis: Ipsilateral TIA or stroke 120 days or greater prior to procedure or any prior contralateral carotid territory or vertebrobasilar TIA or stroke (NMA-No Measure Associated)**
0.00 0.00 **FUD** XXX M

0042T

0042T **Cerebral perfusion analysis using computed tomography with contrast administration, including post-processing of parametric maps with determination of cerebral blood flow, cerebral blood volume, and mean transit time**
0.00 0.00 FUD XXX N 80
AMA: 2003,Nov,5

0054T-0055T

\+ 0054T **Computer-assisted musculoskeletal surgical navigational orthopedic procedure, with image-guidance based on fluoroscopic images (List separately in addition to code for primary procedure)**
Code first primary procedure
0.00 0.00 FUD XXX N 80
AMA: 2018,Jan,8; 2017,Jan,8; 2016,Jan,13

\+ 0055T **Computer-assisted musculoskeletal surgical navigational orthopedic procedure, with image-guidance based on CT/MRI images (List separately in addition to code for primary procedure)**
INCLUDES Performance both CT and MRI in same session (one unit)
Code first primary procedure
0.00 0.00 FUD XXX N 80
AMA: 2018,Jan,8; 2017,Jan,8; 2016,Jan,13

0071T-0072T

EXCLUDES *Insertion bladder catheter (51702)*
MRI guidance for parenchymal tissue ablation (77022)

0071T **Focused ultrasound ablation of uterine leiomyomata, including MR guidance; total leiomyomata volume less than 200 cc of tissue** ♀
0.00 0.00 FUD XXX J 80
AMA: 2005,Mar,1-6; 2005,Dec,3-6

0072T **total leiomyomata volume greater or equal to 200 cc of tissue** ♀
0.00 0.00 FUD XXX J 80
AMA: 2005,Mar,1-6; 2005,Dec,3-6

0075T-0076T

INCLUDES All diagnostic services for stenting
Ipsilateral extracranial vertebral selective catheterization when confirming need for stenting

EXCLUDES *Selective catheterization and imaging when stenting not required (report only selective catheterization codes)*

0075T **Transcatheter placement of extracranial vertebral artery stent(s), including radiologic supervision and interpretation, open or percutaneous; initial vessel**
0.00 0.00 FUD XXX C 80
AMA: 2018,Jan,8; 2017,Jan,8; 2016,Jan,13

\+ 0076T **each additional vessel (List separately in addition to code for primary procedure)**
Code first (0075T)
0.00 0.00 FUD XXX C 80
AMA: 2018,Jan,8; 2017,Jan,8; 2016,Jan,13

0095T-0098T

INCLUDES Fluoroscopy

\+ 0095T **Removal of total disc arthroplasty (artificial disc), anterior approach, each additional interspace, cervical (List separately in addition to code for primary procedure)**
EXCLUDES *Lumbar disc (0164T)*
Revision total disc arthroplasty, cervical (22861)
Revision total disc arthroplasty, lumbar (22862)
Code first (22864)
0.00 0.00 FUD XXX C 80
AMA: 2006,Feb,1-6; 2005,Jun,6-8

\+ 0098T **Revision including replacement of total disc arthroplasty (artificial disc), anterior approach, each additional interspace, cervical (List separately in addition to code for primary procedure)**
EXCLUDES *Application intervertebral biomechanical device(s) at same level (22853-22854, [22859])*
Removal total disc arthroplasty (0095T)
Spinal cord decompression (63001-63048)
Code first (22861)
0.00 0.00 FUD XXX C 80
AMA: 2006,Feb,1-6; 2005,Jun,6-8

0100T

0100T **Placement of a subconjunctival retinal prosthesis receiver and pulse generator, and implantation of intra-ocular retinal electrode array, with vitrectomy**
EXCLUDES *Evaluation and initial programming implantable retinal electrode array device (0472T)*
0.00 0.00 FUD XXX T J8 80
AMA: 2018,Feb,3; 2018,Jan,8; 2017,Jan,8; 2016,Jan,13

0101T-0513T [0512T, 0513T]

▲ 0101T **Extracorporeal shock wave involving musculoskeletal system, not otherwise specified**
EXCLUDES *Extracorporeal shock wave therapy integumentary system not otherwise specified ([0512T, 0513T])*
0.00 0.00 FUD XXX J G2 80
AMA: 2018,Dec,5; 2018,Dec,5; 2018,Jan,8; 2017,Jan,8; 2016,Jan,13

▲ 0102T **Extracorporeal shock wave performed by a physician, requiring anesthesia other than local, and involving the lateral humeral epicondyle**
0.00 0.00 FUD XXX J G2 80
AMA: 2019,Jun,11; 2018,Dec,5; 2018,Dec,5; 2018,Jan,8; 2017,Jan,8; 2016,Jan,13

▲ # 0512T **Extracorporeal shock wave for integumentary wound healing, including topical application and dressing care; initial wound**
0.00 0.00 FUD YYY R2 80
AMA: 2018,Dec,5; 2018,Dec,5

▲ + # 0513T **each additional wound (List separately in addition to code for primary procedure)**
Code first ([0512T])
0.00 0.00 FUD ZZZ N1 80
AMA: 2018,Dec,5; 2018,Dec,5

0106T-0110T

0106T **Quantitative sensory testing (QST), testing and interpretation per extremity; using touch pressure stimuli to assess large diameter sensation**
0.00 0.00 FUD XXX Q1 80
AMA: 2018,Jan,8; 2017,Jan,8; 2016,Jan,13

0107T **using vibration stimuli to assess large diameter fiber sensation**
0.00 0.00 FUD XXX Q1 80
AMA: 2018,Jan,8; 2017,Jan,8; 2016,Jan,13

0108T **using cooling stimuli to assess small nerve fiber sensation and hyperalgesia**
0.00 0.00 FUD XXX Q1 80
AMA: 2018,Jan,8; 2017,Jan,8; 2016,Jan,13

0109T **using heat-pain stimuli to assess small nerve fiber sensation and hyperalgesia**
0.00 0.00 FUD XXX Q1 80
AMA: 2018,Jan,8; 2017,Jan,8; 2016,Jan,13

0110T **using other stimuli to assess sensation**
0.00 0.00 FUD XXX Q1 80
AMA: 2018,Jan,8; 2017,Jan,8; 2016,Jan,13

0163T-0165T

CMS: 100-03,150.10 Lumbar Artificial Disc Replacement (LADR)

INCLUDES Fluoroscopy

EXCLUDES *Application intervertebral biomechanical device(s) at same level (22853-22854, [22859])*
Cervical disc procedures (22856)
Decompression (63001-63048)
Exploration retroperitoneal area at same level (49010)

\+ **0163T** **Total disc arthroplasty (artificial disc), anterior approach, including discectomy to prepare interspace (other than for decompression), each additional interspace, lumbar (List separately in addition to code for primary procedure)**

Code first (22857)
Facility RVU 0.00 Non-Facility RVU 0.00 **FUD** YYY C 80
AMA: 2018,Jan,8; 2017,Jan,8; 2016,Jan,13

\+ **0164T** **Removal of total disc arthroplasty, (artificial disc), anterior approach, each additional interspace, lumbar (List separately in addition to code for primary procedure)**

Code first (22865)
Facility RVU 0.00 Non-Facility RVU 0.00 **FUD** YYY C 80
AMA: 2018,Jan,8; 2017,Jan,8; 2016,Jan,13

\+ **0165T** **Revision including replacement of total disc arthroplasty (artificial disc), anterior approach, each additional interspace, lumbar (List separately in addition to code for primary procedure)**

Code first (22862)
Facility RVU 0.00 Non-Facility RVU 0.00 **FUD** YYY C 80
AMA: 2018,Jan,8; 2017,Jan,8; 2016,Jan,13

0174T-0175T

\+ **0174T** **Computer-aided detection (CAD) (computer algorithm analysis of digital image data for lesion detection) with further physician review for interpretation and report, with or without digitization of film radiographic images, chest radiograph(s), performed concurrent with primary interpretation (List separately in addition to code for primary procedure)**

Code first (71045-71048)
Facility RVU 0.00 Non-Facility RVU 0.00 **FUD** XXX N 80
AMA: 2018,Apr,7

0175T **Computer-aided detection (CAD) (computer algorithm analysis of digital image data for lesion detection) with further physician review for interpretation and report, with or without digitization of film radiographic images, chest radiograph(s), performed remote from primary interpretation**

INCLUDES Chest x-rays (71045-71048)
Facility RVU 0.00 Non-Facility RVU 0.00 **FUD** XXX N 80
AMA: 2018,Apr,7

0184T

0184T **Excision of rectal tumor, transanal endoscopic microsurgical approach (ie, TEMS), including muscularis propria (ie, full thickness)**

INCLUDES Operating microscope (66990)
Proctosigmoidoscopy (45300, 45308-45309, 45315, 45317, 45320)

EXCLUDES *Nonendoscopic excision rectal tumor (45160, 45171-45172)*

Facility RVU 0.00 Non-Facility RVU 0.00 **FUD** XXX J G2 80
AMA: 2018,Feb,11; 2018,Jan,8; 2017,Jan,8; 2016,Feb,12; 2016,Jan,13

0671T-0253T [0253T, 0376T, 0671T]

● # **0671T** **Insertion of anterior segment aqueous drainage device into the trabecular meshwork, without external reservoir, and without concomitant cataract removal, one or more**

EXCLUDES *Aqueous drainage device insertion, external approach (66183)*
Aqueous drainage device insertion, internal approach:
Subconjunctival space (0449T-0450T)
Suprachoroidal space ([0253T])
Supraciliary space (0474T)
With extracapsular cataract removal and insertion of intraocular prosthesis during same session ([66989], [66987], [66991], [66988])
Extracapsular cataract removal with IOL implant without aqueous drainage device during same session (66982, 66984)

Facility RVU 0.00 Non-Facility RVU 0.00 **FUD** 000

0191T ~~**Insertion of anterior segment aqueous drainage device, without extraocular reservoir, internal approach, into the trabecular meshwork; initial insertion**~~

To report, see ([66989], [66991], [0671T])

0376T ~~**each additional device insertion (List separately in addition to code for primary procedure)**~~

To report, see ([66989], [66991], [0671T])

\# **0253T** **Insertion of anterior segment aqueous drainage device, without extraocular reservoir, internal approach, into the suprachoroidal space**

EXCLUDES *Aqueous drainage device insertion, external approach (66183)*
Aqueous drainage device insertion, internal approach:
Subconjunctival space (0449T-0450T)
Supraciliary space (0474T)
Trabecular meshwork ([0671T])

Facility RVU 0.00 Non-Facility RVU 0.00 **FUD** YYY J J8 80
AMA: 2018,Jul,3

0198T

0198T **Measurement of ocular blood flow by repetitive intraocular pressure sampling, with interpretation and report**

Facility RVU 0.00 Non-Facility RVU 0.00 **FUD** XXX Q1 80
AMA: 2018,Jan,8; 2017,Jan,8; 2016,Jan,13

0200T-0201T

INCLUDES Deep bone biopsy (20225)

0200T **Percutaneous sacral augmentation (sacroplasty), unilateral injection(s), including the use of a balloon or mechanical device, when used, 1 or more needles, includes imaging guidance and bone biopsy, when performed**

Facility RVU 0.00 Non-Facility RVU 0.00 **FUD** XXX J G2 80 50
AMA: 2018,Jan,8; 2017,Jan,8; 2016,Jan,13

0201T **Percutaneous sacral augmentation (sacroplasty), bilateral injections, including the use of a balloon or mechanical device, when used, 2 or more needles, includes imaging guidance and bone biopsy, when performed**

Facility RVU 0.00 Non-Facility RVU 0.00 **FUD** XXX J G2 80
AMA: 2018,Jan,8; 2017,Jan,8; 2016,Jan,13

0202T-0563T [0563T]

0202T **Posterior vertebral joint(s) arthroplasty (eg, facet joint[s] replacement), including facetectomy, laminectomy, foraminotomy, and vertebral column fixation, injection of bone cement, when performed, including fluoroscopy, single level, lumbar spine**

INCLUDES Instrumentation (22840, 22853-22854, [22859])
Laminectomy (63005, 63012, 63017, 63047)
Laminotomy (63030, 63042)
Lumbar arthroplasty (22857)
Percutaneous lumbar vertebral augmentation (22514)
Percutaneous vertebroplasty (22511)
Spinal cord decompression (63056)

Facility RVU 0.00 Non-Facility RVU 0.00 **FUD** XXX C 80

26/TC PC/TC Only | A2-Z3 ASC Payment | 50 Bilateral | ♂ Male Only | ♀ Female Only | Facility RVU | Non-Facility RVU | CCI | CLIA
FUD Follow-up Days | CMS: IOM | AMA: CPT Asst | A-Y OPPSI | 80/80 Surg Assist Allowed / w/Doc | Lab Crosswalk | Radiology Crosswalk

0207T **Evacuation of meibomian glands, automated, using heat and intermittent pressure, unilateral**

EXCLUDES *Evacuation using:*
Heat through wearable device ([0563T])
Manual expression only, report appropriate E/M code

0.00 0.00 FUD XXX Q1 80

AMA: 2018,Jan,8; 2017,Jan,8; 2016,Jan,13

\# **0563T** **Evacuation of meibomian glands, using heat delivered through wearable, open-eye eyelid treatment devices and manual gland expression, bilateral**

EXCLUDES *Evacuation using:*
Heat and intermittent pressure (0207T)
Manual expression only, report appropriate E/M code

0.00 0.00 FUD YYY 80

0208T-0212T

EXCLUDES *Manual audiometric testing by qualified health care professional, using audiometers (92551-92557)*

0208T **Pure tone audiometry (threshold), automated; air only**

0.00 0.00 FUD XXX Q1 80 TC

AMA: 2018,Jan,8; 2017,Jan,8; 2016,Jan,13

0209T **air and bone**

0.00 0.00 FUD XXX Q1 80 TC

AMA: 2018,Jan,8; 2017,Jan,8; 2016,Jan,13

0210T **Speech audiometry threshold, automated;**

0.00 0.00 FUD XXX Q1 80 TC

AMA: 2014,Aug,3

0211T **with speech recognition**

0.00 0.00 FUD XXX Q1 80 TC

AMA: 2018,Jan,8; 2017,Jan,8; 2016,Jan,13

0212T **Comprehensive audiometry threshold evaluation and speech recognition (0209T, 0211T combined), automated**

0.00 0.00 FUD XXX Q1 80 TC

AMA: 2018,Jan,8; 2017,Jan,8; 2016,Jan,13

0213T-0215T

INCLUDES Ultrasound guidance (76942)

0213T **Injection(s), diagnostic or therapeutic agent, paravertebral facet (zygapophyseal) joint (or nerves innervating that joint) with ultrasound guidance, cervical or thoracic; single level**

0.00 0.00 FUD XXX T R2 80 50

AMA: 2018,Jan,8; 2017,Jan,8; 2016,Jan,13

\+ **0214T** **second level (List separately in addition to code for primary procedure)**

EXCLUDES *Reporting with modifier 50. Report once for each side when performed bilaterally*

Code first (0213T)

0.00 0.00 FUD ZZZ N N1 80

AMA: 2018,Jan,8; 2017,Jan,8; 2016,Jan,13

\+ **0215T** **third and any additional level(s) (List separately in addition to code for primary procedure)**

EXCLUDES *Reporting code more than one time per service date*
Reporting with modifier 50. Report once for each side when performed bilaterally

Code first (0213T-0214T)

0.00 0.00 FUD ZZZ N N1 80

AMA: 2018,Jan,8; 2017,Jan,8; 2016,Jan,13

0216T-0218T

INCLUDES Ultrasound guidance (76942)

EXCLUDES *Injection with CT or fluoroscopic guidance (64490-64495)*

0216T **Injection(s), diagnostic or therapeutic agent, paravertebral facet (zygapophyseal) joint (or nerves innervating that joint) with ultrasound guidance, lumbar or sacral; single level**

0.00 0.00 FUD XXX T R2 80 50

AMA: 2018,Jan,8; 2017,Jan,8; 2016,Jan,13

\+ **0217T** **second level (List separately in addition to code for primary procedure)**

EXCLUDES *Reporting with modifier 50. Report once for each side when performed bilaterally*

Code first (0216T)

0.00 0.00 FUD ZZZ N N1 80

AMA: 2018,Jan,8; 2017,Jan,8; 2016,Jan,13

\+ **0218T** **third and any additional level(s) (List separately in addition to code for primary procedure)**

EXCLUDES *Reporting code more than one time per service date*
Reporting with modifier 50. Report once for each side when performed bilaterally

Code first (0216T-0217T)

0.00 0.00 FUD ZZZ N N1 80

AMA: 2018,Jan,8; 2017,Jan,8; 2016,Jan,13

0219T-0222T

INCLUDES Allografts at same level (20930-20931)
Application intervertebral biomechanical device(s) at same level (22853-22854, [22859])
Arthrodesis at same level (22600-22614)
Instrumentation at same level (22840)
Radiologic services

0219T **Placement of a posterior intrafacet implant(s), unilateral or bilateral, including imaging and placement of bone graft(s) or synthetic device(s), single level; cervical**

0.00 0.00 FUD XXX C 80

AMA: 2018,Jan,8; 2017,Jan,8; 2016,Jan,13

0220T **thoracic**

0.00 0.00 FUD XXX C 80

AMA: 2018,Jan,8; 2017,Jan,8; 2016,Jan,13

0221T **lumbar**

0.00 0.00 FUD XXX J G2 80

AMA: 2018,Jan,8; 2017,Jan,8; 2016,Jan,13

\+ **0222T** **each additional vertebral segment (List separately in addition to code for primary procedure)**

Code first (0219T-0221T)

0.00 0.00 FUD ZZZ N 80

AMA: 2018,Jan,8; 2017,Jan,8; 2016,Jan,13

0232T

INCLUDES Arthrocentesis (20600-20611)
Blood collection (36415, 36592)
Fat and other soft tissue grafts ([15769], 15771-15774)
Imaging guidance (76942, 77002, 77012, 77021)
Injections (20550-20551)
Platelet/blood product pooling (86965)

EXCLUDES *Aspiration bone marrow for grafting, biopsy, harvesting for transplant (38220-38221, 38230)*
Injections white cell concentrate (0481T)

0232T **Injection(s), platelet rich plasma, any site, including image guidance, harvesting and preparation when performed**

0.00 0.00 FUD XXX Q1 N1

AMA: 2019,Oct,5; 2019,Apr,10; 2018,May,3; 2018,Jan,8; 2017,Jan,8; 2016,Jan,13

0234T-0253T [0253T]

INCLUDES Atherectomy by any technique in arteries above inguinal ligaments
Radiology supervision and interpretation

EXCLUDES *Accessing and catheterization vessel*
Atherectomy performed below inguinal ligaments (37225, 37227, 37229, 37231, 37233, 37235)
Closure arteriotomy by any technique
Negotiating lesion
Other interventions to same or different vessels
Protection from embolism

0234T **Transluminal peripheral atherectomy, open or percutaneous, including radiological supervision and interpretation; renal artery**

0.00 0.00 FUD YYY J 80

AMA: 2018,Jan,8; 2017,Jan,8; 2016,Jan,13

0235T **visceral artery (except renal), each vessel**

0.00 0.00 FUD YYY C 80

AMA: 2018,Jan,8; 2017,Jan,8; 2016,Jan,13

Category III Codes

0236T—0278T

0236T **abdominal aorta**
0.00 0.00 FUD YYY J 80
AMA: 2018,Jan,8; 2017,Jan,8; 2016,Jan,13

0237T **brachiocephalic trunk and branches, each vessel**
0.00 0.00 FUD YYY J 80
AMA: 2018,Jan,8; 2017,Jan,8; 2016,Jan,13

0238T **iliac artery, each vessel**
0.00 0.00 FUD YYY J J8 80
AMA: 2018,Jan,8; 2017,Jan,8; 2016,Jan,13

0253T **Resequenced code. See code before 0198T.**

0263T-0265T

EXCLUDES *Bone marrow and stem cell services (38204-38242 [38243])*

0263T **Intramuscular autologous bone marrow cell therapy, with preparation of harvested cells, multiple injections, one leg, including ultrasound guidance, if performed; complete procedure including unilateral or bilateral bone marrow harvest**
INCLUDES Duplex scan (93925-93926)
Ultrasound guidance (76942)
0.00 0.00 FUD XXX S G2 80

0264T **complete procedure excluding bone marrow harvest**
INCLUDES Bone marrow harvest only (0265T)
Duplex scan (93925-93926)
Ultrasound guidance (76942)
0.00 0.00 FUD XXX S G2 80

0265T **unilateral or bilateral bone marrow harvest only for intramuscular autologous bone marrow cell therapy**
EXCLUDES *Complete procedure (0263T-0264T)*
0.00 0.00 FUD XXX S G2 80

0266T-0273T

0266T **Implantation or replacement of carotid sinus baroreflex activation device; total system (includes generator placement, unilateral or bilateral lead placement, intra-operative interrogation, programming, and repositioning, when performed)**
INCLUDES Components complete procedure (0267T-0268T)
0.00 0.00 FUD YYY C J8 80

0267T **lead only, unilateral (includes intra-operative interrogation, programming, and repositioning, when performed)**
EXCLUDES *Complete procedure (0266T)*
Device interrogation (0272T-0273T)
Removal/revision device or components (0269T-0271T)
0.00 0.00 FUD YYY T G2 80

0268T **pulse generator only (includes intra-operative interrogation, programming, and repositioning, when performed)**
EXCLUDES *Complete procedure (0266T)*
Device interrogation (0272T-0273T)
Removal/revision device or components (0269T-0271T)
0.00 0.00 FUD YYY J J8 80

0269T **Revision or removal of carotid sinus baroreflex activation device; total system (includes generator placement, unilateral or bilateral lead placement, intra-operative interrogation, programming, and repositioning, when performed)**
EXCLUDES *Device interrogation (0272T-0273T)*
Implantation/replacement device and/or components (0266T-0268T)
Removal/revision device or components (0270T-0271T)
0.00 0.00 FUD XXX Q2 G2 80

0270T **lead only, unilateral (includes intra-operative interrogation, programming, and repositioning, when performed)**
EXCLUDES *Device interrogation (0272T-0273T)*
Implantation/replacement device and/or components (0266T-0269T)
Removal/revision device or components (0271T)
0.00 0.00 FUD XXX Q2 G2 80

0271T **pulse generator only (includes intra-operative interrogation, programming, and repositioning, when performed)**
EXCLUDES *Device interrogation (0272T-0273T)*
Implantation/replacement device and/or components (0266T-0268T)
Removal/revision device or components (0271T-0273T)
0.00 0.00 FUD XXX Q2 G2 80

0272T **Interrogation device evaluation (in person), carotid sinus baroreflex activation system, including telemetric iterative communication with the implantable device to monitor device diagnostics and programmed therapy values, with interpretation and report (eg, battery status, lead impedance, pulse amplitude, pulse width, therapy frequency, pathway mode, burst mode, therapy start/stop times each day);**
EXCLUDES *Device interrogation (0273T)*
Implantation/replacement device and/or components (0266T-0268T)
Removal/revision device or components (0269T-0271T)
0.00 0.00 FUD XXX S 80

0273T **with programming**
EXCLUDES *Device interrogation (0272T)*
Implantation/replacement device and/or components (0266T-0268T)
Removal/revision device or components (0269T-0271T)
0.00 0.00 FUD XXX S 80

0274T-0275T

EXCLUDES *Laminotomy/hemilaminectomy by open and endoscopically assisted approach (63020-63035)*
Percutaneous decompression nucleus pulposus intervertebral disc by needle-based technique (62287)

0274T **Percutaneous laminotomy/laminectomy (interlaminar approach) for decompression of neural elements, (with or without ligamentous resection, discectomy, facetectomy and/or foraminotomy), any method, under indirect image guidance (eg, fluoroscopic, CT), single or multiple levels, unilateral or bilateral; cervical or thoracic**
0.00 0.00 FUD YYY J G2 80
AMA: 2018,Jan,8; 2017,Feb,12; 2017,Jan,8; 2016,Jan,13

0275T **lumbar**
0.00 0.00 FUD YYY J J8 80
AMA: 2018,Jan,8; 2017,Feb,12; 2017,Jan,8; 2016,Jan,13

0278T

0278T **Transcutaneous electrical modulation pain reprocessing (eg, scrambler therapy), each treatment session (includes placement of electrodes)**
0.00 0.00 FUD XXX Q1 N1 80

0290T

~~0290T~~ ~~**Corneal incisions in the recipient cornea created using a laser, in preparation for penetrating or lamellar keratoplasty (List separately in addition to code for primary procedure)**~~
To report, see (66999)

0308T

0308T Insertion of ocular telescope prosthesis including removal of crystalline lens or intraocular lens prosthesis

INCLUDES Injection procedures (66020, 66030)
Iridectomy when performed (66600-66635, 66761)
Operating microscope (69990)
Repositioning intraocular lens (66825)

EXCLUDES *Cataract extraction (66982-66986 [66987, 66988, 66989, 66991])*

0.00 0.00 FUD YYY J J8 50

AMA: 2019,Dec,6; 2018,Jan,8; 2017,Jan,8; 2016,Jan,13

0312T-0317T

EXCLUDES *Analysis and/or programming (or reprogramming) vagus nerve stimulator (95970, 95976-95977)*
Implantation, replacement, removal, and/or revision vagus nerve neurostimulator (electrode array and/or pulse generator) for stimulation vagus nerve other than at esophagogastric junction (64568-64570)

0312T Vagus nerve blocking therapy (morbid obesity); laparoscopic implantation of neurostimulator electrode array, anterior and posterior vagal trunks adjacent to esophagogastric junction (EGJ), with implantation of pulse generator, includes programming

0.00 0.00 FUD XXX J G2 80

AMA: 2018,Jan,8; 2017,Jan,8; 2016,Jan,13

0313T laparoscopic revision or replacement of vagal trunk neurostimulator electrode array, including connection to existing pulse generator

0.00 0.00 FUD XXX T J8 80

AMA: 2018,Jan,8; 2017,Jan,8; 2016,Jan,13

0314T laparoscopic removal of vagal trunk neurostimulator electrode array and pulse generator

0.00 0.00 FUD XXX Q2 G2 80

AMA: 2018,Jan,8; 2017,Jan,8; 2016,Jan,13

0315T removal of pulse generator

EXCLUDES *Removal with replacement pulse generator (0316T)*

0.00 0.00 FUD XXX Q2 G2 80

AMA: 2018,Jan,8; 2017,Jan,8; 2016,Jan,13

0316T replacement of pulse generator

EXCLUDES *Removal without replacement pulse generator (0315T)*

0.00 0.00 FUD XXX J J8 80

AMA: 2018,Jan,8; 2017,Jan,8; 2016,Jan,13

0317T neurostimulator pulse generator electronic analysis, includes reprogramming when performed

EXCLUDES *Analysis and/or programming (or reprogramming) vagus nerve stimulator (95970, 95976-95977)*

0.00 0.00 FUD XXX Q1 80

AMA: 2018,Jan,8; 2017,Jan,8; 2016,Jan,13

0329T-0330T

0329T Monitoring of intraocular pressure for 24 hours or longer, unilateral or bilateral, with interpretation and report

0.00 0.00 FUD YYY E

AMA: 2018,Jan,8; 2017,Jan,8; 2016,Jan,13

0330T Tear film imaging, unilateral or bilateral, with interpretation and report

0.00 0.00 FUD YYY Q1 N1

AMA: 2018,Jan,8; 2017,Jan,8; 2016,Jan,13

0331T-0332T

EXCLUDES *Myocardial infarction avid imaging (78466, 78468, 78469)*

0331T Myocardial sympathetic innervation imaging, planar qualitative and quantitative assessment;

0.00 0.00 FUD YYY S Z2

AMA: 2018,Jan,8; 2017,Jan,8; 2016,Jan,13

0332T with tomographic SPECT

0.00 0.00 FUD YYY S Z2

AMA: 2018,Jan,8; 2017,Jan,8; 2016,Jan,13

0333T-0464T [0464T]

0333T Visual evoked potential, screening of visual acuity, automated, with report

EXCLUDES *Visual evoked potential testing for glaucoma ([0464T])*

0.00 0.00 FUD YYY E

AMA: 2018,Feb,3; 2018,Jan,8; 2017,Jan,8; 2016,Jan,13

0464T Visual evoked potential, testing for glaucoma, with interpretation and report

EXCLUDES *Visual evoked potential for visual acuity (0333T)*

0.00 0.00 FUD YYY S

AMA: 2018,Feb,3

0335T-0511T [0510T, 0511T]

0335T Insertion of sinus tarsi implant

EXCLUDES *Arthroscopic subtalar arthrodesis (29907)*
Open talotarsal joint dislocation repair (28585)
Subtalar arthrodesis (28725)

0.00 0.00 FUD YYY J J8

0510T Removal of sinus tarsi implant

0.00 0.00 FUD YYY G2 50

0511T Removal and reinsertion of sinus tarsi implant

0.00 0.00 FUD YYY J8 50

0338T-0339T

INCLUDES Selective catheter placement renal arteries (36251-36254)

0338T Transcatheter renal sympathetic denervation, percutaneous approach including arterial puncture, selective catheter placement(s) renal artery(ies), fluoroscopy, contrast injection(s), intraprocedural roadmapping and radiological supervision and interpretation, including pressure gradient measurements, flush aortogram and diagnostic renal angiography when performed; unilateral

0.00 0.00 FUD YYY J G2

0339T bilateral

0.00 0.00 FUD YYY J G2

0342T

0342T Therapeutic apheresis with selective HDL delipidation and plasma reinfusion

0.00 0.00 FUD YYY S G2

0345T

0345T Transcatheter mitral valve repair percutaneous approach via the coronary sinus

INCLUDES Coronary angiography (93563-93564)
Fluoroscopy (76000)

EXCLUDES *Diagnostic cardiac catheterization procedures integral to valve procedure (93451-93461, 93593-93598)*
Repair mitral valve including transseptal puncture (33418-33419)
Transcatheter implantation/replacement mitral valve (TMVI) (0483T-0484T)
Transcatheter mitral valve annulus reconstruction (0544T)

Code also diagnostic cardiac catheterization/angiography procedures, and append modifier 59, if patient's condition (clinical indication) changed since intervention or prior study, no available prior catheter-based diagnostic study in treatment zone, or prior study not adequate (93451-93461, 93593-93598)

Code also transvascular ventricular support, when performed:
Balloon pump insertion (33967, 33970, 33973)
Ventricular assist device ([33995], 33990-33993, [33997])

0.00 0.00 FUD YYY C

AMA: 2018,Jan,8; 2017,Jan,8; 2016,Jan,13

0347T

0347T Placement of interstitial device(s) in bone for radiostereometric analysis (RSA)

0.00 0.00 FUD YYY Q1 N1

AMA: 2018,Jan,8; 2017,Jan,8; 2016,Jan,13

0348T-0350T

0348T **Radiologic examination, radiostereometric analysis (RSA); spine, (includes cervical, thoracic and lumbosacral, when performed)**
0.00 0.00 **FUD** YYY
AMA: 2018,Jan,8; 2017,Jan,8; 2016,Jan,13

0349T **upper extremity(ies), (includes shoulder, elbow, and wrist, when performed)**
0.00 0.00 **FUD** YYY
AMA: 2018,Jan,8; 2017,Jan,8; 2016,Jan,13

0350T **lower extremity(ies), (includes hip, proximal femur, knee, and ankle, when performed)**
0.00 0.00 **FUD** YYY
AMA: 2018,Jan,8; 2017,Jan,8; 2016,Jan,13

0351T-0354T

0351T **Optical coherence tomography of breast or axillary lymph node, excised tissue, each specimen; real-time intraoperative**
INCLUDES Interpretation and report (0352T)
0.00 0.00 **FUD** YYY
AMA: 2018,Jan,8; 2017,Jan,8; 2016,Jan,13

0352T **interpretation and report, real-time or referred**
INCLUDES Interpretation and report (0351T)
0.00 0.00 **FUD** YYY
AMA: 2018,Jan,8; 2017,Jan,8; 2016,Jan,13

0353T **Optical coherence tomography of breast, surgical cavity; real-time intraoperative**
INCLUDES Interpretation and report (0354T)
EXCLUDES *Reporting code more than one time per session*
0.00 0.00 **FUD** YYY
AMA: 2018,Jan,8; 2017,Jan,8; 2016,Jan,13

0354T **interpretation and report, real time or referred**
0.00 0.00 **FUD** YYY
AMA: 2018,Jan,8; 2017,Jan,8; 2016,Jan,13

0355T-0358T

0355T ~~**Gastrointestinal tract imaging, intraluminal (eg, capsule endoscopy), colon, with interpretation and report**~~
To report, see ([91113])

0356T ~~**Insertion of drug-eluting implant (including punctal dilation and implant removal when performed) into lacrimal canaliculus, each**~~
To report, see (68841, 0444T-0445T)

0358T **Bioelectrical impedance analysis whole body composition assessment, with interpretation and report**
0.00 0.00 **FUD** YYY

0362T-0376T [0376T]

INCLUDES Only one technician time when more than one technician in attendance
Provided by physician/other qualified healthcare professional while on-site (immediately available during procedure), but does not need to be face-to-face
Provided in environment appropriate for patient
Provided to patients with destructive behaviors

EXCLUDES *Adaptive behavior services ([97153, 97154, 97155, 97156, 97157, 97158])*
Aphasia assessment (96105)
Behavioral/developmental screening/testing (96110-96113, [96127])
Behavior/health assessment (96156-96159 [96164, 96165, 96167, 96168, 96170, 96171])
Cognitive testing ([96125])
Neurobehavioral testing (96116-96121)
Psychiatric evaluations/psychotherapy/interactive complexity (90785-90899)
Psychological/neuropsychological evaluation/testing (96130-96146)

0362T **Behavior identification supporting assessment, each 15 minutes of technicians' time face-to-face with a patient, requiring the following components: administration by the physician or other qualified health care professional who is on site; with the assistance of two or more technicians; for a patient who exhibits destructive behavior; completion in an environment that is customized to the patient's behavior.**
INCLUDES Comprises:
Functional analysis and behavioral assessment
Procedures and instruments to assess functional impairment and behavior levels
Structured observation with data collection not including direct patient involvement
EXCLUDES *Conferences by medical team (99366-99368)*
Occupational therapy evaluation ([97165, 97166, 97167, 97168])
Speech evaluation (92521-92524)
Code also when performed on different days until behavioral and supporting assessments complete
0.00 0.00 **FUD** YYY
AMA: 2018,Nov,3; 2018,Jan,8; 2017,Jan,8; 2016,Jan,13

0373T **Adaptive behavior treatment with protocol modification, each 15 minutes of technicians' time face-to-face with a patient, requiring the following components: administration by the physician or other qualified health care professional who is on site; with the assistance of two or more technicians; for a patient who exhibits destructive behavior; completion in an environment that is customized to the patient's behavior.**
0.00 0.00 **FUD** YYY
AMA: 2018,Nov,3; 2018,Jan,8; 2017,Jan,8; 2016,Jan,13

0378T-0379T

0378T **Visual field assessment, with concurrent real time data analysis and accessible data storage with patient initiated data transmitted to a remote surveillance center for up to 30 days; review and interpretation with report by a physician or other qualified health care professional**
0.00 0.00 **FUD** XXX
AMA: 2018,Jan,8; 2017,Jan,8; 2016,Jan,13

0379T **technical support and patient instructions, surveillance, analysis and transmission of daily and emergent data reports as prescribed by a physician or other qualified health care professional**
0.00 0.00 **FUD** XXX
AMA: 2018,Jan,8; 2017,Jan,8; 2016,Jan,13

0394T-0395T

EXCLUDES *Radiation oncology procedures (77261-77263, 77300, 77306-77307, 77316-77318, 77332-77334, 77336, 77427-77499, 77761-77772, 77778, 77789)*

0394T **High dose rate electronic brachytherapy, skin surface application, per fraction, includes basic dosimetry, when performed**
EXCLUDES *Superficial non-brachytherapy radiation (77401)*
0.00 0.00 **FUD** XXX

0395T **High dose rate electronic brachytherapy, interstitial or intracavitary treatment, per fraction, includes basic dosimetry, when performed**

EXCLUDES *High dose rate skin surface application (0394T)*

0.00 0.00 FUD XXX S Z2 80

0397T-0398T

+ 0397T **Endoscopic retrograde cholangiopancreatography (ERCP), with optical endomicroscopy (List separately in addition to code for primary procedure)**

INCLUDES Optical endomicroscopic image(s) (88375)

EXCLUDES *Reporting code more than one time per operative session*

Code first (43260-43265, [43274], [43275], [43276], [43277], [43278])

0.00 0.00 FUD XXX N N1 80

0398T **Magnetic resonance image guided high intensity focused ultrasound (MRgFUS), stereotactic ablation lesion, intracranial for movement disorder including stereotactic navigation and frame placement when performed**

INCLUDES Application stereotactic headframe (61800)
Stereotactic computer-assisted navigation (61781)

0.00 0.00 FUD XXX S 80

0402T

0402T **Collagen cross-linking of cornea, including removal of the corneal epithelium and intraoperative pachymetry, when performed (Report medication separately)**

INCLUDES Corneal epithelium removal (65435)
Corneal pachymetry (76514)
Operating microscope (69990)

0.00 0.00 FUD XXX J R2 80

AMA: 2018,Jun,11; 2018,Jan,8; 2017,Jan,8; 2016,Feb,12

0403T-0488T [0488T]

INCLUDES Intensive behavioral counseling by trained lifestyle coach
Standardized course with emphasis on weight, exercise, stress management, and nutrition

0403T **Preventive behavior change, intensive program of prevention of diabetes using a standardized diabetes prevention program curriculum, provided to individuals in a group setting, minimum 60 minutes, per day**

EXCLUDES *Online/electronic diabetes prevention program ([0488T])*
Self-management training and education by nonphysician health care professional (98960-98962)

0.00 0.00 FUD XXX E 80

AMA: 2020,Jul,7; 2018,Aug,6

0488T **Preventive behavior change, online/electronic structured intensive program for prevention of diabetes using a standardized diabetes prevention program curriculum, provided to an individual, per 30 days**

INCLUDES In person elements when appropriate

EXCLUDES *Group diabetes prevention program (0403T)*
Self-management training and education by nonphysician health care professional (98960-98962)

0.00 0.00 FUD XXX E

AMA: 2020,Jul,7; 2018,Aug,6

0404T

0404T **Transcervical uterine fibroid(s) ablation with ultrasound guidance, radiofrequency** ♀

0.00 0.00 FUD XXX J J8 80

0408T-0418T

0408T **Insertion or replacement of permanent cardiac contractility modulation system, including contractility evaluation when performed, and programming of sensing and therapeutic parameters; pulse generator with transvenous electrodes**

INCLUDES Device evaluation (93286-93287, 0415T, 0417T-0418T)
Insertion or replacement entire system

EXCLUDES *Cardiac catheterization (93452-93453, 93456-93461)*

Code also removal each electrode when pulse generator and electrodes removed and replaced (0410T-0411T)

0.00 0.00 FUD XXX J J8 80

0409T **pulse generator only**

INCLUDES Device evaluation (93286-93287, 0415T, 0417T-0418T)

EXCLUDES *Cardiac catheterization (93452-93453, 93456-93461)*

0.00 0.00 FUD XXX J J8 80

0410T **atrial electrode only**

INCLUDES Device evaluation (93286-93287, 0415T, 0417T-0418T)
Each atrial electrode inserted or replaced

EXCLUDES *Cardiac catheterization (93452-93453, 93456-93461)*

0.00 0.00 FUD XXX J J8 80

0411T **ventricular electrode only**

INCLUDES Device evaluation (93286-93287, 0415T, 0417T-0418T)
Each ventricular electrode inserted or replaced

EXCLUDES *Cardiac catheterization (93452-93453, 93456-93461)*
Insertion or replacement complete CCM system (0408T)

0.00 0.00 FUD XXX J J8 80

0412T **Removal of permanent cardiac contractility modulation system; pulse generator only**

EXCLUDES *Device evaluation (0417T-0418T)*
Insertion or replacement complete CCM system (0408T)

0.00 0.00 FUD XXX Q2 G2 80

0413T **transvenous electrode (atrial or ventricular)**

INCLUDES Each electrode removed

EXCLUDES *Device evaluation (0417T-0418T)*
Insertion or replacement complete CCM system (0408T)

Code also:
Removal and replacement electrode(s), as appropriate (0410T-0411T)
Removal pulse generator when leads also removed (0412T)

0.00 0.00 FUD XXX Q2 G2 80

0414T **Removal and replacement of permanent cardiac contractility modulation system pulse generator only**

INCLUDES Device evaluation (93286-93287, 0417T-0418T)

EXCLUDES *Cardiac catheterization (93452-93453, 93456-93461)*

Code also replacement pulse generator when leads also removed and replaced (0408T, 0412T-0413T)

0.00 0.00 FUD XXX J J8 80

0415T **Repositioning of previously implanted cardiac contractility modulation transvenous electrode, (atrial or ventricular lead)**

INCLUDES Device evaluation (93286-93287, 0417T-0418T)

EXCLUDES *Cardiac catheterization (93452-93453, 93456-93461)*
Insertion or replacement entire system or components (0408T-0411T)

0.00 0.00 FUD XXX T G2 80

0416T **Relocation of skin pocket for implanted cardiac contractility modulation pulse generator**

0.00 0.00 FUD XXX T G2 80

0417T **Programming device evaluation (in person) with iterative adjustment of the implantable device to test the function of the device and select optimal permanent programmed values with analysis, including review and report, implantable cardiac contractility modulation system**

EXCLUDES *Insertion/replacement/removal/repositioning device or components (0408T-0415T, 0418T)*

0.00 0.00 FUD XXX Q1 80

0418T **Interrogation device evaluation (in person) with analysis, review and report, includes connection, recording and disconnection per patient encounter, implantable cardiac contractility modulation system**

EXCLUDES *Insertion/replacement/removal/repositioning device or components (0408T-0415T, 0417T)*

0.00 0.00 FUD XXX Q1 80

0419T-0420T

EXCLUDES *Neurofibroma excision (64792)*
Reporting code more than one time per session

0419T **Destruction of neurofibroma, extensive (cutaneous, dermal extending into subcutaneous); face, head and neck, greater than 50 neurofibromas**

0.00 0.00 FUD XXX T R2 80

AMA: 2018,Jan,8; 2017,Jan,8; 2016,Apr,3

0420T **trunk and extremities, extensive, greater than 100 neurofibromas**

0.00 0.00 FUD XXX T R2 80

AMA: 2018,Jan,8; 2017,Jan,8; 2016,Apr,3

0421T-0423T

0421T **Transurethral waterjet ablation of prostate, including control of post-operative bleeding, including ultrasound guidance, complete (vasectomy, meatotomy, cystourethroscopy, urethral calibration and/or dilation, and internal urethrotomy are included when performed)** ♂

EXCLUDES *Transrectal ultrasound (76872)*
Transurethral prostate resection (52500, 52630)

0.00 0.00 FUD XXX J G2 80

AMA: 2020,Aug,6

0422T **Tactile breast imaging by computer-aided tactile sensors, unilateral or bilateral**

0.00 0.00 FUD XXX Q1 Z2 80

~~**0423T** **Secretory type II phospholipase A2 (sPLA2-IIA)**~~

To report, see (84999)

0424T-0436T

INCLUDES Phrenic nerve stimulation system includes:
Pulse generator
Sensing lead (placed in azygos vein)
Stimulation lead (placed into right brachiocephalic vein or left pericardiophrenic vein)

0424T **Insertion or replacement of neurostimulator system for treatment of central sleep apnea; complete system (transvenous placement of right or left stimulation lead, sensing lead, implantable pulse generator)**

INCLUDES Device evaluation (0434T-0436T)
Insertion or replacement system components (0425T-0427T)
Repositioning leads (0432T-0433T)

Code also when pulse generator and all leads removed and replaced (0428T-0430T)

0.00 0.00 FUD XXX J G2 80

0425T **sensing lead only**

EXCLUDES *Device evaluation (0434T-0436T)*
Insertion/replacement complete system (0424T)
Repositioning leads (0432T-0433T)

0.00 0.00 FUD XXX J G2 80

0426T **stimulation lead only**

EXCLUDES *Device evaluation (0434T-0436T)*
Insertion/replacement complete system (0424T)
Repositioning leads (0432T-0433T)

0.00 0.00 FUD XXX J G2 80

0427T **pulse generator only**

EXCLUDES *Device evaluation (0434T-0436T)*
Insertion/replacement complete system (0424T)
Repositioning leads (0432T-0433T)

0.00 0.00 FUD XXX J J8 80

0428T **Removal of neurostimulator system for treatment of central sleep apnea; pulse generator only**

EXCLUDES *Device evaluation (0434T-0436T)*
Removal with replacement of pulse generator and all leads (0424T, 0429T-0430T)
Repositioning leads (0432T-0433T)

Code also when lead removed (0429T-0430T)

0.00 0.00 FUD XXX Q2 G2 80

0429T **sensing lead only**

INCLUDES Removal one sensing lead

EXCLUDES *Device evaluation (0434T-0436T)*

0.00 0.00 FUD XXX Q2 G2 80

0430T **stimulation lead only**

INCLUDES Removal one stimulation lead

EXCLUDES *Device evaluation (0434T-0436T)*

0.00 0.00 FUD XXX Q2 G2 80

AMA: 2015,Aug,4

0431T **Removal and replacement of neurostimulator system for treatment of central sleep apnea, pulse generator only**

EXCLUDES *Device evaluation (0434T-0436T)*
Removal with replacement generator and all three leads (0424T, 0428T-0430T)

0.00 0.00 FUD XXX J J8 80

0432T **Repositioning of neurostimulator system for treatment of central sleep apnea; stimulation lead only**

EXCLUDES *Device evaluation (0434T-0436T)*
Insertion/replacement complete system or components (0424T-0427T)

0.00 0.00 FUD XXX T G2 80

0433T **sensing lead only**

EXCLUDES *Device evaluation (0434T-0436T)*
Insertion/replacement complete system or components (0424T-0427T)

0.00 0.00 FUD XXX T G2 80

0434T **Interrogation device evaluation implanted neurostimulator pulse generator system for central sleep apnea**

EXCLUDES *Insertion/replacement complete system or components (0424T-0427T)*
Removal system or components (0428T-0431T)
Repositioning leads (0432T-0433T)

0.00 0.00 FUD XXX S G2 80

0435T **Programming device evaluation of implanted neurostimulator pulse generator system for central sleep apnea; single session**

EXCLUDES *Device evaluation (0436T)*
Insertion/replacement complete system or components (0424T-0427T)
Removal system or components (0428T-0431T)
Repositioning leads (0432T-0433T)

0.00 0.00 FUD XXX S 80

0436T **during sleep study**

EXCLUDES *Device evaluation (0435T)*
Insertion/replacement complete system or components (0424T-0427T)
Removal system or components (0428T-0431T)
Reporting code more than one time for each sleep study
Repositioning leads (0432T-0433T)

0.00 0.00 FUD XXX S 80

0437T-0439T

+ **0437T** **Implantation of non-biologic or synthetic implant (eg, polypropylene) for fascial reinforcement of the abdominal wall (List separately in addition to code for primary procedure)**

EXCLUDES *Implantation mesh, other material for repair incisional or ventral hernia (49560-49561, 49565-49566, 49568)*

Insertion mesh, other material for closure wound caused by necrotizing soft tissue infection (11004-11006, 49568)

Code first primary procedure

0.00 0.00 **FUD** ZZZ N N1 80

+ **0439T** **Myocardial contrast perfusion echocardiography, at rest or with stress, for assessment of myocardial ischemia or viability (List separately in addition to code for primary procedure)**

Code first (93306-93308, 93350-93351)

0.00 0.00 **FUD** ZZZ N N1 80

AMA: 2018,Jan,8; 2017,Jan,8; 2016,Apr,8

0440T-0442T

0440T **Ablation, percutaneous, cryoablation, includes imaging guidance; upper extremity distal/peripheral nerve**

0.00 0.00 **FUD** YYY J G2 80

AMA: 2019,Apr,9; 2018,Jan,8

0441T **lower extremity distal/peripheral nerve**

0.00 0.00 **FUD** YYY J G2 80

AMA: 2019,Apr,9; 2018,Jan,8

0442T **nerve plexus or other truncal nerve (eg, brachial plexus, pudendal nerve)**

0.00 0.00 **FUD** YYY J J8 80

AMA: 2019,Apr,9; 2018,Jan,8

0443T

+ **0443T** **Real-time spectral analysis of prostate tissue by fluorescence spectroscopy, including imaging guidance (List separately in addition to code for primary procedure)** ♂

EXCLUDES *Reporting code more than one time for each session*

Code first (55700)

0.00 0.00 **FUD** ZZZ N N1 80

0444T-0445T

EXCLUDES *Insertion/removal drug-eluting stent into canaliculus (68841)*

0444T **Initial placement of a drug-eluting ocular insert under one or more eyelids, including fitting, training, and insertion, unilateral or bilateral**

0.00 0.00 **FUD** YYY N N1 80

AMA: 2018,Jan,8; 2017,Aug,7

0445T **Subsequent placement of a drug-eluting ocular insert under one or more eyelids, including re-training, and removal of existing insert, unilateral or bilateral**

0.00 0.00 **FUD** YYY N N1 80

AMA: 2018,Jan,8; 2017,Aug,7

0446T-0448T

EXCLUDES *Placement non-implantable interstitial glucose sensor without pocket (95250)*

0446T **Creation of subcutaneous pocket with insertion of implantable interstitial glucose sensor, including system activation and patient training**

EXCLUDES *Interpretation/report ambulatory glucose monitoring interstitial tissue (95251)*

Removal interstitial glucose sensor (0447T-0448T)

0.00 0.00 **FUD** YYY T G2

AMA: 2018,Jun,6

0447T **Removal of implantable interstitial glucose sensor from subcutaneous pocket via incision**

0.00 0.00 **FUD** YYY Q2 G2

0448T **Removal of implantable interstitial glucose sensor with creation of subcutaneous pocket at different anatomic site and insertion of new implantable sensor, including system activation**

EXCLUDES *Initial insertion sensor (0446T)*

Removal sensor (0447T)

0.00 0.00 **FUD** YYY T G2

0449T-0450T

EXCLUDES *Insertion anterior segment aqueous drainage device ([0671T])*

Removal by internal approach aqueous drainage device without extraocular reservoir in subconjunctival space (92499)

0449T **Insertion of aqueous drainage device, without extraocular reservoir, internal approach, into the subconjunctival space; initial device**

0.00 0.00 **FUD** YYY J J8

AMA: 2018,Sep,3; 2018,Jul,3

+ **0450T** **each additional device (List separately in addition to code for primary procedure)**

Code first (0449T)

0.00 0.00 **FUD** YYY N N1

AMA: 2018,Jul,3

0451T-0463T

0451T ~~**Insertion or replacement of a permanently implantable aortic counterpulsation ventricular assist system, endovascular approach, and programming of sensing and therapeutic parameters; complete system (counterpulsation device, vascular graft, implantable vascular hemostatic seal, mechano-electrical skin interface and subcutaneous electrodes)**~~

To report, see (33999)

0452T ~~**aortic counterpulsation device and vascular hemostatic seal**~~

To report, see (33999)

0453T ~~**mechano-electrical skin interface**~~

To report, see (33999)

0454T ~~**subcutaneous electrode**~~

To report, see (33999)

0455T ~~**Removal of permanently implantable aortic counterpulsation ventricular assist system; complete system (aortic counterpulsation device, vascular hemostatic seal, mechano-electrical skin interface and electrodes)**~~

To report, see (33999)

0456T ~~**aortic counterpulsation device and vascular hemostatic seal**~~

To report, see (33999)

0457T ~~**mechano-electrical skin interface**~~

To report, see (33999)

0458T ~~**subcutaneous electrode**~~

To report, see (33999)

0459T ~~**Relocation of skin pocket with replacement of implanted aortic counterpulsation ventricular assist device, mechano-electrical skin interface and electrodes**~~

To report, see (33999)

0460T ~~**Repositioning of previously implanted aortic counterpulsation ventricular assist device; subcutaneous electrode**~~

To report, see (33999)

0461T ~~**aortic counterpulsation device**~~

To report, see (33999)

0462T ~~**Programming device evaluation (in person) with iterative adjustment of the implantable mechano-electrical skin interface and/or external driver to test the function of the device and select optimal permanent programmed values with analysis, including review and report, implantable aortic counterpulsation ventricular assist system, per day**~~

To report, see (33999)

~~0463T Interrogation device evaluation (in person) with analysis, review and report, includes connection, recording and disconnection per patient encounter, implantable aortic counterpulsation ventricular assist system, per day~~

To report, see (33999)

0464T [0464T]

0464T Resequenced code. See code following 0333T.

0465T-0469T

EXCLUDES *Replacement/revision cranial nerve neurostimulator electrode array (64569)*

0465T Suprachoroidal injection of a pharmacologic agent (does not include supply of medication)

EXCLUDES *Intravitreal implantation or injection (67025-67028)*

0.00 0.00 FUD YYY T R2

AMA: 2018,Feb,3

~~0466T Insertion of chest wall respiratory sensor electrode or electrode array, including connection to pulse generator (List separately in addition to code for primary procedure)~~

To report, see (64582-64584)

~~0467T Revision or replacement of chest wall respiratory sensor electrode or electrode array, including connection to existing pulse generator~~

To report, see (64582-64584)

~~0468T Removal of chest wall respiratory sensor electrode or electrode array~~

To report, see (64582-64584)

0469T Retinal polarization scan, ocular screening with on-site automated results, bilateral

INCLUDES Ophthalmic medical services (92002-92014)

EXCLUDES *Ocular screening (99174, [99177])*

0.00 0.00 FUD XXX E

AMA: 2018,Feb,3

0470T-0471T

EXCLUDES *Optical coherence tomography coronary vessel or graft (92978-92979)*
Reflectance confocal microscopy (RCM) for cellular and subcellular skin imaging (96931-96936)

0470T Optical coherence tomography (OCT) for microstructural and morphological imaging of skin, image acquisition, interpretation, and report; first lesion

0.00 0.00 FUD XXX M

\+ **0471T each additional lesion (List separately in addition to code for primary procedure)**

Code first (0470T)

0.00 0.00 FUD XXX N N1

0472T-0474T

0472T Device evaluation, interrogation, and initial programming of intraocular retinal electrode array (eg, retinal prosthesis), in person, with iterative adjustment of the implantable device to test functionality, select optimal permanent programmed values with analysis, including visual training, with review and report by a qualified health care professional

0.00 0.00 FUD XXX Q1

AMA: 2018,Feb,3

0473T Device evaluation and interrogation of intraocular retinal electrode array (eg, retinal prosthesis), in person, including reprogramming and visual training, when performed, with review and report by a qualified health care professional

INCLUDES Reprogramming device (0473T)

EXCLUDES *Placement intraocular retinal electrode display (0100T)*

0.00 0.00 FUD XXX Q1

AMA: 2018,Feb,3

0474T Insertion of anterior segment aqueous drainage device, with creation of intraocular reservoir, internal approach, into the supraciliary space

0.00 0.00 FUD XXX J

AMA: 2018,Dec,8; 2018,Dec,8; 2018,Jul,3; 2018,Feb,3

0475T-0478T

0475T Recording of fetal magnetic cardiac signal using at least 3 channels; patient recording and storage, data scanning with signal extraction, technical analysis and result, as well as supervision, review, and interpretation of report by a physician or other qualified health care professional

0.00 0.00 FUD XXX M

0476T patient recording, data scanning, with raw electronic signal transfer of data and storage

0.00 0.00 FUD XXX Q1

0477T signal extraction, technical analysis, and result

0.00 0.00 FUD XXX Q1

0478T review, interpretation, report by physician or other qualified health care professional

0.00 0.00 FUD XXX M

0479T-0480T

EXCLUDES *Ablative laser treatment for additional square cm open wound (0492T)*
Cicatricial lesion excision (11400-11446)
Reporting code more than one time per day

0479T Fractional ablative laser fenestration of burn and traumatic scars for functional improvement; first 100 cm2 or part thereof, or 1% of body surface area of infants and children

0.00 0.00 FUD 000 T G2

AMA: 2018,Jan,8; 2017,Dec,13

\+ **0480T each additional 100 cm2, or each additional 1% of body surface area of infants and children, or part thereof (List separately in addition to code for primary procedure)**

Code first (0479T)

0.00 0.00 FUD ZZZ N N1

AMA: 2018,Jan,8; 2017,Dec,13

0481T

0481T Injection(s), autologous white blood cell concentrate (autologous protein solution), any site, including image guidance, harvesting and preparation, when performed

INCLUDES Radiologic guidance (76942, 77002, 77012, 77021)

EXCLUDES *Blood collection (36415, 36592)*
Bone marrow procedures (38220-38222, 38230)
Injection platelet rich plasma (0232T)
Injections to tendon, ligament, or fascia (20550-20551)
Joint aspiration or injection (20600-20611)
Other tissue grafts ([15769], 15771-15774)
Pooling platelets (86965)

0.00 0.00 FUD 000 Q1

AMA: 2019,Oct,5

0483T-0484T

INCLUDES Access and closure
Angiography
Balloon valvuloplasty
Contrast injections
Fluoroscopy
Radiological supervision and interpretation
Valve deployment and repositioning
Ventriculography

EXCLUDES *Diagnostic heart catheterization (93451-93453, 93456-93461, 93593-93598)*
Transcatheter mitral valve annulus reconstruction (0544T)
Transcatheter mitral valve repair through coronary sinus (0345T)
Transcatheter mitral valve repair with transseptal puncture, when performed (33418-33419)
Transcatheter tricuspid valve annulus reconstruction (0545T)

Code also:
Cardiopulmonary bypass, when provided (33367-33369)
Diagnostic cardiac catheterization/angiography procedures, and append modifier 59, if patient's condition (clinical indication) changed since intervention or prior study, no available prior catheter-based diagnostic study in treatment zone, or prior study not adequate (93451-93461, 93563-93564, 93593-93598)

0483T Transcatheter mitral valve implantation/replacement (TMVI) with prosthetic valve; percutaneous approach, including transseptal puncture, when performed

0.00 0.00 FUD 000 C 80

0484T **transthoracic exposure (eg, thoracotomy, transapical)**
0.00 0.00 FUD 000 C 80

0485T-0486T

0485T **Optical coherence tomography (OCT) of middle ear, with interpretation and report; unilateral**
0.00 0.00 FUD XXX Q1 50

0486T **bilateral**
0.00 0.00 FUD XXX Q1

0487T-0488T [0488T]

0487T **Biomechanical mapping, transvaginal, with report**
0.00 0.00 FUD XXX Q1 N1

0488T **Resequenced code. See code following 0403T.**

0489T-0490T

EXCLUDES *Joint injection/aspiration (20600, 20604)*
Liposuction procedures (15876-15879)
Tissue grafts ([15769], 15771-15774)

Code also for complete procedure report both codes (0489T-0490T)

0489T **Autologous adipose-derived regenerative cell therapy for scleroderma in the hands; adipose tissue harvesting, isolation and preparation of harvested cells including incubation with cell dissociation enzymes, removal of non-viable cells and debris, determination of concentration and dilution of regenerative cells**
0.00 0.00 FUD 000 E
AMA: 2019,Oct,5; 2018,Sep,12

0490T **multiple injections in one or both hands**
EXCLUDES *Single injections*
0.00 0.00 FUD 000 E
AMA: 2019,Oct,5; 2018,Sep,12

0491T-0642T [0640T, 0641T, 0642T]

0491T **Ablative laser treatment, non-contact, full field and fractional ablation, open wound, per day, total treatment surface area; first 20 sq cm or less**
0.00 0.00 FUD 000 T G2

\+ 0492T **each additional 20 sq cm, or part thereof (List separately in addition to code for primary procedure)**
EXCLUDES *Laser fenestration scars (0479T-0480T)*
Code first (0491T)
0.00 0.00 FUD ZZZ N N1

▲ 0493T **Contact near-infrared spectroscopy studies of lower extremity wounds (eg, for oxyhemoglobin measurement)**
EXCLUDES *Noncontact near-infrared spectroscopy studies ([0640T, 0641T, 0642T])*
0.00 0.00 FUD XXX N N1

● # 0640T **Noncontact near-infrared spectroscopy studies of flap or wound (eg, for measurement of deoxyhemoglobin, oxyhemoglobin, and ratio of tissue oxygenation [StO_2]); image acquisition, interpretation and report, each flap or wound**
INCLUDES All complete test components ([0640T], [0641T], [0642T])
EXCLUDES *Contact near-infrared spectroscopy studies (0493T)*
Image acquisition or interpretation and report only ([0641T], [0642T])
0.00 0.00 FUD XXX 80

● # 0641T **image acquisition only, each flap or wound**
EXCLUDES *Complete noncontact-infrared spectroscopy study ([0640T])*
Contact near-infrared spectroscopy studies (0493T)
Interpretation and report only ([0642T])
0.00 0.00 FUD XXX 80 TC

● # 0642T **interpretation and report only, each flap or wound**
EXCLUDES *Complete noncontact-infrared spectroscopy study ([0640T])*
Contact near-infrared spectroscopy studies (0493T)
Image acquisition only ([0641T])
0.00 0.00 FUD XXX 80 26

0494T-0496T

0494T **Surgical preparation and cannulation of marginal (extended) cadaver donor lung(s) to ex vivo organ perfusion system, including decannulation, separation from the perfusion system, and cold preservation of the allograft prior to implantation, when performed**
0.00 0.00 FUD XXX C 80

0495T **Initiation and monitoring marginal (extended) cadaver donor lung(s) organ perfusion system by physician or qualified health care professional, including physiological and laboratory assessment (eg, pulmonary artery flow, pulmonary artery pressure, left atrial pressure, pulmonary vascular resistance, mean/peak and plateau airway pressure, dynamic compliance and perfusate gas analysis), including bronchoscopy and X ray when performed; first two hours in sterile field**
0.00 0.00 FUD XXX C

\+ 0496T **each additional hour (List separately in addition to code for primary procedure)**
Code first (0495T)
0.00 0.00 FUD ZZZ C

0497T-0498T

EXCLUDES *ECG event monitoring (93268, 93271-93272)*
ECG rhythm strips (93040-93042)
Remote telemetry (93228-93229)

0497T **External patient-activated, physician- or other qualified health care professional-prescribed, electrocardiographic rhythm derived event recorder without 24 hour attended monitoring; in-office connection**
0.00 0.00 FUD XXX Q1 TC
AMA: 2020,Nov,10

0498T **review and interpretation by a physician or other qualified health care professional per 30 days with at least one patient-generated triggered event**
0.00 0.00 FUD XXX M 26
AMA: 2020,Nov,10

0499T-0500T

0499T **Cystourethroscopy, with mechanical dilation and urethral therapeutic drug delivery for urethral stricture or stenosis, including fluoroscopy, when performed**
EXCLUDES *Cystourethroscopy for stricture (52281, 52283)*
0.00 0.00 FUD 000 E G2

0500T **Infectious agent detection by nucleic acid (DNA or RNA), human papillomavirus (HPV) for five or more separately reported high-risk HPV types (eg, 16, 18, 31, 33, 35, 39, 45, 51, 52, 56, 58, 59, 68) (ie, genotyping)**
EXCLUDES *Less than five high-risk HPV types ([87624, 87625])*
0.00 0.00 FUD XXX A

0501T-0523T [0523T, 0623T, 0624T, 0625T, 0626T]

EXCLUDES *Reporting code more than one time for each CT angiogram*

0501T **Noninvasive estimated coronary fractional flow reserve (FFR) derived from coronary computed tomography angiography data using computation fluid dynamics physiologic simulation software analysis of functional data to assess the severity of coronary artery disease; data preparation and transmission, analysis of fluid dynamics and simulated maximal coronary hyperemia, generation of estimated FFR model, with anatomical data review in comparison with estimated FFR model to reconcile discordant data, interpretation and report**

INCLUDES All complete test components (0501T-0504T)

EXCLUDES *Automated coronary plaque characterization/quantification using coronary CT angiography data ([0623T, 0624T, 0625T, 0626T])*

0.00 0.00 **FUD** XXX M

AMA: 2018,Sep,10

0502T **data preparation and transmission**

EXCLUDES *Automated coronary plaque characterization/quantification using coronary CT angiography data ([0623T, 0624T, 0625T, 0626T])*

0.00 0.00 **FUD** XXX N N1 TC

AMA: 2018,Sep,10

0503T **analysis of fluid dynamics and simulated maximal coronary hyperemia, and generation of estimated FFR model**

EXCLUDES *Automated coronary plaque characterization/quantification using coronary CT angiography data ([0623T, 0624T, 0625T, 0626T])*

0.00 0.00 **FUD** XXX S N1 TC

AMA: 2018,Sep,10

0504T **anatomical data review in comparison with estimated FFR model to reconcile discordant data, interpretation and report**

EXCLUDES *Automated coronary plaque characterization/quantification using coronary CT angiography data ([0623T, 0624T, 0625T, 0626T])*

0.00 0.00 **FUD** XXX M 26

AMA: 2018,Sep,10

\# **0623T** **Automated quantification and characterization of coronary atherosclerotic plaque to assess severity of coronary disease, using data from coronary computed tomographic angiography; data preparation and transmission, computerized analysis of data, with review of computerized analysis output to reconcile discordant data, interpretation and report**

INCLUDES All complete test components ([0623T, 0624T, 0625T, 0626T])

EXCLUDES *3D rendering (76376-76377)*

Noninvasive estimated coronary fractional flow reserve (FFR) (0501T-0504T)

Report coronary computed tomographic angiography (CTA) separately from automated analysis (75574)

0.00 0.00 **FUD** XXX 80

\# **0624T** **data preparation and transmission**

EXCLUDES *3D rendering (76376-76377)*

Noninvasive estimated coronary fractional flow reserve (FFR) (0501T-0504T)

0.00 0.00 **FUD** XXX 80 TC

\# **0625T** **computerized analysis of data from coronary computed tomographic angiography**

EXCLUDES *3D rendering (76376-76377)*

Noninvasive estimated coronary fractional flow reserve (FFR) (0501T-0504T)

0.00 0.00 **FUD** XXX 80 TC

\# **0626T** **review of computerized analysis output to reconcile discordant data, interpretation and report**

EXCLUDES *3D rendering (76376-76377)*

Noninvasive estimated coronary fractional flow reserve (FFR) (0501T-0504T)

0.00 0.00 **FUD** XXX 80 26

\+ # **0523T** **Intraprocedural coronary fractional flow reserve (FFR) with 3D functional mapping of color-coded FFR values for the coronary tree, derived from coronary angiogram data, for real-time review and interpretation of possible atherosclerotic stenosis(es) intervention (List separately in addition to code for primary procedure)**

EXCLUDES *3D rendering (76376-76377)*

Coronary artery doppler studies (93571-93572)

Noninvasive estimated coronary fractional flow reserve (FFR) (0501T-0504T)

Procedure reported more than one time each session

Code first (93454-93461)

0.00 0.00 **FUD** ZZZ N1 80

0505T-0514T [0510T, 0511T, 0512T, 0513T, 0620T]

0505T **Endovenous femoral-popliteal arterial revascularization, with transcatheter placement of intravascular stent graft(s) and closure by any method, including percutaneous or open vascular access, ultrasound guidance for vascular access when performed, all catheterization(s) and intraprocedural roadmapping and imaging guidance necessary to complete the intervention, all associated radiological supervision and interpretation, when performed, with crossing of the occlusive lesion in an extraluminal fashion**

INCLUDES All procedures performed on same side:

- Catheterization (arterial and venous)
- Diagnostic imaging for arteriography
- Radiologic supervision and interpretation

Ultrasound guidance (76937)

EXCLUDES *Balloon angioplasty arteries other than dialysis circuit ([37248, 37249])*

Revascularization femoral or popliteal artery (37224-37227)

Venous stenting (37238-37239)

0.00 0.00 **FUD** YYY J8 80

\# **0620T** **Endovascular venous arterialization, tibial or peroneal vein, with transcatheter placement of intravascular stent graft(s) and closure by any method, including percutaneous or open vascular access, ultrasound guidance for vascular access when performed, all catheterization(s) and intraprocedural roadmapping and imaging guidance necessary to complete the intervention, all associated radiological supervision and interpretation, when performed**

INCLUDES All procedures performed on same side:

- Catheterization (arterial and venous)
- Diagnostic imaging for arteriography
- Radiologic supervision and interpretation

EXCLUDES *When performed within tibial-peroneal segment:*

- *Endovascular revascularization procedures (37228-37231)*
- *Transcatheter intravascular stent placement (37238-37239)*
- *Transluminal balloon angioplasty ([37248, 37249])*

0.00 0.00 **FUD** YYY J8 80 50

0506T **Macular pigment optical density measurement by heterochromatic flicker photometry, unilateral or bilateral, with interpretation and report**

0.00 0.00 **FUD** XXX 80

AMA: 2018,Dec,6; 2018,Dec,6

0507T **Near-infrared dual imaging (ie, simultaneous reflective and trans-illuminated light) of meibomian glands, unilateral or bilateral, with interpretation and report**

EXCLUDES *External ocular photography (92285)*

Tear film imaging (0330T)

0.00 0.00 **FUD** XXX 80

0508T **Pulse-echo ultrasound bone density measurement resulting in indicator of axial bone mineral density, tibia**
0.00 0.00 FUD XXX Z2 80

0509T **Electroretinography (ERG) with interpretation and report, pattern (PERG)**
EXCLUDES *Full field ERG (92273)*
Multifocal ERG (92274)
2.24 2.24 FUD XXX 80
AMA: 2019,Jan,12

0510T **Resequenced code. See code following 0335T.**

0511T **Resequenced code. See code following 0335T.**

0512T **Resequenced code. See code following 0102T.**

0513T **Resequenced code. See code following 0102T.**

\+ **0514T** **Intraoperative visual axis identification using patient fixation (List separately in addition to code for primary procedure)**
Code first (66982, 66984)
0.00 0.00 FUD ZZZ N1
AMA: 2018,Dec,6; 2018,Dec,6

0515T-0523T [0523T]

INCLUDES Complete system with two components
Pulse generator including battery and transmitter
Wireless endocardial left ventricular electrode

0515T **Insertion of wireless cardiac stimulator for left ventricular pacing, including device interrogation and programming, and imaging supervision and interpretation, when performed; complete system (includes electrode and generator [transmitter and battery])**
INCLUDES Catheterization (93452-93453, 93458-93461, 93595-93597)
Creation pockets
Electrode insertion
Imaging guidance (76000, 76998, 93303-93355 [93319, 93356])
Insertion complete wireless cardiac stimulator system
Interrogation device (0521T)
Programming device (0522T)
Pulse generator (battery and transmitter) (0517T)
Revision and repositioning
EXCLUDES *Insertion electrode as separate procedure (0516T)*
Removal/replacement device or components (0518T-0520T)
0.00 0.00 FUD YYY J8

0516T **electrode only**
INCLUDES Catheterization (93452-93453, 93458-93461, 93595-93597)
Imaging guidance (76000, 76998, 93303-93355 [93319, 93356])
Interrogation device (0521T)
Programming device (0522T)
EXCLUDES *Removal/replacement device or components (0518T-0520T)*
0.00 0.00 FUD YYY G2

0517T **pulse generator component(s) (battery and/or transmitter) only**
INCLUDES Catheterization (93452-93453, 93458-93461, 93595-93597)
Imaging guidance (76000, 76998, 93303-93355 [93319, 93356])
Interrogation device (0521T)
Programming device (0522T)
EXCLUDES *Removal/replacement device or components (0518T-0520T)*
0.00 0.00 FUD YYY J8

0518T **Removal of only pulse generator component(s) (battery and/or transmitter) of wireless cardiac stimulator for left ventricular pacing**
INCLUDES Catheterization (93452-93453, 93458-93461, 93595-93597)
Imaging guidance (76000, 76998, 93303-93355 [93319, 93356])
Interrogation device (0521T)
Programming device (0522T)
Pulse generator (battery and transmitter) (0517T)
EXCLUDES *Complete procedure (0515T)*
Insertion electrode only (0516T)
Removal/replacement device or components (0519T-0520T)
0.00 0.00 FUD YYY G2

0519T **Removal and replacement of wireless cardiac stimulator for left ventricular pacing; pulse generator component(s) (battery and/or transmitter)**
INCLUDES Catheterization (93452-93453, 93458-93461, 93595-93597)
Imaging guidance (76000, 76998, 93303-93355 [93319, 93356])
Interrogation device (0521T)
Programming device (0522T)
Pulse generator (battery and transmitter) (0517T)
EXCLUDES *Complete procedure (0515T)*
Insertion electrode only (0516T)
Removal/replacement device or components (0518T)
0.00 0.00 FUD YYY J8

0520T **pulse generator component(s) (battery and/or transmitter), including placement of a new electrode**
INCLUDES Catheterization (93452-93453, 93458-93461, 93595-93597)
Imaging guidance (76000, 76998, 93303-93355 [93319, 93356])
Interrogation device (0521T)
Programming device (0522T)
Pulse generator (battery and transmitter) (0517T)
EXCLUDES *Complete procedure (0515T)*
Insertion electrode only (0516T)
Removal only device or components (0518T)
0.00 0.00 FUD YYY J8

0521T **Interrogation device evaluation (in person) with analysis, review and report, includes connection, recording, and disconnection per patient encounter, wireless cardiac stimulator for left ventricular pacing**
INCLUDES Programming device (0522T)
Pulse generator (battery and transmitter) (0517T)
EXCLUDES *Complete procedure (0515T)*
Insertion electrode only (0516T)
Removal/replacement device or components (0518T-0520T)
0.00 0.00 FUD XXX

0522T **Programming device evaluation (in person) with iterative adjustment of the implantable device to test the function of the device and select optimal permanent programmed values with analysis, including review and report, wireless cardiac stimulator for left ventricular pacing**
INCLUDES Interrogation device (0521T)
Pulse generator (battery and transmitter) (0517T)
EXCLUDES *Complete procedure (0515T)*
Insertion electrode only (0516T)
Removal/replacement device or components (0518T-0520T)
0.00 0.00 FUD XXX

0523T **Resequenced code. See code before 0505T.**

0524T

0524T Endovenous catheter directed chemical ablation with balloon isolation of incompetent extremity vein, open or percutaneous, including all vascular access, catheter manipulation, diagnostic imaging, imaging guidance and monitoring

🔧 0.00 ⚕ 0.00 **FUD** YYY   G2 50 ▣

0525T-0532T

0525T Insertion or replacement of intracardiac ischemia monitoring system, including testing of the lead and monitor, initial system programming, and imaging supervision and interpretation; complete system (electrode and implantable monitor)

INCLUDES Electrocardiography (93000, 93005, 93010)
Interrogation device (0529T)
Programming device (0528T)

EXCLUDES Removal intracardiac ischemia monitor or components (0530T-0532T)

🔧 0.00 ⚕ 0.00 **FUD** YYY   J8 ▣

0526T electrode only

INCLUDES Electrocardiography (93000, 93005, 93010)
Interrogation device (0529T)
Programming device (0528T)

EXCLUDES Removal intracardiac ischemia monitor or components (0530T-0532T)

🔧 0.00 ⚕ 0.00 **FUD** YYY   J8 ▣

0527T implantable monitor only

INCLUDES Electrocardiography (93000, 93005, 93010)
Interrogation device (0529T)
Programming device (0528T)

EXCLUDES Removal intracardiac ischemia monitor or components (0530T-0532T)

🔧 0.00 ⚕ 0.00 **FUD** YYY   G2 ▣

0528T Programming device evaluation (in person) of intracardiac ischemia monitoring system with iterative adjustment of programmed values, with analysis, review, and report

INCLUDES Electrocardiography (93000, 93005, 93010)

EXCLUDES Insertion/replacement intracardiac ischemia monitor or components (0525T-0527T)
Interrogation device (0529T)
Removal intracardiac ischemia monitor or components (0530T-0532T)

🔧 0.00 ⚕ 0.00 **FUD** XXX   ▣

0529T Interrogation device evaluation (in person) of intracardiac ischemia monitoring system with analysis, review, and report

INCLUDES Electrocardiography (93000, 93005, 93010)

EXCLUDES Insertion/replacement electrode only (0526T)
Insertion/replacement intracardiac ischemia monitor or components (0525T-0527T)
Programming device (0528T)
Removal intracardiac ischemia monitor or components (0530T-0532T)

🔧 0.00 ⚕ 0.00 **FUD** XXX   ▣

0530T Removal of intracardiac ischemia monitoring system, including all imaging supervision and interpretation; complete system (electrode and implantable monitor)

EXCLUDES Interrogation device (0529T)
Programming device (0528T)

🔧 0.00 ⚕ 0.00 **FUD** YYY   G2 ▣

0531T electrode only

EXCLUDES Interrogation device (0529T)
Programming device (0528T)

🔧 0.00 ⚕ 0.00 **FUD** YYY   G2 ▣

0532T implantable monitor only

EXCLUDES Interrogation device (0529T)
Programming device (0528T)

🔧 0.00 ⚕ 0.00 **FUD** YYY   G2 ▣

0533T-0536T

0533T Continuous recording of movement disorder symptoms, including bradykinesia, dyskinesia, and tremor for 6 days up to 10 days; includes set-up, patient training, configuration of monitor, data upload, analysis and initial report configuration, download review, interpretation and report

🔧 0.00 ⚕ 0.00 **FUD** XXX   ▣

0534T set-up, patient training, configuration of monitor

🔧 0.00 ⚕ 0.00 **FUD** XXX   ▣

0535T data upload, analysis and initial report configuration

🔧 0.00 ⚕ 0.00 **FUD** XXX   ▣

0536T download review, interpretation and report

🔧 0.00 ⚕ 0.00 **FUD** XXX   ▣

0537T-0540T

CMS: 100-04,32,400 Chimeric Antigen Receptor (CAR) T-cell therapy; 100-04,32,400.1 Coverage Requirements; 100-04,32,400.2 Billing Requirements; 100-04,32,400.2.1 A/B Medicare Administrative Contractor (MAC) (A) Bill Types; 100-04,32,400.2.2 A/B MAC (A) Revenue Code; 100-04,32,400.2.3 A/B MAC Billing HCPCS Codes; 100-04,32,400.2.4 A/B MAC Diagnosis Requirements; 100-04,32,400.3 Payment Requirements; 100-04,32,400.4 Claim Adjustment Reason Codes (CARCs), Remittance Advice Remark Codes (RARCs), Group Codes, and Medicare Summary Notice (MSN) Messages; 100-04,32,400.5 Claims Editing

INCLUDES Administration genetically modified cells for treatment serious diseases (e.g., cancer)
Evaluation prior to, during, and after CAR-T cell administration
Infusion fluids and supportive medications provided with administration
Management clinical staff
Management untoward events (e.g., nausea)
Physician certification, processing cells
Physician presence during cell administration

Code also care provided not directly related to CAR-T cell administration (e.g., other medical problems) may be reported separately using appropriate E/M code and appending modifier 25

0537T Chimeric antigen receptor T-cell (CAR-T) therapy; harvesting of blood-derived T lymphocytes for development of genetically modified autologous CAR-T cells, per day

EXCLUDES Reporting more than one time per day despite times cells are collected

🔧 0.00 ⚕ 0.00 **FUD** XXX   ▣

AMA: 2019,Jun,5

0538T preparation of blood-derived T lymphocytes for transportation (eg, cryopreservation, storage)

🔧 0.00 ⚕ 0.00 **FUD** XXX   ▣

AMA: 2019,Jun,5

0539T receipt and preparation of CAR-T cells for administration

🔧 0.00 ⚕ 0.00 **FUD** XXX   ▣

AMA: 2019,Jun,5

0540T CAR-T cell administration, autologous

EXCLUDES Reporting more than one time per day despite units administered

🔧 0.00 ⚕ 0.00 **FUD** YYY   ▣

AMA: 2019,Jun,5

0541T-0542T

0541T Myocardial imaging by magnetocardiography (MCG) for detection of cardiac ischemia, by signal acquisition using minimum 36 channel grid, generation of magnetic-field time-series images, quantitative analysis of magnetic dipoles, machine learning-derived clinical scoring, and automated report generation, single study;

🔧 0.00 ⚕ 0.00 **FUD** XXX   TC ▣

0542T interpretation and report

🔧 0.00 ⚕ 0.00 **FUD** XXX   26 ▣

26/TC PC/TC Only   A2-Z3 ASC Payment   50 Bilateral   ♂ Male Only   ♀ Female Only   🔧 Facility RVU   ⚕ Non-Facility RVU   ▣ CCI   ✖ CLIA
FUD Follow-up Days   CMS: IOM   AMA: CPT Asst   A-Y OPPSI   80/80 Surg Assist Allowed / w/Doc   🔬 Lab Crosswalk   ☢ Radiology Crosswalk

596   CPT © 2021 American Medical Association. All Rights Reserved.   © 2021 Optum360, LLC

0543T

EXCLUDES *Transesophageal echocardiography (93355)*

0543T Transapical mitral valve repair, including transthoracic echocardiography, when performed, with placement of artificial chordae tendineae
0.00 0.00 FUD YYY

0544T-0643T [0643T]

INCLUDES Adjustment/deployment reconstruction device
Catheterization
Fluoroscopic guidance (76000)
Insertion temporary pacemaker
Vascular access and closure

EXCLUDES *Diagnostic cardiac catheterization procedures integral to valve procedure (93451-93461, 93565-93566, 93593-93598)*
Percutaneous mitral valve repair (0345T)

Code also diagnostic cardiac catheterization/angiography procedures, and append modifer 59, if patient's condition (clinical indication) changed since intervention or prior study, no available prior catheter-based diagnostic study in treatment zone, or prior study not adequate (93451-93461, 93563-93564, 93593-93598)
Code also transcatheter implantation/replacement mitral valve (0483T)
Code also when performed:
Balloon pump insertion (33967, 33970, 33973)
Central bypass (33369)
Peripheral bypass (33367-33368)
Ventricular assist device (33990-33993)

0544T Transcatheter mitral valve annulus reconstruction, with implantation of adjustable annulus reconstruction device, percutaneous approach including transseptal puncture
EXCLUDES *Transcatheter mitral valve repair (33418-33419)*
Transcatheter mitral valve repair via coronary sinus (0345T)
0.00 0.00 FUD YYY

0545T Transcatheter tricuspid valve annulus reconstruction with implantation of adjustable annulus reconstruction device, percutaneous approach
EXCLUDES *Left ventricular restoration device not necessitating transseptal puncture ([0643T])*
Repositioning/plication tricuspid valve (33468)
0.00 0.00 FUD YYY

● # **0643T Transcatheter left ventricular restoration device implantation including right and left heart catheterization and left ventriculography when performed, arterial approach**
INCLUDES Guide catheter(s) and snare wire(s), when performed
Left ventriculography (93565)
Primary and contralateral arterial access
EXCLUDES *Transcatheter mitral valve annulus reconstruction (0544T)*
0.00 0.00 FUD YYY

0546T

EXCLUDES *Reporting code for re-excision of site*
Reporting code more than one time per partial mastectomy site

0546T Radiofrequency spectroscopy, real time, intraoperative margin assessment, at the time of partial mastectomy, with report
0.00 0.00 FUD YYY
AMA: 2020,May,9

0547T

0547T Bone-material quality testing by microindentation(s) of the tibia(s), with results reported as a score
0.00 0.00 FUD XXX

0548T-0551T

~~**0548T Transperineal periurethral balloon continence device; bilateral placement, including cystoscopy and fluoroscopy**~~
To report, see (53451-53454)

~~**0549T unilateral placement, including cystoscopy and fluoroscopy**~~
To report, see (53451-53454)

~~**0550T removal, each balloon**~~
To report, see (53451-53454)

~~**0551T adjustment of balloon(s) fluid volume**~~
To report, see (53451-53454)

0552T

0552T Low-level laser therapy, dynamic photonic and dynamic thermokinetic energies, provided by a physician or other qualified health care professional
0.00 0.00 FUD YYY

0553T

EXCLUDES *Angiography extremity (75710)*
Endovascular revascularization (37220-37221, 37224, 37226, 37238)
Injection for venography (36005)
Insertion catheter/needle, upper or lower extremity artery (36140)
Selective catheter placement (36011-36012, 36245-36246)
Transluminal balloon angioplasty ([37248])
Venography (75820)

0553T Percutaneous transcatheter placement of iliac arteriovenous anastomosis implant, inclusive of all radiological supervision and interpretation, intraprocedural roadmapping, and imaging guidance necessary to complete the intervention
0.00 0.00 FUD YYY

0554T-0557T

EXCLUDES *Automated analysis existing CT study for vertebral fracture(s) (0691T)*

0554T Bone strength and fracture risk using finite element analysis of functional data, and bone-mineral density, utilizing data from a computed tomography scan; retrieval and transmission of the scan data, assessment of bone strength and fracture risk and bone mineral density, interpretation and report
INCLUDES Assessment, interpretation and report, and retrieval and transmission of data (0555T-0557T)
0.00 0.00 FUD XXX
AMA: 2020,Sep,11

0555T retrieval and transmission of the scan data
0.00 0.00 FUD XXX
AMA: 2020,Sep,11

0556T assessment of bone strength and fracture risk and bone mineral density
0.00 0.00 FUD XXX
AMA: 2020,Sep,11

0557T interpretation and report
0.00 0.00 FUD XXX
AMA: 2020,Sep,11

0558T

EXCLUDES *Automated analysis existing CT study for vertebral fracture(s) (0691T)*
Computed tomography:
Abdominal aorta (75635)
Abdomen/pelvis (72191-72194, 74150-74178)
Chest/thorax (71250-71270, 71275)
Colonography (74261-74263)
Heart (75571-75574)
Spine (72125-72133)
Whole body (78816)

0558T Computed tomography scan taken for the purpose of biomechanical computed tomography analysis
0.00 0.00 FUD XXX
AMA: 2020,Sep,11

0559T-0562T

EXCLUDES *3D rendering (76376-76377)*

0559T Anatomic model 3D-printed from image data set(s); first individually prepared and processed component of an anatomic structure
INCLUDES 3D printed anatomical model production
0.00 0.00 FUD XXX

\+ **0560T each additional individually prepared and processed component of an anatomic structure (List separately in addition to code for primary procedure)**
INCLUDES 3D printed anatomical model production
Code first (0559T)
0.00 0.00 FUD ZZZ

0561T **Anatomic guide 3D-printed and designed from image data set(s); first anatomic guide**

INCLUDES 3D printed cutting or drilling guides for use during surgery

Facility RVU 0.00 Non-Facility RVU 0.00 FUD XXX 80

\+ **0562T** **each additional anatomic guide (List separately in addition to code for primary procedure)**

INCLUDES 3D printed cutting or drilling guides for use during surgery

Code first (0561T)

Facility RVU 0.00 Non-Facility RVU 0.00 FUD ZZZ 80

0563T-0564T [0563T]

0563T **Resequenced code. See code before code 0207T.**

0564T **Oncology, chemotherapeutic drug cytotoxicity assay of cancer stem cells (CSCs), from cultured CSCs and primary tumor cells, categorical drug response reported based on percent of cytotoxicity observed, a minimum of 14 drugs or drug combinations**

Facility RVU 0.00 Non-Facility RVU 0.00 FUD YYY 80

0565T-0566T

0565T **Autologous cellular implant derived from adipose tissue for the treatment of osteoarthritis of the knees; tissue harvesting and cellular implant creation**

EXCLUDES *Other tissue grafts ([15769], 15771-15774)*

Facility RVU 0.00 Non-Facility RVU 0.00 FUD YYY 80

0566T **injection of cellular implant into knee joint including ultrasound guidance, unilateral**

INCLUDES Guidance for needle placement:
Fluoroscopy (77002)
Ultrasound (76942)

EXCLUDES *Arthrocentesis, with or without imaging guidance (20610-20611)*

Facility RVU 0.00 Non-Facility RVU 0.00 FUD YYY R2 80

0567T-0568T

0567T **Permanent fallopian tube occlusion with degradable biopolymer implant, transcervical approach, including transvaginal ultrasound** ♀

INCLUDES Transvaginal ultrasound (76830)

EXCLUDES *Catheter insertion and introduction saline/contrast for sonohysterography or hysterosalpingography (58340)*
Hysterosalpingography (74740)
Nonobstetric pelvic ultrasound (76856-76857)
Surgical hysteroscopy with bilateral occlusion fallopian tube (58565)
Transcervical catheterization fallopian tube (74742)

Facility RVU 0.00 Non-Facility RVU 0.00 FUD YYY 80

0568T **Introduction of mixture of saline and air for sonosalpingography to confirm occlusion of fallopian tubes, transcervical approach, including transvaginal ultrasound and pelvic ultrasound** ♀

INCLUDES Transvaginal ultrasound (76830)

EXCLUDES *Catheter insertion and introduction saline/contrast for sonohysterography or hysterosalpingography (58340)*
Hysterosalpingography (74740)
Nonobstetric pelvic ultrasound (76856-76857)
Sonohysterography (SIS) (76831)
Surgical hysteroscopy with bilateral occlusion fallopian tube (58565)
Transcervical catheterization fallopian tube (74742)

Facility RVU 0.00 Non-Facility RVU 0.00 FUD YYY 80

0569T-0646T [0646T]

INCLUDES Adjustment/deployment prosthetic device
Catheterization
Fluoroscopic guidance (76000)
Intracardiac echocardiography (93662)
Vascular access and closure

EXCLUDES *Open tricuspid valve procedures (33460, 33463-33465, 33468)*

Code also diagnostic cardiac catheterization/angiography procedures, and append modifer 59, if patient's condition (clinical indication) changed since intervention or prior study, no available prior catheter-based diagnostic study in treatment zone, or prior study not adequate (93451-93461, 93563-93564, 93593-93598)

Code also when performed:
Balloon pump insertion (33967, 33970, 33973)
Central bypass (33369)
Peripheral bypass (33367-33368)
Ventricular assist device (33990-33993)
TEE, when done by different operator (93355)

0569T **Transcatheter tricuspid valve repair, percutaneous approach; initial prosthesis**

EXCLUDES *Reporting code more than once per session*

Facility RVU 0.00 Non-Facility RVU 0.00 FUD YYY 80

\+ **0570T** **each additional prosthesis during same session (List separately in addition to code for primary procedure)**

Code first (0569T)

Facility RVU 0.00 Non-Facility RVU 0.00 FUD ZZZ 80

● # **0646T** **Transcatheter tricuspid valve implantation (TTVI)/replacement with prosthetic valve, percutaneous approach, including right heart catheterization, temporary pacemaker insertion, and selective right ventricular or right atrial angiography, when performed**

INCLUDES Temporary pacemaker insertion (33210-33211)

EXCLUDES *Tricuspid valve:*
Transcatheter,
Reconstruction (0545T)
Repair (0569T-0570T)

Facility RVU 0.00 Non-Facility RVU 0.00 FUD YYY 80

0571T-0614T [0614T]

EXCLUDES *Defibrillator or pacemaker device evaluations (93279-93284, 93285-93289, 93290-93298)*
Implantable defibrillator procedures (33215-33220, 33223-33226, 33240-33249 [33230, 33231, 33262, 33263, 33264])
Pacemaker procedures (33202-33220 [33221], 33222-33226, 33233-33238 [33227, 33228, 33229])
Subcutaneous implantable defibrillator system procedures:
Electrophysiological evaluation (93644)
Insertion electrode ([33271])
Insertion/replacement entire system ([33270])
Interrogation ([93261])
Programming ([93260])
Removal electrode ([33272])
Repositioning electrode ([33273])
Transcatheter permanent leadless pacemaker procedures:
Insertion or replacement ([33274])

0571T **Insertion or replacement of implantable cardioverter-defibrillator system with substernal electrode(s), including all imaging guidance and electrophysiological evaluation (includes defibrillation threshold evaluation, induction of arrhythmia, evaluation of sensing for arrhythmia termination, and programming or reprogramming of sensing or therapeutic parameters), when performed**

INCLUDES Imaging guidance
Programming, interrogation, and electrophysiological evaluations (0575T-0577T)

EXCLUDES *Substernal electrode insertion only (0572T)*

Code also removal implantable cardioverter-defibrillator generator and substernal electrode(s), when total system replaced:
Electrode(s) (0573T)
Generator (0580T)

Facility RVU 0.00 Non-Facility RVU 0.00 FUD YYY 80

0572T Insertion of substernal implantable defibrillator electrode

INCLUDES Imaging guidance

EXCLUDES *Insertion generator and electrode (0571T)*
Programming, interrogation, and electrophysiological evaluations (0575T-0577T)
Removal generator only (0580T)

0.00 0.00 FUD YYY 80

0573T Removal of substernal implantable defibrillator electrode

INCLUDES Imaging guidance

EXCLUDES *Programming, interrogation, and electrophysiological evaluations (0575T-0577T)*

Code also removal implantable cardioverter-defibrillator generator and insertion new generator/electrode, when total system replaced:
Insertion new system (0571T)
Removal generator (0580T)

Code also removal generator when system not replaced (0580T)

0.00 0.00 FUD YYY 80

0574T Repositioning of previously implanted substernal implantable defibrillator-pacing electrode

INCLUDES Imaging guidance

EXCLUDES *Programming, interrogation, and electrophysiological evaluations (0575T-0577T)*
Substernal electrode insertion only (0572T)

0.00 0.00 FUD YYY 80

0575T Programming device evaluation (in person) of implantable cardioverter-defibrillator system with substernal electrode, with iterative adjustment of the implantable device to test the function of the device and select optimal permanent programmed values with analysis, review and report by a physician or other qualified health care professional

EXCLUDES *Interrogation and programming device (93260 [93260], 93282, 93287, 0576T)*
Programming during:
Electrode insertion (0572T)
Electrode removal (0573T)
Electrode repositioning (0574T)
Generator removal (0580T)
Insertion/replacement entire system (0571T)
Removal and replacement generator ([0614T])

0.00 0.00 FUD YYY 80

0576T Interrogation device evaluation (in person) of implantable cardioverter-defibrillator system with substernal electrode, with analysis, review and report by a physician or other qualified health care professional, includes connection, recording and disconnection per patient encounter

EXCLUDES *Interrogation and programming device (93261 [93261], 93289, 0575T)*
Interrogation during:
Electrode insertion (0572T)
Electrode removal (0573T)
Electrode repositioning (0574T)
Generator removal (0580T)
Insertion/replacement entire system (0571T)
Removal and replacement generator ([0614T])

0.00 0.00 FUD YYY 80

0577T Electrophysiologic evaluation of implantable cardioverter-defibrillator system with substernal electrode (includes defibrillation threshold evaluation, induction of arrhythmia, evaluation of sensing for arrhythmia termination, and programming or reprogramming of sensing or therapeutic parameters)

EXCLUDES *Electrophysiologic evaluation during:*
Electrode insertion (0572T)
Electrode removal (0573T)
Electrode repositioning (0574T)
Generator removal (0580T)
Insertion/replacement entire system (0571T)
Removal and replacement generator ([0614T])
Electrophysiologic evaluation of subcutaneous implantable defibrillator (93644)

0.00 0.00 FUD YYY 80

0578T Interrogation device evaluation(s) (remote), up to 90 days, substernal lead implantable cardioverter-defibrillator system with interim analysis, review(s) and report(s) by a physician or other qualified health care professional

EXCLUDES *In person device interrogation (0576T)*
Reporting code more than once per 90 days

0.00 0.00 FUD YYY 80

0579T Interrogation device evaluation(s) (remote), up to 90 days, substernal lead implantable cardioverter-defibrillator system, remote data acquisition(s), receipt of transmissions and technician review, technical support and distribution of results

EXCLUDES *In person device interrogation (0576T)*
Reporting code more than once per 90 days

0.00 0.00 FUD YYY 80

0580T Removal of substernal implantable defibrillator pulse generator only

INCLUDES Removal generator when system not replaced

EXCLUDES *Programming, interrogation, and electrophysiological evaluations (0575T-0577T)*
Removal and replacement generator ([33262])

Code also removal substernal electrode and insertion new generator/electrode, when total system replaced:
Insertion new system (0571T)

0.00 0.00 FUD YYY 80

\# **0614T Removal and replacement of substernal implantable defibrillator pulse generator**

EXCLUDES *Electrode insertion (0572T)*
Insertion/replacement entire system (0571T)
Programming, interrogation, and electrophysiological evaluations (0575T-0577T)
Removal generator only (0580T)
Removal/replacement single lead system ([33262])

0.00 0.00 FUD YYY J8 80

0581T-0582T

0581T Ablation, malignant breast tumor(s), percutaneous, cryotherapy, including imaging guidance when performed, unilateral

INCLUDES Ultrasound for:
Breast imaging (76641-76642)
Monitoring tissue ablation (76940)
Needle placement (76942)

EXCLUDES *Cryoablation for breast fibroadenoma(s) (19105)*
Reporting code more than once per treated breast

0.00 0.00 FUD YYY 80

0582T **Transurethral ablation of malignant prostate tissue by high-energy water vapor thermotherapy, including intraoperative imaging and needle guidance** ♂

INCLUDES 3D rendering (76376-76377)
Cystourethroscopy (52000)
MRI pelvis (72195-72197)
Radiologic guidance for:
Needle placement (76942, 77021)
Tissue ablation monitoring (76940, 77022)
Transrectal ultrasound (76872)

EXCLUDES *Destruction by radiofrequency-generated water vapor thermotherapy for benign prostatic hypertrophy (BPH) (53854)*

0.00 0.00 **FUD** YYY 80

0583T

0583T **Tympanostomy (requiring insertion of ventilating tube), using an automated tube delivery system, iontophoresis local anesthesia**

INCLUDES Binocular microscopy (92504)
Iontophoresis (97033)
Operating microscope (69990)

EXCLUDES *Myringotomy (69420-69421)*
Removal impacted cerumen (69209-69210)
Tympanostomy without automated delivery system (69433, 69436)

0.00 0.00 **FUD** YYY J8 80

0584T-0586T

0584T **Islet cell transplant, includes portal vein catheterization and infusion, including all imaging, including guidance, and radiological supervision and interpretation, when performed; percutaneous**

0.00 0.00 **FUD** YYY 80

0585T **laparoscopic**

0.00 0.00 **FUD** YYY 80

0586T **open**

0.00 0.00 **FUD** YYY 80

0587T-0590T

0587T **Percutaneous implantation or replacement of integrated single device neurostimulation system including electrode array and receiver or pulse generator, including analysis, programming, and imaging guidance when performed, posterior tibial nerve**

INCLUDES Electronic analysis (95970-95972, 0589T-0590T)

EXCLUDES *Insertion other neurostimulator devices (64555, 64566, 64575, 64590)*
Revision or removal integrated neurostimulation system (0588T)

0.00 0.00 **FUD** YYY J8 80

0588T **Revision or removal of integrated single device neurostimulation system including electrode array and receiver or pulse generator, including analysis, programming, and imaging guidance when performed, posterior tibial nerve**

INCLUDES Electronic analysis (95970-95972, 0589T-0590T)

EXCLUDES *Initial insertion or replacement integrated neurostimulation system (0587T)*
Insertion other neurostimulator devices (64555, 64566, 64575, 64590)

0.00 0.00 **FUD** YYY R2 80

0589T **Electronic analysis with simple programming of implanted integrated neurostimulation system (eg, electrode array and receiver), including contact group(s), amplitude, pulse width, frequency (Hz), on/off cycling, burst, dose lockout, patient-selectable parameters, responsive neurostimulation, detection algorithms, closed-loop parameters, and passive parameters, when performed by physician or other qualified health care professional, posterior tibial nerve, 1-3 parameters**

EXCLUDES *Electronic analysis other implanted neurostimulators (95970-95977, [95983, 95984])*
Electronic analysis with complex programming (0590T)
Reporting code during insertion, replacement, revision, or removal integrated neurostimulation system (0587T-0588T)
Reporting code during insertion, replacement, revision, or removal other neurostimulator device (generator and/or electrode) (43647-43648, 43881-43882, 61850-61888, 63650, 63655, 63661-63688, 64553-64595)

0.00 0.00 **FUD** YYY 80

0590T **Electronic analysis with complex programming of implanted integrated neurostimulation system (eg, electrode array and receiver), including contact group(s), amplitude, pulse width, frequency (Hz), on/off cycling, burst, dose lockout, patient-selectable parameters, responsive neurostimulation, detection algorithms, closed-loop parameters, and passive parameters, when performed by physician or other qualified health care professional, posterior tibial nerve, 4 or more parameters**

EXCLUDES *Electronic analysis other implanted neurostimulators (95970-95977, [95983, 95984])*
Electronic analysis with simple programming (0589T)
Reporting code during insertion, replacement, revision, or removal integrated neurostimulation system (0587T-0588T)
Reporting code during insertion, replacement, revision, or removal other neurostimulator device (generator and/or electrode) (43647-43648, 43881-43882, 61850-61888, 63650, 63655, 63661-63688, 64553-64595)

0.00 0.00 **FUD** YYY 80

0591T-0593T

INCLUDES Nonphysician health care professional coach trained to assist patients in obtaining improved health and well-being goals through:
Accountability
Active learning processes
Self-discovery

0591T **Health and well-being coaching face-to-face; individual, initial assessment**

EXCLUDES *Health and well-being coaching, follow-up session (0592T)*
Health and well-being coaching, group session (0593T)

0.00 0.00 **FUD** YYY 80

AMA: 2020,Jul,7

0592T **individual, follow-up session, at least 30 minutes**

EXCLUDES *Diabetic preventative behavior change program ([0488T])*
Education/training for self-management (98960)
Health and well-being coaching, group session (0593T)
Health and well-being coaching, initial session (0591T)
Health behavior assessment/intervention (96156-96159)
Medical nutrition therapy (97802-97804)

0.00 0.00 **FUD** YYY 80

AMA: 2020,Jul,7

0593T **group (2 or more individuals), at least 30 minutes**

EXCLUDES *Diabetic preventative behavior change program (0403T)*
Education/training for self-management (98961-98962)
Group therapy procedure (97150)
Health and well-being coaching, individual (0591T-0592T)
Health behavior assessment/intervention ([96164, 96165])

0.00 0.00 FUD YYY 80

AMA: 2020,Jul,7

0594T

0594T **Osteotomy, humerus, with insertion of an externally controlled intramedullary lengthening device, including intraoperative imaging, initial and subsequent alignment assessments, computations of adjustment schedules, and management of the intramedullary lengthening device**

EXCLUDES *Application multiplane external fixation device (20696)*
Osteoplasty, humerus (24420)
Osteotomy, humerus (24400-24410)
Revision externally controlled intramedullary lengthening device (24999)
Treatment humeral shaft fracture (24516)

0.00 0.00 FUD YYY J8 80

0596T-0597T

EXCLUDES *Bladder irrigation (51700)*
Change cystostomy tube (51705)
Injection retrograde urethrocystography (51610)
Insertion bladder catheter (51701-51703)

0596T **Temporary female intraurethral valve-pump (ie, voiding prosthesis); initial insertion, including urethral measurement** ♀

0.00 0.00 FUD YYY R2 80

0597T **replacement** ♀

0.00 0.00 FUD YYY R2 80

0598T-0599T

0598T **Noncontact real-time fluorescence wound imaging, for bacterial presence, location, and load, per session; first anatomic site (eg, lower extremity)**

0.00 0.00 FUD YYY Z2 80

\+ 0599T **each additional anatomic site (eg, upper extremity) (List separately in addition to code for primary procedure)**

Code first (0598T)

0.00 0.00 FUD YYY N1 80

0600T-0601T

0600T **Ablation, irreversible electroporation; 1 or more tumors per organ, including imaging guidance, when performed, percutaneous**

INCLUDES Radiological guidance (76940, 77002, 77013, 77022)

0.00 0.00 FUD YYY J8 80

0601T **1 or more tumors, including fluoroscopic and ultrasound guidance, when performed, open**

INCLUDES Fluoroscopic guidance (76940)
Ultrasound guidance (77002)

0.00 0.00 FUD YYY J8 80

0602T-0603T

0602T **Glomerular filtration rate (GFR) measurement(s), transdermal, including sensor placement and administration of a single dose of fluorescent pyrazine agent**

EXCLUDES *Glomerular filtration rate (GFR) monitoring (0603T)*

0.00 0.00 FUD YYY 80

0603T **Glomerular filtration rate (GFR) monitoring, transdermal, including sensor placement and administration of more than one dose of fluorescent pyrazine agent, each 24 hours**

EXCLUDES *Glomerular filtration rate (GFR) measurement(s) (0602T)*

0.00 0.00 FUD YYY 80

0604T-0606T

EXCLUDES *Remote physiologic monitoring treament management services ([99457], [99458])*

0604T **Optical coherence tomography (OCT) of retina, remote, patient-initiated image capture and transmission to a remote surveillance center unilateral or bilateral; initial device provision, set-up and patient education on use of equipment**

0.00 0.00 FUD YYY 80

0605T **remote surveillance center technical support, data analyses and reports, with a minimum of 8 daily recordings, each 30 days**

0.00 0.00 FUD YYY 80

0606T **review, interpretation and report by the prescribing physician or other qualified health care professional of remote surveillance center data analyses, each 30 days**

0.00 0.00 FUD YYY 80

0607T-0608T

EXCLUDES *During same monitoring period:*
Cardiac event monitor (93268-93272)
External mobile cardiovascular telemetry (93228-93229)
Holter monitor procedures (93224-93227)
Interrogation cardiovasular physiologic monitoring system (93297)
Remote monitoring pulmonary artery pressure sensor ([93264])

0607T **Remote monitoring of an external continuous pulmonary fluid monitoring system, including measurement of radiofrequency-derived pulmonary fluid levels, heart rate, respiration rate, activity, posture, and cardiovascular rhythm (eg, ECG data), transmitted to a remote 24-hour attended surveillance center; set-up and patient education on use of equipment**

EXCLUDES *Remote monitoring physiologic parameters, initial during same monitoring period ([99453])*

0.00 0.00 FUD YYY 80

0608T **analysis of data received and transmission of reports to the physician or other qualified health care professional**

EXCLUDES *Remote monitoring physiologic parameters, each 30 days, during same monitoring period ([99454])*
Reporting more than once per 30 days

0.00 0.00 FUD YYY 80

0609T-0612T

EXCLUDES *Magnetic resonance angiography, spine (72159)*
Magnetic resonance imaging, spine (72141-72158)
Other magnetic spectroscopy (76390)

0609T **Magnetic resonance spectroscopy, determination and localization of discogenic pain (cervical, thoracic, or lumbar); acquisition of single voxel data, per disc, on biomarkers (ie, lactic acid, carbohydrate, alanine, laal, propionic acid, proteoglycan, and collagen) in at least 3 discs**

0.00 0.00 FUD YYY Z2 80

0610T **transmission of biomarker data for software analysis**

0.00 0.00 FUD YYY 80

0611T **postprocessing for algorithmic analysis of biomarker data for determination of relative chemical differences between discs**

0.00 0.00 FUD YYY Z2 80

0612T **interpretation and report**

0.00 0.00 FUD YYY 80

0613T

EXCLUDES *Heart catheterization (93451-93453, 93456-93462)*
Heart catheterization for congenital defect(s) (93593-93598)
Intracardiac echocardiography (93662)
Transcatheter/transvenous procedures atrial septectomy/septostomy (33741-33746)
Transesophageal echocardiography procedures (93313-93314, 93318, 93355)
Ultrasound guidance (76937)

0613T Percutaneous transcatheter implantation of interatrial septal shunt device, including right and left heart catheterization, intracardiac echocardiography, and imaging guidance by the proceduralist, when performed
0.00 0.00 FUD YYY 80

0614T-0615T [0614T]

0614T **Resequenced code. See code following code 0580T.**

0615T Eye-movement analysis without spatial calibration, with interpretation and report
EXCLUDES *Vestibular function tests (92540-92542, 92544-92547)*
0.00 0.00 FUD YYY 80

0616T-0618T

EXCLUDES *Iridectomy (66600)*
Repair/suture iris (66680, 66682)

0616T Insertion of iris prosthesis, including suture fixation and repair or removal of iris, when performed; without removal of crystalline lens or intraocular lens, without insertion of intraocular lens
0.00 0.00 FUD YYY J8 80

0617T with removal of crystalline lens and insertion of intraocular lens
EXCLUDES *Cataract extraction/removal:*
Extracapsular (66982, 66984)
Intracapsular (66983)
0.00 0.00 FUD YYY J8 80

0618T with secondary intraocular lens placement or intraocular lens exchange
EXCLUDES *Intraocular lens:*
Exchange (66986)
Insertion, secondary implant (66985)
0.00 0.00 FUD YYY J8 80

0619T

INCLUDES Cystourethroscopy (separate procedure) (52000)
EXCLUDES *Cystourethroscopy:*
with insertion transprostatic implant (52441-52442)
with mechanical dilation/drug delivery (0499T)
Laser:
Coagulation (52647)
Enucleation (52649)
Vaporization (52648)
Prostate, transurethral:
Destruction (53850-53854)
Incision (52450)
Resection (52500, 52601, 52630, 52640)
Transrectal ultrasound (76872)

0619T Cystourethroscopy with transurethral anterior prostate commissurotomy and drug delivery, including transrectal ultrasound and fluoroscopy, when performed ♂
0.00 0.00 FUD YYY J8 80

0620T-0622T [0620T]

0620T **Resequenced code. See code following 0505T.**

0621T Trabeculostomy ab interno by laser
EXCLUDES *Gonioscopy (92020)*
0.00 0.00 FUD YYY 80 50

0622T with use of ophthalmic endoscope
EXCLUDES *Gonioscopy (92020)*
0.00 0.00 FUD YYY 80 50

0623T-0626T [0623T, 0624T, 0625T, 0626T]

0623T **Resequenced code. See code following 0504T.**

0624T **Resequenced code. See code following 0504T.**

0625T **Resequenced code. See code following 0504T.**

0626T **Resequenced code. See code following 0504T.**

0627T-0630T

0627T Percutaneous injection of allogeneic cellular and/or tissue-based product, intervertebral disc, unilateral or bilateral injection, with fluoroscopic guidance, lumbar; first level
INCLUDES Fluoroscopic guidance (77003)
0.00 0.00 FUD YYY G2 80

+ **0628T each additional level (List separately in addition to code for primary procedure)**
EXCLUDES *Fluoroscopic guidance (77003)*
Code first (0627T)
0.00 0.00 FUD ZZZ N1 80

0629T Percutaneous injection of allogeneic cellular and/or tissue-based product, intervertebral disc, unilateral or bilateral injection, with CT guidance, lumbar; first level
INCLUDES CT guidance (77012)
0.00 0.00 FUD YYY G2 80

+ **0630T each additional level (List separately in addition to code for primary procedure)**
INCLUDES CT guidance (77012)
Code first (0629T)
0.00 0.00 FUD ZZZ N1 80

0631T

EXCLUDES *Pulse oximetry (94760-94762)*
Transcutaneous biomarker measurement (0061U)

0631T Transcutaneous visible light hyperspectral imaging measurement of oxyhemoglobin, deoxyhemoglobin, and tissue oxygenation, with interpretation and report, per extremity
0.00 0.00 FUD XXX 80

0632T

0632T Percutaneous transcatheter ultrasound ablation of nerves innervating the pulmonary arteries, including right heart catheterization, pulmonary artery angiography, and all imaging guidance
INCLUDES Heart catheterization (93451, 93453, 93456, 93460, 93593-93594, 93596-93597)
Pulmonary artery angiography/injection (75741, 75743, 75746, 93568)
Pulmonary artery catheterization (36013-36015)
Swan-Ganz catheter insertion (93503)
EXCLUDES *Endomyocardial biopsy (93505)*
0.00 0.00 FUD YYY J8 80

0633T-0638T

INCLUDES 3D rendering (76376-76377)
EXCLUDES *Diagnostic/interventional CT (76497)*
Limited/localized follow-up CT (76380)

0633T Computed tomography, breast, including 3D rendering, when performed, unilateral; without contrast material
0.00 0.00 FUD XXX Z2 80

0634T with contrast material(s)
0.00 0.00 FUD XXX Z2 80

0635T without contrast, followed by contrast material(s)
0.00 0.00 FUD XXX Z2 80

0636T Computed tomography, breast, including 3D rendering, when performed, bilateral; without contrast material(s)
0.00 0.00 FUD XXX Z2 80

0637T with contrast material(s)
0.00 0.00 FUD XXX Z2 80

0638T without contrast, followed by contrast material(s)
0.00 0.00 FUD XXX Z2 80

0639T

EXCLUDES *Ultrasound guidance (76998-76999)*

0639T **Wireless skin sensor thermal anisotropy measurement(s) and assessment of flow in cerebrospinal fluid shunt, including ultrasound guidance, when performed**
0.00 0.00 FUD XXX 80

0640T-0643T [0640T, 0641T, 0642T, 0643T]

0640T **Resequenced code. See code following 0493T.**
0641T **Resequenced code. See code following 0493T.**
0642T **Resequenced code. See code following 0493T.**
0643T **Resequenced code. See code following 0545T.**

0644T

● 0644T **Transcatheter removal or debulking of intracardiac mass (eg, vegetations, thrombus) via suction (eg, vacuum, aspiration) device, percutaneous approach, with intraoperative reinfusion of aspirated blood, including imaging guidance, when performed**

INCLUDES Access with insertion and positioning of device
Arterial closure device, when used
Blood vessel dilation
Embolic protection, when used
Fluoroscopy (76000)
Imaging guidance
Initial extracorporeal circuit for intraoperative reinfusion aspirated blood
Percutaneous venous thrombectomy (37187-37188)
Selective and nonselective catheterizations

Code also, when performed:
Axillary, femoral, or iliac conduit required for catheter access facilitation (34714, [34833], 34716)
Balloon pump insertion (33967, 33970, 33973)
Central or peripheral bypass (33367-33369)
Extensive repair/replacement blood vessel
Other interventional procedures performed during same operative session (i.e., placement dialysis catheters, removal infected pacemaker wires, removal tunneled catheters, repair/replacement valve)
Prolonged extracorporeal membrane oxygenation (ECMO) or extracorporeal life support (ECLS) required when procedure complete may be separately reported (33946-33947, 33951-33956, [33965], [33966], [33969], [33984], [33985], [33986])
Ventricular assist device (33975-33976, [33995], 33990-33993 [33997], 33999)

0.00 0.00 FUD YYY J8 80

0645T-0646T [0646T]

● 0645T **Transcatheter implantation of coronary sinus reduction device including vascular access and closure, right heart catheterization, venous angiography, coronary sinus angiography, imaging guidance, and supervision and interpretation, when performed**

INCLUDES Access with insertion and positioning of device
Angiography
Arterial closure device, when used
Balloon angioplasty ([37246, 37247])
Coronary sinus catheterization and interventions
Diagnostic right heart catheterization (93451, 93453, 93456-93457, 93460-93461, 93566, 93593-93594, 93596-93597, 93662)
Imaging guidance (76000, 76499, 76937, 77001)
Intracardiac echocardiography (93662)
Intravascular ultrasound during evaluation/intervention (37252-37253)
Introduction/selective catheter placement (36010-36013)
Venography (75827, 75860)

EXCLUDES *Indicator dilution studies (93598)*

Code also, when performed:
Diagnostic right and left heart catheterization and angiography performed:
AND previous study available but documentation states patient's condition changed since previous study; visualization insufficient; or change necessitates re-evaluation; append modifier 59
OR when no previous study available and complete diagnostic study performed; append modifier 59
Code also transesophageal echocardiography by separate operator for guidance, when performed (93355)

0.00 0.00 FUD YYY 80

0646T **Resequenced code. See code following 0570T.**

0647T

● 0647T **Insertion of gastrostomy tube, percutaneous, with magnetic gastropexy, under ultrasound guidance, image documentation and report**

INCLUDES Ultrasound guidance (76942)

0.00 0.00 FUD YYY J8 80

0648T-0698T [0697T, 0698T]

▲ 0648T **Quantitative magnetic resonance for analysis of tissue composition (eg, fat, iron, water content), including multiparametric data acquisition, data preparation and transmission, interpretation and report, obtained without diagnostic MRI examination of the same anatomy (eg, organ, gland, tissue, target structure) during the same session; single organ**

EXCLUDES *Diagnostic MRI on same gland, organ, tissue or target area during same session (70540-70543, 70551-70553, 71550-71552, 72141-72142, 72146-72149, 72156-72158, 72195-72197, 73218-73223, 73718-73723, 74181-74183, 75557-75563, 76498, 77046-77049, 0398T)*
Quantitative magnetic resonance for analysis of tissue composition with MRI (0649T)

0.00 0.00 FUD XXX Z2 80

● # 0697T **multiple organs**
0.00 0.00 FUD 000

▲ + **0649T** **Quantitative magnetic resonance for analysis of tissue composition (eg, fat, iron, water content), including multiparametric data acquisition, data preparation and transmission, interpretation and report, obtained with diagnostic MRI examination of the same anatomy (eg, organ, gland, tissue, target structure); single organ (List separately in addition to code for primary procedure)**

EXCLUDES *Quantitative magnetic resonance for analysis of tissue composition without MRI (0648T)*

Code also diagnostic MRI on same gland, organ, tissue or target area during same session (70540-70543, 70551-70553, 71550-71552, 72141-72142, 72146-72149, 72156-72158, 72195-72197, 73218-73223, 73718-73723, 74181-74183, 75557-75563, 76498, 77046-77049, 0398T)

0.00 0.00 FUD ZZZ 80

● + # **0698T** **multiple organs (List separately in addition to code for primary procedure)**

0.00 0.00 FUD 000

0650T

● **0650T** **Programming device evaluation (remote) of subcutaneous cardiac rhythm monitor system, with iterative adjustment of the implantable device to test the function of the device and select optimal permanently programmed values with analysis, review and report by a physician or other qualified health care professional**

INCLUDES In-person evaluation, interrogation, programming ([93260], 93279-93282, 93284, 93285, 93291)

EXCLUDES *Insertion subcutaneous cardiac rhythm monitor (33285)*

Code also remote interrogation during the 30-day remote interrogation device evaluation period, when performed (93298)

0.00 0.00 FUD XXX 80

0651T

● **0651T** **Magnetically controlled capsule endoscopy, esophagus through stomach, including intraprocedural positioning of capsule, with interpretation and report**

EXCLUDES *Intraluminal gastrointestinal tract imaging (91110, 91111)*

0.00 0.00 FUD YYY J8 80

0652T-0654T

EXCLUDES *Transnasal:*
Diagnostic esophagoscopy, flexible (43197)
Esophagoscopy with biopsy(ies), flexible (43198)
Other esophagogastroduodenoscopy (43499, 43999, 44799)
Transoral:
Esophagoscopy, flexible (43200-43232 [43210, 43211, 43212, 43213, 43214])
Esophagogastroduodenoscopy, rigid (43235-43259 [43233, 43266, 43270])
Esophagoscopy, rigid (43191-43195)

● **0652T** **Esophagogastroduodenoscopy, flexible, transnasal; diagnostic, including collection of specimen(s) by brushing or washing, when performed (separate procedure)**

0.00 0.00 FUD YYY J8

● **0653T** **with biopsy, single or multiple**

0.00 0.00 FUD YYY J8

● **0654T** **with insertion of intraluminal tube or catheter**

0.00 0.00 FUD YYY J8

0655T

● **0655T** **Transperineal focal laser ablation of malignant prostate tissue, including transrectal imaging guidance, with MR-fused images or other enhanced ultrasound imaging** ♂

INCLUDES 3D rendering (76376-76377)
Cystourethroscopy (52000)
Imaging guidance (76872, 76940, 76942, 76998)

0.00 0.00 FUD YYY G2

0656T-0657T

EXCLUDES *Arthrodesis (22800-22812)*
Instrumentation, anterior (22845-22847)
Kyphectomy (22818-22819)

● **0656T** **Vertebral body tethering, anterior; up to 7 vertebral segments**

0.00 0.00 FUD YYY 80

● **0657T** **8 or more vertebral segments**

0.00 0.00 FUD YYY 80

0658T

● **0658T** **Electrical impedance spectroscopy of 1 or more skin lesions for automated melanoma risk score**

0.00 0.00 FUD XXX 80 TC

0659T

● **0659T** **Transcatheter intracoronary infusion of supersaturated oxygen in conjunction with percutaneous coronary revascularization during acute myocardial infarction, including catheter placement, imaging guidance (eg, fluoroscopy), angiography, and radiologic supervision and interpretation**

EXCLUDES *Percutaneous angioplasty or atherectomy ([92920], [92924], [92928], [92933])*
Percutaneous revascularization excluding with acute myocardial infarction ([92937], [92943])

Code also percutaneous coronary revascularization during acute myocardial infarction ([92941])

0.00 0.00 FUD YYY 80

0660T-0661T

Code also drug(s) administered

● **0660T** **Implantation of anterior segment intraocular nonbiodegradable drug-eluting system, internal approach**

0.00 0.00 FUD YYY 50

● **0661T** **Removal and reimplantation of anterior segment intraocular nonbiodegradable drug-eluting implant**

0.00 0.00 FUD YYY 50

0662T-0663T

EXCLUDES *Selective head/total body hypothermia for critically ill neonate (99184)*

● **0662T** **Scalp cooling, mechanical; initial measurement and calibration of cap**

EXCLUDES *Reporting more than one time per chemotherapy treatment period*

0.00 0.00 FUD XXX 80

● + **0663T** **placement of device, monitoring, and removal of device**

EXCLUDES *Reporting more than one time per chemotherapy session*

Code also chemotherapy administration (96409, 96411, 96413, 96415, 96416, 96417)

0.00 0.00 FUD ZZZ 80

0664T-0670T

● **0664T** **Donor hysterectomy (including cold preservation); open, from cadaver donor** ♀

INCLUDES Harvesting uterus allograft from cadaver donor and cold-preservation solution/maintenance

0.00 0.00 FUD XXX

● **0665T** **open, from living donor** ♀

INCLUDES Care for donor
Harvesting uterus allograft from living donor and cold-preservation solution/maintenance

0.00 0.00 FUD XXX

● **0666T** **laparoscopic or robotic, from living donor** ♀

INCLUDES Care for donor
Harvesting uterus allograft from living donor and cold-preservation solution/maintenance

0.00 0.00 FUD XXX

● **0667T** **recipient uterus allograft transplantation from cadaver or living donor** ♀

INCLUDES Care for recipient
Transplantation uterine allograft

0.00 0.00 **FUD** XXX

● **0668T** **Backbench standard preparation of cadaver or living donor uterine allograft prior to transplantation, including dissection and removal of surrounding soft tissues and preparation of uterine vein(s) and uterine artery(ies), as necessary** ♀

INCLUDES Standard preparation cadaver/living uterus allograft (i.e., preparation uterine vein(s) and artery(ies), removal of surrounding soft tissue, as needed)

EXCLUDES *Reconstruction uterine allograft (i.e., venous or arterial anastomosis(es) (0669T-0670T)*

0.00 0.00 **FUD** YYY 80

● **0669T** **Backbench reconstruction of cadaver or living donor uterus allograft prior to transplantation; venous anastomosis, each** ♀

EXCLUDES *Standard preparation cadaver/living uterus allograft (i.e., preparation uterine vein(s) and artery(ies), removal of surrounding soft tissue, as needed) (0668T)*

0.00 0.00 **FUD** YYY 80

● **0670T** **arterial anastomosis, each** ♀

EXCLUDES *Standard preparation cadaver/living uterus allograft (i.e., preparation uterine vein(s) and artery(ies), removal of surrounding soft tissue, as needed) (0668T)*

0.00 0.00 **FUD** YYY 80

0671T-0672T [0671T]

0671T **Resequenced code. See code following 0184T.**

● **0672T** **Endovaginal cryogen-cooled, monopolar radiofrequency remodeling of the tissues surrounding the female bladder neck and proximal urethra for urinary incontinence**

0673T

● **0673T** **Ablation, benign thyroid nodule(s), percutaneous, laser, including imaging guidance**

INCLUDES Radiological guidance for:
Needle placement (76942)
Tissue ablation monitoring (76940, 77013, 77022)

0674T-0685T

● **0674T** **Laparoscopic insertion of new or replacement of permanent implantable synchronized diaphragmatic stimulation system for augmentation of cardiac function, including an implantable pulse generator and diaphragmatic lead(s)**

INCLUDES Complete SDS system insertion/replacement
Device evaluation, interrogation, and programming (0683T-0685T)

EXCLUDES *Diaphragmatic lead(s) only:*
Insertion/replacement (0675T-0676T)
Removal (0679T)
Repositioning/relocation (0677T-0678T)
Pulse generator only:
Insertion/replacement (0680T)
Removal (0682T)
Repositioning/relocation (0681T)

● **0675T** **Laparoscopic insertion of new or replacement of diaphragmatic lead(s), permanent implantable synchronized diaphragmatic stimulation system for augmentation of cardiac function, including connection to an existing pulse generator; first lead**

INCLUDES Device evaluation, interrogation, and programming (0683T-0685T)

EXCLUDES *Diaphragmatic lead:*
Removal (0679T)
Repositioning/relocation (0677T)
Insertion/replacement of complete SDS system (0674T)
Procedures performed on pulse generator only (0680T-0682T)

● + **0676T** **each additional lead (List separately in addition to**

INCLUDES Device evaluation, interrogation, and programming (0683T-0685T)

EXCLUDES *Additional diaphragmatic lead:*
Removal (0679T)
Repositioning/relocation (0678T)

Code first (0675T)

0.00 0.00 **FUD** 000

● **0677T** **Laparoscopic repositioning of diaphragmatic lead(s), permanent implantable synchronized diaphragmatic stimulation system for augmentation of cardiac function, including connection to an existing pulse generator; first repositioned lead**

INCLUDES Device evaluation, interrogation, and programming (0683T-0685T)

EXCLUDES *Diaphragmatic lead:*
Insertion/replacement (0675T)
Removal (0679T)
Insertion/replacement of complete SDS system (0674T)
Procedures performed on pulse generator only (0680T-0682T)

● + **0678T** **each additional repositioned lead (List separately in**

INCLUDES Device evaluation, interrogation, and programming (0683T-0685T)

EXCLUDES *Additional diaphragmatic lead:*
Insertion/replacement (0676T)
Removal (0679T)

Code first (0677T)

0.00 0.00 **FUD** 000

● **0679T** **Laparoscopic removal of diaphragmatic lead(s), permanent implantable synchronized diaphragmatic stimulation system for augmentation of cardiac function**

EXCLUDES *Device evaluation, interrogation, and programming (0683T-0685T)*
Insertion/replacement of complete SDS system (0674T)
Procedures performed on pulse generator only (0680T-0682T)
Reporting more than once when more than one lead removed
Repositioning/relocation of lead (0677T)

● **0680T** **Insertion or replacement of pulse generator only, permanent implantable synchronized diaphragmatic stimulation system for augmentation of cardiac function, with connection to existing lead(s)**

INCLUDES Device evaluation, interrogation, and programming (0683T-0685T)

EXCLUDES *Insertion/replacement of complete SDS system (0674T)*
Procedures performed on diaghragmatic lead(s) only (0675T-0679T)
Pulse generator:
Removal (0682T)
Repositioning/relocation (0681T)

● **0681T** **Relocation of pulse generator only, permanent implantable synchronized diaphragmatic stimulation system for augmentation of cardiac function, with connection to existing dual leads**

INCLUDES Device evaluation, interrogation, and programming (0683T-0685T)

EXCLUDES *Insertion/replacement of complete SDS system (0674T)*
Procedures performed on diaghragmatic lead(s) only (0675T-0679T)
Pulse generator:
Insertion/replacement (0680T)
Removal (0682T)

● **0682T** **Removal of pulse generator only, permanent implantable synchronized diaphragmatic stimulation system for augmentation of cardiac function**

EXCLUDES *Device evaluation, interrogation, and programming (0683T-0685T)*
Insertion/replacement of complete SDS system (0674T)
Procedures performed on diaghragmatic lead(s) only (0675T-0679T)
Pulse generator:
Insertion/replacement (0680T)
Repositioning/relocation (0681T)

● **0683T** **Programming device evaluation (in-person) with iterative adjustment of the implantable device to test the function of the device and select optimal permanent programmed values with analysis, review and report by a physician or other qualified health care professional, permanent implantable synchronized diaphragmatic stimulation system for augmentation of cardiac function**

EXCLUDES *Reporting when performed by the same provider as:*
Complete SDS system or individual component procedures (0674T-0682T)
Device evaluation and programming before and after surgery (0684T)
Device interrogation with analysis (0685T)

● **0684T** **Peri-procedural device evaluation (in-person) and programming of device system parameters before or after a surgery, procedure, or test with analysis, review, and report by a physician or other qualified health care professional, permanent implantable synchronized diaphragmatic stimulation system for augmentation of cardiac function**

EXCLUDES *Reporting when performed by the same provider as:*
Complete SDS system or individual component procedures (0674T-0675T, 0677T, 0679T-0682T)
Device interrogation with analysis (0685T)
Device programming (0683T)

● **0685T** **Interrogation device evaluation (in-person) with analysis, review and report by a physician or other qualified health care professional, including connection, recording and disconnection per patient encounter, permanent implantable synchronized diaphragmatic stimulation system for augmentation of cardiac function**

EXCLUDES *Reporting when performed by the same provider as:*
Complete SDS system or individual component procedures (0674T-0675T, 0677T, 0679T-0682T)
Device evaluation and programming before and after surgery (0684T)
Device programming (0683T)

0686T

● **0686T** **Histotripsy (ie, non-thermal ablation via acoustic energy delivery) of malignant hepatocellular tissue, including image guidance**

0687T-0688T

EXCLUDES *Orthoptic training services on same day (92065)*

● **0687T** **Treatment of amblyopia using an online digital program; device supply, educational set-up, and initial session**

● **0688T** **assessment of patient performance and program data by physician or other qualified health care professional, with report, per calendar month**

0689T-0690T

● **0689T** **Quantitative ultrasound tissue characterization (non-elastographic), including interpretation and report, obtained without diagnostic ultrasound examination of the same anatomy (eg, organ, gland, tissue, target structure)**

EXCLUDES *Quantitative ultrasound with diagnostic ultrasound examination, same anatomy (0690T)*
Ultrasound (76536, 76604, 76641-76642, 76700-76705, 76770-76775, 76830, 76856-76857, 76870, 76872, 76881, 76882, 76981-76983, 76999)
Vascular studies (93880, 93882, 93998)

● + **0690T** **Quantitative ultrasound tissue characterization (non-elastographic), including interpretation and report, obtained with diagnostic ultrasound examination of the same anatomy (eg, organ, gland, tissue, target structure) (List separately in addition to code for primary procedure)**

EXCLUDES *Quantitative ultrasound without diagnostic ultrasound examination, same anatomy (0689T)*
Vascular studies (93880, 93882, 93998)

Code first (76536, 76604, 76641-76642, 76700-76705, 76770-76775, 76830, 76856-76857, 76870, 76872, 76881, 76882, 76981-76982, 76999, 93880, 93882, 93998)

0.00 0.00 **FUD** 000

0691T

● **0691T** **Automated analysis of an existing computed tomography study for vertebral fracture(s), including assessment of bone density when performed, data preparation, interpretation, and report**

EXCLUDES *Computed tomography:*
Abdominal aorta (75635)
Abdomen/pelvis (72191-72194, 74150-74178)
Biomechanical analysis (0558T)
Bone strength and fracture risk analysis (0554T-0557T)
Chest/thorax (71250-71271, 71275)
Colonography (74261-74263)
Heart (75571-75574)
Spine (72125-72133)
Positron emission tomography (PET) with computed tomography (78814-78816)

0692T

● **0692T** **Therapeutic ultrafiltration**

EXCLUDES *Apheresis, therapeutic (36511-36516)*
Dialysis/hemodialysis (90935, 90937, 90945, 90947)
Photophoresis, extracorporeal (36522)
Reporting more than once per day

0693T

● **0693T** **Comprehensive full body computer-based markerless 3D kinematic and kinetic motion analysis and report**

0694T

● **0694T** **3-dimensional volumetric imaging and reconstruction of breast or axillary lymph node tissue, each excised specimen, 3-dimensional automatic specimen reorientation, interpretation and report, real-time intraoperative**

INCLUDES Reporting once per specimen

EXCLUDES *Radiological examination (76098)*

0695T-0696T

● **0695T** **Body surface-activation mapping of pacemaker or pacing cardioverter-defibrillator lead(s) to optimize electrical synchrony, cardiac resynchronization therapy device, including connection, recording, disconnection, review, and report; at time of implant or replacement**

Code also insertion or repositioning pacing electrode for cardiac venous system (33224-33226)

● 0696T **at time of follow-up interrogation or programming device evaluation**

Code also pacemaker/defibrillator device evaluation, programming, interrogation (93281, 93284, 93286-93289)

0697T-0699T [0697T, 0698T]

0697T **Resequenced code. See code following 0648T.**

0698T **Resequenced code. See code following 0649T.**

● 0699T **Injection, posterior chamber of eye, medication**

0700T-0701T

● 0700T **Molecular fluorescent imaging of suspicious nevus; first lesion**

● + 0701T **each additional lesion (List separately in addition to code for primary procedure)**

Code first (0700T)

0.00 0.00 FUD 000

0702T-0703T

EXCLUDES *Behavioral health services:*

Intervention, individual (96158-96159)

Integration ([99484], 99492-99494)

Chronic care management services ([99437])

Collection and interpretation physiologic data ([99091])

Principal care management services ([99424, 99425, 99426, 99427])

Remote physiologic monitoring services ([99453, 99454])

Remote physiologic monitoring treatment management services ([99457, 99458])

Remote therapeutic monitoring (98975-98977)

● 0702T **Remote therapeutic monitoring of a standardized online digital cognitive behavioral therapy program ordered by a physician or other qualified health care professional; supply and technical support, per 30 days**

● 0703T **management services by physician or other qualified health care professional, per calendar month**

0704T-0706T

EXCLUDES *Amblyopia treatment using online digital program during same time period (0687T-0688T)*

Orthoptic training services on same day (92065)

● 0704T **Remote treatment of amblyopia using an eye tracking device; device supply with initial set-up and patient education on use of equipment**

● 0705T **surveillance center technical support including data transmission with analysis, with a minimum of 18 training hours, each 30 days**

● 0706T **interpretation and report by physician or other qualified health care professional, per calendar month**

0707T

● 0707T **Injection(s), bone-substitute material (eg, calcium phosphate) into subchondral bone defect (ie, bone marrow lesion, bone bruise, stress injury, microtrabecular fracture), including imaging guidance and arthroscopic assistance for joint visualization**

INCLUDES Diagnostic arthroscopy of:

Hip (29860)

Knee (29870)

Shoulder (29805)

Fluoroscopy (77002)

0708T-0709T

EXCLUDES *Injection procedure (96372)*

● 0708T **Intradermal cancer immunotherapy; preparation and initial injection**

● + 0709T **each additional injection (List separately in addition to code for primary procedure)**

Code first (0708T)

0.00 0.00 FUD 000

0710T-0713T

EXCLUDES *Automated coronary plaque characterization/quantification using coronary CT angiography data ([0623T, 0624T, 0625T, 0626T])*

Noninvasive estimated coronary fractional flow reserve (FFR) (0501T-0504T)

● 0710T **Noninvasive arterial plaque analysis using software processing of data from non-coronary computerized tomography angiography; including data preparation and transmission, quantification of the structure and composition of the vessel wall and assessment for lipid-rich necrotic core plaque to assess atherosclerotic plaque stability, data review, interpretation and report**

INCLUDES Data preparation/transmission (0711T)

Interpretation and report (0713T)

Vessel wall structure and composition quantification (0712T)

● 0711T **data preparation and transmission**

● 0712T **quantification of the structure and composition of the vessel wall and assessment for lipid-rich necrotic core plaque to assess atherosclerotic plaque stability**

● 0713T **data review, interpretation and report**

Appendix A — Modifiers

CPT Modifiers

A modifier is a two-position alpha or numeric code appended to a CPT® code to clarify the services being billed. Modifiers provide a means by which a service can be altered without changing the procedure code. They add more information, such as the anatomical site, to the code. In addition, they help to eliminate the appearance of duplicate billing and unbundling. Modifiers are used to increase accuracy in reimbursement, coding consistency, editing, and to capture payment data.

22 **Increased Procedural Services:** When the work required to provide a service is substantially greater than typically required, it may be identified by adding modifier 22 to the usual procedure code. Documentation must support the substantial additional work and the reason for the additional work (ie, increased intensity, time, technical difficulty of procedure, severity of patient's condition, physical and mental effort required).
Note: This modifier should not be appended to an E/M service.

23 **Unusual Anesthesia:** Occasionally, a procedure, which usually requires either no anesthesia or local anesthesia, because of unusual circumstances must be done under general anesthesia. This circumstance may be reported by adding modifier 23 to the procedure code of the basic service.

24 **Unrelated Evaluation and Management Service by the Same Physician or Other Qualified Health Care Professional During a Postoperative Period:** The physician or other qualified health care professional may need to indicate that an evaluation and management service was performed during a postoperative period for a reason(s) unrelated to the original procedure. This circumstance may be reported by adding modifier 24 to the appropriate level of E/M service.

25 **Significant, Separately Identifiable Evaluation and Management Service by the Same Physician or Other Qualified Health Care Professional on the Same Day of the Procedure or Other Service:** It may be necessary to indicate that on the day a procedure or service identified by a CPT code was performed, the patient's condition required a significant, separately identifiable E/M service above and beyond the other service provided or beyond the usual preoperative and postoperative care associated with the procedure that was performed. A significant, separately identifiable E/M service is defined or substantiated by documentation that satisfies the relevant criteria for the respective E/M service to be reported (see Evaluation and Management Services Guidelines for instructions on determining level of E/M service). The E/M service may be prompted by the symptom or condition for which the procedure and/or service was provided. As such, different diagnoses are not required for reporting of the E/M services on the same date. This circumstance may be reported by adding modifier 25 to the appropriate level of E/M service.
Note: This modifier is not used to report an E/M service that resulted in a decision to perform surgery. See modifier 57. For significant, separately identifiable non-E/M services, see modifier 59.

26 **Professional Component:** Certain procedures are a combination of a physician or other qualified health care professional component and a technical component. When the physician or other qualified health care professional component is reported separately, the service may be identified by adding modifier 26 to the usual procedure number.

32 **Mandated Services:** Services related to *mandated* consultation and/or related services (eg, third party payer, governmental, legislative or regulatory requirement) may be identified by adding modifier 32 to the basic procedure.

33 **Preventive Services:** When the primary purpose of the service is the delivery of an evidence based service in accordance with a US Preventive Services Task Force A or B rating in effect and other preventive services identified in preventive services mandates (legislative or regulatory), the service may be identified by adding 33 to the procedure. For separately reported services specifically identified as preventive, the modifier should not be used.

47 **Anesthesia by Surgeon:** Regional or general anesthesia provided by the surgeon may be reported by adding modifier 47 to the basic service. (This does not include local anesthesia.)
Note: Modifier 47 would not be used as a modifier for the anesthesia procedures.

50 **Bilateral Procedure:** Unless otherwise identified in the listings, bilateral procedures that are performed at the same session should be identified by adding modifier 50 to the appropriate 5 digit code.
Note: This modifier should not be appended to designated "add-on" codes (see Appendix F).

51 **Multiple Procedures:** When multiple procedures, other than E/M services, Physical Medicine and Rehabilitation services or provision of supplies (eg, vaccines), are performed at the same session by the same individual, the primary procedure or service may be reported as listed. The additional procedure(s) or service(s) may be identified by appending modifier 51 to the additional procedure or service code(s).
Note: This modifier should not be appended to designated "add-on" codes (see Appendix F).

52 **Reduced Services:** Under certain circumstances a service or procedure is partially reduced or eliminated at the discretion of the physician or other qualified health care professional. Under these circumstances the service provided can be identified by its usual procedure number and the addition of modifier 52, signifying that the service is reduced. This provides a means of reporting reduced services without disturbing the identification of the basic service.
Note: For hospital outpatient reporting of a previously scheduled procedure/service that is partially reduced or cancelled as a result of extenuating circumstances or those that threaten the well-being of the patient prior to or after administration of anesthesia, see modifiers 73 and 74 (see modifiers approved for ASC hospital outpatient use).

53 **Discontinued Procedure:** Under certain circumstances, the physician or other qualified health care professional may elect to terminate a surgical or diagnostic procedure. Due to extenuating circumstances or those that threaten the well being of the patient, it may be necessary to indicate that a surgical or diagnostic procedure was started but discontinued. This circumstance may be reported by adding modifier 53 to the code reported by the physician for the discontinued procedure.
Note: This modifier is not used to report the elective cancellation of a procedure prior to the patient's anesthesia induction and/or surgical preparation in the operating suite. For outpatient hospital/ambulatory surgery center (ASC) reporting of a previously scheduled procedure/service that is partially reduced or cancelled as a result of extenuating circumstances or those that threaten the well being of the patient prior to or after administration of anesthesia, see modifiers 73 and 74 (see modifiers approved for ASC hospital outpatient use).

54 **Surgical Care Only:** When 1 physician or other qualified health care professional performs a surgical procedure and another provides preoperative and/or postoperative management, surgical services may be identified by adding modifier 54 to the usual procedure number.

55 **Postoperative Management Only:** When 1 physician or other qualified health care professional performed the postoperative management and another performed the surgical procedure, the postoperative component may be identified by adding modifier 55 to the usual procedure number.

56 **Preoperative Management Only:** When 1 physician or other qualified health care professional performed the preoperative care and evaluation and another performed the surgical procedure, the preoperative component may be identified by adding modifier 56 to the usual procedure number.

57 **Decision for Surgery:** An evaluation and management service that resulted in the initial decision to perform the surgery may be identified by adding modifier 57 to the appropriate level of E/M service.

58 Staged or Related Procedure or Service by the Same Physician or Other Qualified Health Care Professional During the Postoperative Period: It may be necessary to indicate that the performance of a procedure or service during the postoperative period was (a) planned or anticipated (staged); (b) more extensive than the original procedure; or (c) for therapy following a surgical procedure. This circumstance may be reported by adding modifier 58 to the staged or related procedure.
Note: For treatment of a problem that requires a return to the operating/procedure room (eg, unanticipated clinical condition), see modifier 78.

59 Distinct Procedural Service: Under certain circumstances, it may be necessary to indicate that a procedure or service was distinct or independent from other non-E/M services performed on the same day. Modifier 59 is used to identify procedures/services, other than E/M services, that are not normally reported together but are appropriate under the circumstances. Documentation must support a different session, different procedure or surgery, different site or organ system, separate incision/excision, separate lesion, or separate injury (or area of injury in extensive injuries) not ordinarily encountered or performed on the same day by the same individual. However, when another already established modifier is appropriate it should be used rather than modifier 59. Only if no more descriptive modifier is available, and the use of modifier 59 best explains the circumstances, should modifier 59 be used.
Note: Modifier 59 should not be appended to an E/M service. To report a separate and distinct E/M service with a non-E/M service performed on the same date, see modifier 25.

62 Two Surgeons: When 2 surgeons work together as primary surgeons performing distinct part(s) of a procedure, each surgeon should report his/her distinct operative work by adding modifier 62 to the procedure code and any associated add-on code(s) for that procedure as long as both surgeons continue to work together as primary surgeons. Each surgeon should report the co-surgery once using the same procedure code. If additional procedure(s) (including add-on procedure[s]) are performed during the same surgical session, separate code(s) may also be reported with modifier 62 added.
Note: If a co-surgeon acts as an assistant in the performance of additional procedure(s), other than those reported with the modifier 62, during the same surgical session, those services may be reported using separate procedure code(s) with modifier 80 or modifier 82 added, as appropriate.

63 Procedure Performed on Infants less than 4 kg: Procedures performed on neonates and infants up to a present body weight of 4 kg may involve significantly increased complexity and physician or other qualified health care professional work commonly associated with these patients. This circumstance may be reported by adding modifier 63 to the procedure number.
Note: Unless otherwise designated, this modifier may only be appended to procedures/services listed in the 20100-69990 code series and 92920, 92928, 92953, 92960, 92986, 92987, 92990, 92997, 92998, 93312, 93313, 93314, 93315, 93316, 93317, 93318, 93452, 93505, 93563, 93564, 93568, 93580, 93582, 93590, 93591, 93592, 93593, 93594, 93595, 93596, 93597, 93598, 93615, 93616 from the Medicine/Cardiovascular section.

Modifier 63 should not be appended to any CPT codes listed in the Evaluation and Management Services, Anesthesia, Radiology, Pathology/Laboratory, or Medicine sections (other than those identified above from the Medicine/Cardiovascular section).

66 Surgical Team: Under some circumstances, highly complex procedures (requiring the concomitant services of several physicians or other qualified health care professionals, often of different specialties, plus other highly skilled, specially trained personnel, various types of complex equipment) are carried out under the "surgical team" concept. Such circumstances may be identified by each participating individual with the addition of modifier 66 to the basic procedure number used for reporting services.

76 Repeat Procedure or Service by Same Physician or Other Qualified Health Care Professional: It may be necessary to indicate that a procedure or service was repeated by the same physician or other qualified health care professional subsequent to the original procedure or service. This circumstance may be reported by adding modifier 76 to the repeated procedure or service.
Note: This modifier should not be appended to an E/M service.

77 Repeat Procedure by Another Physician or Other Qualified Health Care Professional: It may be necessary to indicate that a basic procedure or service was repeated by another physician or other qualified health care professional subsequent to the original procedure or service. This circumstance may be reported by adding modifier 77 to the repeated procedure or service.
Note: This modifier should not be appended to an E/M service.

78 Unplanned Return to the Operating/Procedure Room by the Same Physician or Other Qualified Health Care Professional Following Initial Procedure for a Related Procedure During the Postoperative Period: It may be necessary to indicate that another procedure was performed during the postoperative period of the initial procedure (unplanned procedure following initial procedure). When this procedure is related to the first, and requires the use of an operating/procedure room, it may be reported by adding modifier 78 to the related procedure. (For repeat procedures, see modifier 76.)

79 Unrelated Procedure or Service by the Same Physician or Other Qualified Health Care Professional During the Postoperative Period: The individual may need to indicate that the performance of a procedure or service during the postoperative period was unrelated to the original procedure. This circumstance may be reported by using modifier 79. (For repeat procedures on the same day, see modifier 76.)

80 Assistant Surgeon: Surgical assistant services may be identified by adding modifier 80 to the usual procedure number(s).

81 Minimum Assistant Surgeon: Minimum surgical assistant services are identified by adding modifier 81 to the usual procedure number.

82 Assistant Surgeon (when qualified resident surgeon not available): The unavailability of a qualified resident surgeon is a prerequisite for use of modifier 82 appended to the usual procedure code number(s).

90 Reference (Outside) Laboratory: When laboratory procedures are performed by a party other than the treating or reporting physician or other qualified health care professional, the procedure may be identified by adding modifier 90 to the usual procedure number.

91 Repeat Clinical Diagnostic Laboratory Test: In the course of treatment of the patient, it may be necessary to repeat the same laboratory test on the same day to obtain subsequent (multiple) test results. Under these circumstances, the laboratory test performed can be identified by its usual procedure number and the addition of modifier 91.
Note: This modifier may not be used when tests are rerun to confirm initial results; due to testing problems with specimens or equipment; or for any other reason when a normal, one-time, reportable result is all that is required. This modifier may not be used when other code(s) describe a series of test results (eg, glucose tolerance tests, evocative/suppression testing). This modifier may only be used for laboratory test(s) performed more than once on the same day on the same patient.

92 Alternative Laboratory Platform Testing: When laboratory testing is being performed using a kit or transportable instrument that wholly or in part consists of a single use, disposable analytical chamber, the service may be identified by adding modifier 92 to the usual laboratory procedure code (HIV testing 86701-86703, and 87389). The test does not require permanent dedicated space, hence by its design may be hand carried or transported to the vicinity of the patient for immediate testing at that site, although location of the testing is not in itself determinative of the use of this modifier.

95 **Synchronous Telemedicine Service Rendered Via a Real-Time Interactive Audio and Video Telecommunications System:** Synchronous telemedicine service is defined as a **real-time** interaction between a physician or other qualified health care professional and a patient who is located at a distant site from the physician or other qualified health care professional. The totality of the communication of information exchanged between the physician or other qualified health care professional and patient during the course of the synchronous telemedicine service must be of an amount and nature that would be sufficient to meet the key components and/or requirements of the same service when rendered via a face-to-face interaction. Modifier 95 may only be appended to the services listed in Appendix F. Appendix F is the list of CPT codes for services that are typically performed face-to-face, but may be rendered via real-time (synchronous) interactive audio and video telecommunications system.

96 **Habilitative Services:** When a service or procedure that may be either habilitative or rehabilitative in nature is provided for habilitative purposes, the physician or other qualified health care professional may add modifier 96 to the service or procedure code to indicate that the service or procedure provided was a habilitative service. Habilitative services help an individual learn skills and functioning for daily living that the individual has not yet developed, and then keep and/or improve those learned skills. Habilitative services also help an individual keep, learn, or improve skills and functioning for daily living.

97 **Rehabilitative Services:** When a service or procedure that may be either habilitative or rehabilitative in nature is provided for rehabilitative purposes, the physician or other qualified health care professional may add modifier 97 to the service or procedure code to indicate that the service or procedure provided was a rehabilitative service. Rehabilitative services help an individual keep, get back, or improve skills and functioning for daily living that have been lost or impaired because the individual was sick, hurt, or disabled.

99 **Multiple Modifiers:** Under certain circumstances 2 or more modifiers may be necessary to completely delineate a service. In such situations modifier 99 should be added to the basic procedure, and other applicable modifiers may be listed as part of the description of the service.

Anesthesia Physical Status Modifiers

All anesthesia services are reported by use of the five-digit anesthesia procedure code with the appropriate physical status modifier appended.

Under certain circumstances, when other modifier(s) are appropriate, they should be reported in addition to the physical status modifier.

P1 A normal healthy patient

P2 A patient with mild systemic disease

P3 A patient with severe systemic disease

P4 A patient with severe systemic disease that is a constant threat to life

P5 A moribund patient who is not expected to survive without the operation

P6 A declared brain-dead patient whose organs are being removed for donor purposes

Modifiers Approved for Ambulatory Surgery Center (ASC) Hospital Outpatient Use

CPT Level I Modifiers

25 **Significant, Separately Identifiable Evaluation and Management Service by the Same Physician or Other Qualified Health Care Professional on the Same Day of the Procedure or Other Service:** It may be necessary to indicate that on the day a procedure or service identified by a CPT code was performed, the patient's condition required a significant, separately identifiable E/M service above and beyond the other service provided or beyond the usual preoperative and postoperative care associated with the procedure that was performed. A significant, separately identifiable E/M service is defined or substantiated by documentation that satisfies the relevant criteria for the respective E/M service to be reported (see Evaluation and Management Services Guidelines for instructions on determining level of E/M service). The E/M service may be prompted by the symptom or condition for which the procedure and/or service was provided. As such, different diagnoses are not required for reporting of the E/M services on the same date. This circumstance may be reported by adding modifier 25 to the appropriate level of E/M service.
Note: This modifier is not used to report an E/M service that resulted in a decision to perform surgery. See modifier 57. For significant, separately identifiable non-E/M services, see modifier 59.

27 **Multiple Outpatient Hospital E/M Encounters on the Same Date:** For hospital outpatient reporting purposes, utilization of hospital resources related to separate and distinct E/M encounters performed in multiple outpatient hospital settings on the same date may be reported by adding modifier 27 to each appropriate level outpatient and/or emergency department E/M code(s). This modifier provides a means of reporting circumstances involving evaluation and management services provided by a physician(s) in more than one (multiple) outpatient hospital setting(s) (eg, hospital emergency department, clinic).
Note: This modifier is not to be used for physician reporting of multiple E/M services performed by the same physician on the same date. For physician reporting of all outpatient evaluation and management services provided by the same physician on the same date and performed in multiple outpatient settings (eg, hospital emergency department, clinic), see Evaluation and Management, Emergency Department, or Preventive Medicine Services codes.

33 **Preventive Services:** When the primary purpose of the service is the delivery of an evidence based service in accordance with a US Preventive Services Task Force A or B rating in effect and other preventive services identified in preventive services mandates (legislative or regulatory), the service may be identified by adding 33 to the procedure. For separately reported services specifically identified as preventive, the modifier should not be used.

50 **Bilateral Procedure:** Unless otherwise identified in the listings, bilateral procedures that are performed at the same session should be identified by adding modifier 50 to the appropriate 5 digit code.
Note: This modifier should not be appended to designated "add-on" codes (see appendix F).

52 **Reduced Services:** Under certain circumstances a service or procedure is partially reduced or eliminated at the discretion of the physician or other qualified health care professional. Under these circumstances the service provided can be identified by its usual procedure number and the addition of modifier 52, signifying that the service is reduced. This provides a means of reporting reduced services without disturbing the identification of the basic service.
Note: For hospital outpatient reporting of a previously scheduled procedure/service that is partially reduced or cancelled as a result of extenuating circumstances or those that threaten the well-being of the patient prior to or after administration of anesthesia, see modifiers 73 and 74 (see modifiers approved for ASC hospital outpatient use).

58 **Staged or Related Procedure or Service by the Same Physician or Other Qualified Health Care Professional During the Postoperative Period:** It may be necessary to indicate that the performance of a procedure or service during the postoperative period was (a) planned or anticipated (staged); (b) more extensive than the original procedure; or (c) for therapy following a surgical procedure. This circumstance may be reported by adding modifier 58 to the staged or related procedure.
Note: For treatment of a problem that requires a return to the operating or procedure room (eg, unanticipated clinical condition), see modifier 78.

59 **Distinct Procedural Service:** Under certain circumstances, it may be necessary to indicate that a procedure or service was distinct or independent from other non-E/M services performed on the same day. Modifier 59 is used to identify procedures/services, other than E/M services, that are not normally reported together but are appropriate under the circumstances. Documentation must support a different session, different procedure or surgery, different site or organ system, separate incision/excision, separate lesion, or

separate injury (or area of injury in extensive injuries) not ordinarily encountered or performed on the same day by the same individual. However, when another already established modifier is appropriate it should be used rather than modifier 59. Only if no more descriptive modifier is available, and the use of modifier 59 best explains the circumstances, should modifier 59 be used.
Note: Modifier 59 should not be appended to an E/M service. To report a separate and distinct E/M service with a non-E/M service performed on the same date, see modifier 25.

73 **Discontinued Out-Patient Hospital/Ambulatory Surgery Center (ASC) Procedure Prior to the Administration of Anesthesia:** Due to extenuating circumstances or those that threaten the well being of the patient, the physician may cancel a surgical or diagnostic procedure subsequent to the patient's surgical preparation (including sedation when provided, and being taken to the room where the procedure is to be performed), but prior to the administration of anesthesia (local, regional block(s) or general). Under these circumstances, the intended service that is prepared for but cancelled can be reported by its usual procedure number and the addition of modifier 73.
Note: The elective cancellation of a service prior to the administration of anesthesia and/or surgical preparation of the patient should not be reported. For physician reporting of a discontinued procedure, see modifier 53.

74 **Discontinued Out-Patient Hospital/Ambulatory Surgery Center (ASC) Procedure After Administration of Anesthesia:** Due to extenuating circumstances or those that threaten the well being of the patient, the physician may terminate a surgical or diagnostic procedure after the administration of anesthesia (local, regional block(s), general) or after the procedure was started (incision made, intubation started, scope inserted, etc.). Under these circumstances, the procedure started but terminated can be reported by its usual procedure number and the addition of modifier 74.
Note: The elective cancellation of a service prior to the administration of anesthesia and/or surgical preparation of the patient should not be reported. For physician reporting of a discontinued procedure, see modifier 53.

76 **Repeat Procedure or Service by Same Physician or Other Qualified Health Care Professional:** It may be necessary to indicate that a procedure or service was repeated by the same physician or other qualified health care professional subsequent to the original procedure or service. This circumstance may be reported by adding modifier 76 to the repeated procedure or service.
Note: This modifier should not be appended to an E/M service.

77 **Repeat Procedure by Another Physician or Other Qualified Health Care Professional:** It may be necessary to indicate that a basic procedure or service was repeated by another physician or other qualified health care professional subsequent to the original procedure or service. This circumstance may be reported by adding modifier 77 to the repeated procedure or service.
Note: This modifier should not be appended to an E/M service.

78 **Unplanned Return to the Operating/Procedure Room by the Same Physician or Other Qualified Health Care Professional Following Initial Procedure for a Related Procedure During the Postoperative Period:** It may be necessary to indicate that another procedure was performed during the postoperative period of the initial procedure (unplanned procedure following initial procedure). When this procedure is related to the first, and requires the use of an operating/procedure room, it may be reported by adding modifier 78 to the related procedure. (For repeat procedures, see modifier 76.)

79 **Unrelated Procedure or Service by the Same Physician During the Postoperative Period:** The individual may need to indicate that the performance of a procedure or service during the postoperative period was unrelated to the original procedure. This circumstance may be reported by using modifier 79. (For repeat procedures on the same day, see modifier 76.)

91 **Repeat Clinical Diagnostic Laboratory Test:** In the course of treatment of the patient, it may be necessary to repeat the same laboratory test on the same day to obtain subsequent (multiple) test results. Under these circumstances, the laboratory test performed can be identified by its usual procedure number and the addition of modifier 91.
Note: This modifier may not be used when tests are rerun to confirm initial results; due to testing problems with specimens or equipment; or for any other reason when a normal, one-time, reportable result is all that is required. This modifier may not be used when other code(s) describe a series of test results (eg, glucose tolerance tests, evocative/suppression testing). This modifier may only be used for laboratory test(s) performed more than once on the same day on the same patient.

Level II (HCPCS/National) Modifiers

The HCPCS Level II modifiers included here are those most commonly used when coding procedures. See your 2022 HCPCS Level II book for a complete listing.

Anatomical Modifiers

E1 Upper left, eyelid
E2 Lower left, eyelid
E3 Upper right, eyelid
E4 Lower right, eyelid
FA Left hand, thumb
F1 Left hand, second digit
F2 Left hand, third digit
F3 Left hand, fourth digit
F4 Left hand, fifth digit
F5 Right hand, thumb
F6 Right hand, second digit
F7 Right hand, third digit
F8 Right hand, fourth digit
F9 Right hand, fifth digit
LT Left side (used to identify procedures performed on the left side of the body)
RT Right side (used to identify procedures performed on the right side of the body)
TA Left foot, great toe
T1 Left foot, second digit
T2 Left foot, third digit
T3 Left foot, fourth digit
T4 Left foot, fifth digit
T5 Right foot, great toe
T6 Right foot, second digit
T7 Right foot, third digit
T8 Right foot, fourth digit
T9 Right foot, fifth digit

Anesthesia Modifiers

AA Anesthesia services performed personally by anesthesiologist
AD Medical supervision by a physician: more than four concurrent anesthesia procedures
G8 Monitored anesthesia care (MAC) for deep complex, complicated, or markedly invasive surgical procedure
G9 Monitored anesthesia care for patient who has history of severe cardiopulmonary condition
QK Medical direction of two, three, or four concurrent anesthesia procedures involving qualified individuals
QS Monitored anesthesiology care service
QX CRNA service: with medical direction by a physician
QY Medical direction of one certified registered nurse anesthetist (CRNA) by an anesthesiologist
QZ CRNA service: without medical direction by a physician

Coronary Artery Modifiers

LC Left circumflex coronary artery

LD Left anterior descending coronary artery

LM Left main coronary artery

RC Right coronary artery

RI Ramus intermedius coronary artery

Other Modifiers

CS Cost-sharing waived for specified COVID-19 testing-related services that result in an order for, or administration of, a COVID-19 test and/or used for cost-sharing waived preventive services furnished via telehealth in Rural Health Clinics and Federally Qualified Health Centers during the COVID-19 public health emergency

CT Computed tomography services furnished using equipment that does not meet each of the attributes of the national electrical manufacturers association (NEMA) XR-29-2013 standard

EA Erythropoetic stimulating agent (ESA) administered to treat anemia due to anticancer chemotherapy

EB Erythropoetic stimulating agent (ESA) administered to treat anemia due to anticancer radiotherapy

EC Erythropoetic stimulating agent (ESA) administered to treat anemia not due to anticancer radiotherapy or anticancer chemotherapy

FP Service provided as part of family planning program

FX X-ray taken using film

G7 Pregnancy resulted from rape or incest or pregnancy certified by physician as life threatening

GA Waiver of liability statement issued as required by payer policy, individual case

GG Performance and payment of a screening mammogram and diagnostic mammogram on the same patient, same day

GH Diagnostic mammogram converted from screening mammogram on same day

GQ Via asynchronous telecommunications system

GT Via interactive audio and video telecommunication systems

GU Waiver of liability statement issued as required by payer policy, routine notice

GX Notice of liability issued, voluntary under payer policy

GY Item or service statutorily excluded, does not meet the definition of any Medicare benefit or, for non-Medicare insurers, is not a contract benefit

GZ Item or service expected to be denied as not reasonable and necessary

PI Positron emission tomography (PET) or PET/computed tomography (CT) to inform the initial treatment strategy of tumors that are biopsy proven or strongly suspected of being cancerous based on other diagnostic testing

PS Positron emission tomography (PET) or PET/computed tomography (CT) to inform the subsequent treatment strategy of cancerous tumors when the beneficiary's treating physician determines that the PET study is needed to inform subsequent antitumor strategy

PT Colorectal cancer screening test; converted to diagnostic test or other procedure

Q7 One Class A finding

Q8 Two Class B findings

Q9 One Class B and two Class C findings

QC Single channel monitoring

QM Ambulance service provided under arrangement by a provider of services

QN Ambulance service furnished directly by a provider of services

QW CLIA waived test

TC Technical component; under certain circumstances, a charge may be made for the technical component alone; under those circumstances the technical component charge is identified by adding modifier TC to the usual procedure number; technical component charges are institutional charges and not billed separately by physicians; however, portable x-ray suppliers only bill for technical component and should utilize modifier TC; the charge data from portable x-ray suppliers will then be used to build customary and prevailing profiles

* **XE** Separate encounter, a service that is distinct because it occurred during a separate encounter

* **XP** Separate practitioner, a service that is distinct because it was performed by a different practitioner

* **XS** Separate structure, a service that is distinct because it was performed on a separate organ/structure

* **XU** Unusual nonoverlapping service, the use of a service that is distinct because it does not overlap usual components of the main service

* CMS instituted additional HCPCS modifiers to define explicit subsets of modifier 59 Distinct Procedural Service.

Category II Modifiers

1P Performance Measure Exclusion Modifier due to Medical Reasons

Reasons include:

- Not indicated (absence of organ/limb, already received/performed, other)
- Contraindicated (patient allergic history, potential adverse drug interaction, other)
- Other medical reasons

2P Performance Measure Exclusion Modifier due to Patient Reasons

Reasons include:

- Patient declined
- Economic, social, or religious reasons
- Other patient reasons

3P Performance Measure Exclusion Modifier due to System Reasons

Reasons include:

- Resources to perform the services not available
- Insurance coverage/payor-related limitations
- Other reasons attributable to health care delivery system

~~Modifier 8P is intended to be used as a "reporting modifier" to allow the reporting of circumstances when an action described in a measure's numerator is not performed and the reason is not otherwise specified.~~

~~8P Performance measure reporting modifier-action not performed, reason not otherwise specified~~

Appendix B — New, Revised, and Deleted Codes

New Codes

01937 Anesthesia for percutaneous image-guided injection, drainage or aspiration procedures on the spine or spinal cord; cervical or thoracic

01938 lumbar or sacral

01939 Anesthesia for percutaneous image-guided destruction procedures by neurolytic agent on the spine or spinal cord; cervical or thoracic

01940 lumbar or sacral

01941 Anesthesia for percutaneous image-guided neuromodulation or intravertebral procedures (eg, kyphoplasty, vertebroplasty) on the spine or spinal cord; cervical or thoracic

01942 lumbar or sacral

33267 Exclusion of left atrial appendage, open, any method (eg, excision, isolation via stapling, oversewing, ligation, plication, clip)

33268 Exclusion of left atrial appendage, open, performed at the time of other sternotomy or thoracotomy procedure(s), any method (eg, excision, isolation via stapling, oversewing, ligation, plication, clip) (List separately in addition to code for primary procedure)

33269 Exclusion of left atrial appendage, thoracoscopic, any method (eg, excision, isolation via stapling, oversewing, ligation, plication, clip)

33370 Transcatheter placement and subsequent removal of cerebral embolic protection device(s), including arterial access, catheterization, imaging, and radiological supervision and interpretation, percutaneous (List separately in addition to code for primary procedure)

33509 Harvest of upper extremity artery, 1 segment, for coronary artery bypass procedure, endoscopic

33894 Endovascular stent repair of coarctation of the ascending, transverse, or descending thoracic or abdominal aorta, involving stent placement; across major side branches

33895 not crossing major side branches

33897 Percutaneous transluminal angioplasty of native or recurrent coarctation of the aorta

42975 Drug-induced sleep endoscopy, with dynamic evaluation of velum, pharynx, tongue base, and larynx for evaluation of sleep-disordered breathing, flexible, diagnostic

43497 Lower esophageal myotomy, transoral (ie, peroral endoscopic myotomy [POEM])

53451 Periurethral transperineal adjustable balloon continence device; bilateral insertion, including cystourethroscopy and imaging guidance

53452 unilateral insertion, including cystourethroscopy and imaging guidance

53453 removal, each balloon

53454 percutaneous adjustment of balloon(s) fluid volume

61736 Laser interstitial thermal therapy (LITT) of lesion, intracranial, including burr hole(s), with magnetic resonance imaging guidance, when performed; single trajectory for 1 simple lesion

61737 multiple trajectories for multiple or complex lesion(s)

63052 Laminectomy, facetectomy, or foraminotomy (unilateral or bilateral with decompression of spinal cord, cauda equina and/or nerve root[s] [eg, spinal or lateral recess stenosis]), during posterior interbody arthrodesis, lumbar; single vertebral segment (List separately in addition to code for primary procedure)

63053 each additional segment (List separately in addition to code for primary procedure)

64582 Open implantation of hypoglossal nerve neurostimulator array, pulse generator, and distal respiratory sensor electrode or electrode array

64583 Revision or replacement of hypoglossal nerve neurostimulator array and distal respiratory sensor electrode or electrode array, including connection to existing pulse generator

64584 Removal of hypoglossal nerve neurostimulator array, pulse generator, and distal respiratory sensor electrode or electrode array

64628 Thermal destruction of intraosseous basivertebral nerve, including all imaging guidance; first 2 vertebral bodies, lumbar or sacral

64629 each additional vertebral body, lumbar or sacral (List separately in addition to code for primary procedure)

66989 with insertion of intraocular (eg, trabecular meshwork, supraciliary, suprachoroidal) anterior segment aqueous drainage device, without extraocular reservoir, internal approach, one or more

66991 with insertion of intraocular (eg, trabecular meshwork, supraciliary, suprachoroidal) anterior segment aqueous drainage device, without extraocular reservoir, internal approach, one or more

68841 Insertion of drug-eluting implant, including punctal dilation when performed, into lacrimal canaliculus, each

69716 with magnetic transcutaneous attachment to external speech processor

69719 with magnetic transcutaneous attachment to external speech processor

69726 Removal, osseointegrated implant, skull; with percutaneous attachment to external speech processor

69727 with magnetic transcutaneous attachment to external speech processor

77089 Trabecular bone score (TBS), structural condition of the bone microarchitecture; using dual X-ray absorptiometry (DXA) or other imaging data on gray-scale variogram, calculation, with interpretation and report on fracture-risk

77090 technical preparation and transmission of data for analysis to be performed elsewhere

77091 technical calculation only

77092 interpretation and report on fracture-risk only by other qualified health care professional

80220 Hydroxychloroquine

80503 Pathology clinical consultation; for a clinical problem, with limited review of patient's history and medical records and straightforward medical decision making

80504 for a moderately complex clinical problem, with review of patient's history and medical records and moderate level of medical decision making

80505 for a highly complex clinical problem, with comprehensive review of patient's history and medical records and high level of medical decision making

80506 prolonged service, each additional 30 minutes (List separately in addition to code for primary procedure)

81349 interrogation of genomic regions for copy number and loss-of-heterozygosity variants, low-pass sequencing analysis

81523 Oncology (breast), mRNA, next-generation sequencing gene profiling of 70 content genes and 31 housekeeping genes, utilizing formalin-fixed paraffin-embedded tissue, algorithm reported as index related to risk to distant metastasis

81560 Transplantation medicine (allograft rejection, pediatric liver and small bowel), measurement of donor and third-party-induced CD154+T-cytotoxic memory cells, utilizing whole peripheral blood, algorithm reported as a rejection risk score

82653 quantitative

83521 Immunoglobulin light chains (ie, kappa, lambda), free, each

83529 Interleukin-6 (IL-6)

86015 Actin (smooth muscle) antibody (ASMA), each

86036 Antineutrophil cytoplasmic antibody (ANCA); screen, each antibody

86037 titer, each antibody

86051 Aquaporin-4 (neuromyelitis optica [NMO]) antibody; enzyme-linked immunosorbent immunoassay (ELISA)

86052 cell-based immunofluorescence assay (CBA), each

86053 flow cytometry (ie, fluorescence-activated cell sorting [FACS]), each

86231 Endomysial antibody (EMA), each immunoglobulin (Ig) class

86258 Gliadin (deamidated) (DGP) antibody, each immunoglobulin (Ig) class

86362 Myelin oligodendrocyte glycoprotein (MOG-IgG1) antibody; cell-based immunofluorescence assay (CBA), each

86363 Myelin oligodendrocyte glycoprotein (MOG-IgG1) antibody; cell-based immunofluorescence assay (CBA), each

86364 Tissue transglutaminase, each immunoglobulin (Ig) class

86381 Mitochondrial antibody (eg, M2), each

86408 Neutralizing antibody, severe acute respiratory syndrome coronavirus 2 (SARS-CoV-2) (coronavirus disease [COVID-19]); screen

86409 titer

86413 Severe acute respiratory syndrome coronavirus 2 (SARS-CoV-2) (coronavirus disease [COVID-19]) antibody, quantitative

86596 Voltage-gated calcium channel antibody, each

87154 identification of blood pathogen and resistance typing, when performed, by nucleic acid (DNA or RNA) probe, multiplexed amplified probe technique including multiplex reverse transcription, when performed, per culture or isolate, 6 or more targets

87428 Infectious agent antigen detection by immunoassay technique, (eg, enzyme immunoassay [EIA], enzyme-linked immunosorbent assay [ELISA], fluorescence immunoassay [FIA], immunochemiluminometric assay [IMCA]) qualitative or semiquantitative; severe acute respiratory syndrome coronavirus (eg, SARS-CoV, SARS-CoV-2 [COVID-19]) and influenza virus types A and B

87636 severe acute respiratory syndrome coronavirus 2 (SARS-CoV-2) (coronavirus disease [COVID-19]) and influenza virus types A and B, multiplex amplified probe technique

87637 severe acute respiratory syndrome coronavirus 2 (SARS-CoV-2) (coronavirus disease [COVID-19]), influenza virus types A and B, and respiratory syncytial virus, multiplex amplified probe technique

87811 severe acute respiratory syndrome coronavirus 2 (SARS-CoV-2) (coronavirus disease [COVID-19])

90626 Tick-borne encephalitis virus vaccine, inactivated; 0.25 mL dosage, for intramuscular use

90627 Tick-borne encephalitis virus vaccine, inactivated; 0.5 mL dosage, for intramuscular use

90671 Pneumococcal conjugate vaccine, 15 valent (PCV15), for intramuscular use

90677 Pneumococcal conjugate vaccine, 20 valent (PCV20), for intramuscular use

90758 Zaire ebolavirus vaccine, live, for intramuscular use

90759 Hepatitis B vaccine (HepB), 3-antigen (S, Pre-S1, Pre-S2), 10 mcg dosage, 3 dose schedule, for intramuscular use

91113 Gastrointestinal tract imaging, intraluminal (eg, capsule endoscopy), colon, with interpretation and report

91300 Severe acute respiratory syndrome coronavirus 2 (SARS-CoV-2) (coronavirus disease [COVID-19]) vaccine, mRNA-LNP, spike protein, preservative free, 30 mcg/0.3.mL dosage, diluent reconstituted, for intramuscular use

91301 Severe acute respiratory syndrome coronavirus 2 (SARS-CoV-2) (coronavirus disease [COVID-19]) vaccine, mRNA-LNP, spike protein, preservative free, 100 mcg/0.5mL dosage, for intramuscular use

91302 Severe acute respiratory syndrome coronavirus 2 (SARS-CoV-2) (coronavirus disease [COVID-19]) vaccine, DNA, spike protein, chimpanzee adenovirus Oxford 1 (ChAdOx1) vector, preservative free, $5x10^{10}$ viral particles/0.5mL dosage, for intramuscular use

91303 Severe acute respiratory syndrome coronavirus 2 (SARS-CoV-2) (coronavirus disease [COVID-19]) vaccine, DNA, spike protein, adenovirus type 26 (Ad26) vector, preservative free, $5x10^{10}$ viral particles/0.5mL dosage, for intramuscular use

91304 Severe acute respiratory syndrome coronavirus 2 (SARS-CoV-2) (coronavirus disease [COVID-19]) vaccine, recombinant spike protein nanoparticle, saponin-based adjuvant, preservative free, 5 mcg/0.5mL dosage, for intramuscular use

93319 3D echocardiographic imaging and postprocessing during transesophageal echocardiography, or during transthoracic echocardiography for congenital cardiac anomalies, for the assessment of cardiac structure(s) (eg, cardiac chambers and valves, left atrial appendage, interatrial septum, interventricular septum) and function, when performed (List separately in addition to code for echocardiographic imaging)

93593 Right heart catheterization for congenital heart defect(s) including imaging guidance by the proceduralist to advance the catheter to the target zone; normal native connections

93594 abnormal native connections

93595 Left heart catheterization for congenital heart defect(s) including imaging guidance by the proceduralist to advance the catheter to the target zone, normal or abnormal native connections

93596 Right and left heart catheterization for congenital heart defect(s) including imaging guidance by the proceduralist to advance the catheter to the target zone(s); normal native connections

93597 abnormal native connections

93598 Cardiac output measurement(s), thermodilution or other indicator dilution method, performed during cardiac catheterization for the evaluation of congenital heart defects (List separately in addition to code for primary procedure)

94625 Physician or other qualified health care professional services for outpatient pulmonary rehabilitation; without continuous oximetry monitoring (per session)

94626 with continuous oximetry monitoring (per session)

98975 Remote therapeutic monitoring (eg, respiratory system status, musculoskeletal system status, therapy adherence, therapy response); initial set-up and patient education on use of equipment

98976 device(s) supply with scheduled (eg, daily) recording(s) and/or programmed alert(s) transmission to monitor respiratory system, each 30 days

98977 device(s) supply with scheduled (eg, daily) recording(s) and/or programmed alert(s) transmission to monitor musculoskeletal system, each 30 days

98980 Remote therapeutic monitoring treatment management services, physician or other qualified health care professional time in a calendar month requiring at least one interactive communication with the patient or caregiver during the calendar month; first 20 minutes

98981 each additional 20 minutes (List separately in addition to code for primary procedure)

99072 Additional supplies, materials, and clinical staff time over and above those usually included in an office visit or other nonfacility service(s), when performed during a Public Health Emergency, as defined by law, due to respiratory-transmitted infectious disease

99424 Principal care management services, for a single high-risk disease, with the following required elements: one complex chronic condition expected to last at least 3 months, and that places the patient at significant risk of hospitalization, acute exacerbation/decompensation, functional decline, or death, the condition requires development, monitoring, or revision of disease-specific care plan, the condition requires frequent adjustments in the medication regimen and/or the management of the condition is unusually complex due to comorbidities, ongoing communication and care coordination between relevant practitioners furnishing care; first 30 minutes provided personally by a physician or other qualified health care professional, per calendar month.

99425 each additional 30 minutes provided personally by a physician or other qualified health care professional, per calendar month (List separately in addition to code for primary procedure)

99426 Principal care management services, for a single high-risk disease, with the following required elements: one complex chronic condition expected to last at least 3 months, and that places the patient at significant risk of hospitalization, acute exacerbation/decompensation, functional decline, or death, the condition requires development, monitoring, or revision of disease-specific care plan, the condition requires frequent adjustments in the medication regimen and/or the management of the condition is unusually complex due to comorbidities, ongoing communication and care coordination between relevant practitioners furnishing care; first 30 minutes of clinical staff time directed by physician or other qualified health care professional, per calendar month.

99427 each additional 30 minutes of clinical staff time directed by a physician or other qualified health care professional, per calendar month (List separately in addition to code for primary procedure)

99437 Chronic care management services with the following required elements: multiple (two or more) chronic conditions expected to last at least 12 months, or until the death of the patient, chronic conditions that place the patient at significant risk of death, acute exacerbation/decompensation, or functional decline, comprehensive care plan established, implemented, revised, or monitored; each additional 30 minutes by a physician or other qualified health care professional, per calendar month (List separately in addition to code for primary procedure)

0001A Immunization administration by intramuscular injection of severe acute respiratory syndrome coronavirus 2 (SARS-CoV-2) (coronavirus disease [COVID-19]) vaccine, mRNA-LNP, spike protein, preservative free, 30 mcg/0.3mL dosage, diluent reconstituted; first dose

0002A Immunization administration by intramuscular injection of severe acute respiratory syndrome coronavirus 2 (SARS-CoV-2) (coronavirus disease [COVID-19]) vaccine, mRNA-LNP, spike protein, preservative free, 30 mcg/0.3mL dosage, diluent reconstituted; second dose

0011A Immunization administration by intramuscular injection of severe acute respiratory syndrome coronavirus 2 (SARS-CoV-2) (coronavirus disease [COVID-19]) vaccine, mRNA-LNP, spike protein, preservative free, 100 mcg/0.5mL dosage; first dose

0012A Immunization administration by intramuscular injection of severe acute respiratory syndrome coronavirus 2 (SARS-CoV-2) (coronavirus disease [COVID-19] vaccine, mRNA-LNP, spike protein, preservative free, 100 mcg/0.5mL dosage; second dose

0021A Immunization administration by intramuscular injection of severe acute respiratory syndrome coronavirus 2 (SARS-CoV-2) (coronavirus disease [COVID-19]) vaccine, DNA, spike protein, chimpanzee adenovirus Oxford 1 (ChAdOx1) vector, preservative free, $5x10^{10}$ viral particles/0.5mL dosage; first dose

0022A Immunization administration by intramuscular injection of severe acute respiratory syndrome coronavirus 2 (SARS-CoV-2) (coronavirus disease [COVID-19]) vaccine, DNA, spike protein, chimpanzee adenovirus Oxford 1 (ChAdOx1) vector, preservative free, $5x10^{10}$ viral particles/0.5mL dosage; second dose

0031A Immunization administration by intramuscular injection of severe acute respiratory syndrome coronavirus 2 (SARS-CoV-2) (coronavirus disease [COVID-19]) vaccine, DNA, spike protein, adenovirus type 26 (Ad26) vector, preservative free, $5x10^{10}$ viral particles/0.5mL dosage, single dose

0041A Immunization administration by intramuscular injection of severe acute respiratory syndrome coronavirus 2 (SARS-CoV-2) (coronavirus disease [COVID-19]) vaccine, recombinant spike protein nanoparticle, saponin-based adjuvant, preservative free, 5 mcg/0.5mL dosage; first dose

0042A Immunization administration by intramuscular injection of severe acute respiratory syndrome coronavirus 2 (SARS-CoV-2) (coronavirus disease [COVID-19]) vaccine, recombinant spike protein nanoparticle, saponin-based adjuvant, preservative free, 5 mcg/0.5mL dosage; second dose

0223U Infectious disease (bacterial or viral respiratory tract infection), pathogen-specific nucleic acid (DNA or RNA), 22 targets including severe acute respiratory syndrome coronavirus 2 (SARS-CoV-2), qualitative RT-PCR, nasopharyngeal swab, each pathogen reported as detected or not detected

0224U Antibody, severe acute respiratory syndrome coronavirus 2 (SARS-CoV-2) (coronavirus disease [COVID-19]), includes titer(s), when performed

0225U Infectious disease (bacterial or viral respiratory tract infection) pathogen-specific DNA and RNA, 21 targets, including severe acute respiratory syndrome coronavirus 2 (SARS-CoV-2), amplified probe technique, including multiplex reverse transcription for RNA targets, each analyte reported as detected or not detected

0226U Surrogate viral neutralization test (sVNT), severe acute respiratory syndrome coronavirus 2 (SARS-CoV-2) (coronavirus disease [COVID-19]), ELISA, plasma, serum

0227U Drug assay, presumptive, 30 or more drugs or metabolites, urine, liquid chromatography with tandem mass spectrometry (LC-MS/MS) using multiple reaction monitoring (MRM), with drug or metabolite description, includes sample validation

0228U Oncology (prostate), multianalyte molecular profile by photometric detection of macromolecules adsorbed on nanosponge array slides with machine learning, utilizing first morning voided urine, algorithm reported as likelihood of prostate cancer

0229U BCAT1 (Branched chain amino acid transaminase 1) or IKZF1 (IKAROS family zinc finger 1) (eg, colorectal cancer) promoter methylation analysis

0230U AR (androgen receptor) (eg, spinal and bulbar muscular atrophy, Kennedy disease, X chromosome inactivation), full sequence analysis, including small sequence changes in exonic and intronic regions, deletions, duplications, short tandem repeat (STR) expansions, mobile element insertions, and variants in non-uniquely mappable regions

0231U CACNA1A (calcium voltage-gated channel subunit alpha 1A) (eg, spinocerebellar ataxia), full gene analysis, including small sequence changes in exonic and intronic regions, deletions, duplications, short tandem repeat (STR) gene expansions, mobile element insertions, and variants in non-uniquely mappable regions

0232U CSTB (cystatin B) (eg, progressive myoclonic epilepsy type 1A, Unverricht-Lundborg disease), full gene analysis, including small sequence changes in exonic and intronic regions, deletions, duplications, short tandem repeat (STR) expansions, mobile element insertions, and variants in non-uniquely mappable regions

0233U FXN (frataxin) (eg, Friedreich ataxia), gene analysis, including small sequence changes in exonic and intronic regions, deletions, duplications, short tandem repeat (STR) expansions, mobile element insertions, and variants in non-uniquely mappable regions

0234U MECP2 (methyl CpG binding protein 2) (eg, Rett syndrome), full gene analysis, including small sequence changes in exonic and intronic regions, deletions, duplications, mobile element insertions, and variants in non-uniquely mappable regions

0235U PTEN (phosphatase and tensin homolog) (eg, Cowden syndrome, PTEN hamartoma tumor syndrome), full gene analysis, including small sequence changes in exonic and intronic regions, deletions, duplications, mobile element insertions, and variants in non-uniquely mappable regions

0236U SMN1 (survival of motor neuron 1, telomeric) and SMN2 (survival of motor neuron 2, centromeric) (eg, spinal muscular atrophy) full gene analysis, including small sequence changes in exonic and intronic regions, duplications, deletions, and mobile element insertions

0237U Cardiac ion channelopathies (eg, Brugada syndrome, long QT syndrome, short QT syndrome, catecholaminergic polymorphic ventricular tachycardia), genomic sequence analysis panel including ANK2, CASQ2, CAV3, KCNE1, KCNE2, KCNH2, KCNJ2, KCNQ1, RYR2, and SCN5A, including small sequence changes in exonic and intronic regions, deletions, duplications, mobile element insertions, and variants in non-uniquely mappable regions

0238U Oncology (Lynch syndrome), genomic DNA sequence analysis of MLH1, MSH2, MSH6, PMS2, and EPCAM, including small sequence changes in exonic and intronic regions, deletions, duplications, mobile element insertions, and variants in non-uniquely mappable regions

0239U Targeted genomic sequence analysis panel, solid organ neoplasm, cell-free DNA, analysis of 311 or more genes, interrogation for sequence variants, including substitutions, insertions, deletions, select rearrangements, and copy number variations

0240U Infectious disease (viral respiratory tract infection), pathogen-specific RNA, 3 targets (severe acute respiratory syndrome coronavirus 2 [SARS-CoV-2], influenza A, influenza B), upper respiratory specimen, each pathogen reported as detected or not detected

0241U Infectious disease (viral respiratory tract infection), pathogen-specific RNA, 4 targets (severe acute respiratory syndrome coronavirus 2 [SARS-CoV-2], influenza A, influenza B, respiratory syncytial virus [RSV]), upper respiratory specimen, each pathogen reported as detected or not detected

0242U Targeted genomic sequence analysis panel, solid organ neoplasm, cell-free circulating DNA analysis of 55-74 genes, interrogation for sequence variants, gene copy number amplifications, and gene rearrangements

0243U Obstetrics (preeclampsia), biochemical assay of placental-growth factor, time-resolved fluorescence immunoassay, maternal serum, predictive algorithm reported as a risk score for preeclampsia

0244U Oncology (solid organ), DNA, comprehensive genomic profiling, 257 genes, interrogation for single-nucleotide variants, insertions/deletions, copy number alterations, gene rearrangements, tumor-mutational burden and microsatellite instability, utilizing formalin-fixed paraffin-embedded tumor tissue

0245U Oncology (thyroid), mutation analysis of 10 genes and 37 RNA fusions and expression of 4 mRNA markers using next-generation sequencing, fine needle aspirate, report includes associated risk of malignancy expressed as a percentage

0246U Red blood cell antigen typing, DNA, genotyping of at least 16 blood groups with phenotype prediction of at least 51 red blood cell antigens

0247U Obstetrics (preterm birth), insulin-like growth factor–binding protein 4 (IBP4), sex hormone–binding globulin (SHBG), quantitative measurement by LC-MS/MS, utilizing maternal serum, combined with clinical data, reported as predictive-risk stratification for spontaneous preterm birth

0248U Oncology (brain), spheroid cell culture in a 3D microenvironment, 12 drug panel, tumor-response prediction for each drug

0249U Oncology (breast), semiquantitative analysis of 32 phosphoproteins and protein analytes, includes laser capture microdissection, with algorithmic analysis and interpretative report

0250U Oncology (solid organ neoplasm), targeted genomic sequence DNA analysis of 505 genes, interrogation for somatic alterations (SNVs [single nucleotide variant], small insertions and deletions, one amplification, and four translocations), microsatellite instability and tumor-mutation burden

0251U Hepcidin-25, enzyme-linked immunosorbent assay (ELISA), serum or plasma

0252U Fetal aneuploidy short tandem–repeat comparative analysis, fetal DNA from products of conception, reported as normal (euploidy), monosomy, trisomy, or partial deletion/duplications, mosaicism, and segmental aneuploidy

0253U Reproductive medicine (endometrial receptivity analysis), RNA gene expression profile, 238 genes by next-generation sequencing, endometrial tissue, predictive algorithm reported as endometrial window of implantation (eg, pre-receptive, receptive, post-receptive)

0254U Reproductive medicine (preimplantation genetic assessment), analysis of 24 chromosomes using embryonic DNA genomic sequence analysis for aneuploidy, and a mitochondrial DNA score in euploid embryos, results reported as normal (euploidy), monosomy, trisomy, or partial deletion/duplications, mosaicism, and segmental aneuploidy, per embryo tested

0255U Andrology (infertility), sperm-capacitation assessment of ganglioside GM1 distribution patterns, fluorescence microscopy, fresh or frozen specimen, reported as percentage of capacitated sperm and probability of generating a pregnancy score

0256U Trimethylamine/trimethylamine N-oxide (TMA/TMAO) profile, tandem mass spectrometry (MS/MS), urine, with algorithmic analysis and interpretive report

0257U Very long chain acyl-coenzyme A (CoA) dehydrogenase (VLCAD), leukocyte enzyme activity, whole blood

0258U Autoimmune (psoriasis), mRNA, next-generation sequencing, gene expression profiling of 50-100 genes, skin-surface collection using adhesive patch, algorithm reported as likelihood of response to psoriasis biologics

0259U Nephrology (chronic kidney disease), nuclear magnetic resonance spectroscopy measurement of myo-inositol, valine, and creatinine, algorithmically combined with cystatin C (by immunoassay) and demographic data to determine estimated glomerular filtration rate (GFR), serum, quantitative

0260U Rare diseases (constitutional/heritable disorders), identification of copy number variations, inversions, insertions, translocations, and other structural variants by optical genome mapping

0261U Oncology (colorectal cancer), image analysis with artificial intelligence assessment of 4 histologic and immunohistochemical features (CD3 and CD8 within tumor-stroma border and tumor core), tissue, reported as immune response and recurrence-risk score

0262U Oncology (solid tumor), gene expression profiling by real-time RT-PCR of 7 gene pathways (ER, AR, PI3K, MAPK, HH, TGFB, Notch), formalin-fixed paraffin-embedded (FFPE), algorithm reported as gene pathway activity score

0263U Neurology (autism spectrum disorder [ASD]), quantitative measurements of 16 central carbon metabolites (ie, α-ketoglutarate, alanine, lactate, phenylalanine, pyruvate, succinate, carnitine, citrate, fumarate, hypoxanthine, inosine, malate, S-sulfocysteine, taurine, urate, and xanthine), liquid chromatography tandem mass spectrometry (LC-MS/MS), plasma, algorithmic analysis with result reported as negative or positive (with metabolic subtypes of ASD)

0264U Rare diseases (constitutional/heritable disorders), identification of copy number variations, inversions, insertions, translocations, and other structural variants by optical genome mapping

0265U Rare constitutional and other heritable disorders, whole genome and mitochondrial DNA sequence analysis, blood, frozen and formalin-fixed paraffin-embedded (FFPE) tissue, saliva, buccal swabs or cell lines, identification of single nucleotide and copy number variants

0266U Unexplained constitutional or other heritable disorders or syndromes, tissue-specific gene expression by whole-transcriptome and next-generation sequencing, blood, formalin-fixed paraffin-embedded (FFPE) tissue or fresh frozen tissue, reported as presence or absence of splicing or expression changes

0267U Rare constitutional and other heritable disorders, identification of copy number variations, inversions, insertions, translocations, and other structural variants by optical genome mapping and whole genome sequencing

0268U Hematology (atypical hemolytic uremic syndrome [aHUS]), genomic sequence analysis of 15 genes, blood, buccal swab, or amniotic fluid

0269U Hematology (autosomal dominant congenital thrombocytopenia), genomic sequence analysis of 14 genes, blood, buccal swab, or amniotic fluid

0270U Hematology (congenital coagulation disorders), genomic sequence analysis of 20 genes, blood, buccal swab, or amniotic fluid

0271U Hematology (congenital neutropenia), genomic sequence analysis of 23 genes, blood, buccal swab, or amniotic fluid

0272U Hematology (genetic bleeding disorders), genomic sequence analysis of 51 genes, blood, buccal swab, or amniotic fluid, comprehensive

0273U Hematology (genetic hyperfibrinolysis, delayed bleeding), genomic sequence analysis of 8 genes (F13A1, F13B, FGA, FGB, FGG, SERPINA1, SERPINE1, SERPINF2, PLAU), blood, buccal swab, or amniotic fluid

0274U Hematology (genetic platelet disorders), genomic sequence analysis of 43 genes, blood, buccal swab, or amniotic fluid

0275U Hematology (heparin-induced thrombocytopenia), platelet antibody reactivity by flow cytometry, serum

0276U Hematology (inherited thrombocytopenia), genomic sequence analysis of 23 genes, blood, buccal swab, or amniotic fluid

0277U Hematology (genetic platelet function disorder), genomic sequence analysis of 31 genes, blood, buccal swab, or amniotic fluid

0278U Hematology (genetic thrombosis), genomic sequence analysis of 12 genes, blood, buccal swab, or amniotic fluid

0279U Hematology (von Willebrand disease [VWD]), von Willebrand factor (VWF) and collagen III binding by enzyme-linked immunosorbent assays (ELISA), plasma, report of collagen III binding

0280U Hematology (von Willebrand disease [VWD]), von Willebrand factor (VWF) and collagen IV binding by enzyme-linked immunosorbent assays (ELISA), plasma, report of collagen IV binding

0281U Hematology (von Willebrand disease [VWD]), von Willebrand propeptide, enzyme-linked immunosorbent assays (ELISA), plasma, diagnostic report of von Willebrand factor (VWF) propeptide antigen level

0282U Red blood cell antigen typing, DNA, genotyping of 12 blood group system genes to predict 44 red blood cell antigen phenotypes

0283U von Willebrand factor (VWF), type 2B, platelet-binding evaluation, radioimmunoassay, plasma

0284U von Willebrand factor (VWF), type 2N, factor VIII and VWF binding evaluation, enzyme-linked immunosorbent assays (ELISA), plasma

0640T Noncontact near-infrared spectroscopy studies of flap or wound (eg, for measurement of deoxyhemoglobin, oxyhemoglobin, and ratio of tissue oxygenation [StO2]); image acquisition, interpretation and report, each flap or wound

0641T Noncontact near-infrared spectroscopy studies of flap or wound (eg, for measurement of deoxyhemoglobin, oxyhemoglobin, and ratio of tissue oxygenation [StO2]); image acquisition only, each flap or wound

0642T Noncontact near-infrared spectroscopy studies of flap or wound (eg, for measurement of deoxyhemoglobin, oxyhemoglobin, and ratio of tissue oxygenation [StO2]); interpretation and report only, each flap or wound

0643T Transcatheter left ventricular restoration device implantation including right and left heart catheterization and left ventriculography when performed, arterial approach

0644T Transcatheter removal or debulking of intracardiac mass (eg, vegetations, thrombus) via suction (eg, vacuum, aspiration) device, percutaneous approach, with intraoperative reinfusion of aspirated blood, including imaging guidance, when performed

0645T Transcatheter implantation of coronary sinus reduction device including vascular access and closure, right heart catheterization, venous angiography, coronary sinus angiography, imaging guidance, and supervision and interpretation, when performed

0646T Transcatheter tricuspid valve implantation/replacement (TTVI) with prosthetic valve, percutaneous approach, including right heart catheterization, temporary pacemaker insertion, and selective right ventricular or right atrial angiography, when performed

0647T Insertion of gastrostomy tube, percutaneous, with magnetic gastropexy, under ultrasound guidance, image documentation and report

0648T Quantitative magnetic resonance for analysis of tissue composition (eg, fat, iron, water content), including multiparametric data acquisition, data preparation and transmission, interpretation and report, obtained without diagnostic MRI examination of the same anatomy (eg, organ, gland, tissue, target structure) during the same session

0649T Quantitative magnetic resonance for analysis of tissue composition (eg, fat, iron, water content), including multiparametric data acquisition, data preparation and transmission, interpretation and report, obtained with diagnostic MRI examination of the same anatomy (eg, organ, gland, tissue, target structure) (List separately in addition to code for primary procedure)

0650T Programming device evaluation (remote) of subcutaneous cardiac rhythm monitor system, with iterative adjustment of the implantable device to test the function of the device and select optimal permanently programmed values with analysis, review and report by a physician or other qualified health care professional

0651T Magnetically controlled capsule endoscopy, esophagus through stomach, including intraprocedural positioning of capsule, with interpretation and report

0652T Esophagogastroduodenoscopy, flexible, transnasal; diagnostic, including collection of specimen(s) by brushing or washing, when performed (separate procedure)

0653T Esophagogastroduodenoscopy, flexible, transnasal; with biopsy, single or multiple

0654T Esophagogastroduodenoscopy, flexible, transnasal; with insertion of intraluminal tube or catheter

0655T Transperineal focal laser ablation of malignant prostate tissue, including transrectal imaging guidance, with MR-fused images or other enhanced ultrasound imaging

0656T Vertebral body tethering, anterior; up to 7 vertebral segments

0657T Vertebral body tethering, anterior; 8 or more vertebral segments

0658T Electrical impedance spectroscopy of 1 or more skin lesions for automated melanoma risk score

0659T Transcatheter intracoronary infusion of supersaturated oxygen in conjunction with percutaneous coronary revascularization during acute myocardial infarction, including catheter placement, imaging guidance (eg, fluoroscopy), angiography, and radiologic supervision and interpretation

0660T Implantation of anterior segment intraocular nonbiodegradable drug-eluting system, internal approach

0661T Removal and reimplantation of anterior segment intraocular nonbiodegradable drug-eluting implant

0662T Scalp cooling, mechanical; initial measurement and calibration of cap

0663T Scalp cooling, mechanical; placement of device, monitoring, and removal of device (List separately in addition to code for primary procedure)

0664T Donor hysterectomy (including cold preservation); open, from cadaver donor

0665T Donor hysterectomy (including cold preservation); open, from living donor

0666T Donor hysterectomy (including cold preservation); laparoscopic or robotic, from living donor

0667T Donor hysterectomy (including cold preservation); recipient uterus allograft transplantation from cadaver or living donor

0668T Backbench standard preparation of cadaver or living donor uterine allograft prior to transplantation, including dissection and removal of surrounding soft tissues and preparation of uterine vein(s) and uterine artery(ies), as necessary

0669T Backbench reconstruction of cadaver or living donor uterus allograft prior to transplantation; venous anastomosis, each

0670T Backbench reconstruction of cadaver or living donor uterus allograft prior to transplantation; arterial anastomosis, each

0671T Insertion of anterior segment aqueous drainage device into the trabecular meshwork, without external reservoir, and without concomitant cataract removal, one or more

0672T Endovaginal cryogen-cooled, monopolar radiofrequency remodeling of the tissues surrounding the female bladder neck and proximal urethra for urinary incontinence

0673T Ablation, benign thyroid nodule(s), percutaneous, laser, including imaging guidance

0674T Laparoscopic insertion of new or replacement of permanent implantable synchronized diaphragmatic stimulation system for augmentation of cardiac function, including an implantable pulse generator and diaphragmatic lead(s)

0675T Laparoscopic insertion of new or replacement of diaphragmatic lead(s), permanent implantable synchronized diaphragmatic stimulation system for augmentation of cardiac function, including connection to an existing pulse generator; first lead

0676T Laparoscopic insertion of new or replacement of diaphragmatic lead(s), permanent implantable synchronized diaphragmatic stimulation system for augmentation of cardiac function, including connection to an existing pulse generator; each additional lead (List separately in addition to code for primary procedure)

0677T Laparoscopic repositioning of diaphragmatic lead(s), permanent implantable synchronized diaphragmatic stimulation system for augmentation of cardiac function, including connection to an existing pulse generator; first repositioned lead

0678T Laparoscopic repositioning of diaphragmatic lead(s), permanent implantable synchronized diaphragmatic stimulation system for augmentation of cardiac function, including connection to an existing pulse generator; each additional repositioned lead (List separately in addition to code for primary procedure)

0679T Laparoscopic removal of diaphragmatic lead(s), permanent implantable synchronized diaphragmatic stimulation system for augmentation of cardiac function

0680T Insertion or replacement of pulse generator only, permanent implantable synchronized diaphragmatic stimulation system for augmentation of cardiac function, with connection to existing lead(s)

0681T Relocation of pulse generator only, permanent implantable synchronized diaphragmatic stimulation system for augmentation of cardiac function, with connection to existing dual leads

0682T Removal of pulse generator only, permanent implantable synchronized diaphragmatic stimulation system for augmentation of cardiac function

0683T Programming device evaluation (in-person) with iterative adjustment of the implantable device to test the function of the device and select optimal permanent programmed values with analysis, review and report by a physician or other qualified health care professional, permanent implantable synchronized diaphragmatic stimulation system for augmentation of cardiac function

0684T Peri-procedural device evaluation (in-person) and programming of device system parameters before or after a surgery, procedure, or test with analysis, review, and report by a physician or other qualified health care professional, permanent implantable synchronized diaphragmatic stimulation system for augmentation of cardiac function

0685T Interrogation device evaluation (in-person) with analysis, review and report by a physician or other qualified health care professional, including connection, recording and disconnection per patient encounter, permanent implantable synchronized diaphragmatic stimulation system for augmentation of cardiac function

0686T Histotripsy (ie, non-thermal ablation via acoustic energy delivery) of malignant hepatocellular tissue, including image guidance

0687T Treatment of amblyopia using an online digital program; device supply, educational set-up, and initial session

0688T Treatment of amblyopia using an online digital program; assessment of patient performance and program data by physician or other qualified health care professional, with report, per calendar month

0689T Quantitative ultrasound tissue characterization (non-elastographic), including interpretation and report, obtained without diagnostic ultrasound examination of the same anatomy (eg, organ, gland, tissue, target structure)

0690T Quantitative ultrasound tissue characterization (non-elastographic), including interpretation and report, obtained with diagnostic ultrasound examination of the same anatomy (eg, organ, gland, tissue, target structure) (List separately in addition to code for primary procedure)

0691T Automated analysis of an existing computed tomography study for vertebral fracture(s), including assessment of bone density when performed, data preparation, interpretation, and report

0692T Therapeutic ultrafiltration

0693T Comprehensive full body computer-based markerless 3D kinematic and kinetic motion analysis and report

0694T 3-dimensional volumetric imaging and reconstruction of breast or axillary lymph node tissue, each excised specimen, 3-dimensional automatic specimen reorientation, interpretation and report, real-time intraoperative

0695T Body surface–activation mapping of pacemaker or pacing cardioverter-defibrillator lead(s) to optimize electrical synchrony, cardiac resynchronization therapy device, including connection, recording, disconnection, review, and report; at time of implant or replacement

0696T Body surface–activation mapping of pacemaker or pacing cardioverter-defibrillator lead(s) to optimize electrical synchrony, cardiac resynchronization therapy device, including connection, recording, disconnection, review, and report; at time of follow-up interrogation or programming device evaluation

0697T multiple organs

0698T multiple organs (List separately in addition to code for primary procedure)

0699T Injection, posterior chamber of eye, medication

0700T Molecular fluorescent imaging of suspicious nevus; first lesion

0701T Molecular fluorescent imaging of suspicious nevus; each additional lesion (List separately in addition to code for primary procedure)

0702T Remote therapeutic monitoring of a standardized online digital cognitive behavioral therapy program ordered by a physician or other qualified health care professional; supply and technical support, per 30 days

0703T Remote therapeutic monitoring of a standardized online digital cognitive behavioral therapy program ordered by a physician or other qualified health care professional; management services by physician or other qualified health care professional, per calendar month

0704T Remote treatment of amblyopia using an eye tracking device; device supply with initial set-up and patient education on use of equipment

0705T Remote treatment of amblyopia using an eye tracking device; surveillance center technical support including data transmission with analysis, with a minimum of 18 training hours, each 30 days

0706T Remote treatment of amblyopia using an eye tracking device; interpretation and report by physician or other qualified health care professional, per calendar month

0707T Injection(s), bone substitute material (eg, calcium phosphate) into subchondral bone defect (ie, bone marrow lesion, bone bruise, stress injury, microtrabecular fracture), including imaging guidance and arthroscopic assistance for joint visualization

0708T Intradermal cancer immunotherapy; preparation and initial injection

0709T Intradermal cancer immunotherapy; each additional injection (List separately in addition to code for primary procedure)

0710T Noninvasive arterial plaque analysis using software processing of data from non-coronary computerized tomography angiography; including data preparation and transmission, quantification of the structure and composition of the vessel wall and assessment for lipid-rich necrotic core plaque to assess atherosclerotic plaque stability, data review, interpretation and report

0711T Noninvasive arterial plaque analysis using software processing of data from non-coronary computerized tomography angiography; data preparation and transmission

0712T Noninvasive arterial plaque analysis using software processing of data from non-coronary computerized tomography angiography; quantification of the structure and composition of the vessel wall and assessment for lipid-rich necrotic core plaque to assess atherosclerotic plaque stability

0713T Noninvasive arterial plaque analysis using software processing of data from non-coronary computerized tomography angiography; data review, interpretation and report

0017M Oncology (diffuse large B-cell lymphoma [DLBCL]), mRNA, gene expression profiling by fluorescent probe hybridization of 20 genes, formalin-fixed paraffin-embedded tissue, algorithm reported as cell of origin

0018M Transplantation medicine (allograft rejection, renal), measurement of donor and third-party-induced CD154+T-cytotoxic memory cells, utilizing whole peripheral blood, algorithm reported as a rejection risk score

Revised Codes

11981 Insertion, ~~non-biodegradable~~ drug-delivery implant (ie, bioresorbable, biodegradable, non-biodegradable)

21315 Closed treatment of nasal bone fracture with manipulation; without stabilization

21320 Closed treatment of nasal bone fracture with manipulation; with~~out~~ stabilization

22600 Arthrodesis, posterior or posterolateral technique, single ~~level~~ interspace; cervical below C2 segment

22610 Arthrodesis, posterior or posterolateral technique, single ~~level~~ interspace; thoracic (with lateral transverse technique, when performed)

22612 Arthrodesis, posterior or posterolateral technique, single ~~level~~ interspace; lumbar (with lateral transverse technique, when performed)

22614 Arthrodesis, posterior or posterolateral technique, single level interspace; each additional ~~vertebral segment~~ interspace (List separately in addition to code for primary procedure)

22633 Arthrodesis, combined posterior or posterolateral technique with posterior interbody technique including laminectomy and/or discectomy sufficient to prepare interspace (other than for decompression), single interspace ~~and segment~~; lumbar

22634 Arthrodesis, combined posterior or posterolateral technique with posterior interbody technique including laminectomy and/or discectomy sufficient to prepare interspace (other than for decompression), single interspace and segment; each additional interspace ~~and segment~~ (List separately in addition to code for primary procedure)

33471 Valvotomy, pulmonary valve, closed heart~~;~~, via pulmonary artery

35600 Harvest of upper extremity artery, 1 segment, for coronary artery bypass procedure, open ~~(List separately in addition to code for primary procedure)~~

54340 Repair of hypospadias complication(s) (ie, fistula, stricture, diverticula); by closure, incision, or excision, simple

54344 Repair of hypospadias complication(s) (ie, fistula, stricture, diverticula); requiring mobilization of skin flaps and urethroplasty with flap or patch graft

54348 Repair of hypospadias complication(s) (ie, fistula, stricture, diverticula); requiring extensive dissection, and urethroplasty with flap, patch or tubed graft (include inges urinary diversion, when performed)

54352 Revision of prior hypospadias repair~~Repair of hypospadias cripple~~ requiring extensive dissection and excision of previously constructed structures including re-release of chordee and reconstruction of urethra and penis by use of local skin as grafts and island flaps and skin brought in as flaps or grafts

63048 Laminectomy, facetectomy and foraminotomy (unilateral or bilateral with decompression of spinal cord, cauda equina and/or nerve root[s], [eg, spinal or lateral recess stenosis]), single vertebral segment; each additional vertebral segment, cervical, thoracic, or lumbar (List separately in addition to code for primary procedure)

63197 Laminectomy with cordotomy, with section of both spinothalamic tracts, 1 stage~~;~~, thoracic

64568 ~~Incision for~~ Open implantation of cranial nerve (eg, vagus nerve) neurostimulator electrode array and pulse generator

64575 ~~Incision for~~ Open implantation of neurostimulator electrode array; peripheral nerve (excludes sacral nerve)

64580 ~~Incision for~~ Open implantation of neurostimulator electrode array; neuromuscular

64581 ~~Incision for~~ Open implantation of neurostimulator electrode array; sacral nerve (transforaminal placement)

67141 Prophylaxis of retinal detachment (eg, retinal break, lattice degeneration) without drainage, ~~1 or more sessions~~; cryotherapy, diathermy

67145 Prophylaxis of retinal detachment (eg, retinal break, lattice degeneration) without drainage, ~~1 or more sessions~~; photocoagulation ~~(laser or xenon arc)~~

69714 Implantation, osseointegrated implant, ~~temporal bone~~ skull~~, with percutaneous attachment to external speech processor/cochlear stimulator;without mastoidectomy~~ with percutaneous attachment to external speech processor

69717 Revision or r~~R~~eplacement (including removal of existing device), osseointegrated implant, ~~temporal bone~~ skull, ~~with percutaneous attachment to external speech processor/cochlear stimulator;~~ with percutaneous attachment to external speech processor~~without mastoidectomy~~

75573 Computed tomography, heart, with contrast material, for evaluation of cardiac structure and morphology in the setting of congenital heart disease (including 3D image postprocessing, assessment of left ventricular [LV] cardiac function, right ventricular [RV] structure and function and evaluation of ~~venous~~ vascular structures, if performed)

81228 Cytogenomic ~~constitutional~~ (genome-wide) ~~microarray~~ analysis for constitutional chromosomal abnormalities; interrogation of genomic regions for copy number variants~~, (eg, bacterial artificial chromosome [BAC] or oligo-based comparative~~ genomic hybridization (~~[~~CGH~~]~~) microarray analysis)

81229 Cytogenomic ~~constitutional~~ (genome-wide) ~~microarray~~ analysis for constitutional chromosomal abnormalities; interrogation of genomic regions for copy number and single nucleotide polymorphism (SNP) variants~~, for chromosomal abnormalities~~ comparative genomic hybridization (CGH) microarray analysis

81405 Molecular pathology procedure, Level 6 (eg, analysis of 6-10 exons by DNA sequence analysis, mutation scanning or duplication/deletion variants of 11-25 exons, regionally targeted cytogenomic array analysis)

82656 Elastase, pancreatic (EL-1), fecal~~, qualitative or semi-quantitative~~ ; qualitative or semi-quantitative

87301 Infectious agent antigen detection by immunoassay technique, (eg, enzyme immunoassay [EIA], enzyme-linked immunosorbent assay [ELISA], fluorescence immunoassay [FIA], immunochemiluminometric assay [IMCA]), qualitative or semiquantitative, ~~multiple-step method~~; adenovirus enteric types 40/41

87305 Infectious agent antigen detection by immunoassay technique, (eg, enzyme immunoassay [EIA], enzyme-linked immunosorbent assay [ELISA], fluorescence immunoassay [FIA], immunochemiluminometric assay [IMCA]), qualitative or semiquantitative~~, multiple-step method~~; Aspergillus

87320 Infectious agent antigen detection by immunoassay technique, (eg, enzyme immunoassay [EIA], enzyme-linked immunosorbent assay [ELISA], fluorescence immunoassay [FIA], immunochemiluminometric assay [IMCA]), qualitative or semiquantitative~~, multiple-step method~~; Chlamydia trachomatis

87324 Infectious agent antigen detection by immunoassay technique, (eg, enzyme immunoassay [EIA], enzyme-linked immunosorbent assay [ELISA], fluorescence immunoassay [FIA], immunochemiluminometric assay [IMCA]), qualitative or semiquantitative~~, multiple-step method~~; Clostridium difficile toxin(s)

87327 Infectious agent antigen detection by immunoassay technique, (eg, enzyme immunoassay [EIA], enzyme-linked immunosorbent assay [ELISA], fluorescence immunoassay [FIA], immunochemiluminometric assay [IMCA]), qualitative or semiquantitative~~, multiple-step method~~; Cryptococcus neoformans

87328 Infectious agent antigen detection by immunoassay technique, (eg, enzyme immunoassay [EIA], enzyme-linked immunosorbent assay [ELISA], fluorescence immunoassay [FIA], immunochemiluminometric assay [IMCA]), qualitative or semiquantitative~~, multiple-step method~~; cryptosporidium

87329 Infectious agent antigen detection by immunoassay technique, (eg, enzyme immunoassay [EIA], enzyme-linked immunosorbent assay [ELISA], fluorescence immunoassay [FIA], immunochemiluminometric assay [IMCA]), qualitative or semiquantitative~~, multiple-step method~~; giardia

87332 Infectious agent antigen detection by immunoassay technique, (eg, enzyme immunoassay [EIA], enzyme-linked immunosorbent assay [ELISA], fluorescence immunoassay [FIA], immunochemiluminometric assay [IMCA]), qualitative or semiquantitative~~, multiple-step method~~; cytomegalovirus

87335 Infectious agent antigen detection by immunoassay technique, (eg, enzyme immunoassay [EIA], enzyme-linked immunosorbent assay [ELISA], fluorescence immunoassay [FIA], immunochemiluminometric assay [IMCA]), qualitative or semiquantitative~~, multiple-step method~~; Escherichia coli 0157

87336 Infectious agent antigen detection by immunoassay technique, (eg, enzyme immunoassay [EIA], enzyme-linked immunosorbent assay [ELISA], fluorescence immunoassay [FIA], immunochemiluminometric assay [IMCA]), qualitative or semiquantitative~~, multiple-step method~~; Entamoeba histolytica dispar group

87337 Infectious agent antigen detection by immunoassay technique, (eg, enzyme immunoassay [EIA], enzyme-linked immunosorbent assay [ELISA], fluorescence immunoassay [FIA], immunochemiluminometric assay [IMCA]), qualitative or semiquantitative~~, multiple-step method~~; Entamoeba histolytica group

87338 Infectious agent antigen detection by immunoassay technique, (eg, enzyme immunoassay [EIA], enzyme-linked immunosorbent assay [ELISA], fluorescence immunoassay [FIA], immunochemiluminometric assay [IMCA]), qualitative or semiquantitative~~, multiple-step method~~; Helicobacter pylori, stool

87339 Infectious agent antigen detection by immunoassay technique, (eg, enzyme immunoassay [EIA], enzyme-linked immunosorbent assay [ELISA], fluorescence immunoassay [FIA], immunochemiluminometric assay [IMCA]), qualitative or semiquantitative~~, multiple-step method~~; Helicobacter pylori

87340 Infectious agent antigen detection by immunoassay technique, (eg, enzyme immunoassay [EIA], enzyme-linked immunosorbent assay [ELISA], fluorescence immunoassay [FIA], immunochemiluminometric assay [IMCA]), qualitative or semiquantitative~~, multiple-step method~~; hepatitis B surface antigen (HBsAg)

87341 Infectious agent antigen detection by immunoassay technique, (eg, enzyme immunoassay [EIA], enzyme-linked immunosorbent assay [ELISA], fluorescence immunoassay [FIA], immunochemiluminometric assay [IMCA]), qualitative or semiquantitative~~, multiple-step method~~; hepatitis B surface antigen (HBsAg) neutralization

87350 Infectious agent antigen detection by immunoassay technique, (eg, enzyme immunoassay [EIA], enzyme-linked immunosorbent assay [ELISA], fluorescence immunoassay [FIA], immunochemiluminometric assay [IMCA]), qualitative or semiquantitative~~, multiple-step method~~; hepatitis Be antigen (HBeAg)

87380 Infectious agent antigen detection by immunoassay technique, (eg, enzyme immunoassay [EIA], enzyme-linked immunosorbent assay [ELISA], fluorescence immunoassay [FIA], immunochemiluminometric assay [IMCA]), qualitative or semiquantitative~~, multiple-step method~~; hepatitis, delta agent

87385 Infectious agent antigen detection by immunoassay technique, (eg, enzyme immunoassay [EIA], enzyme-linked immunosorbent assay [ELISA], fluorescence immunoassay [FIA], immunochemiluminometric assay [IMCA]), qualitative or semiquantitative~~, multiple-step method~~; Histoplasma capsulatum

87389 Infectious agent antigen detection by immunoassay technique, (eg, enzyme immunoassay [EIA], enzyme-linked immunosorbent assay [ELISA], fluorescence immunoassay [FIA], immunochemiluminometric assay [IMCA]), qualitative or semiquantitative~~, multiple-step method~~; HIV-1 antigen(s), with HIV-1 and HIV-2 antibodies, single result

87390 Infectious agent antigen detection by immunoassay technique, (eg, enzyme immunoassay [EIA], enzyme-linked immunosorbent assay [ELISA], fluorescence immunoassay [FIA], immunochemiluminometric assay [IMCA]), qualitative or semiquantitative~~, multiple-step method~~; HIV-1

87391 Infectious agent antigen detection by immunoassay technique, (eg, enzyme immunoassay [EIA], enzyme-linked immunosorbent assay [ELISA], fluorescence immunoassay [FIA], immunochemiluminometric assay [IMCA]), qualitative or semiquantitative~~, multiple-step method~~; HIV-2

87400 Infectious agent antigen detection by immunoassay technique, (eg, enzyme immunoassay [EIA], enzyme-linked immunosorbent assay [ELISA], fluorescence immunoassay [FIA], immunochemiluminometric assay [IMCA]), qualitative or semiquantitative~~, multiple-step method~~; Influenza, A or B, each

87420 Infectious agent antigen detection by immunoassay technique, (eg, enzyme immunoassay [EIA], enzyme-linked immunosorbent assay [ELISA], fluorescence immunoassay [FIA], immunochemiluminometric assay [IMCA]), qualitative or semiquantitative~~, multiple-step method~~; respiratory syncytial virus

87425 Infectious agent antigen detection by immunoassay technique, (eg, enzyme immunoassay [EIA], enzyme-linked immunosorbent assay [ELISA], fluorescence immunoassay [FIA], immunochemiluminometric assay [IMCA]), qualitative or semiquantitative~~, multiple-step method~~; rotavirus

87426 Infectious agent antigen detection by immunoassay technique, (eg, enzyme immunoassay [EIA], enzyme-linked immunosorbent assay [ELISA], fluorescence immunoassay [FIA], immunochemiluminometric assay [IMCA]), qualitative or semiquantitative~~, multiple-step method~~; severe acute respiratory syndrome coronavirus (eg, SARS-CoV, SARS-CoV-2 [COVID-19])

87427 Infectious agent antigen detection by immunoassay technique, (eg, enzyme immunoassay [EIA], enzyme-linked immunosorbent assay [ELISA], fluorescence immunoassay [FIA], immunochemiluminometric assay [IMCA]), qualitative or semiquantitative~~, multiple-step method~~; Shiga-like toxin

87430 Infectious agent antigen detection by immunoassay technique, (eg, enzyme immunoassay [EIA], enzyme-linked immunosorbent assay [ELISA], fluorescence immunoassay [FIA], immunochemiluminometric assay [IMCA]), qualitative or semiquantitative~~, multiple-step method~~; Streptococcus, group A

87449 ~~Infectious agent antigen detection by immunoassay technique, (eg, enzyme immunoassay [EIA], enzymelinked immunosorbent assay [ELISA], immunochemiluminometric assay [IMCA]), qualitative or semiquantitative; multiple-step method,~~; not otherwise specified, each organism

87451 ~~Infectious agent antigen detection by immunoassay technique, (eg, enzyme immunoassay [EIA], enzymelinked immunosorbent assay [ELISA], immunochemiluminometric assay [IMCA]), qualitative or semiquantitative; multiple-step method,~~; polyvalent for multiple organisms, each polyvalent antiserum

87802 Infectious agent antigen detection by immunoassay with direct optical (ie, visual) observation; Streptococcus, group B

87803 Infectious agent antigen detection by immunoassay with direct optical (ie, visual) observation; Clostridium difficile toxin A

87804 Infectious agent antigen detection by immunoassay with direct optical (ie, visual) observation; Influenza

87806 Infectious agent antigen detection by immunoassay with direct optical (ie, visual) observation; HIV-1 antigen(s), with HIV-1 and HIV-2 antibodies

87807 Infectious agent antigen detection by immunoassay with direct optical (ie, visual) observation; respiratory syncytial virus

87808 Infectious agent antigen detection by immunoassay with direct optical (ie, visual) observation; Trichomonas vaginalis

87809 Infectious agent antigen detection by immunoassay with direct optical (ie, visual) observation; adenovirus

87810 Infectious agent antigen detection by immunoassay with direct optical (ie, visual) observation; Chlamydia trachomatis

87850 Infectious agent antigen detection by immunoassay with direct optical (ie, visual) observation; Neisseria gonorrhoeae

87880 Infectious agent antigen detection by immunoassay with direct optical (ie, visual) observation; Streptococcus, group A

87899 Infectious agent antigen detection by immunoassay with direct optical (ie, visual) observation; not otherwise specified

92065 Orthoptic ~~and/or pleoptic~~ training~~, with continuing medical direction and evaluation~~

93653 Comprehensive electrophysiologic evaluation ~~including~~ with insertion and repositioning of multiple electrode catheters, ~~with~~ induction or attempted induction of an arrhythmia with right atrial pacing and recording and catheter ablation of arrhythmogenic focus, including intracardiac electrophysiologic 3-dimensional mapping, right ventricular pacing and recording ~~(when necessary)~~, left atrial pacing and recording from coronary sinus or left atrium, and His bundle recording , when performed ~~(when necessary) with intracardiac catheter ablation of arrhythmogenic focus~~; with treatment of supraventricular tachycardia by ablation of fast or slow atrioventricular pathway, accessory atrioventricular connection, cavo-tricuspid isthmus or other single atrial focus or source of atrial re-entry

93654 Comprehensive electrophysiologic evaluation ~~including~~ with insertion and repositioning of multiple electrode catheters, ~~with~~ induction or attempted induction of an arrhythmia with right atrial pacing and recording and catheter ablation of arrhythmogenic focus, including intracardiac electrophysiologic 3-dimensional mapping, right ventricular pacing and recording ~~(when necessary)~~, left atrial pacing and recording from coronary sinus or left atrium, and His bundle recording , when performed ~~(when necessary) with intracardiac catheter ablation of arrhythmogenic focus~~; with treatment of ventricular tachycardia or focus of ventricular ectopy including ~~intracardiac electrophysiologic 3D mapping, when performed, and~~ left ventricular pacing and recording, when performed

93656 Comprehensive electrophysiologic evaluation including transseptal catheterizations, insertion and repositioning of multiple electrode catheters with intracardiac catheter ablation of atrial fibrillation by pulmonary vein isolation, including intracardiac electrophysiologic 3-dimensional mapping, intracardiac echocardiography including imaging supervision and interpretation, induction or attempted induction of an arrhythmia including left or right atrial pacing/recording when necessary, right ventricular pacing/recording ~~when necessary~~, and His bundle recording, when ~~necessary~~ performed~~with intracardiac catheter ablation of atrial fibrillation by pulmonary vein isolation~~

99072 Additional supplies, materials, and clinical staff time over and above those usually included in an office visit or other nonfacility service(s), when performed during a Public Health Emergency, as defined by law, due to respiratory-transmitted infectious disease

99211 Office or other outpatient visit for the evaluation and management of an established patient, that may not require the presence of a physician or other qualified health care professional. ~~Usually, the presenting problem(s) are minimal.~~

99439 Chronic care management services with the following required elements: multiple (two or more) chronic conditions expected to last at least 12 months, or until the death of the patient, chronic conditions that place the patient at significant risk of death, acute exacerbation/decompensation, or functional decline, comprehensive care plan established, implemented, revised, or monitored; each additional 20 minutes of clinical staff time directed by a physician or other qualified health care professional, per calendar month (List separately in addition to code for primary procedure)

99483 Assessment of and care planning for a patient with cognitive impairment, requiring an independent historian, in the office or other outpatient, home or domiciliary or rest home, with all of the following required elements: Cognition-focused evaluation including a pertinent history and examination~~,~~; Medical decision making of moderate or high complexity~~,~~; Functional assessment (eg, basic and instrumental activities of daily living), including decision-making capacity~~,~~; Use of standardized instruments for staging of dementia (eg, functional assessment staging test [FAST], clinical dementia rating [CDR])~~,~~; Medication reconciliation and review for high-risk medications~~,~~; Evaluation for neuropsychiatric and behavioral symptoms, including depression, including use of standardized screening instrument(s) ~~,~~; Evaluation of safety (eg, home), including motor vehicle operation~~,~~; Identification of caregiver(s), caregiver knowledge, caregiver needs, social supports, and the willingness of caregiver to take on caregiving tasks~~,~~; Development, updating or revision, or review of an Advance Care Plan~~,~~; Creation of a written care plan, including initial plans to address any neuropsychiatric symptoms, neuro-cognitive symptoms, functional limitations, and referral to community resources as needed (eg, rehabilitation services, adult day programs, support groups) shared with the patient and/or caregiver with initial education and support. Typically, 50 minutes are spent face-to-face with the patient and/or family or caregiver.

99484 Care management services for behavioral health conditions, at least 20 minutes of clinical staff time, directed by a physician or other qualified health care professional, per calendar month, with the following required elements: initial assessment or follow-up monitoring, including the use of applicable validated rating scales~~,~~; behavioral health care planning in relation to behavioral/psychiatric health problems, including revision for patients who are not progressing or whose status changes~~,~~; facilitating and coordinating treatment such as psychotherapy, pharmacotherapy, counseling and/or psychiatric consultation~~,~~; and continuity of care with a designated member of the care team.

99487 Complex chronic care management services with the following required elements: multiple (two or more) chronic conditions expected to last at least 12 months, or until the death of the patient, chronic conditions that place the patient at significant risk of death, acute exacerbation/decompensation, or functional decline, comprehensive care plan established, implemented, revised, or monitored, moderate or high complexity medical decision making; first 60 minutes of clinical staff time directed by a physician or other qualified health care professional, per calendar month.

99489 Complex chronic care management services with the following required elements: multiple (two or more) chronic conditions expected to last at least 12 months, or until the death of the patient, chronic conditions that place the patient at significant risk of death, acute exacerbation/decompensation, or functional decline, comprehensive care plan established, implemented, revised, or monitored, moderate or high complexity medical decision making; each additional 30 minutes of clinical staff time directed by a physician or other qualified health care professional, per calendar month (List separately in addition to code for primary procedure)

99490 Chronic care management services with the following required elements: multiple (two or more) chronic conditions expected to last at least 12 months, or until the death of the patient, chronic conditions that place the patient at significant risk of death, acute exacerbation/decompensation, or functional decline, comprehensive care plan established, implemented, revised, or monitored; first 20 minutes of clinical staff time directed by a physician or other qualified health care professional, per calendar month.

99491 Chronic care management services, ~~provided personally by a physician or other qualified health care professional, at least 30 minutes of physician or other qualified health care professional time, per calendar month,~~ with the following required elements: multiple (two or more) chronic conditions expected to last at least 12 months, or until the death of the patient]~~),~~; chronic conditions that place the patient at significant risk of death, acute exacerbation/decompensation, or functional decline~~,~~ ; comprehensive care plan established, implemented, revised, or monitored])~~,~~ ; first 30 minutes provided personally by a physician or other qualified health care professional, per calendar month.

99492 Initial psychiatric collaborative care management, first 70 minutes in the first calendar month of behavioral health care manager activities, in consultation with a psychiatric consultant, and directed by the treating physician or other qualified health care professional, with the following required elements: outreach to and engagement in treatment of a patient directed by the treating physician or other qualified health care professional])~~,~~ ; initial assessment of the patient, including administration of validated rating scales, with the development of an individualized treatment plan~~,~~ ; review by the psychiatric consultant with modifications of the plan if recommended])~~,~~ ; entering patient in a registry and tracking patient follow-up and progress using the registry, with appropriate documentation, and participation in weekly caseload consultation with the psychiatric consultant])~~,~~ ; and provision of brief interventions using evidence-based techniques such as behavioral activation, motivational interviewing, and other focused treatment strategies.

99493 Subsequent psychiatric collaborative care management, first 60 minutes in a subsequent month of behavioral health care manager activities, in consultation with a psychiatric consultant, and directed by the treating physician or other qualified health care professional, with the following required elements: tracking patient follow-up and progress using the registry, with appropriate documentation])~~,~~ ; participation in weekly caseload consultation with the psychiatric consultant~~,~~ ; ongoing collaboration with and coordination of the patient's mental health care with the treating physician or other qualified health care professional and any other treating mental health providers~~,~~ ; additional review of progress and recommendations for changes in treatment, as indicated, including medications, based on recommendations provided by the psychiatric consultant~~,~~ ; provision of brief interventions using evidence-based techniques such as behavioral activation, motivational interviewing, and other focused treatment strategies~~,~~ ; monitoring of patient outcomes using validated rating scales~~,~~ ; and relapse prevention planning with patients as they achieve remission of symptoms and/or other treatment goals and are prepared for discharge from active treatment.

0101T Extracorporeal shock wave involving musculoskeletal system, not otherwise specified~~, high energy~~

0102T Extracorporeal shock wave~~, high energy,~~ performed by a physician, requiring anesthesia other than local, and involving the lateral humeral epicondyle

0493T Contact ~~N~~ near-infrared spectroscopy studies of lower extremity wounds (eg, for oxyhemoglobin measurement)

0512T Extracorporeal shock wave for integumentary wound healing , ~~high energy,~~ including topical application and dressing care; initial wound

0513T Extracorporeal shock wave for integumentary wound healing, ~~high energy,~~ including topical application and dressing care; each additional wound (List separately in addition to code for primary procedure)

0646T Transcatheter tricuspid valve implantation (TTVI)/replacement ~~(TTVI)~~ with prosthetic valve, percutaneous approach, including right heart catheterization, temporary pacemaker insertion, and selective right ventricular or right atrial angiography, when performed

0648T Quantitative magnetic resonance for analysis of tissue composition (eg, fat, iron, water content), including multiparametric data acquisition, data preparation and transmission, interpretation and report, obtained without diagnostic MRI examination of the same anatomy (eg, organ, gland, tissue, target structure) during the same session; single organ

0649T Quantitative magnetic resonance for analysis of tissue composition (eg, fat, iron, water content), including multiparametric data acquisition, data preparation and transmission, interpretation and report, obtained with diagnostic MRI examination of the same anatomy (eg, organ, gland, tissue, target structure); single organ (List separately in addition to code for primary procedure)

0051U Prescription drug monitoring, evaluation of drugs present by liquid chromatography tandem mass spectrometry (LC-MS/MS),urine or blood, 31 drug panel, reported as quantitative results, detected or not detected, per date of service

0152U Infectious disease (bacteria, fungi, parasites, and DNA viruses), microbial cell-free DNA, ~~PCR and~~ plasma, untargeted next-generation sequencing, ~~plasma, detection of >1,000 potential microbial organisms~~ report for significant positive pathogens

Deleted Codes

01935	01936	21310	33470	33722	43850	43855
59135	63194	63195	63196	63198	63199	69715
69718	72275	76101	76102	80500	80502	87450
92559	92560	92561	92564	93530	93531	93532
92533	93561	93562	95943	0191T	0290T	0355T
0356T	0376T	0423T	0451T	0452T	0453T	0454T
0455T	0456T	0457T	0458T	0459T	0460T	0461T
0462T	0463T	0466T	0467T	0468T	0548T	0549T
0550T	0551T	0098U	0099U	0100U	0139U	0168U

Resequenced Icon Added

33267	33268	33269	63052	63053	64628	64629
66989	66991	69714	69716	69717	69719	69726
69727	80220	81349	82653	83529	86015	86051
86052	86053	86362	86363	86364	86408	86409
86413	87154	87428	87806	87811	90626	90627
90677	90758	90759	91113	91300	91301	91302
91303	91304	91305	91306	91307	93319	99424
99425	99426	99427	99437	0640T	0641T	0642T
0643T	0646T	0671T	0697T	0698T		

Web Release New, Revised, and Deleted Codes

Codes indicated as "Web Release" codes indicate CPT codes that are in *Current Procedural Coding Expert* for the current year, but will not be in the AMA CPT book until the following year. This can also include those codes designated by the AMA as new or revised for 2022 but that actually appeared in the 2021 Optum360 book. These codes will have the appropriate new or revised icon appended to match the CPT code book, however. See the complete list that follows:

New codes, deleted codes, and revisions to codes in the 2022 *Current Procedural Coding Expert* that will not appear in the CPT code book until 2023

These codes are indicated with the following icons: ● ▲ These icons will be green in the body of the book.

New Codes

0285U Oncology, response to radiation, cell-free DNA, quantitative branched chain DNA amplification, plasma, reported as a radiation toxicity score

0286U *CEP72 (centrosomal protein, 72-KDa), NUDT15 (nudix hydrolase 15)* and *TPMT (thiopurine S-methyltransferase)* (eg, drug metabolism) gene analysis, common variants

0287U Oncology (thyroid), DNA and mRNA, next-generation sequencing analysis of 112 genes, fine needle aspirate or formalin-fixed paraffin-embedded (FFPE) tissue, algorithmic prediction of cancer recurrence, reported as a categorical risk result (low, intermediate, high)

0288U Oncology (lung), mRNA, quantitative PCR analysis of 11 genes *(BAG1, BRCA1, CDC6, CDK2AP1, ERBB3, FUT3, IL11, LCK, RND3, SH3BGR, WNT3A)* and 3 reference genes *(ESD, TBP, YAP1)*, formalin-fixed paraffin-embedded (FFPE) tumor tissue, algorithmic interpretation reported as a recurrence risk score

0289U Neurology (Alzheimer disease), mRNA, gene expression profiling by RNA sequencing of 24 genes, whole blood, algorithm reported as predictive risk score

0290U Pain management, mRNA, gene expression profiling by RNA sequencing of 36 genes, whole blood, algorithm reported as predictive risk score

0291U Psychiatry (mood disorders), mRNA, gene expression profiling by RNA sequencing of 144 genes, whole blood, algorithm reported as predictive risk score

0292U Psychiatry (stress disorders), mRNA, gene expression profiling by RNA sequencing of 72 genes, whole blood, algorithm reported as predictive risk score

0293U Psychiatry (suicidal ideation), mRNA, gene expression profiling by RNA sequencing of 54 genes, whole blood, algorithm reported as predictive risk score

0294U Longevity and mortality risk, mRNA, gene expression profiling by RNA sequencing of 18 genes, whole blood, algorithm reported as predictive risk score

0295U Oncology (breast ductal carcinoma in situ), protein expression profiling by immunohistochemistry of 7 proteins (COX2, FOXA1, HER2, Ki-67, p16, PR, SIAH2), with 4 clinicopathologic factors (size, age, margin status, palpability), utilizing formalin-fixed paraffin-embedded (FFPE) tissue, algorithm reported as a recurrence risk score

0296U Oncology (oral and/or oropharyngeal cancer), gene expression profiling by RNA sequencing at least 20 molecular features (eg, human and/or microbial mRNA), saliva, algorithm reported as positive or negative for signature associated with malignancy

0297U Oncology (pan tumor), whole genome sequencing of paired malignant and normal DNA specimens, fresh or formalin-fixed paraffin-embedded (FFPE) tissue, blood or bone marrow, comparative sequence analyses and variant identification

0298U Oncology (pan tumor), whole transcriptome sequencing of paired malignant and normal RNA specimens, fresh or formalin-fixed paraffin-embedded (FFPE) tissue, blood or bone marrow, comparative sequence analyses and expression level and chimeric transcript identification

0299U Oncology (pan tumor), whole genome optical genome mapping of paired malignant and normal DNA specimens, fresh frozen tissue, blood, or bone marrow, comparative structural variant identification

0300U Oncology (pan tumor), whole genome sequencing and optical genome mapping of paired malignant and normal DNA specimens, fresh tissue, blood, or bone marrow, comparative sequence analyses and variant identification

0301U Infectious agent detection by nucleic acid (DNA or RNA), Bartonella henselae and Bartonella quintana, droplet digital PCR (ddPCR);

0302U following liquid enhancement

0303U Hematology, red blood cell (RBC) adhesion to endothelial/subendothelial adhesion molecules, functional assessment, whole blood, with algorithmic analysis and result reported as an RBC adhesion index; hypoxic

0304U normoxic

0305U Hematology, red blood cell (RBC) functionality and deformity as a function of shear stress, whole blood, reported as a maximum elongation index

91305 Severe acute respiratory syndrome coronavirus 2 (SARS-CoV-2) (coronavirus disease [COVID-19]) vaccine, mRNA-LNP, spike protein, preservative free, 30 mcg/0.3 mL dosage, tris-sucrose formulation, for intramuscular use

91306 Severe acute respiratory syndrome coronavirus 2 (SARS-CoV-2) (coronavirus disease [COVID-19]) vaccine, mRNA-LNP, spike protein, preservative free, 50 mcg/0.25 mL dosage, for intramuscular use

91307 Severe acute respiratory syndrome coronavirus 2 (SARS-CoV-2) (coronavirus disease [COVID-19]) vaccine, mRNA-LNP, spike protein, preservative free, 10 mcg/0.2 mL dosage, diluent reconstituted, tris-sucrose formulation, for intramuscular use

0003A third dose

0004A booster dose

0013A third dose

0034A booster dose

0051A Immunization administration by intramuscular injection of severe acute respiratory syndrome coronavirus 2 (SARS-CoV-2) (coronavirus disease [COVID-19]) vaccine, mRNA-LNP, spike protein, preservative free, 30 mcg/0.3 mL dosage, tris-sucrose formulation; first dose

0052A second dose

0053A third dose

0054A booster dose

0064A Immunization administration by intramuscular injection of severe acute respiratory syndrome coronavirus 2 (SARS-CoV-2) (coronavirus disease [COVID-19]) vaccine, mRNA-LNP, spike protein, preservative free, 50 mcg/0.25 mL dosage, booster dose

0071A Immunization administration by intramuscular injection of severe acute respiratory syndrome coronavirus 2 (SARS-CoV-2) (coronavirus disease [COVID-19]) vaccine, mRNA-LNP, spike protein, preservative free, 10 mcg/0.2 mL dosage, diluent reconstituted, tris-sucrose formulation; first dose

0072A second dose

Revised Codes

0090U Oncology (cutaneous melanoma), mRNA gene expression profiling by RT-PCR of 23 genes (14 content and 9 housekeeping), utilizing formalin-fixed paraffin-embedded (FFPE) tissue, algorithm reported as a categorical result (ie, benign, ~~indeterminate~~ intermediate, malignant)

Deleted Codes

0208U Oncology (medullary thyroid carcinoma), mRNA, gene expression analysis of 108 genes, utilizing fine needle aspirate, algorithm reported as positive or negative for medullary thyroid carcinoma

[illegible]

New Codes

[illegible]

Deleted Codes

[illegible]

Appendix C — Evaluation and Management Extended Guidelines

This appendix provides an overview of evaluation and management (E/M) services, tables that identify the documentation elements associated with each code, the 2021 changes to some E/M services, and the federal documentation guidelines with emphasis on the 1997 exam guidelines. The 1997 version identifies both general multi-system physical examinations and single-system examinations, but providers may also use the original 1995 version of the E/M guidelines; both are currently supported by the Centers for Medicare and Medicaid Services (CMS) for audit purposes when reporting 99217–99499.

The levels of E/M services define the wide variations in skill, effort, and time and are required for preventing and/or diagnosing and treating illness or injury, and promoting optimal health. These codes are intended to represent physician work, and because much of this work involves the amount of training, experience, expertise, and knowledge that a provider may employ when treating a given patient, the true indications of the level of this work may be difficult to recognize without some explanation.

Providers

The AMA advises coders that while a particular service or procedure may be assigned to a specific section, the service or procedure itself is not limited to use only by that specialty group (see paragraphs 2 and 3 under "Instructions for Use of the CPT® Codebook" on page xiv of the AMA CPT book). Additionally, the procedures and services listed throughout the book are for use by any qualified physician or other qualified health care professional or entity (e.g., hospitals, laboratories, or home health agencies).

The use of the phrase "physician or other qualified health care professional" (OQHCP) was adopted to identify a health care provider other than a physician. This type of provider is further described in CPT as an individual "qualified by education, training, licensure/regulation (when applicable), and facility privileging (when applicable)." State licensure guidelines determine the scope of practice and an OQHCP must practice within these guidelines, even if more restrictive than the CPT guidelines. The OQHCP may report services independently or under incident-to guidelines. The professionals within this definition are separate from "clinical staff" and are able to practice independently. CPT defines clinical staff as "a person who works under the supervision of a physician or OQHCP and who is allowed, by law, regulation, and facility policy to perform or assist in the performance of a specified professional service, but who does not individually report that professional service." Keep in mind that there may be other policies or guidance that can affect who may report a specific service.

Types of E/M Services

When approaching E/M, the first choice that a provider must make is what type of code to use. The following tables outline the E/M codes for different levels of care for:

- Office or other outpatient services—new patient
- Office or other outpatient services—established patient
- Hospital observation services—initial care, subsequent, and discharge
- Hospital inpatient services—initial care, subsequent, and discharge
- Observation or inpatient care (including admission and discharge services)
- Consultations—office or other outpatient
- Consultations—inpatient
- Emergency department services
- Critical care
- Nursing facility—initial services
- Nursing facility—subsequent services
- Nursing facility—discharge and annual assessment
- Domiciliary, rest home, or custodial care—new patient
- Domiciliary, rest home, or custodial care—established patient
- Home services—new patient
- Home services—established patient
- Newborn care services
- Neonatal and pediatric interfacility transport
- Neonatal and pediatric critical care—inpatient
- Neonate and infant intensive care services—initial and continuing
- Care management

The specifics of the code components that determine code selection are listed in the table and discussed in the next section. Before a level of service is decided upon, the correct type of service is identified.

A new patient is a patient who has not received any face-to-face professional services from the physician or OQHCP within the past three years. An established patient is a patient who has received face-to-face professional services from the physician or OQHCP within the past three years. In the case of group practices, if a physician or OQHCP of the exact same specialty or subspecialty has seen the patient within three years, the patient is considered established.

If a physician or OQHCP is on call or covering for another physician or OQHCP, the patient's encounter is classified as it would have been by the physician or OQHCP who is not available. Thus, a locum tenens physician or OQHCP who sees a patient on behalf of the patient's attending physician or OQHCP may not bill a new patient code unless the attending physician or OQHCP has not seen the patient for any problem within three years.

Office or other outpatient services are E/M services provided in the physician or OQHCP office, the outpatient area, or other ambulatory facility. Until the patient is admitted to a health care facility, he/she is considered to be an outpatient. Hospital observation services are E/M services provided to patients who are designated or admitted as "observation status" in a hospital.

Codes 99218-99220 are used to indicate initial observation care. These codes include the initiation of the observation status, supervision of patient care including writing orders, and the performance of periodic reassessments. These codes are used only by the provider "admitting" the patient for observation.

Codes 99234-99236 are used to indicate evaluation and management services to a patient who is admitted to and discharged from observation status or hospital inpatient on the same day. If the patient is admitted as an inpatient from observation on the same day, use the appropriate level of Initial Hospital Care (99221-99223).

Code 99217 indicates discharge from observation status. It includes the final physical examination of the patient, instructions, and preparation of the discharge records. It should not be used when admission and discharge are on the same date of service. As mentioned above, report codes 99234-99236 to appropriately describe same day observation services.

If a patient is in observation longer than one day, subsequent observation care codes 99224-99226 should be reported. If the patient is discharged on the second day, observation discharge code 99217 should be reported. If the patient status is changed to inpatient on a subsequent date, the appropriate inpatient code, 99221-99233, should be reported.

Initial hospital care is defined as E/M services provided during the first hospital inpatient encounter with the patient by the admitting provider. (If a physician other than the admitting physician performs the initial inpatient encounter, refer to consultations or subsequent hospital care in the CPT book.) Subsequent hospital care includes all follow-up encounters with the patient by all physicians or OQHCP. As there may only be one admitting physician, HCPCS Level II modifier AI Principal physician of record, should be appended to the initial hospital care code by the attending physician or OQHCP.

A consultation is the provision of a physician or OQHCP's opinion or advice about a patient for a specific problem at the request of another physician or other appropriate source. CPT also states that a consultation may be performed when a physician or OQHCP is determining whether to accept the transfer of patient care at the request of another physician or appropriate source. An office or other outpatient consultation is a consultation provided in the consultant's office, in the emergency department, or in an outpatient or other ambulatory facility including hospital observation services, home services, domiciliary, rest home, or custodial care. An inpatient consultation is a consultation provided in the hospital or partial hospital nursing facility setting. Report only one inpatient consultation by a consultant for each admission to the hospital or nursing facility.

If a consultant participates in the patient's management after the opinion or advice is provided, use codes for subsequent hospital or observation care or for office or other outpatient services (established patient), as appropriate.

Under CMS guidelines, the inpatient and office/outpatient consultation codes contained in the CPT manual are not covered services.

All outpatient consultation services should be reported for Medicare using the appropriate new or established evaluation and management (E/M) codes. Inpatient consultation services for the initial encounter should be reported by the physician providing the service using initial hospital care codes 99221–99223, and subsequent inpatient care codes 99231–99233.

Codes 99439, 99487, 99489, 99490, 99491, and 99347 are used to report evaluation and management services for chronic care management. These codes represent management and support services provided by clinical staff, under the direction of a physician or OQHCP, to patients residing at home or in a domiciliary, rest home, or assisted living facility. The qualified provider oversees the management and/or coordination of services for all medical conditions, psychosocial needs, and activities of daily living. These codes are reported only once per calendar month and have specific time-based thresholds.

Codes 99424–99427 are used to report principal care management services for complex chronic conditions for medical and/or psychological needs. These codes represent management and support services provided by clinical staff, a physician, or OQHCP for patients with a single, complex chronic condition that is expected to last at least three months. The qualified provider oversees the establishment, implementation, revision, or monitoring of a specific plan of care for that single condition. These codes are reported only once per month and have specific time-based thresholds.

Codes 99497-99498 are used to report the discussion and explanation of advanced directives by a physician or OQHCP. These codes represent a face-to-face service between the provider and a patient, family member, or surrogate. These codes are time-based codes and, since no active management of the problem(s) is undertaken during this time, may be reported on the same day as another E/M service.

Certain codes that CPT considers appropriate telehealth services are identified with the ★ icon and reported with modifier 95 Synchronous telemedicine service rendered via a real-time interactive audio and video telecommunications system. Medicare recognizes certain CPT and HCPCS Level II G codes as telehealth services reported with modifier GT. Check with individual payers for telehealth modifier guidance.

E/M Code	History	Exam	Medical Decision Making	Time Spent Face-to-Face (avg.)
99202	Medically appropriate	Medically appropriate	Straightforward	15–29 min.
99203	Medically appropriate	Medically appropriate	Low	30–44 min.
99204	Medically appropriate	Medically appropriate	Moderate	45–59 min.
99205	Medically appropriate	Medically appropriate	High	60–74 min.

Office or Other Outpatient Services—Established Patient[1]

E/M Code	History	Exam	Medical Decision Making	Time Spent Face-to-Face (avg.)
99211	—	—	Physician supervision, but presence not required	—
99212	Medically appropriate	Medically appropriate	Straightforward	10–19 min.
99213	Medically appropriate	Medically appropriate	Low	20–29 min.
99214	Medically appropriate	Medically appropriate	Moderate	30–39 min.
99215	Medically appropriate	Medically appropriate	High	40–54 min.

1 Includes follow-up, periodic reevaluation, and evaluation and management of new problems.

Hospital Observation Services

E/M Code	History[1]	Exam[1]	Medical Decision Making[1]	Problem Severity	Coordination of Care; Counseling	Time Spent Bedside and on Unit/Floor (avg.)
99217	Observation care discharge day management					
99218	Detailed or comprehensive	Detailed or comprehensive	Straightforward or low complexity	Low	Consistent with problem(s) and patient's needs	30 min.
99219	Comprehensive	Comprehensive	Moderate complexity	Moderate	Consistent with problem(s) and patient's needs	50 min.
99220	Comprehensive	Comprehensive	High complexity	High	Consistent with problem(s) and patient's needs	70 min.

1 Key component. All three components (history, exam, and medical decision making) are crucial for selecting the correct code.

Subsequent Hospital Observation Services[1]

E/M Code[2]	History[3]	Exam[3]	Medical Decision Making[3]	Problem Severity	Coordination of Care; Counseling	Time Spent Bedside and on Unit/Floor (avg.)
99224	Problem-focused interval	Problem-focused	Straightforward or low complexity	Stable, recovering, or improving	Consistent with problem(s) and patient's needs	15 min.
99225	Expanded problem-focused interval	Expanded problem-focused	Moderate complexity	Inadequate response to treatment; minor complications	Consistent with problem(s) and patient's needs	25 min.
99226	Detailed interval	Detailed	High complexity	Unstable; significant new problem or significant complication	Consistent with problem(s) and patient's needs	35 min.

1 All subsequent levels of service include reviewing the medical record, diagnostic studies, and changes in the patient's status, such as history, physical condition, and response to treatment since the last assessment.
2 These codes are resequenced in CPT and are printed following codes 99217-99220.
3 Key component. For subsequent care, at least two of the three components (history, exam, and medical decision making) are needed to select the correct code.

Hospital Inpatient Services—Initial Care[1]

E/M Code	History[2]	Exam[2]	Medical Decision Making[2]	Problem Severity	Coordination of Care; Counseling	Time Spent Bedside and on Unit/Floor (avg.)
99221	Detailed or comprehensive	Detailed or comprehensive	Straightforward or low complexity	Low	Consistent with problem(s) and patient's needs	30 min.
99222	Comprehensive	Comprehensive	Moderate complexity	Moderate	Consistent with problem(s) and patient's needs	50 min.
99223	Comprehensive	Comprehensive	High complexity	High	Consistent with problem(s) and patient's needs	70 min.

1 The admitting physician should append modifier AI, Principal physician of record, for Medicare patients
2 Key component. For initial care, all three components (history, exam, and medical decision making) are crucial for selecting the correct code.

Hospital Inpatient Services—Subsequent Care[1]

E/M Code	History[2]	Exam[2]	Medical Decision Making[2]	Problem Severity	Coordination of Care; Counseling	Time Spent Bedside and on Unit/Floor (avg.)
99231	Problem-focused interval	Problem-focused	Straightforward or low complexity	Stable, recovering or Improving	Consistent with problem(s) and patient's needs	15 min.
99232	Expanded problem-focused interval	Expanded problem-focused	Moderate complexity	Inadequate response to treatment; minor complications	Consistent with problem(s) and patient's needs	25 min.
99233	Detailed interval	Detailed	High complexity	Unstable; significant new problem or significant complication	Consistent with problem(s) and patient's needs	35 min.
99238	Hospital discharge day management					30 min. or less
99239	Hospital discharge day management					> 30 min.

1 All subsequent levels of service include reviewing the medical record, diagnostic studies, and changes in the patient's status, such as history, physical condition, and response to treatment since the last assessment.
2 Key component. For subsequent care, at least two of the three components (history, exam, and medical decision making) are needed to select the correct code.

Appendix C — Evaluation and Management Extended Guidelines

Observation or Inpatient Care Services (Including Admission and Discharge Services)

E/M Code	History[1]	Exam[1]	Medical Decision Making[1]	Problem Severity	Coordination of Care; Counseling	Time
99234	Detailed or comprehensive	Detailed or comprehensive	Straightforward or low complexity	Low	Consistent with problem(s) and patient's needs	40 min.
99235	Comprehensive	Comprehensive	Moderate	Moderate	Consistent with problem(s) and patient's needs	50 min.
99236	Comprehensive	Comprehensive	High	High	Consistent with problem(s) and patient's needs	55 min.

1 Key component. All three components (history, exam, and medical decision making) are crucial for selecting the correct code.

Consultations—Office or Other Outpatient

E/M Code	History[1]	Exam[1]	Medical Decision Making[1]	Problem Severity	Coordination of Care; Counseling	Time Spent Face-to-Face (avg.)
99241	Problem-focused	Problem-focused	Straightforward	Minor or self-limited	Consistent with problem(s) and patient's needs	15 min.
99242	Expanded problem-focused	Expanded problem-focused	Straightforward	Low	Consistent with problem(s) and patient's needs	30 min.
99243	Detailed	Detailed	Low complexity	Moderate	Consistent with problem(s) and patient's needs	40 min.
99244	Comprehensive	Comprehensive	Moderate complexity	Moderate to high	Consistent with problem(s) and patient's needs	60 min.
99245	Comprehensive	Comprehensive	High complexity	Moderate to high	Consistent with problem(s) and patient's needs	80 min.

1 Key component. For office or other outpatient consultations, all three components (history, exam, and medical decision making) are crucial for selecting the correct code.

Consultations—Inpatient[1]

E/M Code	History[2]	Exam[2]	Medical Decision Making[2]	Problem Severity	Coordination of Care; Counseling	Time Spent Bedside and on Unit/Floor (avg.)
99251	Problem-focused	Problem-focused	Straightforward	Minor or self-limited	Consistent with problem(s) and patient's needs	20 min.
99252	Expanded problem-focused	Expanded problem-focused	Straightforward	Low	Consistent with problem(s) and patient's needs	40 min.
99253	Detailed	Detailed	Low complexity	Moderate	Consistent with problem(s) and patient's needs	55 min.
99254	Comprehensive	Comprehensive	Moderate complexity	Moderate to high	Consistent with problem(s) and patient's needs	80 min.
99255	Comprehensive	Comprehensive	High complexity	Moderate to high	Consistent with problem(s) and patient's needs	110 min.

1 These codes are used for hospital inpatients, residents of nursing facilities or patients in a partial hospital setting.
2 Key component. For initial inpatient consultations, all three components (history, exam, and medical decision making) are crucial for selecting the correct code.

Emergency Department Services, New or Established Patient

E/M Code	History[1]	Exam[1]	Medical Decision Making[1]	Problem Severity[3]	Coordination of Care; Counseling	Time Spent[2] Face-to-Face (avg.)
99281	Problem-focused	Problem-focused	Straightforward	Minor or self-limited	Consistent with problem(s) and patient's needs	N/A
99282	Expanded problem-focused	Expanded problem-focused	Low complexity	Low to moderate	Consistent with problem(s) and patient's needs	N/A
99283	Expanded problem-focused	Expanded problem-focused	Moderate complexity	Moderate	Consistent with problem(s) and patient's needs	N/A
99284	Detailed	Detailed	Moderate complexity	High; requires urgent evaluation	Consistent with problem(s) and patient's needs	N/A
99285	Comprehensive	Comprehensive	High complexity	High; poses immediate/significant threat to life or physiologic function	Consistent with problem(s) and patient's needs	N/A
99288[4]			High complexity			N/A

1 Key component. For emergency department services, all three components (history, exam, and medical decision making) are crucial for selecting the correct code and must be adequately documented in the medical record to substantiate the level of service reported.

2 Typical times have not been established for this category of services.

3 NOTE: The severity of the patient's problem, while taken into consideration when evaluating and treating the patient, does not automatically determine the level of E/M service unless the medical record documentation reflects the severity of the patient's illness, injury, or condition in the details of the history, physical examination, and medical decision making process. Federal auditors will "downcode" the level of E/M service despite the nature of the patient's problem when the documentation does not support the E/M code reported.

4 Code 99288 is used to report two-way communication with emergency medical services personnel in the field.

Critical Care

E/M Code	Patient Status	Physician Attendance	Time[1]
99291	Critically ill or critically injured	Constant	First 30–74 minutes
99292	Critically ill or critically injured	Constant	Each additional 30 minutes beyond the first 74 minutes

1 Per the guidelines for time in *CPT 2016 page xv*, "A unit of time is attained when the mid-point is passed. For example, an hour is attained when 31 minutes have elapsed (more than midway between zero and 60 minutes)."

Nursing Facility Services—Initial Nursing Facility Care[1]

E/M Code	History[1]	Exam[1]	Medical Decision Making[1]	Problem Severity	Coordination of Care; Counseling
99304	Detailed or comprehensive	Detailed or comprehensive	Straightforward or low complexity	Low	25 min.
99305	Comprehensive	Comprehensive	Moderate complexity	Moderate	35 min.
99306	Comprehensive	Comprehensive	High complexity	High	45 min.

1 These services must be performed by the physician. See CPT Corrections Document – CPT 2013 page 3 or guidelines CPT 2016 page 26.

2 Key component. For new patients, all three components (history, exam, and medical decision making) are crucial for selecting the correct code.

Nursing Facility Services—Subsequent Nursing Facility Care

E/M Code	History[1]	Exam[1]	Medical Decision Making[2]	Problem Severity	Coordination of Care; Counseling
99307	Problem-focused interval	Problem-focused	Straightforward	Stable, recovering or improving	10 min.
99308	Expanded problem-focused interval	Expanded problem-focused	Low complexity	Responding inadequately or has developed a minor complication	15 min.
99309	Detailed interval	Detailed	Moderate complexity	Significant complication or a significant new problem	25 min.
99310	Comprehensive interval	Comprehensive	High complexity	Developed a significant new problem requiring immediate attention	35 min.

1 Key component. For established patients, at least two of the three components (history, exam, and medical decision making) are needed for selecting the correct code.

Nursing Facility Discharge and Annual Assessment

E/M Code	History[1]	Exam[1]	Medical Decision Making[1]	Problem Severity	Time Spent Bedside and on Unit/Floor (avg.)
99315	Nursing facility discharge day management				30 min. or less
99316	Nursing facility discharge day management				more than 30 min.
99318	Detailed interval	Comprehensive	Low to moderate complexity	Stable, recovering or improving	30 min.

1 Key component. For annual nursing facility assessment, all three components (history, exam, and medical decision making) are crucial for selecting the correct code.

Domiciliary, Rest Home (e.g., Boarding Home) or Custodial Care Services—New Patient

E/M Code	History[1]	Exam[1]	Medical Decision Making[1]	Problem Severity	Coordination of Care; Counseling	Time Spent Face-to-Face (avg.)
99324	Problem-focused	Problem-focused	Straightforward	Low	Consistent with problem(s) and patient's needs	20 min.
99325	Expanded problem-focused	Expanded problem-focused	Low complexity	Moderate	Consistent with problem(s) and patient's needs	30 min.
99326	Detailed	Detailed	Moderate complexity	Moderate to high	Consistent with problem(s) and patient's needs	45 min.
99327	Comprehensive	Comprehensive	Moderate complexity	High	Consistent with problem(s) and patient's needs	60 min.
99328	Comprehensive	Comprehensive	High complexity	Unstable or developed a new problem requiring immediate physician attention	Consistent with problem(s) and patient's needs	75 min.

1 Key component. For new patients, all three components (history, exam, and medical decision making) are crucial for selecting the correct code and must be adequately documented in the medical record to substantiate the level of service reported.

Domiciliary, Rest Home (e.g., Boarding Home) or Custodial Care Services— Established Patient

E/M Code	History[1]	Exam[1]	Medical Decision Making[1]	Problem Severity	Coordination of Care; Counseling	Time Spent Face-to-Face (avg.)
99334	Problem-focused interval	Problem-focused	Straightforward	Minor or self-limited	Consistent with problem(s) and patient's needs	15 min.
99335	Expanded problem-focused interval	Expanded problem-focused	Low complexity	Low to moderate	Consistent with problem(s) and patient's needs	25 min.
99336	Detailed interval	Detailed	Moderate complexity	Moderate to high	Consistent with problem(s) and patient's needs	40 min.
99337	Comprehensive interval	Comprehensive	Moderate to high complexity	Moderate to high	Consistent with problem(s) and patient's needs	60 min.

1 Key component. For established patients, at least two of the three components (history, exam, and medical decision making) are needed for selecting the correct code.

Domiciliary, Rest Home (e.g., Assisted Living Facility), or Home Care Plan Oversight Services

E/M Code	Intent of Service	Presence of Patient	Time
99339	Individual physician supervision of a patient (patient not present) in home, domiciliary or rest home (e.g., assisted living facility) requiring complex and multidisciplinary care modalities involving regular physician development and/or revision of care plans, review of subsequent reports of patient status, review of related laboratory and other studies, communication (including telephone calls) for purposes of assessment or care decisions with health care professional(s), family member(s), surrogate decision maker(s) (e.g., legal guardian) and/or key caregiver(s) involved in patient's care, integration of new information into the medical treatment plan and/or adjustment of medical therapy, within a calendar month	Patient not present	15–29 min.
99340	Same as 99339	Patient not present	30 min. or more

Home Services—New Patient

E/M Code	History[1]	Exam[1]	Medical Decision Making[1]	Problem Severity	Coordination of Care; Counseling	Time Spent Face-to-Face (avg.)
99341	Problem-focused	Problem-focused	Straightforward complexity	Low	Consistent with problem(s) and patient's needs	20 min.
99342	Expanded problem-focused	Expanded problem-focused	Low complexity	Moderate	Consistent with problem(s) and patient's needs	30 min.
99343	Detailed	Detailed	Moderate complexity	Moderate to high	Consistent with problem(s) and patient's needs	45 min.
99344	Comprehensive	Comprehensive	Moderate complexity	High	Consistent with problem(s) and patient's needs	60 min.
99345	Comprehensive	Comprehensive	High complexity	Usually the patient has developed a significant new problem requiring immediate physician attention	Consistent with problem(s) and patient's needs	75 min.

1 Key component. For new patients, all three components (history, exam, and medical decision making) are crucial for selecting the correct code and must be adequately documented in the medical record to substantiate the level of service reported.

Home Services—Established Patient

E/M Code	History[1]	Exam[1]	Medical Decision Making[1]	Problem Severity	Coordination of Care; Counseling	Time Spent Face-to-Face (avg.)
99347	Problem-focused interval	Problem-focused	Straightforward	Minor or self-limited	Consistent with problem(s) and patient's needs	15 min.
99348	Expanded problem-focused interval	Expanded problem-focused	Low complexity	Low to moderate	Consistent with problem(s) and patient's needs	25 min.
99349	Detailed interval	Detailed	Moderate complexity	Moderate to high	Consistent with problem(s) and patient's needs	40 min.
99350	Comprehensive interval	Comprehensive	Moderate to high complexity	Moderate to high Usually the patient has developed a significant new problem requiring immediate physician attention	Consistent with problem(s) and patient's needs	60 min.

1 Key component. For established patients, at least two of the three components (history, exam, and medical decision making) are needed for selecting the correct code.

Newborn Care Services

E/M Code	Patient Status	Type of Visit
99460	Normal newborn	Inpatient initial inpatient hospital or birthing center per day
99461	Normal newborn	Inpatient initial treatment not in hospital or birthing center per day
99462	Normal newborn	Inpatient subsequent per day
99463	Normal newborn	Inpatient initial inpatient and discharge in hospital or birthing center per day
99464	Unstable newborn	Attendance at delivery
99465	High-risk newborn at delivery	Resuscitation, ventilation, and cardiac treatment

Neonatal and Pediatric Interfacility Transportation

E/M Code	Patient Status	Type of Visit
99466	Critically ill or injured infant or young child, to 24 months	Face-to-face transportation from one facility to another, initial 30-74 minutes
99467	Critically ill or injured infant or young child, to 24 months	Face-to-face transportation from one facility to another, each additional 30 minutes
99485[1]	Critically ill or injured infant or young child, to 24 months	Supervision of patient transport from one facility to another, initial 30 minutes
99486[1]	Critically ill or injured infant or young child, to 24 months	Supervision of patient transport from one facility to another, each additional 30 minutes

1 These codes are resequenced in CPT and are printed following codes 99466-99467.

Inpatient Neonatal and Pediatric Critical Care

E/M Code	Patient Status	Type of Visit
99468[1]	Critically ill neonate, aged 28 days or less	Inpatient initial per day
99469[2]	Critically ill neonate, aged 28 days or less	Inpatient subsequent per day
99471	Critically ill infant or young child, aged 29 days to 24 months	Inpatient initial per day
99472	Critically ill infant or young child, aged 29 days to 24 months	Inpatient subsequent per day
99475	Critically ill infant or young child, 2 to 5 years[3]	Inpatient initial per day
99476	Critically ill infant or young child, 2 to 5 years	Inpatient subsequent per day

1 Codes 99468, 99471, and 99475 may be reported only once per admission.
2 Codes 99469, 99472, and 99476 may be reported only once per day and by only one provider.
3 See 99291-99292 for patients 6 years of age and older.

Neonate and Infant Initial and Continuing Intensive Care Services

E/M Code	Patient Status	Type of Visit
99477	Neonate, aged 28 days or less	Inpatient initial per day
99478	Infant with present body weight of less than 1500 grams, no longer critically ill	Inpatient subsequent per day
99479	Infant with present body weight of 1500-2500 grams, no longer critically ill	Inpatient subsequent per day
99480	Infant with present body weight of 2501-5000 grams, no longer critically ill	Inpatient subsequent per day

Reporting Levels of E/M Services Codes 99202–99215

A medically appropriate history and physical examination, as determined by the treating provider, should be documented. The level of history and physical examination are no longer used when determining the level of service. Codes should be selected based upon the CPT 2022 Medical Decision Making (MDM) table or time as documented in the patient record.

The 2022 Medical Decision Making (MDM) table requires two of three levels of the three elements be met or exceeded to determine the level of code reported. The three elements are:

- Number and complexity of problems addressed at the encounter
- Amount and/or complexity of data to be reviewed and analyzed
- Risk of complications and/or morbidity or mortality of patient management

Instructions and examples of each element are given in the table to enable accurate selection of the level of MDM and E/M service to be reported for codes 99202–99215.

Alternately time alone may be used to select the appropriate level of service. Total time for reporting these services included face-to-face and non-face-to-face time personally spent by the physician or other qualified health care professional on the date of the encounter. The E/M codes 99202–99205 and 99212–99215 include specific time ranges used to select the appropriate code. Report 99417 for prolonged services when the time for code 99205 or 99215 is exceeded. Report 99417 for each minimum of 15 minutes additional prolonged services.

Code 99211 is used to report the E/M service that does not require the presence of the physician or other qualified health care professional.

Levels of E/M Services Codes 99217–99499

Confusion may be experienced when first approaching E/M codes 99217–99499 due to the way that each description of a code component or element seems to have another layer of description beneath. The three key components—history, exam, and decision making—are each comprised of elements that combine to create varying levels of that component.

For example, an expanded problem-focused history includes the chief complaint, a brief history of the present illness, and a system review focusing on the patient's problems. The level of exam is not made up of different elements but rather distinguished by the extent of exam across body areas or organ systems.

The single largest source of confusion are the "labels" or names applied to the varying degrees of history, exam, and decision-making. Terms such as expanded problem-focused, detailed, and comprehensive are somewhat meaningless unless they are defined. The lack of definition in CPT guidelines relative to these terms is precisely what caused the first set of federal guidelines to be developed in 1995 and again in 1997.

Documentation Guidelines for Evaluation and Management Services

Both versions of the federal guidelines go well beyond CPT guidelines in defining specific code requirements. The current version of the CPT guidelines does not explain the number of history of present illness (HPI) elements or the specific number of organ systems or body areas to be examined as they are in the federal guidelines. Adherence to some version of the guidelines is required when billing E/M to federal payers, but at this time, the CPT guidelines do not incorporate this level of detail into the code definitions. Although that could be interpreted to mean that non-governmental payers have a lesser documentation standard, it is best to adopt one set of the federal versions for all payer types for both consistency and ease of use.

The 1997 guidelines supply a great amount of detail relative to history and exam and will give the provider clear direction to follow when documenting elements. With that stated, the 1995 guidelines are equally valid and place a lesser documentation burden on the provider in regard to the physical exam.

The 1995 guidelines ask only for a notation of "normal" on systems with normal findings. The only narrative required is for abnormal findings. The 1997 version calls for much greater detail, or an "elemental" or "bullet-point" approach to organ systems, although a notation of normal is sufficient when addressing the elements within a system. The 1997 version works well in a template or electronic health record (EHR) format for recording E/M services.

The 1997 version did produce the single system specialty exam guidelines. When reviewing the complete guidelines listed below, note the differences between exam requirements in the 1995 and 1997 versions.

A Comparison of 1995 and 1997 Exam Guidelines

There are four types of exams indicated in the levels of E/M codes. Although the descriptors or labels are the same under 1995 and 1997 guidelines, the degree of detail required is different. The remaining content on this topic references the 1997 general multi-system specialty examination, at the end of this chapter.

The levels under each set of guidelines are:

1995 Exam Guidelines:

Problem focused:	One body area or system
Expanded problem focused:	Two to seven body areas or organ systems
Detailed:	Two to seven body areas or organ systems
Comprehensive:	Eight or more organ systems or a complete single-system examination

1997 Exam Guidelines:

Problem-focused:	Perform and document examination of one to five bullet point elements in one or more organ systems/body areas from the general multi-system examination
OR	
	Perform or document examination of one to five bullet point elements from one of the 10 single-organ-system examinations, shaded or unshaded boxes
Expanded problem-focused:	Perform and document examination of at least six bullet point elements in one or more organ systems from the general multi-system examination
OR	
	Perform and document examination of at least six bullet point elements from one of the 10 single-organ-system examinations, shaded or unshaded boxes
Detailed:	Perform and document examination of at least six organ systems or body areas, including at least two bullet point elements for each organ system or body area from the general multi-system examination
OR	
	Perform and document examination of at least 12 bullet point elements in two or more organ systems or body areas from the general multisystem examination
OR	
	Perform and document examination of at least 12 bullet elements from one of the single-organ-system examinations, shaded or unshaded boxes
Comprehensive:	Perform and document examination of at least nine organ systems or body areas, with all bullet elements for each organ system or body area (unless specific instructions are expected to limit examination content with at least two bullet elements for each organ system or body area) from the general multi-system examination
OR	
	Perform and document examination of all bullet point elements from one of the 10 single-organ system examinations with documentation of every element in shaded boxes and at least one element in each unshaded box from the single-organ-system examination.

The Documentation Guidelines

The following guidelines were developed jointly by the American Medical Association (AMA) and the Centers for Medicare and Medicaid Services (CMS). Their mutual goal was to provide physicians and claims reviewers with advice about preparing or reviewing documentation for Evaluation and Management (E/M) services.

I. Introduction

What is Documentation and Why Is It Important?

Medical record documentation is required to record pertinent facts, findings, and observations about an individual's health history, including past and present illnesses, examinations, tests, treatments, and outcomes. The medical record chronologically documents the care of the patient and is an important element contributing to high quality care. The medical record facilitates:

- The ability of the physician and other health care professionals to evaluate and plan the patient's immediate treatment and to monitor his/her health care over time
- Communication and continuity of care among physicians and other health care professionals involved in the patient's care
- Accurate and timely claims review and payment
- Appropriate utilization review and quality of care evaluations
- Collection of data that may be useful for research and education

An appropriately documented medical record can reduce many of the problems associated with claims processing and may serve as a legal document to verify the care provided, if necessary.

What Do Payers Want and Why?

Because payers have a contractual obligation to enrollees, they may require reasonable documentation that services are consistent with the insurance coverage provided. They may request information to validate:

- The site of service
- The medical necessity and appropriateness of the diagnostic and/or therapeutic services provided
- Services provided have been accurately reported

II. General Principles of Medical Record Documentation

The principles of documentation listed below are applicable to all types of medical and surgical services in all settings. For Evaluation and Management (E/M) services, the nature and amount of physician work and documentation varies by type of service, place of service, and the patient's status. The general principles listed below may be modified to account for these variable circumstances in providing E/M services.

- The medical record should be complete and legible
- The documentation of each patient encounter should include:

- A reason for the encounter and relevant history, physical examination findings, and prior diagnostic test results
- Assessment, clinical impression, or diagnosis
- Plan for care
- Date and legible identity of the practitioner

- If not documented, the rationale for ordering diagnostic and other ancillary services should be easily inferred
- Past and present diagnoses should be accessible to the treating and/or consulting physician
- Appropriate health risk factors should be identified
- The patient's progress, response to, and changes in treatment and revision of diagnosis should be documented
- The CPT and ICD-9-CM codes reported on the health insurance claim form or billing statement should be supported by the documentation in the medical record

III. *Documentation of E/M Services 1995 and 1997*

The following information provides definitions and documentation guidelines for the three key components of E/M services and for visits that consist predominately of counseling or coordination of care. The three key components—history, examination, and medical decision making—appear in the descriptors for office and other outpatient services, hospital observation services, hospital inpatient services, consultations, emergency department services, nursing facility services, domiciliary care services, and home services. While some of the text of the CPT guidelines has been repeated in this document, the reader should refer to CMS or CPT for the complete descriptors for E/M services and instructions for selecting a level of service. Documentation guidelines are identified by the symbol DG.

The descriptors for the levels of E/M services recognize seven components that are used in defining the levels of E/M services. These components are:

- History
- Examination
- Medical decision making
- Counseling
- Coordination of care
- Nature of presenting problem
- Time

The first three of these components (i.e., history, examination, and medical decision making) are the key components in selecting the level of E/M services. In the case of visits that consist predominately of counseling or coordination of care, time is the key or controlling factor to qualify for a particular level of E/M service.

Because the level of E/M service is dependent on two or three key components, performance and documentation of one component (e.g., examination) at the highest level does not necessarily mean that the encounter in its entirety qualifies for the highest level of E/M service.

These Documentation Guidelines for E/M services reflect the needs of the typical adult population. For certain groups of patients, the recorded information may vary slightly from that described here. Specifically, the medical records of infants, children, adolescents, and pregnant women may have additional or modified information, as appropriate, recorded in each history and examination area.

As an example, newborn records may include under history of the present illness (HPI) the details of the mother's pregnancy and the infant's status at birth; social history will focus on family structure; and family history will focus on congenital anomalies and hereditary disorders in the family. In addition, the content of a pediatric examination will vary with the age and development of the child. Although not specifically defined in these documentation guidelines, these patient group variations on history and examination are appropriate.

A. *Documentation of History*

The levels of E/M services are based on four types of history (Problem Focused, Expanded Problem Focused, Detailed, and Comprehensive). Each type of history includes some or all of the following elements:

- Chief complaint (CC)
- History of present illness (HPI)
- Review of systems (ROS)
- Past, family, and/or social history (PFSH)

The extent of history of present illness, review of systems, and past, family, and/or social history that is obtained and documented is dependent upon clinical judgment and the nature of the presenting problem.

The chart below shows the progression of the elements required for each type of history. To qualify for a given type of history all three elements in the table must be met. (A chief complaint is indicated at all levels.)

- DG: The CC, ROS, and PFSH may be listed as separate elements of history or they may be included in the description of the history of present illness

- DG: A ROS and/or a PFSH obtained during an earlier encounter does not need to be re-recorded if there is evidence that the physician reviewed and updated the previous information. This may occur when a physician updates his/her own record or in an institutional setting or group practice where many physicians use a common record. The review and update may be documented by:
  - Describing any new ROS and/or PFSH information or noting there has been no change in the information
  - Noting the date and location of the earlier ROS and/or PFSH

- DG: The ROS and/or PFSH may be recorded by ancillary staff or on a form completed by the patient. To document that the physician reviewed the information, there must be a notation supplementing or confirming the information recorded by others

- DG: If the physician is unable to obtain a history from the patient or other source, the record should describe the patient's condition or other circumstance that precludes obtaining a history

Definitions and specific documentation guidelines for each of the elements of history are listed below.

Chief Complaint (CC)

The CC is a concise statement describing the symptom, problem, condition, diagnosis, physician recommended return, or other factor that is the reason for the encounter, usually stated in the patient's words.

- DG: The medical record should clearly reflect the chief complaint

History of Present Illness (HPI)

The HPI is a chronological description of the development of the patient's present illness from the first sign and/or symptom or from the previous encounter to the present. It includes the following elements:

- Location
- Quality
- Severity
- Duration
- Timing
- Context
- Modifying factors
- Associated signs and symptoms

Brief and extended HPIs are distinguished by the amount of detail needed to accurately characterize the clinical problem.

A brief HPI consists of one to three elements of the HPI.

- DG: The medical record should describe one to three elements of the present illness (HPI)

An extended HPI consists of at least four elements of the HPI or the status of at least three chronic or inactive conditions.

- DG: The medical record should describe at least four elements of the present illness (HPI) or the status of at least three chronic or inactive conditions

Beginning with services performed on or after September 10, 2013, CMS has stated that physicians and OQHCP will be able to use the 1997 guidelines for an extended history of present illness (HPI) in combination with other elements from the 1995 documentation guidelines to document a particular level of evaluation and management service.

History of Present Illness	Review of systems (ROS)	PFSH	Type of History
Brief	N/A	N/A	Problem-focused
Brief	Problem Pertinent	N/A	Expanded Problem-Focused
Extended	Extended	Pertinent	Detailed
Extended	Complete	Complete	Comprehensive

Review of Systems (ROS)

A ROS is an inventory of body systems obtained through a series of questions seeking to identify signs and/or symptoms that the patient may be experiencing or has experienced. For purposes of ROS, the following systems are recognized:

- Constitutional symptoms (e.g., fever, weight loss)
- Eyes
- Ears, nose, mouth, throat
- Cardiovascular
- Respiratory
- Gastrointestinal
- Genitourinary
- Musculoskeletal
- Integumentary (skin and/or breast)
- Neurological
- Psychiatric
- Endocrine
- Hematologic/lymphatic
- Allergic/immunologic

A problem pertinent ROS inquires about the system directly related to the problem identified in the HPI.

- DG: The patient's positive responses and pertinent negatives for the system related to the problem should be documented

An extended ROS inquires about the system directly related to the problem identified in the HPI and a limited number of additional systems.

- DG: The patient's positive responses and pertinent negatives for two to nine systems should be documented

A complete ROS inquires about the system directly related to the problem identified in the HPI plus all additional body systems.

- DG: At least 10 organ systems must be reviewed. Those systems with positive or pertinent negative responses must be individually documented. For the remaining systems, a notation indicating all other systems are negative is permissible. In the absence of such a notation, at least 10 systems must be individually documented

Past, Family, and/or Social History (PFSH)

The PFSH consists of a review of three areas:

- Past history (the patient's past experiences with illnesses, operations, injuries, and treatment)
- Family history (a review of medical events in the patient's family, including diseases that may be hereditary or place the patient at risk)
- Social history (an age appropriate review of past and current activities)

For certain categories of E/M services that include only an interval history, it is not necessary to record information about the PFSH. Those categories are subsequent hospital care, follow-up inpatient consultations, and subsequent nursing facility care.

A pertinent PFSH is a review of the history area directly related to the problem identified in the HPI.

- DG: At least one specific item from any of the three history areas must be documented for a pertinent PFSH

A complete PFSH is a review of two or all three of the PFSH history areas, depending on the category of the E/M service. A review of all three history areas is required for services that by their nature include a comprehensive assessment or reassessment of the patient. A review of two of the three history areas is sufficient for other services.

- DG: A least one specific item from two of the three history areas must be documented for a complete PFSH for the following categories of E/M services: office or other outpatient services, established patient; emergency department; domiciliary care, established patient; and home care, established patient

- DG: At least one specific item from each of the three history areas must be documented for a complete PFSH for the following categories of E/M services: office or other outpatient services, new patient; hospital observation services; hospital inpatient services, initial care; consultations; comprehensive nursing facility assessments; domiciliary care, new patient; and home care, new patient

B. *Documentation of Examination 1997 Guidelines*

The levels of E/M services are based on four types of examination:

- Problem Focused: A limited examination of the affected body area or organ system
- Expanded Problem Focused: A limited examination of the affected body area or organ system and any other symptomatic or related body area or organ system
- Detailed: An extended examination of the affected body area or organ system and any other symptomatic or related body area or organ system
- Comprehensive: A general multi-system examination or complete examination of a single organ system and other symptomatic or related body area or organ system

These types of examinations have been defined for general multi-system and the following single organ systems:

- Cardiovascular
- Ears, nose, mouth, and throat
- Eyes
- Genitourinary (Female)
- Genitourinary (Male)
- Hematologic/lymphatic/immunologic
- Musculoskeletal
- Neurological
- Psychiatric
- Respiratory
- Skin

Any physician regardless of specialty may perform a general multi-system examination or any of the single organ system examinations. The type (general multi-system or single organ system) and content of examination are selected by the examining physician and are based upon clinical judgment, the patient's history, and the nature of the presenting problem.

The content and documentation requirements for each type and level of examination are summarized below and described in detail in a table found later on in this document. In the table, organ systems and body areas recognized by CPT for purposes of describing examinations are shown in the left column. The content, or individual elements, of the examination pertaining to that body area or organ system are identified by bullets (•) in the right column.

Parenthetical examples "(e.g., ...)," have been used for clarification and to provide guidance regarding documentation. Documentation for each element must satisfy any numeric requirements (such as "Measurement of any three of the following seven...") included in the description of the element. Elements with multiple components but with no specific numeric requirement (such as "Examination of liver and spleen") require documentation of at least one component. It is possible for a given examination to be expanded beyond what is defined here. When that occurs, findings related to the additional systems and/or areas should be documented.

- DG: Specific abnormal and relevant negative findings from the examination of the affected or symptomatic body area or organ system should be documented. A notation of "abnormal" without elaboration is insufficient

- DG: Abnormal or unexpected findings from the examination of any asymptomatic body area or organ system should be described

- DG: A brief statement or notation indicating "negative" or "normal" is sufficient to document normal findings related to an unaffected areas or asymptomatic organ system

General Multi-System Examinations

General multi-system examinations are described in detail later in this document. To qualify for a given level of multi-system examination, the following content and documentation requirements should be met:

- Problem Focused Examination: It should include performance and documentation of one to five elements identified by a bullet (•) in one or more organ systems or body areas
- Expanded Problem Focused Examination: It should include performance and documentation of at least six elements identified by a bullet (•) in one or more organ systems or body areas
- Detailed Examination: It should include at least six organ systems or body areas. For each system/area selected, performance and documentation of at least two elements identified by a bullet (•) is expected. Alternatively, a detailed examination may include performance and documentation of at least 12 elements identified by a bullet (•) in two or more organ systems or body areas
- Comprehensive Examination: It should include at least nine organ systems or body areas. For each system/area selected, all elements of the examination identified by a bullet (•) should be performed, unless specific directions limit the content of the examination. For each area/system, documentation of at least two elements identified by a bullet (•) is expected

Single Organ System Examinations

The single organ system examinations recognized by CMS include eyes; ears, nose, mouth, and throat; cardiovascular; respiratory; genitourinary (male and female); musculoskeletal; neurologic; hematologic, lymphatic, and immunologic; skin; and psychiatric. Note that for each specific single organ examination type, the performance and documentation of the stated number of elements, identified by a bullet (•) should be included, whether in a box with a shaded or unshaded border. The following content and documentation requirements must be met to qualify for a given level:

- Problem Focused Examination: one to five elements
- Expanded Problem Focused Examination: at least six elements
- Detailed Examination: at least 12 elements (other than eye and psychiatric examinations)
- Comprehensive Examination: all elements (Documentation of every element in a box with a shaded border and at least one element in a box with an unshaded border is expected)

Content and Documentation Requirements

General Multisystem Examination 1997

System/Body Area	Elements of Examination
Constitutional	• Measurement of any three of the following seven vital signs: 1) sitting or standing blood pressure, 2) supine blood pressure, 3) pulse rate and regularity, 4) respiration, 5) temperature, 6) height, 7) weight (May be measured and recorded by ancillary staff). • General appearance of patient (e.g., development, nutrition, body habitus, deformities attention to grooming)
Eyes	• Inspection of conjunctivae and lids • Examination of pupils and irises (e.g., reaction to light and accommodation, size and symmetry) • Ophthalmoscopic examination of optic discs (e.g., size, C/D ratio, appearance) and posterior segments (e.g., vessel changes, exudates, hemorrhages)
Ears, nose, mouth, and throat	• External inspection of ears and nose (e.g., overall appearance, scars, lesions, masses) • Otoscopic examination of external auditory canals and tympanic membranes • Assessment of hearing (e.g., whispered voice, finger rub, tuning fork) • Inspection of nasal mucosa, septum and turbinates • Inspection of lips, teeth and gums • Examination of oropharynx: oral mucosa, salivary glands, hard and soft palates, tongue, tonsils and posterior pharynx
Neck	• Examination of neck (e.g., masses, overall appearance, symmetry, tracheal position, crepitus) • Examination of thyroid (e.g., enlargement, tenderness, mass)
Respiratory	• Assessment of respiratory effort (e.g., intercostal retractions, use of accessory muscles, diaphragmatic movement) • Percussion of chest (e.g., dullness, flatness, hyperresonance) • Palpation of chest (e.g., tactile fremitus) • Auscultation of lungs (e.g., breath sounds, adventitious sounds, rubs)
Cardiovascular	• Palpation of heart (e.g., location, size, thrills) • Auscultation of heart with notation of abnormal sounds and murmurs • Examination of: — carotid arteries (e.g., pulse amplitude, bruits) — abdominal aorta (e.g., size, bruits) — femoral arteries (e.g., pulse amplitude, bruits) — pedal pulses (e.g., pulse amplitude) — extremities for edema and/or varicosities
Chest (Breasts)	• Inspection of breasts (e.g., symmetry, nipple discharge) • Palpation of breasts and axillae (e.g., masses or lumps, tenderness)

System/Body Area	Elements of Examination
Gastrointestinal (Abdomen)	• Examination of abdomen with notation of presence of masses or tenderness • Examination of liver and spleen • Examination for presence or absence of hernia • Examination (when indicated) of anus, perineum and rectum, including sphincter tone, presence of hemorrhoids, rectal masses • Obtain stool sample for occult blood test when indicated
Genitourinary	**Male:** • Examination of the scrotal contents (e.g., hydrocele, spermatocele, tenderness of cord, testicular mass) • Examination of the penis • Digital rectal examination of prostate gland (e.g., size, symmetry, nodularity tenderness) **Female:** • Pelvic examination (with or without specimen collection for smears and cultures), including: — examination of external genitalia (e.g., general appearance, hair distribution, lesions) and vagina (e.g., general appearance, estrogen effect, discharge, lesions, pelvic support, cystocele, rectocele) — examination of urethra (e.g., masses, tenderness, scarring) — examination of bladder (e.g., fullness, masses, tenderness) • Cervix (e.g., general appearance, lesions, discharge) • Uterus (e.g., size, contour, position, mobility, tenderness, consistency, descent or support) • Adnexa/parametria (e.g., masses, tenderness)
Lymphatic	Palpation of lymph nodes in **two or more** areas: • Neck • Groin • Axillae • Other
Musculoskeletal	• Examination of gait and station *(if circled, add to total at bottom of column to the left) • Inspection and/or palpation of digits and nails (e.g., clubbing, cyanosis, inflammatory conditions, petechiae, ischemia, infections, nodes) *(if circled, add to total at bottom of column to the left) Examination of joints, bones and muscles of **one or more of the following six** areas: 1) head and neck; 2) spine, ribs, and pelvis; 3) right upper extremity; 4) left upper extremity; 5) right lower extremity; and 6) left lower extremity. The examination of a given area includes: • Inspection and/or palpation with notation of presence of any misalignment, asymmetry, crepitation, defects, tenderness, masses, effusions • Assessment of range of motion with notation of any pain, crepitation or contracture • Assessment of stability with notation of any dislocation (luxation), subluxation, or laxity • Assessment of muscle strength and tone (e.g., flaccid, cog wheel, spastic) with notation of any atrophy or abnormal movements
Skin	• Inspection of skin and subcutaneous tissue (e.g., rashes, lesions, ulcers) • Palpation of skin and subcutaneous tissue (e.g., induration, subcutaneous nodules, tightening)
Neurologic	• Test cranial nerves with notation of any deficits • Examination of deep tendon reflexes with notation of pathological reflexes (e.g., Babinski) • Examination of sensation (e.g., by touch, pin, vibration, proprioception)
Psychiatric	• Description of patient's judgment and insight • Brief assessment of mental status including: — Orientation to time, place and person — Recent and remote memory — Mood and affect (e.g., depression, anxiety, agitation)

Content and Documentation Requirements

Level of exam	Perform and document
Problem focused	**One to five** elements identified by a bullet
Expanded problem focused	**At least six** elements identified by a bullet
Detailed	**At least 12** elements identified by a bullet, whether in a box with a shaded or unshaded border
Comprehensive	Performance of **all** elements identified by a bullet; whether in a box or with a shaded or unshaded box. Documentation of every element in each with a shaded border and at least one element in a box with an unshaded border is expected

Number of Diagnoses or Management Options	Amount and/or Complexity of Data to be Reviewed	Risk of Complications and/or Morbidity or Mortality	Type of Decision Making
Minimal	Minimal or None	Minimal	Straightforward
Limited	Limited	Low	Low Complexity
Multiple	Moderate	Moderate	Moderate Complexity
Extensive	Extensive	High	High Complexity

C. *Documentation of the Complexity of Medical Decision Making 1995 and 1997*

The levels of E/M services recognize four types of medical decision-making (straightforward, low complexity, moderate complexity, and high complexity). Medical decision-making refers to the complexity of establishing a diagnosis and/or selecting a management option as measured by:

- The number of possible diagnoses and/or the number of management options that must be considered
- The amount and/or complexity of medical records, diagnostic tests, and/or other information that must be obtained, reviewed, and analyzed
- The risk of significant complications, morbidity, and/or mortality, as well as comorbidities, associated with the patient's presenting problem, the diagnostic procedure, and/or the possible management options

The following chart shows the progression of the elements required for each level of medical decision-making. To qualify for a given type of decision-making, two of the three elements in the table must be either met or exceeded.

Each of the elements of medical decision-making is described below.

Number of Diagnoses or Management Options

The number of possible diagnoses and/or the number of management options that must be considered is based on the number and types of problems addressed during the encounter, the complexity of establishing a diagnosis, and the management decisions that are made by the physician.

Generally, decision making with respect to a diagnosed problem is easier than that for an identified but undiagnosed problem. The number and type of diagnostic tests employed may be an indicator of the number of possible diagnoses. Problems that are improving or resolving are less complex than those that are worsening or failing to change as expected. The need to seek advice from others is another indicator of complexity of diagnostic or management problems.

- DG: For each encounter, an assessment, clinical impression, or diagnosis should be documented. It may be explicitly stated or implied in documented decisions regarding management plans and/or further evaluation
  - For a presenting problem with an established diagnosis, the record should reflect whether the problem is: a) improved, well controlled, resolving, or resolved; or b) inadequately controlled, worsening, or failing to change as expected
  - For a presenting problem without an established diagnosis, the assessment or clinical impression may be stated in the form of a differential diagnosis or as a "possible," "probable," or "rule-out" (R/O) diagnosis
- DG: The initiation of, or changes in, treatment should be documented. Treatment includes a wide range of management options including patient instructions, nursing instructions, therapies, and medications
- DG: If referrals are made, consultations requested, or advice sought, the record should indicate to whom or where the referral or consultation is made or from whom the advice is requested

Amount and/or Complexity of Data to be Reviewed

The amount and complexity of data to be reviewed is based on the types of diagnostic testing ordered or reviewed. A decision to obtain and review old medical records and/or obtain history from sources other than the patient increases the amount and complexity of data to be reviewed.

Discussion of contradictory or unexpected test results with the physician who performed or interpreted the test is an indication of the complexity of data being reviewed. On occasion, the physician who ordered a test may personally review the image, tracing, or specimen to supplement information from the physician who prepared the test report or interpretation; this is another indication of the complexity of data being reviewed.

- DG: If a diagnostic service (test or procedure) is ordered, planned, scheduled, or performed at the time of the E/M encounter, the type of service (e.g., lab or x-ray) should be documented
- DG: The review of lab, radiology, and/or other diagnostic tests should be documented. A simple notation such as WBC elevated" or "chest x-ray unremarkable" is acceptable. Alternatively, the review may be documented by initialing and dating the report containing the test results
- DG: A decision to obtain old records or a decision to obtain additional history from the family, caretaker, or other source to supplement that obtained from the patient should be documented
- DG: Relevant findings from the review of old records and/or the receipt of additional history from the family, caretaker, or other source to supplement that obtained from the patient should be documented. If there is no relevant information beyond that already obtained, that fact should be documented. A notation of "old records reviewed" or "additional history obtained from family" without elaboration is insufficient
- DG: The results of discussion of laboratory, radiology, or other diagnostic tests with the physician who performed or interpreted the study should be documented
- DG: The direct visualization and independent interpretation of an image, tracing, or specimen previously or subsequently interpreted by another physician should be documented

Risk of Significant Complications, Morbidity, and/or Mortality

The risk of significant complications, morbidity, and/or mortality is based on the risks associated with the presenting problem, the diagnostic procedure, and the possible management options.

- DG: Comorbidities/underlying disease or other factors that increase the complexity of medical decision making by increasing the risk of complications, morbidity, and/or mortality should be documented
- DG: If a surgical or invasive diagnostic procedure is ordered, planned, or scheduled at the time of the E/M encounter, the type of procedure (e.g., laparoscopy) should be documented
- DG: If a surgical or invasive diagnostic procedure is performed at the time of the E/M encounter, the specific procedure should be documented
- DG: The referral for or decision to perform a surgical or invasive diagnostic procedure on an urgent basis should be documented or implied

The following Table of Risk may be used to help determine whether the risk of significant complications, morbidity, and/or mortality is minimal, low, moderate, or high. Because the determination of risk is complex and not readily quantifiable, the table includes common clinical examples rather than absolute measures of risk. The assessment of risk of the presenting problem is based on the risk related to the disease process anticipated between the present encounter and the next one. The assessment of risk of selecting diagnostic procedures and management options is based on the risk during and immediately following any procedures or treatment. The highest level of risk in any one category (presenting problem, diagnostic procedure, or management options) determines the overall risk.

Table of Risk

Level of Risk	Presenting Problem(s)	Diagnostic Procedure(s) Ordered	Management Options Selected
Minimal	One self-limited or minor problem (e.g., cold, insect bite, tinea corporis)	Laboratory test requiring venipuncture Chest x-rays EKG/EEG Urinalysis Ultrasound (e.g., echocardiography) KOH prep	Rest Gargles Elastic bandages Superficial dressings
Low	Two or more self-limited or minor problems One stable chronic illness (e.g., well controlled hypertension, non-insulin dependent diabetes, cataract, BPH) Acute, uncomplicated illness or injury (e.g., cystitis, allergic rhinitis, simple sprain)	Physiologic tests not under stress (e.g., pulmonary function tests) Non-cardiovascular imaging studies with contrast (e.g., barium enema) Superficial needle biopsies Clinical laboratory tests requiring arterial puncture Skin biopsies	Over-the-counter drugs Minor surgery with no identified risk factors Physical therapy Occupational therapy IV fluids without additives
Moderate	One or more chronic illnesses with mild exacerbation, progression or side effects of treatment Two or more stable chronic illnesses Undiagnosed new problem with uncertain prognosis (e.g., lump in breast) Acute illness with systemic symptoms (e.g., pyelonephritis, pneumonitis, colitis) Acute complicated injury (e.g., head injury with brief loss of consciousness)	Physiologic tests not under stress (e.g., cardiac stress test, fetal contraction stress test) Diagnostic endoscopies with no identified risk factors Deep needle or incisional biopsy Cardiovascular imaging studies with contrast and no identified risk factors (e.g., arteriogram, cardiac catheterization) Obtain fluid from body cavity (e.g., lumbar puncture, thoracentesis, culdocentesis)	Minor surgery with identified risk factors Effective major surgery (open, percutaneous or endoscopic) with no identified risk factors Prescription drug management Therapeutic nuclear medicine IV fluids with additives Closed treatment of fracture or dislocation without manipulation
High	One or more chronic illnesses with severe exacerbation, progression or side effects of treatment Acute/chronic illnesses that may pose a threat to life or bodily function (e.g., multiple trauma, acute MI, pulmonary embolus, severe respiratory distress, progressive severe rheumatoid arthritis, psychiatric illness with potential threat to self or others, peritonitis, acute renal failure An abrupt change in neurologic status (e.g., seizure, TIA, weakness or sensory loss)	Cardiovascular imaging studies with contrast with identified risk factors Cardiac electrophysiological tests Diagnostic endoscopies with identified risk factors Discography	Elective major surgery (open, percutaneous or endoscopic) with identified risk factors Emergency major surgery (open, percutaneous or endoscopic) Parenteral controlled substances Drug therapy requiring intensive monitoring for toxicity Decision not to resuscitate or to de-escalate care because of poor prognosis

D. Documentation of an Encounter Dominated by Counseling or Coordination of Care

In the case where counseling and/or coordination of care dominates (more than 50 percent) the physician/patient and/or family encounter (face-to-face time in the office or other outpatient setting or floor-unit time in the hospital or nursing facility), time is considered the key or controlling factor to qualify for a particular level of E/M service.

- DG: If the physician elects to report the level of service based on counseling and/or coordination of care, the total length of time of the encounter (face-to-face or floor time, as appropriate) should be documented and the record should describe the counseling and/or activities to coordinate care

Appendix D — Crosswalk of Deleted Codes

The deleted code crosswalk is meant to be used as a reference tool to find active codes that could be used in place of the deleted code. This will not always be an exact match. Please review the code descriptions and guidelines before selecting a code.

Code	Cross reference
01935	To report, see 01937, 01938, 01939, 01940, 01941, 01942
01936	To report, see 01937, 01938, 01939, 01940, 01941, 01942
69715	To report, see 69501-69530, 69535-69554, 69601-69604, 69610-69646, 69650-69662, 69666-69676
69718	To report, see 69501-69530, 69535-69554, 69601-69604, 69610-69646, 69650-69662, 69666-69676
72275	To report, see 62281, 62282, 62321, 62323, 62325, 62327, 64479, 64480, 64483, 64484
80500	To report, see 80503, 80504, 80505, 80506
80502	To report, see 80503, 80504, 80505, 80506
87450	To report, see 87301-87451, 87802-87899
92559	To report, see 92700
92560	To report, see 92700
92561	To report, see 92700
92564	To report, see 92700
93530	To report, see 93593, 93594
93531	To report, see 93462, 93596, 93597
93532	To report, see 93462, 93596, 93597
93533	To report, see 93462, 93596, 93597
93561	To report, see 93598
93562	To report, see 93598
95943	To report, see 95999
0191T	To report, see [66989], [66991], [0671T]
0290T	To report, see 66999
0355T	To report, see [91113]
0356T	To report, see 68841
0376T	To report, see [66989], [66991], [0671T]
0423T	To report, see 84999
0451T	To report, see 33999
0452T	To report, see 33999
0453T	To report, see 33999
0454T	To report, see 33999
0454T	To report, see 33999
0455T	To report, see 33999
0456T	To report, see 33999
0457T	To report, see 33999
0458T	To report, see 33999
0459T	To report, see 33999
0460T	To report, see 33999
0461T	To report, see 33999
0462T	To report, see 33999
0463T	To report, see 33999
0466T	To report, see 64582-64584
0467T	To report, see 64582-64584
0468T	To report, see 64582-64584
0548T	To report, see 53451-53454
0549T	To report, see 53451-53454
0550T	To report, see 53451-53454
0551T	To report, see 53451-53454

Appendix E — Resequenced Codes

This appendix contains a list of codes that are not in numeric order in the book. AMA resequenced some code numbers to relocate codes in the same category but not in numeric sequence. In addition to the list of resequenced codes, the page number where the code may be found is provided for ease of use.

Code	Page	Reference
10004	13	See code following 10021.
10005	13	See code following 10021.
10006	13	See code following 10021.
10007	13	See code following 10021.
10008	13	See code following 10021.
10009	13	See code following 10021.
10010	13	See code following 10021.
10011	13	See code following 10021.
10012	13	See code following 10021.
11045	15	See code following 11042.
11046	15	See code following 11043.
15769	27	See code following 15770.
20560	38	See code following 20553.
20561	38	See code before 20555.
21552	49	See code following 21555.
21554	49	See code following 21556.
22858	58	See code following 22856.
22859	58	See code following 22854.
23071	60	See code following 23075.
23073	60	See code following 23076.
24071	63	See code following 24075.
24073	64	See code following 24076.
25071	68	See code following 25075.
25073	68	See code following 25076.
26111	73	See code following 26115.
26113	73	See code following 26116.
27043	79	See code following 27047.
27045	79	See code following 27048.
27059	79	See code following 27049.
27329	85	See code following 27360.
27337	84	See code following 27327.
27339	84	See code before 27330.
27632	90	See code following 27618.
27634	90	See code following 27619.
28039	94	See code following 28043.
28041	94	See code following 28045.
28295	97	See code following 28296.
29914	103	See code following 29863.
29915	103	See code following 29863.
29916	103	See code before 29866.
31253	110	See code following 31255.
31257	110	See code following 31255.
31259	110	See code following 31255.
31551	114	See code following 31580.
31552	114	See code following 31580.
31553	114	See code following 31580.
31554	114	See code following 31580.
31572	114	See code following 31578.
31573	114	See code following 31578.
31574	114	See code following 31578.
31651	116	See code following 31647.
32994	122	See code following 32998.
33221	125	See code following 33213.
33227	126	See code following 33233.
33228	126	See code following 33233.
33229	126	See code before 33234.
33230	127	See code following 33240.
33231	127	See code before 33241.
33262	128	See code following 33241.
33263	128	See code following 33241.
33264	128	See code before 33243.
33267	130	See code following 33261.
33268	130	See code following 33261.
33269	131	See code following 33261.
33270	129	See code following 33249.
33271	129	See code following 33249.
33272	129	See code following 33249.
33273	129	See code following 33249.
33274	129	See code following 33249.
33275	129	See code following 33249.
33440	133	See code following 33410.
33962	144	See code following 33959.
33963	145	See code following 33959.
33964	145	See code following 33959.
33965	145	See code following 33959.
33966	145	See code following 33959.
33969	145	See code following 33959.
33984	145	See code following 33959.
33985	145	See code following 33959.
33986	145	See code following 33959.
33987	145	See code following 33959.
33988	145	See code following 33959.
33989	145	See code following 33959.
33995	147	See code following 33983.
33997	147	See code following 33992.
34717	149	See code following 34708.
34718	149	See code following 34709.
34812	150	See code following 34713.
34820	150	See code following 34714.
34833	150	See code following 34714.
34834	150	See code following 34714.
36465	162	See code following 36471.
36466	162	See code following 36471.
36482	163	See code following 36479.
36483	163	See code following 36479.
36572	165	See code following 36569.
36573	165	See code following 36569.
37246	172	See code following 37235.
37247	173	See code following 37235.
37248	173	See code following 37235.
37249	173	See code following 37235.
38243	177	See code following 38241.
43210	194	See code following 43259.
43211	190	See code following 43217.
43212	190	See code following 43217.
43213	190	See code following 43220.
43214	190	See code following 43220.
43233	193	See code following 43249.
43266	194	See code following 43255.
43270	194	See code following 43257.
43274	195	See code following numeric code 43270.
43275	195	See code following numeric code 43270.
43276	195	See code following numeric code 43270.
43277	195	See code following numeric code 43270.
43278	195	See code following numeric code 43270.
44381	206	See code following 44382.
44401	206	See code following 44392.
45346	210	See code following 45338.
45388	211	See code following 45382.
45390	212	See code following 45392.
45398	212	See code following 45393.
45399	213	See code before 45990.
46220	214	See code before 46230.
46320	214	See code following 46230.
46945	214	See code following 46221.
46946	214	See code following resequenced code 46945.
46947	216	See code following 46761.
46948	214	See code before resequenced code 46220.
50430	231	See code following 50396.
50431	231	See code following 50396.
50432	232	See code following 50396.
50433	232	See code following 50396.
50434	232	See code following 50396.
50435	232	See code following 50396.
50436	231	See code following 50391.
50437	231	See code following 50391.
51797	238	See code following 51729.
52356	242	See code following 52353.
58674	260	See code before 58541.

Code	Page	Reference
62328	283	See code following 62270.
62329	283	See code following 62272.
63052	286	See code following 63048.
63053	286	See code following 63048.
64461	292	See code following 64484.
64462	292	See code following 64484.
64463	292	See code following 64484.
64624	294	See code following 64610.
64625	294	See code before 64611.
64628	294	See code before 64611.
64629	294	See code before 64611.
64633	295	See code following 64620.
64634	295	See code following 64620.
64635	295	See code following 64620.
64636	295	See code before 64630.
66987	306	See code following 66982. Resequenced code. See code following resequenced code 66989.
66988	307	See code following 66984. Resequenced code. See code following resequenced code 66991.
66989	306	See code following 66982.
66991	307	See code following 66984.
67810	311	See code following 67715.
69714	317	See code following 69676.
69716	317	See code following 69676.
69717	317	See code following 69676.
69719	317	See code following 69676.
69726	317	See code following 69676.
69727	317	See code following 69676.
77085	344	See code following 77081.
77086	344	See code before 77084.
77295	344	See code before 77300.
77385	346	See code following 77417.
77386	346	See code following 77417.
77387	346	See code following 77417.
77424	346	See code following 77417.
77425	346	See code following 77417.
78429	350	See code following 78459.
78430	350	See code following 78491.
78431	351	See code following 78492.
78432	351	See code following 78492.
78433	351	See code following 78492.
78434	351	See code following 78492.
78804	352	See code following 78802.
78830	352	See code following numeric code 78804.
78831	353	See code following numeric code 78804.
78832	353	See code following numeric code 78804.
78835	353	See code following numeric code 78804.
80081	357	See code following 80055.
80161	360	See code following 80157.
80164	361	See code following 80201.
80165	361	See code following 80201.
80167	360	See code following 80169.
80171	360	See code before 80170.
80176	361	See code following 80177.
80179	361	See code before 80195.
80181	360	See code following resequenced code 80167.
80189	360	See code following resequenced code 80230.
80193	360	See code before 80177.
80204	361	See code following 80178.
80210	361	See code following 80194.
80220	360	See code following 80173.
80230	360	See code following 80173.
80235	360	See code before 80175.
80280	361	See code following 80202.
80285	361	See code before 80203.
80305	358	See code before 80143.
80306	358	See code before 80143.
80307	358	See code before 80143.
80320	358	See code before 80143.
80321	358	See code before 80143.
80322	358	See code before 80143.
80323	358	See code before 80143.
80324	358	See code before 80143.
80325	358	See code before 80143.
80326	358	See code before 80143.
80327	358	See code before 80143.
80328	358	See code before 80143.
80329	358	See code before 80143.
80330	358	See code before 80143.
80331	358	See code before 80143.
80332	358	See code before 80143.
80333	359	See code before 80143.
80334	359	See code before 80143.
80335	359	See code before 80143.
80336	359	See code before 80143.
80337	359	See code before 80143.
80338	359	See code before 80143.
80339	359	See code before 80143.
80340	359	See code following resequenced code 80339.
80341	359	See code before 80143.
80342	359	See code before 80143.
80343	359	See code before 80143.
80344	359	See code before 80143.
80345	359	See code before 80143.
80346	359	See code before 80143.
80347	359	See code before 80143.
80348	359	See code before 80143.
80349	359	See code before 80143.
80350	359	See code before 80143.
80351	359	See code before 80143.
80352	359	See code before 80143.
80353	359	See code before 80143.
80354	359	See code before 80143.
80355	359	See code before 80143.
80356	359	See code before 80143.
80357	359	See code before 80143.
80358	359	See code before 80143.
80359	359	See code before 80143.
80360	359	See code before 80143.
80361	359	See code before 80143.
80362	359	See code before 80143.
80363	359	See code before 80143.
80364	359	See code before 80143.
80365	359	See code before 80143.
80366	359	See code before 80143.
80367	359	See code before 80143.
80368	359	See code before 80143.
80369	359	See code before 80143.
80370	359	See code before 80143.
80371	360	See code before 80143.
80372	360	See code before 80143.
80373	360	See code before 80143.
80374	360	See code before 80143.
80375	360	See code before 80143.
80376	360	See code before 80143.
80377	360	See code before 80143.
81105	369	See code before 81260.
81106	370	See code before 81260.
81107	370	See code before 81260.
81108	370	See code before 81260.
81109	370	See code before 81260.
81110	370	See code before 81260.
81111	370	See code before 81260.
81112	370	See code before 81260.
81120	370	See code before 81260.
81121	370	See code before 81260.
81161	368	See code following numeric code 81231.
81162	366	See code following resequenced code 81210.
81163	366	See code following resequenced code 81210.
81164	366	See code before 81212.
81165	366	See code following 81212.
81166	366	See code following 81212.
81167	366	See code following 81216.
81168	367	See code before 81218.
81173	365	See code following resequenced code 81204.
81174	365	See code following resequenced code 81204.
81184	367	See code following resequenced code 81233.
81185	367	See code following resequenced code 81233.
81186	367	See code following resequenced code 81233.

Code	Page	Reference
81187	367	See code following resequenced code 81268.
81188	367	See code following resequenced code 81266.
81189	367	See code following resequenced code 81266.
81190	367	See code following resequenced code 81266.
81191	372	See code following numeric code 81312.
81192	372	See code following numeric code 81312.
81193	372	See code following numeric code 81312.
81194	372	See code following numeric code 81312.
81200	365	See code before 81175.
81201	365	See code following numeric code 81174.
81202	365	See code following numeric code 81174.
81203	365	See code following numeric code 81174.
81204	365	See code following numeric code 81174.
81205	366	See code following numeric code 81210.
81206	366	See code following numeric code 81210.
81207	366	See code following numeric code 81210.
81208	366	See code following numeric code 81210.
81209	366	See code following numeric code 81210.
81210	366	See code following numeric code 81210.
81219	367	See code before 81218.
81227	367	See code before 81225.
81230	367	See code following numeric code 81227.
81231	367	See code following numeric code 81227.
81233	366	See code following 81217.
81234	368	See code following numeric code 81231.
81238	368	See code following 81241.
81239	368	See code before 81232.
81245	368	See code following 81242.
81246	368	See code following 81242.
81250	369	See code before 81247.
81257	369	See code following 81254.
81258	369	See code following 81254.
81259	369	See code following 81254.
81261	370	See code before 81260.
81262	370	See code before 81260.
81263	370	See code before 81260.
81264	370	See code before 81260.
81265	367	See code following resequenced code 81187.
81266	367	See code following resequenced code 81265.
81267	367	See code following 81224.
81268	367	See code following 81224.
81269	369	See code following resequenced code 81259.
81271	369	See code following numeric code 81259.
81274	369	See code following resequenced code 81271.
81277	368	See code following 81229.
81278	370	See code following resequenced code 81263.
81279	370	See code following 81270.
81283	370	See code following resequenced code 81121.
81284	369	See code following numeric code 81246.
81285	369	See code following numeric code 81246.
81286	369	See code following numeric code 81246.
81287	371	See code following resequenced code 81304.
81288	371	See code following resequenced code 81292.
81289	369	See code following numeric code 81246.
81291	371	See code before 81305.
81292	371	See code before numeric code 81291.
81293	371	See code before numeric code 81291.
81294	371	See code before numeric code 81291.
81295	371	See code before numeric code 81291.
81301	371	See code following resequenced code 81287.
81302	371	See code following 81290.
81303	371	See code following 81290.
81304	371	See code following 81290.
81306	372	See code following resequenced code 81194.
81307	372	See code before 81313.
81308	372	See code before 81313.
81309	372	See code following 81314.
81312	372	See code before resequenced code 81307.
81320	372	See code before 81315.
81324	372	See code following 81316.
81325	372	See code following 81316.
81326	372	See code following 81316.
81332	373	See code following 81327.
81334	373	See code following numeric code 81326.
81336	373	See code following 81329.
81337	373	See code following 81329.
81338	371	See code following resequenced code 81294.
81339	371	See code before resequenced code 81295.
81343	372	See code following numeric code 81320.
81344	373	See code following numeric code 81332.
81345	373	See code following numeric code 81332.
81347	373	See code before 81328.
81348	373	See code following numeric code 81332.
81349	368	See code following 81229.
81351	373	See code before 81335.
81352	373	See code before 81335.
81353	373	See code before 81335.
81357	374	See code before 81350.
81361	369	See code following 81254.
81362	369	See code following 81254.
81363	369	See code following 81254.
81364	369	See code following 81254.
81419	386	See code following 81414.
81443	386	See code following 81422.
81448	387	See code following 81438.
81479	386	See code following 81408.
81500	389	See code following 81538.
81503	389	See code before 81539.
81504	390	See code following resequenced code 81546.
81522	389	See code following 81518.
81540	390	See code before 81552.
81546	390	See code following 81551.
81595	388	See code following 81490.
81596	389	See code following 81514.
82042	391	See code following 82045.
82652	393	See code following 82306.
82653	395	See code following 82656.
82681	396	See code following 82670.
83529	399	See code following 83527.
83992	359	See code following resequenced code 80365.
86015	409	See code before 86000.
86051	409	See code following 86063.
86052	409	See code following 86063.
86053	409	See code following 86063.
86152	410	See code following 86147.
86153	410	See code before 86148.
86328	411	See code following 86318.
86362	411	See code following 86356.
86363	411	See code following 86356.
86364	411	See code following 86357.
86408	412	See code following 86382.
86409	412	See code following 86382.
86413	412	See code following resequenced code 86409.

Code	Page	Reference
87154	419	See code following 87150.
87428	422	See code following 87426.
87623	424	See code following 87539.
87624	424	See code following 87539.
87625	424	See code before 87540.
87806	426	See code following 87803.
87811	426	See code following 87807.
87906	426	See code following 87901.
87910	426	See code following 87900.
87912	426	See code before 87902.
88177	428	See code following 88173.
88341	432	See code following 88342.
88350	432	See code following 88346.
88364	433	See code following 88365.
88373	433	See code following 88367.
88374	433	See code following 88367.
88377	433	See code following 88369.
0051A	454	See code following 0004A.
0052A	454	See code following 0004A.
0053A	454	See code following 0004A.
0054A	454	See code following 0004A.
0064A	454	See code following 0013A.
0071A	454	See code following 0004A.
0072A	454	See code following 0004A.
90619	459	See code following 90734.
90620	459	See code following 90734.
90621	460	See code following 90734.
90625	459	See code following 90723.
90626	459	See code following 90715.
90627	459	See code following 90715.
90630	457	See code following 90654.
90644	459	See code following 90732.
90672	457	See code following 90660.
90673	457	See code before 90662.
90674	457	See code following 90661.
90677	458	See code following 90671.
90694	458	See code following 90689.
90750	460	See code following 90736.
90756	457	See code following 90661.
90758	460	See code following 90748.
90759	460	See code following 90746.
91113	466	See code following 91111.
91300	455	See code before 90476.
91301	456	See code before 90476.
91302	456	See code before 90476.
91303	456	See code before 90476.
91304	456	See code before 90476.
91305	456	See code following resequenced code 91300.
91306	456	See code following resequenced code 91301.
91307	456	See code following resequenced code 91305.
92517	472	See code following 92549.
92518	472	See code following 92549.
92519	472	See code following 92549.
92558	473	See code before 92587.
92597	473	See code following 92604.
92618	473	See code following 92605.
92650	473	See code following 92584.
92651	473	See code following 92584.
92652	473	See code following 92584.
92653	473	See code following 92584.
92920	476	See code following 92998.
92921	476	See code following 92998.
92924	476	See code following 92998.
92925	476	See code following 92998.
92928	476	See code following 92998.
92929	476	See code following 92998.
92933	476	See code following 92998.
92934	477	See code following 92998.
92937	477	See code following 92998.
92938	477	See code following 92998.
92941	477	See code following 92998.
92943	477	See code following 92998.
92944	477	See code following 92998.
92973	477	See code following 92998.
92974	477	See code following 92998.
92975	477	See code following 92998.
92977	477	See code following 92998.
92978	477	See code following 92998.
92979	477	See code following 92998.
93241	479	See code following 93227.
93242	479	See code following 93227.
93243	479	See code following 93227.
93244	479	See code following 93227.
93245	479	See code following 93227.
93246	479	See code following 93227.
93247	479	See code following 93227.
93248	479	See code following 93227.
93260	481	See code following 93284.
93261	482	See code following 93289.
93264	480	See code before 93279.
93319	484	See code following 93317.
93356	484	See code following 93351.
94619	497	See code following 94617.
95249	501	See code following 95250.
95700	508	See code following 95967.
95705	508	See code following 95967.
95706	508	See code following 95967.
95707	508	See code following 95967.
95708	508	See code following 95967.
95709	508	See code following 95967.
95710	508	See code following 95967.
95711	508	See code following 95967.
95712	509	See code following 95967.
95713	509	See code following 95967.
95714	509	See code following 95967.
95715	509	See code following 95967.
95716	509	See code following 95967.
95717	509	See code following 95967.
95718	509	See code following 95967.
95719	509	See code following 95967.
95720	509	See code following 95967.
95721	509	See code following 95967.
95722	509	See code following 95967.
95723	509	See code following 95967.
95724	509	See code following 95967.
95725	509	See code following 95967.
95726	509	See code following 95967.
95782	502	See code following 95811.
95783	502	See code following 95811.
95800	502	See code following 95806.
95801	502	See code following 95806.
95829	503	See code following 95830.
95836	504	See code following 95830.
95885	504	See code following 95872.
95886	505	See code following 95872.
95887	505	See code before 95873.
95938	507	See code following 95926.
95939	507	See code following 95929.
95940	506	See code following 95913.
95941	506	See code following 95913.
95983	510	See code following 95977.
95984	510	See code following 95977.
96125	513	See code following 96105.
96127	513	See code following 96113.
96164	514	See code following 96159.
96165	514	See code following 96159.
96167	514	See code following 96159.
96168	514	See code following 96159.
96170	514	See code following 96159.
96171	514	See code following 96159.
97151	511	See code following 96040.
97152	512	See code following 96040.
97153	512	See code following 96040.
97154	512	See code following 96040.
97155	512	See code following 96040.
97156	512	See code following 96040.
97157	512	See code following 96040.
97158	513	See code following 96040.
97161	521	See code before 97010.
97162	522	See code before 97010.
97163	522	See code before 97010.
97164	522	See code before 97010.
97165	522	See code before 97010.
97166	522	See code before 97010.
97167	523	See code before 97010.
97168	523	See code before 97010.
97169	523	See code before 97010.
97170	523	See code before 97010.
97171	523	See code before 97010.
97172	523	See code before 97010.

Code	Page	Reference
99091	559	See code following resequenced code 99454.
99177	532	See code following 99174.
99224	545	See code following 99220.
99225	545	See code following 99220.
99226	546	See code following 99220.
99415	555	See code following 99359.
99416	555	See code following 99359.
99417	555	See code following resequenced code 99416.
99421	558	See code following 99443.
99422	558	See code following 99443.
99423	558	See code following 99443.
99424	564	See code following 99489.
99425	564	See code following 99489.
99426	564	See code following 99489.
99427	564	See code following 99489.
99437	563	See code following resequenced code 99491.
99439	563	See code following resequenced code 99490.
99451	558	See code following 99449.

Code	Page	Reference
99452	559	See code following 99449.
99453	559	See code following 99449.
99454	559	See code following 99449.
99457	560	See code before 99450.
99458	560	See code before 99450.
99473	559	See code before 99450.
99474	559	See code before 99450.
99484	565	See code following 99498.
99485	561	See code following 99467.
99486	561	See code following 99467.
99490	563	See code before 99487.
99491	563	See code before 99487.
2033F	571	See code following 2026F.
3051F	572	See code following 3044F.
3052F	572	See code before 3046F.
0253T	584	See code before 0198T.
0464T	587	See code following 0333T.
0488T	589	See code following 0403T.
0510T	587	See code following 0335T.
0511T	587	See code following 0335T.
0512T	583	See code following 0102T.

Code	Page	Reference
0513T	583	See code following 0102T.
0523T	594	See code before 0505T.
0563T	585	See code following 0207T.
0614T	599	See code following 0580T.
0620T	594	See code following 0505T.
0623T	594	See code following 0504T.
0624T	594	See code following 0504T.
0625T	594	See code following 0504T.
0626T	594	See code following 0504T.
0640T	593	See code following 0493T
0641T	593	See code following 0493T
0642T	593	See code following 0493T
0643T	597	See code following 0545T
0646T	598	See code following 0570T
0671T	584	See code following 0184T.
0697T	603	See code following 0648T.
0698T	604	See code following 0649T.

Appendix F — Add-on Codes, Optum Modifier 50 Exempt, Modifier 51 Exempt, Optum Modifier 51 Exempt, Modifier 63 Exempt, and Modifier 95 Telemedicine Services

Codes specified as add-on, exempt from modifiers 50, 51 and 63, and modifier 95 (telemedicine services) are listed. The lists are designed to be read left to right rather than vertically.

Add-on Codes

0054T	0055T	0076T	0095T	0098T	0163T	0164T
0165T	0174T	0214T	0215T	0217T	0218T	0222T
0397T	0437T	0439T	0443T	0450T	0471T	0480T
0492T	0496T	0513T	0514T	0523T	0560T	0562T
0570T	0599T	0628T	0630T	0649T	0663T	0676T
0678T	0690T	0698T	0701T	0709T	0071U	0072U
0073U	0074U	0075U	0076U	0130U	0131U	0132U
0133U	0134U	0135U	0136U	0137U	0138U	0157U
0158U	0159U	0160U	0161U	0162U	0207U	01953
01968	01969	10004	10006	10008	10010	10012
10036	11001	11008	11045	11046	11047	11103
11105	11107	11201	11732	11922	13102	13122
13133	13153	14302	15003	15005	15101	15111
15116	15121	15131	15136	15151	15152	15156
15157	15201	15221	15241	15261	15272	15274
15276	15278	15772	15774	15777	15787	15847
16036	17003	17312	17314	17315	19001	19082
19084	19086	19126	19282	19284	19286	19288
19294	19297	20700	20701	20702	20703	20704
20705	20930	20931	20932	20933	20934	20936
20937	20938	20939	20985	22103	22116	22208
22216	22226	22328	22512	22515	22527	22534
22552	22585	22614	22632	22634	22840	22841
22842	22843	22844	22845	22846	22847	22848
22853	22854	22858	22859	22868	22870	26125
26861	26863	27358	27692	29826	31627	31632
31633	31637	31649	31651	31654	32501	32506
32507	32667	32668	32674	33141	33225	33257
33258	33259	33268	33367	33368	33369	33370
33419	33508	33517	33518	33519	33521	33522
33523	33530	33572	33746	33768	33866	33884
33924	33929	33987	34709	34711	34713	34714
34715	34716	34717	34808	34812	34813	34820
34833	34834	35306	35390	35400	35500	35572
35681	35682	35683	35685	35686	35697	35700
36218	36227	36228	36248	36474	36476	36479
36483	36907	36908	36909	37185	37186	37222
37223	37232	37233	37234	37235	37237	37239
37247	37249	37252	37253	38102	38746	38747
38900	43273	43283	43338	43635	44015	44121
44128	44139	44203	44213	44701	44955	47001
47542	47543	47544	47550	48400	49326	49327
49412	49435	49568	49905	50606	50705	50706
51797	52442	56606	57267	57465	58110	58611
59525	60512	61316	61517	61611	61641	61642
61651	61781	61782	61783	61797	61799	61800
61864	61868	62148	62160	63035	63043	63044
63048	63052	63053	63057	63066	63076	63078
63082	63086	63088	63091	63103	63295	63308
63621	64421	64462	64480	64484	64491	64492
64494	64495	64629	64634	64636	64643	64645
64727	64778	64783	64787	64832	64837	64859
64872	64874	64876	64901	64902	64913	65757
66990	67225	67320	67331	67332	67334	67335
67340	69990	74248	74301	74713	75565	75774
76125	76802	76810	76812	76814	76937	76979
76983	77001	77002	77003	77063	77293	78020
78434	78496	78730	78835	80506	81266	81416
81426	81536	82952	86826	87187	87503	87904
88155	88177	88185	88311	88314	88332	88334
88341	88350	88364	88369	88373	88388	90461
90472	90474	90785	90833	90836	90838	90840
90863	90913	91013	92547	92608	92618	92621
92627	92921	92925	92929	92934	92938	92944
92973	92974	92978	92979	92998	93319	93320
93321	93325	93352	93356	93462	93463	93464
93563	93564	93565	93566	93567	93568	93571
93572	93592	93598	93609	93613	93621	93622
93623	93655	93657	93662	94645	94729	94781
95079	95873	95874	95885	95886	95887	95940
95941	95962	95967	95984	96113	96121	96131
96133	96137	96139	96159	96165	96168	96171
96361	96366	96367	96368	96370	96371	96375
96376	96411	96415	96417	96423	96570	96571
96934	96935	96936	97130	97546	97598	97811
97814	98981	99100	99116	99135	99140	99153
99157	99292	99354	99355	99356	99357	99359
99415	99416	99417	99425	99427	99437	99439
99458	99467	99486	99489	99494	99498	99602
99607						

Optum Modifier 50 Exempt Codes

0214T	0215T	0217T	0218T	15777	20939	34713
34714	34715	34716	34717	34812	34820	34833
34834	35572	49568	63035	63043	63044	64421
64480	64484	64491	64492	64494	64495	64634
64636						

AMA Modifier 51 Exempt Codes

20697	20974	20975	33509	35600	44500	61107
93600	93602	93603	93610	93612	93615	93616
93618	94610	95905	99151	99152		

Optum Modifier 51 Exempt Codes

22585	22614	22632	69990	90281	90283	90284
90287	90288	90291	90296	90371	90375	90376
90377	90378	90384	90385	90386	90389	90393
90396	90399	90476	90477	90581	90585	90586
90587	90619	90620	90621	90625	90630	90632
90633	90634	90636	90644	90647	90648	90649
90650	90651	90653	90654	90655	90656	90657
90658	90660	90661	90662	90664	90666	90667
90668	90670	90672	90673	90674	90675	90676
90680	90681	90682	90685	90686	90687	90688
90689	90690	90691	90694	90696	90697	90698
90700	90702	90707	90710	90713	90714	90715
90716	90717	90723	90732	90733	90734	90736
90738	90739	90740	90743	90744	90746	90747
90748	90749	90750	90756	97010	97012	97014
97016	97018	97022	97024	97026	97028	97032
97033	97034	97035	97036	97110	97112	97113
97116	97124	97129	97130	97140	97150	97161
97162	97163	97164	97165	97166	97167	97168
97169	97170	97171	97172	97530	97533	97535
97537	97542	97545	97546	97597	97598	97602
97605	97606	97607	97608	97610	97750	97755
97760	97761	97763	99050	99051	99053	99056
99058	99060					

Modifier 63 Exempt Codes

30540	30545	31520	33502	33503	33505	33506
33610	33611	33619	33647	33670	33690	33694
33730	33732	33735	33736	33741	33750	33755
33762	33778	33786	33922	33946	33947	33948

33949	36415	36420	36450	36456	36460	36510
36660	39503	43313	43314	43520	43831	44055
44126	44127	44128	46070	46705	46715	46716
46730	46735	46740	46742	46744	47700	47701
49215	49491	49492	49495	49496	49600	49605
49606	49610	49611	53025	54000	54150	54160
63700	63702	63704	63706	65820		

Telemedicine Services Codes

The codes on the following list may be used to report telemedicine services when modifier 95 Synchronous Telemedicine Service Rendered via a Real-Time Interactive Audio and Visual Telecommunications System, is appended.

90785	90791	90792	90832	90833	90834	90836
90837	90838	90839	90840	90845	90846	90847
90863	90951	90952	90954	90955	90957	90958
90960	90961	90963	90964	90965	90966	90967
90968	90969	90970	92227	92228	93228	93229
93268	93270	93271	93272	96040	96116	96160
96161	97110	97112	97116	97161	97162	97165
97166	97530	97535	97750	97755	97760	97761
97802	97803	97804	98960	98961	98962	99202
99203	99204	99205	99211	99212	99213	99214
99215	99231	99232	99233	*99241	*99242	*99243
*99244	*99245	*99251	*99252	*99253	*99254	*99255
99307	99308	99309	99310	99354	99355	99356
99357	99406	99407	99408	99409	99417	99495
99496	99497	99498				

* Consultations are noncovered by Medicare

Appendix G — Medicare Internet-only Manuals (IOMs)

The Centers for Medicare and Medicaid Services restructured its paper-based manual system as a web-based system on October 1, 2003. Called the online CMS manual system, it combines all of the various program instructions into internet-only manuals (IOMs), which are used by all CMS programs and contractors. In many instances, the references from the online manuals in appendix G contain a mention of the old paper manuals from which the current information was obtained when the manuals were converted. This information is shown in the header of the text, in the following format, when applicable, as A3-3101, HO-210, and B3-2049.

Effective with implementation of the IOMs, the former method of publishing program memoranda (PMs) to communicate program instructions was replaced by the following four templates:

- One-time notification
- Manual revisions
- Business requirements
- Confidential requirements

The web-based system has been organized by functional area (e.g., eligibility, entitlement, claims processing, benefit policy, program integrity) in an effort to eliminate redundancy within the manuals, simplify updating, and make CMS program instructions available more quickly. The web-based system contains the functional areas included below:

Pub. 100	Introduction
Pub. 100-01	Medicare General Information, Eligibility and Entitlement Manual
Pub. 100-02	Medicare Benefit Policy Manual
Pub. 100-03	Medicare National Coverage Determinations (NCD) Manual
Pub. 100-04	Medicare Claims Processing Manual
Pub. 100-05	Medicare Secondary Payer Manual
Pub. 100-06	Medicare Financial Management Manual
Pub. 100-07	State Operations Manual
Pub. 100-08	Medicare Program Integrity Manual
Pub. 100-09	Medicare Contractor Beneficiary and Provider Communications Manual
Pub. 100-10	Quality Improvement Organization Manual
Pub. 100-11	Programs of All-Inclusive Care for the Elderly (PACE) Manual
Pub. 100-12	State Medicaid Manual (under development)
Pub. 100-13	Medicaid State Children's Health Insurance Program (under development)
Pub. 100-14	Medicare ESRD Network Organizations Manual
Pub. 100-15	Medicaid Integrity Program (MIP)
Pub. 100-16	Medicare Managed Care Manual
Pub. 100-17	CMS/Business Partners Systems Security Manual
Pub. 100-18	Medicare Prescription Drug Benefit Manual
Pub. 100-19	Demonstrations
Pub. 100-20	One-Time Notification
Pub. 100-21	Reserved
Pub. 100-22	Medicare Quality Reporting Incentive Programs Manual
Pub. 100-24	State Buy-In Manual
Pub. 100-25	Information Security Acceptable Risk Safeguards Manual

A brief description of the Medicare manuals primarily used for *CPC Expert* follows:

The ***National Coverage Determinations Manual*** (NCD), is organized according to categories such as diagnostic services, supplies, and medical procedures. The table of contents lists each category and subject within that category. Revision transmittals identify any new or background material, recap the changes, and provide an effective date for the change. The manual contains four sections and is organized in accordance with CPT category sequence and contains a list of HCPCS codes related to coverage determinations, where appropriate.

The ***Medicare Benefit Policy Manual*** contains Medicare general coverage instructions that are not national coverage determinations. As a general rule, in the past these instructions have been found in chapter II of the ***Medicare Carriers Manual,*** the ***Medicare Intermediary Manual***, other provider manuals, and program memoranda.

The ***Medicare Claims Processing Manual*** contains instructions for processing claims for contractors and providers.

The ***Medicare Program Integrity Manual*** communicates the priorities and standards for the Medicare integrity programs.

Medicare IOM References

A printed version of the Medicare IOM references will no longer be published in Optum360's *Current Procedural Coding* product. Complete versions of all the manuals can be found online at https://www.cms.gov/Regulations-and-Guidance/Guidance/Manuals/Internet-Only-Manuals-IOMs.

Appendix H — Quality Payment Program

In 2015, Congress passed the Medicare Access and CHIP Reauthorization Act (MACRA), which included sweeping changes for practitioners who provide services reimbursed under the Medicare physician fee schedule (MPFS). The act focused on repealing the faulty Medicare sustainable growth rate, focusing on quality of patient outcomes, and controlling Medicare spending.

A MACRA final rule in October 2016 established the Quality Payment Program (QPP), which was effective January 1, 2017. This value-based payment model rewards eligible clinicians (ECs) who provide high-quality care and reduce the payments for those who fail to meet specific performance standards.

ECs can receive incentives under the QPP. Once the performance threshold is established, all ECs who score above that threshold are eligible to receive a positive payment adjustment. Keep in mind that the key requirement is that an EC **submit data** to avoid the negative payment adjustment and receive the incentives. The Centers for Medicare and Medicaid Services (CMS) has redesigned the scoring so that clinicians are able to know how well they are doing in the program, as benchmarks are known in advance of participating.

The QPP consists of two tracks that clinicians may choose from based on their practice size, location, specialty, or patient population:

- The merit-based incentive payment system (MIPS)
- Alternative payment models (APMs)

The 2017 QPP final rule established regulations for MIPS and APMs as well as related policies applicable to eligible clinicians who participate in the Shared Savings Program. These policies included requirements for Shared Savings Program accountable care organizations (ACOs) regarding reporting for the MIPS Quality performance category and a policy that gave ACOs full credit for the MIPS Improvement Activities performance category based on their participation in the Shared Savings Program. Since that time, revisions and modifications have been made to allow more focus on measurement efforts and to reduce barriers to entry into advanced APMs. Refinements will continue in order to reduce reporting burden and focus on patient outcomes.

MIPS provides specified performance categories under which payment adjustments may be earned for Part B covered professional services. Eligible clinicians can obtain a composite performance score (CPS) of up to 100 points from these weighted performance categories, which focus on patient care quality and cost, improvements in patient engagement and clinical care processes, and use of certified electronic health record technology (CEHRT). This performance score then defines the payment adjustments in the second calendar year after the year the score is obtained. For instance, the score obtained for the 2020 performance year is linked to payment for Medicare Part B services in 2022.

ECs currently have three available reporting frameworks, depending on individual needs and eligibility—traditional MIPS, MIPS Value Pathways (MVPs), and the alternative payment model (APM) performance pathway (APP). The majority of the proposed updates for CY 2022 focus on MIPS.

Traditional MIPS currently consists of the following performance categories:

- Quality
- Improvement Activities
- Promoting Interoperability (PI)
- Cost

MVPs, which were added as a result of complaints by some physicians of confusing quality measures, allow clinicians to report only on those measures that apply to their specialty. The CY 2022 proposed rule includes seven MVPs for the 2023 performance year related to the following clinical areas: anesthesia, chronic disease management, emergency medicine, heart disease, lower extremity joint repair, rheumatology, and stroke care and prevention. Additional MVPs will gradually be implemented for more specialties and subspecialties that participate in the program.

The APP is intended for MIPS-eligible ECs who also participate in MIPS APMs. Performance is measured across three areas (Quality, Improvement Activities, and Promoting Interoperability) in this reporting and scoring pathway, which aims to decrease reporting burden, encourage APM participation, and create new opportunities for scoring for existing MIPS APM participants. For performance year 2021, the APP Quality performance category accounted for 50 percent of the MIPS final score; the PI performance category weight was 30 percent; and the Improvement Activities performance category weight was 20 percent.

Proposed 2022/2023 Changes

As noted earlier, the majority of the proposed updates for CY 2022 focus on MIPS. In addition to the seven MVPs proposed for the 2023 performance year, other proposals in the CY 2022 proposed rule include:

- Additions to the MVP development criteria beginning with the 2022 performance year/2024 payment year related to relevant outcome measures, high-priority measures, outcomes-based administrative claims measures, and a qualified clinical data registry (QCDR) measure
- Timelines for transitioning to MVPs and for participant registration
- Establishment of subgroup reporting to provide more granular and comprehensive information that will be more clinically meaningful. Subgroup reporting is proposed to be limited to only those clinicians reporting through MVPs or APP
- MVP scoring policies by performance category and updating of the scoring hierarchy to include subgroups
- Revision of the definition of an MIPS-eligible clinician to include certified nurse midwives and clinical social workers
- Revision of the performance threshold
- Revisions and updates to the existing performance categories included in the traditional MIPS framework
- Proposals specific to the transition timeframe of accountable care organizations (ACOs) for reporting specific quality measures

Additionally, a request for public comments was made regarding an incremental timeline to transition to mandatory MVP reporting that will coincide with the sunset of traditional MIPS. The timeline currently being considered is the end of the CY 2027 performance period/2029 MIPS payment year, although this is not an official proposal at this time.

Detailed information regarding the Quality Payment Program may be found at https://qpp.cms.gov/. This website will also announce the final CMS determinations of advanced APMs and MIPS APMs for the 2022 performance period.

Appendix H — Quality Payment Program

Appendix I — Medically Unlikely Edits (MUEs)

The Centers for Medicare & Medicaid Services (CMS) began to publish many of the edits used in the medically unlikely edits (MUE) program for the first time effective October 2008. What follows below is a list of the published CPT codes that have MUEs assigned to them and the number of units allowed with each code. CMS publishes the updates on a quarterly basis. Not all MUEs will be published, however. MUEs intended to detect and discourage any questionable payments will not be published as the agency feels the efficacy of these edits would be compromised. CMS added another component to the MUEs—the MUE Adjudication Indicator (MAI). The appropriate MAI can be found in parentheses following the MUE in this table and specify the maximum units of service (UOS) for a CPT/HCPCS code for the service. The MAI designates whether the UOS edit is applied to the line or claim.

The three MAIs are defined as follows:

MAI 1 (Line Edit) This MAI will continue to be adjudicated as the line edit on the claim and is auto-adjudicated by the contractor.

MAI 2 (Date of Service Edit, Policy) This MAI is considered to be the "absolute date of service edit" and is based on policy. The total unit of services (UOS) for that CPT code and that date of service (DOS) are combined for this edit. Medicare contractors are required to review all claims for the same patient, same date of service, and same provider.

MAI 3 (Date of Service Edit: Clinical) This MAI is also a date-of-service edit but is based upon clinical standards. The review takes current and previously submitted claims for the same patient, same date of service, and same provider into account. When medical necessity is clearly documented, the edit may be bypassed or the claim resubmitted.

The quarterly updates are published on the CMS website at https://www.cms.gov/Medicare/Coding/NationalCorrectCodInitEd/MUE. The following was updated on 10/01/2021.

Practitioner

CPT	MUE	CPT	MUE	CPT	MUE	CPT	MUE	CPT	MUE	CPT	MUE	CPT	MUE	CPT	MUE
0001A	1(2)	0032U	1(2)	0071U	1(2)	0109U	1(3)	0157U	1(2)	0209T	1(3)	0237T	2(3)	0345T	1(2)
0001U	1(2)	0033U	1(2)	0072T	1(2)	0110T	4(2)	0158U	1(2)	0209U	1(2)	0237U	1(2)	0347T	1(3)
0002A	1(2)	0034U	1(2)	0072U	1(2)	0110U	1(2)	0159U	1(2)	0210T	1(3)	0238T	2(3)	0348T	1(3)
0002M	1(3)	0035U	1(2)	0073U	1(2)	0111U	1(2)	0160U	1(2)	0210U	2(3)	0238U	1(2)	0349T	1(3)
0002U	1(2)	0036U	1(3)	0074U	1(2)	0112U	1(3)	0161U	1(2)	0211T	1(3)	0239U	1(2)	0350T	1(3)
0003M	1(3)	0037U	1(3)	0075T	1(2)	0113U	1(2)	0162U	1(2)	0211U	2(3)	0240U	1(3)	0351T	5(3)
0003U	1(2)	0038U	1(2)	0075U	1(2)	0114U	1(2)	0163T	1(3)	0212T	1(3)	0241U	1(3)	0352T	5(3)
0004M	1(2)	0039U	1(2)	0076T	1(2)	0115U	1(3)	0163U	0(3)	0212U	1(2)	0242U	1(2)	0353T	2(3)
0005U	1(2)	0040U	1(2)	0076U	1(2)	0116U	1(2)	0164T	4(2)	0213T	1(2)	0243U	1(2)	0354T	2(3)
0006M	1(2)	0041A	1(2)	0077U	2(2)	0117U	1(2)	0164U	1(2)	0213U	1(3)	0244U	1(3)	0355T	1(2)
0007M	1(2)	0041U	1(2)	0078U	1(2)	0118U	1(2)	0165T	4(2)	0214T	1(2)	0245U	2(3)	0356T	4(2)
0007U	1(2)	0042A	1(2)	0079U	0(3)	0119U	1(2)	0165U	1(2)	0214U	1(2)	0247U	1(2)	0358T	1(2)
0008U	1(3)	0042T	1(3)	0080U	1(2)	0120U	1(2)	0166U	1(2)	0215T	1(2)	0253T	1(3)	0362T	16(3)
0009U	2(3)	0042U	1(2)	0082U	1(2)	0121U	1(2)	0167U	1(2)	0215U	1(3)	0263T	1(3)	0373T	24(3)
0010U	2(3)	0043U	1(2)	0083U	1(3)	0122U	1(2)	0168U	1(2)	0216T	1(2)	0264T	1(3)	0376T	2(3)
0011A	1(2)	0044U	1(2)	0084U	1(2)	0123U	1(2)	0169U	1(2)	0216U	1(2)	0265T	1(3)	0378T	1(2)
0011M	1(2)	0045U	1(3)	0086U	1(3)	0129U	1(2)	0170U	1(2)	0217T	1(2)	0266T	1(2)	0379T	1(2)
0011U	1(2)	0046U	1(3)	0087U	1(2)	0130U	1(2)	0171U	1(2)	0217U	1(2)	0267T	1(3)	0394T	2(3)
0012A	1(2)	0047U	1(3)	0088U	1(2)	0131U	1(2)	0172U	1(2)	0218T	1(2)	0268T	1(3)	0395T	2(3)
0012M	1(2)	0048U	1(3)	0089U	1(3)	0132U	1(2)	0173U	1(2)	0218U	1(2)	0269T	1(2)	0397T	1(3)
0012U	1(2)	0049U	1(3)	0090U	1(2)	0133U	1(2)	0174T	1(3)	0219T	1(2)	0270T	1(3)	0398T	1(3)
0013M	1(2)	0050U	1(3)	0091U	1(2)	0134U	1(2)	0174U	1(2)	0219U	1(2)	0271T	1(3)	0402T	2(2)
0013U	1(3)	0051U	1(2)	0092U	1(2)	0135U	1(2)	0175T	1(3)	0220T	1(2)	0272T	1(3)	0403T	1(2)
0014M	1(2)	0052U	1(2)	0093U	1(2)	0136U	1(2)	0175U	1(2)	0220U	1(2)	0273T	1(3)	0404T	1(2)
0014U	1(3)	0053U	1(3)	0094U	1(2)	0137U	1(2)	0176U	1(3)	0221T	1(2)	0274T	1(2)	0408T	1(3)
0015M	1(2)	0054T	1(3)	0095T	1(3)	0138U	1(2)	0177U	1(3)	0222T	1(3)	0275T	1(2)	0409T	1(3)
0016M	2(3)	0054U	1(2)	0095U	1(2)	0139U	1(2)	0178U	1(2)	0223U	1(3)	0278T	1(3)	0410T	1(3)
0016U	1(3)	0055T	1(3)	0096U	1(2)	0140U	1(2)	0179U	1(3)	0224U	3(3)	0290T	1(3)	0411T	1(3)
0017U	1(3)	0055U	1(2)	0097U	1(2)	0141U	1(2)	0184T	1(3)	0225U	1(3)	0308T	1(3)	0412T	1(2)
0018U	2(3)	0056U	1(3)	0098T	2(3)	0142U	1(2)	0191T	2(2)	0226U	1(3)	0312T	1(3)	0413T	1(3)
0019U	1(3)	0058U	1(2)	0100T	1(2)	0143U	1(2)	0198T	2(2)	0227U	1(2)	0313T	1(3)	0414T	1(2)
0021A	1(2)	0059U	1(2)	0101T	1(3)	0144U	1(2)	01996	1(2)	0228U	1(2)	0314T	1(3)	0415T	1(3)
0021U	1(2)	0060U	1(2)	0101U	1(2)	0145U	1(2)	0200T	1(2)	0229U	1(2)	0315T	1(3)	0416T	1(3)
0022A	1(2)	0061U	2(3)	0102T	2(2)	0146U	1(2)	0201T	1(2)	0230U	1(2)	0316T	1(3)	0417T	1(3)
0022U	2(3)	0062U	1(2)	0102U	1(2)	0147U	1(2)	0202T	1(3)	0231U	1(2)	0317T	1(3)	0418T	1(3)
0023U	1(2)	0063U	1(2)	0103U	1(2)	0148U	1(2)	0202U	1(3)	0232T	1(3)	0329T	1(2)	0419T	1(2)
0024U	1(2)	0064U	2(3)	0105U	1(2)	0149U	1(2)	0203U	1(2)	0232U	1(2)	0330T	1(2)	0420T	1(2)
0025U	1(2)	0065U	2(3)	0106T	4(2)	0150U	1(2)	0204U	1(3)	0233U	1(2)	0331T	1(3)	0421T	1(2)
0026U	2(3)	0066U	1(3)	0106U	1(2)	0151U	1(2)	0205U	1(2)	0234T	2(2)	0332T	1(3)	0422T	1(3)
0027U	1(2)	0067U	2(3)	0107T	4(2)	0152U	1(2)	0206U	1(3)	0234U	1(2)	0333T	1(2)	0423T	1(3)
0029U	1(2)	0068U	1(3)	0107U	1(3)	0153U	1(2)	0207T	2(2)	0235T	2(3)	0335T	2(2)	0424T	1(3)
0030U	1(2)	0069U	1(3)	0108T	4(2)	0154U	1(2)	0207U	1(2)	0235U	1(2)	0338T	1(2)	0425T	1(3)
0031A	1(2)	0070U	1(2)	0108U	1(2)	0155U	1(2)	0208T	1(3)	0236T	1(2)	0339T	1(2)	0426T	1(3)
0031U	1(2)	0071T	1(2)	0109T	4(2)	0156U	1(2)	0208U	1(3)	0236U	1(2)	0342T	1(3)	0427T	1(3)

CPT	MUE
0428T	1(2)
0429T	1(2)
0430T	1(2)
0431T	1(2)
0432T	1(3)
0433T	1(3)
0434T	1(3)
0435T	1(3)
0436T	1(3)
0437T	1(3)
0439T	1(3)
0440T	3(3)
0441T	3(3)
0442T	3(3)
0443T	1(2)
0444T	1(2)
0445T	1(2)
0446T	1(3)
0447T	1(3)
0448T	1(3)
0449T	1(2)
0450T	1(3)
0451T	1(3)
0452T	1(3)
0453T	1(3)
0454T	3(3)
0455T	1(3)
0456T	1(3)
0457T	1(3)
0458T	3(3)
0459T	1(3)
0460T	3(3)
0461T	1(3)
0462T	1(2)
0463T	1(2)
0464T	1(2)
0465T	1(3)
0466T	1(3)
0467T	1(3)
0468T	1(3)
0469T	1(2)
0470T	1(2)
0471T	2(1)
0472T	1(2)
0473T	1(2)
0474T	2(2)
0475T	1(3)
0476T	1(3)
0477T	1(3)
0478T	1(3)
0479T	1(2)
0480T	4(1)
0481T	1(3)
0483T	1(2)
0484T	1(2)
0485T	1(2)
0486T	1(2)
0487T	1(3)
0488T	1(2)
0489T	1(2)
0490T	1(2)
0491T	1(2)
0492T	4(3)
0493T	1(3)
0494T	1(2)
0495T	1(2)

CPT	MUE
0496T	4(3)
0497T	1(3)
0498T	1(2)
0499T	1(2)
0500T	1(3)
0501T	1(2)
0502T	1(2)
0503T	1(2)
0504T	1(2)
0505T	1(3)
0506T	1(2)
0507T	1(2)
0508T	1(3)
0509T	1(2)
0510T	1(2)
0511T	1(2)
0512T	1(2)
0513T	2(3)
0514T	2(2)
0515T	1(3)
0516T	1(3)
0517T	1(3)
0518T	1(3)
0519T	1(3)
0520T	1(3)
0521T	1(3)
0522T	1(3)
0523T	1(3)
0524T	3(3)
0525T	1(3)
0526T	1(3)
0527T	1(3)
0528T	1(3)
0529T	1(3)
0530T	1(3)
0531T	1(3)
0532T	1(3)
0533T	1(2)
0534T	1(2)
0535T	1(2)
0536T	1(2)
0537T	1(3)
0538T	1(3)
0539T	1(3)
0540T	1(3)
0541T	1(3)
0542T	1(3)
0543T	1(2)
0544T	1(2)
0545T	1(2)
0546T	2(2)
0547T	1(2)
0548T	1(2)
0549T	1(2)
0550T	2(3)
0551T	1(2)
0552T	1(3)
0553T	2(2)
0554T	1(2)
0555T	1(2)
0556T	1(2)
0557T	1(2)
0558T	1(2)
0559T	1(2)
0560T	1(3)
0561T	1(2)

CPT	MUE
0562T	1(3)
0563T	1(2)
0564T	1(2)
0565T	1(2)
0566T	1(2)
0567T	1(2)
0568T	1(2)
0569T	1(2)
0570T	1(3)
0571T	1(2)
0572T	1(2)
0573T	1(2)
0574T	1(2)
0575T	1(2)
0576T	1(2)
0577T	1(2)
0578T	1(2)
0579T	1(2)
0580T	1(2)
0581T	0(3)
0582T	0(3)
0583T	2(2)
0584T	1(2)
0585T	1(2)
0586T	1(2)
0587T	1(2)
0588T	1(2)
0589T	1(2)
0590T	1(2)
0591T	1(2)
0592T	1(2)
0593T	1(2)
0594T	2(2)
0596T	1(2)
0597T	1(2)
0598T	1(2)
0599T	1(3)
0600T	3(3)
0601T	3(3)
0602T	1(2)
0603T	1(2)
0604T	1(2)
0605T	1(2)
0606T	1(2)
0607T	1(2)
0608T	1(2)
0609T	1(3)
0610T	1(3)
0611T	1(3)
0612T	1(2)
0613T	1(2)
0614T	1(3)
0615T	1(3)
0616T	2(2)
0617T	2(2)
0618T	2(2)
0619T	1(2)
0620T	2(2)
0621T	2(2)
0622T	2(2)
0623T	1(2)
0624T	1(2)
0625T	1(2)
0626T	1(2)
0627T	1(2)
0628T	4(2)

CPT	MUE
0629T	1(2)
0630T	4(2)
0631T	4(2)
0632T	1(2)
0633T	1(2)
0634T	1(2)
0635T	1(2)
0636T	1(2)
0637T	1(2)
0638T	1(2)
0639T	1(3)
10004	3(3)
10005	1(2)
10006	3(3)
10007	1(2)
10008	2(3)
10009	1(2)
10010	3(3)
10011	1(2)
10012	3(3)
10021	1(2)
10030	2(3)
10035	1(2)
10036	2(3)
10040	1(2)
10060	1(2)
10061	1(2)
10080	1(3)
10081	1(3)
10120	3(3)
10121	2(3)
10140	2(3)
10160	3(3)
10180	2(3)
11000	1(2)
11001	1(3)
11004	1(2)
11005	1(2)
11006	1(2)
11008	1(2)
11010	2(3)
11011	2(3)
11012	2(3)
11042	1(2)
11043	1(2)
11044	1(2)
11045	12(3)
11046	10(3)
11047	10(3)
11055	1(2)
11056	1(2)
11057	1(2)
11102	1(2)
11103	6(3)
11104	1(2)
11105	3(3)
11106	1(2)
11107	2(3)
11200	1(2)
11201	1(3)
11300	5(3)
11301	6(3)
11302	4(3)
11303	3(3)
11305	4(3)
11306	4(3)

CPT	MUE
11307	3(3)
11308	2(3)
11310	4(3)
11311	4(3)
11312	3(3)
11313	3(3)
11400	3(3)
11401	3(3)
11402	3(3)
11403	2(3)
11404	2(3)
11406	2(3)
11420	3(3)
11421	3(3)
11422	3(3)
11423	2(3)
11424	2(3)
11426	2(3)
11440	4(3)
11441	3(3)
11442	3(3)
11443	2(3)
11444	2(3)
11446	2(3)
11450	1(2)
11451	1(2)
11462	1(2)
11463	1(2)
11470	3(2)
11471	2(3)
11600	2(3)
11601	2(3)
11602	3(3)
11603	2(3)
11604	2(3)
11606	2(3)
11620	2(3)
11621	2(3)
11622	2(3)
11623	2(3)
11624	2(3)
11626	2(3)
11640	2(3)
11641	2(3)
11642	3(3)
11643	2(3)
11644	2(3)
11646	2(3)
11719	1(2)
11720	1(2)
11721	1(2)
11730	1(2)
11732	4(3)
11740	2(3)
11750	6(3)
11755	2(3)
11760	4(3)
11762	2(3)
11765	4(3)
11770	1(3)
11771	1(3)
11772	1(3)
11900	1(2)
11901	1(2)
11920	1(2)
11921	1(2)

CPT	MUE
11922	1(3)
11950	1(2)
11951	1(2)
11952	1(2)
11954	1(3)
11960	2(3)
11970	2(3)
11971	2(3)
11976	1(2)
11980	1(2)
11981	1(3)
11982	1(3)
11983	1(3)
12001	1(2)
12002	1(2)
12004	1(2)
12005	1(2)
12006	1(2)
12007	1(2)
12011	1(2)
12013	1(2)
12014	1(2)
12015	1(2)
12016	1(2)
12017	1(2)
12018	1(2)
12020	2(3)
12021	3(3)
12031	1(2)
12032	1(2)
12034	1(2)
12035	1(2)
12036	1(2)
12037	1(2)
12041	1(2)
12042	1(2)
12044	1(2)
12045	1(2)
12046	1(2)
12047	1(2)
12051	1(2)
12052	1(2)
12053	1(2)
12054	1(2)
12055	1(2)
12056	1(2)
12057	1(2)
13100	1(2)
13101	1(2)
13102	9(3)
13120	1(2)
13121	1(2)
13122	9(3)
13131	1(2)
13132	1(2)
13133	7(3)
13151	1(2)
13152	1(2)
13153	2(3)
13160	2(3)
14000	2(3)
14001	2(3)
14020	2(3)
14021	2(3)
14040	2(3)
14041	3(3)

CPT	MUE
14060	2(3)
14061	2(3)
14301	2(3)
14302	8(3)
14350	2(3)
15002	1(2)
15003	60(3)
15004	1(2)
15005	19(3)
15040	1(2)
15050	1(3)
15100	1(2)
15101	40(3)
15110	1(2)
15111	5(3)
15115	1(2)
15116	2(3)
15120	1(2)
15121	8(3)
15130	1(2)
15131	2(3)
15135	1(2)
15136	1(3)
15150	1(2)
15151	1(2)
15152	5(3)
15155	1(2)
15156	1(2)
15157	1(3)
15200	1(2)
15201	7(3)
15220	1(2)
15221	9(3)
15240	1(2)
15241	9(3)
15260	1(2)
15261	6(3)
15271	1(2)
15272	3(3)
15273	1(2)
15274	60(3)
15275	1(2)
15276	3(2)
15277	1(2)
15278	15(3)
15570	2(3)
15572	2(3)
15574	2(3)
15576	2(3)
15600	2(3)
15610	2(3)
15620	2(3)
15630	2(3)
15650	1(3)
15730	1(3)
15731	1(3)
15733	2(3)
15734	4(3)
15736	2(3)
15738	3(3)
15740	2(3)
15750	2(3)
15756	2(3)
15757	2(3)
15758	2(3)
15760	2(3)

CPT	MUE
15769	1(3)
15770	2(3)
15771	1(2)
15772	9(3)
15773	1(2)
15774	3(3)
15775	1(2)
15776	1(2)
15777	1(3)
15780	1(2)
15781	1(3)
15782	1(3)
15783	1(3)
15786	1(2)
15787	2(3)
15788	1(2)
15789	1(2)
15792	1(3)
15793	1(3)
15819	1(2)
15820	1(2)
15821	1(2)
15822	1(2)
15823	1(2)
15824	1(2)
15825	1(2)
15826	1(2)
15828	1(2)
15829	1(2)
15830	1(2)
15832	1(2)
15833	1(2)
15834	1(2)
15835	1(3)
15836	1(2)
15837	2(3)
15838	1(2)
15839	2(3)
15840	1(3)
15841	2(3)
15842	2(3)
15845	2(3)
15847	1(2)
15850	0(3)
15851	1(2)
15852	1(3)
15860	1(3)
15876	1(2)
15877	1(2)
15878	1(2)
15879	1(2)
15920	1(3)
15922	1(3)
15931	1(3)
15933	1(3)
15934	1(3)
15935	1(3)
15936	1(3)
15937	1(3)
15940	2(3)
15941	2(3)
15944	2(3)
15945	2(3)
15946	2(3)
15950	2(3)
15951	2(3)

CPT	MUE
15952	2(3)
15953	2(3)
15956	2(3)
15958	2(3)
15999	1(3)
16000	1(2)
16020	1(3)
16025	1(3)
16030	1(3)
16035	1(2)
16036	8(3)
17000	1(2)
17003	13(2)
17004	1(2)
17106	1(2)
17107	1(2)
17108	1(2)
17110	1(2)
17111	1(2)
17250	4(3)
17260	7(3)
17261	7(3)
17262	6(3)
17263	3(3)
17264	3(3)
17266	2(3)
17270	6(3)
17271	4(3)
17272	5(3)
17273	4(3)
17274	2(3)
17276	2(3)
17280	6(3)
17281	5(3)
17282	4(3)
17283	4(3)
17284	2(3)
17286	2(3)
17311	4(3)
17312	6(3)
17313	3(3)
17314	4(3)
17315	15(3)
17340	1(2)
17360	1(2)
17380	1(3)
17999	1(3)
19000	2(3)
19001	5(3)
19020	2(3)
19030	1(2)
19081	1(2)
19082	2(3)
19083	1(2)
19084	2(3)
19085	1(2)
19086	2(3)
19100	4(3)
19101	3(3)
19105	2(3)
19110	1(3)
19112	2(3)
19120	1(2)
19125	1(2)
19126	3(3)
19281	1(2)

CPT	MUE
19282	2(3)
19283	1(2)
19284	2(3)
19285	1(2)
19286	2(3)
19287	1(2)
19288	2(3)
19294	2(3)
19296	1(3)
19297	2(3)
19298	1(2)
19300	1(2)
19301	1(3)
19302	1(2)
19303	1(2)
19305	1(2)
19306	1(2)
19307	1(2)
19316	1(2)
19318	1(2)
19325	1(2)
19328	1(2)
19330	1(2)
19340	1(2)
19342	1(2)
19350	1(2)
19355	1(2)
19357	1(2)
19361	1(2)
19364	1(3)
19367	1(2)
19368	1(2)
19369	1(2)
19370	1(2)
19371	1(2)
19380	1(2)
19396	1(2)
19499	1(3)
20100	2(3)
20101	2(3)
20102	3(3)
20103	3(3)
20150	2(3)
20200	2(3)
20205	3(3)
20206	3(3)
20220	3(3)
20225	2(3)
20240	4(3)
20245	3(3)
20250	1(3)
20251	2(3)
20500	2(3)
20501	2(3)
20520	2(3)
20525	4(3)
20526	1(2)
20527	2(3)
20550	5(3)
20551	5(3)
20552	1(2)
20553	1(2)
20555	1(3)
20560	1(2)
20561	1(2)
20600	6(3)

CPT	MUE
20604	4(3)
20605	2(3)
20606	2(3)
20610	2(3)
20611	2(3)
20612	2(3)
20615	1(3)
20650	4(3)
20660	1(2)
20661	1(2)
20662	1(2)
20663	1(2)
20664	1(2)
20665	1(2)
20670	3(3)
20680	3(3)
20690	2(3)
20692	2(3)
20693	2(3)
20694	2(3)
20696	2(3)
20697	4(3)
20700	1(3)
20701	1(3)
20702	1(3)
20703	1(3)
20704	1(3)
20705	1(3)
20802	1(2)
20805	1(2)
20808	1(2)
20816	3(3)
20822	3(3)
20824	1(2)
20827	1(2)
20838	1(2)
20900	2(3)
20902	2(3)
20910	1(3)
20912	1(3)
20920	1(3)
20922	1(3)
20924	2(3)
20930	0(3)
20931	1(2)
20932	1(3)
20933	1(3)
20934	1(3)
20936	0(3)
20937	1(2)
20938	1(2)
20939	1(3)
20950	2(3)
20955	1(3)
20956	1(3)
20957	1(3)
20962	1(3)
20969	2(3)
20970	1(3)
20972	2(3)
20973	1(2)
20974	1(3)
20975	1(3)
20979	1(3)
20982	1(2)
20983	1(2)

CPT	MUE
20985	2(3)
20999	1(3)
21010	1(2)
21011	4(3)
21012	3(3)
21013	2(3)
21014	2(3)
21015	1(3)
21016	2(3)
21025	2(3)
21026	2(3)
21029	1(3)
21030	1(3)
21031	2(3)
21032	1(3)
21034	1(3)
21040	2(3)
21044	1(3)
21045	1(3)
21046	2(3)
21047	2(3)
21048	2(3)
21049	1(3)
21050	1(2)
21060	1(2)
21070	1(2)
21073	1(2)
21076	1(2)
21077	1(2)
21079	1(2)
21080	1(2)
21081	1(2)
21082	1(2)
21083	1(2)
21084	1(2)
21085	1(3)
21086	1(2)
21087	1(2)
21088	1(2)
21089	1(3)
21100	1(2)
21110	2(3)
21116	1(2)
21120	1(2)
21121	1(2)
21122	1(2)
21123	1(2)
21125	2(2)
21127	2(3)
21137	1(2)
21138	1(2)
21139	1(2)
21141	1(2)
21142	1(2)
21143	1(2)
21145	1(2)
21146	1(2)
21147	1(2)
21150	1(2)
21151	1(2)
21154	1(2)
21155	1(2)
21159	1(2)
21160	1(2)
21172	1(3)
21175	1(2)

CPT	MUE
21179	1(2)
21180	1(2)
21181	1(3)
21182	1(2)
21183	1(2)
21184	1(2)
21188	1(2)
21193	1(2)
21194	1(2)
21195	1(2)
21196	1(2)
21198	1(3)
21199	1(2)
21206	1(3)
21208	1(3)
21209	1(3)
21210	2(3)
21215	2(3)
21230	2(3)
21235	2(3)
21240	1(2)
21242	1(2)
21243	1(2)
21244	1(2)
21245	2(3)
21246	1(3)
21247	1(2)
21248	2(3)
21249	2(3)
21255	1(2)
21256	1(2)
21260	1(2)
21261	1(2)
21263	1(2)
21267	1(2)
21268	1(2)
21270	1(2)
21275	1(2)
21280	1(2)
21282	1(2)
21295	1(2)
21296	1(2)
21299	1(3)
21310	1(2)
21315	1(2)
21320	1(2)
21325	1(2)
21330	1(2)
21335	1(2)
21336	1(2)
21337	1(2)
21338	1(2)
21339	1(2)
21340	1(2)
21343	1(2)
21344	1(2)
21345	1(2)
21346	1(2)
21347	1(2)
21348	1(2)
21355	1(2)
21356	1(2)
21360	1(2)
21365	1(2)
21366	1(2)
21385	1(2)

CPT	MUE
21386	1(2)
21387	1(2)
21390	1(2)
21395	1(2)
21400	1(2)
21401	1(2)
21406	1(2)
21407	1(2)
21408	1(2)
21421	1(2)
21422	1(2)
21423	1(2)
21431	1(2)
21432	1(2)
21433	1(2)
21435	1(2)
21436	1(2)
21440	2(3)
21445	2(3)
21450	1(2)
21451	1(2)
21452	1(2)
21453	1(2)
21454	1(2)
21461	1(2)
21462	1(2)
21465	1(2)
21470	1(2)
21480	1(2)
21485	1(2)
21490	1(2)
21497	1(2)
21499	1(3)
21501	3(3)
21502	1(3)
21510	1(3)
21550	2(3)
21552	2(3)
21554	2(3)
21555	2(3)
21556	2(3)
21557	1(3)
21558	1(3)
21600	5(3)
21601	2(3)
21602	1(3)
21603	1(3)
21610	1(3)
21615	1(2)
21616	1(2)
21620	1(2)
21627	1(2)
21630	1(2)
21632	1(2)
21685	1(2)
21700	1(2)
21705	1(2)
21720	1(3)
21725	1(3)
21740	1(2)
21742	1(2)
21743	1(2)
21750	1(2)
21811	1(2)
21812	1(2)
21813	1(2)

CPT	MUE
21820	1(2)
21825	1(2)
21899	1(3)
21920	2(3)
21925	2(3)
21930	5(3)
21931	3(3)
21932	2(3)
21933	2(3)
21935	1(3)
21936	1(3)
22010	2(3)
22015	2(3)
22100	1(2)
22101	1(2)
22102	1(2)
22103	3(3)
22110	1(2)
22112	1(2)
22114	1(2)
22116	3(3)
22206	1(2)
22207	1(2)
22208	5(3)
22210	1(2)
22212	1(2)
22214	1(2)
22216	6(3)
22220	1(2)
22222	1(2)
22224	1(2)
22226	4(3)
22310	1(2)
22315	1(2)
22318	1(2)
22319	1(2)
22325	1(2)
22326	1(2)
22327	1(2)
22328	6(3)
22505	1(2)
22510	1(2)
22511	1(2)
22512	3(3)
22513	1(2)
22514	1(2)
22515	4(3)
22526	0(3)
22527	0(3)
22532	1(2)
22533	1(2)
22534	3(3)
22548	1(2)
22551	1(2)
22552	5(3)
22554	1(2)
22556	1(2)
22558	1(2)
22585	5(3)
22586	1(2)
22590	1(2)
22595	1(2)
22600	1(2)
22610	1(2)
22612	1(2)
22614	13(3)

CPT	MUE
22630	1(2)
22632	4(2)
22633	1(2)
22634	4(2)
22800	1(2)
22802	1(2)
22804	1(2)
22808	1(2)
22810	1(2)
22812	1(2)
22818	1(2)
22819	1(2)
22830	1(2)
22840	1(3)
22841	1(2)
22842	1(3)
22843	1(3)
22844	1(3)
22845	1(3)
22846	1(3)
22847	1(3)
22848	1(2)
22849	1(2)
22850	1(2)
22852	1(2)
22853	4(3)
22854	4(3)
22855	1(2)
22856	1(2)
22857	1(2)
22858	1(2)
22859	4(3)
22861	1(2)
22862	1(2)
22864	1(2)
22865	1(2)
22867	1(2)
22868	1(2)
22869	1(2)
22870	1(2)
22899	1(3)
22900	3(3)
22901	2(3)
22902	4(3)
22903	3(3)
22904	1(3)
22905	1(3)
22999	1(3)
23000	1(2)
23020	1(2)
23030	2(3)
23031	1(3)
23035	1(3)
23040	1(2)
23044	1(3)
23065	2(3)
23066	2(3)
23071	2(3)
23073	2(3)
23075	2(3)
23076	2(3)
23077	1(3)
23078	1(3)
23100	1(2)
23101	1(3)
23105	1(2)

CPT	MUE
23106	1(2)
23107	1(2)
23120	1(2)
23125	1(2)
23130	1(2)
23140	1(3)
23145	1(3)
23146	1(3)
23150	1(3)
23155	1(3)
23156	1(3)
23170	1(3)
23172	1(3)
23174	1(3)
23180	1(3)
23182	1(3)
23184	1(3)
23190	1(3)
23195	1(2)
23200	1(3)
23210	1(3)
23220	1(3)
23330	2(3)
23333	1(3)
23334	1(2)
23335	1(2)
23350	1(2)
23395	1(2)
23397	1(3)
23400	1(2)
23405	2(3)
23406	1(3)
23410	1(2)
23412	1(2)
23415	1(2)
23420	1(2)
23430	1(2)
23440	1(2)
23450	1(2)
23455	1(2)
23460	1(2)
23462	1(2)
23465	1(2)
23466	1(2)
23470	1(2)
23472	1(2)
23473	1(2)
23474	1(2)
23480	1(2)
23485	1(2)
23490	1(2)
23491	1(2)
23500	1(2)
23505	1(2)
23515	1(2)
23520	1(2)
23525	1(2)
23530	1(2)
23532	1(2)
23540	1(2)
23545	1(2)
23550	1(2)
23552	1(2)
23570	1(2)
23575	1(2)
23585	1(2)

CPT	MUE
23600	1(2)
23605	1(2)
23615	1(2)
23616	1(2)
23620	1(2)
23625	1(2)
23630	1(2)
23650	1(2)
23655	1(2)
23660	1(2)
23665	1(2)
23670	1(2)
23675	1(2)
23680	1(2)
23700	1(2)
23800	1(2)
23802	1(2)
23900	1(2)
23920	1(2)
23921	1(2)
23929	1(3)
23930	2(3)
23931	2(3)
23935	2(3)
24000	1(2)
24006	1(2)
24065	2(3)
24066	2(3)
24071	2(3)
24073	2(3)
24075	5(3)
24076	4(3)
24077	1(3)
24079	1(3)
24100	1(2)
24101	1(2)
24102	1(2)
24105	1(2)
24110	1(3)
24115	1(3)
24116	1(3)
24120	1(3)
24125	1(3)
24126	1(3)
24130	1(2)
24134	1(3)
24136	1(3)
24138	1(3)
24140	1(3)
24145	1(3)
24147	1(2)
24149	1(2)
24150	1(3)
24152	1(3)
24155	1(2)
24160	1(2)
24164	1(2)
24200	3(3)
24201	3(3)
24220	1(2)
24300	1(2)
24301	2(3)
24305	4(3)
24310	2(3)
24320	2(3)
24330	1(3)

CPT	MUE
24331	1(3)
24332	1(2)
24340	1(2)
24341	2(3)
24342	2(3)
24343	1(2)
24344	1(2)
24345	1(2)
24346	1(2)
24357	1(3)
24358	1(3)
24359	2(3)
24360	1(2)
24361	1(2)
24362	1(2)
24363	1(2)
24365	1(2)
24366	1(2)
24370	1(2)
24371	1(2)
24400	1(3)
24410	1(2)
24420	1(2)
24430	1(3)
24435	1(3)
24470	1(2)
24495	1(2)
24498	1(2)
24500	1(2)
24505	1(2)
24515	1(2)
24516	1(2)
24530	1(2)
24535	1(2)
24538	1(2)
24545	1(2)
24546	1(2)
24560	1(3)
24565	1(3)
24566	1(3)
24575	1(3)
24576	1(3)
24577	1(3)
24579	1(3)
24582	1(3)
24586	1(3)
24587	1(2)
24600	1(2)
24605	1(2)
24615	1(2)
24620	1(2)
24635	1(2)
24640	1(2)
24650	1(2)
24655	1(2)
24665	1(2)
24666	1(2)
24670	1(2)
24675	1(2)
24685	1(2)
24800	1(2)
24802	1(2)
24900	1(2)
24920	1(2)
24925	1(2)
24930	1(2)

CPT	MUE
24931	1(2)
24935	1(2)
24940	1(2)
24999	1(3)
25000	2(3)
25001	1(3)
25020	1(2)
25023	1(2)
25024	1(2)
25025	1(2)
25028	4(3)
25031	2(3)
25035	2(3)
25040	1(3)
25065	2(3)
25066	2(3)
25071	3(3)
25073	2(3)
25075	6(3)
25076	3(3)
25077	1(3)
25078	1(3)
25085	1(2)
25100	1(2)
25101	1(2)
25105	1(2)
25107	1(2)
25109	4(3)
25110	2(3)
25111	1(3)
25112	1(3)
25115	1(3)
25116	1(3)
25118	5(3)
25119	1(2)
25120	1(3)
25125	1(3)
25126	1(3)
25130	1(3)
25135	1(3)
25136	1(3)
25145	1(3)
25150	1(3)
25151	1(3)
25170	1(3)
25210	2(3)
25215	1(2)
25230	1(2)
25240	1(2)
25246	1(2)
25248	3(3)
25250	1(2)
25251	1(2)
25259	1(2)
25260	9(3)
25263	4(3)
25265	4(3)
25270	8(3)
25272	4(3)
25274	4(3)
25275	2(3)
25280	9(3)
25290	10(3)
25295	9(3)
25300	1(2)
25301	1(2)

CPT	MUE
25310	5(3)
25312	4(3)
25315	1(3)
25316	1(3)
25320	1(2)
25332	1(2)
25335	1(2)
25337	1(2)
25350	1(3)
25355	1(3)
25360	1(3)
25365	1(3)
25370	1(2)
25375	1(2)
25390	1(2)
25391	1(2)
25392	1(2)
25393	1(2)
25394	1(3)
25400	1(2)
25405	1(2)
25415	1(2)
25420	1(2)
25425	1(2)
25426	1(2)
25430	1(3)
25431	1(3)
25440	1(2)
25441	1(2)
25442	1(2)
25443	1(2)
25444	1(2)
25445	1(2)
25446	1(2)
25447	4(3)
25449	1(2)
25450	1(2)
25455	1(2)
25490	1(2)
25491	1(2)
25492	1(2)
25500	1(2)
25505	1(2)
25515	1(2)
25520	1(2)
25525	1(2)
25526	1(2)
25530	1(2)
25535	1(2)
25545	1(2)
25560	1(2)
25565	1(2)
25574	1(2)
25575	1(2)
25600	1(2)
25605	1(2)
25606	1(2)
25607	1(2)
25608	1(2)
25609	1(2)
25622	1(2)
25624	1(2)
25628	1(2)
25630	1(3)
25635	1(3)
25645	1(3)

CPT	MUE
25650	1(2)
25651	1(2)
25652	1(2)
25660	1(2)
25670	1(2)
25671	1(2)
25675	1(2)
25676	1(2)
25680	1(2)
25685	1(2)
25690	1(2)
25695	1(2)
25800	1(2)
25805	1(2)
25810	1(2)
25820	1(2)
25825	1(2)
25830	1(2)
25900	1(2)
25905	1(2)
25907	1(2)
25909	1(2)
25915	1(2)
25920	1(2)
25922	1(2)
25924	1(2)
25927	1(2)
25929	1(2)
25931	1(2)
25999	1(3)
26010	2(3)
26011	3(3)
26020	4(3)
26025	1(2)
26030	1(2)
26034	2(3)
26035	1(3)
26037	1(3)
26040	1(2)
26045	1(2)
26055	5(3)
26060	5(3)
26070	2(3)
26075	3(3)
26080	3(3)
26100	1(3)
26105	2(3)
26110	2(3)
26111	4(3)
26113	3(3)
26115	4(3)
26116	2(3)
26117	2(3)
26118	1(3)
26121	1(2)
26123	1(2)
26125	4(3)
26130	1(3)
26135	4(3)
26140	2(3)
26145	6(3)
26160	4(3)
26170	4(3)
26180	4(3)
26185	1(3)
26200	2(3)

CPT	MUE
26205	1(3)
26210	2(3)
26215	2(3)
26230	2(3)
26235	2(3)
26236	2(3)
26250	2(3)
26260	1(3)
26262	1(3)
26320	4(3)
26340	4(3)
26341	2(3)
26350	6(3)
26352	2(3)
26356	4(3)
26357	2(3)
26358	2(3)
26370	3(3)
26372	1(3)
26373	2(3)
26390	2(3)
26392	2(3)
26410	4(3)
26412	3(3)
26415	2(3)
26416	2(3)
26418	4(3)
26420	3(3)
26426	4(3)
26428	2(3)
26432	2(3)
26433	2(3)
26434	2(3)
26437	4(3)
26440	6(3)
26442	5(3)
26445	5(3)
26449	5(3)
26450	6(3)
26455	6(3)
26460	4(3)
26471	4(3)
26474	4(3)
26476	4(3)
26477	2(3)
26478	6(3)
26479	4(3)
26480	4(3)
26483	4(3)
26485	4(3)
26489	2(3)
26490	3(3)
26492	2(3)
26494	1(3)
26496	1(3)
26497	2(3)
26498	1(3)
26499	2(3)
26500	3(3)
26502	2(3)
26508	1(2)
26510	4(3)
26516	1(2)
26517	1(2)
26518	1(2)
26520	4(3)

CPT	MUE
26525	4(3)
26530	4(3)
26531	4(3)
26535	3(3)
26536	4(3)
26540	4(3)
26541	4(3)
26542	4(3)
26545	4(3)
26546	2(3)
26548	3(3)
26550	1(2)
26551	1(2)
26553	1(3)
26554	1(3)
26555	2(3)
26556	2(3)
26560	2(3)
26561	2(3)
26562	2(3)
26565	2(3)
26567	3(3)
26568	2(3)
26580	1(2)
26587	2(3)
26590	2(3)
26591	4(3)
26593	8(3)
26596	1(3)
26600	2(3)
26605	3(3)
26607	2(3)
26608	4(3)
26615	3(3)
26641	1(2)
26645	1(2)
26650	1(2)
26665	1(2)
26670	2(3)
26675	1(3)
26676	2(3)
26685	3(3)
26686	3(3)
26700	2(3)
26705	3(3)
26706	2(3)
26715	3(3)
26720	4(3)
26725	3(3)
26727	3(3)
26735	4(3)
26740	3(3)
26742	3(3)
26746	3(3)
26750	3(3)
26755	2(3)
26756	2(3)
26765	3(3)
26770	3(3)
26775	2(3)
26776	4(3)
26785	3(3)
26820	1(2)
26841	1(2)
26842	1(2)
26843	2(3)

CPT	MUE
26844	2(3)
26850	5(3)
26852	2(3)
26860	1(2)
26861	4(3)
26862	1(2)
26863	2(3)
26910	4(3)
26951	8(3)
26952	4(3)
26989	1(3)
26990	2(3)
26991	1(3)
26992	2(3)
27000	1(3)
27001	1(3)
27003	1(2)
27005	1(2)
27006	1(2)
27025	1(3)
27027	1(2)
27030	1(2)
27033	1(2)
27035	1(2)
27036	1(2)
27040	2(3)
27041	3(3)
27043	2(3)
27045	3(3)
27047	2(3)
27048	2(3)
27049	1(3)
27050	1(2)
27052	1(2)
27054	1(2)
27057	1(2)
27059	1(3)
27060	1(2)
27062	1(2)
27065	1(3)
27066	1(3)
27067	1(3)
27070	1(3)
27071	1(3)
27075	1(3)
27076	1(2)
27077	1(2)
27078	1(2)
27080	1(2)
27086	1(3)
27087	1(3)
27090	1(2)
27091	1(2)
27093	1(2)
27095	1(2)
27096	1(2)
27097	1(3)
27098	1(2)
27100	1(2)
27105	1(3)
27110	1(2)
27111	1(2)
27120	1(2)
27122	1(2)
27125	1(2)
27130	1(2)

CPT	MUE
27132	1(2)
27134	1(2)
27137	1(2)
27138	1(2)
27140	1(2)
27146	1(3)
27147	1(3)
27151	1(3)
27156	1(2)
27158	1(2)
27161	1(2)
27165	1(2)
27170	1(2)
27175	1(2)
27176	1(2)
27177	1(2)
27178	1(2)
27179	1(2)
27181	1(2)
27185	1(2)
27187	1(2)
27197	1(2)
27198	1(2)
27200	1(2)
27202	1(2)
27215	0(3)
27216	0(3)
27217	0(3)
27218	0(3)
27220	1(2)
27222	1(2)
27226	1(2)
27227	1(2)
27228	1(2)
27230	1(2)
27232	1(2)
27235	1(2)
27236	1(2)
27238	1(2)
27240	1(2)
27244	1(2)
27245	1(2)
27246	1(2)
27248	1(2)
27250	1(2)
27252	1(2)
27253	1(2)
27254	1(2)
27256	1(2)
27257	1(2)
27258	1(2)
27259	1(2)
27265	1(2)
27266	1(2)
27267	1(2)
27268	1(2)
27269	1(2)
27275	2(2)
27279	1(2)
27280	1(2)
27282	1(2)
27284	1(2)
27286	1(2)
27290	1(2)
27295	1(2)
27299	1(3)

CPT	MUE
27301	3(3)
27303	2(3)
27305	1(2)
27306	1(2)
27307	1(2)
27310	1(2)
27323	2(3)
27324	3(3)
27325	1(2)
27326	1(2)
27327	5(3)
27328	3(3)
27329	1(3)
27330	1(2)
27331	1(2)
27332	1(2)
27333	1(2)
27334	1(2)
27335	1(2)
27337	3(3)
27339	4(3)
27340	1(2)
27345	1(2)
27347	1(2)
27350	1(2)
27355	1(3)
27356	1(3)
27357	1(3)
27358	1(3)
27360	2(3)
27364	1(3)
27365	1(3)
27369	1(2)
27372	2(3)
27380	1(2)
27381	1(2)
27385	2(3)
27386	2(3)
27390	1(2)
27391	1(2)
27392	1(2)
27393	1(2)
27394	1(2)
27395	1(2)
27396	1(2)
27397	1(2)
27400	1(2)
27403	1(3)
27405	1(3)
27407	1(3)
27409	1(2)
27412	1(2)
27415	1(2)
27416	1(2)
27418	1(2)
27420	1(2)
27422	1(2)
27424	1(2)
27425	1(2)
27427	1(2)
27428	1(2)
27429	1(2)
27430	1(2)
27435	1(2)
27437	1(2)
27438	1(2)

CPT	MUE
27440	1(2)
27441	1(2)
27442	1(2)
27443	1(2)
27445	1(2)
27446	1(2)
27447	1(2)
27448	1(3)
27450	1(3)
27454	1(2)
27455	1(3)
27457	1(3)
27465	1(2)
27466	1(2)
27468	1(2)
27470	1(2)
27472	1(2)
27475	1(2)
27477	1(2)
27479	1(2)
27485	1(2)
27486	1(2)
27487	1(2)
27488	1(2)
27495	1(2)
27496	1(2)
27497	1(2)
27498	1(2)
27499	1(2)
27500	1(2)
27501	1(2)
27502	1(2)
27503	1(2)
27506	1(2)
27507	1(2)
27508	1(2)
27509	1(2)
27510	1(2)
27511	1(2)
27513	1(2)
27514	1(2)
27516	1(2)
27517	1(2)
27519	1(2)
27520	1(2)
27524	1(2)
27530	1(2)
27532	1(2)
27535	1(2)
27536	1(2)
27538	1(2)
27540	1(2)
27550	1(2)
27552	1(2)
27556	1(2)
27557	1(2)
27558	1(2)
27560	1(2)
27562	1(2)
27566	1(2)
27570	1(2)
27580	1(2)
27590	1(2)
27591	1(2)
27592	1(2)
27594	1(2)

CPT	MUE
27596	1(2)
27598	1(2)
27599	1(3)
27600	1(2)
27601	1(2)
27602	1(2)
27603	2(3)
27604	2(3)
27605	1(2)
27606	1(2)
27607	2(3)
27610	1(2)
27612	1(2)
27613	3(3)
27614	3(3)
27615	1(3)
27616	1(3)
27618	3(3)
27619	2(3)
27620	1(2)
27625	1(2)
27626	1(2)
27630	2(3)
27632	3(3)
27634	2(3)
27635	1(3)
27637	1(3)
27638	1(3)
27640	1(3)
27641	1(3)
27645	1(3)
27646	1(3)
27647	1(3)
27648	1(2)
27650	1(2)
27652	1(2)
27654	1(2)
27656	1(3)
27658	2(3)
27659	2(3)
27664	2(3)
27665	2(3)
27675	1(2)
27676	1(2)
27680	2(3)
27681	1(2)
27685	2(3)
27686	3(3)
27687	1(2)
27690	2(3)
27691	2(3)
27692	4(3)
27695	1(2)
27696	1(2)
27698	2(2)
27700	1(2)
27702	1(2)
27703	1(2)
27704	1(2)
27705	1(3)
27707	1(3)
27709	1(3)
27712	1(2)
27715	1(2)
27720	1(2)
27722	1(2)

CPT	MUE
27724	1(2)
27725	1(2)
27726	1(2)
27727	1(2)
27730	1(2)
27732	1(2)
27734	1(2)
27740	1(2)
27742	1(2)
27745	1(2)
27750	1(2)
27752	1(2)
27756	1(2)
27758	1(2)
27759	1(2)
27760	1(2)
27762	1(2)
27766	1(2)
27767	1(2)
27768	1(2)
27769	1(2)
27780	1(2)
27781	1(2)
27784	1(2)
27786	1(2)
27788	1(2)
27792	1(2)
27808	1(2)
27810	1(2)
27814	1(2)
27816	1(2)
27818	1(2)
27822	1(2)
27823	1(2)
27824	1(2)
27825	1(2)
27826	1(2)
27827	1(2)
27828	1(2)
27829	1(2)
27830	1(2)
27831	1(2)
27832	1(2)
27840	1(2)
27842	1(2)
27846	1(2)
27848	1(2)
27860	1(2)
27870	1(2)
27871	1(3)
27880	1(2)
27881	1(2)
27882	1(2)
27884	1(2)
27886	1(2)
27888	1(2)
27889	1(2)
27892	1(2)
27893	1(2)
27894	1(2)
27899	1(3)
28001	2(3)
28002	3(3)
28003	2(3)
28005	3(3)
28008	2(3)

CPT	MUE
28010	4(3)
28011	4(3)
28020	2(3)
28022	3(3)
28024	4(3)
28035	1(2)
28039	2(3)
28041	2(3)
28043	4(3)
28045	4(3)
28046	1(3)
28047	1(3)
28050	2(3)
28052	2(3)
28054	2(3)
28055	1(3)
28060	1(2)
28062	1(2)
28070	2(3)
28072	4(3)
28080	3(3)
28086	2(3)
28088	2(3)
28090	2(3)
28092	2(3)
28100	1(3)
28102	1(3)
28103	1(3)
28104	2(3)
28106	1(3)
28107	1(3)
28108	2(3)
28110	1(2)
28111	1(2)
28112	4(3)
28113	1(2)
28114	1(2)
28116	1(2)
28118	1(2)
28119	1(2)
28120	2(3)
28122	4(3)
28124	4(3)
28126	4(3)
28130	1(2)
28140	3(3)
28150	4(3)
28153	4(3)
28160	5(3)
28171	1(3)
28173	2(3)
28175	2(3)
28190	3(3)
28192	2(3)
28193	2(3)
28200	4(3)
28202	2(3)
28208	4(3)
28210	2(3)
28220	1(2)
28222	1(2)
28225	1(2)
28226	1(2)
28230	1(2)
28232	6(3)
28234	6(3)

CPT	MUE
28238	1(2)
28240	1(2)
28250	1(2)
28260	1(2)
28261	1(3)
28262	1(2)
28264	1(2)
28270	6(3)
28272	6(3)
28280	1(2)
28285	4(3)
28286	1(2)
28288	4(3)
28289	1(2)
28291	1(2)
28292	1(2)
28295	1(2)
28296	1(2)
28297	1(2)
28298	1(2)
28299	1(2)
28300	1(3)
28302	1(2)
28304	1(3)
28305	1(3)
28306	1(2)
28307	1(2)
28308	4(3)
28309	1(2)
28310	1(2)
28312	4(3)
28313	4(3)
28315	1(2)
28320	1(2)
28322	2(3)
28340	2(3)
28341	2(3)
28344	1(2)
28345	2(3)
28360	1(2)
28400	1(2)
28405	1(2)
28406	1(2)
28415	1(2)
28420	1(2)
28430	1(2)
28435	1(2)
28436	1(2)
28445	1(2)
28446	1(2)
28450	2(3)
28455	3(3)
28456	2(3)
28465	3(3)
28470	2(3)
28475	5(3)
28476	4(3)
28485	5(3)
28490	1(2)
28495	1(2)
28496	1(2)
28505	1(2)
28510	4(3)
28515	4(3)
28525	4(3)
28530	1(2)

CPT	MUE
28531	1(2)
28540	1(3)
28545	1(3)
28546	1(3)
28555	1(3)
28570	1(2)
28575	1(2)
28576	1(2)
28585	1(3)
28600	2(3)
28605	2(3)
28606	3(3)
28615	5(3)
28630	2(3)
28635	2(3)
28636	4(3)
28645	4(3)
28660	4(3)
28665	3(3)
28666	4(3)
28675	3(3)
28705	1(2)
28715	1(2)
28725	1(2)
28730	1(2)
28735	1(2)
28737	1(2)
28740	1(2)
28750	1(2)
28755	1(2)
28760	1(2)
28800	1(2)
28805	1(2)
28810	5(3)
28820	6(3)
28825	8(3)
28890	1(2)
28899	1(3)
29000	1(3)
29010	1(3)
29015	1(3)
29035	1(3)
29040	1(3)
29044	1(3)
29046	1(3)
29049	1(3)
29055	1(3)
29058	1(3)
29065	1(3)
29075	1(3)
29085	1(3)
29086	2(3)
29105	1(2)
29125	1(2)
29126	1(2)
29130	3(3)
29131	2(3)
29200	1(2)
29240	1(2)
29260	1(3)
29280	2(3)
29305	1(3)
29325	1(3)
29345	1(3)
29355	1(3)
29358	1(3)

CPT	MUE
29365	1(3)
29405	1(3)
29425	1(3)
29435	1(3)
29440	1(2)
29445	1(3)
29450	1(3)
29505	1(2)
29515	1(2)
29520	1(2)
29530	1(2)
29540	1(2)
29550	1(2)
29580	1(2)
29581	1(2)
29584	1(2)
29700	2(3)
29705	1(3)
29710	1(2)
29720	1(2)
29730	1(3)
29740	1(3)
29750	1(3)
29799	1(3)
29800	1(2)
29804	1(2)
29805	1(2)
29806	1(2)
29807	1(2)
29819	1(2)
29820	1(2)
29821	1(2)
29822	1(2)
29823	1(2)
29824	1(2)
29825	1(2)
29826	1(2)
29827	1(2)
29828	1(2)
29830	1(2)
29834	1(2)
29835	1(2)
29836	1(2)
29837	1(2)
29838	1(2)
29840	1(2)
29843	1(2)
29844	1(2)
29845	1(2)
29846	1(2)
29847	1(2)
29848	1(2)
29850	1(2)
29851	1(2)
29855	1(2)
29856	1(2)
29860	1(2)
29861	1(2)
29862	1(2)
29863	1(2)
29866	1(2)
29867	1(2)
29868	1(3)
29870	1(2)
29871	1(2)
29873	1(2)

CPT	MUE
29874	1(2)
29875	1(2)
29876	1(2)
29877	1(2)
29879	1(2)
29880	1(2)
29881	1(2)
29882	1(2)
29883	1(2)
29884	1(2)
29885	1(2)
29886	1(2)
29887	1(2)
29888	1(2)
29889	1(2)
29891	1(2)
29892	1(2)
29893	1(2)
29894	1(2)
29895	1(2)
29897	1(2)
29898	1(2)
29899	1(2)
29900	2(3)
29901	2(3)
29902	2(3)
29904	1(2)
29905	1(2)
29906	1(2)
29907	1(2)
29914	1(2)
29915	1(2)
29916	1(2)
29999	1(3)
30000	1(3)
30020	1(3)
30100	2(3)
30110	1(2)
30115	1(2)
30117	2(3)
30118	1(3)
30120	1(2)
30124	2(3)
30125	1(3)
30130	1(2)
30140	1(2)
30150	1(2)
30160	1(2)
30200	1(2)
30210	1(3)
30220	1(2)
30300	1(3)
30310	1(3)
30320	1(3)
30400	1(2)
30410	1(2)
30420	1(2)
30430	1(2)
30435	1(2)
30450	1(2)
30460	1(2)
30462	1(2)
30465	1(2)
30468	1(2)
30520	1(2)
30540	1(2)

CPT	MUE
30545	1(2)
30560	1(2)
30580	2(3)
30600	1(3)
30620	1(2)
30630	1(2)
30801	1(2)
30802	1(2)
30901	1(3)
30903	1(3)
30905	1(2)
30906	1(3)
30915	1(3)
30920	1(3)
30930	1(2)
30999	1(3)
31000	1(2)
31002	1(2)
31020	1(2)
31030	1(2)
31032	1(2)
31040	1(2)
31050	1(2)
31051	1(2)
31070	1(2)
31075	1(2)
31080	1(2)
31081	1(2)
31084	1(2)
31085	1(2)
31086	1(2)
31087	1(2)
31090	1(2)
31200	1(2)
31201	1(2)
31205	1(2)
31225	1(2)
31230	1(2)
31231	1(2)
31233	1(2)
31235	1(2)
31237	1(2)
31238	1(3)
31239	1(2)
31240	1(2)
31241	1(2)
31253	1(2)
31254	1(2)
31255	1(2)
31256	1(2)
31257	1(2)
31259	1(2)
31267	1(2)
31276	1(2)
31287	1(2)
31288	1(2)
31290	1(2)
31291	1(2)
31292	1(2)
31293	1(2)
31294	1(2)
31295	1(2)
31296	1(2)
31297	1(2)
31298	1(2)
31299	1(3)

CPT	MUE
31300	1(2)
31360	1(2)
31365	1(2)
31367	1(2)
31368	1(2)
31370	1(2)
31375	1(2)
31380	1(2)
31382	1(2)
31390	1(2)
31395	1(2)
31400	1(3)
31420	1(2)
31500	2(3)
31502	1(3)
31505	1(3)
31510	1(2)
31511	1(3)
31512	1(3)
31513	1(3)
31515	1(3)
31520	1(3)
31525	1(3)
31526	1(3)
31527	1(2)
31528	1(2)
31529	1(3)
31530	1(3)
31531	1(3)
31535	1(3)
31536	1(3)
31540	1(3)
31541	1(3)
31545	1(2)
31546	1(2)
31551	1(2)
31552	1(2)
31553	1(2)
31554	1(2)
31560	1(2)
31561	1(2)
31570	1(2)
31571	1(2)
31572	1(2)
31573	1(2)
31574	1(2)
31575	1(3)
31576	1(3)
31577	1(3)
31578	1(3)
31579	1(2)
31580	1(2)
31584	1(2)
31587	1(2)
31590	1(2)
31591	1(2)
31592	1(2)
31599	1(3)
31600	1(2)
31601	1(2)
31603	1(2)
31605	1(2)
31610	1(2)
31611	1(2)
31612	1(3)
31613	1(2)

CPT	MUE
31614	1(2)
31615	1(3)
31622	1(3)
31623	1(3)
31624	1(3)
31625	1(2)
31626	1(2)
31627	1(3)
31628	1(2)
31629	1(2)
31630	1(3)
31631	1(2)
31632	2(3)
31633	2(3)
31634	1(3)
31635	1(3)
31636	1(2)
31637	2(3)
31638	1(3)
31640	1(3)
31641	1(3)
31643	1(2)
31645	1(2)
31646	2(3)
31647	1(2)
31648	1(2)
31649	2(3)
31651	3(3)
31652	1(2)
31653	1(2)
31654	1(3)
31660	1(2)
31661	1(2)
31717	1(3)
31720	1(3)
31725	1(3)
31730	1(3)
31750	1(2)
31755	1(2)
31760	1(2)
31766	1(2)
31770	2(3)
31775	1(3)
31780	1(2)
31781	1(2)
31785	1(3)
31786	1(3)
31800	1(3)
31805	1(3)
31820	1(2)
31825	1(2)
31830	1(2)
31899	1(3)
32035	1(2)
32036	1(3)
32096	1(3)
32097	1(3)
32098	1(2)
32100	1(3)
32110	1(3)
32120	1(3)
32124	1(3)
32140	1(3)
32141	1(3)
32150	1(3)
32151	1(3)

CPT	MUE
32160	1(3)
32200	2(3)
32215	1(2)
32220	1(2)
32225	1(2)
32310	1(3)
32320	1(3)
32400	2(3)
32408	2(3)
32440	1(2)
32442	1(2)
32445	1(2)
32480	1(2)
32482	1(2)
32484	2(3)
32486	1(3)
32488	1(2)
32491	1(2)
32501	1(3)
32503	1(2)
32504	1(2)
32505	1(2)
32506	3(3)
32507	2(3)
32540	1(3)
32550	2(3)
32551	2(3)
32552	2(2)
32553	1(2)
32554	2(3)
32555	2(3)
32556	2(3)
32557	2(3)
32560	1(3)
32561	1(2)
32562	1(2)
32601	1(3)
32604	1(3)
32606	1(3)
32607	1(3)
32608	1(3)
32609	1(3)
32650	1(2)
32651	1(2)
32652	1(2)
32653	1(3)
32654	1(3)
32655	1(3)
32656	1(2)
32658	1(3)
32659	1(2)
32661	1(3)
32662	1(3)
32663	1(3)
32664	1(2)
32665	1(2)
32666	1(3)
32667	3(3)
32668	2(3)
32669	2(3)
32670	1(2)
32671	1(2)
32672	1(3)
32673	1(2)
32674	1(2)
32701	1(2)

CPT	MUE
32800	1(3)
32810	1(3)
32815	1(3)
32820	1(2)
32850	1(2)
32851	1(2)
32852	1(2)
32853	1(2)
32854	1(2)
32855	1(2)
32856	1(2)
32900	1(2)
32905	1(2)
32906	1(2)
32940	1(3)
32960	1(2)
32994	1(2)
32997	1(2)
32998	1(2)
32999	1(3)
33016	1(3)
33017	1(3)
33018	1(3)
33019	1(3)
33020	1(3)
33025	1(2)
33030	1(2)
33031	1(2)
33050	1(2)
33120	1(3)
33130	1(3)
33140	1(2)
33141	1(2)
33202	1(2)
33203	1(2)
33206	1(3)
33207	1(3)
33208	1(3)
33210	1(3)
33211	1(3)
33212	1(3)
33213	1(3)
33214	1(3)
33215	2(3)
33216	1(3)
33217	1(3)
33218	1(3)
33220	1(3)
33221	1(3)
33222	1(3)
33223	1(3)
33224	1(3)
33225	1(3)
33226	1(3)
33227	1(3)
33228	1(3)
33229	1(3)
33230	1(3)
33231	1(3)
33233	1(2)
33234	1(2)
33235	1(2)
33236	1(2)
33237	1(2)
33238	1(2)
33240	1(3)

CPT	MUE
33241	1(2)
33243	1(2)
33244	1(2)
33249	1(3)
33250	1(2)
33251	1(2)
33254	1(2)
33255	1(2)
33256	1(2)
33257	1(2)
33258	1(2)
33259	1(2)
33261	1(2)
33262	1(3)
33263	1(3)
33264	1(3)
33265	1(2)
33266	1(2)
33270	1(3)
33271	1(3)
33272	1(3)
33273	1(3)
33274	1(3)
33275	1(3)
33285	1(3)
33286	1(3)
33289	1(3)
33300	1(3)
33305	1(3)
33310	1(2)
33315	1(2)
33320	1(3)
33321	1(3)
33322	1(3)
33330	1(3)
33335	1(3)
33340	1(2)
33361	1(2)
33362	1(2)
33363	1(2)
33364	1(2)
33365	1(2)
33366	1(3)
33367	1(2)
33368	1(2)
33369	1(2)
33390	1(2)
33391	1(2)
33404	1(2)
33405	1(2)
33406	1(2)
33410	1(2)
33411	1(2)
33412	1(2)
33413	1(2)
33414	1(2)
33415	1(2)
33416	1(2)
33417	1(2)
33418	1(3)
33419	1(2)
33420	1(2)
33422	1(2)
33425	1(2)
33426	1(2)
33427	1(2)

CPT	MUE
33430	1(2)
33440	1(2)
33460	1(2)
33463	1(2)
33464	1(2)
33465	1(2)
33468	1(2)
33470	1(2)
33471	1(2)
33474	1(2)
33475	1(2)
33476	1(2)
33477	1(2)
33478	1(2)
33496	1(3)
33500	1(3)
33501	1(3)
33502	1(3)
33503	1(3)
33504	1(3)
33505	1(3)
33506	1(3)
33507	1(3)
33508	1(2)
33510	1(2)
33511	1(2)
33512	1(2)
33513	1(2)
33514	1(2)
33516	1(2)
33517	1(2)
33518	1(2)
33519	1(2)
33521	1(2)
33522	1(2)
33523	1(2)
33530	1(2)
33533	1(2)
33534	1(2)
33535	1(2)
33536	1(2)
33542	1(2)
33545	1(2)
33548	1(2)
33572	3(2)
33600	1(3)
33602	1(3)
33606	1(2)
33608	1(2)
33610	1(2)
33611	1(2)
33612	1(2)
33615	1(2)
33617	1(2)
33619	1(2)
33620	1(2)
33621	1(3)
33622	1(2)
33641	1(2)
33645	1(2)
33647	1(2)
33660	1(2)
33665	1(2)
33670	1(2)
33675	1(2)
33676	1(2)

CPT	MUE
33677	1(2)
33681	1(2)
33684	1(2)
33688	1(2)
33690	1(2)
33692	1(2)
33694	1(2)
33697	1(2)
33702	1(2)
33710	1(2)
33720	1(2)
33722	1(3)
33724	1(2)
33726	1(2)
33730	1(2)
33732	1(2)
33735	1(2)
33736	1(2)
33737	1(2)
33741	1(3)
33745	2(2)
33746	1(3)
33750	1(3)
33755	1(2)
33762	1(2)
33764	1(3)
33766	1(2)
33767	1(2)
33768	1(2)
33770	1(2)
33771	1(2)
33774	1(2)
33775	1(2)
33776	1(2)
33777	1(2)
33778	1(2)
33779	1(2)
33780	1(2)
33781	1(2)
33782	1(2)
33783	1(2)
33786	1(2)
33788	1(2)
33800	1(2)
33802	1(3)
33803	1(3)
33813	1(2)
33814	1(2)
33820	1(2)
33822	1(2)
33824	1(2)
33840	1(2)
33845	1(2)
33851	1(2)
33852	1(2)
33853	1(2)
33858	1(2)
33859	1(2)
33863	1(2)
33864	1(2)
33866	1(2)
33871	1(2)
33875	1(2)
33877	1(2)
33880	1(2)
33881	1(2)

CPT	MUE
33883	1(2)
33884	2(3)
33886	1(2)
33889	1(2)
33891	1(2)
33910	1(3)
33915	1(3)
33916	1(3)
33917	1(2)
33920	1(2)
33922	1(2)
33924	1(2)
33925	1(2)
33926	1(2)
33927	1(3)
33928	1(3)
33929	1(3)
33930	1(2)
33933	1(2)
33935	1(2)
33940	1(2)
33944	1(2)
33945	1(2)
33946	1(2)
33947	1(2)
33948	1(2)
33949	1(2)
33951	1(3)
33952	1(3)
33953	1(3)
33954	1(3)
33955	1(3)
33956	1(3)
33957	1(3)
33958	1(3)
33959	1(3)
33962	1(3)
33963	1(3)
33964	1(3)
33965	1(3)
33966	1(3)
33967	1(3)
33968	1(3)
33969	1(3)
33970	1(3)
33971	1(3)
33973	1(3)
33974	1(3)
33975	1(3)
33976	1(3)
33977	1(3)
33978	1(3)
33979	1(3)
33980	1(3)
33981	1(3)
33982	1(3)
33983	1(3)
33984	1(3)
33985	1(3)
33986	1(3)
33987	1(3)
33988	1(3)
33989	1(3)
33990	1(3)
33991	1(3)
33992	1(2)

CPT	MUE
33993	1(3)
33995	1(3)
33997	1(3)
33999	1(3)
34001	1(3)
34051	1(3)
34101	1(3)
34111	2(3)
34151	1(3)
34201	1(3)
34203	1(2)
34401	1(3)
34421	1(3)
34451	1(3)
34471	1(2)
34490	1(2)
34501	1(2)
34502	1(2)
34510	2(3)
34520	1(3)
34530	1(2)
34701	1(2)
34702	1(2)
34703	1(2)
34704	1(2)
34705	1(2)
34706	1(2)
34707	1(2)
34708	1(2)
34709	3(3)
34710	1(2)
34711	2(3)
34712	1(2)
34713	1(2)
34714	1(2)
34715	1(2)
34716	1(2)
34717	2(2)
34718	2(2)
34808	1(3)
34812	1(2)
34813	1(2)
34820	1(2)
34830	1(2)
34831	1(2)
34832	1(2)
34833	1(2)
34834	1(2)
34839	1(2)
34841	1(2)
34842	1(2)
34843	1(2)
34844	1(2)
34845	1(2)
34846	1(2)
34847	1(2)
34848	1(2)
35001	1(2)
35002	1(2)
35005	1(2)
35011	1(2)
35013	1(2)
35021	1(2)
35022	1(2)
35045	1(3)
35081	1(2)

CPT	MUE
35082	1(2)
35091	1(2)
35092	1(2)
35102	1(2)
35103	1(2)
35111	1(2)
35112	1(2)
35121	1(3)
35122	1(3)
35131	1(2)
35132	1(2)
35141	1(2)
35142	1(2)
35151	1(2)
35152	1(2)
35180	2(3)
35182	2(3)
35184	2(3)
35188	2(3)
35189	1(3)
35190	2(3)
35201	2(3)
35206	2(3)
35207	3(3)
35211	3(3)
35216	2(3)
35221	3(3)
35226	3(3)
35231	2(3)
35236	2(3)
35241	2(3)
35246	2(3)
35251	2(3)
35256	2(3)
35261	1(3)
35266	2(3)
35271	2(3)
35276	2(3)
35281	2(3)
35286	2(3)
35301	2(3)
35302	1(2)
35303	1(2)
35304	1(2)
35305	1(2)
35306	2(3)
35311	1(2)
35321	1(2)
35331	1(2)
35341	3(3)
35351	1(3)
35355	1(2)
35361	1(2)
35363	1(2)
35371	1(2)
35372	1(2)
35390	1(3)
35400	1(3)
35500	2(3)
35501	1(3)
35506	1(3)
35508	1(3)
35509	1(3)
35510	1(3)
35511	1(3)
35512	1(3)

CPT	MUE
35515	1(3)
35516	1(3)
35518	1(3)
35521	1(3)
35522	1(3)
35523	1(3)
35525	1(3)
35526	1(3)
35531	1(3)
35533	1(3)
35535	1(3)
35536	1(3)
35537	1(3)
35538	1(3)
35539	1(3)
35540	1(3)
35556	1(3)
35558	1(3)
35560	1(3)
35563	1(3)
35565	1(3)
35566	1(3)
35570	1(3)
35571	1(3)
35572	2(3)
35583	1(2)
35585	2(3)
35587	1(3)
35600	2(3)
35601	1(3)
35606	1(3)
35612	1(3)
35616	1(3)
35621	1(3)
35623	1(3)
35626	3(3)
35631	4(3)
35632	1(3)
35633	1(3)
35634	1(3)
35636	1(3)
35637	1(3)
35638	1(3)
35642	1(3)
35645	1(3)
35646	1(3)
35647	1(3)
35650	1(3)
35654	1(3)
35656	1(3)
35661	1(3)
35663	1(3)
35665	1(3)
35666	2(3)
35671	2(3)
35681	1(3)
35682	1(2)
35683	1(2)
35685	2(3)
35686	1(3)
35691	1(3)
35693	1(3)
35694	1(3)
35695	1(3)
35697	2(3)
35700	2(3)

CPT	MUE
35701	1(2)
35702	2(2)
35703	2(2)
35800	2(3)
35820	2(3)
35840	2(3)
35860	2(3)
35870	1(3)
35875	2(3)
35876	2(3)
35879	2(3)
35881	1(3)
35883	1(3)
35884	1(3)
35901	1(3)
35903	2(3)
35905	1(3)
35907	1(3)
36000	4(3)
36002	2(3)
36005	2(3)
36010	2(3)
36011	4(3)
36012	4(3)
36013	2(3)
36014	2(3)
36015	4(3)
36100	2(3)
36140	3(3)
36160	2(3)
36200	2(3)
36215	6(3)
36216	4(3)
36217	2(3)
36218	6(3)
36221	1(3)
36222	1(3)
36223	1(3)
36224	1(3)
36225	1(3)
36226	1(3)
36227	2(2)
36228	4(3)
36245	6(3)
36246	4(3)
36247	3(3)
36248	6(3)
36251	1(3)
36252	1(3)
36253	1(3)
36254	1(3)
36260	1(2)
36261	1(2)
36262	1(2)
36299	1(3)
36400	1(3)
36405	1(3)
36406	1(3)
36410	3(3)
36415	2(3)
36416	0(3)
36420	2(3)
36425	2(3)
36430	1(3)
36440	1(3)
36450	1(3)

CPT	MUE
36455	1(3)
36456	1(3)
36460	2(3)
36465	1(2)
36466	1(2)
36468	2(3)
36470	1(2)
36471	1(2)
36473	1(3)
36474	1(3)
36475	1(3)
36476	2(3)
36478	1(3)
36479	2(3)
36481	1(3)
36482	1(3)
36483	2(3)
36500	4(3)
36510	1(3)
36511	1(3)
36512	1(3)
36513	1(3)
36514	1(3)
36516	1(3)
36522	1(3)
36555	2(3)
36556	2(3)
36557	2(3)
36558	2(3)
36560	2(3)
36561	2(3)
36563	1(3)
36565	1(3)
36566	1(3)
36568	2(3)
36569	2(3)
36570	2(3)
36571	2(3)
36572	1(3)
36573	1(3)
36575	2(3)
36576	2(3)
36578	2(3)
36580	2(3)
36581	2(3)
36582	2(3)
36583	2(3)
36584	2(3)
36585	2(3)
36589	2(3)
36590	2(3)
36591	2(3)
36592	1(3)
36593	2(3)
36595	2(3)
36596	2(3)
36597	2(3)
36598	2(3)
36600	4(3)
36620	3(3)
36625	2(3)
36640	1(3)
36660	1(3)
36680	1(3)
36800	1(3)
36810	1(3)

CPT	MUE
36815	1(3)
36818	1(3)
36819	1(3)
36820	1(3)
36821	2(3)
36823	1(3)
36825	1(3)
36830	2(3)
36831	1(3)
36832	2(3)
36833	1(3)
36835	1(3)
36838	1(3)
36860	2(3)
36861	2(3)
36901	1(3)
36902	1(3)
36903	1(3)
36904	1(3)
36905	1(3)
36906	1(3)
36907	1(3)
36908	1(3)
36909	1(3)
37140	1(2)
37145	1(3)
37160	1(3)
37180	1(2)
37181	1(2)
37182	1(2)
37183	1(2)
37184	1(2)
37185	2(3)
37186	2(3)
37187	1(3)
37188	1(3)
37191	1(3)
37192	1(3)
37193	1(3)
37195	1(3)
37197	2(3)
37200	2(3)
37211	1(2)
37212	1(2)
37213	1(2)
37214	1(2)
37215	1(2)
37216	0(3)
37217	1(2)
37218	1(2)
37220	1(2)
37221	1(2)
37222	2(2)
37223	2(2)
37224	1(2)
37225	1(2)
37226	1(2)
37227	1(2)
37228	1(2)
37229	1(2)
37230	1(2)
37231	1(2)
37232	2(3)
37233	2(3)
37234	2(3)
37235	2(3)

CPT	MUE
37236	1(2)
37237	2(3)
37238	1(2)
37239	2(3)
37241	2(3)
37242	2(3)
37243	1(3)
37244	2(3)
37246	1(2)
37247	2(3)
37248	1(2)
37249	3(3)
37252	1(2)
37253	5(3)
37500	1(3)
37501	1(3)
37565	1(2)
37600	1(3)
37605	1(3)
37606	1(3)
37607	1(3)
37609	1(2)
37615	2(3)
37616	1(3)
37617	3(3)
37618	2(3)
37619	1(2)
37650	1(2)
37660	1(2)
37700	1(2)
37718	1(2)
37722	1(2)
37735	1(2)
37760	1(2)
37761	1(2)
37765	1(2)
37766	1(2)
37780	1(2)
37785	1(2)
37788	1(2)
37790	1(2)
37799	1(3)
38100	1(2)
38101	1(3)
38102	1(2)
38115	1(3)
38120	1(2)
38129	1(3)
38200	1(3)
38204	0(3)
38205	1(3)
38206	1(3)
38207	0(3)
38208	0(3)
38209	0(3)
38210	0(3)
38211	0(3)
38212	0(3)
38213	0(3)
38214	0(3)
38215	0(3)
38220	1(3)
38221	1(3)
38222	1(2)
38230	1(2)
38232	1(2)

CPT	MUE
38240	1(3)
38241	1(2)
38242	1(2)
38243	1(3)
38300	1(3)
38305	1(3)
38308	1(3)
38380	1(2)
38381	1(2)
38382	1(2)
38500	2(3)
38505	2(3)
38510	1(2)
38520	1(2)
38525	1(2)
38530	1(2)
38531	1(2)
38542	1(2)
38550	1(3)
38555	1(3)
38562	1(2)
38564	1(2)
38570	1(2)
38571	1(2)
38572	1(2)
38573	1(2)
38589	1(3)
38700	1(2)
38720	1(2)
38724	1(2)
38740	1(2)
38745	1(2)
38746	1(2)
38747	1(2)
38760	1(2)
38765	1(2)
38770	1(2)
38780	1(2)
38790	1(2)
38792	1(3)
38794	1(2)
38900	1(3)
38999	1(3)
39000	1(2)
39010	1(2)
39200	1(2)
39220	1(2)
39401	1(3)
39402	1(3)
39499	1(3)
39501	1(3)
39503	1(2)
39540	1(2)
39541	1(2)
39545	1(2)
39560	1(3)
39561	1(3)
39599	1(3)
40490	2(3)
40500	2(3)
40510	2(3)
40520	2(3)
40525	2(3)
40527	2(3)
40530	2(3)
40650	2(3)

CPT	MUE
40652	2(3)
40654	2(3)
40700	1(2)
40701	1(2)
40702	1(2)
40720	1(2)
40761	1(2)
40799	1(3)
40800	2(3)
40801	2(3)
40804	1(3)
40805	2(3)
40806	2(2)
40808	2(3)
40810	2(3)
40812	2(3)
40814	4(3)
40816	2(3)
40818	2(3)
40819	2(2)
40820	2(3)
40830	2(3)
40831	2(3)
40840	1(2)
40842	1(2)
40843	1(2)
40844	1(2)
40845	1(3)
40899	1(3)
41000	1(3)
41005	1(3)
41006	2(3)
41007	2(3)
41008	2(3)
41009	2(3)
41010	1(2)
41015	2(3)
41016	1(3)
41017	2(3)
41018	2(3)
41019	1(2)
41100	2(3)
41105	2(3)
41108	2(3)
41110	2(3)
41112	2(3)
41113	2(3)
41114	2(3)
41115	1(2)
41116	2(3)
41120	1(2)
41130	1(2)
41135	1(2)
41140	1(2)
41145	1(2)
41150	1(2)
41153	1(2)
41155	1(2)
41250	2(3)
41251	2(3)
41252	2(3)
41510	1(2)
41512	1(2)
41520	1(3)
41530	1(3)
41599	1(3)

CPT	MUE
41800	2(3)
41805	1(3)
41806	1(3)
41820	4(2)
41821	2(3)
41822	1(2)
41823	1(2)
41825	2(3)
41826	2(3)
41827	2(3)
41828	4(2)
41830	2(3)
41850	2(3)
41870	2(3)
41872	4(2)
41874	4(2)
41899	1(3)
42000	1(3)
42100	2(3)
42104	2(3)
42106	2(3)
42107	2(3)
42120	1(2)
42140	1(2)
42145	1(2)
42160	1(3)
42180	1(3)
42182	1(3)
42200	1(2)
42205	1(2)
42210	1(2)
42215	1(2)
42220	1(2)
42225	1(2)
42226	1(2)
42227	1(2)
42235	1(2)
42260	1(3)
42280	1(2)
42281	1(2)
42299	1(3)
42300	2(3)
42305	2(3)
42310	2(3)
42320	2(3)
42330	1(3)
42335	2(2)
42340	1(2)
42400	2(3)
42405	2(3)
42408	1(3)
42409	1(3)
42410	1(2)
42415	1(2)
42420	1(2)
42425	1(2)
42426	1(2)
42440	1(2)
42450	1(3)
42500	2(3)
42505	2(3)
42507	1(2)
42509	1(2)
42510	1(2)
42550	2(3)
42600	1(3)

CPT	MUE
42650	2(3)
42660	2(3)
42665	2(3)
42699	1(3)
42700	2(3)
42720	1(3)
42725	1(3)
42800	3(3)
42804	1(3)
42806	1(3)
42808	2(3)
42809	1(3)
42810	1(3)
42815	1(3)
42820	1(2)
42821	1(2)
42825	1(2)
42826	1(2)
42830	1(2)
42831	1(2)
42835	1(2)
42836	1(2)
42842	1(3)
42844	1(3)
42845	1(3)
42860	1(3)
42870	1(3)
42890	1(2)
42892	1(3)
42894	1(3)
42900	1(3)
42950	1(2)
42953	1(3)
42955	1(2)
42960	1(3)
42961	1(3)
42962	1(3)
42970	1(3)
42971	1(3)
42972	1(3)
42999	1(3)
43020	1(2)
43030	1(2)
43045	1(2)
43100	1(3)
43101	1(3)
43107	1(2)
43108	1(2)
43112	1(2)
43113	1(2)
43116	1(2)
43117	1(2)
43118	1(2)
43121	1(2)
43122	1(2)
43123	1(2)
43124	1(2)
43130	1(3)
43135	1(3)
43180	1(2)
43191	1(3)
43192	1(3)
43193	1(3)
43194	1(3)
43195	1(3)
43196	1(3)

CPT	MUE
43197	1(3)
43198	1(3)
43200	1(3)
43201	1(2)
43202	1(2)
43204	1(2)
43205	1(2)
43206	1(2)
43210	1(2)
43211	1(3)
43212	1(3)
43213	1(2)
43214	1(3)
43215	1(3)
43216	1(2)
43217	1(2)
43220	1(3)
43226	1(3)
43227	1(3)
43229	1(3)
43231	1(2)
43232	1(2)
43233	1(3)
43235	1(3)
43236	1(2)
43237	1(2)
43238	1(2)
43239	1(2)
43240	1(2)
43241	1(3)
43242	1(2)
43243	1(2)
43244	1(2)
43245	1(2)
43246	1(2)
43247	1(2)
43248	1(3)
43249	1(3)
43250	1(2)
43251	1(2)
43252	1(2)
43253	1(3)
43254	1(3)
43255	2(3)
43257	1(2)
43259	1(2)
43260	1(3)
43261	1(2)
43262	2(2)
43263	1(2)
43264	1(2)
43265	1(2)
43266	1(3)
43270	1(3)
43273	1(2)
43274	2(3)
43275	1(3)
43276	2(3)
43277	3(3)
43278	1(3)
43279	1(2)
43280	1(2)
43281	1(2)
43282	1(2)
43283	1(2)
43284	1(2)

CPT	MUE
43285	1(2)
43286	1(2)
43287	1(2)
43288	1(2)
43289	1(3)
43300	1(2)
43305	1(2)
43310	1(2)
43312	1(2)
43313	1(2)
43314	1(2)
43320	1(2)
43325	1(2)
43327	1(2)
43328	1(2)
43330	1(2)
43331	1(2)
43332	1(2)
43333	1(2)
43334	1(2)
43335	1(2)
43336	1(2)
43337	1(2)
43338	1(2)
43340	1(2)
43341	1(2)
43351	1(2)
43352	1(2)
43360	1(2)
43361	1(2)
43400	1(2)
43405	1(2)
43410	1(3)
43415	1(3)
43420	1(3)
43425	1(3)
43450	1(3)
43453	1(3)
43460	1(3)
43496	1(3)
43499	1(3)
43500	1(2)
43501	1(3)
43502	1(2)
43510	1(2)
43520	1(2)
43605	1(2)
43610	2(3)
43611	2(3)
43620	1(2)
43621	1(2)
43622	1(2)
43631	1(2)
43632	1(2)
43633	1(2)
43634	1(2)
43635	1(2)
43640	1(2)
43641	1(2)
43644	1(2)
43645	1(2)
43647	1(2)
43648	1(2)
43651	1(2)
43652	1(2)
43653	1(2)

CPT	MUE
43659	1(3)
43752	2(3)
43753	1(3)
43754	1(3)
43755	1(3)
43756	1(2)
43757	1(2)
43761	2(3)
43762	2(3)
43763	2(3)
43770	1(2)
43771	1(2)
43772	1(2)
43773	1(2)
43774	1(2)
43775	1(2)
43800	1(2)
43810	1(2)
43820	1(2)
43825	1(2)
43830	1(2)
43831	1(2)
43832	1(2)
43840	2(3)
43842	0(3)
43843	1(2)
43845	1(2)
43846	1(2)
43847	1(2)
43848	1(2)
43850	1(2)
43855	1(2)
43860	1(2)
43865	1(2)
43870	1(2)
43880	1(3)
43881	1(3)
43882	1(3)
43886	1(2)
43887	1(2)
43888	1(2)
43999	1(3)
44005	1(2)
44010	1(2)
44015	1(2)
44020	2(3)
44021	1(3)
44025	1(3)
44050	1(2)
44055	1(2)
44100	1(2)
44110	1(2)
44111	1(2)
44120	1(2)
44121	2(3)
44125	1(2)
44126	1(2)
44127	1(2)
44128	2(3)
44130	2(3)
44132	1(2)
44133	1(2)
44135	1(2)
44136	1(2)
44137	1(2)
44139	1(2)

CPT	MUE
44140	2(3)
44141	1(3)
44143	1(2)
44144	1(3)
44145	1(2)
44146	1(2)
44147	1(3)
44150	1(2)
44151	1(2)
44155	1(2)
44156	1(2)
44157	1(2)
44158	1(2)
44160	1(2)
44180	1(2)
44186	1(2)
44187	1(3)
44188	1(3)
44202	1(2)
44203	2(3)
44204	2(3)
44205	1(2)
44206	1(2)
44207	1(2)
44208	1(2)
44210	1(2)
44211	1(2)
44212	1(2)
44213	1(2)
44227	1(3)
44238	1(3)
44300	1(3)
44310	2(3)
44312	1(2)
44314	1(2)
44316	1(2)
44320	1(2)
44322	1(2)
44340	1(2)
44345	1(2)
44346	1(2)
44360	1(3)
44361	1(2)
44363	1(3)
44364	1(2)
44365	1(2)
44366	1(3)
44369	1(2)
44370	1(2)
44372	1(2)
44373	1(2)
44376	1(3)
44377	1(2)
44378	1(3)
44379	1(2)
44380	1(3)
44381	1(3)
44382	1(2)
44384	1(3)
44385	1(3)
44386	1(2)
44388	1(3)
44389	1(2)
44390	1(3)
44391	1(3)
44392	1(2)

CPT	MUE
44394	1(2)
44401	1(2)
44402	1(3)
44403	1(3)
44404	1(3)
44405	1(3)
44406	1(3)
44407	1(2)
44408	1(3)
44500	1(3)
44602	1(2)
44603	1(2)
44604	1(2)
44605	1(2)
44615	3(3)
44620	2(3)
44625	1(3)
44626	1(3)
44640	2(3)
44650	2(3)
44660	1(3)
44661	1(3)
44680	1(3)
44700	1(2)
44701	1(2)
44705	1(3)
44715	1(2)
44720	2(3)
44721	2(3)
44799	1(3)
44800	1(3)
44820	1(3)
44850	1(3)
44899	1(3)
44900	1(2)
44950	1(2)
44955	1(2)
44960	1(2)
44970	1(2)
44979	1(3)
45000	1(3)
45005	1(3)
45020	1(3)
45100	2(3)
45108	1(2)
45110	1(2)
45111	1(2)
45112	1(2)
45113	1(2)
45114	1(2)
45116	1(2)
45119	1(2)
45120	1(2)
45121	1(2)
45123	1(2)
45126	1(2)
45130	1(2)
45135	1(2)
45136	1(2)
45150	1(2)
45160	1(3)
45171	2(3)
45172	2(3)
45190	1(3)
45300	1(3)
45303	1(3)

CPT	MUE
45305	1(2)
45307	1(3)
45308	1(2)
45309	1(2)
45315	1(2)
45317	1(3)
45320	1(2)
45321	1(2)
45327	1(2)
45330	1(3)
45331	1(2)
45332	1(3)
45333	1(2)
45334	1(3)
45335	1(2)
45337	1(2)
45338	1(2)
45340	1(2)
45341	1(2)
45342	1(2)
45346	1(2)
45347	1(3)
45349	1(3)
45350	1(2)
45378	1(3)
45379	1(3)
45380	1(2)
45381	1(2)
45382	1(3)
45384	1(2)
45385	1(2)
45386	1(2)
45388	1(2)
45389	1(3)
45390	1(3)
45391	1(2)
45392	1(2)
45393	1(3)
45395	1(2)
45397	1(2)
45398	1(2)
45399	1(3)
45400	1(2)
45402	1(2)
45499	1(3)
45500	1(2)
45505	1(2)
45520	1(2)
45540	1(2)
45541	1(2)
45550	1(2)
45560	1(2)
45562	1(2)
45563	1(2)
45800	1(3)
45805	1(3)
45820	1(3)
45825	1(3)
45900	1(2)
45905	1(2)
45910	1(2)
45915	1(2)
45990	1(2)
45999	1(3)
46020	2(3)
46030	1(3)

CPT	MUE
46040	2(3)
46045	2(3)
46050	2(3)
46060	2(3)
46070	1(2)
46080	1(2)
46083	2(3)
46200	1(3)
46220	1(2)
46221	1(2)
46230	1(2)
46250	1(2)
46255	1(2)
46257	1(2)
46258	1(2)
46260	1(2)
46261	1(2)
46262	1(2)
46270	1(3)
46275	1(3)
46280	1(2)
46285	1(3)
46288	1(3)
46320	2(3)
46500	1(2)
46505	1(2)
46600	1(3)
46601	1(3)
46604	1(2)
46606	1(2)
46607	1(2)
46608	1(3)
46610	1(2)
46611	1(2)
46612	1(2)
46614	1(3)
46615	1(2)
46700	1(2)
46705	1(2)
46706	1(3)
46707	1(3)
46710	1(3)
46712	1(3)
46715	1(2)
46716	1(2)
46730	1(2)
46735	1(2)
46740	1(2)
46742	1(2)
46744	1(2)
46746	1(2)
46748	1(2)
46750	1(2)
46751	1(2)
46753	1(2)
46754	1(3)
46760	1(2)
46761	1(2)
46900	1(2)
46910	1(2)
46916	1(2)
46917	1(2)
46922	1(2)
46924	1(2)
46930	1(2)
46940	1(2)

CPT	MUE
46942	1(3)
46945	1(2)
46946	1(2)
46947	1(2)
46948	1(2)
46999	1(3)
47000	3(3)
47001	3(3)
47010	1(3)
47015	1(2)
47100	3(3)
47120	2(3)
47122	1(2)
47125	1(2)
47130	1(2)
47133	1(2)
47135	1(2)
47140	1(2)
47141	1(2)
47142	1(2)
47143	1(2)
47144	1(2)
47145	1(2)
47146	2(3)
47147	1(3)
47300	2(3)
47350	1(3)
47360	1(3)
47361	1(3)
47362	1(3)
47370	1(2)
47371	1(2)
47379	1(3)
47380	1(2)
47381	1(2)
47382	1(2)
47383	1(2)
47399	1(3)
47400	1(3)
47420	1(2)
47425	1(2)
47460	1(2)
47480	1(2)
47490	1(2)
47531	2(3)
47532	1(3)
47533	1(3)
47534	2(3)
47535	1(3)
47536	2(3)
47537	1(3)
47538	2(3)
47539	2(3)
47540	2(3)
47541	1(3)
47542	2(3)
47543	1(3)
47544	1(3)
47550	1(3)
47552	1(3)
47553	1(2)
47554	1(3)
47555	1(2)
47556	1(2)
47562	1(2)
47563	1(2)

CPT	MUE
47564	1(2)
47570	1(2)
47579	1(3)
47600	1(2)
47605	1(2)
47610	1(2)
47612	1(2)
47620	1(2)
47700	1(2)
47701	1(2)
47711	1(2)
47712	1(2)
47715	1(2)
47720	1(2)
47721	1(2)
47740	1(2)
47741	1(2)
47760	1(2)
47765	1(2)
47780	1(2)
47785	1(2)
47800	1(2)
47801	1(3)
47802	1(2)
47900	1(2)
47999	1(3)
48000	1(2)
48001	1(2)
48020	1(3)
48100	1(3)
48102	1(3)
48105	1(2)
48120	1(3)
48140	1(2)
48145	1(2)
48146	1(2)
48148	1(2)
48150	1(2)
48152	1(2)
48153	1(2)
48154	1(2)
48155	1(2)
48160	0(3)
48400	1(3)
48500	1(3)
48510	1(3)
48520	1(3)
48540	1(3)
48545	1(3)
48547	1(2)
48548	1(2)
48550	1(2)
48551	1(2)
48552	2(3)
48554	1(2)
48556	1(2)
48999	1(3)
49000	1(2)
49002	1(3)
49010	1(3)
49013	1(2)
49014	1(3)
49020	2(3)
49040	2(3)
49060	2(3)
49062	1(3)

CPT	MUE
49082	1(3)
49083	2(3)
49084	1(3)
49180	2(3)
49185	2(3)
49203	1(2)
49204	1(2)
49205	1(2)
49215	1(2)
49250	1(2)
49255	1(2)
49320	1(3)
49321	1(2)
49322	1(2)
49323	1(2)
49324	1(2)
49325	1(2)
49326	1(2)
49327	1(2)
49329	1(3)
49400	1(3)
49402	1(3)
49405	2(3)
49406	2(3)
49407	1(3)
49411	1(2)
49412	1(2)
49418	1(3)
49419	1(2)
49421	1(2)
49422	1(2)
49423	2(3)
49424	3(3)
49425	1(2)
49426	1(3)
49427	1(3)
49428	1(2)
49429	1(2)
49435	1(2)
49436	1(2)
49440	1(3)
49441	1(3)
49442	1(3)
49446	1(2)
49450	1(3)
49451	1(3)
49452	1(3)
49460	1(3)
49465	1(3)
49491	1(2)
49492	1(2)
49495	1(2)
49496	1(2)
49500	1(2)
49501	1(2)
49505	1(2)
49507	1(2)
49520	1(2)
49521	1(2)
49525	1(2)
49540	1(2)
49550	1(2)
49553	1(2)
49555	1(2)
49557	1(2)
49560	2(3)

CPT	MUE
49561	1(3)
49565	2(3)
49566	2(3)
49568	2(3)
49570	1(3)
49572	1(3)
49580	1(2)
49582	1(2)
49585	1(2)
49587	1(2)
49590	1(2)
49600	1(2)
49605	1(2)
49606	1(2)
49610	1(2)
49611	1(2)
49650	1(2)
49651	1(2)
49652	2(3)
49653	2(3)
49654	1(3)
49655	1(3)
49656	1(3)
49657	1(3)
49659	1(3)
49900	1(3)
49904	1(3)
49905	1(3)
49906	1(3)
49999	1(3)
50010	1(2)
50020	1(3)
50040	1(2)
50045	1(2)
50060	1(2)
50065	1(2)
50070	1(2)
50075	1(2)
50080	1(2)
50081	1(2)
50100	1(2)
50120	1(2)
50125	1(2)
50130	1(2)
50135	1(2)
50200	1(3)
50205	1(3)
50220	1(2)
50225	1(2)
50230	1(2)
50234	1(2)
50236	1(2)
50240	1(2)
50250	1(3)
50280	1(2)
50290	1(3)
50300	1(2)
50320	1(2)
50323	1(2)
50325	1(2)
50327	2(3)
50328	1(3)
50329	1(3)
50340	1(2)
50360	1(2)
50365	1(2)

CPT	MUE
50370	1(2)
50380	1(2)
50382	1(3)
50384	1(3)
50385	1(3)
50386	1(3)
50387	1(3)
50389	1(3)
50390	2(3)
50391	1(3)
50396	1(3)
50400	1(2)
50405	1(2)
50430	2(3)
50431	2(3)
50432	2(3)
50433	2(3)
50434	2(3)
50435	2(3)
50436	1(3)
50437	1(3)
50500	1(3)
50520	1(3)
50525	1(3)
50526	1(3)
50540	1(2)
50541	1(2)
50542	1(2)
50543	1(2)
50544	1(2)
50545	1(2)
50546	1(2)
50547	1(2)
50548	1(2)
50549	1(3)
50551	1(3)
50553	1(3)
50555	1(2)
50557	1(2)
50561	1(2)
50562	1(3)
50570	1(3)
50572	1(3)
50574	1(2)
50575	1(2)
50576	1(2)
50580	1(2)
50590	1(2)
50592	1(2)
50593	1(2)
50600	1(3)
50605	1(3)
50606	1(3)
50610	1(2)
50620	1(2)
50630	1(2)
50650	1(2)
50660	1(3)
50684	1(3)
50686	2(3)
50688	2(3)
50690	2(3)
50693	2(3)
50694	2(3)
50695	2(3)
50700	1(2)

CPT	MUE
50705	2(3)
50706	2(3)
50715	1(2)
50722	1(2)
50725	1(3)
50727	1(3)
50728	1(3)
50740	1(2)
50750	1(2)
50760	1(2)
50770	1(2)
50780	1(2)
50782	1(2)
50783	1(2)
50785	1(2)
50800	1(2)
50810	1(3)
50815	1(2)
50820	1(2)
50825	1(3)
50830	1(3)
50840	1(2)
50845	1(2)
50860	1(2)
50900	1(3)
50920	2(3)
50930	2(3)
50940	1(2)
50945	1(2)
50947	1(2)
50948	1(2)
50949	1(3)
50951	1(3)
50953	1(3)
50955	1(2)
50957	1(2)
50961	1(2)
50970	1(3)
50972	1(3)
50974	1(2)
50976	1(2)
50980	1(2)
51020	1(2)
51030	1(2)
51040	1(3)
51045	2(3)
51050	1(3)
51060	1(3)
51065	1(3)
51080	1(3)
51100	1(3)
51101	1(3)
51102	1(3)
51500	1(2)
51520	1(2)
51525	1(2)
51530	1(2)
51535	1(2)
51550	1(2)
51555	1(2)
51565	1(2)
51570	1(2)
51575	1(2)
51580	1(2)
51585	1(2)
51590	1(2)

CPT	MUE
51595	1(2)
51596	1(2)
51597	1(2)
51600	1(3)
51605	1(3)
51610	1(3)
51700	1(3)
51701	2(3)
51702	2(3)
51703	2(3)
51705	1(3)
51710	1(3)
51715	1(2)
51720	1(3)
51725	1(3)
51726	1(3)
51727	1(3)
51728	1(3)
51729	1(3)
51736	1(3)
51741	1(3)
51784	1(3)
51785	1(3)
51792	1(3)
51797	1(3)
51798	1(3)
51800	1(2)
51820	1(2)
51840	1(2)
51841	1(2)
51845	1(2)
51860	1(3)
51865	1(3)
51880	1(2)
51900	1(3)
51920	1(3)
51925	1(2)
51940	1(2)
51960	1(2)
51980	1(2)
51990	1(2)
51992	1(2)
51999	1(3)
52000	1(3)
52001	1(3)
52005	2(3)
52007	1(2)
52010	1(2)
52204	1(2)
52214	1(2)
52224	1(2)
52234	1(2)
52235	1(2)
52240	1(2)
52250	1(2)
52260	1(2)
52265	1(2)
52270	1(2)
52275	1(2)
52276	1(2)
52277	1(2)
52281	1(2)
52282	1(2)
52283	1(2)
52285	1(2)
52287	1(2)

CPT	MUE
52290	1(2)
52300	1(2)
52301	1(2)
52305	1(2)
52310	1(3)
52315	2(3)
52317	1(3)
52318	1(3)
52320	1(2)
52325	1(3)
52327	1(2)
52330	1(2)
52332	1(2)
52334	1(2)
52341	1(2)
52342	1(2)
52343	1(2)
52344	1(2)
52345	1(2)
52346	1(2)
52351	1(3)
52352	1(2)
52353	1(2)
52354	1(3)
52355	1(3)
52356	1(2)
52400	1(2)
52402	1(2)
52441	1(2)
52442	6(3)
52450	1(2)
52500	1(2)
52601	1(2)
52630	1(2)
52640	1(2)
52647	1(2)
52648	1(2)
52649	1(2)
52700	1(3)
53000	1(2)
53010	1(2)
53020	1(2)
53025	1(2)
53040	1(3)
53060	1(3)
53080	1(3)
53085	1(3)
53200	1(3)
53210	1(2)
53215	1(2)
53220	1(3)
53230	1(3)
53235	1(3)
53240	1(3)
53250	1(3)
53260	1(2)
53265	1(3)
53270	1(2)
53275	1(2)
53400	1(2)
53405	1(2)
53410	1(2)
53415	1(2)
53420	1(2)
53425	1(2)
53430	1(2)

CPT	MUE
53431	1(2)
53440	1(2)
53442	1(2)
53444	1(3)
53445	1(2)
53446	1(2)
53447	1(2)
53448	1(2)
53449	1(2)
53450	1(2)
53460	1(2)
53500	1(2)
53502	1(3)
53505	1(3)
53510	1(3)
53515	1(3)
53520	1(3)
53600	1(3)
53601	1(3)
53605	1(3)
53620	1(2)
53621	1(3)
53660	1(2)
53661	1(3)
53665	1(3)
53850	1(2)
53852	1(2)
53854	1(2)
53855	1(2)
53860	1(2)
53899	1(3)
54000	1(2)
54001	1(2)
54015	1(3)
54050	1(2)
54055	1(2)
54056	1(2)
54057	1(2)
54060	1(2)
54065	1(2)
54100	2(3)
54105	2(3)
54110	1(2)
54111	1(2)
54112	1(3)
54115	1(3)
54120	1(2)
54125	1(2)
54130	1(2)
54135	1(2)
54150	1(2)
54160	1(2)
54161	1(2)
54162	1(2)
54163	1(2)
54164	1(2)
54200	1(2)
54205	1(2)
54220	1(3)
54230	1(3)
54231	1(3)
54235	1(3)
54240	1(2)
54250	1(2)
54300	1(2)
54304	1(2)

CPT	MUE
54308	1(2)
54312	1(2)
54316	1(2)
54318	1(2)
54322	1(2)
54324	1(2)
54326	1(2)
54328	1(2)
54332	1(2)
54336	1(2)
54340	1(2)
54344	1(2)
54348	1(2)
54352	1(2)
54360	1(2)
54380	1(2)
54385	1(2)
54390	1(2)
54400	1(2)
54401	1(2)
54405	1(2)
54406	1(2)
54408	1(2)
54410	1(2)
54411	1(2)
54415	1(2)
54416	1(2)
54417	1(2)
54420	1(2)
54430	1(2)
54435	1(2)
54437	1(2)
54438	1(2)
54440	1(2)
54450	1(2)
54500	1(3)
54505	1(3)
54512	1(3)
54520	1(2)
54522	1(2)
54530	1(2)
54535	1(2)
54550	1(2)
54560	1(2)
54600	1(2)
54620	1(2)
54640	1(2)
54650	1(2)
54660	1(2)
54670	1(3)
54680	1(2)
54690	1(2)
54692	1(2)
54699	1(3)
54700	1(3)
54800	1(2)
54830	1(2)
54840	1(2)
54860	1(2)
54861	1(2)
54865	1(3)
54900	1(2)
54901	1(2)
55000	1(3)
55040	1(2)
55041	1(2)

CPT	MUE	CPT	MUE	CPT	MUE	CPT	MUE	CPT	MUE	CPT	MUE	CPT	MUE	CPT	MUE
55060	1(2)	56637	1(2)	57415	1(3)	58400	1(3)	58957	1(2)	59870	1(2)	61330	1(2)	61600	1(3)
55100	2(3)	56640	1(2)	57420	1(3)	58410	1(2)	58958	1(2)	59871	1(2)	61333	1(2)	61601	1(3)
55110	1(2)	56700	1(2)	57421	1(3)	58520	1(2)	58960	1(2)	59897	1(3)	61340	1(2)	61605	1(3)
55120	1(3)	56740	1(3)	57423	1(2)	58540	1(3)	58970	1(3)	59898	1(3)	61343	1(2)	61606	1(3)
55150	1(2)	56800	1(2)	57425	1(2)	58541	1(3)	58974	1(3)	59899	1(3)	61345	1(3)	61607	1(3)
55175	1(2)	56805	1(2)	57426	1(2)	58542	1(2)	58976	2(3)	60000	1(3)	61450	1(3)	61608	1(3)
55180	1(2)	56810	1(2)	57452	1(3)	58543	1(3)	58999	1(3)	60100	3(3)	61458	1(2)	61611	1(3)
55200	1(2)	56820	1(2)	57454	1(3)	58544	1(2)	59000	2(3)	60200	2(3)	61460	1(2)	61613	1(3)
55250	1(2)	56821	1(2)	57455	1(3)	58545	1(2)	59001	2(3)	60210	1(2)	61500	1(3)	61615	1(3)
55300	1(2)	57000	1(3)	57456	1(3)	58546	1(2)	59012	2(3)	60212	1(2)	61501	1(3)	61616	1(3)
55400	1(2)	57010	1(3)	57460	1(3)	58548	1(2)	59015	2(3)	60220	1(3)	61510	1(3)	61618	2(3)
55500	1(2)	57020	1(3)	57461	1(3)	58550	1(3)	59020	2(3)	60225	1(2)	61512	1(3)	61619	2(3)
55520	1(2)	57022	1(3)	57465	1(3)	58552	1(3)	59025	2(3)	60240	1(2)	61514	2(3)	61623	2(3)
55530	1(2)	57023	1(3)	57500	1(3)	58553	1(3)	59030	2(3)	60252	1(2)	61516	1(3)	61624	2(3)
55535	1(2)	57061	1(2)	57505	1(3)	58554	1(2)	59050	2(3)	60254	1(2)	61517	1(3)	61626	2(3)
55540	1(2)	57065	1(2)	57510	1(3)	58555	1(3)	59051	2(3)	60260	1(2)	61518	1(3)	61630	1(3)
55550	1(2)	57100	2(3)	57511	1(3)	58558	1(3)	59070	2(3)	60270	1(2)	61519	1(3)	61635	2(3)
55559	1(3)	57105	2(3)	57513	1(3)	58559	1(3)	59072	2(3)	60271	1(2)	61520	1(3)	61640	0(3)
55600	1(2)	57106	1(2)	57520	1(3)	58560	1(3)	59074	2(3)	60280	1(3)	61521	1(3)	61641	0(3)
55605	1(2)	57107	1(2)	57522	1(3)	58561	1(3)	59076	2(3)	60281	1(3)	61522	1(3)	61642	0(3)
55650	1(2)	57109	1(2)	57530	1(3)	58562	1(3)	59100	1(2)	60300	2(3)	61524	2(3)	61645	1(3)
55680	1(3)	57110	1(2)	57531	1(2)	58563	1(3)	59120	1(3)	60500	1(2)	61526	1(3)	61650	1(2)
55700	1(2)	57111	1(2)	57540	1(2)	58565	1(2)	59121	1(3)	60502	1(3)	61530	1(3)	61651	2(2)
55705	1(2)	57120	1(2)	57545	1(3)	58570	1(3)	59130	1(3)	60505	1(3)	61531	1(2)	61680	1(3)
55706	1(2)	57130	1(2)	57550	1(3)	58571	1(2)	59135	1(3)	60512	1(3)	61533	2(3)	61682	1(3)
55720	1(3)	57135	2(3)	57555	1(2)	58572	1(3)	59136	1(3)	60520	1(2)	61534	1(3)	61684	1(3)
55725	1(3)	57150	1(3)	57556	1(2)	58573	1(2)	59140	1(2)	60521	1(2)	61535	2(3)	61686	1(3)
55801	1(2)	57155	1(3)	57558	1(3)	58575	1(2)	59150	1(3)	60522	1(2)	61536	1(3)	61690	1(3)
55810	1(2)	57156	1(3)	57700	1(3)	58578	1(3)	59151	1(3)	60540	1(2)	61537	1(3)	61692	1(3)
55812	1(2)	57160	1(2)	57720	1(3)	58579	1(3)	59160	1(2)	60545	1(2)	61538	1(2)	61697	2(3)
55815	1(2)	57170	1(2)	57800	1(3)	58600	1(2)	59200	1(3)	60600	1(3)	61539	1(3)	61698	1(3)
55821	1(2)	57180	1(3)	58100	1(3)	58605	1(2)	59300	1(2)	60605	1(3)	61540	1(3)	61700	2(3)
55831	1(2)	57200	1(3)	58110	1(3)	58611	1(2)	59320	1(2)	60650	1(2)	61541	1(2)	61702	1(3)
55840	1(2)	57210	1(3)	58120	1(3)	58615	1(2)	59325	1(2)	60659	1(3)	61543	1(2)	61703	1(3)
55842	1(2)	57220	1(2)	58140	1(3)	58660	1(2)	59350	1(2)	60699	1(3)	61544	1(3)	61705	1(3)
55845	1(2)	57230	1(2)	58145	1(3)	58661	1(2)	59400	1(2)	61000	1(2)	61545	1(2)	61708	1(3)
55860	1(2)	57240	1(2)	58146	1(3)	58662	1(2)	59409	2(3)	61001	1(2)	61546	1(2)	61710	1(3)
55862	1(2)	57250	1(2)	58150	1(3)	58670	1(2)	59410	1(2)	61020	2(3)	61548	1(2)	61711	1(3)
55865	1(2)	57260	1(2)	58152	1(2)	58671	1(2)	59412	1(3)	61026	2(3)	61550	1(2)	61720	1(3)
55866	1(2)	57265	1(2)	58180	1(3)	58672	1(2)	59414	1(3)	61050	1(3)	61552	1(2)	61735	1(3)
55870	1(2)	57267	2(3)	58200	1(2)	58673	1(2)	59425	1(2)	61055	1(3)	61556	1(3)	61750	2(3)
55873	1(2)	57268	1(2)	58210	1(2)	58674	1(2)	59426	1(2)	61070	2(3)	61557	1(2)	61751	2(3)
55874	1(2)	57270	1(2)	58240	1(2)	58679	1(3)	59430	1(2)	61105	1(3)	61558	1(3)	61760	1(2)
55875	1(2)	57280	1(2)	58260	1(3)	58700	1(2)	59510	1(2)	61107	1(3)	61559	1(3)	61770	1(2)
55876	1(2)	57282	1(2)	58262	1(3)	58720	1(2)	59514	1(3)	61108	1(3)	61563	2(3)	61781	1(3)
55880	1(2)	57283	1(2)	58263	1(2)	58740	1(2)	59515	1(2)	61120	1(3)	61564	1(2)	61782	1(3)
55899	1(3)	57284	1(2)	58267	1(2)	58750	1(2)	59525	1(2)	61140	1(3)	61566	1(3)	61783	1(3)
55920	1(2)	57285	1(2)	58270	1(2)	58752	1(2)	59610	1(2)	61150	1(3)	61567	1(2)	61790	1(2)
55970	1(2)	57287	1(2)	58275	1(2)	58760	1(2)	59612	2(3)	61151	1(3)	61570	1(3)	61791	1(2)
55980	1(2)	57288	1(2)	58280	1(2)	58770	1(2)	59614	1(2)	61154	1(3)	61571	1(3)	61796	1(2)
56405	2(3)	57289	1(2)	58285	1(3)	58800	1(2)	59618	1(2)	61156	1(3)	61575	1(2)	61797	4(3)
56420	1(3)	57291	1(2)	58290	1(3)	58805	1(2)	59620	1(2)	61210	1(3)	61576	1(2)	61798	1(2)
56440	1(3)	57292	1(2)	58291	1(2)	58820	1(3)	59622	1(2)	61215	1(3)	61580	1(2)	61799	4(3)
56441	1(2)	57295	1(2)	58292	1(2)	58822	1(3)	59812	1(2)	61250	1(3)	61581	1(2)	61800	1(2)
56442	1(2)	57296	1(2)	58294	1(2)	58825	1(2)	59820	1(2)	61253	1(3)	61582	1(2)	61850	1(3)
56501	1(2)	57300	1(3)	58300	0(3)	58900	1(2)	59821	1(2)	61304	1(3)	61583	1(2)	61860	1(3)
56515	1(2)	57305	1(3)	58301	1(3)	58920	1(2)	59830	1(2)	61305	1(3)	61584	1(2)	61863	1(2)
56605	1(2)	57307	1(3)	58321	1(2)	58925	1(3)	59840	1(2)	61312	2(3)	61585	1(2)	61864	1(3)
56606	6(3)	57308	1(3)	58322	1(2)	58940	1(2)	59841	1(2)	61313	2(3)	61586	1(3)	61867	1(2)
56620	1(2)	57310	1(3)	58323	1(3)	58943	1(2)	59850	1(2)	61314	2(3)	61590	1(2)	61868	2(3)
56625	1(2)	57311	1(3)	58340	1(3)	58950	1(2)	59851	1(2)	61315	1(3)	61591	1(2)	61880	1(2)
56630	1(2)	57320	1(3)	58345	1(3)	58951	1(2)	59852	1(2)	61316	1(3)	61592	1(2)	61885	1(3)
56631	1(2)	57330	1(3)	58346	1(2)	58952	1(2)	59855	1(2)	61320	2(3)	61595	1(2)	61886	1(3)
56632	1(2)	57335	1(2)	58350	1(2)	58953	1(2)	59856	1(2)	61321	1(3)	61596	1(2)	61888	1(3)
56633	1(2)	57400	1(2)	58353	1(3)	58954	1(2)	59857	1(2)	61322	1(3)	61597	1(2)	62000	1(3)
56634	1(2)	57410	1(2)	58356	1(3)	58956	1(2)	59866	1(2)	61323	1(3)	61598	1(3)	62005	1(3)

CPT	MUE
62010	1(3)
62100	1(3)
62115	1(2)
62117	1(2)
62120	1(2)
62121	1(2)
62140	1(3)
62141	1(3)
62142	2(3)
62143	2(3)
62145	2(3)
62146	2(3)
62147	1(3)
62148	1(3)
62160	1(3)
62161	1(3)
62162	1(3)
62164	1(3)
62165	1(2)
62180	1(3)
62190	1(3)
62192	1(3)
62194	1(3)
62200	1(2)
62201	1(2)
62220	1(3)
62223	1(3)
62225	2(3)
62230	2(3)
62252	2(3)
62256	1(3)
62258	1(3)
62263	1(2)
62264	1(2)
62267	2(3)
62268	1(3)
62269	2(3)
62270	2(3)
62272	1(3)
62273	2(3)
62280	1(3)
62281	1(3)
62282	1(3)
62284	1(3)
62287	1(2)
62290	5(2)
62291	4(3)
62292	1(2)
62294	1(3)
62302	1(3)
62303	1(3)
62304	1(3)
62305	1(3)
62320	1(3)
62321	1(3)
62322	1(3)
62323	1(3)
62324	1(3)
62325	1(3)
62326	1(3)
62327	1(3)
62328	2(3)
62329	1(3)
62350	1(3)
62351	1(3)
62355	1(3)

CPT	MUE
62360	1(2)
62361	1(2)
62362	1(2)
62365	1(2)
62367	1(3)
62368	1(3)
62369	1(3)
62370	1(3)
62380	2(3)
63001	1(2)
63003	1(2)
63005	1(2)
63011	1(2)
63012	1(2)
63015	1(2)
63016	1(2)
63017	1(2)
63020	1(2)
63030	1(2)
63035	4(3)
63040	1(2)
63042	1(2)
63043	4(3)
63044	4(2)
63045	1(2)
63046	1(2)
63047	1(2)
63048	5(3)
63050	1(2)
63051	1(2)
63055	1(2)
63056	1(2)
63057	3(3)
63064	1(2)
63066	1(3)
63075	1(2)
63076	3(3)
63077	1(2)
63078	3(3)
63081	1(2)
63082	6(2)
63085	1(2)
63086	2(3)
63087	1(2)
63088	3(3)
63090	1(2)
63091	3(3)
63101	1(2)
63102	1(2)
63103	3(3)
63170	1(3)
63172	1(3)
63173	1(3)
63185	1(2)
63190	1(2)
63191	1(2)
63194	1(2)
63195	1(2)
63196	1(2)
63197	1(2)
63198	1(2)
63199	1(2)
63200	1(2)
63250	1(3)
63251	1(3)
63252	1(3)

CPT	MUE
63265	1(3)
63266	1(3)
63267	1(3)
63268	1(3)
63270	1(3)
63271	1(3)
63272	1(3)
63273	1(3)
63275	1(3)
63276	1(3)
63277	1(3)
63278	1(3)
63280	1(3)
63281	1(3)
63282	1(3)
63283	1(3)
63285	1(3)
63286	1(3)
63287	1(3)
63290	1(3)
63295	1(2)
63300	1(2)
63301	1(2)
63302	1(2)
63303	1(2)
63304	1(2)
63305	1(2)
63306	1(2)
63307	1(2)
63308	3(3)
63600	2(3)
63610	1(3)
63620	1(2)
63621	2(2)
63650	2(3)
63655	1(3)
63661	1(2)
63662	1(2)
63663	1(3)
63664	1(3)
63685	1(3)
63688	1(3)
63700	1(3)
63702	1(3)
63704	1(3)
63706	1(3)
63707	1(3)
63709	1(3)
63710	1(3)
63740	1(3)
63741	1(3)
63744	1(3)
63746	1(2)
64400	4(3)
64405	1(3)
64408	1(3)
64415	1(3)
64416	1(2)
64417	1(3)
64418	1(3)
64420	2(2)
64421	3(3)
64425	1(3)
64430	1(3)
64435	1(3)
64445	1(3)

CPT	MUE
64446	1(2)
64447	1(3)
64448	1(2)
64449	1(2)
64450	10(3)
64451	2(2)
64454	2(2)
64455	1(2)
64461	1(2)
64462	1(2)
64463	1(3)
64479	1(2)
64480	4(3)
64483	1(2)
64484	4(3)
64486	1(3)
64487	1(2)
64488	1(3)
64489	1(2)
64490	1(2)
64491	1(2)
64492	1(2)
64493	1(2)
64494	1(2)
64495	1(2)
64505	1(3)
64510	1(3)
64517	1(3)
64520	1(3)
64530	1(3)
64553	1(3)
64555	2(3)
64561	1(3)
64566	1(3)
64568	1(3)
64569	1(3)
64570	1(3)
64575	2(3)
64580	2(3)
64581	2(3)
64585	2(3)
64590	1(3)
64595	1(3)
64600	2(3)
64605	1(2)
64610	1(2)
64611	1(2)
64612	1(2)
64615	1(2)
64616	1(2)
64617	1(2)
64620	5(3)
64624	2(2)
64625	2(2)
64630	1(3)
64632	1(2)
64633	1(2)
64634	4(3)
64635	1(2)
64636	4(3)
64640	5(3)
64642	1(2)
64643	3(2)
64644	1(2)
64645	3(2)
64646	1(2)

CPT	MUE
64647	1(2)
64650	1(2)
64653	1(2)
64680	1(2)
64681	1(2)
64702	2(3)
64704	4(3)
64708	3(3)
64712	1(2)
64713	1(2)
64714	1(2)
64716	2(3)
64718	1(2)
64719	1(2)
64721	1(2)
64722	4(3)
64726	2(3)
64727	2(3)
64732	1(2)
64734	1(2)
64736	1(2)
64738	1(2)
64740	1(2)
64742	1(2)
64744	1(2)
64746	1(2)
64755	1(2)
64760	1(2)
64763	1(2)
64766	1(2)
64771	2(3)
64772	2(3)
64774	2(3)
64776	1(2)
64778	1(3)
64782	2(2)
64783	2(3)
64784	3(3)
64786	1(3)
64787	4(3)
64788	5(3)
64790	1(3)
64792	2(3)
64795	2(3)
64802	1(2)
64804	1(2)
64809	1(2)
64818	1(2)
64820	4(3)
64821	1(2)
64822	1(2)
64823	1(2)
64831	1(2)
64832	3(3)
64834	1(2)
64835	1(2)
64836	1(2)
64837	2(3)
64840	1(2)
64856	2(3)
64857	2(3)
64858	1(2)
64859	2(3)
64861	1(2)
64862	1(2)
64864	2(3)

CPT	MUE
64865	1(3)
64866	1(3)
64868	1(3)
64872	1(3)
64874	1(3)
64876	1(3)
64885	1(3)
64886	1(3)
64890	2(3)
64891	2(3)
64892	2(3)
64893	2(3)
64895	2(3)
64896	2(3)
64897	2(3)
64898	2(3)
64901	2(3)
64902	1(3)
64905	1(3)
64907	1(3)
64910	3(3)
64911	2(3)
64912	3(3)
64913	3(3)
64999	1(3)
65091	1(2)
65093	1(2)
65101	1(2)
65103	1(2)
65105	1(2)
65110	1(2)
65112	1(2)
65114	1(2)
65125	1(2)
65130	1(2)
65135	1(2)
65140	1(2)
65150	1(2)
65155	1(2)
65175	1(2)
65205	1(3)
65210	1(3)
65220	1(3)
65222	1(3)
65235	1(3)
65260	1(3)
65265	1(3)
65270	1(3)
65272	1(3)
65273	1(3)
65275	1(3)
65280	1(3)
65285	1(3)
65286	1(3)
65290	1(3)
65400	1(3)
65410	1(3)
65420	1(2)
65426	1(2)
65430	1(2)
65435	1(2)
65436	1(2)
65450	1(3)
65600	1(2)
65710	1(2)
65730	1(2)

CPT	MUE
65750	1(2)
65755	1(2)
65756	1(2)
65757	1(3)
65760	0(3)
65765	0(3)
65767	0(3)
65770	1(2)
65771	0(3)
65772	1(2)
65775	1(2)
65778	1(2)
65779	1(2)
65780	1(2)
65781	1(2)
65782	1(2)
65785	1(2)
65800	1(2)
65810	1(2)
65815	1(3)
65820	1(2)
65850	1(2)
65855	1(2)
65860	1(2)
65865	1(2)
65870	1(2)
65875	1(2)
65880	1(2)
65900	1(3)
65920	1(2)
65930	1(3)
66020	1(3)
66030	1(3)
66130	1(3)
66150	1(2)
66155	1(2)
66160	1(2)
66170	1(2)
66172	1(2)
66174	1(2)
66175	1(2)
66179	1(2)
66180	1(2)
66183	1(3)
66184	1(2)
66185	1(2)
66225	1(2)
66250	1(2)
66500	1(2)
66505	1(2)
66600	1(2)
66605	1(2)
66625	1(2)
66630	1(2)
66635	1(2)
66680	1(2)
66682	1(2)
66700	1(2)
66710	1(2)
66711	1(2)
66720	1(2)
66740	1(2)
66761	1(2)
66762	1(2)
66770	1(3)
66820	1(2)

CPT	MUE
66821	1(2)
66825	1(2)
66830	1(2)
66840	1(2)
66850	1(2)
66852	1(2)
66920	1(2)
66930	1(2)
66940	1(2)
66982	1(2)
66983	1(2)
66984	1(2)
66985	1(2)
66986	1(2)
66987	2(2)
66988	2(2)
66990	1(3)
66999	1(3)
67005	1(2)
67010	1(2)
67015	1(2)
67025	1(2)
67027	1(2)
67028	1(3)
67030	1(2)
67031	1(2)
67036	1(2)
67039	1(2)
67040	1(2)
67041	1(2)
67042	1(2)
67043	1(2)
67101	1(2)
67105	1(2)
67107	1(2)
67108	1(2)
67110	1(2)
67113	1(2)
67115	1(2)
67120	1(2)
67121	1(2)
67141	1(2)
67145	1(2)
67208	1(2)
67210	1(2)
67218	1(2)
67220	1(2)
67221	1(2)
67225	1(2)
67227	1(2)
67228	1(2)
67229	1(2)
67250	1(2)
67255	1(2)
67299	1(3)
67311	1(2)
67312	1(2)
67314	1(2)
67316	1(2)
67318	1(2)
67320	2(3)
67331	1(2)
67332	1(2)
67334	1(2)
67335	1(2)
67340	2(2)

CPT	MUE
67343	1(2)
67345	1(3)
67346	1(3)
67399	1(3)
67400	1(2)
67405	1(2)
67412	1(2)
67413	1(2)
67414	1(2)
67415	1(3)
67420	1(2)
67430	1(2)
67440	1(2)
67445	1(2)
67450	1(2)
67500	1(3)
67505	1(3)
67515	1(3)
67550	1(2)
67560	1(2)
67570	1(2)
67599	1(3)
67700	2(3)
67710	1(2)
67715	1(3)
67800	1(2)
67801	1(2)
67805	1(2)
67808	1(2)
67810	2(3)
67820	1(2)
67825	1(2)
67830	1(2)
67835	1(2)
67840	3(3)
67850	3(3)
67875	1(2)
67880	1(2)
67882	1(2)
67900	1(2)
67901	1(2)
67902	1(2)
67903	1(2)
67904	1(2)
67906	1(2)
67908	1(2)
67909	1(2)
67911	2(3)
67912	1(2)
67914	2(3)
67915	2(3)
67916	2(3)
67917	2(3)
67921	2(3)
67922	2(3)
67923	2(3)
67924	2(3)
67930	2(3)
67935	2(3)
67938	2(3)
67950	2(2)
67961	2(3)
67966	2(3)
67971	1(2)
67973	1(2)
67974	1(2)
67975	1(2)
67999	1(3)
68020	1(3)
68040	1(2)
68100	1(3)
68110	1(3)
68115	1(3)
68130	1(3)
68135	1(3)
68200	1(3)
68320	1(2)
68325	1(2)
68326	1(2)
68328	1(2)
68330	1(3)
68335	1(3)
68340	1(3)
68360	1(3)
68362	1(3)
68371	1(3)
68399	1(3)
68400	1(2)
68420	1(2)
68440	2(3)
68500	1(2)
68505	1(2)
68510	1(2)
68520	1(2)
68525	1(2)
68530	1(2)
68540	1(2)
68550	1(2)
68700	1(2)
68705	2(3)
68720	1(2)
68745	1(2)
68750	1(2)
68760	4(2)
68761	4(2)
68770	1(3)
68801	4(2)
68810	1(2)
68811	1(2)
68815	1(2)
68816	1(2)
68840	1(2)
68850	1(3)
68899	1(3)
69000	1(3)
69005	1(3)
69020	1(3)
69090	0(3)
69100	3(3)
69105	1(3)
69110	1(2)
69120	1(3)
69140	1(2)
69145	1(3)
69150	1(3)
69155	1(3)
69200	1(2)
69205	1(3)
69209	1(2)
69210	1(2)
69220	1(2)
69222	1(2)
69300	1(2)
69310	1(2)
69320	1(2)
69399	1(3)
69420	1(2)
69421	1(2)
69424	1(2)
69433	1(2)
69436	1(2)
69440	1(2)
69450	1(2)
69501	1(3)
69502	1(2)
69505	1(2)
69511	1(2)
69530	1(2)
69535	1(2)
69540	1(3)
69550	1(3)
69552	1(2)
69554	1(2)
69601	1(2)
69602	1(2)
69603	1(2)
69604	1(2)
69610	1(2)
69620	1(2)
69631	1(2)
69632	1(3)
69633	1(2)
69635	1(3)
69636	1(3)
69637	1(3)
69641	1(2)
69642	1(2)
69643	1(2)
69644	1(2)
69645	1(2)
69646	1(2)
69650	1(2)
69660	1(2)
69661	1(2)
69662	1(2)
69666	1(2)
69667	1(2)
69670	1(2)
69676	1(2)
69700	1(3)
69705	1(2)
69706	1(2)
69710	0(3)
69711	1(2)
69714	1(2)
69715	1(3)
69717	1(2)
69718	1(2)
69720	1(2)
69725	1(2)
69740	1(2)
69745	1(2)
69799	1(3)
69801	1(3)
69805	1(3)
69806	1(3)
69905	1(2)
69910	1(2)
69915	1(3)
69930	1(2)
69949	1(3)
69950	1(2)
69955	1(2)
69960	1(2)
69970	1(3)
69979	1(3)
69990	1(3)
70010	1(3)
70015	1(3)
70030	2(2)
70100	2(3)
70110	2(3)
70120	1(3)
70130	1(3)
70134	1(3)
70140	2(3)
70150	1(3)
70160	1(3)
70170	2(2)
70190	1(2)
70200	2(3)
70210	1(3)
70220	1(3)
70240	1(2)
70250	2(3)
70260	1(3)
70300	1(3)
70310	1(3)
70320	1(3)
70328	1(3)
70330	1(3)
70332	2(3)
70336	1(3)
70350	1(3)
70355	1(3)
70360	2(3)
70370	1(3)
70371	1(2)
70380	2(3)
70390	2(3)
70450	3(3)
70460	1(3)
70470	2(3)
70480	1(3)
70481	1(3)
70482	1(3)
70486	1(3)
70487	1(3)
70488	1(3)
70490	1(3)
70491	1(3)
70492	1(3)
70496	2(3)
70498	2(3)
70540	1(3)
70542	1(3)
70543	1(3)
70544	2(3)
70545	1(3)
70546	1(3)
70547	1(3)
70548	1(3)
70549	1(3)
70551	2(3)
70552	2(3)
70553	2(3)
70554	1(3)
70555	1(3)
70557	1(3)
70558	1(3)
70559	1(3)
71045	4(3)
71046	2(3)
71047	1(3)
71048	1(3)
71100	2(3)
71101	2(3)
71110	1(3)
71111	1(3)
71120	1(3)
71130	1(3)
71250	2(3)
71260	2(3)
71270	1(3)
71271	1(2)
71275	1(3)
71550	1(3)
71551	1(3)
71552	1(3)
71555	1(3)
72020	4(3)
72040	3(3)
72050	1(3)
72052	1(3)
72070	1(3)
72072	1(3)
72074	1(3)
72080	1(3)
72081	1(3)
72082	1(3)
72083	1(3)
72084	1(3)
72100	2(3)
72110	1(3)
72114	1(3)
72120	1(3)
72125	1(3)
72126	1(3)
72127	1(3)
72128	1(3)
72129	1(3)
72130	1(3)
72131	1(3)
72132	1(3)
72133	1(3)
72141	1(3)
72142	1(3)
72146	1(3)
72147	1(3)
72148	1(3)
72149	1(3)
72156	1(3)
72157	1(3)
72158	1(3)
72159	1(3)
72170	2(3)
72190	1(3)
72191	1(3)
72192	1(3)
72193	1(3)
72194	1(3)
72195	1(3)
72196	1(3)
72197	1(3)
72198	1(3)
72200	2(3)
72202	1(3)
72220	1(3)
72240	1(2)
72255	1(2)
72265	1(2)
72270	1(2)
72275	1(3)
72285	4(3)
72295	5(3)
73000	2(3)
73010	2(3)
73020	2(3)
73030	4(3)
73040	2(2)
73050	1(3)
73060	2(3)
73070	2(3)
73080	2(3)
73085	2(2)
73090	2(3)
73092	2(3)
73100	2(3)
73110	3(3)
73115	2(2)
73120	2(3)
73130	3(3)
73140	3(3)
73200	2(3)
73201	2(3)
73202	2(3)
73206	2(3)
73218	2(3)
73219	2(3)
73220	2(3)
73221	2(3)
73222	2(3)
73223	2(3)
73225	2(3)
73501	2(3)
73502	2(3)
73503	2(3)
73521	2(3)
73522	2(3)
73523	2(3)
73525	2(2)
73551	2(3)
73552	2(3)
73560	4(3)
73562	3(3)
73564	4(3)
73565	1(3)
73580	2(2)
73590	3(3)
73592	2(3)
73600	2(3)
73610	3(3)
73615	2(2)
73620	2(3)
73630	3(3)
73650	2(3)
73660	2(3)
73700	2(3)
73701	2(3)
73702	2(3)
73706	2(3)
73718	2(3)
73719	2(3)
73720	2(3)
73721	3(3)
73722	2(3)
73723	2(3)
73725	2(3)
74018	3(3)
74019	2(3)
74021	2(3)
74022	2(3)
74150	1(3)
74160	1(3)
74170	1(3)
74174	1(3)
74175	1(3)
74176	2(3)
74177	2(3)
74178	1(3)
74181	1(3)
74182	1(3)
74183	1(3)
74185	1(3)
74190	1(3)
74210	1(3)
74220	1(3)
74221	1(3)
74230	1(3)
74235	1(3)
74240	2(3)
74246	1(3)
74248	1(2)
74250	1(3)
74251	1(3)
74261	1(2)
74262	1(2)
74263	0(3)
74270	1(3)
74280	1(3)
74283	1(3)
74290	1(3)
74300	1(3)
74301	1(3)
74328	1(3)
74329	1(3)
74330	1(3)
74340	1(3)
74355	1(3)
74360	1(3)
74363	2(3)
74400	1(3)
74410	1(3)
74415	1(3)
74420	2(3)
74425	2(3)
74430	1(3)
74440	1(2)
74445	1(2)
74450	1(3)
74455	1(3)
74470	2(2)
74485	2(3)
74710	1(3)
74712	1(3)
74713	2(3)
74740	1(3)
74742	2(2)
74775	1(2)
75557	1(3)
75559	1(3)
75561	1(3)
75563	1(3)
75565	1(3)
75571	1(3)
75572	1(3)
75573	1(3)
75574	1(3)
75600	1(3)
75605	1(3)
75625	1(3)
75630	1(3)
75635	1(3)
75705	20(3)
75710	2(3)
75716	1(3)
75726	3(3)
75731	1(3)
75733	1(3)
75736	2(3)
75741	1(3)
75743	1(3)
75746	1(3)
75756	2(3)
75774	7(3)
75801	1(3)
75803	1(3)
75805	1(2)
75807	1(2)
75809	1(3)
75810	1(3)
75820	2(3)
75822	1(3)
75825	1(3)
75827	1(3)
75831	1(3)
75833	1(3)
75840	1(3)
75842	1(3)
75860	2(3)
75870	1(3)
75872	1(3)
75880	1(3)
75885	1(3)
75887	1(3)
75889	1(3)
75891	1(3)
75893	2(3)
75894	2(3)
75898	2(3)
75901	1(3)
75902	2(3)
75956	1(2)
75957	1(2)
75958	2(3)
75959	1(2)
75970	1(3)
75984	2(3)

CPT	MUE	CPT	MUE	CPT	MUE	CPT	MUE	CPT	MUE	CPT	MUE	CPT	MUE	CPT	MUE
75989	2(3)	76873	1(2)	77299	1(3)	78020	1(3)	78466	1(3)	80047	2(3)	80307	1(2)	80415	1(3)
76000	3(3)	76881	2(3)	77300	10(3)	78070	1(2)	78468	1(3)	80048	2(3)	80320	1(3)	80416	1(3)
76010	2(3)	76882	2(3)	77301	1(3)	78071	1(3)	78469	1(3)	80050	0(3)	80321	1(3)	80417	1(3)
76080	3(3)	76885	1(2)	77306	1(3)	78072	1(3)	78472	1(2)	80051	2(3)	80322	1(3)	80418	1(3)
76098	3(3)	76886	1(2)	77307	1(3)	78075	1(2)	78473	1(2)	80053	1(3)	80323	1(3)	80420	1(2)
76100	2(3)	76932	1(2)	77316	1(3)	78099	1(3)	78481	1(2)	80055	1(3)	80324	1(3)	80422	1(3)
76101	1(3)	76936	1(3)	77317	1(3)	78102	1(2)	78483	1(2)	80061	1(3)	80325	1(3)	80424	1(3)
76102	1(3)	76937	2(3)	77318	1(3)	78103	1(2)	78491	1(3)	80069	1(3)	80326	1(3)	80426	1(3)
76120	1(3)	76940	1(3)	77321	1(2)	78104	1(2)	78492	1(2)	80074	1(2)	80327	1(3)	80428	1(3)
76125	1(3)	76941	3(3)	77331	3(3)	78110	1(2)	78494	1(3)	80076	1(3)	80328	1(3)	80430	1(3)
76140	0(3)	76942	1(3)	77332	4(3)	78111	1(2)	78496	1(3)	80081	1(2)	80329	1(3)	80432	1(3)
76145	1(2)	76945	1(3)	77333	2(3)	78120	1(2)	78499	1(3)	80143	2(3)	80330	1(3)	80434	1(3)
76376	2(3)	76946	1(3)	77334	10(3)	78121	1(2)	78579	1(3)	80145	1(3)	80331	1(3)	80435	1(3)
76377	2(3)	76948	1(2)	77336	1(2)	78122	1(2)	78580	1(3)	80150	2(3)	80332	1(3)	80436	1(3)
76380	2(3)	76965	2(3)	77338	1(3)	78130	1(2)	78582	1(3)	80151	1(3)	80333	1(3)	80438	1(3)
76390	1(3)	76975	1(3)	77370	1(3)	78140	1(3)	78597	1(3)	80155	1(3)	80334	1(3)	80439	1(3)
76391	1(3)	76977	1(2)	77371	1(2)	78185	1(2)	78598	1(3)	80156	2(3)	80335	1(3)	80500	1(3)
76496	1(3)	76978	1(2)	77372	1(2)	78191	1(2)	78599	1(3)	80157	2(3)	80336	1(3)	80502	1(3)
76497	1(3)	76979	3(3)	77373	1(3)	78195	1(2)	78600	1(3)	80158	1(3)	80337	1(3)	81000	2(3)
76498	1(3)	76981	1(3)	77385	1(3)	78199	1(3)	78601	1(3)	80159	2(3)	80338	1(3)	81001	2(3)
76499	1(3)	76982	1(2)	77386	1(3)	78201	1(3)	78605	1(3)	80161	1(3)	80339	1(3)	81002	2(3)
76506	1(2)	76983	2(3)	77387	1(3)	78202	1(3)	78606	1(3)	80162	2(3)	80340	1(3)	81003	2(3)
76510	2(2)	76998	1(3)	77399	1(3)	78215	1(3)	78608	1(3)	80163	1(3)	80341	1(3)	81005	2(3)
76511	2(2)	76999	1(3)	77401	1(2)	78216	1(3)	78609	0(3)	80164	2(3)	80342	1(3)	81007	1(3)
76512	2(2)	77001	2(3)	77402	2(3)	78226	1(3)	78610	1(3)	80165	1(3)	80343	1(3)	81015	2(3)
76513	1(2)	77002	1(3)	77407	2(3)	78227	1(3)	78630	1(3)	80167	1(3)	80344	1(3)	81020	1(3)
76514	1(2)	77003	1(3)	77412	2(3)	78230	1(3)	78635	1(3)	80168	2(3)	80345	1(3)	81025	1(3)
76516	1(2)	77011	1(3)	77417	1(2)	78231	1(3)	78645	1(3)	80169	1(3)	80346	1(3)	81050	2(3)
76519	2(2)	77012	1(3)	77423	1(3)	78232	1(3)	78650	1(3)	80170	2(3)	80347	1(3)	81099	1(3)
76529	2(2)	77013	1(3)	77424	1(2)	78258	1(2)	78660	1(2)	80171	1(3)	80348	1(3)	81105	1(2)
76536	1(3)	77014	2(3)	77425	1(3)	78261	1(2)	78699	1(3)	80173	2(3)	80349	1(3)	81106	1(2)
76604	1(3)	77021	1(3)	77427	1(2)	78262	1(2)	78700	1(3)	80175	1(3)	80350	1(3)	81107	1(2)
76641	2(2)	77022	1(3)	77431	1(2)	78264	1(2)	78701	1(3)	80176	1(3)	80351	1(3)	81108	1(2)
76642	2(2)	77046	1(2)	77432	1(2)	78265	1(2)	78707	1(2)	80177	1(3)	80352	1(3)	81109	1(2)
76700	1(3)	77047	1(2)	77435	1(2)	78266	1(2)	78708	1(2)	80178	2(3)	80353	1(3)	81110	1(2)
76705	2(3)	77048	1(2)	77469	1(2)	78267	1(2)	78709	1(2)	80179	2(3)	80354	1(3)	81111	1(2)
76706	1(2)	77049	1(2)	77470	1(2)	78268	1(2)	78725	1(3)	80180	1(3)	80355	1(3)	81112	1(2)
76770	1(3)	77053	2(2)	77499	1(3)	78278	2(3)	78730	1(2)	80181	1(3)	80356	1(3)	81120	1(3)
76775	2(3)	77054	2(2)	77520	1(3)	78282	1(2)	78740	1(2)	80183	1(3)	80357	1(3)	81121	1(3)
76776	2(3)	77061	1(2)	77522	1(3)	78290	1(3)	78761	1(2)	80184	2(3)	80358	1(3)	81161	1(3)
76800	1(3)	77062	1(2)	77523	1(3)	78291	1(3)	78799	1(3)	80185	2(3)	80359	1(3)	81162	1(2)
76801	1(2)	77063	1(2)	77525	1(3)	78299	1(3)	78800	1(2)	80186	2(3)	80360	1(3)	81163	1(2)
76802	2(3)	77065	1(2)	77600	1(3)	78300	1(2)	78801	1(2)	80187	1(3)	80361	1(3)	81164	1(2)
76805	1(2)	77066	1(2)	77605	1(3)	78305	1(2)	78802	1(2)	80188	2(3)	80362	1(3)	81165	1(2)
76810	2(3)	77067	1(2)	77610	1(3)	78306	1(2)	78803	1(2)	80189	1(3)	80363	1(3)	81166	1(2)
76811	1(2)	77071	1(3)	77615	1(3)	78315	1(2)	78804	1(2)	80190	2(3)	80364	1(3)	81167	1(2)
76812	2(3)	77072	1(2)	77620	1(3)	78350	0(3)	78808	1(2)	80192	2(3)	80365	1(3)	81168	1(3)
76813	1(2)	77073	1(2)	77750	1(3)	78351	0(3)	78811	1(2)	80193	1(3)	80366	1(3)	81170	1(2)
76814	2(3)	77074	1(2)	77761	1(3)	78399	1(3)	78812	1(2)	80194	2(3)	80367	1(3)	81171	1(2)
76815	1(2)	77075	1(2)	77762	1(3)	78414	1(2)	78813	1(2)	80195	2(3)	80368	1(3)	81172	1(2)
76816	2(3)	77076	1(2)	77763	1(3)	78428	1(3)	78814	1(2)	80197	2(3)	80369	1(3)	81173	1(2)
76817	1(3)	77077	1(2)	77767	2(3)	78429	1(2)	78815	1(2)	80198	2(3)	80370	1(3)	81174	1(2)
76818	2(3)	77078	1(2)	77768	2(3)	78430	1(2)	78816	1(2)	80199	1(3)	80371	1(3)	81175	1(3)
76819	2(3)	77080	1(2)	77770	2(3)	78431	1(2)	78830	1(2)	80200	2(3)	80372	1(3)	81176	1(3)
76820	3(3)	77081	1(2)	77771	2(3)	78432	1(2)	78831	1(2)	80201	2(3)	80373	1(3)	81177	1(2)
76821	2(3)	77084	1(2)	77772	2(3)	78433	1(2)	78832	1(2)	80202	2(3)	80374	1(3)	81178	1(2)
76825	2(3)	77085	1(2)	77778	1(3)	78434	1(2)	78835	4(3)	80203	1(3)	80375	1(3)	81179	1(2)
76826	2(3)	77086	1(2)	77789	2(3)	78445	1(3)	78999	1(3)	80204	1(3)	80376	1(3)	81180	1(2)
76827	2(3)	77261	1(3)	77790	1(3)	78451	1(2)	79005	1(3)	80210	1(3)	80377	1(3)	81181	1(2)
76828	2(3)	77262	1(3)	77799	1(3)	78452	1(2)	79101	1(3)	80230	1(3)	80400	1(3)	81182	1(2)
76830	1(3)	77263	1(3)	78012	1(3)	78453	1(2)	79200	1(3)	80235	1(3)	80402	1(3)	81183	1(2)
76831	1(3)	77280	2(3)	78013	1(3)	78454	1(2)	79300	1(3)	80280	1(3)	80406	1(3)	81184	1(2)
76856	1(3)	77285	1(3)	78014	1(2)	78456	1(3)	79403	1(3)	80285	1(3)	80408	1(3)	81185	1(2)
76857	1(3)	77290	1(3)	78015	1(3)	78457	1(2)	79440	1(3)	80299	3(3)	80410	1(3)	81186	1(2)
76870	1(2)	77293	1(3)	78016	1(3)	78458	1(2)	79445	1(3)	80305	1(2)	80412	1(3)	81187	1(2)
76872	1(3)	77295	1(3)	78018	1(2)	78459	1(3)	79999	1(3)	80306	1(2)	80414	1(3)	81188	1(2)

CPT	MUE	CPT	MUE	CPT	MUE	CPT	MUE	CPT	MUE	CPT	MUE	CPT	MUE	CPT	MUE
81189	1(2)	81263	1(3)	81332	1(3)	81431	1(2)	82043	1(3)	82390	1(2)	82760	1(3)	83505	1(3)
81190	1(2)	81264	1(3)	81333	1(2)	81432	1(2)	82044	1(3)	82397	3(3)	82775	1(3)	83516	4(3)
81191	1(3)	81265	1(3)	81334	1(3)	81433	1(2)	82045	1(3)	82415	1(3)	82776	1(2)	83518	1(3)
81192	1(3)	81266	2(3)	81335	1(2)	81434	1(2)	82075	2(3)	82435	1(3)	82777	1(3)	83519	5(3)
81193	1(3)	81267	1(3)	81336	1(2)	81435	1(2)	82077	1(3)	82436	1(3)	82784	6(3)	83520	9(3)
81194	1(3)	81268	4(3)	81337	1(2)	81436	1(2)	82085	1(3)	82438	1(3)	82785	1(3)	83525	4(3)
81200	1(2)	81269	1(2)	81338	1(3)	81437	1(2)	82088	2(3)	82441	1(2)	82787	4(3)	83527	1(3)
81201	1(2)	81270	1(2)	81339	1(2)	81438	1(2)	82103	1(3)	82465	1(3)	82800	1(3)	83528	1(3)
81202	1(3)	81271	1(2)	81340	1(3)	81439	1(2)	82104	1(2)	82480	2(3)	82803	2(3)	83540	2(3)
81203	1(3)	81272	1(3)	81341	1(3)	81440	1(2)	82105	1(3)	82482	1(3)	82805	2(3)	83550	1(3)
81204	1(2)	81273	1(3)	81342	1(3)	81442	1(2)	82106	2(3)	82485	1(3)	82810	2(3)	83570	1(3)
81205	1(3)	81274	1(2)	81343	1(2)	81443	1(2)	82107	1(3)	82495	1(2)	82820	1(3)	83582	1(3)
81206	1(3)	81275	1(3)	81344	1(2)	81445	1(2)	82108	1(3)	82507	1(3)	82930	1(3)	83586	1(3)
81207	1(3)	81276	1(3)	81345	1(3)	81448	1(2)	82120	1(3)	82523	1(3)	82938	1(3)	83593	1(3)
81208	1(3)	81277	1(2)	81346	1(2)	81450	1(2)	82127	1(3)	82525	2(3)	82941	1(3)	83605	1(3)
81209	1(3)	81278	1(3)	81347	1(2)	81455	1(2)	82128	2(3)	82528	1(3)	82943	1(3)	83615	2(3)
81210	1(3)	81279	1(2)	81348	1(2)	81460	1(2)	82131	2(3)	82530	4(3)	82945	4(3)	83625	1(3)
81212	1(2)	81283	1(2)	81350	1(3)	81465	1(2)	82135	1(3)	82533	5(3)	82946	1(2)	83630	1(3)
81215	1(2)	81284	1(2)	81351	1(2)	81470	1(2)	82136	2(3)	82540	1(3)	82947	5(3)	83631	1(3)
81216	1(2)	81285	1(2)	81352	1(2)	81471	1(2)	82139	2(3)	82542	6(3)	82948	2(3)	83632	1(3)
81217	1(2)	81286	1(2)	81353	1(2)	81479	3(3)	82140	2(3)	82550	3(3)	82950	3(3)	83633	1(3)
81218	1(3)	81287	1(3)	81355	1(3)	81490	1(2)	82143	2(3)	82552	3(3)	82951	1(2)	83655	2(3)
81219	1(3)	81288	1(3)	81357	1(2)	81493	1(2)	82150	2(3)	82553	3(3)	82952	3(3)	83661	3(3)
81220	1(3)	81289	1(2)	81360	1(2)	81500	1(2)	82154	1(3)	82554	1(3)	82955	1(2)	83662	4(3)
81221	1(3)	81290	1(3)	81361	1(2)	81503	1(2)	82157	1(3)	82565	2(3)	82960	1(2)	83663	3(3)
81222	1(3)	81291	1(3)	81362	1(2)	81504	1(2)	82160	1(3)	82570	3(3)	82962	2(3)	83664	3(3)
81223	1(2)	81292	1(2)	81363	1(2)	81506	1(2)	82163	1(3)	82575	1(3)	82963	1(3)	83670	1(3)
81224	1(3)	81293	1(3)	81364	1(2)	81507	1(2)	82164	1(3)	82585	1(2)	82965	1(3)	83690	2(3)
81225	1(3)	81294	1(3)	81370	1(2)	81508	1(2)	82172	2(3)	82595	1(3)	82977	1(3)	83695	1(3)
81226	1(3)	81295	1(2)	81371	1(2)	81509	1(2)	82175	2(3)	82600	1(3)	82978	1(3)	83698	1(3)
81227	1(3)	81296	1(3)	81372	1(2)	81510	1(2)	82180	1(2)	82607	1(2)	82979	1(3)	83700	1(2)
81228	1(3)	81297	1(3)	81373	2(2)	81511	1(2)	82190	2(3)	82608	1(2)	82985	1(3)	83701	1(3)
81229	1(3)	81298	1(2)	81374	1(3)	81512	1(2)	82232	2(3)	82610	1(3)	83001	1(3)	83704	1(3)
81230	1(2)	81299	1(3)	81375	1(2)	81513	1(2)	82239	1(3)	82615	1(3)	83002	1(3)	83718	1(3)
81231	1(2)	81300	1(3)	81376	5(3)	81514	1(2)	82240	1(3)	82626	1(3)	83003	5(3)	83719	1(3)
81232	1(2)	81301	1(3)	81377	2(3)	81518	1(2)	82247	2(3)	82627	1(3)	83006	1(2)	83721	1(3)
81233	1(3)	81302	1(3)	81378	1(2)	81519	1(2)	82248	2(3)	82633	1(3)	83009	1(3)	83722	1(2)
81234	1(2)	81303	1(3)	81379	1(2)	81520	1(2)	82252	1(3)	82634	1(3)	83010	1(3)	83727	1(3)
81235	1(3)	81304	1(3)	81380	2(2)	81521	1(2)	82261	1(3)	82638	1(3)	83012	1(2)	83735	4(3)
81236	1(3)	81305	1(3)	81381	3(3)	81522	1(2)	82270	1(3)	82642	1(2)	83013	1(3)	83775	1(3)
81237	1(3)	81306	1(2)	81382	6(3)	81525	1(2)	82271	1(3)	82652	1(2)	83014	1(2)	83785	1(3)
81238	1(2)	81307	1(2)	81383	2(3)	81528	1(2)	82272	1(3)	82656	1(3)	83015	1(2)	83789	4(3)
81239	1(2)	81308	1(2)	81400	2(3)	81529	1(2)	82274	1(3)	82657	2(3)	83018	4(3)	83825	2(3)
81240	1(2)	81309	1(2)	81401	2(3)	81535	1(2)	82286	1(3)	82658	2(3)	83020	2(3)	83835	2(3)
81241	1(2)	81310	1(3)	81402	1(3)	81536	11(3)	82300	1(3)	82664	2(3)	83021	2(3)	83857	1(3)
81242	1(3)	81311	1(3)	81403	4(3)	81538	1(2)	82306	1(2)	82668	1(3)	83026	1(3)	83861	2(2)
81243	1(3)	81312	1(2)	81404	5(3)	81539	1(2)	82308	1(3)	82670	1(3)	83030	1(3)	83864	1(2)
81244	1(3)	81313	1(3)	81405	2(3)	81540	1(2)	82310	2(3)	82671	1(3)	83033	1(3)	83872	2(3)
81245	1(3)	81314	1(3)	81406	2(3)	81541	1(2)	82330	2(3)	82672	1(3)	83036	1(2)	83873	1(3)
81246	1(3)	81315	1(3)	81407	1(3)	81542	1(2)	82331	1(3)	82677	1(3)	83037	1(2)	83874	2(3)
81247	1(2)	81316	1(2)	81408	2(3)	81546	2(3)	82340	1(3)	82679	1(3)	83045	1(3)	83876	1(3)
81248	1(2)	81317	1(2)	81410	1(2)	81551	1(2)	82355	2(3)	82681	1(3)	83050	1(3)	83880	1(3)
81249	1(2)	81318	1(3)	81411	1(2)	81552	1(2)	82360	2(3)	82693	2(3)	83051	1(3)	83883	4(3)
81250	1(3)	81319	1(2)	81412	1(2)	81554	1(2)	82365	2(3)	82696	1(3)	83060	1(3)	83885	2(3)
81251	1(3)	81320	1(3)	81413	1(2)	81595	1(2)	82370	2(3)	82705	1(3)	83065	1(2)	83915	1(3)
81252	1(3)	81321	1(3)	81414	1(2)	81596	1(2)	82373	1(3)	82710	1(3)	83068	1(2)	83916	2(3)
81253	1(3)	81322	1(3)	81415	1(2)	81599	1(3)	82374	1(3)	82715	3(3)	83069	1(3)	83918	2(3)
81254	1(3)	81323	1(3)	81416	2(3)	82009	1(3)	82375	1(3)	82725	1(3)	83070	1(2)	83919	1(3)
81255	1(3)	81324	1(3)	81417	1(3)	82010	1(3)	82376	1(3)	82726	1(3)	83080	2(3)	83921	2(3)
81256	1(2)	81325	1(3)	81419	1(2)	82013	1(3)	82378	1(3)	82728	1(3)	83088	1(3)	83930	2(3)
81257	1(2)	81326	1(3)	81420	1(2)	82016	1(3)	82379	1(3)	82731	1(3)	83090	2(3)	83935	2(3)
81258	1(2)	81327	1(2)	81422	1(2)	82017	1(3)	82380	1(3)	82735	1(3)	83150	1(3)	83937	1(3)
81259	1(2)	81328	1(2)	81425	1(2)	82024	4(3)	82382	1(2)	82746	1(2)	83491	1(3)	83945	2(3)
81260	1(3)	81329	1(2)	81426	2(3)	82030	1(3)	82383	1(3)	82747	1(2)	83497	1(3)	83950	1(2)
81261	1(3)	81330	1(3)	81427	1(3)	82040	1(3)	82384	2(3)	82757	1(2)	83498	2(3)	83951	1(2)
81262	1(3)	81331	1(3)	81430	1(2)	82042	2(3)	82387	1(3)	82759	1(3)	83500	1(3)	83970	2(3)

CPT	MUE
83986	2(3)
83987	1(3)
83992	2(3)
83993	1(3)
84030	1(2)
84035	1(2)
84060	1(3)
84066	1(3)
84075	2(3)
84078	1(2)
84080	1(3)
84081	1(3)
84085	1(2)
84087	1(3)
84100	2(3)
84105	1(3)
84106	1(2)
84110	1(3)
84112	1(3)
84119	1(2)
84120	1(3)
84126	1(3)
84132	2(3)
84133	2(3)
84134	1(3)
84135	1(3)
84138	1(3)
84140	1(3)
84143	2(3)
84144	1(3)
84145	1(3)
84146	3(3)
84150	2(3)
84152	1(2)
84153	1(2)
84154	1(2)
84155	1(3)
84156	1(3)
84157	2(3)
84160	2(3)
84163	1(3)
84165	1(2)
84166	2(3)
84181	3(3)
84182	6(3)
84202	1(2)
84203	1(2)
84206	1(2)
84207	1(2)
84210	1(3)
84220	1(3)
84228	1(3)
84233	1(3)
84234	1(3)
84235	1(3)
84238	3(3)
84244	2(3)
84252	1(2)
84255	2(3)
84260	1(3)
84270	1(3)
84275	1(3)
84285	1(3)
84295	1(3)
84300	2(3)
84302	1(3)

CPT	MUE
84305	1(3)
84307	1(3)
84311	2(3)
84315	1(3)
84375	1(3)
84376	1(3)
84377	1(3)
84378	2(3)
84379	1(3)
84392	1(3)
84402	1(3)
84403	2(3)
84410	1(2)
84425	1(2)
84430	1(3)
84431	1(3)
84432	1(2)
84436	1(2)
84437	1(2)
84439	1(2)
84442	1(2)
84443	4(2)
84445	1(2)
84446	1(2)
84449	1(3)
84450	1(3)
84460	1(3)
84466	1(3)
84478	1(3)
84479	1(2)
84480	1(2)
84481	1(2)
84482	1(2)
84484	2(3)
84485	1(3)
84488	1(3)
84490	1(2)
84510	1(3)
84512	1(3)
84520	1(3)
84525	1(3)
84540	2(3)
84545	1(3)
84550	1(3)
84560	2(3)
84577	1(3)
84578	1(3)
84580	1(3)
84583	1(3)
84585	1(2)
84586	1(2)
84588	1(3)
84590	1(2)
84591	1(3)
84597	1(3)
84600	2(3)
84620	1(2)
84630	2(3)
84681	1(3)
84702	2(3)
84703	1(3)
84704	1(3)
84830	1(2)
84999	1(3)
85002	1(3)
85004	1(3)

CPT	MUE
85007	1(3)
85008	1(3)
85009	1(3)
85013	1(3)
85014	2(3)
85018	2(3)
85025	2(3)
85027	2(3)
85032	1(3)
85041	1(3)
85044	1(2)
85045	1(2)
85046	1(2)
85048	2(3)
85049	2(3)
85055	1(3)
85060	1(3)
85097	2(3)
85130	1(3)
85170	1(3)
85175	1(3)
85210	2(3)
85220	2(3)
85230	2(3)
85240	2(3)
85244	1(3)
85245	2(3)
85246	2(3)
85247	2(3)
85250	2(3)
85260	2(3)
85270	2(3)
85280	2(3)
85290	2(3)
85291	1(3)
85292	1(3)
85293	1(3)
85300	2(3)
85301	1(3)
85302	1(3)
85303	2(3)
85305	2(3)
85306	2(3)
85307	2(3)
85335	2(3)
85337	1(3)
85345	1(3)
85347	3(3)
85348	1(3)
85360	1(3)
85362	2(3)
85366	1(3)
85370	1(3)
85378	1(3)
85379	2(3)
85380	1(3)
85384	2(3)
85385	1(3)
85390	3(3)
85396	1(2)
85397	2(3)
85400	1(3)
85410	1(3)
85415	2(3)
85420	2(3)
85421	1(3)

CPT	MUE
85441	1(2)
85445	1(2)
85460	1(3)
85461	1(2)
85475	1(3)
85520	1(3)
85525	2(3)
85530	1(3)
85536	1(2)
85540	1(2)
85547	1(2)
85549	1(3)
85555	1(2)
85557	1(2)
85576	7(3)
85597	1(3)
85598	1(3)
85610	4(3)
85611	2(3)
85612	1(3)
85613	3(3)
85635	1(3)
85651	1(2)
85652	1(2)
85660	2(3)
85670	2(3)
85675	1(3)
85705	1(3)
85730	4(3)
85732	4(3)
85810	2(3)
85999	1(3)
86000	6(3)
86001	20(3)
86005	2(3)
86008	20(3)
86021	1(2)
86022	1(2)
86023	3(3)
86038	1(3)
86039	1(3)
86060	1(3)
86063	1(3)
86077	1(2)
86078	1(3)
86079	1(3)
86140	1(2)
86141	1(2)
86146	3(3)
86147	4(3)
86148	3(3)
86152	1(3)
86153	1(3)
86155	1(3)
86156	1(2)
86157	1(2)
86160	4(3)
86161	2(3)
86162	1(2)
86171	2(3)
86200	1(3)
86215	1(3)
86225	1(3)
86226	1(3)
86235	10(3)
86255	5(3)

CPT	MUE
86256	9(3)
86277	1(3)
86280	1(3)
86294	1(3)
86300	2(3)
86301	1(2)
86304	1(2)
86305	1(2)
86308	1(2)
86309	1(2)
86310	1(2)
86316	2(3)
86317	6(3)
86318	2(3)
86320	1(2)
86325	2(3)
86327	1(3)
86328	3(3)
86329	3(3)
86331	12(3)
86332	1(3)
86334	2(2)
86335	2(3)
86336	1(3)
86337	1(2)
86340	1(2)
86341	4(3)
86343	1(3)
86344	1(2)
86352	1(3)
86353	7(3)
86355	1(2)
86356	7(3)
86357	1(2)
86359	1(2)
86360	1(2)
86361	1(2)
86367	1(3)
86376	2(3)
86382	3(3)
86384	1(3)
86386	1(2)
86403	2(3)
86406	2(3)
86408	1(3)
86409	1(3)
86413	3(3)
86430	2(3)
86431	2(3)
86480	1(3)
86481	1(3)
86485	1(2)
86486	2(3)
86490	1(2)
86510	1(2)
86580	1(2)
86590	1(3)
86592	2(3)
86593	2(3)
86602	3(3)
86603	2(3)
86609	14(3)
86611	4(3)
86612	2(3)
86615	6(3)
86617	2(3)

CPT	MUE
86618	2(3)
86619	2(3)
86622	2(3)
86625	1(3)
86628	3(3)
86631	6(3)
86632	3(3)
86635	4(3)
86638	6(3)
86641	2(3)
86644	2(3)
86645	1(3)
86648	2(3)
86651	2(3)
86652	2(3)
86653	2(3)
86654	2(3)
86658	12(3)
86663	2(3)
86664	2(3)
86665	2(3)
86666	4(3)
86668	2(3)
86671	3(3)
86674	3(3)
86677	3(3)
86682	2(3)
86684	2(3)
86687	1(3)
86688	1(3)
86689	2(3)
86692	2(3)
86694	2(3)
86695	2(3)
86696	2(3)
86698	3(3)
86701	1(3)
86702	2(3)
86703	1(2)
86704	1(2)
86705	1(2)
86706	2(3)
86707	1(3)
86708	1(2)
86709	1(2)
86710	4(3)
86711	2(3)
86713	3(3)
86717	8(3)
86720	2(3)
86723	2(3)
86727	2(3)
86732	2(3)
86735	2(3)
86738	2(3)
86741	2(3)
86744	2(3)
86747	2(3)
86750	4(3)
86753	3(3)
86756	2(3)
86757	6(3)
86759	2(3)
86762	2(3)
86765	2(3)
86768	5(3)

CPT	MUE
86769	3(3)
86771	2(3)
86774	2(3)
86777	2(3)
86778	2(3)
86780	2(3)
86784	1(3)
86787	2(3)
86788	2(3)
86789	2(3)
86790	4(3)
86793	2(3)
86794	1(3)
86800	1(3)
86803	1(3)
86804	1(2)
86805	2(3)
86806	2(3)
86807	2(3)
86808	1(3)
86812	1(2)
86813	1(2)
86816	1(2)
86817	1(2)
86821	1(3)
86825	1(3)
86826	2(3)
86828	1(3)
86829	1(3)
86830	2(3)
86831	2(3)
86832	2(3)
86833	1(3)
86834	1(3)
86835	1(3)
86849	1(3)
86850	3(3)
86860	2(3)
86870	2(3)
86880	4(3)
86885	2(3)
86886	3(3)
86890	1(3)
86891	1(3)
86900	1(3)
86901	1(3)
86902	6(3)
86904	2(3)
86905	8(3)
86906	1(2)
86910	0(3)
86911	0(3)
86920	9(3)
86921	2(3)
86922	5(3)
86923	10(3)
86927	2(3)
86930	0(3)
86931	1(3)
86932	1(3)
86940	1(3)
86941	1(3)
86945	2(3)
86950	1(3)
86960	1(3)
86965	1(3)

CPT	MUE
86970	1(3)
86971	1(3)
86972	1(3)
86975	1(3)
86976	1(3)
86977	1(3)
86978	1(3)
86985	1(3)
86999	1(3)
87003	1(3)
87015	3(3)
87040	2(3)
87045	3(3)
87046	6(3)
87070	3(3)
87071	2(3)
87073	2(3)
87075	6(3)
87076	2(3)
87077	4(3)
87081	2(3)
87084	1(3)
87086	3(3)
87088	3(3)
87101	2(3)
87102	4(3)
87103	2(3)
87106	3(3)
87107	4(3)
87109	2(3)
87110	2(3)
87116	2(3)
87118	3(3)
87140	3(3)
87143	2(3)
87149	4(3)
87150	12(3)
87152	1(3)
87153	3(3)
87158	1(3)
87164	2(3)
87166	2(3)
87168	2(3)
87169	2(3)
87172	1(3)
87176	2(3)
87177	3(3)
87181	12(3)
87184	8(3)
87185	4(3)
87186	12(3)
87187	3(3)
87188	6(3)
87190	9(3)
87197	1(3)
87205	3(3)
87206	6(3)
87207	3(3)
87209	4(3)
87210	4(3)
87220	3(3)
87230	2(3)
87250	1(3)
87252	2(3)
87253	2(3)
87254	7(3)

CPT	MUE
87255	2(3)
87260	1(3)
87265	1(3)
87267	1(3)
87269	1(3)
87270	1(3)
87271	1(3)
87272	1(3)
87273	1(3)
87274	1(3)
87275	1(3)
87276	1(3)
87278	1(3)
87279	1(3)
87280	1(3)
87281	1(3)
87283	1(3)
87285	1(3)
87290	1(3)
87299	1(3)
87300	2(3)
87301	1(3)
87305	1(3)
87320	1(3)
87324	2(3)
87327	1(3)
87328	2(3)
87329	2(3)
87332	1(3)
87335	1(3)
87336	1(3)
87337	1(3)
87338	1(3)
87339	1(3)
87340	1(2)
87341	1(2)
87350	1(2)
87380	1(2)
87385	2(3)
87389	1(3)
87390	1(3)
87391	1(3)
87400	2(3)
87420	1(3)
87425	1(3)
87426	3(3)
87427	2(3)
87428	3(3)
87430	1(3)
87449	3(3)
87450	2(3)
87451	2(3)
87471	1(3)
87472	1(3)
87475	1(3)
87476	1(3)
87480	1(3)
87481	5(3)
87482	1(3)
87483	1(2)
87485	1(3)
87486	1(3)
87487	1(3)
87490	1(3)
87491	3(3)
87492	1(3)

CPT	MUE
87493	2(3)
87495	1(3)
87496	1(3)
87497	2(3)
87498	1(3)
87500	1(3)
87501	1(3)
87502	1(3)
87503	1(3)
87505	1(2)
87506	1(2)
87507	1(2)
87510	1(3)
87511	1(3)
87512	1(3)
87516	1(3)
87517	1(3)
87520	1(3)
87521	1(3)
87522	1(3)
87525	1(3)
87526	1(3)
87527	1(3)
87528	1(3)
87529	2(3)
87530	2(3)
87531	1(3)
87532	1(3)
87533	1(3)
87534	1(3)
87535	1(3)
87536	1(3)
87537	1(3)
87538	1(3)
87539	1(3)
87540	1(3)
87541	1(3)
87542	1(3)
87550	1(3)
87551	2(3)
87552	1(3)
87555	1(3)
87556	1(3)
87557	1(3)
87560	1(3)
87561	1(3)
87562	1(3)
87563	3(3)
87580	1(3)
87581	1(3)
87582	1(3)
87590	1(3)
87591	3(3)
87592	1(3)
87623	1(2)
87624	1(3)
87625	1(3)
87631	1(3)
87632	1(3)
87633	1(3)
87634	1(3)
87635	2(3)
87636	3(3)
87637	3(3)
87640	1(3)
87641	1(3)

CPT	MUE
87650	1(3)
87651	1(3)
87652	1(3)
87653	1(3)
87660	1(3)
87661	1(3)
87662	2(3)
87797	3(3)
87798	13(3)
87799	3(3)
87800	2(3)
87801	3(3)
87802	2(3)
87803	3(3)
87804	3(3)
87806	1(2)
87807	2(3)
87808	1(3)
87809	2(3)
87810	2(3)
87811	3(3)
87850	1(3)
87880	2(3)
87899	4(3)
87900	1(2)
87901	1(2)
87902	1(2)
87903	1(2)
87904	14(3)
87905	2(3)
87906	2(3)
87910	1(3)
87912	1(3)
87999	1(3)
88000	0(3)
88005	0(3)
88007	0(3)
88012	0(3)
88014	0(3)
88016	0(3)
88020	0(3)
88025	0(3)
88027	0(3)
88028	0(3)
88029	0(3)
88036	0(3)
88037	0(3)
88040	0(3)
88045	0(3)
88099	0(3)
88104	5(3)
88106	5(3)
88108	6(3)
88112	6(3)
88120	2(3)
88121	2(3)
88125	1(3)
88130	1(2)
88140	1(2)
88141	1(3)
88142	1(3)
88143	1(3)
88147	1(3)
88148	1(3)
88150	1(3)
88152	1(3)

CPT	MUE
88153	1(3)
88155	1(3)
88160	4(3)
88161	4(3)
88162	3(3)
88164	1(3)
88165	1(3)
88166	1(3)
88167	1(3)
88172	5(3)
88173	5(3)
88174	1(3)
88175	1(3)
88177	6(3)
88182	2(3)
88184	2(3)
88185	35(3)
88187	2(3)
88188	2(3)
88189	2(3)
88199	1(3)
88230	2(3)
88233	2(3)
88235	2(3)
88237	4(3)
88239	3(3)
88240	1(3)
88241	3(3)
88245	1(2)
88248	1(2)
88249	1(2)
88261	2(3)
88262	2(3)
88263	1(3)
88264	1(3)
88267	2(3)
88269	2(3)
88271	16(3)
88272	12(3)
88273	3(3)
88274	5(3)
88275	12(3)
88280	1(3)
88283	5(3)
88285	10(3)
88289	1(3)
88291	1(3)
88299	1(3)
88300	4(3)
88302	4(3)
88304	5(3)
88305	16(3)
88307	8(3)
88309	3(3)
88311	4(3)
88312	9(3)
88313	8(3)
88314	6(3)
88319	11(3)
88321	1(2)
88323	1(2)
88325	1(2)
88329	2(3)
88331	11(3)
88332	13(3)
88333	4(3)

CPT	MUE
88334	5(3)
88341	13(3)
88342	4(3)
88344	6(3)
88346	2(3)
88348	1(3)
88350	9(3)
88355	1(3)
88356	3(3)
88358	2(3)
88360	6(3)
88361	6(3)
88362	1(3)
88363	2(3)
88364	3(3)
88365	4(3)
88366	2(3)
88367	3(3)
88368	3(3)
88369	3(3)
88371	1(3)
88372	1(3)
88373	3(3)
88374	5(3)
88375	1(3)
88377	5(3)
88380	1(3)
88381	1(3)
88387	2(3)
88388	1(3)
88399	1(3)
88720	1(3)
88738	1(3)
88740	1(2)
88741	1(2)
88749	1(3)
89049	1(3)
89050	2(3)
89051	2(3)
89055	2(3)
89060	2(3)
89125	2(3)
89160	1(3)
89190	1(3)
89220	2(3)
89230	1(2)
89240	1(3)
89250	1(2)
89251	1(2)
89253	1(3)
89254	1(3)
89255	1(3)
89257	1(3)
89258	1(2)
89259	1(2)
89260	1(2)
89261	1(2)
89264	1(3)
89268	1(2)
89272	1(2)
89280	1(2)
89281	1(2)
89290	1(2)
89291	1(2)
89300	1(2)
89310	1(2)

CPT	MUE
89320	1(2)
89321	1(2)
89322	1(2)
89325	1(2)
89329	1(2)
89330	1(2)
89331	1(2)
89335	1(3)
89337	1(2)
89342	1(2)
89343	1(2)
89344	1(2)
89346	1(2)
89352	1(2)
89353	1(3)
89354	1(3)
89356	2(3)
89398	1(3)
90281	0(3)
90283	0(3)
90284	0(3)
90287	0(3)
90288	0(3)
90291	0(3)
90296	1(2)
90371	10(3)
90375	20(3)
90376	20(3)
90377	20(3)
90378	4(3)
90384	0(3)
90385	1(2)
90386	0(3)
90389	0(3)
90393	1(2)
90396	1(2)
90399	0(3)
90460	9(3)
90461	8(3)
90471	1(2)
90472	8(3)
90473	1(2)
90474	1(3)
90476	1(2)
90477	1(2)
90581	1(2)
90585	1(2)
90586	1(2)
90587	1(2)
90619	1(2)
90620	1(2)
90621	1(2)
90625	1(2)
90630	1(2)
90632	1(2)
90633	1(2)
90634	1(2)
90636	1(2)
90644	1(2)
90647	1(2)
90648	1(2)
90649	1(2)
90650	1(2)
90651	1(2)
90653	1(2)
90654	1(2)

CPT	MUE
90655	1(2)
90656	1(2)
90657	1(2)
90658	1(2)
90660	1(2)
90661	1(2)
90662	1(2)
90664	1(2)
90666	1(2)
90667	1(2)
90668	1(2)
90670	1(2)
90672	1(2)
90673	1(2)
90674	1(2)
90675	1(2)
90676	1(2)
90680	1(2)
90681	1(2)
90682	1(2)
90685	1(2)
90686	1(2)
90687	1(2)
90688	1(2)
90689	1(2)
90690	1(2)
90691	1(2)
90694	1(2)
90696	1(2)
90697	1(2)
90698	1(2)
90700	1(2)
90702	1(2)
90707	1(2)
90710	1(2)
90713	1(2)
90714	1(2)
90715	1(2)
90716	1(2)
90717	1(2)
90723	0(3)
90732	1(2)
90733	1(2)
90734	1(2)
90736	1(2)
90738	1(2)
90739	1(2)
90740	1(2)
90743	1(2)
90744	1(2)
90746	1(2)
90747	1(2)
90748	0(3)
90749	1(3)
90750	1(2)
90756	1(2)
90785	3(3)
90791	1(3)
90792	1(3)
90832	2(3)
90833	2(3)
90834	2(3)
90836	2(3)
90837	2(3)
90838	2(3)
90839	1(2)

CPT	MUE
90840	3(3)
90845	1(2)
90846	1(3)
90847	1(3)
90849	1(3)
90853	1(3)
90863	1(3)
90865	1(3)
90867	1(2)
90868	1(3)
90869	1(3)
90870	2(3)
90875	1(3)
90876	0(3)
90880	1(3)
90882	0(3)
90885	0(3)
90887	0(3)
90889	0(3)
90899	1(3)
90901	1(3)
90912	1(2)
90913	3(3)
90935	1(3)
90937	1(3)
90940	1(3)
90945	1(3)
90947	1(3)
90951	1(2)
90952	1(2)
90953	1(2)
90954	1(2)
90955	1(2)
90956	1(2)
90957	1(2)
90958	1(2)
90959	1(2)
90960	1(2)
90961	1(2)
90962	1(2)
90963	1(2)
90964	1(2)
90965	1(2)
90966	1(2)
90967	1(2)
90968	1(2)
90969	1(2)
90970	1(2)
90989	1(2)
90993	1(3)
90997	1(3)
90999	1(3)
91010	1(2)
91013	1(3)
91020	1(2)
91022	1(2)
91030	1(2)
91034	1(2)
91035	1(2)
91037	1(2)
91038	1(2)
91040	1(2)
91065	2(2)
91110	1(2)
91111	1(2)
91112	1(3)

CPT	MUE
91117	1(2)
91120	1(2)
91122	1(2)
91132	1(3)
91133	1(3)
91200	1(2)
91299	1(3)
91300	1(2)
91301	1(2)
91302	1(2)
91303	1(2)
91304	1(2)
92002	1(2)
92004	1(2)
92012	1(3)
92014	1(3)
92015	0(3)
92018	1(2)
92019	1(2)
92020	1(2)
92025	1(2)
92060	1(2)
92065	1(2)
92071	2(2)
92072	1(2)
92081	1(2)
92082	1(2)
92083	1(2)
92100	1(2)
92132	1(2)
92133	1(2)
92134	1(2)
92136	2(2)
92145	1(2)
92201	1(2)
92202	1(2)
92227	1(2)
92228	1(2)
92229	1(2)
92230	2(2)
92235	1(2)
92240	1(2)
92242	1(2)
92250	1(2)
92260	1(2)
92265	1(2)
92270	1(2)
92273	1(2)
92274	1(2)
92283	1(2)
92284	1(2)
92285	1(2)
92286	1(2)
92287	1(2)
92310	0(3)
92311	1(2)
92312	1(2)
92313	1(3)
92314	0(3)
92315	1(2)
92316	1(2)
92317	1(3)
92325	1(3)
92326	2(2)
92340	0(3)
92341	0(3)

CPT	MUE
92342	0(3)
92352	0(3)
92353	0(3)
92354	0(3)
92355	0(3)
92358	0(3)
92370	0(3)
92371	0(3)
92499	1(3)
92502	1(3)
92504	1(3)
92507	1(3)
92508	1(3)
92511	1(3)
92512	1(2)
92516	1(3)
92517	1(2)
92518	1(2)
92519	1(2)
92520	1(2)
92521	1(2)
92522	1(2)
92523	1(2)
92524	1(2)
92526	1(2)
92531	0(3)
92532	0(3)
92533	0(3)
92534	0(3)
92537	1(2)
92538	1(2)
92540	1(3)
92541	1(3)
92542	1(3)
92544	1(3)
92545	1(3)
92546	1(3)
92547	1(3)
92548	1(3)
92549	1(3)
92550	1(2)
92551	0(3)
92552	1(2)
92553	1(2)
92555	1(2)
92556	1(2)
92557	1(2)
92558	0(3)
92559	0(3)
92560	0(3)
92561	1(2)
92562	1(2)
92563	1(2)
92564	1(2)
92565	1(2)
92567	1(2)
92568	1(2)
92570	1(2)
92571	1(2)
92572	1(2)
92575	1(2)
92576	1(2)
92577	1(2)
92579	1(2)
92582	1(2)
92583	1(2)

CPT	MUE
92584	1(2)
92587	1(2)
92588	1(2)
92590	0(3)
92591	0(3)
92592	0(3)
92593	0(3)
92594	0(3)
92595	0(3)
92596	1(2)
92597	1(3)
92601	1(3)
92602	1(3)
92603	1(3)
92604	1(3)
92605	0(3)
92606	0(3)
92607	1(3)
92608	4(3)
92609	1(3)
92610	1(2)
92611	1(3)
92612	1(3)
92613	1(2)
92614	1(3)
92615	1(2)
92616	1(3)
92617	1(2)
92618	1(3)
92620	1(2)
92621	2(3)
92625	1(2)
92626	1(2)
92627	6(3)
92630	0(3)
92633	0(3)
92640	1(3)
92650	1(2)
92651	1(2)
92652	1(2)
92653	1(2)
92700	1(3)
92920	3(3)
92921	6(2)
92924	2(3)
92925	6(2)
92928	3(3)
92929	2(3)
92933	2(3)
92934	2(3)
92937	2(3)
92938	2(3)
92941	1(3)
92943	2(3)
92944	2(3)
92950	2(3)
92953	2(3)
92960	2(3)
92961	1(3)
92970	1(3)
92971	1(3)
92973	2(3)
92974	1(3)
92975	1(3)
92977	1(3)
92978	1(3)

CPT	MUE
92979	2(3)
92986	1(2)
92987	1(2)
92990	1(2)
92997	1(2)
92998	2(3)
93000	3(3)
93005	3(3)
93010	5(3)
93015	1(3)
93016	1(3)
93017	1(3)
93018	1(3)
93024	1(3)
93025	1(2)
93040	3(3)
93041	2(3)
93042	3(3)
93050	1(3)
93224	1(2)
93225	1(2)
93226	1(2)
93227	1(2)
93228	1(2)
93229	1(2)
93241	1(2)
93242	1(2)
93243	1(2)
93244	1(2)
93245	1(2)
93246	1(2)
93247	1(2)
93248	1(2)
93260	1(2)
93261	1(3)
93264	1(2)
93268	1(2)
93270	1(2)
93271	1(2)
93272	1(2)
93278	1(3)
93279	1(3)
93280	1(3)
93281	1(3)
93282	1(3)
93283	1(3)
93284	1(3)
93285	1(3)
93286	2(3)
93287	2(3)
93288	1(3)
93289	1(3)
93290	1(3)
93291	1(3)
93292	1(3)
93293	1(2)
93294	1(2)
93295	1(2)
93296	1(2)
93297	1(2)
93298	1(2)
93303	1(3)
93304	1(3)
93306	1(3)
93307	1(3)
93308	1(3)

CPT	MUE
93312	1(3)
93313	1(3)
93314	1(3)
93315	1(3)
93316	1(3)
93317	1(3)
93318	1(3)
93320	2(3)
93321	1(3)
93325	2(3)
93350	1(2)
93351	1(2)
93352	1(3)
93355	1(3)
93356	1(3)
93451	1(3)
93452	1(3)
93453	1(3)
93454	1(3)
93455	1(3)
93456	1(3)
93457	1(3)
93458	1(3)
93459	1(3)
93460	1(3)
93461	1(3)
93462	1(3)
93463	1(3)
93464	1(3)
93503	2(3)
93505	1(2)
93530	1(3)
93531	1(3)
93532	1(3)
93533	1(3)
93561	1(3)
93562	1(3)
93563	1(3)
93564	1(3)
93565	1(3)
93566	1(3)
93567	1(3)
93568	1(3)
93571	1(3)
93572	2(3)
93580	1(3)
93581	1(3)
93582	1(2)
93583	1(2)
93590	1(2)
93591	1(2)
93592	2(3)
93600	1(3)
93602	1(3)
93603	1(3)
93609	1(3)
93610	1(3)
93612	1(3)
93613	1(3)
93615	1(3)
93616	1(3)
93618	1(3)
93619	1(3)
93620	1(3)
93621	1(3)
93622	1(3)

CPT	MUE
93623	1(3)
93624	1(3)
93631	1(3)
93640	1(3)
93641	1(2)
93642	1(3)
93644	1(3)
93650	1(2)
93653	1(3)
93654	1(3)
93655	2(3)
93656	1(3)
93657	2(3)
93660	1(3)
93662	1(3)
93668	1(3)
93701	1(2)
93702	1(2)
93724	1(3)
93740	0(3)
93745	1(2)
93750	4(3)
93770	0(3)
93784	1(2)
93786	1(2)
93788	1(2)
93790	1(2)
93792	1(2)
93793	1(2)
93797	2(2)
93798	2(2)
93799	1(3)
93880	1(3)
93882	1(3)
93886	1(3)
93888	1(3)
93890	1(3)
93892	1(3)
93893	1(3)
93895	1(3)
93922	2(2)
93923	2(2)
93924	1(2)
93925	1(3)
93926	1(3)
93930	1(3)
93931	1(3)
93970	1(3)
93971	1(3)
93975	1(3)
93976	1(3)
93978	1(3)
93979	1(3)
93980	1(3)
93981	1(3)
93985	1(3)
93986	1(3)
93990	2(3)
93998	1(3)
94002	1(2)
94003	1(2)
94004	1(2)
94005	1(3)
94010	1(3)
94011	1(3)
94012	1(3)

CPT	MUE
94013	1(3)
94014	1(2)
94015	1(2)
94016	1(2)
94060	1(3)
94070	1(2)
94150	0(3)
94200	1(3)
94375	1(3)
94450	1(3)
94452	1(2)
94453	1(2)
94610	2(3)
94617	1(3)
94618	1(3)
94619	1(3)
94621	1(3)
94640	4(3)
94642	1(3)
94644	1(2)
94645	2(3)
94660	1(2)
94662	1(2)
94664	1(3)
94667	1(2)
94668	2(3)
94669	2(3)
94680	1(3)
94681	1(3)
94690	1(3)
94726	1(3)
94727	1(3)
94728	1(3)
94729	1(3)
94760	1(3)
94761	1(2)
94762	1(2)
94772	1(2)
94774	1(2)
94775	1(2)
94776	1(2)
94777	1(2)
94780	1(2)
94781	2(3)
94799	1(3)
95004	80(3)
95012	2(3)
95017	27(3)
95018	19(3)
95024	40(3)
95027	90(3)
95028	30(3)
95044	80(3)
95052	20(3)
95056	1(2)
95060	1(2)
95065	1(3)
95070	1(3)
95076	1(2)
95079	2(3)
95115	1(2)
95117	1(2)
95120	0(3)
95125	0(3)
95130	0(3)
95131	0(3)

CPT	MUE
95132	0(3)
95133	0(3)
95134	0(3)
95144	30(3)
95145	10(3)
95146	10(3)
95147	10(3)
95148	10(3)
95149	10(3)
95165	30(3)
95170	10(3)
95180	6(3)
95199	1(3)
95249	1(2)
95250	1(2)
95251	1(2)
95700	1(2)
95705	1(2)
95706	1(2)
95707	1(2)
95708	4(3)
95709	4(3)
95710	4(3)
95711	1(2)
95712	1(2)
95713	1(2)
95714	4(3)
95715	4(3)
95716	4(3)
95717	1(2)
95718	1(2)
95719	1(2)
95720	1(2)
95721	1(2)
95722	1(2)
95723	1(2)
95724	1(2)
95725	1(2)
95726	1(2)
95782	1(2)
95783	1(2)
95800	1(2)
95801	1(2)
95803	1(2)
95805	1(2)
95806	1(2)
95807	1(2)
95808	1(2)
95810	1(2)
95811	1(2)
95812	1(3)
95813	1(3)
95816	1(3)
95819	1(3)
95822	1(3)
95824	1(3)
95829	1(3)
95830	1(3)
95836	1(2)
95851	3(3)
95852	1(3)
95857	1(2)
95860	1(3)
95861	1(3)
95863	1(3)
95864	1(3)

CPT	MUE
95865	1(3)
95866	1(3)
95867	1(3)
95868	1(3)
95869	1(3)
95870	4(3)
95872	4(3)
95873	1(2)
95874	1(2)
95875	2(3)
95885	4(2)
95886	4(2)
95887	1(2)
95905	2(3)
95907	1(2)
95908	1(2)
95909	1(2)
95910	1(2)
95911	1(2)
95912	1(2)
95913	1(2)
95921	1(3)
95922	1(3)
95923	1(3)
95924	1(3)
95925	1(3)
95926	1(3)
95927	1(3)
95928	1(3)
95929	1(3)
95930	1(3)
95933	1(3)
95937	4(3)
95938	1(3)
95939	1(3)
95940	32(3)
95941	0(3)
95943	1(3)
95954	1(3)
95955	1(3)
95957	1(3)
95958	1(3)
95961	1(2)
95962	5(3)
95965	1(3)
95966	1(3)
95967	3(3)
95970	1(3)
95971	1(3)
95972	1(3)
95976	1(3)
95977	1(3)
95980	1(3)
95981	1(3)
95982	1(3)
95983	1(2)
95984	11(3)
95990	1(3)
95991	1(3)
95992	1(2)
95999	1(3)
96000	1(2)
96001	1(2)
96002	1(3)
96003	1(3)
96004	1(2)

CPT	MUE
96020	1(2)
96040	4(3)
96105	3(3)
96110	3(3)
96112	1(2)
96113	6(3)
96116	1(2)
96121	3(3)
96125	2(3)
96127	2(3)
96130	1(2)
96131	7(3)
96132	1(2)
96133	7(3)
96136	1(2)
96137	11(3)
96138	1(2)
96139	11(3)
96146	1(2)
96156	1(3)
96158	1(2)
96159	4(3)
96160	3(3)
96161	1(3)
96164	1(2)
96165	6(3)
96167	1(2)
96168	6(3)
96170	1(3)
96171	2(3)
96360	1(3)
96361	8(3)
96365	1(3)
96366	8(3)
96367	4(3)
96368	1(2)
96369	1(2)
96370	3(3)
96371	1(3)
96372	4(3)
96373	2(3)
96374	1(3)
96375	6(3)
96376	0(3)
96377	1(3)
96379	1(3)
96401	3(3)
96402	2(3)
96405	1(2)
96406	1(2)
96409	1(3)
96411	3(3)
96413	1(3)
96415	8(3)
96416	1(3)
96417	3(3)
96420	1(3)
96422	2(3)
96423	1(3)
96425	1(3)
96440	1(3)
96446	1(3)
96450	1(3)
96521	2(3)
96522	1(3)
96523	1(3)

CPT	MUE
96542	1(3)
96549	1(3)
96567	1(3)
96570	1(2)
96571	2(3)
96573	1(2)
96574	1(2)
96900	1(3)
96902	0(3)
96904	1(2)
96910	1(3)
96912	1(3)
96913	1(3)
96920	1(2)
96921	1(2)
96922	1(2)
96931	1(2)
96932	1(2)
96933	1(2)
96934	2(3)
96935	2(3)
96936	2(3)
96999	1(3)
97010	0(3)
97012	1(3)
97014	0(3)
97016	1(3)
97018	1(3)
97022	1(3)
97024	1(3)
97026	1(3)
97028	1(3)
97032	4(3)
97033	4(3)
97034	2(3)
97035	2(3)
97036	3(3)
97039	1(3)
97110	6(3)
97112	4(3)
97113	6(3)
97116	4(3)
97124	4(3)
97129	1(2)
97130	7(3)
97139	1(3)
97140	6(3)
97150	1(3)
97151	8(3)
97152	16(3)
97153	32(3)
97154	18(3)
97155	24(3)
97156	16(3)
97157	16(3)
97158	16(3)
97161	1(2)
97162	1(2)
97163	1(2)
97164	1(2)
97165	1(2)
97166	1(2)
97167	1(2)
97168	1(2)
97169	0(3)
97170	0(3)

CPT	MUE
97171	0(3)
97172	0(3)
97530	6(3)
97533	4(3)
97535	8(3)
97537	6(3)
97542	8(3)
97545	1(2)
97546	2(3)
97597	1(3)
97598	8(3)
97602	0(3)
97605	1(3)
97606	1(3)
97607	1(3)
97608	1(3)
97610	1(2)
97750	8(3)
97755	8(3)
97760	6(3)
97761	6(3)
97763	6(3)
97799	1(3)
97802	8(3)
97803	8(3)
97804	6(3)
97810	1(2)
97811	2(3)
97813	1(2)
97814	2(3)
98925	1(2)
98926	1(2)
98927	1(2)
98928	1(2)
98929	1(2)
98940	1(2)
98941	1(2)
98942	1(2)
98943	0(3)
98960	0(3)
98961	0(3)
98962	0(3)
98966	1(2)
98967	1(2)
98968	1(2)
98970	1(2)
98971	1(2)
98972	1(2)
99000	0(3)
99001	0(3)
99002	0(3)
99024	1(3)
99026	0(3)
99027	0(3)
99050	0(3)
99051	0(3)
99053	0(3)
99056	0(3)
99058	0(3)
99060	0(3)
99070	0(3)
99071	0(3)
99075	0(3)
99078	0(3)
99080	0(3)
99082	1(3)

CPT	MUE
99091	1(2)
99100	1(3)
99116	0(3)
99135	0(3)
99140	0(3)
99151	1(3)
99152	2(3)
99153	9(3)
99155	1(3)
99156	1(3)
99157	6(3)
99170	1(3)
99172	0(3)
99173	0(3)
99174	0(3)
99175	1(3)
99177	1(2)
99183	1(3)
99184	1(2)
99188	1(2)
99190	1(3)
99191	1(3)
99192	1(3)
99195	2(3)
99199	1(3)
99202	1(2)
99203	1(2)
99204	1(2)
99205	1(2)
99211	1(3)
99212	2(3)
99213	2(3)
99214	2(3)
99215	1(3)
99217	1(2)
99218	1(2)
99219	1(2)
99220	1(2)
99221	1(3)
99222	1(3)
99223	1(3)
99224	1(2)
99225	1(2)
99226	1(2)
99231	1(3)
99232	1(3)
99233	1(3)
99234	1(3)
99235	1(3)
99236	1(3)
99238	1(3)
99239	1(3)
99241	0(3)
99242	0(3)
99243	0(3)
99244	0(3)
99245	0(3)
99251	0(3)
99252	0(3)
99253	0(3)
99254	0(3)
99255	0(3)
99281	1(3)
99282	1(3)
99283	1(3)
99284	1(3)

CPT	MUE
99285	1(3)
99288	0(3)
99291	1(2)
99292	8(3)
99304	1(2)
99305	1(2)
99306	1(2)
99307	1(2)
99308	1(2)
99309	1(2)
99310	1(2)
99315	1(2)
99316	1(2)
99318	1(2)
99324	1(2)
99325	1(2)
99326	1(2)
99327	1(2)
99328	1(2)
99334	1(3)
99335	1(3)
99336	1(3)
99337	1(3)
99339	0(3)
99340	0(3)
99341	1(2)
99342	1(2)
99343	1(2)
99344	1(2)
99345	1(2)
99347	1(3)
99348	1(3)
99349	1(3)
99350	1(3)
99354	1(2)
99355	4(3)
99356	1(2)
99357	4(3)
99358	1(2)
99359	2(3)
99360	1(3)
99366	0(3)
99367	0(3)
99368	0(3)
99374	0(3)
99375	0(3)
99377	0(3)
99378	0(3)
99379	0(3)
99380	0(3)
99381	0(3)
99382	0(3)
99383	0(3)
99384	0(3)
99385	0(3)
99386	0(3)
99387	0(3)
99391	0(3)
99392	0(3)
99393	0(3)
99394	0(3)
99395	0(3)
99396	0(3)
99397	0(3)
99401	0(3)
99402	0(3)

CPT	MUE
99403	0(3)
99404	0(3)
99406	1(2)
99407	1(2)
99408	0(3)
99409	0(3)
99411	0(3)
99412	0(3)
99415	1(2)
99416	3(3)
99417	4(3)
99421	1(2)
99422	1(2)
99423	1(2)
99429	0(3)
99439	2(2)
99441	1(2)
99442	1(2)
99443	1(2)
99446	1(2)
99447	1(2)
99448	1(2)
99449	1(2)
99450	0(3)
99451	1(2)
99452	1(2)
99453	1(2)
99454	1(2)
99455	1(3)
99456	1(3)
99457	1(2)
99458	3(3)
99460	1(2)
99461	1(2)
99462	1(2)
99463	1(2)
99464	1(2)
99465	1(2)
99466	1(2)
99467	4(3)
99468	1(2)
99469	1(2)
99471	1(2)
99472	1(2)
99473	1(2)
99474	1(2)
99475	1(2)
99476	1(2)
99477	1(2)
99478	1(2)
99479	1(2)
99480	1(2)
99483	1(2)
99484	1(2)
99485	1(3)
99486	4(1)
99487	1(2)
99489	10(3)
99490	1(2)
99491	1(2)
99492	1(2)
99493	1(2)
99494	2(3)
99495	1(2)
99496	1(2)
99497	1(2)

CPT	MUE
99498	3(3)
99499	1(3)
99500	0(3)
99501	0(3)
99502	0(3)
99503	0(3)
99504	0(3)
99505	0(3)
99506	0(3)
99507	0(3)
99509	0(3)
99510	0(3)
99511	0(3)
99512	0(3)
99600	0(3)
99601	0(3)
99602	0(3)
99605	0(2)
99606	0(3)
99607	0(3)
A0021	0(3)
A0080	0(3)
A0090	0(3)
A0100	0(3)
A0110	0(3)
A0120	0(3)
A0130	0(3)
A0140	0(3)
A0160	0(3)
A0170	0(3)
A0180	0(3)
A0190	0(3)
A0200	0(3)
A0210	0(3)
A0225	0(3)
A0380	0(3)
A0382	0(3)
A0384	0(3)
A0390	0(3)
A0392	0(3)
A0394	0(3)
A0396	0(3)
A0398	0(3)
A0420	0(3)
A0422	0(3)
A0424	0(3)
A0425	250(1)
A0426	2(3)
A0427	2(3)
A0428	2(3)
A0429	2(3)
A0430	1(3)
A0431	1(3)
A0432	1(3)
A0433	1(3)
A0434	2(3)
A0435	999(3)
A0436	300(3)
A0888	0(3)
A0998	0(3)
A0999	1(3)
A4206	0(3)
A4207	0(3)
A4208	0(3)
A4209	0(3)
A4210	0(3)

CPT	MUE
A4211	0(3)
A4212	0(3)
A4213	0(3)
A4215	0(3)
A4216	0(3)
A4217	0(3)
A4218	0(3)
A4220	1(3)
A4221	0(3)
A4222	0(3)
A4223	0(3)
A4224	0(3)
A4225	0(3)
A4226	0(3)
A4230	0(3)
A4231	0(3)
A4232	0(3)
A4233	0(3)
A4234	0(3)
A4235	0(3)
A4236	0(3)
A4244	0(3)
A4245	0(3)
A4246	0(3)
A4247	0(3)
A4248	0(3)
A4250	0(3)
A4252	0(3)
A4253	0(3)
A4255	0(3)
A4256	0(3)
A4257	0(3)
A4258	0(3)
A4259	0(3)
A4261	0(3)
A4262	0(3)
A4263	0(3)
A4264	0(3)
A4265	0(3)
A4266	0(3)
A4267	0(3)
A4268	0(3)
A4269	0(3)
A4270	0(3)
A4280	0(3)
A4281	0(3)
A4282	0(3)
A4283	0(3)
A4284	0(3)
A4285	0(3)
A4286	0(3)
A4290	2(3)
A4300	0(3)
A4301	1(2)
A4305	0(3)
A4306	0(3)
A4310	0(3)
A4311	0(3)
A4312	0(3)
A4313	0(3)
A4314	0(3)
A4315	0(3)
A4316	0(3)
A4320	0(3)
A4321	1(3)
A4322	0(3)

CPT	MUE
A4326	0(3)
A4327	0(3)
A4328	0(3)
A4330	0(3)
A4331	1(3)
A4332	2(3)
A4333	1(3)
A4334	2(3)
A4335	0(3)
A4336	1(3)
A4337	0(3)
A4338	0(3)
A4340	0(3)
A4344	0(3)
A4346	0(3)
A4349	1(3)
A4351	0(3)
A4352	0(3)
A4353	1(3)
A4354	0(3)
A4355	0(3)
A4356	0(3)
A4357	0(3)
A4358	0(3)
A4360	1(3)
A4361	0(3)
A4362	0(3)
A4363	1(3)
A4364	0(3)
A4366	1(3)
A4367	0(3)
A4368	1(3)
A4369	1(3)
A4371	1(3)
A4372	1(3)
A4373	1(3)
A4375	2(3)
A4376	2(3)
A4377	2(3)
A4378	2(3)
A4379	2(3)
A4380	2(3)
A4381	2(3)
A4382	2(3)
A4383	2(3)
A4384	2(3)
A4385	2(3)
A4387	1(3)
A4388	1(3)
A4389	2(3)
A4390	1(3)
A4391	1(3)
A4392	2(3)
A4393	1(3)
A4394	1(3)
A4395	3(3)
A4396	2(3)
A4397	0(3)
A4398	0(3)
A4399	0(3)
A4400	0(3)
A4402	0(3)
A4404	0(3)
A4405	1(3)
A4406	1(3)
A4407	2(3)

CPT	MUE
A4408	1(3)
A4409	1(3)
A4410	2(3)
A4411	1(3)
A4412	1(3)
A4413	2(3)
A4414	1(3)
A4415	1(3)
A4416	2(3)
A4417	2(3)
A4418	2(3)
A4419	2(3)
A4420	1(3)
A4422	7(3)
A4423	2(3)
A4424	1(3)
A4425	1(3)
A4426	2(3)
A4427	1(3)
A4428	1(3)
A4429	2(3)
A4430	1(3)
A4431	1(3)
A4432	2(3)
A4433	1(3)
A4434	1(3)
A4435	2(3)
A4450	0(3)
A4452	0(3)
A4455	0(3)
A4458	0(3)
A4459	0(3)
A4461	2(3)
A4463	0(3)
A4465	0(3)
A4467	0(3)
A4470	0(3)
A4480	0(3)
A4481	0(3)
A4483	0(3)
A4490	0(3)
A4495	0(3)
A4500	0(3)
A4510	0(3)
A4520	0(3)
A4550	0(3)
A4553	0(3)
A4554	0(3)
A4555	0(3)
A4556	0(3)
A4557	0(3)
A4558	0(3)
A4559	0(3)
A4561	1(3)
A4562	1(3)
A4563	1(2)
A4565	2(3)
A4566	0(3)
A4570	0(3)
A4575	0(3)
A4580	0(3)
A4590	0(3)
A4595	0(3)
A4600	0(3)
A4601	0(3)
A4602	0(3)

CPT	MUE
A4604	0(3)
A4605	0(3)
A4606	0(3)
A4608	0(3)
A4611	0(3)
A4612	0(3)
A4613	0(3)
A4614	0(3)
A4615	0(3)
A4616	0(3)
A4617	0(3)
A4618	1(3)
A4619	0(3)
A4620	0(3)
A4623	0(3)
A4624	0(3)
A4625	30(3)
A4626	0(3)
A4627	0(3)
A4628	0(3)
A4629	0(3)
A4630	0(3)
A4633	0(3)
A4634	0(3)
A4635	0(3)
A4636	0(3)
A4637	0(3)
A4638	0(3)
A4639	0(3)
A4640	0(3)
A4642	1(3)
A4648	5(3)
A4649	1(3)
A4650	3(3)
A4651	0(3)
A4652	0(3)
A4653	0(3)
A4657	0(3)
A4660	0(3)
A4663	0(3)
A4670	0(3)
A4671	0(3)
A4672	0(3)
A4673	0(3)
A4674	0(3)
A4680	0(3)
A4690	0(3)
A4706	0(3)
A4707	0(3)
A4708	0(3)
A4709	0(3)
A4714	0(3)
A4719	0(3)
A4720	0(3)
A4721	0(3)
A4722	0(3)
A4723	0(3)
A4724	0(3)
A4725	0(3)
A4726	0(3)
A4728	0(3)
A4730	0(3)
A4736	0(3)
A4737	0(3)
A4740	0(3)
A4750	0(3)

CPT	MUE
A4755	0(3)
A4760	0(3)
A4765	0(3)
A4766	0(3)
A4770	0(3)
A4771	0(3)
A4772	0(3)
A4773	0(3)
A4774	0(3)
A4802	0(3)
A4860	0(3)
A4870	0(3)
A4890	0(3)
A4911	0(3)
A4913	0(3)
A4918	0(3)
A4927	0(3)
A4928	0(3)
A4929	0(3)
A4930	0(3)
A4931	0(3)
A4932	0(3)
A5051	0(3)
A5052	0(3)
A5053	0(3)
A5054	0(3)
A5055	0(3)
A5056	90(3)
A5057	90(3)
A5061	0(3)
A5062	0(3)
A5063	0(3)
A5071	0(3)
A5072	0(3)
A5073	0(3)
A5081	0(3)
A5082	0(3)
A5083	5(3)
A5093	0(3)
A5102	0(3)
A5105	0(3)
A5112	0(3)
A5113	0(3)
A5114	0(3)
A5120	150(3)
A5121	0(3)
A5122	0(3)
A5126	0(3)
A5131	0(3)
A5200	2(3)
A5500	0(3)
A5501	0(3)
A5503	0(3)
A5504	0(3)
A5505	0(3)
A5506	0(3)
A5507	0(3)
A5508	0(3)
A5510	0(3)
A5512	0(3)
A5513	0(3)
A5514	0(3)
A6000	0(3)
A6010	0(3)
A6011	0(3)
A6021	0(3)

CPT	MUE
A6022	0(3)
A6023	0(3)
A6024	0(3)
A6025	0(3)
A6154	0(3)
A6196	0(3)
A6197	0(3)
A6198	0(3)
A6199	0(3)
A6203	0(3)
A6204	0(3)
A6205	0(3)
A6206	0(3)
A6207	0(3)
A6208	0(3)
A6209	0(3)
A6210	0(3)
A6211	0(3)
A6212	0(3)
A6213	0(3)
A6214	0(3)
A6215	0(3)
A6216	0(3)
A6217	0(3)
A6218	0(3)
A6219	0(3)
A6220	0(3)
A6221	0(3)
A6222	0(3)
A6223	0(3)
A6224	0(3)
A6228	0(3)
A6229	0(3)
A6230	0(3)
A6231	0(3)
A6232	0(3)
A6233	0(3)
A6234	0(3)
A6235	0(3)
A6236	0(3)
A6237	0(3)
A6238	0(3)
A6239	0(3)
A6240	0(3)
A6241	0(3)
A6242	0(3)
A6243	0(3)
A6244	0(3)
A6245	0(3)
A6246	0(3)
A6247	0(3)
A6248	0(3)
A6250	0(3)
A6251	0(3)
A6252	0(3)
A6253	0(3)
A6254	0(3)
A6255	0(3)
A6256	0(3)
A6257	0(3)
A6258	0(3)
A6259	0(3)
A6260	0(3)
A6261	0(3)
A6262	0(3)
A6266	0(3)

CPT	MUE
A6402	0(3)
A6403	0(3)
A6404	0(3)
A6407	0(3)
A6410	2(3)
A6411	0(3)
A6412	0(3)
A6413	0(3)
A6441	0(3)
A6442	0(3)
A6443	0(3)
A6444	0(3)
A6445	0(3)
A6446	0(3)
A6447	0(3)
A6448	0(3)
A6449	0(3)
A6450	0(3)
A6451	0(3)
A6452	0(3)
A6453	0(3)
A6454	0(3)
A6455	0(3)
A6456	0(3)
A6457	0(3)
A6460	1(1)
A6461	1(1)
A6501	0(3)
A6502	0(3)
A6503	0(3)
A6504	0(3)
A6505	0(3)
A6506	0(3)
A6507	0(3)
A6508	0(3)
A6509	0(3)
A6510	0(3)
A6511	0(3)
A6513	0(3)
A6530	0(3)
A6531	0(3)
A6532	0(3)
A6533	0(3)
A6534	0(3)
A6535	0(3)
A6536	0(3)
A6537	0(3)
A6538	0(3)
A6539	0(3)
A6540	0(3)
A6541	0(3)
A6544	0(3)
A6545	0(3)
A6549	0(3)
A6550	0(3)
A7000	0(3)
A7001	0(3)
A7002	0(3)
A7003	0(3)
A7004	0(3)
A7005	0(3)
A7006	0(3)
A7007	0(3)
A7008	0(3)
A7009	0(3)
A7010	0(3)

CPT	MUE
A7012	0(3)
A7013	0(3)
A7014	0(3)
A7015	0(3)
A7016	0(3)
A7017	0(3)
A7018	0(3)
A7020	0(3)
A7025	0(3)
A7026	0(3)
A7027	0(3)
A7028	0(3)
A7029	0(3)
A7030	0(3)
A7031	0(3)
A7032	0(3)
A7033	0(3)
A7034	0(3)
A7035	0(3)
A7036	0(3)
A7037	0(3)
A7038	0(3)
A7039	0(3)
A7040	2(3)
A7041	2(3)
A7044	0(3)
A7045	0(3)
A7046	0(3)
A7047	0(3)
A7048	2(3)
A7501	0(3)
A7502	0(3)
A7503	0(3)
A7504	0(3)
A7505	0(3)
A7506	0(3)
A7507	0(3)
A7508	0(3)
A7509	0(3)
A7520	0(3)
A7521	0(3)
A7522	0(3)
A7523	0(3)
A7524	0(3)
A7525	8(3)
A7526	0(3)
A7527	0(3)
A8000	0(3)
A8001	0(3)
A8002	0(3)
A8003	0(3)
A8004	0(3)
A9152	0(3)
A9153	0(3)
A9155	1(3)
A9180	0(3)
A9270	0(3)
A9272	0(3)
A9273	0(3)
A9274	0(3)
A9275	0(3)
A9276	0(3)
A9277	0(3)
A9278	0(3)
A9279	0(3)
A9280	0(3)

CPT	MUE
A9281	0(3)
A9282	0(3)
A9283	0(3)
A9284	0(3)
A9285	0(3)
A9286	0(3)
A9300	0(3)
A9500	3(3)
A9501	1(3)
A9502	3(3)
A9503	1(3)
A9504	1(3)
A9505	4(3)
A9507	1(3)
A9508	2(3)
A9509	5(3)
A9510	1(3)
A9512	30(3)
A9513	200(3)
A9515	1(3)
A9516	4(3)
A9517	200(3)
A9520	1(3)
A9521	2(3)
A9524	10(3)
A9526	2(3)
A9527	195(3)
A9528	10(3)
A9529	10(3)
A9530	200(3)
A9531	100(3)
A9532	10(3)
A9536	1(3)
A9537	1(3)
A9538	1(3)
A9539	2(3)
A9540	2(3)
A9541	1(3)
A9542	1(3)
A9543	1(3)
A9546	1(3)
A9547	2(3)
A9548	2(3)
A9550	1(3)
A9551	1(3)
A9552	1(3)
A9553	1(3)
A9554	1(3)
A9555	2(3)
A9556	10(3)
A9557	2(3)
A9558	7(3)
A9559	1(3)
A9560	2(3)
A9561	1(3)
A9562	2(3)
A9563	10(3)
A9564	20(3)
A9566	1(3)
A9567	2(3)
A9568	0(3)
A9569	1(3)
A9570	1(3)
A9571	1(3)
A9572	1(3)
A9575	300(3)

CPT	MUE
A9576	40(3)
A9577	50(3)
A9578	50(3)
A9579	100(3)
A9580	1(3)
A9581	20(3)
A9582	1(3)
A9583	18(3)
A9584	1(3)
A9585	300(3)
A9586	1(3)
A9587	54(3)
A9588	10(3)
A9589	1(3)
A9590	675(3)
A9591	6(3)
A9600	7(3)
A9604	1(3)
A9606	224(3)
A9698	2(3)
A9700	2(3)
A9900	1(3)
A9901	0(3)
A9999	1(3)
B4034	0(3)
B4035	0(3)
B4036	0(3)
B4081	0(3)
B4082	0(3)
B4083	0(3)
B4087	0(3)
B4088	0(3)
B4100	0(3)
B4102	0(3)
B4103	0(3)
B4104	0(3)
B4149	0(3)
B4150	0(3)
B4152	0(3)
B4153	0(3)
B4154	0(3)
B4155	0(3)
B4157	0(3)
B4158	0(3)
B4159	0(3)
B4160	0(3)
B4161	0(3)
B4162	0(3)
B4164	0(3)
B4168	0(3)
B4172	0(3)
B4176	0(3)
B4178	0(3)
B4180	0(3)
B4185	0(3)
B4187	0(3)
B4189	0(3)
B4193	0(3)
B4197	0(3)
B4199	0(3)
B4216	0(3)
B4220	0(3)
B4222	0(3)
B4224	0(3)
B5000	0(3)
B5100	0(3)

CPT	MUE
B5200	0(3)
B9002	0(3)
B9004	0(3)
B9006	0(3)
B9998	0(3)
B9999	0(3)
C1052	1(3)
C1062	2(3)
C1713	20(3)
C1714	4(3)
C1715	45(3)
C1716	4(3)
C1717	10(3)
C1719	99(3)
C1721	1(3)
C1722	1(3)
C1724	5(3)
C1725	9(3)
C1726	5(3)
C1727	4(3)
C1728	5(3)
C1729	6(3)
C1730	4(3)
C1731	2(3)
C1732	3(3)
C1733	3(3)
C1734	2(3)
C1748	1(3)
C1749	1(3)
C1750	2(3)
C1751	3(3)
C1752	2(3)
C1753	2(3)
C1754	2(3)
C1755	2(3)
C1756	2(3)
C1757	6(3)
C1758	2(3)
C1759	2(3)
C1760	4(3)
C1762	4(3)
C1763	4(3)
C1764	1(3)
C1765	4(3)
C1766	4(3)
C1767	2(3)
C1768	3(3)
C1769	9(3)
C1770	3(3)
C1771	1(3)
C1772	1(3)
C1773	3(3)
C1776	10(3)
C1777	2(3)
C1778	4(3)
C1779	2(3)
C1780	2(3)
C1781	4(3)
C1782	1(3)
C1783	2(3)
C1784	2(3)
C1785	1(3)
C1786	1(3)
C1787	2(3)
C1788	2(3)
C1789	2(3)

CPT	MUE
C1813	1(3)
C1814	2(3)
C1815	1(3)
C1816	2(3)
C1817	1(3)
C1818	2(3)
C1819	4(3)
C1820	2(3)
C1821	4(3)
C1822	1(3)
C1823	1(3)
C1824	1(2)
C1825	1(2)
C1830	2(3)
C1839	2(2)
C1840	1(3)
C1841	1(2)
C1842	1(2)
C1874	5(3)
C1875	4(3)
C1876	5(3)
C1877	5(3)
C1878	2(3)
C1880	2(3)
C1881	2(3)
C1882	1(3)
C1883	4(3)
C1884	4(3)
C1885	2(3)
C1886	1(3)
C1887	7(3)
C1888	2(3)
C1889	1(3)
C1890	1(3)
C1891	1(3)
C1892	6(3)
C1893	6(3)
C1894	6(3)
C1895	2(3)
C1896	2(3)
C1897	2(3)
C1898	2(3)
C1899	2(3)
C1900	1(3)
C1982	1(3)
C2596	1(3)
C2613	2(3)
C2614	3(3)
C2615	2(3)
C2616	1(3)
C2617	4(3)
C2618	4(3)
C2619	1(3)
C2620	1(3)
C2621	1(3)
C2622	1(3)
C2623	2(3)
C2624	1(3)
C2625	4(3)
C2626	1(3)
C2627	2(3)
C2628	4(3)
C2629	4(3)
C2630	3(3)
C2631	1(3)
C2634	24(3)

CPT	MUE
C2635	124(3)
C2636	690(3)
C2637	0(3)
C2638	150(3)
C2639	150(3)
C2640	150(3)
C2641	150(3)
C2642	120(3)
C2643	120(3)
C2644	500(1)
C2645	4608(3)
C5271	1(2)
C5272	3(2)
C5273	1(2)
C5274	35(3)
C5275	1(2)
C5276	3(2)
C5277	1(2)
C5278	15(3)
C8900	1(3)
C8901	1(3)
C8902	1(3)
C8903	1(3)
C8905	1(3)
C8906	1(3)
C8908	1(3)
C8909	1(3)
C8910	1(3)
C8911	1(3)
C8912	1(3)
C8913	1(3)
C8914	1(3)
C8918	1(3)
C8919	1(3)
C8920	1(3)
C8921	1(3)
C8922	1(3)
C8923	1(3)
C8924	1(3)
C8925	1(3)
C8926	1(3)
C8927	1(3)
C8928	1(2)
C8929	1(3)
C8930	1(2)
C8931	1(3)
C8932	1(3)
C8933	1(3)
C8934	2(3)
C8935	2(3)
C8936	2(3)
C8937	2(2)
C8957	2(3)
C9046	160(3)
C9047	22(3)
C9065	40(3)
C9067	500(3)
C9113	10(3)
C9132	5500(3)
C9248	25(3)
C9250	1(3)
C9254	400(3)
C9257	10(2)
C9285	2(3)
C9290	266(3)
C9293	700(3)

CPT	MUE
C9352	3(3)
C9353	4(3)
C9354	300(3)
C9355	3(3)
C9356	125(3)
C9358	800(3)
C9359	30(3)
C9360	300(3)
C9361	10(3)
C9362	60(3)
C9363	500(3)
C9364	600(3)
C9460	1(3)
C9462	600(3)
C9482	150(3)
C9488	20(3)
C9600	3(3)
C9601	2(3)
C9602	2(3)
C9603	2(3)
C9604	2(3)
C9605	2(3)
C9606	1(3)
C9607	2(3)
C9608	2(3)
C9725	1(3)
C9726	2(3)
C9727	1(2)
C9728	1(2)
C9733	1(3)
C9734	1(3)
C9738	1(3)
C9739	1(2)
C9740	1(2)
C9751	1(3)
C9752	1(2)
C9753	3(3)
C9756	1(3)
C9757	2(2)
C9758	1(2)
C9759	1(3)
C9760	1(2)
C9761	2(2)
C9762	1(3)
C9763	1(3)
C9764	2(3)
C9765	2(3)
C9766	2(3)
C9767	2(3)
C9768	1(3)
C9769	1(2)
C9770	2(2)
C9771	1(2)
C9772	2(2)
C9773	2(2)
C9774	2(2)
C9775	2(2)
C9803	2(3)
D0150	1(3)
D0240	1(3)
D0250	2(3)
D0270	1(3)
D0272	1(3)
D0274	1(3)
D0277	1(3)
D0412	0(3)

CPT	MUE
D0416	1(3)
D0431	1(3)
D0460	1(2)
D0484	1(2)
D0485	1(2)
D0601	1(2)
D0602	1(2)
D0603	1(2)
D1510	2(2)
D1516	1(2)
D1517	1(2)
D1520	2(2)
D1526	1(2)
D1527	1(2)
D1551	1(2)
D1552	1(2)
D1553	2(2)
D1575	4(2)
D4260	4(2)
D4263	4(2)
D4264	3(3)
D4270	4(3)
D4273	1(2)
D4277	1(2)
D4278	3(3)
D4355	1(2)
D4381	12(3)
D5282	0(3)
D5283	0(3)
D5876	0(3)
D5911	1(3)
D5912	1(2)
D5983	1(3)
D5984	1(3)
D5985	1(3)
D7111	20(3)
D7140	32(2)
D7210	32(2)
D7220	6(3)
D7230	6(3)
D7240	6(3)
D7241	6(3)
D7250	32(2)
D7260	1(3)
D7261	1(3)
D7283	4(3)
D7288	2(3)
D7321	4(2)
D9110	1(3)
D9130	0(3)
D9230	1(3)
D9248	1(3)
D9613	0(3)
D9930	1(2)
D9944	0(3)
D9945	0(3)
D9946	0(3)
D9950	1(3)
D9951	1(3)
D9952	1(3)
D9961	0(3)
D9990	0(3)
E0100	0(3)
E0105	0(3)
E0110	0(3)
E0111	0(3)

CPT	MUE
E0112	0(3)
E0113	0(3)
E0114	0(3)
E0116	0(3)
E0117	0(3)
E0118	0(3)
E0130	0(3)
E0135	0(3)
E0140	0(3)
E0141	0(3)
E0143	0(3)
E0144	0(3)
E0147	0(3)
E0148	0(3)
E0149	0(3)
E0153	0(3)
E0154	0(3)
E0155	0(3)
E0156	0(3)
E0157	0(3)
E0158	0(3)
E0159	2(2)
E0160	0(3)
E0161	0(3)
E0162	0(3)
E0163	0(3)
E0165	0(3)
E0167	0(3)
E0168	0(3)
E0170	0(3)
E0171	0(3)
E0172	0(3)
E0175	0(3)
E0181	0(3)
E0182	0(3)
E0184	0(3)
E0185	0(3)
E0186	0(3)
E0187	0(3)
E0188	0(3)
E0189	0(3)
E0190	0(3)
E0191	0(3)
E0193	0(3)
E0194	0(3)
E0196	0(3)
E0197	0(3)
E0198	0(3)
E0199	0(3)
E0200	0(3)
E0202	0(3)
E0203	0(3)
E0205	0(3)
E0210	0(3)
E0215	0(3)
E0217	0(3)
E0218	0(3)
E0221	0(3)
E0225	0(3)
E0231	0(3)
E0232	0(3)
E0235	0(3)
E0236	0(3)
E0239	0(3)
E0240	0(3)
E0241	0(3)

CPT	MUE	CPT	MUE	CPT	MUE	CPT	MUE	CPT	MUE	CPT	MUE	CPT	MUE	CPT	MUE
E0242	0(3)	E0446	0(3)	E0657	0(3)	E0935	0(3)	E1037	0(3)	E1355	0(3)	E2204	0(3)	E2371	0(3)
E0243	0(3)	E0447	0(3)	E0660	0(3)	E0936	0(3)	E1038	0(3)	E1356	0(3)	E2205	0(3)	E2372	0(3)
E0244	0(3)	E0455	0(3)	E0665	0(3)	E0940	0(3)	E1039	0(3)	E1357	0(3)	E2206	0(3)	E2373	0(3)
E0245	0(3)	E0457	0(3)	E0666	0(3)	E0941	0(3)	E1050	0(3)	E1358	0(3)	E2207	0(3)	E2374	0(3)
E0246	0(3)	E0459	0(3)	E0667	0(3)	E0942	0(3)	E1060	0(3)	E1372	0(3)	E2208	0(3)	E2375	0(3)
E0247	0(3)	E0462	0(3)	E0668	0(3)	E0944	0(3)	E1070	0(3)	E1390	0(3)	E2209	0(3)	E2376	0(3)
E0248	0(3)	E0465	0(3)	E0669	0(3)	E0945	0(3)	E1083	0(3)	E1391	0(3)	E2210	0(3)	E2377	0(3)
E0249	0(3)	E0466	0(3)	E0670	0(3)	E0946	0(3)	E1084	0(3)	E1392	0(3)	E2211	0(3)	E2378	0(3)
E0250	0(3)	E0467	0(3)	E0671	0(3)	E0947	0(3)	E1085	0(3)	E1399	1(3)	E2212	0(3)	E2381	0(3)
E0251	0(3)	E0470	0(3)	E0672	0(3)	E0948	0(3)	E1086	0(3)	E1405	0(3)	E2213	0(3)	E2382	0(3)
E0255	0(3)	E0471	0(3)	E0673	0(3)	E0950	0(3)	E1087	0(3)	E1406	0(3)	E2214	0(3)	E2383	0(3)
E0256	0(3)	E0472	0(3)	E0675	0(3)	E0951	0(3)	E1088	0(3)	E1500	0(3)	E2215	0(3)	E2384	0(3)
E0260	0(3)	E0480	0(3)	E0676	1(3)	E0952	0(3)	E1089	0(3)	E1510	0(3)	E2216	0(3)	E2385	0(3)
E0261	0(3)	E0481	0(3)	E0691	0(3)	E0953	0(3)	E1090	0(3)	E1520	0(3)	E2217	0(3)	E2386	0(3)
E0265	0(3)	E0482	0(3)	E0692	0(3)	E0954	0(3)	E1092	0(3)	E1530	0(3)	E2218	0(3)	E2387	0(3)
E0266	0(3)	E0483	0(3)	E0693	0(3)	E0955	0(3)	E1093	0(3)	E1540	0(3)	E2219	0(3)	E2388	0(3)
E0270	0(3)	E0484	0(3)	E0694	0(3)	E0956	0(3)	E1100	0(3)	E1550	0(3)	E2220	0(3)	E2389	0(3)
E0271	0(3)	E0485	0(3)	E0700	0(3)	E0957	0(3)	E1110	0(3)	E1560	0(3)	E2221	0(3)	E2390	0(3)
E0272	0(3)	E0486	0(3)	E0705	0(3)	E0958	0(3)	E1130	0(3)	E1570	0(3)	E2222	0(3)	E2391	0(3)
E0273	0(3)	E0487	0(3)	E0710	0(3)	E0959	0(3)	E1140	0(3)	E1575	0(3)	E2224	0(3)	E2392	0(3)
E0274	0(3)	E0500	0(3)	E0720	0(3)	E0960	0(3)	E1150	0(3)	E1580	0(3)	E2225	0(3)	E2394	0(3)
E0275	0(3)	E0550	0(3)	E0730	0(3)	E0961	0(3)	E1160	0(3)	E1590	0(3)	E2226	0(3)	E2395	0(3)
E0276	0(3)	E0555	0(3)	E0731	0(3)	E0966	0(3)	E1161	0(3)	E1592	0(3)	E2227	0(3)	E2396	0(3)
E0277	0(3)	E0560	0(3)	E0740	0(3)	E0967	0(3)	E1170	0(3)	E1594	0(3)	E2228	0(3)	E2397	0(3)
E0280	0(3)	E0561	0(3)	E0744	0(3)	E0968	0(3)	E1171	0(3)	E1600	0(3)	E2230	0(3)	E2398	0(3)
E0290	0(3)	E0562	0(3)	E0745	0(3)	E0969	0(3)	E1172	0(3)	E1610	0(3)	E2231	0(3)	E2402	0(3)
E0291	0(3)	E0565	0(3)	E0746	1(3)	E0970	0(3)	E1180	0(3)	E1615	0(3)	E2291	1(2)	E2500	0(3)
E0292	0(3)	E0570	0(3)	E0747	0(3)	E0971	0(3)	E1190	0(3)	E1620	0(3)	E2292	1(2)	E2502	0(3)
E0293	0(3)	E0572	0(3)	E0748	0(3)	E0973	0(3)	E1195	0(3)	E1625	0(3)	E2293	1(2)	E2504	0(3)
E0294	0(3)	E0574	0(3)	E0749	1(3)	E0974	0(3)	E1200	0(3)	E1630	0(3)	E2294	1(2)	E2506	0(3)
E0295	0(3)	E0575	0(3)	E0755	0(3)	E0978	0(3)	E1220	0(3)	E1632	0(3)	E2295	0(3)	E2508	0(3)
E0296	0(3)	E0580	0(3)	E0760	0(3)	E0980	0(3)	E1221	0(3)	E1634	0(3)	E2300	0(3)	E2510	0(3)
E0297	0(3)	E0585	0(3)	E0761	0(3)	E0981	0(3)	E1222	0(3)	E1635	0(3)	E2301	0(3)	E2511	0(3)
E0300	0(3)	E0600	0(3)	E0762	0(3)	E0982	0(3)	E1223	0(3)	E1636	0(3)	E2310	0(3)	E2512	0(3)
E0301	0(3)	E0601	0(3)	E0764	0(3)	E0983	0(3)	E1224	0(3)	E1637	0(3)	E2311	0(3)	E2599	0(3)
E0302	0(3)	E0602	0(3)	E0765	0(3)	E0984	0(3)	E1225	0(3)	E1639	0(3)	E2312	0(3)	E2601	0(3)
E0303	0(3)	E0603	0(3)	E0766	0(3)	E0985	0(3)	E1226	0(3)	E1699	0(3)	E2313	0(3)	E2602	0(3)
E0304	0(3)	E0604	0(3)	E0769	0(3)	E0986	0(3)	E1227	0(3)	E1700	0(3)	E2321	0(3)	E2603	0(3)
E0305	0(3)	E0605	0(3)	E0770	1(3)	E0988	0(3)	E1228	0(3)	E1701	0(3)	E2322	0(3)	E2604	0(3)
E0310	0(3)	E0606	0(3)	E0776	0(3)	E0990	0(3)	E1229	0(3)	E1702	0(3)	E2323	0(3)	E2605	0(3)
E0315	0(3)	E0607	0(3)	E0779	0(3)	E0992	0(3)	E1230	0(3)	E1800	0(3)	E2324	0(3)	E2606	0(3)
E0316	0(3)	E0610	0(3)	E0780	0(3)	E0994	0(3)	E1231	0(3)	E1801	0(3)	E2325	0(3)	E2607	0(3)
E0325	0(3)	E0615	0(3)	E0781	1(2)	E0995	0(3)	E1232	0(3)	E1802	0(3)	E2326	0(3)	E2608	0(3)
E0326	0(3)	E0616	1(2)	E0782	1(2)	E1002	0(3)	E1233	0(3)	E1805	0(3)	E2327	0(3)	E2609	0(3)
E0328	0(3)	E0617	0(3)	E0783	1(2)	E1003	0(3)	E1234	0(3)	E1806	0(3)	E2328	0(3)	E2610	0(3)
E0329	0(3)	E0618	0(3)	E0784	0(3)	E1004	0(3)	E1235	0(3)	E1810	0(3)	E2329	0(3)	E2611	0(3)
E0350	0(3)	E0619	0(3)	E0785	1(2)	E1005	0(3)	E1236	0(3)	E1811	0(3)	E2330	0(3)	E2612	0(3)
E0352	0(3)	E0620	0(3)	E0786	1(2)	E1006	0(3)	E1237	0(3)	E1812	0(3)	E2331	0(3)	E2613	0(3)
E0370	0(3)	E0621	0(3)	E0787	0(3)	E1007	0(3)	E1238	0(3)	E1815	0(3)	E2340	0(3)	E2614	0(3)
E0371	0(3)	E0625	0(3)	E0791	0(3)	E1008	0(3)	E1239	0(3)	E1816	0(3)	E2341	0(3)	E2615	0(3)
E0372	0(3)	E0627	0(3)	E0830	0(3)	E1009	0(3)	E1240	0(3)	E1818	0(3)	E2342	0(3)	E2616	0(3)
E0373	0(3)	E0629	0(3)	E0840	0(3)	E1010	0(3)	E1250	0(3)	E1820	0(3)	E2343	0(3)	E2617	0(3)
E0424	0(3)	E0630	0(3)	E0849	0(3)	E1011	0(3)	E1260	0(3)	E1821	0(3)	E2351	0(3)	E2619	0(3)
E0425	0(3)	E0635	0(3)	E0850	0(3)	E1012	0(3)	E1270	0(3)	E1825	0(3)	E2358	0(3)	E2620	0(3)
E0430	0(3)	E0636	0(3)	E0855	0(3)	E1014	0(3)	E1280	0(3)	E1830	0(3)	E2359	0(3)	E2621	0(3)
E0431	0(3)	E0637	0(3)	E0856	0(3)	E1015	0(3)	E1285	0(3)	E1831	0(3)	E2360	0(3)	E2622	0(3)
E0433	0(3)	E0638	0(3)	E0860	0(3)	E1016	0(3)	E1290	0(3)	E1840	0(3)	E2361	0(3)	E2623	0(3)
E0434	0(3)	E0639	0(3)	E0870	0(3)	E1017	0(3)	E1295	0(3)	E1841	0(3)	E2362	0(3)	E2624	0(3)
E0435	0(3)	E0640	0(3)	E0880	0(3)	E1018	0(3)	E1296	0(3)	E1902	0(3)	E2363	0(3)	E2625	0(3)
E0439	0(3)	E0641	0(3)	E0890	0(3)	E1020	0(3)	E1297	0(3)	E2000	0(3)	E2364	0(3)	E2626	0(3)
E0440	0(3)	E0642	0(3)	E0900	0(3)	E1028	0(3)	E1298	0(3)	E2100	0(3)	E2365	0(3)	E2627	0(3)
E0441	0(3)	E0650	0(3)	E0910	0(3)	E1029	0(3)	E1300	0(3)	E2101	0(3)	E2366	0(3)	E2628	0(3)
E0442	0(3)	E0651	0(3)	E0911	0(3)	E1030	0(3)	E1310	0(3)	E2120	0(3)	E2367	0(3)	E2629	0(3)
E0443	0(3)	E0652	0(3)	E0912	0(3)	E1031	0(3)	E1352	0(3)	E2201	0(3)	E2368	0(3)	E2630	0(3)
E0444	0(3)	E0655	0(3)	E0920	0(3)	E1035	0(3)	E1353	0(3)	E2202	0(3)	E2369	0(3)	E2631	0(3)
E0445	0(3)	E0656	0(3)	E0930	0(3)	E1036	0(3)	E1354	0(3)	E2203	0(3)	E2370	0(3)	E2632	0(3)

CPT	MUE
E2633	0(3)
E8000	0(3)
E8001	0(3)
E8002	0(3)
G0008	1(2)
G0009	1(2)
G0010	1(3)
G0027	1(2)
G0071	1(3)
G0076	1(3)
G0077	1(3)
G0078	1(3)
G0079	1(3)
G0080	1(3)
G0081	1(3)
G0082	1(3)
G0083	1(3)
G0084	1(3)
G0085	1(3)
G0086	1(3)
G0087	1(3)
G0101	1(2)
G0102	1(2)
G0103	1(2)
G0104	1(2)
G0105	1(2)
G0106	1(2)
G0108	6(3)
G0109	12(3)
G0117	1(2)
G0118	1(2)
G0120	1(2)
G0121	1(2)
G0122	0(3)
G0123	1(3)
G0124	1(3)
G0127	1(2)
G0128	1(3)
G0130	1(2)
G0141	1(3)
G0143	1(3)
G0144	1(3)
G0145	1(3)
G0147	1(3)
G0148	1(3)
G0166	2(3)
G0168	2(3)
G0175	1(3)
G0177	0(3)
G0179	1(2)
G0180	1(2)
G0181	1(2)
G0182	1(2)
G0186	1(2)
G0219	0(3)
G0235	1(3)
G0237	8(3)
G0238	8(3)
G0239	1(3)
G0245	1(2)
G0246	1(2)
G0247	1(2)
G0248	1(2)
G0249	3(3)
G0250	1(2)
G0252	0(3)

CPT	MUE
G0255	0(3)
G0257	0(3)
G0259	2(3)
G0260	2(3)
G0268	1(2)
G0269	0(3)
G0270	8(3)
G0271	4(3)
G0276	1(3)
G0277	5(3)
G0278	1(2)
G0279	1(2)
G0281	1(3)
G0282	0(3)
G0283	1(3)
G0288	1(2)
G0289	1(2)
G0293	1(2)
G0294	1(2)
G0295	0(3)
G0296	1(2)
G0302	1(2)
G0303	1(2)
G0304	1(2)
G0305	1(2)
G0306	1(3)
G0307	1(3)
G0328	1(2)
G0329	1(3)
G0333	0(3)
G0337	1(2)
G0339	1(2)
G0340	1(3)
G0341	1(2)
G0342	1(2)
G0343	1(2)
G0372	1(2)
G0378	0(3)
G0379	0(3)
G0380	0(3)
G0381	0(3)
G0382	0(3)
G0383	0(3)
G0384	0(3)
G0390	0(3)
G0396	1(2)
G0397	1(2)
G0398	1(2)
G0399	1(2)
G0400	1(2)
G0402	1(2)
G0403	1(2)
G0404	1(2)
G0405	1(2)
G0406	1(3)
G0407	1(3)
G0408	1(3)
G0410	4(3)
G0411	4(3)
G0412	1(2)
G0413	1(2)
G0414	1(2)
G0415	1(2)
G0416	1(2)
G0420	2(3)
G0421	2(3)

CPT	MUE
G0422	6(2)
G0423	6(2)
G0424	2(2)
G0425	1(3)
G0426	1(3)
G0427	1(3)
G0428	0(3)
G0429	1(2)
G0432	1(2)
G0433	1(2)
G0435	1(2)
G0438	1(2)
G0439	1(2)
G0442	1(2)
G0443	1(2)
G0444	1(2)
G0445	1(2)
G0446	1(3)
G0447	2(3)
G0448	1(3)
G0451	1(3)
G0452	6(3)
G0453	40(3)
G0454	1(2)
G0455	1(2)
G0458	1(3)
G0459	1(3)
G0460	1(3)
G0463	0(3)
G0466	1(2)
G0467	1(3)
G0468	1(2)
G0469	1(2)
G0470	1(3)
G0471	2(3)
G0472	1(2)
G0473	1(3)
G0475	1(2)
G0476	1(2)
G0480	1(2)
G0481	1(2)
G0482	1(2)
G0483	1(2)
G0490	1(3)
G0491	1(3)
G0492	1(3)
G0493	1(3)
G0494	1(3)
G0495	1(3)
G0496	1(3)
G0498	1(2)
G0499	1(2)
G0500	1(3)
G0501	0(3)
G0506	1(2)
G0508	1(2)
G0509	1(2)
G0511	1(2)
G0512	1(2)
G0513	1(2)
G0514	1(1)
G0516	1(2)
G0517	1(2)
G0518	1(2)
G0659	1(2)
G2000	1(3)

CPT	MUE
G2001	1(3)
G2002	1(3)
G2003	1(3)
G2004	1(3)
G2005	1(3)
G2006	1(3)
G2007	1(3)
G2008	1(3)
G2009	1(3)
G2010	1(3)
G2011	1(2)
G2012	1(3)
G2013	1(3)
G2014	1(3)
G2015	1(3)
G2023	2(3)
G2024	2(3)
G2025	1(3)
G2064	1(2)
G2065	1(2)
G2066	1(2)
G2067	1(2)
G2068	1(2)
G2069	1(2)
G2070	1(2)
G2071	1(2)
G2072	1(2)
G2073	1(2)
G2074	1(2)
G2075	1(2)
G2076	1(2)
G2078	3(3)
G2079	3(3)
G2081	1(2)
G2082	1(2)
G2083	1(2)
G2086	1(3)
G2087	2(3)
G2170	1(3)
G2171	1(3)
G2212	4(3)
G2213	1(2)
G2214	1(2)
G2250	1(2)
G2251	1(2)
G2252	1(2)
G6001	2(3)
G6002	2(3)
G6003	2(3)
G6004	2(3)
G6005	2(3)
G6006	2(3)
G6007	2(3)
G6008	2(3)
G6009	2(3)
G6010	2(3)
G6011	2(3)
G6012	2(3)
G6013	2(3)
G6014	2(3)
G6015	2(3)
G6016	2(3)
G6017	2(3)
G9143	1(2)
G9147	0(3)
G9148	1(3)

CPT	MUE
G9149	1(3)
G9150	1(3)
G9151	1(3)
G9152	1(3)
G9153	1(3)
G9156	1(2)
G9157	1(2)
G9187	1(3)
G9480	1(3)
G9481	1(3)
G9482	1(3)
G9483	1(3)
G9484	1(3)
G9485	1(3)
G9486	1(3)
G9487	1(3)
G9488	1(3)
G9489	1(3)
G9490	1(3)
G9678	1(2)
G9685	1(3)
G9978	1(3)
G9979	1(3)
G9980	1(3)
G9981	1(3)
G9982	1(3)
G9983	1(3)
G9984	1(3)
G9985	1(3)
G9986	1(3)
G9987	1(3)
J0120	1(3)
J0121	200(3)
J0122	300(3)
J0129	100(3)
J0130	4(3)
J0131	400(3)
J0132	12(3)
J0133	1200(3)
J0135	8(3)
J0153	180(3)
J0171	20(3)
J0178	4(2)
J0179	12(2)
J0180	140(3)
J0185	130(3)
J0190	0(3)
J0200	0(3)
J0202	12(3)
J0205	0(3)
J0207	4(3)
J0210	4(3)
J0215	30(3)
J0220	1(3)
J0221	250(3)
J0222	300(3)
J0223	756(3)
J0256	1600(3)
J0257	1400(3)
J0270	32(3)
J0275	1(3)
J0278	15(3)
J0280	7(3)
J0282	5(3)
J0285	5(3)
J0287	50(3)

CPT	MUE
J0288	0(3)
J0289	50(3)
J0290	24(3)
J0291	500(3)
J0295	12(3)
J0300	8(3)
J0330	10(3)
J0348	200(3)
J0350	0(3)
J0360	2(3)
J0364	6(3)
J0365	0(3)
J0380	1(3)
J0390	0(3)
J0395	0(3)
J0400	39(3)
J0401	400(3)
J0456	4(3)
J0461	200(3)
J0470	2(3)
J0475	8(3)
J0476	2(3)
J0480	1(3)
J0485	1500(3)
J0490	160(3)
J0500	4(3)
J0515	3(3)
J0517	30(3)
J0520	0(3)
J0558	24(3)
J0561	24(3)
J0565	200(3)
J0567	300(3)
J0570	4(3)
J0571	0(3)
J0572	0(3)
J0573	0(3)
J0574	0(3)
J0575	0(3)
J0583	250(3)
J0584	90(3)
J0585	600(3)
J0586	300(3)
J0587	300(3)
J0588	600(3)
J0591	100(3)
J0592	6(3)
J0593	300(3)
J0594	320(3)
J0595	8(3)
J0596	840(3)
J0597	250(3)
J0598	100(3)
J0599	900(3)
J0600	3(3)
J0606	150(3)
J0610	15(3)
J0620	1(3)
J0630	1(3)
J0636	100(3)
J0637	20(3)
J0638	300(3)
J0640	24(3)
J0641	1200(3)
J0642	1200(3)
J0670	10(3)

CPT	MUE
J0690	12(3)
J0691	300(3)
J0692	12(3)
J0693	1600(3)
J0694	8(3)
J0695	60(3)
J0696	16(3)
J0697	4(3)
J0698	10(3)
J0702	18(3)
J0706	1(3)
J0710	0(3)
J0712	120(3)
J0713	12(3)
J0714	12(3)
J0715	0(3)
J0716	4(3)
J0717	400(3)
J0720	15(3)
J0725	10(3)
J0735	50(3)
J0740	2(3)
J0742	500(3)
J0743	16(3)
J0744	6(3)
J0745	2(3)
J0770	5(3)
J0775	180(3)
J0780	4(3)
J0791	160(3)
J0795	100(3)
J0800	3(3)
J0834	3(3)
J0840	6(3)
J0841	20(3)
J0850	9(3)
J0875	300(3)
J0878	1500(3)
J0881	500(3)
J0882	300(3)
J0883	1125(3)
J0884	1125(3)
J0885	60(3)
J0887	360(3)
J0888	360(3)
J0890	0(3)
J0894	100(3)
J0895	12(3)
J0896	1100(3)
J0897	120(3)
J0945	4(3)
J1000	1(3)
J1020	8(3)
J1030	8(3)
J1040	4(3)
J1050	1000(3)
J1071	400(3)
J1094	0(3)
J1095	1034(2)
J1096	8(2)
J1097	4(3)
J1100	120(3)
J1110	3(3)
J1120	2(3)
J1130	300(3)
J1160	2(3)

CPT	MUE
J1162	1(3)
J1165	50(3)
J1170	350(3)
J1180	0(3)
J1190	8(3)
J1200	8(3)
J1201	20(3)
J1205	4(3)
J1212	1(3)
J1230	3(3)
J1240	6(3)
J1245	10(3)
J1250	2(3)
J1260	2(3)
J1265	20(3)
J1267	150(3)
J1270	8(3)
J1290	30(3)
J1300	120(3)
J1301	60(3)
J1303	360(3)
J1320	0(3)
J1322	150(3)
J1324	108(3)
J1325	1(3)
J1327	1(3)
J1330	1(3)
J1335	2(3)
J1364	2(3)
J1380	4(3)
J1410	4(3)
J1428	450(3)
J1429	450(3)
J1430	10(3)
J1435	1(3)
J1436	0(3)
J1437	100(3)
J1438	2(3)
J1439	750(3)
J1442	1500(3)
J1443	272(3)
J1444	272(3)
J1447	960(3)
J1450	4(3)
J1451	1(3)
J1452	0(3)
J1453	150(3)
J1454	1(3)
J1455	18(3)
J1457	0(3)
J1458	100(3)
J1459	300(3)
J1460	10(2)
J1554	240(3)
J1555	480(3)
J1556	300(3)
J1557	300(3)
J1558	480(3)
J1559	300(3)
J1560	1(2)
J1561	300(3)
J1562	0(3)
J1566	300(3)
J1568	300(3)
J1569	300(3)
J1570	4(3)

CPT	MUE
J1571	20(3)
J1572	300(3)
J1573	130(3)
J1575	650(3)
J1580	9(3)
J1595	1(3)
J1599	300(3)
J1600	2(3)
J1602	300(3)
J1610	2(3)
J1620	0(3)
J1626	30(3)
J1627	100(3)
J1628	100(3)
J1630	5(3)
J1631	9(3)
J1632	700(3)
J1640	672(3)
J1642	100(3)
J1644	40(3)
J1645	10(3)
J1650	30(3)
J1652	20(3)
J1655	0(3)
J1670	1(3)
J1675	0(3)
J1700	0(3)
J1710	0(3)
J1720	10(3)
J1726	28(3)
J1729	25(3)
J1730	0(3)
J1738	30(3)
J1740	3(3)
J1741	8(3)
J1742	2(3)
J1743	66(3)
J1744	30(3)
J1745	150(3)
J1746	200(3)
J1750	45(3)
J1756	500(3)
J1786	680(3)
J1790	2(3)
J1800	6(3)
J1810	0(3)
J1815	8(3)
J1817	0(3)
J1823	300(3)
J1826	1(3)
J1830	1(3)
J1833	372(3)
J1835	0(3)
J1840	3(3)
J1850	4(3)
J1885	8(3)
J1890	0(3)
J1930	120(3)
J1931	377(3)
J1940	6(3)
J1943	675(3)
J1944	1064(3)
J1945	0(3)
J1950	12(3)
J1953	300(3)
J1955	11(3)

CPT	MUE
J1956	4(3)
J1960	0(3)
J1980	2(3)
J1990	0(3)
J2001	60(3)
J2010	10(3)
J2020	6(3)
J2060	4(3)
J2062	10(3)
J2150	8(3)
J2170	8(3)
J2175	4(3)
J2180	0(3)
J2182	300(3)
J2185	60(3)
J2186	600(3)
J2210	1(3)
J2212	240(3)
J2248	150(3)
J2250	22(3)
J2260	4(3)
J2265	400(3)
J2270	9(3)
J2274	250(3)
J2278	1000(3)
J2280	4(3)
J2300	4(3)
J2310	4(3)
J2315	380(3)
J2320	4(3)
J2323	300(3)
J2325	0(3)
J2326	120(3)
J2350	600(3)
J2353	60(3)
J2354	60(3)
J2355	2(3)
J2357	120(3)
J2358	405(3)
J2360	2(3)
J2370	2(3)
J2400	4(3)
J2405	64(3)
J2407	120(3)
J2410	2(3)
J2425	125(3)
J2426	819(3)
J2430	3(3)
J2440	4(3)
J2460	0(3)
J2469	10(3)
J2501	2(3)
J2502	60(3)
J2503	2(3)
J2504	15(3)
J2505	1(3)
J2507	8(3)
J2510	4(3)
J2513	1(3)
J2515	1(3)
J2540	75(3)
J2543	16(3)
J2545	1(3)
J2547	600(3)
J2550	3(3)
J2560	1(3)

CPT	MUE
J2562	48(3)
J2590	3(3)
J2597	45(3)
J2650	0(3)
J2670	0(3)
J2675	1(3)
J2680	4(3)
J2690	4(3)
J2700	48(3)
J2704	80(3)
J2710	2(3)
J2720	5(3)
J2724	3500(3)
J2725	0(3)
J2730	2(3)
J2760	2(3)
J2765	10(3)
J2770	6(3)
J2778	10(2)
J2780	16(3)
J2783	60(3)
J2785	4(3)
J2786	500(3)
J2787	2(3)
J2788	1(3)
J2790	1(3)
J2791	15(3)
J2792	450(3)
J2793	320(3)
J2794	100(3)
J2795	200(3)
J2796	150(3)
J2797	333(3)
J2798	240(3)
J2800	3(3)
J2805	3(3)
J2810	5(3)
J2820	15(3)
J2840	160(3)
J2850	16(3)
J2860	170(3)
J2910	0(3)
J2916	20(3)
J2920	25(3)
J2930	25(3)
J2940	0(3)
J2941	8(3)
J2950	0(3)
J2993	2(3)
J2995	0(3)
J2997	8(3)
J3000	2(3)
J3010	100(3)
J3030	1(3)
J3031	675(3)
J3032	300(3)
J3060	760(3)
J3070	3(3)
J3090	200(3)
J3095	150(3)
J3101	50(3)
J3105	2(3)
J3110	2(3)
J3111	210(3)
J3121	400(3)
J3145	750(3)

CPT	MUE
J3230	2(3)
J3240	1(3)
J3241	300(3)
J3243	150(3)
J3245	100(3)
J3246	1(3)
J3250	2(3)
J3260	8(3)
J3262	800(3)
J3265	0(3)
J3280	0(3)
J3285	1(3)
J3300	160(3)
J3301	16(3)
J3302	0(3)
J3303	24(3)
J3304	64(2)
J3305	0(3)
J3310	0(3)
J3315	6(3)
J3316	6(3)
J3320	0(3)
J3350	0(3)
J3355	1(3)
J3357	90(3)
J3358	520(3)
J3360	6(3)
J3364	0(3)
J3365	0(3)
J3370	12(3)
J3380	300(3)
J3385	80(3)
J3396	150(3)
J3397	600(3)
J3398	150(2)
J3399	1(3)
J3400	0(3)
J3410	8(3)
J3411	4(3)
J3415	6(3)
J3420	1(3)
J3430	25(3)
J3465	40(3)
J3470	3(3)
J3471	999(1)
J3472	2(3)
J3473	450(3)
J3475	20(3)
J3480	40(3)
J3485	160(3)
J3486	4(3)
J3489	5(3)
J3520	0(3)
J3530	0(3)
J3535	0(3)
J3570	0(3)
J7030	5(3)
J7040	6(3)
J7042	6(3)
J7050	10(3)
J7060	10(3)
J7070	4(3)
J7100	2(3)
J7110	2(3)
J7120	4(3)
J7121	4(3)

CPT	MUE
J7131	500(3)
J7169	180(3)
J7170	1800(3)
J7175	9000(1)
J7177	10500(3)
J7178	7700(1)
J7179	7500(1)
J7180	6000(1)
J7181	3850(1)
J7182	22000(1)
J7183	7500(1)
J7185	22000(1)
J7186	7500(1)
J7187	7500(1)
J7188	22000(1)
J7189	13000(1)
J7190	22000(1)
J7191	0(3)
J7192	22000(1)
J7193	4000(1)
J7194	9000(1)
J7195	6000(1)
J7196	175(3)
J7197	6300(1)
J7198	6000(1)
J7200	20000(1)
J7201	9000(1)
J7202	11550(1)
J7203	12000(1)
J7204	19500(1)
J7205	9750(1)
J7207	22500(1)
J7208	12000(1)
J7209	7500(1)
J7210	22000(1)
J7211	22000(1)
J7212	90000(1)
J7296	0(3)
J7297	0(3)
J7298	0(3)
J7300	0(3)
J7301	0(3)
J7303	0(3)
J7304	0(3)
J7306	0(3)
J7307	0(3)
J7308	3(3)
J7309	1(3)
J7310	0(3)
J7311	118(2)
J7312	14(2)
J7313	38(2)
J7314	36(2)
J7315	2(3)
J7316	3(3)
J7318	120(3)
J7320	50(3)
J7321	2(2)
J7322	48(3)
J7323	2(2)
J7324	2(2)
J7325	96(3)
J7326	2(2)
J7327	2(2)
J7328	336(3)
J7329	50(2)

CPT	MUE
J7330	1(3)
J7331	40(3)
J7332	40(3)
J7336	1120(3)
J7340	1(3)
J7342	10(3)
J7345	200(3)
J7351	20(2)
J7352	16(3)
J7500	0(3)
J7501	1(3)
J7502	0(3)
J7503	0(3)
J7504	15(3)
J7505	1(3)
J7507	0(3)
J7508	0(3)
J7509	0(3)
J7510	0(3)
J7511	9(3)
J7512	0(3)
J7513	0(3)
J7515	0(3)
J7516	1(3)
J7517	0(3)
J7518	0(3)
J7520	0(3)
J7525	2(3)
J7527	0(3)
J7599	1(3)
J7604	0(3)
J7605	2(3)
J7606	2(3)
J7607	0(3)
J7608	3(3)
J7609	0(3)
J7610	0(3)
J7611	10(3)
J7612	10(3)
J7613	10(3)
J7614	10(3)
J7615	0(3)
J7620	6(3)
J7622	0(3)
J7624	0(3)
J7626	2(3)
J7627	0(3)
J7628	0(3)
J7629	0(3)
J7631	4(3)
J7632	0(3)
J7633	0(3)
J7634	0(3)
J7635	0(3)
J7636	0(3)
J7637	0(3)
J7638	0(3)
J7639	3(3)
J7640	0(3)
J7641	0(3)
J7642	0(3)
J7643	0(3)
J7644	3(3)
J7645	0(3)
J7647	0(3)
J7648	0(3)

CPT	MUE
J7649	0(3)
J7650	0(3)
J7657	0(3)
J7658	0(3)
J7659	0(3)
J7660	0(3)
J7665	0(3)
J7667	0(3)
J7668	0(3)
J7669	0(3)
J7670	0(3)
J7674	100(3)
J7676	0(3)
J7677	175(3)
J7680	0(3)
J7681	0(3)
J7682	2(3)
J7683	0(3)
J7684	0(3)
J7685	0(3)
J7686	1(3)
J7699	1(3)
J7799	2(3)
J7999	2(3)
J8498	0(3)
J8499	0(3)
J8501	0(3)
J8510	0(3)
J8515	0(3)
J8520	0(3)
J8521	0(3)
J8530	0(3)
J8540	0(3)
J8560	0(3)
J8562	0(3)
J8565	0(3)
J8597	0(3)
J8600	0(3)
J8610	0(3)
J8650	0(3)
J8655	1(3)
J8670	0(3)
J8700	0(3)
J8705	0(3)
J8999	0(3)
J9000	20(3)
J9015	1(3)
J9017	30(3)
J9019	60(3)
J9020	0(3)
J9022	168(3)
J9023	140(3)
J9025	300(3)
J9027	100(3)
J9030	50(3)
J9032	300(3)
J9033	300(3)
J9034	360(3)
J9035	180(3)
J9036	360(3)
J9039	210(3)
J9040	4(3)
J9041	35(3)
J9042	200(3)
J9043	60(3)
J9044	35(3)

CPT	MUE
J9045	22(3)
J9047	160(3)
J9050	6(3)
J9055	150(3)
J9057	60(3)
J9060	24(3)
J9065	100(3)
J9070	55(3)
J9098	5(3)
J9100	120(3)
J9118	750(3)
J9119	350(3)
J9120	5(3)
J9130	24(3)
J9144	180(3)
J9145	240(3)
J9150	12(3)
J9151	12(3)
J9153	132(3)
J9155	240(3)
J9160	7(3)
J9165	0(3)
J9171	240(3)
J9173	150(3)
J9175	10(3)
J9176	3000(3)
J9177	520(3)
J9178	150(3)
J9179	50(3)
J9181	100(3)
J9185	2(3)
J9190	20(3)
J9198	38(3)
J9200	5(3)
J9201	20(3)
J9202	3(3)
J9203	180(3)
J9204	160(3)
J9205	215(3)
J9206	42(3)
J9207	90(3)
J9208	15(3)
J9209	55(3)
J9210	1500(3)
J9211	6(3)
J9212	0(3)
J9213	12(3)
J9214	100(3)
J9215	0(3)
J9216	2(3)
J9217	6(3)
J9218	1(3)
J9219	1(3)
J9223	120(3)
J9225	1(3)
J9226	1(3)
J9227	150(3)
J9228	1100(3)
J9229	27(3)
J9230	5(3)
J9245	9(3)
J9246	300(3)
J9250	25(3)
J9260	20(3)
J9261	80(3)
J9262	700(3)

CPT	MUE
J9263	700(3)
J9264	600(3)
J9266	2(3)
J9267	750(3)
J9268	1(3)
J9269	200(3)
J9270	0(3)
J9271	400(3)
J9280	12(3)
J9281	80(3)
J9285	200(3)
J9293	8(3)
J9295	800(3)
J9299	480(3)
J9301	100(3)
J9302	200(3)
J9303	90(3)
J9304	150(3)
J9305	150(3)
J9306	840(3)
J9307	60(3)
J9308	280(3)
J9309	280(3)
J9311	160(3)
J9312	150(3)
J9313	600(3)
J9315	40(3)
J9316	120(3)
J9317	648(3)
J9320	4(3)
J9325	400(3)
J9328	400(3)
J9330	50(3)
J9340	4(3)
J9351	120(3)
J9352	40(3)
J9354	600(3)
J9355	105(3)
J9356	60(3)
J9357	4(3)
J9358	900(3)
J9360	40(3)
J9370	4(3)
J9371	5(3)
J9390	36(3)
J9395	20(3)
J9400	500(3)
J9600	4(3)
K0001	0(3)
K0002	0(3)
K0003	0(3)
K0004	0(3)
K0005	0(3)
K0006	0(3)
K0007	0(3)
K0008	0(3)
K0009	0(3)
K0010	0(3)
K0011	0(3)
K0012	0(3)
K0013	0(3)
K0014	0(3)
K0015	0(3)
K0017	0(3)
K0018	0(3)
K0019	0(3)

CPT	MUE
K0020	0(3)
K0037	0(3)
K0038	0(3)
K0039	0(3)
K0040	0(3)
K0041	0(3)
K0042	0(3)
K0043	0(3)
K0044	0(3)
K0045	0(3)
K0046	0(3)
K0047	0(3)
K0050	0(3)
K0051	0(3)
K0052	0(3)
K0053	0(3)
K0056	0(3)
K0065	0(3)
K0069	0(3)
K0070	0(3)
K0071	0(3)
K0072	0(3)
K0073	0(3)
K0077	0(3)
K0098	0(3)
K0105	0(3)
K0108	0(3)
K0195	0(3)
K0455	0(3)
K0462	0(3)
K0553	0(3)
K0554	0(3)
K0602	0(3)
K0604	0(3)
K0605	0(3)
K0606	0(3)
K0607	0(3)
K0608	0(3)
K0609	0(3)
K0669	0(3)
K0672	0(3)
K0730	0(3)
K0733	0(3)
K0738	0(3)
K0740	0(3)
K0743	0(3)
K0744	0(3)
K0745	0(3)
K0746	0(3)
K0800	0(3)
K0801	0(3)
K0802	0(3)
K0806	0(3)
K0807	0(3)
K0808	0(3)
K0812	0(3)
K0813	0(3)
K0814	0(3)
K0815	0(3)
K0816	0(3)
K0820	0(3)
K0821	0(3)
K0822	0(3)
K0823	0(3)
K0824	0(3)
K0825	0(3)

CPT	MUE
K0826	0(3)
K0827	0(3)
K0828	0(3)
K0829	0(3)
K0830	0(3)
K0831	0(3)
K0835	0(3)
K0836	0(3)
K0837	0(3)
K0838	0(3)
K0839	0(3)
K0840	0(3)
K0841	0(3)
K0842	0(3)
K0843	0(3)
K0848	0(3)
K0849	0(3)
K0850	0(3)
K0851	0(3)
K0852	0(3)
K0853	0(3)
K0854	0(3)
K0855	0(3)
K0856	0(3)
K0857	0(3)
K0858	0(3)
K0859	0(3)
K0860	0(3)
K0861	0(3)
K0862	0(3)
K0863	0(3)
K0864	0(3)
K0868	0(3)
K0869	0(3)
K0870	0(3)
K0871	0(3)
K0877	0(3)
K0878	0(3)
K0879	0(3)
K0880	0(3)
K0884	0(3)
K0885	0(3)
K0886	0(3)
K0890	0(3)
K0891	0(3)
K0898	1(2)
K0899	0(3)
K0900	0(3)
K1001	1(3)
K1002	1(3)
K1003	1(3)
K1004	1(3)
K1005	1(3)
K1006	1(2)
K1007	1(2)
K1009	1(2)
K1013	1(3)
K1014	1(3)
K1015	2(2)
K1016	1(2)
K1017	3(2)
K1018	1(2)
K1019	3(2)
K1020	1(2)
L0112	0(3)
L0113	0(3)

CPT	MUE
L0120	0(3)
L0130	0(3)
L0140	0(3)
L0150	0(3)
L0160	0(3)
L0170	0(3)
L0172	0(3)
L0174	0(3)
L0180	0(3)
L0190	0(3)
L0200	0(3)
L0220	0(3)
L0450	0(3)
L0452	0(3)
L0454	0(3)
L0455	0(3)
L0456	0(3)
L0457	0(3)
L0458	0(3)
L0460	0(3)
L0462	0(3)
L0464	0(3)
L0466	0(3)
L0467	0(3)
L0468	0(3)
L0469	0(3)
L0470	0(3)
L0472	0(3)
L0480	0(3)
L0482	0(3)
L0484	0(3)
L0486	0(3)
L0488	0(3)
L0490	0(3)
L0491	0(3)
L0492	0(3)
L0621	0(3)
L0622	0(3)
L0623	0(3)
L0624	0(3)
L0625	0(3)
L0626	0(3)
L0627	0(3)
L0628	0(3)
L0629	0(3)
L0630	0(3)
L0631	0(3)
L0632	0(3)
L0633	0(3)
L0634	0(3)
L0635	0(3)
L0636	0(3)
L0637	0(3)
L0638	0(3)
L0639	0(3)
L0640	0(3)
L0641	0(3)
L0642	0(3)
L0643	0(3)
L0648	0(3)
L0649	0(3)
L0650	0(3)
L0651	0(3)
L0700	0(3)
L0710	0(3)
L0810	0(3)

CPT	MUE
L0820	0(3)
L0830	0(3)
L0859	0(3)
L0861	0(3)
L0970	0(3)
L0972	0(3)
L0974	0(3)
L0976	0(3)
L0978	0(3)
L0980	0(3)
L0982	0(3)
L0984	0(3)
L0999	0(3)
L1000	0(3)
L1001	0(3)
L1005	0(3)
L1010	0(3)
L1020	0(3)
L1025	0(3)
L1030	0(3)
L1040	0(3)
L1050	0(3)
L1060	0(3)
L1070	0(3)
L1080	0(3)
L1085	0(3)
L1090	0(3)
L1100	0(3)
L1110	0(3)
L1120	0(3)
L1200	0(3)
L1210	0(3)
L1220	0(3)
L1230	0(3)
L1240	0(3)
L1250	0(3)
L1260	0(3)
L1270	0(3)
L1280	0(3)
L1290	0(3)
L1300	0(3)
L1310	0(3)
L1499	1(3)
L1600	0(3)
L1610	0(3)
L1620	0(3)
L1630	0(3)
L1640	0(3)
L1650	0(3)
L1652	0(3)
L1660	0(3)
L1680	0(3)
L1685	0(3)
L1686	0(3)
L1690	0(3)
L1700	0(3)
L1710	0(3)
L1720	0(3)
L1730	0(3)
L1755	0(3)
L1810	0(3)
L1812	0(3)
L1820	0(3)
L1830	0(3)
L1831	0(3)
L1832	0(3)

CPT	MUE
L1833	0(3)
L1834	0(3)
L1836	0(3)
L1840	0(3)
L1843	0(3)
L1844	0(3)
L1845	0(3)
L1846	0(3)
L1847	0(3)
L1848	0(3)
L1850	0(3)
L1851	0(3)
L1852	0(3)
L1860	0(3)
L1900	0(3)
L1902	0(3)
L1904	0(3)
L1906	0(3)
L1907	0(3)
L1910	0(3)
L1920	0(3)
L1930	0(3)
L1932	0(3)
L1940	0(3)
L1945	0(3)
L1950	0(3)
L1951	0(3)
L1960	0(3)
L1970	0(3)
L1971	0(3)
L1980	0(3)
L1990	0(3)
L2000	0(3)
L2005	0(3)
L2006	0(3)
L2010	0(3)
L2020	0(3)
L2030	0(3)
L2034	0(3)
L2035	0(3)
L2036	0(3)
L2037	0(3)
L2038	0(3)
L2040	0(3)
L2050	0(3)
L2060	0(3)
L2070	0(3)
L2080	0(3)
L2090	0(3)
L2106	0(3)
L2108	0(3)
L2112	0(3)
L2114	0(3)
L2116	0(3)
L2126	0(3)
L2128	0(3)
L2132	0(3)
L2134	0(3)
L2136	0(3)
L2180	0(3)
L2182	0(3)
L2184	0(3)
L2186	0(3)
L2188	0(3)
L2190	0(3)
L2192	0(3)

CPT	MUE
L2200	0(3)
L2210	0(3)
L2220	0(3)
L2230	0(3)
L2232	0(3)
L2240	0(3)
L2250	0(3)
L2260	0(3)
L2265	0(3)
L2270	0(3)
L2275	0(3)
L2280	0(3)
L2300	0(3)
L2310	0(3)
L2320	0(3)
L2330	0(3)
L2335	0(3)
L2340	0(3)
L2350	0(3)
L2360	0(3)
L2370	0(3)
L2375	0(3)
L2380	0(3)
L2385	0(3)
L2387	0(3)
L2390	0(3)
L2395	0(3)
L2397	0(3)
L2405	0(3)
L2415	0(3)
L2425	0(3)
L2430	0(3)
L2492	0(3)
L2500	0(3)
L2510	0(3)
L2520	0(3)
L2525	0(3)
L2526	0(3)
L2530	0(3)
L2540	0(3)
L2550	0(3)
L2570	0(3)
L2580	0(3)
L2600	0(3)
L2610	0(3)
L2620	0(3)
L2622	0(3)
L2624	0(3)
L2627	0(3)
L2628	0(3)
L2630	0(3)
L2640	0(3)
L2650	0(3)
L2660	0(3)
L2670	0(3)
L2680	0(3)
L2750	0(3)
L2755	0(3)
L2760	0(3)
L2768	0(3)
L2780	0(3)
L2785	0(3)
L2795	0(3)
L2800	0(3)
L2810	0(3)
L2820	0(3)

CPT	MUE
L2830	0(3)
L2840	0(3)
L2850	0(3)
L2861	0(3)
L2999	0(3)
L3000	0(3)
L3001	0(3)
L3002	0(3)
L3003	0(3)
L3010	0(3)
L3020	0(3)
L3030	0(3)
L3031	0(3)
L3040	0(3)
L3050	0(3)
L3060	0(3)
L3070	0(3)
L3080	0(3)
L3090	0(3)
L3100	0(3)
L3140	0(3)
L3150	0(3)
L3160	0(3)
L3170	0(3)
L3201	0(3)
L3202	0(3)
L3203	0(3)
L3204	0(3)
L3206	0(3)
L3207	0(3)
L3208	0(3)
L3209	0(3)
L3211	0(3)
L3212	0(3)
L3213	0(3)
L3214	0(3)
L3215	0(3)
L3216	0(3)
L3217	0(3)
L3219	0(3)
L3221	0(3)
L3222	0(3)
L3224	0(3)
L3225	0(3)
L3230	0(3)
L3250	0(3)
L3251	0(3)
L3252	0(3)
L3253	0(3)
L3254	0(3)
L3255	0(3)
L3257	0(3)
L3260	0(3)
L3265	0(3)
L3300	0(3)
L3310	0(3)
L3320	0(3)
L3330	0(3)
L3332	0(3)
L3334	0(3)
L3340	0(3)
L3350	0(3)
L3360	0(3)
L3370	0(3)
L3380	0(3)
L3390	0(3)

CPT	MUE
L3400	0(3)
L3410	0(3)
L3420	0(3)
L3430	0(3)
L3440	0(3)
L3450	0(3)
L3455	0(3)
L3460	0(3)
L3465	0(3)
L3470	0(3)
L3480	0(3)
L3485	0(3)
L3500	0(3)
L3510	0(3)
L3520	0(3)
L3530	0(3)
L3540	0(3)
L3550	0(3)
L3560	0(3)
L3570	0(3)
L3580	0(3)
L3590	0(3)
L3595	0(3)
L3600	0(3)
L3610	0(3)
L3620	0(3)
L3630	0(3)
L3640	0(3)
L3649	0(3)
L3650	0(3)
L3660	0(3)
L3670	0(3)
L3671	0(3)
L3674	0(3)
L3675	0(3)
L3677	0(3)
L3678	0(3)
L3702	0(3)
L3710	0(3)
L3720	0(3)
L3730	0(3)
L3740	0(3)
L3760	0(3)
L3761	0(3)
L3762	0(3)
L3763	0(3)
L3764	0(3)
L3765	0(3)
L3766	0(3)
L3806	0(3)
L3807	0(3)
L3808	0(3)
L3809	0(3)
L3891	0(3)
L3900	0(3)
L3901	0(3)
L3904	0(3)
L3905	0(3)
L3906	0(3)
L3908	0(3)
L3912	0(3)
L3913	0(3)
L3915	0(3)
L3916	0(3)
L3917	0(3)
L3918	0(3)

CPT	MUE
L3919	0(3)
L3921	0(3)
L3923	0(3)
L3924	0(3)
L3925	0(3)
L3927	0(3)
L3929	0(3)
L3930	0(3)
L3931	0(3)
L3933	0(3)
L3935	0(3)
L3956	0(3)
L3960	0(3)
L3961	0(3)
L3962	0(3)
L3967	0(3)
L3971	0(3)
L3973	0(3)
L3975	0(3)
L3976	0(3)
L3977	0(3)
L3978	0(3)
L3980	0(3)
L3981	0(3)
L3982	0(3)
L3984	0(3)
L3995	0(3)
L3999	0(3)
L4000	0(3)
L4002	0(3)
L4010	0(3)
L4020	0(3)
L4030	0(3)
L4040	0(3)
L4045	0(3)
L4050	0(3)
L4055	0(3)
L4060	0(3)
L4070	0(3)
L4080	0(3)
L4090	0(3)
L4100	0(3)
L4110	0(3)
L4130	0(3)
L4205	0(3)
L4210	0(3)
L4350	0(3)
L4360	0(3)
L4361	0(3)
L4370	0(3)
L4386	0(3)
L4387	0(3)
L4392	0(3)
L4394	0(3)
L4396	0(3)
L4397	0(3)
L4398	0(3)
L4631	0(3)
L5000	0(3)
L5010	0(3)
L5020	0(3)
L5050	0(3)
L5060	0(3)
L5100	0(3)
L5105	0(3)
L5150	0(3)

CPT	MUE
L5160	0(3)
L5200	0(3)
L5210	0(3)
L5220	0(3)
L5230	0(3)
L5250	0(3)
L5270	0(3)
L5280	0(3)
L5301	0(3)
L5312	0(3)
L5321	0(3)
L5331	0(3)
L5341	0(3)
L5400	0(3)
L5410	0(3)
L5420	0(3)
L5430	0(3)
L5450	0(3)
L5460	0(3)
L5500	0(3)
L5505	0(3)
L5510	0(3)
L5520	0(3)
L5530	0(3)
L5535	0(3)
L5540	0(3)
L5560	0(3)
L5570	0(3)
L5580	0(3)
L5585	0(3)
L5590	0(3)
L5595	0(3)
L5600	0(3)
L5610	0(3)
L5611	0(3)
L5613	0(3)
L5614	0(3)
L5616	0(3)
L5617	0(3)
L5618	0(3)
L5620	0(3)
L5622	0(3)
L5624	0(3)
L5626	0(3)
L5628	0(3)
L5629	0(3)
L5630	0(3)
L5631	0(3)
L5632	0(3)
L5634	0(3)
L5636	0(3)
L5637	0(3)
L5638	0(3)
L5639	0(3)
L5640	0(3)
L5642	0(3)
L5643	0(3)
L5644	0(3)
L5645	0(3)
L5646	0(3)
L5647	0(3)
L5648	0(3)
L5649	0(3)
L5650	0(3)
L5651	0(3)
L5652	0(3)

CPT	MUE
L5653	0(3)
L5654	0(3)
L5655	0(3)
L5656	0(3)
L5658	0(3)
L5661	0(3)
L5665	0(3)
L5666	0(3)
L5668	0(3)
L5670	0(3)
L5671	0(3)
L5672	0(3)
L5673	0(3)
L5676	0(3)
L5677	0(3)
L5678	0(3)
L5679	0(3)
L5680	0(3)
L5681	0(3)
L5682	0(3)
L5683	0(3)
L5684	0(3)
L5685	0(3)
L5686	0(3)
L5688	0(3)
L5690	0(3)
L5692	0(3)
L5694	0(3)
L5695	0(3)
L5696	0(3)
L5697	0(3)
L5698	0(3)
L5699	0(3)
L5700	0(3)
L5701	0(3)
L5702	0(3)
L5703	0(3)
L5704	0(3)
L5705	0(3)
L5706	0(3)
L5707	0(3)
L5710	0(3)
L5711	0(3)
L5712	0(3)
L5714	0(3)
L5716	0(3)
L5718	0(3)
L5722	0(3)
L5724	0(3)
L5726	0(3)
L5728	0(3)
L5780	0(3)
L5781	0(3)
L5782	0(3)
L5785	0(3)
L5790	0(3)
L5795	0(3)
L5810	0(3)
L5811	0(3)
L5812	0(3)
L5814	0(3)
L5816	0(3)
L5818	0(3)
L5822	0(3)
L5824	0(3)
L5826	0(3)

CPT	MUE
L5828	0(3)
L5830	0(3)
L5840	0(3)
L5845	0(3)
L5848	0(3)
L5850	0(3)
L5855	0(3)
L5856	0(3)
L5857	0(3)
L5858	0(3)
L5859	0(3)
L5910	0(3)
L5920	0(3)
L5925	0(3)
L5930	0(3)
L5940	0(3)
L5950	0(3)
L5960	0(3)
L5961	0(3)
L5962	0(3)
L5964	0(3)
L5966	0(3)
L5968	0(3)
L5969	0(3)
L5970	0(3)
L5971	0(3)
L5972	0(3)
L5973	0(3)
L5974	0(3)
L5975	0(3)
L5976	0(3)
L5978	0(3)
L5979	0(3)
L5980	0(3)
L5981	0(3)
L5982	0(3)
L5984	0(3)
L5985	0(3)
L5986	0(3)
L5987	0(3)
L5988	0(3)
L5990	0(3)
L5999	0(3)
L6000	0(3)
L6010	0(3)
L6020	0(3)
L6026	0(3)
L6050	0(3)
L6055	0(3)
L6100	0(3)
L6110	0(3)
L6120	0(3)
L6130	0(3)
L6200	0(3)
L6205	0(3)
L6250	0(3)
L6300	0(3)
L6310	0(3)
L6320	0(3)
L6350	0(3)
L6360	0(3)
L6370	0(3)
L6380	0(3)
L6382	0(3)
L6384	0(3)
L6386	0(3)

CPT	MUE
L6388	0(3)
L6400	0(3)
L6450	0(3)
L6500	0(3)
L6550	0(3)
L6570	0(3)
L6580	0(3)
L6582	0(3)
L6584	0(3)
L6586	0(3)
L6588	0(3)
L6590	0(3)
L6600	0(3)
L6605	0(3)
L6610	0(3)
L6611	0(3)
L6615	0(3)
L6616	0(3)
L6620	0(3)
L6621	0(3)
L6623	0(3)
L6624	0(3)
L6625	0(3)
L6628	0(3)
L6629	0(3)
L6630	0(3)
L6632	0(3)
L6635	0(3)
L6637	0(3)
L6638	0(3)
L6640	0(3)
L6641	0(3)
L6642	0(3)
L6645	0(3)
L6646	0(3)
L6647	0(3)
L6648	0(3)
L6650	0(3)
L6655	0(3)
L6660	0(3)
L6665	0(3)
L6670	0(3)
L6672	0(3)
L6675	0(3)
L6676	0(3)
L6677	0(3)
L6680	0(3)
L6682	0(3)
L6684	0(3)
L6686	0(3)
L6687	0(3)
L6688	0(3)
L6689	0(3)
L6690	0(3)
L6691	0(3)
L6692	0(3)
L6693	0(3)
L6694	0(3)
L6695	0(3)
L6696	0(3)
L6697	0(3)
L6698	0(3)
L6703	0(3)
L6704	0(3)
L6706	0(3)
L6707	0(3)

CPT	MUE
L6708	0(3)
L6709	0(3)
L6711	0(3)
L6712	0(3)
L6713	0(3)
L6714	0(3)
L6715	0(3)
L6721	0(3)
L6722	0(3)
L6805	0(3)
L6810	0(3)
L6880	0(3)
L6881	0(3)
L6882	0(3)
L6883	0(3)
L6884	0(3)
L6885	0(3)
L6890	0(3)
L6895	0(3)
L6900	0(3)
L6905	0(3)
L6910	0(3)
L6915	0(3)
L6920	0(3)
L6925	0(3)
L6930	0(3)
L6935	0(3)
L6940	0(3)
L6945	0(3)
L6950	0(3)
L6955	0(3)
L6960	0(3)
L6965	0(3)
L6970	0(3)
L6975	0(3)
L7007	0(3)
L7008	0(3)
L7009	0(3)
L7040	0(3)
L7045	0(3)
L7170	0(3)
L7180	0(3)
L7181	0(3)
L7185	0(3)
L7186	0(3)
L7190	0(3)
L7191	0(3)
L7259	0(3)
L7360	0(3)
L7362	0(3)
L7364	0(3)
L7366	0(3)
L7367	0(3)
L7368	0(3)
L7400	0(3)
L7401	0(3)
L7402	0(3)
L7403	0(3)
L7404	0(3)
L7405	0(3)
L7499	0(3)
L7510	4(3)
L7600	0(3)
L7700	0(3)
L7900	0(3)
L7902	0(3)

CPT	MUE
L8000	0(3)
L8001	0(3)
L8002	0(3)
L8010	0(3)
L8015	0(3)
L8020	0(3)
L8030	0(3)
L8031	0(3)
L8032	0(3)
L8033	0(3)
L8035	0(3)
L8039	0(3)
L8040	0(3)
L8041	0(3)
L8042	0(3)
L8043	0(3)
L8044	0(3)
L8045	0(3)
L8046	0(3)
L8047	0(3)
L8048	1(3)
L8049	0(3)
L8300	0(3)
L8310	0(3)
L8320	0(3)
L8330	0(3)
L8400	0(3)
L8410	0(3)
L8415	0(3)
L8417	0(3)
L8420	0(3)
L8430	0(3)
L8435	0(3)
L8440	0(3)
L8460	0(3)
L8465	0(3)
L8470	0(3)
L8480	0(3)
L8485	0(3)
L8499	1(3)
L8500	0(3)
L8501	0(3)
L8505	0(3)
L8507	0(3)
L8509	1(3)
L8510	0(3)
L8511	1(3)
L8512	1(3)
L8513	1(3)
L8514	1(3)
L8515	1(3)
L8600	2(3)
L8603	4(3)
L8604	3(3)
L8605	4(3)
L8606	5(3)
L8607	20(3)
L8609	1(3)
L8610	1(3)
L8612	1(3)
L8613	1(3)
L8614	1(3)
L8615	2(3)
L8616	2(3)
L8617	2(3)
L8618	2(3)

CPT	MUE
L8619	2(3)
L8621	360(3)
L8622	2(3)
L8625	1(3)
L8627	2(2)
L8628	2(2)
L8629	2(2)
L8631	1(3)
L8641	4(3)
L8642	2(3)
L8658	2(3)
L8659	2(3)
L8670	2(3)
L8679	1(3)
L8681	1(3)
L8682	2(3)
L8683	1(3)
L8684	1(3)
L8685	1(3)
L8686	2(3)
L8687	1(3)
L8688	1(3)
L8689	1(3)
L8690	2(2)
L8691	1(3)
L8692	0(3)
L8693	1(3)
L8694	1(3)
L8695	1(3)
L8696	1(3)
L8701	0(3)
L8702	0(3)
M0075	0(3)
M0076	0(3)
M0100	0(3)
M0201	1(2)
M0243	1(2)
M0244	1(2)
M0245	1(2)
M0246	1(2)
M0247	1(2)
M0248	1(2)
M0300	0(3)
M0301	0(3)
P2028	1(2)
P2029	1(2)
P2031	0(3)
P2033	1(2)
P2038	1(2)
P3000	1(3)
P3001	1(3)
P7001	0(3)
P9010	2(3)
P9011	2(3)
P9012	8(3)
P9016	3(3)
P9017	2(3)
P9019	2(3)
P9020	2(3)

CPT	MUE
P9021	3(3)
P9022	2(3)
P9023	2(3)
P9031	12(3)
P9032	12(3)
P9033	12(3)
P9034	2(3)
P9035	2(3)
P9036	2(3)
P9037	2(3)
P9038	2(3)
P9039	2(3)
P9040	3(3)
P9041	5(3)
P9043	5(3)
P9044	10(3)
P9045	20(3)
P9046	25(3)
P9047	20(3)
P9048	1(3)
P9050	1(3)
P9051	2(3)
P9052	2(3)
P9053	2(3)
P9054	2(3)
P9055	2(3)
P9056	2(3)
P9057	2(3)
P9058	2(3)
P9059	2(3)
P9060	2(3)
P9070	2(3)
P9071	2(3)
P9073	2(3)
P9099	1(3)
P9100	2(3)
P9603	300(3)
P9604	2(3)
P9612	1(3)
P9615	1(3)
Q0035	1(3)
Q0081	1(3)
Q0083	1(3)
Q0084	1(3)
Q0085	1(3)
Q0091	1(3)
Q0111	2(3)
Q0112	3(3)
Q0113	1(3)
Q0114	1(3)
Q0115	1(3)
Q0138	510(3)
Q0139	510(3)
Q0144	0(3)
Q0161	0(3)
Q0162	0(3)
Q0163	0(3)
Q0164	0(3)
Q0166	0(3)

CPT	MUE
Q0167	0(3)
Q0169	0(3)
Q0173	0(3)
Q0174	0(3)
Q0175	0(3)
Q0177	0(3)
Q0180	0(3)
Q0181	0(3)
Q0243	1(3)
Q0244	1(3)
Q0245	1(3)
Q0247	1(2)
Q0477	1(1)
Q0478	1(3)
Q0479	1(3)
Q0480	1(3)
Q0481	1(2)
Q0482	1(3)
Q0483	1(3)
Q0484	1(3)
Q0485	1(3)
Q0486	1(3)
Q0487	1(3)
Q0488	1(3)
Q0489	1(3)
Q0490	1(3)
Q0491	1(3)
Q0492	1(3)
Q0493	1(3)
Q0494	1(3)
Q0495	1(3)
Q0496	1(3)
Q0497	2(3)
Q0498	1(3)
Q0499	1(3)
Q0501	1(3)
Q0502	1(3)
Q0503	3(3)
Q0504	1(3)
Q0506	8(3)
Q0507	1(3)
Q0508	4(3)
Q0509	2(3)
Q0510	0(3)
Q0511	0(3)
Q0512	0(3)
Q0513	0(3)
Q0514	0(3)
Q0515	0(3)
Q1004	2(2)
Q1005	2(2)
Q2004	1(3)
Q2009	100(3)
Q2017	12(3)
Q2026	30(3)
Q2028	1470(3)
Q2034	1(2)
Q2035	1(2)
Q2036	1(2)

CPT	MUE
Q2037	1(2)
Q2038	1(2)
Q2039	1(2)
Q2043	1(2)
Q2049	10(3)
Q2050	14(3)
Q2052	1(3)
Q3014	1(3)
Q3027	30(3)
Q3028	0(3)
Q3031	1(3)
Q4001	1(3)
Q4002	1(3)
Q4003	2(3)
Q4004	2(3)
Q4012	2(3)
Q4013	2(3)
Q4014	2(3)
Q4018	2(3)
Q4021	2(3)
Q4025	1(3)
Q4026	1(3)
Q4027	1(3)
Q4028	1(3)
Q4030	2(3)
Q4037	2(3)
Q4042	2(3)
Q4046	2(3)
Q4050	2(3)
Q4051	2(3)
Q4074	3(3)
Q4081	100(3)
Q5101	1500(3)
Q5103	150(3)
Q5104	150(3)
Q5105	100(3)
Q5106	60(3)
Q5107	170(3)
Q5108	12(3)
Q5109	150(3)
Q5110	1500(3)
Q5111	12(3)
Q5112	120(3)
Q5113	120(3)
Q5114	120(3)
Q5115	150(3)
Q5116	120(3)
Q5117	120(3)
Q5118	230(3)
Q5119	150(3)
Q5120	12(3)
Q5121	150(3)
Q5122	12(3)
Q9001	1(3)
Q9002	1(3)
Q9003	1(3)
Q9950	5(3)
Q9951	0(3)
Q9953	10(3)

CPT	MUE
Q9954	18(3)
Q9955	0(3)
Q9956	9(3)
Q9957	3(3)
Q9958	300(3)
Q9959	0(3)
Q9960	250(3)
Q9961	200(3)
Q9962	150(3)
Q9963	240(3)
Q9964	0(3)
Q9966	250(3)
Q9967	300(3)
Q9969	3(3)
Q9982	1(3)
Q9983	1(3)
Q9991	1(2)
Q9992	1(2)
R0070	2(3)
R0075	2(3)
R0076	1(3)
U0001	2(3)
U0002	2(3)
U0003	2(3)
U0004	2(3)
U0005	1(3)
V2020	0(3)
V2025	0(3)
V2100	0(3)
V2101	0(3)
V2102	0(3)
V2103	0(3)
V2104	0(3)
V2105	0(3)
V2106	0(3)
V2107	0(3)
V2108	0(3)
V2109	0(3)
V2110	0(3)
V2111	0(3)
V2112	0(3)
V2113	0(3)
V2114	0(3)
V2115	0(3)
V2118	0(3)
V2121	0(3)
V2199	2(3)
V2200	0(3)
V2201	0(3)
V2202	0(3)
V2203	0(3)
V2204	0(3)
V2205	0(3)
V2206	0(3)
V2207	0(3)
V2208	0(3)
V2209	0(3)
V2210	0(3)
V2211	0(3)

CPT	MUE
V2212	0(3)
V2213	0(3)
V2214	0(3)
V2215	0(3)
V2218	0(3)
V2219	0(3)
V2220	0(3)
V2221	0(3)
V2299	0(3)
V2300	0(3)
V2301	0(3)
V2302	0(3)
V2303	0(3)
V2304	0(3)
V2305	0(3)
V2306	0(3)
V2307	0(3)
V2308	0(3)
V2309	0(3)
V2310	0(3)
V2311	0(3)
V2312	0(3)
V2313	0(3)
V2314	0(3)
V2315	0(3)
V2318	0(3)
V2319	0(3)
V2320	0(3)
V2321	0(3)
V2399	0(3)
V2410	0(3)
V2430	0(3)
V2499	2(3)
V2500	0(3)
V2501	0(3)
V2502	0(3)
V2503	0(3)
V2510	0(3)
V2511	0(3)
V2512	0(3)
V2513	0(3)
V2520	2(3)
V2521	2(3)
V2522	2(3)
V2523	2(3)
V2524	2(3)
V2530	0(3)
V2531	0(3)
V2599	2(3)
V2600	0(2)
V2610	0(2)
V2615	0(2)
V2623	0(3)
V2624	0(3)
V2625	0(3)
V2626	0(3)
V2627	0(3)
V2628	0(3)
V2629	0(3)

CPT	MUE
V2630	2(2)
V2631	2(2)
V2632	2(2)
V2700	0(3)
V2702	0(3)
V2710	0(3)
V2715	0(3)
V2718	0(3)
V2730	0(3)
V2744	0(3)
V2745	0(3)
V2750	0(3)
V2755	0(3)
V2756	0(3)
V2760	0(3)
V2761	0(2)
V2762	0(3)
V2770	0(3)
V2780	0(3)
V2781	0(2)
V2782	0(3)
V2783	0(3)
V2784	0(3)
V2785	2(2)
V2786	0(3)
V2787	0(3)
V2788	0(3)
V2790	1(3)
V2797	0(3)
V5008	0(3)
V5010	0(3)
V5011	0(3)
V5014	0(3)
V5020	0(3)
V5030	0(3)
V5040	0(3)
V5050	0(3)
V5060	0(3)
V5070	0(3)
V5080	0(3)
V5090	0(3)
V5095	0(3)
V5100	0(3)
V5110	0(3)
V5120	0(3)
V5130	0(3)
V5140	0(3)
V5150	0(3)
V5160	0(3)
V5171	0(3)
V5172	0(3)
V5181	0(3)
V5190	0(3)
V5200	0(3)
V5211	0(3)
V5212	0(3)
V5213	0(3)
V5214	0(3)
V5215	0(3)

CPT	MUE
V5221	0(3)
V5230	0(3)
V5240	0(3)
V5241	0(3)
V5242	0(3)
V5243	0(3)
V5244	0(3)
V5245	0(3)
V5246	0(3)
V5247	0(3)
V5248	0(3)
V5249	0(3)
V5250	0(3)
V5251	0(3)
V5252	0(3)
V5253	0(3)
V5254	0(3)
V5255	0(3)
V5256	0(3)
V5257	0(3)
V5258	0(3)
V5259	0(3)
V5260	0(3)
V5261	0(3)
V5262	0(3)
V5263	0(3)
V5264	0(3)
V5265	0(3)
V5266	0(3)
V5267	0(3)
V5268	0(3)
V5269	0(3)
V5270	0(3)
V5271	0(3)
V5272	0(3)
V5273	0(3)
V5274	0(3)
V5275	0(3)
V5281	0(3)
V5282	0(3)
V5283	0(3)
V5284	0(3)
V5285	0(3)
V5286	0(3)
V5287	0(3)
V5288	0(3)
V5289	0(3)
V5290	0(3)
V5298	0(3)
V5299	1(3)
V5336	0(3)
V5362	0(3)
V5363	0(3)
V5364	0(3)

OPPS

CPT	MUE
0001A	1(2)
0001U	1(2)
0002A	1(2)
0002M	1(3)
0002U	1(2)
0003M	1(3)
0003U	1(2)
0004M	1(2)
0005U	1(2)
0006M	1(2)
0007M	1(2)
0007U	1(2)
0008U	1(3)
0009U	2(3)
0010U	2(3)
0011A	1(2)
0011M	1(2)
0011U	1(2)
0012A	1(2)
0012M	1(2)
0012U	1(2)
0013M	1(2)
0013U	1(3)
0014M	1(2)
0014U	1(3)
0015M	1(2)
0016M	2(3)
0016U	1(3)
0017U	1(3)
0018U	2(3)
0019U	1(3)
0021A	1(2)
0021U	1(2)
0022A	1(2)
0022U	2(3)
0023U	1(2)
0024U	1(2)
0025U	1(2)
0026U	2(3)
0027U	1(2)
0029U	1(2)
0030U	1(2)
0031A	1(2)
0031U	1(2)
0032U	1(2)
0033U	1(2)
0034U	1(2)
0035U	1(2)
0036U	1(3)
0037U	1(3)
0038U	1(2)
0039U	1(2)
0040U	1(2)
0041A	1(2)
0041U	1(2)
0042A	1(2)
0042T	1(3)
0042U	1(2)
0043U	1(2)
0044U	1(2)
0045U	1(3)
0046U	1(3)
0047U	1(3)
0048U	1(3)
0049U	1(3)

CPT	MUE
0050U	1(3)
0051U	1(2)
0052U	1(2)
0053U	1(3)
0054T	1(3)
0054U	1(2)
0055T	1(3)
0055U	1(2)
0056U	1(3)
0058U	1(2)
0059U	1(2)
0060U	1(2)
0061U	2(3)
0062U	1(2)
0063U	1(2)
0064U	2(3)
0065U	2(3)
0066U	1(3)
0067U	2(3)
0068U	1(3)
0069U	1(3)
0070U	1(2)
0071T	1(2)
0071U	1(2)
0072T	1(2)
0072U	1(2)
0073U	1(2)
0074U	1(2)
0075T	1(2)
0075U	1(2)
0076T	1(2)
0076U	1(2)
0077U	2(2)
0078U	1(2)
0079U	0(3)
0080U	1(2)
0082U	1(2)
0083U	1(3)
0084U	1(2)
0086U	1(3)
0087U	1(2)
0088U	1(2)
0089U	1(3)
0090U	1(2)
0091U	1(2)
0092U	1(2)
0093U	1(2)
0094U	1(2)
0095T	1(3)
0095U	1(2)
0096U	1(2)
0097U	1(2)
0098T	2(3)
0100T	1(2)
0101T	1(3)
0101U	1(2)
0102T	2(2)
0102U	1(2)
0103U	1(2)
0105U	1(2)
0106T	4(2)
0106U	1(2)
0107T	4(2)
0107U	1(3)
0108T	4(2)

CPT	MUE
0108U	1(2)
0109T	4(2)
0109U	1(3)
0110T	4(2)
0110U	1(2)
0111U	1(2)
0112U	1(3)
0113U	1(2)
0114U	1(2)
0115U	1(3)
0116U	1(2)
0117U	1(2)
0118U	1(2)
0119U	1(2)
0120U	1(2)
0121U	1(2)
0122U	1(2)
0123U	1(2)
0129U	1(2)
0130U	1(2)
0131U	1(2)
0132U	1(2)
0133U	1(2)
0134U	1(2)
0135U	1(2)
0136U	1(2)
0137U	1(2)
0138U	1(2)
0139U	1(2)
0140U	1(2)
0141U	1(2)
0142U	1(2)
0143U	1(2)
0144U	1(2)
0145U	1(2)
0146U	1(2)
0147U	1(2)
0148U	1(2)
0149U	1(2)
0150U	1(2)
0151U	1(2)
0152U	1(2)
0153U	1(2)
0154U	1(2)
0155U	1(2)
0156U	1(2)
0157U	1(2)
0158U	1(2)
0159U	1(2)
0160U	1(2)
0161U	1(2)
0162U	1(2)
0163T	1(3)
0163U	0(3)
0164T	4(2)
0164U	1(2)
0165T	4(2)
0165U	1(2)
0166U	1(2)
0167U	1(2)
0168U	1(2)
0169U	1(2)
0170U	1(2)
0171U	1(2)
0172U	1(2)

CPT	MUE
0173U	1(2)
0174T	1(3)
0174U	1(2)
0175T	1(3)
0175U	1(2)
0176U	1(3)
0177U	1(3)
0178U	1(2)
0179U	1(3)
0184T	1(3)
0191T	2(2)
0198T	2(2)
01996	1(2)
0200T	1(2)
0201T	1(2)
0202T	1(3)
0202U	1(3)
0203U	1(2)
0204U	1(3)
0205U	1(2)
0206U	1(3)
0207T	2(2)
0207U	1(2)
0208T	1(3)
0208U	1(3)
0209T	1(3)
0209U	1(2)
0210T	1(3)
0210U	2(3)
0211T	1(3)
0211U	2(3)
0212T	1(3)
0212U	1(2)
0213T	1(2)
0213U	1(3)
0214T	1(2)
0214U	1(2)
0215T	1(2)
0215U	1(3)
0216T	1(2)
0216U	1(2)
0217T	1(2)
0217U	1(2)
0218T	1(2)
0218U	1(2)
0219T	1(2)
0219U	1(2)
0220T	1(2)
0220U	1(2)
0221T	1(2)
0222T	1(3)
0223U	1(3)
0224U	3(3)
0225U	1(3)
0226U	1(3)
0227U	1(2)
0228U	1(2)
0229U	1(2)
0230U	1(2)
0231U	1(2)
0232T	1(3)
0232U	1(2)
0233U	1(2)
0234T	2(2)
0234U	1(2)

CPT	MUE
0235T	2(3)
0235U	1(2)
0236T	1(2)
0236U	1(2)
0237T	2(3)
0237U	1(2)
0238T	2(3)
0238U	1(2)
0239U	1(2)
0240U	1(3)
0241U	1(3)
0242U	1(2)
0243U	1(2)
0244U	1(3)
0245U	2(3)
0247U	1(2)
0253T	1(3)
0263T	1(3)
0264T	1(3)
0265T	1(3)
0266T	1(2)
0267T	1(3)
0268T	1(3)
0269T	1(2)
0270T	1(3)
0271T	1(3)
0272T	1(3)
0273T	1(3)
0274T	1(2)
0275T	1(2)
0278T	1(3)
0290T	1(3)
0308T	1(3)
0312T	1(3)
0313T	1(3)
0314T	1(3)
0315T	1(3)
0316T	1(3)
0317T	1(3)
0329T	0(3)
0330T	1(2)
0331T	1(3)
0332T	1(3)
0333T	0(3)
0335T	2(2)
0338T	1(2)
0339T	1(2)
0342T	1(3)
0345T	1(2)
0347T	1(3)
0348T	1(3)
0349T	1(3)
0350T	1(3)
0351T	5(3)
0352T	5(3)
0353T	2(3)
0354T	2(3)
0355T	1(2)
0356T	4(2)
0358T	1(2)
0362T	16(3)
0373T	24(3)
0376T	2(3)
0378T	1(2)
0379T	1(2)

CPT	MUE
0394T	2(3)
0395T	2(3)
0397T	1(3)
0398T	1(3)
0402T	2(2)
0403T	0(3)
0404T	1(2)
0408T	1(3)
0409T	1(3)
0410T	1(3)
0411T	1(3)
0412T	1(2)
0413T	1(3)
0414T	1(2)
0415T	1(3)
0416T	1(3)
0417T	1(3)
0418T	1(3)
0419T	1(2)
0420T	1(2)
0421T	1(2)
0422T	1(3)
0423T	1(3)
0424T	1(3)
0425T	1(3)
0426T	1(3)
0427T	1(3)
0428T	1(2)
0429T	1(2)
0430T	1(2)
0431T	1(2)
0432T	1(3)
0433T	1(3)
0434T	1(3)
0435T	1(3)
0436T	1(3)
0437T	1(3)
0439T	1(3)
0440T	3(3)
0441T	3(3)
0442T	3(3)
0443T	1(2)
0444T	1(2)
0445T	1(2)
0446T	1(3)
0447T	1(3)
0448T	1(3)
0449T	1(2)
0450T	1(3)
0451T	1(3)
0452T	1(3)
0453T	1(3)
0454T	3(3)
0455T	1(3)
0456T	1(3)
0457T	1(3)
0458T	3(3)
0459T	1(3)
0460T	3(3)
0461T	1(3)
0462T	1(2)
0463T	1(2)
0464T	1(2)
0465T	1(3)
0466T	1(3)

CPT	MUE
0467T	1(3)
0468T	1(3)
0469T	1(2)
0470T	1(2)
0471T	2(1)
0472T	1(2)
0473T	1(2)
0474T	0(3)
0475T	1(3)
0476T	1(3)
0477T	1(3)
0478T	1(3)
0479T	1(2)
0480T	4(1)
0481T	1(3)
0483T	1(2)
0484T	1(2)
0485T	1(2)
0486T	1(2)
0487T	1(3)
0488T	1(2)
0489T	1(2)
0490T	1(2)
0491T	1(2)
0492T	4(3)
0493T	1(3)
0494T	1(2)
0495T	1(2)
0496T	4(3)
0497T	1(3)
0498T	1(2)
0499T	1(2)
0500T	1(3)
0501T	1(2)
0502T	1(2)
0503T	1(2)
0504T	1(2)
0505T	1(3)
0506T	1(2)
0507T	1(2)
0508T	1(3)
0509T	1(2)
0510T	1(2)
0511T	1(2)
0512T	1(2)
0513T	2(3)
0514T	2(2)
0515T	1(3)
0516T	1(3)
0517T	1(3)
0518T	1(3)
0519T	1(3)
0520T	1(3)
0521T	1(3)
0522T	1(3)
0523T	1(3)
0524T	3(3)
0525T	1(3)
0526T	1(3)
0527T	1(3)
0528T	1(3)
0529T	1(3)
0530T	1(3)
0531T	1(3)
0532T	1(3)

CPT	MUE
0533T	1(2)
0534T	1(2)
0535T	1(2)
0536T	1(2)
0537T	1(3)
0538T	1(3)
0539T	1(3)
0540T	1(3)
0541T	1(3)
0542T	1(3)
0543T	1(2)
0544T	1(2)
0545T	1(2)
0546T	2(2)
0547T	1(2)
0548T	1(2)
0549T	1(2)
0550T	2(3)
0551T	1(2)
0552T	0(3)
0553T	0(3)
0554T	0(3)
0555T	1(2)
0556T	1(2)
0557T	0(3)
0558T	1(2)
0559T	1(2)
0560T	1(3)
0561T	1(2)
0562T	1(3)
0563T	1(2)
0564T	1(2)
0565T	1(2)
0566T	1(2)
0567T	1(2)
0568T	1(2)
0569T	1(2)
0570T	1(3)
0571T	1(2)
0572T	1(2)
0573T	1(2)
0574T	1(2)
0575T	1(2)
0576T	1(2)
0577T	1(2)
0578T	1(2)
0579T	1(2)
0580T	1(2)
0581T	0(3)
0582T	0(3)
0583T	2(2)
0584T	1(2)
0585T	1(2)
0586T	1(2)
0587T	1(2)
0588T	1(2)
0589T	1(2)
0590T	1(2)
0591T	1(2)
0592T	1(2)
0593T	1(2)
0594T	2(2)
0596T	1(2)
0597T	1(2)
0598T	1(2)

CPT	MUE
0599T	1(3)
0600T	3(3)
0601T	3(3)
0602T	1(2)
0603T	1(2)
0604T	1(2)
0605T	1(2)
0606T	0(3)
0607T	1(2)
0608T	1(2)
0609T	1(3)
0610T	1(3)
0611T	1(3)
0612T	0(3)
0613T	0(3)
0614T	1(3)
0615T	1(3)
0616T	2(2)
0617T	2(2)
0618T	2(2)
0619T	1(2)
0620T	2(2)
0621T	2(2)
0622T	2(2)
0623T	1(2)
0624T	1(2)
0625T	1(2)
0626T	1(2)
0627T	1(2)
0628T	4(2)
0629T	1(2)
0630T	4(2)
0631T	4(2)
0632T	1(2)
0633T	1(2)
0634T	1(2)
0635T	1(2)
0636T	1(2)
0637T	1(2)
0638T	1(2)
0639T	1(3)
10004	3(3)
10005	1(2)
10006	3(3)
10007	1(2)
10008	2(3)
10009	1(2)
10010	3(3)
10011	1(2)
10012	3(3)
10021	1(2)
10030	2(3)
10035	1(2)
10036	3(3)
10040	1(2)
10060	1(2)
10061	1(2)
10080	1(3)
10081	1(3)
10120	3(3)
10121	2(3)
10140	2(3)
10160	3(3)
10180	2(3)
11000	1(2)
11001	1(3)

CPT	MUE
11004	1(2)
11005	1(2)
11006	1(2)
11008	1(2)
11010	2(3)
11011	2(3)
11012	2(3)
11042	1(2)
11043	1(2)
11044	1(2)
11045	12(3)
11046	4(3)
11047	4(3)
11055	1(2)
11056	1(2)
11057	1(2)
11102	1(2)
11103	6(3)
11104	1(2)
11105	3(3)
11106	1(2)
11107	2(3)
11200	1(2)
11201	1(3)
11300	5(3)
11301	6(3)
11302	4(3)
11303	3(3)
11305	4(3)
11306	4(3)
11307	3(3)
11308	2(3)
11310	4(3)
11311	4(3)
11312	3(3)
11313	3(3)
11400	3(3)
11401	3(3)
11402	3(3)
11403	2(3)
11404	2(3)
11406	2(3)
11420	3(3)
11421	3(3)
11422	3(3)
11423	2(3)
11424	2(3)
11426	2(3)
11440	4(3)
11441	3(3)
11442	3(3)
11443	2(3)
11444	2(3)
11446	2(3)
11450	1(2)
11451	1(2)
11462	1(2)
11463	1(2)
11470	3(2)
11471	2(3)
11600	2(3)
11601	2(3)
11602	3(3)
11603	2(3)
11604	2(3)
11606	2(3)

CPT	MUE
11620	2(3)
11621	2(3)
11622	2(3)
11623	2(3)
11624	2(3)
11626	2(3)
11640	2(3)
11641	2(3)
11642	3(3)
11643	2(3)
11644	2(3)
11646	2(3)
11719	1(2)
11720	1(2)
11721	1(2)
11730	1(2)
11732	4(3)
11740	2(3)
11750	6(3)
11755	2(3)
11760	4(3)
11762	2(3)
11765	4(3)
11770	1(3)
11771	1(3)
11772	1(3)
11900	1(2)
11901	1(2)
11920	1(2)
11921	1(2)
11922	1(3)
11950	1(2)
11951	1(2)
11952	1(2)
11954	1(3)
11960	2(3)
11970	2(3)
11971	2(3)
11976	1(2)
11980	1(2)
11981	1(3)
11982	1(3)
11983	1(3)
12001	1(2)
12002	1(2)
12004	1(2)
12005	1(2)
12006	1(2)
12007	1(2)
12011	1(2)
12013	1(2)
12014	1(2)
12015	1(2)
12016	1(2)
12017	1(2)
12018	1(2)
12020	2(3)
12021	3(3)
12031	1(2)
12032	1(2)
12034	1(2)
12035	1(2)
12036	1(2)
12037	1(2)
12041	1(2)
12042	1(2)

CPT	MUE
12044	1(2)
12045	1(2)
12046	1(2)
12047	1(2)
12051	1(2)
12052	1(2)
12053	1(2)
12054	1(2)
12055	1(2)
12056	1(2)
12057	1(2)
13100	1(2)
13101	1(2)
13102	9(3)
13120	1(2)
13121	1(2)
13122	9(3)
13131	1(2)
13132	1(2)
13133	7(3)
13151	1(2)
13152	1(2)
13153	2(3)
13160	2(3)
14000	2(3)
14001	2(3)
14020	2(3)
14021	2(3)
14040	2(3)
14041	3(3)
14060	2(3)
14061	2(3)
14301	2(3)
14302	8(3)
14350	2(3)
15002	1(2)
15003	9(3)
15004	1(2)
15005	2(3)
15040	1(2)
15050	1(3)
15100	1(2)
15101	9(3)
15110	1(2)
15111	2(3)
15115	1(2)
15116	2(3)
15120	1(2)
15121	5(3)
15130	1(2)
15131	2(3)
15135	1(2)
15136	1(3)
15150	1(2)
15151	1(2)
15152	2(3)
15155	1(2)
15156	1(2)
15157	1(3)
15200	1(2)
15201	7(3)
15220	1(2)
15221	9(3)
15240	1(2)
15241	9(3)
15260	1(2)

CPT	MUE
15261	6(3)
15271	1(2)
15272	3(3)
15273	1(2)
15274	6(3)
15275	1(2)
15276	3(2)
15277	1(2)
15278	3(3)
15570	2(3)
15572	2(3)
15574	2(3)
15576	2(3)
15600	2(3)
15610	2(3)
15620	2(3)
15630	2(3)
15650	1(3)
15730	1(3)
15731	1(3)
15733	2(3)
15734	4(3)
15736	2(3)
15738	3(3)
15740	2(3)
15750	2(3)
15756	2(3)
15757	2(3)
15758	2(3)
15760	2(3)
15769	1(3)
15770	2(3)
15771	1(2)
15772	9(3)
15773	1(2)
15774	3(3)
15775	1(2)
15776	1(2)
15777	1(3)
15780	1(2)
15781	1(3)
15782	1(3)
15783	1(3)
15786	1(2)
15787	2(3)
15788	1(2)
15789	1(2)
15792	1(3)
15793	1(3)
15819	1(2)
15820	1(2)
15821	1(2)
15822	1(2)
15823	1(2)
15824	1(2)
15825	1(2)
15826	1(2)
15828	1(2)
15829	1(2)
15830	1(2)
15832	1(2)
15833	1(2)
15834	1(2)
15835	1(3)
15836	1(2)
15837	2(3)

CPT	MUE
15838	1(2)
15839	2(3)
15840	1(3)
15841	2(3)
15842	2(3)
15845	2(3)
15847	1(2)
15850	1(2)
15851	1(2)
15852	1(3)
15860	1(3)
15876	1(2)
15877	1(2)
15878	1(2)
15879	1(2)
15920	1(3)
15922	1(3)
15931	1(3)
15933	1(3)
15934	1(3)
15935	1(3)
15936	1(3)
15937	1(3)
15940	2(3)
15941	2(3)
15944	2(3)
15945	2(3)
15946	2(3)
15950	2(3)
15951	2(3)
15952	2(3)
15953	2(3)
15956	2(3)
15958	2(3)
15999	1(3)
16000	1(2)
16020	1(3)
16025	1(3)
16030	1(3)
16035	1(2)
16036	2(3)
17000	1(2)
17003	13(2)
17004	1(2)
17106	1(2)
17107	1(2)
17108	1(2)
17110	1(2)
17111	1(2)
17250	4(3)
17260	7(3)
17261	7(3)
17262	6(3)
17263	3(3)
17264	3(3)
17266	2(3)
17270	6(3)
17271	4(3)
17272	5(3)
17273	4(3)
17274	2(3)
17276	2(3)
17280	6(3)
17281	5(3)
17282	4(3)
17283	4(3)

CPT	MUE
17284	2(3)
17286	2(3)
17311	4(3)
17312	6(3)
17313	3(3)
17314	4(3)
17315	15(3)
17340	1(2)
17360	1(2)
17380	1(3)
17999	1(3)
19000	2(3)
19001	5(3)
19020	2(3)
19030	1(2)
19081	1(2)
19082	2(3)
19083	1(2)
19084	2(3)
19085	1(2)
19086	2(3)
19100	4(3)
19101	3(3)
19105	2(3)
19110	1(3)
19112	2(3)
19120	1(2)
19125	1(2)
19126	3(3)
19281	1(2)
19282	2(3)
19283	1(2)
19284	2(3)
19285	1(2)
19286	2(3)
19287	1(2)
19288	2(3)
19294	2(3)
19296	1(3)
19297	2(3)
19298	1(2)
19300	1(2)
19301	1(3)
19302	1(2)
19303	1(2)
19305	1(2)
19306	1(2)
19307	1(2)
19316	1(2)
19318	1(2)
19325	1(2)
19328	1(2)
19330	1(2)
19340	1(2)
19342	1(2)
19350	1(2)
19355	1(2)
19357	1(2)
19361	1(2)
19364	1(3)
19367	1(2)
19368	1(2)
19369	1(2)
19370	1(2)
19371	1(2)
19380	1(2)

CPT	MUE
19396	1(2)
19499	1(3)
20100	2(3)
20101	2(3)
20102	3(3)
20103	3(3)
20150	2(3)
20200	2(3)
20205	3(3)
20206	3(3)
20220	3(3)
20225	2(3)
20240	4(3)
20245	3(3)
20250	1(3)
20251	2(3)
20500	2(3)
20501	2(3)
20520	2(3)
20525	4(3)
20526	1(2)
20527	2(3)
20550	5(3)
20551	5(3)
20552	1(2)
20553	1(2)
20555	1(3)
20560	1(2)
20561	1(2)
20600	6(3)
20604	4(3)
20605	2(3)
20606	2(3)
20610	2(3)
20611	2(3)
20612	2(3)
20615	1(3)
20650	4(3)
20660	1(2)
20661	1(2)
20662	1(2)
20663	1(2)
20664	1(2)
20665	1(2)
20670	3(3)
20680	3(3)
20690	2(3)
20692	2(3)
20693	2(3)
20694	2(3)
20696	2(3)
20697	4(3)
20700	1(3)
20701	1(3)
20702	1(3)
20703	1(3)
20704	1(3)
20705	1(3)
20802	1(2)
20805	1(2)
20808	1(2)
20816	3(3)
20822	3(3)
20824	1(2)
20827	1(2)
20838	1(2)

CPT	MUE
20900	2(3)
20902	2(3)
20910	1(3)
20912	1(3)
20920	1(3)
20922	1(3)
20924	2(3)
20930	1(3)
20931	1(2)
20932	1(3)
20933	1(3)
20934	1(3)
20936	1(3)
20937	1(2)
20938	1(2)
20939	1(3)
20950	2(3)
20955	1(3)
20956	1(3)
20957	1(3)
20962	1(3)
20969	2(3)
20970	1(3)
20972	2(3)
20973	1(2)
20974	1(3)
20975	1(3)
20979	1(3)
20982	1(2)
20983	1(2)
20985	2(3)
20999	1(3)
21010	1(2)
21011	4(3)
21012	3(3)
21013	2(3)
21014	2(3)
21015	1(3)
21016	2(3)
21025	2(3)
21026	2(3)
21029	1(3)
21030	1(3)
21031	2(3)
21032	1(3)
21034	1(3)
21040	2(3)
21044	1(3)
21045	1(3)
21046	2(3)
21047	2(3)
21048	2(3)
21049	1(3)
21050	1(2)
21060	1(2)
21070	1(2)
21073	1(2)
21076	1(2)
21077	1(2)
21079	1(2)
21080	1(2)
21081	1(2)
21082	1(2)
21083	1(2)
21084	1(2)
21085	1(3)

CPT	MUE
21086	1(2)
21087	1(2)
21088	1(2)
21089	1(3)
21100	1(2)
21110	2(3)
21116	1(2)
21120	1(2)
21121	1(2)
21122	1(2)
21123	1(2)
21125	2(2)
21127	2(3)
21137	1(2)
21138	1(2)
21139	1(2)
21141	1(2)
21142	1(2)
21143	1(2)
21145	1(2)
21146	1(2)
21147	1(2)
21150	1(2)
21151	1(2)
21154	1(2)
21155	1(2)
21159	1(2)
21160	1(2)
21172	1(3)
21175	1(2)
21179	1(2)
21180	1(2)
21181	1(3)
21182	1(2)
21183	1(2)
21184	1(2)
21188	1(2)
21193	1(2)
21194	1(2)
21195	1(2)
21196	1(2)
21198	1(3)
21199	1(2)
21206	1(3)
21208	1(3)
21209	1(3)
21210	2(3)
21215	2(3)
21230	2(3)
21235	2(3)
21240	1(2)
21242	1(2)
21243	1(2)
21244	1(2)
21245	2(3)
21246	1(3)
21247	1(2)
21248	2(3)
21249	2(3)
21255	1(2)
21256	1(2)
21260	1(2)
21261	1(2)
21263	1(2)
21267	1(2)
21268	1(2)

CPT	MUE
21270	1(2)
21275	1(2)
21280	1(2)
21282	1(2)
21295	1(2)
21296	1(2)
21299	1(3)
21310	1(2)
21315	1(2)
21320	1(2)
21325	1(2)
21330	1(2)
21335	1(2)
21336	1(2)
21337	1(2)
21338	1(2)
21339	1(2)
21340	1(2)
21343	1(2)
21344	1(2)
21345	1(2)
21346	1(2)
21347	1(2)
21348	1(2)
21355	1(2)
21356	1(2)
21360	1(2)
21365	1(2)
21366	1(2)
21385	1(2)
21386	1(2)
21387	1(2)
21390	1(2)
21395	1(2)
21400	1(2)
21401	1(2)
21406	1(2)
21407	1(2)
21408	1(2)
21421	1(2)
21422	1(2)
21423	1(2)
21431	1(2)
21432	1(2)
21433	1(2)
21435	1(2)
21436	1(2)
21440	2(3)
21445	2(3)
21450	1(2)
21451	1(2)
21452	1(2)
21453	1(2)
21454	1(2)
21461	1(2)
21462	1(2)
21465	1(2)
21470	1(2)
21480	1(2)
21485	1(2)
21490	1(2)
21497	1(2)
21499	1(3)
21501	3(3)
21502	1(3)
21510	1(3)

CPT	MUE
21550	2(3)
21552	2(3)
21554	2(3)
21555	2(3)
21556	2(3)
21557	1(3)
21558	1(3)
21600	5(3)
21601	2(3)
21602	1(3)
21603	1(3)
21610	1(3)
21615	1(2)
21616	1(2)
21620	1(2)
21627	1(2)
21630	1(2)
21632	1(2)
21685	1(2)
21700	1(2)
21705	1(2)
21720	1(3)
21725	1(3)
21740	1(2)
21742	1(2)
21743	1(2)
21750	1(2)
21811	1(2)
21812	1(2)
21813	1(2)
21820	1(2)
21825	1(2)
21899	1(3)
21920	2(3)
21925	2(3)
21930	5(3)
21931	3(3)
21932	2(3)
21933	2(3)
21935	1(3)
21936	1(3)
22010	2(3)
22015	2(3)
22100	1(2)
22101	1(2)
22102	1(2)
22103	3(3)
22110	1(2)
22112	1(2)
22114	1(2)
22116	3(3)
22206	1(2)
22207	1(2)
22208	5(3)
22210	1(2)
22212	1(2)
22214	1(2)
22216	6(3)
22220	1(2)
22222	1(2)
22224	1(2)
22226	4(3)
22310	1(2)
22315	1(2)
22318	1(2)
22319	1(2)

CPT	MUE
22325	1(2)
22326	1(2)
22327	1(2)
22328	6(3)
22505	1(2)
22510	1(2)
22511	1(2)
22512	3(3)
22513	1(2)
22514	1(2)
22515	4(3)
22526	0(3)
22527	0(3)
22532	1(2)
22533	1(2)
22534	3(3)
22548	1(2)
22551	1(2)
22552	5(3)
22554	1(2)
22556	1(2)
22558	1(2)
22585	5(3)
22586	1(2)
22590	1(2)
22595	1(2)
22600	1(2)
22610	1(2)
22612	1(2)
22614	13(3)
22630	1(2)
22632	4(2)
22633	1(2)
22634	4(2)
22800	1(2)
22802	1(2)
22804	1(2)
22808	1(2)
22810	1(2)
22812	1(2)
22818	1(2)
22819	1(2)
22830	1(2)
22840	1(3)
22841	1(2)
22842	1(3)
22843	1(3)
22844	1(3)
22845	1(3)
22846	1(3)
22847	1(3)
22848	1(2)
22849	1(2)
22850	1(2)
22852	1(2)
22853	4(3)
22854	4(3)
22855	1(2)
22856	1(2)
22857	1(2)
22858	1(2)
22859	4(3)
22861	1(2)
22862	1(2)
22864	1(2)
22865	1(2)

CPT	MUE
22867	1(2)
22868	1(2)
22869	1(2)
22870	1(2)
22899	1(3)
22900	3(3)
22901	2(3)
22902	4(3)
22903	3(3)
22904	1(3)
22905	1(3)
22999	1(3)
23000	1(2)
23020	1(2)
23030	2(3)
23031	1(3)
23035	1(3)
23040	1(2)
23044	1(3)
23065	2(3)
23066	2(3)
23071	2(3)
23073	2(3)
23075	2(3)
23076	2(3)
23077	1(3)
23078	1(3)
23100	1(2)
23101	1(3)
23105	1(2)
23106	1(2)
23107	1(2)
23120	1(2)
23125	1(2)
23130	1(2)
23140	1(3)
23145	1(3)
23146	1(3)
23150	1(3)
23155	1(3)
23156	1(3)
23170	1(3)
23172	1(3)
23174	1(3)
23180	1(3)
23182	1(3)
23184	1(3)
23190	1(3)
23195	1(2)
23200	1(3)
23210	1(3)
23220	1(3)
23330	2(3)
23333	1(3)
23334	1(2)
23335	1(2)
23350	1(2)
23395	1(2)
23397	1(3)
23400	1(2)
23405	2(3)
23406	1(3)
23410	1(2)
23412	1(2)
23415	1(2)
23420	1(2)

CPT	MUE
23430	1(2)
23440	1(2)
23450	1(2)
23455	1(2)
23460	1(2)
23462	1(2)
23465	1(2)
23466	1(2)
23470	1(2)
23472	1(2)
23473	1(2)
23474	1(2)
23480	1(2)
23485	1(2)
23490	1(2)
23491	1(2)
23500	1(2)
23505	1(2)
23515	1(2)
23520	1(2)
23525	1(2)
23530	1(2)
23532	1(2)
23540	1(2)
23545	1(2)
23550	1(2)
23552	1(2)
23570	1(2)
23575	1(2)
23585	1(2)
23600	1(2)
23605	1(2)
23615	1(2)
23616	1(2)
23620	1(2)
23625	1(2)
23630	1(2)
23650	1(2)
23655	1(2)
23660	1(2)
23665	1(2)
23670	1(2)
23675	1(2)
23680	1(2)
23700	1(2)
23800	1(2)
23802	1(2)
23900	1(2)
23920	1(2)
23921	1(2)
23929	1(3)
23930	2(3)
23931	2(3)
23935	2(3)
24000	1(2)
24006	1(2)
24065	2(3)
24066	2(3)
24071	2(3)
24073	2(3)
24075	5(3)
24076	4(3)
24077	1(3)
24079	1(3)
24100	1(2)
24101	1(2)

CPT	MUE
24102	1(2)
24105	1(2)
24110	1(3)
24115	1(3)
24116	1(3)
24120	1(3)
24125	1(3)
24126	1(3)
24130	1(2)
24134	1(3)
24136	1(3)
24138	1(3)
24140	1(3)
24145	1(3)
24147	1(2)
24149	1(2)
24150	1(3)
24152	1(3)
24155	1(2)
24160	1(2)
24164	1(2)
24200	3(3)
24201	3(3)
24220	1(2)
24300	1(2)
24301	2(3)
24305	4(3)
24310	2(3)
24320	2(3)
24330	1(3)
24331	1(3)
24332	1(2)
24340	1(2)
24341	2(3)
24342	2(3)
24343	1(2)
24344	1(2)
24345	1(2)
24346	1(2)
24357	1(3)
24358	1(3)
24359	2(3)
24360	1(2)
24361	1(2)
24362	1(2)
24363	1(2)
24365	1(2)
24366	1(2)
24370	1(2)
24371	1(2)
24400	1(3)
24410	1(2)
24420	1(2)
24430	1(3)
24435	1(3)
24470	1(2)
24495	1(2)
24498	1(2)
24500	1(2)
24505	1(2)
24515	1(2)
24516	1(2)
24530	1(2)
24535	1(2)
24538	1(2)
24545	1(2)

CPT	MUE
24546	1(2)
24560	1(3)
24565	1(3)
24566	1(3)
24575	1(3)
24576	1(3)
24577	1(3)
24579	1(3)
24582	1(3)
24586	1(3)
24587	1(2)
24600	1(2)
24605	1(2)
24615	1(2)
24620	1(2)
24635	1(2)
24640	1(2)
24650	1(2)
24655	1(2)
24665	1(2)
24666	1(2)
24670	1(2)
24675	1(2)
24685	1(2)
24800	1(2)
24802	1(2)
24900	1(2)
24920	1(2)
24925	1(2)
24930	1(2)
24931	1(2)
24935	1(2)
24940	1(2)
24999	1(3)
25000	2(3)
25001	1(3)
25020	1(2)
25023	1(2)
25024	1(2)
25025	1(2)
25028	4(3)
25031	2(3)
25035	2(3)
25040	1(3)
25065	2(3)
25066	2(3)
25071	3(3)
25073	2(3)
25075	6(3)
25076	3(3)
25077	1(3)
25078	1(3)
25085	1(2)
25100	1(2)
25101	1(2)
25105	1(2)
25107	1(2)
25109	4(3)
25110	2(3)
25111	1(3)
25112	1(3)
25115	1(3)
25116	1(3)
25118	5(3)
25119	1(2)
25120	1(3)

CPT	MUE
25125	1(3)
25126	1(3)
25130	1(3)
25135	1(3)
25136	1(3)
25145	1(3)
25150	1(3)
25151	1(3)
25170	1(3)
25210	2(3)
25215	1(2)
25230	1(2)
25240	1(2)
25246	1(2)
25248	3(3)
25250	1(2)
25251	1(2)
25259	1(2)
25260	7(3)
25263	4(3)
25265	4(3)
25270	8(3)
25272	4(3)
25274	4(3)
25275	2(3)
25280	9(3)
25290	10(3)
25295	9(3)
25300	1(2)
25301	1(2)
25310	5(3)
25312	4(3)
25315	1(3)
25316	1(3)
25320	1(2)
25332	1(2)
25335	1(2)
25337	1(2)
25350	1(3)
25355	1(3)
25360	1(3)
25365	1(3)
25370	1(2)
25375	1(2)
25390	1(2)
25391	1(2)
25392	1(2)
25393	1(2)
25394	1(3)
25400	1(2)
25405	1(2)
25415	1(2)
25420	1(2)
25425	1(2)
25426	1(2)
25430	1(3)
25431	1(3)
25440	1(2)
25441	1(2)
25442	1(2)
25443	1(2)
25444	1(2)
25445	1(2)
25446	1(2)
25447	4(3)
25449	1(2)

CPT	MUE
25450	1(2)
25455	1(2)
25490	1(2)
25491	1(2)
25492	1(2)
25500	1(2)
25505	1(2)
25515	1(2)
25520	1(2)
25525	1(2)
25526	1(2)
25530	1(2)
25535	1(2)
25545	1(2)
25560	1(2)
25565	1(2)
25574	1(2)
25575	1(2)
25600	1(2)
25605	1(2)
25606	1(2)
25607	1(2)
25608	1(2)
25609	1(2)
25622	1(2)
25624	1(2)
25628	1(2)
25630	1(3)
25635	1(3)
25645	1(3)
25650	1(2)
25651	1(2)
25652	1(2)
25660	1(2)
25670	1(2)
25671	1(2)
25675	1(2)
25676	1(2)
25680	1(2)
25685	1(2)
25690	1(2)
25695	1(2)
25800	1(2)
25805	1(2)
25810	1(2)
25820	1(2)
25825	1(2)
25830	1(2)
25900	1(2)
25905	1(2)
25907	1(2)
25909	1(2)
25915	1(2)
25920	1(2)
25922	1(2)
25924	1(2)
25927	1(2)
25929	1(2)
25931	1(2)
25999	1(3)
26010	2(3)
26011	3(3)
26020	4(3)
26025	1(2)
26030	1(2)
26034	2(3)

CPT	MUE
26035	1(3)
26037	1(3)
26040	1(2)
26045	1(2)
26055	5(3)
26060	5(3)
26070	2(3)
26075	3(3)
26080	3(3)
26100	1(3)
26105	2(3)
26110	2(3)
26111	4(3)
26113	3(3)
26115	4(3)
26116	2(3)
26117	2(3)
26118	1(3)
26121	1(2)
26123	1(2)
26125	4(3)
26130	1(3)
26135	4(3)
26140	2(3)
26145	6(3)
26160	4(3)
26170	4(3)
26180	4(3)
26185	1(3)
26200	2(3)
26205	1(3)
26210	2(3)
26215	2(3)
26230	2(3)
26235	2(3)
26236	2(3)
26250	2(3)
26260	1(3)
26262	1(3)
26320	4(3)
26340	4(3)
26341	2(3)
26350	6(3)
26352	2(3)
26356	4(3)
26357	2(3)
26358	2(3)
26370	3(3)
26372	1(3)
26373	2(3)
26390	2(3)
26392	2(3)
26410	4(3)
26412	3(3)
26415	2(3)
26416	2(3)
26418	4(3)
26420	3(3)
26426	4(3)
26428	2(3)
26432	2(3)
26433	2(3)
26434	2(3)
26437	4(3)
26440	6(3)
26442	5(3)

CPT	MUE
26445	5(3)
26449	5(3)
26450	6(3)
26455	6(3)
26460	4(3)
26471	4(3)
26474	4(3)
26476	4(3)
26477	2(3)
26478	6(3)
26479	4(3)
26480	4(3)
26483	4(3)
26485	4(3)
26489	2(3)
26490	3(3)
26492	2(3)
26494	1(3)
26496	1(3)
26497	2(3)
26498	1(3)
26499	2(3)
26500	3(3)
26502	2(3)
26508	1(2)
26510	4(3)
26516	1(2)
26517	1(2)
26518	1(2)
26520	4(3)
26525	4(3)
26530	4(3)
26531	4(3)
26535	3(3)
26536	4(3)
26540	4(3)
26541	4(3)
26542	4(3)
26545	4(3)
26546	2(3)
26548	3(3)
26550	1(2)
26551	1(2)
26553	1(3)
26554	1(3)
26555	2(3)
26556	2(3)
26560	2(3)
26561	2(3)
26562	2(3)
26565	2(3)
26567	3(3)
26568	2(3)
26580	1(2)
26587	2(3)
26590	2(3)
26591	4(3)
26593	8(3)
26596	1(3)
26600	2(3)
26605	3(3)
26607	2(3)
26608	4(3)
26615	3(3)
26641	1(2)
26645	1(2)

CPT	MUE
26650	1(2)
26665	1(2)
26670	2(3)
26675	1(3)
26676	2(3)
26685	3(3)
26686	3(3)
26700	2(3)
26705	3(3)
26706	2(3)
26715	3(3)
26720	4(3)
26725	3(3)
26727	3(3)
26735	4(3)
26740	3(3)
26742	3(3)
26746	3(3)
26750	3(3)
26755	2(3)
26756	2(3)
26765	3(3)
26770	3(3)
26775	2(3)
26776	4(3)
26785	3(3)
26820	1(2)
26841	1(2)
26842	1(2)
26843	2(3)
26844	2(3)
26850	5(3)
26852	2(3)
26860	1(2)
26861	4(3)
26862	1(2)
26863	2(3)
26910	4(3)
26951	8(3)
26952	4(3)
26989	1(3)
26990	2(3)
26991	1(3)
26992	2(3)
27000	1(3)
27001	1(3)
27003	1(2)
27005	1(2)
27006	1(2)
27025	1(3)
27027	1(2)
27030	1(2)
27033	1(2)
27035	1(2)
27036	1(2)
27040	2(3)
27041	3(3)
27043	2(3)
27045	3(3)
27047	2(3)
27048	2(3)
27049	1(3)
27050	1(2)
27052	1(2)
27054	1(2)
27057	1(2)

CPT	MUE
27059	1(3)
27060	1(2)
27062	1(2)
27065	1(3)
27066	1(3)
27067	1(3)
27070	1(3)
27071	1(3)
27075	1(3)
27076	1(2)
27077	1(2)
27078	1(2)
27080	1(2)
27086	1(3)
27087	1(3)
27090	1(2)
27091	1(2)
27093	1(2)
27095	1(2)
27096	1(2)
27097	1(3)
27098	1(2)
27100	1(2)
27105	1(3)
27110	1(2)
27111	1(2)
27120	1(2)
27122	1(2)
27125	1(2)
27130	1(2)
27132	1(2)
27134	1(2)
27137	1(2)
27138	1(2)
27140	1(2)
27146	1(3)
27147	1(3)
27151	1(3)
27156	1(2)
27158	1(2)
27161	1(2)
27165	1(2)
27170	1(2)
27175	1(2)
27176	1(2)
27177	1(2)
27178	1(2)
27179	1(2)
27181	1(2)
27185	1(2)
27187	1(2)
27197	1(2)
27198	1(2)
27200	1(2)
27202	1(2)
27215	0(3)
27216	0(3)
27217	0(3)
27218	0(3)
27220	1(2)
27222	1(2)
27226	1(2)
27227	1(2)
27228	1(2)
27230	1(2)
27232	1(2)

CPT	MUE
27235	1(2)
27236	1(2)
27238	1(2)
27240	1(2)
27244	1(2)
27245	1(2)
27246	1(2)
27248	1(2)
27250	1(2)
27252	1(2)
27253	1(2)
27254	1(2)
27256	1(2)
27257	1(2)
27258	1(2)
27259	1(2)
27265	1(2)
27266	1(2)
27267	1(2)
27268	1(2)
27269	1(2)
27275	2(2)
27279	1(2)
27280	1(2)
27282	1(2)
27284	1(2)
27286	1(2)
27290	1(2)
27295	1(2)
27299	1(3)
27301	3(3)
27303	2(3)
27305	1(2)
27306	1(2)
27307	1(2)
27310	1(2)
27323	2(3)
27324	3(3)
27325	1(2)
27326	1(2)
27327	5(3)
27328	3(3)
27329	1(3)
27330	1(2)
27331	1(2)
27332	1(2)
27333	1(2)
27334	1(2)
27335	1(2)
27337	3(3)
27339	4(3)
27340	1(2)
27345	1(2)
27347	1(2)
27350	1(2)
27355	1(3)
27356	1(3)
27357	1(3)
27358	1(3)
27360	2(3)
27364	1(3)
27365	1(3)
27369	1(2)
27372	2(3)
27380	1(2)
27381	1(2)

CPT	MUE
27385	2(3)
27386	2(3)
27390	1(2)
27391	1(2)
27392	1(2)
27393	1(2)
27394	1(2)
27395	1(2)
27396	1(2)
27397	1(2)
27400	1(2)
27403	1(3)
27405	1(3)
27407	1(3)
27409	1(2)
27412	1(2)
27415	1(2)
27416	1(2)
27418	1(2)
27420	1(2)
27422	1(2)
27424	1(2)
27425	1(2)
27427	1(2)
27428	1(2)
27429	1(2)
27430	1(2)
27435	1(2)
27437	1(2)
27438	1(2)
27440	1(2)
27441	1(2)
27442	1(2)
27443	1(2)
27445	1(2)
27446	1(2)
27447	1(2)
27448	1(3)
27450	1(3)
27454	1(2)
27455	1(3)
27457	1(3)
27465	1(2)
27466	1(2)
27468	1(2)
27470	1(2)
27472	1(2)
27475	1(2)
27477	1(2)
27479	1(2)
27485	1(2)
27486	1(2)
27487	1(2)
27488	1(2)
27495	1(2)
27496	1(2)
27497	1(2)
27498	1(2)
27499	1(2)
27500	1(2)
27501	1(2)
27502	1(2)
27503	1(2)
27506	1(2)
27507	1(2)
27508	1(2)

CPT	MUE
27509	1(2)
27510	1(2)
27511	1(2)
27513	1(2)
27514	1(2)
27516	1(2)
27517	1(2)
27519	1(2)
27520	1(2)
27524	1(2)
27530	1(2)
27532	1(2)
27535	1(2)
27536	1(2)
27538	1(2)
27540	1(2)
27550	1(2)
27552	1(2)
27556	1(2)
27557	1(2)
27558	1(2)
27560	1(2)
27562	1(2)
27566	1(2)
27570	1(2)
27580	1(2)
27590	1(2)
27591	1(2)
27592	1(2)
27594	1(2)
27596	1(2)
27598	1(2)
27599	1(3)
27600	1(2)
27601	1(2)
27602	1(2)
27603	2(3)
27604	2(3)
27605	1(2)
27606	1(2)
27607	2(3)
27610	1(2)
27612	1(2)
27613	3(3)
27614	3(3)
27615	1(3)
27616	1(3)
27618	3(3)
27619	2(3)
27620	1(2)
27625	1(2)
27626	1(2)
27630	2(3)
27632	3(3)
27634	2(3)
27635	1(3)
27637	1(3)
27638	1(3)
27640	1(3)
27641	1(3)
27645	1(3)
27646	1(3)
27647	1(3)
27648	1(2)
27650	1(2)
27652	1(2)

CPT	MUE
27654	1(2)
27656	1(3)
27658	2(3)
27659	2(3)
27664	2(3)
27665	2(3)
27675	1(2)
27676	1(2)
27680	2(3)
27681	1(2)
27685	2(3)
27686	3(3)
27687	1(2)
27690	2(3)
27691	2(3)
27692	4(3)
27695	1(2)
27696	1(2)
27698	2(2)
27700	1(2)
27702	1(2)
27703	1(2)
27704	1(2)
27705	1(3)
27707	1(3)
27709	1(3)
27712	1(2)
27715	1(2)
27720	1(2)
27722	1(2)
27724	1(2)
27725	1(2)
27726	1(2)
27727	1(2)
27730	1(2)
27732	1(2)
27734	1(2)
27740	1(2)
27742	1(2)
27745	1(2)
27750	1(2)
27752	1(2)
27756	1(2)
27758	1(2)
27759	1(2)
27760	1(2)
27762	1(2)
27766	1(2)
27767	1(2)
27768	1(2)
27769	1(2)
27780	1(2)
27781	1(2)
27784	1(2)
27786	1(2)
27788	1(2)
27792	1(2)
27808	1(2)
27810	1(2)
27814	1(2)
27816	1(2)
27818	1(2)
27822	1(2)
27823	1(2)
27824	1(2)
27825	1(2)

CPT	MUE
27826	1(2)
27827	1(2)
27828	1(2)
27829	1(2)
27830	1(2)
27831	1(2)
27832	1(2)
27840	1(2)
27842	1(2)
27846	1(2)
27848	1(2)
27860	1(2)
27870	1(2)
27871	1(3)
27880	1(2)
27881	1(2)
27882	1(2)
27884	1(2)
27886	1(2)
27888	1(2)
27889	1(2)
27892	1(2)
27893	1(2)
27894	1(2)
27899	1(3)
28001	2(3)
28002	3(3)
28003	2(3)
28005	3(3)
28008	2(3)
28010	4(3)
28011	4(3)
28020	2(3)
28022	3(3)
28024	4(3)
28035	1(2)
28039	2(3)
28041	2(3)
28043	4(3)
28045	4(3)
28046	1(3)
28047	1(3)
28050	2(3)
28052	2(3)
28054	2(3)
28055	1(3)
28060	1(2)
28062	1(2)
28070	2(3)
28072	4(3)
28080	3(3)
28086	2(3)
28088	2(3)
28090	2(3)
28092	2(3)
28100	1(3)
28102	1(3)
28103	1(3)
28104	2(3)
28106	1(3)
28107	1(3)
28108	2(3)
28110	1(2)
28111	1(2)
28112	4(3)
28113	1(2)

CPT	MUE
28114	1(2)
28116	1(2)
28118	1(2)
28119	1(2)
28120	2(3)
28122	4(3)
28124	4(3)
28126	4(3)
28130	1(2)
28140	3(3)
28150	4(3)
28153	4(3)
28160	5(3)
28171	1(3)
28173	2(3)
28175	2(3)
28190	3(3)
28192	2(3)
28193	2(3)
28200	4(3)
28202	2(3)
28208	4(3)
28210	2(3)
28220	1(2)
28222	1(2)
28225	1(2)
28226	1(2)
28230	1(2)
28232	6(3)
28234	6(3)
28238	1(2)
28240	1(2)
28250	1(2)
28260	1(2)
28261	1(3)
28262	1(2)
28264	1(2)
28270	6(3)
28272	6(3)
28280	1(2)
28285	4(3)
28286	1(2)
28288	4(3)
28289	1(2)
28291	1(2)
28292	1(2)
28295	1(2)
28296	1(2)
28297	1(2)
28298	1(2)
28299	1(2)
28300	1(3)
28302	1(2)
28304	1(3)
28305	1(3)
28306	1(2)
28307	1(2)
28308	4(3)
28309	1(2)
28310	1(2)
28312	4(3)
28313	4(3)
28315	1(2)
28320	1(2)
28322	2(3)
28340	2(3)

CPT	MUE
28341	2(3)
28344	1(2)
28345	2(3)
28360	1(2)
28400	1(2)
28405	1(2)
28406	1(2)
28415	1(2)
28420	1(2)
28430	1(2)
28435	1(2)
28436	1(2)
28445	1(2)
28446	1(2)
28450	2(3)
28455	3(3)
28456	2(3)
28465	3(3)
28470	2(3)
28475	5(3)
28476	4(3)
28485	5(3)
28490	1(2)
28495	1(2)
28496	1(2)
28505	1(2)
28510	4(3)
28515	4(3)
28525	4(3)
28530	1(2)
28531	1(2)
28540	1(3)
28545	1(3)
28546	1(3)
28555	1(3)
28570	1(2)
28575	1(2)
28576	1(2)
28585	1(3)
28600	2(3)
28605	2(3)
28606	3(3)
28615	5(3)
28630	2(3)
28635	2(3)
28636	4(3)
28645	4(3)
28660	4(3)
28665	3(3)
28666	4(3)
28675	3(3)
28705	1(2)
28715	1(2)
28725	1(2)
28730	1(2)
28735	1(2)
28737	1(2)
28740	1(2)
28750	1(2)
28755	1(2)
28760	1(2)
28800	1(2)
28805	1(2)
28810	5(3)
28820	6(3)
28825	8(3)

CPT	MUE
28890	1(2)
28899	1(3)
29000	1(3)
29010	1(3)
29015	1(3)
29035	1(3)
29040	1(3)
29044	1(3)
29046	1(3)
29049	1(3)
29055	1(3)
29058	1(3)
29065	1(3)
29075	1(3)
29085	1(3)
29086	2(3)
29105	1(2)
29125	1(2)
29126	1(2)
29130	3(3)
29131	2(3)
29200	1(2)
29240	1(2)
29260	1(3)
29280	2(3)
29305	1(3)
29325	1(3)
29345	1(3)
29355	1(3)
29358	1(3)
29365	1(3)
29405	1(3)
29425	1(3)
29435	1(3)
29440	1(2)
29445	1(3)
29450	1(3)
29505	1(2)
29515	1(2)
29520	1(2)
29530	1(2)
29540	1(2)
29550	1(2)
29580	1(2)
29581	1(2)
29584	1(2)
29700	2(3)
29705	1(3)
29710	1(2)
29720	1(2)
29730	1(3)
29740	1(3)
29750	1(3)
29799	1(3)
29800	1(2)
29804	1(2)
29805	1(2)
29806	1(2)
29807	1(2)
29819	1(2)
29820	1(2)
29821	1(2)
29822	1(2)
29823	1(2)
29824	1(2)
29825	1(2)

CPT	MUE
29826	1(2)
29827	1(2)
29828	1(2)
29830	1(2)
29834	1(2)
29835	1(2)
29836	1(2)
29837	1(2)
29838	1(2)
29840	1(2)
29843	1(2)
29844	1(2)
29845	1(2)
29846	1(2)
29847	1(2)
29848	1(2)
29850	1(2)
29851	1(2)
29855	1(2)
29856	1(2)
29860	1(2)
29861	1(2)
29862	1(2)
29863	1(2)
29866	1(2)
29867	1(2)
29868	1(3)
29870	1(2)
29871	1(2)
29873	1(2)
29874	1(2)
29875	1(2)
29876	1(2)
29877	1(2)
29879	1(2)
29880	1(2)
29881	1(2)
29882	1(2)
29883	1(2)
29884	1(2)
29885	1(2)
29886	1(2)
29887	1(2)
29888	1(2)
29889	1(2)
29891	1(2)
29892	1(2)
29893	1(2)
29894	1(2)
29895	1(2)
29897	1(2)
29898	1(2)
29899	1(2)
29900	2(3)
29901	2(3)
29902	2(3)
29904	1(2)
29905	1(2)
29906	1(2)
29907	1(2)
29914	1(2)
29915	1(2)
29916	1(2)
29999	1(3)
30000	1(3)
30020	1(3)

CPT	MUE	CPT	MUE	CPT	MUE	CPT	MUE	CPT	MUE	CPT	MUE	CPT	MUE	CPT	MUE
30100	2(3)	31225	1(2)	31552	1(2)	31730	1(3)	32601	1(3)	33207	1(3)	33340	1(2)	33530	1(2)
30110	1(2)	31230	1(2)	31553	1(2)	31750	1(2)	32604	1(3)	33208	1(3)	33361	1(2)	33533	1(2)
30115	1(2)	31231	1(2)	31554	1(2)	31755	1(2)	32606	1(3)	33210	1(3)	33362	1(2)	33534	1(2)
30117	2(3)	31233	1(2)	31560	1(2)	31760	1(2)	32607	1(3)	33211	1(3)	33363	1(2)	33535	1(2)
30118	1(3)	31235	1(2)	31561	1(2)	31766	1(2)	32608	1(3)	33212	1(3)	33364	1(2)	33536	1(2)
30120	1(2)	31237	1(2)	31570	1(2)	31770	2(3)	32609	1(3)	33213	1(3)	33365	1(2)	33542	1(2)
30124	2(3)	31238	1(3)	31571	1(2)	31775	1(3)	32650	1(2)	33214	1(3)	33366	1(3)	33545	1(2)
30125	1(3)	31239	1(2)	31572	1(2)	31780	1(2)	32651	1(2)	33215	2(3)	33367	1(2)	33548	1(2)
30130	1(2)	31240	1(2)	31573	1(2)	31781	1(2)	32652	1(2)	33216	1(3)	33368	1(2)	33572	3(2)
30140	1(2)	31241	1(2)	31574	1(2)	31785	1(3)	32653	1(3)	33217	1(3)	33369	1(2)	33600	1(3)
30150	1(2)	31253	1(2)	31575	1(3)	31786	1(3)	32654	1(3)	33218	1(3)	33390	1(2)	33602	1(3)
30160	1(2)	31254	1(2)	31576	1(3)	31800	1(3)	32655	1(3)	33220	1(3)	33391	1(2)	33606	1(2)
30200	1(2)	31255	1(2)	31577	1(3)	31805	1(3)	32656	1(2)	33221	1(3)	33404	1(2)	33608	1(2)
30210	1(3)	31256	1(2)	31578	1(3)	31820	1(2)	32658	1(3)	33222	1(3)	33405	1(2)	33610	1(2)
30220	1(2)	31257	1(2)	31579	1(2)	31825	1(2)	32659	1(2)	33223	1(3)	33406	1(2)	33611	1(2)
30300	1(3)	31259	1(2)	31580	1(2)	31830	1(2)	32661	1(3)	33224	1(3)	33410	1(2)	33612	1(2)
30310	1(3)	31267	1(2)	31584	1(2)	31899	1(3)	32662	1(3)	33225	1(3)	33411	1(2)	33615	1(2)
30320	1(3)	31276	1(2)	31587	1(2)	32035	1(2)	32663	1(3)	33226	1(3)	33412	1(2)	33617	1(2)
30400	1(2)	31287	1(2)	31590	1(2)	32036	1(3)	32664	1(2)	33227	1(3)	33413	1(2)	33619	1(2)
30410	1(2)	31288	1(2)	31591	1(2)	32096	1(3)	32665	1(2)	33228	1(3)	33414	1(2)	33620	1(2)
30420	1(2)	31290	1(2)	31592	1(2)	32097	1(3)	32666	1(3)	33229	1(3)	33415	1(2)	33621	1(3)
30430	1(2)	31291	1(2)	31599	1(3)	32098	1(2)	32667	3(3)	33230	1(3)	33416	1(2)	33622	1(2)
30435	1(2)	31292	1(2)	31600	1(2)	32100	1(3)	32668	2(3)	33231	1(3)	33417	1(2)	33641	1(2)
30450	1(2)	31293	1(2)	31601	1(2)	32110	1(3)	32669	2(3)	33233	1(2)	33418	1(3)	33645	1(2)
30460	1(2)	31294	1(2)	31603	1(2)	32120	1(3)	32670	1(2)	33234	1(2)	33419	1(2)	33647	1(2)
30462	1(2)	31295	1(2)	31605	1(2)	32124	1(3)	32671	1(2)	33235	1(2)	33420	1(2)	33660	1(2)
30465	1(2)	31296	1(2)	31610	1(2)	32140	1(3)	32672	1(3)	33236	1(2)	33422	1(2)	33665	1(2)
30468	1(2)	31297	1(2)	31611	1(2)	32141	1(3)	32673	1(2)	33237	1(2)	33425	1(2)	33670	1(2)
30520	1(2)	31298	1(2)	31612	1(3)	32150	1(3)	32674	1(2)	33238	1(2)	33426	1(2)	33675	1(2)
30540	1(2)	31299	1(3)	31613	1(2)	32151	1(3)	32701	1(2)	33240	1(3)	33427	1(2)	33676	1(2)
30545	1(2)	31300	1(2)	31614	1(2)	32160	1(3)	32800	1(3)	33241	1(2)	33430	1(2)	33677	1(2)
30560	1(2)	31360	1(2)	31615	1(3)	32200	2(3)	32810	1(3)	33243	1(2)	33440	1(2)	33681	1(2)
30580	2(3)	31365	1(2)	31622	1(3)	32215	1(2)	32815	1(3)	33244	1(2)	33460	1(2)	33684	1(2)
30600	1(3)	31367	1(2)	31623	1(3)	32220	1(2)	32820	1(2)	33249	1(3)	33463	1(2)	33688	1(2)
30620	1(2)	31368	1(2)	31624	1(3)	32225	1(2)	32850	1(2)	33250	1(2)	33464	1(2)	33690	1(2)
30630	1(2)	31370	1(2)	31625	1(2)	32310	1(3)	32851	1(2)	33251	1(2)	33465	1(2)	33692	1(2)
30801	1(2)	31375	1(2)	31626	1(2)	32320	1(3)	32852	1(2)	33254	1(2)	33468	1(2)	33694	1(2)
30802	1(2)	31380	1(2)	31627	1(3)	32400	2(3)	32853	1(2)	33255	1(2)	33470	1(2)	33697	1(2)
30901	1(3)	31382	1(2)	31628	1(2)	32408	2(3)	32854	1(2)	33256	1(2)	33471	1(2)	33702	1(2)
30903	1(3)	31390	1(2)	31629	1(2)	32440	1(2)	32855	1(2)	33257	1(2)	33474	1(2)	33710	1(2)
30905	1(2)	31395	1(2)	31630	1(3)	32442	1(2)	32856	1(2)	33258	1(2)	33475	1(2)	33720	1(2)
30906	1(3)	31400	1(3)	31631	1(2)	32445	1(2)	32900	1(2)	33259	1(2)	33476	1(2)	33722	1(3)
30915	1(3)	31420	1(2)	31632	2(3)	32480	1(2)	32905	1(2)	33261	1(2)	33477	1(2)	33724	1(2)
30920	1(3)	31500	2(3)	31633	2(3)	32482	1(2)	32906	1(2)	33262	1(3)	33478	1(2)	33726	1(2)
30930	1(2)	31502	1(3)	31634	1(3)	32484	2(3)	32940	1(3)	33263	1(3)	33496	1(3)	33730	1(2)
30999	1(3)	31505	1(3)	31635	1(3)	32486	1(3)	32960	1(2)	33264	1(3)	33500	1(3)	33732	1(2)
31000	1(2)	31510	1(2)	31636	1(2)	32488	1(2)	32994	1(2)	33265	1(2)	33501	1(3)	33735	1(2)
31002	1(2)	31511	1(3)	31637	2(3)	32491	1(2)	32997	1(2)	33266	1(2)	33502	1(3)	33736	1(2)
31020	1(2)	31512	1(3)	31638	1(3)	32501	1(3)	32998	1(2)	33270	1(3)	33503	1(3)	33737	1(2)
31030	1(2)	31513	1(3)	31640	1(3)	32503	1(2)	32999	1(3)	33271	1(3)	33504	1(3)	33741	1(3)
31032	1(2)	31515	1(3)	31641	1(3)	32504	1(2)	33016	1(3)	33272	1(3)	33505	1(3)	33745	2(2)
31040	1(2)	31520	1(3)	31643	1(2)	32505	1(2)	33017	1(3)	33273	1(3)	33506	1(3)	33746	1(3)
31050	1(2)	31525	1(3)	31645	1(2)	32506	3(3)	33018	1(3)	33274	1(3)	33507	1(3)	33750	1(3)
31051	1(2)	31526	1(3)	31646	2(3)	32507	2(3)	33019	1(3)	33275	1(3)	33508	1(2)	33755	1(2)
31070	1(2)	31527	1(2)	31647	1(2)	32540	1(3)	33020	1(3)	33285	1(3)	33510	1(2)	33762	1(2)
31075	1(2)	31528	1(2)	31648	1(2)	32550	2(3)	33025	1(2)	33286	1(3)	33511	1(2)	33764	1(3)
31080	1(2)	31529	1(3)	31649	2(3)	32551	2(3)	33030	1(2)	33289	1(3)	33512	1(2)	33766	1(2)
31081	1(2)	31530	1(3)	31651	3(3)	32552	2(2)	33031	1(2)	33300	1(3)	33513	1(2)	33767	1(2)
31084	1(2)	31531	1(3)	31652	1(2)	32553	1(2)	33050	1(2)	33305	1(3)	33514	1(2)	33768	1(2)
31085	1(2)	31535	1(3)	31653	1(2)	32554	2(3)	33120	1(3)	33310	1(2)	33516	1(2)	33770	1(2)
31086	1(2)	31536	1(3)	31654	1(3)	32555	2(3)	33130	1(3)	33315	1(2)	33517	1(2)	33771	1(2)
31087	1(2)	31540	1(3)	31660	1(2)	32556	2(3)	33140	1(2)	33320	1(3)	33518	1(2)	33774	1(2)
31090	1(2)	31541	1(3)	31661	1(2)	32557	2(3)	33141	1(2)	33321	1(3)	33519	1(2)	33775	1(2)
31200	1(2)	31545	1(2)	31717	1(3)	32560	1(3)	33202	1(2)	33322	1(3)	33521	1(2)	33776	1(2)
31201	1(2)	31546	1(2)	31720	3(3)	32561	1(2)	33203	1(2)	33330	1(3)	33522	1(2)	33777	1(2)
31205	1(2)	31551	1(2)	31725	1(3)	32562	1(2)	33206	1(3)	33335	1(3)	33523	1(2)	33778	1(2)

CPT	MUE	CPT	MUE	CPT	MUE	CPT	MUE	CPT	MUE	CPT	MUE	CPT	MUE	CPT	MUE
33779	1(2)	33962	1(3)	34716	1(2)	35271	2(3)	35631	4(3)	36222	1(3)	36570	2(3)	37191	1(3)
33780	1(2)	33963	1(3)	34717	2(2)	35276	2(3)	35632	1(3)	36223	1(3)	36571	2(3)	37192	1(3)
33781	1(2)	33964	1(3)	34718	2(2)	35281	2(3)	35633	1(3)	36224	1(3)	36572	1(3)	37193	1(3)
33782	1(2)	33965	1(3)	34808	1(3)	35286	2(3)	35634	1(3)	36225	1(3)	36573	1(3)	37195	1(3)
33783	1(2)	33966	1(3)	34812	1(2)	35301	2(3)	35636	1(3)	36226	1(3)	36575	2(3)	37197	2(3)
33786	1(2)	33967	1(3)	34813	1(2)	35302	1(2)	35637	1(3)	36227	2(2)	36576	2(3)	37200	2(3)
33788	1(2)	33968	1(3)	34820	1(2)	35303	1(2)	35638	1(3)	36228	2(3)	36578	2(3)	37211	1(2)
33800	1(2)	33969	1(3)	34830	1(2)	35304	1(2)	35642	1(3)	36245	3(3)	36580	2(3)	37212	1(2)
33802	1(3)	33970	1(3)	34831	1(2)	35305	1(2)	35645	1(3)	36246	4(3)	36581	2(3)	37213	1(2)
33803	1(3)	33971	1(3)	34832	1(2)	35306	2(3)	35646	1(3)	36247	2(3)	36582	2(3)	37214	1(2)
33813	1(2)	33973	1(3)	34833	1(2)	35311	1(2)	35647	1(3)	36248	2(3)	36583	2(3)	37215	1(2)
33814	1(2)	33974	1(3)	34834	1(2)	35321	1(2)	35650	1(3)	36251	1(3)	36584	2(3)	37216	0(3)
33820	1(2)	33975	1(3)	34839	1(2)	35331	1(2)	35654	1(3)	36252	1(3)	36585	2(3)	37217	1(2)
33822	1(2)	33976	1(3)	34841	1(2)	35341	3(3)	35656	1(3)	36253	1(3)	36589	2(3)	37218	1(2)
33824	1(2)	33977	1(3)	34842	1(2)	35351	1(3)	35661	1(3)	36254	1(3)	36590	2(3)	37220	1(2)
33840	1(2)	33978	1(3)	34843	1(2)	35355	1(2)	35663	1(3)	36260	1(2)	36591	2(3)	37221	1(2)
33845	1(2)	33979	1(3)	34844	1(2)	35361	1(2)	35665	1(3)	36261	1(2)	36592	1(3)	37222	2(2)
33851	1(2)	33980	1(3)	34845	1(2)	35363	1(2)	35666	2(3)	36262	1(2)	36593	2(3)	37223	2(2)
33852	1(2)	33981	1(3)	34846	1(2)	35371	1(2)	35671	2(3)	36299	1(3)	36595	2(3)	37224	1(2)
33853	1(2)	33982	1(3)	34847	1(2)	35372	1(2)	35681	1(3)	36400	1(3)	36596	2(3)	37225	1(2)
33858	1(2)	33983	1(3)	34848	1(2)	35390	1(3)	35682	1(2)	36405	1(3)	36597	2(3)	37226	1(2)
33859	1(2)	33984	1(3)	35001	1(2)	35400	1(3)	35683	1(2)	36406	1(3)	36598	2(3)	37227	1(2)
33863	1(2)	33985	1(3)	35002	1(2)	35500	2(3)	35685	2(3)	36410	3(3)	36600	4(3)	37228	1(2)
33864	1(2)	33986	1(3)	35005	1(2)	35501	1(3)	35686	1(3)	36415	2(3)	36620	3(3)	37229	1(2)
33866	1(2)	33987	1(3)	35011	1(2)	35506	1(3)	35691	1(3)	36416	6(3)	36625	2(3)	37230	1(2)
33871	1(2)	33988	1(3)	35013	1(2)	35508	1(3)	35693	1(3)	36420	2(3)	36640	1(3)	37231	1(2)
33875	1(2)	33989	1(3)	35021	1(2)	35509	1(3)	35694	1(3)	36425	2(3)	36660	1(3)	37232	2(3)
33877	1(2)	33990	1(3)	35022	1(2)	35510	1(3)	35695	1(3)	36430	1(3)	36680	1(3)	37233	2(3)
33880	1(2)	33991	1(3)	35045	1(3)	35511	1(3)	35697	2(3)	36440	1(3)	36800	1(3)	37234	2(3)
33881	1(2)	33992	1(2)	35081	1(2)	35512	1(3)	35700	2(3)	36450	1(3)	36810	1(3)	37235	2(3)
33883	1(2)	33993	1(3)	35082	1(2)	35515	1(3)	35701	1(2)	36455	1(3)	36815	1(3)	37236	1(2)
33884	2(3)	33995	1(3)	35091	1(2)	35516	1(3)	35702	2(2)	36456	1(3)	36818	1(3)	37237	2(3)
33886	1(2)	33997	1(3)	35092	1(2)	35518	1(3)	35703	2(2)	36460	2(3)	36819	1(3)	37238	1(2)
33889	1(2)	33999	1(3)	35102	1(2)	35521	1(3)	35800	2(3)	36465	1(2)	36820	1(3)	37239	2(3)
33891	1(2)	34001	1(3)	35103	1(2)	35522	1(3)	35820	2(3)	36466	1(2)	36821	2(3)	37241	2(3)
33910	1(3)	34051	1(3)	35111	1(2)	35523	1(3)	35840	2(3)	36468	2(3)	36823	1(3)	37242	2(3)
33915	1(3)	34101	1(3)	35112	1(2)	35525	1(3)	35860	2(3)	36470	1(2)	36825	1(3)	37243	1(3)
33916	1(3)	34111	2(3)	35121	1(3)	35526	1(3)	35870	1(3)	36471	1(2)	36830	2(3)	37244	2(3)
33917	1(2)	34151	1(3)	35122	1(3)	35531	1(3)	35875	2(3)	36473	1(3)	36831	1(3)	37246	1(2)
33920	1(2)	34201	1(3)	35131	1(2)	35533	1(3)	35876	2(3)	36474	1(3)	36832	2(3)	37247	2(3)
33922	1(2)	34203	1(2)	35132	1(2)	35535	1(3)	35879	2(3)	36475	1(3)	36833	1(3)	37248	1(2)
33924	1(2)	34401	1(3)	35141	1(2)	35536	1(3)	35881	1(3)	36476	2(3)	36835	1(3)	37249	3(3)
33925	1(2)	34421	1(3)	35142	1(2)	35537	1(3)	35883	1(3)	36478	1(3)	36838	1(3)	37252	1(2)
33926	1(2)	34451	1(3)	35151	1(2)	35538	1(3)	35884	1(3)	36479	2(3)	36860	2(3)	37253	5(3)
33927	1(3)	34471	1(2)	35152	1(2)	35539	1(3)	35901	1(3)	36481	1(3)	36861	2(3)	37500	1(3)
33928	1(3)	34490	1(2)	35180	2(3)	35540	1(3)	35903	2(3)	36482	1(3)	36901	1(3)	37501	1(3)
33929	1(3)	34501	1(2)	35182	2(3)	35556	1(3)	35905	1(3)	36483	2(3)	36902	1(3)	37565	1(2)
33930	1(2)	34502	1(2)	35184	2(3)	35558	1(3)	35907	1(3)	36500	4(3)	36903	1(3)	37600	1(3)
33933	1(2)	34510	2(3)	35188	2(3)	35560	1(3)	36000	4(3)	36510	1(3)	36904	1(3)	37605	1(3)
33935	1(2)	34520	1(3)	35189	1(3)	35563	1(3)	36002	2(3)	36511	1(3)	36905	1(3)	37606	1(3)
33940	1(2)	34530	1(2)	35190	2(3)	35565	1(3)	36005	2(3)	36512	1(3)	36906	1(3)	37607	1(3)
33944	1(2)	34701	1(2)	35201	2(3)	35566	1(3)	36010	2(3)	36513	1(3)	36907	1(3)	37609	1(2)
33945	1(2)	34702	1(2)	35206	2(3)	35570	1(3)	36011	4(3)	36514	1(3)	36908	1(3)	37615	2(3)
33946	1(2)	34703	1(2)	35207	3(3)	35571	1(3)	36012	4(3)	36516	1(3)	36909	1(3)	37616	1(3)
33947	1(2)	34704	1(2)	35211	3(3)	35572	2(3)	36013	2(3)	36522	1(3)	37140	1(2)	37617	3(3)
33948	1(2)	34705	1(2)	35216	2(3)	35583	1(2)	36014	2(3)	36555	2(3)	37145	1(3)	37618	2(3)
33949	1(2)	34706	1(2)	35221	3(3)	35585	2(3)	36015	4(3)	36556	2(3)	37160	1(3)	37619	1(2)
33951	1(3)	34707	1(2)	35226	3(3)	35587	1(3)	36100	2(3)	36557	2(3)	37180	1(2)	37650	1(2)
33952	1(3)	34708	1(2)	35231	2(3)	35600	2(3)	36140	3(3)	36558	2(3)	37181	1(2)	37660	1(2)
33953	1(3)	34709	3(3)	35236	2(3)	35601	1(3)	36160	2(3)	36560	2(3)	37182	1(2)	37700	1(2)
33954	1(3)	34710	1(2)	35241	2(3)	35606	1(3)	36200	2(3)	36561	2(3)	37183	1(2)	37718	1(2)
33955	1(3)	34711	2(3)	35246	2(3)	35612	1(3)	36215	2(3)	36563	1(3)	37184	1(2)	37722	1(2)
33956	1(3)	34712	1(2)	35251	2(3)	35616	1(3)	36216	2(3)	36565	1(3)	37185	2(3)	37735	1(2)
33957	1(3)	34713	1(2)	35256	2(3)	35621	1(3)	36217	2(3)	36566	1(3)	37186	2(3)	37760	1(2)
33958	1(3)	34714	1(2)	35261	1(3)	35623	1(3)	36218	2(3)	36568	2(3)	37187	1(3)	37761	1(2)
33959	1(3)	34715	1(2)	35266	2(3)	35626	3(3)	36221	1(3)	36569	2(3)	37188	1(3)	37765	1(2)

CPT	MUE
37766	1(2)
37780	1(2)
37785	1(2)
37788	1(2)
37790	1(2)
37799	1(3)
38100	1(2)
38101	1(3)
38102	1(2)
38115	1(3)
38120	1(2)
38129	1(3)
38200	1(3)
38204	1(2)
38205	1(3)
38206	1(3)
38207	1(3)
38208	1(3)
38209	1(3)
38210	1(3)
38211	1(3)
38212	1(3)
38213	1(3)
38214	1(3)
38215	1(3)
38220	1(3)
38221	1(3)
38222	1(2)
38230	1(2)
38232	1(2)
38240	1(3)
38241	1(2)
38242	1(2)
38243	1(3)
38300	1(3)
38305	1(3)
38308	1(3)
38380	1(2)
38381	1(2)
38382	1(2)
38500	2(3)
38505	2(3)
38510	1(2)
38520	1(2)
38525	1(2)
38530	1(2)
38531	1(2)
38542	1(2)
38550	1(3)
38555	1(3)
38562	1(2)
38564	1(2)
38570	1(2)
38571	1(2)
38572	1(2)
38573	1(2)
38589	1(3)
38700	1(2)
38720	1(2)
38724	1(2)
38740	1(2)
38745	1(2)
38746	1(2)
38747	1(2)
38760	1(2)
38765	1(2)

CPT	MUE
38770	1(2)
38780	1(2)
38790	1(2)
38792	1(3)
38794	1(2)
38900	1(3)
38999	1(3)
39000	1(2)
39010	1(2)
39200	1(2)
39220	1(2)
39401	1(3)
39402	1(3)
39499	1(3)
39501	1(3)
39503	1(2)
39540	1(2)
39541	1(2)
39545	1(2)
39560	1(3)
39561	1(3)
39599	1(3)
40490	2(3)
40500	2(3)
40510	2(3)
40520	2(3)
40525	2(3)
40527	2(3)
40530	2(3)
40650	2(3)
40652	2(3)
40654	2(3)
40700	1(2)
40701	1(2)
40702	1(2)
40720	1(2)
40761	1(2)
40799	1(3)
40800	2(3)
40801	2(3)
40804	1(3)
40805	2(3)
40806	2(2)
40808	2(3)
40810	2(3)
40812	2(3)
40814	4(3)
40816	2(3)
40818	2(3)
40819	2(2)
40820	2(3)
40830	2(3)
40831	2(3)
40840	1(2)
40842	1(2)
40843	1(2)
40844	1(2)
40845	1(3)
40899	1(3)
41000	1(3)
41005	1(3)
41006	2(3)
41007	2(3)
41008	2(3)
41009	2(3)
41010	1(2)

CPT	MUE
41015	2(3)
41016	1(3)
41017	2(3)
41018	2(3)
41019	1(2)
41100	2(3)
41105	2(3)
41108	2(3)
41110	2(3)
41112	2(3)
41113	2(3)
41114	2(3)
41115	1(2)
41116	2(3)
41120	1(2)
41130	1(2)
41135	1(2)
41140	1(2)
41145	1(2)
41150	1(2)
41153	1(2)
41155	1(2)
41250	2(3)
41251	2(3)
41252	2(3)
41510	1(2)
41512	1(2)
41520	1(3)
41530	1(3)
41599	1(3)
41800	2(3)
41805	1(3)
41806	1(3)
41820	4(2)
41821	2(3)
41822	1(2)
41823	1(2)
41825	2(3)
41826	2(3)
41827	2(3)
41828	4(2)
41830	2(3)
41850	2(3)
41870	2(3)
41872	4(2)
41874	4(2)
41899	1(3)
42000	1(3)
42100	2(3)
42104	2(3)
42106	2(3)
42107	2(3)
42120	1(2)
42140	1(2)
42145	1(2)
42160	1(3)
42180	1(3)
42182	1(3)
42200	1(2)
42205	1(2)
42210	1(2)
42215	1(2)
42220	1(2)
42225	1(2)
42226	1(2)
42227	1(2)

CPT	MUE
42235	1(2)
42260	1(3)
42280	1(2)
42281	1(2)
42299	1(3)
42300	2(3)
42305	2(3)
42310	2(3)
42320	2(3)
42330	1(3)
42335	2(2)
42340	1(2)
42400	2(3)
42405	2(3)
42408	1(3)
42409	1(3)
42410	1(2)
42415	1(2)
42420	1(2)
42425	1(2)
42426	1(2)
42440	1(2)
42450	1(3)
42500	2(3)
42505	2(3)
42507	1(2)
42509	1(2)
42510	1(2)
42550	2(3)
42600	1(3)
42650	2(3)
42660	2(3)
42665	2(3)
42699	1(3)
42700	2(3)
42720	1(3)
42725	1(3)
42800	3(3)
42804	1(3)
42806	1(3)
42808	2(3)
42809	1(3)
42810	1(3)
42815	1(3)
42820	1(2)
42821	1(2)
42825	1(2)
42826	1(2)
42830	1(2)
42831	1(2)
42835	1(2)
42836	1(2)
42842	1(3)
42844	1(3)
42845	1(3)
42860	1(3)
42870	1(3)
42890	1(2)
42892	1(3)
42894	1(3)
42900	1(3)
42950	1(2)
42953	1(3)
42955	1(2)
42960	1(3)
42961	1(3)

CPT	MUE
42962	1(3)
42970	1(3)
42971	1(3)
42972	1(3)
42999	1(3)
43020	1(2)
43030	1(2)
43045	1(2)
43100	1(3)
43101	1(3)
43107	1(2)
43108	1(2)
43112	1(2)
43113	1(2)
43116	1(2)
43117	1(2)
43118	1(2)
43121	1(2)
43122	1(2)
43123	1(2)
43124	1(2)
43130	1(3)
43135	1(3)
43180	1(2)
43191	1(3)
43192	1(3)
43193	1(3)
43194	1(3)
43195	1(3)
43196	1(3)
43197	1(3)
43198	1(3)
43200	1(3)
43201	1(2)
43202	1(2)
43204	1(2)
43205	1(2)
43206	1(2)
43210	1(2)
43211	1(3)
43212	1(3)
43213	1(2)
43214	1(3)
43215	1(3)
43216	1(2)
43217	1(2)
43220	1(3)
43226	1(3)
43227	1(3)
43229	1(3)
43231	1(2)
43232	1(2)
43233	1(3)
43235	1(3)
43236	1(2)
43237	1(2)
43238	1(2)
43239	1(2)
43240	1(2)
43241	1(3)
43242	1(2)
43243	1(2)
43244	1(2)
43245	1(2)
43246	1(2)
43247	1(2)

CPT	MUE
43248	1(3)
43249	1(3)
43250	1(2)
43251	1(2)
43252	1(2)
43253	1(3)
43254	1(3)
43255	2(3)
43257	1(2)
43259	1(2)
43260	1(3)
43261	1(2)
43262	2(2)
43263	1(2)
43264	1(2)
43265	1(2)
43266	1(3)
43270	1(3)
43273	1(2)
43274	2(3)
43275	1(3)
43276	2(3)
43277	3(3)
43278	1(3)
43279	1(2)
43280	1(2)
43281	1(2)
43282	1(2)
43283	1(2)
43284	1(2)
43285	1(2)
43286	1(2)
43287	1(2)
43288	1(2)
43289	1(3)
43300	1(2)
43305	1(2)
43310	1(2)
43312	1(2)
43313	1(2)
43314	1(2)
43320	1(2)
43325	1(2)
43327	1(2)
43328	1(2)
43330	1(2)
43331	1(2)
43332	1(2)
43333	1(2)
43334	1(2)
43335	1(2)
43336	1(2)
43337	1(2)
43338	1(2)
43340	1(2)
43341	1(2)
43351	1(2)
43352	1(2)
43360	1(2)
43361	1(2)
43400	1(2)
43405	1(2)
43410	1(3)
43415	1(3)
43420	1(3)
43425	1(3)

CPT	MUE
43450	1(3)
43453	1(3)
43460	1(3)
43496	1(3)
43499	1(3)
43500	1(2)
43501	1(3)
43502	1(2)
43510	1(2)
43520	1(2)
43605	1(2)
43610	2(3)
43611	2(3)
43620	1(2)
43621	1(2)
43622	1(2)
43631	1(2)
43632	1(2)
43633	1(2)
43634	1(2)
43635	1(2)
43640	1(2)
43641	1(2)
43644	1(2)
43645	1(2)
43647	1(2)
43648	1(2)
43651	1(2)
43652	1(2)
43653	1(2)
43659	1(3)
43752	2(3)
43753	1(3)
43754	1(3)
43755	1(3)
43756	1(2)
43757	1(2)
43761	2(3)
43762	2(3)
43763	2(3)
43770	1(2)
43771	1(2)
43772	1(2)
43773	1(2)
43774	1(2)
43775	1(2)
43800	1(2)
43810	1(2)
43820	1(2)
43825	1(2)
43830	1(2)
43831	1(2)
43832	1(2)
43840	2(3)
43842	0(3)
43843	1(2)
43845	1(2)
43846	1(2)
43847	1(2)
43848	1(2)
43850	1(2)
43855	1(2)
43860	1(2)
43865	1(2)
43870	1(2)
43880	1(3)

CPT	MUE
43881	1(3)
43882	1(3)
43886	1(2)
43887	1(2)
43888	1(2)
43999	1(3)
44005	1(2)
44010	1(2)
44015	1(2)
44020	2(3)
44021	1(3)
44025	1(3)
44050	1(2)
44055	1(2)
44100	1(2)
44110	1(2)
44111	1(2)
44120	1(2)
44121	2(3)
44125	1(2)
44126	1(2)
44127	1(2)
44128	2(3)
44130	2(3)
44132	1(2)
44133	1(2)
44135	1(2)
44136	1(2)
44137	1(2)
44139	1(2)
44140	2(3)
44141	1(3)
44143	1(2)
44144	1(3)
44145	1(2)
44146	1(2)
44147	1(3)
44150	1(2)
44151	1(2)
44155	1(2)
44156	1(2)
44157	1(2)
44158	1(2)
44160	1(2)
44180	1(2)
44186	1(2)
44187	1(3)
44188	1(3)
44202	1(2)
44203	2(3)
44204	2(3)
44205	1(2)
44206	1(2)
44207	1(2)
44208	1(2)
44210	1(2)
44211	1(2)
44212	1(2)
44213	1(2)
44227	1(3)
44238	1(3)
44300	1(3)
44310	2(3)
44312	1(2)
44314	1(2)
44316	1(2)

CPT	MUE
44320	1(2)
44322	1(2)
44340	1(2)
44345	1(2)
44346	1(2)
44360	1(3)
44361	1(2)
44363	1(3)
44364	1(2)
44365	1(2)
44366	1(3)
44369	1(2)
44370	1(2)
44372	1(2)
44373	1(2)
44376	1(3)
44377	1(2)
44378	1(3)
44379	1(2)
44380	1(3)
44381	1(3)
44382	1(2)
44384	1(3)
44385	1(3)
44386	1(2)
44388	1(3)
44389	1(2)
44390	1(3)
44391	1(3)
44392	1(2)
44394	1(2)
44401	1(2)
44402	1(3)
44403	1(3)
44404	1(3)
44405	1(3)
44406	1(3)
44407	1(2)
44408	1(3)
44500	1(3)
44602	1(2)
44603	1(2)
44604	1(2)
44605	1(2)
44615	3(3)
44620	2(3)
44625	1(3)
44626	1(3)
44640	2(3)
44650	2(3)
44660	1(3)
44661	1(3)
44680	1(3)
44700	1(2)
44701	1(2)
44705	1(3)
44715	1(2)
44720	2(3)
44721	2(3)
44799	1(3)
44800	1(3)
44820	1(3)
44850	1(3)
44899	1(3)
44900	1(2)
44950	1(2)

CPT	MUE
44955	1(2)
44960	1(2)
44970	1(2)
44979	1(3)
45000	1(3)
45005	1(3)
45020	1(3)
45100	2(3)
45108	1(2)
45110	1(2)
45111	1(2)
45112	1(2)
45113	1(2)
45114	1(2)
45116	1(2)
45119	1(2)
45120	1(2)
45121	1(2)
45123	1(2)
45126	1(2)
45130	1(2)
45135	1(2)
45136	1(2)
45150	1(2)
45160	1(3)
45171	2(3)
45172	2(3)
45190	1(3)
45300	1(3)
45303	1(3)
45305	1(2)
45307	1(3)
45308	1(2)
45309	1(2)
45315	1(2)
45317	1(3)
45320	1(2)
45321	1(2)
45327	1(2)
45330	1(3)
45331	1(2)
45332	1(3)
45333	1(2)
45334	1(3)
45335	1(2)
45337	1(2)
45338	1(2)
45340	1(2)
45341	1(2)
45342	1(2)
45346	1(2)
45347	1(3)
45349	1(3)
45350	1(2)
45378	1(3)
45379	1(3)
45380	1(2)
45381	1(2)
45382	1(3)
45384	1(2)
45385	1(2)
45386	1(2)
45388	1(2)
45389	1(3)
45390	1(3)
45391	1(2)

CPT	MUE
45392	1(2)
45393	1(3)
45395	1(2)
45397	1(2)
45398	1(2)
45399	1(3)
45400	1(2)
45402	1(2)
45499	1(3)
45500	1(2)
45505	1(2)
45520	1(2)
45540	1(2)
45541	1(2)
45550	1(2)
45560	1(2)
45562	1(2)
45563	1(2)
45800	1(3)
45805	1(3)
45820	1(3)
45825	1(3)
45900	1(2)
45905	1(2)
45910	1(2)
45915	1(2)
45990	1(2)
45999	1(3)
46020	2(3)
46030	1(3)
46040	2(3)
46045	2(3)
46050	2(3)
46060	2(3)
46070	1(2)
46080	1(2)
46083	2(3)
46200	1(3)
46220	1(2)
46221	1(2)
46230	1(2)
46250	1(2)
46255	1(2)
46257	1(2)
46258	1(2)
46260	1(2)
46261	1(2)
46262	1(2)
46270	1(3)
46275	1(3)
46280	1(2)
46285	1(3)
46288	1(3)
46320	2(3)
46500	1(2)
46505	1(2)
46600	1(3)
46601	1(3)
46604	1(2)
46606	1(2)
46607	1(2)
46608	1(3)
46610	1(2)
46611	1(2)
46612	1(2)
46614	1(3)

CPT	MUE
46615	1(2)
46700	1(2)
46705	1(2)
46706	1(3)
46707	1(3)
46710	1(3)
46712	1(3)
46715	1(2)
46716	1(2)
46730	1(2)
46735	1(2)
46740	1(2)
46742	1(2)
46744	1(2)
46746	1(2)
46748	1(2)
46750	1(2)
46751	1(2)
46753	1(2)
46754	1(3)
46760	1(2)
46761	1(2)
46900	1(2)
46910	1(2)
46916	1(2)
46917	1(2)
46922	1(2)
46924	1(2)
46930	1(2)
46940	1(2)
46942	1(3)
46945	1(2)
46946	1(2)
46947	1(2)
46948	1(2)
46999	1(3)
47000	3(3)
47001	3(3)
47010	1(3)
47015	1(2)
47100	3(3)
47120	2(3)
47122	1(2)
47125	1(2)
47130	1(2)
47133	1(2)
47135	1(2)
47140	1(2)
47141	1(2)
47142	1(2)
47143	1(2)
47144	1(2)
47145	1(2)
47146	2(3)
47147	1(3)
47300	2(3)
47350	1(3)
47360	1(3)
47361	1(3)
47362	1(3)
47370	1(2)
47371	1(2)
47379	1(3)
47380	1(2)
47381	1(2)
47382	1(2)

CPT	MUE
47383	1(2)
47399	1(3)
47400	1(3)
47420	1(2)
47425	1(2)
47460	1(2)
47480	1(2)
47490	1(2)
47531	2(3)
47532	1(3)
47533	1(3)
47534	2(3)
47535	1(3)
47536	2(3)
47537	1(3)
47538	2(3)
47539	2(3)
47540	2(3)
47541	1(3)
47542	2(3)
47543	1(3)
47544	1(3)
47550	1(3)
47552	1(3)
47553	1(2)
47554	1(3)
47555	1(2)
47556	1(2)
47562	1(2)
47563	1(2)
47564	1(2)
47570	1(2)
47579	1(3)
47600	1(2)
47605	1(2)
47610	1(2)
47612	1(2)
47620	1(2)
47700	1(2)
47701	1(2)
47711	1(2)
47712	1(2)
47715	1(2)
47720	1(2)
47721	1(2)
47740	1(2)
47741	1(2)
47760	1(2)
47765	1(2)
47780	1(2)
47785	1(2)
47800	1(2)
47801	1(3)
47802	1(2)
47900	1(2)
47999	1(3)
48000	1(2)
48001	1(2)
48020	1(3)
48100	1(3)
48102	1(3)
48105	1(2)
48120	1(3)
48140	1(2)
48145	1(2)
48146	1(2)

CPT	MUE
48148	1(2)
48150	1(2)
48152	1(2)
48153	1(2)
48154	1(2)
48155	1(2)
48160	0(3)
48400	1(3)
48500	1(3)
48510	1(3)
48520	1(3)
48540	1(3)
48545	1(3)
48547	1(2)
48548	1(2)
48550	1(2)
48551	1(2)
48552	2(3)
48554	1(2)
48556	1(2)
48999	1(3)
49000	1(2)
49002	1(3)
49010	1(3)
49013	1(2)
49014	1(3)
49020	2(3)
49040	2(3)
49060	2(3)
49062	1(3)
49082	1(3)
49083	2(3)
49084	1(3)
49180	2(3)
49185	2(3)
49203	1(2)
49204	1(2)
49205	1(2)
49215	1(2)
49250	1(2)
49255	1(2)
49320	1(3)
49321	1(2)
49322	1(2)
49323	1(2)
49324	1(2)
49325	1(2)
49326	1(2)
49327	1(2)
49329	1(3)
49400	1(3)
49402	1(3)
49405	2(3)
49406	2(3)
49407	1(3)
49411	1(2)
49412	1(2)
49418	1(3)
49419	1(2)
49421	1(2)
49422	1(2)
49423	2(3)
49424	3(3)
49425	1(2)
49426	1(3)
49427	1(3)

CPT	MUE
49428	1(2)
49429	1(2)
49435	1(2)
49436	1(2)
49440	1(3)
49441	1(3)
49442	1(3)
49446	1(2)
49450	1(3)
49451	1(3)
49452	1(3)
49460	1(3)
49465	1(3)
49491	1(2)
49492	1(2)
49495	1(2)
49496	1(2)
49500	1(2)
49501	1(2)
49505	1(2)
49507	1(2)
49520	1(2)
49521	1(2)
49525	1(2)
49540	1(2)
49550	1(2)
49553	1(2)
49555	1(2)
49557	1(2)
49560	2(3)
49561	1(3)
49565	2(3)
49566	2(3)
49568	2(3)
49570	1(3)
49572	1(3)
49580	1(2)
49582	1(2)
49585	1(2)
49587	1(2)
49590	1(2)
49600	1(2)
49605	1(2)
49606	1(2)
49610	1(2)
49611	1(2)
49650	1(2)
49651	1(2)
49652	2(3)
49653	2(3)
49654	1(3)
49655	1(3)
49656	1(3)
49657	1(3)
49659	1(3)
49900	1(3)
49904	1(3)
49905	1(3)
49906	1(3)
49999	1(3)
50010	1(2)
50020	1(3)
50040	1(2)
50045	1(2)
50060	1(2)
50065	1(2)

CPT	MUE
50070	1(2)
50075	1(2)
50080	1(2)
50081	1(2)
50100	1(2)
50120	1(2)
50125	1(2)
50130	1(2)
50135	1(2)
50200	1(3)
50205	1(3)
50220	1(2)
50225	1(2)
50230	1(2)
50234	1(2)
50236	1(2)
50240	1(2)
50250	1(3)
50280	1(2)
50290	1(3)
50300	1(2)
50320	1(2)
50323	1(2)
50325	1(2)
50327	2(3)
50328	1(3)
50329	1(3)
50340	1(2)
50360	1(2)
50365	1(2)
50370	1(2)
50380	1(2)
50382	1(3)
50384	1(3)
50385	1(3)
50386	1(3)
50387	1(3)
50389	1(3)
50390	2(3)
50391	1(3)
50396	1(3)
50400	1(2)
50405	1(2)
50430	2(3)
50431	2(3)
50432	2(3)
50433	2(3)
50434	2(3)
50435	2(3)
50436	1(3)
50437	1(3)
50500	1(3)
50520	1(3)
50525	1(3)
50526	1(3)
50540	1(2)
50541	1(2)
50542	1(2)
50543	1(2)
50544	1(2)
50545	1(2)
50546	1(2)
50547	1(2)
50548	1(2)
50549	1(3)
50551	1(3)

CPT	MUE
50553	1(3)
50555	1(2)
50557	1(2)
50561	1(2)
50562	1(3)
50570	1(3)
50572	1(3)
50574	1(2)
50575	1(2)
50576	1(2)
50580	1(2)
50590	1(2)
50592	1(2)
50593	1(2)
50600	1(3)
50605	1(3)
50606	1(3)
50610	1(2)
50620	1(2)
50630	1(2)
50650	1(2)
50660	1(3)
50684	1(3)
50686	2(3)
50688	2(3)
50690	2(3)
50693	2(3)
50694	2(3)
50695	2(3)
50700	1(2)
50705	2(3)
50706	2(3)
50715	1(2)
50722	1(2)
50725	1(3)
50727	1(3)
50728	1(3)
50740	1(2)
50750	1(2)
50760	1(2)
50770	1(2)
50780	1(2)
50782	1(2)
50783	1(2)
50785	1(2)
50800	1(2)
50810	1(3)
50815	1(2)
50820	1(2)
50825	1(3)
50830	1(3)
50840	1(2)
50845	1(2)
50860	1(2)
50900	1(3)
50920	2(3)
50930	2(3)
50940	1(2)
50945	1(2)
50947	1(2)
50948	1(2)
50949	1(3)
50951	1(3)
50953	1(3)
50955	1(2)
50957	1(2)

CPT	MUE
50961	1(2)
50970	1(3)
50972	1(3)
50974	1(2)
50976	1(2)
50980	1(2)
51020	1(2)
51030	1(2)
51040	1(3)
51045	2(3)
51050	1(3)
51060	1(3)
51065	1(3)
51080	1(3)
51100	1(3)
51101	1(3)
51102	1(3)
51500	1(2)
51520	1(2)
51525	1(2)
51530	1(2)
51535	1(2)
51550	1(2)
51555	1(2)
51565	1(2)
51570	1(2)
51575	1(2)
51580	1(2)
51585	1(2)
51590	1(2)
51595	1(2)
51596	1(2)
51597	1(2)
51600	1(3)
51605	1(3)
51610	1(3)
51700	1(3)
51701	2(3)
51702	2(3)
51703	2(3)
51705	2(3)
51710	1(3)
51715	1(2)
51720	1(3)
51725	1(3)
51726	1(3)
51727	1(3)
51728	1(3)
51729	1(3)
51736	1(3)
51741	1(3)
51784	1(3)
51785	1(3)
51792	1(3)
51797	1(3)
51798	1(3)
51800	1(2)
51820	1(2)
51840	1(2)
51841	1(2)
51845	1(2)
51860	1(3)
51865	1(3)
51880	1(2)
51900	1(3)
51920	1(3)

CPT	MUE
51925	1(2)
51940	1(2)
51960	1(2)
51980	1(2)
51990	1(2)
51992	1(2)
51999	1(3)
52000	1(3)
52001	1(3)
52005	2(3)
52007	1(2)
52010	1(2)
52204	1(2)
52214	1(2)
52224	1(2)
52234	1(2)
52235	1(2)
52240	1(2)
52250	1(2)
52260	1(2)
52265	1(2)
52270	1(2)
52275	1(2)
52276	1(2)
52277	1(2)
52281	1(2)
52282	1(2)
52283	1(2)
52285	1(2)
52287	1(2)
52290	1(2)
52300	1(2)
52301	1(2)
52305	1(2)
52310	1(3)
52315	2(3)
52317	1(3)
52318	1(3)
52320	1(2)
52325	1(3)
52327	1(2)
52330	1(2)
52332	1(2)
52334	1(2)
52341	1(2)
52342	1(2)
52343	1(2)
52344	1(2)
52345	1(2)
52346	1(2)
52351	1(3)
52352	1(2)
52353	1(2)
52354	1(3)
52355	1(3)
52356	1(2)
52400	1(2)
52402	1(2)
52441	1(2)
52442	6(3)
52450	1(2)
52500	1(2)
52601	1(2)
52630	1(2)
52640	1(2)
52647	1(2)

CPT	MUE
52648	1(2)
52649	1(2)
52700	1(3)
53000	1(2)
53010	1(2)
53020	1(2)
53025	1(2)
53040	1(3)
53060	1(3)
53080	1(3)
53085	1(3)
53200	1(3)
53210	1(2)
53215	1(2)
53220	1(3)
53230	1(3)
53235	1(3)
53240	1(3)
53250	1(3)
53260	1(2)
53265	1(3)
53270	1(2)
53275	1(2)
53400	1(2)
53405	1(2)
53410	1(2)
53415	1(2)
53420	1(2)
53425	1(2)
53430	1(2)
53431	1(2)
53440	1(2)
53442	1(2)
53444	1(3)
53445	1(2)
53446	1(2)
53447	1(2)
53448	1(2)
53449	1(2)
53450	1(2)
53460	1(2)
53500	1(2)
53502	1(3)
53505	1(3)
53510	1(3)
53515	1(3)
53520	1(3)
53600	1(3)
53601	1(3)
53605	1(3)
53620	1(2)
53621	1(3)
53660	1(2)
53661	1(3)
53665	1(3)
53850	1(2)
53852	1(2)
53854	1(2)
53855	1(2)
53860	1(2)
53899	1(3)
54000	1(2)
54001	1(2)
54015	1(3)
54050	1(2)
54055	1(2)

CPT	MUE
54056	1(2)
54057	1(2)
54060	1(2)
54065	1(2)
54100	2(3)
54105	2(3)
54110	1(2)
54111	1(2)
54112	1(3)
54115	1(3)
54120	1(2)
54125	1(2)
54130	1(2)
54135	1(2)
54150	1(2)
54160	1(2)
54161	1(2)
54162	1(2)
54163	1(2)
54164	1(2)
54200	1(2)
54205	1(2)
54220	1(3)
54230	1(3)
54231	1(3)
54235	1(3)
54240	1(2)
54250	1(2)
54300	1(2)
54304	1(2)
54308	1(2)
54312	1(2)
54316	1(2)
54318	1(2)
54322	1(2)
54324	1(2)
54326	1(2)
54328	1(2)
54332	1(2)
54336	1(2)
54340	1(2)
54344	1(2)
54348	1(2)
54352	1(2)
54360	1(2)
54380	1(2)
54385	1(2)
54390	1(2)
54400	1(2)
54401	1(2)
54405	1(2)
54406	1(2)
54408	1(2)
54410	1(2)
54411	1(2)
54415	1(2)
54416	1(2)
54417	1(2)
54420	1(2)
54430	1(2)
54435	1(2)
54437	1(2)
54438	1(2)
54440	1(2)
54450	1(2)
54500	1(3)

CPT	MUE
54505	1(3)
54512	1(3)
54520	1(2)
54522	1(2)
54530	1(2)
54535	1(2)
54550	1(2)
54560	1(2)
54600	1(2)
54620	1(2)
54640	1(2)
54650	1(2)
54660	1(2)
54670	1(3)
54680	1(2)
54690	1(2)
54692	1(2)
54699	1(3)
54700	1(3)
54800	1(2)
54830	1(2)
54840	1(2)
54860	1(2)
54861	1(2)
54865	1(3)
54900	1(2)
54901	1(2)
55000	1(3)
55040	1(2)
55041	1(2)
55060	1(2)
55100	2(3)
55110	1(2)
55120	1(3)
55150	1(2)
55175	1(2)
55180	1(2)
55200	1(2)
55250	1(2)
55300	1(2)
55400	1(2)
55500	1(2)
55520	1(2)
55530	1(2)
55535	1(2)
55540	1(2)
55550	1(2)
55559	1(3)
55600	1(2)
55605	1(2)
55650	1(2)
55680	1(3)
55700	1(2)
55705	1(2)
55706	1(2)
55720	1(3)
55725	1(3)
55801	1(2)
55810	1(2)
55812	1(2)
55815	1(2)
55821	1(2)
55831	1(2)
55840	1(2)
55842	1(2)
55845	1(2)

CPT	MUE
55860	1(2)
55862	1(2)
55865	1(2)
55866	1(2)
55870	1(2)
55873	1(2)
55874	1(2)
55875	1(2)
55876	1(2)
55880	1(2)
55899	1(3)
55920	1(2)
55970	1(2)
55980	1(2)
56405	2(3)
56420	1(3)
56440	1(3)
56441	1(2)
56442	1(2)
56501	1(2)
56515	1(2)
56605	1(2)
56606	6(3)
56620	1(2)
56625	1(2)
56630	1(2)
56631	1(2)
56632	1(2)
56633	1(2)
56634	1(2)
56637	1(2)
56640	1(2)
56700	1(2)
56740	1(3)
56800	1(2)
56805	1(2)
56810	1(2)
56820	1(2)
56821	1(2)
57000	1(3)
57010	1(3)
57020	1(3)
57022	1(3)
57023	1(3)
57061	1(2)
57065	1(2)
57100	2(3)
57105	2(3)
57106	1(2)
57107	1(2)
57109	1(2)
57110	1(2)
57111	1(2)
57120	1(2)
57130	1(2)
57135	2(3)
57150	1(3)
57155	1(3)
57156	1(3)
57160	1(2)
57170	1(2)
57180	1(3)
57200	1(3)
57210	1(3)
57220	1(2)
57230	1(2)

CPT	MUE
57240	1(2)
57250	1(2)
57260	1(2)
57265	1(2)
57267	2(3)
57268	1(2)
57270	1(2)
57280	1(2)
57282	1(2)
57283	1(2)
57284	1(2)
57285	1(2)
57287	1(2)
57288	1(2)
57289	1(2)
57291	1(2)
57292	1(2)
57295	1(2)
57296	1(2)
57300	1(3)
57305	1(3)
57307	1(3)
57308	1(3)
57310	1(3)
57311	1(3)
57320	1(3)
57330	1(3)
57335	1(2)
57400	1(2)
57410	1(2)
57415	1(3)
57420	1(3)
57421	1(3)
57423	1(2)
57425	1(2)
57426	1(2)
57452	1(3)
57454	1(3)
57455	1(3)
57456	1(3)
57460	1(3)
57461	1(3)
57465	1(3)
57500	1(3)
57505	1(3)
57510	1(3)
57511	1(3)
57513	1(3)
57520	1(3)
57522	1(3)
57530	1(3)
57531	1(2)
57540	1(2)
57545	1(3)
57550	1(3)
57555	1(2)
57556	1(2)
57558	1(3)
57700	1(3)
57720	1(3)
57800	1(3)
58100	1(3)
58110	1(3)
58120	1(3)
58140	1(3)
58145	1(3)

CPT	MUE
58146	1(3)
58150	1(3)
58152	1(2)
58180	1(3)
58200	1(2)
58210	1(2)
58240	1(2)
58260	1(3)
58262	1(3)
58263	1(2)
58267	1(2)
58270	1(2)
58275	1(2)
58280	1(2)
58285	1(3)
58290	1(3)
58291	1(2)
58292	1(2)
58294	1(2)
58300	0(3)
58301	1(3)
58321	1(2)
58322	1(2)
58323	1(3)
58340	1(3)
58345	1(3)
58346	1(2)
58350	1(2)
58353	1(3)
58356	1(3)
58400	1(3)
58410	1(2)
58520	1(2)
58540	1(3)
58541	1(3)
58542	1(2)
58543	1(3)
58544	1(2)
58545	1(2)
58546	1(2)
58548	1(2)
58550	1(3)
58552	1(3)
58553	1(3)
58554	1(2)
58555	1(3)
58558	1(3)
58559	1(3)
58560	1(3)
58561	1(3)
58562	1(3)
58563	1(3)
58565	1(2)
58570	1(3)
58571	1(2)
58572	1(3)
58573	1(2)
58575	1(2)
58578	1(3)
58579	1(3)
58600	1(2)
58605	1(2)
58611	1(2)
58615	1(2)
58660	1(2)
58661	1(2)

CPT	MUE
58662	1(2)
58670	1(2)
58671	1(2)
58672	1(2)
58673	1(2)
58674	1(2)
58679	1(3)
58700	1(2)
58720	1(2)
58740	1(2)
58750	1(2)
58752	1(2)
58760	1(2)
58770	1(2)
58800	1(2)
58805	1(2)
58820	1(3)
58822	1(3)
58825	1(2)
58900	1(2)
58920	1(2)
58925	1(3)
58940	1(2)
58943	1(2)
58950	1(2)
58951	1(2)
58952	1(2)
58953	1(2)
58954	1(2)
58956	1(2)
58957	1(2)
58958	1(2)
58960	1(2)
58970	1(3)
58974	1(3)
58976	2(3)
58999	1(3)
59000	2(3)
59001	2(3)
59012	2(3)
59015	2(3)
59020	2(3)
59025	2(3)
59030	2(3)
59050	2(3)
59051	2(3)
59070	2(3)
59072	2(3)
59074	2(3)
59076	2(3)
59100	1(2)
59120	1(3)
59121	1(3)
59130	1(3)
59135	1(3)
59136	1(3)
59140	1(2)
59150	1(3)
59151	1(3)
59160	1(2)
59200	1(3)
59300	1(2)
59320	1(2)
59325	1(2)
59350	1(2)
59400	1(2)

CPT	MUE
59409	2(3)
59410	1(2)
59412	1(3)
59414	1(3)
59425	1(2)
59426	1(2)
59430	1(2)
59510	1(2)
59514	1(3)
59515	1(2)
59525	1(2)
59610	1(2)
59612	2(3)
59614	1(2)
59618	1(2)
59620	1(2)
59622	1(2)
59812	1(2)
59820	1(2)
59821	1(2)
59830	1(2)
59840	1(2)
59841	1(2)
59850	1(2)
59851	1(2)
59852	1(2)
59855	1(2)
59856	1(2)
59857	1(2)
59866	1(2)
59870	1(2)
59871	1(2)
59897	1(3)
59898	1(3)
59899	1(3)
60000	1(3)
60100	3(3)
60200	2(3)
60210	1(2)
60212	1(2)
60220	1(3)
60225	1(2)
60240	1(2)
60252	1(2)
60254	1(2)
60260	1(2)
60270	1(2)
60271	1(2)
60280	1(3)
60281	1(3)
60300	2(3)
60500	1(2)
60502	1(3)
60505	1(3)
60512	1(3)
60520	1(2)
60521	1(2)
60522	1(2)
60540	1(2)
60545	1(2)
60600	1(3)
60605	1(3)
60650	1(2)
60659	1(3)
60699	1(3)
61000	1(2)

CPT	MUE
61001	1(2)
61020	2(3)
61026	2(3)
61050	1(3)
61055	1(3)
61070	2(3)
61105	1(3)
61107	1(3)
61108	1(3)
61120	1(3)
61140	1(3)
61150	1(3)
61151	1(3)
61154	1(3)
61156	1(3)
61210	1(3)
61215	1(3)
61250	1(3)
61253	1(3)
61304	1(3)
61305	1(3)
61312	2(3)
61313	2(3)
61314	2(3)
61315	1(3)
61316	1(3)
61320	2(3)
61321	1(3)
61322	1(3)
61323	1(3)
61330	1(2)
61333	1(2)
61340	1(2)
61343	1(2)
61345	1(3)
61450	1(3)
61458	1(2)
61460	1(2)
61500	1(3)
61501	1(3)
61510	1(3)
61512	1(3)
61514	2(3)
61516	1(3)
61517	1(3)
61518	1(3)
61519	1(3)
61520	1(3)
61521	1(3)
61522	1(3)
61524	2(3)
61526	1(3)
61530	1(3)
61531	1(2)
61533	2(3)
61534	1(3)
61535	2(3)
61536	1(3)
61537	1(3)
61538	1(2)
61539	1(3)
61540	1(3)
61541	1(2)
61543	1(2)
61544	1(3)
61545	1(2)

CPT	MUE
61546	1(2)
61548	1(2)
61550	1(2)
61552	1(2)
61556	1(3)
61557	1(2)
61558	1(3)
61559	1(3)
61563	2(3)
61564	1(2)
61566	1(3)
61567	1(2)
61570	1(3)
61571	1(3)
61575	1(2)
61576	1(2)
61580	1(2)
61581	1(2)
61582	1(2)
61583	1(2)
61584	1(2)
61585	1(2)
61586	1(3)
61590	1(2)
61591	1(2)
61592	1(2)
61595	1(2)
61596	1(2)
61597	1(2)
61598	1(3)
61600	1(3)
61601	1(3)
61605	1(3)
61606	1(3)
61607	1(3)
61608	1(3)
61611	1(3)
61613	1(3)
61615	1(3)
61616	1(3)
61618	2(3)
61619	2(3)
61623	2(3)
61624	2(3)
61626	2(3)
61630	1(3)
61635	2(3)
61640	0(3)
61641	0(3)
61642	0(3)
61645	1(3)
61650	1(2)
61651	2(2)
61680	1(3)
61682	1(3)
61684	1(3)
61686	1(3)
61690	1(3)
61692	1(3)
61697	2(3)
61698	1(3)
61700	2(3)
61702	1(3)
61703	1(3)
61705	1(3)
61708	1(3)

CPT	MUE
61710	1(3)
61711	1(3)
61720	1(3)
61735	1(3)
61750	2(3)
61751	2(3)
61760	1(2)
61770	1(2)
61781	1(3)
61782	1(3)
61783	1(3)
61790	1(2)
61791	1(2)
61796	1(2)
61797	4(3)
61798	1(2)
61799	4(3)
61800	1(2)
61850	1(3)
61860	1(3)
61863	1(2)
61864	1(3)
61867	1(2)
61868	2(3)
61880	1(2)
61885	1(3)
61886	1(3)
61888	1(3)
62000	1(3)
62005	1(3)
62010	1(3)
62100	1(3)
62115	1(2)
62117	1(2)
62120	1(2)
62121	1(2)
62140	1(3)
62141	1(3)
62142	2(3)
62143	2(3)
62145	2(3)
62146	2(3)
62147	1(3)
62148	1(3)
62160	1(3)
62161	1(3)
62162	1(3)
62164	1(3)
62165	1(2)
62180	1(3)
62190	1(3)
62192	1(3)
62194	1(3)
62200	1(2)
62201	1(2)
62220	1(3)
62223	1(3)
62225	2(3)
62230	2(3)
62252	2(3)
62256	1(3)
62258	1(3)
62263	1(2)
62264	1(2)
62267	2(3)
62268	1(3)

CPT	MUE
62269	2(3)
62270	2(3)
62272	2(3)
62273	2(3)
62280	1(3)
62281	1(3)
62282	1(3)
62284	1(3)
62287	1(2)
62290	5(2)
62291	4(3)
62292	1(2)
62294	1(3)
62302	1(3)
62303	1(3)
62304	1(3)
62305	1(3)
62320	1(3)
62321	1(3)
62322	1(3)
62323	1(3)
62324	1(3)
62325	1(3)
62326	1(3)
62327	1(3)
62328	2(3)
62329	1(3)
62350	1(3)
62351	1(3)
62355	1(3)
62360	1(2)
62361	1(2)
62362	1(2)
62365	1(2)
62367	1(3)
62368	1(3)
62369	1(3)
62370	1(3)
62380	2(3)
63001	1(2)
63003	1(2)
63005	1(2)
63011	1(2)
63012	1(2)
63015	1(2)
63016	1(2)
63017	1(2)
63020	1(2)
63030	1(2)
63035	4(3)
63040	1(2)
63042	1(2)
63043	4(3)
63044	4(2)
63045	1(2)
63046	1(2)
63047	1(2)
63048	5(3)
63050	1(2)
63051	1(2)
63055	1(2)
63056	1(2)
63057	3(3)
63064	1(2)
63066	1(3)
63075	1(2)

CPT	MUE
63076	3(3)
63077	1(2)
63078	3(3)
63081	1(2)
63082	6(2)
63085	1(2)
63086	2(3)
63087	1(2)
63088	3(3)
63090	1(2)
63091	3(3)
63101	1(2)
63102	1(2)
63103	3(3)
63170	1(3)
63172	1(3)
63173	1(3)
63185	1(2)
63190	1(2)
63191	1(2)
63194	1(2)
63195	1(2)
63196	1(2)
63197	1(2)
63198	1(2)
63199	1(2)
63200	1(2)
63250	1(3)
63251	1(3)
63252	1(3)
63265	1(3)
63266	1(3)
63267	1(3)
63268	1(3)
63270	1(3)
63271	1(3)
63272	1(3)
63273	1(3)
63275	1(3)
63276	1(3)
63277	1(3)
63278	1(3)
63280	1(3)
63281	1(3)
63282	1(3)
63283	1(3)
63285	1(3)
63286	1(3)
63287	1(3)
63290	1(3)
63295	1(2)
63300	1(2)
63301	1(2)
63302	1(2)
63303	1(2)
63304	1(2)
63305	1(2)
63306	1(2)
63307	1(2)
63308	3(3)
63600	2(3)
63610	1(3)
63620	1(2)
63621	2(2)
63650	2(3)
63655	1(3)

CPT	MUE	CPT	MUE	CPT	MUE	CPT	MUE	CPT	MUE	CPT	MUE	CPT	MUE	CPT	MUE
63661	1(2)	64570	1(3)	64783	2(3)	65140	1(2)	66160	1(2)	67110	1(2)	67875	1(2)	68750	1(2)
63662	1(2)	64575	2(3)	64784	3(3)	65150	1(2)	66170	1(2)	67113	1(2)	67880	1(2)	68760	4(2)
63663	1(3)	64580	2(3)	64786	1(3)	65155	1(2)	66172	1(2)	67115	1(2)	67882	1(2)	68761	4(2)
63664	1(3)	64581	2(3)	64787	4(3)	65175	1(2)	66174	1(2)	67120	1(2)	67900	1(2)	68770	1(3)
63685	1(3)	64585	2(3)	64788	5(3)	65205	1(3)	66175	1(2)	67121	1(2)	67901	1(2)	68801	4(2)
63688	1(3)	64590	1(3)	64790	1(3)	65210	1(3)	66179	1(2)	67141	1(2)	67902	1(2)	68810	1(2)
63700	1(3)	64595	1(3)	64792	2(3)	65220	1(3)	66180	1(2)	67145	1(2)	67903	1(2)	68811	1(2)
63702	1(3)	64600	2(3)	64795	2(3)	65222	1(3)	66183	1(3)	67208	1(2)	67904	1(2)	68815	1(2)
63704	1(3)	64605	1(2)	64802	1(2)	65235	1(3)	66184	1(2)	67210	1(2)	67906	1(2)	68816	1(2)
63706	1(3)	64610	1(2)	64804	1(2)	65260	1(3)	66185	1(2)	67218	1(2)	67908	1(2)	68840	1(2)
63707	1(3)	64611	1(2)	64809	1(2)	65265	1(3)	66225	1(2)	67220	1(2)	67909	1(2)	68850	1(3)
63709	1(3)	64612	1(2)	64818	1(2)	65270	1(3)	66250	1(2)	67221	1(2)	67911	2(3)	68899	1(3)
63710	1(3)	64615	1(2)	64820	4(3)	65272	1(3)	66500	1(2)	67225	1(2)	67912	1(2)	69000	1(3)
63740	1(3)	64616	1(2)	64821	1(2)	65273	1(3)	66505	1(2)	67227	1(2)	67914	2(3)	69005	1(3)
63741	1(3)	64617	1(2)	64822	1(2)	65275	1(3)	66600	1(2)	67228	1(2)	67915	2(3)	69020	1(3)
63744	1(3)	64620	5(3)	64823	1(2)	65280	1(3)	66605	1(2)	67229	1(2)	67916	2(3)	69090	0(3)
63746	1(2)	64624	2(2)	64831	1(2)	65285	1(3)	66625	1(2)	67250	1(2)	67917	2(3)	69100	3(3)
64400	4(3)	64625	2(2)	64832	3(3)	65286	1(3)	66630	1(2)	67255	1(2)	67921	2(3)	69105	1(3)
64405	1(3)	64630	1(3)	64834	1(2)	65290	1(3)	66635	1(2)	67299	1(3)	67922	2(3)	69110	1(2)
64408	1(3)	64632	1(2)	64835	1(2)	65400	1(3)	66680	1(2)	67311	1(2)	67923	2(3)	69120	1(3)
64415	1(3)	64633	1(2)	64836	1(2)	65410	1(3)	66682	1(2)	67312	1(2)	67924	2(3)	69140	1(2)
64416	1(2)	64634	4(3)	64837	2(3)	65420	1(2)	66700	1(2)	67314	1(2)	67930	2(3)	69145	1(3)
64417	1(3)	64635	1(2)	64840	1(2)	65426	1(2)	66710	1(2)	67316	1(2)	67935	2(3)	69150	1(3)
64418	1(3)	64636	4(3)	64856	2(3)	65430	1(2)	66711	1(2)	67318	1(2)	67938	2(3)	69155	1(3)
64420	2(2)	64640	5(3)	64857	2(3)	65435	1(2)	66720	1(2)	67320	2(3)	67950	2(2)	69200	1(2)
64421	3(3)	64642	1(2)	64858	1(2)	65436	1(2)	66740	1(2)	67331	1(2)	67961	2(3)	69205	1(3)
64425	1(3)	64643	3(2)	64859	2(3)	65450	1(3)	66761	1(2)	67332	1(2)	67966	2(3)	69209	1(2)
64430	1(3)	64644	1(2)	64861	1(2)	65600	1(2)	66762	1(2)	67334	1(2)	67971	1(2)	69210	1(2)
64435	1(3)	64645	3(2)	64862	1(2)	65710	1(2)	66770	1(3)	67335	1(2)	67973	1(2)	69220	1(2)
64445	1(3)	64646	1(2)	64864	2(3)	65730	1(2)	66820	1(2)	67340	2(2)	67974	1(2)	69222	1(2)
64446	1(2)	64647	1(2)	64865	1(3)	65750	1(2)	66821	1(2)	67343	1(2)	67975	1(2)	69300	1(2)
64447	1(3)	64650	1(2)	64866	1(3)	65755	1(2)	66825	1(2)	67345	1(3)	67999	1(3)	69310	1(2)
64448	1(2)	64653	1(2)	64868	1(3)	65756	1(2)	66830	1(2)	67346	1(3)	68020	1(3)	69320	1(2)
64449	1(2)	64680	1(2)	64872	1(3)	65757	1(3)	66840	1(2)	67399	1(3)	68040	1(2)	69399	1(3)
64450	10(3)	64681	1(2)	64874	1(3)	65760	0(3)	66850	1(2)	67400	1(2)	68100	1(3)	69420	1(2)
64451	2(2)	64702	2(3)	64876	1(3)	65765	0(3)	66852	1(2)	67405	1(2)	68110	1(3)	69421	1(2)
64454	2(2)	64704	4(3)	64885	1(3)	65767	0(3)	66920	1(2)	67412	1(2)	68115	1(3)	69424	1(2)
64455	1(2)	64708	3(3)	64886	1(3)	65770	1(2)	66930	1(2)	67413	1(2)	68130	1(3)	69433	1(2)
64461	1(2)	64712	1(2)	64890	2(3)	65771	0(3)	66940	1(2)	67414	1(2)	68135	1(3)	69436	1(2)
64462	1(2)	64713	1(2)	64891	2(3)	65772	1(2)	66982	1(2)	67415	1(3)	68200	1(3)	69440	1(2)
64463	1(3)	64714	1(2)	64892	2(3)	65775	1(2)	66983	1(2)	67420	1(2)	68320	1(2)	69450	1(2)
64479	1(2)	64716	2(3)	64893	2(3)	65778	1(2)	66984	1(2)	67430	1(2)	68325	1(2)	69501	1(3)
64480	4(3)	64718	1(2)	64895	2(3)	65779	1(2)	66985	1(2)	67440	1(2)	68326	1(2)	69502	1(2)
64483	1(2)	64719	1(2)	64896	2(3)	65780	1(2)	66986	1(2)	67445	1(2)	68328	1(2)	69505	1(2)
64484	4(3)	64721	1(2)	64897	2(3)	65781	1(2)	66987	2(2)	67450	1(2)	68330	1(3)	69511	1(2)
64486	1(3)	64722	4(3)	64898	2(3)	65782	1(2)	66988	2(2)	67500	1(3)	68335	1(3)	69530	1(2)
64487	1(2)	64726	2(3)	64901	2(3)	65785	1(2)	66990	1(3)	67505	1(3)	68340	1(3)	69535	1(2)
64488	1(3)	64727	2(3)	64902	1(3)	65800	1(2)	66999	1(3)	67515	1(3)	68360	1(3)	69540	1(3)
64489	1(2)	64732	1(2)	64905	1(3)	65810	1(2)	67005	1(2)	67550	1(2)	68362	1(3)	69550	1(3)
64490	1(2)	64734	1(2)	64907	1(3)	65815	1(3)	67010	1(2)	67560	1(2)	68371	1(3)	69552	1(2)
64491	1(2)	64736	1(2)	64910	3(3)	65820	1(2)	67015	1(2)	67570	1(2)	68399	1(3)	69554	1(2)
64492	1(2)	64738	1(2)	64911	2(3)	65850	1(2)	67025	1(2)	67599	1(3)	68400	1(2)	69601	1(2)
64493	1(2)	64740	1(2)	64912	3(3)	65855	1(2)	67027	1(2)	67700	2(3)	68420	1(2)	69602	1(2)
64494	1(2)	64742	1(2)	64913	3(3)	65860	1(2)	67028	1(3)	67710	1(2)	68440	2(3)	69603	1(2)
64495	1(2)	64744	1(2)	64999	1(3)	65865	1(2)	67030	1(2)	67715	1(3)	68500	1(2)	69604	1(2)
64505	1(3)	64746	1(2)	65091	1(2)	65870	1(2)	67031	1(2)	67800	1(2)	68505	1(2)	69610	1(2)
64510	1(3)	64755	1(2)	65093	1(2)	65875	1(2)	67036	1(2)	67801	1(2)	68510	1(2)	69620	1(2)
64517	1(3)	64760	1(2)	65101	1(2)	65880	1(2)	67039	1(2)	67805	1(2)	68520	1(2)	69631	1(2)
64520	1(3)	64763	1(2)	65103	1(2)	65900	1(3)	67040	1(2)	67808	1(2)	68525	1(2)	69632	1(3)
64530	1(3)	64766	1(2)	65105	1(2)	65920	1(2)	67041	1(2)	67810	2(3)	68530	1(2)	69633	1(2)
64553	1(3)	64771	2(3)	65110	1(2)	65930	1(3)	67042	1(2)	67820	1(2)	68540	1(2)	69635	1(3)
64555	2(3)	64772	2(3)	65112	1(2)	66020	1(3)	67043	1(2)	67825	1(2)	68550	1(2)	69636	1(3)
64561	1(3)	64774	2(3)	65114	1(2)	66030	1(3)	67101	1(2)	67830	1(2)	68700	1(2)	69637	1(3)
64566	1(3)	64776	1(2)	65125	1(2)	66130	1(3)	67105	1(2)	67835	1(2)	68705	2(3)	69641	1(2)
64568	1(3)	64778	1(3)	65130	1(2)	66150	1(2)	67107	1(2)	67840	3(3)	68720	1(2)	69642	1(2)
64569	1(3)	64782	2(2)	65135	1(2)	66155	1(2)	67108	1(2)	67850	3(3)	68745	1(2)	69643	1(2)

CPT	MUE
69644	1(2)
69645	1(2)
69646	1(2)
69650	1(2)
69660	1(2)
69661	1(2)
69662	1(2)
69666	1(2)
69667	1(2)
69670	1(2)
69676	1(2)
69700	1(3)
69705	1(2)
69706	1(2)
69710	0(3)
69711	1(2)
69714	1(2)
69715	1(3)
69717	1(2)
69718	1(2)
69720	1(2)
69725	1(2)
69740	1(2)
69745	1(2)
69799	1(3)
69801	1(3)
69805	1(3)
69806	1(3)
69905	1(2)
69910	1(2)
69915	1(3)
69930	1(2)
69949	1(3)
69950	1(2)
69955	1(2)
69960	1(2)
69970	1(3)
69979	1(3)
69990	1(3)
70010	1(3)
70015	1(3)
70030	2(2)
70100	2(3)
70110	2(3)
70120	1(3)
70130	1(3)
70134	1(3)
70140	2(3)
70150	1(3)
70160	1(3)
70170	2(2)
70190	1(2)
70200	2(3)
70210	1(3)
70220	1(3)
70240	1(2)
70250	2(3)
70260	1(3)
70300	1(3)
70310	1(3)
70320	1(3)
70328	1(3)
70330	1(3)
70332	2(3)
70336	1(3)
70350	1(3)

CPT	MUE
70355	1(3)
70360	2(3)
70370	1(3)
70371	1(2)
70380	2(3)
70390	2(3)
70450	3(3)
70460	1(3)
70470	2(3)
70480	1(3)
70481	1(3)
70482	1(3)
70486	1(3)
70487	1(3)
70488	1(3)
70490	1(3)
70491	1(3)
70492	1(3)
70496	2(3)
70498	2(3)
70540	1(3)
70542	1(3)
70543	1(3)
70544	2(3)
70545	1(3)
70546	1(3)
70547	1(3)
70548	1(3)
70549	1(3)
70551	2(3)
70552	2(3)
70553	2(3)
70554	1(3)
70555	1(3)
70557	1(3)
70558	1(3)
70559	1(3)
71045	4(3)
71046	3(3)
71047	2(3)
71048	1(3)
71100	2(3)
71101	2(3)
71110	1(3)
71111	1(3)
71120	1(3)
71130	1(3)
71250	2(3)
71260	2(3)
71270	1(3)
71271	1(2)
71275	1(3)
71550	1(3)
71551	1(3)
71552	1(3)
71555	1(3)
72020	4(3)
72040	3(3)
72050	1(3)
72052	1(3)
72070	1(3)
72072	1(3)
72074	1(3)
72080	1(3)
72081	1(3)
72082	1(3)

CPT	MUE
72083	1(3)
72084	1(3)
72100	2(3)
72110	1(3)
72114	1(3)
72120	1(3)
72125	1(3)
72126	1(3)
72127	1(3)
72128	1(3)
72129	1(3)
72130	1(3)
72131	1(3)
72132	1(3)
72133	1(3)
72141	1(3)
72142	1(3)
72146	1(3)
72147	1(3)
72148	1(3)
72149	1(3)
72156	1(3)
72157	1(3)
72158	1(3)
72159	1(3)
72170	2(3)
72190	1(3)
72191	1(3)
72192	1(3)
72193	1(3)
72194	1(3)
72195	1(3)
72196	1(3)
72197	1(3)
72198	1(3)
72200	2(3)
72202	1(3)
72220	1(3)
72240	1(2)
72255	1(2)
72265	1(2)
72270	1(2)
72275	1(3)
72285	4(3)
72295	5(3)
73000	2(3)
73010	2(3)
73020	2(3)
73030	4(3)
73040	2(2)
73050	1(3)
73060	2(3)
73070	2(3)
73080	2(3)
73085	2(2)
73090	2(3)
73092	2(3)
73100	2(3)
73110	3(3)
73115	2(2)
73120	2(3)
73130	3(3)
73140	3(3)
73200	2(3)
73201	2(3)
73202	2(3)

CPT	MUE
73206	2(3)
73218	2(3)
73219	2(3)
73220	2(3)
73221	2(3)
73222	2(3)
73223	2(3)
73225	2(3)
73501	2(3)
73502	2(3)
73503	2(3)
73521	2(3)
73522	2(3)
73523	2(3)
73525	2(2)
73551	2(3)
73552	2(3)
73560	4(3)
73562	3(3)
73564	4(3)
73565	1(3)
73580	2(2)
73590	3(3)
73592	2(3)
73600	2(3)
73610	3(3)
73615	2(2)
73620	2(3)
73630	3(3)
73650	2(3)
73660	2(3)
73700	2(3)
73701	2(3)
73702	2(3)
73706	2(3)
73718	2(3)
73719	2(3)
73720	2(3)
73721	3(3)
73722	2(3)
73723	2(3)
73725	2(3)
74018	3(3)
74019	2(3)
74021	2(3)
74022	2(3)
74150	1(3)
74160	1(3)
74170	1(3)
74174	1(3)
74175	1(3)
74176	2(3)
74177	2(3)
74178	1(3)
74181	1(3)
74182	1(3)
74183	1(3)
74185	1(3)
74190	1(3)
74210	1(3)
74220	1(3)
74221	1(3)
74230	1(3)
74235	1(3)
74240	2(3)
74246	1(3)

CPT	MUE
74248	1(2)
74250	1(3)
74251	1(3)
74261	1(2)
74262	1(2)
74263	0(3)
74270	1(3)
74280	1(3)
74283	1(3)
74290	1(3)
74300	1(3)
74301	1(3)
74328	1(3)
74329	1(3)
74330	1(3)
74340	1(3)
74355	1(3)
74360	1(3)
74363	2(3)
74400	1(3)
74410	1(3)
74415	1(3)
74420	2(3)
74425	2(3)
74430	1(3)
74440	1(2)
74445	1(2)
74450	1(3)
74455	1(3)
74470	2(2)
74485	2(3)
74710	1(3)
74712	1(3)
74713	2(3)
74740	1(3)
74742	2(2)
74775	1(2)
75557	1(3)
75559	1(3)
75561	1(3)
75563	1(3)
75565	1(3)
75571	1(3)
75572	1(3)
75573	1(3)
75574	1(3)
75600	1(3)
75605	1(3)
75625	1(3)
75630	1(3)
75635	1(3)
75705	20(3)
75710	2(3)
75716	1(3)
75726	3(3)
75731	1(3)
75733	1(3)
75736	2(3)
75741	1(3)
75743	1(3)
75746	1(3)
75756	2(3)
75774	7(3)
75801	1(3)
75803	1(3)
75805	1(2)

CPT	MUE
75807	1(2)
75809	1(3)
75810	1(3)
75820	2(3)
75822	1(3)
75825	1(3)
75827	1(3)
75831	1(3)
75833	1(3)
75840	1(3)
75842	1(3)
75860	2(3)
75870	1(3)
75872	1(3)
75880	1(3)
75885	1(3)
75887	1(3)
75889	1(3)
75891	1(3)
75893	2(3)
75894	2(3)
75898	2(3)
75901	1(3)
75902	2(3)
75956	1(2)
75957	1(2)
75958	2(3)
75959	1(2)
75970	1(3)
75984	2(3)
75989	2(3)
76000	3(3)
76010	2(3)
76080	3(3)
76098	3(3)
76100	2(3)
76101	1(3)
76102	1(3)
76120	1(3)
76125	1(3)
76140	0(3)
76145	1(2)
76376	2(3)
76377	2(3)
76380	2(3)
76390	1(3)
76391	1(3)
76496	1(3)
76497	1(3)
76498	1(3)
76499	1(3)
76506	1(2)
76510	2(2)
76511	2(2)
76512	2(2)
76513	1(2)
76514	1(2)
76516	1(2)
76519	1(3)
76529	2(2)
76536	1(3)
76604	1(3)
76641	2(2)
76642	2(2)
76700	1(3)
76705	2(3)

CPT	MUE
76706	1(2)
76770	1(3)
76775	2(3)
76776	2(3)
76800	1(3)
76801	1(2)
76802	2(3)
76805	1(2)
76810	2(3)
76811	1(2)
76812	2(3)
76813	1(2)
76814	2(3)
76815	1(2)
76816	2(3)
76817	1(3)
76818	2(3)
76819	2(3)
76820	3(3)
76821	2(3)
76825	2(3)
76826	2(3)
76827	2(3)
76828	2(3)
76830	1(3)
76831	1(3)
76856	1(3)
76857	1(3)
76870	1(2)
76872	1(3)
76873	1(2)
76881	2(3)
76882	2(3)
76885	1(2)
76886	1(2)
76932	1(2)
76936	1(3)
76937	2(3)
76940	1(3)
76941	3(3)
76942	1(3)
76945	1(3)
76946	1(3)
76948	1(2)
76965	2(3)
76975	1(3)
76977	1(2)
76978	1(2)
76979	3(3)
76981	1(3)
76982	1(2)
76983	2(3)
76998	1(3)
76999	1(3)
77001	2(3)
77002	1(3)
77003	1(3)
77011	1(3)
77012	1(3)
77013	1(3)
77014	2(3)
77021	1(3)
77022	1(3)
77046	1(2)
77047	1(2)
77048	1(2)

CPT	MUE
77049	1(2)
77053	2(2)
77054	2(2)
77061	1(2)
77062	1(2)
77063	1(2)
77065	1(2)
77066	1(2)
77067	1(2)
77071	1(3)
77072	1(2)
77073	1(2)
77074	1(2)
77075	1(2)
77076	1(2)
77077	1(2)
77078	1(2)
77080	1(2)
77081	1(2)
77084	1(2)
77085	1(2)
77086	1(2)
77261	1(3)
77262	1(3)
77263	1(3)
77280	2(3)
77285	1(3)
77290	1(3)
77293	1(3)
77295	1(3)
77299	1(3)
77300	10(3)
77301	1(3)
77306	1(3)
77307	1(3)
77316	1(3)
77317	1(3)
77318	1(3)
77321	1(2)
77331	3(3)
77332	4(3)
77333	2(3)
77334	10(3)
77336	1(2)
77338	1(3)
77370	1(3)
77371	1(2)
77372	1(2)
77373	1(3)
77385	2(3)
77386	2(3)
77387	2(3)
77399	1(3)
77401	1(2)
77402	2(3)
77407	2(3)
77412	2(3)
77417	1(2)
77423	1(3)
77424	1(2)
77425	1(3)
77427	1(2)
77431	1(2)
77432	1(2)
77435	1(2)
77469	1(2)

CPT	MUE	CPT	MUE	CPT	MUE	CPT	MUE	CPT	MUE	CPT	MUE	CPT	MUE	CPT	MUE
77470	1(2)	78268	1(2)	78725	1(3)	80180	1(3)	80355	1(3)	81112	1(2)	81233	1(3)	81302	1(3)
77499	1(3)	78278	2(3)	78730	1(2)	80181	1(3)	80356	1(3)	81120	1(3)	81234	1(2)	81303	1(3)
77520	2(3)	78282	1(2)	78740	1(2)	80183	1(3)	80357	1(3)	81121	1(3)	81235	1(3)	81304	1(3)
77522	2(3)	78290	1(3)	78761	1(2)	80184	2(3)	80358	1(3)	81161	1(3)	81236	1(3)	81305	1(3)
77523	2(3)	78291	1(3)	78799	1(3)	80185	2(3)	80359	1(3)	81162	1(2)	81237	1(3)	81306	1(2)
77525	2(3)	78299	1(3)	78800	1(2)	80186	2(3)	80360	1(3)	81163	1(2)	81238	1(2)	81307	1(2)
77600	1(3)	78300	1(2)	78801	1(2)	80187	1(3)	80361	2(3)	81164	1(2)	81239	1(2)	81308	1(2)
77605	1(3)	78305	1(2)	78802	1(2)	80188	2(3)	80362	1(3)	81165	1(2)	81240	1(2)	81309	1(2)
77610	1(3)	78306	1(2)	78803	1(2)	80189	1(3)	80363	1(3)	81166	1(2)	81241	1(2)	81310	1(3)
77615	1(3)	78315	1(2)	78804	1(2)	80190	2(3)	80364	1(3)	81167	1(2)	81242	1(3)	81311	1(3)
77620	1(3)	78350	0(3)	78808	1(2)	80192	2(3)	80365	2(3)	81168	1(3)	81243	1(3)	81312	1(2)
77750	1(3)	78351	0(3)	78811	1(2)	80193	1(3)	80366	1(3)	81170	1(2)	81244	1(3)	81313	1(3)
77761	1(3)	78399	1(3)	78812	1(2)	80194	2(3)	80367	1(3)	81171	1(2)	81245	1(3)	81314	1(3)
77762	1(3)	78414	1(2)	78813	1(2)	80195	2(3)	80368	1(3)	81172	1(2)	81246	1(3)	81315	1(3)
77763	1(3)	78428	1(3)	78814	1(2)	80197	2(3)	80369	1(3)	81173	1(2)	81247	1(2)	81316	1(2)
77767	2(3)	78429	1(2)	78815	1(2)	80198	2(3)	80370	1(3)	81174	1(2)	81248	1(2)	81317	1(2)
77768	2(3)	78430	1(2)	78816	1(2)	80199	1(3)	80371	1(3)	81175	1(3)	81249	1(2)	81318	1(3)
77770	2(3)	78431	1(2)	78830	1(2)	80200	2(3)	80372	1(3)	81176	1(3)	81250	1(3)	81319	1(2)
77771	2(3)	78432	1(2)	78831	1(2)	80201	2(3)	80373	1(3)	81177	1(2)	81251	1(3)	81320	1(3)
77772	2(3)	78433	1(2)	78832	1(2)	80202	2(3)	80374	1(3)	81178	1(2)	81252	1(3)	81321	1(3)
77778	1(3)	78434	1(2)	78835	4(3)	80203	1(3)	80375	1(3)	81179	1(2)	81253	1(3)	81322	1(3)
77789	2(3)	78445	1(3)	78999	1(3)	80204	1(3)	80376	1(3)	81180	1(2)	81254	1(3)	81323	1(3)
77790	1(3)	78451	1(2)	79005	1(3)	80210	1(3)	80377	1(3)	81181	1(2)	81255	1(3)	81324	1(3)
77799	1(3)	78452	1(2)	79101	1(3)	80230	1(3)	80400	1(3)	81182	1(2)	81256	1(2)	81325	1(3)
78012	1(3)	78453	1(2)	79200	1(3)	80235	1(3)	80402	1(3)	81183	1(2)	81257	1(2)	81326	1(3)
78013	1(3)	78454	1(2)	79300	1(3)	80280	1(3)	80406	1(3)	81184	1(2)	81258	1(2)	81327	1(2)
78014	1(2)	78456	1(3)	79403	1(3)	80285	1(3)	80408	1(3)	81185	1(2)	81259	1(2)	81328	1(2)
78015	1(3)	78457	1(2)	79440	1(3)	80299	3(3)	80410	1(3)	81186	1(2)	81260	1(3)	81329	1(2)
78016	1(3)	78458	1(2)	79445	1(3)	80305	1(2)	80412	1(3)	81187	1(2)	81261	1(3)	81330	1(3)
78018	1(2)	78459	1(3)	79999	1(3)	80306	1(2)	80414	1(3)	81188	1(2)	81262	1(3)	81331	1(3)
78020	1(3)	78466	1(3)	80047	2(3)	80307	1(2)	80415	1(3)	81189	1(2)	81263	1(3)	81332	1(3)
78070	1(2)	78468	1(3)	80048	2(3)	80320	2(3)	80416	1(3)	81190	1(2)	81264	1(3)	81333	1(2)
78071	1(3)	78469	1(3)	80050	0(3)	80321	1(3)	80417	1(3)	81191	1(3)	81265	1(3)	81334	1(3)
78072	1(3)	78472	1(2)	80051	4(3)	80322	1(3)	80418	1(3)	81192	1(3)	81266	2(3)	81335	1(2)
78075	1(2)	78473	1(2)	80053	1(3)	80323	1(3)	80420	1(2)	81193	1(3)	81267	1(3)	81336	1(2)
78099	1(3)	78481	1(2)	80055	1(3)	80324	1(3)	80422	1(3)	81194	1(3)	81268	4(3)	81337	1(2)
78102	1(2)	78483	1(2)	80061	1(3)	80325	1(3)	80424	1(3)	81200	1(2)	81269	1(2)	81338	1(3)
78103	1(2)	78491	1(3)	80069	1(3)	80326	1(3)	80426	1(3)	81201	1(2)	81270	1(2)	81339	1(2)
78104	1(2)	78492	1(2)	80074	1(2)	80327	1(3)	80428	1(3)	81202	1(3)	81271	1(2)	81340	1(3)
78110	1(2)	78494	1(3)	80076	1(3)	80328	1(3)	80430	1(3)	81203	1(3)	81272	1(3)	81341	1(3)
78111	1(2)	78496	1(3)	80081	1(2)	80329	2(3)	80432	1(3)	81204	1(2)	81273	1(3)	81342	1(3)
78120	1(2)	78499	1(3)	80143	2(3)	80330	1(3)	80434	1(3)	81205	1(3)	81274	1(2)	81343	1(2)
78121	1(2)	78579	1(3)	80145	1(3)	80331	1(3)	80435	1(3)	81206	1(3)	81275	1(3)	81344	1(2)
78122	1(2)	78580	1(3)	80150	2(3)	80332	1(3)	80436	1(3)	81207	1(3)	81276	1(3)	81345	1(3)
78130	1(2)	78582	1(3)	80151	1(3)	80333	1(3)	80438	1(3)	81208	1(3)	81277	1(2)	81346	1(2)
78140	1(3)	78597	1(3)	80155	1(3)	80334	1(3)	80439	1(3)	81209	1(3)	81278	1(3)	81347	1(2)
78185	1(2)	78598	1(3)	80156	2(3)	80335	1(3)	80500	1(3)	81210	1(3)	81279	1(2)	81348	1(2)
78191	1(2)	78599	1(3)	80157	2(3)	80336	1(3)	80502	1(3)	81212	1(2)	81283	1(2)	81350	1(3)
78195	1(2)	78600	1(3)	80158	2(3)	80337	1(3)	81000	2(3)	81215	1(2)	81284	1(2)	81351	1(2)
78199	1(3)	78601	1(3)	80159	2(3)	80338	1(3)	81001	2(3)	81216	1(2)	81285	1(2)	81352	1(2)
78201	1(3)	78605	1(3)	80161	1(3)	80339	2(3)	81002	2(3)	81217	1(2)	81286	1(2)	81353	1(2)
78202	1(3)	78606	1(3)	80162	2(3)	80340	1(3)	81003	2(3)	81218	1(3)	81287	1(3)	81355	1(3)
78215	1(3)	78608	1(3)	80163	1(3)	80341	1(3)	81005	2(3)	81219	1(3)	81288	1(3)	81357	1(2)
78216	1(3)	78609	0(3)	80164	2(3)	80342	1(3)	81007	1(3)	81220	1(3)	81289	1(2)	81360	1(2)
78226	1(3)	78610	1(3)	80165	1(3)	80343	1(3)	81015	2(3)	81221	1(3)	81290	1(3)	81361	1(2)
78227	1(3)	78630	1(3)	80167	1(3)	80344	1(3)	81020	1(3)	81222	1(3)	81291	1(3)	81362	1(2)
78230	1(3)	78635	1(3)	80168	2(3)	80345	2(3)	81025	1(3)	81223	1(2)	81292	1(2)	81363	1(2)
78231	1(3)	78645	1(3)	80169	2(3)	80346	1(3)	81050	2(3)	81224	1(3)	81293	1(3)	81364	1(2)
78232	1(3)	78650	1(3)	80170	2(3)	80347	1(3)	81099	1(3)	81225	1(3)	81294	1(3)	81370	1(2)
78258	1(2)	78660	1(2)	80171	1(3)	80348	1(3)	81105	1(2)	81226	1(3)	81295	1(2)	81371	1(2)
78261	1(2)	78699	1(3)	80173	2(3)	80349	1(3)	81106	1(2)	81227	1(3)	81296	1(3)	81372	1(2)
78262	1(2)	78700	1(3)	80175	1(3)	80350	1(3)	81107	1(2)	81228	1(3)	81297	1(3)	81373	2(2)
78264	1(2)	78701	1(3)	80176	1(3)	80351	1(3)	81108	1(2)	81229	1(3)	81298	1(2)	81374	1(3)
78265	1(2)	78707	1(2)	80177	1(3)	80352	1(3)	81109	1(2)	81230	1(2)	81299	1(3)	81375	1(2)
78266	1(2)	78708	1(2)	80178	2(3)	80353	1(3)	81110	1(2)	81231	1(2)	81300	1(3)	81376	5(3)
78267	1(2)	78709	1(2)	80179	2(3)	80354	1(3)	81111	1(2)	81232	1(2)	81301	1(3)	81377	2(3)

CPT	MUE
81378	1(2)
81379	1(2)
81380	2(2)
81381	3(3)
81382	6(3)
81383	2(3)
81400	2(3)
81401	3(3)
81402	1(3)
81403	3(3)
81404	3(3)
81405	2(3)
81406	3(3)
81407	1(3)
81408	1(3)
81410	1(2)
81411	1(2)
81412	1(2)
81413	1(2)
81414	1(2)
81415	1(2)
81416	2(3)
81417	1(3)
81419	1(2)
81420	1(2)
81422	1(2)
81425	1(2)
81426	2(3)
81427	1(3)
81430	1(2)
81431	1(2)
81432	1(2)
81433	1(2)
81434	1(2)
81435	1(2)
81436	1(2)
81437	1(2)
81438	1(2)
81439	1(2)
81440	1(2)
81442	1(2)
81443	1(2)
81445	1(2)
81448	1(2)
81450	1(2)
81455	1(2)
81460	1(2)
81465	1(2)
81470	1(2)
81471	1(2)
81479	3(3)
81490	1(2)
81493	1(2)
81500	1(2)
81503	1(2)
81504	1(2)
81506	1(2)
81507	1(2)
81508	1(2)
81509	1(2)
81510	1(2)
81511	1(2)
81512	1(2)
81513	1(2)
81514	1(2)
81518	1(2)

CPT	MUE
81519	1(2)
81520	1(2)
81521	1(2)
81522	1(2)
81525	1(2)
81528	1(2)
81529	1(2)
81535	1(2)
81536	11(3)
81538	1(2)
81539	1(2)
81540	1(2)
81541	1(2)
81542	1(2)
81546	2(3)
81551	1(2)
81552	1(2)
81554	1(2)
81595	1(2)
81596	1(2)
81599	1(3)
82009	3(3)
82010	3(3)
82013	1(3)
82016	1(3)
82017	1(3)
82024	4(3)
82030	1(3)
82040	1(3)
82042	2(3)
82043	1(3)
82044	1(3)
82045	1(3)
82075	2(3)
82077	1(3)
82085	1(3)
82088	2(3)
82103	1(3)
82104	1(2)
82105	1(3)
82106	2(3)
82107	1(3)
82108	1(3)
82120	1(3)
82127	1(3)
82128	2(3)
82131	2(3)
82135	1(3)
82136	2(3)
82139	2(3)
82140	2(3)
82143	2(3)
82150	4(3)
82154	1(3)
82157	1(3)
82160	1(3)
82163	1(3)
82164	1(3)
82172	2(3)
82175	2(3)
82180	1(2)
82190	2(3)
82232	2(3)
82239	1(3)
82240	1(3)
82247	2(3)

CPT	MUE
82248	2(3)
82252	1(3)
82261	1(3)
82270	1(3)
82271	3(3)
82272	1(3)
82274	1(3)
82286	1(3)
82300	1(3)
82306	1(2)
82308	1(3)
82310	4(3)
82330	4(3)
82331	1(3)
82340	1(3)
82355	2(3)
82360	2(3)
82365	2(3)
82370	2(3)
82373	1(3)
82374	2(3)
82375	4(3)
82376	2(3)
82378	1(3)
82379	1(3)
82380	1(3)
82382	1(2)
82383	1(3)
82384	2(3)
82387	1(3)
82390	1(2)
82397	4(3)
82415	1(3)
82435	2(3)
82436	1(3)
82438	1(3)
82441	1(2)
82465	1(3)
82480	2(3)
82482	1(3)
82485	1(3)
82495	1(2)
82507	1(3)
82523	1(3)
82525	2(3)
82528	1(3)
82530	4(3)
82533	5(3)
82540	1(3)
82542	6(3)
82550	3(3)
82552	3(3)
82553	3(3)
82554	2(3)
82565	2(3)
82570	3(3)
82575	1(3)
82585	1(2)
82595	1(3)
82600	1(3)
82607	1(2)
82608	1(2)
82610	1(3)
82615	1(3)
82626	1(3)
82627	1(3)

CPT	MUE
82633	1(3)
82634	1(3)
82638	1(3)
82642	1(2)
82652	1(2)
82656	1(3)
82657	2(3)
82658	2(3)
82664	2(3)
82668	1(3)
82670	1(3)
82671	1(3)
82672	1(3)
82677	1(3)
82679	1(3)
82681	1(3)
82693	2(3)
82696	1(3)
82705	1(3)
82710	1(3)
82715	3(3)
82725	1(3)
82726	1(3)
82728	1(3)
82731	1(3)
82735	1(3)
82746	1(2)
82747	1(2)
82757	1(2)
82759	1(3)
82760	1(3)
82775	1(3)
82776	1(2)
82777	1(3)
82784	6(3)
82785	1(3)
82787	4(3)
82800	2(3)
82805	3(3)
82810	4(3)
82820	1(3)
82930	1(3)
82938	1(3)
82941	1(3)
82943	1(3)
82945	4(3)
82946	1(2)
82947	5(3)
82950	3(3)
82951	1(2)
82952	3(3)
82955	1(2)
82960	1(2)
82963	1(3)
82965	1(3)
82977	1(3)
82978	1(3)
82979	1(3)
82985	1(3)
83001	1(3)
83002	1(3)
83003	5(3)
83006	1(2)
83009	1(3)
83010	1(3)
83012	1(2)

CPT	MUE
83013	1(3)
83014	1(2)
83015	1(2)
83018	4(3)
83020	2(3)
83021	2(3)
83026	1(3)
83030	1(3)
83033	1(3)
83036	1(2)
83037	1(2)
83045	1(3)
83050	2(3)
83051	1(3)
83060	1(3)
83065	1(2)
83068	1(2)
83069	1(3)
83070	1(2)
83080	2(3)
83088	1(3)
83090	2(3)
83150	1(3)
83491	1(3)
83497	1(3)
83498	2(3)
83500	1(3)
83505	1(3)
83516	5(3)
83518	1(3)
83519	5(3)
83520	9(3)
83525	4(3)
83527	1(3)
83528	1(3)
83540	2(3)
83550	1(3)
83570	1(3)
83582	1(3)
83586	1(3)
83593	1(3)
83605	2(3)
83615	3(3)
83625	1(3)
83630	1(3)
83631	1(3)
83632	1(3)
83633	1(3)
83655	2(3)
83661	3(3)
83662	4(3)
83663	3(3)
83664	3(3)
83670	1(3)
83690	2(3)
83695	1(3)
83698	1(3)
83700	1(2)
83701	1(3)
83704	1(3)
83718	1(3)
83719	1(3)
83721	1(3)
83722	1(2)
83727	1(3)
83735	4(3)

CPT	MUE
83775	1(3)
83785	1(3)
83789	4(3)
83825	2(3)
83835	2(3)
83857	1(3)
83861	2(2)
83864	1(2)
83872	2(3)
83873	1(3)
83874	4(3)
83876	1(3)
83880	1(3)
83883	4(3)
83885	2(3)
83915	1(3)
83916	2(3)
83918	2(3)
83919	1(3)
83921	2(3)
83930	2(3)
83935	2(3)
83937	1(3)
83945	2(3)
83950	1(2)
83951	1(2)
83970	4(3)
83986	2(3)
83987	1(3)
83992	2(3)
83993	1(3)
84030	1(2)
84035	1(2)
84060	1(3)
84066	1(3)
84075	2(3)
84078	1(2)
84080	1(3)
84081	1(3)
84085	1(2)
84087	1(3)
84100	2(3)
84105	1(3)
84106	1(2)
84110	1(3)
84112	1(3)
84119	1(2)
84120	1(3)
84126	1(3)
84132	3(3)
84133	2(3)
84134	1(3)
84135	1(3)
84138	1(3)
84140	1(3)
84143	2(3)
84144	1(3)
84145	1(3)
84146	3(3)
84150	2(3)
84152	1(2)
84153	1(2)
84154	1(2)
84155	1(3)
84156	1(3)
84157	2(3)

CPT	MUE
84160	2(3)
84163	1(3)
84165	1(2)
84166	2(3)
84181	3(3)
84182	6(3)
84202	1(2)
84203	1(2)
84206	1(2)
84207	1(2)
84210	1(3)
84220	1(3)
84228	1(3)
84233	1(3)
84234	1(3)
84235	1(3)
84238	3(3)
84244	2(3)
84252	1(2)
84255	2(3)
84260	1(3)
84270	1(3)
84275	1(3)
84285	1(3)
84295	2(3)
84300	2(3)
84302	1(3)
84305	1(3)
84307	1(3)
84311	2(3)
84315	1(3)
84375	1(3)
84376	1(3)
84377	1(3)
84378	2(3)
84379	1(3)
84392	1(3)
84402	1(3)
84403	2(3)
84410	1(2)
84425	1(2)
84430	1(3)
84431	1(3)
84432	1(2)
84436	1(2)
84437	1(2)
84439	1(2)
84442	1(2)
84443	4(2)
84445	1(2)
84446	1(2)
84449	1(3)
84450	1(3)
84460	1(3)
84466	1(3)
84478	1(3)
84479	1(2)
84480	1(2)
84481	1(2)
84482	1(2)
84484	4(3)
84485	1(3)
84488	1(3)
84490	1(2)
84510	1(3)
84512	3(3)

CPT	MUE
84520	2(3)
84525	1(3)
84540	2(3)
84545	1(3)
84550	1(3)
84560	2(3)
84577	1(3)
84578	1(3)
84580	1(3)
84583	1(3)
84585	1(2)
84586	1(2)
84588	1(3)
84590	1(2)
84591	1(3)
84597	1(3)
84600	2(3)
84620	1(2)
84630	2(3)
84681	1(3)
84702	2(3)
84703	1(3)
84704	1(3)
84830	1(2)
84999	1(3)
85002	1(3)
85004	2(3)
85007	1(3)
85008	1(3)
85009	1(3)
85013	1(3)
85014	4(3)
85018	4(3)
85025	4(3)
85027	4(3)
85032	2(3)
85041	1(3)
85044	1(2)
85045	1(2)
85046	1(2)
85048	2(3)
85049	2(3)
85055	1(3)
85060	1(3)
85097	2(3)
85130	1(3)
85170	1(3)
85175	1(3)
85210	2(3)
85220	2(3)
85230	2(3)
85240	2(3)
85244	1(3)
85245	2(3)
85246	2(3)
85247	2(3)
85250	2(3)
85260	2(3)
85270	2(3)
85280	2(3)
85290	2(3)
85291	1(3)
85292	1(3)
85293	1(3)
85300	2(3)
85301	1(3)

CPT	MUE	CPT	MUE	CPT	MUE	CPT	MUE
85302	1(3)	86038	1(3)	86382	3(3)	86704	1(2)
85303	2(3)	86039	1(3)	86384	1(3)	86705	1(2)
85305	2(3)	86060	1(3)	86386	1(2)	86706	2(3)
85306	2(3)	86063	1(3)	86403	3(3)	86707	1(3)
85307	2(3)	86077	1(2)	86406	2(3)	86708	1(2)
85335	2(3)	86078	1(3)	86408	1(3)	86709	1(2)
85337	1(3)	86079	1(3)	86409	1(3)	86710	4(3)
85345	1(3)	86140	1(2)	86413	3(3)	86711	2(3)
85347	9(3)	86141	1(2)	86430	2(3)	86713	3(3)
85348	4(3)	86146	3(3)	86431	2(3)	86717	8(3)
85360	1(3)	86147	4(3)	86480	1(3)	86720	2(3)
85362	2(3)	86148	3(3)	86481	1(3)	86723	2(3)
85366	1(3)	86152	1(3)	86485	1(2)	86727	2(3)
85370	1(3)	86153	1(3)	86486	2(3)	86732	2(3)
85378	2(3)	86155	1(3)	86490	1(2)	86735	2(3)
85379	2(3)	86156	1(2)	86510	1(2)	86738	2(3)
85380	2(3)	86157	1(2)	86580	1(2)	86741	2(3)
85384	2(3)	86160	4(3)	86590	1(3)	86744	2(3)
85385	1(3)	86161	2(3)	86592	2(3)	86747	2(3)
85390	3(3)	86162	1(2)	86593	2(3)	86750	4(3)
85396	1(2)	86171	2(3)	86602	3(3)	86753	3(3)
85397	2(3)	86200	1(3)	86603	2(3)	86756	2(3)
85400	1(3)	86215	1(3)	86609	14(3)	86757	6(3)
85410	1(3)	86225	1(3)	86611	4(3)	86759	2(3)
85415	2(3)	86226	1(3)	86612	2(3)	86762	2(3)
85420	2(3)	86235	10(3)	86615	6(3)	86765	2(3)
85421	1(3)	86255	5(3)	86617	2(3)	86768	5(3)
85441	1(2)	86256	9(3)	86618	2(3)	86769	3(3)
85445	1(2)	86277	1(3)	86619	2(3)	86771	2(3)
85460	1(3)	86280	1(3)	86622	2(3)	86774	2(3)
85461	1(2)	86294	1(3)	86625	1(3)	86777	2(3)
85475	1(3)	86300	2(3)	86628	3(3)	86778	2(3)
85520	3(3)	86301	1(2)	86631	6(3)	86780	2(3)
85525	2(3)	86304	1(2)	86632	3(3)	86784	1(3)
85530	1(3)	86305	1(2)	86635	4(3)	86787	2(3)
85536	1(2)	86308	1(2)	86638	6(3)	86788	2(3)
85540	1(2)	86309	1(2)	86641	2(3)	86789	2(3)
85547	1(2)	86310	1(2)	86644	2(3)	86790	4(3)
85549	1(3)	86316	2(3)	86645	1(3)	86793	2(3)
85555	1(2)	86317	6(3)	86648	2(3)	86794	1(3)
85557	1(2)	86318	2(3)	86651	2(3)	86800	1(3)
85576	7(3)	86320	1(2)	86652	2(3)	86803	1(3)
85597	1(3)	86325	2(3)	86653	2(3)	86804	1(2)
85598	1(3)	86327	1(3)	86654	2(3)	86805	12(3)
85610	4(3)	86328	3(3)	86658	12(3)	86806	2(3)
85611	2(3)	86329	3(3)	86663	2(3)	86807	2(3)
85612	1(3)	86331	12(3)	86664	2(3)	86808	1(3)
85613	3(3)	86332	1(3)	86665	2(3)	86812	1(2)
85635	1(3)	86334	2(2)	86666	4(3)	86813	1(2)
85651	1(2)	86335	2(3)	86668	2(3)	86816	1(2)
85652	1(2)	86336	1(3)	86671	3(3)	86817	1(2)
85660	2(3)	86337	1(2)	86674	3(3)	86821	1(3)
85670	2(3)	86340	1(2)	86677	3(3)	86825	1(3)
85675	1(3)	86341	4(3)	86682	2(3)	86826	8(3)
85705	1(3)	86343	1(3)	86684	2(3)	86828	2(3)
85730	4(3)	86344	1(2)	86687	1(3)	86829	2(3)
85732	4(3)	86352	1(3)	86688	1(3)	86830	2(3)
85810	2(3)	86353	7(3)	86689	2(3)	86831	2(3)
85999	1(3)	86355	1(2)	86692	2(3)	86832	2(3)
86000	6(3)	86356	7(3)	86694	2(3)	86833	1(3)
86001	20(3)	86357	1(2)	86695	2(3)	86834	1(3)
86005	6(3)	86359	1(2)	86696	2(3)	86835	1(3)
86008	20(3)	86360	1(2)	86698	3(3)	86849	1(3)
86021	1(2)	86361	1(2)	86701	1(3)	86850	3(3)
86022	1(2)	86367	2(3)	86702	2(3)	86860	2(3)
86023	3(3)	86376	2(3)	86703	1(2)	86870	6(3)

CPT	MUE	CPT	MUE	CPT	MUE	CPT	MUE
86880	4(3)	87185	4(3)	87450	2(3)	87582	1(3)
86885	3(3)	87186	12(3)	87451	2(3)	87590	1(3)
86886	3(3)	87187	3(3)	87471	1(3)	87591	3(3)
86890	2(3)	87188	14(3)	87472	1(3)	87592	1(3)
86891	2(3)	87190	10(3)	87475	1(3)	87623	1(2)
86900	3(3)	87197	1(3)	87476	1(3)	87624	1(3)
86901	3(3)	87206	6(3)	87480	1(3)	87625	1(3)
86902	40(3)	87207	3(3)	87481	6(3)	87631	1(3)
86905	28(3)	87209	4(3)	87482	1(3)	87632	1(3)
86906	1(2)	87210	4(3)	87483	1(2)	87633	1(3)
86910	0(3)	87220	3(3)	87485	1(3)	87634	1(3)
86911	0(3)	87230	2(3)	87486	1(3)	87635	2(3)
86920	19(3)	87250	1(3)	87487	1(3)	87636	3(3)
86922	10(3)	87252	4(3)	87490	1(3)	87637	3(3)
86923	10(3)	87253	3(3)	87491	3(3)	87640	1(3)
86930	3(3)	87254	10(3)	87492	1(3)	87641	1(3)
86931	4(3)	87255	2(3)	87493	2(3)	87650	1(3)
86940	3(3)	87260	1(3)	87495	1(3)	87651	1(3)
86941	3(3)	87265	1(3)	87496	1(3)	87652	1(3)
86945	5(3)	87267	1(3)	87497	2(3)	87653	1(3)
86950	1(3)	87269	1(3)	87498	1(3)	87660	1(3)
86960	3(3)	87270	1(3)	87500	1(3)	87661	1(3)
86965	4(3)	87271	1(3)	87501	1(3)	87662	2(3)
86971	6(3)	87272	1(3)	87502	1(3)	87797	3(3)
86972	2(3)	87273	1(3)	87503	1(3)	87798	21(3)
86975	2(3)	87274	1(3)	87505	1(2)	87799	3(3)
86976	2(3)	87275	1(3)	87506	1(2)	87800	2(3)
86977	2(3)	87276	1(3)	87507	1(2)	87801	3(3)
86999	1(3)	87278	1(3)	87510	1(3)	87802	2(3)
87003	1(3)	87279	1(3)	87511	1(3)	87803	3(3)
87015	3(3)	87280	1(3)	87512	1(3)	87804	3(3)
87040	4(3)	87281	1(3)	87516	1(3)	87806	1(2)
87045	3(3)	87283	1(3)	87517	1(3)	87807	2(3)
87046	6(3)	87285	1(3)	87520	1(3)	87808	1(3)
87071	2(3)	87290	1(3)	87521	1(3)	87809	2(3)
87073	2(3)	87299	1(3)	87522	1(3)	87810	2(3)
87075	6(3)	87300	2(3)	87525	1(3)	87811	3(3)
87076	4(3)	87301	1(3)	87526	1(3)	87850	1(3)
87077	6(3)	87305	1(3)	87527	1(3)	87880	2(3)
87081	4(3)	87320	1(3)	87528	1(3)	87899	6(3)
87084	1(3)	87324	2(3)	87529	2(3)	87900	1(2)
87086	3(3)	87327	1(3)	87530	2(3)	87901	1(2)
87088	3(3)	87328	2(3)	87531	1(3)	87902	1(2)
87101	3(3)	87329	2(3)	87532	1(3)	87903	1(2)
87102	4(3)	87332	1(3)	87533	1(3)	87904	14(3)
87103	2(3)	87335	1(3)	87534	1(3)	87905	2(3)
87106	4(3)	87336	1(3)	87535	1(3)	87906	2(3)
87107	4(3)	87337	1(3)	87536	1(3)	87910	1(3)
87109	2(3)	87338	1(3)	87537	1(3)	87912	1(3)
87110	2(3)	87339	1(3)	87538	1(3)	87999	1(3)
87118	3(3)	87340	1(2)	87539	1(3)	88000	0(3)
87140	3(3)	87341	1(2)	87540	1(3)	88005	0(3)
87143	2(3)	87350	1(2)	87541	1(3)	88007	0(3)
87149	11(3)	87380	1(2)	87542	1(3)	88012	0(3)
87150	12(3)	87385	2(3)	87550	1(3)	88014	0(3)
87152	1(3)	87389	1(3)	87551	2(3)	88016	0(3)
87153	3(3)	87390	1(3)	87552	1(3)	88020	0(3)
87164	2(3)	87391	1(3)	87555	1(3)	88025	0(3)
87166	2(3)	87400	2(3)	87556	1(3)	88027	0(3)
87168	2(3)	87420	1(3)	87557	1(3)	88028	0(3)
87169	2(3)	87425	1(3)	87560	1(3)	88029	0(3)
87172	1(3)	87426	3(3)	87561	1(3)	88036	0(3)
87176	3(3)	87427	2(3)	87562	1(3)	88037	0(3)
87177	3(3)	87428	3(3)	87563	3(3)	88040	0(3)
87181	12(3)	87430	1(3)	87580	1(3)	88045	0(3)
87184	8(3)	87449	3(3)	87581	1(3)	88099	0(3)

CPT	MUE
88104	5(3)
88106	5(3)
88108	6(3)
88112	6(3)
88120	2(3)
88121	2(3)
88125	1(3)
88130	1(2)
88140	1(2)
88141	1(3)
88142	1(3)
88143	1(3)
88147	1(3)
88148	1(3)
88150	1(3)
88152	1(3)
88153	1(3)
88155	1(3)
88160	4(3)
88161	4(3)
88162	3(3)
88164	1(3)
88165	1(3)
88166	1(3)
88167	1(3)
88172	7(3)
88173	7(3)
88174	1(3)
88175	1(3)
88177	6(3)
88182	2(3)
88184	2(3)
88185	35(3)
88187	2(3)
88188	2(3)
88189	2(3)
88199	1(3)
88230	2(3)
88233	2(3)
88235	2(3)
88237	4(3)
88239	3(3)
88240	3(3)
88241	3(3)
88245	1(2)
88248	1(2)
88249	1(2)
88261	2(3)
88262	2(3)
88263	1(3)
88264	1(3)
88267	2(3)
88269	2(3)
88271	16(3)
88272	12(3)
88273	3(3)
88274	5(3)
88275	12(3)
88280	1(3)
88283	5(3)
88285	10(3)
88289	1(3)
88291	0(3)
88299	1(3)
88300	4(3)
88302	4(3)

CPT	MUE
88304	5(3)
88305	16(3)
88307	8(3)
88309	3(3)
88311	4(3)
88312	9(3)
88313	8(3)
88314	6(3)
88319	11(3)
88321	1(2)
88323	1(2)
88325	1(2)
88329	2(3)
88331	11(3)
88332	13(3)
88333	4(3)
88334	5(3)
88341	13(3)
88342	4(3)
88344	6(3)
88346	2(3)
88348	1(3)
88350	9(3)
88355	1(3)
88356	3(3)
88358	2(3)
88360	6(3)
88361	6(3)
88362	1(3)
88363	2(3)
88364	3(3)
88365	4(3)
88366	2(3)
88367	3(3)
88368	3(3)
88369	3(3)
88371	1(3)
88372	1(3)
88373	3(3)
88374	5(3)
88375	1(3)
88377	5(3)
88380	1(3)
88381	1(3)
88387	2(3)
88388	1(3)
88399	1(3)
88720	1(3)
88738	1(3)
88740	1(2)
88741	1(2)
88749	1(3)
89049	1(3)
89050	2(3)
89051	2(3)
89055	2(3)
89060	2(3)
89125	2(3)
89160	1(3)
89190	1(3)
89220	2(3)
89230	1(2)
89240	1(3)
89250	1(2)
89251	1(2)
89253	1(3)

CPT	MUE
89254	1(3)
89255	1(3)
89257	1(3)
89258	1(2)
89259	1(2)
89260	1(2)
89261	1(2)
89264	1(3)
89268	1(2)
89272	1(2)
89280	1(2)
89281	1(2)
89290	1(2)
89291	1(2)
89300	1(2)
89310	1(2)
89320	1(2)
89321	1(2)
89322	1(2)
89325	1(2)
89329	1(2)
89330	1(2)
89331	1(2)
89335	1(3)
89337	1(2)
89342	1(2)
89343	1(2)
89344	1(2)
89346	1(2)
89352	1(2)
89353	1(3)
89354	1(3)
89356	2(3)
89398	1(3)
90281	0(3)
90283	0(3)
90284	0(3)
90287	0(3)
90288	0(3)
90291	0(3)
90296	1(2)
90371	10(3)
90375	20(3)
90376	20(3)
90377	20(3)
90378	4(3)
90384	0(3)
90385	1(2)
90386	0(3)
90389	0(3)
90393	1(2)
90396	1(2)
90399	0(3)
90460	9(3)
90461	8(3)
90471	1(2)
90472	8(3)
90473	1(2)
90474	1(3)
90476	1(2)
90477	1(2)
90581	1(2)
90585	1(2)
90586	1(2)
90587	1(2)
90619	1(2)

CPT	MUE
90620	1(2)
90621	1(2)
90625	1(2)
90630	1(2)
90632	1(2)
90633	1(2)
90634	1(2)
90636	1(2)
90644	1(2)
90647	1(2)
90648	1(2)
90649	1(2)
90650	1(2)
90651	1(2)
90653	1(2)
90654	1(2)
90655	1(2)
90656	1(2)
90657	1(2)
90658	1(2)
90660	1(2)
90661	1(2)
90662	1(2)
90664	1(2)
90666	1(2)
90667	1(2)
90668	1(2)
90670	1(2)
90672	1(2)
90673	1(2)
90674	1(2)
90675	1(2)
90676	1(2)
90680	1(2)
90681	1(2)
90682	1(2)
90685	1(2)
90686	1(2)
90687	1(2)
90688	1(2)
90689	1(2)
90690	1(2)
90691	1(2)
90694	1(2)
90696	1(2)
90697	1(2)
90698	1(2)
90700	1(2)
90702	1(2)
90707	1(2)
90710	1(2)
90713	1(2)
90714	1(2)
90715	1(2)
90716	1(2)
90717	1(2)
90723	0(3)
90732	1(2)
90733	1(2)
90734	1(2)
90736	1(2)
90738	1(2)
90739	1(2)
90740	1(2)
90743	1(2)
90744	1(2)

CPT	MUE
90746	1(2)
90747	1(2)
90748	0(3)
90749	1(3)
90750	1(2)
90756	1(2)
90785	3(3)
90791	1(3)
90792	2(3)
90832	3(3)
90833	3(3)
90834	3(3)
90836	3(3)
90837	3(3)
90838	3(3)
90839	1(2)
90840	4(3)
90845	1(2)
90846	2(3)
90847	2(3)
90849	2(3)
90853	4(3)
90863	1(3)
90865	1(3)
90867	1(2)
90868	1(3)
90869	1(3)
90870	2(3)
90875	1(3)
90876	0(3)
90880	1(3)
90882	0(3)
90885	1(3)
90887	1(3)
90889	1(3)
90899	1(3)
90901	1(3)
90912	1(2)
90913	3(3)
90935	1(3)
90937	1(3)
90940	1(3)
90945	1(3)
90947	1(3)
90951	1(2)
90952	1(2)
90953	1(2)
90954	1(2)
90955	1(2)
90956	1(2)
90957	1(2)
90958	1(2)
90959	1(2)
90960	1(2)
90961	1(2)
90962	1(2)
90963	1(2)
90964	1(2)
90965	1(2)
90966	1(2)
90967	1(2)
90968	1(2)
90969	1(2)
90970	1(2)
90989	1(2)
90993	1(3)

CPT	MUE
90997	1(3)
90999	1(3)
91010	1(2)
91013	1(3)
91020	1(2)
91022	1(2)
91030	1(2)
91034	1(2)
91035	1(2)
91037	1(2)
91038	1(2)
91040	1(2)
91065	2(2)
91110	1(2)
91111	1(2)
91112	1(3)
91117	1(2)
91120	1(2)
91122	1(2)
91132	1(3)
91133	1(3)
91200	1(2)
91299	1(3)
91300	1(2)
91301	1(2)
91302	1(2)
91303	1(2)
91304	1(2)
92002	1(2)
92004	1(2)
92012	1(3)
92014	1(3)
92015	0(3)
92018	1(2)
92019	1(2)
92020	1(2)
92025	1(2)
92060	1(2)
92065	1(2)
92071	2(2)
92072	1(2)
92081	1(2)
92082	1(2)
92083	1(2)
92100	1(2)
92132	1(2)
92133	1(2)
92134	1(2)
92136	1(3)
92145	1(2)
92201	1(2)
92202	1(2)
92227	1(2)
92228	1(2)
92229	1(2)
92230	2(2)
92235	1(2)
92240	1(2)
92242	1(2)
92250	1(2)
92260	1(2)
92265	1(2)
92270	1(2)
92273	1(2)
92274	1(2)
92283	1(2)

CPT	MUE
92284	1(2)
92285	1(2)
92286	1(2)
92287	1(2)
92310	0(3)
92311	1(2)
92312	1(2)
92313	1(3)
92314	0(3)
92315	1(2)
92316	1(2)
92317	1(3)
92325	1(3)
92326	2(2)
92340	0(3)
92341	0(3)
92342	0(3)
92352	1(3)
92353	1(3)
92354	1(3)
92355	1(3)
92358	1(3)
92370	0(3)
92371	1(3)
92499	1(3)
92502	1(3)
92504	1(3)
92507	1(3)
92508	1(3)
92511	1(3)
92512	1(2)
92516	1(3)
92517	1(2)
92518	1(2)
92519	1(2)
92520	1(2)
92521	1(2)
92522	1(2)
92523	1(2)
92524	1(2)
92526	1(2)
92531	1(3)
92532	1(3)
92533	4(2)
92534	1(3)
92537	1(2)
92538	1(2)
92540	1(3)
92541	1(3)
92542	1(3)
92544	1(3)
92545	1(3)
92546	1(3)
92547	1(3)
92548	1(3)
92549	1(3)
92550	1(2)
92551	0(3)
92552	1(2)
92553	1(2)
92555	1(2)
92556	1(2)
92557	1(2)
92558	0(3)
92559	0(3)
92560	0(3)

CPT	MUE
92561	1(2)
92562	1(2)
92563	1(2)
92564	1(2)
92565	1(2)
92567	1(2)
92568	1(2)
92570	1(2)
92571	1(2)
92572	1(2)
92575	1(2)
92576	1(2)
92577	1(2)
92579	1(2)
92582	1(2)
92583	1(2)
92584	1(2)
92587	1(2)
92588	1(2)
92590	0(3)
92591	0(3)
92592	0(3)
92593	0(3)
92594	0(3)
92595	0(3)
92596	1(2)
92597	1(3)
92601	1(3)
92602	1(3)
92603	1(3)
92604	1(3)
92605	1(2)
92606	1(2)
92607	1(3)
92608	4(3)
92609	1(3)
92610	1(2)
92611	1(3)
92612	1(3)
92613	1(2)
92614	1(3)
92615	1(2)
92616	1(3)
92617	1(2)
92618	1(3)
92620	1(2)
92621	4(3)
92625	1(2)
92626	1(2)
92627	6(3)
92630	0(3)
92633	0(3)
92640	1(3)
92650	1(2)
92651	1(2)
92652	1(2)
92653	1(2)
92700	1(3)
92920	3(3)
92921	6(2)
92924	2(3)
92925	6(2)
92928	3(3)
92929	2(3)
92933	2(3)
92934	2(3)

CPT	MUE	CPT	MUE	CPT	MUE	CPT	MUE	CPT	MUE	CPT	MUE	CPT	MUE	CPT	MUE
92937	2(3)	93288	1(3)	93591	1(2)	93976	1(3)	95027	90(3)	95812	1(3)	95976	1(3)	96409	1(3)
92938	2(3)	93289	1(3)	93592	2(3)	93978	1(3)	95028	30(3)	95813	1(3)	95977	1(3)	96411	3(3)
92941	1(3)	93290	1(3)	93600	1(3)	93979	1(3)	95044	80(3)	95816	1(3)	95980	1(3)	96413	1(3)
92943	2(3)	93291	1(3)	93602	1(3)	93980	1(3)	95052	20(3)	95819	1(3)	95981	1(3)	96415	8(3)
92944	2(3)	93292	1(3)	93603	1(3)	93981	1(3)	95056	1(2)	95822	1(3)	95982	1(3)	96416	1(3)
92950	2(3)	93293	1(2)	93609	1(3)	93985	1(3)	95060	1(2)	95824	1(3)	95983	1(2)	96417	3(3)
92953	2(3)	93294	1(2)	93610	1(3)	93986	1(3)	95065	1(3)	95829	1(3)	95984	11(3)	96420	2(3)
92960	2(3)	93295	1(2)	93612	1(3)	93990	2(3)	95070	1(3)	95830	1(3)	95990	1(3)	96422	2(3)
92961	1(3)	93296	1(2)	93613	1(3)	93998	1(3)	95076	1(2)	95836	1(2)	95991	1(3)	96423	2(3)
92970	1(3)	93297	1(2)	93615	1(3)	94002	1(2)	95079	2(3)	95851	3(3)	95992	1(2)	96425	1(3)
92971	1(3)	93298	1(2)	93616	1(3)	94003	1(2)	95115	1(2)	95852	1(3)	95999	1(3)	96440	1(3)
92973	2(3)	93303	1(3)	93618	1(3)	94004	1(2)	95117	1(2)	95857	1(2)	96000	1(2)	96446	1(3)
92974	1(3)	93304	1(3)	93619	1(3)	94005	1(3)	95120	0(3)	95860	1(3)	96001	1(2)	96450	1(3)
92975	1(3)	93306	1(3)	93620	1(3)	94010	1(3)	95125	0(3)	95861	1(3)	96002	1(3)	96521	2(3)
92977	1(3)	93307	1(3)	93621	1(3)	94011	1(3)	95130	0(3)	95863	1(3)	96003	1(3)	96522	1(3)
92978	1(3)	93308	1(3)	93622	1(3)	94012	1(3)	95131	0(3)	95864	1(3)	96004	1(2)	96523	2(3)
92979	2(3)	93312	1(3)	93623	1(3)	94013	1(3)	95132	0(3)	95865	1(3)	96020	1(2)	96542	1(3)
92986	1(2)	93313	1(3)	93624	1(3)	94014	1(2)	95133	0(3)	95866	1(3)	96040	4(3)	96549	1(3)
92987	1(2)	93314	1(3)	93631	1(3)	94015	1(2)	95134	0(3)	95867	1(3)	96105	3(3)	96567	1(3)
92990	1(2)	93315	1(3)	93640	1(3)	94016	1(2)	95144	30(3)	95868	1(3)	96110	3(3)	96570	1(2)
92997	1(2)	93316	1(3)	93641	1(2)	94060	1(3)	95145	10(3)	95869	1(3)	96112	1(2)	96571	2(3)
92998	2(3)	93317	1(3)	93642	1(3)	94070	1(2)	95146	10(3)	95870	4(3)	96113	6(3)	96573	1(2)
93000	3(3)	93318	1(3)	93644	1(3)	94150	2(3)	95147	10(3)	95872	4(3)	96116	1(2)	96574	1(2)
93005	5(3)	93320	2(3)	93650	1(2)	94200	1(3)	95148	10(3)	95873	1(2)	96121	3(3)	96900	1(3)
93010	5(3)	93321	1(3)	93653	1(3)	94375	1(3)	95149	10(3)	95874	1(2)	96125	2(3)	96902	1(3)
93015	1(3)	93325	2(3)	93654	1(3)	94450	1(3)	95165	30(3)	95875	2(3)	96127	2(3)	96904	1(2)
93016	1(3)	93350	1(2)	93655	2(3)	94452	1(2)	95170	10(3)	95885	4(2)	96130	1(2)	96910	1(3)
93017	1(3)	93351	1(2)	93656	1(3)	94453	1(2)	95180	8(3)	95886	4(2)	96131	7(3)	96912	1(3)
93018	1(3)	93352	1(3)	93657	2(3)	94610	2(3)	95199	1(3)	95887	1(2)	96132	1(2)	96913	1(3)
93024	1(3)	93355	1(3)	93660	1(3)	94617	1(3)	95249	1(2)	95905	2(3)	96133	7(3)	96920	1(2)
93025	1(2)	93356	1(3)	93662	1(3)	94618	1(3)	95250	1(2)	95907	1(2)	96136	1(2)	96921	1(2)
93040	3(3)	93451	1(3)	93668	1(3)	94619	1(3)	95251	1(2)	95908	1(2)	96137	11(3)	96922	1(2)
93041	3(3)	93452	1(3)	93701	1(2)	94621	1(3)	95700	1(2)	95909	1(2)	96138	1(2)	96931	1(2)
93042	3(3)	93453	1(3)	93702	1(2)	94640	1(3)	95705	1(2)	95910	1(2)	96139	11(3)	96932	1(2)
93050	1(3)	93454	1(3)	93724	1(3)	94642	1(3)	95706	1(2)	95911	1(2)	96146	1(2)	96933	1(2)
93224	1(2)	93455	1(3)	93740	1(3)	94644	1(2)	95707	1(2)	95912	1(2)	96156	1(3)	96934	2(3)
93225	1(2)	93456	1(3)	93745	1(2)	94645	4(3)	95708	4(3)	95913	1(2)	96158	1(2)	96935	2(3)
93226	1(2)	93457	1(3)	93750	1(3)	94660	1(2)	95709	4(3)	95921	1(3)	96159	4(3)	96936	2(3)
93227	1(2)	93458	1(3)	93770	1(3)	94662	1(2)	95710	4(3)	95922	1(3)	96160	3(3)	96999	1(3)
93228	1(2)	93459	1(3)	93784	1(2)	94664	1(3)	95711	1(2)	95923	1(3)	96161	1(3)	97010	1(3)
93229	1(2)	93460	1(3)	93786	1(2)	94667	1(2)	95712	1(2)	95924	1(3)	96164	1(2)	97012	1(3)
93241	1(2)	93461	1(3)	93788	1(2)	94668	5(3)	95713	1(2)	95925	1(3)	96165	6(3)	97014	0(3)
93242	1(2)	93462	1(3)	93790	1(2)	94669	4(3)	95714	4(3)	95926	1(3)	96167	1(2)	97016	1(3)
93243	1(2)	93463	1(3)	93792	1(2)	94680	1(3)	95715	4(3)	95927	1(3)	96168	6(3)	97018	1(3)
93244	1(2)	93464	1(3)	93793	1(2)	94681	1(3)	95716	4(3)	95928	1(3)	96170	1(3)	97022	1(3)
93245	1(2)	93503	2(3)	93797	2(2)	94690	1(3)	95717	1(2)	95929	1(3)	96171	2(3)	97024	1(3)
93246	1(2)	93505	1(2)	93798	2(2)	94726	1(3)	95718	1(2)	95930	1(3)	96360	2(3)	97026	1(3)
93247	1(2)	93530	1(3)	93799	1(3)	94727	1(3)	95719	1(2)	95933	1(3)	96361	24(3)	97028	1(3)
93248	1(2)	93531	1(3)	93880	1(3)	94728	1(3)	95720	1(2)	95937	4(3)	96365	2(3)	97032	4(3)
93260	1(2)	93532	1(3)	93882	1(3)	94729	1(3)	95721	1(2)	95938	1(3)	96366	24(3)	97033	4(3)
93261	1(3)	93533	1(3)	93886	1(3)	94760	1(3)	95722	1(2)	95939	1(3)	96367	4(3)	97034	2(3)
93264	1(2)	93561	1(3)	93888	1(3)	94761	1(2)	95723	1(2)	95940	20(3)	96368	1(2)	97035	2(3)
93268	1(2)	93562	1(3)	93890	1(3)	94762	1(2)	95724	1(2)	95941	8(3)	96369	1(2)	97036	3(3)
93270	1(2)	93563	1(3)	93892	1(3)	94772	1(2)	95725	1(2)	95943	1(3)	96370	3(3)	97039	1(3)
93271	1(2)	93564	1(3)	93893	1(3)	94774	1(2)	95726	1(2)	95954	1(3)	96371	1(3)	97110	8(3)
93272	1(2)	93565	1(3)	93895	1(3)	94775	1(2)	95782	1(2)	95955	1(3)	96372	5(3)	97112	6(3)
93278	1(3)	93566	1(3)	93922	2(2)	94776	1(2)	95783	1(2)	95957	1(3)	96373	3(3)	97113	6(3)
93279	1(3)	93567	1(3)	93923	2(2)	94777	1(2)	95800	1(2)	95958	1(3)	96374	1(3)	97116	4(3)
93280	1(3)	93568	1(3)	93924	1(2)	94780	1(2)	95801	1(2)	95961	1(2)	96375	6(3)	97124	4(3)
93281	1(3)	93571	1(3)	93925	1(3)	94781	2(3)	95803	1(2)	95962	3(3)	96376	10(3)	97129	1(2)
93282	1(3)	93572	2(3)	93926	1(3)	94799	1(3)	95805	1(2)	95965	1(3)	96377	1(3)	97130	7(3)
93283	1(3)	93580	1(3)	93930	1(3)	95004	80(3)	95806	1(2)	95966	1(3)	96379	2(3)	97139	1(3)
93284	1(3)	93581	1(3)	93931	1(3)	95012	2(3)	95807	1(2)	95967	3(3)	96401	4(3)	97140	6(3)
93285	1(3)	93582	1(2)	93970	1(3)	95017	27(3)	95808	1(2)	95970	1(3)	96402	2(3)	97150	2(3)
93286	2(3)	93583	1(2)	93971	1(3)	95018	19(3)	95810	1(2)	95971	1(3)	96405	1(2)	97151	8(3)
93287	2(3)	93590	1(2)	93975	1(3)	95024	40(3)	95811	1(2)	95972	1(3)	96406	1(2)	97152	16(3)

CPT	MUE
97153	32(3)
97154	18(3)
97155	24(3)
97156	16(3)
97157	16(3)
97158	16(3)
97161	1(2)
97162	1(2)
97163	1(2)
97164	1(2)
97165	1(2)
97166	1(2)
97167	1(2)
97168	1(2)
97169	0(3)
97170	0(3)
97171	0(3)
97172	0(3)
97530	6(3)
97533	4(3)
97535	8(3)
97537	8(3)
97542	8(3)
97545	1(2)
97546	2(3)
97597	1(3)
97598	8(3)
97602	1(3)
97605	1(3)
97606	1(3)
97607	1(3)
97608	1(3)
97610	1(2)
97750	8(3)
97755	8(3)
97760	6(3)
97761	6(3)
97763	6(3)
97799	1(3)
97802	8(3)
97803	8(3)
97804	6(3)
97810	1(2)
97811	2(3)
97813	1(2)
97814	2(3)
98925	1(2)
98926	1(2)
98927	1(2)
98928	1(2)
98929	1(2)
98940	1(2)
98941	1(2)
98942	1(2)
98943	0(3)
98960	0(3)
98961	0(3)
98962	0(3)
98966	1(2)
98967	1(2)
98968	1(2)
98970	1(2)
98971	1(2)
98972	1(2)
99000	0(3)
99001	0(3)

CPT	MUE
99002	1(3)
99024	1(3)
99026	0(3)
99027	0(3)
99050	1(3)
99051	1(3)
99053	1(3)
99056	1(3)
99058	1(3)
99060	1(3)
99070	1(3)
99071	1(3)
99075	0(3)
99078	3(3)
99080	1(3)
99082	1(3)
99091	1(2)
99100	1(3)
99116	1(3)
99135	1(3)
99140	2(3)
99151	1(3)
99152	2(3)
99153	12(3)
99155	1(3)
99156	1(3)
99157	6(3)
99170	1(3)
99172	0(3)
99173	0(3)
99174	0(3)
99175	1(3)
99177	1(2)
99183	1(3)
99184	1(2)
99188	1(2)
99190	1(3)
99191	1(3)
99192	1(3)
99195	2(3)
99199	1(3)
99202	1(2)
99203	1(2)
99204	1(2)
99205	1(2)
99211	2(3)
99212	2(3)
99213	2(3)
99214	2(3)
99215	2(3)
99217	1(2)
99218	1(2)
99219	1(2)
99220	1(2)
99221	0(3)
99222	0(3)
99223	0(3)
99224	1(2)
99225	1(2)
99226	1(2)
99231	0(3)
99232	0(3)
99233	0(3)
99234	1(3)
99235	1(3)
99236	1(3)

CPT	MUE
99238	0(3)
99239	0(3)
99241	0(3)
99242	0(3)
99243	0(3)
99244	0(3)
99245	0(3)
99251	0(3)
99252	0(3)
99253	0(3)
99254	0(3)
99255	0(3)
99281	2(3)
99282	2(3)
99283	2(3)
99284	2(3)
99285	2(3)
99288	1(3)
99291	1(2)
99292	8(3)
99304	1(2)
99305	1(2)
99306	1(2)
99307	1(2)
99308	1(2)
99309	1(2)
99310	1(2)
99315	1(2)
99316	1(2)
99318	1(2)
99324	1(2)
99325	1(2)
99326	1(2)
99327	1(2)
99328	1(2)
99334	1(3)
99335	1(3)
99336	1(3)
99337	1(3)
99339	1(2)
99340	1(2)
99341	1(2)
99342	1(2)
99343	1(2)
99344	1(2)
99345	1(2)
99347	1(3)
99348	1(3)
99349	1(3)
99350	1(3)
99354	1(2)
99355	4(3)
99356	1(2)
99357	1(3)
99358	1(2)
99359	1(3)
99360	1(3)
99366	2(3)
99367	1(3)
99368	2(3)
99374	1(2)
99375	0(3)
99377	1(2)
99378	0(3)
99379	1(2)
99380	1(2)

CPT	MUE
99381	0(3)
99382	0(3)
99383	0(3)
99384	0(3)
99385	0(3)
99386	0(3)
99387	0(3)
99391	0(3)
99392	0(3)
99393	0(3)
99394	0(3)
99395	0(3)
99396	0(3)
99397	0(3)
99401	0(3)
99402	0(3)
99403	0(3)
99404	0(3)
99406	1(2)
99407	1(2)
99408	0(3)
99409	0(3)
99411	0(3)
99412	0(3)
99415	1(2)
99416	3(3)
99417	4(3)
99421	1(2)
99422	1(2)
99423	1(2)
99429	0(3)
99439	2(2)
99441	1(2)
99442	1(2)
99443	1(2)
99446	1(2)
99447	1(2)
99448	1(2)
99449	1(2)
99450	0(3)
99451	1(2)
99452	1(2)
99453	1(2)
99454	1(2)
99455	1(3)
99456	1(3)
99457	1(2)
99458	3(3)
99460	1(2)
99461	1(2)
99462	1(2)
99463	1(2)
99464	1(2)
99465	1(2)
99466	1(2)
99467	4(3)
99468	1(2)
99469	1(2)
99471	1(2)
99472	1(2)
99473	1(2)
99474	1(2)
99475	1(2)
99476	1(2)
99477	1(2)
99478	1(2)

CPT	MUE
99479	1(2)
99480	1(2)
99483	1(2)
99484	1(2)
99485	1(3)
99486	4(1)
99487	1(2)
99489	4(3)
99490	1(2)
99491	1(2)
99492	1(2)
99493	1(2)
99494	2(3)
99495	1(2)
99496	1(2)
99497	1(2)
99498	3(3)
99499	1(3)
99500	0(3)
99501	0(3)
99502	0(3)
99503	0(3)
99504	0(3)
99505	0(3)
99506	0(3)
99507	0(3)
99509	0(3)
99510	0(3)
99511	0(3)
99512	0(3)
99600	0(3)
99601	0(3)
99602	0(3)
99605	0(2)
99606	0(3)
99607	0(3)
A0021	0(3)
A0080	0(3)
A0090	0(3)
A0100	0(3)
A0110	0(3)
A0120	0(3)
A0130	0(3)
A0140	0(3)
A0160	0(3)
A0170	0(3)
A0180	0(3)
A0190	0(3)
A0200	0(3)
A0210	0(3)
A0225	0(3)
A0380	0(3)
A0382	0(3)
A0384	0(3)
A0390	0(3)
A0392	0(3)
A0394	0(3)
A0396	0(3)
A0398	0(3)
A0420	0(3)
A0422	0(3)
A0424	0(3)
A0425	250(1)
A0426	2(3)
A0427	2(3)
A0428	2(3)

CPT	MUE
A0429	2(3)
A0430	1(3)
A0431	1(3)
A0432	1(3)
A0433	1(3)
A0434	2(3)
A0435	999(3)
A0436	300(3)
A0888	0(3)
A0998	0(3)
A0999	1(3)
A4206	1(3)
A4207	1(3)
A4208	4(3)
A4209	6(3)
A4210	0(3)
A4211	1(3)
A4212	2(3)
A4213	5(3)
A4215	9(3)
A4216	25(3)
A4217	4(3)
A4218	20(3)
A4220	1(3)
A4221	1(3)
A4222	2(3)
A4223	1(3)
A4224	1(2)
A4225	1(3)
A4226	0(3)
A4230	1(3)
A4231	1(3)
A4232	0(3)
A4233	0(3)
A4234	0(3)
A4235	1(3)
A4236	0(3)
A4244	1(3)
A4245	1(3)
A4246	1(3)
A4247	1(3)
A4248	10(3)
A4250	0(3)
A4252	0(3)
A4253	0(3)
A4255	0(3)
A4256	1(3)
A4257	0(3)
A4258	0(3)
A4259	0(3)
A4261	0(3)
A4262	4(2)
A4263	4(2)
A4264	0(3)
A4265	1(3)
A4266	0(3)
A4267	0(3)
A4268	0(3)
A4269	0(3)
A4270	3(3)
A4280	1(3)
A4281	0(3)
A4282	0(3)
A4283	0(3)
A4284	0(3)
A4285	0(3)

CPT	MUE
A4286	0(3)
A4290	2(3)
A4300	4(3)
A4301	1(2)
A4305	2(3)
A4306	2(3)
A4310	2(3)
A4311	2(3)
A4312	1(3)
A4313	1(3)
A4314	2(3)
A4315	2(3)
A4316	1(3)
A4320	2(3)
A4321	1(3)
A4322	2(3)
A4326	1(3)
A4327	2(3)
A4328	1(3)
A4330	1(3)
A4331	3(3)
A4332	2(3)
A4334	3(3)
A4335	1(3)
A4336	1(3)
A4337	2(3)
A4338	3(3)
A4340	2(3)
A4344	2(3)
A4346	2(3)
A4351	2(3)
A4352	2(3)
A4353	3(3)
A4354	2(3)
A4355	2(3)
A4356	2(3)
A4357	2(3)
A4358	6(3)
A4360	1(3)
A4361	1(3)
A4362	2(3)
A4363	0(3)
A4364	2(3)
A4366	1(3)
A4367	1(3)
A4368	1(3)
A4369	1(3)
A4371	1(3)
A4372	1(3)
A4373	1(3)
A4375	2(3)
A4376	2(3)
A4377	2(3)
A4378	2(3)
A4379	2(3)
A4380	2(3)
A4381	2(3)
A4382	2(3)
A4383	2(3)
A4384	2(3)
A4385	2(3)
A4387	1(3)
A4388	1(3)
A4389	2(3)
A4390	1(3)
A4391	1(3)

CPT	MUE
A4392	2(3)
A4393	1(3)
A4394	1(3)
A4395	3(3)
A4396	2(3)
A4397	1(3)
A4398	2(3)
A4399	1(3)
A4400	1(3)
A4402	1(3)
A4404	1(3)
A4405	1(3)
A4406	1(3)
A4407	2(3)
A4408	1(3)
A4409	1(3)
A4410	2(3)
A4411	1(3)
A4412	1(3)
A4413	2(3)
A4414	1(3)
A4415	1(3)
A4416	2(3)
A4417	2(3)
A4418	2(3)
A4419	2(3)
A4420	1(3)
A4423	2(3)
A4424	1(3)
A4425	1(3)
A4426	2(3)
A4427	1(3)
A4428	1(3)
A4429	2(3)
A4430	1(3)
A4431	1(3)
A4432	2(3)
A4433	1(3)
A4434	1(3)
A4435	2(3)
A4450	20(3)
A4452	4(3)
A4455	1(3)
A4458	1(3)
A4459	1(3)
A4461	2(3)
A4463	2(3)
A4465	1(3)
A4467	0(3)
A4470	1(3)
A4480	1(3)
A4481	2(3)
A4483	1(3)
A4490	0(3)
A4495	0(3)
A4500	0(3)
A4510	0(3)
A4520	0(3)
A4550	3(3)
A4553	0(3)
A4554	0(3)
A4555	0(3)
A4556	2(3)
A4557	2(3)
A4558	1(3)
A4559	1(3)

CPT	MUE
A4561	1(3)
A4562	1(3)
A4563	1(2)
A4565	2(3)
A4566	0(3)
A4570	0(3)
A4575	0(3)
A4580	0(3)
A4590	0(3)
A4595	2(3)
A4600	0(3)
A4601	0(3)
A4602	1(3)
A4604	1(3)
A4605	1(3)
A4606	1(3)
A4608	1(3)
A4611	0(3)
A4612	0(3)
A4613	0(3)
A4614	1(2)
A4615	2(3)
A4616	1(3)
A4617	1(3)
A4618	1(3)
A4619	1(3)
A4620	1(3)
A4623	10(3)
A4624	2(3)
A4625	30(3)
A4626	1(3)
A4627	0(3)
A4628	1(3)
A4629	1(3)
A4630	0(3)
A4633	0(3)
A4634	1(3)
A4635	0(3)
A4636	0(3)
A4637	0(3)
A4638	0(3)
A4639	0(3)
A4640	0(3)
A4642	1(3)
A4648	3(3)
A4650	3(3)
A4651	2(3)
A4652	2(3)
A4653	0(3)
A4657	0(3)
A4660	0(3)
A4663	0(3)
A4670	0(3)
A4671	0(3)
A4672	0(3)
A4673	0(3)
A4674	0(3)
A4680	0(3)
A4690	0(3)
A4706	0(3)
A4707	0(3)
A4708	0(3)
A4709	0(3)
A4714	0(3)
A4719	0(3)
A4720	0(3)

CPT	MUE
A4721	0(3)
A4722	0(3)
A4723	0(3)
A4724	0(3)
A4725	0(3)
A4726	0(3)
A4728	0(3)
A4730	0(3)
A4736	0(3)
A4737	0(3)
A4740	0(3)
A4750	0(3)
A4755	0(3)
A4760	0(3)
A4765	0(3)
A4766	0(3)
A4770	0(3)
A4771	0(3)
A4772	0(3)
A4773	0(3)
A4774	0(3)
A4802	0(3)
A4860	0(3)
A4870	0(3)
A4890	0(3)
A4911	0(3)
A4913	0(3)
A4918	0(3)
A4927	0(3)
A4928	0(3)
A4929	0(3)
A4930	0(3)
A4931	0(3)
A4932	0(3)
A5051	1(3)
A5052	1(3)
A5053	2(3)
A5054	1(3)
A5055	1(3)
A5056	90(3)
A5057	90(3)
A5061	2(3)
A5062	1(3)
A5063	1(3)
A5071	2(3)
A5072	1(3)
A5073	1(3)
A5081	2(3)
A5082	1(3)
A5083	5(3)
A5093	2(3)
A5102	1(3)
A5105	1(3)
A5112	2(3)
A5113	0(3)
A5114	0(3)
A5120	150(3)
A5121	1(3)
A5122	1(3)
A5126	2(3)
A5131	1(3)
A5200	2(3)
A5500	0(3)
A5501	0(3)
A5503	0(3)
A5504	0(3)

CPT	MUE
A5505	0(3)
A5506	0(3)
A5507	0(3)
A5508	0(3)
A5510	0(3)
A5512	0(3)
A5513	0(3)
A5514	0(3)
A6000	0(3)
A6010	3(3)
A6011	20(3)
A6024	1(3)
A6025	4(3)
A6154	1(3)
A6205	1(3)
A6221	9(3)
A6228	2(3)
A6230	1(3)
A6236	1(3)
A6238	3(3)
A6239	1(3)
A6240	2(3)
A6241	1(3)
A6244	1(3)
A6246	3(3)
A6247	2(3)
A6250	1(3)
A6256	3(3)
A6259	3(3)
A6261	3(3)
A6262	3(3)
A6404	2(3)
A6407	4(3)
A6410	2(3)
A6411	2(3)
A6412	2(3)
A6413	0(3)
A6441	8(3)
A6442	8(3)
A6443	8(3)
A6444	4(3)
A6445	8(3)
A6446	14(3)
A6447	6(3)
A6448	24(3)
A6449	12(3)
A6450	8(3)
A6451	8(3)
A6452	22(3)
A6453	6(3)
A6454	25(3)
A6455	4(3)
A6456	20(3)
A6457	12(3)
A6460	1(1)
A6461	1(1)
A6501	1(3)
A6502	1(3)
A6503	1(3)
A6504	2(3)
A6505	2(3)
A6506	2(3)
A6507	2(3)
A6508	2(3)
A6509	1(3)
A6510	1(3)

CPT	MUE
A6511	1(3)
A6513	1(3)
A6530	0(3)
A6531	2(3)
A6532	2(3)
A6533	0(3)
A6534	0(3)
A6535	0(3)
A6536	0(3)
A6537	0(3)
A6538	0(3)
A6539	0(3)
A6540	0(3)
A6541	0(3)
A6544	0(3)
A6545	2(3)
A6549	0(3)
A6550	1(3)
A7000	0(3)
A7001	0(3)
A7002	0(3)
A7003	0(3)
A7004	0(3)
A7005	0(3)
A7006	0(3)
A7007	0(3)
A7008	0(3)
A7009	0(3)
A7010	0(3)
A7012	0(3)
A7013	0(3)
A7014	0(3)
A7015	0(3)
A7016	0(3)
A7017	0(3)
A7018	0(3)
A7020	0(3)
A7025	0(3)
A7026	0(3)
A7027	0(3)
A7028	0(3)
A7029	0(3)
A7030	0(3)
A7031	0(3)
A7032	0(3)
A7033	0(3)
A7034	0(3)
A7035	0(3)
A7036	0(3)
A7037	0(3)
A7038	0(3)
A7039	0(3)
A7040	2(3)
A7041	2(3)
A7044	0(3)
A7045	0(3)
A7046	0(3)
A7047	1(3)
A7048	2(3)
A7501	1(3)
A7502	1(3)
A7503	1(3)
A7504	180(3)
A7505	1(3)
A7506	0(3)
A7507	200(3)

CPT	MUE
A7508	0(3)
A7509	0(3)
A7520	1(3)
A7521	1(3)
A7522	0(3)
A7523	0(3)
A7524	1(3)
A7525	8(3)
A7526	0(3)
A7527	1(3)
A8000	0(3)
A8001	0(3)
A8002	0(3)
A8003	0(3)
A8004	0(3)
A9152	0(3)
A9153	0(3)
A9155	1(3)
A9180	0(3)
A9270	0(3)
A9272	0(3)
A9273	0(3)
A9274	0(3)
A9275	0(3)
A9276	0(3)
A9277	0(3)
A9278	0(3)
A9279	0(3)
A9280	0(3)
A9281	0(3)
A9282	0(3)
A9283	0(3)
A9284	0(3)
A9285	0(3)
A9286	0(3)
A9300	0(3)
A9500	3(3)
A9501	1(3)
A9502	3(3)
A9503	1(3)
A9504	1(3)
A9505	4(3)
A9507	1(3)
A9508	2(3)
A9509	5(3)
A9510	1(3)
A9512	30(3)
A9513	200(3)
A9515	1(3)
A9516	4(3)
A9517	200(3)
A9520	1(3)
A9521	2(3)
A9524	10(3)
A9526	2(3)
A9527	195(3)
A9528	10(3)
A9529	10(3)
A9530	200(3)
A9531	100(3)
A9532	10(3)
A9536	1(3)
A9537	1(3)
A9538	1(3)
A9539	2(3)
A9540	2(3)

CPT	MUE
A9541	1(3)
A9542	1(3)
A9543	1(3)
A9546	1(3)
A9547	2(3)
A9548	2(3)
A9550	1(3)
A9551	1(3)
A9552	1(3)
A9553	1(3)
A9554	1(3)
A9555	2(3)
A9556	10(3)
A9557	2(3)
A9558	7(3)
A9559	1(3)
A9560	2(3)
A9561	1(3)
A9562	2(3)
A9563	10(3)
A9564	0(3)
A9566	1(3)
A9567	2(3)
A9568	0(3)
A9569	1(3)
A9570	1(3)
A9571	1(3)
A9572	1(3)
A9575	300(3)
A9576	100(3)
A9577	50(3)
A9578	50(3)
A9579	100(3)
A9580	1(3)
A9581	20(3)
A9582	1(3)
A9583	18(3)
A9584	1(3)
A9585	300(3)
A9586	1(3)
A9587	54(3)
A9588	10(3)
A9589	1(3)
A9590	675(3)
A9591	6(3)
A9600	7(3)
A9604	1(3)
A9606	224(3)
A9698	3(3)
A9700	2(3)
A9900	0(3)
A9901	0(3)
A9999	0(3)
B4034	0(3)
B4035	0(3)
B4036	0(3)
B4081	0(3)
B4082	0(3)
B4083	0(3)
B4087	0(3)
B4088	0(3)
B4100	0(3)
B4102	0(3)
B4103	0(3)
B4104	0(3)
B4149	0(3)

CPT	MUE
B4150	0(3)
B4152	0(3)
B4153	0(3)
B4154	0(3)
B4155	0(3)
B4157	0(3)
B4158	0(3)
B4159	0(3)
B4160	0(3)
B4161	0(3)
B4162	0(3)
B4164	0(3)
B4168	0(3)
B4172	0(3)
B4176	0(3)
B4178	0(3)
B4180	0(3)
B4185	0(3)
B4187	0(3)
B4189	0(3)
B4193	0(3)
B4197	0(3)
B4199	0(3)
B4216	0(3)
B4220	0(3)
B4222	0(3)
B4224	0(3)
B5000	0(3)
B5100	0(3)
B5200	0(3)
B9002	0(3)
B9004	0(3)
B9006	0(3)
B9998	0(3)
B9999	0(3)
C1052	1(3)
C1062	2(3)
C1713	20(3)
C1714	4(3)
C1715	45(3)
C1716	4(3)
C1717	10(3)
C1719	99(3)
C1721	1(3)
C1722	1(3)
C1724	5(3)
C1725	9(3)
C1726	5(3)
C1727	4(3)
C1728	5(3)
C1729	6(3)
C1730	4(3)
C1731	2(3)
C1732	3(3)
C1733	3(3)
C1734	2(3)
C1748	1(3)
C1749	1(3)
C1750	2(3)
C1751	3(3)
C1752	2(3)
C1753	2(3)
C1754	2(3)
C1755	2(3)
C1756	2(3)
C1757	6(3)

CPT	MUE
C1758	2(3)
C1759	2(3)
C1760	4(3)
C1762	4(3)
C1763	4(3)
C1764	1(3)
C1765	4(3)
C1766	4(3)
C1767	2(3)
C1768	3(3)
C1769	9(3)
C1770	3(3)
C1771	1(3)
C1772	1(3)
C1773	3(3)
C1776	10(3)
C1777	2(3)
C1778	4(3)
C1779	2(3)
C1780	2(3)
C1781	4(3)
C1782	1(3)
C1783	2(3)
C1784	2(3)
C1785	1(3)
C1786	1(3)
C1787	2(3)
C1788	2(3)
C1789	2(3)
C1813	1(3)
C1814	2(3)
C1815	1(3)
C1816	2(3)
C1817	1(3)
C1818	2(3)
C1819	4(3)
C1820	2(3)
C1821	4(3)
C1822	1(3)
C1823	1(3)
C1824	1(2)
C1825	1(2)
C1830	2(3)
C1839	2(2)
C1840	1(3)
C1841	1(2)
C1842	1(2)
C1874	5(3)
C1875	4(3)
C1876	5(3)
C1877	5(3)
C1878	2(3)
C1880	2(3)
C1881	2(3)
C1882	1(3)
C1883	4(3)
C1884	4(3)
C1885	2(3)
C1886	1(3)
C1887	7(3)
C1888	2(3)
C1889	2(3)
C1890	1(3)
C1891	1(3)
C1892	6(3)
C1893	6(3)

CPT	MUE
C1894	6(3)
C1895	2(3)
C1896	2(3)
C1897	2(3)
C1898	2(3)
C1899	2(3)
C1900	1(3)
C1982	1(3)
C2596	1(3)
C2613	2(3)
C2614	3(3)
C2615	2(3)
C2616	1(3)
C2617	4(3)
C2618	4(3)
C2619	1(3)
C2620	1(3)
C2621	1(3)
C2622	1(3)
C2623	4(3)
C2624	1(3)
C2625	4(3)
C2626	1(3)
C2627	2(3)
C2628	4(3)
C2629	4(3)
C2630	3(3)
C2631	1(3)
C2634	24(3)
C2635	124(3)
C2636	690(3)
C2637	0(3)
C2638	150(3)
C2639	150(3)
C2640	150(3)
C2641	150(3)
C2642	120(3)
C2643	120(3)
C2644	0(3)
C2645	4608(3)
C5271	1(2)
C5272	3(2)
C5273	1(2)
C5274	35(3)
C5275	1(2)
C5276	3(2)
C5277	1(2)
C5278	15(3)
C8900	1(3)
C8901	1(3)
C8902	1(3)
C8903	1(3)
C8905	1(3)
C8906	1(3)
C8908	1(3)
C8909	1(3)
C8910	1(3)
C8911	1(3)
C8912	1(3)
C8913	1(3)
C8914	1(3)
C8918	1(3)
C8919	1(3)
C8920	1(3)
C8921	1(3)
C8922	1(3)

CPT	MUE
C8923	1(3)
C8924	1(3)
C8925	1(3)
C8926	1(3)
C8927	1(3)
C8928	1(2)
C8929	1(3)
C8930	1(2)
C8931	1(3)
C8932	1(3)
C8933	1(3)
C8934	2(3)
C8935	2(3)
C8936	2(3)
C8937	2(2)
C8957	2(3)
C9046	160(3)
C9047	22(3)
C9065	40(3)
C9067	500(3)
C9113	10(3)
C9132	5500(3)
C9248	25(3)
C9250	5(3)
C9254	400(3)
C9257	10(2)
C9285	2(3)
C9290	266(3)
C9293	700(3)
C9352	3(3)
C9353	4(3)
C9354	300(3)
C9355	3(3)
C9356	125(3)
C9358	800(3)
C9359	30(3)
C9360	300(3)
C9361	10(3)
C9362	60(3)
C9363	500(3)
C9364	600(3)
C9460	100(3)
C9462	600(3)
C9482	300(3)
C9488	40(3)
C9600	3(3)
C9601	2(3)
C9602	2(3)
C9603	2(3)
C9604	2(3)
C9605	2(3)
C9606	1(3)
C9607	2(3)
C9608	2(3)
C9725	1(3)
C9726	2(3)
C9727	1(2)
C9728	1(2)
C9733	1(3)
C9734	1(3)
C9738	1(3)
C9739	1(2)
C9740	1(2)
C9751	1(3)
C9752	1(2)
C9753	3(3)

CPT	MUE
C9756	1(3)
C9757	2(2)
C9758	1(2)
C9759	1(3)
C9760	1(2)
C9761	2(2)
C9762	1(3)
C9763	1(3)
C9764	2(3)
C9765	2(3)
C9766	2(3)
C9767	2(3)
C9768	1(3)
C9769	1(2)
C9770	2(2)
C9771	1(2)
C9772	2(2)
C9773	2(2)
C9774	2(2)
C9775	2(2)
C9803	2(3)
C9898	1(3)
D0150	1(3)
D0240	1(3)
D0250	2(3)
D0270	1(3)
D0272	1(3)
D0274	1(3)
D0277	1(3)
D0412	0(3)
D0416	1(3)
D0431	1(3)
D0460	1(2)
D0484	1(2)
D0485	1(2)
D0601	0(3)
D0602	0(3)
D0603	0(3)
D1510	2(2)
D1516	1(2)
D1517	1(2)
D1520	2(2)
D1526	1(2)
D1527	1(2)
D1551	1(2)
D1552	1(2)
D1553	2(2)
D1575	4(2)
D1999	0(3)
D4260	4(2)
D4263	4(2)
D4264	3(3)
D4270	4(3)
D4273	1(2)
D4277	0(3)
D4278	0(3)
D4355	1(2)
D4381	12(3)
D5282	0(3)
D5283	0(3)
D5876	0(3)
D5911	1(3)
D5912	1(2)
D5951	0(3)
D5983	1(3)
D5984	1(3)

CPT	MUE
D5985	1(3)
D6052	0(3)
D7111	20(3)
D7140	32(2)
D7210	32(2)
D7220	6(3)
D7230	6(3)
D7240	6(3)
D7241	6(3)
D7250	32(2)
D7260	1(3)
D7261	1(3)
D7283	4(3)
D7288	2(3)
D7321	4(2)
D9110	1(3)
D9130	0(3)
D9230	1(3)
D9248	1(3)
D9613	0(3)
D9930	1(2)
D9944	2(2)
D9945	2(2)
D9946	2(2)
D9950	1(3)
D9951	1(3)
D9952	1(3)
D9961	0(3)
D9990	0(3)
E0100	0(3)
E0105	0(3)
E0110	0(3)
E0111	0(3)
E0112	0(3)
E0113	0(3)
E0114	0(3)
E0116	0(3)
E0117	0(3)
E0118	0(3)
E0130	0(3)
E0135	0(3)
E0140	0(3)
E0141	0(3)
E0143	0(3)
E0144	0(3)
E0147	0(3)
E0148	0(3)
E0149	0(3)
E0153	0(3)
E0154	0(3)
E0155	0(3)
E0156	0(3)
E0157	0(3)
E0158	0(3)
E0159	1(3)
E0160	0(3)
E0161	0(3)
E0162	0(3)
E0163	0(3)
E0165	0(3)
E0167	0(3)
E0168	0(3)
E0170	0(3)
E0171	0(3)
E0172	0(3)
E0175	0(3)

CPT	MUE
E0181	0(3)
E0182	0(3)
E0184	0(3)
E0185	0(3)
E0186	0(3)
E0187	0(3)
E0188	0(3)
E0189	0(3)
E0190	0(3)
E0191	0(3)
E0193	0(3)
E0194	0(3)
E0196	0(3)
E0197	0(3)
E0198	0(3)
E0199	0(3)
E0200	0(3)
E0202	0(3)
E0203	0(3)
E0205	0(3)
E0210	0(3)
E0215	0(3)
E0217	0(3)
E0218	0(3)
E0221	0(3)
E0225	0(3)
E0231	0(3)
E0232	0(3)
E0235	0(3)
E0236	0(3)
E0239	0(3)
E0240	0(3)
E0241	0(3)
E0242	0(3)
E0243	0(3)
E0244	0(3)
E0245	0(3)
E0246	0(3)
E0247	0(3)
E0248	0(3)
E0249	0(3)
E0250	0(3)
E0251	0(3)
E0255	0(3)
E0256	0(3)
E0260	0(3)
E0261	0(3)
E0265	0(3)
E0266	0(3)
E0270	0(3)
E0271	0(3)
E0272	0(3)
E0273	0(3)
E0274	0(3)
E0275	0(3)
E0276	0(3)
E0277	0(3)
E0280	0(3)
E0290	0(3)
E0291	0(3)
E0292	0(3)
E0293	0(3)
E0294	0(3)
E0295	0(3)
E0296	0(3)
E0297	0(3)

CPT	MUE
E0300	0(3)
E0301	0(3)
E0302	0(3)
E0303	0(3)
E0304	0(3)
E0305	0(3)
E0310	0(3)
E0315	0(3)
E0316	0(3)
E0325	0(3)
E0326	0(3)
E0328	0(3)
E0329	0(3)
E0350	0(3)
E0352	0(3)
E0370	0(3)
E0371	0(3)
E0372	0(3)
E0373	0(3)
E0424	0(3)
E0425	0(3)
E0430	0(3)
E0431	0(3)
E0433	0(3)
E0434	0(3)
E0435	0(3)
E0439	0(3)
E0440	0(3)
E0441	0(3)
E0442	0(3)
E0443	0(3)
E0444	0(3)
E0445	0(3)
E0446	0(3)
E0447	0(3)
E0455	0(3)
E0457	0(3)
E0459	0(3)
E0462	0(3)
E0465	0(3)
E0466	0(3)
E0467	0(3)
E0470	0(3)
E0471	0(3)
E0472	0(3)
E0480	0(3)
E0481	0(3)
E0482	0(3)
E0483	0(3)
E0484	0(3)
E0485	0(3)
E0486	0(3)
E0487	0(3)
E0500	0(3)
E0550	0(3)
E0555	0(3)
E0560	0(3)
E0561	0(3)
E0562	0(3)
E0565	0(3)
E0570	0(3)
E0572	0(3)
E0574	0(3)
E0575	0(3)
E0580	0(3)
E0585	0(3)

CPT	MUE
E0600	0(3)
E0601	0(3)
E0602	0(3)
E0603	0(3)
E0604	0(3)
E0605	0(3)
E0606	0(3)
E0607	0(3)
E0610	0(3)
E0615	0(3)
E0616	1(2)
E0617	0(3)
E0618	0(3)
E0619	0(3)
E0620	0(3)
E0621	0(3)
E0625	0(3)
E0627	0(3)
E0629	0(3)
E0630	0(3)
E0635	0(3)
E0636	0(3)
E0637	0(3)
E0638	0(3)
E0639	0(3)
E0640	0(3)
E0641	0(3)
E0642	0(3)
E0650	0(3)
E0651	0(3)
E0652	0(3)
E0655	0(3)
E0656	0(3)
E0657	0(3)
E0660	0(3)
E0665	0(3)
E0666	0(3)
E0667	0(3)
E0668	0(3)
E0669	0(3)
E0670	0(3)
E0671	0(3)
E0672	0(3)
E0673	0(3)
E0675	0(3)
E0676	1(3)
E0691	0(3)
E0692	0(3)
E0693	0(3)
E0694	0(3)
E0700	0(3)
E0705	1(2)
E0710	0(3)
E0720	0(3)
E0730	0(3)
E0731	0(3)
E0740	0(3)
E0744	0(3)
E0745	0(3)
E0746	1(3)
E0747	0(3)
E0748	0(3)
E0749	1(3)
E0755	0(3)
E0760	0(3)
E0761	0(3)

CPT	MUE
E0762	1(3)
E0764	0(3)
E0765	0(3)
E0766	0(3)
E0769	0(3)
E0770	1(3)
E0776	0(3)
E0779	0(3)
E0780	0(3)
E0781	1(3)
E0782	1(2)
E0783	1(2)
E0784	0(3)
E0785	1(2)
E0786	1(2)
E0787	0(3)
E0791	0(3)
E0830	0(3)
E0840	0(3)
E0849	0(3)
E0850	0(3)
E0855	0(3)
E0856	0(3)
E0860	0(3)
E0870	0(3)
E0880	0(3)
E0890	0(3)
E0900	0(3)
E0910	0(3)
E0911	0(3)
E0912	0(3)
E0920	0(3)
E0930	0(3)
E0935	0(3)
E0936	0(3)
E0940	0(3)
E0941	0(3)
E0942	0(3)
E0944	0(3)
E0945	0(3)
E0946	0(3)
E0947	0(3)
E0948	0(3)
E0950	0(3)
E0951	0(3)
E0952	0(3)
E0953	0(3)
E0954	0(3)
E0955	0(3)
E0956	0(3)
E0957	0(3)
E0958	0(3)
E0959	2(2)
E0960	0(3)
E0961	2(2)
E0966	1(2)
E0967	0(3)
E0968	0(3)
E0969	0(3)
E0970	0(3)
E0971	2(3)
E0973	2(2)
E0974	2(2)
E0978	1(3)
E0980	0(3)
E0981	0(3)

CPT	MUE	CPT	MUE	CPT	MUE	CPT	MUE	CPT	MUE	CPT	MUE	CPT	MUE	CPT	MUE
E0982	0(3)	E1223	0(3)	E1636	0(3)	E2310	0(3)	E2512	0(3)	G0122	0(3)	G0339	1(2)	G0469	1(2)
E0983	0(3)	E1224	0(3)	E1637	0(3)	E2311	0(3)	E2599	0(3)	G0123	1(3)	G0340	1(3)	G0470	1(3)
E0984	0(3)	E1225	0(3)	E1639	0(3)	E2312	0(3)	E2601	0(3)	G0124	1(3)	G0341	1(2)	G0471	2(3)
E0985	0(3)	E1226	1(2)	E1699	1(3)	E2313	0(3)	E2602	0(3)	G0127	1(2)	G0342	1(2)	G0472	1(2)
E0986	0(3)	E1227	0(3)	E1700	0(3)	E2321	0(3)	E2603	0(3)	G0128	1(3)	G0343	1(2)	G0473	1(3)
E0988	0(3)	E1228	0(3)	E1701	0(3)	E2322	0(3)	E2604	0(3)	G0129	6(3)	G0372	1(2)	G0475	1(2)
E0990	2(2)	E1229	0(3)	E1702	0(3)	E2323	0(3)	E2605	0(3)	G0130	1(2)	G0379	1(2)	G0476	1(2)
E0992	1(2)	E1230	0(3)	E1800	0(3)	E2324	0(3)	E2606	0(3)	G0141	1(3)	G0380	2(3)	G0480	1(2)
E0994	0(3)	E1231	0(3)	E1801	0(3)	E2325	0(3)	E2607	0(3)	G0143	1(3)	G0381	2(3)	G0481	1(2)
E0995	2(2)	E1232	0(3)	E1802	0(3)	E2326	0(3)	E2608	0(3)	G0144	1(3)	G0382	2(3)	G0482	1(2)
E1002	0(3)	E1233	0(3)	E1805	0(3)	E2327	0(3)	E2609	0(3)	G0145	1(3)	G0383	2(3)	G0483	1(2)
E1003	0(3)	E1234	0(3)	E1806	0(3)	E2328	0(3)	E2610	1(3)	G0147	1(3)	G0384	2(3)	G0490	1(3)
E1004	0(3)	E1235	0(3)	E1810	0(3)	E2329	0(3)	E2611	0(3)	G0148	1(3)	G0390	1(2)	G0491	1(3)
E1005	0(3)	E1236	0(3)	E1811	0(3)	E2330	0(3)	E2612	0(3)	G0166	2(3)	G0396	1(2)	G0492	1(3)
E1006	0(3)	E1237	0(3)	E1812	0(3)	E2331	0(3)	E2613	0(3)	G0168	2(3)	G0397	1(2)	G0493	1(3)
E1007	0(3)	E1238	0(3)	E1815	0(3)	E2340	0(3)	E2614	0(3)	G0175	1(3)	G0398	1(2)	G0494	1(3)
E1008	0(3)	E1239	0(3)	E1816	0(3)	E2341	0(3)	E2615	0(3)	G0176	5(3)	G0399	1(2)	G0495	1(3)
E1009	0(3)	E1240	0(3)	E1818	0(3)	E2342	0(3)	E2616	0(3)	G0177	5(3)	G0400	1(2)	G0496	1(3)
E1010	0(3)	E1250	0(3)	E1820	0(3)	E2343	0(3)	E2617	0(3)	G0179	1(2)	G0402	1(2)	G0498	1(2)
E1011	0(3)	E1260	0(3)	E1821	0(3)	E2351	0(3)	E2619	0(3)	G0180	1(2)	G0403	1(2)	G0499	1(2)
E1012	0(3)	E1270	0(3)	E1825	0(3)	E2358	0(3)	E2620	0(3)	G0181	1(2)	G0404	1(2)	G0500	1(3)
E1014	0(3)	E1280	0(3)	E1830	0(3)	E2359	0(3)	E2621	0(3)	G0182	1(2)	G0405	1(2)	G0501	1(3)
E1015	0(3)	E1285	0(3)	E1831	0(3)	E2360	0(3)	E2622	0(3)	G0186	1(2)	G0406	1(3)	G0506	1(2)
E1016	0(3)	E1290	0(3)	E1840	0(3)	E2361	0(3)	E2623	0(3)	G0219	0(3)	G0407	1(3)	G0508	1(2)
E1017	0(3)	E1295	0(3)	E1841	0(3)	E2362	0(3)	E2624	0(3)	G0235	1(3)	G0408	1(3)	G0509	1(2)
E1018	0(3)	E1296	0(3)	E1902	0(3)	E2363	0(3)	E2625	0(3)	G0237	8(3)	G0410	6(3)	G0511	1(2)
E1020	0(3)	E1297	0(3)	E2000	0(3)	E2364	0(3)	E2626	0(3)	G0238	8(3)	G0411	6(3)	G0512	1(2)
E1028	0(3)	E1298	0(3)	E2100	0(3)	E2365	0(3)	E2627	0(3)	G0239	2(3)	G0412	1(2)	G0513	1(2)
E1029	0(3)	E1300	0(3)	E2101	0(3)	E2366	0(3)	E2628	0(3)	G0245	1(2)	G0413	1(2)	G0514	1(1)
E1030	0(3)	E1310	0(3)	E2120	0(3)	E2367	0(3)	E2629	0(3)	G0246	1(2)	G0414	1(2)	G0516	1(2)
E1031	0(3)	E1352	0(3)	E2201	0(3)	E2368	0(3)	E2630	0(3)	G0247	1(2)	G0415	1(2)	G0517	1(2)
E1035	0(3)	E1353	0(3)	E2202	0(3)	E2369	0(3)	E2631	0(3)	G0248	1(2)	G0416	1(2)	G0518	1(2)
E1036	0(3)	E1354	0(3)	E2203	0(3)	E2370	0(3)	E2632	0(3)	G0249	3(3)	G0420	2(3)	G0659	1(2)
E1037	0(3)	E1355	0(3)	E2204	0(3)	E2371	0(3)	E2633	0(3)	G0250	1(2)	G0421	2(3)	G2000	1(3)
E1038	0(3)	E1356	0(3)	E2205	0(3)	E2372	0(3)	E8000	0(3)	G0252	0(3)	G0422	6(2)	G2001	1(3)
E1039	0(3)	E1357	0(3)	E2206	0(3)	E2373	0(3)	E8001	0(3)	G0255	0(3)	G0423	6(2)	G2002	1(3)
E1050	0(3)	E1358	0(3)	E2207	0(3)	E2374	0(3)	E8002	0(3)	G0257	1(3)	G0424	2(2)	G2003	1(3)
E1060	0(3)	E1372	0(3)	E2208	0(3)	E2375	0(3)	G0008	1(2)	G0259	2(3)	G0425	1(3)	G2004	1(3)
E1070	0(3)	E1390	0(3)	E2209	0(3)	E2376	0(3)	G0009	1(2)	G0260	2(3)	G0426	1(3)	G2005	1(3)
E1083	0(3)	E1391	0(3)	E2210	0(3)	E2377	0(3)	G0010	1(3)	G0268	1(2)	G0427	1(3)	G2006	1(3)
E1084	0(3)	E1392	0(3)	E2211	0(3)	E2378	0(3)	G0027	1(2)	G0269	2(3)	G0428	0(3)	G2007	1(3)
E1085	0(3)	E1399	0(3)	E2212	0(3)	E2381	0(3)	G0071	1(3)	G0270	8(3)	G0429	1(2)	G2008	1(3)
E1086	0(3)	E1405	0(3)	E2213	0(3)	E2382	0(3)	G0076	1(3)	G0271	4(3)	G0432	1(2)	G2009	1(3)
E1087	0(3)	E1406	0(3)	E2214	0(3)	E2383	0(3)	G0077	1(3)	G0276	1(3)	G0433	1(2)	G2010	1(3)
E1088	0(3)	E1500	0(3)	E2215	0(3)	E2384	0(3)	G0078	1(3)	G0277	5(3)	G0435	1(2)	G2011	1(2)
E1089	0(3)	E1510	0(3)	E2216	0(3)	E2385	0(3)	G0079	1(3)	G0278	1(2)	G0438	1(2)	G2012	1(3)
E1090	0(3)	E1520	0(3)	E2217	0(3)	E2386	0(3)	G0080	1(3)	G0279	1(2)	G0439	1(2)	G2013	1(3)
E1092	0(3)	E1530	0(3)	E2218	0(3)	E2387	0(3)	G0081	1(3)	G0281	1(3)	G0442	1(2)	G2014	1(3)
E1093	0(3)	E1540	0(3)	E2219	0(3)	E2388	0(3)	G0082	1(3)	G0282	0(3)	G0443	1(2)	G2015	1(3)
E1100	0(3)	E1550	0(3)	E2220	0(3)	E2389	0(3)	G0083	1(3)	G0283	1(3)	G0444	1(2)	G2023	2(3)
E1110	0(3)	E1560	0(3)	E2221	0(3)	E2390	0(3)	G0084	1(3)	G0288	1(2)	G0445	1(2)	G2024	2(3)
E1130	0(3)	E1570	0(3)	E2222	0(3)	E2391	0(3)	G0085	1(3)	G0289	1(2)	G0446	1(3)	G2025	1(3)
E1140	0(3)	E1575	0(3)	E2224	0(3)	E2392	0(3)	G0086	1(3)	G0293	1(2)	G0447	2(3)	G2064	1(2)
E1150	0(3)	E1580	0(3)	E2225	0(3)	E2394	0(3)	G0087	1(3)	G0294	1(2)	G0448	1(3)	G2065	1(2)
E1160	0(3)	E1590	0(3)	E2226	0(3)	E2395	0(3)	G0101	1(2)	G0295	0(3)	G0451	1(3)	G2066	1(2)
E1161	0(3)	E1592	0(3)	E2227	0(3)	E2396	0(3)	G0102	1(2)	G0296	1(2)	G0452	1(3)	G2067	1(2)
E1170	0(3)	E1594	0(3)	E2228	0(3)	E2397	0(3)	G0103	1(2)	G0302	1(2)	G0453	10(3)	G2068	1(2)
E1171	0(3)	E1600	0(3)	E2230	0(3)	E2398	0(3)	G0104	1(2)	G0303	1(2)	G0454	1(2)	G2069	1(2)
E1172	0(3)	E1610	0(3)	E2231	0(3)	E2402	0(3)	G0105	1(2)	G0304	1(2)	G0455	1(2)	G2070	1(2)
E1180	0(3)	E1615	0(3)	E2291	1(2)	E2500	0(3)	G0106	1(2)	G0305	1(2)	G0458	1(3)	G2071	1(2)
E1190	0(3)	E1620	0(3)	E2292	1(2)	E2502	0(3)	G0108	8(3)	G0306	4(3)	G0459	1(3)	G2072	1(2)
E1195	0(3)	E1625	0(3)	E2293	1(2)	E2504	0(3)	G0109	12(3)	G0307	4(3)	G0460	1(3)	G2073	1(2)
E1200	0(3)	E1630	0(3)	E2294	1(2)	E2506	0(3)	G0117	1(2)	G0328	1(2)	G0463	4(3)	G2074	1(2)
E1220	0(3)	E1632	0(3)	E2295	0(3)	E2508	0(3)	G0118	1(2)	G0329	1(3)	G0466	1(2)	G2075	1(2)
E1221	0(3)	E1634	0(3)	E2300	0(3)	E2510	0(3)	G0120	1(2)	G0333	0(3)	G0467	1(3)	G2076	1(2)
E1222	0(3)	E1635	0(3)	E2301	0(3)	E2511	0(3)	G0121	1(2)	G0337	1(2)	G0468	1(2)	G2078	3(3)

CPT	MUE	CPT	MUE	CPT	MUE	CPT	MUE	CPT	MUE	CPT	MUE	CPT	MUE	CPT	MUE
G2079	3(3)	J0121	200(3)	J0567	300(3)	J0834	3(3)	J1429	450(3)	J1738	30(3)	J2326	120(3)	J2797	333(3)
G2081	1(2)	J0122	300(3)	J0570	4(3)	J0840	18(3)	J1430	10(3)	J1740	3(3)	J2350	600(3)	J2798	240(3)
G2082	1(2)	J0129	100(3)	J0571	0(3)	J0841	24(3)	J1435	0(3)	J1741	32(3)	J2353	60(3)	J2800	3(3)
G2083	1(2)	J0130	6(3)	J0572	0(3)	J0850	9(3)	J1436	0(3)	J1742	4(3)	J2354	60(3)	J2805	3(3)
G2086	1(3)	J0131	400(3)	J0573	0(3)	J0875	300(3)	J1437	100(3)	J1743	66(3)	J2355	2(3)	J2810	20(3)
G2087	2(3)	J0132	300(3)	J0574	0(3)	J0878	1500(3)	J1438	2(3)	J1744	90(3)	J2357	120(3)	J2820	10(3)
G2170	1(3)	J0133	1200(3)	J0575	0(3)	J0881	500(3)	J1439	750(3)	J1745	150(3)	J2358	405(3)	J2840	160(3)
G2171	1(3)	J0135	8(3)	J0583	1250(3)	J0882	300(3)	J1442	1500(3)	J1746	200(3)	J2360	3(3)	J2850	48(3)
G2212	4(3)	J0153	180(3)	J0584	90(3)	J0883	1250(3)	J1443	0(3)	J1750	45(3)	J2370	30(3)	J2860	170(3)
G2213	1(2)	J0171	120(3)	J0585	600(3)	J0884	1250(3)	J1444	272(3)	J1756	500(3)	J2400	4(3)	J2910	0(3)
G2214	1(2)	J0178	4(2)	J0586	300(3)	J0885	60(3)	J1447	960(3)	J1786	680(3)	J2405	64(3)	J2916	20(3)
G2250	1(2)	J0179	12(2)	J0587	300(3)	J0887	360(3)	J1450	4(3)	J1790	2(3)	J2407	120(3)	J2920	25(3)
G2251	1(2)	J0180	140(3)	J0588	600(3)	J0888	360(3)	J1451	200(3)	J1800	12(3)	J2410	2(3)	J2930	25(3)
G2252	1(2)	J0185	130(3)	J0591	100(3)	J0890	0(3)	J1452	0(3)	J1810	0(3)	J2425	125(3)	J2940	0(3)
G6001	2(3)	J0190	0(3)	J0592	12(3)	J0894	100(3)	J1453	150(3)	J1815	200(3)	J2426	819(3)	J2941	8(3)
G6002	2(3)	J0200	0(3)	J0593	300(3)	J0895	12(3)	J1454	1(3)	J1817	0(3)	J2430	3(3)	J2950	0(3)
G6003	2(3)	J0202	12(3)	J0594	320(3)	J0896	1100(3)	J1455	18(3)	J1823	300(3)	J2440	4(3)	J2993	2(3)
G6004	2(3)	J0205	0(3)	J0595	12(3)	J0897	120(3)	J1457	0(3)	J1826	1(3)	J2460	0(3)	J2995	0(3)
G6005	2(3)	J0207	4(3)	J0596	840(3)	J0945	4(3)	J1458	100(3)	J1830	1(3)	J2469	10(3)	J2997	100(3)
G6006	2(3)	J0210	16(3)	J0597	250(3)	J1000	1(3)	J1459	300(3)	J1833	1116(3)	J2501	25(3)	J3000	2(3)
G6007	2(3)	J0215	0(3)	J0598	100(3)	J1020	8(3)	J1460	10(2)	J1835	0(3)	J2502	60(3)	J3010	100(3)
G6008	2(3)	J0220	20(3)	J0599	900(3)	J1030	8(3)	J1554	240(3)	J1840	3(3)	J2503	2(3)	J3030	2(3)
G6009	2(3)	J0221	300(3)	J0600	3(3)	J1040	4(3)	J1555	480(3)	J1850	14(3)	J2504	15(3)	J3031	675(3)
G6010	2(3)	J0222	300(3)	J0606	150(3)	J1050	1000(3)	J1556	300(3)	J1885	8(3)	J2505	1(3)	J3032	300(3)
G6011	2(3)	J0223	756(3)	J0610	15(3)	J1071	400(3)	J1557	300(3)	J1890	0(3)	J2507	8(3)	J3060	760(3)
G6012	2(3)	J0256	1600(3)	J0620	1(3)	J1094	0(3)	J1558	480(3)	J1930	120(3)	J2510	4(3)	J3070	3(3)
G6013	2(3)	J0257	1400(3)	J0630	8(3)	J1095	1034(2)	J1559	300(3)	J1931	609(3)	J2513	1(3)	J3090	200(3)
G6014	2(3)	J0270	32(3)	J0636	100(3)	J1096	8(2)	J1560	1(2)	J1940	10(3)	J2515	8(3)	J3095	150(3)
G6015	2(3)	J0275	1(3)	J0637	20(3)	J1097	4(3)	J1561	300(3)	J1943	675(3)	J2540	75(3)	J3101	50(3)
G6016	2(3)	J0278	15(3)	J0638	300(3)	J1100	120(3)	J1562	0(3)	J1944	1064(3)	J2543	20(3)	J3105	4(3)
G6017	2(3)	J0280	10(3)	J0640	24(3)	J1110	3(3)	J1566	300(3)	J1945	0(3)	J2545	1(3)	J3110	2(3)
G9143	1(2)	J0282	70(3)	J0641	1200(3)	J1120	2(3)	J1568	300(3)	J1950	12(3)	J2547	600(3)	J3111	210(3)
G9147	0(3)	J0285	5(3)	J0642	1200(3)	J1130	300(3)	J1569	300(3)	J1953	300(3)	J2550	3(3)	J3121	400(3)
G9148	0(3)	J0287	60(3)	J0670	10(3)	J1160	3(3)	J1570	4(3)	J1955	11(3)	J2560	16(3)	J3145	750(3)
G9149	0(3)	J0288	0(3)	J0690	16(3)	J1162	10(3)	J1571	20(3)	J1956	4(3)	J2562	48(3)	J3230	6(3)
G9150	0(3)	J0289	115(3)	J0691	300(3)	J1165	50(3)	J1572	300(3)	J1960	0(3)	J2590	15(3)	J3240	1(3)
G9151	0(3)	J0290	24(3)	J0692	12(3)	J1170	50(3)	J1573	130(3)	J1980	8(3)	J2597	45(3)	J3241	300(3)
G9152	0(3)	J0291	500(3)	J0693	1600(3)	J1180	0(3)	J1575	650(3)	J1990	0(3)	J2650	0(3)	J3243	200(3)
G9153	0(3)	J0295	12(3)	J0694	12(3)	J1190	8(3)	J1580	9(3)	J2001	400(3)	J2670	0(3)	J3245	100(3)
G9156	1(2)	J0300	8(3)	J0695	60(3)	J1200	8(3)	J1595	2(3)	J2010	10(3)	J2675	1(3)	J3246	100(3)
G9157	1(2)	J0330	50(3)	J0696	16(3)	J1201	20(3)	J1599	300(3)	J2020	6(3)	J2680	4(3)	J3250	4(3)
G9187	0(3)	J0348	200(3)	J0697	12(3)	J1205	4(3)	J1600	0(3)	J2060	10(3)	J2690	4(3)	J3260	12(3)
G9480	1(3)	J0350	0(3)	J0698	12(3)	J1212	1(3)	J1602	300(3)	J2062	10(3)	J2700	48(3)	J3262	800(3)
G9481	2(3)	J0360	6(3)	J0702	20(3)	J1230	5(3)	J1610	3(3)	J2150	8(3)	J2704	400(3)	J3265	0(3)
G9482	2(3)	J0364	6(3)	J0706	16(3)	J1240	6(3)	J1620	0(3)	J2170	8(3)	J2710	10(3)	J3280	0(3)
G9483	2(3)	J0365	0(3)	J0710	0(3)	J1245	10(3)	J1626	30(3)	J2175	6(3)	J2720	10(3)	J3285	9(3)
G9484	2(3)	J0380	1(3)	J0712	180(3)	J1250	4(3)	J1627	100(3)	J2180	0(3)	J2724	3500(3)	J3300	160(3)
G9485	2(3)	J0390	0(3)	J0713	12(3)	J1260	2(3)	J1628	100(3)	J2182	300(3)	J2725	0(3)	J3301	16(3)
G9486	2(3)	J0395	0(3)	J0714	12(3)	J1265	100(3)	J1630	7(3)	J2185	60(3)	J2730	2(3)	J3302	0(3)
G9487	2(3)	J0400	120(3)	J0715	0(3)	J1267	150(3)	J1631	9(3)	J2186	600(3)	J2760	2(3)	J3303	24(3)
G9488	2(3)	J0401	400(3)	J0716	4(1)	J1270	16(3)	J1632	700(3)	J2210	5(3)	J2765	18(3)	J3304	64(2)
G9489	2(3)	J0456	4(3)	J0717	400(3)	J1290	60(3)	J1640	672(3)	J2212	240(3)	J2770	7(3)	J3305	0(3)
G9490	2(3)	J0461	800(3)	J0720	15(3)	J1300	120(3)	J1642	150(3)	J2248	300(3)	J2778	10(2)	J3310	0(3)
G9678	1(2)	J0470	2(3)	J0725	10(3)	J1301	60(3)	J1644	50(3)	J2250	30(3)	J2780	16(3)	J3315	6(3)
G9685	1(3)	J0475	8(3)	J0735	50(3)	J1303	360(3)	J1645	10(3)	J2260	16(3)	J2783	60(3)	J3316	6(3)
G9978	2(3)	J0476	2(3)	J0740	2(3)	J1320	0(3)	J1650	30(3)	J2265	400(3)	J2785	4(3)	J3320	0(3)
G9979	2(3)	J0480	1(3)	J0742	500(3)	J1322	150(3)	J1652	20(3)	J2270	15(3)	J2786	500(3)	J3350	0(3)
G9980	2(3)	J0485	1500(3)	J0743	16(3)	J1324	0(3)	J1655	0(3)	J2274	100(3)	J2787	2(3)	J3355	0(3)
G9981	2(3)	J0490	160(3)	J0744	8(3)	J1325	18(3)	J1670	2(3)	J2278	1000(3)	J2788	1(3)	J3357	90(3)
G9982	2(3)	J0500	4(3)	J0745	8(3)	J1327	99(3)	J1675	0(3)	J2280	8(3)	J2790	3(3)	J3358	520(3)
G9983	2(3)	J0515	6(3)	J0770	5(3)	J1330	0(3)	J1700	0(3)	J2300	10(3)	J2791	15(3)	J3360	6(3)
G9984	2(3)	J0517	30(3)	J0775	180(3)	J1335	2(3)	J1710	0(3)	J2310	10(3)	J2792	450(3)	J3364	0(3)
G9985	2(3)	J0520	0(3)	J0780	10(3)	J1364	8(3)	J1720	10(3)	J2315	380(3)	J2793	320(3)	J3365	0(3)
G9986	2(3)	J0558	24(3)	J0791	160(3)	J1380	4(3)	J1726	28(3)	J2320	4(3)	J2794	100(3)	J3370	12(3)
G9987	2(3)	J0561	24(3)	J0795	100(3)	J1410	4(3)	J1729	25(3)	J2323	300(3)	J2795	2400(3)	J3380	300(3)
J0120	1(3)	J0565	200(3)	J0800	3(3)	J1428	450(3)	J1730	0(3)	J2325	34(3)	J2796	150(3)	J3385	80(3)

CPT	MUE
J3396	150(3)
J3397	600(3)
J3398	150(2)
J3399	1(3)
J3400	0(3)
J3410	16(3)
J3411	8(3)
J3415	6(3)
J3420	1(3)
J3430	50(3)
J3465	120(3)
J3470	3(3)
J3471	999(1)
J3472	2(3)
J3473	450(3)
J3475	80(3)
J3480	200(3)
J3485	160(3)
J3486	4(3)
J3489	5(3)
J3520	0(3)
J3530	0(3)
J3535	0(3)
J3570	0(3)
J7030	20(3)
J7040	12(3)
J7042	12(3)
J7050	20(3)
J7060	10(3)
J7070	7(3)
J7100	2(3)
J7110	3(3)
J7120	20(3)
J7121	5(3)
J7131	500(3)
J7169	180(3)
J7170	1800(3)
J7175	9000(1)
J7177	10500(3)
J7178	7700(1)
J7179	9600(1)
J7180	6000(1)
J7181	3850(1)
J7182	22000(1)
J7183	9600(1)
J7185	22000(1)
J7186	9600(1)
J7187	9600(1)
J7188	22000(1)
J7189	26000(1)
J7190	22000(1)
J7191	0(3)
J7192	22000(1)
J7193	20000(1)
J7194	9000(1)
J7195	20000(1)
J7196	175(3)
J7197	6300(1)
J7198	30000(1)
J7200	20000(1)
J7201	9000(1)
J7202	11550(1)
J7203	12000(1)
J7204	19500(1)
J7205	9750(1)
J7207	22500(1)

CPT	MUE
J7208	18000(1)
J7209	7500(1)
J7210	22000(1)
J7211	22000(1)
J7212	90000(1)
J7296	0(3)
J7297	0(3)
J7298	0(3)
J7300	0(3)
J7301	0(3)
J7303	0(3)
J7304	0(3)
J7306	0(3)
J7307	0(3)
J7308	3(3)
J7309	0(3)
J7310	0(3)
J7311	118(2)
J7312	14(2)
J7313	38(2)
J7314	36(2)
J7315	2(3)
J7316	3(3)
J7318	120(3)
J7320	50(3)
J7321	2(2)
J7322	48(3)
J7323	2(2)
J7324	2(2)
J7325	96(3)
J7326	2(2)
J7327	2(2)
J7328	336(3)
J7329	50(2)
J7330	1(3)
J7331	40(3)
J7332	40(3)
J7336	1120(3)
J7340	1(3)
J7342	10(3)
J7345	200(3)
J7351	20(2)
J7352	16(3)
J7500	15(3)
J7501	8(3)
J7502	60(3)
J7503	120(3)
J7504	15(3)
J7505	1(3)
J7507	40(3)
J7508	300(3)
J7509	60(3)
J7510	60(3)
J7511	9(3)
J7512	300(3)
J7513	0(3)
J7515	90(3)
J7516	4(3)
J7517	16(3)
J7518	12(3)
J7520	40(3)
J7525	2(3)
J7527	20(3)
J7599	1(3)
J7604	0(3)
J7605	0(3)

CPT	MUE
J7606	0(3)
J7607	0(3)
J7608	0(3)
J7609	0(3)
J7610	0(3)
J7611	0(3)
J7612	0(3)
J7613	0(3)
J7614	0(3)
J7615	0(3)
J7620	0(3)
J7622	0(3)
J7624	0(3)
J7626	0(3)
J7627	0(3)
J7628	0(3)
J7629	0(3)
J7631	0(3)
J7632	0(3)
J7633	0(3)
J7634	0(3)
J7635	0(3)
J7636	0(3)
J7637	0(3)
J7638	0(3)
J7639	0(3)
J7640	0(3)
J7641	0(3)
J7642	0(3)
J7643	0(3)
J7644	0(3)
J7645	0(3)
J7647	0(3)
J7648	0(3)
J7649	0(3)
J7650	0(3)
J7657	0(3)
J7658	0(3)
J7659	0(3)
J7660	0(3)
J7665	0(3)
J7667	0(3)
J7668	0(3)
J7669	0(3)
J7670	0(3)
J7674	100(3)
J7676	0(3)
J7677	175(3)
J7680	0(3)
J7681	0(3)
J7682	0(3)
J7683	0(3)
J7684	0(3)
J7685	0(3)
J7686	0(3)
J7699	0(3)
J7799	2(3)
J7999	6(3)
J8498	1(3)
J8499	0(3)
J8501	57(3)
J8510	5(3)
J8515	0(3)
J8520	50(3)
J8521	15(3)
J8530	60(3)

CPT	MUE
J8540	48(3)
J8560	6(3)
J8562	12(3)
J8565	0(3)
J8597	4(3)
J8600	40(3)
J8610	20(3)
J8650	0(3)
J8655	1(3)
J8670	180(3)
J8700	120(3)
J8705	22(3)
J8999	2(3)
J9000	20(3)
J9015	1(3)
J9017	30(3)
J9019	60(3)
J9020	0(3)
J9022	168(3)
J9023	140(3)
J9025	300(3)
J9027	100(3)
J9030	50(3)
J9032	300(3)
J9033	300(3)
J9034	360(3)
J9035	180(3)
J9036	360(3)
J9039	210(3)
J9040	4(3)
J9041	35(3)
J9042	200(3)
J9043	60(3)
J9044	35(3)
J9045	22(3)
J9047	160(3)
J9050	6(3)
J9055	150(3)
J9057	60(3)
J9060	24(3)
J9065	100(3)
J9070	55(3)
J9098	5(3)
J9100	120(3)
J9118	750(3)
J9119	350(3)
J9120	5(3)
J9130	24(3)
J9144	180(3)
J9145	240(3)
J9150	12(3)
J9151	12(3)
J9153	132(3)
J9155	240(3)
J9160	0(3)
J9165	0(3)
J9171	240(3)
J9173	150(3)
J9175	10(3)
J9176	3000(3)
J9177	520(3)
J9178	150(3)
J9179	50(3)
J9181	100(3)
J9185	2(3)
J9190	20(3)

CPT	MUE
J9198	38(3)
J9200	20(3)
J9201	20(3)
J9202	3(3)
J9203	180(3)
J9204	160(3)
J9205	215(3)
J9206	42(3)
J9207	90(3)
J9208	15(3)
J9209	55(3)
J9210	1500(3)
J9211	6(3)
J9212	0(3)
J9213	12(3)
J9214	100(3)
J9215	0(3)
J9216	0(3)
J9217	6(3)
J9218	1(3)
J9219	0(3)
J9223	120(3)
J9225	1(3)
J9226	1(3)
J9227	150(3)
J9228	1100(3)
J9229	27(3)
J9230	5(3)
J9245	11(3)
J9246	300(3)
J9250	50(3)
J9260	20(3)
J9261	80(3)
J9262	700(3)
J9263	700(3)
J9264	600(3)
J9266	2(3)
J9267	750(3)
J9268	1(3)
J9269	200(3)
J9270	0(3)
J9271	400(3)
J9280	12(3)
J9281	80(3)
J9285	200(3)
J9293	8(3)
J9295	800(3)
J9299	480(3)
J9301	100(3)
J9302	200(3)
J9303	90(3)
J9304	150(3)
J9305	150(3)
J9306	840(3)
J9307	80(3)
J9308	280(3)
J9309	280(3)
J9311	160(3)
J9312	150(3)
J9313	600(3)
J9315	40(3)
J9316	120(3)
J9317	648(3)
J9320	4(3)
J9325	400(3)
J9328	400(3)

CPT	MUE
J9330	50(3)
J9340	4(3)
J9351	120(3)
J9352	40(3)
J9354	600(3)
J9355	105(3)
J9356	60(3)
J9357	4(3)
J9358	900(3)
J9360	40(3)
J9370	4(3)
J9371	5(3)
J9390	36(3)
J9395	20(3)
J9400	500(3)
J9600	4(3)
K0001	0(3)
K0002	0(3)
K0003	0(3)
K0004	0(3)
K0005	0(3)
K0006	0(3)
K0007	0(3)
K0008	0(3)
K0009	0(3)
K0010	0(3)
K0011	0(3)
K0012	0(3)
K0013	0(3)
K0014	0(3)
K0015	0(3)
K0017	0(3)
K0018	0(3)
K0019	0(3)
K0020	0(3)
K0037	0(3)
K0038	0(3)
K0039	0(3)
K0040	0(3)
K0041	0(3)
K0042	0(3)
K0043	0(3)
K0044	0(3)
K0045	0(3)
K0046	0(3)
K0047	0(3)
K0050	0(3)
K0051	0(3)
K0052	0(3)
K0053	0(3)
K0056	0(3)
K0065	0(3)
K0069	0(3)
K0070	0(3)
K0071	0(3)
K0072	0(3)
K0073	0(3)
K0077	0(3)
K0098	0(3)
K0105	0(3)
K0108	0(3)
K0195	0(3)
K0455	0(3)
K0462	0(3)
K0552	0(3)
K0553	0(3)

CPT	MUE
K0554	0(3)
K0601	0(3)
K0602	0(3)
K0603	0(3)
K0604	0(3)
K0605	0(3)
K0606	0(3)
K0607	0(3)
K0608	0(3)
K0609	0(3)
K0669	0(3)
K0672	4(3)
K0730	0(3)
K0733	0(3)
K0738	0(3)
K0740	0(3)
K0743	0(3)
K0800	0(3)
K0801	0(3)
K0802	0(3)
K0806	0(3)
K0807	0(3)
K0808	0(3)
K0812	0(3)
K0813	0(3)
K0814	0(3)
K0815	0(3)
K0816	0(3)
K0820	0(3)
K0821	0(3)
K0822	0(3)
K0823	0(3)
K0824	0(3)
K0825	0(3)
K0826	0(3)
K0827	0(3)
K0828	0(3)
K0829	0(3)
K0830	0(3)
K0831	0(3)
K0835	0(3)
K0836	0(3)
K0837	0(3)
K0838	0(3)
K0839	0(3)
K0840	0(3)
K0841	0(3)
K0842	0(3)
K0843	0(3)
K0848	0(3)
K0849	0(3)
K0850	0(3)
K0851	0(3)
K0852	0(3)
K0853	0(3)
K0854	0(3)
K0855	0(3)
K0856	0(3)
K0857	0(3)
K0858	0(3)
K0859	0(3)
K0860	0(3)
K0861	0(3)
K0862	0(3)
K0863	0(3)
K0864	0(3)

CPT	MUE
K0868	0(3)
K0869	0(3)
K0870	0(3)
K0871	0(3)
K0877	0(3)
K0878	0(3)
K0879	0(3)
K0880	0(3)
K0884	0(3)
K0885	0(3)
K0886	0(3)
K0890	0(3)
K0891	0(3)
K0898	1(2)
K0899	0(3)
K0900	0(3)
K1001	1(3)
K1002	1(3)
K1003	1(3)
K1004	1(3)
K1005	1(3)
K1006	1(2)
K1007	1(2)
K1009	1(2)
K1013	1(3)
K1014	1(3)
K1015	2(2)
K1016	1(2)
K1017	3(2)
K1018	1(2)
K1019	3(2)
K1020	1(2)
L0112	1(2)
L0113	1(2)
L0120	1(2)
L0130	1(2)
L0140	1(2)
L0150	1(2)
L0160	1(2)
L0170	1(2)
L0172	1(2)
L0174	1(2)
L0180	1(2)
L0190	1(2)
L0200	1(2)
L0220	1(3)
L0450	1(2)
L0452	1(2)
L0454	1(2)
L0455	1(2)
L0456	1(2)
L0457	1(2)
L0458	1(2)
L0460	1(2)
L0462	1(2)
L0464	1(2)
L0466	1(2)
L0467	1(2)
L0468	1(2)
L0469	1(2)
L0470	1(2)
L0472	1(2)
L0480	1(2)
L0482	1(2)
L0484	1(2)
L0486	1(2)

CPT	MUE
L0488	1(2)
L0490	1(2)
L0491	1(2)
L0492	1(2)
L0621	1(2)
L0622	1(2)
L0623	1(2)
L0624	1(2)
L0625	1(2)
L0626	1(2)
L0627	1(2)
L0628	1(2)
L0629	1(2)
L0630	1(2)
L0631	1(2)
L0632	1(2)
L0633	1(2)
L0634	1(2)
L0635	1(2)
L0636	1(2)
L0637	1(2)
L0638	1(2)
L0639	1(2)
L0640	1(2)
L0641	1(2)
L0642	1(2)
L0643	1(2)
L0648	1(2)
L0649	1(2)
L0650	1(2)
L0651	1(2)
L0700	1(2)
L0710	1(2)
L0810	1(2)
L0820	1(2)
L0830	1(2)
L0859	1(2)
L0861	1(2)
L0970	1(2)
L0972	1(2)
L0974	1(2)
L0976	1(2)
L0978	2(3)
L0980	1(2)
L0982	1(3)
L0984	3(3)
L0999	1(3)
L1000	1(2)
L1001	1(2)
L1005	1(2)
L1010	2(2)
L1020	2(3)
L1025	1(3)
L1030	1(3)
L1040	1(3)
L1050	1(3)
L1060	1(3)
L1070	2(2)
L1080	2(2)
L1085	1(2)
L1090	1(3)
L1100	2(2)
L1110	2(2)
L1120	3(3)
L1200	1(2)
L1210	2(3)

CPT	MUE
L1220	1(3)
L1230	1(2)
L1240	1(3)
L1250	2(3)
L1260	1(3)
L1270	3(3)
L1280	2(3)
L1290	2(3)
L1300	1(2)
L1310	1(2)
L1499	1(3)
L1600	1(2)
L1610	1(2)
L1620	1(2)
L1630	1(2)
L1640	1(2)
L1650	1(2)
L1652	1(2)
L1660	1(2)
L1680	1(2)
L1685	1(2)
L1686	1(3)
L1690	1(2)
L1700	1(2)
L1710	1(2)
L1720	2(2)
L1730	1(2)
L1755	2(2)
L1810	2(2)
L1812	2(2)
L1820	2(2)
L1830	2(2)
L1831	2(2)
L1832	2(2)
L1833	2(2)
L1834	2(2)
L1836	2(2)
L1840	2(2)
L1843	2(2)
L1844	2(2)
L1845	2(2)
L1846	2(2)
L1847	2(2)
L1848	2(2)
L1850	2(2)
L1851	2(2)
L1852	2(2)
L1860	2(2)
L1900	2(2)
L1902	2(2)
L1904	2(2)
L1906	2(2)
L1907	2(2)
L1910	2(2)
L1920	2(2)
L1930	2(2)
L1932	2(2)
L1940	2(2)
L1945	2(2)
L1950	2(2)
L1951	2(2)
L1960	2(2)
L1970	2(2)
L1971	2(2)
L1980	2(2)
L1990	2(2)

CPT	MUE
L2000	2(2)
L2005	2(2)
L2006	0(3)
L2010	2(2)
L2020	2(2)
L2030	2(2)
L2034	2(2)
L2035	2(2)
L2036	2(2)
L2037	2(2)
L2038	2(2)
L2040	1(2)
L2050	1(2)
L2060	1(2)
L2070	1(2)
L2080	1(2)
L2090	1(2)
L2106	2(2)
L2108	2(2)
L2112	2(2)
L2114	2(2)
L2116	2(2)
L2126	2(2)
L2128	2(2)
L2132	2(2)
L2134	2(2)
L2136	2(2)
L2180	2(2)
L2182	4(2)
L2184	4(2)
L2186	4(2)
L2188	2(2)
L2190	2(2)
L2192	2(2)
L2200	4(2)
L2210	4(2)
L2220	4(2)
L2230	2(2)
L2232	2(2)
L2240	2(2)
L2250	2(2)
L2260	2(2)
L2265	2(2)
L2270	2(3)
L2275	2(3)
L2280	2(2)
L2300	1(2)
L2310	1(2)
L2320	2(3)
L2330	2(3)
L2335	2(2)
L2340	2(2)
L2350	2(2)
L2360	2(2)
L2370	2(2)
L2375	2(2)
L2380	2(3)
L2385	4(2)
L2387	4(2)
L2390	4(2)
L2395	4(2)
L2397	4(3)
L2405	4(2)
L2415	4(2)
L2425	4(2)
L2430	4(2)

CPT	MUE
L2492	4(2)
L2500	2(2)
L2510	2(2)
L2520	2(2)
L2525	2(2)
L2526	2(2)
L2530	2(2)
L2540	2(2)
L2550	2(2)
L2570	2(2)
L2580	2(2)
L2600	2(2)
L2610	2(2)
L2620	2(2)
L2622	2(2)
L2624	2(2)
L2627	1(3)
L2628	1(3)
L2630	1(2)
L2640	1(2)
L2650	2(3)
L2660	1(3)
L2670	2(3)
L2680	2(3)
L2750	8(3)
L2755	8(3)
L2760	8(2)
L2768	4(2)
L2780	8(3)
L2785	4(2)
L2795	2(2)
L2800	2(2)
L2810	4(2)
L2820	2(3)
L2830	2(3)
L2861	0(3)
L2999	2(3)
L3000	2(3)
L3001	2(3)
L3002	2(3)
L3003	2(3)
L3010	2(3)
L3020	2(3)
L3030	2(3)
L3031	2(3)
L3040	2(3)
L3050	2(3)
L3060	2(3)
L3070	2(3)
L3080	2(3)
L3090	2(3)
L3100	2(2)
L3140	1(2)
L3150	1(2)
L3160	2(2)
L3170	2(2)
L3201	1(3)
L3202	1(3)
L3203	1(3)
L3204	1(3)
L3206	1(3)
L3207	1(3)
L3208	1(3)
L3209	1(3)
L3211	1(3)
L3212	1(3)

CPT	MUE
L3213	1(3)
L3214	1(3)
L3215	0(3)
L3216	0(3)
L3217	0(3)
L3219	0(3)
L3221	0(3)
L3222	0(3)
L3224	2(2)
L3225	2(2)
L3230	2(2)
L3250	2(2)
L3251	2(2)
L3252	2(2)
L3253	2(2)
L3254	1(3)
L3255	1(3)
L3257	1(3)
L3260	0(3)
L3265	1(3)
L3300	4(3)
L3310	4(3)
L3330	2(2)
L3332	2(2)
L3334	4(3)
L3340	2(2)
L3350	2(2)
L3360	2(2)
L3370	2(2)
L3380	2(2)
L3390	2(2)
L3400	2(2)
L3410	2(2)
L3420	2(2)
L3430	2(2)
L3440	2(2)
L3450	2(2)
L3455	2(2)
L3460	2(2)
L3465	2(2)
L3470	2(2)
L3480	2(2)
L3485	2(2)
L3500	2(2)
L3510	2(2)
L3520	2(2)
L3530	2(2)
L3540	2(2)
L3550	2(2)
L3560	2(2)
L3570	2(2)
L3580	2(2)
L3590	2(2)
L3595	2(2)
L3600	2(2)
L3610	2(2)
L3620	2(2)
L3630	2(2)
L3640	1(2)
L3649	2(3)
L3650	1(2)
L3660	1(2)
L3670	1(3)
L3671	1(3)
L3674	1(3)
L3675	1(2)

CPT	MUE
L3677	1(2)
L3678	1(2)
L3702	2(2)
L3710	2(2)
L3720	2(2)
L3730	2(2)
L3740	2(2)
L3760	2(2)
L3761	2(2)
L3762	2(2)
L3763	2(2)
L3764	2(2)
L3765	2(2)
L3766	2(2)
L3806	2(2)
L3807	2(2)
L3808	2(2)
L3809	2(2)
L3891	0(3)
L3900	2(2)
L3901	2(2)
L3904	2(2)
L3905	2(2)
L3906	2(2)
L3908	2(2)
L3912	2(3)
L3913	2(2)
L3915	2(2)
L3916	2(3)
L3917	2(2)
L3918	2(2)
L3919	2(2)
L3921	2(2)
L3923	2(2)
L3924	2(2)
L3925	4(3)
L3927	4(3)
L3929	2(2)
L3930	2(2)
L3931	2(2)
L3933	3(3)
L3935	3(3)
L3956	4(3)
L3960	1(3)
L3961	1(3)
L3962	1(3)
L3967	1(3)
L3971	1(3)
L3973	1(3)
L3975	1(3)
L3976	1(3)
L3977	1(3)
L3978	1(3)
L3980	2(2)
L3981	2(2)
L3982	2(2)
L3984	2(2)
L3999	2(3)
L4000	1(2)
L4002	4(3)
L4010	2(2)
L4020	2(2)
L4030	2(2)
L4040	2(2)
L4045	2(2)
L4050	2(2)

CPT	MUE
L4055	2(2)
L4060	2(2)
L4070	2(3)
L4080	2(2)
L4090	4(2)
L4100	2(2)
L4110	4(2)
L4130	2(2)
L4205	8(3)
L4210	4(3)
L4350	2(2)
L4360	2(2)
L4361	2(2)
L4370	2(2)
L4386	2(2)
L4387	2(2)
L4392	2(3)
L4394	2(3)
L4396	2(2)
L4397	2(2)
L4398	2(2)
L4631	2(2)
L5000	2(3)
L5010	2(2)
L5020	2(2)
L5050	2(2)
L5060	2(2)
L5100	2(2)
L5105	2(2)
L5150	2(2)
L5160	2(2)
L5200	2(2)
L5210	2(2)
L5220	2(2)
L5230	2(2)
L5250	2(2)
L5270	2(2)
L5280	2(2)
L5301	2(2)
L5312	2(2)
L5321	2(2)
L5331	2(2)
L5341	2(2)
L5400	2(2)
L5410	2(2)
L5420	2(2)
L5430	2(2)
L5450	2(2)
L5460	2(2)
L5500	2(2)
L5505	2(2)
L5510	2(2)
L5520	2(2)
L5530	2(2)
L5535	2(2)
L5540	2(2)
L5560	2(2)
L5570	2(2)
L5580	2(2)
L5585	2(2)
L5590	2(2)
L5595	2(2)
L5600	2(2)
L5610	2(2)
L5611	2(2)
L5613	2(2)

CPT	MUE
L5614	2(2)
L5616	2(2)
L5617	2(3)
L5618	4(3)
L5620	4(3)
L5622	4(3)
L5624	4(3)
L5626	4(3)
L5628	2(3)
L5629	2(2)
L5630	2(2)
L5631	2(2)
L5632	2(2)
L5634	2(2)
L5636	2(2)
L5637	2(2)
L5638	2(2)
L5639	2(2)
L5640	2(2)
L5642	2(2)
L5643	2(2)
L5644	2(2)
L5645	2(2)
L5646	2(2)
L5647	2(2)
L5648	2(2)
L5649	2(2)
L5650	2(2)
L5651	2(2)
L5652	2(2)
L5653	2(2)
L5654	2(2)
L5655	2(2)
L5656	2(2)
L5658	2(2)
L5661	2(2)
L5665	2(2)
L5666	2(2)
L5668	2(2)
L5670	2(2)
L5671	2(2)
L5672	2(2)
L5673	4(3)
L5676	2(2)
L5677	2(2)
L5678	2(2)
L5679	4(3)
L5680	2(2)
L5681	2(2)
L5682	2(2)
L5683	2(2)
L5684	2(3)
L5685	4(3)
L5686	2(2)
L5688	2(3)
L5690	2(3)
L5692	2(2)
L5694	2(2)
L5695	2(3)
L5696	2(2)
L5697	2(2)
L5698	2(2)
L5699	2(3)
L5700	2(2)
L5701	2(2)
L5702	2(2)

CPT	MUE
L5703	2(2)
L5704	2(2)
L5705	2(2)
L5706	2(2)
L5707	2(2)
L5710	2(2)
L5711	2(2)
L5712	2(2)
L5714	2(2)
L5716	2(2)
L5718	2(2)
L5722	2(2)
L5724	2(2)
L5726	2(2)
L5728	2(2)
L5780	2(2)
L5781	2(2)
L5782	2(2)
L5785	2(2)
L5790	2(2)
L5795	2(2)
L5810	2(2)
L5811	2(2)
L5812	2(2)
L5814	2(2)
L5816	2(2)
L5818	2(2)
L5822	2(2)
L5824	2(2)
L5826	2(2)
L5828	2(2)
L5830	2(2)
L5840	2(2)
L5845	2(2)
L5848	2(2)
L5850	2(2)
L5855	2(2)
L5856	2(2)
L5857	2(2)
L5858	2(2)
L5859	2(2)
L5910	2(2)
L5920	2(2)
L5925	2(3)
L5930	2(2)
L5940	2(2)
L5950	2(2)
L5960	2(2)
L5961	1(3)
L5962	2(2)
L5964	2(2)
L5966	2(2)
L5968	2(2)
L5969	0(3)
L5970	2(2)
L5971	2(2)
L5972	2(2)
L5973	2(3)
L5974	2(2)
L5975	2(2)
L5976	2(2)
L5978	2(2)
L5979	2(2)
L5980	2(2)
L5981	2(2)
L5982	2(2)

CPT	MUE
L5984	2(2)
L5985	2(2)
L5986	2(2)
L5987	2(2)
L5988	2(2)
L5990	2(2)
L5999	2(3)
L6000	2(2)
L6010	2(2)
L6020	2(2)
L6026	2(2)
L6050	2(2)
L6055	2(2)
L6100	2(2)
L6110	2(2)
L6120	2(2)
L6130	2(2)
L6200	2(2)
L6205	2(2)
L6250	2(2)
L6300	2(2)
L6310	2(2)
L6320	2(2)
L6350	2(2)
L6360	2(2)
L6370	2(2)
L6380	2(2)
L6382	2(2)
L6384	2(2)
L6386	2(2)
L6388	2(2)
L6400	2(2)
L6450	2(2)
L6500	2(2)
L6550	2(2)
L6570	2(2)
L6580	2(2)
L6582	2(2)
L6584	2(2)
L6586	2(2)
L6588	2(2)
L6590	2(2)
L6600	2(2)
L6605	2(2)
L6610	2(2)
L6611	2(3)
L6615	2(2)
L6616	2(2)
L6620	2(2)
L6621	2(2)
L6623	2(2)
L6624	2(2)
L6625	2(2)
L6628	2(2)
L6629	2(2)
L6630	2(2)
L6632	4(3)
L6635	2(2)
L6637	2(2)
L6638	2(2)
L6640	2(2)
L6641	2(3)
L6642	2(3)
L6645	2(2)
L6646	2(2)
L6647	2(2)

CPT	MUE
L6648	2(2)
L6650	2(2)
L6655	4(3)
L6660	4(3)
L6665	4(3)
L6670	2(2)
L6672	2(2)
L6675	2(2)
L6676	2(2)
L6677	2(2)
L6680	4(3)
L6682	4(3)
L6684	4(3)
L6686	2(2)
L6687	2(2)
L6688	2(2)
L6689	2(2)
L6690	2(2)
L6691	2(3)
L6692	2(3)
L6693	2(2)
L6694	2(3)
L6695	2(3)
L6696	2(2)
L6697	2(2)
L6698	2(2)
L6703	2(2)
L6704	2(2)
L6706	2(2)
L6707	2(2)
L6708	2(2)
L6709	2(2)
L6711	2(2)
L6712	2(2)
L6713	2(2)
L6714	2(2)
L6715	5(3)
L6721	2(2)
L6722	2(2)
L6805	2(2)
L6810	2(3)
L6880	2(2)
L6881	2(2)
L6882	2(2)
L6883	2(2)
L6884	2(2)
L6885	2(2)
L6890	2(3)
L6895	2(3)
L6900	2(2)
L6905	2(2)
L6910	2(2)
L6915	2(2)
L6920	2(2)
L6925	2(2)
L6930	2(2)
L6935	2(2)
L6940	2(2)
L6945	2(2)
L6950	2(2)
L6955	2(2)
L6960	2(2)
L6965	2(2)
L6970	2(2)
L6975	2(2)
L7007	2(2)

CPT	MUE
L7008	2(2)
L7009	2(2)
L7040	2(2)
L7045	2(2)
L7170	2(2)
L7180	2(2)
L7181	2(2)
L7185	2(2)
L7186	2(2)
L7190	2(2)
L7191	2(2)
L7259	2(2)
L7360	1(3)
L7362	1(2)
L7364	1(3)
L7366	1(2)
L7367	2(3)
L7368	1(2)
L7400	2(2)
L7401	2(2)
L7402	2(2)
L7403	2(2)
L7404	2(2)
L7405	2(2)
L7499	2(3)
L7510	4(3)
L7600	0(3)
L7700	2(1)
L7900	0(3)
L7902	0(3)
L8000	6(3)
L8001	4(3)
L8002	4(3)
L8010	4(3)
L8015	4(3)
L8020	4(3)
L8030	2(3)
L8031	2(3)
L8032	2(2)
L8033	0(3)
L8035	2(3)
L8039	2(3)
L8040	1(2)
L8041	1(2)
L8042	2(2)
L8043	1(2)
L8044	1(2)
L8045	2(2)
L8046	1(3)
L8047	1(2)
L8048	1(3)
L8049	6(3)
L8300	1(3)
L8310	1(3)
L8320	2(3)
L8330	2(3)
L8400	12(3)
L8410	12(3)
L8415	6(3)
L8417	12(3)
L8420	14(3)
L8430	12(3)
L8435	12(3)
L8440	4(3)
L8460	4(3)
L8465	4(3)

CPT	MUE
L8470	14(3)
L8480	12(3)
L8485	12(3)
L8499	1(3)
L8500	1(2)
L8501	2(3)
L8507	3(3)
L8509	1(3)
L8510	1(2)
L8511	1(3)
L8512	1(3)
L8513	1(3)
L8514	1(3)
L8515	1(3)
L8600	2(3)
L8603	4(3)
L8604	3(3)
L8605	4(3)
L8606	5(3)
L8607	20(3)
L8609	1(3)
L8610	2(3)
L8612	1(3)
L8613	2(3)
L8614	2(3)
L8615	2(3)
L8616	2(3)
L8617	2(3)
L8618	2(3)
L8619	2(3)
L8621	360(3)
L8622	2(3)
L8625	1(3)
L8627	2(2)
L8628	2(2)
L8629	2(2)
L8631	2(3)
L8641	4(3)
L8642	2(3)
L8658	3(3)
L8659	4(3)
L8670	3(3)
L8679	3(3)
L8680	0(3)
L8681	1(3)
L8682	2(3)
L8683	1(3)
L8684	1(3)
L8685	0(3)
L8686	0(3)
L8687	0(3)
L8688	0(3)
L8689	1(3)
L8690	2(2)
L8691	1(3)
L8692	0(3)
L8693	1(3)
L8694	1(3)
L8695	1(3)
L8696	1(3)
L8701	1(3)
L8702	1(3)
M0075	0(3)
M0076	0(3)
M0100	0(3)
M0201	1(2)

CPT	MUE
M0243	1(2)
M0244	1(2)
M0245	1(2)
M0246	1(2)
M0247	1(2)
M0248	1(2)
M0300	0(3)
M0301	0(3)
P2028	1(2)
P2029	1(2)
P2031	0(3)
P2033	1(2)
P2038	1(2)
P3000	1(3)
P3001	1(3)
P7001	0(3)
P9010	4(3)
P9011	4(3)
P9012	12(3)
P9016	12(3)
P9017	24(3)
P9019	12(3)
P9020	5(3)
P9021	8(3)
P9022	12(3)
P9023	15(3)
P9031	12(3)
P9032	12(3)
P9033	12(3)
P9034	4(3)
P9035	4(3)
P9036	4(3)
P9037	4(3)
P9038	4(3)
P9039	2(3)
P9040	8(3)
P9041	100(3)
P9043	10(3)
P9044	20(3)
P9045	20(3)
P9046	40(3)
P9047	20(3)
P9048	2(3)
P9050	1(3)
P9051	4(3)
P9052	3(3)
P9053	3(3)
P9054	2(3)
P9055	2(3)
P9056	3(3)
P9057	4(3)
P9058	4(3)
P9059	15(3)
P9060	4(3)
P9070	15(3)
P9071	15(3)
P9073	4(3)
P9099	1(3)
P9100	12(3)
P9603	100(3)
P9604	2(3)
P9612	1(3)
P9615	1(3)
Q0035	1(3)
Q0081	2(3)
Q0083	2(3)

CPT	MUE
Q0084	2(3)
Q0085	2(3)
Q0091	1(3)
Q0092	2(3)
Q0111	2(3)
Q0112	3(3)
Q0113	1(3)
Q0114	1(3)
Q0115	1(3)
Q0138	510(3)
Q0139	510(3)
Q0144	0(3)
Q0161	66(3)
Q0162	24(3)
Q0163	6(3)
Q0164	8(3)
Q0166	2(3)
Q0167	108(3)
Q0169	12(3)
Q0173	5(3)
Q0174	0(3)
Q0175	6(3)
Q0177	16(3)
Q0180	1(3)
Q0181	2(3)
Q0243	1(3)
Q0244	1(3)
Q0245	1(3)
Q0247	1(2)
Q0477	1(1)
Q0478	1(3)
Q0479	1(3)
Q0480	1(3)
Q0481	1(2)
Q0482	1(3)
Q0483	1(3)
Q0484	1(3)
Q0485	1(3)
Q0486	1(3)
Q0487	1(3)
Q0488	1(3)
Q0489	1(3)
Q0490	1(3)
Q0491	1(3)
Q0492	1(3)
Q0493	1(3)
Q0494	1(3)
Q0495	1(3)
Q0497	2(3)
Q0498	1(3)
Q0499	1(3)
Q0501	1(3)
Q0502	1(3)
Q0503	3(3)
Q0504	1(3)
Q0506	8(3)
Q0507	1(3)
Q0508	24(3)
Q0509	2(3)
Q0510	1(2)
Q0511	1(2)
Q0512	4(3)
Q0513	1(2)
Q0514	1(2)
Q0515	0(3)
Q1004	0(3)

CPT	MUE
Q1005	0(3)
Q2004	1(3)
Q2009	100(3)
Q2017	12(3)
Q2026	30(3)
Q2028	1470(3)
Q2034	1(2)
Q2035	1(2)
Q2036	1(2)
Q2037	1(2)
Q2038	1(2)
Q2039	1(2)
Q2043	1(2)
Q2049	10(3)
Q2050	20(3)
Q2052	0(3)
Q3014	2(3)
Q3027	30(3)
Q3028	0(3)
Q3031	1(3)
Q4001	1(3)
Q4002	1(3)
Q4003	2(3)
Q4004	2(3)
Q4012	2(3)
Q4013	2(3)
Q4014	2(3)
Q4018	2(3)
Q4021	2(3)
Q4025	1(3)
Q4026	1(3)
Q4027	1(3)
Q4028	1(3)
Q4030	2(3)
Q4037	2(3)
Q4042	2(3)
Q4046	2(3)
Q4050	2(3)
Q4051	2(3)
Q4074	0(3)
Q4081	400(3)
Q5101	1500(3)
Q5103	150(3)
Q5104	150(3)
Q5105	400(3)
Q5106	60(3)
Q5107	170(3)
Q5108	12(3)
Q5109	150(3)
Q5110	1500(3)
Q5111	12(3)
Q5112	120(3)
Q5113	120(3)
Q5114	120(3)
Q5115	150(3)
Q5116	120(3)
Q5117	120(3)
Q5118	230(3)
Q5119	150(3)
Q5120	12(3)
Q5121	150(3)
Q5122	12(3)
Q9001	1(3)
Q9002	1(3)
Q9003	1(3)
Q9950	5(3)

CPT	MUE
Q9951	0(3)
Q9953	10(3)
Q9954	18(3)
Q9955	0(3)
Q9956	9(3)
Q9957	3(3)
Q9958	600(3)
Q9959	0(3)
Q9960	250(3)
Q9961	200(3)
Q9962	200(3)
Q9963	240(3)
Q9964	0(3)
Q9966	250(3)
Q9967	300(3)
Q9969	3(3)
Q9982	1(3)
Q9983	1(3)
Q9991	1(2)
Q9992	1(2)
R0070	2(3)
R0075	2(3)
R0076	1(3)
U0001	2(3)
U0002	2(3)
U0003	2(3)
U0004	2(3)
U0005	1(3)
V2020	1(3)
V2025	0(3)

CPT	MUE
V2100	2(3)
V2101	2(3)
V2102	2(3)
V2103	2(3)
V2104	2(3)
V2105	2(3)
V2106	2(3)
V2107	2(3)
V2108	2(3)
V2109	2(3)
V2110	2(3)
V2111	2(3)
V2112	2(3)
V2113	2(3)
V2114	2(3)
V2115	2(3)
V2118	2(3)
V2121	2(3)
V2199	2(3)
V2200	2(3)
V2201	2(3)
V2202	2(3)
V2203	2(3)
V2204	2(3)
V2205	2(3)
V2206	2(3)
V2207	2(3)
V2208	2(3)
V2209	2(3)
V2210	2(3)

CPT	MUE
V2211	2(3)
V2212	2(3)
V2213	2(3)
V2214	2(3)
V2215	2(3)
V2218	2(3)
V2219	2(3)
V2220	2(3)
V2221	2(3)
V2299	2(3)
V2300	2(3)
V2301	2(3)
V2302	2(3)
V2303	2(3)
V2304	2(3)
V2305	2(3)
V2306	2(3)
V2307	2(3)
V2308	2(3)
V2309	2(3)
V2310	2(3)
V2311	2(3)
V2312	2(3)
V2313	2(3)
V2314	2(3)
V2315	2(3)
V2318	2(3)
V2319	2(3)
V2320	2(3)
V2321	2(3)

CPT	MUE
V2399	2(3)
V2410	2(3)
V2430	2(3)
V2499	2(3)
V2500	2(3)
V2501	2(3)
V2502	2(3)
V2503	2(3)
V2510	2(3)
V2511	2(3)
V2512	2(3)
V2513	2(3)
V2520	2(3)
V2521	2(3)
V2522	2(3)
V2523	2(3)
V2524	2(3)
V2530	2(3)
V2531	2(3)
V2599	2(3)
V2600	0(2)
V2610	0(2)
V2615	0(2)
V2623	2(2)
V2624	2(2)
V2625	2(2)
V2626	2(2)
V2627	2(2)
V2628	2(3)
V2629	2(2)

CPT	MUE
V2630	2(2)
V2631	2(2)
V2632	2(2)
V2700	2(3)
V2702	0(3)
V2710	2(3)
V2715	4(3)
V2718	2(3)
V2730	2(3)
V2744	2(3)
V2745	2(3)
V2750	2(3)
V2755	2(3)
V2756	0(3)
V2760	0(3)
V2761	0(2)
V2762	0(3)
V2770	2(3)
V2780	2(3)
V2781	0(2)
V2782	2(3)
V2783	2(3)
V2784	2(3)
V2785	2(2)
V2786	0(3)
V2787	0(3)
V2788	0(3)
V2790	1(3)
V2797	0(3)
V5008	0(3)

CPT	MUE
V5010	0(3)
V5011	0(3)
V5014	0(3)
V5020	0(3)
V5030	0(3)
V5040	0(3)
V5050	0(3)
V5060	0(3)
V5070	0(3)
V5080	0(3)
V5090	0(3)
V5095	0(3)
V5100	0(3)
V5110	0(3)
V5120	0(3)
V5130	0(3)
V5140	0(3)
V5150	0(3)
V5160	0(3)
V5171	0(3)
V5172	0(3)
V5181	0(3)
V5190	0(3)
V5200	0(3)
V5211	0(3)
V5212	0(3)
V5213	0(3)
V5214	0(3)
V5215	0(3)
V5221	0(3)

CPT	MUE
V5230	0(3)
V5240	0(3)
V5241	0(3)
V5242	0(3)
V5243	0(3)
V5244	0(3)
V5245	0(3)
V5246	0(3)
V5247	0(3)
V5248	0(3)
V5249	0(3)
V5250	0(3)
V5251	0(3)
V5252	0(3)
V5253	0(3)
V5254	0(3)
V5255	0(3)
V5256	0(3)
V5257	0(3)
V5258	0(3)
V5259	0(3)
V5260	0(3)
V5261	0(3)
V5262	0(3)
V5263	0(3)
V5264	0(3)
V5265	0(3)
V5266	0(3)
V5267	0(3)
V5268	0(3)

CPT	MUE
V5269	0(3)
V5270	0(3)
V5271	0(3)
V5272	0(3)
V5273	0(3)
V5274	0(3)
V5275	0(3)
V5281	0(3)
V5282	0(3)
V5283	0(3)
V5284	0(3)
V5285	0(3)
V5286	0(3)
V5287	0(3)
V5288	0(3)
V5289	0(3)
V5290	0(3)
V5298	0(3)
V5299	1(3)
V5336	0(3)
V5362	0(3)
V5363	0(3)
V5364	0(3)

Appendix J — Inpatient-Only Procedures

Inpatient Only Procedures—This appendix identifies services with the status indicator C. Medicare will not pay an OPPS hospital or ASC when they are performed on a Medicare patient as an outpatient. Physicians should refer to this list when scheduling Medicare patients for surgical procedures. CMS updates this list quarterly. The following was updated 10/01/2021.

00176 Anesth pharyngeal surgery
00211 Anesth cran surg hematoma
00214 Anesth skull drainage
00215 Anesth skull repair/fract
00474 Anesth surgery of rib
00524 Anesth chest drainage
00540 Anesth chest surgery
00542 Anesthesia removal pleura
00546 Anesth lung chest wall surg
00560 Anesth heart surg w/o pump
00561 Anesth heart surg <1 yr
00562 Anesth hrt surg w/pmp age 1+
00567 Anesth CABG w/pump
00580 Anesth heart/lung transplnt
00632 Anesth removal of nerves
0075T Perq stent/chest vert art
0076T S&i stent/chest vert art
00792 Anesth hemorr/excise liver
00794 Anesth pancreas removal
00796 Anesth for liver transplant
00844 Anesth pelvis surgery
00846 Anesth hysterectomy
00848 Anesth pelvic organ surg
00864 Anesth removal of bladder
00866 Anesth removal of adrenal
00868 Anesth kidney transplant
00882 Anesth major vein ligation
00908 Anesth removal of prostate
00932 Anesth amputation of penis
00934 Anesth penis nodes removal
00936 Anesth penis nodes removal
01272 Anesth femoral artery surg
01442 Anesth knee artery surg
01444 Anesth knee artery repair
01502 Anesth lwr leg embolectomy
01652 Anesth shoulder vessel surg
01654 Anesth shoulder vessel surg
01656 Anesth arm-leg vessel surg
01990 Support for organ donor
0235T Trluml perip athrc visceral
0345T Transcath mtral vlve repair
0451T Insj/rplcmt aortic ventr sys
0452T Insj/rplcmt dev vasc seal
0455T Remvl aortic ventr cmpl sys
0456T Remvl aortic dev vasc seal
0459T Relocaj rplcmt aortic ventr
0461T Repos aortic contrpulsj dev
0483T Tmvi percutaneous approach
0484T Tmvi transthoracic exposure
0494T Prep & cannulj cdvr don lung
0495T Mntr cdvr don lng 1st 2 hrs
0496T Mntr cdvr don lng ea addl hr
0543T Ta mv rpr w/artif chord tend
0544T Tcat mv annulus rcnstj
0545T Tcat tv annulus rcnstj
0569T Ttvr perq appr 1st prosth
0570T Ttvr perq ea addl prosth
0584T Perq islet cell transplant
0585T Laps islet cell transplant
0586T Open islet cell transplant
11004 Debride genitalia & perineum
11005 Debride abdom wall
11006 Debride genit/per/abdom wall
11008 Remove mesh from abd wall
15756 Free myo/skin flap microvasc
15757 Free skin flap microvasc
15758 Free fascial flap microvasc
16036 Escharotomy addl incision
19305 Mast radical
19306 Mast rad urban type
19361 Breast reconstr w/lat flap
19364 Breast reconstruction
19367 Breast reconstruction
19368 Breast reconstruction
19369 Breast reconstruction
31225 Removal of upper jaw
31230 Removal of upper jaw
31290 Nasal/sinus endoscopy surg
31291 Nasal/sinus endoscopy surg
31360 Removal of larynx
31365 Removal of larynx
31367 Partial removal of larynx
31368 Partial removal of larynx
31370 Partial removal of larynx
31375 Partial removal of larynx
31380 Partial removal of larynx
31382 Partial removal of larynx
31390 Removal of larynx & pharynx
31395 Reconstruct larynx & pharynx
31725 Clearance of airways
31760 Repair of windpipe
31766 Reconstruction of windpipe
31770 Repair/graft of bronchus
31775 Reconstruct bronchus
31780 Reconstruct windpipe
31781 Reconstruct windpipe
31786 Remove windpipe lesion
31800 Repair of windpipe injury
31805 Repair of windpipe injury
32035 Thoracostomy w/rib resection
32036 Thoracostomy w/flap drainage
32096 Open wedge/bx lung infiltr
32097 Open wedge/bx lung nodule
32098 Open biopsy of lung pleura
32100 Exploration of chest
32110 Explore/repair chest
32120 Re-exploration of chest
32124 Explore chest free adhesions
32140 Removal of lung lesion(s)
32141 Remove/treat lung lesions
32150 Removal of lung lesion(s)
32151 Remove lung foreign body
32160 Open chest heart massage
32200 Drain open lung lesion
32215 Treat chest lining
32220 Release of lung
32225 Partial release of lung
32310 Removal of chest lining
32320 Free/remove chest lining
32440 Remove lung pneumonectomy
32442 Sleeve pneumonectomy
32445 Removal of lung extrapleural
32480 Partial removal of lung
32482 Bilobectomy
32484 Segmentectomy
32486 Sleeve lobectomy
32488 Completion pneumonectomy
32491 Lung volume reduction
32501 Repair bronchus add-on
32503 Resect apical lung tumor
32504 Resect apical lung tum/chest
32505 Wedge resect of lung initial
32506 Wedge resect of lung add-on
32507 Wedge resect of lung diag
32540 Removal of lung lesion
32650 Thoracoscopy w/pleurodesis
32651 Thoracoscopy remove cortex
32652 Thoracoscopy rem totl cortex
32653 Thoracoscopy remov fb/fibrin
32654 Thoracoscopy contrl bleeding
32655 Thoracoscopy resect bullae
32656 Thoracoscopy w/pleurectomy
32658 Thoracoscopy w/sac fb remove
32659 Thoracoscopy w/sac drainage
32661 Thoracoscopy w/pericard exc
32662 Thoracoscopy w/mediast exc
32663 Thoracoscopy w/lobectomy
32664 Thoracoscopy w/ th nrv exc
32665 Thoracoscop w/esoph musc exc
32666 Thoracoscopy w/wedge resect
32667 Thoracoscopy w/w resect addl
32668 Thoracoscopy w/w resect diag
32669 Thoracoscopy remove segment
32670 Thoracoscopy bilobectomy
32671 Thoracoscopy pneumonectomy
32672 Thoracoscopy for lvrs
32673 Thoracoscopy w/thymus resect
32674 Thoracoscopy lymph node exc
32800 Repair lung hernia
32810 Close chest after drainage
32815 Close bronchial fistula
32820 Reconstruct injured chest
32850 Donor pneumonectomy
32851 Lung transplant single
32852 Lung transplant with bypass

32853	Lung transplant double
32854	Lung transplant with bypass
32855	Prepare donor lung single
32856	Prepare donor lung double
32900	Removal of rib(s)
32905	Revise & repair chest wall
32906	Revise & repair chest wall
32940	Revision of lung
32997	Total lung lavage
33017	Prcrd drg 6yr+ w/o cgen car
33018	Prcrd drg 0-5yr or w/anomly
33019	Perq prcrd drg insj cath ct
33020	Incision of heart sac
33025	Incision of heart sac
33030	Partial removal of heart sac
33031	Partial removal of heart sac
33050	Resect heart sac lesion
33120	Removal of heart lesion
33130	Removal of heart lesion
33140	Heart revascularize (tmr)
33141	Heart tmr w/other procedure
33202	Insert epicard eltrd open
33203	Insert epicard eltrd endo
33236	Remove electrode/thoracotomy
33237	Remove electrode/thoracotomy
33238	Remove electrode/thoracotomy
33243	Remove eltrd/thoracotomy
33250	Ablate heart dysrhythm focus
33251	Ablate heart dysrhythm focus
33254	Ablate atria lmtd
33255	Ablate atria w/o bypass ext
33256	Ablate atria w/bypass exten
33257	Ablate atria lmtd add-on
33258	Ablate atria x10sv add-on
33259	Ablate atria w/bypass add-on
33261	Ablate heart dysrhythm focus
33265	Ablate atria lmtd endo
33266	Ablate atria x10sv endo
33300	Repair of heart wound
33305	Repair of heart wound
33310	Exploratory heart surgery
33315	Exploratory heart surgery
33320	Repair major blood vessel(s)
33321	Repair major vessel
33322	Repair major blood vessel(s)
33330	Insert major vessel graft
33335	Insert major vessel graft
33340	Perq clsr tcat l atr apndge
33361	Replace aortic valve perq
33362	Replace aortic valve open
33363	Replace aortic valve open
33364	Replace aortic valve open
33365	Replace aortic valve open
33366	Trcath replace aortic valve
33367	Replace aortic valve w/byp
33368	Replace aortic valve w/byp
33369	Replace aortic valve w/byp
33390	Valvuloplasty aortic valve
33391	Valvuloplasty aortic valve
33404	Prepare heart-aorta conduit
33405	Replacement of aortic valve
33406	Replacement of aortic valve
33410	Replacement of aortic valve
33411	Replacement of aortic valve
33412	Replacement of aortic valve
33413	Replacement of aortic valve
33414	Repair of aortic valve
33415	Revision subvalvular tissue
33416	Revise ventricle muscle
33417	Repair of aortic valve
33418	Repair tcat mitral valve
33420	Revision of mitral valve
33422	Revision of mitral valve
33425	Repair of mitral valve
33426	Repair of mitral valve
33427	Repair of mitral valve
33430	Replacement of mitral valve
33440	Rplcmt a-valve tlcj autol pv
33460	Revision of tricuspid valve
33463	Valvuloplasty tricuspid
33464	Valvuloplasty tricuspid
33465	Replace tricuspid valve
33468	Revision of tricuspid valve
33470	Revision of pulmonary valve
33471	Valvotomy pulmonary valve
33474	Revision of pulmonary valve
33475	Replacement pulmonary valve
33476	Revision of heart chamber
33477	Implant tcat pulm vlv perq
33478	Revision of heart chamber
33496	Repair prosth valve clot
33500	Repair heart vessel fistula
33501	Repair heart vessel fistula
33502	Coronary artery correction
33503	Coronary artery graft
33504	Coronary artery graft
33505	Repair artery w/tunnel
33506	Repair artery translocation
33507	Repair art intramural
33510	Cabg vein single
33511	Cabg vein two
33512	Cabg vein three
33513	Cabg vein four
33514	Cabg vein five
33516	Cabg vein six or more
33517	Cabg artery-vein single
33518	Cabg artery-vein two
33519	Cabg artery-vein three
33521	Cabg artery-vein four
33522	Cabg artery-vein five
33523	Cabg art-vein six or more
33530	Coronary artery bypass/reop
33533	Cabg arterial single
33534	Cabg arterial two
33535	Cabg arterial three
33536	Cabg arterial four or more
33542	Removal of heart lesion
33545	Repair of heart damage
33548	Restore/remodel ventricle
33572	Open coronary endarterectomy
33600	Closure of valve
33602	Closure of valve
33606	Anastomosis/artery-aorta
33608	Repair anomaly w/conduit
33610	Repair by enlargement
33611	Repair double ventricle
33612	Repair double ventricle
33615	Repair modified fontan
33617	Repair single ventricle
33619	Repair single ventricle
33620	Apply r&l pulm art bands
33621	Transthor cath for stent
33622	Redo compl cardiac anomaly
33641	Repair heart septum defect
33645	Revision of heart veins
33647	Repair heart septum defects
33660	Repair of heart defects
33665	Repair of heart defects
33670	Repair of heart chambers
33675	Close mult vsd
33676	Close mult vsd w/resection
33677	Cl mult vsd w/rem pul band
33681	Repair heart septum defect
33684	Repair heart septum defect
33688	Repair heart septum defect
33690	Reinforce pulmonary artery
33692	Repair of heart defects
33694	Repair of heart defects
33697	Repair of heart defects
33702	Repair of heart defects
33710	Repair of heart defects
33720	Repair of heart defect
33722	Repair of heart defect
33724	Repair venous anomaly
33726	Repair pul venous stenosis
33730	Repair heart-vein defect(s)
33732	Repair heart-vein defect
33735	Revision of heart chamber
33736	Revision of heart chamber
33737	Revision of heart chamber
33741	Tas congenital car anomal
33745	Tis cgen car anomal 1st shnt
33746	Tis cgen car anomal ea addl
33750	Major vessel shunt
33755	Major vessel shunt
33762	Major vessel shunt
33764	Major vessel shunt & graft
33766	Major vessel shunt
33767	Major vessel shunt
33768	Cavopulmonary shunting
33770	Repair great vessels defect
33771	Repair great vessels defect
33774	Repair great vessels defect
33775	Repair great vessels defect
33776	Repair great vessels defect
33777	Repair great vessels defect
33778	Repair great vessels defect
33779	Repair great vessels defect
33780	Repair great vessels defect
33781	Repair great vessels defect
33782	Nikaidoh proc
33783	Nikaidoh proc w/ostia implt
33786	Repair arterial trunk

33788	Revision of pulmonary artery
33800	Aortic suspension
33802	Repair vessel defect
33803	Repair vessel defect
33813	Repair septal defect
33814	Repair septal defect
33820	Revise major vessel
33822	Revise major vessel
33824	Revise major vessel
33840	Remove aorta constriction
33845	Remove aorta constriction
33851	Remove aorta constriction
33852	Repair septal defect
33853	Repair septal defect
33858	As-aort grf f/aortic dsj
33859	As-aort grf f/ds oth/thn dsj
33863	Ascending aortic graft
33864	Ascending aortic graft
33871	Transvrs a-arch grf hypthrm
33875	Thoracic aortic graft
33877	Thoracoabdominal graft
33880	Endovasc taa repr incl subcl
33881	Endovasc taa repr w/o subcl
33883	Insert endovasc prosth taa
33884	Endovasc prosth taa add-on
33886	Endovasc prosth delayed
33889	Artery transpose/endovas taa
33891	Car-car bp grft/endovas taa
33910	Remove lung artery emboli
33915	Remove lung artery emboli
33916	Surgery of great vessel
33917	Repair pulmonary artery
33920	Repair pulmonary atresia
33922	Transect pulmonary artery
33924	Remove pulmonary shunt
33925	Rpr pul art unifocal w/o cpb
33926	Repr pul art unifocal w/cpb
33927	Impltj tot rplcmt hrt sys
33928	Rmvl & rplcmt tot hrt sys
33929	Rmvl rplcmt hrt sys f/trnspl
33930	Removal of donor heart/lung
33933	Prepare donor heart/lung
33935	Transplantation heart/lung
33940	Removal of donor heart
33944	Prepare donor heart
33945	Transplantation of heart
33946	Ecmo/ecls initiation venous
33947	Ecmo/ecls initiation artery
33948	Ecmo/ecls daily mgmt-venous
33949	Ecmo/ecls daily mgmt artery
33951	Ecmo/ecls insj prph cannula
33952	Ecmo/ecls insj prph cannula
33953	Ecmo/ecls insj prph cannula
33954	Ecmo/ecls insj prph cannula
33955	Ecmo/ecls insj ctr cannula
33956	Ecmo/ecls insj ctr cannula
33957	Ecmo/ecls repos perph cnula
33958	Ecmo/ecls repos perph cnula
33959	Ecmo/ecls repos perph cnula
33962	Ecmo/ecls repos perph cnula
33963	Ecmo/ecls repos perph cnula
33964	Ecmo/ecls repos perph cnula
33965	Ecmo/ecls rmvl perph cannula
33966	Ecmo/ecls rmvl prph cannula
33967	Insert i-aort percut device
33968	Remove aortic assist device
33969	Ecmo/ecls rmvl perph cannula
33970	Aortic circulation assist
33971	Aortic circulation assist
33973	Insert balloon device
33974	Remove intra-aortic balloon
33975	Implant ventricular device
33976	Implant ventricular device
33977	Remove ventricular device
33978	Remove ventricular device
33979	Insert intracorporeal device
33980	Remove intracorporeal device
33981	Replace vad pump ext
33982	Replace vad intra w/o bp
33983	Replace vad intra w/bp
33984	Ecmo/ecls rmvl prph cannula
33985	Ecmo/ecls rmvl ctr cannula
33986	Ecmo/ecls rmvl ctr cannula
33987	Artery expos/graft artery
33988	Insertion of left heart vent
33989	Removal of left heart vent
33990	Insert vad artery access
33991	Insert vad art&vein access
33992	Remove vad different session
33993	Reposition vad diff session
33995	Insj perq vad r hrt venous
33997	Rmvl perq right heart vad
34001	Removal of artery clot
34051	Removal of artery clot
34151	Removal of artery clot
34401	Removal of vein clot
34451	Removal of vein clot
34502	Reconstruct vena cava
34701	Evasc rpr a-ao ndgft
34702	Evasc rpr a-ao ndgft rpt
34703	Evasc rpr a-unilac ndgft
34704	Evasc rpr a-unilac ndgft rpt
34705	Evac rpr a-biiliac ndgft
34706	Evasc rpr a-biiliac rpt
34707	Evasc rpr ilio-iliac ndgft
34708	Evasc rpr ilio-iliac rpt
34709	Plmt xtn prosth evasc rpr
34710	Dlyd plmt xtn prosth 1st vsl
34711	Dlyd plmt xtn prosth ea addl
34712	Tcat dlvr enhncd fixj dev
34717	Evasc rpr a-iliac ndgft
34718	Evasc rpr n/a a-iliac ndgft
34808	Endovas iliac a device addon
34812	Xpose for endoprosth femorl
34813	Femoral endovas graft add-on
34820	Xpose for endoprosth iliac
34830	Open aortic tube prosth repr
34831	Open aortoiliac prosth repr
34832	Open aortofemor prosth repr
34833	Xpose for endoprosth iliac
34834	Xpose endoprosth brachial
34841	Endovasc visc aorta 1 graft
34842	Endovasc visc aorta 2 graft
34843	Endovasc visc aorta 3 graft
34844	Endovasc visc aorta 4 graft
34845	Visc & infraren abd 1 prosth
34846	Visc & infraren abd 2 prosth
34847	Visc & infraren abd 3 prosth
34848	Visc & infraren abd 4+ prost
35001	Repair defect of artery
35002	Repair artery rupture neck
35005	Repair defect of artery
35013	Repair artery rupture arm
35021	Repair defect of artery
35022	Repair artery rupture chest
35081	Repair defect of artery
35082	Repair artery rupture aorta
35091	Repair defect of artery
35092	Repair artery rupture aorta
35102	Repair defect of artery
35103	Repair artery rupture aorta
35111	Repair defect of artery
35112	Repair artery rupture spleen
35121	Repair defect of artery
35122	Repair artery rupture belly
35131	Repair defect of artery
35132	Repair artery rupture groin
35141	Repair defect of artery
35142	Repair artery rupture thigh
35151	Repair defect of artery
35152	Repair ruptd popliteal art
35182	Repair blood vessel lesion
35189	Repair blood vessel lesion
35211	Repair blood vessel lesion
35216	Repair blood vessel lesion
35221	Repair blood vessel lesion
35241	Repair blood vessel lesion
35246	Repair blood vessel lesion
35251	Repair blood vessel lesion
35271	Repair blood vessel lesion
35276	Repair blood vessel lesion
35281	Repair blood vessel lesion
35301	Rechanneling of artery
35302	Rechanneling of artery
35303	Rechanneling of artery
35304	Rechanneling of artery
35305	Rechanneling of artery
35306	Rechanneling of artery
35311	Rechanneling of artery
35331	Rechanneling of artery
35341	Rechanneling of artery
35351	Rechanneling of artery
35355	Rechanneling of artery
35361	Rechanneling of artery
35363	Rechanneling of artery
35371	Rechanneling of artery
35390	Reoperation carotid add-on
35400	Angioscopy
35501	Art byp grft ipsilat carotid
35506	Art byp grft subclav-carotid
35508	Art byp grft carotid-vertbrl
35509	Art byp grft contral carotid
35510	Art byp grft carotid-brchial

35511	Art byp grft subclav-subclav	35694	Art trnsposj subclav carotid	42426	Excise parotid gland/lesion
35512	Art byp grft subclav-brchial	35695	Art trnsposj carotid subclav	42845	Extensive surgery of throat
35515	Art byp grft subclav-vertbrl	35697	Reimplant artery each	42894	Revision of pharyngeal walls
35516	Art byp grft subclav-axilary	35700	Reoperation bypass graft	42953	Repair throat esophagus
35518	Art byp grft axillary-axilry	35701	Exploration carotid artery	42961	Control throat bleeding
35521	Art byp grft axill-femoral	35702	Expl n/flwd surg uxtr art	42971	Control nose/throat bleeding
35522	Art byp grft axill-brachial	35703	Expl n/flwd surg lxtr art	43045	Incision of esophagus
35523	Art byp grft brchl-ulnr-rdl	35820	Explore chest vessels	43100	Excision of esophagus lesion
35525	Art byp grft brachial-brchl	35840	Explore abdominal vessels	43101	Excision of esophagus lesion
35526	Art byp grft aor/carot/innom	35870	Repair vessel graft defect	43107	Removal of esophagus
35531	Art byp grft aorcel/aormesen	35901	Excision graft neck	43108	Removal of esophagus
35533	Art byp grft axill/fem/fem	35905	Excision graft thorax	43112	Removal of esophagus
35535	Art byp grft hepatorenal	35907	Excision graft abdomen	43113	Removal of esophagus
35536	Art byp grft splenorenal	36660	Insertion catheter artery	43116	Partial removal of esophagus
35537	Art byp grft aortoiliac	36823	Insertion of cannula(s)	43117	Partial removal of esophagus
35538	Art byp grft aortobi-iliac	37140	Revision of circulation	43118	Partial removal of esophagus
35539	Art byp grft aortofemoral	37145	Revision of circulation	43121	Partial removal of esophagus
35540	Art byp grft aortbifemoral	37160	Revision of circulation	43122	Partial removal of esophagus
35556	Art byp grft fem-popliteal	37180	Revision of circulation	43123	Partial removal of esophagus
35558	Art byp grft fem-femoral	37181	Splice spleen/kidney veins	43124	Removal of esophagus
35560	Art byp grft aortorenal	37215	Transcath stent cca w/eps	43135	Removal of esophagus pouch
35563	Art byp grft ilioiliac	37217	Stent placemt retro carotid	43279	Lap myotomy heller
35565	Art byp grft iliofemoral	37218	Stent placemt ante carotid	43283	Lap esoph lengthening
35566	Art byp fem-ant-post tib/prl	37616	Ligation of chest artery	43286	Esphg tot w/laps moblj
35570	Art byp tibial-tib/peroneal	37618	Ligation of extremity artery	43287	Esphg dstl 2/3 w/laps moblj
35571	Art byp pop-tibl-prl-other	37660	Revision of major vein	43288	Esphg thrsc moblj
35583	Vein byp grft fem-popliteal	37788	Revascularization penis	43300	Repair of esophagus
35585	Vein byp fem-tibial peroneal	38100	Removal of spleen total	43305	Repair esophagus and fistula
35587	Vein byp pop-tibl peroneal	38101	Removal of spleen partial	43310	Repair of esophagus
35600	Harvest art for cabg add-on	38102	Removal of spleen total	43312	Repair esophagus and fistula
35601	Art byp common ipsi carotid	38115	Repair of ruptured spleen	43313	Esophagoplasty congenital
35606	Art byp carotid-subclavian	38380	Thoracic duct procedure	43314	Tracheo-esophagoplasty cong
35612	Art byp subclav-subclavian	38381	Thoracic duct procedure	43320	Fuse esophagus & stomach
35616	Art byp subclav-axillary	38382	Thoracic duct procedure	43325	Revise esophagus & stomach
35621	Art byp axillary-femoral	38564	Removal abdomen lymph nodes	43327	Esoph fundoplasty lap
35623	Art byp axillary-pop-tibial	38724	Removal of lymph nodes neck	43328	Esoph fundoplasty thor
35626	Art byp aorsubcl/carot/innom	38746	Remove thoracic lymph nodes	43330	Esophagomyotomy abdominal
35631	Art byp aor-celiac-msn-renal	38747	Remove abdominal lymph nodes	43331	Esophagomyotomy thoracic
35632	Art byp ilio-celiac	38765	Remove groin lymph nodes	43332	Transab esoph hiat hern rpr
35633	Art byp ilio-mesenteric	38770	Remove pelvis lymph nodes	43333	Transab esoph hiat hern rpr
35634	Art byp iliorenal	38780	Remove abdomen lymph nodes	43334	Transthor diaphrag hern rpr
35636	Art byp spenorenal	39000	Exploration of chest	43335	Transthor diaphrag hern rpr
35637	Art byp aortoiliac	39010	Exploration of chest	43336	Thorabd diaphr hern repair
35638	Art byp aortobi-iliac	39200	Resect mediastinal cyst	43337	Thorabd diaphr hern repair
35642	Art byp carotid-vertebral	39220	Resect mediastinal tumor	43338	Esoph lengthening
35645	Art byp subclav-vertebrl	39499	Chest procedure	43340	Fuse esophagus & intestine
35646	Art byp aortobifemoral	39501	Repair diaphragm laceration	43341	Fuse esophagus & intestine
35647	Art byp aortofemoral	39503	Repair of diaphragm hernia	43351	Surgical opening esophagus
35650	Art byp axillary-axillary	39540	Repair of diaphragm hernia	43352	Surgical opening esophagus
35654	Art byp axill-fem-femoral	39541	Repair of diaphragm hernia	43360	Gastrointestinal repair
35656	Art byp femoral-popliteal	39545	Revision of diaphragm	43361	Gastrointestinal repair
35661	Art byp femoral-femoral	39560	Resect diaphragm simple	43400	Ligate esophagus veins
35663	Art byp ilioiliac	39561	Resect diaphragm complex	43405	Ligate/staple esophagus
35665	Art byp iliofemoral	39599	Diaphragm surgery procedure	43410	Repair esophagus wound
35666	Art byp fem-ant-post tib/prl	41130	Partial removal of tongue	43415	Repair esophagus wound
35671	Art byp pop-tibl-prl-other	41135	Tongue and neck surgery	43425	Repair esophagus opening
35681	Composite byp grft pros&vein	41140	Removal of tongue	43460	Pressure treatment esophagus
35682	Composite byp grft 2 veins	41145	Tongue removal neck surgery	43496	Free jejunum flap microvasc
35683	Composite byp grft 3/> segmt	41150	Tongue mouth jaw surgery	43500	Surgical opening of stomach
35691	Art trnsposj vertbrl carotid	41153	Tongue mouth neck surgery	43501	Surgical repair of stomach
35693	Art trnsposj subclavian	41155	Tongue jaw & neck surgery	43502	Surgical repair of stomach

43520	Incision of pyloric muscle
43605	Biopsy of stomach
43610	Excision of stomach lesion
43611	Excision of stomach lesion
43620	Removal of stomach
43621	Removal of stomach
43622	Removal of stomach
43631	Removal of stomach partial
43632	Removal of stomach partial
43633	Removal of stomach partial
43634	Removal of stomach partial
43635	Removal of stomach partial
43640	Vagotomy & pylorus repair
43641	Vagotomy & pylorus repair
43644	Lap gastric bypass/roux-en-y
43645	Lap gastr bypass incl smll i
43771	Lap revise gastr adj device
43775	Lap sleeve gastrectomy
43800	Reconstruction of pylorus
43810	Fusion of stomach and bowel
43820	Fusion of stomach and bowel
43825	Fusion of stomach and bowel
43832	Place gastrostomy tube
43843	Gastroplasty w/o v-band
43845	Gastroplasty duodenal switch
43846	Gastric bypass for obesity
43847	Gastric bypass incl small i
43848	Revision gastroplasty
43850	Revise stomach-bowel fusion
43855	Revise stomach-bowel fusion
43860	Revise stomach-bowel fusion
43865	Revise stomach-bowel fusion
43880	Repair stomach-bowel fistula
43881	Impl/redo electrd antrum
43882	Revise/remove electrd antrum
44005	Freeing of bowel adhesion
44010	Incision of small bowel
44015	Insert needle cath bowel
44020	Explore small intestine
44021	Decompress small bowel
44025	Incision of large bowel
44050	Reduce bowel obstruction
44055	Correct malrotation of bowel
44110	Excise intestine lesion(s)
44111	Excision of bowel lesion(s)
44120	Removal of small intestine
44121	Removal of small intestine
44125	Removal of small intestine
44126	Enterectomy w/o taper cong
44127	Enterectomy w/taper cong
44128	Enterectomy cong add-on
44130	Bowel to bowel fusion
44132	Enterectomy cadaver donor
44133	Enterectomy live donor
44135	Intestine transplnt cadaver
44136	Intestine transplant live
44137	Remove intestinal allograft
44139	Mobilization of colon
44140	Partial removal of colon
44141	Partial removal of colon
44143	Partial removal of colon
44144	Partial removal of colon
44145	Partial removal of colon
44146	Partial removal of colon
44147	Partial removal of colon
44150	Removal of colon
44151	Removal of colon/ileostomy
44155	Removal of colon/ileostomy
44156	Removal of colon/ileostomy
44157	Colectomy w/ileoanal anast
44158	Colectomy w/neo-rectum pouch
44160	Removal of colon
44187	Lap ileo/jejuno-stomy
44188	Lap colostomy
44202	Lap enterectomy
44203	Lap resect s/intestine addl
44204	Laparo partial colectomy
44205	Lap colectomy part w/ileum
44206	Lap part colectomy w/stoma
44207	L colectomy/coloproctostomy
44208	L colectomy/coloproctostomy
44210	Laparo total proctocolectomy
44211	Lap colectomy w/proctectomy
44212	Laparo total proctocolectomy
44213	Lap mobil splenic fl add-on
44227	Lap close enterostomy
44310	Ileostomy/jejunostomy
44316	Devise bowel pouch
44320	Colostomy
44322	Colostomy with biopsies
44603	Suture small intestine
44604	Suture large intestine
44605	Repair of bowel lesion
44615	Intestinal stricturoplasty
44620	Repair bowel opening
44625	Repair bowel opening
44626	Repair bowel opening
44640	Repair bowel-skin fistula
44650	Repair bowel fistula
44660	Repair bowel-bladder fistula
44661	Repair bowel-bladder fistula
44680	Surgical revision intestine
44700	Suspend bowel w/prosthesis
44715	Prepare donor intestine
44720	Prep donor intestine/venous
44721	Prep donor intestine/artery
44800	Excision of bowel pouch
44820	Excision of mesentery lesion
44850	Repair of mesentery
44899	Bowel surgery procedure
44900	Drain appendix abscess open
44960	Appendectomy
45110	Removal of rectum
45111	Partial removal of rectum
45112	Removal of rectum
45113	Partial proctectomy
45114	Partial removal of rectum
45116	Partial removal of rectum
45119	Remove rectum w/reservoir
45120	Removal of rectum
45121	Removal of rectum and colon
45123	Partial proctectomy
45126	Pelvic exenteration
45130	Excision of rectal prolapse
45135	Excision of rectal prolapse
45136	Excise ileoanal reservior
45395	Lap removal of rectum
45397	Lap remove rectum w/pouch
45400	Laparoscopic proc
45402	Lap proctopexy w/sig resect
45540	Correct rectal prolapse
45550	Repair rectum/remove sigmoid
45562	Exploration/repair of rectum
45563	Exploration/repair of rectum
45800	Repair rect/bladder fistula
45805	Repair fistula w/colostomy
45820	Repair rectourethral fistula
45825	Repair fistula w/colostomy
46705	Repair of anal stricture
46710	Repr per/vag pouch sngl proc
46712	Repr per/vag pouch dbl proc
46715	Rep perf anoper fistu
46716	Rep perf anoper/vestib fistu
46730	Construction of absent anus
46735	Construction of absent anus
46740	Construction of absent anus
46742	Repair of imperforated anus
46744	Repair of cloacal anomaly
46746	Repair of cloacal anomaly
46748	Repair of cloacal anomaly
46751	Repair of anal sphincter
47010	Open drainage liver lesion
47015	Inject/aspirate liver cyst
47100	Wedge biopsy of liver
47120	Partial removal of liver
47122	Extensive removal of liver
47125	Partial removal of liver
47130	Partial removal of liver
47133	Removal of donor liver
47135	Transplantation of liver
47140	Partial removal donor liver
47141	Partial removal donor liver
47142	Partial removal donor liver
47143	Prep donor liver whole
47144	Prep donor liver 3-segment
47145	Prep donor liver lobe split
47146	Prep donor liver/venous
47147	Prep donor liver/arterial
47300	Surgery for liver lesion
47350	Repair liver wound
47360	Repair liver wound
47361	Repair liver wound
47362	Repair liver wound
47380	Open ablate liver tumor rf
47381	Open ablate liver tumor cryo
47400	Incision of liver duct
47420	Incision of bile duct
47425	Incision of bile duct
47460	Incise bile duct sphincter
47480	Incision of gallbladder
47550	Bile duct endoscopy add-on
47570	Laparo cholecystoenterostomy
47600	Removal of gallbladder

47605	Removal of gallbladder
47610	Removal of gallbladder
47612	Removal of gallbladder
47620	Removal of gallbladder
47700	Exploration of bile ducts
47701	Bile duct revision
47711	Excision of bile duct tumor
47712	Excision of bile duct tumor
47715	Excision of bile duct cyst
47720	Fuse gallbladder & bowel
47721	Fuse upper gi structures
47740	Fuse gallbladder & bowel
47741	Fuse gallbladder & bowel
47760	Fuse bile ducts and bowel
47765	Fuse liver ducts & bowel
47780	Fuse bile ducts and bowel
47785	Fuse bile ducts and bowel
47800	Reconstruction of bile ducts
47801	Placement bile duct support
47802	Fuse liver duct & intestine
47900	Suture bile duct injury
48000	Drainage of abdomen
48001	Placement of drain pancreas
48020	Removal of pancreatic stone
48100	Biopsy of pancreas open
48105	Resect/debride pancreas
48120	Removal of pancreas lesion
48140	Partial removal of pancreas
48145	Partial removal of pancreas
48146	Pancreatectomy
48148	Removal of pancreatic duct
48150	Partial removal of pancreas
48152	Pancreatectomy
48153	Pancreatectomy
48154	Pancreatectomy
48155	Removal of pancreas
48400	Injection intraop add-on
48500	Surgery of pancreatic cyst
48510	Drain pancreatic pseudocyst
48520	Fuse pancreas cyst and bowel
48540	Fuse pancreas cyst and bowel
48545	Pancreatorrhaphy
48547	Duodenal exclusion
48548	Fuse pancreas and bowel
48551	Prep donor pancreas
48552	Prep donor pancreas/venous
48554	Transpl allograft pancreas
48556	Removal allograft pancreas
49000	Exploration of abdomen
49002	Reopening of abdomen
49013	Prpertl pel pack hemrrg trma
49014	Reexploration pelvic wound
49020	Drainage abdom abscess open
49040	Drain open abdom abscess
49060	Drain open retroperi abscess
49062	Drain to peritoneal cavity
49203	Exc abd tum 5 cm or less
49204	Exc abd tum over 5 cm
49205	Exc abd tum over 10 cm
49215	Excise sacral spine tumor
49412	Ins device for rt guide open
49425	Insert abdomen-venous drain
49428	Ligation of shunt
49605	Repair umbilical lesion
49606	Repair umbilical lesion
49610	Repair umbilical lesion
49611	Repair umbilical lesion
49900	Repair of abdominal wall
49904	Omental flap extra-abdom
49905	Omental flap intra-abdom
49906	Free omental flap microvasc
50010	Exploration of kidney
50040	Drainage of kidney
50045	Exploration of kidney
50060	Removal of kidney stone
50065	Incision of kidney
50070	Incision of kidney
50075	Removal of kidney stone
50100	Revise kidney blood vessels
50120	Exploration of kidney
50125	Explore and drain kidney
50130	Removal of kidney stone
50135	Exploration of kidney
50205	Renal biopsy open
50220	Remove kidney open
50225	Removal kidney open complex
50230	Removal kidney open radical
50234	Removal of kidney & ureter
50236	Removal of kidney & ureter
50240	Partial removal of kidney
50250	Cryoablate renal mass open
50280	Removal of kidney lesion
50290	Removal of kidney lesion
50300	Remove cadaver donor kidney
50320	Remove kidney living donor
50323	Prep cadaver renal allograft
50325	Prep donor renal graft
50327	Prep renal graft/venous
50328	Prep renal graft/arterial
50329	Prep renal graft/ureteral
50340	Removal of kidney
50360	Transplantation of kidney
50365	Transplantation of kidney
50370	Remove transplanted kidney
50380	Reimplantation of kidney
50400	Revision of kidney/ureter
50405	Revision of kidney/ureter
50500	Repair of kidney wound
50520	Close kidney-skin fistula
50525	Close nephrovisceral fistula
50526	Close nephrovisceral fistula
50540	Revision of horseshoe kidney
50545	Laparo radical nephrectomy
50546	Laparoscopic nephrectomy
50547	Laparo removal donor kidney
50548	Laparo remove w/ureter
50600	Exploration of ureter
50605	Insert ureteral support
50610	Removal of ureter stone
50620	Removal of ureter stone
50630	Removal of ureter stone
50650	Removal of ureter
50660	Removal of ureter
50700	Revision of ureter
50715	Release of ureter
50722	Release of ureter
50725	Release/revise ureter
50728	Revise ureter
50740	Fusion of ureter & kidney
50750	Fusion of ureter & kidney
50760	Fusion of ureters
50770	Splicing of ureters
50780	Reimplant ureter in bladder
50782	Reimplant ureter in bladder
50783	Reimplant ureter in bladder
50785	Reimplant ureter in bladder
50800	Implant ureter in bowel
50810	Fusion of ureter & bowel
50815	Urine shunt to intestine
50820	Construct bowel bladder
50825	Construct bowel bladder
50830	Revise urine flow
50840	Replace ureter by bowel
50845	Appendico-vesicostomy
50860	Transplant ureter to skin
50900	Repair of ureter
50920	Closure ureter/skin fistula
50930	Closure ureter/bowel fistula
50940	Release of ureter
51525	Removal of bladder lesion
51530	Removal of bladder lesion
51550	Partial removal of bladder
51555	Partial removal of bladder
51565	Revise bladder & ureter(s)
51570	Removal of bladder
51575	Removal of bladder & nodes
51580	Remove bladder/revise tract
51585	Removal of bladder & nodes
51590	Remove bladder/revise tract
51595	Remove bladder/revise tract
51596	Remove bladder/create pouch
51597	Removal of pelvic structures
51800	Revision of bladder/urethra
51820	Revision of urinary tract
51841	Attach bladder/urethra
51865	Repair of bladder wound
51900	Repair bladder/vagina lesion
51920	Close bladder-uterus fistula
51925	Hysterectomy/bladder repair
51940	Correction of bladder defect
51960	Revision of bladder & bowel
51980	Construct bladder opening
53415	Reconstruction of urethra
53448	Remov/replc ur sphinctr comp
54125	Removal of penis
54130	Remove penis & nodes
54135	Remove penis & nodes
54390	Repair penis and bladder
54430	Revision of penis
54438	Replantation of penis
55605	Incise sperm duct pouch
55650	Remove sperm duct pouch
55801	Removal of prostate

55810	Extensive prostate surgery
55812	Extensive prostate surgery
55815	Extensive prostate surgery
55821	Removal of prostate
55831	Removal of prostate
55840	Extensive prostate surgery
55842	Extensive prostate surgery
55845	Extensive prostate surgery
55862	Extensive prostate surgery
55865	Extensive prostate surgery
56631	Extensive vulva surgery
56632	Extensive vulva surgery
56633	Extensive vulva surgery
56634	Extensive vulva surgery
56637	Extensive vulva surgery
56640	Extensive vulva surgery
57110	Remove vagina wall complete
57111	Remove vagina tissue compl
57270	Repair of bowel pouch
57280	Suspension of vagina
57296	Revise vag graft open abd
57305	Repair rectum-vagina fistula
57307	Fistula repair & colostomy
57308	Fistula repair transperine
57311	Repair urethrovaginal lesion
57531	Removal of cervix radical
57540	Removal of residual cervix
57545	Remove cervix/repair pelvis
58140	Myomectomy abdom method
58146	Myomectomy abdom complex
58150	Total hysterectomy
58152	Total hysterectomy
58180	Partial hysterectomy
58200	Extensive hysterectomy
58210	Extensive hysterectomy
58240	Removal of pelvis contents
58267	Vag hyst w/urinary repair
58275	Hysterectomy/revise vagina
58280	Hysterectomy/revise vagina
58285	Extensive hysterectomy
58400	Suspension of uterus
58410	Suspension of uterus
58520	Repair of ruptured uterus
58540	Revision of uterus
58548	Lap radical hyst
58575	Laps tot hyst resj mal
58605	Division of fallopian tube
58611	Ligate oviduct(s) add-on
58700	Removal of fallopian tube
58720	Removal of ovary/tube(s)
58740	Adhesiolysis tube ovary
58750	Repair oviduct
58752	Revise ovarian tube(s)
58760	Fimbrioplasty
58822	Drain ovary abscess percut
58825	Transposition ovary(s)
58940	Removal of ovary(s)
58943	Removal of ovary(s)
58950	Resect ovarian malignancy
58951	Resect ovarian malignancy
58952	Resect ovarian malignancy
58953	Tah rad dissect for debulk
58954	Tah rad debulk/lymph remove
58956	Bso omentectomy w/tah
58957	Resect recurrent gyn mal
58958	Resect recur gyn mal w/lym
58960	Exploration of abdomen
59120	Treat ectopic pregnancy
59121	Treat ectopic pregnancy
59130	Treat ectopic pregnancy
59135	Treat ectopic pregnancy
59136	Treat ectopic pregnancy
59140	Treat ectopic pregnancy
59325	Revision of cervix
59350	Repair of uterus
59514	Cesarean delivery only
59525	Remove uterus after cesarean
59620	Attempted vbac delivery only
59830	Treat uterus infection
59850	Abortion
59851	Abortion
59852	Abortion
59855	Abortion
59856	Abortion
59857	Abortion
60254	Extensive thyroid surgery
60270	Removal of thyroid
60505	Explore parathyroid glands
60521	Removal of thymus gland
60522	Removal of thymus gland
60540	Explore adrenal gland
60545	Explore adrenal gland
60600	Remove carotid body lesion
60605	Remove carotid body lesion
60650	Laparoscopy adrenalectomy
61105	Twist drill hole
61107	Drill skull for implantation
61108	Drill skull for drainage
61120	Burr hole for puncture
61140	Pierce skull for biopsy
61150	Pierce skull for drainage
61151	Pierce skull for drainage
61154	Pierce skull & remove clot
61156	Pierce skull for drainage
61210	Pierce skull implant device
61250	Pierce skull & explore
61253	Pierce skull & explore
61304	Open skull for exploration
61305	Open skull for exploration
61312	Open skull for drainage
61313	Open skull for drainage
61314	Open skull for drainage
61315	Open skull for drainage
61316	Implt cran bone flap to abdo
61320	Open skull for drainage
61321	Open skull for drainage
61322	Decompressive craniotomy
61323	Decompressive lobectomy
61333	Explore orbit/remove lesion
61340	Subtemporal decompression
61343	Incise skull (press relief)
61345	Relieve cranial pressure
61450	Incise skull for surgery
61458	Incise skull for brain wound
61460	Incise skull for surgery
61500	Removal of skull lesion
61501	Remove infected skull bone
61510	Removal of brain lesion
61512	Remove brain lining lesion
61514	Removal of brain abscess
61516	Removal of brain lesion
61517	Implt brain chemotx add-on
61518	Removal of brain lesion
61519	Remove brain lining lesion
61520	Removal of brain lesion
61521	Removal of brain lesion
61522	Removal of brain abscess
61524	Removal of brain lesion
61526	Removal of brain lesion
61530	Removal of brain lesion
61531	Implant brain electrodes
61533	Implant brain electrodes
61534	Removal of brain lesion
61535	Remove brain electrodes
61536	Removal of brain lesion
61537	Removal of brain tissue
61538	Removal of brain tissue
61539	Removal of brain tissue
61540	Removal of brain tissue
61541	Incision of brain tissue
61543	Removal of brain tissue
61544	Remove & treat brain lesion
61545	Excision of brain tumor
61546	Removal of pituitary gland
61548	Removal of pituitary gland
61550	Release of skull seams
61552	Release of skull seams
61556	Incise skull/sutures
61557	Incise skull/sutures
61558	Excision of skull/sutures
61559	Excision of skull/sutures
61563	Excision of skull tumor
61564	Excision of skull tumor
61566	Removal of brain tissue
61567	Incision of brain tissue
61570	Remove foreign body brain
61571	Incise skull for brain wound
61575	Skull base/brainstem surgery
61576	Skull base/brainstem surgery
61580	Craniofacial approach skull
61581	Craniofacial approach skull
61582	Craniofacial approach skull
61583	Craniofacial approach skull
61584	Orbitocranial approach/skull
61585	Orbitocranial approach/skull
61586	Resect nasopharynx skull
61590	Infratemporal approach/skull
61591	Infratemporal approach/skull
61592	Orbitocranial approach/skull
61595	Transtemporal approach/skull
61596	Transcochlear approach/skull
61597	Transcondylar approach/skull
61598	Transpetrosal approach/skull

61600	Resect/excise cranial lesion
61601	Resect/excise cranial lesion
61605	Resect/excise cranial lesion
61606	Resect/excise cranial lesion
61607	Resect/excise cranial lesion
61608	Resect/excise cranial lesion
61611	Transect artery sinus
61613	Remove aneurysm sinus
61615	Resect/excise lesion skull
61616	Resect/excise lesion skull
61618	Repair dura
61619	Repair dura
61630	Intracranial angioplasty
61635	Intracran angioplsty w/stent
61645	Perq art m-thrombect &/nfs
61650	Evasc prlng admn rx agnt 1st
61651	Evasc prlng admn rx agnt add
61680	Intracranial vessel surgery
61682	Intracranial vessel surgery
61684	Intracranial vessel surgery
61686	Intracranial vessel surgery
61690	Intracranial vessel surgery
61692	Intracranial vessel surgery
61697	Brain aneurysm repr complx
61698	Brain aneurysm repr complx
61700	Brain aneurysm repr simple
61702	Inner skull vessel surgery
61703	Clamp neck artery
61705	Revise circulation to head
61708	Revise circulation to head
61710	Revise circulation to head
61711	Fusion of skull arteries
61735	Incise skull/brain surgery
61750	Incise skull/brain biopsy
61751	Brain biopsy w/ct/mr guide
61760	Implant brain electrodes
61850	Implant neuroelectrodes
61860	Implant neuroelectrodes
61863	Implant neuroelectrode
61864	Implant neuroelectrde addl
61867	Implant neuroelectrode
61868	Implant neuroelectrde addl
62005	Treat skull fracture
62010	Treatment of head injury
62100	Repair brain fluid leakage
62115	Reduction of skull defect
62117	Reduction of skull defect
62120	Repair skull cavity lesion
62121	Incise skull repair
62140	Repair of skull defect
62141	Repair of skull defect
62142	Remove skull plate/flap
62143	Replace skull plate/flap
62145	Repair of skull & brain
62146	Repair of skull with graft
62147	Repair of skull with graft
62148	Retr bone flap to fix skull
62161	Dissect brain w/scope
62162	Remove colloid cyst w/scope
62164	Remove brain tumor w/scope
62165	Remove pituit tumor w/scope
62180	Establish brain cavity shunt
62190	Establish brain cavity shunt
62192	Establish brain cavity shunt
62200	Establish brain cavity shunt
62201	Brain cavity shunt w/scope
62220	Establish brain cavity shunt
62223	Establish brain cavity shunt
62256	Remove brain cavity shunt
62258	Replace brain cavity shunt
63050	Cervical laminoplsty 2/> seg
63051	C-laminoplasty w/graft/plate
63077	Spine disk surgery thorax
63078	Spine disk surgery thorax
63081	Remove vert body dcmprn crvl
63082	Remove vertebral body add-on
63085	Remove vert body dcmprn thrc
63086	Remove vertebral body add-on
63087	Remov vertbr dcmprn thrclmbr
63088	Remove vertebral body add-on
63090	Remove vert body dcmprn lmbr
63091	Remove vertebral body add-on
63101	Remove vert body dcmprn thrc
63102	Remove vert body dcmprn lmbr
63103	Remove vertebral body add-on
63170	Incise spinal cord tract(s)
63172	Drainage of spinal cyst
63173	Drainage of spinal cyst
63185	Incise spine nrv half segmnt
63190	Incise spine nrv >2 segmnts
63191	Incise spine accessory nerve
63194	Incise spine & cord cervical
63195	Incise spine & cord thoracic
63196	Incise spine&cord 2 trx crvl
63197	Incise spine&cord 2 trx thrc
63198	Incise spin&cord 2 stgs crvl
63199	Incise spin&cord 2 stgs thrc
63200	Release spinal cord lumbar
63250	Revise spinal cord vsls crvl
63251	Revise spinal cord vsls thrc
63252	Revise spine cord vsl thrlmb
63270	Excise intrspinl lesion crvl
63271	Excise intrspinl lesion thrc
63272	Excise intrspinl lesion lmbr
63273	Excise intrspinl lesion scrl
63275	Bx/exc xdrl spine lesn crvl
63276	Bx/exc xdrl spine lesn thrc
63277	Bx/exc xdrl spine lesn lmbr
63278	Bx/exc xdrl spine lesn scrl
63280	Bx/exc idrl spine lesn crvl
63281	Bx/exc idrl spine lesn thrc
63282	Bx/exc idrl spine lesn lmbr
63283	Bx/exc idrl spine lesn scrl
63285	Bx/exc idrl imed lesn cervl
63286	Bx/exc idrl imed lesn thrc
63287	Bx/exc idrl imed lesn thrlmb
63290	Bx/exc xdrl/idrl lsn any lvl
63295	Repair laminectomy defect
63300	Remove vert xdrl body crvcl
63301	Remove vert xdrl body thrc
63302	Remove vert xdrl body thrlmb
63303	Remov vert xdrl bdy lmbr/sac
63304	Remove vert idrl body crvcl
63305	Remove vert idrl body thrc
63306	Remov vert idrl bdy thrclmbr
63307	Remov vert idrl bdy lmbr/sac
63308	Remove vertebral body add-on
63700	Repair of spinal herniation
63702	Repair of spinal herniation
63704	Repair of spinal herniation
63706	Repair of spinal herniation
63707	Repair spinal fluid leakage
63709	Repair spinal fluid leakage
63710	Graft repair of spine defect
63740	Install spinal shunt
64755	Incision of stomach nerves
64760	Incision of vagus nerve
64809	Remove sympathetic nerves
64818	Remove sympathetic nerves
64866	Fusion of facial/other nerve
64868	Fusion of facial/other nerve
65273	Repair of eye wound
69155	Extensive ear/neck surgery
69535	Remove part of temporal bone
69554	Remove ear lesion
69950	Incise inner ear nerve
75956	Xray endovasc thor ao repr
75957	Xray endovasc thor ao repr
75958	Xray place prox ext thor ao
75959	Xray place dist ext thor ao
92941	Prq card revasc mi 1 vsl
92970	Cardioassist internal
92971	Cardioassist external
92975	Dissolve clot heart vessel
93583	Perq transcath septal reduxn
99184	Hypothermia ill neonate
99190	Special pump services
99191	Special pump services
99192	Special pump services
99356	Prolonged service inpatient
99357	Prolonged service inpatient
99462	Sbsq nb em per day hosp
99468	Neonate crit care initial
99469	Neonate crit care subsq
99471	Ped critical care initial
99472	Ped critical care subsq
99475	Ped crit care age 2-5 init
99476	Ped crit care age 2-5 subsq
99477	Init day hosp neonate care
99478	Ic lbw inf < 1500 gm subsq
99479	Ic lbw inf 1500-2500 g subsq
99480	Ic inf pbw 2501-5000 g subsq
C9606	PC H rev ac tot/subtot occl 1 ves
G0341	Percutaneous islet celltrans
G0342	Laparoscopy islet cell trans
G0343	Laparotomy islet cell transp
0656T	Vrt bdy tethering ant
0657T	Vrt bdy tethering ant 8+ seg
0659T	Tcat intra-c nfs supersat o2

Appendix K — Place of Service and Type of Service

Place-of-Service Codes for Professional Claims

Listed below are place of service codes and descriptions. These codes should be used on professional claims to specify the entity where service(s) were rendered. Check with individual payers (e.g., Medicare, Medicaid, other private insurance) for reimbursement policies regarding these codes. Comments or questions regarding place-of-service codes or descriptions should be directed to your Medicare administrative contractor (MAC).

01	Pharmacy	A facility or location where drugs and other medically related items and services are sold, dispensed, or otherwise provided directly to patients.
02	Telehealth Provided Other than in Patient's Home	The location where health services and health related services are provided or received, through telecommunication technology. Patient is not located in their home when receiving health services or health related services through telecommunication technology.
03	School	A facility whose primary purpose is education.
04	Homeless Shelter	A facility or location whose primary purpose is to provide temporary housing to homeless individuals (e.g., emergency shelters, individual or family shelters).
05	Indian Health Service Free-Standing Facility	A facility or location, owned and operated by the Indian Health Service, which provides diagnostic, therapeutic (surgical and non-surgical), and rehabilitation services to American Indians and Alaska Natives who do not require hospitalization.
06	Indian Health Service Provider-based Facility	A facility or location, owned and operated by the Indian Health Service, which provides diagnostic, therapeutic (surgical and nonsurgical), and rehabilitation services rendered by, or under the supervision of, physicians to American Indians and Alaska Natives admitted as inpatients or outpatients.
07	Tribal 638 Free-Standing Facility	A facility or location owned and operated by a federally recognized American Indian or Alaska Native tribe or tribal organization under a 638 agreement, which provides diagnostic, therapeutic (surgical and nonsurgical), and rehabilitation services to tribal members who do not require hospitalization.
08	Tribal 638 Provider-based Facility	A facility or location owned and operated by a federally recognized American Indian or Alaska Native tribe or tribal organization under a 638 agreement, which provides diagnostic, therapeutic (surgical and nonsurgical), and rehabilitation services to tribal members admitted as inpatients or outpatients.
09	Prison/Correctional Facility	A prison, jail, reformatory, work farm, detention center, or any other similar facility maintained by either Federal, State or local authorities for the purpose of confinement or rehabilitation of adult or juvenile criminal offenders.
10	Telehealth Provided in Patient's Home	The location where health services and health related services are provided or received, through telecommunication technology. Patient is located in their home (which is a location other than a hospital or other facility where the patient receives care in a private residence) when receiving health services or health related services through telecommunication technology.
11	Office	Location, other than a hospital, skilled nursing facility (SNF), military treatment facility, community health center, State or local public health clinic, or intermediate care facility (ICF), where the health professional routinely provides health examinations, diagnosis, and treatment of illness or injury on an ambulatory basis.
12	Home	Location, other than a hospital or other facility, where the patient receives care in a private residence.
13	Assisted Living Facility	Congregate residential facility with self-contained living units providing assessment of each resident's needs and on-site support 24 hours a day, 7 days a week, with the capacity to deliver or arrange for services including some health care and other services.
14	Group Home	A residence, with shared living areas, where clients receive supervision and other services such as social and/or behavioral services, custodial service, and minimal services (e.g., medication administration).
15	Mobile Unit	A facility/unit that moves from place-to-place equipped to provide preventive, screening, diagnostic, and/or treatment services.
16	Temporary Lodging	A short-term accommodation such as a hotel, campground, hostel, cruise ship or resort where the patient receives care, and which is not identified by any other POS code.
17	Walk-in Retail Health Clinic	A walk-in health clinic, other than an office, urgent care facility, pharmacy, or independent clinic and not described by any other place of service code, that is located within a retail operation and provides, on an ambulatory basis, preventive and primary care services.
18	Place of Employment-Worksite	A location, not described by any other POS code, owned or operated by a public or private entity where the patient is employed, and where a health professional provides on-going or episodic occupational medical, therapeutic or rehabilitative services to the individual.

19	Off Campus-Outpatient Hospital	A portion of an off-campus hospital provider based department which provides diagnostic, therapeutic (both surgical and nonsurgical), and rehabilitation services to sick or injured persons who do not require hospitalization or institutionalization.
20	Urgent Care Facility	Location, distinct from a hospital emergency room, an office, or a clinic, whose purpose is to diagnose and treat illness or injury for unscheduled, ambulatory patients seeking immediate medical attention.
21	Inpatient Hospital	A facility, other than psychiatric, which primarily provides diagnostic, therapeutic (both surgical and nonsurgical), and rehabilitation services by, or under, the supervision of physicians to patients admitted for a variety of medical conditions.
22	On Campus-Outpatient Hospital	A portion of a hospital's main campus which provides diagnostic, therapeutic (both surgical and nonsurgical), and rehabilitation services to sick or injured persons who do not require hospitalization or institutionalization.
23	Emergency Room—Hospital	A portion of a hospital where emergency diagnosis and treatment of illness or injury is provided.
24	Ambulatory Surgical Center	A freestanding facility, other than a physician's office, where surgical and diagnostic services are provided on an ambulatory basis.
25	Birthing Center	A facility, other than a hospital's maternity facilities or a physician's office, which provides a setting for labor, delivery, and immediate post-partum care as well as immediate care of new born infants.
26	Military Treatment Facility	A medical facility operated by one or more of the Uniformed Services. Military Treatment Facility (MTF) also refers to certain former U.S. Public Health Service (USPHS) facilities now designated as Uniformed Service Treatment Facilities (USTF).
27-30	Unassigned	N/A
31	Skilled Nursing Facility	A facility which primarily provides inpatient skilled nursing care and related services to patients who require medical, nursing, or rehabilitative services but does not provide the level of care or treatment available in a hospital.
32	Nursing Facility	A facility which primarily provides to residents skilled nursing care and related services for the rehabilitation of injured, disabled, or sick persons, or, on a regular basis, health-related care services above the level of custodial care to individuals other than those with intellectual disabilities.
33	Custodial Care Facility	A facility which provides room, board, and other personal assistance services, generally on a long-term basis, and which does not include a medical component.
34	Hospice	A facility, other than a patient's home, in which palliative and supportive care for terminally ill patients and their families is provided.
35-40	Unassigned	N/A
41	Ambulance—Land	A land vehicle specifically designed, equipped and staffed for lifesaving and transporting the sick or injured.
42	Ambulance—Air or Water	An air or water vehicle specifically designed, equipped and staffed for lifesaving and transporting the sick or injured.
43-48	Unassigned	N/A
49	Independent Clinic	A location, not part of a hospital and not described by any other Place of Service code, that is organized and operated to provide preventive, diagnostic, therapeutic, rehabilitative, or palliative services to outpatients only.
50	Federally Qualified Health Center	A facility located in a medically underserved area that provides Medicare beneficiaries with preventive primary medical care under the general direction of a physician.
51	Inpatient Psychiatric Facility	A facility that provides inpatient psychiatric services for the diagnosis and treatment of mental illness on a 24-hour basis, by or under the supervision of a physician.
52	Psychiatric Facility-Partial Hospitalization	A facility for the diagnosis and treatment of mental illness that provides a planned therapeutic program for patients who do not require full time hospitalization, but who need broader programs than are possible from outpatient visits to a hospital-based or hospital-affiliated facility.
53	Community Mental Health Center	A facility that provides the following services: outpatient services, including specialized outpatient services for children, the elderly, individuals who are chronically ill, and residents of the CMHC's mental health services area who have been discharged from inpatient treatment at a mental health facility; 24 hour a day emergency care services; day treatment, other partial hospitalization services, or psychosocial rehabilitation services; screening for patients being considered for admission to State mental health facilities to determine the appropriateness of such admission; and consultation and education services.
54	Intermediate Care Facility/Individuals with Intellectual Disabilities	A facility which primarily provides health-related care and services above the level of custodial care to individuals but does not provide the level of care or treatment available in a hospital or SNF.
55	Residential Substance Abuse Treatment Facility	A facility which provides treatment for substance (alcohol and drug) abuse to live-in residents who do not require acute medical care. Services include individual and group therapy and counseling, family counseling, laboratory tests, drugs and supplies, psychological testing, and room and board.
56	Psychiatric Residential Treatment Center	A facility or distinct part of a facility for psychiatric care which provides a total 24-hour therapeutically planned and professionally staffed group living and learning environment.

57	Non-residential Substance Abuse Treatment Facility	A location which provides treatment for substance (alcohol and drug) abuse on an ambulatory basis. Services include individual and group therapy and counseling, family counseling, laboratory tests, drugs and supplies, and psychological testing.
58	Non-residential Opioid Treatment Facility	A location that provides treatment for opioid use disorder on an ambulatory basis. Services include methadone and other forms of Medication Assisted Treatment (MAT).
59	Unassigned	N/A
60	Mass Immunization Center	A location where providers administer pneumococcal pneumonia and influenza virus vaccinations and submit these services as electronic media claims, paper claims, or using the roster billing method. This generally takes place in a mass immunization setting, such as, a public health center, pharmacy, or mall but may include a physician office setting.
61	Comprehensive Inpatient Rehabilitation Facility	A facility that provides comprehensive rehabilitation services under the supervision of a physician to inpatients with physical disabilities. Services include physical therapy, occupational therapy, speech pathology, social or psychological services, and orthotics and prosthetics services.
62	Comprehensive Outpatient Rehabilitation Facility	A facility that provides comprehensive rehabilitation services under the supervision of a physician to outpatients with physical disabilities. Services include physical therapy, occupational therapy, and speech pathology services.
63-64	Unassigned	N/A
65	End-Stage Renal Disease Treatment Facility	A facility other than a hospital, which provides dialysis treatment, maintenance, and/or training to patients or caregivers on an ambulatory or home-care basis.
66-70	Unassigned	N/A
71	Public Health Clinic	A facility maintained by either State or local health departments that provides ambulatory primary medical care under the general direction of a physician.
72	Rural Health Clinic	A certified facility which is located in a rural medically underserved area that provides ambulatory primary medical care under the general direction of a physician.
73-80	Unassigned	N/A
81	Independent Laboratory	A laboratory certified to perform diagnostic and/or clinical tests independent of an institution or a physician's office.
82-98	Unassigned	N/A
99	Other Place of Service	Other place of service not identified above.

Type of Service

Common Working File Type of Service (TOS) Indicators

For submitting a claim to the Common Working File (CWF), use the following table to assign the proper TOS. Some procedures may have more than one applicable TOS. CWF will reject codes with incorrect TOS designations. CWF will produce alerts on codes with incorrect TOS designations.

The only exceptions to this annual update are:

- Surgical services billed for dates of service through December 31, 2007, containing the ASC facility service modifier SG must be reported as TOS F. Effective for services on or after January 1, 2008, the SG modifier is no longer applicable for Medicare services. ASC providers should discontinue applying the SG modifier on ASC facility claims. The indicator F does not appear in the TOS table because its use depends upon claims submitted with POS 24 (ASC facility) from an ASC (specialty 49). This became effective for dates of service January 1, 2008, or after.
- Surgical services billed with an assistant-at-surgery modifier (80-82, AS) must be reported with TOS 8. The 8 indicator does not appear on the TOS table because its use is dependent upon the use of the appropriate modifier. (See Pub. 100-4 *Medicare Claims Processing Manual,* chapter 12, "Physician/Practitioner Billing," for instructions on when assistant-at-surgery is allowable.)
- TOS H appears in the list of descriptors. However, it does not appear in the table. In CWF, "H" is used only as an indicator for hospice. The contractor should not submit TOS H to CWF at this time.
- For outpatient services, when a transfusion medicine code appears on a claim that also contains a blood product, the service is paid under reasonable charge at 80 percent; coinsurance and deductible apply. When transfusion medicine codes are paid under the clinical laboratory fee schedule they are paid at 100 percent; coinsurance and deductible do not apply.

Note: For injection codes with more than one possible TOS designation, use the following guidelines when assigning the TOS:

When the choice is L or 1:

- Use TOS L when the drug is used related to ESRD; or
- Use TOS 1 when the drug is not related to ESRD and is administered in the office.

When the choice is G or 1:

- Use TOS G when the drug is an immunosuppressive drug; or
- Use TOS 1 when the drug is used for other than immunosuppression.

When the choice is P or 1:

- Use TOS P if the drug is administered through durable medical equipment (DME); or
- Use TOS 1 if the drug is administered in the office.

The place of service or diagnosis may be considered when determining the appropriate TOS. The descriptors for each of the TOS codes listed in the annual HCPCS update are:

0	Whole blood
1	Medical care
2	Surgery
3	Consultation
4	Diagnostic radiology
5	Diagnostic laboratory
6	Therapeutic radiology
7	Anesthesia
8	Assistant at surgery
9	Other medical items or services
A	Used durable medical equipment (DME)
D	Ambulance
E	Enteral/parenteral nutrients/supplies
F	Ambulatory surgical center (facility usage for surgical services)
G	Immunosuppressive drugs
J	Diabetic shoes
K	Hearing items and services
L	ESRD supplies
M	Monthly capitation payment for dialysis
N	Kidney donor

P Lump sum purchase of DME, prosthetics, orthotics

Q Vision items or services

R Rental of DME

S Surgical dressings or other medical supplies

T Outpatient mental health limitation

U Occupational therapy

V Pneumococcal/flu vaccine

W Physical therapy

Appendix L — Multianalyte Assays with Algorithmic Analyses

The following tables contain the Administrative Codes for Multianalyte Assays with Algorithmic Analyses (MAAA), Category I codes for MAAA and the most current list of Proprietary Laboratory Analysis (PLA) codes.

The following is a list of MAAA procedures that are usually exclusive to one single clinical laboratory or manufacturer. These tests use the results from several different assays, including molecular pathology assays, fluorescent in situ hybridization assays, and nonnucleic acid-based assays (e.g., proteins, polypeptides, lipids, and carbohydrates) to perform an algorithmic analysis that is reported as a numeric score or probability. Although the laboratory report may list results of individual component tests of the MAAAs, these assays are not separately reportable.

The following list includes the proprietary name and clinical laboratory/manufacturer, an alphanumeric code, and the code descriptor.

The format for the code descriptor usually includes:

- Type of disease (e.g., oncology, autoimmune, tissue rejection)
- Chemical(s) analyzed (e.g., DNA, RNA, protein, antibody)
- Number of markers (e.g., number of genes, number of proteins)
- Methodology(s) (e.g., microarray, real-time [RT]-PCR, in situ hybridization [ISH], enzyme linked immunosorbent assays [ELISA])
- Number of functional domains (when indicated)
- Type of specimen (e.g., blood, fresh tissue, formalin-fixed paraffin embedded)
- Type of algorithm result (e.g., prognostic, diagnostic)
- Report (e.g., probability index, risk score)

MAAA procedures with a Category I code are noted on the following list and can also be found in code range 81500–81599 in the pathology and laboratory chapter. If a specific MAAA test does not have a Category I code, it is denoted with a four-digit number and the letter M. Use code 81599 if an MAAA test is not included on the following list or in the Category I codes. The codes on the list are exclusive to the assays identified by proprietary name. Report code 81599 also when an analysis is performed that may possibly fall within a specific descriptor but the proprietary name is not included in the list. The list does not contain all MAAA procedures.

Proprietary Name/Clinical Laboratory/Manufacturer	Code	Descriptor
Administrative Codes for Multianalyte Assays with Algorithmic Analyses (MAAA)		
ASH FibroSURE™, BioPredictive S.A.S	0002M	Liver disease, ten biochemical assays (ALT, A2-macroglobulin, apolipoprotein A-1, total bilirubin, GGT, haptoglobin, AST, glucose, total cholesterol and triglycerides) utilizing serum, prognostic algorithm reported as quantitative scores for fibrosis, steatosis and alcoholic steatohepatitis (ASH)
NASH FibroSURE™, BioPredictive S.A.S	0003M	Liver disease, ten biochemical assays (ALT, A2-macroglobulin, apolipoprotein A-1, total bilirubin, GGT, haptoglobin, AST, glucose, total cholesterol and triglycerides) utilizing serum, prognostic algorithm reported as quantitative scores for fibrosis, steatosis and nonalcoholic steatohepatitis (NASH)
ScoliScore™ Transgenomic	0004M	Scoliosis, DNA analysis of 53 single nucleotide polymorphisms (SNPs), using saliva, prognostic algorithm reported as a risk score
HeproDX™, GoPath Laboratories, LLC	0006M	Oncology (hepatic), mRNA expression levels of 161 genes, utilizing fresh hepatocellular carcinoma tumor tissue, with alpha-fetoprotein level, algorithm reported as a risk classifier
NETest, Wren Laboratories, LLC	0007M	Oncology (gastrointestinal neuroendocrine tumors), real-time PCR expression analysis of 51 genes, utilizing whole peripheral blood, algorithm reported as a nomogram of tumor disease index
	(0009M has been deleted)	
NeoLAB™ Prostate Liquid Biopsy, NeoGenomics Laboratories	0011M	Oncology, prostate cancer, mRNA expression assay of 12 genes (10 content and 2 housekeeping), RT-PCR test utilizing blood plasma and urine, algorithms to predict high-grade prostate cancer risk
Cxbladder™ Detect, Pacific Edge Diagnostics USA, Ltd	0012M	Oncology (urothelial), mRNA, gene expression profiling by real-time quantitative PCR of five genes (*MDK, HOXA13, CDC2 [CDK1], IGFBP5*, and *CXCR2*), utilizing urine, algorithm reported as a risk score for having urothelial carcinoma
Cxbladder™ Monitor, Pacific Edge Diagnostics USA, Ltd	0013M	Oncology (urothelial), mRNA, gene expression profiling by real-time quantitative PCR of five genes (*MDK, HOXA13, CDC2 [CDK1], IGFBP5*, and *CXCR2*), utilizing urine, algorithm reported as a risk score for having recurrent urothelial carcinoma
Enhanced Liver Fibrosis™ (ELF™) Test, Siemens Healthcare Diagnostics Inc/Siemens Healthcare Laboratory LLC	0014M	Liver disease, analysis of 3 biomarkers (hyaluronic acid [HA], procollagen III amino terminal peptide [PIIINP], tissue inhibitor of metalloproteinase 1 [TIMP-1]), using immunoassays, utilizing serum, prognostic algorithm reported as a risk score and risk of liver fibrosis and liver-related clinical events within 5 years
Adrenal Mass Panel, 24 Hour, Urine, Mayo Clinic Laboratories (MCL), Mayo Clinic	0015M	Adrenal cortical tumor, biochemical assay of 25 steroid markers, utilizing 24-hour urine specimen and clinical parameters, prognostic algorithm reported as a clinical risk and integrated clinical steroid risk for adrenal cortical carcinoma, adenoma, or other adrenal malignancy
Decipher Bladder TURBT®, Decipher Biosciences, Inc	0016M	Oncology (bladder), mRNA, microarray gene expression profiling of 209 genes, utilizing formalin fixed paraffin-embedded tissue, algorithm reported as molecular subtype (luminal, luminal infiltrated, basal, basal claudin-low, neuroendocrine-like)
Lymph2Cx, Mayo Clinic Arizona Molecular Diagnostics Laboratory CPT Excludes: Lymph3Cx Lymphoma Molecular Subtyping Assay, Mayo Clinic, Laboratory Developed Test (0120U)	● 0017M	Oncology (diffuse large B-cell lymphoma [DLBCL]), mRNA, gene expression profiling by fluorescent probe hybridization of 20 genes, formalin-fixed paraffin-embedded tissue, algorithm reported as cell of origin

Proprietary Name/Clinical Laboratory/Manufacturer	Code	Descriptor
Pleximark™ Plexision, Inc CPT Excludes: Blood count (85032); Cryopreservation (88240); Flow cytometry (88184-88185, 88187); HLA typing (86821); Lymphocyte transformation, mitogen, antigen induced blastogenesis (86353); Thawing, expansion frozen cells (88241); Tissue cultures, nonneoplastic disorders (88230); Transplantation rejection risk score (81560)	● 0018M	Transplantation medicine (allograft rejection, renal), measurement of donor and third-party-induced CD154+T-cytotoxic memory cells, utilizing whole peripheral blood, algorithm reported as a rejection risk score
Category I Codes for Multianalyte Assays with Algorithmic Analyses (MAAA)		
Vectra® DA, Crescendo Bioscience, Inc	81490	Autoimmune (rheumatoid arthritis), analysis of 12 biomarkers using immunoassays, utilizing serum, prognostic algorithm reported as a disease activity score
AlloMap®, CareDx, Inc	# 81595	Cardiology (heart transplant), mRNA, gene expression profiling by real-time quantitative PCR of 20 genes (11 content and 9 housekeeping), utilizing subfraction of peripheral blood, algorithm reported as a rejection risk score
Corus® CAD, CardioDx, Inc	81493	Coronary artery disease, mRNA, gene expression profiling by real-time RT-PCR of 23 genes, utilizing whole peripheral blood, algorithm reported as a risk score
PreDx Diabetes Risk Score™, Tethys Clinical Laboratory	81506	Endocrinology (type 2 diabetes), biochemical assays of seven analytes (glucose, HbA1c, insulin, hs-CRP, adiponectin, ferritin, interleukin 2-receptor alpha), utilizing serum or plasma, algorithm reporting a risk score
Harmony™ Prenatal Test, Ariosa Diagnostics	81507	Fetal aneuploidy (trisomy 21, 18, and 13) DNA sequence analysis of selected regions using maternal plasma, algorithm reported as a risk score for each trisomy
No proprietary name and clinical laboratory or manufacturer. Maternal serum screening procedures are performed by many labs and are not exclusive to a single facility.	81508	Fetal congenital abnormalities, biochemical assays of two proteins (PAPP-A, hCG [any form]), utilizing maternal serum, algorithm reported as a risk score
	81509	Fetal congenital abnormalities, biochemical assays of three proteins (PAPP-A, hCG [any form], DIA), utilizing maternal serum, algorithm reported as a risk score
	81510	Fetal congenital abnormalities, biochemical assays of three analytes (AFP, uE3, hCG [any form]), utilizing maternal serum, algorithm reported as a risk score
	81511	Fetal congenital abnormalities, biochemical assays of four analytes (AFP, uE3, hCG [any form], DIA) utilizing maternal serum, algorithm reported as a risk score (may include additional results from previous biochemical testing)
	81512	Fetal congenital abnormalities, biochemical assays of five analytes (AFP, uE3, total hCG, hyperglycosylated hCG, DIA) utilizing maternal serum, algorithm reported as a risk score
Aptima® BV Assay, Hologic, Inc	81513	Infectious disease, bacterial vaginosis, quantitative real-time amplification of RNA markers for Atopobium vaginae, Gardnerella vaginalis, and Lactobacillus species, utilizing vaginal-fluid specimens, algorithm reported as a positive or negative result for bacterial vaginosis
BD MAX™ Vaginal Panel, Becton Dickson and Company	81514	Infectious disease, bacterial vaginosis and vaginitis, quantitative real-time amplification of DNA markers for Gardnerella vaginalis, Atopobium vaginae, Megasphaera type 1, Bacterial Vaginosis Associated Bacteria-2 (BVAB-2), and Lactobacillus species (L. crispatus and L. jensenii), utilizing vaginal-fluid specimens, algorithm reported as a positive or negative for high likelihood of bacterial vaginosis, includes separate detection of Trichomonas vaginalis and/or Candida species (C. albicans, C. tropicalis, C. parapsilosis, C. dubliniensis), Candida glabrata, Candida krusei, when reported
HCV FibroSURE™, FibroTest™, BioPredictive S.A.S.	# 81596	Infectious disease, chronic hepatitis C virus (HCV) infection, six biochemical assays (ALT, A2-macroglobulin, apolipoprotein A-1, total bilirubin, GGT, and haptoglobin) utilizing serum, prognostic algorithm reported as scores for fibrosis and necroinflammatory activity in liver
Breast Cancer Index, Biotheranostics, Inc	81518	Oncology (breast), mRNA, gene expression profiling by real-time RT-PCR of 11 genes (7 content and 4 housekeeping), utilizing formalin-fixed paraffin-embedded tissue, algorithms reported as percentage risk for metastatic recurrence and likelihood of benefit from extended endocrine therapy
EndoPredict®, Myriad Genetic Laboratories, Inc	# 81522	Oncology (breast), mRNA, gene expression profiling by RT-PCR of 12 genes (8 content and 4 housekeeping), utilizing formalin-fixed paraffin-embedded tissue, algorithm reported as recurrence risk score
Oncotype DX® Genomic Health	81519	Oncology (breast), mRNA, gene expression profiling by real-time RT-PCR of 21 genes, utilizing formalin-fixed paraffin embedded tissue, algorithm reported as recurrence score
Prosigna® Breast Cancer Assay, NanoString Technologies, Inc	81520	Oncology (breast), mRNA gene expression profiling by hybrid capture of 58 genes (50 content and 8 housekeeping), utilizing formalin-fixed paraffin-embedded tissue, algorithm reported as a recurrence risk score
MammaPrint®, Agendia, Inc	81521	Oncology (breast), mRNA, microarray gene expression profiling of 70 content genes and 465 housekeeping genes, utilizing fresh frozen or formalin-fixed paraffin-embedded tissue, algorithm reported as index related to risk of distant metastasis
MammaPrint®, Agendia, Inc	● 81523	Oncology (breast), mRNA, next-generation sequencing gene expression profiling of 70 content genes and 31 housekeeping genes, utilizing formalin-fixed paraffin-embedded tissue, algorithm reported as index related to risk to distant metastasis

Proprietary Name/Clinical Laboratory/Manufacturer	Code	Descriptor
Oncotype DX® Colon Cancer Assay, Genomic Health CPT Excludes: Oncology (breast), mRNA, next-generation sequencing gene expression profiling, when performed on same specimen (81523).	81525	Oncology (colon), mRNA, gene expression profiling by real-time RT-PCR of 12 genes (7 content and 5 housekeeping), utilizing formalin-fixed paraffin-embedded tissue, algorithm reported as a recurrence score
Cologuard™, Exact Sciences, Inc	81528	Oncology (colorectal) screening, quantitative real-time target and signal amplification of 10 DNA markers (*KRAS* mutations, promoter methylation of *NDRG4* and *BMP3*) and fecal hemoglobin, utilizing stool, algorithm reported as a positive or negative result
DecisionDx® Melanoma, Castle Biosciences, Inc	81529	Oncology (cutaneous melanoma), mRNA, gene expression profiling by real-time RT-PCR of 31 genes (28 content and 3 housekeeping), utilizing formalin-fixed paraffin-embedded tissue, algorithm reported as recurrence risk, including likelihood of sentinel lymph node metastasis
ChemoFX®, Helomics, Corp	81535	Oncology (gynecologic), live tumor cell culture and chemotherapeutic response by DAPI stain and morphology, predictive algorithm reported as a drug response score; first single drug or drug combination
ChemoFX®, Helomics, Corp	+ 81536	each additional single drug or drug combination (List separately in addition to code for primary procedure)
VeriStrat, Biodesix, Inc	81538	Oncology (lung), mass spectrometric 8-protein signature, including amyloid A, utilizing serum, prognostic and predictive algorithm reported as good versus poor overall survival
Risk of Ovarian Malignancy Algorithm (ROMA)™, Fujirebio Diagnostics	# 81500	Oncology (ovarian), biochemical assays of two proteins (CA-125 and HE4), utilizing serum, with menopausal status, algorithm reported as a risk score
OVA1™, Vermillion, Inc	# 81503	Oncology (ovarian), biochemical assays of five proteins (CA-125, apolipoprotein A1, beta-2 microglobulin, transferrin, and pre-albumin), utilizing serum, algorithm reported as a risk score
4Kscore test, OPKO Health, Inc	81539	Oncology (high-grade prostate cancer), biochemical assay of four proteins (Total PSA, Free PSA, Intact PSA, and human kallikrein-2 [hK2]), utilizing plasma or serum, prognostic algorithm reported as a probability score
Prolaris®, Myriad Genetic Laboratories, Inc	81541	Oncology (prostate), mRNA gene expression profiling by real-time RT-PCR of 46 genes (31 content and 15 housekeeping), utilizing formalin-fixed paraffin-embedded tissue, algorithm reported as a disease-specific mortality risk score
Decipher® Prostate, Decipher® Biosciences	81542	Oncology (prostate), mRNA, microarray gene expression profiling of 22 content genes, utilizing formalin-fixed paraffin-embedded tissue, algorithm reported as metastasis risk score
	(81545 has been deleted)	
ConfirmMDx® for Prostate Cancer, MDxHealth, Inc	81551	Oncology (prostate), promoter methylation profiling by real-time PCR of 3 genes (*GSTP1, APC, RASSF1*), utilizing formalin-fixed paraffin-embedded tissue, algorithm reported as a likelihood of prostate cancer detection on repeat biopsy
Afirma® Genomic Sequencing Classifier, Veracyte, Inc	# 81546	Oncology (thyroid), mRNA, gene expression analysis of 10,196 genes, utilizing fine needle aspirate, algorithm reported as a categorical result (eg, benign or suspicious)
Tissue of Origin Test, Kit-FFPE, Cancer Genetics, Inc	# 81504	Oncology (tissue of origin), microarray gene expression profiling of >2000 genes, utilizing formalin-fixed paraffin-embedded tissue, algorithm reported as tissue similarity scores
CancerTYPE ID, bioTheranostics, Inc	# 81540	Oncology (tumor of unknown origin), mRNA, gene expression profiling by real-time RT-PCR of 92 genes (87 content and 5 housekeeping) to classify tumor into main cancer type and subtype, utilizing formalin-fixed paraffin-embedded tissue, algorithm reported as a probability of a predicted main cancer type and subtype
DecisionDx®-UM test, Castle Biosciences, Inc	81552	Oncology (uveal melanoma), mRNA, gene expression profiling by real-time RT-PCR of 15 genes (12 content and 3 housekeeping), utilizing fine needle aspirate or formalin-fixed paraffin-embedded tissue, algorithm reported as risk of metastasis
Envisia® Genomic Classifier, Veracyte, Inc	81554	Pulmonary disease (idiopathic pulmonary fibrosis [IPF]), mRNA, gene expression analysis of 190 genes, utilizing transbronchial biopsies, diagnostic algorithm reported as categorical result (eg, positive or negative for high probability of usual interstitial pneumonia [UIP])
Pleximmune™; Plexision, Inc	● 81560	Transplantation medicine (allograft rejection, pediatric liver and small bowel), measurement of donor and third-party-induced CD154+T-cytotoxic memory cells, utilizing whole peripheral blood, algorithm reported as a rejection risk score
	81599	Unlisted multianalyte assay with algorithmic analysis
Proprietary Laboratory Analyses (PLA)		
PreciseType® HEA Test, Immucor, Inc	0001U	Red blood cell antigen typing, DNA, human erythrocyte antigen gene analysis of 35 antigens from 11 blood groups, utilizing whole blood, common RBC alleles reported
PolypDX™, Atlantic Diagnostic Laboratories, LLC, Metabolomic Technologies, Inc	0002U	Oncology (colorectal), quantitative assessment of three urine metabolites (ascorbic acid, succinic acid and carnitine) by liquid chromatography with tandem mass spectrometry (LC-MS/MS) using multiple reaction monitoring acquisition, algorithm reported as likelihood of adenomatous polyps

Proprietary Name/Clinical Laboratory/Manufacturer	Code	Descriptor
Overa (OVA1 Next Generation), Aspira Labs, Inc, Vermillion, Inc	0003U	Oncology (ovarian) biochemical assays of five proteins (apolipoprotein A-1, CA 125 II, follicle stimulating hormone, human epididymis protein 4, transferrin), utilizing serum, algorithm reported as a likelihood score
ExosomeDx®, Prostate (IntelliScore), Exosome Diagnostics, Inc, Exosome Diagnostics, Inc	0005U	Oncology (prostate) gene expression profile by real-time RT-PCR of 3 genes *ERG*, *PCA3*, and *SPDEF*), urine, algorithm reported as risk score
	(0006U has been deleted)	
ToxProtect, Genotox Laboratories LTD	0007U	Drug test(s), presumptive, with definitive confirmation of positive results, any number of drug classes, urine, includes specimen verification including DNA authentication in comparison to buccal DNA, per date of service.
AmHPR® H. pylori Antibiotic Resistance Panel, American Molecular Laboratories, Inc	0008U	Helicobacter pylori detection and antibiotic resistance, DNA, 16S and 23S rRNA, gyrA, pbp1,rdxA and rpoB, next generation sequencing, formalin-fixed paraffin-embedded or fresh tissue or fecal sample, predictive, reported as positive or negative for resistance to clarithromycin, fluoroquinolones, metronidazole, amoxicillin, tetracycline, and rifabutin
DEPArray™ HER2, PacificDx	0009U	Oncology (breast cancer), *ERBB2* (HER2) copy number by FISH, tumor cells from formalin-fixed paraffin-embedded tissue isolated using image-based dielectrophoresis (DEP) sorting, reported as *ERBB2* gene amplified or non-amplified
Bacterial Typing by Whole Genome Sequencing, Mayo Clinic	0010U	Infectious disease (bacterial), strain typing by whole genome sequencing, phylogenetic-based report of strain relatedness, per submitted isolate
Cordant CORE™, Cordant Health Solutions	0011U	Prescription drug monitoring, evaluation of drugs present by LC-MS/MS, using oral fluid, reported as a comparison to an estimated steady-state range, per date of service including all drug compounds and metabolites
MatePair Targeted Rearrangements, Congenital, Mayo Clinic	0012U	Germline disorders, gene rearrangement detection by whole genome next-generation sequencing, DNA, whole blood, report of specific gene rearrangement(s)
MatePair Targeted Rearrangements, Oncology, Mayo Clinic	0013U	Oncology (solid organ neoplasia), gene rearrangement detection by whole genome next-generation sequencing, DNA, fresh or frozen tissue or cells, report of specific gene rearrangement(s)
MatePair Targeted Rearrangements, Hematologic, Mayo Clinic	0014U	Hematology (hematolymphoid neoplasia), gene rearrangement detection by whole genome next-generation sequencing, DNA, whole blood or bone marrow, report of specific gene rearrangement(s)
BCR-ABL1 major and minor breakpoint fusion transcripts, University of Iowa, Department of Pathology, Asuragen	0016U	Oncology (hematolymphoid neoplasia), RNA, *BCR/ABL1* major and minor breakpoint fusion transcripts, quantitative PCR amplification, blood or bone marrow, report of fusion not detected or detected with quantitation
JAK2 Mutation, University of Iowa, Department of Pathology	0017U	Oncology (hematolymphoid neoplasia), *JAK2* mutation, DNA, PCR amplification of exons 12-14 and sequence analysis, blood or bone marrow, report of *JAK2* mutation not detected or detected
ThyraMIR™, Interpace Diagnostics	0018U	Oncology (thyroid), microRNA profiling by RT-PCR of 10 microRNA sequences, utilizing fine needle aspirate, algorithm reported as a positive or negative result for moderate to high risk of malignancy
OncoTarget/OncoTreat, Columbia University Department of Pathology and Cell Biology, Darwin Health	0019U	Oncology, RNA, gene expression by whole transcriptome sequencing, formalin-fixed paraffin embedded tissue or fresh frozen tissue, predictive algorithm reported as potential targets for therapeutic agents
	(0020U has been deleted)	
Apifiny®, Armune BioScience, Inc	0021U	Oncology (prostate), detection of 8 autoantibodies (ARF 6, NKX3-1, 5'-UTR-BMI1, CEP 164, 3'-UTR-Ropporin, Desmocollin, AURKAIP-1, CSNK2A2), multiplexed immunoassay and flow cytometry serum, algorithm reported as risk score
Oncomine™ Dx Target Test, Thermo Fisher Scientific	0022U	Targeted genomic sequence analysis panel, non-small cell lung neoplasia, DNA and RNA analysis, 23 genes, interrogation for sequence variants and rearrangements, reported as presence/absence of variants and associated therapy(ies) to consider
LeukoStrat® CDx *FLT3* Mutation Assay, LabPMM LLC, an Invivoscribe Technologies, Inc Company, Invivoscribe Technologies, Inc	0023U	Oncology (acute myelogenous leukemia), DNA, genotyping of internal tandem duplication, p.D835, p.I836, using mononuclear cells, reported as detection or non-detection of *FLT3* mutation and indication for or against the use of midostaurin
GlycA, Laboratory Corporation of America, Laboratory Corporation of America	0024U	Glycosylated acute phase proteins (GlycA), nuclear magnetic resonance spectroscopy, quantitative
UrSure Tenofovir Quantification Test, Synergy Medical Laboratories, UrSure Inc	0025U	Tenofovir, by liquid chromatography with tandem mass spectrometry (LC-MS/MS), urine, quantitative
Thyroseq Genomic Classifier, CBLPath, Inc, University of Pittsburgh Medical Center	0026U	Oncology (thyroid), DNA and mRNA of 112 genes, next-generation sequencing, fine needle aspirate of thyroid nodule, algorithmic analysis reported as a categorical result ("Positive, high probability of malignancy" or "Negative, low probability of malignancy")
JAK2 Exons 12 to 15 Sequencing, Mayo Clinic, Mayo Clinic	0027U	*JAK2 (Janus kinase 2)* (eg, myeloproliferative disorder) gene analysis, targeted sequence analysis exons 12-15
	(0028U has been deleted)	
Focused Pharmacogenomics Panel, Mayo Clinic, Mayo Clinic	0029U	Drug metabolism (adverse drug reactions and drug response), targeted sequence analysis (ie, *CYP1A2*, *CYP2C19*, *CYP2C9*, *CYP2D6*, *CYP3A4*, *CYP3A5*, *CYP4F2*, *SLCO1B1*, *VKORC1* and rs12777823)

Proprietary Name/Clinical Laboratory/Manufacturer	Code	Descriptor
Warfarin Response Genotype, Mayo Clinic, Mayo Clinic	0030U	Drug metabolism (warfarin drug response), targeted sequence analysis (i.e., *CYP2C9, CYP4F2, VKORC1*, rs12777823)
Cytochrome P450 1A2 Genotype, Mayo Clinic, Mayo Clinic	0031U	*CYP1A2 (cytochrome P450 family 1, subfamily A, member 2)* (eg, drug metabolism) gene analysis, common variants (ie, *1F, *1K, *6, *7)
Catechol-O-Methyltransferase *(COMT)* Genotype, Mayo Clinic, Mayo Clinic	0032U	*COMT (catechol-O-methyltransferase)* (eg, drug metabolism) gene analysis, c.472G>A (rs4680) variant
Serotonin Receptor Genotype *(HTR2A* and *HTR2C)*, Mayo Clinic, Mayo Clinic	0033U	*HTR2A (5-hydroxytryptamine receptor 2A), HTR2C (5-hydroxytryptamine receptor 2C)* (eg, citalopram metabolism) gene analysis, common variants (i.e., *HTR2A* rs7997012 [c.614-2211T>C], *HTR2C* rs3813929 [c.- 759C>T] and rs1414334 [c.551-3008C>G])
Thiopurine Methyltransferase *(TPMT)* and Nudix Hydrolase *(NUDT15)* Genotyping, Mayo Clinic, Mayo Clinic	0034U	*TPMT (thiopurine S-methyltransferase), NUDT15 (nudix hydroxylase 15)* (eg, thiopurine metabolism) gene analysis, common variants (i.e., *TPMT* *2, *3A, *3B, *3C, *4, *5, *6, *8, *12; *NUDT15* *3, *4, *5)
Real-time quaking-induced conversion for prion detection (RT QuIC), National Prion Disease Pathology Surveillance Center	0035U	Neurology (prion disease), cerebrospinal fluid, detection of prion protein by quaking induced conformational conversion, qualitative
EXaCT-1 Whole Exome Testing, Lab of Oncology-Molecular Detection, Weill Cornell Medicine- Clinical Genomics Laboratory	0036U	Exome (ie, somatic mutations), paired formalin-fixed paraffin-embedded tumor tissue and normal specimen, sequence analyses
FoundationOne CDx™ (F1CDx), Foundation Medicine, Inc, Foundation Medicine, Inc	0037U	Targeted genomic sequence analysis, solid organ neoplasm, DNA analysis of 324 genes, interrogation for sequence variants, gene copy number amplifications, gene rearrangements, microsatellite instability and tumor mutational burden
Sensieva ™ Droplet 25OH Vitamin D2/D3 Microvolume LC/MS Assay, InSource Diagnostics, InSource Diagnostics	0038U	Vitamin D, 25 hydroxy D2 and D3, by LC- MS/MS, serum microsample, quantitative
Anti-dsDNA, High Salt/Avidity, University of Washington, Department of Laboratory Medicine, Bio-Rad	0039U	Deoxyribonucleic acid (DNA) antibody, double stranded, high avidity
MRDx BCR-ABL Test, MolecularMD, MolecularMD	0040U	*BCR/ABL1 (t(9;22))* (eg, chronic myelogenous leukemia) translocation analysis, major breakpoint, quantitative
Lyme ImmunoBlot IgM, IGeneX Inc, ID-FISH Technology Inc (ASR) (Lyme ImmunoBlot IgM Strips Only)	0041U	Borrelia burgdorferi, antibody detection of 5 recombinant protein groups, by immunoblot, IgM
Lyme ImmunoBlot IgG, IGeneX Inc, ID-FISH Technology Inc (ASR) (Lyme ImmunoBlot IgG Strips Only)	0042U	Borrelia burgdorferi, antibody detection of 12 recombinant protein groups, by immunoblot, IgG
Tick-Borne Relapsing Fever (TBRF) Borrelia ImmunoBlots IgM Test, IGeneX Inc, ID-FISH Technology Inc (Provides TBRF ImmunoBlot IgM Strips)	0043U	Tick-borne relapsing fever Borrelia group, antibody detection to 4 recombinant protein groups, by immunoblot, IgM
Tick-Borne Relapsing Fever (TBRF) Borrelia ImmunoBlots IgG Test, IGeneX Inc, ID-FISH Technology Inc (Provides TBRF ImmunoBlot IgG Strips)	0044U	Tick-borne relapsing fever Borrelia group, antibody detection to 4 recombinant protein groups, by immunoblot, IgG
The Oncotype DX® Breast DCIS Score™ Test, Genomic Health, Inc, Genomic Health, Inc	0045U	Oncology (breast ductal carcinoma in situ), mRNA, gene expression profiling by real- time RT-PCR of 12 genes (7 content and 5 housekeeping), utilizing formalin-fixed paraffin-embedded tissue, algorithm reported as recurrence score
FLT3 ITD MRD by NGS, LabPMM LLC, an Invivoscribe Technologies, Inc Company	0046U	*FLT3 (fms-related tyrosine kinase 3)* (eg, acute myeloid leukemia) internal tandem duplication (ITD) variants, quantitative
Oncotype DX Genomic Prostate Score, Genomic Health, Inc, Genomic Health, Inc	0047U	Oncology (prostate), mRNA, gene expression profiling by real-time RT-PCR of 17 genes (12 content and 5 housekeeping), utilizing formalin-fixed paraffin-embedded tissue, algorithm reported as a risk score
MSK-IMPACT (Integrated Mutation Profiling of Actionable Cancer Targets), Memorial Sloan Kettering Cancer Center	0048U	Oncology (solid organ neoplasia), DNA, targeted sequencing of protein-coding exons of 468 cancer-associated genes, including interrogation for somatic mutations and microsatellite instability, matched with normal specimens, utilizing formalin-fixed paraffin-embedded tumor tissue, report of clinically significant mutation(s)
NPM1 MRD by NGS, LabPMM LLC, an Invivoscribe Technologies, Inc Company	0049U	*NPM1 (nucleophosmin)* (eg, acute myeloid leukemia) gene analysis, quantitative
MyAML NGS Panel, LabPMM LLC, an Invivoscribe Technologies, Inc Company	0050U	Targeted genomic sequence analysis panel, acute myelogenous leukemia, DNA analysis, 194 genes, interrogation for sequence variants, copy number variants or rearrangements
UCompliDx, Elite Medical Laboratory Solutions, LLC, Elite Medical Laboratory Solutions, LLC (LDT)	▲ 0051U	Prescription drug monitoring, evaluation of drugs present by liquid chromatography tandem mass spectrometry (LC-MS/MS), urine or blood, 31 drug panel, reported as quantitative results, detected or not detected, per date of service
VAP Cholesterol Test, VAP Diagnostics Laboratory, Inc, VAP Diagnostics Laboratory, Inc	0052U	Lipoprotein, blood, high resolution fractionation and quantitation of lipoproteins, including all five major lipoprotein classes and subclasses of HDL, LDL, and VLDL by vertical auto profile ultracentrifugation
Prostate Cancer Risk Panel, Mayo Clinic, Laboratory Developed Test	0053U	Oncology (prostate cancer), FISH analysis of 4 genes (*ASAP1, HDAC9, CHD1 and PTEN*), needle biopsy specimen, algorithm reported as probability of higher tumor grade
AssuranceRx Micro Serum, Firstox Laboratories, LLC, Firstox Laboratories, LLC	0054U	Prescription drug monitoring, 14 or more classes of drugs and substances, definitive tandem mass spectrometry with chromatography, capillary blood, quantitative report with therapeutic and toxic ranges, including steady-state range for the prescribed dose when detected, per date of service

Proprietary Name/Clinical Laboratory/Manufacturer	Code	Descriptor
myTAIHEART, TAI Diagnostics, Inc, TAI Diagnostics, Inc	0055U	Cardiology (heart transplant), cell-free DNA, PCR assay of 96 DNA target sequences (94 single nucleotide polymorphism targets and two control targets), plasma
MatePair Acute Myeloid Leukemia Panel, Mayo Clinic, Laboratory Developed Test	0056U	Hematology (acute myelogenous leukemia), DNA, whole genome next- generation sequencing to detect gene rearrangement(s), blood or bone marrow, report of specific gene rearrangement(s)
	(0057U has been deleted)	
Merkel SmT Oncoprotein Antibody Titer, University of Washington, Department of Laboratory Medicine	0058U	Oncology (Merkel cell carcinoma), detection of antibodies to the Merkel cell polyoma virus oncoprotein (small T antigen), serum, quantitative
Merkel Virus VP1 Capsid Antibody, University of Washington, Department of Laboratory Medicine	0059U	Oncology (Merkel cell carcinoma), detection of antibodies to the Merkel cell polyoma virus capsid protein (VP1), serum, reported as positive or negative
Twins Zygosity PLA, Natera, Inc, Natera, Inc	0060U	Twin zygosity, genomic-targeted sequence analysis of chromosome 2, using circulating cell-free fetal DNA in maternal blood
Transcutaneous multispectral measurement of tissue oxygenation and hemoglobin using spatial frequency domain imaging (SFDI), Modulated Imaging, Inc, Modulated Imaging, Inc	0061U	Transcutaneous measurement of five biomarkers (tissue oxygenation [StO2], oxyhemoglobin [ctHbO2], deoxyhemoglobin [ctHbR], papillary and reticular dermal hemoglobin concentrations [ctHb1 and ctHb2]), using spatial frequency domain imaging (SFDI) and multi-spectral analysis
SLE-key® Rule Out, Veracis Inc, Veracis Inc	0062U	Autoimmune (systemic lupus erythematosus), IgG and IgM analysis of 80 biomarkers, utilizing serum, algorithm reported with a risk score
NPDX ASD ADM Panel I, Stemina Biomarker Discovery, Inc, Stemina Biomarker Discovery, Inc d/b/a NeuroPointDX	0063U	Neurology (autism), 32 amines by LC-MS/MS, using plasma, algorithm reported as metabolic signature associated with autism spectrum disorder
BioPlex 2200 Syphilis Total & RPR Assay, Bio-Rad Laboratories, Bio-Rad Laboratories	0064U	Antibody, Treponema pallidum, total and rapid plasma reagin (RPR), immunoassay, qualitative
BioPlex 2200 RPR Assay, Bio-Rad Laboratories, Bio-Rad Laboratories	0065U	Syphilis test, non-treponemal antibody, immunoassay, qualitative (RPR)
PartoSure™ Test, Parsagen Diagnostics, Inc, Parsagen Diagnostics, Inc, a QIAGEN Company	0066U	Placental alpha-micro globulin-1 (PAMG-1), immunoassay with direct optical observation, cervico-vaginal fluid, each specimen
BBDRisk Dx™, Silbiotech, Inc, Silbiotech, Inc	0067U	Oncology (breast), immunohistochemistry, protein expression profiling of 4 biomarkers (matrix metalloproteinase-1 [MMP-1], carcinoembryonic antigen-related cell adhesion molecule 6 [CEACAM6], hyaluronoglucosaminidase [HYAL1], highly expressed in cancer protein [HEC1]), formalin-fixed paraffin-embedded precancerous breast tissue, algorithm reported as carcinoma risk score
MYCODART-PCR™ Dual Amplification Real Time PCR Panel for 6 Candida species, RealTime Laboratories, Inc/MycoDART, Inc, RealTime Laboratories, Inc	0068U	Candida species panel *(C. albicans, C. glabrata, C. parapsilosis, C. kruseii, C tropicalis, and C. auris)*, amplified probe technique with qualitative report of the presence or absence of each species
miR-31now™, GoPath Laboratories, GoPath Laboratories	0069U	Oncology (colorectal), microRNA, RT-PCR expression profiling of miR-31-3p, formalin-fixed paraffin-embedded tissue, algorithm reported as an expression score
CYP2D6 Common Variants and Copy Number, Mayo Clinic, Laboratory Developed Test	0070U	*CYP2D6 (cytochrome P450, family 2, subfamily D, polypeptide 6)* (eg, drug metabolism) gene analysis, common and select rare variants (ie, *2, *3, *4, *4N, *5, *6, *7, *8, *9, *10, *11, *12, *13, *14A, *14B, *15, *17, *29, *35, *36, *41, *57, *61, *63, *68, *83, *xN)
CYP2D6 Full Gene Sequencing, Mayo Clinic, Laboratory Developed Test	+ 0071U	*CYP2D6 (cytochrome P450, family 2, subfamily D, polypeptide 6)* (eg, drug metabolism) gene analysis, full gene sequence (List separately in addition to code for primary procedure)
CYP2D6-2D7 Hybrid Gene Targeted Sequence Analysis, Mayo Clinic, Laboratory Developed Test	+ 0072U	*CYP2D6 (cytochrome P450, family 2, subfamily D, polypeptide 6)* (eg, drug metabolism) gene analysis, targeted sequence analysis (ie, CYP2D6-2D7 hybrid gene) (List separately in addition to code for primary procedure)
CYP2D7-2D6 Hybrid Gene Targeted Sequence Analysis, Mayo Clinic, Laboratory Developed Test	+ 0073U	*CYP2D6 (cytochrome P450, family 2, subfamily D, polypeptide 6)* (eg, drug metabolism) gene analysis, targeted sequence analysis (ie, CYP2D7-2D6 hybrid gene) (List separately in addition to code for primary procedure)
CYP2D6 trans-duplication/multiplication non-duplicated gene targeted sequence analysis, Mayo Clinic, Laboratory Developed Test	+ 0074U	*CYP2D6 (cytochrome P450, family 2, subfamily D, polypeptide 6)* (eg, drug metabolism) gene analysis, targeted sequence analysis (ie, non-duplicated gene when duplication/multiplication is trans) (List separately in addition to code for primary procedure)
CYP2D6 5' gene duplication/multiplication targeted sequence analysis, Mayo Clinic, Laboratory Developed Test	+ 0075U	*CYP2D6 (cytochrome P450, family 2, subfamily D, polypeptide 6)* (eg, drug metabolism) gene analysis, targeted sequence analysis (ie, 5' gene duplication/multiplication) (List separately in addition to code for primary procedure)
CYP2D6 3' gene duplication/multiplication targeted sequence analysis, Mayo Clinic, Laboratory Developed Test	+ 0076U	*CYP2D6 (cytochrome P450, family 2, subfamily D, polypeptide 6)* (eg, drug metabolism) gene analysis, targeted sequence analysis (ie, 3' gene duplication/multiplication) (List separately in addition to code for primary procedure)
M-Protein Detection and Isotyping by MALDI-TOF Mass Spectrometry, Mayo Clinic, Laboratory Developed Test	0077U	Immunoglobulin paraprotein (M-protein), qualitative, immunoprecipitation and mass spectrometry, blood or urine, including isotype
INFINITI® Neural Response Panel, PersonalizeDx Labs, AutoGenomics Inc	0078U	Pain management (opioid-use disorder) genotyping panel, 16 common variants (ie, *ABCB1, COMT, DAT1, DBH, DOR, DRD1, DRD2, DRD4, GABA, GAL, HTR2A, HTTLPR, MTHFR, MUOR, OPRK1, OPRM1*), buccal swab or other germline tissue sample, algorithm reported as positive or negative risk of opioid-use disorder
ToxLok™, InSource Diagnostics, InSource Diagnostics	0079U	Comparative DNA analysis using multiple selected single-nucleotide polymorphisms (SNPs), urine and buccal DNA, for specimen identity verification

Proprietary Name/Clinical Laboratory/Manufacturer	Code	Descriptor
BDX-XL2, Biodesix®, Inc, Biodesix®, Inc	0080U	Oncology (lung), mass spectrometric analysis of galectin-3-binding protein and scavenger receptor cysteine-rich type 1 protein M130, with five clinical risk factors (age, smoking status, nodule diameter, nodule-spiculation status and nodule location), utilizing plasma, algorithm reported as a categorical probability of malignancy
	(0081U has been deleted. To report, use 81552)	
NextGen Precision™ Testing, Precision Diagnostics, Precision Diagnostics LBN Precision Toxicology, LLC	0082U	Drug test(s), definitive, 90 or more drugs or substances, definitive chromatography with mass spectrometry, and presumptive, any number of drug classes, by instrument chemistry analyzer (utilizing immunoassay), urine, report of presence or absence of each drug, drug metabolite or substance with description and severity of significant interactions per date of service
Onco4D™, Animated Dynamics, Inc, Animated Dynamics, Inc	0083U	Oncology, response to chemotherapy drugs using motility contrast tomography, fresh or frozen tissue, reported as likelihood of sensitivity or resistance to drugs or drug combinations
BLOODchip®, ID CORE XT™, Grifols Diagnostic Solutions Inc	0084U	Red blood cell antigen typing, DNA, genotyping of 10 blood groups with phenotype prediction of 37 red blood cell antigens
	(0085U has been deleted)	
Accelerate PhenoTest™ BC kit, Accelerate Diagnostics, Inc	0086U	Infectious disease (bacterial and fungal), organism identification, blood culture, using rRNA FISH, 6 or more organism targets, reported as positive or negative with phenotypic minimum inhibitory concentration (MIC)-based antimicrobial susceptibility
Molecular Microscope® MMDx—Heart, Kashi Clinical Laboratories	0087U	Cardiology (heart transplant), mRNA gene expression profiling by microarray of 1283 genes, transplant biopsy tissue, allograft rejection and injury algorithm reported as a probability score
Molecular Microscope® MMDx—Kidney, Kashi Clinical Laboratories	0088U	Transplantation medicine (kidney allograft rejection), microarray gene expression profiling of 1494 genes, utilizing transplant biopsy tissue, algorithm reported as a probability score for rejection
Pigmented Lesion Assay (PLA), DermTech	0089U	Oncology (melanoma), gene expression profiling by RTqPCR, *PRAME* and *LINC00518*, superficial collection using adhesive patch(es)
myPath® Melanoma, Myriad Genetic Laboratories	0090U	Oncology (cutaneous melanoma), mRNA gene expression profiling by RT-PCR of 23 genes (14 content and 9 housekeeping), utilizing formalin-fixed paraffin-embedded tissue, algorithm reported as a categorical result (ie, benign, indeterminate, malignant)
FirstSight^{CRC}, CellMax Life	0091U	Oncology (colorectal) screening, cell enumeration of circulating tumor cells, utilizing whole blood, algorithm, for the presence of adenoma or cancer, reported as a positive or negative result
REVEAL Lung Nodule Characterization, MagArray, Inc	0092U	Oncology (lung), three protein biomarkers, immunoassay using magnetic nanosensor technology, plasma, algorithm reported as risk score for likelihood of malignancy
ComplyRX, Claro Labs	0093U	Prescription drug monitoring, evaluation of 65 common drugs by LC-MS/MS, urine, each drug reported detected or not detected
RCIGM Rapid Whole Genome Sequencing, Rady Children's Institute for Genomic Medicine (RCIGM)	0094U	Genome (eg, unexplained constitutional or heritable disorder or syndrome), rapid sequence analysis
Esophageal String Test™ (EST), Cambridge Biomedical, Inc	0095U	Inflammation (eosinophilic esophagitis), ELISA analysis of eotaxin-3 (*CCL26 [C-C motif chemokine ligand 26]*) and major basic protein (*PRG2 [proteoglycan 2, pro eosinophil major basic protein]*), specimen obtained by swallowed nylon string, algorithm reported as predictive probability index for active eosinophilic esophagitis
HPV, High-Risk, Male Urine, Molecular Testing Labs	0096U	Human papillomavirus (HPV), high-risk types (ie, 16, 18, 31, 33, 35, 39, 45, 51, 52, 56, 58, 59, 66, 68), male urine
BioFire® FilmArray® Gastrointestinal (GI) Panel, BioFire® Diagnostics	0097U	Gastrointestinal pathogen, multiplex reverse transcription and multiplex amplified probe technique, multiple types or subtypes, 22 targets (Campylobacter [C. jejuni/C. coli/C. upsaliensis], Clostridium difficile [C. difficile] toxin A/B, Plesiomonas shigelloides, Salmonella, Vibrio [V. parahaemolyticus/V. vulnificus/V. cholerae], including specific identification of Vibrio cholerae, Yersinia enterocolitica, Enteroaggregative Escherichia coli [EAEC], Enteropathogenic Escherichia coli [EPEC], Enterotoxigenic Escherichia coli [ETEC] lt/st, Shiga-like toxin-producing Escherichia coli [STEC] stx1/stx2 [including specific identification of the E. coli O157 serogroup within STEC], Shigella/Enteroinvasive Escherichia coli [EIEC], Cryptosporidium, Cyclospora cayetanensis, Entamoeba histolytica, Giardia lamblia [also known as G. intestinalis and G. duodenalis], adenovirus F 40/41, astrovirus, norovirus GI/GII, rotavirus A, sapovirus [Genogroups I, II, IV, and V])
	(0098U has been deleted)	
	(0099U has been deleted)	
	(0100U has been deleted)	
ColoNext®, Ambry Genetics®, Ambry Genetics®	0101U	Hereditary colon cancer disorders (eg, Lynch syndrome, *PTEN* hamartoma syndrome, Cowden syndrome, familial adenomatosis polyposis), genomic sequence analysis panel utilizing a combination of NGS, Sanger, MLPA, and array CGH, with MRNA analytics to resolve variants of unknown significance when indicated (15 genes [sequencing and deletion/duplication], *EPCAM* and *GREM1* [deletion/duplication only])

Proprietary Name/Clinical Laboratory/Manufacturer	Code	Descriptor
BreastNext®, Ambry Genetics®, Ambry Genetics®	0102U	Hereditary breast cancer-related disorders (eg, hereditary breast cancer, hereditary ovarian cancer, hereditary endometrial cancer), genomic sequence analysis panel utilizing a combination of NGS, Sanger, MLPA, and array CGH, with MRNA analytics to resolve variants of unknown significance when indicated (17 genes [sequencing and deletion/duplication])
OvaNext®, Ambry Genetics®, Ambry Genetics®	0103U	Hereditary ovarian cancer (eg, hereditary ovarian cancer, hereditary endometrial cancer), genomic sequence analysis panel utilizing a combination of NGS, Sanger, MLPA, and array CGH, with MRNA analytics to resolve variants of unknown significance when indicated (24 genes [sequencing and deletion/duplication], *EPCAM* [deletion/duplication only])
	(0104U has been deleted)	
KidneyIntelX™, RenalytixAI, RenalytixAI	0105U	Nephrology (chronic kidney disease), multiplex electrochemiluminescent immunoassay (ECLIA) of tumor necrosis factor receptor 1A, receptor superfamily 2 *(TNFR1, TNFR2)*, and kidney injury molecule-1 (KIM-1) combined with longitudinal clinical data, including *APOL1* genotype if available, and plasma (isolated fresh or frozen), algorithm reported as probability score for rapid kidney function decline (RKFD)
13C-Spirulina Gastric Emptying Breath Test (GEBT), Cairn Diagnostics d/b/a Advanced Breath Diagnostics, LLC, Cairn Diagnostics d/b/a Advanced Breath Diagnostics, LLC	0106U	Gastric emptying, serial collection of 7 timed breath specimens, non-radioisotope carbon-13(^{13}C) spirulina substrate, analysis of each specimen by gas isotope ratio mass spectrometry, reported as rate of $^{13}CO_2$ excretion
Singulex Clarity C.diff toxins A/B Assay, Singulex	0107U	Clostridium difficile toxin(s) antigen detection by immunoassay technique, stool, qualitative, multiple-step method
TissueCypher® Barrett's Esophagus Assay, Cernostics, Cernostics	0108U	Gastroenterology (Barrett's esophagus), whole slide-digital imaging, including morphometric analysis, computer-assisted quantitative immunolabeling of 9 protein biomarkers (p16, AMACR, p53, CD68, COX-2, CD45RO, HIF1a, HER-2, K20) and morphology, formalin-fixed paraffin-embedded tissue, algorithm reported as risk of progression to high-grade dysplasia or cancer
MYCODART Dual Amplification Real Time PCR Panel for 4 Aspergillus species, RealTime Laboratories, Inc/MycoDART, Inc	0109U	Infectious disease (Aspergillus species), real-time PCR for detection of DNA from 4 species *(A. fumigatus, A. terreus, A. niger,* and *A. flavus)*, blood, lavage fluid, or tissue, qualitative reporting of presence or absence of each species
Oral OncolyticAssuranceRX, Firstox Laboratories, LLC, Firstox Laboratories, LLC	0110U	Prescription drug monitoring, one or more oral oncology drug(s) and substances, definitive tandem mass spectrometry with chromatography, serum or plasma from capillary blood or venous blood, quantitative report with steady-state range for the prescribed drug(s) when detected
Praxis™ Extended RAS Panel, Illumina, Illumina	0111U	Oncology (colon cancer), targeted *KRAS* (codons 12, 13, and 61) and *NRAS* (codons 12, 13, and 61) gene analysis utilizing formalin-fixed paraffin-embedded tissue
MicroGenDX qPCR & NGS For Infection, MicroGenDX, MicroGenDX	0112U	Infectious agent detection and identification, targeted sequence analysis (16S and 18S rRNA genes) with drug-resistance gene
MiPS (Mi-Prostate Score), MLabs, MLabs	0113U	Oncology (prostate), measurement of *PCA3* and *TMPRSS2-ERG* in urine and PSA in serum following prostatic massage, by RNA amplification and fluorescence-based detection, algorithm reported as risk score
EsoGuard™, Lucid Diagnostics, Lucid Diagnostics	0114U	Gastroenterology (Barrett's esophagus), *VIM* and *CCNA1* methylation analysis, esophageal cells, algorithm reported as likelihood for Barrett's esophagus
ePlex Respiratory Pathogen (RP) Panel, GenMark Diagnostics, Inc, GenMark Diagnostics, Inc	0115U	Respiratory infectious agent detection by nucleic acid (DNA and RNA), 18 viral types and subtypes and 2 bacterial targets, amplified probe technique, including multiplex reverse transcription for RNA targets, each analyte reported as detected or not detected
Snapshot Oral Fluid Compliance, Ethos Laboratories	0116U	Prescription drug monitoring, enzyme immunoassay of 35 or more drugs confirmed with LC-MS/MS, oral fluid, algorithm results reported as a patient-compliance measurement with risk of drug to drug interactions for prescribed medications
Foundation PI℠, Ethos Laboratories	0117U	Pain management, analysis of 11 endogenous analytes (methylmalonic acid, xanthurenic acid, homocysteine, pyroglutamic acid, vanilmandelate, 5-hydroxyindoleacetic acid, hydroxymethylglutarate, ethylmalonate, 3-hydroxypropyl mercapturic acid (3-HPMA), quinolinic acid, kynurenic acid), LC-MS/MS, urine, algorithm reported as a pain-index score with likelihood of atypical biochemical function associated with pain
Viracor TRAC™ dd-cfDNA, Viracor Eurofins, Viracor Eurofins	0118U	Transplantation medicine, quantification of donor-derived cell-free DNA using whole genome next-generation sequencing, plasma, reported as percentage of donor-derived cell-free DNA in the total cell-free DNA
MI-HEART Ceramides, Plasma, Mayo Clinic, Laboratory Developed Test	0119U	Cardiology, ceramides by liquid chromatography-tandem mass spectrometry, plasma, quantitative report with risk score for major cardiovascular events
Lymph3Cx Lymphoma Molecular Subtyping Assay, Mayo Clinic, Laboratory Developed Test CPT Excludes: Oncology (diffuse large B-cell lymphoma [DLBCL]), mRNA, gene expression profiling by fluorescent probe hybridization of 20 genes (0017M)	0120U	Oncology (B-cell lymphoma classification), mRNA, gene expression profiling by fluorescent probe hybridization of 58 genes (45 content and 13 housekeeping genes), formalin-fixed paraffin-embedded tissue, algorithm reported as likelihood for primary mediastinal B-cell lymphoma (PMBCL) and diffuse large B-cell lymphoma (DLBCL) with cell of origin subtyping in the latter
Flow Adhesion of Whole Blood on VCAM-1 (FAB-V), Functional Fluidics, Functional Fluidics	0121U	Sickle cell disease, microfluidic flow adhesion (VCAM-1), whole blood
Flow Adhesion of Whole Blood to P-SELECTIN (WB-PSEL), Functional Fluidics, Functional Fluidics	0122U	Sickle cell disease, microfluidic flow adhesion (P-Selectin), whole blood

Proprietary Name/Clinical Laboratory/Manufacturer	Code	Descriptor
Mechanical Fragility, RBC by shear stress profiling and spectral analysis, Functional Fluidics, Functional Fluidics	0123U	Mechanical fragility, RBC, shear stress and spectral analysis profiling
	(0124U has been deleted)	
	(0125U has been deleted)	
	(0126U has been deleted)	
	(0127U has been deleted)	
	(0128U has been deleted)	
BRCAplus, Ambry Genetics	0129U	Hereditary breast cancer-related disorders (eg, hereditary breast cancer, hereditary ovarian cancer, hereditary endometrial cancer), genomic sequence analysis and deletion/duplication analysis panel (*ATM, BRCA1, BRCA2, CDH1, CHEK2, PALB2, PTEN,* and *TP53)*
+RNAinsight™ for ColoNext®, Ambry Genetics	+ 0130U	Hereditary colon cancer disorders (eg, Lynch syndrome, PTEN hamartoma syndrome, Cowden syndrome, familial adenomatosis polyposis), targeted mRNA sequence analysis panel *(APC, CDH1, CHEK2, MLH1, MSH2, MSH6, MUTYH, PMS2, PTEN,* and *TP53)* (List separately in addition to code for primary procedure)
+RNAinsight™ for BreastNext®, Ambry Genetics	+ 0131U	Hereditary breast cancer-related disorders (eg, hereditary breast cancer, hereditary ovarian cancer, hereditary endometrial cancer), targeted mRNA sequence analysis panel (13 genes) (List separately in addition to code for primary procedure)
+RNAinsight™ for OvaNext®, Ambry Genetics	+ 0132U	Hereditary ovarian cancer-related disorders (eg, hereditary breast cancer, hereditary ovarian cancer, hereditary endometrial cancer), targeted mRNA sequence analysis panel (17 genes) (List separately in addition to code for primary procedure)
+RNAinsight™ for ProstateNext®, Ambry Genetics	+ 0133U	Hereditary prostate cancer-related disorders, targeted mRNA sequence analysis panel (11 genes) (List separately in addition to code for primary procedure)
+RNAinsight™ for CancerNext®, Ambry Genetics	+ 0134U	Hereditary pan cancer (eg, hereditary breast and ovarian cancer, hereditary endometrial cancer, hereditary colorectal cancer), targeted mRNA sequence analysis panel (18 genes) (List separately in addition to code for primary procedure)
+RNAinsight™ for GYNPlus®, Ambry Genetics	+ 0135U	Hereditary gynecological cancer (eg, hereditary breast and ovarian cancer, hereditary endometrial cancer, hereditary colorectal cancer), targeted mRNA sequence analysis panel (12 genes) (List separately in addition to code for primary procedure)
+RNAinsight™ for *ATM*, Ambry Genetics	+ 0136U	*ATM (ataxia telangiectasia mutated)* (eg, ataxia telangiectasia) mRNA sequence analysis (List separately in addition to code for primary procedure)
+RNAinsight™ for *PALB2*, Ambry Genetics	+ 0137U	*PALB2 (partner and localizer of BRCA2)* (eg, breast and pancreatic cancer) mRNA sequence analysis (List separately in addition to code for primary procedure)
+RNAinsight™ for *BRCA1/2*, Ambry Genetics	+ 0138U	*BRCA1 (BRCA1, DNA repair associated), BRCA2 (BRCA2, DNA repair associated)* (eg, hereditary breast and ovarian cancer) mRNA sequence analysis (List separately in addition to code for primary procedure)
	(0139U has been deleted)	
ePlex® BCID Fungal Pathogens Panel, GenMark Diagnostics, Inc, GenMark Diagnostics, Inc	0140U	Infectious disease (fungi), fungal pathogen identification, DNA (15 fungal targets), blood culture, amplified probe technique, each target reported as detected or not detected
ePlex® BCID Gram-Positive Panel, GenMark Diagnostics, Inc, GenMark Diagnostics, Inc	0141U	Infectious disease (bacteria and fungi), gram-positive organism identification and drug resistance element detection, DNA (20 gram-positive bacterial targets, 4 resistance genes, 1 pan gram-negative bacterial target, 1 pan Candida target), blood culture, amplified probe technique, each target reported as detected or not detected
ePlex® BCID Gram-Negative Panel, GenMark Diagnostics, Inc, GenMark Diagnostics, Inc	0142U	Infectious disease (bacteria and fungi), gram-negative bacterial identification and drug resistance element detection, DNA (21 gram-negative bacterial targets, 6 resistance genes, 1 pan gram-positive bacterial target, 1 pan Candida target), amplified probe technique, each target reported as detected or not detected
CareViewRx, Newstar Medical Laboratories, LLC, Newstar Medical Laboratories, LLC CPT Excludes: PsychViewRx Plus analysis by Newstar Medical Laboratories, LLC. (0150U)	0143U	Drug assay, definitive, 120 or more drugs or metabolites, urine, quantitative liquid chromatography with tandem mass spectrometry (LC-MS/MS) using multiple reaction monitoring (MRM), with drug or metabolite description, comments including sample validation, per date of service
CareViewRx Plus, Newstar Medical Laboratories, LLC, Newstar Medical Laboratories, LLC	0144U	Drug assay, definitive, 160 or more drugs or metabolites, urine, quantitative liquid chromatography with tandem mass spectrometry (LC-MS/MS) using multiple reaction monitoring (MRM), with drug or metabolite description, comments including sample validation, per date of service
PainViewRx, Newstar Medical Laboratories, LLC, Newstar Medical Laboratories, LLC	0145U	Drug assay, definitive, 65 or more drugs or metabolites, urine, quantitative liquid chromatography with tandem mass spectrometry (LC-MS/MS) using multiple reaction monitoring (MRM), with drug or metabolite description, comments including sample validation, per date of service
PainViewRx Plus, Newstar Medical Laboratories, LLC, Newstar Medical Laboratories, LLC	0146U	Drug assay, definitive, 80 or more drugs or metabolites, urine, by quantitative liquid chromatography with tandem mass spectrometry (LC-MS/MS) using multiple reaction monitoring (MRM), with drug or metabolite description, comments including sample validation, per date of service

Proprietary Name/Clinical Laboratory/Manufacturer	Code	Descriptor
RiskViewRx, Newstar Medical Laboratories, LLC, Newstar Medical Laboratories, LLC	0147U	Drug assay, definitive, 85 or more drugs or metabolites, urine, quantitative liquid chromatography with tandem mass spectrometry (LC-MS/MS) using multiple reaction monitoring (MRM), with drug or metabolite description, comments including sample validation, per date of service
RiskViewRx Plus, Newstar Medical Laboratories, LLC, Newstar Medical Laboratories, LLC	0148U	Drug assay, definitive, 100 or more drugs or metabolites, urine, quantitative liquid chromatography with tandem mass spectrometry (LC-MS/MS) using multiple reaction monitoring (MRM), with drug or metabolite description, comments including sample validation, per date of service
PsychViewRx, Newstar Medical Laboratories, LLC, Newstar Medical Laboratories, LLC	0149U	Drug assay, definitive, 60 or more drugs or metabolites, urine, quantitative liquid chromatography with tandem mass spectrometry (LC-MS/MS) using multiple reaction monitoring (MRM), with drug or metabolite description, comments including sample validation, per date of service
PsychViewRx Plus, Newstar Medical Laboratories, LLC, Newstar Medical Laboratories, LLC CPT Excludes: CareViewRx analysis by Newstar Medical Laboratories, LLC. (0143U)	0150U	Drug assay, definitive, 120 or more drugs or metabolites, urine, quantitative liquid chromatography with tandem mass spectrometry (LC-MS/MS) using multiple reaction monitoring (MRM), with drug or metabolite description, comments including sample validation, per date of service
BioFire® FilmArray® Pneumonia Panel, BioFire® Diagnostics, BioFire® Diagnostics	0151U	Infectious disease (bacterial or viral respiratory tract infection), pathogen specific nucleic acid (DNA or RNA), 33 targets, real-time semi-quantitative PCR, bronchoalveolar lavage, sputum, or endotracheal aspirate, detection of 33 organismal and antibiotic resistance genes with limited semi-quantitative results
Karius® Test, Karius Inc, Karius Inc	▲ 0152U	Infectious disease (bacteria, fungi, parasites, and DNA viruses), microbial cell-free DNA, plasma, untargeted next-generation sequencing, report for significant positive pathogens
Insight TNBCtype™, Insight Molecular Labs	0153U	Oncology (breast), mRNA, gene expression profiling by next-generation sequencing of 101 genes, utilizing formalin-fixed paraffin-embedded tissue, algorithm reported as a triple negative breast cancer clinical subtype(s) with information on immune cell involvement
therascreen® *FGFR* RGQ RT-PCR Kit, QIAGEN, QIAGEN GmbH	0154U	Oncology (urothelial cancer), RNA, analysis by real-time RT-PCR of the *FGFR3 (fibroblast growth factor receptor3)* gene analysis (ie, p.R248C [c.742C>T], p.S249C [c.746C>G], p.G370C [c.1108G>T], p.Y373C [c.1118A>G], FGFR3-TACC3v1, and FGFR3-TACC3v3) utilizing formalin-fixed paraffin-embedded urothelial cancer tumor tissue, reported as *FGFR* gene alteration status
therascreen *PIK3CA* RGQ PCR Kit, QIAGEN, QIAGEN GmbH	0155U	Oncology (breast cancer), DNA, *PIK3CA (phosphatidylinositol-4,5-bisphosphate 3-kinase, catalytic subunit alpha)* (eg, breast cancer) gene analysis (ie, p.C420R, p.E542K, p.E545A, p.E545D [g.1635G>T only], p.E545G, p.E545K, p.Q546E, p.Q546R, p.H1047L, p.H1047R, p.H1047Y), utilizing formalin-fixed paraffin-embedded breast tumor tissue, reported as *PIK3CA* gene mutation status
SMASH™, New York Genome Center, Marvel Genomics™	0156U	Copy number (eg, intellectual disability, dysmorphology), sequence analysis
CustomNext + RNA: APC, Ambry Genetics®, Ambry Genetics®	+ 0157U	*APC (APC regulator of WNT signaling pathway)* (eg, familial adenomatosis polyposis [FAP]) mRNA sequence analysis (List separately in addition to code for primary procedure)
CustomNext + RNA: *MLH1,* Ambry Genetics®, Ambry Genetics®	+ 0158U	*MLH1 (mutL homolog 1)* (eg, hereditary non-polyposis colorectal cancer, Lynch syndrome) mRNA sequence analysis (List separately in addition to code for primary procedure)
CustomNext + RNA: *MSH2,* Ambry Genetics®, Ambry Genetics®	+ 0159U	*MSH2 (mutS homolog 2)* (eg, hereditary colon cancer, Lynch syndrome) mRNA sequence analysis (List separately in addition to code for primary procedure)
CustomNext + RNA: *MSH6,* Ambry Genetics®, Ambry Genetics®	+ 0160U	*MSH6 (mutS homolog 6)* (eg, hereditary colon cancer, Lynch syndrome) mRNA sequence analysis (List separately in addition to code for primary procedure)
CustomNext + RNA: *PMS2,* Ambry Genetics®, Ambry Genetics®	+ 0161U	*PMS2 (PMS1 homolog 2, mismatch repair system component)* (eg, hereditary non-polyposis colorectal cancer, Lynch syndrome) mRNA sequence analysis (List separately in addition to code for primary procedure)
CustomNext + RNA: Lynch *(MLH1, MSH2, MSH6, PMS2),* Ambry Genetics®, Ambry Genetics®	+ 0162U	Hereditary colon cancer (Lynch syndrome), targeted mRNA sequence analysis panel *(MLH1, MSH2, MSH6, PMS2)* (List separately in addition to code for primary procedure)
BeScreened™-CRC, Beacon Biomedical Inc, Beacon Biomedical Inc	0163U	Oncology (colorectal) screening, biochemical enzyme-linked immunosorbent assay (ELISA) of 3 plasma or serum proteins (teratocarcinoma derived growth factor-1 [TDGF-1, Cripto-1], carcinoembryonic antigen [CEA], extracellular matrix protein [ECM]), with demographic data (age, gender, CRC-screening compliance) using a proprietary algorithm and reported as likelihood of CRC or advanced adenomas
ibs-smart™, Gemelli Biotech, Gemelli Biotech	0164U	Gastroenterology (irritable bowel syndrome [IBS]), immunoassay for anti-CdtB and anti-vinculin antibodies, utilizing plasma, algorithm for elevated or not elevated qualitative results
VeriMAP™ Peanut Dx—Bead-based Epitope Assay, AllerGenis™ Clinical Laboratory, AllerGenis™ LLC	0165U	Peanut allergen-specific quantitative assessment of multiple epitopes using enzyme-linked immunosorbent assay (ELISA), blood, individual epitope results and interpretation probability of peanut allergy
LiverFASt™, Fibronostics, Fibronostics	0166U	Liver disease, 10 biochemical assays (a2-macroglobulin, haptoglobin, apolipoprotein A1, bilirubin, GGT, ALT, AST, triglycerides, cholesterol, fasting glucose) and biometric and demographic data, utilizing serum, algorithm reported as scores for fibrosis, necroinflammatory activity, and steatosis with a summary interpretation
ADEXUSDx hCG Test, NOWDiagnostics, NOWDiagnostics	0167U	Gonadotropin, chorionic (hCG), immunoassay with direct optical observation, blood

Proprietary Name/Clinical Laboratory/Manufacturer	Code	Descriptor
	(0168U has been deleted)	
NT (*NUDT15* and *TPMT*) genotyping panel, RPRD Diagnostics	0169U	*NUDT15 (nudix hydrolase 15)* and *TPMT (thiopurine S-methyltransferase)* (eg, drug metabolism) gene analysis, common variants
Clarifi™, Quadrant Biosciences, Inc, Quadrant Biosciences, Inc	0170U	Neurology (autism spectrum disorder [ASD]), RNA, next-generation sequencing, saliva, algorithmic analysis, and results reported as predictive probability of ASD diagnosis
MyMRD® NGS Panel, Laboratory for Personalized Molecular Medicine, Laboratory for Personalized Molecular Medicine	0171U	Targeted genomic sequence analysis panel, acute myeloid leukemia, myelodysplastic syndrome, and myeloproliferative neoplasms, DNA analysis, 23 genes, interrogation for sequence variants, rearrangements and minimal residual disease, reported as presence/absence
myChoice® CDx, Myriad Genetics Laboratories, Inc, Myriad Genetics Laboratories, Inc	0172U	Oncology (solid tumor as indicated by the label), somatic mutation analysis of *BRCA1 (BRCA1, DNA repair associated), BRCA2 (BRCA2, DNA repair associated)* and analysis of homologous recombination deficiency pathways, DNA, formalin-fixed paraffin-embedded tissue, algorithm quantifying tumor genomic instability score
Psych HealthPGx Panel, RPRD Diagnostics, RPRD Diagnostics	0173U	Psychiatry (ie, depression, anxiety), genomic analysis panel, includes variant analysis of 14 genes
LC-MS/MS Targeted Proteomic Assay, OncoOmicDx Laboratory, LDT	0174U	Oncology (solid tumor), mass spectrometric 30 protein targets, formalin-fixed paraffin-embedded tissue, prognostic and predictive algorithm reported as likely, unlikely, or uncertain benefit of 39 chemotherapy and targeted therapeutic oncology agents
Genomind® Professional PGx Express™ CORE, Genomind, Inc, Genomind, Inc	0175U	Psychiatry (eg, depression, anxiety), genomic analysis panel, variant analysis of 15 genes
IBSchek®, Commonwealth Diagnostics International, Inc, Commonwealth Diagnostics International, Inc	0176U	Cytolethal distending toxin B (CdtB) and vinculin IgG antibodies by immunoassay (ie, ELISA)
therascreen® *PIK3CA* RGQ PCR Kit, QIAGEN, QIAGEN GmbH	0177U	Oncology (breast cancer), DNA, *PIK3CA (phosphatidylinositol-4,5-bisphosphate 3-kinase catalytic subunit alpha)* gene analysis of 11 gene variants utilizing plasma, reported as PIK3CA gene mutation status
VeriMAP™ Peanut Reactivity Threshold Bead Based Epitope Assay, AllerGenis™ Clinical Laboratory, AllerGenis™ LLC	0178U	Peanut allergen-specific quantitative assessment of multiple epitopes using enzyme-linked immunosorbent assay (ELISA), blood, report of minimum eliciting exposure for a clinical reaction
Resolution ctDx Lung™, Resolution Bioscience, Resolution Bioscience, Inc	0179U	Oncology (non-small cell lung cancer), cell-free DNA, targeted sequence analysis of 23 genes (single nucleotide variations, insertions and deletions, fusions without prior knowledge of partner/breakpoint, copy number variations), with report of significant mutation(s)
Navigator ABO Sequencing, Grifols Immunohematology Center, Grifols Immunohematology Center	0180U	Red cell antigen (ABO blood group) genotyping *(ABO), gene analysis Sanger/chain termination/conventional sequencing, ABO (ABO, alpha 1-3-N-acetylgalactosaminyltransferase and alpha 1-3-galactosyltransferase)* gene, including subtyping, 7 exons
Navigator CO Sequencing, Grifols Immunohematology Center, Grifols Immunohematology Center	0181U	Red cell antigen (Colton blood group) genotyping (CO), gene analysis, *AQP1 (aquaporin 1 [Colton blood group])* exon 1
Navigator CROM Sequencing, Grifols Immunohematology Center, Grifols Immunohematology Center	0182U	Red cell antigen (Cromer blood group) genotyping (CROM), gene analysis, *CD55 (CD55 molecule [Cromer blood group])* exons 1-10
Navigator DI Sequencing, Grifols Immunohematology Center, Grifols Immunohematology Center	0183U	Red cell antigen (Diego blood group) genotyping (DI), gene analysis, *SLC4A1 (solute carrier family 4 member 1 [Diego blood group])* exon 19
Navigator DO Sequencing, Grifols Immunohematology Center, Grifols Immunohematology Center	0184U	Red cell antigen (Dombrock blood group) genotyping (DO), gene analysis, *ART4 (ADP-ribosyltransferase 4 [Dombrock blood group])* exon 2
Navigator FUT1 Sequencing, Grifols Immunohematology Center, Grifols Immunohematology Center	0185U	Red cell antigen (H blood group) genotyping (FUT1), gene analysis, *FUT1 (fucosyltransferase 1 [H blood group])* exon 4
Navigator FUT2 Sequencing, Grifols Immunohematology Center, Grifols Immunohematology Center	0186U	Red cell antigen (H blood group) genotyping (FUT2), gene analysis, *FUT2 (fucosyltransferase 2)* exon 2
Navigator FY Sequencing, Grifols Immunohematology Center, Grifols Immunohematology Center	0187U	Red cell antigen (Duffy blood group) genotyping (FY), gene analysis, *ACKR1 (atypical chemokine receptor 1 [Duffy blood group])* exons 1-2
Navigator GE Sequencing, Grifols Immunohematology Center, Grifols Immunohematology Center	0188U	Red cell antigen (Gerbich blood group) genotyping (GE), gene analysis, *GYPC (glycophorin C [Gerbich blood group])* exons 1-4
Navigator GYPA Sequencing, Grifols Immunohematology Center, Grifols Immunohematology Center	0189U	Red cell antigen (MNS blood group) genotyping (GYPA), gene analysis, *GYPA (glycophorin A [MNS blood group])* introns 1, 5, exon 2
Navigator GYPB Sequencing, Grifols Immunohematology Center, Grifols Immunohematology Center	0190U	Red cell antigen (MNS blood group) genotyping (GYPB), gene analysis, *GYPB (glycophorin B [MNS blood group])* introns 1, 5, pseudoexon 3
Navigator IN Sequencing, Grifols Immunohematology Center, Grifols Immunohematology Center	0191U	Red cell antigen (Indian blood group) genotyping (IN), gene analysis, *CD44 (CD44 molecule [Indian blood group])* exons 2, 3, 6
Navigator JK Sequencing, Grifols Immunohematology Center, Grifols Immunohematology Center	0192U	Red cell antigen (Kidd blood group) genotyping (JK), gene analysis, *SLC14A1 (solute carrier family 14 member 1 [Kidd blood group])* gene promoter, exon 9
Navigator JR Sequencing, Grifols Immunohematology Center, Grifols Immunohematology Center	0193U	Red cell antigen (JR blood group) genotyping (JR), gene analysis, *ABCG2 (ATP binding cassette subfamily G member 2 [Junior blood group])* exons 2-26
Navigator KEL Sequencing, Grifols Immunohematology Center, Grifols Immunohematology Center	0194U	Red cell antigen (Kell blood group) genotyping (KEL), gene analysis, *KEL (Kell metallo-endopeptidase [Kell blood group])* exon 8
Navigator *KLF1* Sequencing, Grifols Immunohematology Center, Grifols Immunohematology Center	0195U	*KLF1 (Kruppel-like factor 1)*, targeted sequencing (ie, exon 13)

Proprietary Name/Clinical Laboratory/Manufacturer	Code	Descriptor
Navigator LU Sequencing, Grifols Immunohematology Center, Grifols Immunohematology Center	0196U	Red cell antigen (Lutheran blood group) genotyping (LU), gene analysis, *BCAM (basal cell adhesion molecule [Lutheran blood group])* exon 3
Navigator LW Sequencing, Grifols Immunohematology Center, Grifols Immunohematology Center	0197U	Red cell antigen (Landsteiner-Wiener blood group) genotyping (LW), gene analysis, *ICAM4 (intercellular adhesion molecule 4 [Landsteiner-Wiener blood group])* exon 1
Navigator RHD/CE Sequencing, Grifols Immunohematology Center, Grifols Immunohematology Center	0198U	Red cell antigen (RH blood group) genotyping (RHD and RHCE), gene analysis Sanger/chain termination/conventional sequencing, *RHD (Rh blood group D antigen)* exons 1-10 and *RHCE (Rh blood group CcEe antigens)* exon 5
Navigator SC Sequencing, Grifols Immunohematology Center, Grifols Immunohematology Center	0199U	Red cell antigen (Scianna blood group) genotyping (SC), gene analysis, *ERMAP (erythroblast membrane associated protein [Scianna blood group])* exons 4, 12
Navigator XK Sequencing, Grifols Immunohematology Center, Grifols Immunohematology Center	0200U	Red cell antigen (Kx blood group) genotyping (XK), gene analysis, *XK (X-linked Kx blood group)* exons 1-3
Navigator YT Sequencing, Grifols Immunohematology Center, Grifols Immunohematology Center	0201U	Red cell antigen (Yt blood group) genotyping (YT), gene analysis, *ACHE (acetylcholinesterase [Cartwright blood group])* exon 2
BioFire® Respiratory Panel 2.1 (RP2.1), BioFire® Diagnostics, BioFire® Diagnostics, LLC CPT Excludes: QIAstat-Dx Respiratory SARS CoV-2 Panel, QIAGEN Sciences, QIAGEN GmbH. (0223U)	0202U	Infectious disease (bacterial or viral respiratory tract infection), pathogen-specific nucleic acid (DNA or RNA), 22 targets including severe acute respiratory syndrome coronavirus 2 (SARS-CoV-2), qualitative RT-PCR, nasopharyngeal swab, each pathogen reported as detected or not detected
PredictSURE IBD™ Test, KSL Diagnostics, PredictImmune Ltd	0203U	Autoimmune (inflammatory bowel disease), mRNA, gene expression profiling by quantitative RT-PCR, 17 genes (15 target and 2 reference genes), whole blood, reported as a continuous risk score and classification of inflammatory bowel disease aggressiveness
Afirma Xpression Atlas, Veracyte, Inc, Veracyte, Inc	0204U	Oncology (thyroid), mRNA, gene expression analysis of 593 genes (including *BRAF, RAS, RET, PAX8,* and *NTRK*) for sequence variants and rearrangements, utilizing fine needle aspirate, reported as detected or not detected
Vita Risk®, Arctic Medical Laboratories, Arctic Medical Laboratories	0205U	Ophthalmology (age-related macular degeneration), analysis of 3 gene variants (2 *CFH* gene, 1 *ARMS2* gene), using PCR and MALDI-TOF, buccal swab, reported as positive or negative for neovascular age-related macular-degeneration risk associated with zinc supplements
DISCERN™, NeuroDiagnostics, NeuroDiagnostics	0206U	Neurology (Alzheimer disease); cell aggregation using morphometric imaging and protein kinase C-epsilon (PKCe) concentration in response to amylospheroid treatment by ELISA, cultured skin fibroblasts, each reported as positive or negative for Alzheimer disease
DISCERN™, NeuroDiagnostics, NeuroDiagnostics	+ 0207U	quantitative imaging of phosphorylated *ERK1* and *ERK2* in response to bradykinin treatment by in situ immunofluorescence, using cultured skin fibroblasts, reported as a probability index for Alzheimer disease (List separately in addition to code for primary procedure)
Afirma Medullary Thyroid Carcinoma (MTC) Classifier, Veracyte, Inc, Veracyte, Inc	0208U	Oncology (medullary thyroid carcinoma), mRNA, gene expression analysis of 108 genes, utilizing fine needle aspirate, algorithm reported as positive or negative for medullary thyroid carcinoma
CNGnome™, PerkinElmer Genomics, PerkinElmer Genomics	0209U	Cytogenomic constitutional (genome-wide) analysis, interrogation of genomic regions for copy number, structural changes and areas of homozygosity for chromosomal abnormalities
BioPlex 2200 RPR Assay - Quantitative, Bio-Rad Laboratories, Bio-Rad Laboratories	0210U	Syphilis test, non-treponemal antibody, immunoassay, quantitative (RPR)
MI Cancer Seek™ - NGS Analysis, Caris MPI d/b/a Caris Life Sciences, Caris MPI d/b/a Caris Life Sciences	0211U	Oncology (pan-tumor), DNA and RNA by next-generation sequencing, utilizing formalin-fixed paraffin-embedded tissue, interpretative report for single nucleotide variants, copy number alterations, tumor mutational burden, and microsatellite instability, with therapy association
Genomic Unity® Whole Genome Analysis—Proband, Variantyx Inc, Variantyx Inc	0212U	Rare diseases (constitutional/heritable disorders), whole genome and mitochondrial DNA sequence analysis, including small sequence changes, deletions, duplications, short tandem repeat gene expansions, and variants in non-uniquely mappable regions, blood or saliva, identification and categorization of genetic variants, proband
Genomic Unity® Whole Genome Analysis - Comparator, Variantyx Inc, Variantyx Inc	0213U	Rare diseases (constitutional/heritable disorders), whole genome and mitochondrial DNA sequence analysis, including small sequence changes, deletions, duplications, short tandem repeat gene expansions, and variants in non-uniquely mappable regions, blood or saliva, identification and categorization of genetic variants, each comparator genome (eg, parent, sibling)
Genomic Unity® Exome Plus Analysis - Proband, Variantyx Inc, Variantyx Inc	0214U	Rare diseases (constitutional/heritable disorders), whole exome and mitochondrial DNA sequence analysis, including small sequence changes, deletions, duplications, short tandem repeat gene expansions, and variants in non-uniquely mappable regions, blood or saliva, identification and categorization of genetic variants, proband
Genomic Unity® Exome Plus Analysis - Comparator, Variantyx Inc, Variantyx Inc	0215U	Rare diseases (constitutional/heritable disorders), whole exome and mitochondrial DNA sequence analysis, including small sequence changes, deletions, duplications, short tandem repeat gene expansions, and variants in non-uniquely mappable regions, blood or saliva, identification and categorization of genetic variants, each comparator exome (eg, parent, sibling)
Genomic Unity® Ataxia Repeat Expansion and Sequence Analysis, Variantyx Inc, Variantyx Inc	0216U	Neurology (inherited ataxias), genomic DNA sequence analysis of 12 common genes including small sequence changes, deletions, duplications, short tandem repeat gene expansions, and variants in non-uniquely mappable regions, blood or saliva, identification and categorization of genetic variants

Proprietary Name/Clinical Laboratory/Manufacturer	Code	Descriptor
Genomic Unity® Comprehensive Ataxia Repeat Expansion and Sequence Analysis, Variantyx Inc, Variantyx Inc	0217U	Neurology (inherited ataxias), genomic DNA sequence analysis of 51 genes including small sequence changes, deletions, duplications, short tandem repeat gene expansions, and variants in non-uniquely mappable regions, blood or saliva, identification and categorization of genetic variants
Genomic Unity® DMD Analysis, Variantyx Inc, Variantyx Inc	0218U	Neurology (muscular dystrophy), *DMD* gene sequence analysis, including small sequence changes, deletions, duplications, and variants in non-uniquely mappable regions, blood or saliva, identification and characterization of genetic variants
Sentosa® SQ HIV-1 Genotyping Assay, Vela Diagnostics USA, Inc, Vela Operations Singapore Pte Ltd	0219U	Infectious agent (human immunodeficiency virus), targeted viral next-generation sequence analysis (ie, protease [PR], reverse transcriptase [RT], integrase [INT]), algorithm reported as prediction of antiviral drug susceptibility
PreciseDx™ Breast Cancer Test, PreciseDx, PreciseDx	0220U	Oncology (breast cancer), image analysis with artificial intelligence assessment of 12 histologic and immunohistochemical features, reported as a recurrence score
Navigator ABO Blood Group NGS, Grifols Immunohematology Center, Grifols Immunohematology Center	0221U	Red cell antigen (ABO blood group) genotyping (ABO), gene analysis, next-generation sequencing, *ABO (ABO, alpha 1-3-N-acetylgalactosaminyltransferase and alpha 1-3-galactosyltransferase)* gene
Navigator Rh Blood Group NGS, Grifols Immunohematology Center, Grifols Immunohematology Center	0222U	Red cell antigen (RH blood group) genotyping (RHD and RHCE), gene analysis, next-generation sequencing, RH proximal promoter, exons 1-10, portions of introns 2-3
QIAstat-Dx Respiratory SARS CoV-2 Panel, QIAGEN Sciences, QIAGEN GmbH CPT Excludes: BioFire® Respiratory Panel 2.1 (RP2.1), BioFire® Diagnostics, BioFire® Diagnostics, LLC. (0202U)	● 0223U	Infectious disease (bacterial or viral respiratory tract infection), pathogen-specific nucleic acid (DNA or RNA), 22 targets including severe acute respiratory syndrome coronavirus 2 (SARS-CoV-2), qualitative RT-PCR, nasopharyngeal swab, each pathogen reported as detected or not detected
COVID-19 Antibody Test, Mt Sinai, Mount Sinai Laboratory	● 0224U	Antibody, severe acute respiratory syndrome coronavirus 2 (SARS-CoV-2) (Coronavirus disease [COVID-19]), includes titer(s), when performed
ePlex® Respiratory Pathogen Panel 2, GenMark Dx, GenMark Diagnostics, Inc	● 0225U	Infectious disease (bacterial or viral respiratory tract infection) pathogen-specific DNA and RNA, 21 targets, including severe acute respiratory syndrome coronavirus 2 (SARS-CoV-2), amplified probe technique, including multiplex reverse transcription for RNA targets, each analyte reported as detected or not detected
Tru-Immune™, Ethos Laboratories, GenScript® USA Inc	● 0226U	Surrogate viral neutralization test (sVNT), severe acute respiratory syndrome coronavirus 2 (SARS-CoV-2) (Coronavirus disease [COVID-19]), ELISA, plasma, serum
Comprehensive Screen, Aspenti Health	● 0227U	Drug assay, presumptive, 30 or more drugs or metabolites, urine, liquid chromatography with tandem mass spectrometry (LC-MS/MS) using multiple reaction monitoring (MRM), with drug or metabolite description, includes sample validation
PanGIA Prostate, Genetics Institute of America, Entopsis, LLC	● 0228U	Oncology (prostate), multianalyte molecular profile by photometric detection of macromolecules adsorbed on nanosponge array slides with machine learning, utilizing first morning voided urine, algorithm reported as likelihood of prostate cancer
Colvera®, Clinical Genomic Pathology Inc	● 0229U	*BCAT1 (Branched chain amino acid transaminase 1) or IKZF1 (IKAROS family zinc finger 1)* (eg, colorectal cancer) promoter methylation analysis
Genomic Unity® AR Analysis, Variantyx Inc, Variantyx Inc	● 0230U	*AR (androgen receptor)* (eg, spinal and bulbar muscular atrophy, Kennedy disease, X chromosome inactivation), full sequence analysis, including small sequence changes in exonic and intronic regions, deletions, duplications, short tandem repeat (STR) expansions, mobile element insertions, and variants in non-uniquely mappable regions
Genomic Unity® CACNA1A Analysis, Variantyx Inc, Variantyx Inc	● 0231U	*CACNA1A (calcium voltage-gated channel subunit alpha 1A)* (eg, spinocerebellar ataxia), full gene analysis, including small sequence changes in exonic and intronic regions, deletions, duplications, short tandem repeat (STR) gene expansions, mobile element insertions, and variants in non-uniquely mappable regions
Genomic Unity® CSTB Analysis, Variantyx Inc, Variantyx Inc	● 0232U	*CSTB (cystatin B)* (eg, progressive myoclonic epilepsy type 1A, Unverricht-Lundborg disease), full gene analysis, including small sequence changes in exonic and intronic regions, deletions, duplications, short tandem repeat (STR) expansions, mobile element insertions, and variants in non-uniquely mappable regions
Genomic Unity® FXN Analysis, Variantyx Inc, Variantyx Inc	● 0233U	*FXN (frataxin)* (eg, Friedreich ataxia), gene analysis, including small sequence changes in exonic and intronic regions, deletions, duplications, short tandem repeat (STR) expansions, mobile element insertions, and variants in non-uniquely mappable regions
Genomic Unity® MECP2 Analysis, Variantyx Inc, Variantyx Inc	● 0234U	*MECP2 (methyl CpG binding protein 2)* (eg, Rett syndrome), full gene analysis, including small sequence changes in exonic and intronic regions, deletions, duplications, mobile element insertions, and variants in non-uniquely mappable regions
Genomic Unity® PTEN Analysis, Variantyx Inc, Variantyx Inc	● 0235U	*PTEN (phosphatase and tensin homolog)* (eg, Cowden syndrome, PTEN hamartoma tumor syndrome), full gene analysis, including small sequence changes in exonic and intronic regions, deletions, duplications, mobile element insertions, and variants in non-uniquely mappable regions
Genomic Unity® SMN1/2 Analysis, Variantyx Inc, Variantyx Inc	● 0236U	*SMN1 (survival of motor neuron 1, telomeric)* and *SMN2 (survival of motor neuron 2, centromeric)* (eg, spinal muscular atrophy) full gene analysis, including small sequence changes in exonic and intronic regions, duplications, deletions, and mobile element insertions

Proprietary Name/Clinical Laboratory/Manufacturer	Code	Descriptor
Genomic Unity® Cardiac Ion Channelopathies Analysis, Variantyx Inc, Variantyx Inc	● 0237U	Cardiac ion channelopathies (eg, Brugada syndrome, long QT syndrome, short QT syndrome, catecholaminergic polymorphic ventricular tachycardia), genomic sequence analysis panel including *ANK2, CASQ2, CAV3, KCNE1, KCNE2, KCNH2, KCNJ2, KCNQ1, RYR2*, and *SCN5A*, including small sequence changes in exonic and intronic regions, deletions, duplications, mobile element insertions, and variants in non-uniquely mappable regions
Genomic Unity® Lynch Syndrome Analysis, Variantyx Inc, Variantyx Inc	● 0238U	Oncology (Lynch syndrome), genomic DNA sequence analysis of *MLH1, MSH2, MSH6, PMS2*, and *EPCAM*, including small sequence changes in exonic and intronic regions, deletions, duplications, mobile element insertions, and variants in non-uniquely mappable regions
FoundationOne® Liquid CDx, Foundation Medicine Inc, Foundation Medicine Inc	● 0239U	Targeted genomic sequence analysis panel, solid organ neoplasm, cell-free DNA, analysis of 311 or more genes, interrogation for sequence variants, including substitutions, insertions, deletions, select rearrangements, and copy number variations
Xpert® Xpress SARS-CoV-2/Flu/RSV (SARS-CoV-2 & Flu targets only), Cepheid	● 0240U	Infectious disease (viral respiratory tract infection), pathogen-specific RNA, 3 targets (severe acute respiratory syndrome coronavirus 2 [SARS-CoV-2], influenza A, influenza B), upper respiratory specimen, each pathogen reported as detected or not detected
Xpert® Xpress SARS-CoV-2/Flu/RSV (all targets), Cepheid	● 0241U	Infectious disease (viral respiratory tract infection), pathogen-specific RNA, 4 targets (severe acute respiratory syndrome coronavirus 2 [SARS-CoV-2], influenza A, influenza B, respiratory syncytial virus [RSV]), upper respiratory specimen, each pathogen reported as detected or not detected
Guardant360® CDx, Guardant Health Inc, Guardant Health Inc	● 0242U	Targeted genomic sequence analysis panel, solid organ neoplasm, cell-free circulating DNA analysis of 55-74 genes, interrogation for sequence variants, gene copy number amplifications, and gene rearrangements
PlGF Preeclampsia Screen, PerkinElmer Genetics, PerkinElmer Genetics, Inc	● 0243U	Obstetrics (preeclampsia), biochemical assay of placental-growth factor, time-resolved fluorescence immunoassay, maternal serum, predictive algorithm reported as a risk score for preeclampsia
Oncotype MAP™ Pan-Cancer Tissue Test, Paradigm Diagnostics, Inc, Paradigm Diagnostics, Inc	● 0244U	Oncology (solid organ), DNA, comprehensive genomic profiling, 257 genes, interrogation for single-nucleotide variants, insertions/deletions, copy number alterations, gene rearrangements, tumor-mutational burden and microsatellite instability, utilizing formalin-fixed paraffin-embedded tumor tissue
ThyGeNEXT® Thyroid Oncogene Panel, Interpace Diagnostics, Interpace Diagnostics	● 0245U	Oncology (thyroid), mutation analysis of 10 genes and 37 RNA fusions and expression of 4 mRNA markers using next-generation sequencing, fine needle aspirate, report includes associated risk of malignancy expressed as a percentage
PrecisionBlood™, San Diego Blood Bank, San Diego Blood Bank	● 0246U	Red blood cell antigen typing, DNA, genotyping of at least 16 blood groups with phenotype prediction of at least 51 red blood cell antigens
PreTRM®, Sera Prognostics, Sera Prognostics, Inc®	● 0247U	Obstetrics (preterm birth), insulin-like growth factor-binding protein 4 (IBP4), sex hormone-binding globulin (SHBG), quantitative measurement by LC-MS/MS, utilizing maternal serum, combined with clinical data, reported as predictive-risk stratification for spontaneous preterm birth
3D Predict Glioma, KIYATEC®, Inc	● 0248U	Oncology (brain), spheroid cell culture in a 3D microenvironment, 12 drug panel, tumor-response prediction for each drug
Theralink® Reverse Phase Protein Array (RPPA), Theralink® Technologies, Inc, Theralink® Technologies, Inc	● 0249U	Oncology (breast), semiquantitative analysis of 32 phosphoproteins and protein analytes, includes laser capture microdissection, with algorithmic analysis and interpretative report
PGDx elio™ tissue complete, Personal Genome Diagnostics, Inc, Personal Genome Diagnostics, Inc	● 0250U	Oncology (solid organ neoplasm), targeted genomic sequence DNA analysis of 505 genes, interrogation for somatic alterations (SNVs [single nucleotide variant], small insertions and deletions, one amplification, and four translocations), microsatellite instability and tumor-mutation burden
Intrinsic Hepcidin IDx™ Test, IntrinsicDx, Intrinsic LifeSciences™ LLC	● 0251U	Hepcidin-25, enzyme-linked immunosorbent assay (ELISA), serum or plasma
POC (Products of Conception), Igenomix®, Igenomix® USA	● 0252U	Fetal aneuploidy short tandem-repeat comparative analysis, fetal DNA from products of conception, reported as normal (euploidy), monosomy, trisomy, or partial deletion/duplications, mosaicism, and segmental aneuploidy
ERA® (Endometrial Receptivity Analysis), Igenomix®, Igenomix® USA	● 0253U	Reproductive medicine (endometrial receptivity analysis), RNA gene expression profile, 238 genes by next-generation sequencing, endometrial tissue, predictive algorithm reported as endometrial window of implantation (eg, pre-receptive, receptive, post-receptive)
SMART PGT-A (Pre-implantation Genetic Testing — Aneuploidy), Igenomix®, Igenomix® USA	● 0254U	Reproductive medicine (preimplantation genetic assessment), analysis of 24 chromosomes using embryonic DNA genomic sequence analysis for aneuploidy, and a mitochondrial DNA score in euploid embryos, results reported as normal (euploidy), monosomy, trisomy, or partial deletion/duplications, mosaicism, and segmental aneuploidy, per embryo tested
Cap-Score™ Test, Androvia LifeSciences, Avantor Clinical Services (previously known as Therapak)	● 0255U	Andrology (infertility), sperm-capacitation assessment of ganglioside GM1 distribution patterns, fluorescence microscopy, fresh or frozen specimen, reported as percentage of capacitated sperm and probability of generating a pregnancy score
Trimethylamine (TMA) and TMA N-Oxide, Children's Hospital Colorado Laboratory	● 0256U	Trimethylamine/trimethylamine N-oxide (TMA/TMAO) profile, tandem mass spectrometry (MS/MS), urine, with algorithmic analysis and interpretive report
Very-Long Chain Acyl-CoA Dehydrogenase (VLCAD) Enzyme Activity, Children's Hospital Colorado Laboratory	● 0257U	Very long chain acyl-coenzyme A (CoA) dehydrogenase (VLCAD), leukocyte enzyme activity, whole blood

Proprietary Name/Clinical Laboratory/Manufacturer	Code	Descriptor
Mind.Px, Mindera, Mindera Corporation	● 0258U	Autoimmune (psoriasis), mRNA, nextgeneration sequencing, gene expression profiling of 50-100 genes, skin-surface collection using adhesive patch, algorithm reported as likelihood of response to psoriasis biologics
GFR by NMR, Labtech™ Diagnostics	● 0259U	Nephrology (chronic kidney disease), nuclear magnetic resonance spectroscopy measurement of myo-inositol, valine, and creatinine, algorithmically combined with cystatin C (by immunoassay) and demographic data to determine estimated glomerular filtration rate (GFR), serum, quantitative
Augusta Optical Genome Mapping, Georgia Esoteric and Molecular (GEM) CPT Excludes: Praxis Optical Genome Mapping, Praxis Genomics LLC (0264U)	● 0260U	Rare diseases (constitutional/heritable disorders), identification of copy number variations, inversions, insertions, translocations, and other structural variants by optical genome mapping
Immunoscore®, HalioDx, HalioDx	● 0261U	Oncology (colorectal cancer), image analysis with artificial intelligence assessment of 4 histologic and immunohistochemical features (CD3 and CD8 within tumor-stroma border and tumor core), tissue, reported as immune response and recurrence-risk score
OncoSignal 7 Pathway Signal, Protean BioDiagnostics, Philips Electronics Nederland BV	● 0262U	Oncology (solid tumor), gene expression profiling by real-time RT-PCR of 7 gene pathways *(ER, AR, PI3K, MAPK, HH, TGFB,* Notch), formalin-fixed paraffin-embedded (FFPE), algorithm reported as gene pathway activity score
NPDX ASD and Central Carbon Energy Metabolism, Stemina Biomarker Discovery, Inc, Stemina Biomarker Discovery, Inc	● 0263U	Neurology (autism spectrum disorder [ASD]), quantitative measurements of 16 central carbon metabolites (ie, a-ketoglutarate, alanine, lactate, phenylalanine, pyruvate, succinate, carnitine, citrate, fumarate, hypoxanthine, inosine, malate, S-sulfocysteine, taurine, urate, and xanthine), liquid chromatography tandem mass spectrometry (LC-MS/MS), plasma, algorithmic analysis with result reported as negative or positive (with metabolic subtypes of ASD)
Praxis Optical Genome Mapping, Praxis Genomics LLC CPT Excludes: Augusta Optical Genome Mapping, Georgia Esoteric and Molecular (GEM) Laboratory, LLC, Bionano Genomics Inc (0260U)	● 0264U	Rare diseases (constitutional/heritable disorders), identification of copy number variations, inversions, insertions, translocations, and other structural variants by optical genome mapping
Praxis Whole Genome Sequencing, Praxis Genomics LLC	● 0265U	Rare constitutional and other heritable disorders, whole genome and mitochondrial DNA sequence analysis, blood, frozen and formalin-fixed paraffin-embedded (FFPE) tissue, saliva, buccal swabs or cell lines, identification of single nucleotide and copy number variants
Praxis Transcriptome, Praxis Genomics LLC	● 0266U	Unexplained constitutional or other heritable disorders or syndromes, tissue-specific gene expression by whole-transcriptome and next-generation sequencing, blood, formalin-fixed paraffin-embedded (FFPE) tissue or fresh frozen tissue, reported as presence or absence of splicing or expression changes
Praxis Combined Whole Genome Sequencing and Optical Genome Mapping, Praxis Genomics LLC	● 0267U	Rare constitutional and other heritable disorders, identification of copy number variations, inversions, insertions, translocations, and other structural variants by optical genome mapping and whole genome sequencing
Versiti™ aHUS Genetic Evaluation, Versiti™ Diagnostic Laboratories, Versiti™	● 0268U	Hematology (atypical hemolytic uremic syndrome [aHUS]), genomic sequence analysis of 15 genes, blood, buccal swab, or amniotic fluid
Versiti™ Autosomal Dominant Thrombocytopenia Panel, Versiti™ Diagnostic Laboratories, Versiti™	● 0269U	Hematology (autosomal dominant congenital thrombocytopenia), genomic sequence analysis of 14 genes, blood, buccal swab, or amniotic fluid
Versiti™ Coagulation Disorder Panel, Versiti™ Diagnostic Laboratories, Versiti™	● 0270U	Hematology (congenital coagulation disorders), genomic sequence analysis of 20 genes, blood, buccal swab, or amniotic fluid
Versiti™ Congenital Neutropenia Panel, Versiti™ Diagnostic Laboratories, Versiti™	● 0271U	Hematology (congenital neutropenia), genomic sequence analysis of 23 genes, blood, buccal swab, or amniotic fluid
Versiti™ Comprehensive Bleeding Disorder Panel, Versiti™ Diagnostic Laboratories, Versiti™	● 0272U	Hematology (genetic bleeding disorders), genomic sequence analysis of 51 genes, blood, buccal swab, or amniotic fluid, comprehensive
Versiti™ Fibrinolytic Disorder Panel, Versiti™ Diagnostic Laboratories, Versiti™	● 0273U	Hematology (genetic hyperfibrinolysis, delayed bleeding), genomic sequence analysis of 8 genes *(F13A1, F13B, FGA, FGB, FGG, SERPINA1, SERPINE1, SERPINF2, PLAU),* blood, buccal swab, or amniotic fluid
Versiti™ Comprehensive Platelet Disorder Panel, Versiti™ Diagnostic Laboratories, Versiti™	● 0274U	Hematology (genetic platelet disorders), genomic sequence analysis of 43 genes, blood, buccal swab, or amniotic fluid
Versiti™ Heparin-Induced Thrombocytopenia Evaluation — PEA, Versiti™ Diagnostic Laboratories, Versiti™	● 0275U	Hematology (heparin-induced thrombocytopenia), platelet antibody reactivity by flow cytometry, serum
Versiti™ Inherited Thrombocytopenia Panel, Versiti™ Diagnostic Laboratories, Versiti™	● 0276U	Hematology (inherited thrombocytopenia), genomic sequence analysis of 23 genes, blood, buccal swab, or amniotic fluid
Versiti™ Platelet Function Disorder Panel, Versiti™ Diagnostic Laboratories, Versiti™	● 0277U	Hematology (genetic platelet function disorder), genomic sequence analysis of 31 genes, blood, buccal swab, or amniotic fluid
Versiti™ Thrombosis Panel, Versiti™ Diagnostic Laboratories, Versiti™	● 0278U	Hematology (genetic thrombosis), genomic sequence analysis of 12 genes, blood, buccal swab, or amniotic fluid
Versiti™ VWF Collagen III Binding, Versiti™ Diagnostic Laboratories, Versiti™	● 0279U	Hematology (von Willebrand disease [VWD]), von Willebrand factor (VWF) and collagen III binding by enzyme-linked immunosorbent assays (ELISA), plasma, report of collagen III binding
Versiti™ VWF Collagen IV Binding, Versiti™ Diagnostic Laboratories, Versiti™	● 0280U	Hematology (von Willebrand disease [VWD]), von Willebrand factor (VWF) and collagen IV binding by enzyme-linked immunosorbent assays (ELISA), plasma, report of collagen IV binding

Proprietary Name/Clinical Laboratory/Manufacturer	Code	Descriptor
Versiti™ VWF Propeptide Antigen, Versiti™ Diagnostic Laboratories, Versiti™	● 0281U	Hematology (von Willebrand disease [VWD]), von Willebrand propeptide, enzyme-linked immunosorbent assays (ELISA), plasma, diagnostic report of von Willebrand factor (VWF) propeptide antigen level
Versiti™ Red Cell Genotyping Panel, Versiti™ Diagnostic Laboratories, Versiti™	● 0282U	Red blood cell antigen typing, DNA, genotyping of 12 blood group system genes to predict 44 red blood cell antigen phenotypes
Versiti™ VWD Type 2B Evaluation, Versiti™ Diagnostic Laboratories, Versiti™	● 0283U	von Willebrand factor (VWF), type 2B, platelet-binding evaluation, radioimmunoassay, plasma
Versiti™ VWD Type 2N Binding, Versiti™ Diagnostic Laboratories, Versiti™	● 0284U	von Willebrand factor (VWF), type 2N, factor VIII and VWF binding evaluation, enzyme-linked immunosorbent assays (ELISA), plasma
RadTox™ cfDNA test, DiaCarta Clinical Lab, DiaCarta Inc	● 0285U	Oncology, response to radiation, cell-free DNA, quantitative branched chain DNA amplification, plasma, reported as a radiation toxicity score
CNT *CEP72, TPMT and NUDT15)* genotyping panel, RPRD Diagnostics	● 0286U	*CEP72 (centrosomal protein, 72-KDa), NUDT15 (nudix hydrolase 15)* and *TPMT (thiopurine S-methyltransferase)* (eg, drug metabolism) gene analysis, common variants
ThyroSeq® CRC, CBLPath, Inc, University of Pittsburgh Medical Center	● 0287U	Oncology (thyroid), DNA and mRNA, next-generation sequencing analysis of 112 genes, fine needle aspirate or formalin-fixed paraffin-embedded (FFPE) tissue, algorithmic prediction of cancer recurrence, reported as a categorical risk result (low, intermediate, high)
DetermaRx™, Oncocyte Corporation	● 0288U	Oncology (lung), mRNA, quantitative PCR analysis of 11 genes *(BAG1, BRCA1, CDC6, CDK2AP1, ERBB3, FUT3, IL11, LCK, RND3, SH3BGR, WNT3A)* and 3 reference genes *(ESD, TBP, YAP1)*, formalin-fixed paraffin-embedded (FFPE) tumor tissue, algorithmic interpretation reported as a recurrence risk score
MindX Blood Test™ — Memory/Alzheimer's, MindX Sciences™ Laboratory, MindX Sciences™ Inc	● 0289U	Neurology (Alzheimer disease), mRNA, gene expression profiling by RNA sequencing of 24 genes, whole blood, algorithm reported as predictive risk score
MindX Blood Test™ — Pain, MindX Sciences™ Laboratory, MindX Sciences™ Inc	● 0290U	Pain management, mRNA, gene expression profiling by RNA sequencing of 36 genes, whole blood, algorithm reported as predictive risk score
MindX Blood Test™ — Mood, MindX Sciences™ Laboratory, MindX Sciences™ Inc	● 0291U	Psychiatry (mood disorders), mRNA, gene expression profiling by RNA sequencing of 144 genes, whole blood, algorithm reported as predictive risk score
MindX Blood Test™ — Stress, MindX Sciences™ Laboratory, MindX Sciences™ Inc	● 0292U	Psychiatry (stress disorders), mRNA, gene expression profiling by RNA sequencing of 72 genes, whole blood, algorithm reported as predictive risk score
MindX Blood Test™ — Suicidality, MindX Sciences™ Laboratory, MindX Sciences™ Inc	● 0293U	Psychiatry (suicidal ideation), mRNA, gene expression profiling by RNA sequencing of 54 genes, whole blood, algorithm reported as predictive risk score
MindX Blood Test™ — Longevity, MindX Sciences™ Laboratory, MindX Sciences™ Inc	● 0294U	Longevity and mortality risk, mRNA, gene expression profiling by RNA sequencing of 18 genes, whole blood, algorithm reported as predictive risk score
DCISionRT®, PreludeDx™, Prelude Corporation	● 0295U	Oncology (breast ductal carcinoma in situ), protein expression profiling by immunohistochemistry of 7 proteins (COX2, FOXA1, HER2, Ki-67, p16, PR, SIAH2), with 4 clinicopathologic factors (size, age, margin status, palpability), utilizing formalin-fixed paraffin-embedded (FFPE) tissue, algorithm reported as a recurrence risk score
mRNA CancerDetect™, Viome Life Sciences, Inc, Viome Life Sciences, Inc	● 0296U	Oncology (oral and/or oropharyngeal cancer), gene expression profiling by RNA sequencing at least 20 molecular features (eg, human and/or microbial mRNA), saliva, algorithm reported as positive or negative for signature associated with malignancy
Praxis Somatic Whole Genome Sequencing, Praxis Genomics LLC	● 0297U	Oncology (pan tumor), whole genome sequencing of paired malignant and normal DNA specimens, fresh or formalin-fixed paraffin-embedded (FFPE) tissue, blood or bone marrow, comparative sequence analyses and variant identification
Praxis Somatic Transcriptome, Praxis Genomics LLC	● 0298U	Oncology (pan tumor), whole transcriptome sequencing of paired malignant and normal RNA specimens, fresh or formalin-fixed paraffin-embedded (FFPE) tissue, blood or bone marrow, comparative sequence analyses and expression level and chimeric transcript identification
Praxis Somatic Optical Genome Mapping, Praxis Genomics LLC	● 0299U	Oncology (pan tumor), whole genome optical genome mapping of paired malignant and normal DNA specimens, fresh frozen tissue, blood, or bone marrow, comparative structural variant identification
Praxis Somatic Combined Whole Genome Sequencing and Optical Genome Mapping, Praxis Genomics LLC	● 0300U	Oncology (pan tumor), whole genome sequencing and optical genome mapping of paired malignant and normal DNA specimens, fresh tissue, blood, or bone marrow, comparative sequence analyses and variant identification
Bartonella ddPCR, Galaxy Diagnostics Inc	● 0301U	Infectious agent detection by nucleic acid (DNA or RNA), Bartonella henselae and Bartonella quintana, droplet digital PCR (ddPCR);
Bartonella Digital ePCR™, Galaxy Diagnostics Inc	● 0302U	following liquid enhancement
Hypoxic BioChip Adhesion, BioChip Labs™, BioChip Labs™	● 0303U	Hematology, red blood cell (RBC) adhesion to endothelial/subendothelial adhesion molecules, functional assessment, whole blood, with algorithmic analysis and result reported as an RBC adhesion index; hypoxic
Normoxic BioChip Adhesion, BioChip Labs™, BioChip Labs™	● 0304U	normoxic
Ektacytometry, BioChip Labs™, BioChip Labs™	● 0305U	Hematology, red blood cell (RBC) functionality and deformity as a function of shear stress, whole blood, reported as a maximum elongation index

Appendix M — Glossary

-centesis. Puncture, as with a needle, trocar, or aspirator; often done for withdrawing fluid from a cavity.

-ectomy. Excision, removal.

-orrhaphy. Suturing.

-ostomy. Indicates a surgically created artificial opening.

-otomy. Making an incision or opening.

-plasty. Indicates surgically formed or molded.

abdominal lymphadenectomy. Surgical removal of the abdominal lymph nodes grouping, with or without para-aortic and vena cava nodes.

ablation. Removal or destruction of a body part or tissue or its function. Ablation may be performed by surgical means, hormones, drugs, radiofrequency, heat, chemical application, or other methods.

abnormal alleles. Form of gene that includes disease-related variations.

absorbable sutures. Strands prepared from collagen or a synthetic polymer and capable of being absorbed by tissue over time. Examples include surgical gut and collagen sutures; or synthetics like polydioxanone (PDS), polyglactin 910 (Vicryl), poliglecaprone 25 (Monocryl), polyglyconate (Maxon), and polyglycolic acid (Dexon).

acetabuloplasty. Surgical repair or reconstruction of the large cup-shaped socket in the hipbone (acetabulum) with which the head of the femur articulates.

Achilles tendon. Tendon attached to the back of the heel bone (calcaneus) that flexes the foot downward.

acromioclavicular joint. Junction between the clavicle and the scapula. The acromion is the projection from the back of the scapula that forms the highest point of the shoulder and connects with the clavicle. Trauma or injury to the acromioclavicular joint is often referred to as a dislocation of the shoulder. This is not correct, however, as a dislocation of the shoulder is a disruption of the glenohumeral joint.

acromionectomy. Surgical treatment for acromioclavicular arthritis in which the distal portion of the acromion process is removed.

acromioplasty. Repair of the part of the shoulder blade that connects to the deltoid muscles and clavicle.

actigraphy. Science of monitoring activity levels, particularly during sleep. In most cases, the patient wears a wristband that records motion while sleeping. The data are recorded, analyzed, and interpreted to study sleep/wake patterns and circadian rhythms.

air conduction. Transportation of sound from the air, through the external auditory canal, to the tympanic membrane and ossicular chain. Air conduction hearing is tested by presenting an acoustic stimulus through earphones or a loudspeaker to the ear.

air puff device. Instrument that measures intraocular pressure by evaluating the force of a reflected amount of air blown against the cornea.

alleles. Form of gene usually arising from a mutation responsible for a hereditary variation.

allogeneic collection. Collection of blood or blood components from one person for the use of another. Allogeneic collection was formerly termed homologous collection.

allograft. Graft from one individual to another of the same species.

amniocentesis. Surgical puncture through the abdominal wall, with a specialized needle and under ultrasonic guidance, into the interior of the pregnant uterus and directly into the amniotic sac to collect fluid for diagnostic analysis or therapeutic reduction of fluid levels.

anastomosis. Surgically created connection between ducts, blood vessels, or bowel segments to allow flow from one to the other.

anesthesia time. Time period factored into anesthesia procedures beginning with the anesthesiologist preparing the patient for surgery and ending when the patient is turned over to the recovery department.

Angelman syndrome. Early childhood emergence of a pattern of interrupted development, stiff, jerky gait, absence or impairment of speech, excessive laughter, and seizures.

angioplasty. Reconstruction or repair of a diseased or damaged blood vessel.

annuloplasty. Surgical plication of weakened tissue of the heart, to improve its muscular function. Annuli are thick, fibrous rings and one is found surrounding each of the cardiac chambers. The atrial and ventricular muscle fibers attach to the annuli. In annuloplasty, weakened annuli may be surgically plicated, or tucked, to improve muscular functions.

anorectal anometry. Measurement of pressure generated by anal sphincter to diagnose incontinence.

anterior chamber lenses. Lenses inserted into the anterior chamber following intracapsular cataract extraction.

applanation tonometer. Instrument that measures intraocular pressure by recording the force required to flatten an area of the cornea.

appropriateness of care. Proper setting of medical care that best meets the patient's care or diagnosis, as defined by a health care plan or other legal entity.

aqueous humor. Fluid within the anterior and posterior chambers of the eye that is continually replenished as it diffuses out into the blood. When the flow of aqueous is blocked, a build-up of fluid in the eye causes increased intraocular pressure and leads to glaucoma and blindness.

arteriogram. Radiograph of arteries.

arteriovenous fistula. Connecting passage between an artery and a vein.

arteriovenous malformation. Connecting passage between an artery and a vein.

arthrotomy. Surgical incision into a joint that may include exploration, drainage, or removal of a foreign body.

ASA. 1) Acetylsalicylic acid. Synonym(s): aspirin. 2) American Society of Anesthesiologists. National organization for anesthesiology that maintains and publishes the guidelines and relative values for anesthesia coding.

aspirate. To withdraw fluid or air from a body cavity by suction.

assay. Chemical analysis of a substance to establish the presence and strength of its components. A therapeutic drug assay is used to determine if a drug is within the expected therapeutic range for a patient.

asynchronous services. Those that allow a physician or other qualified health care professional (QHP) to share a patient's clinical data, medical history, radiographic images, laboratory results, and/or pathology reports with a specialist physician in order to obtain their expertise in diagnosis and treatment. They also allow the patient to share health information with their physician or other QHP. These services utilize an electronic health record (EHR), encrypted email, a secure Web server, or specially designed software (store-and-forward).

atrial septal defect. Cardiac anomaly consisting of a patent opening in the atrial septum due to a fusion failure, classified as ostium secundum type, ostium primum defect, or endocardial cushion defect.

attended surveillance. Ability of a technician at a remote surveillance center or location to respond immediately to patient transmissions regarding rhythm or device alerts as they are produced and received at the remote location. These transmissions may originate from wearable or implanted therapy or monitoring devices.

auricle. External ear, which is a single elastic cartilage covered in skin and normal adnexal features (hair follicles, sweat glands, and sebaceous glands), shaped to channel sound waves into the acoustic meatus.

autogenous transplant. Tissue, such as bone, that is harvested from the patient and used for transplantation back into the same patient.

autograft. Any tissue harvested from one anatomical site of a person and grafted to another anatomical site of the same person. Most commonly, blood vessels, skin, tendons, fascia, and bone are used as autografts.

autologous. Tissue, cells, or structure obtained from the same individual.

AVF. Arteriovenous fistula.

AVM. Arteriovenous malformation. Clusters of abnormal blood vessels that grow in the brain comprised of a blood vessel "nidus" or nest through which arteries and veins connect directly without going through the capillaries. As time passes, the nidus may enlarge resulting in the formation of a mass that may bleed. AVMs are more prone to bleeding in patients ages 10 to 55. Once older than age 55, the possibility of bleeding is reduced dramatically.

backbench preparation. Procedures performed on a donor organ following procurement to prepare the organ for transplant into the recipient. Excess fat and other tissue may be removed, the organ may be perfused, and vital arteries may be sized, repaired, or modified to fit the patient. These procedures are done on a back table in the operating room before transplantation can begin.

Bartholin's gland. Mucous-producing gland found in the vestibular bulbs on either side of the vaginal orifice and connected to the mucosal membrane at the opening by a duct.

Bartholin's gland abscess. Pocket of pus and surrounding cellulitis caused by infection of the Bartholin's gland and causing localized swelling and pain in the posterior labia majora that may extend into the lower vagina.

basic value. Relative weighted value based upon the usual anesthesia services and the relative work or cost of the specific anesthesia service assigned to each anesthesia-specific procedure code.

Berman locator. Small, sensitive tool used to detect the location of a metallic foreign body in the eye.

bifurcated. Having two branches or divisions, such as the left pulmonary veins that split off from the left atrium to carry oxygenated blood away from the heart.

Billroth's operation. Anastomosis of the stomach to the duodenum or jejunum.

bioprosthetic heart valve. Replacement cardiac valve made of biological tissue. Allograft, xenograft or engineered tissue.

biopsy. Tissue or fluid removed for diagnostic purposes through analysis of the cells in the biopsy material.

Blalock-Hanlon procedure. Atrial septectomy procedure to allow free mixing of the blood from the right and left atria.

Blalock-Taussig procedure. Anastomosis of the left subclavian artery to the left pulmonary artery or the right subclavian artery to the right pulmonary artery in order to shunt some of the blood flow from the systemic to the pulmonary circulation.

blepharochalasis. Loss of elasticity and relaxation of skin of the eyelid, thickened or indurated skin on the eyelid associated with recurrent episodes of edema, and intracellular atrophy.

blepharoplasty. Plastic surgery of the eyelids to remove excess fat and redundant skin weighting down the lid. The eyelid is pulled tight and sutured to support sagging muscles.

blepharoptosis. Droop or displacement of the upper eyelid, caused by paralysis, muscle problems, or outside mechanical forces.

blepharorrhaphy. Suture of a portion or all of the opposing eyelids to shorten the palpebral fissure or close it entirely.

bone conduction. Transportation of sound through the bones of the skull to the inner ear.

bone mass measurement. Radiologic or radioisotopic procedure or other procedure approved by the FDA for identifying bone mass, detecting bone loss, or determining bone quality. The procedure includes a physician's interpretation of the results. Qualifying individuals must be an estrogen-deficient woman at clinical risk for osteoporosis with vertebral abnormalities.

brachytherapy. Form of radiation therapy in which radioactive pellets or seeds are implanted directly into the tissue being treated to deliver their dose of radiation in a more directed fashion. Brachytherapy provides radiation to the prescribed body area while minimizing exposure to normal tissue.

breakpoint. Point at which a chromosome breaks.

Bristow procedure. Anterior capsulorrhaphy prevents chronic separation of the shoulder. In this procedure, the bone block is affixed to the anterior glenoid rim with a screw.

buccal mucosa. Tissue from the mucous membrane on the inside of the cheek.

bundle of His. Bundle of modified cardiac fibers that begins at the atrioventricular node and passes through the right atrioventricular fibrous ring to the interventricular septum, where it divides into two branches. Bundle of His recordings are taken for intracardiac electrograms.

Caldwell-Luc operation. Intraoral antrostomy approach into the maxillary sinus for the removal of tooth roots or tissue, or for packing the sinus to reduce zygomatic fractures by creating a window above the teeth in the canine fossa area.

canthorrhaphy. Suturing of the palpebral fissure, the juncture between the eyelids, at either end of the eye.

canthotomy. Horizontal incision at the canthus (junction of upper and lower eyelids) to divide the outer canthus and enlarge lid margin separation.

cardio-. Relating to the heart.

cardiopulmonary bypass. Venous blood is diverted to a heart-lung machine, which mechanically pumps and oxygenates the blood temporarily so the heart can be bypassed while an open procedure on the heart or coronary arteries is performed. During bypass, the lungs are deflated and immobile.

cardioverter-defibrillator. Device that uses both low energy cardioversion or defibrillating shocks and antitachycardia pacing to treat ventricular tachycardia or ventricular fibrillation.

care plan oversight services. Physician's ongoing review and revision of a patient's care plan involving complex or multidisciplinary care modalities.

case management services. Physician case management is a process of involving direct patient care as well as coordinating and controlling access to the patient or initiating and/or supervising other necessary health care services.

cataract extraction. Surgical removal of the cataract or cloudy lens. Anterior chamber lenses are inserted in conjunction with intracapsular cataract extraction and posterior chamber lenses are inserted in conjunction with extracapsular cataract extraction.

catheter. Flexible tube inserted into an area of the body for introducing or withdrawing fluid.

Centers for Medicare and Medicaid Services. Federal agency that oversees the administration of the public health programs such as Medicare, Medicaid, and State Children's Insurance Program.

certified nurse midwife. Registered nurse who has successfully completed a program of study and clinical experience or has been certified by a recognized organization for the care of pregnant or delivering patients.

CFR. Code of Federal Regulations.

CGMS. Continuous glucose monitoring system.

CHAMPUS. Civilian Health and Medical Program of the Uniformed Services. See Tricare.

CHAMPVA. Civilian Health and Medical Program of the Department of Veterans Affairs.

chemodenervation. Chemical destruction of nerves. A substance, for example, Botox, is used to temporarily inhibit the transfer of chemicals at the presynaptic membrane, blocking the neuromuscular junctions.

chemoembolization. Administration of chemotherapeutic agents directly to a tumor in combination with the percutaneous administration of an occlusive substance into a vessel to deprive the tumor of its blood supply. This ensures a prolonged level of therapy directed at the tumor. Chemoembolization is primarily being used for cancers of the liver and endocrine system.

chemosurgery. Application of chemical agents to destroy tissue, originally referring to the in situ chemical fixation of premalignant or malignant lesions to facilitate surgical excision.

Chiari osteotomy. Top of the femur is altered to correct a dislocated hip caused by congenital conditions or cerebral palsy. Plate and screws are often used.

chimera. Organ or anatomic structure consisting of tissues of diverse genetic constitution.

choanal atresia. Congenital, membranous, or bony closure of one or both posterior nostrils due to failure of the embryonic bucconasal membrane to rupture and open up the nasal passageway.

chondromalacia. Condition in which the articular cartilage softens, seen in various body sites but most often in the patella, and may be congenital or acquired.

chorionic villus sampling. Aspiration of a placental sample through a catheter, under ultrasonic guidance. The specialized needle is placed transvaginally through the cervix or transabdominally into the uterine cavity.

chronic pain management services. Distinct services frequently performed by anesthesiologists who have additional training in pain management procedures. Pain management services include initial and subsequent evaluation and management (E/M) services, trigger point injections, spine and spinal cord injections, and nerve blocks.

cineplastic amputation. Amputation in which muscles and tendons of the remaining portion of the extremity are arranged so that they may be utilized for motor functions. Following this type of amputation, a specially constructed prosthetic device allows the individual to execute more complex movements because the muscles and tendons are able to communicate independent movements to the device.

circadian. Relating to a cyclic, 24-hour period.

CLIA. Clinical Laboratory Improvement Amendments. Requirements set in 1988, CLIA imposes varying levels of federal regulations on clinical procedures. Few laboratories, including those in physician offices, are exempt. Adopted by Medicare and Medicaid, CLIA regulations redefine laboratory testing in regard to laboratory certification and accreditation, proficiency testing, quality assurance, personnel standards, and program administration.

clinical social worker. Individual who possesses a master's or doctor's degree in social work and, after obtaining the degree, has performed at least two years of supervised clinical social work. A clinical social worker must be licensed by the state or, in the case of states without licensure, must completed at least two years or 3,000 hours of post-master's degree supervised clinical social work practice under the supervision of a master's level social worker.

clinical staff. Someone who works for, or under, the direction of a physician or qualified health care professional and does not bill services separately. The person may be licensed or regulated to help the physician perform specific duties.

clonal. Originating from one cell.

CMS. Centers for Medicare and Medicaid Services. Federal agency that administers the public health programs.

CO_2 laser. Carbon dioxide laser that emits an invisible beam and vaporizes water-rich tissue. The vapor is suctioned from the site.

codons. Series of three adjoining bases in one polynucleotide chain of a DNA or RNA molecule that provides the codes for a specific amino acid.

cognitive. Being aware by drawing from knowledge, such as judgment, reason, perception, and memory.

colostomy. Artificial surgical opening anywhere along the length of the colon to the skin surface for the diversion of feces.

commissurotomy. Surgical division or disruption of any two parts that are joined to form a commissure in order to increase the opening. The procedure most often refers to opening the adherent leaflet bands of fibrous tissue in a stenosed mitral valve.

common variants. Nucleotide sequence differences associated with abnormal gene function. Tests are usually performed in a single series of laboratory testing (in a single, typically multiplex, assay arrangement or using more than one assay to include all variants to be examined). Variants are representative of a mutation that mainly causes a single disease, such as cystic fibrosis. Other uncommon variants could provide additional information. Tests may be performed based on society recommendations and guidelines.

community mental health center. Facility providing outpatient mental health day treatment, assessments, and education as appropriate to community members.

component code. In the National Correct Coding Initiative (NCCI), the column II code that cannot be charged to Medicare when the column I code is reported.

comprehensive code. In the National Correct Coding Initiative (NCCI), the column I code that is reported to Medicare and precludes reporting column II codes.

computerized corneal topography. Digital imaging and analysis by computer of the shape of the corneal.

conjunctiva. Mucous membrane lining of the eyelids and covering of the exposed, anterior sclera.

conjunctivodacryocystostomy. Surgical connection of the lacrimal sac directly to the conjunctival sac.

conjunctivorhinostomy. Correction of an obstruction of the lacrimal canal achieved by suturing the posterior flaps and removing any lacrimal obstruction, preserving the conjunctiva.

constitutional. Cells containing genetic code that may be passed down to future generations. May also be referred to as germline.

consultation. Advice or opinion regarding diagnosis and treatment or determination to accept transfer of care of a patient rendered by a medical professional at the request of the primary care provider.

continuous positive airway pressure device. Pressurized device used to maintain the patient's airway for spontaneous or mechanically aided breathing. Often used for patients with mild to moderate sleep apnea.

core needle biopsy. Large-bore biopsy needle inserted into a mass and a core of tissue is removed for diagnostic study.

corpectomy. Removal of the body of a bone, such as a vertebra.

costochondral. Pertaining to the ribs and the scapula.

COTD. Cardiac output thermodilution. Cardiac output measured by thermodilution method that requires heart catheterization and then injection of a thermal indicator, usually iced saline. A computer calculates the cardiac output using an equation that incorporates body temperature, injectate volume and temperature, time, and other calculated ratios over a denominator of the integral of the change in blood temperature during the cold injection, reflected by the area of the inscribed curve.

CPT. 1) Chest physical therapy. 2) Cold pressor test. 3) Current Procedural Terminology.

craniosynostosis. Congenital condition in which one or more of the cranial sutures fuse prematurely, creating a deformed or aberrant head shape.

craterization. Excision of a portion of bone creating a crater-like depression to facilitate drainage from infected areas of bone.

cricoid. Circular cartilage around the trachea.

CRNA. Certified registered nurse anesthetist. Nurse trained and specializing in the administration of anesthesia.

cryolathe. Tool used for reshaping a button of corneal tissue.

cryosurgery. Application of intense cold, usually produced using liquid nitrogen, to locally freeze diseased or unwanted tissue and induce tissue necrosis without causing harm to adjacent tissue.

CT. Computed tomography.

cutdown. Small, incised opening in the skin to expose a blood vessel, especially over a vein (venous cutdown) to allow venipuncture and permit a needle or cannula to be inserted for the withdrawal of blood or administration of fluids.

cyclophotocoagulation. Procedure done to prevent vision loss from glaucoma in which a neodymium: YAG laser is used to burn and destroy a portion of the ciliary body in order to decrease the amount of aqueous humor being produced in the eye. This procedure is only done when creating a drain for aqueous humor to reduce intraocular pressure would not be successful. Destroying portions of the ciliary body reduces the amount of fluid present in the eye.

cytogenetic studies. Procedures in CPT that are related to the branch of genetics that studies cellular (cyto) structure and function as it relates to heredity (genetics). White blood cells, specifically T-lymphocytes, are the most commonly used specimen for chromosome analysis.

cytogenomic. Chromosomic evaluation using molecular methods.

dacryocystotome. Instrument used for incising the lacrimal duct strictures.

DBS. Deep brain stimulation. Treatment for disabling neurological symptoms associated with diseases including Parkinson's. DBS requires three components: the implanted electrode, extension, and neurostimulator. Electrical impulses are sent from the neurostimulator to the implant to block tremors.

debride. To remove all foreign objects and devitalized or infected tissue from a burn or wound to prevent infection and promote healing.

definitive drug testing. Drug tests used to further analyze or confirm the presence or absence of specific drugs or classes of drugs used by the patient. These tests are able to provide more conclusive information regarding the concentration of the drug and their metabolites. May be used for medical, workplace, or legal purposes.

definitive identification. Identification of microorganisms using additional tests to specify the genus or species (e.g., slide cultures or biochemical panels).

dentoalveolar structure. Area of alveolar bone surrounding the teeth and adjacent tissue.

Department of Health and Human Services. Cabinet department that oversees the operating divisions of the federal government responsible for health and welfare. HHS oversees the Centers for Medicare and Medicaid Services, Food and Drug Administration, Public Health Service, and other such entities.

Department of Justice. Attorneys from the DOJ and the United States Attorney's Office have, under the memorandum of understanding, the same direct access to contractor data and records as the OIG and the Federal Bureau of Investigation (FBI). DOJ is responsible for prosecution of fraud and civil or criminal cases presented.

dermis. Skin layer found under the epidermis that contains a papillary upper layer and the deep reticular layer of collagen, vascular bed, and nerves.

dermis graft. Skin graft that has been separated from the epidermal tissue and the underlying subcutaneous fat, used primarily as a substitute for fascia grafts in plastic surgery.

desensitization. 1) Administration of extracts of allergens periodically to build immunity in the patient. 2) Application of medication to decrease the symptoms, usually pain, associated with a dental condition or disease.

destruction. Ablation or eradication of a structure or tissue.

diabetes outpatient self-management training services. Educational and training services furnished by a certified provider in an outpatient setting. The physician managing the individual's diabetic condition must certify that the services are needed under a comprehensive plan of care and provide the patient with the skills and knowledge necessary for therapeutic program compliance (including skills related to the self-administration of injectable drugs). The provider must meet applicable standards established by the National Diabetes Advisory or be recognized by an organization that represents individuals with diabetes as meeting standards for furnishing the services.

diagnostic procedures. Procedure performed on a patient to obtain information to assess the medical condition of the patient or to identify a disease and to determine the nature and severity of an illness or injury.

dialysis. Artificial filtering of the blood to remove contaminating waste elements and restore normal balance.

diaphragm. 1) Muscular wall separating the thorax and its structures from the abdomen. 2) Flexible disk inserted into the vagina and against the cervix as a method of birth control.

diaphysectomy. Surgical removal of a portion of the shaft of a long bone, often done to facilitate drainage from infected bone.

diathermy. Applying heat to body tissues by various methods for therapeutic treatment or surgical purposes to coagulate and seal tissue.

digital medicine services. Those that utilize technology in various forms to provide patient health services.

dilation. Artificial increase in the diameter of an opening or lumen made by medication or by instrumentation.

dissect. Cut apart or separate tissue for surgical purposes or for visual or microscopic study.

DNA. Deoxyribonucleic acid. Chemical containing the genetic information necessary to produce and propagate living organisms. Molecules are comprised of two twisting paired strands, called a double helix.

DNA marker. Specific gene sequence within a chromosome indicating the inheritance of a certain trait.

dorsal. Pertaining to the back or posterior aspect.

drugs and biologicals. Drugs and biologicals included - or approved for inclusion - in the United States Pharmacopoeia, the National Formulary, the United States Homeopathic Pharmacopoeia, in New Drugs or Accepted Dental Remedies, or approved by the pharmacy and drug therapeutics committee of the medical staff of the hospital. Also included are medically accepted and FDA approved drugs used in an anticancer chemotherapeutic regimen. The carrier determines medical acceptance based on supportive clinical evidence.

dual-lead device. Implantable cardiac device (pacemaker or implantable cardioverter-defibrillator [ICD]) in which pacing and sensing components are placed in only two chambers of the heart.

duplex scan. Noninvasive vascular diagnostic technique that uses ultrasonic scanning to identify the pattern and direction of blood flow within arteries or veins displayed in real time images. Duplex scanning combines B-mode two-dimensional pictures of the vessel structure with spectra and/or color flow Doppler mapping or imaging of the blood as it moves through the vessels.

duplication/deletion (DUP/DEL). Term used in molecular testing which examines genomic regions to determine if there are extra chromosomes (duplication) or missing chromosomes (deletions). Normal gene dosage is two copies per cell except for the sex chromosomes which have one per cell.

DuToit staple capsulorrhaphy. Reattachment of the capsule of the shoulder and glenoid labrum to the glenoid lip using staples to anchor the avulsed capsule and glenoid labrum.

Dx. Diagnosis.

DXA. Dual energy x-ray absorptiometry. Radiological technique for bone density measurement using a two-dimensional projection system in which two x-ray beams with different levels of energy are pulsed alternately and the results are given in two scores, reported as standard deviations from peak bone mass density.

dynamic mutation. Unstable or changing polynucleotides resulting in repeats related to genes that can undergo disease-producing increases or decreases in the repeats that differ within tissues or over generations.

ECMO. Extracorporeal membrane oxygenation.

ectropion. Drooping of the lower eyelid away from the eye or outward turning or eversion of the edge of the eyelid, exposing the palpebral conjunctiva and causing irritation.

Eden-Hybinette procedure. Anterior shoulder repair using an anterior bone block to augment the bony anterior glenoid lip.

EDTA. Drug used to inhibit damage to the cornea by collagenase. EDTA is especially effective in alkali burns as it neutralizes soluble alkali, including lye.

effusion. Escape of fluid from within a body cavity.

electrocardiographic rhythm derived. Analysis of data obtained from readings of the heart's electrical activation, including heart rate and rhythm, variability of heart rate, ST analysis, and T-wave alternans. Other data may also be assessed when warranted.

electrocautery. Division or cutting of tissue using high-frequency electrical current to produce heat, which destroys cells.

electrode array. Electronic device containing more than one contact whose function can be adjusted during programming services. Electrodes are specialized for a particular electrochemical reaction that acts as a medium between a body surface and another instrument.

electromyography. Test that measures muscle response to nerve stimulation determining if muscle weakness is present and if it is related to the muscles themselves or a problem with the nerves that supply the muscles.

electrooculogram (EOG). Record of electrical activity associated with eye movements.

electrophysiologic studies. Electrical stimulation and monitoring to diagnose heart conduction abnormalities that predispose patients to bradyarrhythmias and to determine a patient's chance for developing ventricular and supraventricular tachyarrhythmias.

embolization. Placement of a clotting agent, such as a coil, plastic particles, gel, foam, etc., into an area of hemorrhage to stop the bleeding or to block blood flow to a problem area, such as an aneurysm or a tumor.

emergency. Serious medical condition or symptom (including severe pain) resulting from injury, sickness, or mental illness that arises suddenly and requires immediate care and treatment, generally received within 24 hours of onset, to avoid jeopardy to the life, limb, or health of a covered person.

empyema. Accumulation of pus within the respiratory, or pleural, cavity.

EMTALA. Emergency Medical Treatment and Active Labor Act.

end-stage renal disease. Chronic, advanced kidney disease requiring renal dialysis or a kidney transplant to prevent imminent death.

endarterectomy. Removal of the thickened, endothelial lining of a diseased or damaged artery.

endomicroscopy. Diagnostic technology that allows for the examination of tissue at the cellular level during endoscopy. The technology decreases the need for biopsy with histological examination for some types of lesions.

endovascular embolization. Procedure whereby vessels are occluded by a variety of therapeutic substances for the treatment of abnormal blood vessels by inhibiting the flow of blood to a tumor, arteriovenous malformations, lymphatic malformation, and to prevent or stop hemorrhage.

entropion. Inversion of the eyelid, turning the edge in toward the eyeball and causing irritation from contact of the lashes with the surface of the eye.

enucleation. Removal of a growth or organ cleanly so as to extract it in one piece.

enzyme immunoassay. Any of several diagnostic immunoassay methods in which an enzyme is bound to an antigen or antibody and acts as a label.

enzyme-linked immunosorbent assay. A laboratory immunoassay technique used in the diagnosis of certain diseases in which antibodies bound to enzymes reveal and quantify the amount of a substance in a solution, such as serum. It is performed using a solid surface to which the antibodies and other molecules adhere. In the last step, an enzymatic reaction occurs that results in a color change that can be read using a specialized instrument.

epidermis. Outermost, nonvascular layer of skin that contains four to five differentiated layers depending on its body location: stratum corneum, lucidum, granulosum, spinosum, and basale.

epiphysiodesis. Surgical fusion of an epiphysis performed to prematurely stop further bone growth.

escharotomy. Surgical incision into the scab or crust resulting from a severe burn in order to relieve constriction and allow blood flow to the distal unburned tissue.

established patient. 1) Patient who has received professional services in a face-to-face setting within the last three years from the same physician/qualified health care professional or another physician/qualified health care professional of the exact same specialty and subspecialty who belongs to the same group practice. 2) For OPPS hospitals, patient who has been registered as an inpatient or outpatient in a hospital's provider-based clinic or emergency department within the past three years.

evacuation. Removal or purging of waste material.

evaluation and management codes. Assessment and management of a patient's health care.

evaluation and management service components. Key components of history, examination, and medical decision making that are key to selecting the correct E/M codes. Other non-key components include counseling, coordination of care, nature of presenting problem, and time.

event recorder. Portable, ambulatory heart monitor worn by the patient that makes electrocardiographic recordings of the length and frequency of aberrant cardiac rhythm to help diagnose heart conditions and to assess pacemaker functioning or programming.

exenteration. Surgical removal of the entire contents of a body cavity, such as the pelvis or orbit.

exon. One of multiple nucleic acid sequences used to encode information for a gene polypeptide or protein. Exons are separated from other exons by non-protein-coding sequences known as introns.

extended care services. Items and services provided to an inpatient of a skilled nursing facility, including nursing care, physical or occupational therapy, speech pathology, drugs and supplies, and medical social services.

external electrical capacitor device. External electrical stimulation device designed to promote bone healing. This device may also promote neural regeneration, revascularization, epiphyseal growth, and ligament maturation.

external pulsating electromagnetic field. External stimulation device designed to promote bone healing. This device may also promote neural regeneration, revascularization, epiphyseal growth, and ligament maturation.

extracorporeal. Located or taking place outside the body.

Eyre-Brook capsulorrhaphy. Reattachment of the capsule of the shoulder and glenoid labrum to the glenoid lip.

False Claims Act. Governs civil actions for filing false claims. Liability under this act pertains to any person who knowingly presents or causes to be presented a false or fraudulent claim to the government for payment or approval.

fascia. Fibrous sheet or band of tissue that envelops organs, muscles, and groupings of muscles.

fasciectomy. Excision of fascia or strips of fascial tissue.

fasciotomy. Incision or transection of fascial tissue.

fat graft. Graft composed of fatty tissue completely freed from surrounding tissue that is used primarily to fill in depressions.

FDA. Food and Drug Administration. Federal agency responsible for protecting public health by substantiating the safety, efficacy, and security of human and veterinary drugs, biological products, medical devices, national food supply, cosmetics, and items that give off radiation.

filtered speech test. Test most commonly used to identify central auditory dysfunction in which the patient is presented monosyllabic words that are low pass filtered, allowing only the parts of each word below a certain pitch to be presented. A score is given on the number of correct responses. This may be a subset of a standard battery of tests provided during a single encounter.

fissure. Deep furrow, groove, or cleft in tissue structures.

fistulization. Creation of a communication between two structures that were not previously connected.

flexor digitorum profundus tendon. Tendon originating in the proximal forearm and extending to the index finger and wrist. A thickened FDP sheath, usually caused by age, illness, or injury, can fill the carpal canal and lead to impingement of the median nerve.

fluorescence immunoassay. A form of immunoassay that uses a fluorescent compound as the detection reagent. This compound absorbs light or energy at a particular wavelength and then emits light or energy at a different wavelength.

fluoroscopy. Radiology technique that allows visual examination of part of the body or a function of an organ using a device that projects an x-ray image on a fluorescent screen.

focal length. Distance between the object in focus and the lens.

focused medical review. Process of targeting and directing medical review efforts on Medicare claims where the greatest risk of inappropriate program payment exists. The goal is to reduce the number of noncovered claims or unnecessary services. CMS analyzes national data such as internal billing, utilization, and payment data and provides its findings to the FI. Local medical review policies are developed identifying aberrances, abuse, and overutilized services. Providers are responsible for knowing national Medicare coverage and billing guidelines and local medical review policies, and for determining whether the services provided to Medicare beneficiaries are covered by Medicare.

fragile X syndrome. Intellectual disabilities, enlarged testes, big jaw, high forehead, and long ears in males. In females, fragile X presents with mild intellectual disabilities and heterozygous sexual structures. In some families, males have shown no symptoms but carry the gene.

free flap. Tissue that is completely detached from the donor site and transplanted to the recipient site, receiving its blood supply from capillary ingrowth at the recipient site.

free microvascular flap. Tissue that is completely detached from the donor site following careful dissection and preservation of the blood vessels, then attached to the recipient site with the transferred blood vessels anastomosed to the vessels in the recipient bed.

fulguration. Destruction of living tissue by using sparks from a high-frequency electric current.

gas tamponade. Absorbable gas may be injected to force the retina against the choroid. Common gases include room air, short-acting sulfahexafluoride, intermediate-acting perfluoroethane, or long-acting perfluorooctane.

Gaucher disease. Genetic metabolic disorder in which fat deposits may accumulate in the spleen, liver, lungs, bone marrow, and brain.

gene. Basic unit of heredity that contains nucleic acid. Genes are arranged in different and unique sequences or strings that determine the gene's function. Human genes usually include multiple protein coding regions such as exons separated by introns which are nonprotein coding sections.

genome. Complete set of DNA of an organism. Each cell in the human body is comprised of a complete copy of the approximately three billion DNA base pairs that constitute the human genome.

habilitative services. Procedures or services provided to assist a patient in learning, keeping, and improving new skills needed to perform daily living activities. Habilitative services assist patients in acquiring a skill for the first time.

HCPCS. Healthcare Common Procedure Coding System.

HCPCS Level I. Healthcare Common Procedure Coding System Level I. Numeric coding system used by physicians, facility outpatient departments, and ambulatory surgery centers (ASC) to code ambulatory, laboratory, radiology, and other diagnostic services for Medicare billing. This coding system contains only the American Medical Association's Physicians' Current Procedural Terminology (CPT) codes. The AMA updates codes annually.

HCPCS Level II. Healthcare Common Procedure Coding System Level II. National coding system, developed by CMS, that contains alphanumeric codes for physician and nonphysician services not included in the CPT coding system. HCPCS Level II covers such things as ambulance services, durable medical equipment, and orthotic and prosthetic devices.

HCPCS modifiers. Two-character code (AA-ZZ) that identifies circumstances that alter or enhance the description of a service or supply. They are recognized by carriers nationally and are updated annually by CMS.

Hct. Hematocrit.

health care provider. Entity that administers diagnostic and therapeutic services.

hemilaminectomy. Excision of a portion of the vertebral lamina.

hemodialysis. Cleansing of wastes and contaminating elements from the blood by virtue of different diffusion rates through a semipermeable membrane, which separates blood from a filtration solution that diffuses other elements out of the blood. The blood is slowly filtered extracorporeally through special dialysis equipment and returned to the body. Synonym(s): renal dialysis.

hemodialysis. Cleansing of wastes and contaminating elements from the blood by virtue of different diffusion rates through a semipermeable membrane, which separates blood from a filtration solution that diffuses other elements out of the blood.

hemoperitoneum. Effusion of blood into the peritoneal cavity, the space between the continuous membrane lining the abdominopelvic walls and encasing the visceral organs.

heterograft. Surgical graft of tissue from one animal species to a different animal species. A common type of heterograft is porcine (pig) tissue, used for temporary wound closure.

heterotopic transplant. Tissue transplanted from a different anatomical site for usage as is natural for that tissue, for example, buccal mucosa to a conjunctival site.

HGNC. HUGO gene nomenclature committee.

HGVS. Human genome variation society.

Hickman catheter. Central venous catheter used for long-term delivery of medications, such as antibiotics, nutritional substances, or chemotherapeutic agents.

HLA. Human leukocyte antigen.

home health services. Services furnished to patients in their homes under the care of physicians. These services include part-time or intermittent skilled nursing care, physical therapy, medical social services, medical supplies, and some rehabilitation equipment. Home health supplies and services must be prescribed by a physician, and the beneficiary must be confined at home in order for Medicare to pay the benefits in full.

homograft. Graft from one individual to another of the same species.

hospice care. Items and services provided to a terminally ill individual by a hospice program under a written plan established and periodically reviewed by the individual's attending physician and by the medical director: Nursing care provided by or under the supervision of a registered professional nurse; Physical or occupational therapy or speech-language pathology services; Medical social services under the direction of a physician; Services of a home health aide who has successfully completed a training program; Medical supplies (including drugs and biologicals) and the use of medical appliances; Physicians' services; Short-term inpatient care (including both respite care and procedures necessary for pain control and acute and chronic symptom management) in an inpatient facility on an intermittent basis and not consecutively over longer than five days; Counseling (including dietary counseling) with respect to care of the terminally ill individual and adjustment to his death; Any item or service which is specified in the plan and for which payment may be made.

hospital. Institution that provides, under the supervision of physicians, diagnostic, therapeutic, and rehabilitation services for medical diagnosis, treatment, and care of patients. Hospitals receiving federal funds must maintain clinical records on all patients, provide 24-hour nursing services, and have a discharge planning process in place. The term "hospital" also includes religious nonmedical health care institutions and facilities of 50 beds or less located in rural areas.

HUGO. Human genome organization

IA. Intra-arterial.

ICD. Implantable cardioverter defibrillator.

ICD-10-CM. International Classification of Diseases, 10th Revision, Clinical Modification. Clinical modification of the alphanumeric classification of diseases used by the World Health Organization, already in use in much of the world, and used for mortality reporting in the United States. The implementation date for ICD-10-CM diagnostic coding system to replace ICD-9-CM in the United States was October 1, 2015.

ICD-10-PCS. International Classification of Diseases, 10th Revision, Procedure Coding System. Beginning October 1, 2015, inpatient hospital services and surgical procedures must be coded using ICD-10-PCS codes, replacing ICD-9-CM, Volume 3 for procedures.

ICM. Implantable cardiovascular monitor.

ileostomy. Artificial surgical opening that brings the end of the ileum out through the abdominal wall to the skin surface for the diversion of feces through a stoma.

iliopsoas tendon. Fibrous tissue that connects muscle to bone in the pelvic region, common to the iliacus and psoas major.

ILR. Implantable loop recorder.

IM. 1) Infectious mononucleosis. 2) Internal medicine. 3) Intramuscular.

immunochemiluminometric assay. A form of immunoassay in which the antigen-antibody complex is measured using light emission produced from a chemical reaction.

immunotherapy. Therapeutic use of serum or gamma globulin.

implant. Material or device inserted or placed within the body for therapeutic, reconstructive, or diagnostic purposes.

implantable cardiovascular monitor. Implantable electronic device that stores cardiovascular physiologic data such as intracardiac pressure waveforms collected from internal sensors or data such as weight and blood pressure collected from external sensors. The information stored in these devices is used as an aid in managing patients with heart failure and other cardiac conditions that are non-rhythm related. The data may be transmitted via local telemetry or remotely to a surveillance technician or an internet-based file server.

implantable cardioverter-defibrillator. Implantable electronic cardiac device used to control rhythm abnormalities such as tachycardia, fibrillation, or bradycardia by producing high- or low-energy stimulation and pacemaker functions. It may also have the capability to provide the functions of an implantable loop recorder or implantable cardiovascular monitor.

implantable loop recorder. Implantable electronic cardiac device that constantly monitors and records electrocardiographic rhythm. It may be triggered by the patient when a symptomatic episode occurs or activated automatically by rapid or slow heart rates. This may be the sole purpose of the device or it may be a component of another cardiac device, such as a pacemaker or implantable cardioverter-defibrillator. The data can be transmitted via local telemetry or remotely to a surveillance technician or an internet-based file server.

implantable venous access device. Catheter implanted for continuous access to the venous system for long-term parenteral feeding or for the administration of fluids or medications.

IMRT. Intensity modulated radiation therapy. External beam radiation therapy delivery using computer planning to specify the target dose and to modulate the radiation intensity, usually as a treatment for a malignancy. The delivery system approaches the patient from multiple angles, minimizing damage to normal tissue.

in situ. Located in the natural position or contained within the origin site, not spread into neighboring tissue.

incontinence. Inability to control urination or defecation.

infundibulectomy. Excision of the anterosuperior portion of the right ventricle of the heart.

internal direct current stimulator. Electrostimulation device placed directly into the surgical site designed to promote bone regeneration by encouraging cellular healing response in bone and ligaments.

interrogation device evaluation. Assessment of an implantable cardiac device (pacemaker, cardioverter-defibrillator, cardiovascular monitor, or loop recorder) in which collected data about the patient's heart rate and rhythm, battery and pulse generator function, and any leads or sensors present, are retrieved and evaluated. Determinations regarding device programming and appropriate treatment settings are made based on the findings. CPT provides required components for evaluation of the various types of devices.

intramedullary implants. Nail, rod, or pin placed into the intramedullary canal at the fracture site. Intramedullary implants not only provide a method of aligning the fracture, they also act as a splint and may reduce fracture pain. Implants may be rigid or flexible. Rigid implants are preferred for prophylactic treatment of diseased bone, while flexible implants are preferred for traumatic injuries.

intraocular lens. Artificial lens implanted into the eye to replace a damaged natural lens or cataract.

intravenous. Within a vein or veins.

introducer. Instrument, such as a catheter, needle, or tube, through which another instrument or device is introduced into the body.

intron. Nonprotein section of a gene that separates exons in human genes. Contains vital sequences that allow splicing of exons to produce a functional protein from a gene. Sometimes referred to as intervening sequences (IVS).

IP. 1) Interphalangeal. 2) Intraperitoneal.

irrigation. To wash out or cleanse a body cavity, wound, or tissue with water or other fluid.

Kayser-Fleischer ring. Condition found in Wilson's disease in which deposits of copper cause a pigmented ring around the cornea's outer border in the deep epithelial layers.

keratoprosthesis. Surgical procedure in which the physician creates a new anterior chamber with a plastic optical implant to replace a severely damaged cornea that cannot be repaired.

keratotomy. Surgical incision of the cornea.

krypton laser. Laser light energy that uses ionized krypton by electric current as the active source, has a radiation beam between the visible yellow-red spectrum, and is effective in photocoagulation of retinal bleeding, macular lesions, and vessel aberrations of the choroid.

lacrimal. Tear-producing gland or ducts that provides lubrication and flushing of the eyes and nasal cavities.

lacrimal punctum. Opening of the lacrimal papilla of the eyelid through which tears flow to the canaliculi to the lacrimal sac.

lacrimotome. Knife for cutting the lacrimal sac or duct.

lacrimotomy. Incision of the lacrimal sac or duct.

laparotomy. Incision through the flank or abdomen for therapeutic or diagnostic purposes.

laryngoscopy. Examination of the hypopharynx, larynx, and tongue base with an endoscope.

larynx. Musculocartilaginous structure between the trachea and the pharynx that functions as the valve preventing food and other particles from entering the respiratory tract, as well as the voice mechanism. Also called the voicebox, the larynx is composed of three single cartilages: cricoid, epiglottis, and thyroid; and three paired cartilages: arytenoid, corniculate, and cuneiform.

laser surgery. Use of concentrated, sharply defined light beams to cut, cauterize, coagulate, seal, or vaporize tissue.

LEEP. Loop electrode excision procedure. Biopsy specimen or cone shaped wedge of cervical tissue is removed using a hot cautery wire loop with an electrical current running through it.

levonorgestrel. Drug inhibiting ovulation and preventing sperm from penetrating cervical mucus. It is delivered subcutaneously in polysiloxone capsules. The capsules can be effective for up to five years, and provide a cumulative pregnancy rate of less than 2 percent. The capsules are not biodegradable, and therefore must be removed. Removal is more difficult than insertion of levonorgestrel capsules because fibrosis develops around the capsules. Normal hormonal activity and a return to fertility begins immediately upon removal.

ligament. Band or sheet of fibrous tissue that connects the articular surfaces of bones or supports visceral organs.

ligation. Tying off a blood vessel or duct with a suture or a soft, thin wire.

light chains. Proteins produced by plasma (immune) cells; also called kappa and lambda light chains.

lymphadenectomy. Dissection of lymph nodes free from the vessels and removal for examination by frozen section in a separate procedure to detect early-stage metastases.

lysis. Destruction, breakdown, dissolution, or decomposition of cells or substances by a specific catalyzing agent.

Magnuson-Stack procedure. Treatment for recurrent anterior dislocation of the shoulder that involves tightening and realigning the subscapularis tendon.

maintenance of wakefulness test. Attended study determining the patient's ability to stay awake.

Manchester operation. Preservation of the uterus following prolapse by amputating the vaginal portion of the cervix, shortening the cardinal ligaments, and performing a colpoperineorrhaphy posteriorly.

mapping. Multidimensional depiction of a tachycardia that identifies its site of origin and its electrical conduction pathway after tachycardia has been induced. The recording is made from multiple catheter sites within the heart, obtaining electrograms simultaneously or sequentially.

marsupialization. Creation of a pouch in surgical treatment of a cyst in which one wall is resected and the remaining cut edges are sutured to adjacent tissue creating an open pouch of the previously enclosed cyst.

mastectomy. Surgical removal of one or both breasts.

McDonald procedure. Polyester tape is placed around the cervix with a running stitch to assist in the prevention of pre-term delivery. Tape is removed at term for vaginal delivery.

MCP. Metacarpophalangeal.

medial. Middle or midline.

mediastinotomy. Incision into the mediastinum for purposes of exploration, foreign body removal, drainage, or biopsy.

medical review. Review by a Medicare administrative contractor, carrier, and/or quality improvement organization (QIO) of services and items provided by physicians, other health care practitioners, and providers of health care services under Medicare. The review determines if the items and services are reasonable and necessary and meet Medicare coverage requirements, whether the quality meets professionally recognized standards of health care, and whether the services are medically appropriate in an inpatient, outpatient, or other setting as supported by documentation.

Medicare contractor. Medicare Part A fiscal intermediary, Medicare Part B carrier, Medicare administrative contractor (MAC), or a durable medical equipment Medicare administrative contractor (DME MAC).

Medicare physician fee schedule. List of payments Medicare allows by procedure or service. Payments may vary through geographic adjustments. The MPFS is based on the resource-based relative value scale (RBRVS). A national total relative value unit (RVU) is given to each procedure (HCPCS Level I CPT, Level II national codes). Each total RVU has three components: physician work, practice expense, and malpractice insurance.

meibomian gland. Sebaceous gland located in the tarsal plates along the eyelid margins that produces the lipid components found in tears.

metabolite. Chemical compound resulting from the natural process of metabolism. In drug testing, the metabolite of the drug may endure in a higher concentration or for a longer duration than the initial "parent" drug.

methylation. Mechanism used to regulate genes and protect DNA from some types of cleavage.

microarray. Small surface onto which multiple specific nucleic acid sequences can be attached to be used for analysis. Microarray may also be known as a gene chip or DNA chip. Tests can be run on the sequences for any variants that may be present.

mitral valve. Valve with two cusps that is between the left atrium and left ventricle of the heart.

moderate sedation. Medically controlled state of depressed consciousness, with or without analgesia, while maintaining the patient's airway, protective reflexes, and ability to respond to stimulation or verbal commands.

Mohs micrographic surgery. Special technique used to treat complex or ill-defined skin cancer and requires a single physician to provide two distinct services. The first service is surgical and involves the destruction of the lesion by a combination of chemosurgery and excision. The second service is that of a pathologist and includes mapping, color coding of specimens, microscopic examination of specimens, and complete histopathologic preparation.

monitored anesthesia care. Sedation, with or without analgesia, used to achieve a medically controlled state of depressed consciousness while maintaining the patient's airway, protective reflexes, and ability to respond to stimulation or verbal commands. In dental conscious sedation, the patient is rendered free of fear, apprehension, and anxiety through the use of pharmacological agents.

monoclonal. Relating to a single clone of cells.

mosaicplasty. Multiple, small grafts composed of bone and cartilage placed to treat osteochondral defects of the knee. The grafts are cylindrical in shape and are placed in corresponding size holes made to the desired depth to fill the defect and allow for a more naturally shaped reconstruction.

multiple sleep latency test (MSLT). Attended study to determine the tendency of the patient to fall asleep.

multiple-lead device. Implantable cardiac device (pacemaker or implantable cardioverter-defibrillator [ICD]) in which pacing and sensing components are placed in at least three chambers of the heart.

Mustard procedure. Corrective measure for transposition of great vessels involves an intra-atrial baffle made of pericardial tissue or synthetic material. The baffle is secured between pulmonary veins and mitral valve and between mitral and tricuspid valves. The baffle directs systemic venous flow into the left ventricle and lungs and pulmonary venous flow into the right ventricle and aorta.

mutation. Alteration in gene function that results in changes to a gene or chromosome. Can cause deficits or disease that can be inherited, can have beneficial effects, or result in no noticeable change.

mutation scanning. Process normally used on multiple polymerase chain reaction (PCR) amplicons to determine DNA sequence variants by differences in characteristics compared to normal. Specific DNA variants can then be studied further.

myotomy. Surgical cutting of a muscle to gain access to underlying tissues or for therapeutic reasons.

myringotomy. Incision in the eardrum done to prevent spontaneous rupture precipitated by fluid pressure build-up behind the tympanic membrane and to prevent stagnant infection and erosion of the ossicles.

nasal polyp. Fleshy outgrowth projecting from the mucous membrane of the nose or nasal sinus cavity that may obstruct ventilation or affect the sense of smell.

nasal sinus. Air-filled cavities in the cranial bones lined with mucous membrane and continuous with the nasal cavity, draining fluids through the nose.

nasogastric tube. Long, hollow, cylindrical catheter made of soft rubber or plastic that is inserted through the nose down into the stomach, and is used for feeding, instilling medication, or withdrawing gastric contents.

nasolacrimal punctum. Opening of the lacrimal duct near the nose.

nasopharynx. Membranous passage above the level of the soft palate.

Nd:YAG laser. Laser light energy that uses an yttrium, aluminum, and garnet crystal doped with neodymium ions as the active source, has a radiation beam nearing the infrared spectrum, and is effective in photocoagulation, photoablation, cataract extraction, and lysis of vitreous strands.

nebulizer. Latin for mist, a device that converts liquid into a fine spray and is commonly used to deliver medicine to the upper respiratory, bronchial, and lung areas.

nerve conduction study. Diagnostic test performed to assess muscle or nerve damage. Nerves are stimulated with electric shocks along the course of the muscle. Sensors are utilized to measure and record nerve functions, including conduction and velocity.

neurectomy. Excision of all or a portion of a nerve.

neuromuscular junction. Nerve synapse at the meeting point between the terminal end of a nerve (motor neuron) and a muscle fiber.

neuropsychological testing. Evaluation of a patient's behavioral abilities wherein a physician or other health care professional administers a series of tests in thinking, reasoning, and judgment.

new patient. Patient who is receiving face-to-face care from a provider/qualified health care professional or another physician/qualified health care professional of the exact same specialty and subspecialty who belongs to the same group practice for the first time in three years. For OPPS hospitals, a patient who has not been registered as an inpatient or outpatient, including off-campus provider based clinic or emergency department, within the past three years.

Niemann-Pick syndrome. Accumulation of phospholipid in histiocytes in the bone marrow, liver, lymph nodes, and spleen, cerebral involvement, and red macular spots similar to Tay-Sachs disease. Most commonly found in Jewish infants.

Nissen fundoplasty. Surgical repair technique that involves the fundus of the stomach being wrapped around the lower end of the esophagus to treat reflux esophagitis.

nonabsorbable sutures. Strands of natural or synthetic material that resist absorption into living tissue and are removed once healing is under way. Nonabsorbable sutures are commonly used to close skin wounds and repair tendons or collagenous tissue.

obturator. Prosthesis used to close an acquired or congenital opening in the palate that aids in speech and chewing.

obturator nerve. Lumbar plexus nerve with anterior and posterior divisions that innervate the adductor muscles (e.g., adductor longus, adductor brevis) of the leg and the skin over the medial area of the thigh or a sacral plexus nerve with anterior and posterior divisions that innervate the superior gemellus muscles.

occult blood test. Chemical or microscopic test to determine the presence of blood in a specimen.

ocular implant. Implant inside muscular cone.

oophorectomy. Surgical removal of all or part of one or both ovaries, either as open procedure or laparoscopically. Menstruation and childbearing ability continues when one ovary is removed.

orthosis. Derived from a Greek word meaning "to make straight," it is an artificial appliance that supports, aligns, or corrects an anatomical deformity or improves the use of a moveable body part. Unlike a prosthesis, an orthotic device is always functional in nature.

osteo-. Having to do with bone.

osteogenesis stimulator. Device used to stimulate the growth of bone by electrical impulses or ultrasound.

osteotomy. Surgical cutting of a bone.

ostomy. Artificial (surgical) opening in the body used for drainage or for delivery of medications or nutrients.

pacemaker. Implantable cardiac device that controls the heart's rhythm and maintains regular beats by artificial electric discharges. This device consists of the pulse generator with a battery and the electrodes, or leads, which are placed in single or dual chambers of the heart, usually transvenously.

palmaris longus tendon. Tendon located in the hand that flexes the wrist joint.

paracentesis. Surgical puncture of a body cavity with a specialized needle or hollow tubing to aspirate fluid for diagnostic or therapeutic reasons.

paratenon graft. Graft composed of the fatty tissue found between a tendon and its sheath.

passive mobilization. Pressure, movement, or pulling of a limb or body part utilizing an apparatus or device.

pedicle flap. Full-thickness skin and subcutaneous tissue for grafting that remains partially attached to the donor site by a pedicle or stem in which the blood vessels supplying the flap remain intact.

Pemberton osteotomy. Osteotomy is performed to position triradiate cartilage as a hinge for rotating the acetabular roof in cases of dysplasia of the hip in children.

penetrance. Being formed by, or pertaining to, a single clone.

percutaneous intradiscal electrothermal annuloplasty. Procedure corrects tears in the vertebral annulus by applying heat to the collagen disc walls percutaneously through a catheter. The heat contracts and thickens the wall, which may contract and close any annular tears.

percutaneous skeletal fixation. Treatment that is neither open nor closed and the injury site is not directly visualized. Fixation devices (pins, screws) are placed through the skin to stabilize the dislocation using x-ray guidance.

pericardium. Thin and slippery case in which the heart lies that is lined with fluid so that the heart is free to pulse and move as it beats.

peripheral arterial tonometry (PAT). Pulsatile volume changes in a digit are measured to determine activity in the sympathetic nervous system for respiratory analysis.

peritoneal. Space between the lining of the abdominal wall, or parietal peritoneum, and the surface layer of the abdominal organs, or visceral peritoneum. It contains a thin, watery fluid that keeps the peritoneal surfaces moist.

peritoneal dialysis. Dialysis that filters waste from blood inside the body using the peritoneum, the natural lining of the abdomen, as the semipermeable membrane across which ultrafiltration is accomplished. A special catheter is inserted into the abdomen and a dialysis solution is drained into the abdomen. This solution extracts fluids and wastes, which are then discarded when the fluid is drained. Various forms of peritoneal dialysis include CAPD, CCPD, and NIDP.

peritoneal effusion. Persistent escape of fluid within the peritoneal cavity.

pessary. Device placed in the vagina to support and reposition a prolapsing or retropositioned uterus, rectum, or vagina.

phacoemulsification. Cataract extraction in which the lens is fragmented by ultrasonic vibrations and simultaneously irrigated and aspirated.

phenotype. Physical expression of a trait or characteristic as determined by an individual's genetic makeup or genotype.

photocoagulation. Application of an intense laser beam of light to disrupt tissue and condense protein material to a residual mass, used especially for treating ocular conditions.

physical status modifiers. Alphanumeric modifier used to identify the patient's health status as it affects the work related to providing the anesthesia service.

physical therapy modality. Therapeutic agent or regimen applied or used to provide appropriate treatment of the musculoskeletal system.

physician. Legally authorized practitioners including a doctor of medicine or osteopathy, a doctor of dental surgery or of dental medicine, a doctor of podiatric medicine, a doctor of optometry, and a chiropractor only with respect to treatment by means of manual manipulation of the spine (to correct a subluxation).

PICC. Peripherally inserted central catheter. PICC is inserted into one of the large veins of the arm and threaded through the vein until the tip sits in a large vein just above the heart.

PKR. Photorefractive therapy. Procedure involving the removal of the surface layer of the cornea (epithelium) by gentle scraping and use of a computer-controlled excimer laser to reshape the stroma.

plasma. The liquid portion of normal unclotted blood that contains red cells, white cells, and platelets.

pleurodesis. Injection of a sclerosing agent into the pleural space for creating adhesions between the parietal and the visceral pleura to treat a collapsed lung caused by air trapped in the pleural cavity, or severe cases of pleural effusion.

plication. Surgical technique involving folding, tucking, or pleating to reduce the size of a hollow structure or organ.

polyclonal. Containing one or more cells.

polymorphism. Genetic variation in the same species that does not harm the gene function or create disease.

polypeptide. Chain of amino acids held together by covalent bonds. Proteins are made up of amino acids.

polysomnography. Test involving monitoring of respiratory, cardiac, muscle, brain, and ocular function during sleep.

Potts-Smith-Gibson procedure. Side-to-side anastomosis of the aorta and left pulmonary artery creating a shunt that enlarges as the child grows.

Prader-Willi syndrome. Rounded face, almond-shaped eyes, strabismus, low forehead, hypogonadism, hypotonia, intellectual disabilities, and an insatiable appetite.

presumptive drug testing. Drug screening tests to identify the presence or absence of drugs in a patient's system. Tests are usually able to identify low concentrations of the drug. These tests may be used for medical, workplace, or legal purposes.

presumptive identification. Identification of microorganisms using media growth, colony morphology, gram stains, or up to three specific tests (e.g., catalase, indole, oxidase, urease).

professional component. Portion of a charge for health care services that represents the physician's (or other practitioner's) work in providing the service, including interpretation and report of the procedure. This component of the service usually is charged for and billed separately from the inpatient hospital charges.

profunda. Denotes a part of a structure that is deeper from the surface of the body than the rest of the structure.

prolonged physician services. Extended pre- or post-service care provided to a patient whose condition requires services beyond the usual.

prostate. Male gland surrounding the bladder neck and urethra that secretes a substance into the seminal fluid.

prosthetic. Device that replaces all or part of an internal body organ or body part, or that replaces part of the function of a permanently inoperable or malfunctioning internal body organ or body part.

provider of services. Institution, individual, or organization that provides health care.

proximal. Located closest to a specified reference point, usually the midline or trunk.

psychiatric hospital. Specialized institution that provides, under the supervision of physicians, services for the diagnosis and treatment of mentally ill persons.

pterygium. Benign, wedge-shaped, conjunctival thickening that advances from the inner corner of the eye toward the cornea.

pterygomaxillary fossa. Wide depression on the external surface of the maxilla above and to the side of the canine tooth socket.

pulmonary artery banding. Surgical constriction of the pulmonary artery to prevent irreversible pulmonary vascular obstructive changes and overflow into the left ventricle.

Putti-Platt procedure. Realignment of the subscapularis tendon to treat recurrent anterior dislocation, thereby partially eliminating external rotation. The anterior capsule is also tightened and reinforced.

pyloroplasty. Enlargement and reconstruction of the lower portion of the stomach opening into the duodenum performed after vagotomy to speed gastric emptying and treat duodenal ulcers.

qualified health care professional. Educated, licensed or certified, and regulated professional operating under a specified scope of practice to provide patient services that are separate and distinct from other clinical staff. Services may be billed independently or under the facility's services.

RAC. Recovery audit contractor. National program using CMS-affiliated contractors to review claims prior to payment as well as for payments on claims already processed, including overpayments and underpayments.

radiation therapy simulation. Radiation therapy simulation. Procedure by which the specific body area to be treated with radiation is defined and marked. A CT scan is performed to define the body contours and these images are used to create a plan customized treatment for the patient, targeting the area to be treated while sparing adjacent tissue. The center of the area to be treated is marked and an immobilization device (e.g., cradle, mold) is created to make sure the patient is in the same position each time for treatment. Complexity of treatment depends on the number of treatment areas and the use of tools to isolate the area of treatment.

radioactive substances. Materials used in the diagnosis and treatment of disease that emit high-speed particles and energy-containing rays.

radiology services. Services that include diagnostic and therapeutic radiology, nuclear medicine, CT scan procedures, magnetic resonance imaging services, ultrasound, and other imaging procedures.

radiotherapy afterloading. Part of the radiation therapy process in which the chemotherapy agent is actually instilled into the tumor area subsequent to surgery and placement of an expandable catheter into the void remaining after tumor excision. The specialized catheter remains in place and the patient may come in for multiple treatments with radioisotope placed to treat the margin of tissue surrounding the excision. After the radiotherapy is completed, the patient returns to have the catheter emptied and removed. This is a new therapy in breast cancer treatment.

Rashkind procedure. Transvenous balloon atrial septectomy or septostomy performed by cardiac catheterization. A balloon catheter is inserted into the heart either to create or enlarge an opening in the interatrial septal wall.

rehabilitation services. Therapy services provided primarily for assisting in a rehabilitation program of evaluation and service including cardiac rehabilitation, medical social services, occupational therapy, physical therapy, respiratory therapy, skilled nursing, speech therapy, psychiatric rehabilitation, and alcohol and substance abuse rehabilitation.

respiratory airflow (ventilation). Assessment of air movement during inhalation and exhalation as measured by nasal pressure sensors and thermistor.

respiratory analysis. Assessment of components of respiration obtained by other methods such as airflow or peripheral arterial tone.

respiratory effort. Measurement of diaphragm and/or intercostal muscle for airflow using transducers to estimate thoracic and abdominal motion.

respiratory movement. Measurement of chest and abdomen movement during respiration.

ribbons. In oncology, small plastic tubes containing radioactive sources for interstitial placement that may be cut into specific lengths tailored to the size of the area receiving ionizing radiation treatment.

Ridell sinusotomy. Frontal sinus tissue is destroyed to eliminate tumors.

RNA. Ribonucleic acid.

rural health clinic. Clinic in an area where there is a shortage of health services staffed by a nurse practitioner, physician assistant, or certified nurse midwife under physician direction that provides routine diagnostic services, including clinical laboratory services, drugs, and biologicals and that has prompt access to additional diagnostic services from facilities meeting federal requirements.

Salter osteotomy. Innominate bone of the hip is cut, removed, and repositioned to repair a congenital dislocation, subluxation, or deformity.

saucerization. Creation of a shallow, saucer-like depression in the bone to facilitate drainage of infected areas.

Schiotz tonometer. Instrument that measures intraocular pressure by recording the depth of an indentation on the cornea by a plunger of known weight.

screening mammography. Radiologic images taken of the female breast for the early detection of breast cancer.

screening pap smear. Diagnostic laboratory test consisting of a routine exfoliative cytology test (Papanicolaou test) provided to a woman for the early detection of cervical or vaginal cancer. The exam includes a clinical breast examination and a physician's interpretation of the results.

seeds. Small (1 mm or less) sources of radioactive material that are permanently placed directly into tumors.

Senning procedure. Flaps of intra-atrial septum and right atrial wall are used to create two interatrial channels to divert the systemic and pulmonary venous circulation.

sensitivity tests. Number of methods of applying selective suspected allergens to the skin or mucous.

sensorineural conduction. Transportation of sound from the cochlea to the acoustic nerve and central auditory pathway to the brain.

sentinel lymph node. First node to which lymph drainage and metastasis from a cancer can occur.

separate procedures. Services commonly carried out as a fundamental part of a total service and, as such, do not usually warrant separate identification. These services are identified in CPT with the parenthetical phrase (separate procedure) at the end of the description and are payable only when performed alone.

septectomy. 1) Surgical removal of all or part of the nasal septum. 2) Submucosal resection of the nasal septum.

serum. The clear liquid portion of the blood that remains after the clotting proteins and blood cells have been removed.

Shirodkar procedure. Treatment of an incompetent cervical os by placing nonabsorbent suture material in purse-string sutures as a cerclage to support the cervix.

short tandem repeat (STR). Short sequences of a DNA pattern that are repeated. Can be used as genetic markers for human identity testing.

sialodochoplasty. Surgical repair of a salivary gland duct.

single-lead device. Implantable cardiac device (pacemaker or implantable cardioverter-defibrillator [ICD]) in which pacing and sensing components are placed in only one chamber of the heart.

single-nucleotide polymorphism (SNP). Single nucleotide (A, T, C, or G that is different in a DNA sequence. This difference occurs at a significant frequency in the population.

sinus of Valsalva. Any of three sinuses corresponding to the individual cusps of the aortic valve, located in the most proximal part of the aorta just above the cusps. These structures are contained within the pericardium and appear as distinct but subtle outpouchings or dilations of the aortic wall between each of the semilunar cusps of the valve.

sleep apnea. Intermittent cessation of breathing during sleep that may cause hypoxemia and pulmonary arterial hypertension.

sleep latency. Time period between lying down in bed and the onset of sleep.

sleep staging. Determination of the separate levels of sleep according to physiological measurements.

somatic. 1) Pertaining to the body or trunk. 2) In genetics acquired or occurring after birth.

SPECT. Single photon emission computerized tomography. SPECT images are taken after the injection of a radionuclide using a special camera containing a detector crystal, usually sodium iodide. Images are captured as the gamma radiation from the radionuclide scintillates or gives off its energy in a flash of light when coming in contact with the crystal. This type of imaging is reported for the anatomical area and purpose such as detecting liver function or myocardial perfusion after an ischemic event.

speculoscopy. Viewing the cervix utilizing a magnifier and a special wavelength of light, allowing detection of abnormalities that may not be discovered on a routine Pap smear.

speech-language pathology services. Speech, language, and related function assessment and rehabilitation service furnished by a qualified speech-language pathologist. Audiology services include hearing and balance assessment services furnished by a qualified audiologist. A qualified speech pathologist and audiologist must have a master's or doctoral degree in their respective fields and be licensed to serve in the state. Speech pathologists and audiologists practicing in states without licensure must complete 350 hours of supervised clinical work and perform at least nine months of supervised full-time service after earning their degrees.

sphincteroplasty. Surgical repair done to correct, augment, or improve the muscular function of a sphincter, such as the anus or intestines.

spirometry. Measurement of the lungs' breathing capacity.

splint. Brace or support. 1) dynamic splint: brace that permits movement of an anatomical structure such as a hand, wrist, foot, or other part of the body after surgery or injury. 2) static splint: brace that prevents movement and maintains support and position for an anatomical structure after surgery or injury.

stent. Tube to provide support in a body cavity or lumen.

stereotactic radiosurgery. Delivery of externally-generated ionizing radiation to specific targets for destruction or inactivation. Most often utilized in the treatment of brain or spinal tumors, high-resolution stereotactic imaging is used to identify the target and then deliver the treatment. Computer-assisted planning may also be employed. Simple and complex cranial lesions and spinal lesions are typically treated in a single planning and treatment session, although a maximum of five sessions may be required. No incision is made for stereotactic radiosurgery procedures.

stereotaxis. Three-dimensional method for precisely locating structures.

Stoffel rhizotomy. Nerve roots are sectioned to relieve pain or spastic paralysis.

strabismus. Misalignment of the eyes due to an imbalance in extraocular muscles.

surgical package. Normal, uncomplicated performance of specific surgical services, with the assumption that, on average, all surgical procedures of a given type are similar with respect to skill level, duration, and length of normal follow-up care.

symblepharopterygium. Adhesion in which the eyelid is adhered to the eyeball by a band that resembles a pterygium.

sympathectomy. Surgical interruption or transection of a sympathetic nervous system pathway.

synchronous services. Those that entail real-time communication between the patient and/or family and a physician or other qualified health care professional (QHP) when both are located at different physical sites.

tarso-. 1) Relating to the foot. 2) Relating to the margin of the eyelid.

tarsocheiloplasty. Plastic operation upon the edge of the eyelid for the treatment of trichiasis.

tarsorrhaphy. Suture of a portion or all of the opposing eyelids together for the purpose of shortening the palpebral fissure or closing it entirely.

technical component. Portion of a health care service that identifies the provision of the equipment, supplies, technical personnel, and costs attendant to the performance of the procedure other than the professional services.

tendon. Fibrous tissue that connects muscle to bone, consisting primarily of collagen and containing little vasculature.

tendon allograft. Allografts are tissues obtained from another individual of the same species. Tendon allografts are usually obtained from cadavers and frozen or freeze dried for later use in soft tissue repairs where the physician elects not to obtain an autogenous graft (a graft obtained from the individual on whom the surgery is being performed).

tendon suture material. Tendons are composed of fibrous tissue consisting primarily of collagen and containing few cells or blood vessels. This tissue heals more slowly than tissues with more vascularization. Because of this, tendons are usually repaired with nonabsorbable suture material. Examples include surgical silk, surgical cotton, linen, stainless steel, surgical nylon, polyester fiber, polybutester (Novafil), polyethylene (Dermalene), and polypropylene (Prolene, Surilene).

tendon transplant. Replacement of a tendon with another tendon.

tenon's capsule. Connective tissue that forms the capsule enclosing the posterior eyeball, extending from the conjunctival fornix and continuous with the muscular fascia of the eye.

tenonectomy. Excision of a portion of a tendon to make it shorter.

tenotomy. Cutting into a tendon.

TENS. Transcutaneous electrical nerve stimulator. TENS is applied by placing electrode pads over the area to be stimulated and connecting the electrodes to a transmitter box, which sends a current through the skin to sensory nerve fibers to help decrease pain in that nerve distribution.

tensilon. Edrophonium chloride. Agent used for evaluation and treatment of myasthenia gravis.

terminally ill. Individual whose medical prognosis for life expectancy is six months or less.

tetralogy of Fallot. Specific combination of congenital cardiac defects: obstruction of the right ventricular outflow tract with pulmonary stenosis, interventricular septal defect, malposition of the aorta, overriding the interventricular septum and receiving blood from both the venous and arterial systems, and enlargement of the right ventricle.

therapeutic services. Services performed for treatment of a specific diagnosis. These services include performance of the procedure, various incidental elements, and normal, related follow-up care.

thoracentesis. Surgical puncture of the chest cavity with a specialized needle or hollow tubing to aspirate fluid from within the pleural space for diagnostic or therapeutic reasons.

thoracic lymphadenectomy. Procedure to cut out the lymph nodes near the lungs, around the heart, and behind the trachea.

thoracostomy. Creation of an opening in the chest wall for drainage.

thyroglossal duct. Embryonic duct at the front of the neck, which becomes the pyramidal lobe of the thyroid gland with obliteration of the remaining duct, but may form a cyst or sinus in adulthood if it persists.

total disc arthroplasty with artificial disc. Removal of an intravertebral disc and its replacement with an implant. The implant is an artificial disc consisting of two metal plates with a weight-bearing surface of polyethylene between the plates. The plates are anchored to the vertebral immediately above and below the affected disc.

total shoulder replacement. Prosthetic replacement of the entire shoulder joint, including the humeral head and the glenoid fossa.

trabeculae carneae cordis. Bands of muscular tissue that line the walls of the ventricles in the heart.

trabeculectomy. Surgical incision between the anterior portion of the eye and the canal of Schlemm to drain the aqueous humor.

tracheostomy. Formation of a tracheal opening on the neck surface with tube insertion to allow for respiration in cases of obstruction or decreased patency. A tracheostomy may be planned or performed on an emergency basis for temporary or long-term use.

tracheotomy. Formation of a tracheal opening on the neck surface with tube insertion to allow for respiration in cases of obstruction or decreased patency. A tracheotomy may be planned or performed on an emergency basis for temporary or long-term use.

traction. Drawing out or holding tension on an area by applying a direct therapeutic pulling force.

transcranial magnetic stimulation. Application of electromagnetic energy to the brain through a coil placed on the scalp. The procedure stimulates cortical neurons and is intended to activate and normalize their processes.

transcription. Process by which messenger RNA is synthesized from a DNA template resulting in the transfer of genetic information from the DNA molecule to the messenger RNA.

translocation. Disconnection of all or part of a chromosome that reattaches to another position in the DNA sequence of the same or another chromosome. Often results in a reciprocal exchange of DNA sequences between two differently numbered chromosomes. May or may not result in a clinically significant loss of DNA.

trephine. 1) Specialized round saw for cutting circular holes in bone, especially the skull. 2) Instrument that removes small disc-shaped buttons of corneal tissue for transplanting.

tricuspid atresia. Congenital absence of the valve that may occur with other defects, such as atrial septal defect, pulmonary atresia, and transposition of great vessels.

turbinates. Scroll or shell-shaped elevations from the wall of the nasal cavity, the inferior turbinate being a separate bone, while the superior and middle turbinates are of the ethmoid bone.

tympanic membrane. Thin, sensitive membrane across the entrance to the middle ear that vibrates in response to sound waves, allowing the waves to be transmitted via the ossicular chain to the internal ear.

tympanoplasty. Surgical repair of the structures of the middle ear, including the eardrum and the three small bones, or ossicles.

unlisted procedure. Procedural descriptions used when the overall procedure and outcome of the procedure are not adequately described by an existing procedure code. Such codes are used as a last resort and only when there is not a more appropriate procedure code.

ureterorrhaphy. Surgical repair using sutures to close an open wound or injury of the ureter.

vagotomy. Division of the vagus nerves, interrupting impulses resulting in lower gastric acid production and hastening gastric emptying. Used in the treatment of chronic gastric, pyloric, and duodenal ulcers that can cause severe pain and difficulties in eating and sleeping.

variant. Nucleotide deviation from the normal sequence of a region. Variations are usually either substitutions or deletions. Substitution variations are the result of one nucleotide taking the place of another. A deletion occurs when one or more nucleotides are left out. In some cases, several in a reasonably close proximity on the same chromosome in a DNA strand. These variations result in amino acid changes in the protein made by the gene. However, the term variant does not itself imply a functional change. Intron variations are usually described in one of two ways: 1) the changed nucleotide is defined by a plus or a minus sign indicating the position relative to the first or last nucleotide to the intron, or 2) the second variant description is indicated relative to the last nucleotide of the preceding exon or first nucleotide of the following exon.

vascular family. Group of vessels (family) that branch from the aorta or vena cava. At each branching, the vascular order increases by one. The first order vessel is the primary branch off the aorta or vena cava. The second order vessel branches from the first order, the third order branches from the second order, and any further branching is beyond the third order. For example, for the inferior vena cava, the common iliac artery is a first order vessel. The internal and external iliac arteries are second order vessels, as they each originate from the first order common iliac artery. The external iliac artery extends directly from the common iliac artery and the internal iliac artery bifurcates from the common iliac artery. A third order vessel from the external iliac artery is the inferior epigastric artery and a third order vessel from the internal iliac artery is the obturator artery. Note orders are not always identical bilaterally (e.g., the left common carotid artery is a first order and the right common carotid is a second order. Synonym(s): vascular origins and distributions.

vasectomy. Surgical procedure involving the removal of all or part of the vas deferens, usually performed for sterilization or in conjunction with a prostatectomy.

vena cava interruption. Procedure that places a filter device, called an umbrella or sieve, within the large vein returning deoxygenated blood to the heart to prevent pulmonary embolism caused by clots.

ventricular assist device. Temporary measure used to support the heart by substituting for left and/or right heart function. The device replaces the work of the left and/or right ventricle when a patient has a damaged or weakened heart. A left ventricular assist device (VAD) helps the heart pump blood through the rest of the body. A right VAD helps the heart pump blood to the lungs to become oxygenated again. Catheters are inserted to circulate the blood through external tubing to a pump machine located outside of the body and back to the correct artery.

ventricular septal defect. Congenital cardiac anomaly resulting in a continual opening in the septum between the ventricles that, in severe cases, causes oxygenated blood to flow back into the lungs, resulting in pulmonary hypertension.

vertebral interspace. Non-bony space between two adjacent vertebral bodies that contains the cushioning intervertebral disk.

volar. Palm of the hand (palmar) or sole of the foot (plantar).

Waterston procedure. Type of aortopulmonary shunting done to increase pulmonary blood flow. The ascending aorta is anastomosed to the right pulmonary artery.

Wharton's ducts. Salivary ducts below the mandible.

wick catheter. Device used to monitor interstitial fluid pressure, and sometimes used intraoperatively during fasciotomy procedures to evaluate the effectiveness of the decompression.

wound closure. Closure or repair of a wound created surgically or due to trauma (e.g., laceration). The closure technique depends on the type, site, and depth of the defect. Consideration is also given to cosmetic and functional outcome. A single layer closure involves approximation of the edges of the wound. The second type of closure involves closing the one or more deeper layers of tissue prior to skin closure. The most complex type of closure may include techniques such as debridement or undermining, which involves manipulation of tissue around the wound to allow the skin to cover the wound. The AMA CPT® book defines these as Simple, Intermediate and Complex repair.

xenograft. Tissue that is nonhuman and harvested from one species and grafted to another. Pigskin is the most common xenograft for human skin and is applied to a wound as a temporary closure until a permanent option is performed.

z-plasty. Plastic surgery technique used primarily to release tension or elongate contractured scar tissue in which a Z-shaped incision is made with the middle line of the Z crossing the area of greatest tension. The triangular flaps are then rotated so that they cross the incision line in the opposite direction, creating a reversed Z.

ZPIC. Zone Program Integrity Contractor. CMS contractor that replaced the existing Program Safeguard Contractors (PSC). Contractors are responsible for ensuring the integrity of all Medicare-related claims under Parts A and B (hospital, skilled nursing, home health, provider, and durable medical equipment claims), Part C (Medicare Advantage health plans), Part D (prescription drug plans), and coordination of Medicare-Medicaid data matches (Medi-Medi).

Appendix N — Listing of Sensory, Motor, and Mixed Nerves

This list contains the sensory, motor, and mixed nerves assigned to each nerve conduction study to improve coding accuracy. Each nerve makes up one single unit of service.

Motor Nerves Assigned to Codes 95907-95913

I. Upper extremity, cervical plexus, and brachial plexus motor nerves
  A. Axillary motor nerve to the deltoid
  B. Long thoracic motor nerve to the serratus anterior
  C. Median nerve
    1. Median motor nerve to the abductor pollicis brevis
    2. Median motor nerve, anterior interosseous branch, to the flexor pollicis longus
    3. Median motor nerve, anterior interosseous branch, to the pronator quadratus
    4. Median motor nerve to the first lumbrical
    5. Median motor nerve to the second lumbrical
  D. Musculocutaneous motor nerve to the biceps brachii
  E. Radial nerve
    1. Radial motor nerve to the extensor carpi ulnaris
    2. Radial motor nerve to the extensor digitorum communis
    3. Radial motor nerve to the extensor indicis proprius
    4. Radial motor nerve to the brachioradialis
  F. Suprascapular nerve
    1. Suprascapular motor nerve to the supraspinatus
    2. Suprascapular motor nerve to the infraspinatus
  G. Thoracodorsal motor nerve to the latissimus dorsi
  H. Ulnar nerve
    1. Ulnar motor nerve to the abductor digiti minimi
    2. Ulnar motor nerve to the palmar interosseous
    3. Ulnar motor nerve to the first dorsal interosseous
    4. Ulnar motor nerve to the flexor carpi ulnaris
  I. Other

II. Lower extremity motor nerves
  A. Femoral motor nerve to the quadriceps
    1. Femoral motor nerve to vastus medialis
    2. Femoral motor nerve to vastus lateralis
    3. Femoral motor nerve to vastus intermedius
    4. Femoral motor nerve to rectus femoris
  B. Ilioinguinal motor nerve
  C. Peroneal (fibular) nerve
    1. Peroneal motor nerve to the extensor digitorum brevis
    2. Peroneal motor nerve to the peroneus brevis
    3. Peroneal motor nerve to the peroneus longus
    4. Peroneal motor nerve to the tibialis anterior
  D. Plantar motor nerve
  E. Sciatic nerve
  F. Tibial nerve
    1. Tibial motor nerve, inferior calcaneal branch, to the abductor digiti minimi
    2. Tibial motor nerve, medial plantar branch, to the abductor hallucis
    3. Tibial motor nerve, lateral plantar branch, to the flexor digiti minimi brevis
  G. Other

III. Cranial nerves and trunk
  A. Cranial nerve VII (facial motor nerve)
    1. Facial nerve to the frontalis
    2. Facial nerve to the nasalis
    3. Facial nerve to the orbicularis oculi
    4. Facial nerve to the orbicularis oris
  B. Cranial nerve XI (spinal accessory motor nerve)
  C. Cranial nerve XII (hypoglossal motor nerve)
  D. Intercostal motor nerve
  E. Phrenic motor nerve to the diaphragm
  F. Recurrent laryngeal nerve
  G. Other

IV. Nerve Roots
  A. Cervical nerve root stimulation
    1. Cervical level 5 (C5)
    2. Cervical level 6 (C6)
    3. Cervical level 7 (C7)
    4. Cervical level 8 (C8)
  B. Thoracic nerve root stimulation
    1. Thoracic level 1 (T1)
    2. Thoracic level 2 (T2)
    3. Thoracic level 3 (T3)
    4. Thoracic level 4 (T4)
    5. Thoracic level 5 (T5)
    6. Thoracic level 6 (T6)
    7. Thoracic level 7 (T7)
    8. Thoracic level 8 (T8)
    9. Thoracic level 9 (T9)
    10. Thoracic level 10 (T10)
    11. Thoracic level 11 (T11)
    12. Thoracic level 12 (T12)
  C. Lumbar nerve root stimulation
    1. Lumbar level 1 (L1)
    2. Lumbar level 2 (L2)
    3. Lumbar level 3 (L3)
    4. Lumbar level 4 (L4)
    5. Lumbar level 5 (L5)
  D. Sacral nerve root stimulation
    1. Sacral level 1 (S1)
    2. Sacral level 2 (S2)
    3. Sacral level 3 (S3)
    4. Sacral level 4 (S4)

Sensory and Mixed Nerves Assigned to Codes 95907–95913

I. Upper extremity sensory and mixed nerves
   A. Lateral antebrachial cutaneous sensory nerve
   B. Medial antebrachial cutaneous sensory nerve
   C. Medial brachial cutaneous sensory nerve
   D. Median nerve
      1. Median sensory nerve to the first digit
      2. Median sensory nerve to the second digit
      3. Median sensory nerve to the third digit
      4. Median sensory nerve to the fourth digit
      5. Median palmar cutaneous sensory nerve
      6. Median palmar mixed nerve
   E. Posterior antebrachial cutaneous sensory nerve
   F. Radial sensory nerve
      1. Radial sensory nerve to the base of the thumb
      2. Radial sensory nerve to digit 1
   G. Ulnar nerve
      1. Ulnar dorsal cutaneous sensory nerve
      2. Ulnar sensory nerve to the fourth digit
      3. Ulnar sensory nerve to the fifth digit
      4. Ulnar palmar mixed nerve
   H. Intercostal sensory nerve
   I. Other

II. Lower extremity sensory and mixed nerves
   A. Lateral femoral cutaneous sensory nerve
   B. Medical calcaneal sensory nerve
   C. Medial femoral cutaneous sensory nerve
   D. Peroneal nerve
      1. Deep peroneal sensory nerve
      2. Superficial peroneal sensory nerve, medial dorsal cutaneous branch
      3. Superficial peroneal sensory nerve, intermediate dorsal cutaneous branch
   E. Posterior femoral cutaneous sensory nerve
   F. Saphenous nerve
      1. Saphenous sensory nerve (distal technique)
      2. Saphenous sensory nerve (proximal technique)
   G. Sural nerve
      1. Sural sensory nerve, lateral dorsal cutaneous branch
      2. Sural sensory nerve
   H. Tibial sensory nerve (digital nerve to toe 1)
   I. Tibial sensory nerve (medial plantar nerve)
   J. Tibial sensory nerve (lateral plantar nerve)
   K. Other

III. Head and trunk sensory nerves
   A. Dorsal nerve of the penis
   B. Greater auricular nerve
   C. Ophthalmic branch of the trigeminal nerve
   D. Pudendal sensory nerve
   E. Suprascapular sensory nerves
   F. Other

In the following table, the reasonable maximum number of studies per diagnostic category is listed that allows for a physician or other qualified health care professional to obtain a diagnosis for 90 percent of patients with that same final diagnosis. The numbers denote the suggested number of studies, although the decision is up to the provider.

Type of Study/Maximum Number of Studies

Indication	Limbs Studied by Needle EMG (95860–95864, 95867–95870, 95885–95887)	Nerve Conduction Studies (Total nerves studied, 95907-95913)	Neuromuscular Junction Testing (Repetitive Stimulation 95937)
Carpal Tunnel (Unilateral)	1	7	—
Carpal Tunnel (Bilateral)	2	10	—
Radiculopathy	2	7	2
Mononeuropathy	1	8	—
Polyneuropathy/Mononeuropathy Multiplex	3	10	—
Myopathy	2	4	2
Motor Neuronopathy (e.g., ALS)	4	6	2
Plexopathy	2	12	—
Neuromuscular Junction	2	4	3
Tarsal Tunnel Syndrome (Unilateral)	1	8	—
Tarsal Tunnel Syndrome (Bilateral)	2	11	—
Weakness, Fatigue, Cramps, or Twitching (Focal)	2	7	2
Weakness, Fatigue, Cramps, or Twitching (General)	4	8	2
Pain, Numbness, or Tingling (Unilateral)	1	9	—
Pain, Numbness, or Tingling (Bilateral)	2	12	—

Appendix O — Vascular Families

This table assumes that the starting point is aortic, vena cava, pulmonary artery, or portal vein catheterization. This categorization would not be accurate if, for instance, a femoral or carotid artery were catheterized with the blood's flow. The names of the arteries appearing in bold face type in the following table indicate those arteries that are most often the subject of arteriographic procedures.

Arterial Vascular Family

	First Order	Second Order	Third Order	Beyond Third Order
• **Thoracic aorta**	• Right and left coronary			
	• Innominate (brachiocephalic)	• Right common carotid	• Right internal carotid	• Right vidian • Right caroticotympanic • Right meningohypophyseal trunk • Right inferolateral trunk • Right inferior hypophyseal • Right ophthalmic • Right superior hypophyseal • Right anterior choroidal • Right posterior communicating • Right middle cerebral • Right anterior cerebral
			• Right external carotid	• Right superior thyroid • Right ascending pharyngeal • Right lingual • Right facial • Right occipital • Right posterior auricular • Right superficial temporal • Right internal maxillary – Right middle meningeal
		• Right subclavian	• Right vertebral	• Basilar and branches • Posterior cerebral
			• Right internal thoracic (internal mammary)	• Right superior epigastric
			• Right thyrocervical trunk	• Right inferior thyroid • Right ascending cervical • Right transverse cervical • Right suprascapular
			• Right costocervical trunk	• Right deep cervical • Right supreme intercostal
		Right subclavian and right axillary considered 1 vessel for coding purposes • Right axillary	• Right superior thoracic • Right thoracoacromial • Right lateral thoracic • Right anterior & posterior circumflex humeral • Right subscapular	• Right circumflex scapular • Right thoracodorsal
			• Right brachial	• Right profunda brachii • Right ulnar – Right common interosseous • Right radial – Right deep palmar arch – Right superficial palmar arch – Right metacarpal(s) – Right digital(s)
	• Left common carotid	• Left internal carotid	• Left vidian • Left caroticotympanic • Left meningohypophyseal trunk • Left inferolateral trunk • Left inferior hypophyseal • Left ophthalmic • Left superior hypophyseal • Left anterior choroidal • Left posterior communicating • Left middle cerebral • Left anterior cerebral	
		• Left external carotid	• Left superior thyroid • Left ascending pharyngeal • Left lingual • Left facial • Left occipital • Left posterior auricular • Left superficial temporal • Left internal maxillary	• Left middle meningeal

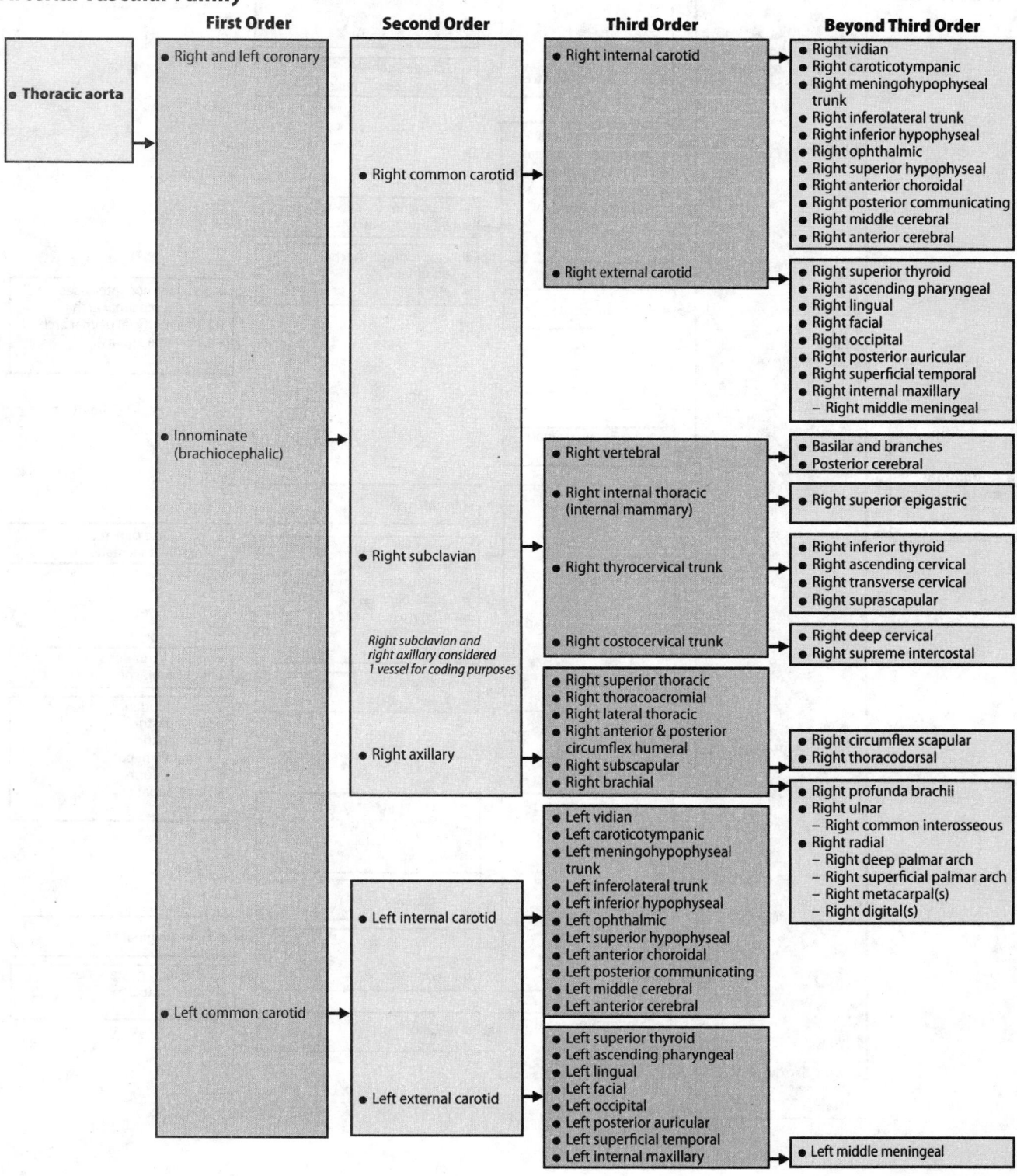

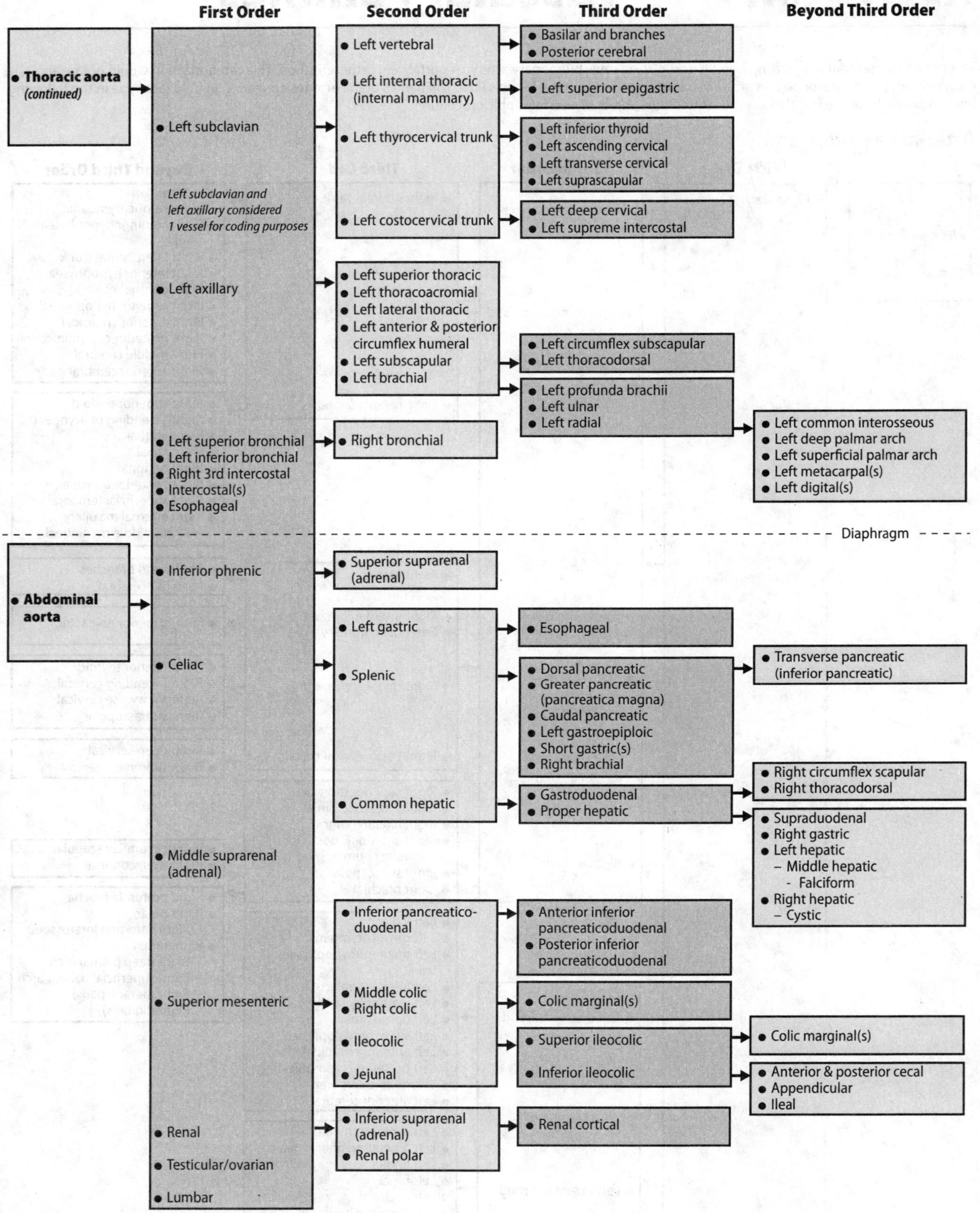
First Order
Second Order
Third Order
Beyond Third Order
Thoracic aorta (continued)
Left subclavian
Left subclavian and left axillary considered 1 vessel for coding purposes
Left axillary
Left superior bronchial
Left inferior bronchial
Right 3rd intercostal
Intercostal(s)
Esophageal
Left vertebral
Left internal thoracic (internal mammary)
Left thyrocervical trunk
Left costocervical trunk
Basilar and branches
Posterior cerebral
Left superior epigastric
Left inferior thyroid
Left ascending cervical
Left transverse cervical
Left suprascapular
Left deep cervical
Left supreme intercostal
Left superior thoracic
Left thoracoacromial
Left lateral thoracic
Left anterior & posterior circumflex humeral
Left subscapular
Left brachial
Left circumflex subscapular
Left thoracodorsal
Left profunda brachii
Left ulnar
Left radial
Left common interosseous
Left deep palmar arch
Left superficial palmar arch
Left metacarpal(s)
Left digital(s)
Right bronchial
Diaphragm
Abdominal aorta
Inferior phrenic
Celiac
Middle suprarenal (adrenal)
Superior mesenteric
Renal
Testicular/ovarian
Lumbar
Superior suprarenal (adrenal)
Left gastric
Splenic
Common hepatic
Esophageal
Dorsal pancreatic
Greater pancreatic (pancreatica magna)
Caudal pancreatic
Left gastroepiploic
Short gastric(s)
Right brachial
Transverse pancreatic (inferior pancreatic)
Right circumflex scapular
Right thoracodorsal
Gastroduodenal
Proper hepatic
Supraduodenal
Right gastric
Left hepatic
– Middle hepatic
- Falciform
Right hepatic
– Cystic
Inferior pancreatico-duodenal
Middle colic
Right colic
Ileocolic
Jejunal
Anterior inferior pancreaticoduodenal
Posterior inferior pancreaticoduodenal
Colic marginal(s)
Superior ileocolic
Inferior ileocolic
Colic marginal(s)
Anterior & posterior cecal
Appendicular
Ileal
Inferior suprarenal (adrenal)
Renal polar
Renal cortical

	First Order	Second Order	Third Order	Beyond Third Order
• **Abdominal aorta** *(continued)*	• Inferior mesenteric	• Left colic • Sigmoid • Superior rectal	• Ascending left colic • Ascending left colic	• Colic marginal(s)
	• Middle (median) sacral			
	• Common iliac	• Internal iliac	• Posterior division	• Iliolumbar • Lateral sacral • Superior gluteal
			• Anterior division	• Obturator • Umbilical – Superior vesical • Uterine • Vaginal • Inferior vesical • Middle rectal – Prostate • Internal pudendal – Inferior rectal • Inferior gluteal
		• External iliac	• Deep circumflex iliac • Inferior epigastric	• Cremasteric
		External iliac and common femoral considered 1 vessel for coding purposes • Common femoral	• Profunda femoris • Deep external pudendal • Superficial external pudendal	• Medial femoral circumflex • Lateral femoral circumflex
			• Superficial femoral *Superficial femoral and popliteal considered 1 vessel for coding purposes* • Popliteal	• Geniculate • Anterior tibial • Posterior tibial • Peroneal • Pedal arch • Digital(s)

Venous Vascular Family

	First Order	Second Order	Beyond Second Order
• **Superior vena cava**	• Innominate (Right brachiocephalic)	• Right internal jugular	• Right inferior petrosal sinus • Right sigmoid sinus • Retromandibular • Facial • Lingual • Superior thyroid • Middle thyroid • Pharyngeal
		• Right subclavian	• Right exterior jugular
		Right subclavian and right axillary considered 1 vessel for coding purposes • Right axillary	• Shoulder and arm veins (eg, brachial, basilic, ulnar, radial)
	• Left brachiocephalic	• Left internal jugular	• Left inferior petrosal sinus • Left sigmoid sinus • Retromandibular • Facial • Lingual • Superior thyroid • Middle thyroid • Pharyngeal
		• Left subclavian	• Left exterior jugular
		Right subclavian and right axillary considered 1 vessel for coding purposes • Left axillary	• Shoulder & arm veins (e.g. brachial, basilic, ulnar, radial)
	• Azygos	• Intercostal(s) • Hemiazygos • Right ascending lumbar	• Left ascending lumbar

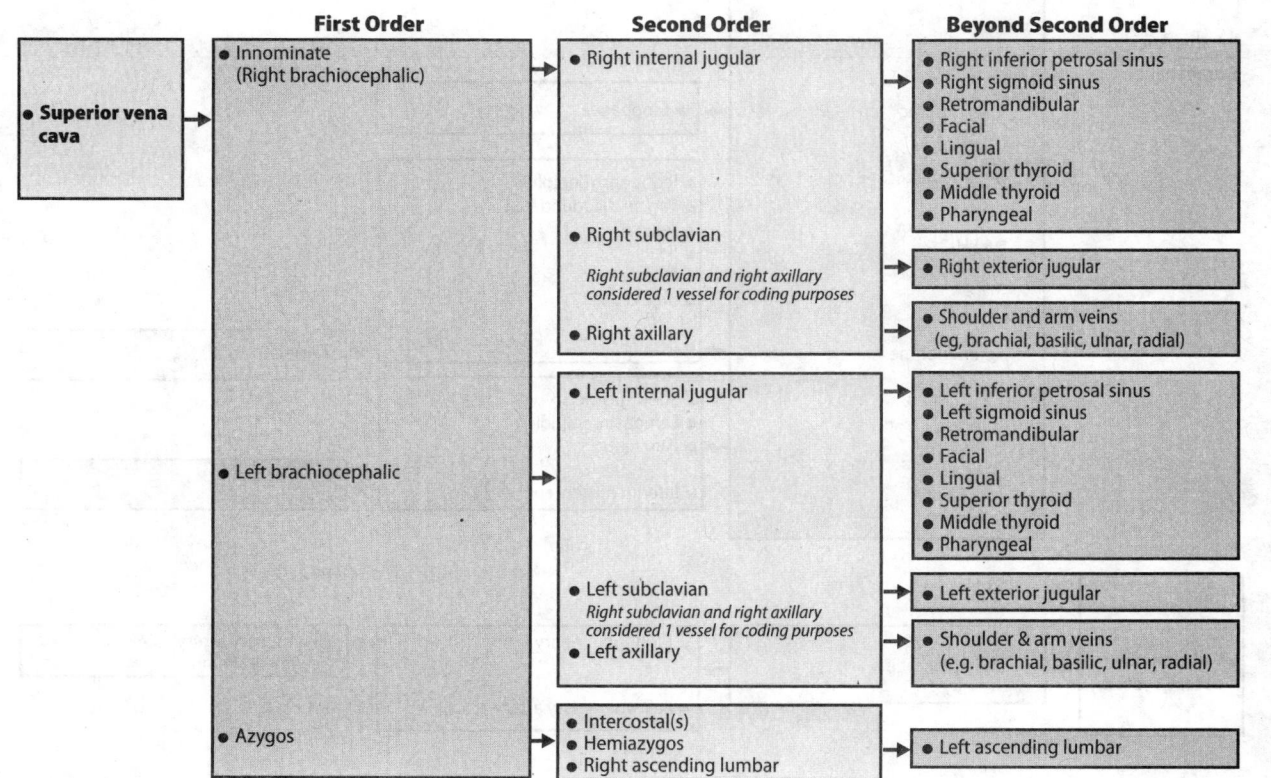

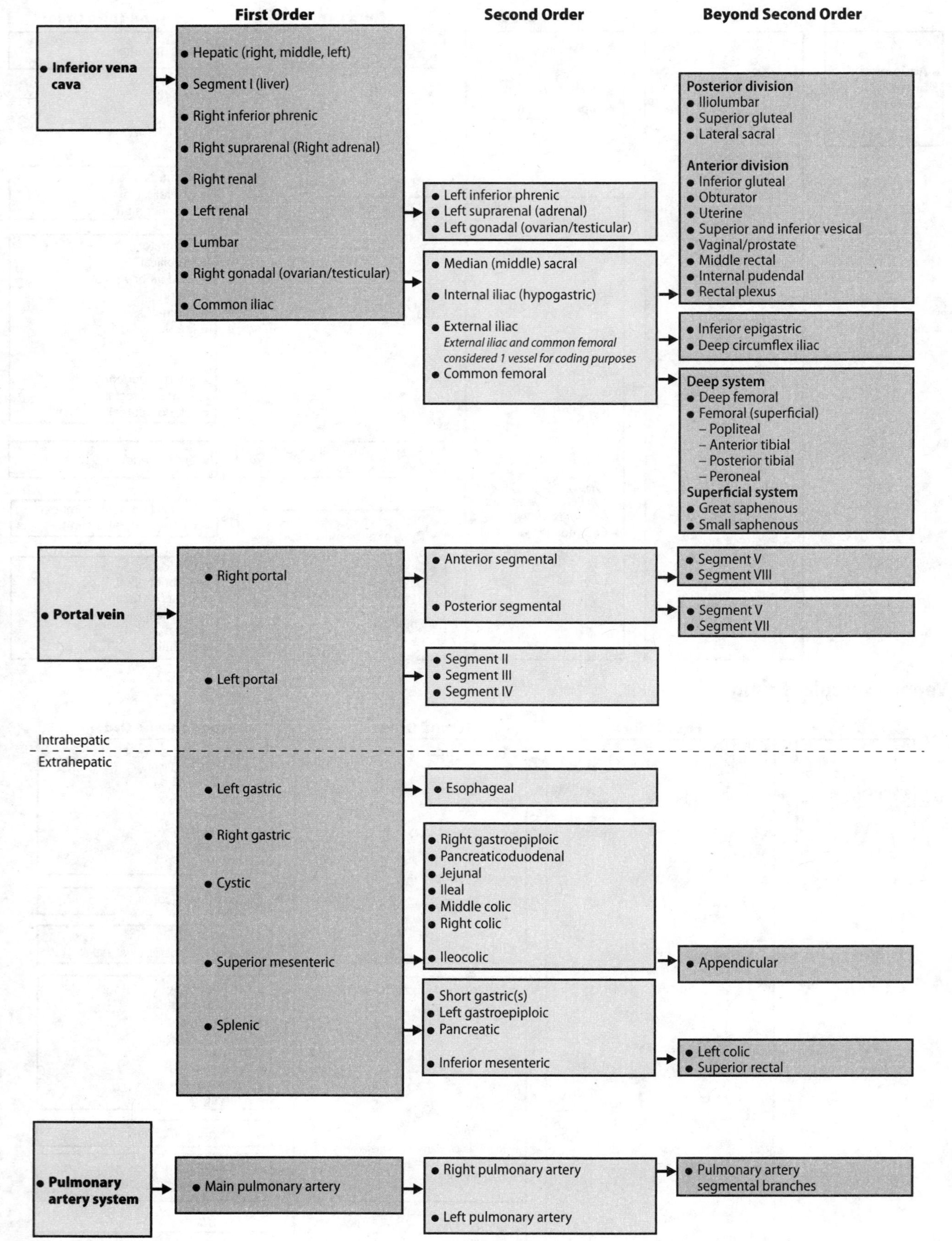
First Order
Second Order
Beyond Second Order
Inferior vena cava
Hepatic (right, middle, left)
Segment I (liver)
Right inferior phrenic
Right suprarenal (Right adrenal)
Right renal
Left renal
Lumbar
Right gonadal (ovarian/testicular)
Common iliac
Left inferior phrenic
Left suprarenal (adrenal)
Left gonadal (ovarian/testicular)
Median (middle) sacral
Internal iliac (hypogastric)
External iliac
External iliac and common femoral considered 1 vessel for coding purposes
Common femoral
Posterior division
Iliolumbar
Superior gluteal
Lateral sacral
Anterior division
Inferior gluteal
Obturator
Uterine
Superior and inferior vesical
Vaginal/prostate
Middle rectal
Internal pudendal
Rectal plexus
Inferior epigastric
Deep circumflex iliac
Deep system
Deep femoral
Femoral (superficial)
– Popliteal
– Anterior tibial
– Posterior tibial
– Peroneal
Superficial system
Great saphenous
Small saphenous
Portal vein
Right portal
Left portal
Anterior segmental
Posterior segmental
Segment V
Segment VIII
Segment V
Segment VII
Segment II
Segment III
Segment IV
Intrahepatic
Extrahepatic
Left gastric
Right gastric
Cystic
Superior mesenteric
Splenic
Esophageal
Right gastroepiploic
Pancreaticoduodenal
Jejunal
Ileal
Middle colic
Right colic
Ileocolic
Appendicular
Short gastric(s)
Left gastroepiploic
Pancreatic
Inferior mesenteric
Left colic
Superior rectal
Pulmonary artery system
Main pulmonary artery
Right pulmonary artery
Left pulmonary artery
Pulmonary artery segmental branches

Appendix P — Interventional Radiology Illustrations

Internal Carotid and Vertebral Arterial Anatomy

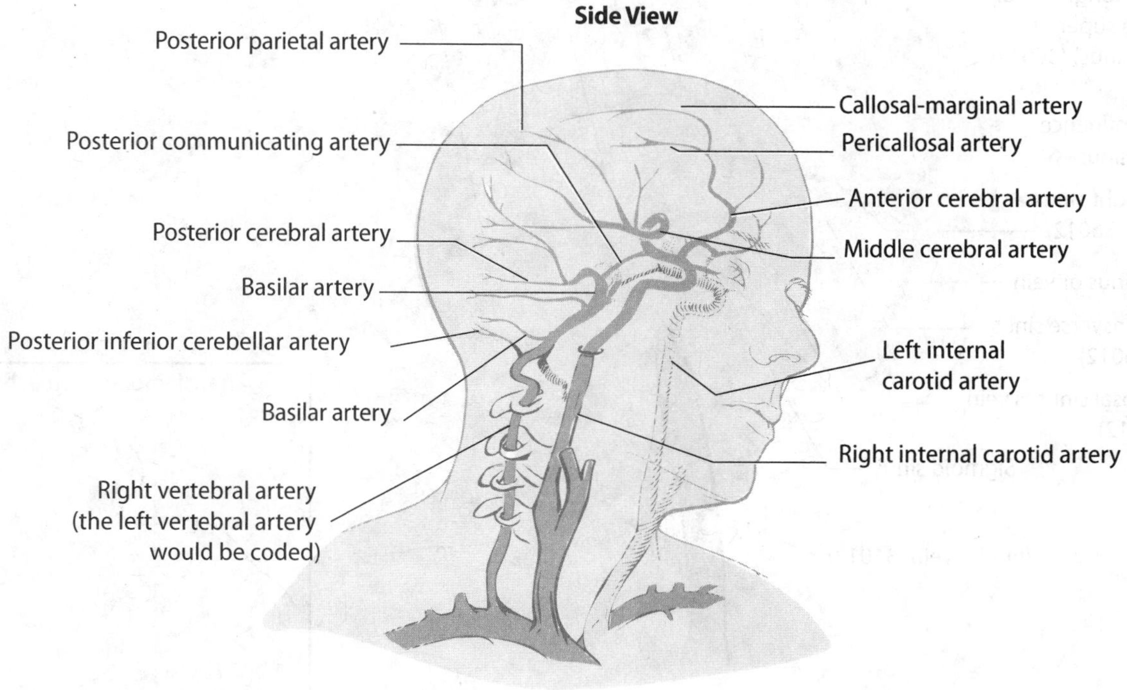

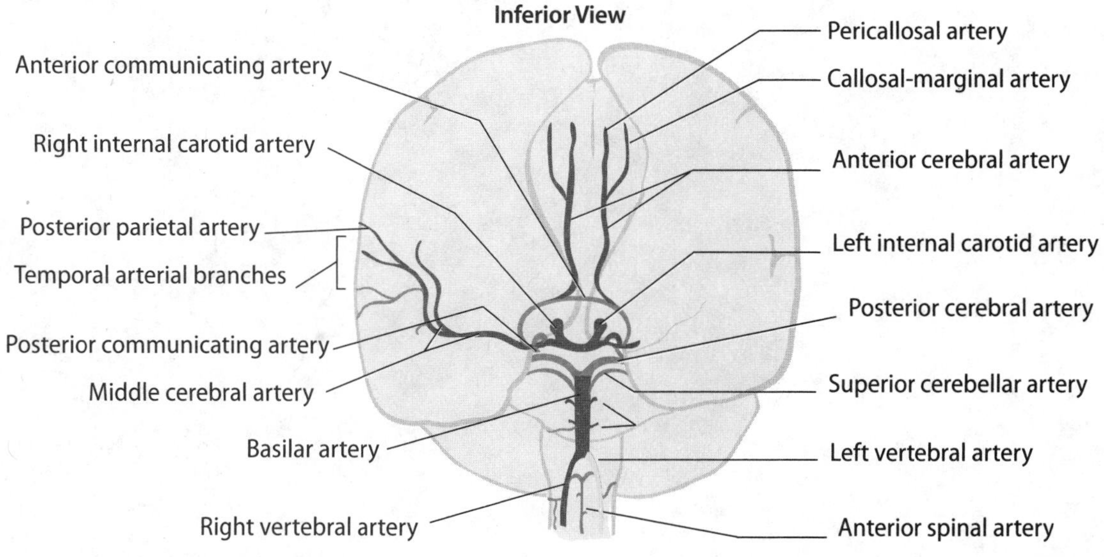

Cerebral Venous Anatomy

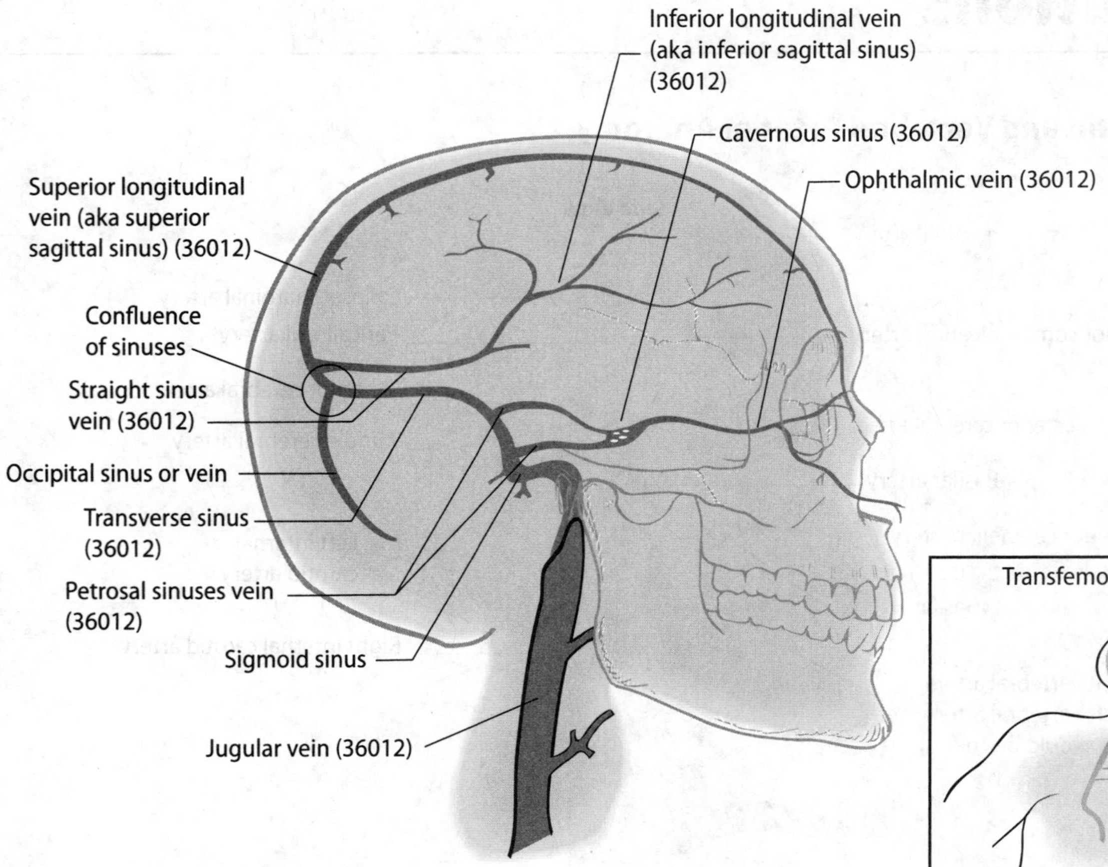
Inferior longitudinal vein
(aka inferior sagittal sinus)
(36012)
Cavernous sinus (36012)
Ophthalmic vein (36012)
Superior longitudinal
vein (aka superior
sagittal sinus) (36012)
Confluence
of sinuses
Straight sinus
vein (36012)
Occipital sinus or vein
Transverse sinus
(36012)
Petrosal sinuses vein
(36012)
Sigmoid sinus
Jugular vein (36012)

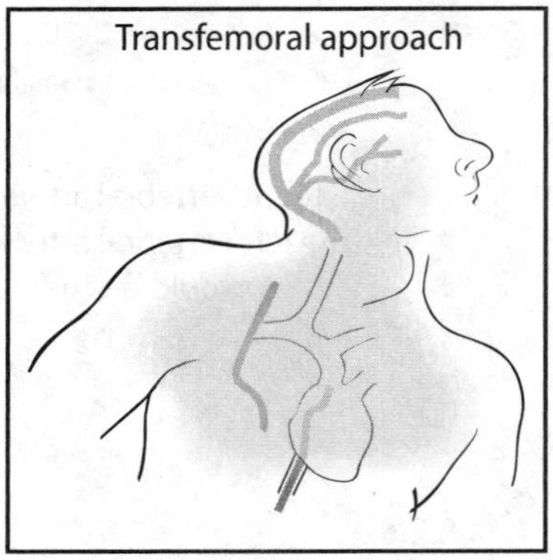
Transfemoral approach

Normal Aortic Arch and Branch Anatomy—Transfemoral Approach

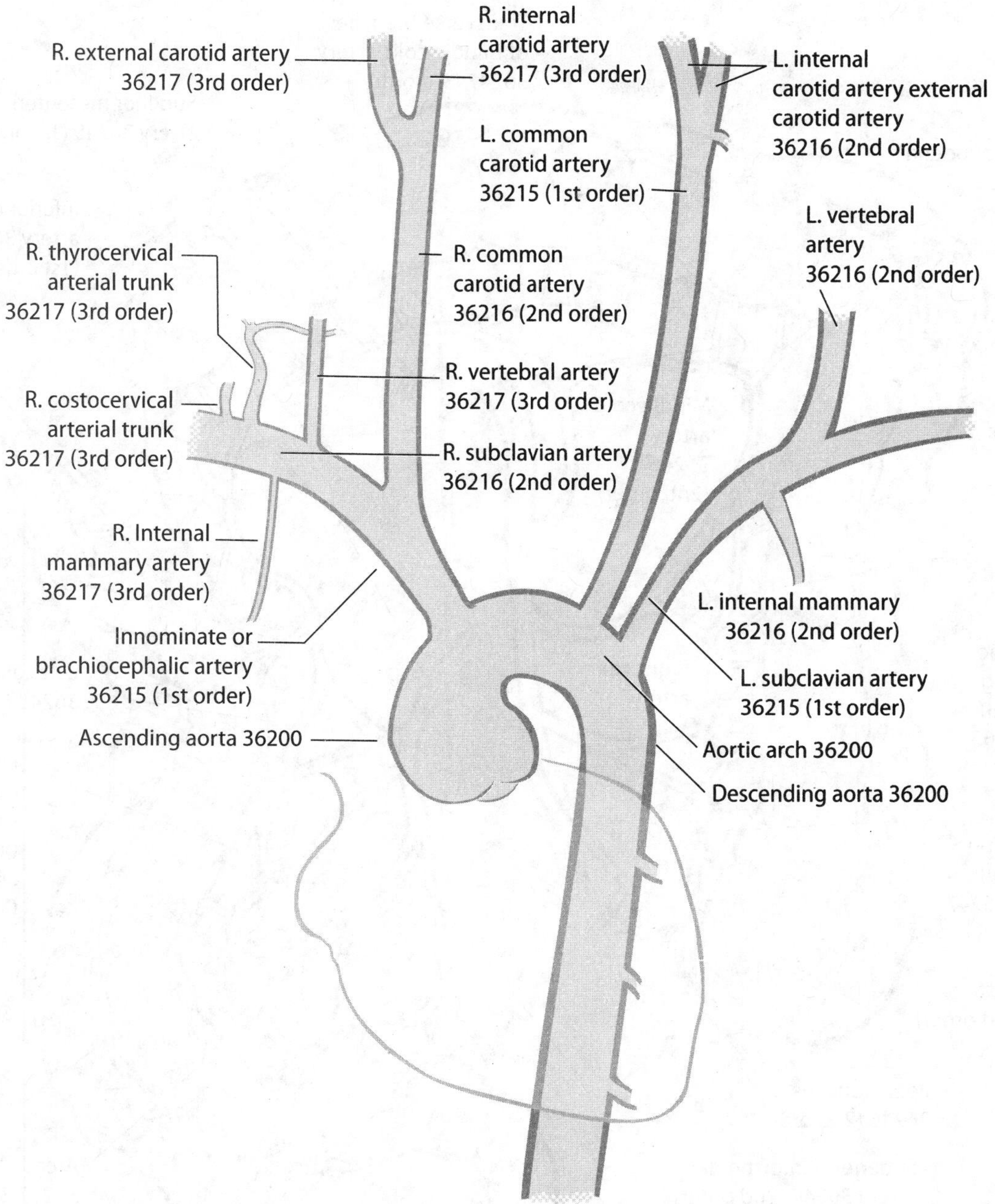
R. external carotid artery 36217 (3rd order)
R. internal carotid artery 36217 (3rd order)
L. internal carotid artery external carotid artery 36216 (2nd order)
L. common carotid artery 36215 (1st order)
L. vertebral artery 36216 (2nd order)
R. thyrocervical arterial trunk 36217 (3rd order)
R. common carotid artery 36216 (2nd order)
R. vertebral artery 36217 (3rd order)
R. costocervical arterial trunk 36217 (3rd order)
R. subclavian artery 36216 (2nd order)
R. Internal mammary artery 36217 (3rd order)
L. internal mammary 36216 (2nd order)
Innominate or brachiocephalic artery 36215 (1st order)
L. subclavian artery 36215 (1st order)
Ascending aorta 36200
Aortic arch 36200
Descending aorta 36200

Superior and Inferior Mesenteric Arteries and Branches

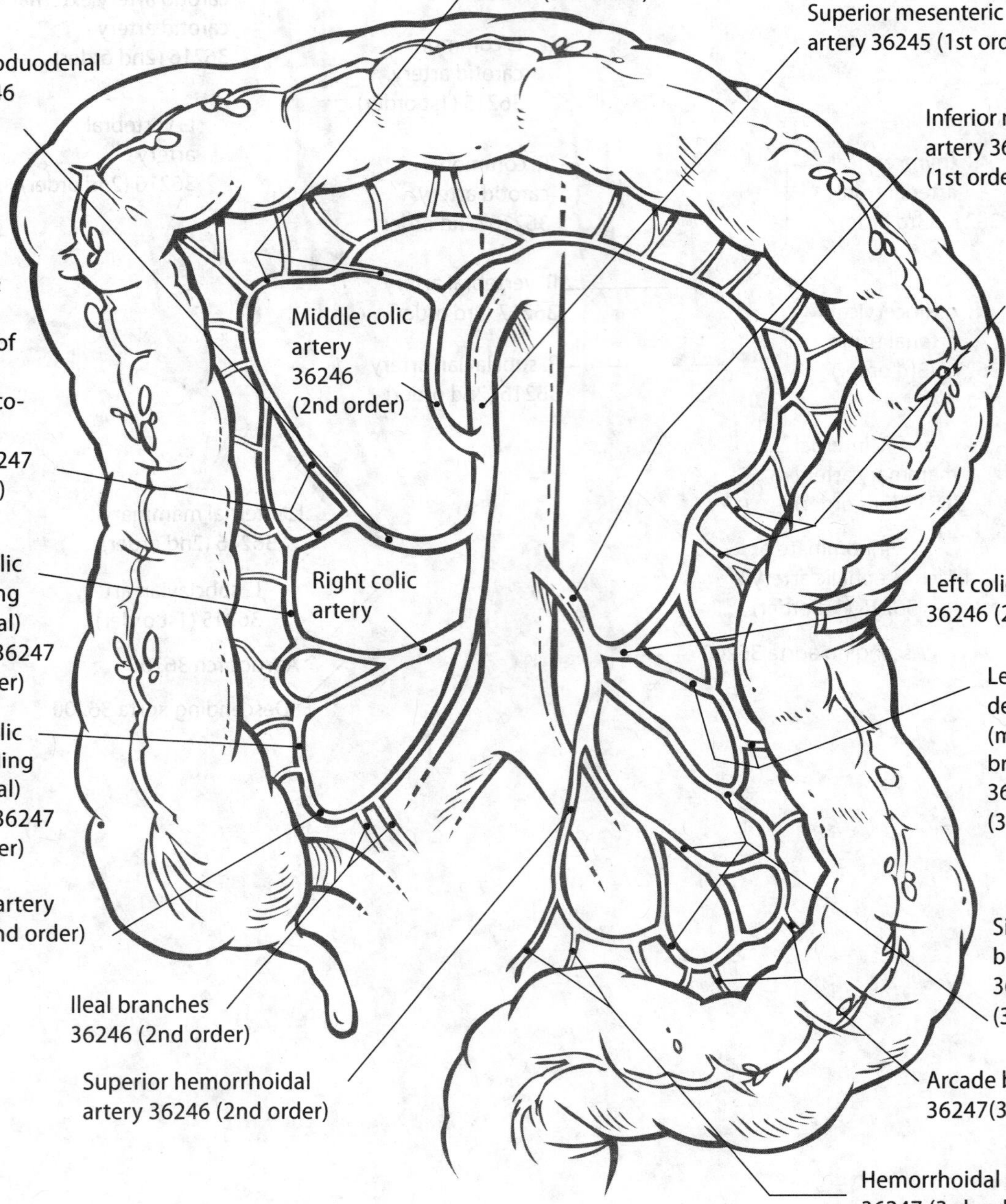
Transverse branches of middle colic artery 36247 (3rd order)
Superior mesenteric artery 36245 (1st order)
Inferior pancreaticoduodenal artery 36246 (2nd order)
Inferior mesenteric artery 36245 (1st order)
Left colic ascending (marginal) branches 36247 (3rd order)
Anterior & posterior branches of inferior pancreatico-duodenal arcade 36247 (3rd order)
Middle colic artery 36246 (2nd order)
Right colic ascending (marginal) branch 36247 (3rd order)
Right colic artery
Left colic artery 36246 (2nd order)
Left colic descending (marginal) branches 36247 (3rd order)
Right colic descending (marginal) branch 36247 (3rd order)
Ileocolic artery 36246 (2nd order)
Sigmoid branches 36247 (3rd order)
Ileal branches 36246 (2nd order)
Superior hemorrhoidal artery 36246 (2nd order)
Arcade branches 36247(3rd order)
Hemorrhoidal branches 36247 (3rd order)

Renal Artery Anatomy—Femoral Approach

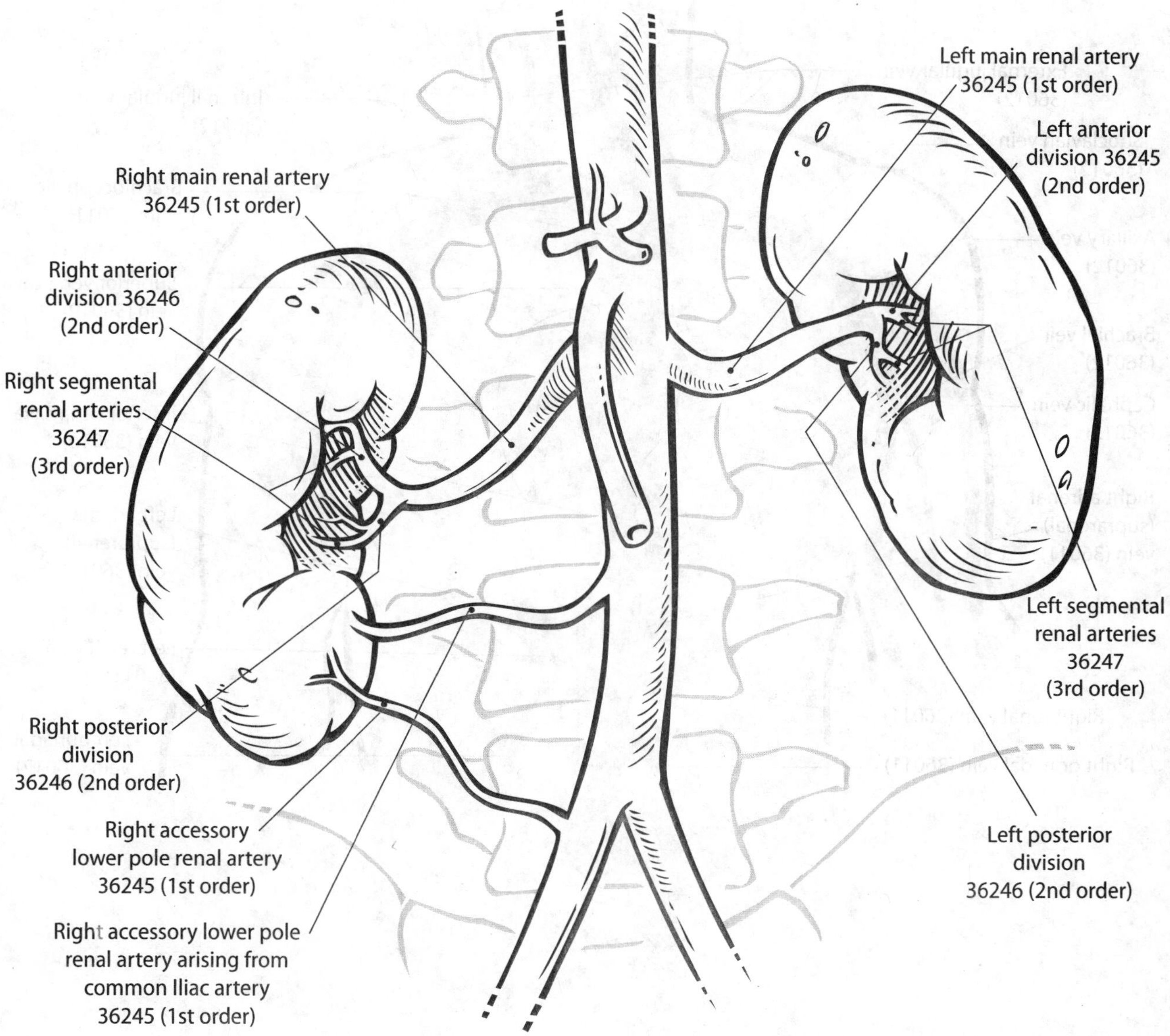
Left main renal artery 36245 (1st order)
Left anterior division 36245 (2nd order)
Right main renal artery 36245 (1st order)
Right anterior division 36246 (2nd order)
Right segmental renal arteries 36247 (3rd order)
Left segmental renal arteries 36247 (3rd order)
Right posterior division 36246 (2nd order)
Right accessory lower pole renal artery 36245 (1st order)
Left posterior division 36246 (2nd order)
Right accessory lower pole renal artery arising from common Iliac artery 36245 (1st order)

Central Venous Anatomy

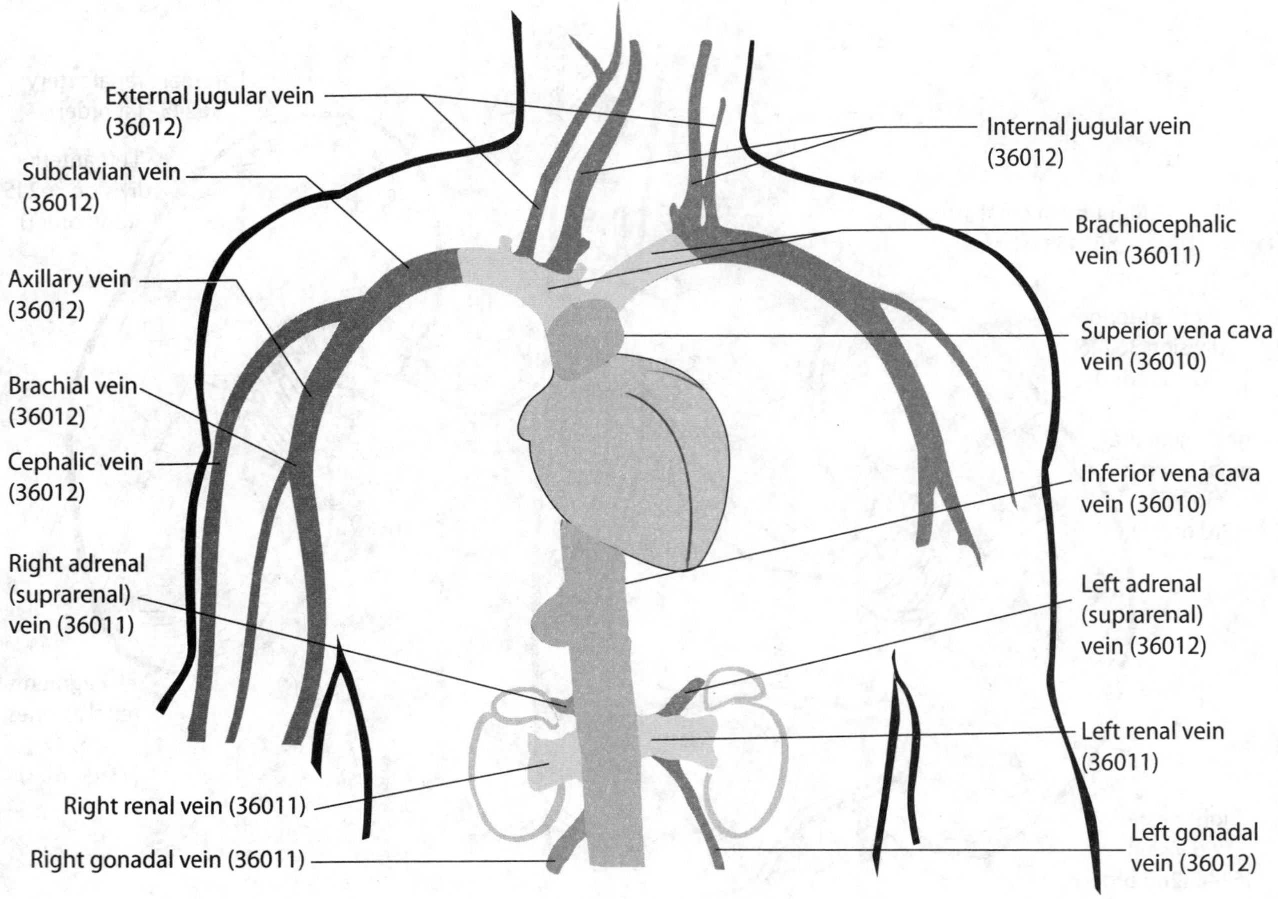
External jugular vein (36012)
Subclavian vein (36012)
Axillary vein (36012)
Brachial vein (36012)
Cephalic vein (36012)
Right adrenal (suprarenal) vein (36011)
Right renal vein (36011)
Right gonadal vein (36011)
Internal jugular vein (36012)
Brachiocephalic vein (36011)
Superior vena cava vein (36010)
Inferior vena cava vein (36010)
Left adrenal (suprarenal) vein (36012)
Left renal vein (36011)
Left gonadal vein (36012)

Portal System (Arterial)

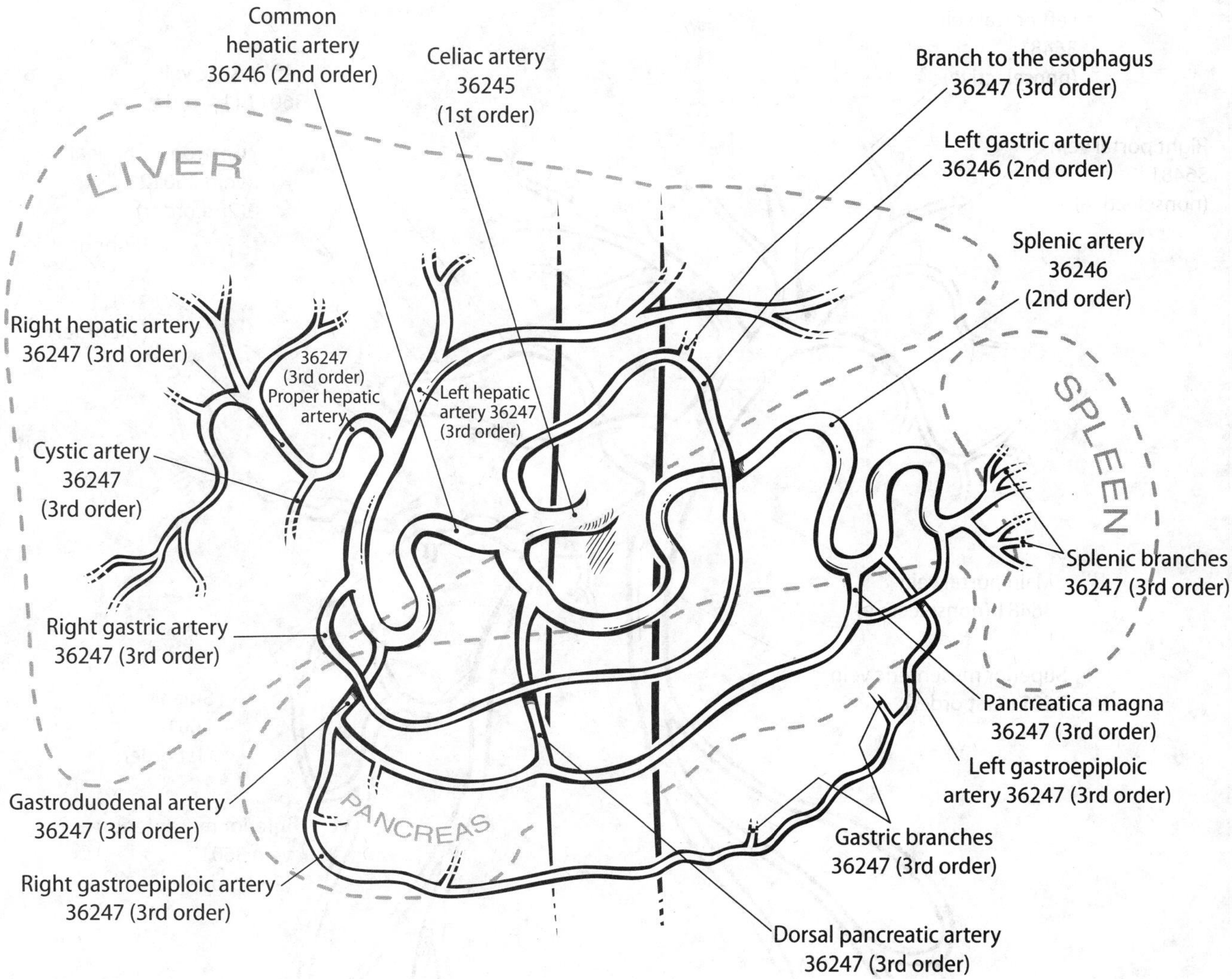
Common
hepatic artery
36246 (2nd order)
Celiac artery
36245
(1st order)
Branch to the esophagus
36247 (3rd order)
Left gastric artery
36246 (2nd order)
LIVER
Splenic artery
36246
(2nd order)
Right hepatic artery
36247 (3rd order)
36247
(3rd order)
Proper hepatic
artery
Left hepatic
artery 36247
(3rd order)
SPLEEN
Cystic artery
36247
(3rd order)
Splenic branches
36247 (3rd order)
Right gastric artery
36247 (3rd order)
Pancreatica magna
36247 (3rd order)
Left gastroepiploic
artery 36247 (3rd order)
Gastroduodenal artery
36247 (3rd order)
PANCREAS
Gastric branches
36247 (3rd order)
Right gastroepiploic artery
36247 (3rd order)
Dorsal pancreatic artery
36247 (3rd order)

Portal System (Venous)

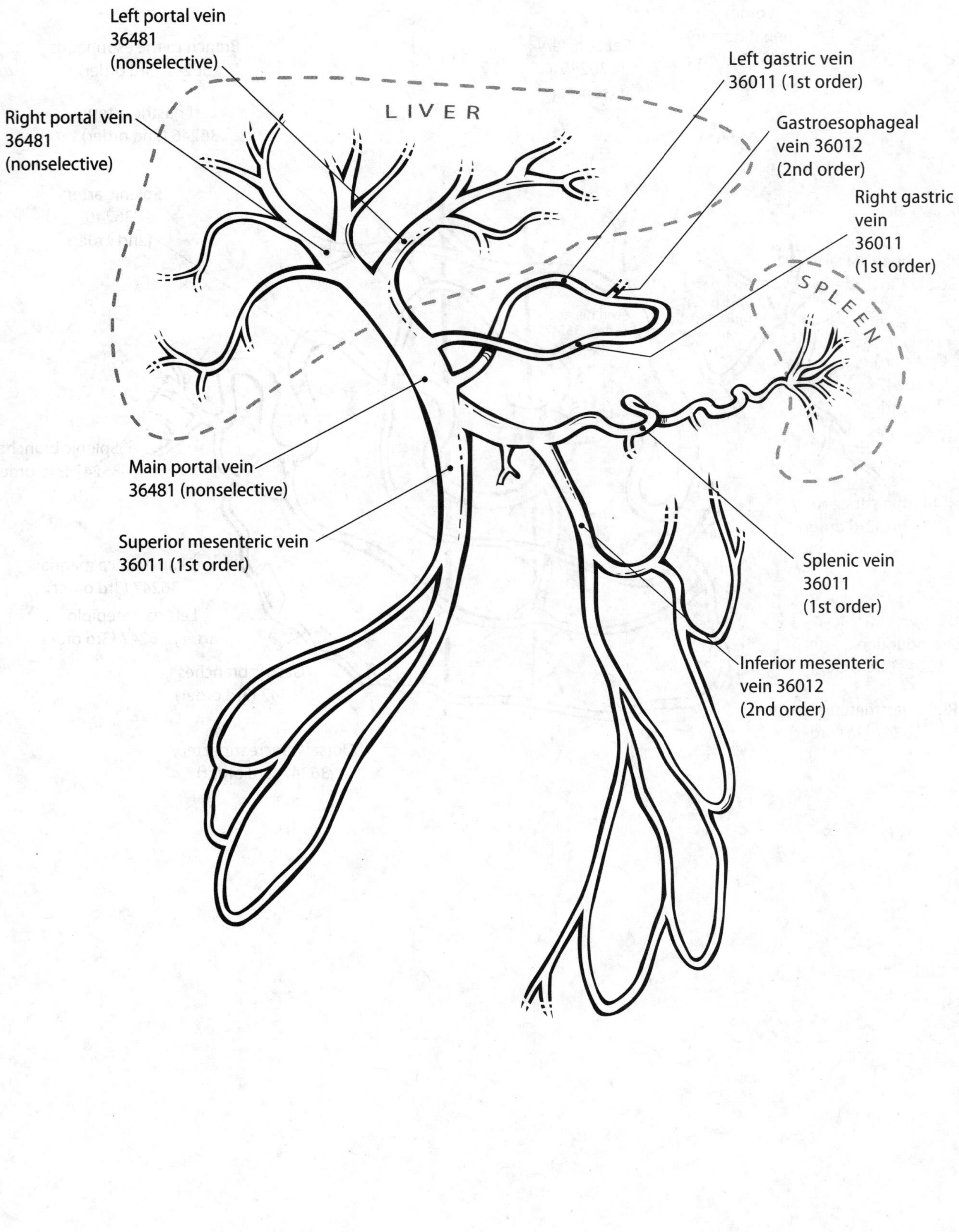
Left portal vein
36481
(nonselective)
Right portal vein
36481
(nonselective)
LIVER
Left gastric vein
36011 (1st order)
Gastroesophageal
vein 36012
(2nd order)
Right gastric
vein
36011
(1st order)
SPLEEN
Main portal vein
36481 (nonselective)
Superior mesenteric vein
36011 (1st order)
Splenic vein
36011
(1st order)
Inferior mesenteric
vein 36012
(2nd order)

Pulmonary Artery Angiography

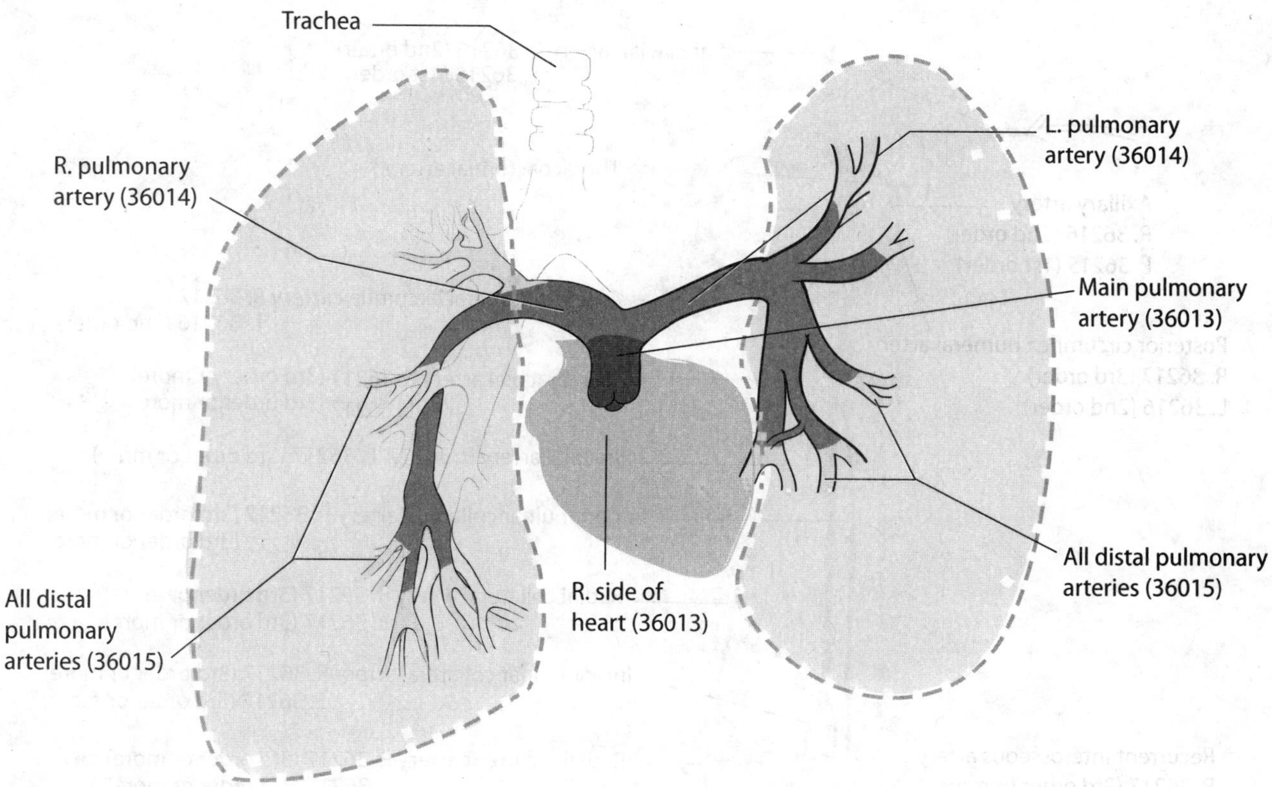

Upper Extremity Arterial Anatomy—Transfemoral or Contralateral Approach

Subclavian artery R. 36216 (2nd order)
L. 36215 (1st order)

Thoracoacromial artery

Axillary artery
R. 36216 (2nd order)
L. 36215 (1st order)

Anterior humeral circumflex artery R. 36217
L. 36216 (2nd order)

Posterior circumflex humeral artery
R. 36217 (3rd order)
L. 36216 (2nd order)

Deep brachial artery R. 36217 (3rd order or more)
L. 36217 (3rd order or more)

Brachial artery R. 36217, L. 36217 (3rd order or more)

Superior ulnar collateral artery R. 36217 (3rd order or more)
L. 36217 (3rd order or more)

Radial collateral artery R. 36217 (3rd order or more)
L. 36217 (3rd order or more)

Inferior ulnar collateral artery R. 36217 (3rd order or more)
L. 36217 (3rd order or more)

Recurrent interosseous artery
R. 36217 (3rd order or more)
L. 36217 (3rd order or more)

Radial recurrent artery R. 36217 (3rd order or more)
L. 36217 (3rd order or more)

Common interosseous artery R. 36217 (3rd order or more)
L. 36217 (3rd order or more)

Anterior interosseous artery R. 36217 (3rd order or more)
L. 36217 (3rd order or more)

Ulnar artery
R. 36217 (3rd order or more)
L. 36217 (3rd order or more)

Radial artery R. 36217 (3rd order or more)
L. 36217 (3rd order or more)

Posterior interosseous artery R. 36217 (3rd order or more)
L. 36217 (3rd order or more)

Superficial palmar branch
of radial artery R. 36217 (3rd order or more)
L. 36217 (3rd order or more)

Deep palmar arch R. 36217 (3rd order or more)
L. 36217 (3rd order or more)

Digital arteries

Appendix P — Interventional Radiology Illustrations

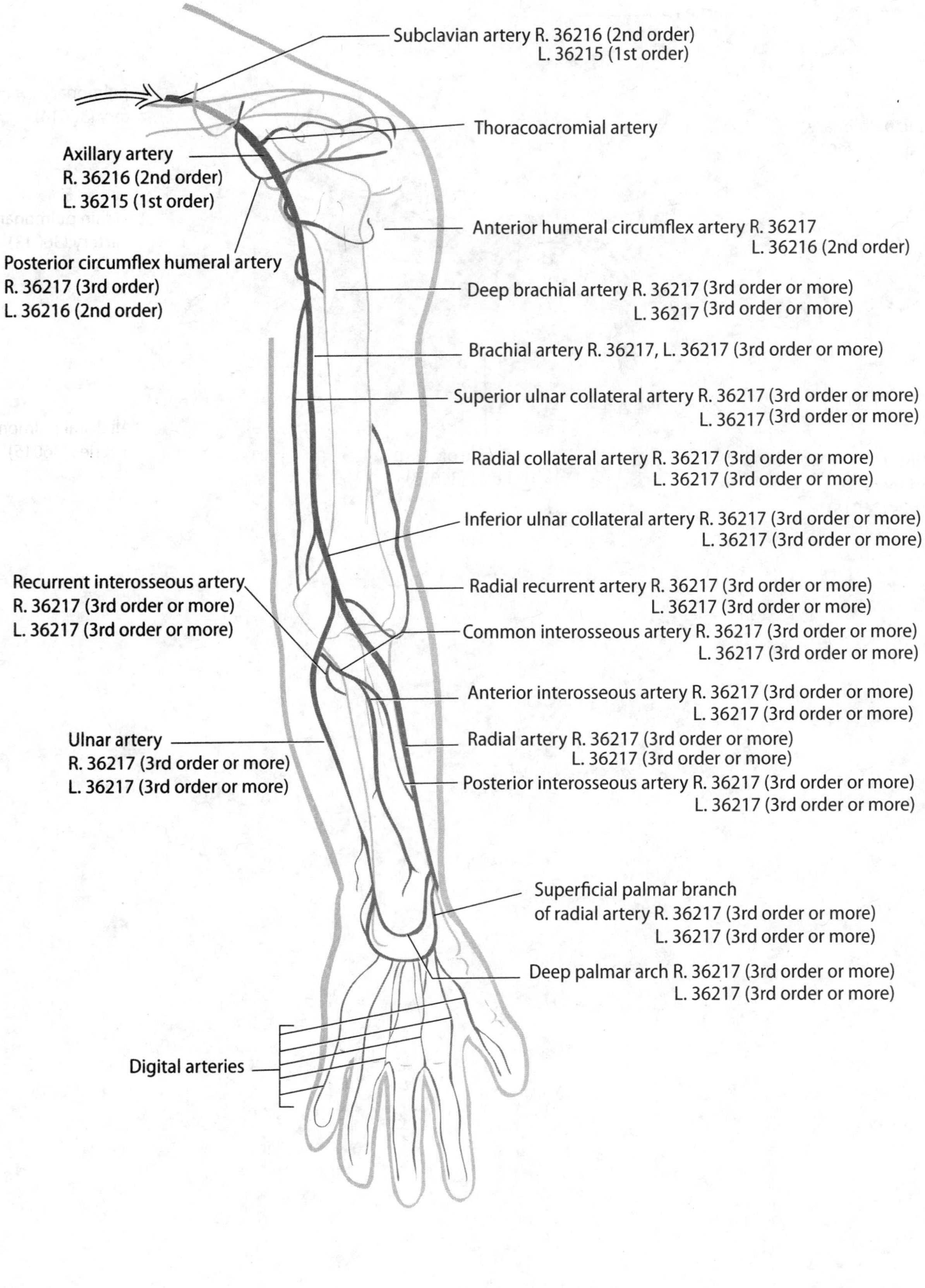

Lower Extremity Arterial Anatomy—Contralateral, Axillary or Brachial Approach

Common iliac artery
36245 (1st order)

External iliac artery
36246 (2nd order)

Aorta 36200

Internal iliac artery
(aka hypogastric)
36246 (2nd order)

Common femoral
artery 36246 (2nd order)

Profunda femoris
36247 artery
(3rd order)

Perforating artery
branches 36247
(3rd order)

Superficial femoral artery
36247 (3rd order)

Superior lateral
genicular artery
36247 (3rd order)

Superior medial
genicular artery
36247 (3rd order)

Popliteal artery
36247 (3rd order)

Inferior lateral
genicular artery
36247 (3rd order)

Inferior medial
genicular artery
36247 (3rd order)

Peroneal artery
36247 (3rd order)

Posterior tibial
artery 36247
(3rd order)

Popliteal artery
36247 (3rd order)

Anterior tibial
artery 36247
(3rd order)

Anterior tibial artery
36247 (3rd order)

Posterior
tibial artery
36247 (3rd order)

Lateral anterior
malleolar artery 36247
(3rd order)

Medial anterior
malleolar artery
36247 (3rd order)

Peroneal artery
36247 (3rd order)

Pedis dorsalis artery
36247 (3rd order)

Posterior view
of right leg

© 2021 Optum360, LLC

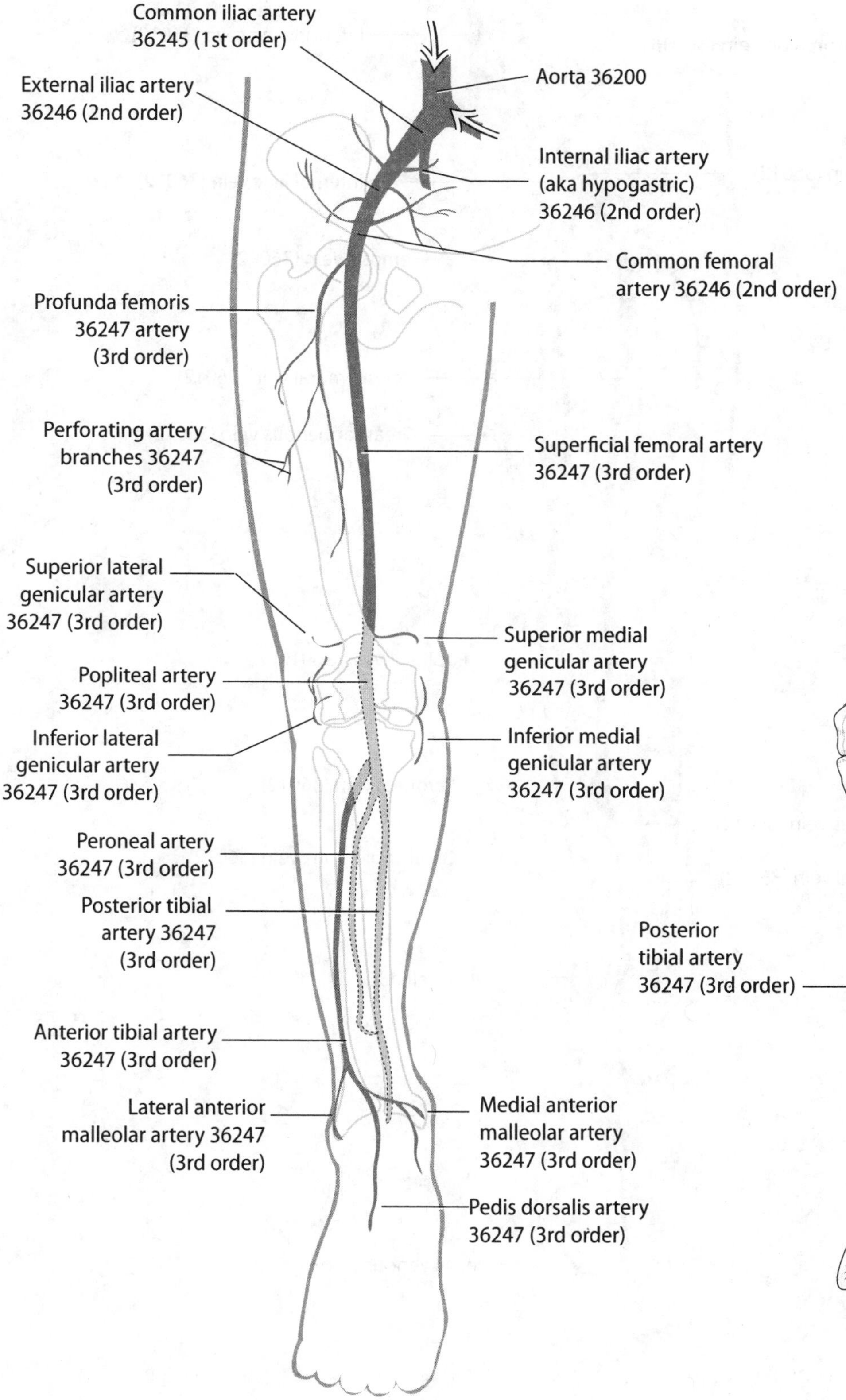

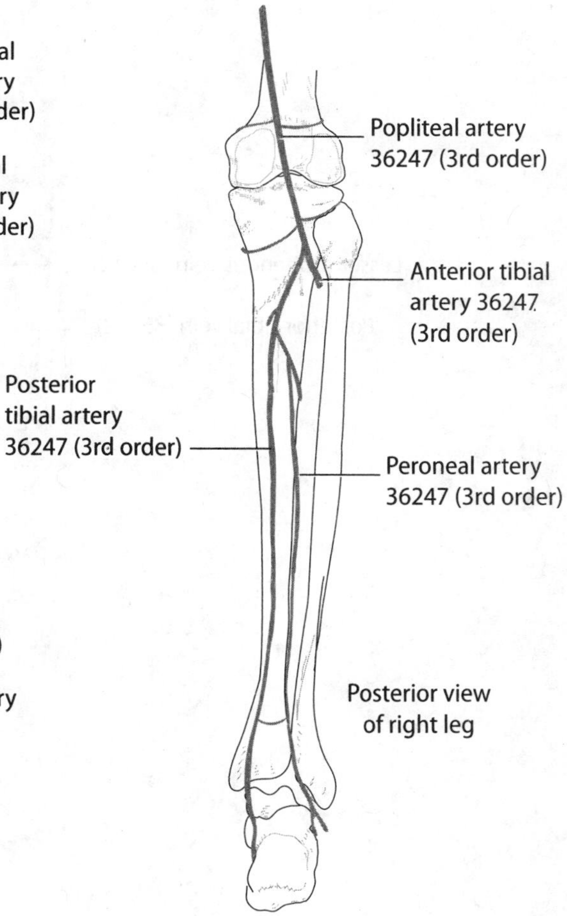

Lower Extremity Venous Anatomy

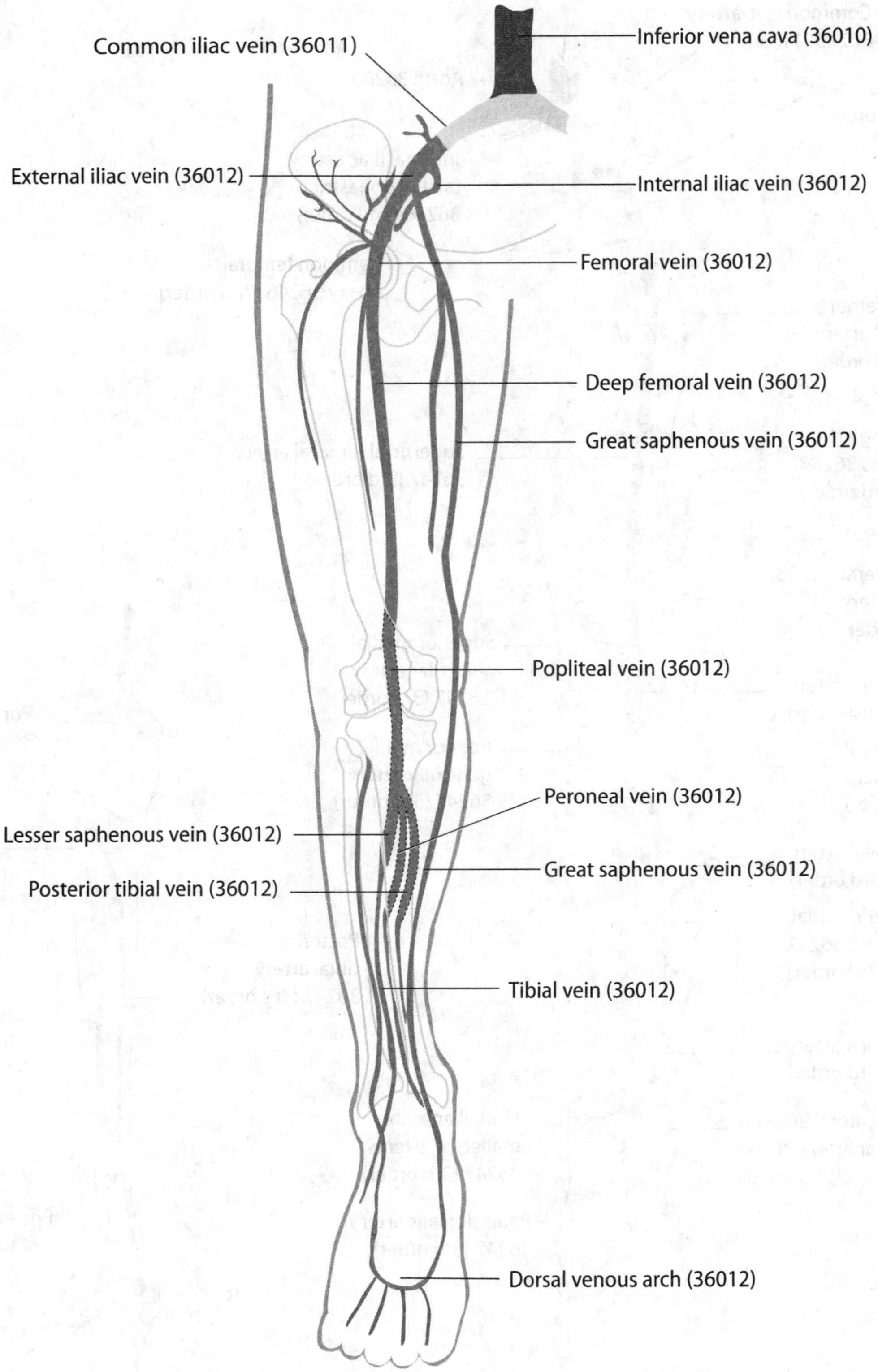
Common iliac vein (36011)
Inferior vena cava (36010)
External iliac vein (36012)
Internal iliac vein (36012)
Femoral vein (36012)
Deep femoral vein (36012)
Great saphenous vein (36012)
Popliteal vein (36012)
Peroneal vein (36012)
Lesser saphenous vein (36012)
Great saphenous vein (36012)
Posterior tibial vein (36012)
Tibial vein (36012)
Dorsal venous arch (36012)

Coronary Arteries Anterior View

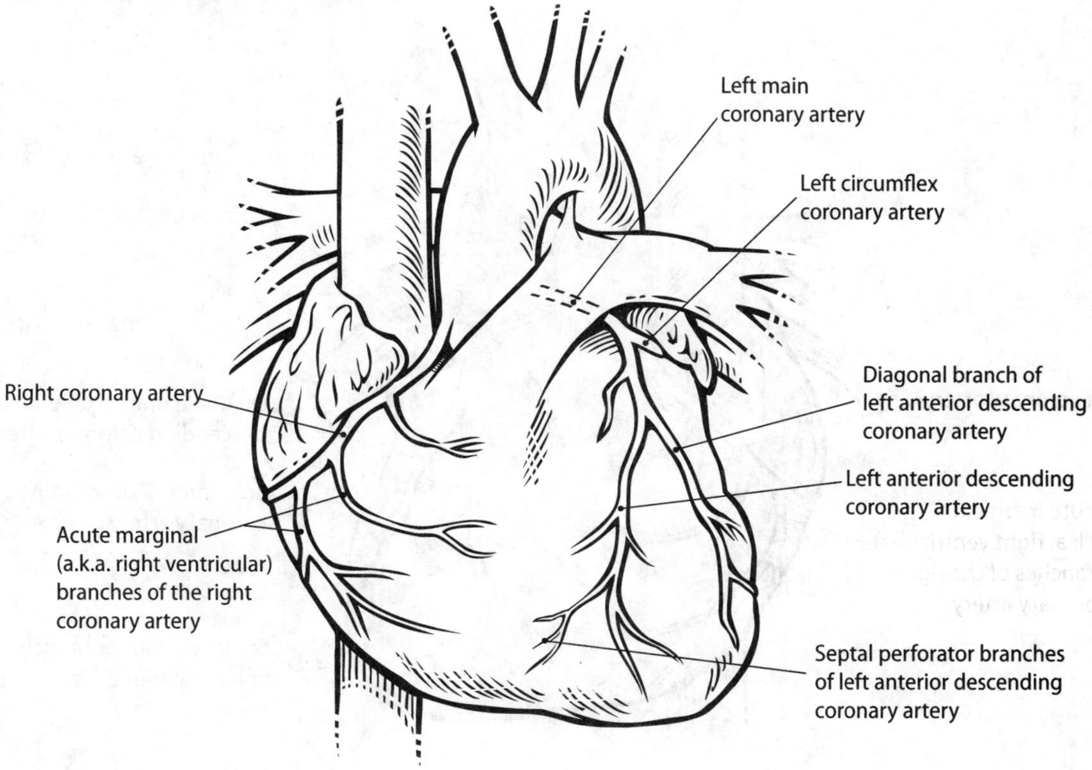

Left Heart Catheterization

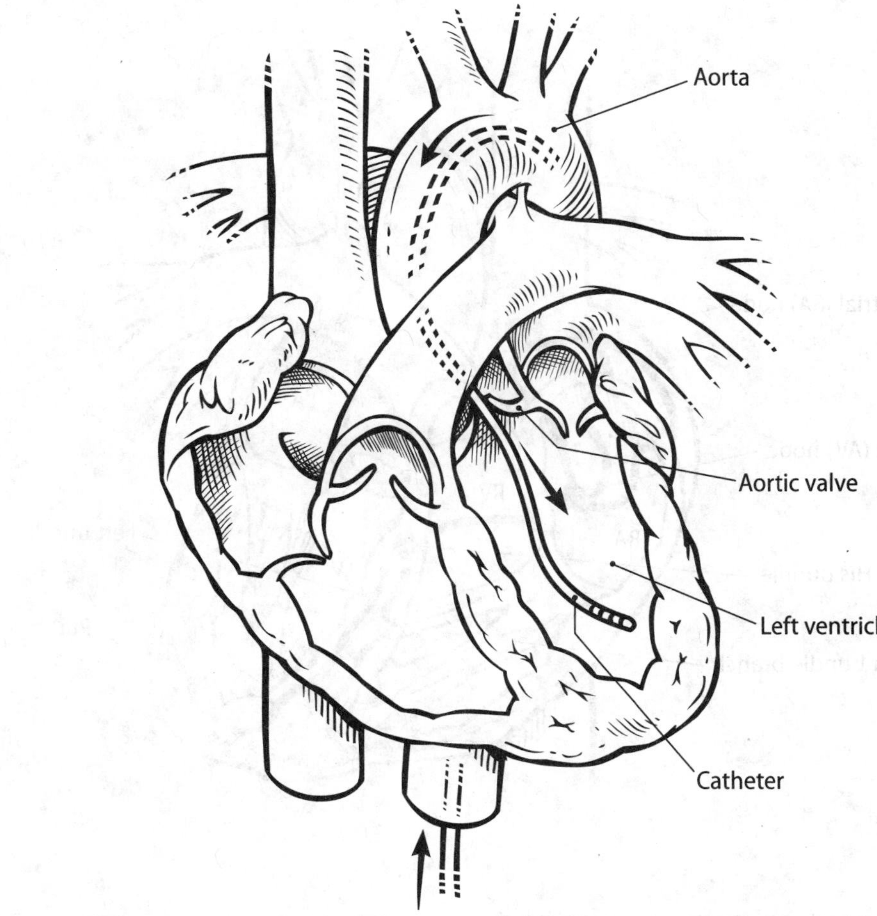

Right Heart Catheterization

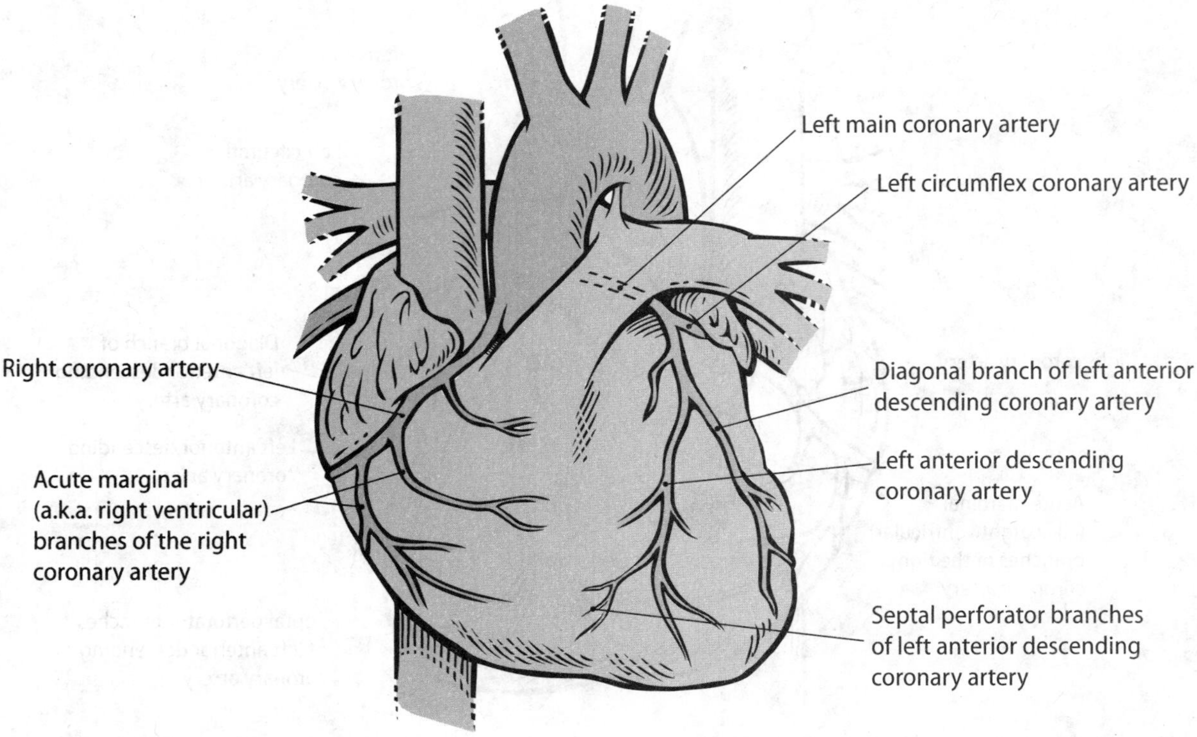

Heart Conduction System

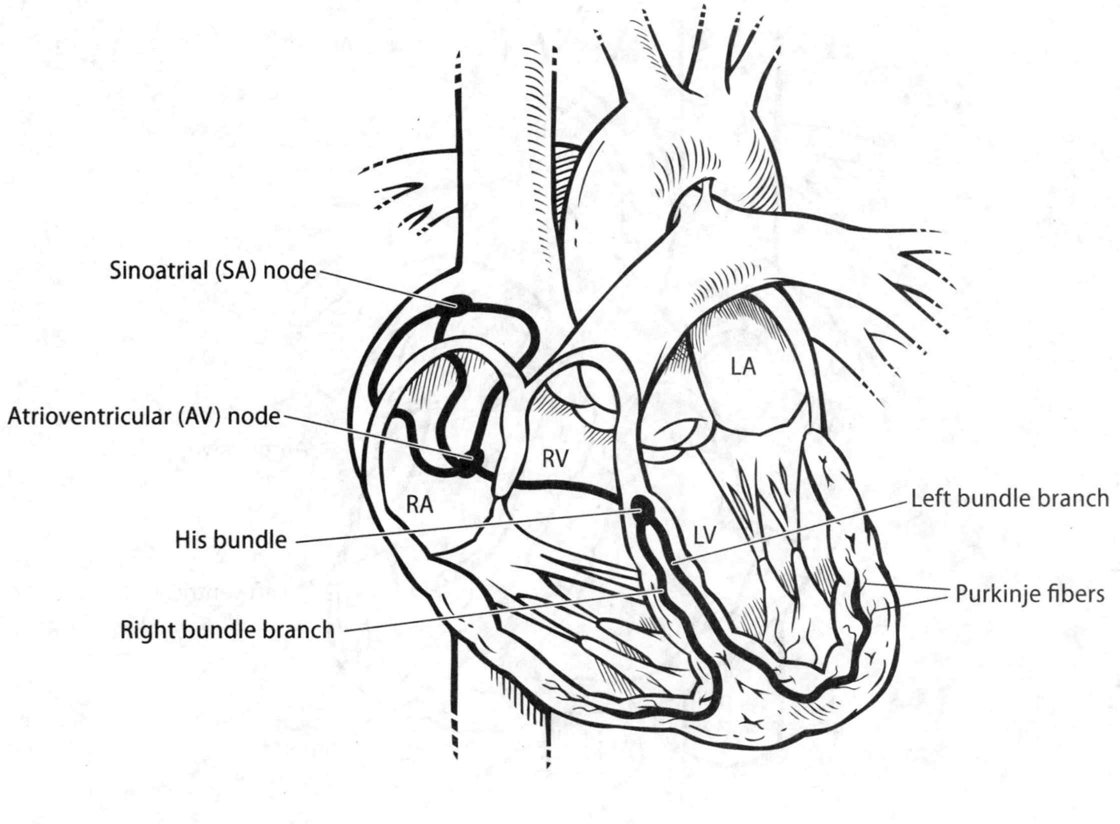

Appendix Q — Severe Acute Respiratory Syndrome Coronavirus 2 (SARS-CoV-2) (coronavirus disease [COVID-19]) Vaccine and Administration Codes

The following table provides a link between each individual severe acute respiratory syndrome coronavirus 2 (SARS-CoV-2) (coronavirus disease [COVID-19]) vaccine code and its corresponding vaccine administration code, along with the vaccine manufacturer name, vaccine name, National Drug Code (NDC) Labeler Product ID number(s), the recommended interval between vaccine doses, and the emergency use authorization (EUA)or Federal Drug Administration (FDA) approval dates (when received). These resequenced codes are located in the Medicine section. Additional instructional notes can be found with the codes in the appropriate code ranges or at https://www.ama-assn.org/practice-management/cpt/covid-19-cpt-vaccine-and-immunization-codes. Information regarding FDA EUA processes and dates can be found at https://www.fda.gov/emergency-preparedness-and-response/mcm-legal-regulatory-and-policy-framework/emergency-use-authorization#vaccines.

Vaccine Code	Long Descriptor	Administration Code(s)	Manufacturer	Vaccine Name(s)	NDC 10/NDC 11 Labeler Product ID (vial)	Dosing Interval	Location in the Optum360 coding products
#● 91300	Severe acute respiratory syndrome coronavirus 2 (SARS-CoV-2) (coronavirus disease [COVID-19]) vaccine, mRNA-LNP, spike protein, preservative free, 30 mcg/0.3mL dosage, diluent reconstituted, for intramuscular use	● 0001A (1st dose) ● 0002A (2nd dose) ● 0003A (3rd dose) ● 0004A (booster dose)	Pfizer, Inc	Pfizer-BioNTech COVID-19 Vaccine; Comirnaty	59267-1000-1 59267-1000-01	1st to 2nd dose: 21 days 2nd to 3rd dose: 28 or more days Booster: See FDA/CDC Guidance	[91300]—Before code 90476
#● ⚡ 91305	Severe acute respiratory syndrome coronavirus 2 (SARS-CoV-2) (coronavirus disease [C OVID-19]) vaccine, mRNA-LNP, spike protein, preservative free, 30 mcg/0.3 mL dosage, tris-sucrose formulation, for intramuscular use	#● 0051A (1st dose) #● 0052A (2nd dose) #● 0053A(3rd dose) #● 0054A (booster dose)	Pfizer, Inc	Pfizer-BioNTech COVID-19 Vaccine	59267-1025-1 59267-1025-01	1st to 2nd dose: 21 days 2nd to 3rd dose: 28 or more days Booster: See FDA/CDC Guidance	[91305]—Following resequenced code 91300
#● ⚡ 91307	Severe acute respiratory syndrome coronavirus 2 (SARS-CoV-2) (coronavirus disease [COVID-19]) vaccine, mRNA-LNP, spike protein, preservative free, 10 mcg/0.2 mL dosage, diluent reconstituted, tris-sucrose formulation, for intramuscular use	#● 0071A (1st dose) #● 0072A (2nd dose)	Pfizer, Inc	Pfizer-BioNTech COVID-19 Vaccine	59267-1055-1 59267-1055-01	1st to 2nd dose: 21 days	[91307]—Following resequenced code 91305
#● 91301	Severe acute respiratory syndrome coronavirus 2 (SARS-CoV-2) (coronavirus disease [COVID-19]) vaccine, mRNA-LNP, spike protein, preservative free, 100 mcg/0.5mL dosage, for intramuscular use	● 0011A (1st dose) ● 0012A (2nd dose) ● 0013A (3rd dose)	Moderna, Inc	Moderna COVID-19 Vaccine	80777-273-10 80777-0273-10	1st to 2nd dose: 28 days 2nd to 3rd dose: 28 or more days See FDA/CDC Guidance	[91301]—Before code 90476
#● 91306	Severe acute respiratory syndrome coronavirus 2 (SARS-CoV-2) (coronavirus disease [COVID-19]) vaccine, mRNA-LNP, spike protein, preservative free, 50 mcg/0.25 mL dosage, for intramuscular use	#● 0064A (booster dose)	Moderna, Inc	Moderna COVID-19 Vaccine	80777-273-10 80777-0273-10	See FDA/CDC Guidance	[91306]—Following resequenced code 91301

Notes:

COVID-19 vaccine drug codes [91300, 91301, 91302, 91303, 91304, 91305, 91306, 91307] are exempt from reporting with modifier 51.

COVID-19 vaccine administration codes 0001A-0004A, 0011A-0013A, 0021A-0022A, 0031A, 0034A, 0041A-0042A, [0051A-0054A], [0064A], [0071A-0072A] should be reported with vaccine codes [91300, 91301, 91302, 91303, 91304, 91305, 91306, 91307] *only*. All other vaccines should be reported with [90460-90461], 90476-90749. COVID-19 vaccine administration codes should not be reported with other immunization administration codes unless an additional vaccine/toxoid is administered during the same visit.

Vaccine Code	Long Descriptor	Administration Code(s)	Manufacturer	Vaccine Name(s)	NDC 10/NDC 11 Labeler Product ID (vial)	Dosing Interval	Location in the Optum360 coding products
#● ✓ 91302	Severe acute respiratory syndrome coronavirus 2 (SARS-CoV-2) (coronavirus disease [COVID-19]) vaccine, DNA, spike protein, chimpanzee adenovirus Oxford 1 (ChAdOx1) vector, preservative free, $5x10^{10}$ viral particles/0.5mL dosage, for intramuscular use	● 0021A (1st dose) ● 0022A (2nd dose)	AstraZeneca, Plc	AstraZeneca COVID-19 Vaccine	0310-1222-10 00310-1222-10	28 days	[91302]—Before code 90476
#● 91303	Severe acute respiratory syndrome coronavirus 2 (SARS-CoV-2) (coronavirus disease [COVID-19]) vaccine, DNA, spike protein, adenovirus type 26 (Ad26) vector, preservative free, $5x10^{10}$ viral particles/0.5mL dosage, for intramuscular use	● 0031A (single dose) ● 0034A (booster dose)	Janssen	Janssen COVID-19 Vaccine	59676-580-05 59676-0580-05	N/A	[91303]—Before code 90476
#● ✓ 91304	Severe acute respiratory syndrome coronavirus 2 (SARS-CoV-2) (coronavirus disease [COVID-19]) vaccine, recombinant spike protein nanoparticle, saponin-based adjuvant, preservative free, 5 mcg/0.5mL dosage, for intramuscular use	● 0041A (1st dose) ● 0042A (2nd dose)	Novavax, Inc	Novavax COVID-19 Vaccine	80631-100-01 80631-1000-01	21 days	[91304]—Before code 90476

Notes:

COVID-19 vaccine drug codes [91300, 91301, 91302, 91303, 91304, 91305, 91306, 91307] are exempt from reporting with modifier 51.

COVID-19 vaccine administration codes 0001A-0004A, 0011A-0013A, 0021A-0022A, 0031A, 0034A, 0041A-0042A, [0051A-0054A], [0064A], [0071A-0072A] should be reported with vaccine codes [91300, 91301, 91302, 91303, 91304, 91305, 91306, 91307] *only*. All other vaccines should be reported with [90460-90461], 90476-90749. COVID-19 vaccine administration codes should not be reported with other immunization administration codes unless an additional vaccine/toxoid is administered during the same visit.

Appendix R — Digital Medicine Services

This table defines digital medicine services, classifies related CPT codes to those services, and is designed to support understanding of the approaches to patient care through digital medicine services available throughout the CPT code set. The term "clinician" is defined as a physician or other qualified health care professional (QHP) who may report the indicated code. This is not intended to be a complete list of CPT codes in the digital medicine services category. Coding guidelines from specific CPT code sections should be followed.

	Clinician-to-Patient (Visit)		**Clinician-to-Clinician (Consult)**		**Patient Monitoring/Therapeutic Services**			**Digital Diagnostic**	
	Asynchronous	**Synchronous**	**Asynchronous**	**Synchronous**	**Set-Up and Education (Device/Software)**	**Data Transfer**	**Data Interpretation**	**Patient Directed**	**Image/ Specimen Directed**
Encounter Activity	Digital communication, store-and-forward	Audiovisual interaction, real-time	Consultative digital exchange of clinical information between requesting and consulting clinicians, store-and-forward	Consultative communication between requesting and consulting clinicians, real-time	Communication with patient to support device set-up education/supply, in-person, virtual face-to-face, telephone, or other modalities	Acquisition of patient data for transfer to managing/interpreting physician/QHP/clinical staff	Data review/interpretation and patient management by physician/QHP/clinical staff with patient communication	Algorithmically enabled diagnostic support, automated/autonomous	
CPT Service	Online digital E/M (99421-99423) (98970-98972)	E/M performed as virtual face-to-face visit (append modifier 95)	Consultation, interprofessional telephone, internet, electronic health record (99446-99449, 99451, 99452)	Consultation, interprofessional telephone, internet, electronic health record [typically via telephone] (99446-99449,99451)	Initial set-up/education, remote physiologic monitoring (99453)		Physiologic data collection/interpretation by physician/QHP/ (99091)	Retinopathy screening, automated (92229)	
		Telephone services, audio only (99441-99443)		Transition to virtual face-to-face E/M consultation if patient present at originating site (append modifier 95)		Remote physiologic monitoring device supply (99454)	Physician/QHP/clinical staff treatment management of remote physiologic monitoring (99457-99458)		Multianalyte assays with algorithmic analyses (MAAA)
					Remote therapeutic monitoring, initial set-up/education (98975)	Remote therapeutic monitoring device supply (98976, respiratory) (98977, musculoskeletal)	Remote therapeutic monitoring treatment management by physician/QHP/clinical staff (98980-98981)		
					Treatment management of remote pulmonary artery pressure sensor by physician/QHP (93264)				Computer-aided detection (CAD) imaging (77048-77049, 77065-77067, 0042T, 0174T-0175T)
					Continuous glucose monitoring hook-up/education/recording print-out, ambulatory (95250, office equipped) (95249, patient equipped)		Continuous glucose monitoring analysis, ambulatory (95251)		
					Electrocardiographic recording, external (including recording, scanning analysis with report, review, and interpretation) (93224, 93241, 93245)			External electrocardiographic recording (autonomous algorithms used to analyze and create report) (93241-93243, 93245-93247)	
					External electrocardiographic, recording only (93224-93225, 93241-93242, 93245-93246)	External electrocardiographic recording, scanning analysis with report only (93226, 93241, 93243, 93247)	External electrocardiographic recording, review and interpretation only (93224, 93227, 93241, 93244, 93245, 93248)		
					External mobile cardiovascular telemetry technical support (93229)		External mobile cardiovascular telemetry review and interpretation (93228)		
					Remote monitoring digital cognitive behavioral therapy program, supply/technical support (0702T)		Remote monitoring treatment management by physician/QHP (0703T)		
					Digital amblyopia services (0704T, initial set-up/education) (0705T, surveillance center technical support, including data transmission)		Digital amblyopia services, assessment of patient performance/program data (0706T)		
						CT study, automated analysis including data preparation, interpretation and report (0691T)			

Notes

Notes